OPERATIVE TECHNIQUES IN ORTHOPAEDIC TRAUMA SURGERY

Third Edition

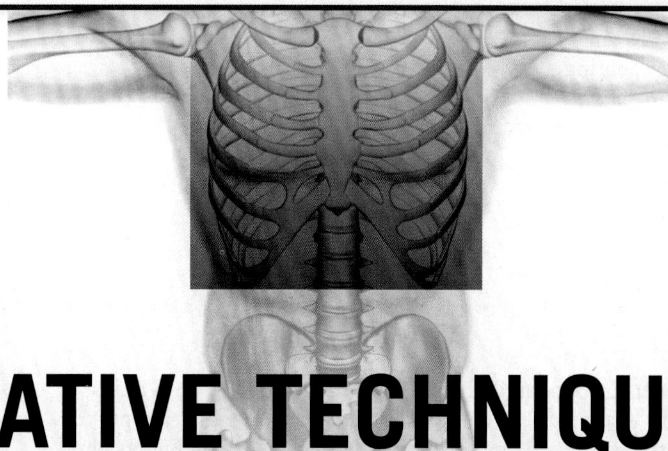

OPERATIVE TECHNIQUES IN ORTHOPAEDIC TRAUMA SURGERY

Third Edition

Paul Tornetta III, MD
Professor and Chair, Department of Orthopaedic Surgery
Boston University Medical Center
Boston, Massachusetts

EDITORS-IN-CHIEF

Sam W. Wiesel, MD
Chairman and Professor
Department of Orthopaedic Surgery
Georgetown University Medical School
Washington, District of Columbia

Todd J. Albert, MD
Surgeon in Chief Emeritus
Hospital for Special Surgery
Professor of Orthopaedics
Weill Cornell Medical College
New York, New York

With select chapters from:

Adult Reconstruction edited by
Edwin P. Su, MD
Seth Jerabek, MD

Hand, Wrist, and Forearm edited by
Thomas R. Hunt III, MD, DSc
Jerry I. Huang, MD

Oncology edited by
Martin M. Malawer, MD, FACS
James C. Wittig, MD
Jacob Bickels, MD

Shoulder and Elbow edited by
Gerald R. Williams, Jr., MD
Matthew L. Ramsey, MD
Brent B. Wiesel, MD
Surena Namdari, MD

Sports Medicine edited by
Mark D. Miller, MD

Wolters Kluwer

Philadelphia • Baltimore • New York • London
Buenos Aires • Hong Kong • Sydney • Tokyo

Director, Medical Practice: Brian Brown
Senior Development Editor: Stacey Sebring
Marketing Manager: Kristin Ciotto
Production Project Manager: Bridgett Dougherty
Design Coordinator: Steve Druding
Manufacturing Coordinator: Beth Welsh
Prepress Vendor: Absolute Service, Inc.

3rd edition

9 8 7 6 5 4 3 2 1

Printed in China

Library of Congress Cataloging-in-Publication Data

Library of Congress Control Number: 2021937314

shop.lww.com

CCS0521

EDITORS-IN-CHIEF – DEDICATIONS

We would like to dedicate this Volume to the memory of Richard H. Rothman, MD, PhD whose guidance and mentorship is responsible for our success and that of generations of orthopaedic surgeons. That influence also has led to improvements in the lives of thousands of his patients and those of his orthopaedic offspring.

Sam W. Wiesel, MD and Todd J. Albert, MD
January 5, 2021

DEDICATION

To my mother, Phyllis, who found the best in people, had compassion for all, and whose insight, guidance, and love have always made me believe that anything is possible.

—PT3

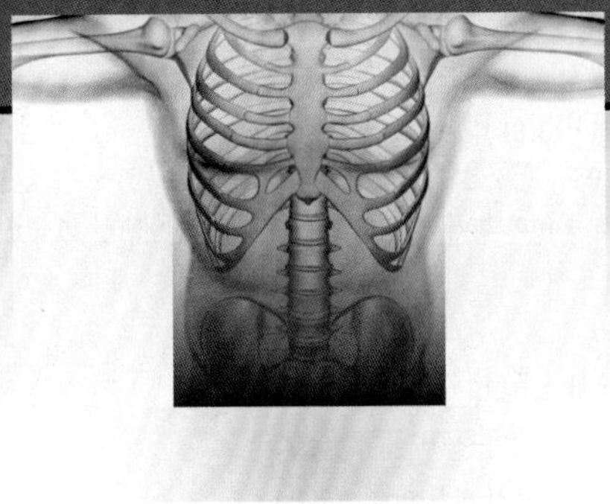

Contents

SECTION III Pelvis and Hip

SECTION IV Femur and Knee

SECTION V Leg

SECTION VI Foot and Ankle

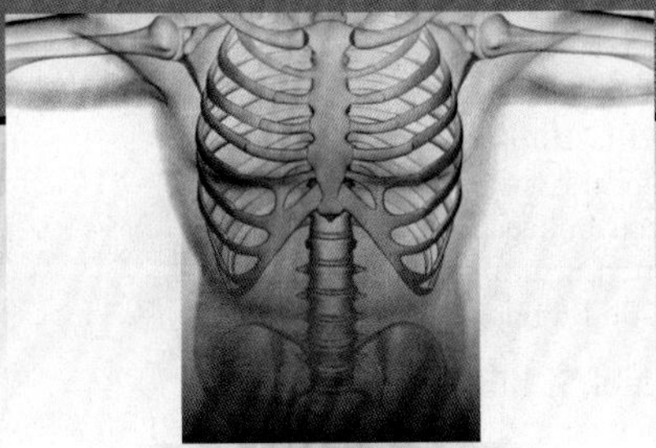

Contributors

Abed Abdelaziz, MD, MPH
Resident
Department of Orthopedic Surgery
Dell Medical School
Austin, Texas

Animesh Agarwal, MD
Professor and Director of Orthopaedic Trauma
Department of Orthopaedics
University of Texas Health Science Center at San Antonio
San Antonio, Texas

Ram K. Alluri
Department of Orthopedic Surgery
University of Southern California
Los Angeles, California

Paul Andrzejowski, BMedSci(Hons), BMBS, MRCS(Ed)
Specialty Registrar in Trauma and Orthopaedics
Leeds Teaching Hospitals
Department of Trauma and Orthopaedics
Leeds General Infirmary
Leeds, South Yorkshire, United Kingdom

Jeff Anglen, MD
Orthopedic Trauma Surgeon
Sadhana Boneworks
Indianapolis, Indiana

Luke Austin, MD
Associate Professor of Orthopaedic Surgery
Shoulder and Elbow Surgery
Rothman Orthopaedic Institute
Sewell, New Jersey

Carl Basamania, MD
Orthopedic Surgeon
Providence Health
Seattle, Washington

Hari P. Bezwada, MD
Orthopaedic Surgeon
University Medical Center of Princeton at Plainsboro
Princeton Orthopaedic Associates
Princeton, New Jersey

Jacob Bickels, MD
Director of Orthopedic Oncology
Division of Orthopedic Surgery
Hillel-Yaffe Medical Center
Hadera, Israel
Professor, Orthopedic Surgery
Director, Orthopedic Surgery
Rappaport Faculty of Medicine
Technion
Haifa, Israel

Eric M. Black
Orthopedic Surgeon
Summit Medical Group
Florham Park, New Jersey

Kamal I. Bohsali, MD
Chairman, Department of Surgery
Shoulder and Elbow Service
Jacksonville Orthopaedic Institute
Jacksonville Beach, Florida

Christopher Born, MD
Emeritus Director of Orthopedic Trauma
Community College of Rhode Hospital
Providence, Rhode Island

David J. Bozentka, MD
Chief of Hand Surgery
Department of Orthopaedics
Hospital of the University of Pennsylvania
Philadelphia, Pennsylvania

Daniel Bravin, MD
Assistant Professor
Department of Orthopaedic Surgery
University of Missouri Columbia School of Medicine
Columbia, Missouri

Sean T. Campbell, MD
Resident
Department of Orthopaedic Surgery
Stanford University
Redwood City, California

Kevin Chan, MD, MSc, FRCSC
Clinical Assistant Professor
Department of Orthopaedics
Spectrum Health Medical Group
Grand Rapids, Michigan

Christopher Chiodo, MD
Chief, Foot and Ankle Surgery Service
Department of Orthopaedic Surgery
Brigham and Women's Hospital
Jamaica Plain, Massachusetts

Ryan Churchill, MD
Orthopedic Shoulder and Elbow Surgeon
New England Orthopedic Specialists
Peabody, Massachusetts

Michael P. Clare, MD
Orthopedic Surgeon
360 Orthopedics
Bradenton, Florida

Patrick K. Cronin, MD
Resident
Department of Orthopaedic Surgery
Massachusetts General Hospital
Boston, Massachusetts

Brian M. Culp, MD
Orthopaedic Surgeon
University Medical Center of Princeton at Plainsboro
Princeton Orthopaedic Associates
Princeton, New Jersey

Malcolm R. DeBaun, MD
Resident
Department of Orthopaedic Surgery
Stanford University
Redwood City, California

Steven F. DeFroda, MD, ME
Fellow
Department of Orthopedics
Brown University
Providence, Rhode Island

Christopher Del Balso, MBBS, MSc, FRCSC
Physician and Lecturer
Department of Surgery
Western University
London Health Sciences Centre
Victoria Hospital
London, Ontario, Canada

Mihir J. Desai, MD
Department of Orthopaedic Surgery
Vanderbilt University Medical Center
Nashville, Tennessee

Seth D. Dodds, MD
Associate Professor, Hand and Upper Extremity Surgery
Department of Orthopaedic Hand Surgery
University of Miami School of Medicine
Miami, Florida

Alex Doermann, MD
Orthopaedic Surgery Resident
University of California Irvine
Orange, California

Derek J. Donegan, MD
Assistant Professor of Orthopaedic Surgery
Hospital of the University of Pennsylvania
Philadelphia, Pennsylvania

David Donohue, MD
Assistant Professor
Department of Orthopaedics
Florida Orthopaedic Institute
University of South Florida
Tampa, Florida

Christopher Doumas, MD
Hand Surgeon
Department of Orthopedics
Robert Wood Johnson University Hospital
New Brunswick, New Jersey

Israel Dudkiewicz, MD
Professor
Department of Orthopaedic Surgery
Rabin Medical Center
Tel Aviv, Israel

Thomas J. Ergen, MD
Resident
Department of Orthopedics
Prisma Health Midlands
Columbia, South Carolina

John G. Esposito, MD
Orthopaedic Trauma Surgeon
Massachusetts General Hospital
Boston, Massachusetts

John J. Fernandez, MD, FAAOS
Assistant Professor of Orthopaedics
Midwest Orthopaedics at Rush
Rush University Medical Center
Chicago, Illinois

Reza Firoozabadi, MD
Associate Professor
Orthopaedics and Sports Medicine
Harborview Medical Center
Seattle, Washington

Evan L. Flatow, MD
President, Mount Sinai West Hospital
Department of Orthopedic Surgery
Icahn School of Medicine at Mount Sinai
New York, New York

Mark A. Frankle, MD
Chief, Shoulder and Elbow Service
Florida Orthopaedic Institute
Tampa, Florida

Andrew Furey, MD, FRCSC
Orthopedic Surgeon
14th Premier of Newfoundland and Labrador
St. John's, Newfoundland, Canada

Leesa M. Galatz, MD
Chair, Department of Orthopedic Surgery
Icahn School of Medicine at Mount Sinai
New York, New York

Matthew J. Garberina, MD
Orthopedic Surgeon
Summit Medical Group
Florham Park, New Jersey

Michael J. Gardner, MD
Chief of Orthopaedic Trauma
Department of Orthopaedic Surgery
Stanford University
Redwood City, California

Brandon J. Gaston, BS
Researcher
Department of Orthopaedic Surgery
Cedars-Sinai
Los Angeles, California

R. Glenn Gaston, MD
Hand Fellowship Director and Chief of Hand Surgery
Department of Orthopedic Surgery
OrthoCarolina
Charlotte, North Carolina

Charles L. Getz, MD
Associate Professor
Division of Shoulder and Elbow Surgery
Department of Orthopaedic Surgery
Sidney Kimmel Medical College
Thomas Jefferson University
Philadelphia, Pennsylvania

Alidad Ghiassi, MD
Assistant Professor of Clinical Orthopaedic Surgery
University of Southern California Health Sciences Center
Los Angeles, California

Peter V. Giannoudis, MD, FACS, FRCS
Professor and Chairman
Department of Trauma and Orthopaedics
University of Leeds School of Medicine
Leeds General Infi rmary University Hospital
Leeds, West Yorkshire, United Kingdom

Thomas Githens, DO
Orthopaedic Trauma Fellow
Department of Orthopaedic Surgery
Stanford University
Redwood City, California

L. Henry Goodnough, MD, PhD
Orthopaedic Surgery Resident
Stanford University
Redwood City, California

Stephen B. Gunther, MD
Orthopedic Surgeon
Sentara Martha Jefferson Hospital
Charlottesville, Virginia

Christina J. Hajewski, MD
Orthopedic Surgeon
University of Iowa
Iowa City, Iowa

Mitchel B. Harris, MD
Chief of Orthopaedic Surgery
Massachusetts General Hospital
Boston, Massachusetts

Levi L. Hinkelman, MD
Clinical Assistant Professor
Spectrum Health Medical Group
Department of Orthopaedics
Grand Rapids, Michigan

Daniel S. Horwitz, MD
Professor and Chief of Orthopaedic Trauma
Department of Orthopaedics
Geisinger Health
Danville, Pennsylvania

Michael M. Hussey, MD
Orthopedic Surgeon
Shoulder and Elbow Service
OrthoArkansas
Little Rock, Arkansas

Lindsay Hussey-Andersen, MD
Fellow
Department of Orthopedic Surgery
Icahn School of Medicine at Mount Sinai
New York, New York

Asif M. Ilyas, MD
Professor and Program Director of Orthopaedics and Hand Surgery
Rothman Institute at Thomas Jefferson University
Philadelphia, Pennsylvania

John M. Itamura, MD
Orthopaedic Surgeon
Shoulder and Elbow Surgery
Cedars-Sinai Kerlan-Jobe Institute
Los Angeles, California

Peter J.L. Jebson, MD
Associate Professor
Michigan State College of Human Medicine
Clinical Instructor
Department of Orthopaedic Surgery
Grand Rapids Medical Education Partners
Spectrum Health Medical Group
Grand Rapids, Michigan

Clifford B. Jones, MD, FACS, FAAOS, FAOA
Chief, Department of Orthopaedic Surgery
Dignity Health — Phoenix
Phoenix, Arizona

Marci D. Jones, MD
Associate Professor of Orthopedic Surgery
University of Massachusetts Medical School
Worcester, Massachusetts

Michael S.H. Kain, MD
Assistant Professor
Department of Orthopaedic Surgery
Boston Medical Center
Boston, Massachusetts

Steven P. Kalandiak, MD
Assistant Professor of Clinical Orthopaedics
University of Miami Health Systems
Miami, Florida

Amir Khoshbin, MD, FRCSC
Assistant Professor
Department of Surgery
University of Toronto
Toronto, Ontario, Canada

Richard Kim, MD
Hand Surgeon
Department of Plastic and Reconstructive Surgery
Hackensack University Medical Center
Maywood, New Jersey

Stephen A. Kottmeier, MD
Associate Chairman
Department of Orthopaedics
Stony Brook University Hospital
Stony Brook, New York

James Krieg, MD
Professor and Orthopaedic Trauma Director
Department of Orthopaedic Surgery
Thomas Jefferson University
Philadelphia, Pennsylvania

Erik Noble Kubiak, MD
Chief of Orthopaedic Trauma
Vice Chair, Department of Orthopaedics
University of Nevada Las Vegas
Las Vegas, Nevada

John Y. Kwon, MD
Chief, Orthopaedic Foot and Ankle Service
Beth Israel Deaconess Medical Center
Boston, Massachusetts

Joseph T. Labrum IV, MD
Department of Orthopaedic Surgery
Vanderbilt University Medical Center
Nashville, Tennessee

Phillip Langer, MD, MS
Medical Director
Department of Orthopedic Surgery Sports Medicine
Ortho Sport and Spine Physicians
Atlanta, Georgia

Joshua R. Langford, MD
Orthopedic Surgeon
Orlando Health Orthopedic Institute
Orlando, Florida

David Lee, MD
Resident
Department of Orthopedics
Robert Wood Johnson University Hospital
New Brunswick, New Jersey

Ross K. Leighton, MD, FACS, FRCS(C)
Professor
Department of Surgery
Dalhousie University
Halifax, Nova Scotia, Canada

Frank A. Liporace, MD
Chairman and Vice President
Department of Orthopaedic Surgery
Jersey City Medical Center
Jersey City, New Jersey

Steven B. Lippitt, MD
Professor
Department of Orthopaedic Surgery
Northeast Ohio Medical University
Akron General Orthopaedics
Cleveland Clinic
Akron, Ohio

Milton Thomas Michael Little, MD
Director, Orthopaedic Trauma Fellowship Program
Cedars-Sinai Orthopaedic Center
Los Angeles, California

Martin M. Malawer, MD, FACS
Director of Orthopedic Oncology
Professor, Orthopedic Surgery
George Washington University School of Medicine
Professor (Clinical Scholar) of Orthopedics and Professor of Pediatrics (Hematology and Oncology)
Georgetown University School of Medicine
Washington, District of Columbia
Consultant, Pediatric and Surgery Branch
National Cancer Institute
National Institutes of Health
Bethesda, Maryland

Elizabeth A. Martin, MD
Orthopaedic Surgeon
Department of Orthopaedic Surgery
Lahey Hospital and Medical Center
Burlington, Massachusetts
Clinical Instructor
Department of Orthopaedic Surgery
Brigham and Women's Hospital
Jamaica Plain, Massachusetts

Natalia Martínez Catalán, MD
Orthopedic Surgeon
Hospital Fundación Jiménez Diaz
Madrid, Spain

Jed I. Maslow, MD
Assistant Professor
Division of Hand and Upper Extremity Surgery
Vanderbilt University Medical Center
Nashville, Tennessee

Robert J. Medoff, MD
Department of Surgery
University of Hawaii
Kailua, Hawaii

Samir Mehta, MD
Chief, Division of Orthopaedic Trauma and Fracture Care
Associate Professor of Orthopaedic Surgery
Hospital of the University of Pennsylvania
Philadelphia, Pennsylvania

Max P. Michalski, MD, MSc
Fellow
Department of Orthopaedic Surgery
Brigham and Women's Hospital
Boston, Massachusetts

Hassan R. Mir, MD
Professor
Department of Orthopaedic Surgery
University of South Florida
Tampa, Florida

Brian Mullis, MD
Professor and Program Director
Department of Orthopaedic Surgery
Indiana University
Indianapolis, Indiana

Sameer Nagda, MD
Orthopaedic Surgeon
Sports Medicine, Shoulder, Elbow, and Knee Surgery
President, Anderson Orthopaedic Clinic
Arlington, Virginia

Aaron Nauth, MD, FRCSC
Associate Professor
Department of Surgery
University of Toronto
Toronto, Ontario, Canada

Michael U. Okoli, MD
Resident
Department of Orthopaedic Surgery
Thomas Jefferson University Hospital
Philadelphia, Pennsylvania

Robert Ostrum, MD
Professor
Department of Orthopaedics
University of North Carolina at Chapel Hill
Chapel Hill, North Carolina

Robert V. O'Toole, MD
Chief of Orthopaedics
R. Adams Cowley Shock Trauma Center
Hansjörg Wyss Medical Foundation Endowed Professor in Orthopaedic Trauma
Division Head, Orthopaedic Traumatology
University of Maryland School of Medicine
Baltimore, Maryland

George Partal, MD
Orthopedic Surgeon
Northern Light Surgery and Trauma
Bangor, Maine

Midhat Patel, MD
Orthopedic Surgeon
Banner Good Samaritan Medical Center
Phoenix, Arizona

Amanda C. Pawlak, MD
Resident
Department of Orthopedics
Stony Brook University Hospital
Stony Brook, New York

E. Scott Paxton, MD
Assistant Professor
Department of Orthopedics
Brown University
Providence, Rhode Island

Michael Quackenbush, DO
Orthopaedic Surgeon
Resurgens Orthopaedics
Roswell, Georgia

Dipak B. Ramkumar, MD, MS
Instructor in Orthopaedic Surgery
Massachusetts General Hospital
Harvard Medical School
Boston, Massachusetts

Niveditta Ramkumar, MPH
Dartmouth Institute for Health Policy and Clinical Practice
Dartmouth College
Lebanon, New Hampshire

Rajesh Rangarajan, MD
Orthopaedic Surgeon
Shoulder and Elbow Surgery
Cedars-Sinai Kerlan-Jobe Institute
Los Angeles, California

Saqib Rehman, MD
Professor
Orthopaedic Surgery
Temple University
Philadelphia, Pennsylvania

William M. Ricci, MD
Chief, Orthopedic Trauma Service
Department of Orthopedic Surgery
Hospital for Special Surgery
New York, New York

Raveesh D. Richard, MD
Orthopedic Surgeon
Centura Orthopedics and Spine
Parker, Colorado

David Ring, MD, PhD
Associate Dean for Comprehensive Care
Department of Surgery and Perioperative Care
Dell Medical School
Austin, Texas

Charles A. Rockwood, MD
Professor and Chairman Emeritus of Orthopaedics
The University of Texas Health Science Center at San Antonio
San Antonio, Texas

Casey M. Sabbag, MD
Hand Surgery Fellow
Department of Orthopedic Surgery
OrthoCarolina
Charlotte, North Carolina

Henry Claude Sagi, MD
Professor
Department of Orthopaedics
University of Cincinnati College of Medicine
Cincinnati, Ohio

Joaquin Sanchez-Sotelo, MD, PhD
Consultant
Department of Orthopedic Surgery
Mayo Clinic Minnesota
Rochester, Minnesota

David W. Sanders, MD, MSc, FRCSC
Professor
Department of Surgery
Western University
London Health Sciences Centre
Victoria Hospital
London, Ontario, Canada

Roy W. Sanders, MD
Director, Orthopaedic Trauma Service
Florida Orthopaedic Institute
Tampa, Florida

Emil H. Schemitsch, MD, FRCSC
Chair and Chief
Department of Surgery
Western University
London, Ontario, Canada

John A. Scolaro, MD
Associate Professor
Department of Orthopaedic Surgery
University of California Irvine
Orange, California

Jodi Siegel, MD
Assistant Professor
Department of Orthopaedics
UMass Memorial Medical Center
Worcester, Massachusetts

Edwin E. Spencer, Jr., MD
Orthopaedic Surgeon
Shoulder and Elbow Center
Knoxville Orthopaedic Clinic
Knoxville, Tennessee

Brandon M. Steen, MD
Shoulder and Elbow Specialist
Florida Orthopaedic Associates
DeLand, Florida

Steven D. Steinlauf, MD
Clinical Assistant Professor
Department of Orthopaedics and Rehabilitation
University of Miami
Miami, Florida

James Stenson, DO
Resident
Department of Orthopedic Surgery
Rowan University School of Osteopathic Medicine
Stratford, New Jersey

Robert J. Strauch, MD
Professor of Orthopedic Surgery
Columbia University Medical Center
New York, New York

Kirsten A. Sumner, MD
Hand Surgery Fellow
Department of Orthopaedic Surgery
University of Miami School of Medicine
Miami, Florida

David C. Templeman, MD
Professor
Department of Orthopedics
Hennepin County Medical Center
Minneapolis, Minnesota

Paul Tornetta III, MD
Professor and Chair, Department of Orthopaedic Surgery
Boston University Medical Center
Boston, Massachusetts

Venus Vakhshori, MD
Department of Orthopaedic Surgery
Keck School of Medicine
University of Southern California
Los Angeles, California

Heather A. Vallier, MD
Professor
Department of Orthopaedic Surgery
Case Western Reserve University
Cleveland, Ohio

Hans P. Van Lancker, MD, FRCSC
Chief of Orthopedic Trauma
Department of Orthopedic Surgery
Saint Elizabeth's Medical Center
Boston, Massachusetts

John J. Walsh IV, MD
Faculty
Department of Orthopedics
University of South Carolina
Columbia, South Carolina

Lance G. Warhold, MD
Department of Orthopaedic Surgery
Dartmouth-Hitchcock Medical Center
Lebanon, New Hampshire

J. Tracy Watson, MD
Professor
Department of Orthopedics
The CORE Institute
Phoenix, Arizona

David J. Wilson, MD, FAAOS
Hand and Elbow Surgeon
Department of Orthopaedic Surgery
US Army Brooke Army Medical Center
Fort Sam Houston, Texas

Michael A. Wirth, MD
Professor
Department of Orthopaedics
Charles A. Rockwood, Jr., MD, Chair of Shoulder Service
University of Texas Health Science Center at San Antonio
San Antonio, Texas

Robert D. Wojahn, MD
Acting Instructor
Orthopaedics and Sports Medicine
Harborview Medical Center
Seattle, Washington

Brian R. Wolf, MD
Professor
Department of Orthopedic Surgery
University of Iowa
Iowa City, Iowa

Philip R. Wolinsky, MD
Professor
Department of Orthopaedic Surgery
University of California Davis
Sacramento, California

Chia H. Wu, MD, MBA
Assistant Professor
Department of Orthopedic Surgery
Baylor College of Medicine
Houston, Texas

Richard S. Yoon, MD
Director, Orthopaedic Research
Department of Orthopaedic Surgery
Jersey City Medical Center
Jersey City, New Jersey

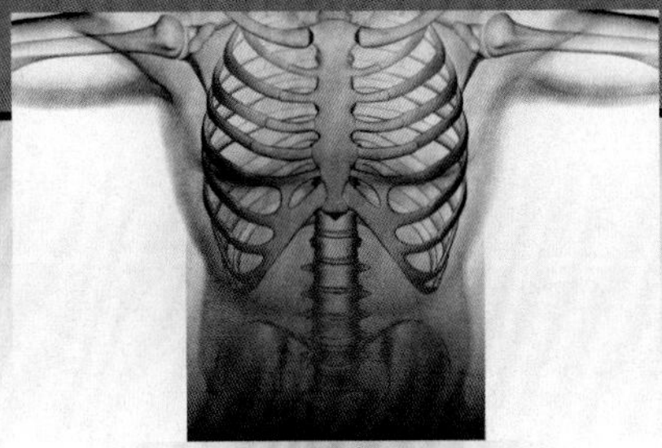

Preface

Techniques in modern orthopaedic surgery continue to evolve at a rapid pace. The principles associated with most modern procedures, however, generally remain rooted in generally sound historical tenets established over the last 150 years.

The goal of the third edition of *Operative Techniques in Orthopaedic Surgery* continues to be to describe in a detailed and step-by-step manner the technical parts of how to do the majority of orthopaedic procedures. The "why" and "when" are covered in outline form at the beginning of each chapter, but it is assumed that the surgeon understands this information. Each of the nine major topics has been revised to include updated procedures. Additionally, the audiovisual part of the text has been increased and continues to evolve. I am very proud of the final text and very grateful to all the section editors and the authors. I have very much enjoyed working with all of them and it has been a great privilege for me.

I would also like to welcome Dr. Todd J. Albert as a Co-Editor-in-Chief for this edition. I have known Todd since he was a resident at Jefferson under Dr. Richard Rothman. He has had an outstanding career. He is an internationally known academic spine surgeon and has had major administrative roles leading the Rothman Orthopaedic Institute in Philadelphia and the Hospital for Special Surgery in New York. Dr. Albert will assume the sole Editor-in-Chief position for the fourth edition. I am absolutely delighted that he has been able to join us.

Finally, I would like to thank all of the people at Wolters Kluwer for their hard work. I can still remember when Bob Hurley, in 2000, proposed the first edition of this text. The first time around it took us 10 years to get it put together. Brian Brown took over as Acquisitions Editor in the middle of the second edition and has been the guiding force for this text since then. I think *Operative Techniques in Orthopaedic Surgery* is in good hands as we look to the future.

Sam W. Wiesel, MD
Washington, DC
January 5, 2021

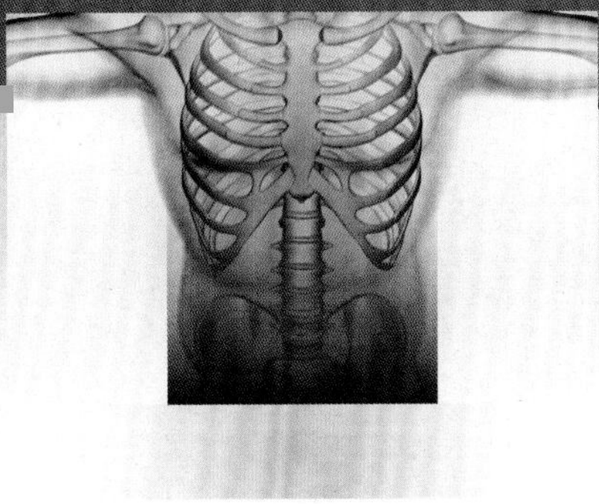

Preface to the Second Edition

The purpose of the second edition of *Operative Techniques in Orthopaedic Surgery* remains the same as the first: to describe in a detailed, step-by-step manner the technical parts of "how to do" the majority of orthopaedic procedures.

It is assumed that the surgeon understands the "why" and the "when," although this information is covered in outline form at the beginning of each procedure.

Each of the nine major sections has been carefully reviewed and updated in both its content and artwork. The second edition has given each section editor the ability to include additional procedures and has also placed more emphasis in creating online content which is easily accessible and fully searchable.

The section editors and chapter authors have done an excellent job. Each has specific expertise and experience in their area and has given their time and effort most generously. It has again been stimulating to interact with these wonderful and talented people, and I am honored to have been able to play a part in this rewarding experience.

I also would like to thank all of the people at Wolters Kluwer. Dave Murphy has been especially helpful and had a great deal of input into this edition, as with the first edition. I would like, as well, to acknowledge Bob Hurley, who was a driving force for the first edition and has been a great resource for this second one as well.

Finally, special thanks goes to Brian Brown, the new acquisitions editor. It has been a wonderful experience to work with Brian who has done an excellent job of bringing this text to completion.

Sam W. Wiesel, MD
Washington, DC
January 2, 2015

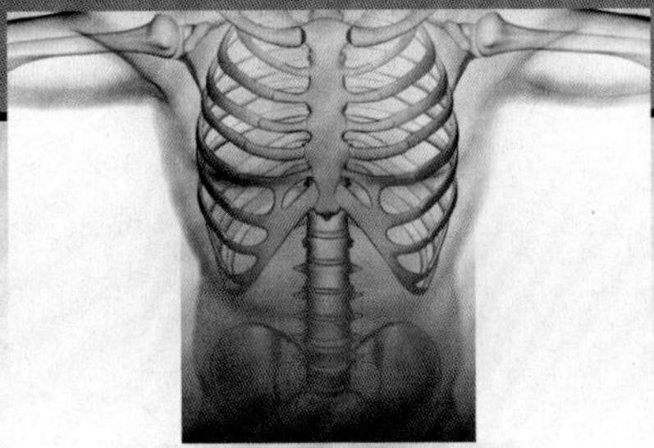

Preface to the First Edition

When a surgeon contemplates performing a procedure, there are three major questions to consider: Why is the surgery being done? When in the course of a disease process should it be performed? And, finally, what are the technical steps involved? The purpose of this text is to describe in a detailed, step-by-step manner the "how to do it" of the vast majority of orthopaedic procedures. The "why" and "when" are covered in outline form at the beginning of each procedure. However, it is assumed that the surgeon understands the basics of "why" and "when," and has made the definitive decision to undertake a specific case. This text is designed to review and make clear the detailed steps of the anticipated operation.

Operative Techniques in Orthopaedic Surgery differs from other books because it is mainly visual. Each procedure is described in a systematic way that makes liberal use of focused, original artwork. It is hoped that the surgeon will be able to visualize each significant step of a procedure as it unfolds during a case.

The text is divided into nine major topics: Adult Reconstruction; Foot and Ankle; Hand, Wrist, and Forearm; Oncology; Pediatrics; Shoulder and Elbow; Sports Medicine; Spine; and Pelvis and Lower Extremity Trauma. Each chapter has been edited by a specialist who has specific expertise and experience in the discipline. It has taken a tremendous amount of work for each editor to enlist talented authors for each procedure and then review the final work. It has been very stimulating to work with all of these wonderful and talented people, and I am honored to have taken part in this rewarding experience.

Finally, I would like to thank everyone who has contributed to the development of this book. Specifically, Grace Caputo at Dovetail Content Solutions, and Dave Murphy and Eileen Wolfberg at Lippincott Williams & Wilkins, who have been very helpful and generous with their input. Special thanks, as well, goes to Bob Hurley at LWW, who has adeptly guided this textbook from original concept to publication.

SWW
January 1, 2010

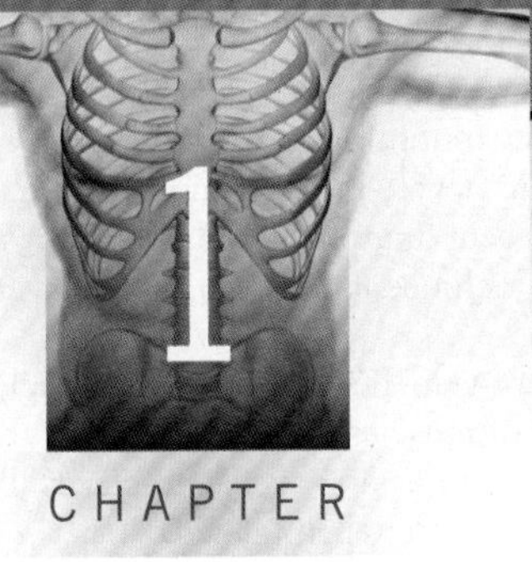

Shoulder and Elbow

Acute Repair and Reconstruction of Sternoclavicular Dislocation

Steven P. Kalandiak, Edwin E. Spencer, Jr., Michael A. Wirth, and Charles A. Rockwood

DEFINITION

- Sternoclavicular dislocation is one of the rarest dislocations but one most shoulder surgeons will encounter several times during a career (more so if they are in a practice with significant exposure to high-energy trauma).
- Sternoclavicular dislocations represented 3% of a series of 1603 injuries of the shoulder girdle reported by Cave.[9]
- The true ratio of anterior to posterior dislocations is unknown because most reports focus on the rarer posterior type. Estimates range from a ratio of 20 anterior dislocations to each posterior by Nettles and Linscheid,[22] in a series of 60 patients (57 anterior and 3 posterior), to a ratio of approximately 3:1 (135 anterior and 50 posterior) in our series[29] of 185 traumatic sternoclavicular injuries.
- Not all sternoclavicular dislocations require surgery. Avoiding inappropriate patient selection, preventing hardware-related complications, and repairing or reconstructing the capsule and the rhomboid ligament if the medial clavicle has been resected require special emphasis.
- Although this region can be intimidating because of the surrounding anatomic structures, a knowledgeable and careful surgeon can treat this joint safely and reliably produce good results.

ANATOMY

- The epiphysis of the medial clavicle is the last epiphysis of the long bones to appear and the last to close. It does not ossify until the 18th to 20th year, and it generally fuses with the shaft of the clavicle around age 23 to 25 years.[17,18] For this reason, many sternoclavicular "dislocations" in young adults are in fact physeal fractures.
- The articular surface of the medial clavicle is much larger than that of the sternum. It is bulbous and concave front to back and convex vertically, creating a saddle-type joint with the curved clavicular notch of the sternum.[17,18]
- A small facet on the inferior aspect of the medial clavicle articulates with the superior aspect of the first rib in 2.5% of subjects.[8]
- There is little congruence and the least bony stability of any major joint in the body. Almost all of the joint's integrity comes from the surrounding ligaments.

Ligaments

- The intra-articular disc ligament is dense and fibrous, arises from the synchondral junction of the first rib to the sternum, passes through the sternoclavicular joint, and divides it into two separate spaces **(FIG 1)**.[17,18] It attaches on the superior and posterior medial clavicle and acts as a checkrein against medial displacement of the inner clavicle.
- The costoclavicular (rhomboid) ligament attaches the upper surface of the medial first rib and upper surface of the first

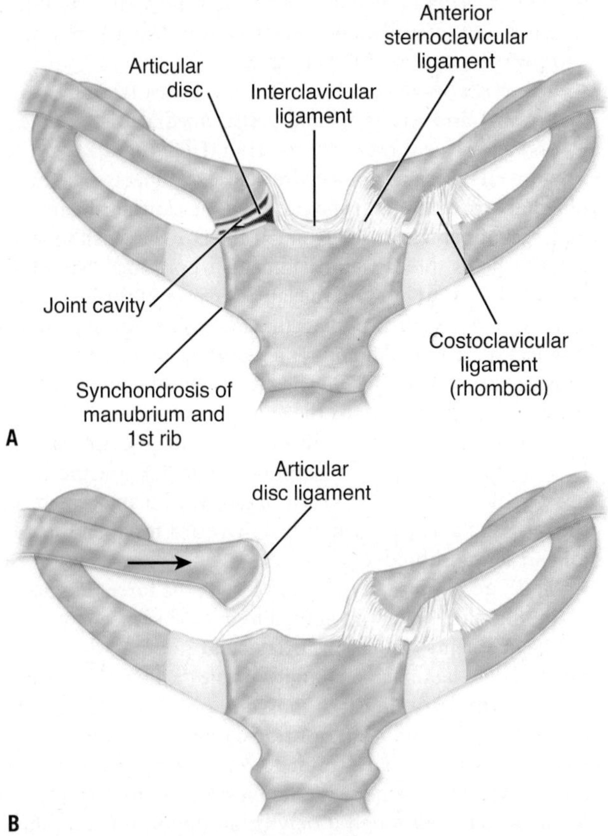

FIG 1 A. Normal anatomy around the sternoclavicular joint. The articular disc ligament divides the sternoclavicular joint cavity into two separate spaces and inserts onto the superior and posterior aspects of the medial clavicle. **B.** The articular disc ligament acts as a checkrein for medial displacement of the proximal clavicle. The *black arrow* represents a medially directed load.

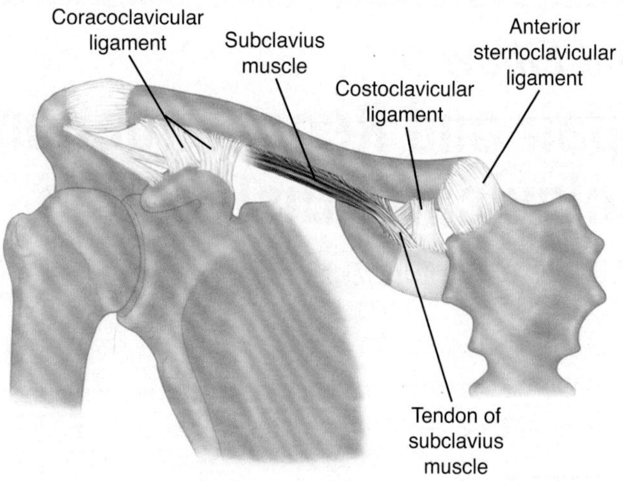

FIG 2 Normal anatomy around the sternoclavicular and acromioclavicular joints. The tendon of the subclavius muscle arises in the vicinity of the costoclavicular ligament from the first rib and has a long tendon structure.

costal cartilage and to the rhomboid fossa on the inferior surface of the medial end of the clavicle.[17,18] It averages 1.3 cm long, 1.9 cm wide, and 1.3 cm thick.[8]

- The anterior fasciculus arises anteromedially, runs upward and laterally, and resists lateral displacement and upward rotation of the clavicle.
- The posterior fasciculus is shorter, arises laterally, runs upward and medially, and resists medial displacement and excessive downward rotation (**FIGS 1** and **2**).[3,8,17]

- The interclavicular ligament (see **FIG 1**) connects the superomedial aspects of each clavicle with the capsular ligaments and the upper sternum. Comparable to the wishbone of birds, it helps the capsular ligaments to produce "shoulder poise"; that is, to hold up the lateral aspect of the clavicle.[18]
- The capsular ligaments cover the anterosuperior and posterior aspects of the joint and represent thickenings of the joint capsule (see **FIGS 1** and **2**). The clavicular attachment of the ligament is primarily onto the epiphysis of the medial clavicle, with some blending of the fibers into the metaphysis.[5,11]
- In sectioning studies, the capsular ligaments are the most important structures in preventing upward displacement of the medial clavicle caused by a downward force on the distal end of the shoulder.[3]
  - This lateral poise of the shoulder (ie, the force that holds the shoulder up) is attributed to a locking mechanism of the ligaments of the sternoclavicular joint.
- Other single ligament sectioning studies[32] have shown that the posterior capsule is the most important primary stabilizer to anterior and posterior translation. The anterior capsule is an important restraint to anterior translation. The costoclavicular ligament is unimportant if the capsule remains intact,[32] although it may be an important secondary restraint if the capsular ligaments are torn, much like the coracoclavicular ligament laterally.

Applied Surgical Anatomy

- A "curtain" of muscles—the sternohyoid, sternothyroid, and scalenus—lies posterior to the sternoclavicular joint and the inner third of the clavicle and blocks the view of vital structures—the innominate artery, innominate vein, vagus nerve, phrenic nerve, internal jugular vein, trachea, and esophagus. A recent anatomic study demonstrated that the closest is the brachiocephalic vein, at an average distance of 6.6 mm.[24]
- The anterior jugular vein lies behind the clavicle and in front of the curtain of muscles. Variable in size and as large as 1.5 cm in diameter, it has no valves and bleeds like someone has opened a floodgate when nicked.
- The surgeon who is considering stabilizing the sternoclavicular joint by running a pin down from the clavicle into the sternum should not do it and should remember that the arch of the aorta, the superior vena cava, and the right pulmonary artery are also very close at hand.

PATHOGENESIS

- Most sternoclavicular joint dislocations result from high-energy trauma, usually a motor vehicle accident. They occasionally result from contact sports.
- A force applied directly to the anteromedial aspect of the clavicle can push the medial clavicle back behind the sternum and into the mediastinum.
- More commonly, a force is applied indirectly, from the lateral aspect of the shoulder. If the shoulder is compressed and rolled forward, a posterior dislocation results; if the shoulder is compressed and rolled backward, an anterior dislocation results.
- As noted earlier, many injuries of the sternoclavicular joint in patients younger than 25 years are, in fact, fractures through the medial physis of the clavicle.

NATURAL HISTORY

- Mild or moderate sprain
  - The mildly sprained sternoclavicular joint is stable but painful.
  - The moderately sprained joint may be slightly subluxated anteriorly or posteriorly and may often be reduced by drawing the shoulders backward as if reducing and holding a fracture of the clavicle.
- Anterior dislocation
  - Although most anterior dislocations are unstable after closed reduction, we still recommend an attempt to reduce the dislocation closed.
  - Occasionally, the clavicle remains reduced, but typically, the clavicle remains unstable after closed reduction. We usually accept the deformity because an anteriorly dislocated sternoclavicular joint typically becomes asymptomatic, and we believe that the deformity is less of a problem than the potential complications of operative fixation.
  - When the entire medial clavicle is stripped out of the deltotrapezial fascia, the deformity can be so severe that it may be poorly tolerated, so we consider primary fixation. In those rare cases when a chronic anterior dislocation is symptomatic, one may perform a capsular reconstruction or a medial clavicle resection and costoclavicular ligament reconstruction.
- Posterior dislocation
  - In contrast to anterior dislocations, the complications of an unreduced posterior dislocation are numerous: thoracic outlet syndrome, vascular compromise, and erosion of the medial clavicle into any of the vital structures that lie posterior to the sternoclavicular joint.

- Closed reduction for acute posterior sternoclavicular dislocation can usually be obtained, and the reduction is generally stable. Often, general anesthesia is necessary. However, when a posterior dislocation is irreducible or the reduction is unstable, an open reduction should be performed.
- When chronic posterior dislocation is present, late complications may arise from mediastinal impingement, so we recommend medial clavicle resection and ligament reconstruction.
- Physeal injuries
  - The typical history for physeal injuries is the same as for other traumatic dislocations. The difference between these injuries and pure dislocations is that most of these injuries will heal with time, without surgical intervention.
  - In very young patients, the remodeling process can eliminate deformity because of the osteogenic potential of an intact periosteal tube. Zaslav et al,[39] Rockwood and Wirth,[29] and Hsu et al[19] have all reported successful treatment of displaced medial clavicle physeal injury in adolescents and provided radiographic evidence of remodeling.
  - Anterior physeal injuries may be reduced, but if reduction cannot be obtained, they can be left alone without problem. Posterior physeal injuries should likewise undergo an attempt at reduction. If a posterior dislocation cannot be reduced closed and the patient is having no significant symptoms, the displacement can be observed while remodeling occurs. Even in older individuals, a posteriorly displaced fracture with moderate displacement and no mediastinal symptoms may be observed, as it usually becomes asymptomatic with fracture healing.
  - However, as with severely displaced dislocations, one may wish to consider operative repair for severely displaced physeal fractures. Suture repair through the medial shaft and the epiphysis and Balser plate fixation have both been successfully used in this situation.[16,34,36]

PATIENT HISTORY AND PHYSICAL FINDINGS

- A history of high-energy trauma is almost a requirement for the diagnosis. Most cases will be due to a motor vehicle accident, a fall from a significant height, or a sports injury.
  - The absence of such a history suggests either an atraumatic instability or some other atraumatic condition of the joint.
- Posterior displacement may be obvious, but anterior fullness can represent either anterior displacement or swelling overlying posterior displacement.
- Careful examination is extremely important. Mediastinal injuries may occur when a traumatic dislocation is posterior, and the physician should seek evidence of damage to the pulmonary and vascular systems, such as hoarseness, venous congestion, and difficulty breathing or swallowing.
- Evaluation should also include the remainder of the thorax, shoulder girdle, and upper extremity as well as the contralateral sternoclavicular joint.

IMAGING AND OTHER DIAGNOSTIC STUDIES

- Plain radiographs
  - Occasionally, routine anteroposterior chest radiographs suggest displacement compared with the normal side. However, these are difficult to interpret.
  - Serendipity view: A 45-degree cephalic tilt view is the most useful and reproducible plain radiograph for the sternoclavicular joint. The tube is centered directly on the sternum, and a nongrid 11 × 14 cassette is placed on the table under the patient's upper shoulders and neck, so the beam will project the medial half of both clavicles onto the film **(FIG 3)**. The technique is the same as a posteroanterior view of the chest.
    - An anteriorly dislocated medial clavicle will appear to ride higher compared to the normal side. The reverse is true if the sternoclavicular joint is dislocated posteriorly **(FIG 4)**.

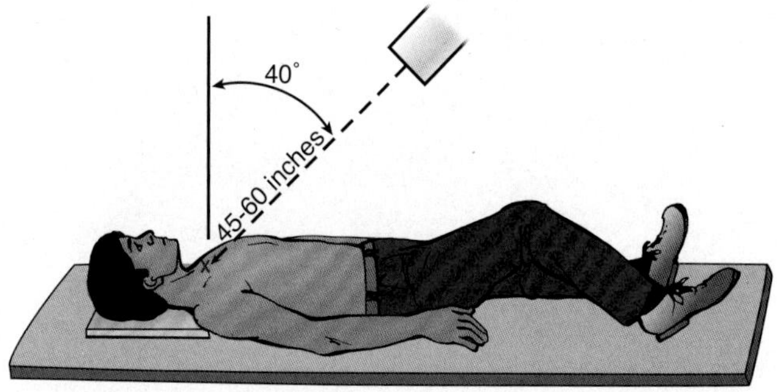

FIG 3 Serendipity view. Positioning of the patient to take the serendipity view of the sternoclavicular joints. The x-ray tube is tilted 40 degrees from the vertical position and aimed directly at the manubrium. The nongrid cassette should be large enough to receive the projected images of the medial halves of both clavicles. In children, the tube distance from the patient should be 45 inches; in thicker chested adults, the distance should be 60 inches.

- More recently, ultrasound has been proposed as an alternate method of making the initial diagnosis of sternoclavicular dislocation.[4]
- In the past, tomograms were useful in distinguishing a sternoclavicular dislocation from a fracture of the medial clavicle and defining questionable anterior and posterior injuries of the sternoclavicular joint. Although they provide more information than plain films, at present, they have been replaced with computed tomography (CT) scans.
- Without question, CT scanning is the best technique to study the sternoclavicular joint. It distinguishes dislocations of the joint from fractures of the medial clavicle and clearly defines minor subluxations **(FIG 5)**. With the increasing presence of O-arms in hospitals, intraoperative CT may

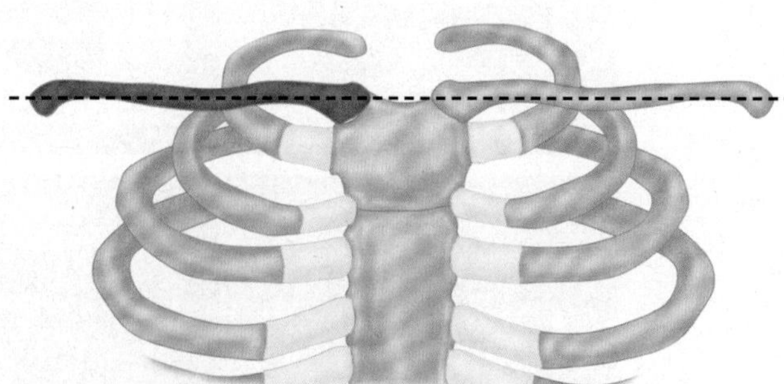

A

FIG 4 Interpretation of the cephalic tilt films of the sternoclavicular joints. **A.** In a normal person, both clavicles appear on the same imaginary line drawn horizontally across the film. *(continued)*

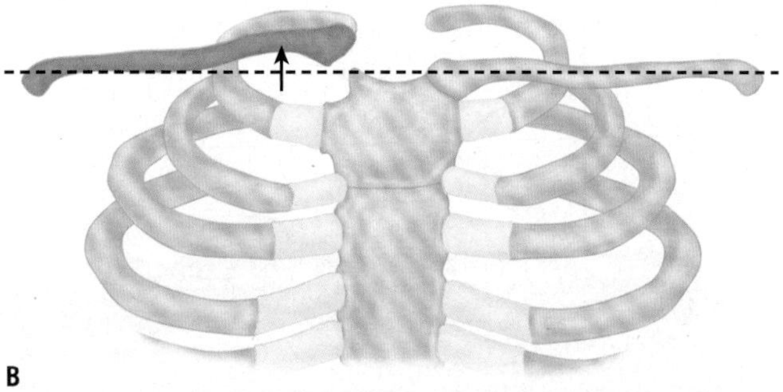

B

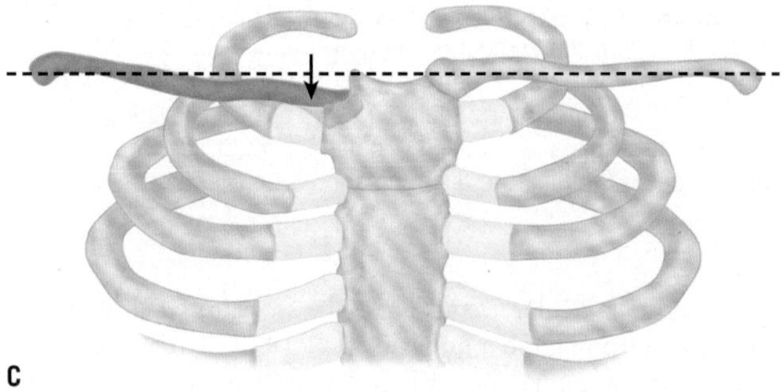

C

FIG 4 *(continued)* **B.** In a patient with anterior dislocation of the right sternoclavicular joint, the medial half of the right clavicle is projected above the imaginary line drawn through the level of the normal left clavicle. **C.** If the patient has a posterior dislocation of the right sternoclavicular joint, the medial half of the right clavicle is displaced below the imaginary line drawn through the normal left clavicle.

become more readily available for both closed and open reductions.[33]

- The patient should lie supine. The scan should include both sternoclavicular joints and the medial halves of both clavicles so that the injured side can be compared with the normal.
- If symptoms of mediastinal compression are present or displacement of the medial clavicle is severe, the use of intravenous contrast will aid in the imaging of the vascular structures in the mediastinum.

DIFFERENTIAL DIAGNOSIS

- Arthritic conditions: sternocostoclavicular hyperostosis, osteitis condensans, Friedrich disease, Tietze syndrome, and osteoarthritis
- Atraumatic (spontaneous) subluxation or dislocation: One or both of the sternoclavicular joints may spontaneously subluxate or dislocate during abduction or flexion during overhead motion. Typically seen in ligamentously lax females in their late teens or early 20s, it is not painful, it is almost always anterior, and it should almost always be managed nonoperatively.[28]
- Congenital or developmental or acquired subluxation or dislocation: Birth trauma, congenital defects with loss of bone substance on either side of the joint, or neuromuscular or other developmental disorders can predispose the patient to subluxation or dislocation.
- Iatrogenic instability may be due to failure to reconstruct the ligaments of the sternoclavicular joint adequately or to an excessive medial clavicle resection. History is significant for a prior procedure on the sternoclavicular joint.

NONOPERATIVE MANAGEMENT

- A mild sprain is stable but painful. We treat mild sprains with a sling, cold packs, and resumption of activity as comfort dictates.
- A moderate sprain may be slightly subluxated anteriorly or posteriorly. Moderate sprains may be reduced by drawing the shoulders backward as if reducing a fracture of the clavicle. This is followed by cold packs and immobilization in a padded figure-8 strap for 4 to 6 weeks and then gradual resumption of activity as comfort dictates.
- Anterior dislocations may undergo closed reduction with either local or general anesthesia, narcotics, or muscle relaxants.
  - The patient is supine on the table, with a 3- to 4-inch thick pad between the shoulders. Direct gentle pressure over the anteriorly displaced clavicle or traction on the outstretched arm combined with pressure on the medial clavicle will generally reduce the dislocation.
- Posterior dislocation in a stoic patient may possibly be reducible under intravenous narcotics and muscle relaxation.

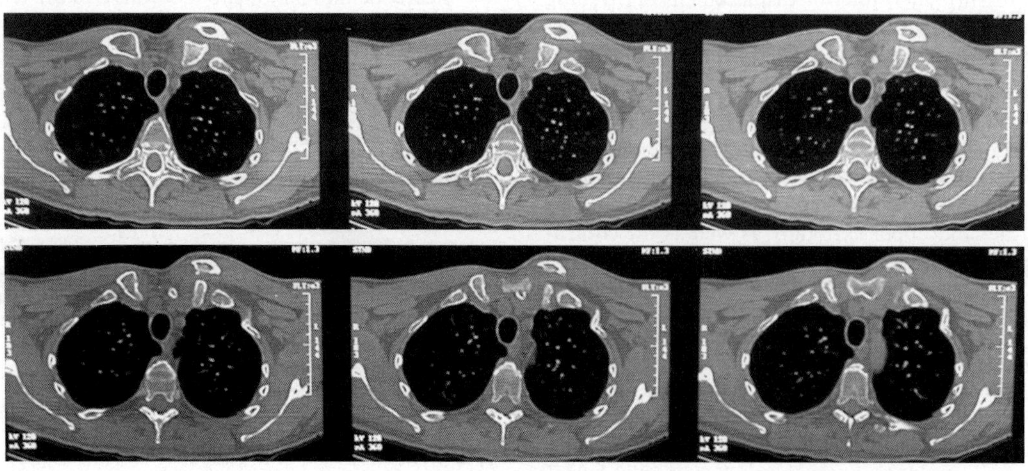

FIG 5 CT scans of a 6-month-old medial clavicle fracture demonstrate anterior displacement without significant healing.

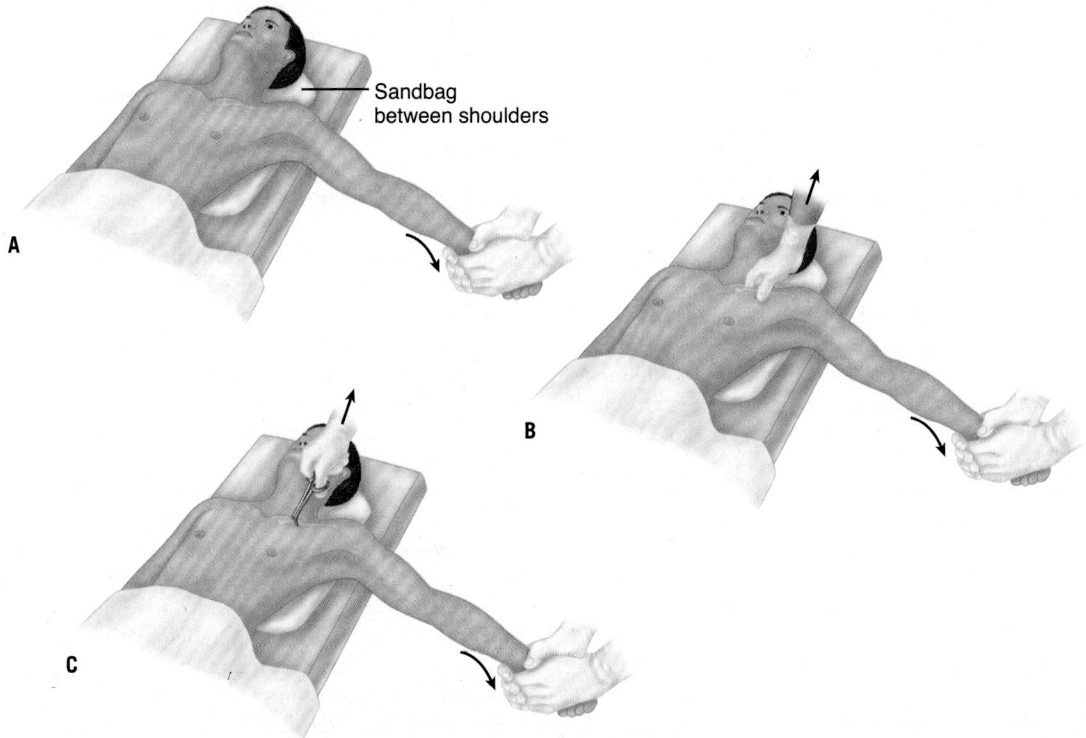

FIG 6 Technique for closed reduction of the sternoclavicular joint. **A.** The patient is positioned supine with a sandbag placed between the two shoulders. Traction is then applied to the arm against countertraction in an abducted and slightly extended position. In anterior dislocations, direct pressure over the medial end of the clavicle may reduce the joint. **B.** In posterior dislocations, in addition to the traction, it may be necessary to manipulate the medial end of the clavicle with the fingers to dislodge the clavicle from behind the manubrium. **C.** In stubborn posterior dislocations, it may be necessary to prepare the medial end of the clavicle sterilely and use a towel clip to grasp around the medial clavicle to lift it back into position.

However, general anesthesia is usually required for reduction of a posterior dislocation because of pain and muscle spasm.

- Our preferred method is the abduction traction technique.
  - The patient is placed supine, with the dislocated side near the edge of the table. A 3- to 4-inch thick sandbag is placed between the scapulae **(FIG 6)**. Lateral traction is applied to the abducted arm, which is then gradually brought back into extension. The clavicle usually reduces with an audible snap or pop, and it is almost always stable. Too much extension can bind the anterior surface of the dislocated medial clavicle on the back of the manubrium.
  - Occasionally, it is necessary to grasp the medial clavicle with one's fingers to dislodge it from behind the sternum. If this fails, the skin is prepared, and a sterile towel clip is used to grasp the medial clavicle to apply lateral and anterior traction (see **FIG 6C**). If the joint is stable after reduction, the shoulders should be held back for 4 to 6 weeks with a figure-8 dressing to allow ligament healing.
- Many investigators have reported that closed reduction usually cannot be accomplished after 48 hours. However, others have reported closed reductions as late as 4 and 5 days after the injury.[6]
- Physeal fractures are reduced in the same manner as dislocations, with immobilization in a figure-8 strap for 4 weeks to protect stable reductions. Fractures that cannot be reduced and are being managed nonoperatively are treated with a figure-8 strap or a sling for comfort and mobilized as symptoms permit.

SURGICAL MANAGEMENT

- A posterior displacement of the medial clavicle that is irreducible or redislocates after closed reduction is a well-accepted surgical indication.
- More controversial is anterior displacement that fails to maintain a stable reduction.
  - The traditional treatment for persistent anterior displacement is nonoperative, which, in the majority of cases, produces excellent function and minimal pain despite the persistent displacement and deformity.
  - However, when the entire medial clavicle is torn out of the deltotrapezial sleeve, the extreme displacement can result in either instability or abundant heterotopic bone formation with accompanying pain and limited motion. As a result, operative treatment for severe anterior displacement is gaining acceptance.

Preoperative Planning

- Careful review of the history and examination for symptoms of mediastinal compression is crucial.
- Review of the CT scan for the direction and degree of displacement and determination of a very medial fracture versus pure dislocation follows.
- If a history or radiographic evidence of mediastinal compromise or potential compromise is present, a cardiothoracic surgeon should be either present or readily available.
- Very medial fractures can occasionally be repaired with independent small fragment lag screws or orthogonal minifragment plates. For pure dislocations, heavy nonabsorbable suture will sometimes suffice. Suture anchors are useful for augmenting ligament repairs. Allograft tendons may be used if the capsule is irreparable and must be reconstructed.
- Closed reduction under anesthesia is then attempted and the stability of the joint is evaluated after reduction.

Positioning

- To begin, the patient is positioned supine on the table, and three or four towels or a sandbag placed between the scapulae.
- The upper extremity should be draped free so that lateral traction can be applied during the open reduction.
- A folded sheet may be left in place around the patient's thorax so that it can be used for countertraction.
- If there is concern regarding the mediastinum, the entire sternum should be draped into the field.

Approach

- An anterior incision that parallels the superior border of the medial 3 to 4 inches of the clavicle and then extends downward over the sternum just medial to the involved sternoclavicular joint is used **(FIG 7A)**.
  - As an alternative, a necklace-type incision may be created in Langer lines, beginning at the midline and sweeping lateral and up along the clavicle.
- Careful subperiosteal dissection around the medial clavicle and onto the surface of the manubrium allows exposure of the articular surfaces.
  - If the medial clavicle is resting posteriorly, it is safer to identify the shaft more laterally and then trace it back medially along the subperiosteal plane **(FIG 7B)**.
- Traction and blunt retractors can then be used to lever the medial clavicle back up into its anatomic location **(FIG 7C)**. These retractors may be used behind the medial clavicle and manubrium to protect the posterior structures.
- If one has chosen to operate on an anterior medial clavicle because of extreme displacement, it may generally be simply pushed back into place.

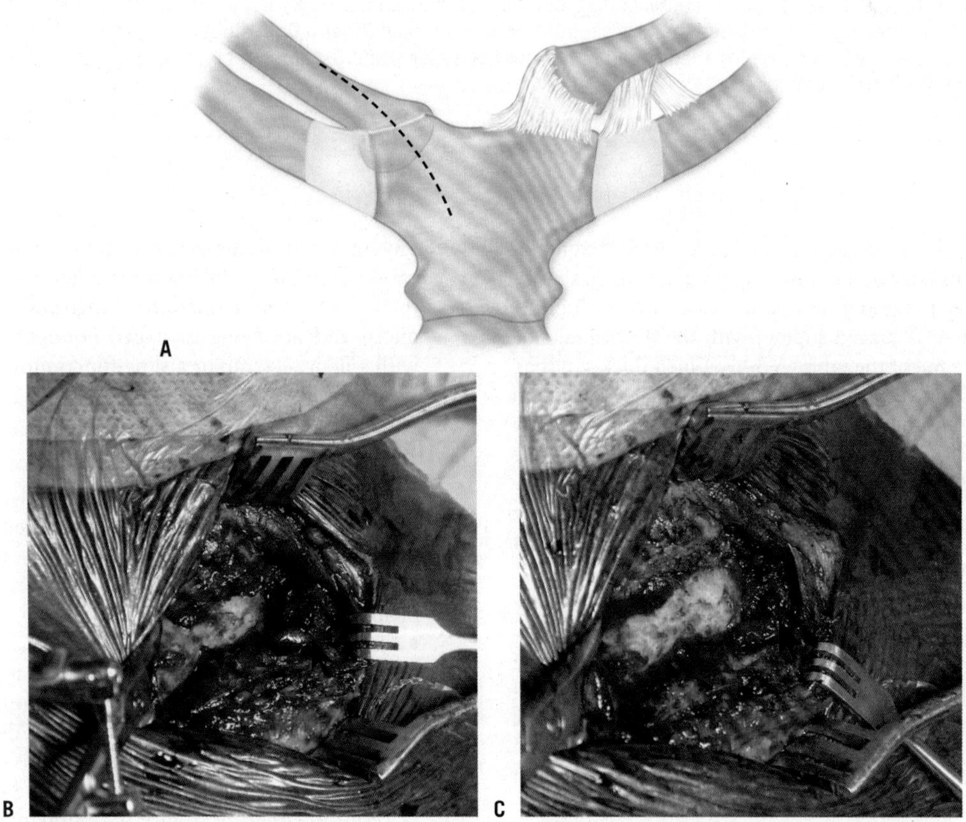

FIG 7 **A.** Proposed skin incision for open reduction of a posterior dislocation. **B.** Subperiosteal exposure of the medial clavicle shows a posteriorly displaced medial clavicular shaft (*left*) resting posterior to the medial clavicular physis (*arrow, right*). **C.** The medial shaft of the clavicle has been lifted anteriorly with a clamp and now rests adjacent to the medial physis (*arrow, right*).

PRIMARY REPAIR: MEDIAL FRACTURE

- In children and in young adults, the dislocation of the medial clavicle may occur through the medial physis or as a fracture, leaving a small amount of bone articulating with the manubrium.
- Because much of the capsule remains intact to this medial fragment, it can serve as an anchor for internal fixation of the medial clavicle shaft. Depending on the amount of bone, the type of fixation will vary.
- The smallest fragments will permit only osseous suture fixation, but the medial clavicle is cancellous bone and heals very quickly **(TECH FIG 1A)**.
- As the fragment gets larger, independent lag screw fixation may be possible **(TECH FIG 1B,C)**.
- For very medial shaft fractures, it may even be possible to use two orthogonal minifragment plates.

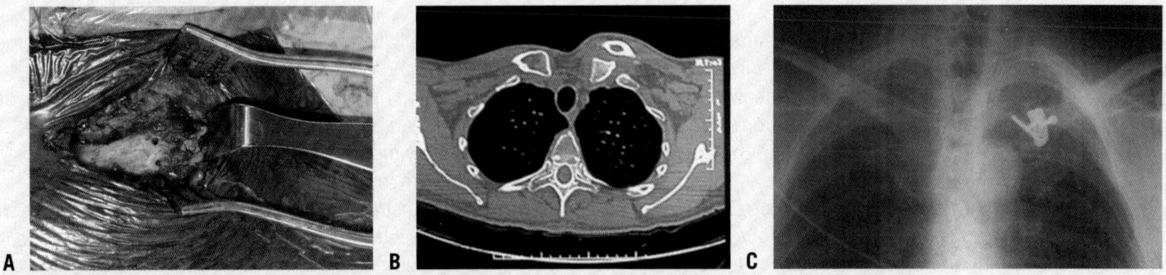

TECH FIG 1 A. Heavy nonabsorbable suture has been placed through drill holes in the medial clavicle and through the physis to secure the fracture shown in **FIG 7B,C**. **B,C.** A symptomatic medial clavicle nonunion had a medial fragment large enough to allow fixation with three cortical lag screws.

PRIMARY REPAIR: CAPSULAR LIGAMENTS AND SUTURE REPAIR

- After reduction, the position of the clavicle may be maintained with either nonabsorbable osseous sutures through drill holes in the medial clavicle and manubrium,[34,36] suture anchors[21] **(TECH FIG 2)**, sutures wrapped around screws placed as anchor points,[7] or sternal cable[20] until tissue healing occurs.
- The ligaments of the anterior and superior capsule may then be repaired primarily with heavy nonabsorbable suture. The costoclavicular ligament may occasionally be repaired primarily as well, but, for obvious reasons, the important posterior capsule cannot be easily repaired.
- These suture techniques were not only initially employed primarily in children but also now used more frequently in adults as well.

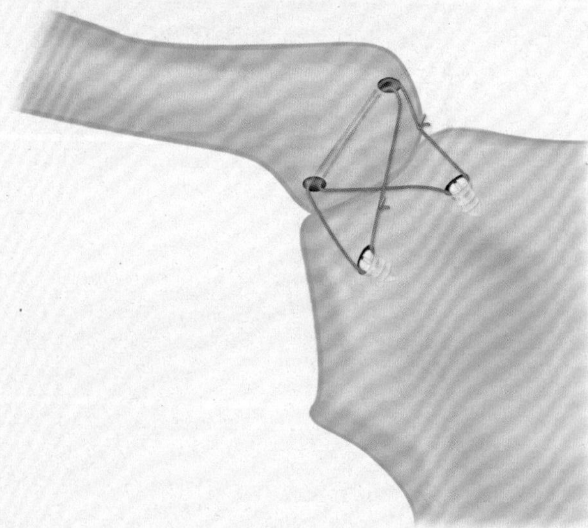

TECH FIG 2 Suture anchors may be used to create a sling to hold the medial clavicle reduced while the capsular ligaments heal.

IMMEDIATE RECONSTRUCTION: CAPSULAR LIGAMENTS

- At times, the joint may be reducible but the ligaments are damaged to the point where primary repair is not feasible. In this circumstance, the ligaments may be immediately reconstructed using tendon graft. Variations of this technique are typically used for chronic instability. Autograft or allograft tendon may be used. Artificial ligaments have also been reported.[25]
- This may be done by passing a tendon in a simple fashion from the front of the sternum, through the articular surfaces and intra-articular disc, and out the front of the medial clavicle and tying the tendon to itself anteriorly.[26] Suture anchors may also be used to anchor the graft.
- The capsule may also be reconstructed in the manner described by Spencer and Kuhn[31] **(TECH FIG 3)**. Since their initial description, numerous variations have been described.
  - Drill holes 4 mm in diameter are created from anterior to posterior through the medial clavicle and the adjacent manubrium.
  - A free semitendinosus tendon graft is woven through the drill holes so the tendon strands are parallel to each other posterior to the joint and cross each other anterior to it.
  - The tendon is tied in a square knot and secured with no. 2 Ethibond suture (Ethicon, Inc., Somerville, NJ).
- This technique has the advantage of reconstructing both the anterior and the posterior ligament in a very strong and secure manner.
- If a resection of the medial clavicle is performed, care should be taken to not excise beyond the rhomboid ligament, which provides security to the medial end of the first rib. If the rhomboid ligament is attenuated or torn, then axial instability can occur. The capsular reconstruction will garner stability in the anteroposterior direction but not longitudinally along the axis of the clavicle. Axial instability results in the medial end of the resected clavicle abutting and grinding on the sternal fossa. This can be mitigated by placing an "anchovy" graft as demonstrated in the video that accompanies this chapter. Fascia lata or the remaining portions of the graft that was used to stabilize the joint can be fashioned in an accordion style to "fill" the gap created by the resection. The author has also used a stemmed radial head implant (off label) for the same purpose.
- Recently, Armstrong and Dias[1] and Uri et al[35] have described the use of the sternocleidomastoid (SCM) tendon to moor the medial clavicle back to the manubrium in cases of sternoclavicular instability. Although their cases were done for more chronic conditions, the SCM tendon would also be readily available for additional stabilization in the acute setting.

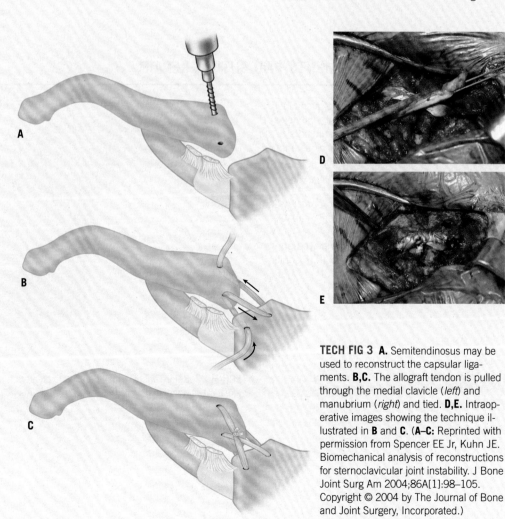

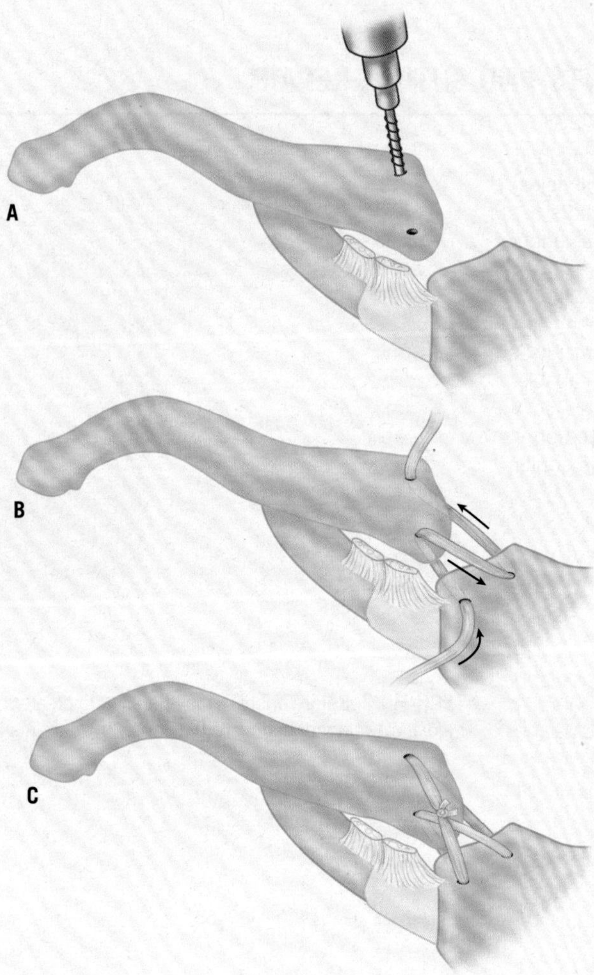

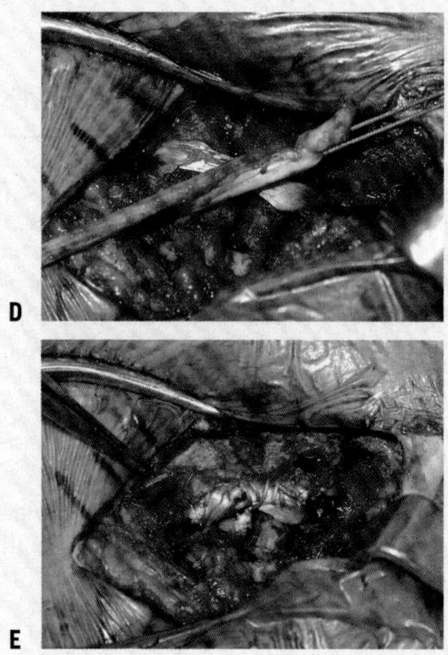

TECH FIG 3 A. Semitendinosus may be used to reconstruct the capsular ligaments. **B,C.** The allograft tendon is pulled through the medial clavicle (*left*) and manubrium (*right*) and tied. **D,E.** Intraoperative images showing the technique illustrated in **B** and **C**. (**A–C:** Reprinted with permission from Spencer EE Jr, Kuhn JE. Biomechanical analysis of reconstructions for sternoclavicular joint instability. J Bone Joint Surg Am 2004;86A[1]:98–105. Copyright © 2004 by The Journal of Bone and Joint Surgery, Incorporated.)

MEDIAL CLAVICLE RESECTION AND LIGAMENT RECONSTRUCTION

- If there is concern about the stability of a reconstruction or repair, if the dislocation is subacute and posterior, or if there is a question of impingement on the mediastinal structures, one may elect to resect the medial clavicle entirely. In this situation, it is important to repair or reconstruct the costoclavicular ligament (akin to a modified Weaver-Dunn procedure).
- The medullary canal can also be used to create an attachment point for an additional medial tether. We prefer to use the patient's own tissue, such as the sternoclavicular ligament, whenever possible **(TECH FIG 4)**.
- The medial clavicle is resected and the canal curetted and prepared with drill holes on the superior surface.
- Grasping suture is woven through the remaining ligament, pulled through the superior drill holes, and tied over bone.
- Heavy nonabsorbable sutures are then passed through the remaining costoclavicular ligament and around the clavicle, and the periosteal tube is closed.
- If adequate local tissue is not present, an allograft such as Achilles tendon may also be used.[2]

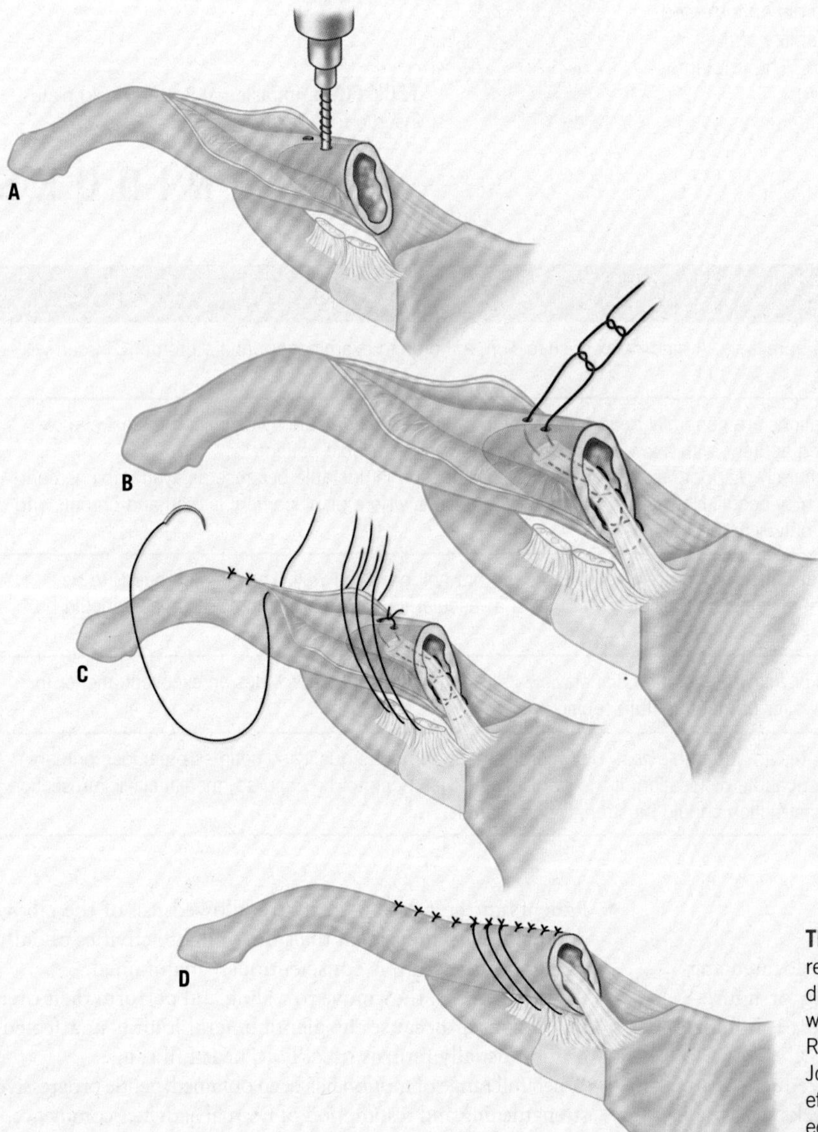

TECH FIG 4 The residual capsule may be used to reconstruct a medial clavicular restraint, akin to a medial Weaver-Dunn procedure, as described by Rockwood and Wirth.[29] (Redrawn from Bois AJ, Wirth MA, Rockwood CA Jr. Disorders of the Sternoclavicular Joint. In: Rockwood CA Jr, Matsen FA III, Wirth MA, et al., eds. Rockwood and Matsen's The Shoulder. 5th ed. Philadelphia: Elsevier; 2017:453-491. Copyright © 2017 Elsevier. With permission.)

REDUCTION AND PLATE FIXATION

- The use of Kirschner wires (K-wires) around the sternoclavicular joint has been routinely condemned, and they should not be used.
  - There are reports, however, of temporary plate fixation from the medial clavicle to the sternum or to the opposite clavicle[23] to maintain a reduced joint while the soft tissues heal. Hook plates, reconstruction plates, and locked plates have all been used. After several months, the hardware is usually removed.
- The Balser plate is a hook plate used in Europe for treatment of acromioclavicular joint separations and distal clavicle fractures. It has been used for sternoclavicular dislocations by placing the hook into the sternum and using screws to fix the plate onto the medial clavicle **(TECH FIG 5)**.
  - Franck et al[15] published good results for 10 patients treated with Balser plates. They thought that the stability of this construct allowed a more rapid rehabilitation. The implant is quite bulky and removal is generally required.

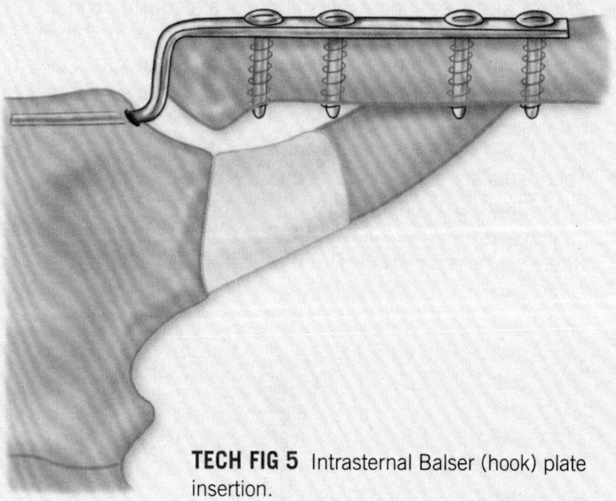

TECH FIG 5 Intrasternal Balser (hook) plate insertion.

TECHNIQUES

Pearls and Pitfalls

Diagnosis	• Conventional studies are unreliable. A high index of suspicion, a thorough examination, and a prompt CT scan will ensure correct diagnosis.
Individualize Treatment When Necessary	• Although anterior dislocations are generally treated nonoperatively, a severely anteriorly displaced medial clavicle may be reduced and fixed acutely, with a low risk of complications, in a reliable patient. • Posterior dislocations generally mandate surgery when closed reduction is unstable because delayed impingement on mediastinal contents may occur. However, there may be situations where displacement is mild and chronic and the risks of surgery may outweigh the benefits.
Prepare for Complications	• Although complications are uncommon, they are spectacular but not in a good way. The surgeon needs to be ready for both pneumothorax and the unlikely possibility of a vascular injury. A cardiothoracic surgeon should be immediately available.
Use the Medial Clavicle	• Even a medial epiphysis or a tiny piece of medial clavicle in its anatomic location provides an excellent anchor for heavy suture or lag screws for primary fracture repair.
Be Flexible Intraoperatively	• Preserving the native joint is an admirable goal, but poor ligament and bone quality sometimes precludes primary repair, especially in the subacute dislocation. If the stability of the joint cannot be ensured, medial clavicle resection and costoclavicular reconstruction should be strongly considered.

POSTOPERATIVE CARE

- For sternoclavicular strains and anteriorly dislocated medial clavicles accepted in this position, a sling or figure-8 strap is prescribed, and the patient is allowed to mobilize the extremity as function permits.
- Medial clavicle fractures that are stable after reduction are immobilized in a figure-8 strap for 4 to 6 weeks and then mobilized as comfort allows.
- Acute dislocations that have been reduced and are stable or have been surgically repaired receive a sling or figure-8 strap for 6 weeks to protect the reduction and allow ligament healing.
- Patients in the figure-8 strap are allowed use of the elbow and hand with the arm at the side for light activities of daily living, but the strap is conscientiously maintained.
- At 4 to 6 weeks, they move to a sling and perform their own mobilization. Because the glenohumeral joint is unaffected, motion usually returns quickly to near full range.
- When full range of motion has been obtained, gentle progressive strengthening and resumption of normal activities commence.
- In general, patients treated with joint preservation can return to all activities, including heavy labor, but we have seen traumatic failure of costoclavicular reconstructions and do ask patients who have undergone medial clavicle resection and ligament reconstruction to avoid heavy overhead labor for their lifetimes.

OUTCOMES

- A recent Medline search for "sternoclavicular" and "dislocation" yielded 550 citations, most dealing with sternoclavicular instability and its sequelae. Most were case reports or a series of three or four patients or a discussion of the complications of the injury or its treatment. There are very few large series, which makes discussing outcomes difficult. However, several themes do emerge.
- The need for proper patient selection becomes evident when one considers that some forms of sternoclavicular instability generally do well when treated without surgery.
  - Sadr and Swann[30] and Rockwood and Odor[28] have both documented the good long-term results obtained with nonoperative treatment of atraumatic sternoclavicular instability.
  - De Jong and Sukul[10] has documented good long-term results in 13 patients with anterior dislocations treated nonoperatively.
- Several larger series[13,14,35,37] have reported on a dozen or more patients treated with open reduction, ligament repair or reconstruction, and fixation with pins or sternoclavicular wiring. Good results were obtained when the medial clavicle was successfully stabilized.
  - Eskola,[12] however, noted a high failure rate if the remaining medial clavicle was not successfully stabilized to the first rib.
  - In a separate study, Rockwood et al[27] reported on seven patients who had previously undergone medial clavicle resection without ligament reconstruction. Six of the seven had worse symptoms than before their index procedure.

COMPLICATIONS

- Complications of injury
  - Anterior dislocation: cosmetic "bump" (which may occasionally be pronounced) and late degenerative changes
  - Posterior dislocation: Great vessel injuries, including laceration, compression, and occlusion; pneumothorax; rupture of the esophagus with abscess and osteomyelitis of the clavicle; fatal tracheoesophageal fistula; brachial plexus compression; stridor and dysphagia; hoarseness of the voice; onset of snoring; and voice changes from normal to falsetto with movement of the arm have all been reported. These all may occur acutely or in a delayed fashion.
  - Worman and Leagus[38] reported that 16 of 60 patients with posterior dislocations had suffered complications of the trachea, esophagus, or great vessels.
- Errors of patient selection
  - Operating in unindicated circumstances introduces another set of complications. Rockwood and Odor[28] reviewed 37 patients with spontaneous atraumatic subluxation.
  - Twenty-nine managed without surgery had no limitations of activity or lifestyle at over 8 years average follow-up. Eight treated (elsewhere) with surgical reconstruction had increased pain, limitation of activity, alteration of lifestyle, persistent instability, and significant scars.
  - Before surgery, most of these patients had minimal discomfort and excellent motion and complained only of a bump that slipped in and out of place with certain motions.
- Intraoperative complications
  - Little has been written about these, but a veritable jungle of vitally important structures lurks immediately behind the sternoclavicular joint. We always perform these operations with an available, in-house cardiothoracic surgeon on notice and request his or her presence in the operating suite for all but the most routine cases.
- Postoperative complications
  - Hardware migration: Because of the motion at the sternoclavicular joint, tremendous leverage is applied to pins that cross it; fatigue breakage of the pins is common. Numerous authors have reported deaths and many near-deaths from K-wires and Steinmann pins migrating into the heart, pulmonary artery, innominate artery, aorta, and elsewhere in the mediastinum. Despite numerous admonitions in the literature regarding the use of sternoclavicular pins, there have been continued reports of K-wire migration to intrathoracic and other remote locations.
  - For this reason, we do not recommend the use of any transfixing pins—large or small, smooth or threaded, bent or straight—across the sternoclavicular joint.
  - Iatrogenic instability: Failure to preserve the costoclavicular ligament when it is intact and failure to reconstruct it when it is deficient both severely compromise the surgical result. As noted earlier, both Rockwood et al[27] and Eskola[12] noted vastly inferior results when the residual medial clavicle was not stabilized to the first rib and an inability to obtain equivalent results when the costoclavicular ligament was reconstructed in a delayed fashion.
  - Iatrogenic instability: An excessive resection that removes bone to a point lateral to the costoclavicular ligament is an extremely difficult problem that is best avoided because there is no reconstructive option. In these difficult cases, we have occasionally performed a subtotal claviculectomy to a point just medial to the coracoclavicular ligaments. This leaves the extremity without a "strut" connecting it to the thorax but can produce substantial relief of pain and improvement in motion and activity.

REFERENCES

1. Armstrong AL, Dias JJ. Reconstruction for instability of the sternoclavicular joint using the tendon of the sternocleidomastoid muscle. J Bone Joint Surg Br 2008;90(5):610–613.
2. Battaglia TC, Pannunzio ME, Chhabra AB, et al. Interposition arthroplasty with bone-tendon allograft: a technique for treatment of the unstable sternoclavicular joint. J Orthop Trauma 2005;19:124–129.
3. Bearn JG. Direct observations on the function of the capsule of the sternoclavicular joint in the clavicular support. J Anat 1967;101:159–170.
4. Blakeley CJ, Harrison HL, Siow S, et al. The use of bedside ultrasound to diagnose posterior sterno-clavicular dislocation. Emerg Med J 2011;28(6):542.
5. Brooks AL, Henning CD. Injury to the proximal clavicular epiphysis [abstract]. J Bone Joint Surg Am 1972;54A:1347–1348.
6. Buckerfield CT, Castle ME. Acute traumatic retrosternal dislocation of the clavicle. J Bone Joint Surg Am 1984;66:379–385.
7. Carpentier E, Rubens-Duval B, Saragaglia D. A simple surgical treatment for acute traumatic sternoclavicular dislocation. Eur J Orthop Surg Traumatol 2013;23(6):719–723.
8. Cave AJE. The nature and morphology of the costoclavicular ligament. J Anat 1961;95:170–179.
9. Cave EF. Fractures and Other Injuries. Chicago: Year Book Medical, 1958.

10. De Jong KP, Sukul DM. Anterior sternoclavicular dislocation: a long-term follow-up study. J Orthop Trauma 1990;4:420–423.
11. Denham RH Jr, Dingley AF Jr. Epiphyseal separation of the medial end of the clavicle. J Bone Joint Surg Am 1967;49:1179–1183.
12. Eskola A. Sternoclavicular dislocation. A plea for open treatment. Acta Orthop Scand 1986;57:227–228.
13. Eskola A, Vainionpää S, Vastamäki M, et al. Operation for old sternoclavicular dislocation. Results in 12 cases. J Bone Joint Surg Br 1989;71:63–65.
14. Ferrandez L, Yubero J, Usabiaga J, et al. Sternoclavicular dislocation. Treatment and complications. Ital J Orthop Traumatol 1988;14:349–355.
15. Franck WM, Jannasch O, Siassi M, et al. Balser plate stabilization: an alternate therapy for traumatic sternoclavicular instability. J Shoulder Elbow Surg 2003;12:276–281.
16. Franck WM, Siassi RM, Hennig FF. Treatment of posterior epiphyseal disruption of the medial clavicle with a modified Balser plate. J Trauma 2003;55:966–968.
17. Grant JCB. Method of Anatomy, ed 7. Baltimore: Williams & Wilkins, 1965.
18. Gray H. Osteology. In: Goss CM, ed. Anatomy of the Human Body, ed 28. Philadelphia: Lea & Febiger, 1966:324–326.
19. Hsu HC, Wu JJ, Lo WH, et al. Epiphyseal fracture-retrosternal dislocation of the medial end of the clavicle: a case report. Zhonghua Yi Xue Za Zhi (Taipei) 1993;52:198–202.
20. Janson JT, Rossouw GJ. A new technique for repair of a dislocated sternoclavicular joint using a sternal tension cable system. Ann Thorac Surg 2013;95(2):e53–e55.
21. Mirza AH, Alam K, Ali A. Posterior sternoclavicular dislocation in a rugby player as a cause of silent vascular compromise: a case report. Br J Sports Med 2005;39:e28.
22. Nettles JL, Linscheid R. Sternoclavicular dislocations. J Trauma 1968;8:158–164.
23. Pensy RA, Eglseder WA. Posterior sternoclavicular fracture-dislocation: a case report and novel treatment method. J Shoulder Elbow Surg 2010;19(4):e5–e8.
24. Ponce BA, Kundukulam JA, Pflugner R, et al. Sternoclavicular joint surgery: how far does danger lurk below? J Shoulder Elbow Surg 2013;22(7):993–999.
25. Quayle JM, Arnander MW, Pennington RG, et al. Artificial ligament reconstruction of sternoclavicular joint instability: report of a novel surgical technique with early results. Tech Hand Up Extrem Surg 2014;18(1):31–35.
26. Qureshi SA, Shah AK, Pruzansky ME. Using the semitendinosus tendon to stabilize sternoclavicular joints in a patient with Ehlers-Danlos syndrome: a case report. Am J Orthop (Belle Mead NJ) 2005;34:315–318.
27. Rockwood CA Jr, Groh GI, Wirth MA, et al. Resection arthroplasty of the sternoclavicular joint. J Bone Joint Surg Am 1997;79:387–393.
28. Rockwood CA Jr, Odor JM. Spontaneous atraumatic anterior subluxation of the sternoclavicular joint. J Bone Joint Surg Am 1989;71:1280–1288.
29. Rockwood CA Jr, Wirth MA. Disorders of the sternoclavicular joint. In: Rockwood CA Jr, Matsen FA III, eds. The Shoulder, ed 2. Philadelphia: WB Saunders, 1998:555–609.
30. Sadr B, Swann M. Spontaneous dislocation of the sterno-clavicular joint. Acta Orthop Scand 1979;50:269–274.
31. Spencer EE Jr, Kuhn JE. Biomechanical analysis of reconstructions for sternoclavicular joint instability. J Bone Joint Surg Am 2004;86:98–105.
32. Spencer EE Jr, Kuhn JE, Huston LJ, et al. Ligamentous restraints to anterior and posterior translation of the sternoclavicular joint. J Shoulder Elbow Surg 2002;11:43–47.
33. Sullivan JP, Warme BA, Wolf BR. Use of an O-arm intraoperative computed tomography scanner for closed reduction of posterior sternoclavicular dislocations. J Shoulder Elbow Surg 2012;21(3):e17–e20.
34. Thacker MM, Patankar JV, Goregaonkar AB. A safe technique for sternoclavicular stabilization. Am J Orthop 2006;35:64–66.
35. Uri O, Barmpagiannis K, Higgs D, et al. Clinical outcome after reconstruction for sternoclavicular joint instability using a sternocleidomastoid tendon graft. J Bone Joint Surg Am 2014;96(5):417–422.
36. Waters PM, Bae DS, Kadiyala RK. Short-term outcomes after surgical treatment of traumatic posterior sternoclavicular fracture-dislocations in children and adolescents. J Pediatr Orthop 2003;23:464–469.
37. Witvoët J, Martinez B. Treatment of anterior sternoclavicular dislocations. Apropos of 18 cases [in French]. Rev Chir Orthop Reparatrice Appar Mot 1982;68(5):311–316.
38. Worman LW, Leagus C. Intrathoracic injury following retrosternal dislocation of the clavicle. J Trauma 1967;7:416–423.
39. Zaslav KR, Ray S, Neer CS 2nd. Conservative management of a displaced medial clavicular physeal injury in an adolescent athlete. Am J Sports Med 1989;17:833–836.

CHAPTER 2

Plate Fixation of Clavicle Fractures

Ryan Churchill and Sameer Nagda

DEFINITION

- Displaced, comminuted fractures of the clavicle are at risk for nonunion and malunion[9,10,12,15,16,20] and can be considered for open reduction and internal fixation with a plate and screws.

ANATOMY

- The clavicle and scapula are tightly linked through the strong coracoclavicular and acromioclavicular ligaments and link the axial skeleton to the upper extremity.
- Clavicles are present only in brachiating animals and apparently serve to help hold the upper limb away from the trunk to enhance more global positioning and use of the limb.
- The clavicle is named for its S-shaped curvature, with an apex anteromedially and an apex posterolaterally, similar to the musical symbol clavicula. The larger medial curvature widens the space for passage of neurovascular structures from the neck into the upper extremity through the costoclavicular interval.
- The clavicle is made up of very dense trabecular bone lacking a well-defined medullary canal. In cross-section, the clavicle changes gradually between a flat lateral aspect, a tubular midportion, and an expanded prismatic medial end.
- The clavicle is subcutaneous throughout its length and makes a prominent aesthetic contribution to the contour of the neck and upper part of the chest.
- The supraclavicular nerves run obliquely across the clavicle just deep to the platysma muscle and should be identified and protected during operative exposure to offset the development of hyperesthesia or dysesthesia over the chest wall.

PATHOGENESIS

- Clavicle fractures represent 2% to 10% of fractures in adults.[2]
- Clavicle fractures usually result from a direct blow to the point of the shoulder.
- This is usually a moderate- to high-energy injury in younger adults but can result from a low-energy fall from a standing height in an older individual.

NATURAL HISTORY

- The overall nonunion rate for diaphyseal clavicle fractures is 4.5%.[16]
- The risk of nonunion increases with age, female gender, displacement (>100%), shortening greater than 2 cm, and comminution.[2,9,16]
- The risk of nonunion for completely displaced (no apposition) and comminuted fractures is between 14% and 24% (**FIG 1**).[20]
- Malunion of the clavicle can result in shoulder girdle deformity and weakness.[7,9,10,12,17,20]
- Malunion and nonunion of the clavicle can result in brachial plexus compression.

PATIENT HISTORY AND PHYSICAL FINDINGS

- The mechanism and date of injury should be elicited.
- A careful neurologic examination should be performed contrast to late dysfunction of the brachial plexus after clavicular fracture, a situation in which medial cord structures are typically involved, acute injury to the brachial plexus at the time of clavicular fracture usually takes the form of a traction injury to the upper cervical roots.
- Vascular status should be assessed carefully for symmetry especially in displaced fractures where a fragment can tent or pierce a vessel.
- "Tenting" of the skin by a fracture fragment is only problematic in patients who cannot protect their skin (eg, patients who are comatose) and represents an impending open fracture without intervention.

IMAGING AND OTHER DIAGNOSTIC STUDIES

- An anteroposterior (AP) radiograph can be supplemented by a 20- to 60-degree cephalad-tilted view.
- The so-called apical oblique view (tilted 45 degrees anterior and 20 degrees cephalad) may facilitate the diagnosis of minimally displaced fractures (eg, birth fractures, fractures in children).
- Standard views in conjunction with 45 degrees cephalic and 45 degrees caudal tilt views can give the surgeon a thorough understanding of the superior–inferior and anterior–posterior displacement.[1]
- The abduction lordotic view taken with the shoulder abducted above 135 degrees and the central ray angled 25 degrees cephalad is useful in evaluating the clavicle after internal fixation. Abduction of the shoulder results

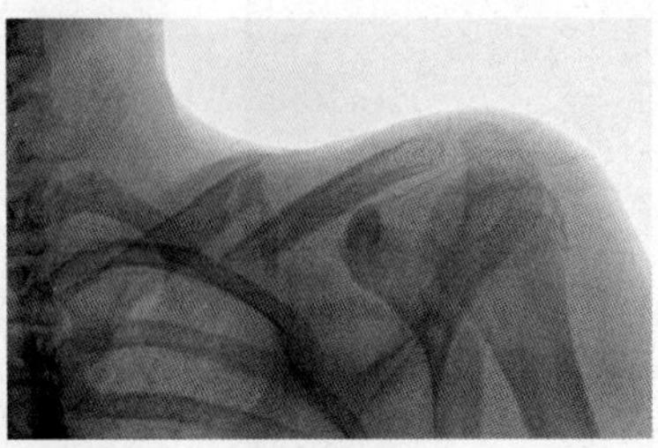

FIG 1 An AP radiograph shows greater than 100% displacement and comminution with a vertical fracture fragment. The clavicle is shortened. (Copyright David Ring, MD.)

in rotation of the clavicle on its longitudinal axis, which causes the plate to rotate superiorly and thereby expose the shaft of the clavicle and the fracture site under the plate.
- Computed tomography with three-dimensional (3-D) reconstructions can help understand 3-D deformity.

DIFFERENTIAL DIAGNOSIS

- Lateral or medial clavicle fracture
- Acromioclavicular or sternoclavicular (SC) dislocation

NONOPERATIVE MANAGEMENT

- Closed reduction of clavicular fractures is rarely attempted because the reduction is usually unstable, and no reliable means of providing external support is available.
- A simple sling provides comfort and limits activity during healing. A figure-8 bandage leaves the arm free, but it cannot improve alignment.
- Shoulder stiffness is not common in isolated clavicle fractures, and patients should be encouraged to keep the arm at the side and limit activity for the first 3 to 6 weeks.
- An increasing number of randomized trials have confirmed that operative treatment of displaced diaphyseal clavicle fractures decreases the rate of nonunion compared to nonoperative treatment, but it is not yet clear that operative treatment provides significantly less disability in the long term.[11,18] Given the risks and inconveniences associated with operative treatment, nonoperative treatment remains an appealing option.

SURGICAL MANAGEMENT

- Intramedullary fixation is an option when comminution is limited, but otherwise, plate-and-screw fixation is preferred.
- Plate fixation techniques consist of superior, anterior–inferior, and dual plating methods.[4,6]

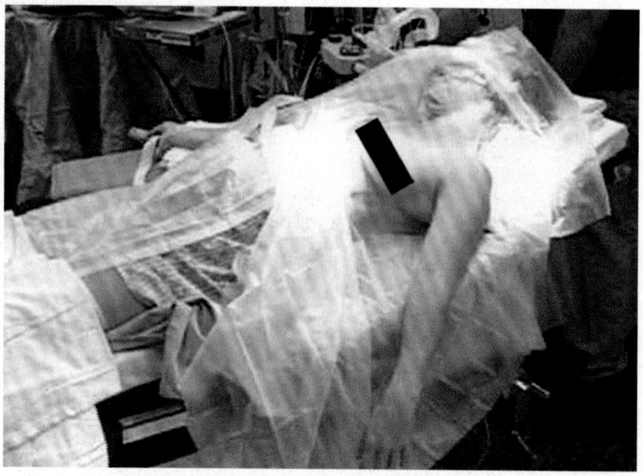

FIG 2 The patient is positioned supine with the head and trunk elevated slightly. (Copyright David Ring, MD.)

Preoperative Planning

- Planning of the surgery using tracings of radiographs helps limit intraoperative decision making and helps the surgeon anticipate problems and contingencies.

Positioning

- The patient is supine with a bump underneath the scapula or in the beach-chair position according to surgeon preference **(FIG 2)**. The arm should be draped free out to the contralateral SC joint.

Approach

- A longitudinal incision is made in line with the clavicle and inferior to it.

TECHNIQUES

SUPERIOR PLATE-AND-SCREW FIXATION

- An incision is made parallel and just inferior to the long axis of the clavicle **(TECH FIG 1A)**. Infiltration with dilute epinephrine can help limit bleeding.
- The crossing supraclavicular nerves are identified under loupe magnification and preserved **(TECH FIG 1B)**.
- Muscle attachments and periosteum are preserved as much as possible.
- Realignment and provisional fixation may be facilitated by the use of a small distractor, Kirschner wires, reduction clamps, and/or placement of 2.0 mm minifragment plate (Synthes, Paoli, PA) **(TECH FIG 1C)**.
- The arm can often be used as a joystick to help manipulate the fracture fragments into correct position for a clamp to be applied.

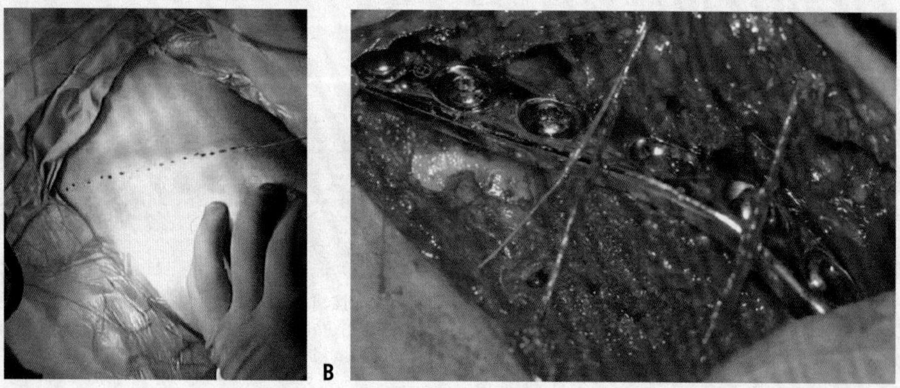

A B

TECH FIG 1 **A.** A straight incision in line with the clavicle and just inferior to it is infiltrated with dilute epinephrine. **B.** The supraclavicular nerves cross the clavicle at the level of the platysma, and an effort should be made to protect them. *(continued)*

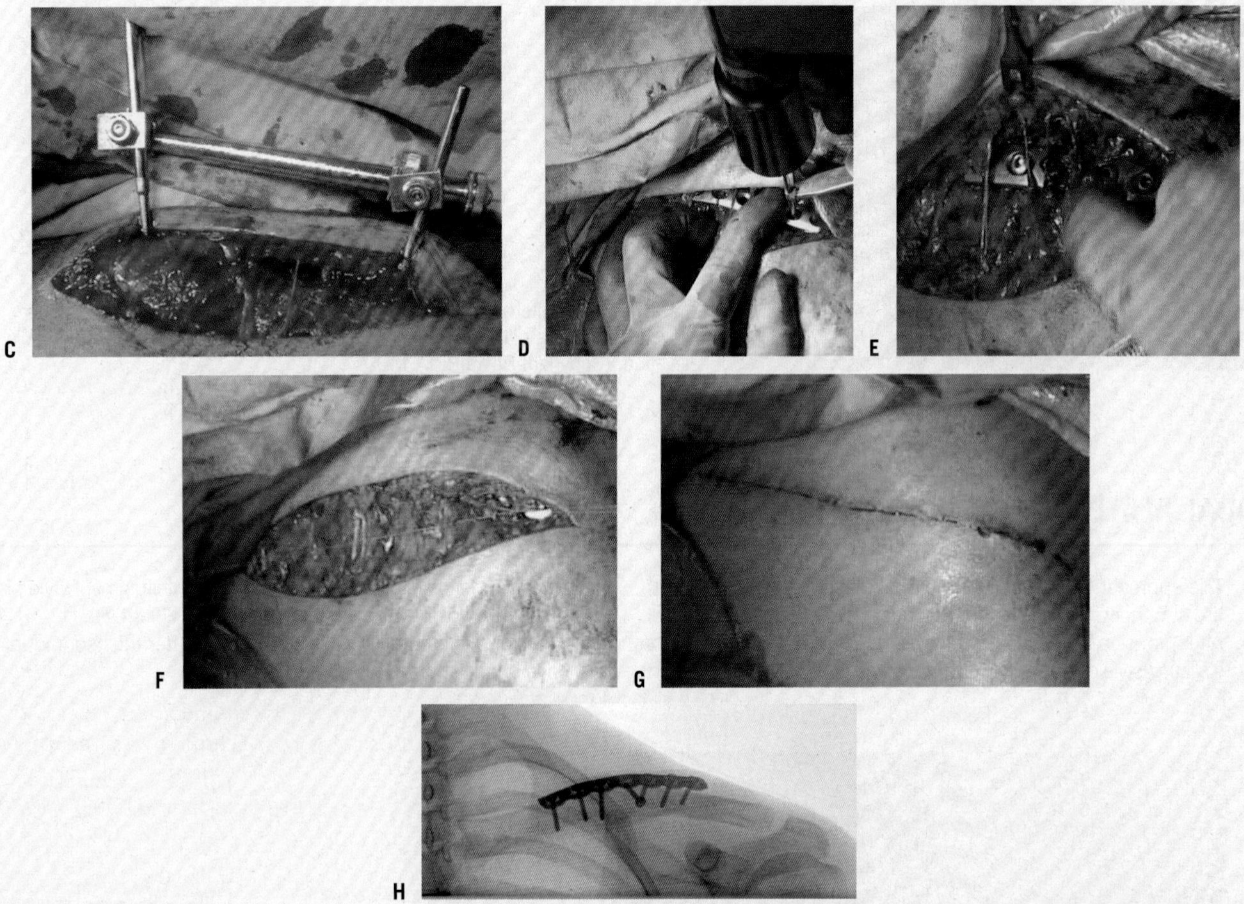

TECH FIG 1 *(continued)* **C.** A small distractor or temporary external fixator can be used to facilitate realignment and provide provisional fixation. **D.** In this patient, a superior 3.5-mm LC-DCP is applied. An oscillating drill is used to limit the risk to nerves. **E.** Final plate placement. **F.** The platysma is sutured closed. **G.** A subcuticular skin closure is used. **H.** Final AP radiograph demonstrates superior plate placement with lag screw fixation of an oblique fracture line. (Copyright David Ring, MD.)

- A 2.7-mm or 3.5-mm limited contact dynamic compression plate (LC-DCP, Synthes, Paoli, PA) or a precontoured plate is applied to the superior aspect of the clavicle **(TECH FIG 1D)**. A minimum of three screws should be placed in each major fragment. If the fracture pattern is amenable, placement of an interfragmentary screw greatly enhances the stability of the construct.
- Care should be taken when drilling holes for plate fixation to avoid injuring structures deep to the clavicle. Retractors can be placed inferiorly to help with this.
- When the vascularity of the fragments has been preserved, no bone graft is needed **(TECH FIG 1E)**. When extensive stripping or gaps have occurred in the cortex opposite the plate, one might consider adding a small amount of autogenous iliac crest cancellous bone graft.
- Close the platysma **(TECH FIG 1F)**.
- If the skin condition is suitable, wound closure is accomplished in atraumatic fashion with a subcuticular suture **(TECH FIG 1G,H)**.

ANTERIOR PLATE-AND-SCREW FIXATION

- The technique is identical for an anterior plate placement with the exception that the origins of the pectoralis major and deltoid are partially extraperiosteally elevated off the anterior clavicle **(TECH FIG 2)**.
- The anterior plate placement may help to decrease hardware prominence, and the drill and screws are directed posterior rather than directly inferior to the clavicle, which may increase the margin of safety as well as result in longer screws traversing the clavicle. This may provide more torsional rigidity.[19]

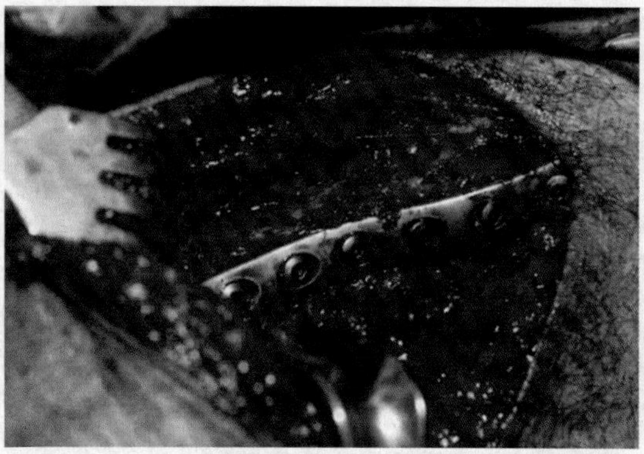

TECH FIG 2 An alternative is to place the plate on the anterior surface of the clavicle. This limits plate prominence but requires greater stripping and muscle elevation. (Copyright David Ring, MD.)

DUAL PLATE-AND-SCREW FIXATION

- The approach is identical for the dual plating technique as with the superior and anterior approaches.
- After provisional reduction is achieved, a 2.7-mm or 3.5-mm reconstruction style or precontoured plate (Synthes, Paoli, PA) is placed anterior–inferior with a 2.0-mm or 2.4-mm minifragment style plate (Synthes, Paoli, PA) placed superiorly **(TECH FIG 3A–F)**.[3,14]
- Rates of symptomatic hardware removal after this technique have been reported between 3% and 4%.[5]

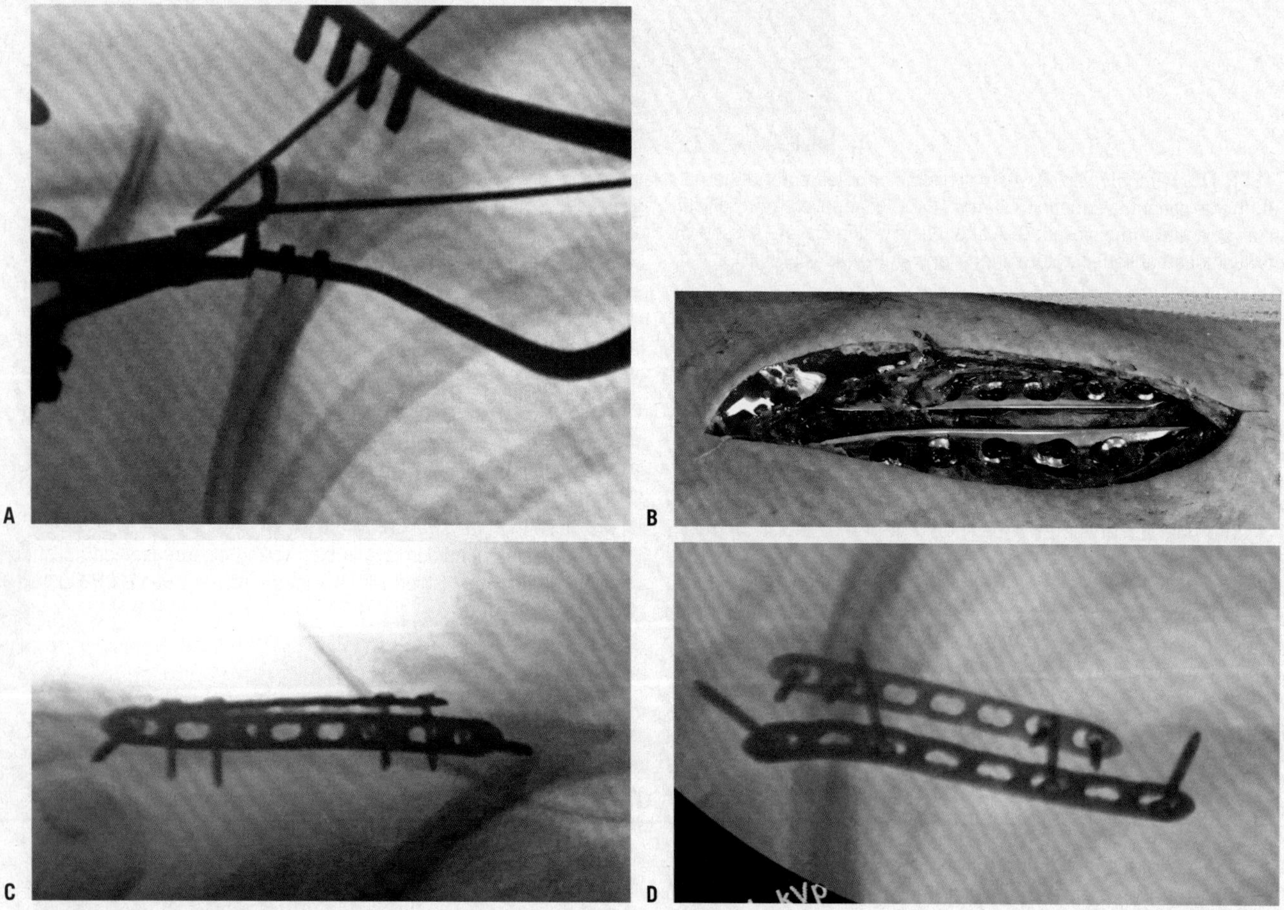

TECH FIG 3 **A.** Intraoperative fluoroscopic images demonstrating provisional reduction with reduction clamps and Kirschner wires of a 17-year-old football player. **B.** Intraoperative image of dual plating technique using a contoured 3.5-mm plate anterior–inferior and a 2.4 mm plate placed superiorly. **C.** Intraoperative AP fluoroscopy image. **D.** Intraoperative fluoroscopy image with cephalad tilt. *(continued)*

E

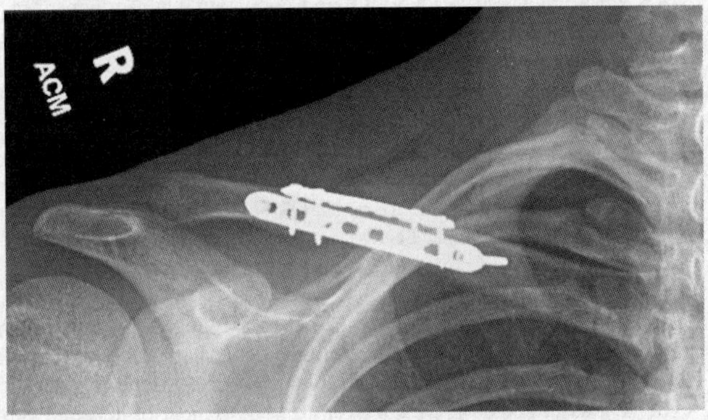

F

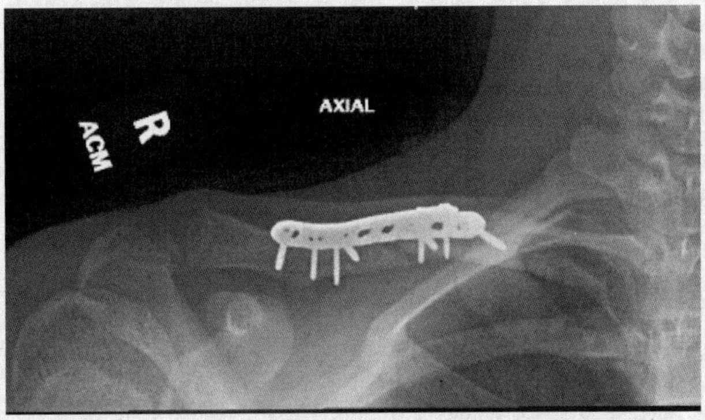

TECH FIG 3 *(continued)* **E,F.** Final radiographs demonstrating dual plate placement. The patient had returned to contact sports at 8 weeks and went on to play collegiate football.

Pearls and Pitfalls

Supraclavicular Nerve Neuroma	• Attempts to identify and protect these nerves are worthwhile.
Brachial Plexus Stretch Injury	• Realignment should be done gradually and can be facilitated by temporary external fixation. Pulling fragments out of the wound (eg, to ream for an intramedullary fixation device) should be limited.
Loosening of Fixation	• A minimum of six cortices of fixation on each side of the fracture should be achieved.
Axial Pullout of Locked Screws	• Locking screws may be troublesome when used on the lateral fragment with the plate in a superior position.
Plate Prominence	• Dual plating or anterior–inferior plating may diminish plate prominence.

POSTOPERATIVE CARE

- Confident use of the hand at the side is encouraged immediately.
- Evaluation and supplementation of metabolic bone status with blood testing of vitamin D levels can help in healing.
- May start passive forward elevation to 90 degrees at 10 to 14 days postoperatively
- At 6 weeks, may start active range of motion of shoulder without restrictions as long as there are signs of radiographic and clinical healing
- May begin weight bearing as tolerated at 3 months
- Most athletes are allowed to return to sport between 4 and 6 months postoperatively.
- Shoulder abduction, cross-body adduction, and handling of more than 15 lb are delayed until early healing is established.
- Shoulder stiffness is unusual and usually responds quickly to exercises. Shoulder exercises can therefore be delayed until healing is established.

OUTCOMES

- Plate loosening and nonunion occur in 3% to 5% of cases.[13]
- Healing leads to good function.

COMPLICATIONS

- Infection and wound complications occur (1% to 3%) but are uncommon.
- Neurovascular injury is very uncommon and pneumothorax has not been described.
- Symptomatic hardware requiring removal in 3.7% to 24.6% of patients[5,8]

REFERENCES

1. Austin LS, O'Brien MJ, Zmistowski B, et al. Additional x-ray views increase decision to treat clavicular fractures surgically. J Shoulder Elbow Surg 2012;21:1263–1268.
2. Canadian Orthopaedic Trauma Society. Nonoperative treatment compared with plate fixation of displaced midshaft clavicular fractures: a multicenter, randomized clinical trial. J Bone Joint Surg Am 2007;89:1–10.
3. Chen X, Shannon SF, Torchia M, et al. Radiographic outcomes of single versus dual plate fixation of acute mid-shaft clavicle fractures. Arch Orthop Trauma Surg 2017;137:749–754.
4. Collinge C, Devinney S, Herscovici D, et al. Anterior-inferior plate fixation of middle-third fractures and nonunions of the clavicle. J Orthop Trauma 2006;20:680–686.
5. Czajka CM, Kay A, Gary JL, et al. Symptomatic implant removal following dual mini-fragment plating for clavicular shaft fractures. J Orthop Trauma 2017;31: 236–240.

6. Kloen P, Sorkin AT, Rubel IF, et al. Anteroinferior plating of midshaft clavicular nonunions. J Orthop Trauma 2002;16:425–430.
7. Lazarides S, Zafiropoulos G. Conservative treatment of fractures at the middle third of the clavicle: the relevance of shortening and clinical outcome. J Shoulder Elbow Surg 2006;15:191–194.
8. Leroux T, Wasserstein D, Henry P, et al. Rate of and risk factors for reoperations after open reduction and internal fixation of midshaft clavicle fractures: a population-based study in Ontario, Canada. J Bone Joint Surg Am 2014;96:1119–1125.
9. McKee MD, Pedersen EM, Jones C, et al. Deficits following nonoperative treatment of displaced midshaft clavicular fractures. J Bone Joint Surg Am 2006;88:35–40.
10. McKee MD, Wild LM, Schemitsch EH. Midshaft malunions of the clavicle. J Bone Joint Surg Am 2003;85:790–797.
11. McKee RC, Whelan DB, Schemitsch EH, et al. Operative versus nonoperative care of displaced midshaft clavicular fractures: a meta-analysis of randomized clinical trials. J Bone Joint Surg Am 2012;94(8):675–684. doi:10.2106/JBJS.J.01364.
12. Nowak J, Holgersson M, Larsson S. Can we predict long-term sequelae after fractures of the clavicle based on initial findings? A prospective study with nine to ten years of follow-up. J Shoulder Elbow Surg 2004;13:479–486.
13. Poigenfürst J, Rappold G, Fischer W. Plating of fresh clavicular fractures: results of 122 operations. Injury 1992;23:237–241.
14. Prasarn ML, Meyers KN, Wilkin G, et al. Dual mini-fragment plating for midshaft clavicle fractures: a clinical and biomechanical investigation. Arch Orthop Trauma Surg 2015;135:1655–1662.
15. Robinson CM. Fractures of the clavicle in the adult. Epidemiology and classification. J Bone Joint Surg Br 1998;80:476–484.
16. Robinson CM, Court-Brown CM, McQueen MM, et al. Estimating the risk of nonunion following nonoperative treatment of a clavicular fracture. J Bone Joint Surg Am 2004;86:1359–1365.
17. Shields E, Behrend C, Beiswenger T, et al. Scapular dyskinesis following displaced fractures of the middle clavicle. J Shoulder Elbow Surg 2015;24:e331–e336.
18. Virtanen KJ, Remes V, Pajarinen J, et al. Sling compared with plate osteosynthesis for treatment of displaced midshaft clavicular fractures: a randomized clinical trial. J Bone Joint Surg Am 2012;94(17):1546–1553.
19. Wiesel B, Nagda S, Mehta S, et al. Management of midshaft clavicle fractures in adults. J Am Acad Orthop Surg 2018;26:e468–e476.
20. Zlowodzki M, Zelle BA, Cole PA, et al. Treatment of acute midshaft clavicle fractures: systematic review of 2144 fractures: on behalf of the Evidence-Based Orthopaedic Trauma Working Group. J Orthop Trauma 2005;19:504–507.

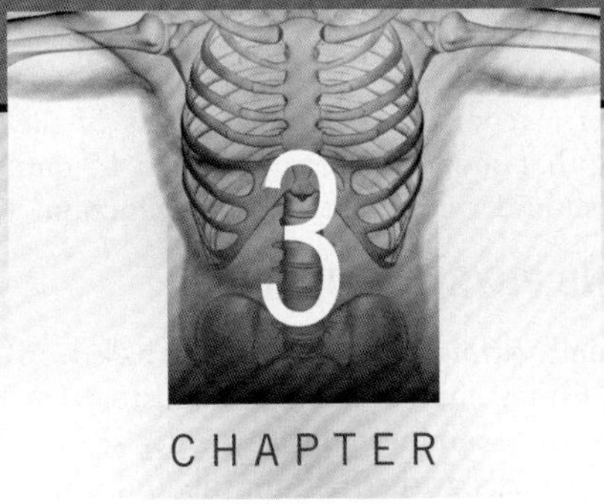

Intramedullary Fixation of Clavicle Fractures

Stephen B. Gunther and Carl Basamania

DEFINITION

- The clavicle is one of the most commonly fractured bones.
- The site on the clavicle most often fractured is the middle third.[10]
  - The midclavicular region is the thinnest and narrowest portion of the bone.
  - It is the only area not supported by ligament or muscle attachments.
  - It represents a transitional region of both cross-sectional anatomy and curvature.
    - It is the transition point between the lateral part, with a flatter cross-section, and the more tubular medial portion of the bone.
- Because the clavicle has an S shape, any axial load creates a very high tensile force along the anterior cortex of the middle third of the clavicle.

ANATOMY

- The clavicle is the only long bone to ossify by a combination of intramembranous and endochondral ossification.[7]
- The clavicle contour is S-shaped, with a double curve. The medial curve is apex anterior and the lateral curve is apex posterior **(FIG 1A)**.
- The larger medial curvature widens the space for the neurovascular structures, providing bony protection.
- The clavicle has very dense trabecular cortical bone. The intramedullary (IM) canal is narrow.
- The cross-sectional anatomy gradually changes from flat laterally to tubular in the midportion to an expanded prism medially.
- The clavicle is subcutaneous throughout, covered by the thin platysma muscle.
- The supraclavicular nerves that provide sensation to the overlying skin of the clavicle are found deep to the platysma muscle.

A

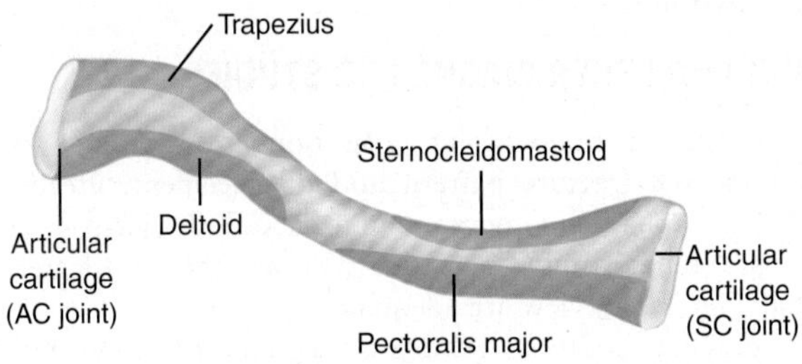

B

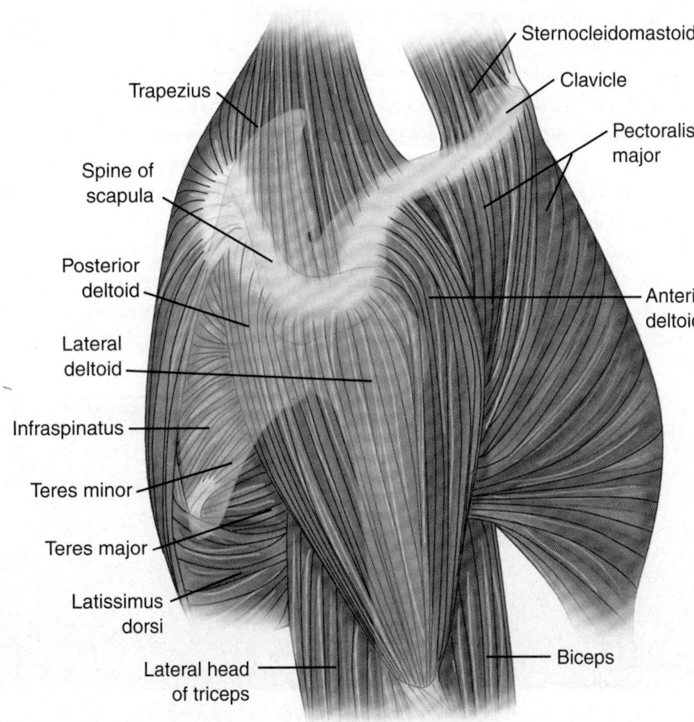

FIG 1 **A.** The clavicle is S-shaped and has a double curve. The medial curve is apex anterior and the lateral curve is apex posterior. **B.** Proximal muscle attachments to the clavicle include the sternocleidomastoid, pectoralis major, and subclavius. Distal muscle attachments to the clavicle include the deltoid and trapezius. *AC*, acromioclavicular; *SC*, sternoclavicular.

- Very strong capsular and extracapsular ligaments attach the medial end to the sternum and first rib, and they attach the lateral end to the acromion and coracoid process.
- Proximal muscle attachments include the sternocleidomastoid, pectoralis major, and subclavius. Lateral muscle attachments include the deltoid and trapezius **(FIG 1B)**.
- The clavicle functions by providing a fixed-length strut through which the muscles attached to the shoulder girdle can generate and transmit large forces to the upper extremity.

PATHOGENESIS

- The mechanism of clavicle fractures in the vast majority of injuries is a direct trauma to the shoulder.[11] Stanley and associates[11] studied 106 injured patients; 87% had fallen onto the shoulder, 7% were injured by a direct blow on the point of the shoulder, and only 6% reported falling onto an outstretched hand.
- Stanley suggests that in the patients who described hitting the ground with an outstretched hand, the shoulder became the next contact point with the ground, causing the fracture. Stanley stated that a compressive force equivalent to body weight would exceed the critical buckling load to cause the clavicle fracture.

NATURAL HISTORY

- In the 1960s, both Neer[8] and Rowe[10] published large series of midclavicle fractures, showing very low nonunion rate (0.1% and 0.8%) with closed treatment and a higher nonunion rate (4.6% and 3.7%) with operative treatment.
- More recent studies have shown that nonunion is more common than previously recognized and that a significant percentage of patients with nonunion are symptomatic.
- Malunion with shortening greater than 15 to 20 mm has also been shown to be associated with significant shoulder dysfunction.
- McKee and colleagues[6] identified 15 patients with malunion of the midclavicle after closed treatment. All patients had shortening of more than 15 mm, all were symptomatic and unsatisfied, and all underwent corrective osteotomy. Postoperatively, all 15 patients demonstrated improved function and satisfaction.
- Hill and associates[5] reviewed 52 completely displaced midshaft clavicle fractures and found that shortening of more than 20 mm had a significant association with nonunion and unsatisfactory results.
- Eskola and coworkers[4] reported on 89 malunions of the midclavicle, showing that shortening of more than 15 mm was associated with shoulder discomfort and dysfunction.

PATIENT HISTORY AND PHYSICAL FINDINGS

- The diagnosis is usually straightforward and is based on obtaining the mechanism of injury from a good history.
- On visual inspection, the examiner will frequently see notable swelling or ecchymosis at the fracture site and possibly deformity of the clavicle, with drooping of the shoulder downward and forward if the fracture is significantly displaced. The skin is inspected for tenting at the fracture site and characteristic bruising and abrasions that might suggest a direct blow or seatbelt shoulder strap injury **(FIG 2A,B)**.
- Palpation over the fracture site will reveal tenderness, and gentle manipulation of the upper extremity or clavicle itself may reveal crepitus and motion at the fracture site.
- The amount of shortening can be identified by clinically measuring the distance of a straight line (in centimeters) from both acromioclavicular (AC) joints to the sternal notch and noting the difference **(FIG 2C)** or by measuring directly on digital x-rays.
- It is important to perform a complete musculoskeletal and neurovascular examination of the upper extremity and auscultation of the chest to identify the rare associated injuries; these are more frequently seen when there is a high-energy mechanism of injuries.
  - Rib and scapula fracture
  - Brachial plexus injury (usually traction to upper cervical root)
  - Vascular injury (subclavian artery or vein injury associated with scapulothoracic dissociation)
  - Pneumothorax and hemothorax

IMAGING AND OTHER DIAGNOSTIC STUDIES

- Two orthogonal radiographic projections are necessary to determine the fracture pattern and displacement, ideally 45-degree cephalic tilt and 45-degree caudal tilt views.
- Usually, a standard anteroposterior (AP) view and a 45-degree cephalic tilt **(FIG 3)** view are adequate.
  - In practice, a 20- to 60-degree cephalic tilt view will minimize interference of thoracic structures.
- The film should be large enough to include the AC and sternoclavicular joints, the scapula, and the upper lung fields to evaluate for associated injuries.

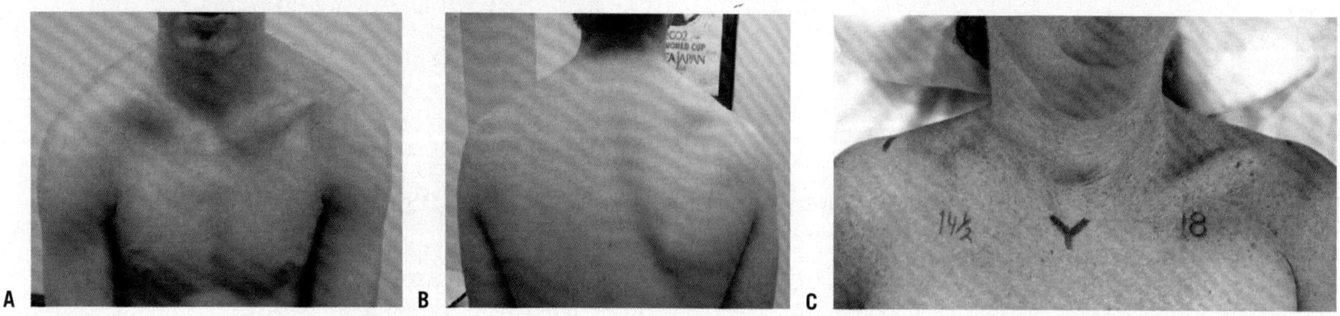

FIG 2 A,B. Anterior and posterior photographs of a displaced right clavicle fracture showing deformity of the clavicle and drooping of the shoulder girdle downward and forward. **C.** Clinical picture of a displaced right clavicle fracture, showing 3.5 cm of shortening, measured from the sternal notch to the AC joint.

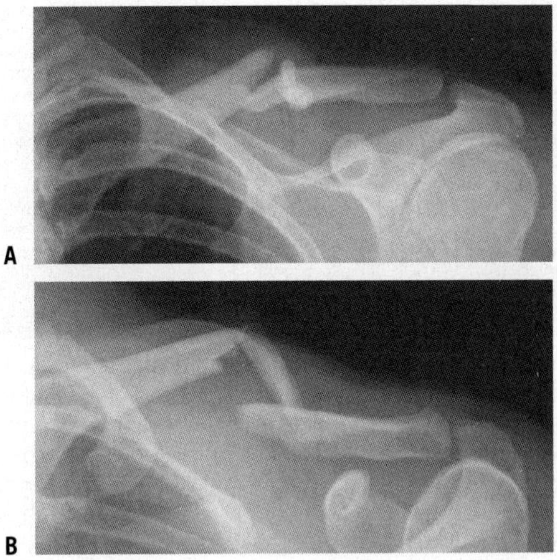

FIG 3 Radiographs of the same displaced left clavicle fracture viewed from a standard AP projection (**A**) and a 45-degree cephalic tilt projection (**B**).

DIFFERENTIAL DIAGNOSIS

- Sprain of AC joint
- Sprain of sternoclavicular joint
- Rib fracture
- Muscle injury
- Kehr sign: referred pain to the left shoulder from irritation of the diaphragm, signaled by the phrenic nerve. Irritation may be caused by diaphragmatic or peridiaphragmatic lesions, renal calculi, splenic injury, or ectopic pregnancy.

NONOPERATIVE MANAGEMENT

- If the clavicle fracture alignment is acceptable, generally a simple configuration with less than 10 to 15 mm of shortening, then standard methods of shoulder immobilization may be adequate: figure-8 harness, sling, or Velpeau dressing.
- Nordqvist and colleagues[9] reported on 35 clavicle fracture malunions with shortening of less than 15 mm. They were all treated nonoperatively in a sling. All 35 had normal mobility, strength, and function compared to the normal shoulder.
- A prospective, randomized study[2] comparing sling versus figure-8 bandage showed that a greater percentage of patients were dissatisfied with the figure-8 bandage, and there was no difference in overall healing and alignment. The study concluded that the figure-8 bandage may not be necessary in most cases.

SURGICAL MANAGEMENT

- Indications for operative treatment of acute midshaft clavicle fractures are as follows:
  - Open fractures
  - Fractures with neurovascular injury
  - Fractures with severe associated chest injury or multiple trauma including patients who require their upper extremity for transfer and ambulation
  - "Floating shoulder"
  - Impending skin necrosis
  - Fracture displacement: more than 15 to 20 mm of shortening (especially if there is associated shoulder girdle protraction and shortening)
- In a multicenter, randomized, prospective clinical trial of displaced midshaft clavicle fractures, Altamimi and McKee[1] showed that operative fixation compared to nonoperative treatment improved functional outcome and had a lower rate of both malunion and nonunion.
- Potential advantages of IM versus plate fixation of the clavicle are as follows:
  - Less soft tissue stripping and therefore potentially better healing
  - Smaller incision
  - Better cosmesis
  - Easier hardware removal
  - Less weakness of bone after hardware removal
- Potential disadvantages of IM fixation of the clavicle are as follows:
  - Less ability to resist torsional forces
  - Pin breakage
  - Pin migration

Preoperative Planning

- After the decision has been made to fix a clavicle fracture, one must evaluate whether the fracture pattern is amenable to IM fixation.
- Fractures in the middle third of the bone are ideal.
- The IM canal must have a large enough central canal to permit passage of the implant. This issue relates mostly to kids.
- Comminution and butterfly fragments (usually anterior) are common and do not preclude IM fixation as long as the medial and distal main fragments have cortical contact.

Positioning

- There are two good options for patient positioning that facilitate use of a C-arm imaging device during the surgery (**FIG 4A,B**).
  - Beach-chair position of the operating room (OR) table, using a shoulder-positioning device, which leaves the posterior shoulder area exposed. This is our preferred position.
  - The C-arm can be brought in from the head of the bed with the gantry rotated upside down and slightly away from the operative shoulder and oriented with a cephalic tilt. Alternatively, the C-arm can be brought in perpendicular from the opposite side of the table, which is out of the way of the surgeon. In small patients, a mini C-arm can be brought in from the surgical side.
  - The arm is prepped free and placed in an arm holder to facilitate fracture reduction.
- The other option is to place the patient supine on a Jackson radiolucent surgical table so the C-arm can be brought in perpendicular from the opposite side of the table (**FIG 4C,D**).
  - A 1-L bag is placed under the affected shoulder, medial to the scapula, to aid in fracture reduction.
  - The arm is also prepped free and placed in an arm holder to facilitate fracture reduction.

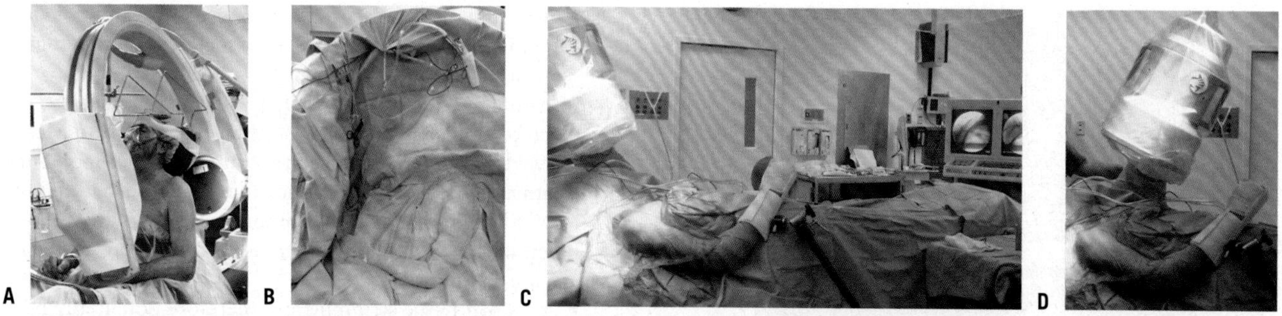

FIG 4 A,B. The patient is placed in the beach-chair position on the OR table, using a radiolucent shoulder-positioning device. **A.** The arm is prepared free and placed in an arm holder to facilitate fracture reduction. The C-arm is brought in from the head of the bed with the gantry rotated upside down and slightly away from the operative shoulder and oriented with a cephalic tilt. **B.** The same beach-chair positioning shown sterilely draped. **C,D.** Alternatively, the patient is placed supine on a Jackson radiolucent surgical table. A 1-L bag is placed under the affected shoulder, medial to the scapula, and the arm is prepared free and placed in an arm holder to aid in fracture reduction. The C-arm can be brought in perpendicular from the opposite side of the table, which is out of the way of the surgeon and facilitates getting orthogonal radiographic views of the fracture: 45-degree caudal tilt view (**C**) and 45-degree cephalic tilt view (**D**).

INCISION AND DISSECTION

- Drape with wide margins around the entire clavicle; mark the clavicle, fracture site, and surrounding anatomy **(TECH FIG 1A)**.
- Use the C-arm to identify the appropriate position for the incision, which should be over the distal end of the medial fragment, in the anatomic Langer skin lines **(TECH FIG 1B)**.
- Make a 2- to 3-cm skin incision over the fracture site.
- Divide the subcutaneous fat down to the platysma muscle **(TECH FIG 1C)**.
- Although there is usually very little subcutaneous fat, gently make full-thickness flaps to include skin and subcutaneous tissue around the entire incision to facilitate exposure.
- Bluntly split the platysma muscle in line of its fibers to identify, protect, and retract the underlying supraclavicular nerves: The middle branches are frequently found near the midclavicle **(TECH FIG 1D,E)**.
- The fracture site is then identified while carefully preserving as much intact periosteum as possible. You may slightly elevate the periosteum at the edges of the fracture site if necessary, but there is no need for extensive periosteal stripping as with plate fixation. Maintaining the intact periosteal blood supply to the fracture fragments is an important advantage of this technique.
- Remove any debris, hematoma, or interposed muscle from the fracture site.
- If there are butterfly fragments, be careful to keep any soft tissue attachments.

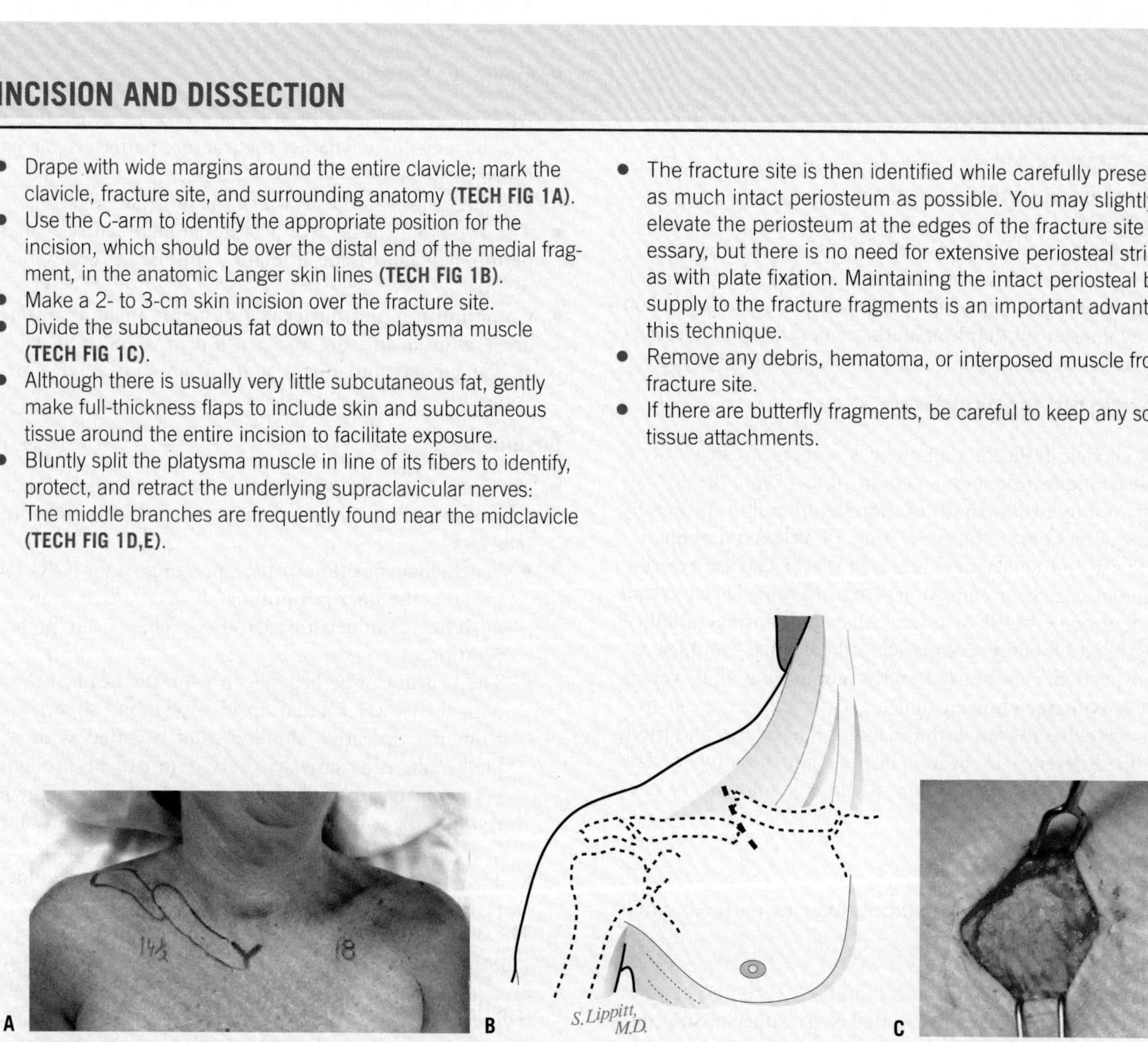

TECH FIG 1 A. Displaced right clavicle fracture, showing the clavicle and fracture site marked out. **B.** A skin incision of about 2 to 3 cm is made over the distal end of the medial clavicular fragment, in the Langer lines of normal skin creases around the neck. **C.** Incision over a clavicle fracture site, showing full-thickness flaps to include skin and subcutaneous tissue around the entire incision. This exposes the fascia that covers the platysma muscle. *(continued)*

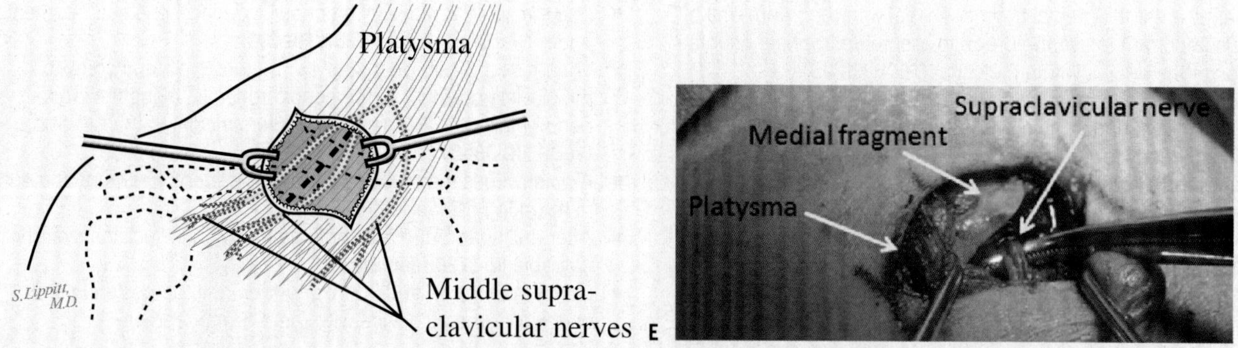

TECH FIG 1 *(continued)* **D.** Skin incision over a displaced clavicle fracture, with underlying platysma muscle and the middle supraclavicular nerves. **E.** Intraoperative photo showing the platysma muscle bluntly split in the line of its fibers to identify an underlying supraclavicular nerve, which is under the clamp. The fracture site is usually easily identifiable in acute injuries because the periosteum is disrupted and usually requires no further division; as shown here, the medial clavicular fragment is easily seen. (**B,D:** Courtesy of Steven B. Lippitt, MD.)

CLAVICLE PREPARATION

- The following technique uses a flexible IM device, which locks medially in a rigid, partially flexed position and locks laterally with a crossing screw **(TECH FIG 2A)**.
- Use a bone-reducing clamp or towel clip to grab and elevate the medial clavicular fragment through the incision **(TECH FIG 2B)**.

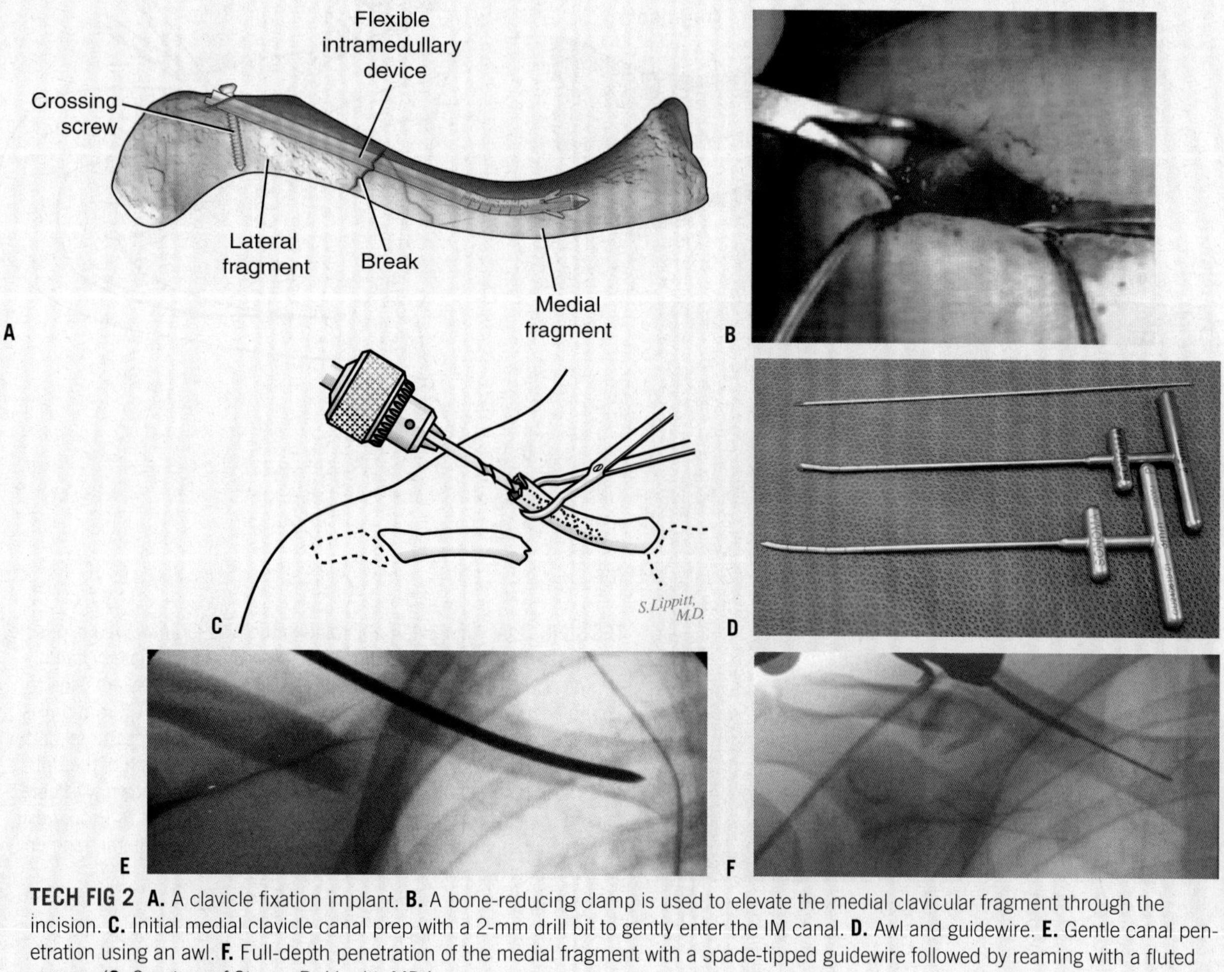

TECH FIG 2 **A.** A clavicle fixation implant. **B.** A bone-reducing clamp is used to elevate the medial clavicular fragment through the incision. **C.** Initial medial clavicle canal prep with a 2-mm drill bit to gently enter the IM canal. **D.** Awl and guidewire. **E.** Gentle canal penetration using an awl. **F.** Full-depth penetration of the medial fragment with a spade-tipped guidewire followed by reaming with a fluted reamer. (**C:** Courtesy of Steven B. Lippitt, MD.)

- Gently enter the medial fragment canal with the 2-mm drill bit. It is important to use the C-arm to assure appropriate orientation of the drill bit within the canal **(TECH FIG 2C)**.
  - The surgeon must be 100% sure that the drill bit does not skive under the clavicle toward the subclavian vein or superiorly toward the neck.
- The medial canal may then be prepared with either a curved awl or a reamer over a spade-tipped guidewire. Be careful to avoid penetrating the anterior cortex **(TECH FIG 2D–F)**.
- Next, elevate the lateral clavicular fragment through the incision. This is facilitated by externally rotating the arm.
- Use the same 2-mm drill bit or awl to enter the lateral fragment under C-arm guidance **(TECH FIG 3A)**.
- Then, use a 3-mm drill bit to exit the posterolateral cortex of the clavicle posterior to the conoid tubercle, along the lateral bend of the clavicle a few centimeters medial to the AC joint **(TECH FIG 3B–D)**.
- A guidewire is then placed through the lateral fragment and out to the skin posterior to the AC joint.
- After drilling through the cortex, make a small incision over the palpable tip **(TECH FIG 3E)**.
- Gently split the deltoid fibers and then drill the posterolateral cortex over the guidewire with the 4.5-mm reamer.

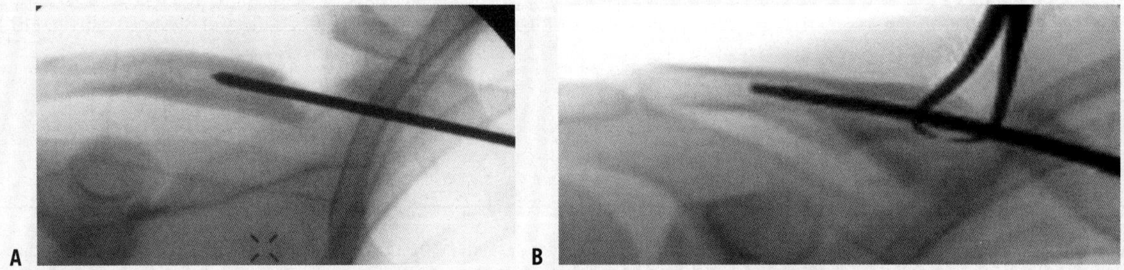

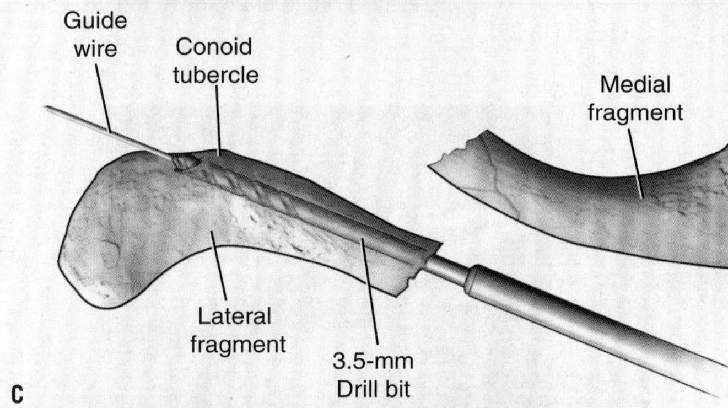

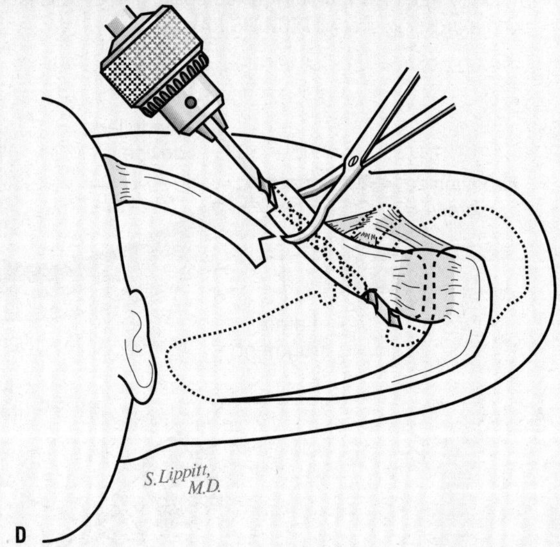

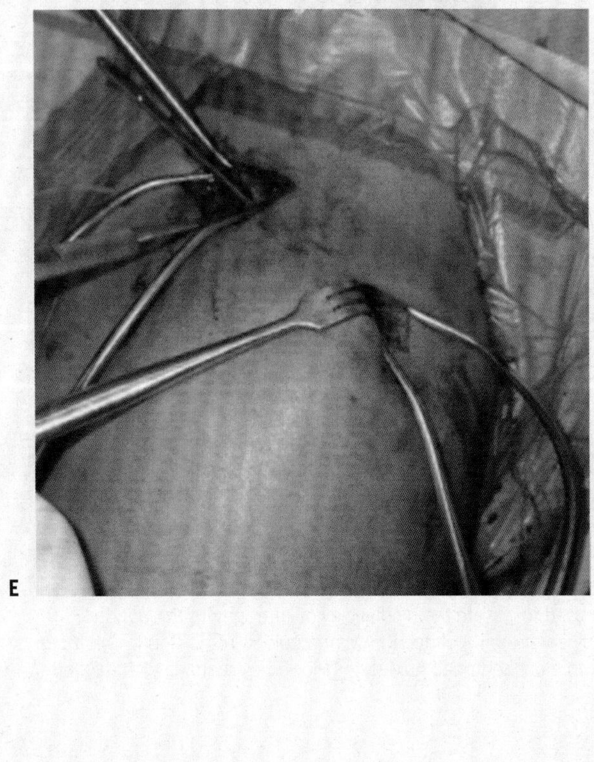

TECH FIG 3 A. After externally rotating the arm for improved exposure, a 2-mm drill bit or straight awl is gently placed into the lateral canal. AP and 45-degree caudal and cephalic tilt C-arm images are used to assure accurate alignment straight down the canal. **B.** A 3-mm drill is then advanced past the conoid tubercle to exit the posterolateral cortex while carefully assuring proper IM alignment. **C.** The path of the drill must reproduce the anatomic IM canal alignment as shown with here with an implant overlying the IM canal of a bone model. **D.** Proper exit point posterior and medial to the AC joint capsule. **E.** Lateral fragment prep through two mini-incisions.

FRACTURE REDUCTION AND IMPLANT FIXATION

- Reduce the fracture site and then pass the guidewire through the fracture and fully into the medial fragment **(TECH FIG 4A)**.
- Then, ream over the guidewire to the full length of the prepared IM canal **(TECH FIG 4B)**. The midpoint marking on the reamer should pass to the most medial aspect of the fracture site or slightly further. Then, measure the implant length with a depth gauge placed over the guidewire **(TECH FIG 4C)**.
- A lateral entry guide is then used **(TECH FIG 4D)**. This is placed over the guidewire. The guidewire is then removed so that the surgeon can slide the implant over the lateral guide sled into the clavicle entry site.
  - Avoid any angular torque on the implant during penetration of the clavicle and do not use a mallet.
- Once the surgeon is satisfied with the fracture reduction and implant alignment (fully seated into the medial clavicle with the flexible implant segment at least 2 cm past the fracture site), the implant is locked in its position with the torque driver. Engaging and turning the torque driver inside the lateral implant opening expands the medial grippers to engage the medial bone and locks the flexible distal section of the implant in a rigid position.
- The lateral screw is then placed through the lateral screw guide and across the implant **(TECH FIG 4E)**.
- Accurate screw placement across the implant can be easily checked by placing the torque driver back in the end of the implant: The torque driver will bump into the cross screw inside the implant if it was placed correctly through the implant.

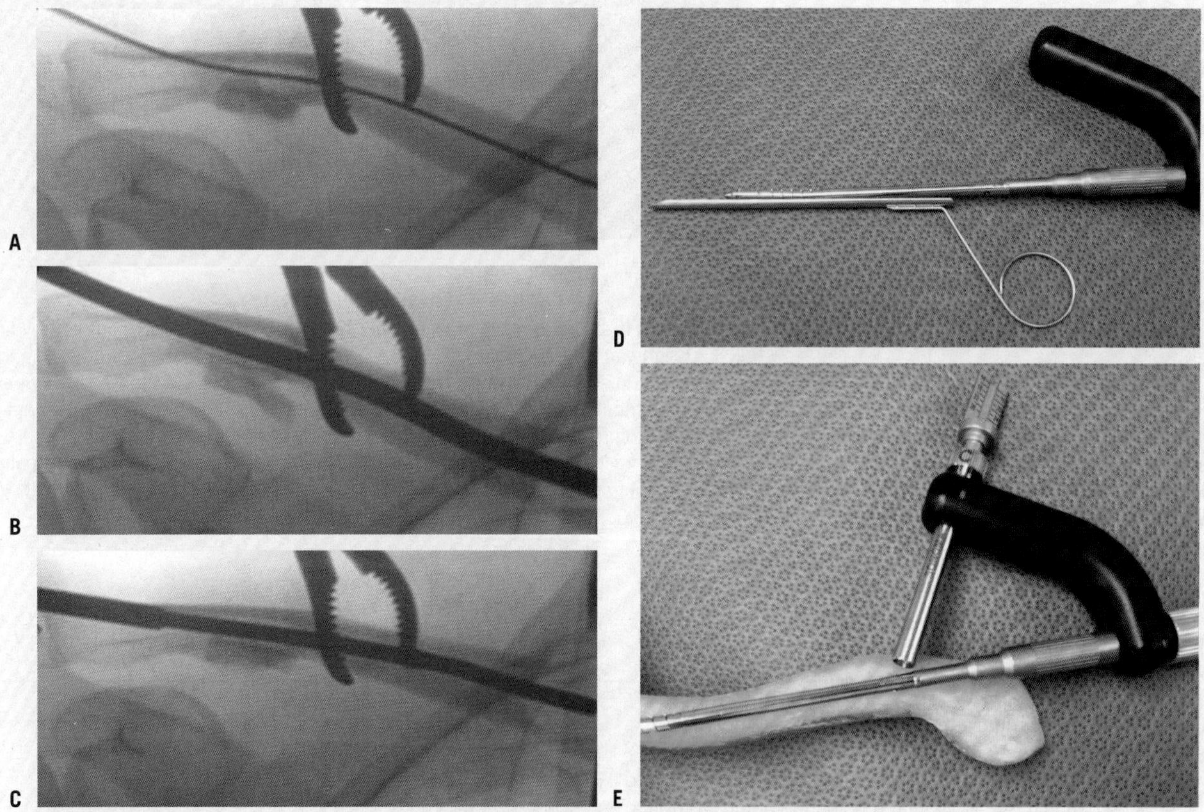

TECH FIG 4 **A.** The fracture is anatomically reduced and held in place with bone reduction clamps while the IM pin is placed all the way across the fracture site deep into the medial clavicle. **B.** The clavicle is then reamed while the reduction is held tight to clear the IM path for the implant. This step assures that the implant does not distract the fracture site during implantation. **C.** Use the depth gauge over the guidewire to measure implant length. Make sure that the flexible section of the implant bypasses the fracture site by at least 2 cm and preferably 3 cm. **D.** Lateral entry guide used to place over guidewire and then allow easy placement of implant into lateral clavicle entry site. **E.** Implant guide with lateral screw sheath overlying clavicle model for demonstration of surgical technique.

BUTTERFLY FRAGMENT MANAGEMENT AND WOUND CLOSURE

- If there is a large butterfly segmental fragment or significant comminution, it can be helpful to extend the fracture site incision posteriorly along the skin lines instead of performing two separate smaller incisions.
- If an anterior butterfly fragment exists, cerclage suture fixation is performed.
  - Pass an elevator under the clavicle to deflect the sutures **(TECH FIG 5A)**.
  - Then, pass a no. 2 suture in a figure-8 manner through the periosteum of the butterfly fragment and around the fragment and the clavicle **(TECH FIG 5B)**.
- Close the periosteum overlying the fracture site with no. 0 absorbable suture in an interrupted figure-8 manner.
- Reapproximate the fascia of the platysma muscle using 2-0 absorbable suture.
- Close the subcutaneous tissue and skin incisions.

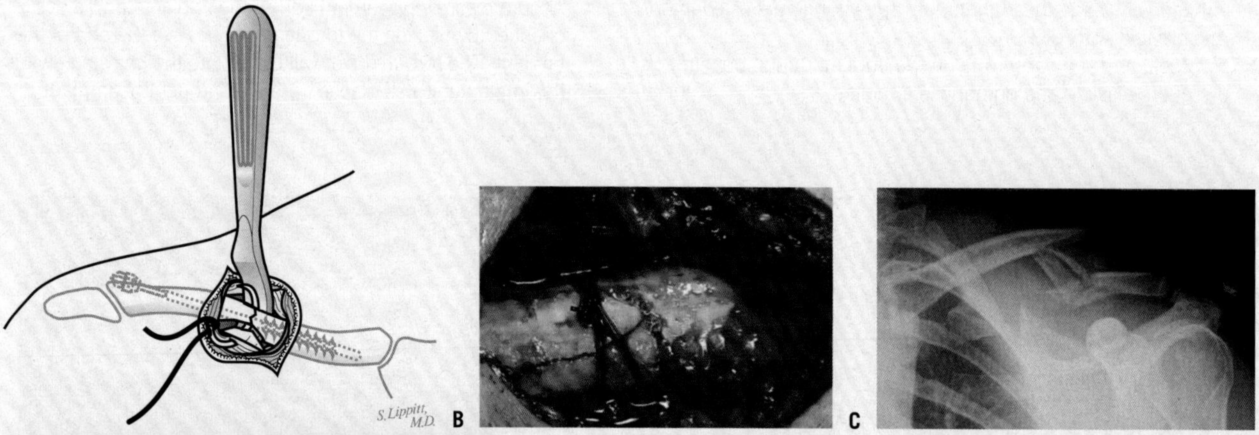

A B C

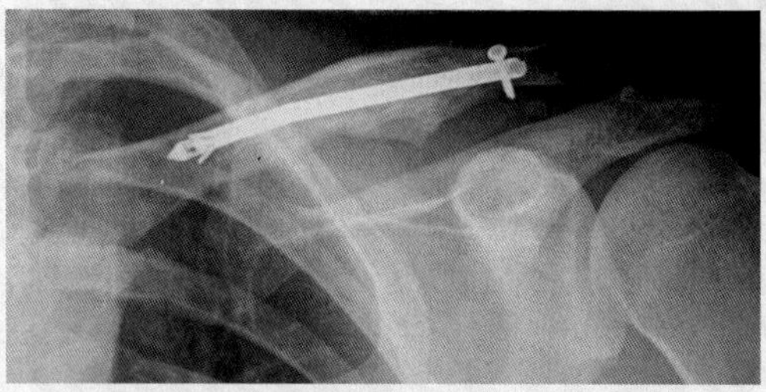

D

TECH FIG 5 **A.** Cerclage of an anterior butterfly fragment is accomplished by first passing an elevator under the clavicle to deflect the sutures and then passing the suture, in a figure-8 manner, through the periosteum of the butterfly fragment and around the fragment and the clavicle. **B.** Operative picture of butterfly fragment cerclage suture fixation. **C.** Radiograph of a comminuted midshaft clavicle fracture with Z-type fracture pattern and two butterfly fragments. **D.** Radiograph of same patient after IM fixation and cerclage suture fixation. (**A:** Courtesy of Steven B. Lippitt, MD.)

IMPLANT REMOVAL

- The implant can be removed at 10 to 12 weeks if the fracture is healed.
- An incision is made over the same previous lateral incision, and the subcutaneous tissue is dissected using the hemostat until the lateral aspect of the implant is identified.
- An insertion/extraction jig is attached to the implant, and then the lateral cross screw is located and removed.
- The torque driver is then engaged inside the implant and turned counterclockwise until the tension in the implant releases the medial gripper and flexible fixation mechanism.
- The implant is then gently pulled or tapped out of the lateral clavicle insertion site **(TECH FIG 6)**.

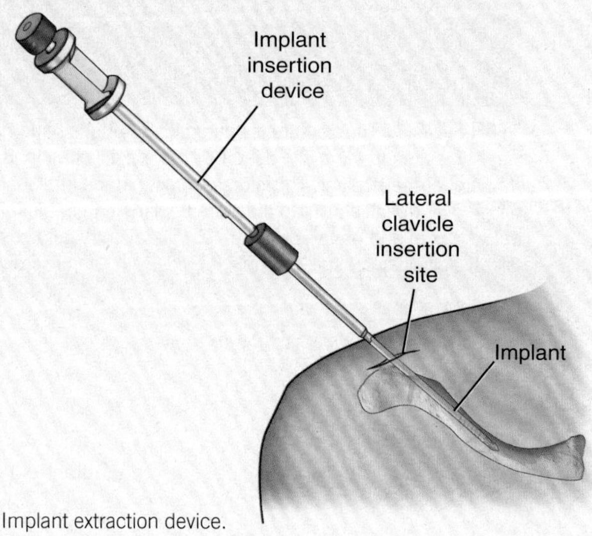

TECH FIG 6 Implant extraction device.

Pearls and Pitfalls

Medial Prep	• First, enter the canal with 2-mm drill bit and check position with orthogonal C-arm images to make 100% sure that drill is fully inside canal. Do not miss the IM canal. • Next, make sure to avoid drilling or reaming out through the medial fragment cortex. This can be accomplished with a gentle twisting of the awl or with the spade-tipped guidewire. Use C-arm imaging. • Finally, ream at least 5 cm into the medial fragment in order to assure adequate fixation.
Lateral Prep	• Enter the canal gently with the 2-mm drill bit and check C-arm images. • When passing a guidewire or 3-mm drill through the posterolateral clavicle cortex, make sure that it exits the posterior cortex adjacent to the conoid tubercle at the curve of the lateral clavicle. This will assure a straight shot down through the fracture and into the medial clavicle when passing the implant antegrade. Check images before exiting lateral cortex.
Implantation	• First, reduce fracture, then place guidewire across fracture fully into medial segment, and ream entire length over guidewire while holding fracture in anatomic reduction. This will assure that the implant does not displace the fracture slightly during the implantation process. • When placing the implant through the lateral entry guide and through the clavicle, gently push and rotate the implant. Do not strike the implant guide with a mallet because that can bend the flexible segment prematurely. • Gently rotate the torque driver as directed. Avoid aggressive torque.
Locking Screw	• Split the deltoid as needed. Avoid bending the screw guide because that can misalign screw placement. • Check final screw placement with C-arm image and check by placing torque driver back through end of implant. The torque driver will bump into the screw if the screw is properly placed through the implant.

POSTOPERATIVE CARE

- A sling is worn for 3 to 4 weeks. During this time, the sling can be removed several times per day for active range of motion of the elbow and active-assisted range of motion of the shoulder to 90 degrees of forward flexion.
- The sling is discontinued at 3 to 4 weeks, and full active range of motion of the shoulder is started if the fracture is healing well.
- Progressive resistance exercises are started at 6 weeks if the patient has achieved full range of motion and there is clinical and radiographic evidence of healing.
- Once the clavicle fracture is fully healed, the implant can be removed at 10 to 12 weeks or it can be left alone.

OUTCOMES

- The authors have fixed several hundred displaced clavicle fractures with this technique. The results are excellent when the aforementioned techniques and principles are followed closely. Comminuted fractures heal very well as long as some cortical contact can be reconstructed. **FIG 5** is a typical illustration of a comminuted fracture treated with this technique.
- In a recent consecutive clinical outcome series by Basamania[3] (160 clavicle fractures: 46% acute fractures, 29% malunions, 25% nonunions), there was only one mechanical hardware failure. The average postoperative American Shoulder and Elbow Surgeons score was 95 in acute fractures and 93 in the combined group.

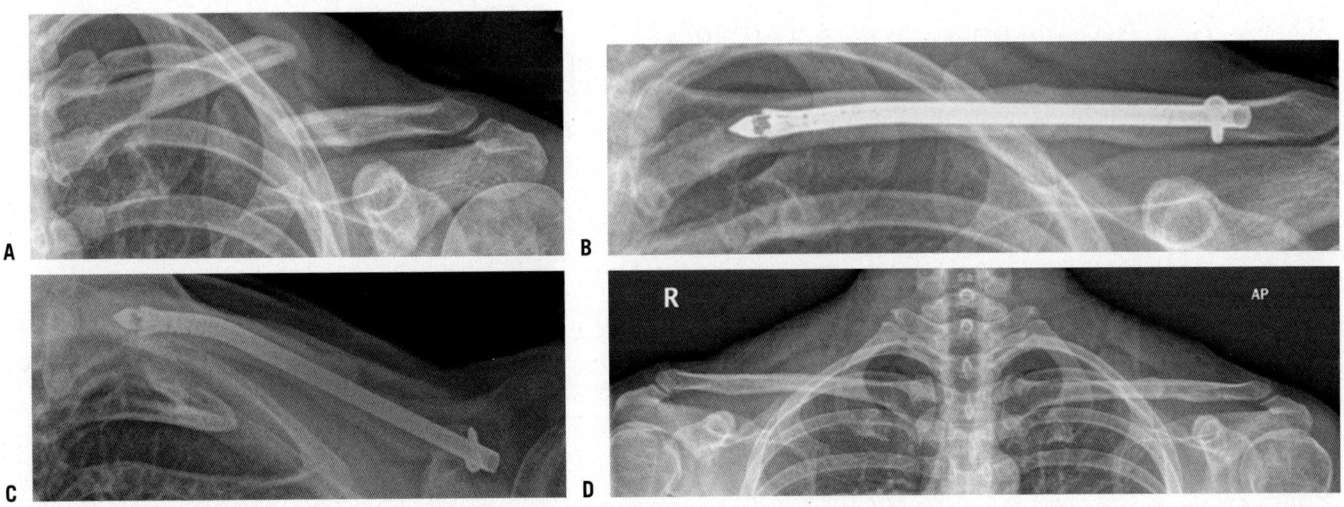

FIG 5 A. Radiograph of displaced midshaft clavicle fracture. **B,C.** Postoperative radiographs of healed clavicle fracture. **D.** AP radiograph of bilateral clavicles after implant removal. *(continued)*

E
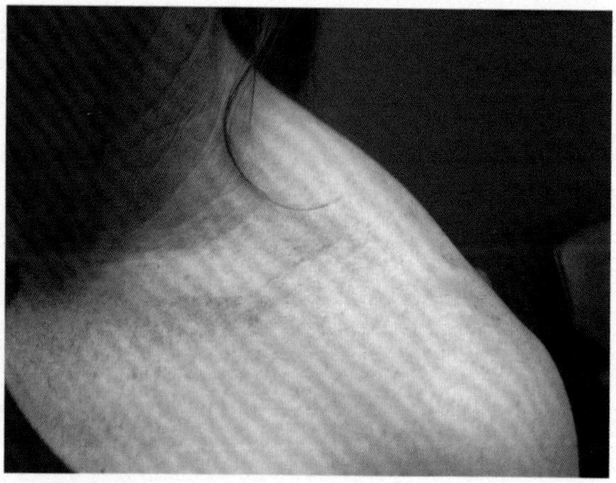

FIG 5 *(continued)* **E.** Picture of healed incision.

COMPLICATIONS

- Nonunion rates are low and can be minimized by avoiding unnecessary periosteal soft tissue stripping, following procedural technical details to obtain proper fracture site compression and alignment, and encouraging patient compliance with the postoperative protocol.
- Neurovascular complications are possible but can be avoided.
  - There is no drilling toward the neurovascular structures with this technique.
  - When exposing the fracture site, the surgeon should stay on bone at all times.
- Infection is rare, especially with this technique, which has a relatively short surgical time and small exposure. Preoperative antibiotics, meticulous handling of the soft tissues, and adequate irrigation should be part of any surgical technique.
- Implant complications can occur, but these are very rare if the implant is fully seated in the medial fragment, fracture site distraction is avoided, the locking screw is properly aligned through the implant, and the patient follows the postoperative protocol.
- As we observe with other minimally invasive surgeries, excellent outcomes depend on the surgeon's attention to detail and respect for the soft tissue envelope.

REFERENCES

1. Altamimi SA, McKee MD. Nonoperative treatment compared with plate fixation of displaced midshaft clavicle fractures. Surgical technique. J Bone Joint Surg Am 2008;90(suppl 2, pt 1):1–8.
2. Andersen K, Jensen PO, Lauritzen J. Treatment of clavicular fractures. Figure-of-eight versus a simple sling. Acta Orthop Scand 1987;58:71–74.
3. Basamania CJ. Intramedullary fixation of clavicle shaft fractures with the Sonoma CRx clavicle fracture nail device: a consecutive case series. Paper presented at: 12th International Congress of Shoulder and Elbow Surgery, Nagoya, Japan, 2013.
4. Eskola A, Vainionpää S, Myllynen P, et al. Outcome of clavicular fracture in 89 patients. Arch Orthop Trauma Surg 1986;105:337–338.
5. Hill JM, McGuire MH, Crosby LA. Closed treatment of displaced middle-third fractures of the clavicle gives poor results. J Bone Joint Surg Br 1997;79(4):537–539.
6. McKee MD, Wild LM, Schemitsch EH. Midshaft malunions of the clavicle. J Bone Joint Surg Am 2003;85(5):790–797.
7. Moseley HF. The clavicle: its anatomy and function. Clin Orthop Relat Res 1968;58:17–27.
8. Neer C. Nonunion of the clavicle. JAMA 1960;172:96–101.
9. Nordqvist A, Redlund-Johnell I, von Scheele A, et al. Shortening of clavicle after fracture. Incidence and clinical significance, a 5-year follow-up of 85 patients. Acta Orthop Scand 1997;68:349–351.
10. Rowe CR. An atlas of anatomy and treatment of midclavicular fractures. Clin Orthop Relat Res 1968;58:29–42.
11. Stanley D, Trowbridge EA, Norris SH. The mechanism of clavicular fracture. A clinical and biomechanical analysis. J Bone Joint Surg Br 1988;70(3):461–464.

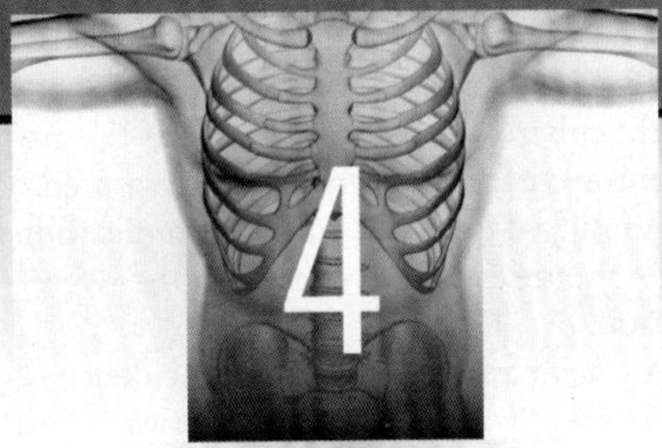

CHAPTER 4

Percutaneous Pinning for Proximal Humerus Fractures

Lindsay Hussey-Andersen, Leesa M. Galatz, and Evan L. Flatow

DEFINITION

- *Proximal humerus fractures* are defined as those of the proximal portion of the humerus involving the shoulder joint.
- *Fracture lines* divide the proximal humerus into "parts" or anatomic structures that arise from early centers of ossification.
  - Codman first recognized that proximal humerus fractures typically occur along physeal lines. This later became the basis for the Neer classification,[9] which is commonly used today.
  - The parts refer to the head of the humerus, the greater tuberosity, the lesser tuberosity, and the shaft **(FIG 1)**.
  - Proximal humerus fractures are classified as two-, three-, or four-part fractures according to the Neer classification.[9]
- In this system, a fracture fragment is classically defined as a "part" if there is 1 cm of displacement or 45 degrees of angulation. Importantly, displacement is not necessarily an indication for surgery but only a criterion for classification.
  - The type of fracture, degree of displacement, and the likelihood of osteonecrosis, as well as patient considerations, all factor into surgical decision making.

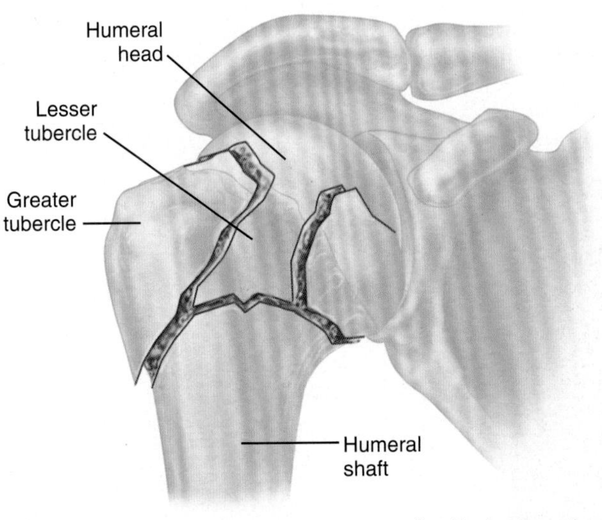

FIG 1 Fractures of the proximal humerus are classified as two-, three-, or four-part fractures based on fracture and degree of displacement of the greater tuberosity, the lesser tuberosity, the humeral head, and the humeral shaft.

ANATOMY

- The proximal humerus arises from four distinct centers of ossification: the humeral head, the greater tuberosity, the lesser tuberosity, and the shaft.
  - The greater tuberosity consists of three facets for the insertion of the supraspinatus, the infraspinatus, and the teres minor muscles of the rotator cuff.
  - The lesser tuberosity is the insertion site for the subscapularis, which is larger than the remaining three rotator cuff muscles combined.
- The pectoralis major muscle inserts on the proximal shaft of the humerus lateral to the long head of the biceps tendon. The latissimus dorsi muscle inserts onto the proximal shaft medial to the biceps groove.
  - In the fracture setting the muscular attachments to the proximal humerus produce deforming forces. An understanding of these forces is critical to understanding fracture morphology and planning reduction and fixation techniques.
- The rotator interval lies between the upper subscapularis and the anterior border of the supraspinatus.
  - The long head of the biceps tendon lies in a shallow groove on the anterior proximal humerus and enters the glenohumeral joint at the rotator interval.
  - The proximal 3 cm of the long head of the biceps tendon lies deep to the interval tissue intra-articularly.
- The blood supply to the proximal humerus comes from the anterior and posterior humeral circumflex vessels, which branch off of the axillary artery.
  - The anterior humeral circumflex artery **(FIG 2)** courses laterally along the inferior subscapularis.
    - The anterolateral branch of the anterior humeral circumflex artery then travels superiorly along the lateral aspect of the biceps groove and enters the humeral head at the proximal aspect of the groove.[1]
  - The posterior humeral circumflex artery travels within the posteromedial capsule and supplies 64% of the humeral head.[4]
- Care must be taken to protect the medial hinge and posteromedial capsule and preserve all soft tissue attachments to the humeral head at the time of surgery to minimize the risk of osteonecrosis.

PATHOGENESIS

- Proximal humerus fractures occur in a bimodal distribution but are most commonly seen in elderly women.
  - Most proximal humerus fractures are fragility fractures in older individuals with age-related osteopenia.

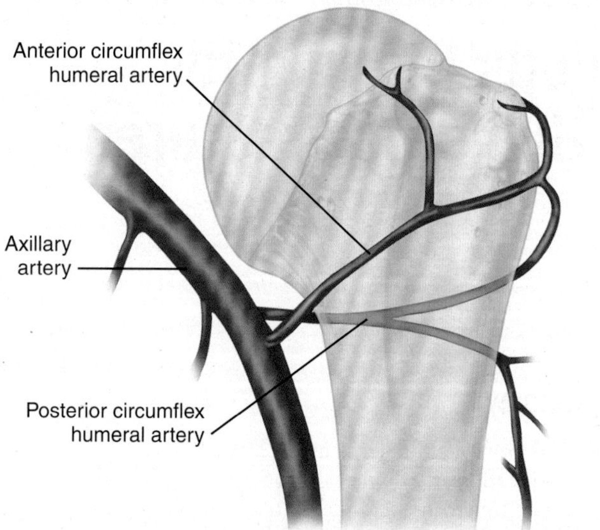

FIG 2 The rotator interval lies between the upper border of the subscapularis and the anterior border of the supraspinatus. The biceps tendon runs deep to the rotator interval tissue. Importantly, the fracture line between the greater and lesser tuberosities lies just posterior to the biceps groove. The posterior humeral circumflex artery provides 64% of the blood supply to the humeral head.

They commonly result from low-energy injuries such as ground-level falls.
- They also occur in younger individuals as the result of high-energy injuries such as motorcycle or automobile accidents.
- Associated nerve injuries can occur and usually resolve spontaneously over the course of several months. Axillary nerve neurapraxia is the most common.

NATURAL HISTORY

- Eighty-five percent of proximal humerus fractures can be treated nonoperatively with early mobilization.[9]
  - Displacement at the surgical neck is better tolerated than displacement at the greater tuberosity.
  - Because of the vast range of motion (ROM) of the shoulder in multiple planes, the arm can compensate for translational displacement or angulation at the surgical neck.
  - Displacement of the tuberosities, however, affects the mechanics of the rotator cuff and is very poorly tolerated.
- Osteonecrosis of the humeral head is a known complication of proximal humerus fractures and is related to the degree of soft tissue disruption.
  - Four-part fractures have an extremely high incidence of avascular necrosis—45% in Neer classic series—with the exception of valgus impacted four-part fractures in which the incidence is only 11%.[10] Disruption of the medial periosteal hinge, and with it branches from the posterior humeral circumflex artery, with medial displacement of the humeral shaft is thought to increase the risk of osteonecrosis.
  - Conversely, the blood supply is maintained in most valgus impacted fractures **(FIG 3)**, making this fracture configuration particularly amenable to fixation.

PATIENT HISTORY AND PHYSICAL FINDINGS

- A complete history of injury is important to determine the mechanism of injury. It is helpful to differentiate low-energy from high-energy injuries.
  - Elderly individuals often sustain proximal humerus fractures as the result of low-energy injuries such as slipping and falling. Many of these injuries are amenable to minimally invasive fixation techniques because the displacement is manageable and the periosteal sleeve between fracture fragments tends to be intact. The rotator cuff is often intact as a sleeve. All these qualities facilitate minimally invasive reduction and fixation techniques.
  - In younger individuals, proximal humerus fractures generally result from higher energy injuries. These fractures commonly have greater fracture fragment displacement, rotator cuff tears between the tuberosities, and disruption of the periosteal sleeve. These factors do not necessarily preclude percutaneous pinning but make it more challenging and should be considered in preoperative planning.
- Other important aspects of the history include the following:
  - Previous history of injury to the affected shoulder
  - Previous shoulder function and functional goals
  - History of numbness or tingling in the affected extremity
- Rule out elbow and wrist fractures, especially in osteoporotic patients with injuries resulting from a fall on an outstretched arm.

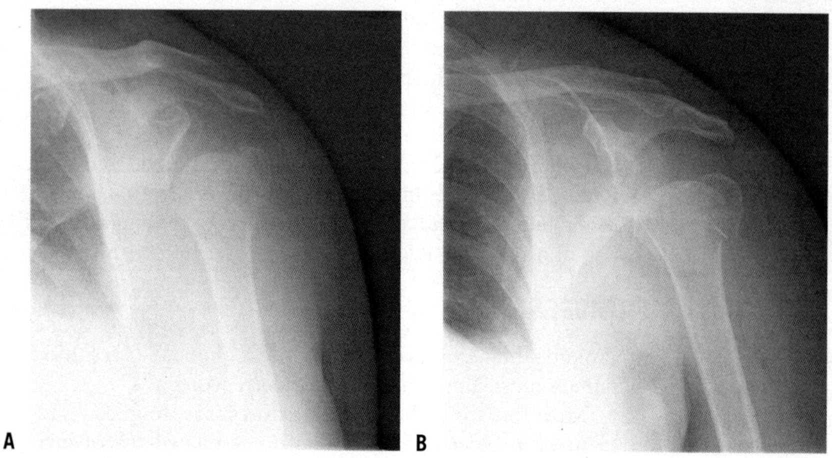

FIG 3 Valgus impacted fractures maintain blood supply to the articular surface via ascending branches off the posterior humeral circumflex artery along the intact medial periosteal hinge.

- Examination should include visual inspection for skin integrity, presence of ecchymosis, downward carriage of shoulder girdle, and deformity consistent with shoulder dislocation or acromioclavicular joint separation.
- Examine for possible associated nerve injury (usually neurapraxia) by testing sensation to light touch in individual nerve distributions, two-point discrimination, and muscle strength (testing is limited to isometric at shoulder because of limited ROM and pain).
- Pay particular attention to axillary nerve function as injuries are common.
- Possible associated vascular injury can be determined by testing radial pulse and capillary refill. An abnormal vascular exam warrants a computed tomography (CT) angiogram.

IMAGING AND OTHER DIAGNOSTIC STUDIES

- A trauma series of radiographs of the shoulder should be obtained **(FIG 4)**.
  - The series includes an anteroposterior (AP) view of the shoulder, a scapular AP or Grashey view, a scapular Y view, and an axillary view. In patients who are unable to tolerate positioning for an axillary view, a Velpeau view may be taken instead.
- Radiographs are used to determine whether the fracture is a two-, three-, or four-part fracture and to assess the degree of displacement. A CT scan is helpful in many cases and should be obtained if there is any question regarding the extent of fracture involvement or the level of displacement of the fragments.
  - Lesser tuberosity fragments are often best seen with CT scan due to their location. Additionally, these fragments often include a portion of the articular surface, which may be missed on plain x-rays.
  - Displaced head split fractures are difficult to treat percutaneously and often warrant CT evaluation.
- A CT scan is also is helpful if there is any question of joint dislocation or glenoid fracture. Three-dimensional reconstructions of the CT scan can be helpful in fracture evaluation but are not routinely required.

DIFFERENTIAL DIAGNOSIS

- Acromioclavicular joint separation
- Glenohumeral joint dislocation
- Humeral shaft fracture
- Scapulothoracic dissociation
- Elbow and wrist fractures (may coexist)

NONOPERATIVE MANAGEMENT

- Minimally displaced fractures can be treated nonoperatively.
- Displacement at the surgical neck is well tolerated.
  - An AP view of the shoulder can be misleading in the case of a surgical neck fracture.
    - In addition to pulling the humeral shaft medially, the pectoralis major muscle exerts an anterior force on the shaft, resulting in anterior displacement of the shaft relative to the humeral head.
  - A scapular Y or axillary view is necessary to appreciate this angular deformity.
- Displacement of the greater tuberosity is less well tolerated.
  - Historically, 1 cm of displacement has been used as the criterion for clinically significant tuberosity displacement.
  - Recently, however, even 5 mm of displacement has been considered an operative indication.
- Patients wear a sling for 2 to 3 weeks or until the proximal humerus feels stable with gentle internal or external rotation of the arm. During that time, they should receive close radiographic follow-up to monitor for progressive displacement.
  - Patients should be instructed to remove the sling for elbow, wrist, and hand ROM to avoid stiffness of these joints.

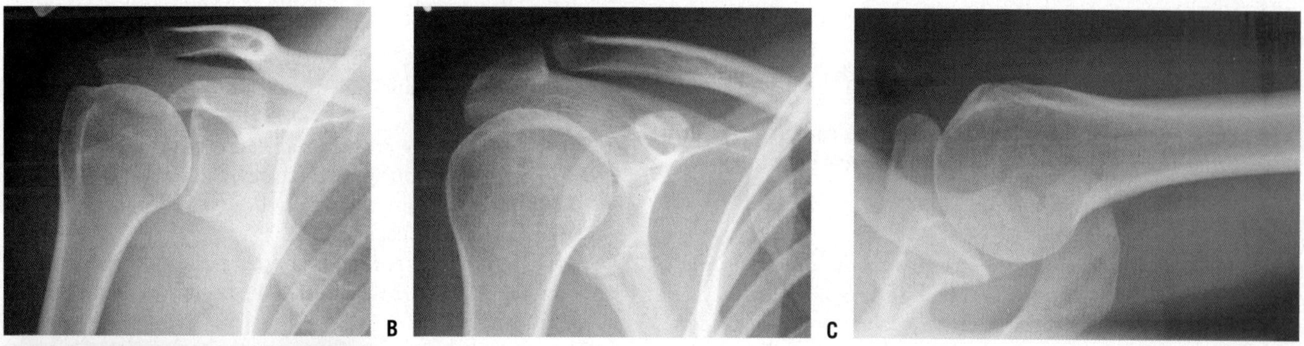

A B C

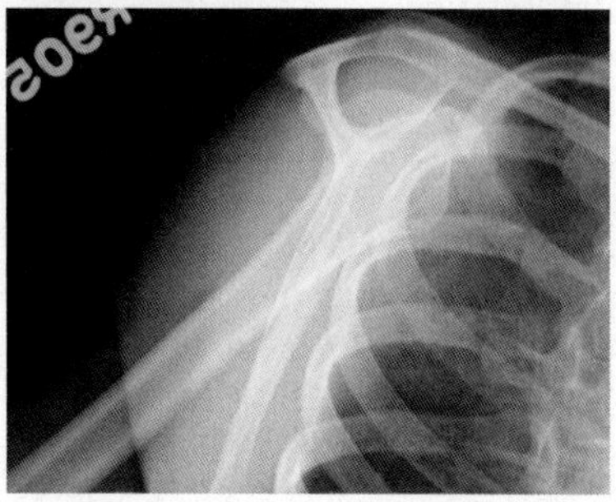

D

FIG 4 A normal trauma series includes a scapular AP radiograph, an AP radiograph of the shoulder, an axillary view, and a Y lateral view. **A.** The scapular AP view is taken, by convention, with the arm in neutral rotation. **B.** The AP view of the shoulder is taken with the arm in internal rotation. **C.** The axillary lateral view is taken with the arm abducted and in neutral rotation. **D.** The Y lateral view often allows the examiner to detect any posterior displacement of subtle greater tuberosity fractures.

- Early signs of healing (eg, callus formation) are also helpful indicators of when it is safe to commence ROM exercises.
- In borderline instances, it is better to err toward a longer period of immobilization to ensure healing because shoulder stiffness is easier to address than a nonunion.
- Therapy begins with passive stretching until 6 weeks when active ROM and strengthening can be started, progressing as tolerated.

SURGICAL MANAGEMENT

Preoperative Planning

- All imaging studies should be reviewed carefully to determine the type of fracture, the degree of displacement, fracture configuration, and bone quality.
- Certain radiographic findings that can suggest that minimally invasive fracture fixation is not appropriate for a given fracture are as follows:
  - Poor bone quality, including severe osteopenia and impaction of the humeral head. The bone may not hold the pins and screws well and may be better treated with a more stable construct.
  - Comminution of the greater tuberosity. A comminuted bone fragment is not amenable to fixation with screws. Fractures with a comminuted greater tuberosity require suture fixation through the tendon–bone junction (requires an open approach).
  - Comminution of the medial calcar region leads to unstable reduction of the head onto the shaft.
- Fractures amenable to minimally invasive fixation are two-part, three-part, and valgus impacted four-part fractures with the following:
  - Good bone quality
  - Substantial fracture fragments with minimal comminution of the tuberosities
  - Minimal or no comminution at the medial calcar region
- Minimally invasive fixation is not appropriate for noncompliant or unreliable patients. This procedure should be performed only in patients committed to consistent follow-up in the postoperative period.
  - The pins require close surveillance in the early postoperative period.
  - Pin migration is possible and must be caught early in order to avoid potential injury to thoracic structures.

Positioning

- Percutaneous pinning is performed with the patient in the 45-degree beach-chair position **(FIG 5)**.
  - This allows easy intraoperative evaluation with C-arm fluoroscopy.
- The C-arm fluoroscope is placed parallel to the patient, extending over the shoulder from the cephalad direction.
  - This position leaves the lateral shoulder completely accessible for instrumentation and pin fixation.
- The patient must be positioned far lateral on the table or on a specialized shoulder surgery positioning device such that the shoulder can be imaged in the AP plane without the table obstructing the view.
  - This image should be checked before prepping and draping to confirm adequate visualization.

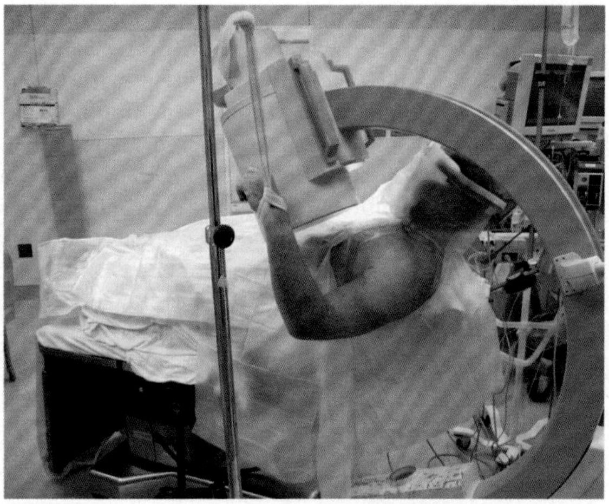

FIG 5 The patient is placed in the supine or gently upright position. The C-arm is brought in parallel to the patient, leaving the lateral aspect of the arm free for instrumentation. The patient should be positioned laterally on the table such that an adequate fluoroscopic view can be obtained.

- The entire upper extremity is draped free to allow for manipulation of the arm.

Approach

- Closed fracture reductions are performed with the aid of a "reduction portal" **(FIG 6)**.[5]
  - The reduction portal is a small incision (similar to an arthroscopic portal) used to access the fracture fragments.
  - Instruments can be introduced through this portal to lever fracture fragments or pull fragments into reduced position.
  - The surgeon also can insert a finger through this portal to palpate fragments.
    - Medially, the biceps tendon can be palpated.
    - The surgical neck fracture is located just deep to the portal.
    - By sweeping posteriorly and superiorly, the greater tuberosity and its extent of displacement can be palpated.
- The location of the reduction portal is critical **(FIG 6B)**.
  - In three- and four-part fractures, the fracture line of the greater tuberosity is reliably 0.5 to 1 cm posterior and lateral to the biceps groove.
  - Therefore, the reduction portal is located at the level of the surgical neck and 1 cm posterior to the biceps groove.
- The arm is held in neutral rotation.
  - The level of the surgical neck is located using fluoroscopic imagery **(FIG 6C,D)**.
  - The location of the biceps tendon is estimated based on surface anatomic landmarks.
- A 2-cm incision is made in the skin **(FIG 6E)**.
  - Subcutaneous tissues and the deltoid muscle are spread bluntly using a straight hemostat to avoid injury to the axillary nerve on the deep surface of the deltoid. Subdeltoid adhesions are gently released by sweeping finger if necessary.

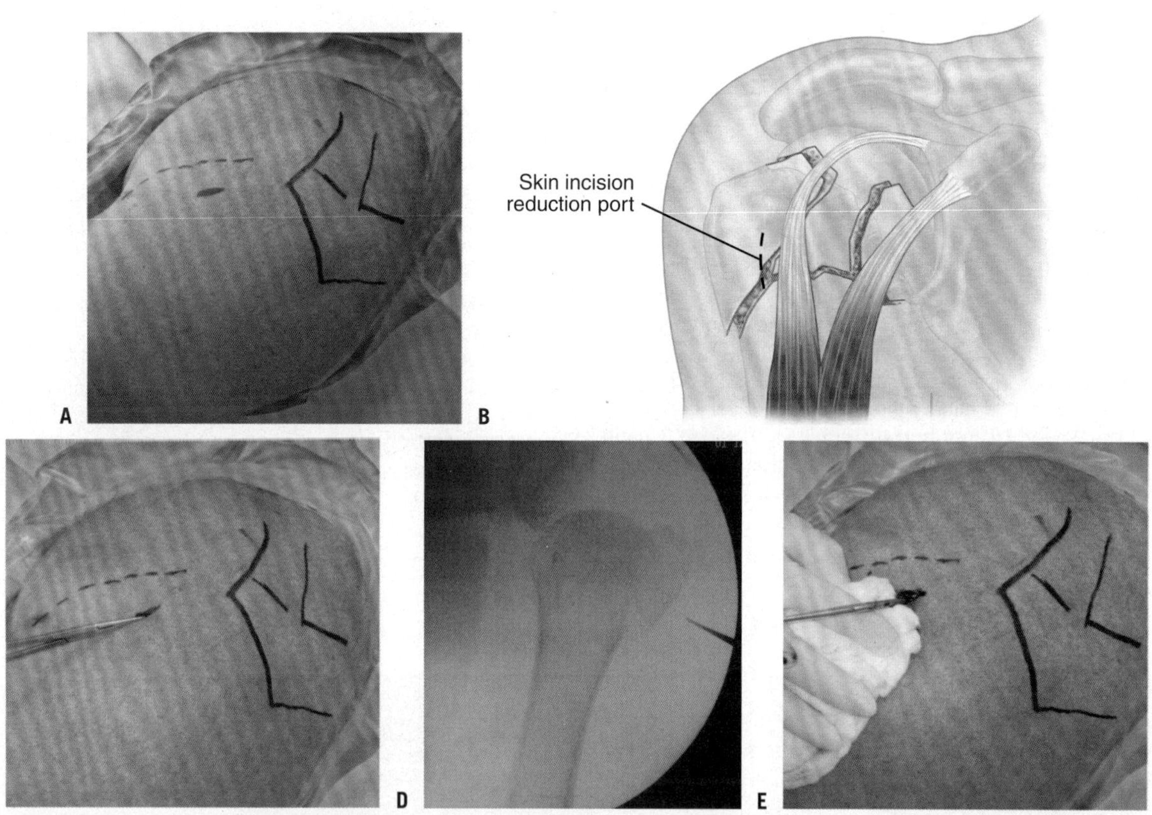

FIG 6 A. The reduction portal is established off the anterolateral corner of the acromion. Instruments can be introduced through this portal to help reduce the fracture. **B.** The reduction portal is located at the level of the surgical neck fracture approximately 0.5 to 1 cm posterior to the biceps groove. The reduction portal is definitively localized using C-arm imagery. A hemostat is applied to the skin (**C**) and then imaged (**D**) to confirm that this portal will be directly at the level of the surgical neck fracture. **E.** A small incision is made in the skin, and the deltoid is spread bluntly to avoid injury to the underlying axillary nerve.

SURGICAL NECK FRACTURE

Reduction

- The pectoralis major muscle provides the major deforming force resulting in displacement of surgical neck fractures. The shaft usually is displaced anteriorly and medially with respect to the head.
- Anterior displacement is best appreciated on an axillary or scapular Y radiograph. The reduction maneuver involves flexion, adduction, and possibly some slight internal rotation to relax the pull of the pectoralis major muscle **(TECH FIG 1)**.[6]
  - Longitudinal traction is applied to the arm, and a posteriorly directed force is applied to the proximal shaft of the humerus.
  - A bump may be placed in the axilla to help lateralize the humeral shaft.
- A blunt instrument can be inserted into the fracture at the surgical neck to lever the head back onto the shaft. This maneuver can be a powerful reduction tool, but care should be used to avoid further damage or fracture to the humeral head during this maneuver, especially on osteopenic patients.
  - The long head of the biceps tendon can become interposed between the fracture fragments, precluding reduction. Therefore, if reduction is not achieved, check the biceps tendon through the reduction portal (or consider open reduction).

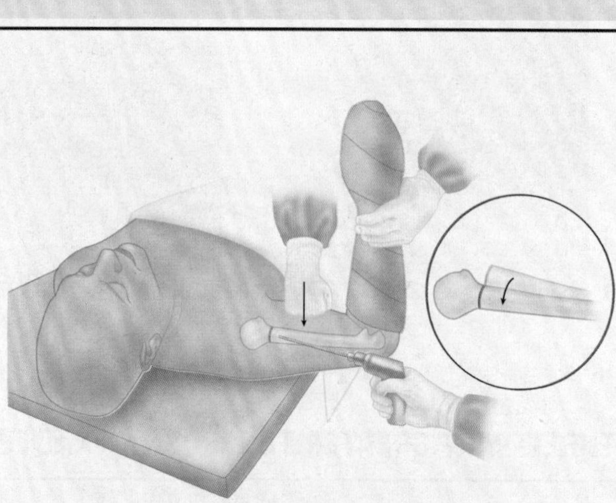

TECH FIG 1 The reduction maneuver for surgical neck fractures involves flexion and internal rotation of the arm to negate the effect of the pectoralis major fragment on the proximal aspect of the shaft. Often, a posterior vector must be applied to the shaft or an instrument can be introduced through the reduction portal to lever the head back onto the shaft.

Fixation

- Two or three retrograde pins are placed from the shaft into the humeral head **(TECH FIG 2)**.
  - The starting point for the pins is approximately 5 to 6 cm distal to the surgical neck fracture line. Pins shoulder be inserted no less than 5 cm from the lateral acromion to avoid the axillary nerve and proximal to the deltoid insertion to protect the radial nerve.
  - The pins must angle steeply to enter the head fragment and not cut out posteriorly **(TECH FIG 2B,C)**.
  - Pins should be smooth to avoid injury to soft tissues upon insertion and terminally threaded to avoid backing out.
  - The 2.5- or 2.7-mm smooth, terminally threaded Schantz pins are commonly found in external fixation instrument sets. Alternatively, the guidewires from a 7.3-mm cannulated screw set may be used.
- The pins should enter at different directions to enhance stability of fixation construct.
  - One pin should enter lateral to the biceps in a primarily anterior to posterior direction.
  - Another pin should enter further laterally in a primarily lateral to medial direction.
  - Avoid placing pins medial to the biceps to protect the musculocutaneous nerve.
- Stability should be checked under fluoroscopic imaging with live, gentle internal and external rotation.
  - Any suggestion of instability or motion at the fracture is an indication for open reduction and plate fixation at that point.
- Pins are cut below the skin to prevent pin site infection **(TECH FIG 2D)**.
- The reduction portal is closed with interrupted absorbable sutures.
- A soft dressing and sling are applied.

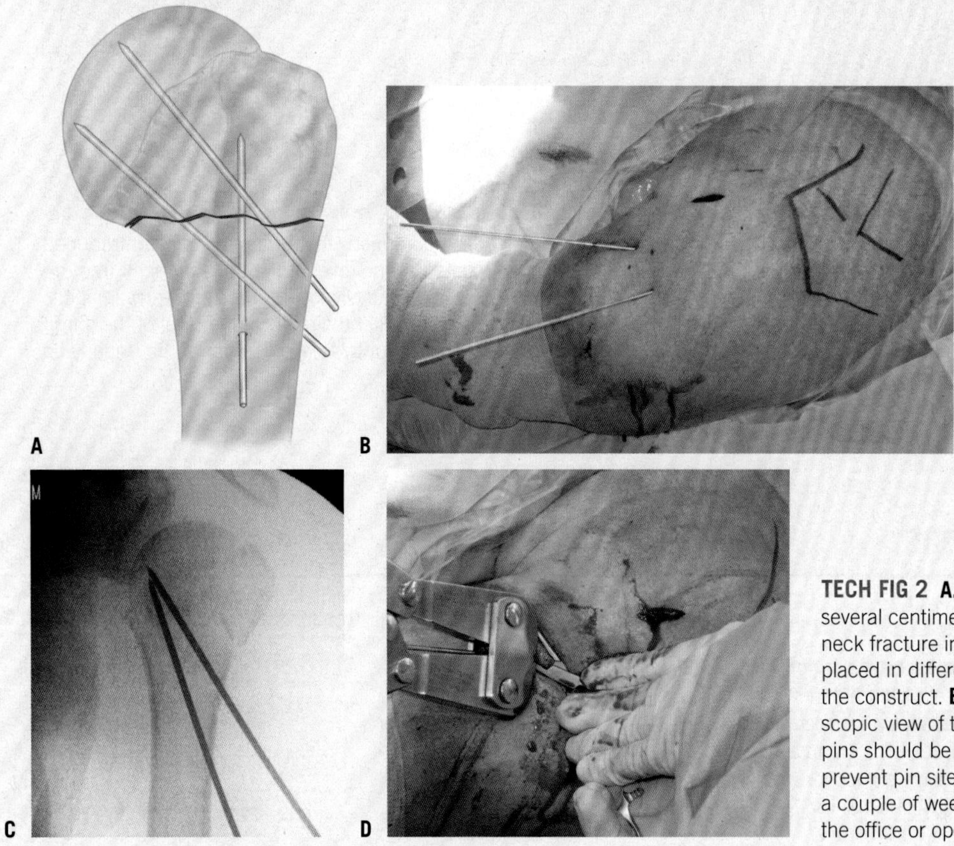

TECH FIG 2 **A.** Retrograde pins are introduced several centimeters below the level of the surgical neck fracture into the head. The pins should be placed in different directions to provide stability to the construct. **B.** Placement of two pins. **C.** Fluoroscopic view of two retrograde pins in place. **D.** The pins should be cut below the skin after insertion to prevent pin site infection. They are easily removed a couple of weeks later with a small procedure in the office or operating room.

THREE-PART GREATER TUBEROSITY FRACTURES

Reduction

- Deforming forces influencing displacement of three-part fractures include the pectoralis major, as described earlier, and the rotator cuff muscles. The rotator cuff pulls the tuberosity medially (to a certain extent) and posteriorly. Posterior displacement and rotation often are underappreciated and must be considered.
- The surgical neck component is addressed first. (See Surgical Neck Fracture earlier in this section.)
- The greater tuberosity fracture is reduced using the "reduction portal." A dental pick or small hooked instrument is inserted through the portal to engage the tuberosity and pull it inferiorly and anteriorly into a reduced position. It should sit roughly 5 mm below the top of the humeral head.

Fixation

- The 4.5-mm cannulated screws are used to fix the tuberosity fragment.
  - The screw is placed through the tuberosity fragment distal to the cuff insertion **(TECH FIG 3A)**. The trajectory of the screw should be such that it exits the medial cortex roughly 2 cm below the articular margin to avoid injury to the axillary nerve.
  - The proper location is confirmed with fluoroscopic imaging.
- The guidewire is first passed through a small incision in the skin just large enough to pass the drill guide and screw through the deltoid **(TECH FIG 3B,C)**.
  - The guidewire is passed through the tuberosity, across the surgical neck fracture, and engages the medial cortex of the proximal humeral shaft.
  - After the guidewire is overdrilled, the screw is passed over the guidewire. We use a partially threaded screw with a washer **(TECH FIG 3D–F)**. Overcompression of this screw can result in fracturing of the fragment.
  - If the greater tuberosity fragment is large enough, a second cancellous screw is directed through the tuberosity fragment, engaging cancellous bone of the humeral head.
- Pins are cut beneath the skin.
- Incisions are closed with nylon interrupted sutures.
- A dressing and sling are applied.

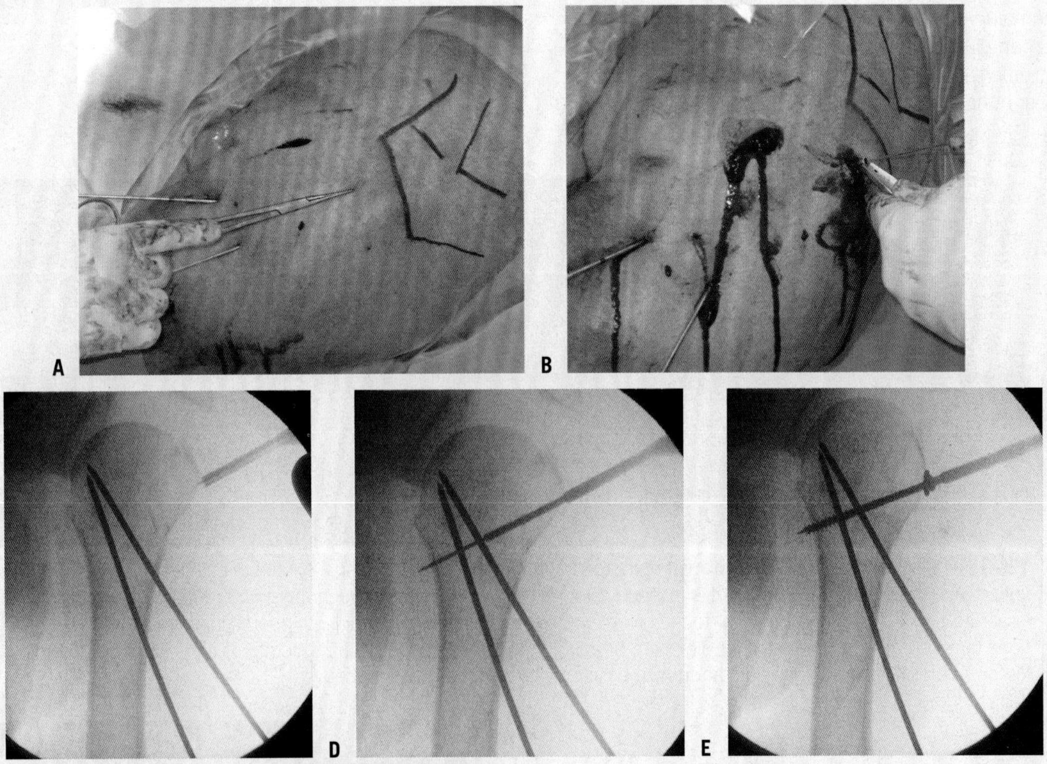

A B C D E

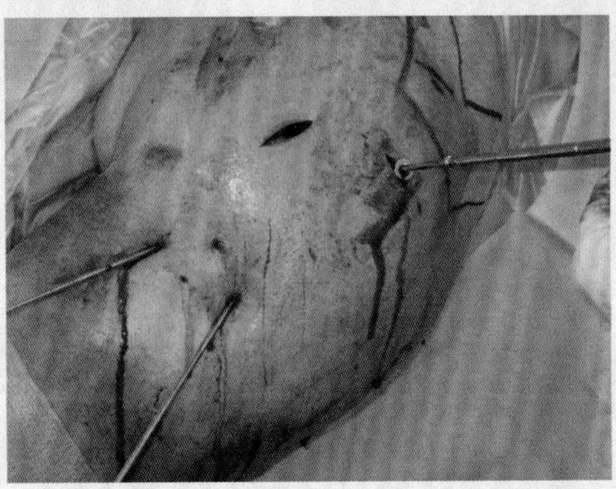

F

TECH FIG 3 **A.** The greater tuberosity is localized under fluoroscopy using a hemostat. **B.** A small incision is made over the greater tuberosity, and a cannulated screw is used for fixation. This photograph demonstrates the drill guide used for soft tissue protection. **C.** The guidewire is aimed to engage the greater tuberosity fragment as well as the medial cortex to provide compression. **D.** This fluoroscopic view demonstrates the screw being inserted over the guidewire. **E.** A washer is used to provide some compression. Overtightening should be avoided to prevent fracture of the greater tuberosity fragment. **F.** Screw and washer insertion.

VALGUS IMPACTED FOUR-PART PROXIMAL HUMERUS FRACTURES

- Valgus impacted fractures are recognized by the 90-degree angle between the long axis of the humeral shaft and the articular surface of the humeral head with loss of the normal neck shaft angle.[7] The tuberosities are displaced laterally from the head of the humerus and slightly proximally.
  - This fracture configuration results in a low incidence of avascular necrosis compared to that of other four-part fractures because the medial periosteal hinge of soft tissues is intact along the medial and posterior anatomic neck, preserving the blood supply provided by the posterior humeral circumflex artery and its ascending vessels.
- The reduction maneuver for this fracture requires raising the humeral head back into its anatomic position.
  - The reduction portal described previously is created, and an instrument such as a blunt elevator or small bone tamp is inserted beneath the humeral head **(TECH FIG 4A,B)**.
  - The instrument passes through the surgical neck fracture and through the fracture line between the tuberosities, which reliably exists 0.5 to 1 cm posterior and lateral to the biceps groove.
- The instrument is tapped with a mallet in a distal to proximal direction, lifting the head fragment into anatomic position **(TECH FIG 4C)**.
- The surgical neck fractures and tuberosity fractures are then fixed using the techniques described earlier.
- In some cases, there may be significant medial displacement of the lesser tuberosity. In these cases, the lesser tuberosity is reduced using the hook through the reduction portal and fixed with a screw placed in the anterior to posterior direction through the tuberosity into the head.
  - In most cases, minimal medial displacement of the lesser tuberosity is well tolerated and no fixation is required.
- Pins are cut beneath the skin.
- Incisions are closed with nylon sutures.
- A dressing and sling are applied.

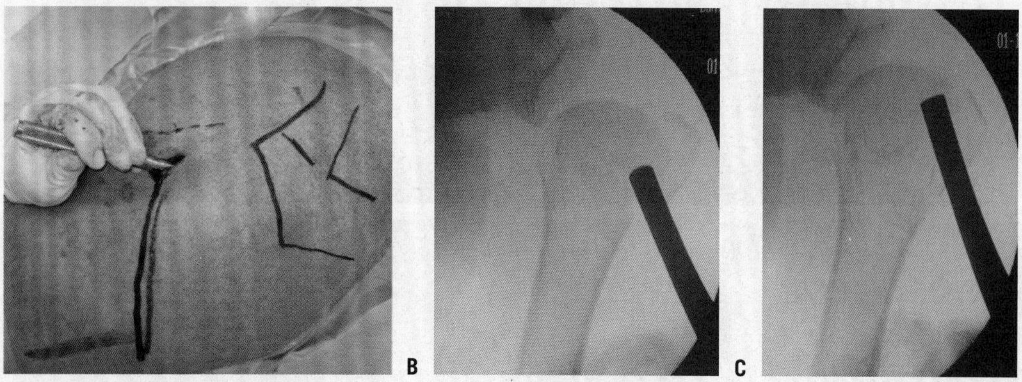

A B C

TECH FIG 4 **A.** Valgus impacted proximal humerus fractures are reduced using a small bone tamp or other blunt-tipped instrument. **B.** The instrument is inserted through the fracture line between the greater tuberosity and the lesser tuberosity, which lies posterior to the biceps groove. Position is confirmed with fluoroscopic imaging. **C.** The bone tamp is impacted in a superior direction, bringing the humeral head into a reduced position. The greater and lesser tuberosities fall naturally into a reduced position after this reduction maneuver.

Pearls and Pitfalls

Indications	• Successful percutaneous pinning depends on appropriate patient selection. Criteria include good bone stock, minimal to no comminution at the greater tuberosity fragment, minimal to no comminution at the medial calcar and proximal shaft, and patient compliance. • Contraindications include poor bone stock that will not hold pins, comminution of greater tuberosity or proximal shaft fragments, and a noncompliant patient with poor follow-up potential.
Positioning	• The patient must be lateral enough on the table to obtain unencumbered access to the shoulder and clear fluoroscopic images.
Reduction Technique	• The location of the reduction portal is critical for maximizing its usefulness during the procedure. • The surgeon must have a thorough understanding of three-dimensional anatomy as well as interpretation and application of two-dimensional fluoroscopic images.

Pin Placement	• Pins should engage the humerus distal to the axillary nerve but proximal to the deltoid insertion to avoid nerve injury. • The angle of insertion is steep to enter the humeral head and avoid cutting out posteriorly. • At least two fluoroscopic images in different planes are necessary to confirm successful pin placement. • A drill guide can be used to protect the soft tissues during pin insertion.
Screw Placement	• The deltoid should be spread bluntly and a drill guide used to prevent injury to the axillary nerve in this location. In most cases, insertion will be proximal to the nerve, but precautionary measures should be taken. • Overtightening the screw with a washer may result in fracture of the greater tuberosity. • Engaging medial cortex of the proximal shaft gives stability to the screw construct.
Intraoperative Assessment of Stability	• The arm should be internally and externally rotated gently under continuous fluoroscopic imagery after completion of hardware placement. Any motion or suggestion of instability is an indication for open reduction and fixation.

POSTOPERATIVE CARE

- The operative arm is immobilized in a sling.
- The patient is instructed to begin active elbow, wrist, and hand ROM exercises.
- Radiographs are checked weekly to monitor for pin migration or loss of fixation.
  - Pins are removed as a short procedure in the office or operating room about 3 to 4 weeks postoperatively or when early signs of healing are evident radiographically.
- Pendulum exercises are initiated 2 to 3 weeks postoperatively, and passive stretching (forward elevation in scapular plane), external rotation, and internal rotation (all in supine position) is initiated when pins are removed.
  - Ideally, pins should be out and motion started no later than 4 weeks postoperatively.
- Active ROM progressing as tolerated to resistance exercises commences at 6 weeks postoperatively.

OUTCOMES

- Jaberg et al[6] reported good to excellent results in 34 of 48 fractures. There were 29 surgical neck, 3 anatomic neck, 8 three-part, and 5 four-part fractures. Four patients required revision percutaneous pinning for loss of fixation and all four of those had good to excellent final results.
- Resch et al[11] reported results of 9 three-part fractures and 18 four-part fractures. In the four-part fractures, the incidence of avascular necrosis was 11%. Good results correlated with anatomic reconstruction.
- Keener et al[8] reported a multicenter study of 35 patients—7 two-part, 8 three-part, and 12 valgus impacted fractures. Average duration of follow-up was 35 months. All fractures healed, and only 1 developed avascular necrosis (4.2%). American Shoulder and Elbow Surgeons (ASES) and Constant scores were 83.4 and 73.9, respectively. Four patients had some residual malunion, and 4 developed posttraumatic arthritis. Neither of these affected outcome at this early follow-up period, however.
- This same group of patients was subsequently followed for an average of 50 months (range, 11 to 101 months).[3] Osteonecrosis was present in 10 (37%) of the patients and was diagnosed an average of 50 months after the index procedure. Only 2 were symptomatic enough to warrant revision to an arthroplasty. Average ASES score was 82 at this intermediate-term follow-up.
- In a recent systematic review comparing operative treatments for proximal humerus fractures, closed reduction and percutaneous pinning had the highest complication rate at 28.4% and higher rates of osteonecrosis than open reduction internal fixation (11.7% vs. 6.4%).[2] However, the lack of randomized trials, reproducible classification systems, and standardized treatment algorithms makes comparison difficult.
- Most studies report satisfactory results with this procedure. Patient selection is critical. In published studies, patients are not randomized to percutaneous pinning, but rather, careful patient selection is left to the treating surgeon. Therefore, it can be concluded that this is an appropriate technique in certain patients who meet the outlined criteria.

COMPLICATIONS

- Nerve injury[12]
- Pin migration
- Loss of fixation
- Malunion
- Nonunion
- Osteonecrosis
- Infection
- Glenohumeral joint stiffness

REFERENCES

1. Gerber C, Schneeberger AG, Vinh TS. The arterial vascularization of the humeral head. An anatomical study. J Bone Joint Surg Am 1990;72A:1486–1494.
2. Gupta AK, Harris JD, Erickson BJ, et al. Surgical management of complex proximal humerus fractures—a systematic review of 92 studies including 4500 patients. J Orthop Trauma 2015;29(1):54–59.
3. Harrison AK, Gruson KI, Zmistowski B, et al. Intermediate outcomes following percutaneous fixation of proximal humeral fractures. J Bone Joint Surg Am 2012;94(13):1223–1228.
4. Hettrich CM, Boraiah S, Dyke JP, et al. Quantitative assessment of the vascularity of the proximal part of the humerus. J Bone Joint Surg Am 2010;92:943–948.
5. Hsu J, Galatz LM. Mini-incision fixation of proximal humeral four-part fractures. In: Scuderi GR, Tria A, Berger RA, eds. MIS Techniques in Orthopedics. New York: Springer, 2006:32–44.
6. Jaberg H, Warner JJ, Jakob RP. Percutaneous stabilization of unstable fractures of the humerus. J Bone Joint Surg Am 1992;74A:508–515.
7. Jakob RP, Miniaci A, Anson PS, et al. Four-part valgus impacted fractures of the proximal humerus. J Bone Joint Surg Br 1991;73B:295–298.
8. Keener J, Parsons BO, Flatow EL, et al. Outcomes after percutaneous reduction and fixation of proximal humeral fractures. J Shoulder Elbow Surg 2007;16:330–338.
9. Neer CS II. Displaced proximal humerus fractures. I. Classification and evaluation. J Bone Joint Surg Am 1970;52A:1077–1089.
10. Resch H, Beck A, Bayley I. Reconstruction of the valgus-impacted humeral head fracture. J Shoulder Elbow Surg 1995;4:73–80.
11. Resch H, Povacz P, Fröhlich R, et al. Percutaneous fixation of three- and four-part fractures of the proximal humerus. J Bone Joint Surg Br 1997;79B:295–300.
12. Rowles DJ, McGrory JE. Percutaneous pinning of the proximal humerus: an anatomic study. J Bone Joint Surg Am 2001;83A:1695–1699.

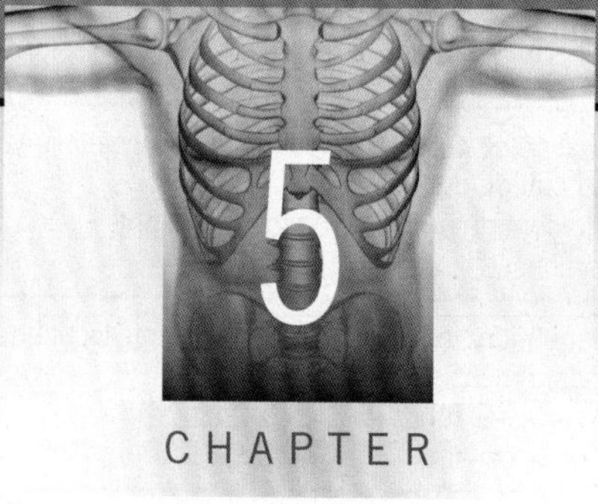

CHAPTER 5

Open Reduction and Internal Fixation of Proximal Humerus Fractures

Steven F. DeFroda and E. Scott Paxton

DEFINITION

- Proximal humerus fractures may involve the surgical neck, the greater tuberosity, and/or the lesser tuberosity.
- The Neer classification, which is most commonly used, categorizes fractures based on the number of displaced parts (**FIG 1**). This classification system involves four segments: the articular surface, the greater tuberosity, the lesser tuberosity, and the humeral shaft. Fracture fragments displaced 1 cm or angulated 45 degrees are considered a displaced part.
- The Association for Osteosynthesis/Association for the Study of Internal Fixation broadly classifies fractures into three types: type 1, unifocal extra-articular; type 2, bifocal extra-articular; and type 3, intra-articular.
  - Each type is then further divided into groups and subgroups.
  - This system places more emphasis on the vascular supply to the humerus, with intra-articular fracture patterns having the highest risk of avascular necrosis.
- Interobserver reliability for both classification systems is not high, however.
- Although not included in Neer original classification, valgus-impacted fractures are a unique entity that are important to recognize because of their unique characteristics as four-part fractures in which the humeral articular surface is impacted on the shaft segment in a valgus position with an intact medial hinge, leading to an increase in the angle between the humeral shaft and the articular surface and spreading of the tuberosities (**FIG 2**).

ANATOMY

- The osseous anatomy of the proximal humerus consists of the greater tuberosity, the lesser tuberosity, and the articular surface.
  - The subscapularis inserts onto the lesser tuberosity, whereas the supraspinatus, infraspinatus, and teres minor insert onto the greater tuberosity.

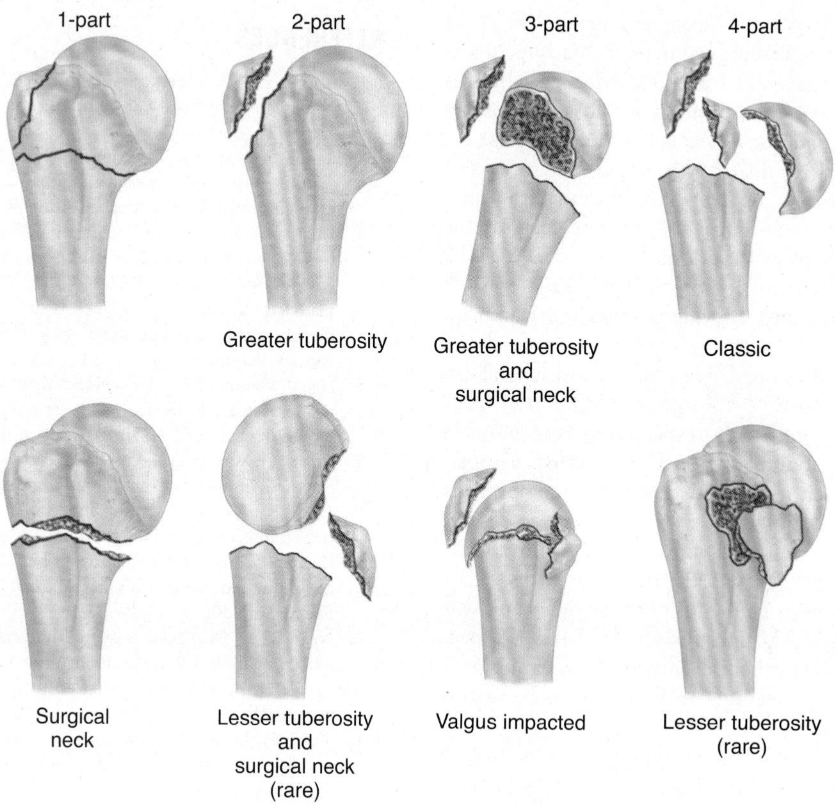

FIG 1 Neer classification of fractures of the proximal humerus.

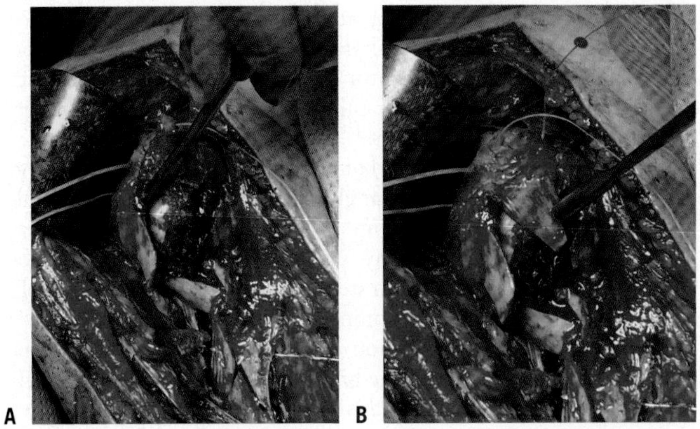

FIG 2 **A.** Valgus-impacted four-part fracture of the left shoulder showing the articular surface laterally, with the tuberosities displaced around the head portion. **B.** This can be reduced by elevating the lateral portion of the head and tying the tuberosities back together underneath via nonabsorbable suture.

- Knowledge of deforming forces associated with humerus fractures allows the surgeon to better treat these fractures by both operative and nonoperative means. The surgeon must understand the deforming forces in order to successfully reduce fragments and counteract the deforming forces.
  - In a two-part surgical neck fracture, the pectoralis major pulls the humeral shaft anteromedial and causes internal rotation. The rotator cuff attachment abducts the proximal segment, typically leading to varus malalignment. If there is significant calcar comminution, the latissimus and teres major may pull medial calcar fragments posteromedially.
  - In a two-part greater tuberosity fracture, the pull of the supraspinatus, infraspinatus, and teres minor tendons displaces the greater tuberosity superomedially.
  - Three-part fractures involving the greater tuberosity result in unopposed subscapularis function, and the humeral articular surface rotates internally.
  - Three-part fractures involving the lesser tuberosity and surgical neck are very rare.
  - Four-part fractures result in displacement of the shaft and both tuberosities, leaving a free head fragment with little soft tissue attachment. The tuberosities displace as a result of the attached rotator cuff muscles.
- An understanding of the vascular anatomy is important in treating proximal humerus fractures in order to avoid further disruption of blood supply to the humeral head, which may help to prevent nonunion or avascular necrosis.
- The proximal humerus receives its blood supply from two branches of the axillary artery: the anterior and posterior circumflex humeral arteries. The main blood supply to the humeral head is from the posterior circumflex humeral artery, supplying approximately 60%.[10]
- The arcuate branch comes from the anterior circumflex and runs just lateral to the tendon of the long head of the biceps in the bicipital groove, enters the humeral head, and becomes interosseous proximally at the transition between the bicipital groove and greater tuberosity and supplies the medial aspect of the humeral head.[10]
- The posterior circumflex humeral artery branches from the axillary artery; travels through the quadrangular space with the axillary nerve; winds superolaterally around the posterior aspect of the humerus; and supplies the superior, lateral, and inferior aspects of the humeral head.[10]
  - Fracture extension of less than 8 mm into the medial humeral head metaphysis has also been shown to be a significant predictor of initial head ischemia (ie, the longer the metaphyseal head extension, the greater the likelihood of perfusion[9]).
  - More recent studies of this population, however, failed to show any relationship between initial head ischemia and later avascular necrosis.[1]

PATHOGENESIS

- Proximal humerus fractures usually result from ground-level, low-energy falls in older patients.
- In contrast, younger patients sustain proximal humerus fractures as the result of high-energy mechanisms such as an automobile collision or a sports-related injury (eg, extreme sports).
- The presence of an associated glenohumeral dislocation can also be present and must be determined at the time of initial evaluation as this could influence management strategy, particularly for irreducible fracture dislocations.

PATIENT HISTORY AND PHYSICAL FINDINGS

- In addition to a standard orthopaedic history, history should include if the injury involves the dominant or nondominant extremity, the mechanism of injury, social situation and support, and preexisting shoulder symptoms, which could indicate rotator cuff pathology or arthritis.
  - History of weight-bearing requirements of the upper extremity secondary to chronic conditions or concomitant lower extremity injuries is important to consider.
- Visual inspection can reveal ecchymosis and swelling of the arm, and palpation generally elicits diffuse pain. It is not uncommon in the first 1 to 2 weeks for the swelling and ecchymosis to involve the entire extremity and even the forearm and hand.
- Assessment of the initial range of motion (ROM) is difficult due to pain and is often unnecessary. However, assessment of fracture stability is important in determining treatment.
  - If the shaft and the proximal portion move as a unit when taken through internal and external rotation, the fracture usually is considered stable. If they do not and crepitus is felt, the fracture is unstable.
  - This is important to evaluate for initiation of ROM in the nonoperative patient or in determining the need for operative intervention.

- If there is an associated dislocation, it may be possible to palpate the humeral head as an anterior or posterior fullness.
- A thorough neurovascular examination is performed to determine the presence of associated injuries.
- Particular attention should be paid to the ability of the patient to contract all three heads of the deltoid to ensure that the axillary nerve is fully functional. However, partial axillary nerve injuries can be impossible to diagnose initially if sensation is intact as full strength testing is not typically possible secondary to the fracture.
- Nerve injuries, usually of the axillary nerve, are not uncommon in the setting of proximal humerus fractures.
  - Low-energy injury can also lead to nerve deficits; Visser et al[25] reported electromyography abnormalities in 67% of patients following this mechanism of injury.
- Although major vascular injury is rare in these fractures, a high index of suspicion should be present when evaluating fractures with significant medial shaft displacement or anterior dislocations. The axillary artery can be injured in these instances, and diminished radial and ulnar pulses should raise suspicion for this injury.[11]
  - Do not be fooled by an intact radial pulse as the upper arm has significant collateral circulation and a palpable pulse does not rule out a vascular injury. The pulse must be compared to the contralateral side with equal pressure. If concern exists, vascular studies should be obtained.

IMAGING AND OTHER DIAGNOSTIC STUDIES

- Initial imaging studies consist of anteroposterior (AP), true AP (Grashey), scapular Y, and axillary views **(FIG 3)**.
  - Additional views may include internal and external rotation views if the fracture pattern is stable. Internal rotation views help to visualize the lesser tuberosity, whereas external rotation shows the greater tuberosity. West Point axillary view may be useful for fracture of the anterior glenoid rim and a Stryker notch view for a Hill-Sachs lesion.
- Attention should be paid not only to fracture pattern but also to bone quality and assessment for any concern of bony lesions that may indicate pathologic fracture.

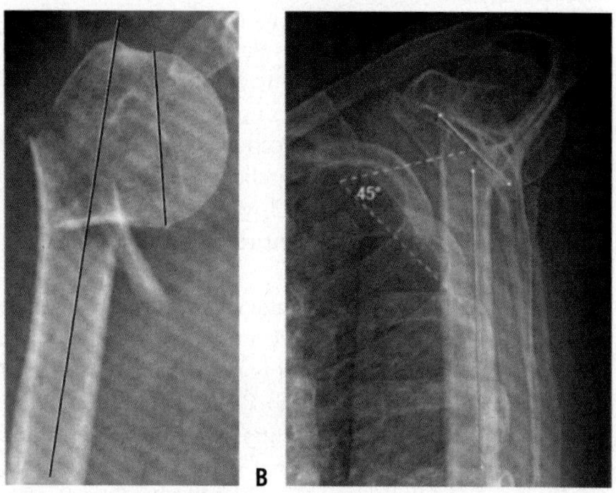

A B

FIG 3 A. True AP radiograph of right shoulder showing a varus angulated proximal humerus fracture with a neck–shaft angle of 95 degrees (normal neck–shaft angle 130 to 135 degrees) and medial comminution (*red lines*). **B.** Scapular Y radiograph demonstrating typical apex anterior sagittal malalignment (*yellow lines*).

- Evidence of preexisting arthritis (eg, subchondral sclerosis, osteophytes) may alter treatment and should be noted as well as signs of rotator cuff disease (acromial spurring, rounding of the greater tuberosity, and wear of the undersurface of the acromion).
- Specific measurements that can be obtained to help decision making are neck–shaft angle, sagittal plane angulation, and displacement of fragments.
- A computed tomography (CT) scan may be helpful if radiographs do not demonstrate the fracture pattern adequately or for preoperative planning.
  - Although the addition of a CT scan may improve intraobserver reproducibility only minimally and not affect interobserver reliability, CT scanning may prove valuable in determining the method of fixation as well as identifying associated injuries such as glenoid fractures.
  - An additional benefit of CT scan is the ability to obtain three-dimensional reconstruction of the fracture, which may better characterize the injury along with evaluation of the rotator cuff musculature to assess for any atrophy, which may indicate preexisting rotator cuff disease.[16]
- Indications for magnetic resonance imaging are limited, and it is very rarely used.

DIFFERENTIAL DIAGNOSIS

- Glenohumeral dislocation
- Scapula fracture
- Clavicle fracture
- Humeral shaft fracture
- Neurovascular injury
- Neuropathic arthropathy

NONOPERATIVE MANAGEMENT

- Operative indications are highly variable regarding fractures involving the surgical neck and often depend as much on patient factors, including age and demand level, as they do on fracture pattern and displacement.
- Recent studies have shown equal outcomes for open reduction and internal fixation (ORIF) and nonoperative treatment of proximal humerus fractures. However, many of these studies do not use strict inclusion criteria and do not assess for the quality of the reduction or fixation.[2,21]
- Nonoperative treatment should be considered when restoring anatomic alignment by correcting the deformity of the proximal humerus fracture is not thought to be beneficial to the patient or would produce undue risk. This may be secondary to only mild displacement, secondary to a low demand level of the patient or unwillingness or inability to participate in postoperative rehabilitation.
- In the case of isolated greater tuberosity fractures, more than 5 mm of displacement may lead to poor functional results.
  - Neer original description called for fixation of greater tuberosity fractures when there was more than 1 cm of displacement.
  - Greater tuberosity displacement of greater than 5 mm may lead to impingement, and displacement of less than 5 mm does not appear to warrant surgery.
- For proximal humerus fractures not involving the humeral shaft, patients initially are immobilized in a simple sling.

- When the fracture is deemed stable (which may be immediately following the fracture for many fracture types), pendulums and passive ROM are started. Passive ROM in all planes is allowed.
- When treating proximal humerus fractures conservatively, physical therapy for passive ROM is important to initiate as soon as possible. Koval et al[13] showed significant improvement with one-part fractures when physical therapy was initiated before 2 weeks.
- Between 6 and 10 weeks, the fracture usually has healed enough that strengthening exercises may be started.[18] However, it is often beneficial to delay strengthening until active ROM has been maximized.
- Studies done before the advent of periarticular locked proximal humeral plating comparing patients treated surgically and nonsurgically have shown no difference in outcome with two-part surgical neck fractures and displaced three- and four-part fractures. It is important to realize the limitations of these early studies when discussing surgical decision making with patients.

SURGICAL MANAGEMENT

- It is imperative that patients have reasonable expectations of their outcome following surgery.
  - A "good" outcome is dependent on these expectations as well as the patients' overall resiliency and coping ability allowing for full participation in rehabilitation.
  - A functional ROM with minimal pain is the goal, with most patients having some degree of motion loss, even with anatomic restoration of the proximal humerus.
- Multiple techniques can be employed for surgical fixation of the proximal humerus. We describe the most common current techniques in the following text. Choice of fixation should be based on the individual patient, the fracture pattern, and the surgeon's own comfort level.
- ORIF involving anatomic plating of the proximal humerus commonly is performed through the deltopectoral interval and requires a locked plate.
  - Strong consideration should be given to use of a variable angle, or polyaxial, locked plate to better accommodate accurate positioning of calcar screws in all patients despite the anatomy of the proximal humerus.[17]
- Intramedullary nailing can also be used for proximal humerus fractures, typically for two-part surgical neck fractures.
  - It has the benefit of being able to be done in a percutaneous fashion, making it very biologically friendly, as the fracture site is not exposed.
  - A short intramedullary device can be used for these fractures unlike the longer intramedullary nails commonly used for humeral shaft fractures.
  - Newer nail designs include a straight nail passed through the superior articular surface unlike older nails that entered through the rotator cuff insertion. The older nails had a high rate of rotator cuff symptoms secondary to this unlike newer designs.[24]

Preoperative Planning

- Acceptable imaging studies, including plain radiographs and often CT scanning, are necessary before proceeding to surgery.
- Each proximal humerus fracture is unique, but certain patterns of fracture are more common and the treating surgeon should be familiar with these. Different types of fractures may be more or less amenable to specific treatment modalities. Consequently, the surgeon should be prepared with an arsenal of different fixation techniques or arthroplasty options.
  - If the fracture is not deemed suitable for internal fixation intraoperatively, the surgeon must be prepared to perform a hemiarthroplasty or a reverse shoulder arthroplasty, but in most cases, this decision can be made preoperatively.
  - In a study of 260,000 proximal humerus "fragility" fractures in Medicare patients from 2005 to 2012, nonoperative management was the most common treatment; within the surgically treated cohort, there was an increase in treatment with arthroplasty including reverse total shoulder arthroplasty, with a low rate of early revisions.[8]

Positioning

- The techniques discussed in this section are easiest to perform with the patient in the beach-chair position, with the use of a pneumatic arm holder.
  - With the patient nearly seated, the hips and knees are flexed.
  - The patient is moved as far laterally as possible on the table to allow full ROM of the shoulder.
- A lateral buttress is used to help keep the patient in position on the table.
- C-arm fluoroscopy is helpful in determining the quality of reduction. The C-arm is best positioned with the machine "flipped," with the intensifier posterior to the shoulder and the arm over the patient **(FIG 4)**.
- A fluoroscopic image is obtained prior to prepping to ensure that the entire fracture can be visualized without obstruction.

Approach

- The deltopectoral approach is most commonly employed. It has the benefit of being the approach that would be used if future arthroplasty were needed.
- A deltoid split may be performed in select fractures.
- Outcomes of these two approaches have been shown to be comparable.[3]

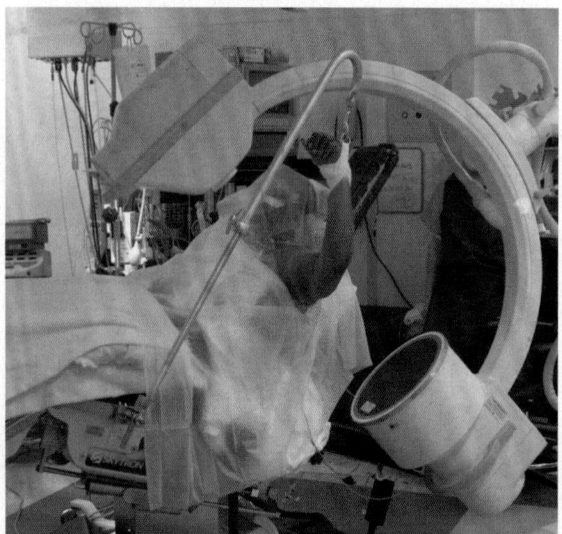

FIG 4 Position of the patient in the beach-chair position with fluoroscopic imaging. The C-arm intensifier should be posterior to allow for ideal visualization.

FIXATION OF ISOLATED TUBEROSITY FRACTURES

Exposure

- The patient is placed in the beach-chair position.
- A deltoid split or a deltopectoral approach may be used.
- Deltoid split: An incision is made from the anterolateral tip of the acromion extending laterally down the arm.
  - Alternatively, an incision can be made parallel to the lateral border of the acromion, as used in open rotator cuff repair.
- Skin flaps are raised.
- The deltoid is split in line with its fibers, and the anterior portion of the deltoid may be detached from the acromion.
  - The deltoid fibers should not be split further than 5 cm below the acromion to prevent damage to the axillary nerve. A suture at the distal aspect of the split can help prevent inadvertent extension.
- As with all open procedures described in this chapter, the fracture should be cleaned of hematoma and any callous to facilitate reduction.

Reduction and Fixation

- The greater tuberosity usually is displaced posteriorly and superiorly. Abducting and externally rotating the shoulder will take tension off the posterosuperior rotator cuff, allowing the greater tuberosity fragment to be more easily reduced.
  - If the fragment is difficult to access, a single-prong skin hook can be used to pull it into the field.
  - Traction sutures in the rotator cuff may prove valuable in obtaining reduction.
  - Provisional fixation can then be obtained with Kirschner wires (K-wires) **(TECH FIG 1A,B)**.

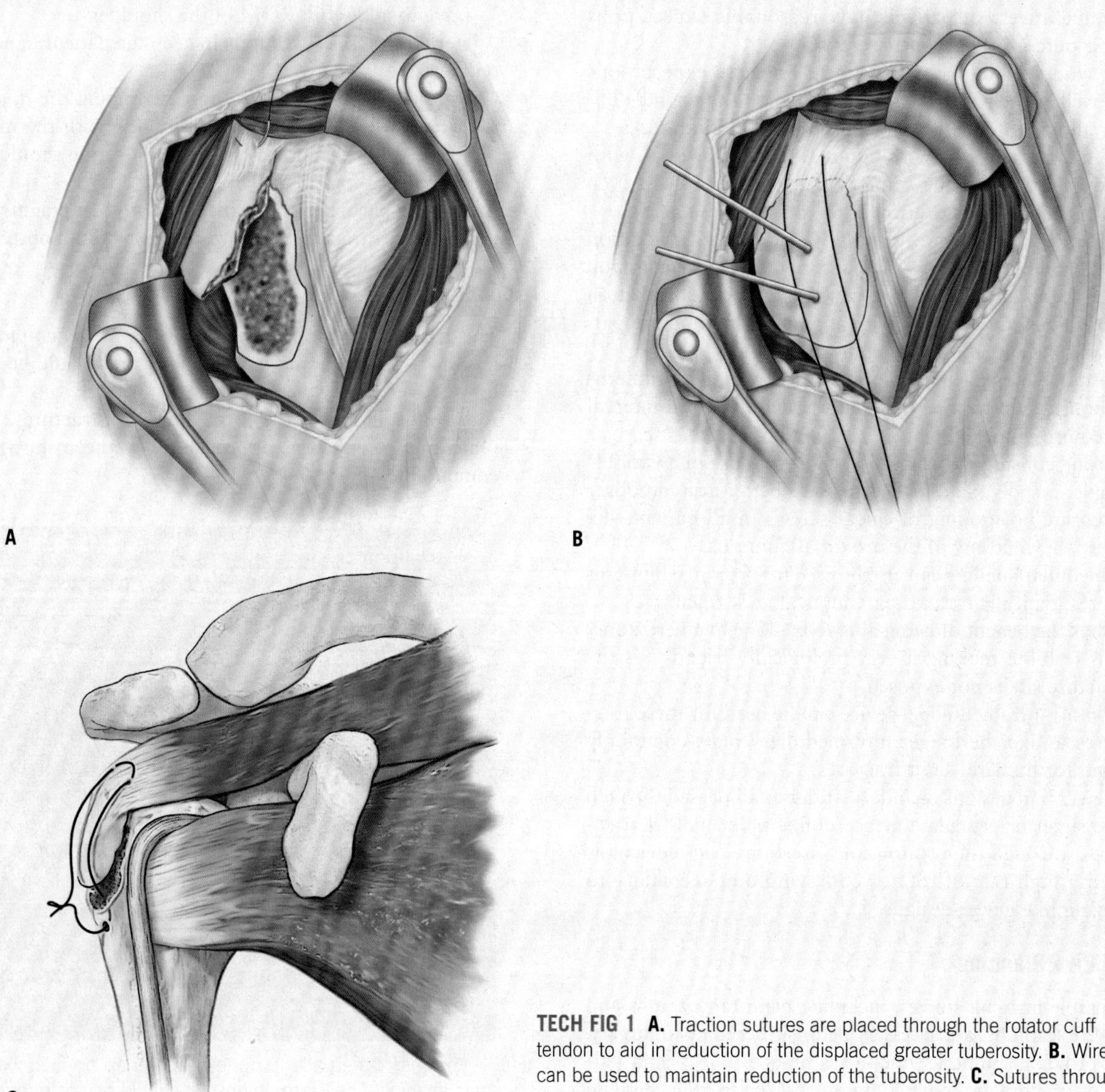

TECH FIG 1 **A.** Traction sutures are placed through the rotator cuff tendon to aid in reduction of the displaced greater tuberosity. **B.** Wires can be used to maintain reduction of the tuberosity. **C.** Sutures through drill holes.

- The most common mistake is to over reduce the fragment distally but under reduce anteriorly, leaving the fragment in a position distal and posterior to the donor site.
- Suture fixation of the greater tuberosity back to the humerus likely provides better fixation than screws in most patients secondary to either comminution or poor bone quality.
  - No. 5 suture is passed through the bone–tendon junction on the superficial surface (it is unnecessary for the suture to exit deep to the fragment and come out through the fracture).
  - These sutures can be fixed either in transosseous fashion through drill holes anterior and distal to the fracture bed **(TECH FIG 1C)** or can be tied around a 3.5-mm bicortical screw with a washer placed anterior and distal to the fracture (exiting inferior to the humeral head at the calcar area) used as a post.
  - K-wires should be used to hold the reduction anatomically and kept in place while the sutures are tied. This prevents overreduction with inadvertent tightening of the rotator cuff and posterosuperior joint capsule.
  - If the fracture was a result of a dislocation, the subscapularis should be palpated or visualized to assure it is not torn.
- If the anterior deltoid was detached during the approach, it must be repaired back to the acromion using transosseous, nonabsorbable sutures. These can pass through the acromion easily.

OPEN REDUCTION AND INTERNAL FIXATION USING LOCKED PLATING

Exposure

- With the patient in the beach-chair position, an incision is made starting from above the coracoid process and extending distally as needed along the deltopectoral groove **(TECH FIG 2A)**.
- The plane between the deltoid and pectoralis major is developed, mobilizing the cephalic vein.
  - Cobb elevators or finger dissection can be used to develop this plane, making it easier for the surgeon to identify and ligate branches of the cephalic vein **(TECH FIG 2B,C)**.
- The underlying clavipectoral fascia is identified and incised laterally to the conjoined tendon.
  - The conjoined tendon is carefully retracted medially with the pectoralis major while the deltoid is retracted laterally.

Reduction

- The fracture and rotator cuff are now visible. With fractures involving displaced tuberosities, we recommend obtaining control of the tuberosities with sutures placed at the bone–tendon interface **(TECH FIG 3A)**.
- Heavy sutures may be placed through the insertions of the cuff tendons and later used as supplemental fixation if necessary.
  - K-wires can be used to hold the greater tuberosity reduced to the humeral head as well. These should be placed at the proximal aspect of the tuberosity as to not interfere with the plate placement.
  - For fractures with minimally displaced tuberosities, sutures may not be needed before a reduction maneuver.
- Radiolucent Brown deltoid retractors and blunt Hohmann and Kobel blades can greatly aid in assessing reduction fluoroscopically while maintaining exposure.
- A Cobb elevator placed in the fracture site will aid in reducing the fracture **(TECH FIG 3B)**.

Plate Placement

- The plate should be placed lateral to the biceps tendon so as not to disrupt the blood supply to the humeral head (arcuate artery) **(TECH FIG 4A)**.
  - It should be approximately 10 to 15 mm distal to the top of the greater tuberosity to prevent impingement.

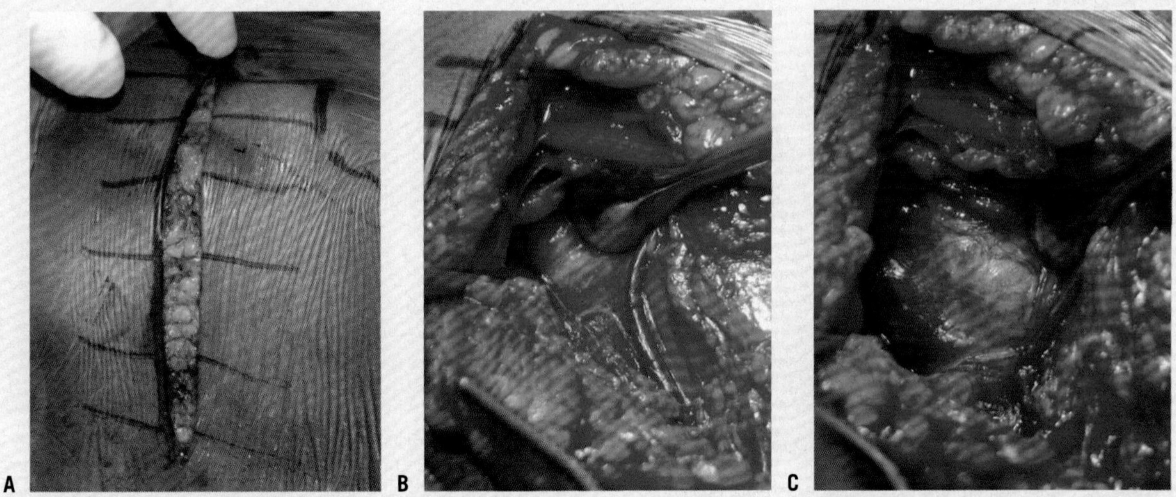

TECH FIG 2 A. The incision is made extending from the coracoid process distally along the deltopectoral groove. **B.** Identifying the interval between the deltoid and pectoralis major. **C.** Using two Cobb elevators to develop the interval, bringing the cephalic vein laterally.

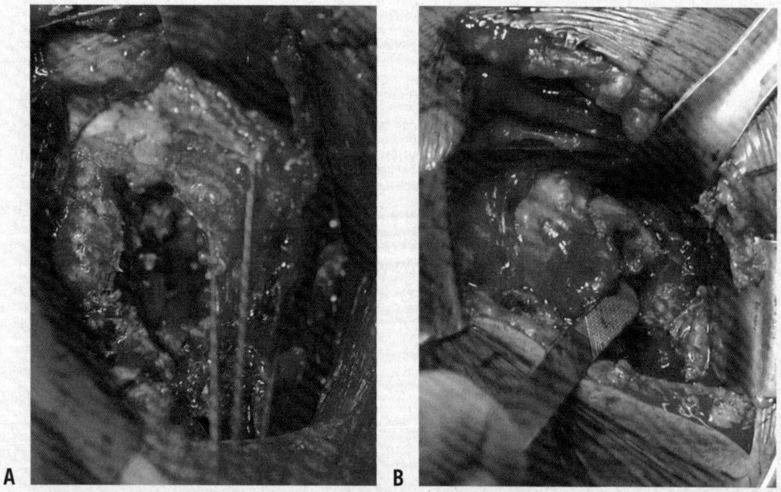

TECH FIG 3 A. Traction sutures through the tendinous attachments of the rotator cuff may be helpful in correcting varus deformity. **B.** Reducing the fracture by elevating the proximal fragment.

- If a nonvariable angled plate is used, the position of the plate will depend on the ability to get calcar screws within the inferior 25% of the humeral head.[19]
- It may be necessary to release a small portion of the anterior deltoid insertion before placing the plate, especially if a longer plate is used.
- Sutures can be preloaded through the plate prior to fixation **(TECH FIG 4B)**.

Provisional Plate Fixation

- Fluoroscopy should be used to confirm the reduction and plate placement, especially in regard to plate height, which is specific to each particular plate.
  - A plate positioned too high or a fracture fixed in varus may result in the plate impinging on the undersurface of the acromion.
- K-wires can be used to temporarily maintain fixation proximally and distally **(TECH FIG 5)**.
  - Alternatively, multiple guidewires can be placed into drill sleeves.
- Confirm plate location again, both proximally and distally, before placing screws.

Screw Placement

- Locking screws usually are placed proximally into the head first, and multiple configurations of screws are possible.
- After the plate is fixed to the head with anatomic neck–shaft angle, sagittal alignment should be confirmed and often the plate can then be used as a reduction aid with a nonlocked screw used into the shaft and tightened until the calcar is restored anatomically, bringing the shaft lateral, as it is often displaced medial as a result of the pectoralis major **(TECH FIG 6A,B)**.
  - Also, a bolster can be placed into the axilla to help lateralize the shaft and counter act deforming forces, especially in more obese patients.
- Once the head is secured to the shaft, distal screws can be placed.
  - The placement of a superiorly directed inferomedial screw to the calcar has been shown to maintain reduction and decrease the risk of postoperative varus collapse.[7,19]
- If there is calcar comminution, a fibular strut can be very helpful to restore alignment.[22] If a fibular allograft is used, it should be kept short (<3 cm) and should not pass the proximal shaft screw.
  - The graft should also be shaped to better recreate the calcar and reduce the overall allograft tissue required **(TECH FIG 6C)**.

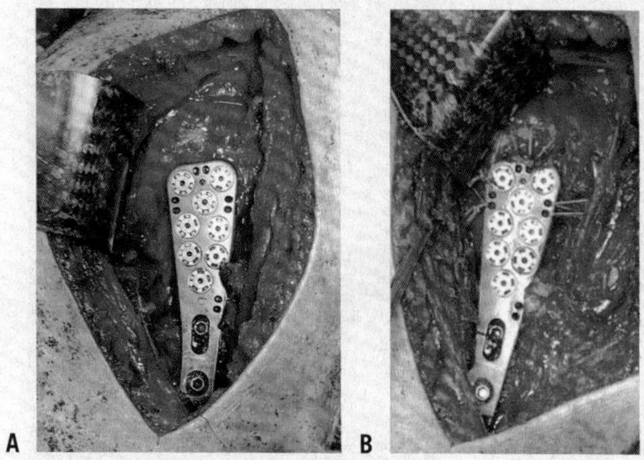

TECH FIG 4 A. Final position of proximal humerus plate posterior to the bicipital groove in the right shoulder. **B.** Heavy nonabsorbable suture passed through the rotator cuff and the plate.

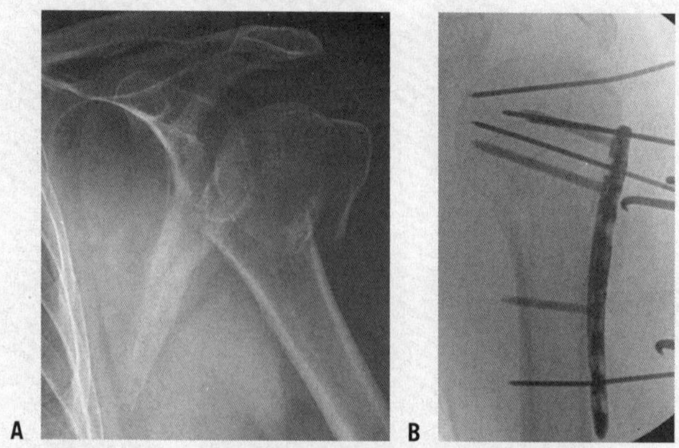

TECH FIG 5 A. AP x-ray of the left shoulder shows a three-part proximal humerus fracture with displaced greater tuberosity and surgical neck. **B.** Intraoperative fluoroscopy showing accurate plate placement at least 1 cm distal to the greater tuberosity with provisional K-wires used to hold reduction while polyaxial locking screws are applied.

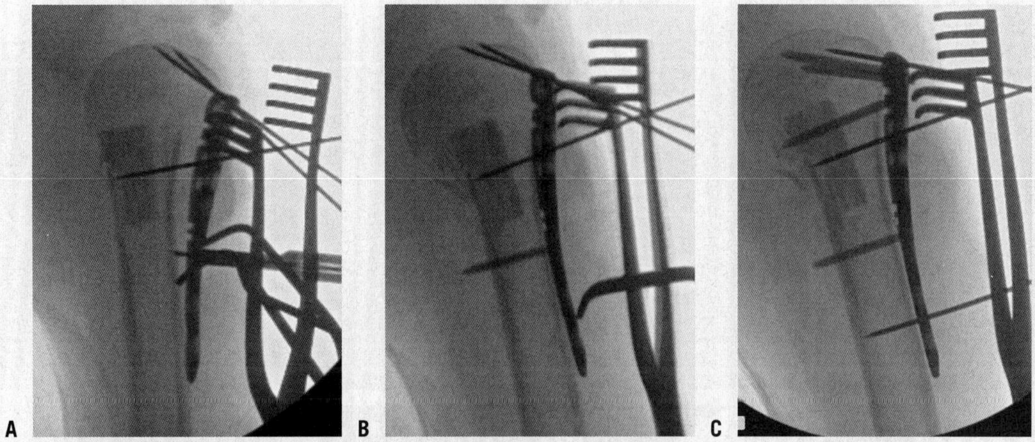

TECH FIG 6 A. Intraoperative fluoroscopic image showing fixation of the plate to the humeral head portion (the plate was purposefully placed more superior than normal secondary to fracture morphology). **B.** A nonlocked screw is placed into the shaft and used to reduce the shaft to the plate and restore the anatomic relationship of the head and shaft and recreate the calcar. **C.** Fluoroscopic image showing screw placement proximal and distal. Note the small contoured fibular graft used to recreate the medial calcar bone.

Completion

- Final plate placement should be confirmed fluoroscopically and the lengths of all screws closely assessed by taking the shoulder through multiple planes of motion with live fluoroscopy **(TECH FIG 7A,B)**.
- Sutures placed through the cuff tendons also are secured to the plate, shaft, or other tuberosity.
- If the biceps is damaged, it can be tenodesed to the pectoralis major tendon, although this is rarely required and care should be taken to avoid dissection about the bicipital groove and transverse humeral ligament, as blood supply to the head may be injured.
- In many cases, a void is left within the humeral head after impaction is reversed. This can be filled with cancellous bone allograft or synthetic bone graft substitute or cement.[4]
- In the case of four-part fractures, a separate anterior to posterior screw can be placed outside the plate to secure the lesser tuberosity, along with heavy sutures through the subscapularis passed through the plate **(TECH FIG 7C)**.

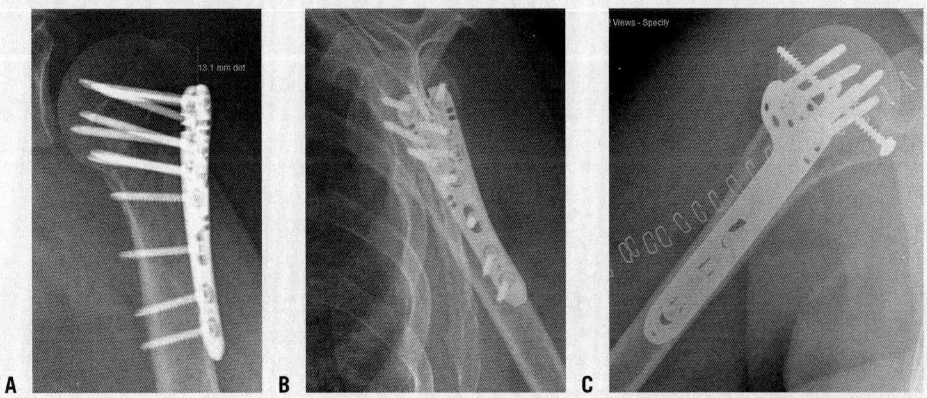

TECH FIG 7 A,B. Final radiographs showing polyaxial locking plate fixation with anatomic reduction of the patient in **TECH FIGS 4** and **5**. **C.** Example of supplemental fixation in the lesser tuberosity from anterior to posterior for a four-part proximal humerus fracture in a different patient.

INTRAMEDULLARY NAILING

- The patient is placed in beach-chair position similar to the aforementioned surgical techniques, with the C-arm placed as previously described.
- The nail may be used as a reduction aid, or the reduction may be obtained prior to nail insertion.
- Most two-part fractures deform into a combination of varus and apex anterior angulation, with variable amounts of shaft displacement anteriorly and/or medially **(TECH FIG 8A)**.
- Reduction can often be obtained with a posterolaterally directed force on the upper arm. A bolster in the axilla is often helpful to lateralize the shaft.
- If the fracture is unstable, the reduction can be held with percutaneous K-wires **(TECH FIG 8B,C)**.

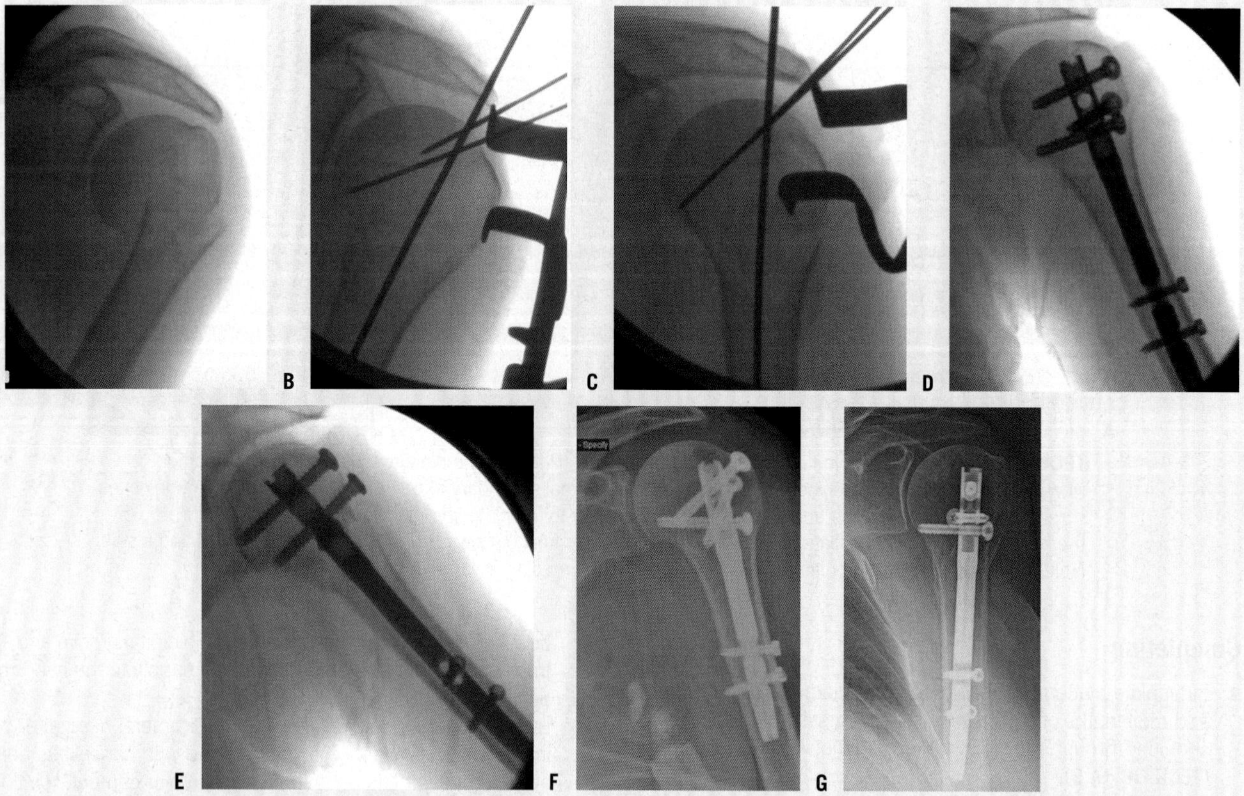

TECH FIG 8 A. Intraoperative fluoroscopic image of a varus displaced surgical neck fracture. **B,C.** With closed reduction techniques, the alignment was improved. The entry K-wire is placed at the superior articular surface in line with the humeral shaft, medial to the rotator cuff insertion. Smaller K-wires have been placed for manipulation of the proximal fragment. **D,E.** Fluoroscopic AP and lateral views with appropriate position of the intramedullary nail 5 mm deep to the articular surface with tuberosity-specific interlocking screws. **F.** Postoperative AP radiograph showing anatomic alignment. **G.** Final radiograph showing healed fracture.

- The incision is only 2 to 3 cm long and over the anterior acromioclavicular joint and anterior deltoid attachment.
  - The deltoid is split in line with fibers and the bursa entered.
  - A small retractor is placed, and a small split in the rotator cuff at the muscle tendon junction is created.
- The start point is obtained at the top of the articular surface and approximately just posterior to the biceps tendon to align with the center of the humeral canal
  - Remember that the center of the humeral head is medial and posterior relative to the center of the canal.
  - The arm needs to be extended and adducted in order to obtain the sufficient starting location. The manufacturers awl can help with controlling the alignment of the head portion.
  - K-wires may also be used in joystick fashion into the head to help control.
  - In more subacute fractures, it may be necessary to make a very small incision over the fracture so a Freer elevator can be inserted into the fracture line to aid in reduction. Often this requires the Freer elevator to be aimed at the posteromedial head and used as a lever to restore alignment.
- Once the guidewire is placed, the opening reamer or awl is used in line with the guidewire.
- The nail is then inserted.
  - Most proximal humerus nails have a guide arm to align the various proximal and distal locking screws so that percutaneous technique can be used to insert these screws.
- The nail is advanced until the proximal tip of the nail seats under the articular surface, generally about 5 mm **(TECH FIG 8D,E)**.
  - Alternatively, the nail can be sunk about 10 mm deep and fixed distally. It can then be backslapped to compress at the surgical neck.
- Locking screws can be inserted proximally as desired into the calcar, greater tuberosity, and lesser tuberosity to achieve proximal stability.
- Nonlocking distal shaft screws are inserted to achieve distal fixation in static or dynamic mode or both **(TECH FIG 8F,G)**.
- During closure, the rotator cuff is once again inspected and repaired if needed and the small deltoid split is repaired in a side-to-side fashion.

Pearls and Pitfalls

Indications	• Appropriate indications for ORIF of a proximal humerus fracture involve assessment of the patient, their demand level, as well as their ability to successfully participate in postoperative rehabilitation. • An understanding of the neurovascular anatomy as well as the deforming forces present in proximal humerus fractures is vital to treating these injuries effectively and understanding which fractures require operative treatment. • There are multiple methods for fracture fixation, we prefer intramedullary nails for the majority of two-part fractures and polyaxial locking plate fixation for three- and four-part fractures.
Exposure	• Avoid devascularizing fracture fragments by minimizing soft tissue of the pieces during exposure and reduction. • Deltoid splitting or deltopectoral approaches have shown equivalent outcomes, although a deltopectoral approach allows later utilization if arthroplasty is required.
Maintaining Fixation	• K-wires are useful for maintaining initial fixation. • Use of fibular allograft can aid in reduction and fixation. Cancellous allograft or bone void filler may also be considered.
Poor Bone Quality	• Screw placement into the inferior–medial head and calcar region is paramount. • Allograft augmentation • Suture augmentation of greater and lesser tuberosity fixation
Superior Impingement	• Avoid placing the locking plate too high on greater tuberosity. This can be avoided with use of a polyaxial plate, allowing more distal placement, even on a smaller patient, while still allowing accurate calcar screw placement.
Screw Placement and Penetration	• Check the lengths of screws in multiple planes to avoid intraoperative screw perforation of the humeral head. • If a fibular allograft is used, it should be kept short (<3 cm) and should not pass the proximal shaft screw. This is important in case later arthroplasty is required **(FIG 5)**.

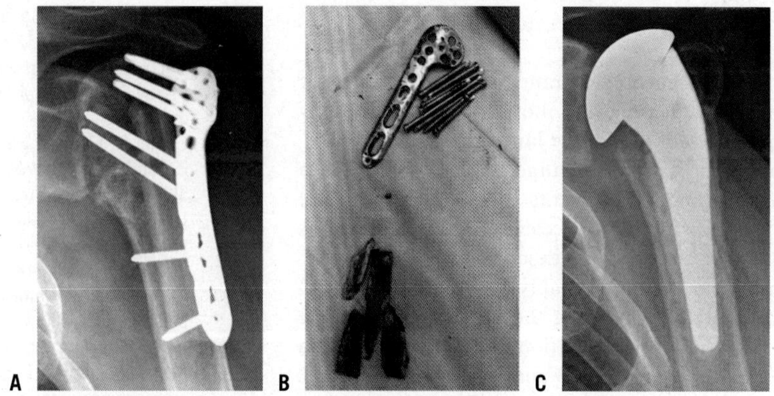

FIG 5 A. True AP radiograph of the left shoulder 18 months after ORIF of a left posterior fracture-dislocation. The fibular strut graft can be seen extending past the most distal screw to the level of the inferior plate. **B.** The fibular allograft tissue removed along with the plate and screws at reoperation show minimal incorporation of the graft after 18 months. **C.** Cemented hemiarthroplasty was required as a result of the damage to the medullary canal caused by removing the excessively long graft.

POSTOPERATIVE CARE

- Stable fixation must be obtained to allow for immediate passive ROM.
- Patients are placed in an abduction or neutral pillow sling to be worn at all times.
- Ideally, the fixation should allow physical therapy consisting of pendulum exercises, passive forward flexion, external rotation, adduction, and extension/internal rotation on the first postoperative day. These should be performed four times a day.
- Between 4 and 6 weeks after surgery, active motion is instituted.
- Formal strengthening with elastic bands is not started until 10 to 12 weeks after surgery, as long as the fracture is healed and motion is acceptable.
- If motion is limited and there is evidence of fracture healing, an intra-articular corticosteroid injection can be very helpful at the 10- to 12-week time point.
- As with nonoperative treatment, active and diligent participation in physical therapy is key to a successful outcome.
- In a recent study looking at fixation of two- and three-part fractures, the only patients with unsatisfactory outcomes were those who were noncompliant with physical therapy.[20]

OUTCOMES

- Flatow et al[6] had excellent or good results in 12 of 16 patients with fixation of greater tuberosity fractures displaced more than 1 cm. Forward elevation averaged 170 degrees, and external rotation averaged 63 degrees.
- Early ORIF with a laterally placed T-plate failed to yield consistently good results, especially for four-part fractures.[14] Other early osteosynthesis techniques include the cloverleaf and the blade plate, but the current trend is toward anatomic locked plating technology.
  - Use of such locking plates shows promise, although this technique is not without complications.
- A meta-analysis by Li et al[15] comparing proximal humeral nailing to plating in 1384 patients found that the nail was superior with regard to incision length, operative time, blood loss, and fracture healing time, with no difference in constant score or postoperative complications. Further prospective studies are needed to determine which method may be truly superior.
- The Proximal Fracture of the Humerus Evaluation by Randomization (PROFHER) study found that there was no significant difference between surgical treatment versus nonsurgical treatment in patient-reported clinical outcomes over 2 years following fracture occurrence.[21]
  - However, most of the injuries in this study were two-part fractures, which may have not otherwise been indicated for surgery.
  - There was a low enrollment rate and no assessment of the quality of reduction, and most cases were done by low-volume surgeons at low-volume sites.
  - Furthermore, indications for surgery were variable, with a significant number of patients excluded early by the treating surgeon for meeting clear surgical indications without further discussion or description.
- Schnetzke et al[23] examined the quality of reduction for proximal humerus fractures involving the anatomic neck (type C according to the AO Foundation/Orthopaedic Trauma Association classification system) and found that anatomic reduction lead to significantly fewer complications than "acceptable" or malreduced fractures fixed with a locking plate.
  - Cranialization of the greater tuberosity of more than 5 mm, head–shaft displacement of more than 5 mm, and valgus head–shaft alignment all increased the relative risk for inferior clinical outcome by two- to threefold.
  - Less than 50% of cases result in anatomic or acceptable reductions, highlighting the difficulty of this technically demanding procedure.

COMPLICATIONS

- Infection
- Stiffness/adhesive capsulitis
- Nonunion
- Malunion
- Avascular necrosis
- Nerve injury
- Impingement secondary to fixation or residual tuberosity displacement
- Screw perforation of the humeral head (due to incorrect length placed at the time of surgery, head settling, or following varus collapse)[12]
- Failure of fixation, including varus malposition and plate fracture following anatomic plating of proximal humerus fractures[5]

REFERENCES

1. Bastian JD, Hertel R. Initial post-fracture humeral head ischemia does not predict development of necrosis. J Shoulder Elbow Surg 2008;17(1):2–8.
2. Beks RB, Ochen Y, Frima H, et al. Operative versus nonoperative treatment of proximal humeral fractures: a systematic review, meta-analysis, and comparison of observational studies and randomized controlled trials. J Shoulder Elbow Surg 2018;27(8): 1526–1534.
3. Buecking B, Mohr J, Bockmann B, et al. Deltoid-split or deltopectoral approaches for the treatment of displaced proximal humeral fractures? Clin Orthop Relat Res 2014;472(5):1576–1585.
4. Euler SA, Kralinger FS, Hengg C, et al. Allograft augmentation in proximal humerus fractures. Oper Orthop Traumatol 2016;28(3):153–163.
5. Fankhauser F, Boldin C, Schippinger G, et al. A new locking plate for unstable fractures of the proximal humerus. Clin Orthop Relat Res 2005;(430):176–181.
6. Flatow EL, Cuomo F, Maday MG, et al. Open reduction and internal fixation of two-part displaced fractures of the greater tuberosity of the proximal part of the humerus. J Bone Joint Surg Am 1991;73(8): 1213–1218.
7. Gardner MJ, Weil Y, Barker JU, et al. The importance of medial support in locked plating of proximal humerus fractures. J Orthop Trauma 2007;21(3):185–191.
8. Han RJ, Sing DC, Feeley BT, et al. Proximal humerus fragility fractures: recent trends in nonoperative and operative treatment in the Medicare population. J Shoulder Elbow Surg 2016;25(2): 256–261.
9. Hertel R, Hempfing A, Stiehler M, et al. Predictors of humeral head ischemia after intracapsular fracture of the proximal humerus. J Shoulder Elbow Surg 2004;13(4):427–433.
10. Hettrich CM, Boraiah S, Dyke JP, et al. Quantitative assessment of the vascularity of the proximal part of the humerus. J Bone Joint Surg Am 2010;92(4):943–948.
11. Hofman M, Grommes J, Krombach GA, et al. Vascular injury accompanying displaced proximal humeral fractures: two cases and a review of the literature. Emerg Med Int 2011;2011:742870.
12. Konrad G, Bayer J, Hepp P, et al. Open reduction and internal fixation of proximal humeral fractures with use of the locking proximal humerus plate. Surgical technique. J Bone Joint Surg Am 2010;92(suppl 1, pt 1):85–95.
13. Koval KJ, Gallagher MA, Marsicano JG, et al. Functional outcome after minimally displaced fractures of the proximal part of the humerus. J Bone Joint Surg Am 1997;79(2):203–207.
14. Kristiansen B, Christensen SW. Plate fixation of proximal humeral fractures. Acta Orthop Scand 1986;57(4):320–323.
15. Li M, Wang Y, Zhang Y, et al. Intramedullary nail versus locking plate for treatment of proximal humeral fractures: a meta-analysis based on 1384 individuals. J Int Med Res 2018;46(11):4363–4376.
16. Matsushigue T, Pagliaro Franco V, Pierami R, et al. Do computed tomography and its 3D reconstruction increase the reproducibility of classifications of fractures of the proximal extremity of the humerus? Rev Bras Ortop 2014;49(2):174–177.
17. McDonald E, Kwiat D, Kandemir U. Geometry of proximal humerus locking plates. J Orthop Trauma 2015;29(11):e425–e430.
18. McKoy BE, Bensen CV, Hartsock LA. Fractures about the shoulder: conservative management. Orthop Clin North Am 2000;31: 205–216.
19. Padegimas EM, Zmistowski B, Lawrence C, et al. Defining optimal calcar screw positioning in proximal humerus fracture fixation. J Shoulder Elbow Surg 2017;26(11):1931–1937.
20. Park MC, Murthi AM, Roth NS, et al. Two-part and three-part fractures of the proximal humerus treated with suture fixation. J Orthop Trauma 2003;17(5):319–325.

21. Rangan A, Handoll H, Brealey S, et al. Surgical vs nonsurgical treatment of adults with displaced fractures of the proximal humerus: the PROFHER randomized clinical trial. JAMA 2015;313(10):1037–1047.
22. Saltzman BM, Erickson BJ, Harris JD, et al. Fibular strut graft augmentation for open reduction and internal fixation of proximal humerus fractures: a systematic review and the authors' preferred surgical technique. Orthop J Sports Med 2016;4(7):2325967116656829.
23. Schnetzke M, Bockmeyer J, Porschke F, et al. Quality of reduction influences outcome after locked-plate fixation of proximal humeral type-C fractures. J Bone Joint Surg Am 2016;98(21):1777–1785.
24. Verdano MA, Pellegrini A, Schiavi P, et al. Humeral shaft fractures treated with antegrade intramedullary nailing: what are the consequences for the rotator cuff? Int Orthop 2013;37(10):2001–2007.
25. Visser CP, Coene LN, Brand R, et al. Nerve lesions in proximal humeral fractures. J Shoulder Elbow Surg 2001;10(5):421–427.

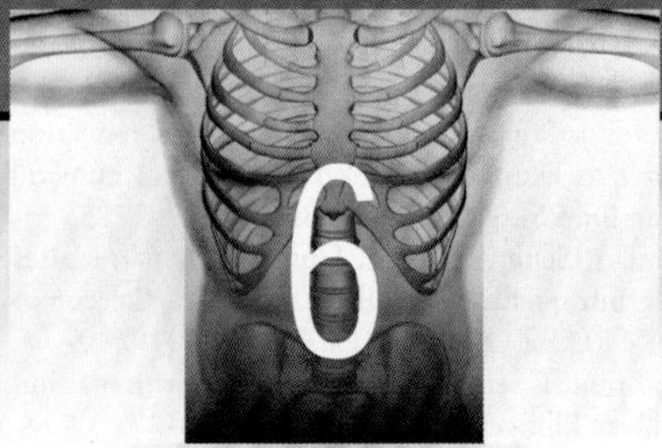

CHAPTER 6

Intramedullary Fixation of Proximal Humerus Fractures

James Krieg

DEFINITION

- Fractures of the proximal humerus can be two-, three-, or four-part according to the Neer modification of the Codman classification **(FIG 1)**.
- Fifty percent to 80% of proximal humerus fractures are nondisplaced or minimally displaced and stable. A short period of immobilization in neutral rotation to avoid fracture malunion followed by early mobilization is usually sufficient to treat fractures and can result in satisfactory outcomes.
- Twenty percent to 50% of patients with displaced, unstable two-, three-, or four-part proximal humerus fractures with a vascularized, attached head fragment may benefit from operative management with reduction and internal fixation.
- There is no clear consensus on surgical indications, with similar long-term data with closed or surgical treatment, in general. What is not known is the short-to-intermediate differences in function and the specific injury and patient populations that benefit from surgery.
- Extensive surgical dissection can further compromise bone healing potential, lead to increased scar tissue formation, and lead to impaired soft tissue function.
- Fracture pattern and comminution, accuracy of reduction, implant placement, and osteopenia are the commonly cited reasons for failure of internal fixation constructs.
- Results of fixation with intramedullary (IM) nails in two- and some three-part fractures have been equivalent in several series to more traditional plate and screw constructs.
- Newer designs of IM nails facilitate stable fixation of the head to the shaft of the humerus while maximizing biomechanical fixation of the tuberosities.
- Improved surgical techniques may facilitate more accurate reduction, improved biomechanical fixation, while maintaining a smaller surgical footprint.

ANATOMY

Osteology

- The proximal humerus includes the humeral head, the lesser tuberosity (LT), the greater tuberosity (GT), and the proximal humeral metaphysis.
- The anatomic relationships between the tuberosities, head, and shaft determine the functionality of the shoulder.
- The humeral head is slightly medial (3 mm) and posterior (7 mm) in relation to the humeral shaft and is retroverted approximately 30 degrees (ranges from 20 to 60) **(FIG 2)**. It functions as a cam.
- The bicipital groove separates the lesser and greater tuberosities. The head is slightly higher than the tuberosities, where the rotator cuff tendons attach.
- The density of bone within the head is greatest in the subchondral zone. It is denser in the superior, posterior part of the head than in lateral parts, including the GT. This difference increases with age, and is more significant in women, with the lateral head and GT losing bone mass quicker.
- The bicipital groove is made of dense bone. As a result, most fractures of the GT occur posterior to the groove. In four-part fractures, the LT fragment often includes the bicipital groove.
- The sulcus at the base of the GT is roughly centered on a tangent to the lateral cortical wall of the shaft.
- The humeral head is largely situated anterior to the acromion, facilitating access to nail entry point **(FIG 3)**.

Vascular Supply of the Proximal Humerus

- The anterior and posterior humeral circumflex arteries are branches of the axillary artery.
  - The arcuate artery, the terminal vessel of the ascending branch of the anterior humeral circumflex artery, supplies much of the humeral head.
    - Avascularity of the humeral head can occur if this vessel is disrupted during a fracture of the anatomic neck or damaged during subsequent surgery.
  - The posterior circumflex artery becomes more important in patients with proximal humerus fractures.
    - It may be the primary source of blood supply to the fractured head, so care should be taken to prevent additional devascularization.
- Traumatic and iatrogenic vascular insult may lead to devascularization of the fracture fragments, resulting in delayed union, nonunion, and avascular necrosis (AVN). Traumatic injury cannot be prevented; well-planned minimally invasive procedures should reduce the risk of further damage.
- The presence of an extra-articular medial spike of bone that is at least 8 mm on the head fragment is a good prognostic indicator of head fragment blood flow.
- There is not a direct correlation between compromised blood flow to the head fragment, eventual AVN, or later collapse due to AVN. However, care should be taken to minimize the vascular insult of surgery.

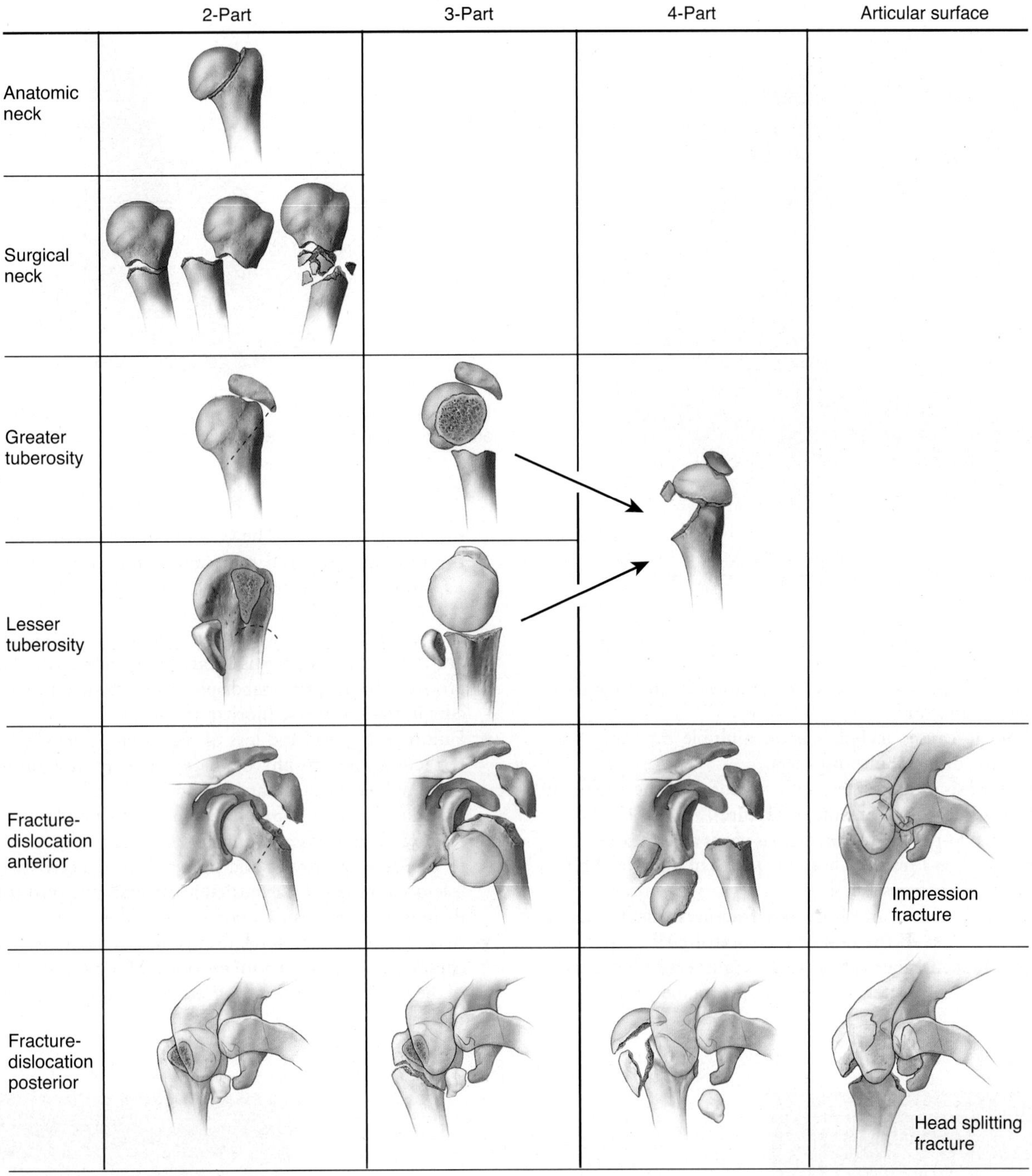

FIG 1 Classification of shoulder fractures according to Neer.

Innervation

- The brachial plexus is at risk in patients with upper extremity injury, and thorough neurologic evaluation is mandatory.
- The axillary nerve courses through the quadrilateral space, where it is at risk during fracture dislocation.
- The axillary nerve courses along the undersurface of the deltoid muscle, 6.5 cm distal to the tip of the acromion. The nerve is at risk of iatrogenic injury from dissection in this area, in particular when placing interlock bolts.

PATHOGENESIS

- A direct blow to lateral upper arm will often result in a relatively high-energy fracture of the proximal humerus. This mechanism is common in younger patients.
- Indirect trauma, usually the result of a fall on an outstretched arm, is most common mechanism in elderly.
  - Fracture pattern and displacement determined by position of the arm and body as well as the direction of the fall
- Violent muscle contractures, as in grand mal seizures and electric shock, are associated with posterior dislocation- and

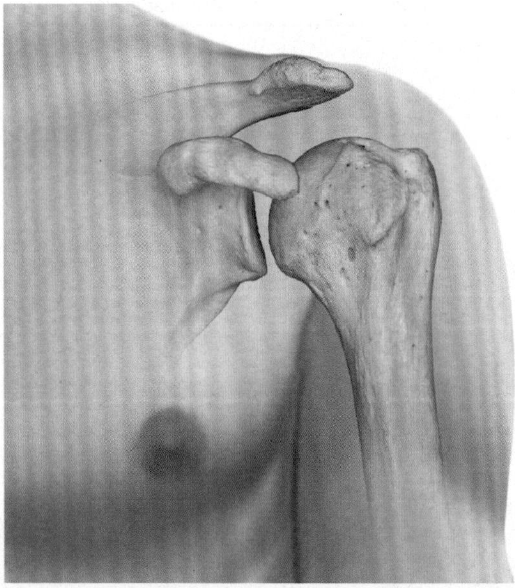

FIG 2 Normal shoulder anatomy. The head is slightly higher than the tuberosities, slightly medial and posterior to the humeral shaft, and retroverted 30 degrees. (Copyright J. Dean Cole, MD.)

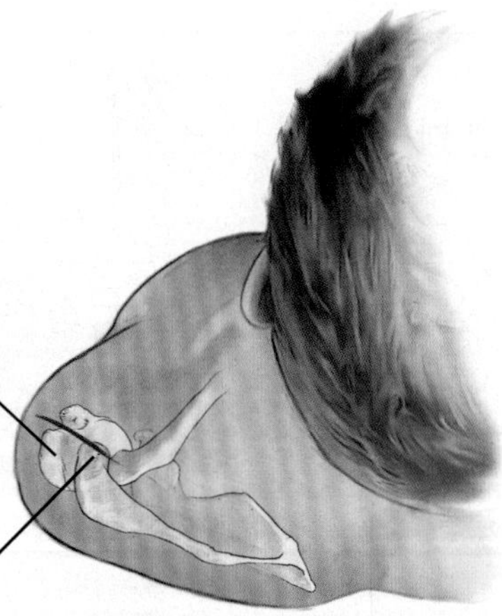

FIG 3 The humeral head is anterior to the acromion, allowing direct access to a starting point centered over the canal.

impaction-type fractures due to overpowering internal rotators and adductors.

- Pathologic causes include tumor, multiple myeloma, and metastatic or metabolic disorders.
- Osteoporosis is associated with fractures of the proximal humerus (more than any other fracture).
- In many two-part fractures, there is varus and apex anterior angulation, as a result of both the forces of injury and muscle deforming forces (**FIG 4**).
- In unstable three- and four-part fractures, displacement occurs because of the pull of the rotator cuff muscles on their attached tuberosities in the transverse plane, widening the gap created by the fracture plane posterior to the bicipital groove. The GT is pulled posteromedially by the infraspinatus and teres minor muscles, whereas the LT is pulled anteromedially by the subscapularis muscle (**FIG 5**).
- In four-part proximal humerus fractures, the fracture separating the tuberosities is located posterior to the bicipital groove, and the principal displacement of such fractures occurs in the transverse (horizontal) plane.
- Failure of fixation and loss of reduction of the GT leads to retraction and atrophy of the external rotator muscles of the shoulder (infraspinatus and teres minor).
  - Results in pseudoparalyzed and stiff shoulder for which surgical options are limited
- In contrast, posttraumatic humeral head necrosis is well tolerated if the GT has healed in an anatomic position, and there is no screw penetration or glenoid erosion.
- Accuracy of reduction relates to construct stability. This includes reduction of the tuberosities. Maintaining reduction of the tuberosities not only affects the long-term function of

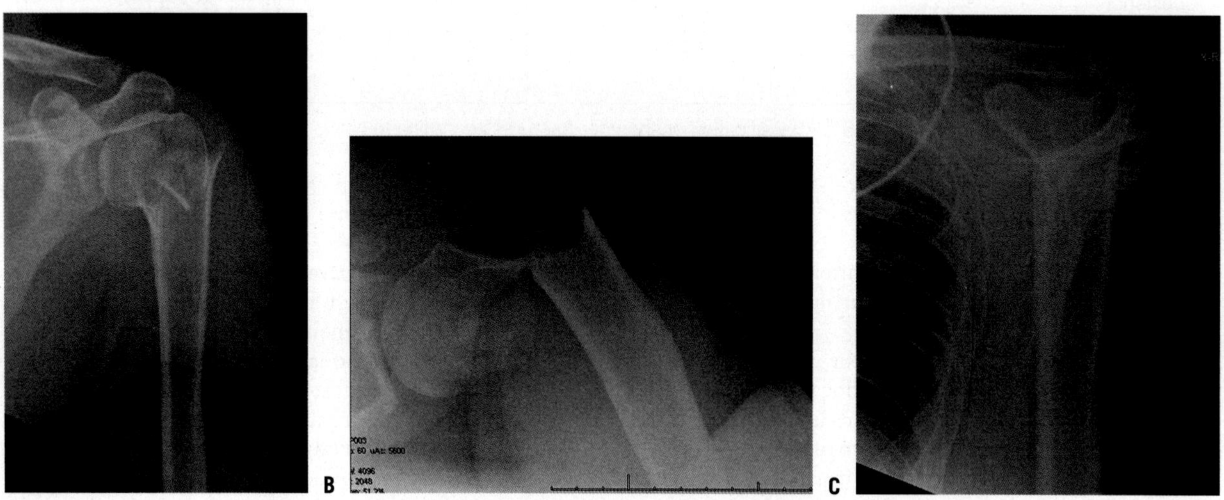

FIG 4 AP (**A**), axillary (**B**), and Y (**C**) views of a two-part surgical next fracture.

A 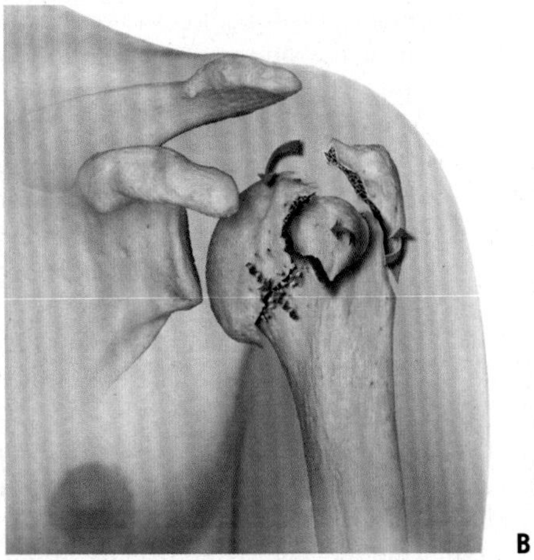 B 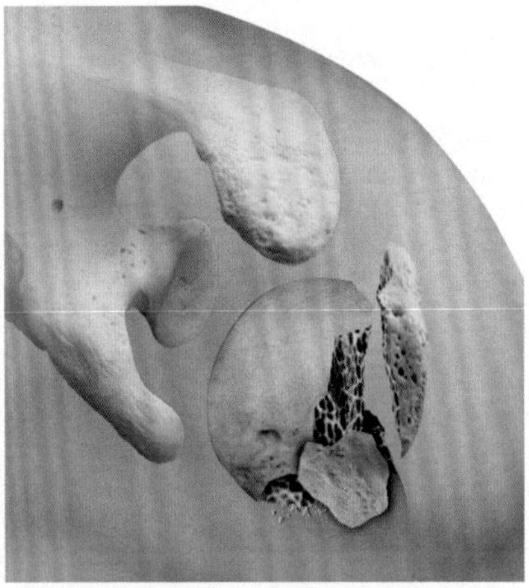

FIG 5 A. Three-part fractures. *Arrows* show typical displacement of fragments. The muscular attachments of the GT and LT will cause abduction, external rotation, and internal rotation, respectively. The head will follow whichever tuberosity is intact. **B.** In four-part fractures, the head often is in a neutrally rotated position. (Copyright J. Dean Cole, MD.)

the muscles attached to them but also relates to the ability to maintain the reduction of the head. The tuberosities support the head.

- IM nails have been designed specifically to optimize tuberosity fragment fixation and provide stable support for the humeral head, improving proximal humerus fixation in osteopenic bone. The design of these nails and these specific techniques have been developed to minimize the common complications of poor reduction and loss of fixation.

NATURAL HISTORY

- Epidemiology
  - 4% to 5% of all fractures
  - Increased incidence due to osteoporosis in elderly and some older middle-age persons (third most common fracture in elderly)
  - In persons older than 50 years of age, the female-to-male ratio is 4:1 (osteoporosis). Minor falls and trauma may cause comminuted fracture.
  - In patients younger than 50 years of age, violent trauma, contact sports, and falls from heights are responsible for fractures.
  - Surgical neck fracture is common.
- Consequences of injury
  - Nondisplaced fractures may heal without major consequences.
  - Acute, recurrent, or chronic dislocation
  - Rotator cuff tears
  - Neurovascular injury: axillary nerve, brachial plexus
  - AVN of the humeral head can result from disruption of the arcuate artery. The axillary artery also may be damaged but less commonly.
- Malunion
  - Malunion of the tuberosities causes poor shoulder function due to altered biomechanics.
  - Shortening may cause poor shoulder function due to changes in the length tension relationship of the deltoid and loss of the cam effect of the humeral head.
- Posttraumatic arthrosis
- Adhesive capsulitis
- Biceps tendinopathy
- Chronic pain

PATIENT HISTORY AND PHYSICAL FINDINGS

- Associated injuries
  - Rotator cuff tears
  - Dislocation
  - Brachial plexus, axillary, and radial and ulnar nerve injuries (5% to 30% of complex proximal humerus fractures)
  - Biceps tendon injury/entrapment
- Medical conditions: surgical risk assessment
- Social history: functional demands and limitations

IMAGING AND OTHER DIAGNOSTIC STUDIES

- Trauma series
  - True anteroposterior (AP) (Grashey/glenoid view)
  - Transscapular Y
  - Axillary
- Computed tomography scanning is very helpful to characterize the fracture fragments and aid in surgical planning.
- Magnetic resonance imaging has a role in determining the integrity of the rotator cuff in candidates for arthroplasty, if the history suggests preexisting cuff dysfunction.

SURGICAL MANAGEMENT

- Indications for IM nailing
  - Displaced or unstable two-part fractures
    - Bridge technique for comminuted fractures
    - Enhanced fixation in osteopenic bone
    - Segmental fractures involving neck and shaft of humerus
  - Can be used for three- and some four-part fractures
    - Technically more challenging; harder to maintain reduction during placement of implant versus plate and screw construct

- Prerequisites
  - Radiolucent table, image intensification, and experienced radiology technician
  - Be mindful of the learning curve.
    - Reduction maneuvers and nail entry are key steps.
    - Have contingency plans, including plate and screws and arthroplasty options.
- Relative contraindications: head-splitting, more complex three- and four-part fractures

Preoperative Planning

- The entire operation is dependent on fluoroscopic imaging. Radiolucent table and proper patient positioning are required.
- Multiple tools and tactics for reduction are essential (eg, joysticks, clamps, cuff sutures, elevators).

Positioning and Imaging

- Positioning on the table must allow for orthogonal views on C-arm. Ideally, this is done without moving the limb.
- Supine position allows for easy imaging, with a small bump under the side in order to allow for some shoulder extension. Extension allows easier access to the entry site, anterior to the acromion.
- The C-arm is positioned on the opposite side of the table and is brought in toward the surgeon. The unaffected arm must be tucked at the side, in order to allow the C-arm to reach the affected shoulder from the opposite side of the bed.
- The C-arm is rolled back from the vertical to obtain a true AP of the shoulder. The limb is held in the neutral position to get a standard view.
- A transscapular Y view can be obtained by rolling the C-arm "over the top" toward the surgeon, without moving the limb.
- Axillary view is obtained by tilting the C-arm sideways, the same direction that one would use to get an inlet view of the pelvis. A small amount of abduction may be necessary to obtain the image **(FIG 6)**.

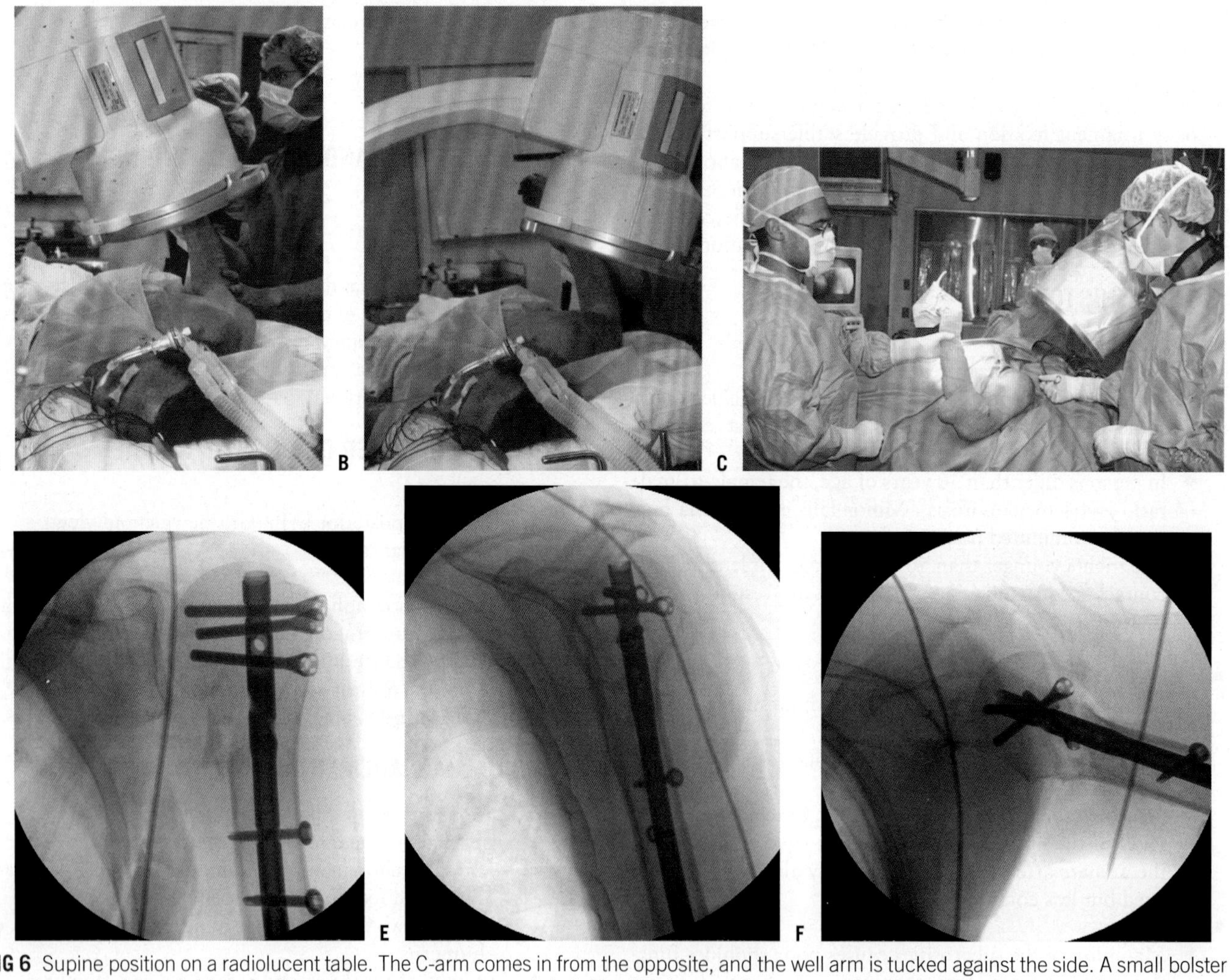

A B C D E F

FIG 6 Supine position on a radiolucent table. The C-arm comes in from the opposite, and the well arm is tucked against the side. A small bolster can elevate the injured side to facilitate some extension as needed. **A.** The AP view requires some rolling back of the C-arm, and the arm is held in neutral. For the Y view (**B**), the C-arm is rolled over the top, and for the axillary (**C**), it is tilted as an inlet view would be. **D–F.** Corresponding images allow for assessment of reduction and implant placement. Note that the image of the axillary view is inverted, and the anterior landmarks are seen at the bottom of the image.

Approach

- Three surgical approaches are possible depending on the fracture type and the surgeon's preference:
  - The percutaneous approach, in which the deltoid muscle and supraspinatus are bluntly split through a superior, 1-cm incision
  - The anterolateral transdeltoid approach, in which the deltoid is split at the junction of anterior and middle thirds
  - The deltopectoral approach
- The approach chosen should take into account the fracture pattern and access to the fragments in a way that facilitates reduction and placement of the implant.
- This chapter describes the anterolateral or transdeltoid approach. Advantages of this approach include direct access to both the head and GT fragments as well as the entry point for nail insertion.
- Although the deltopectoral approach allows for excellent visualization of most of the proximal humerus, the ability to see and control a posteriorly displaced GT fragment is limited. In addition, it can be difficult to retract the deltoid enough to easily access the nail entry point in the humeral head.
- Percutaneous techniques require alternative methods of reduction, which can be challenging.
- IM nailing can put the axillary nerve at risk when interlocking if it is not directly identified and protected.

ANTEROLATERAL TRANSDELTOID APPROACH

Exposure

- An incision is marked out from the anterolateral edge of the acromion.
  - Often, a fluoroscopic view with guidewire held over the skin can help identify the correct placement for the incision. It tends to be more anterior than one might think when looking at the arm **(TECH FIG 1A)**.
  - The acromion may be difficult to palpate, especially with the swelling of the injury. Palpating the scapular spine and tracing it anteriorly to the acromion may help.
  - A mark is made on the incision, 6.5 cm from the tip of the acromion. This will help identify the axillary nerve as it crosses under the deltoid.
- A split is made between the anterior and middle deltoid fibers with cautery and blunt scissor dissection. Often, a tendinous raphe is seen in this internervous interval. As the deltoid is split, the subdeltoid bursa is identified **(TECH FIG 1B,C)**.
- The bursa must be incised. The distal end of the bursa is opened, allowing for careful palpation along the underneath surface of the deltoid.
  - This allows for direct identification of the axillary nerve, as it can easily be discerned from the muscle itself by feel. The nerve almost always crosses at the 6.5-cm mark and must be identified to avoid iatrogenic damage when placing interlock screws.
  - Self-retaining retractors help to facilitate the exposure.
- The bursa is excised to expose the GT, LT, and head fracture fragments. Great care is taken to stay below the deltoid fascia to avoid injury to any branches of the axillary nerve.

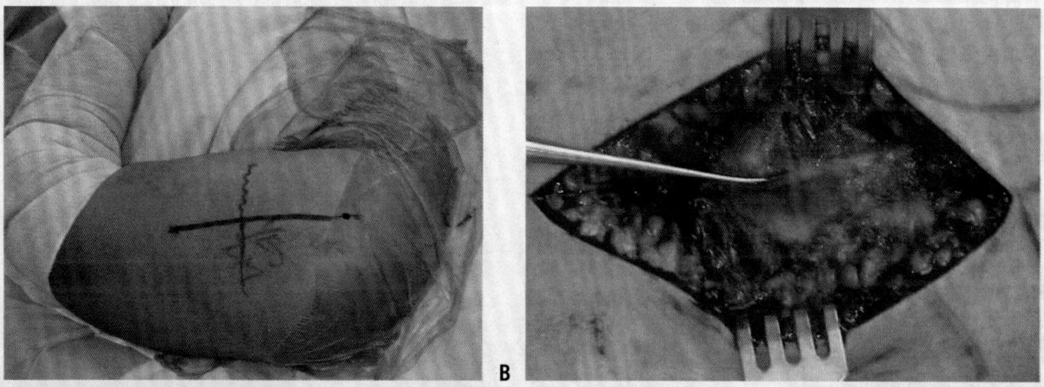
A B

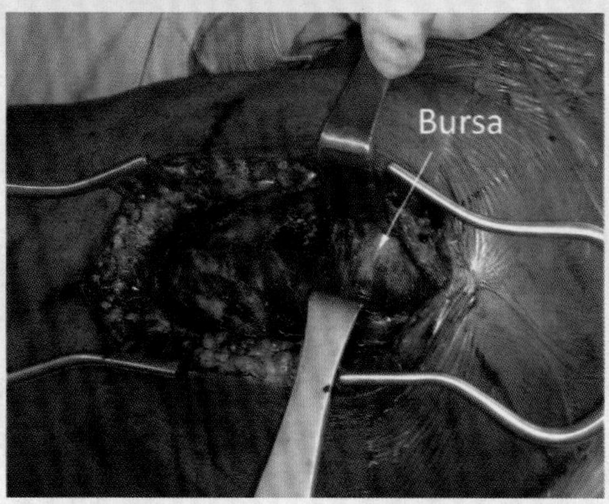

C

TECH FIG 1 **A.** The incision is drawn out from the anterior edge of the acromion. A mark is made 6.5 cm distal to the tip of the acromion to mark the anticipated course of the axillary nerve. The raphe in the deltoid is identified (**B**) and split (**C**). The bursa is exposed (*arrow*) and will be excised.

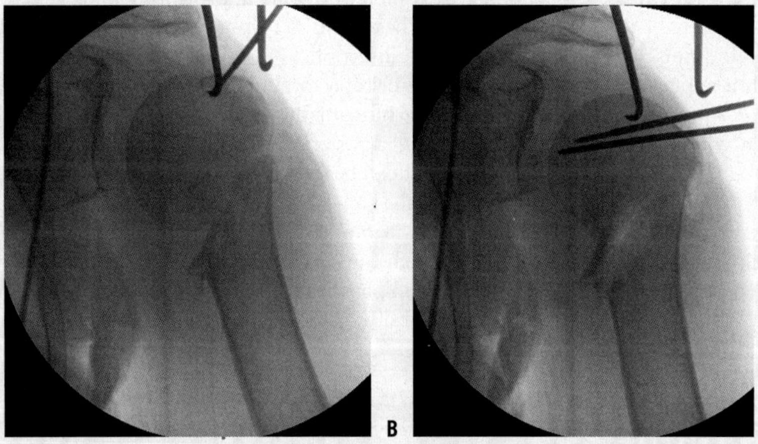

A B

TECH FIG 2 The reduction is performed by placing the Schanz screws in the head (**A**), avoiding the path of the nail and manipulating the head to neutral (**B**).

Fracture Reduction

- The fracture fragments are identified, and control of the head fragment is obtained with one or two terminally threaded 2.5-mm Schanz screws (often found in small external fixator set) **(TECH FIG 2A,B)**.
  - Placement should be in the anterior and/or posterior regions of the head to avoid the path of the nail.
- Reduction is performed by manipulating the head to neutral position with the Schanz screw and then manipulating the arm to reduce the fracture.
  - Most surgical neck fractures have an apex anterior deformity, which is often the plane of deformity that is most easily overlooked.
  - The arm must be brought to neutral rotation. There is a tendency to internal rotation malreduction if the arm is left against the chest. Once the reduction is performed, it can be held in place by an assistant or with multiple Kirschner wires (K-wires).
- Multipart fractures are more challenging to reduce. The head fragment is controlled by the Schanz screws, and the tuberosity fragments can be manipulated with dental pick, clamps, or sutures at the tendon insertion. Often, the head is elevated off the shaft enough to allow for reduction of the tuberosities and then the head is reduced to the tuberosities.
  - Again, multiple K-wires are used for temporary fixation, avoiding the path of the nail.
- It is imperative to assess the reduction on at least two views, including the true AP and an axillary and/or Y view.
  - The advantage of the supine position with the C-arm coming in from the opposite side is that multiple views can be obtained without moving the limb.

Preparation for Nail Placement

- The nail entry point is identified with a guidewire before making an incision in the supraspinatus tendon. The entry point is directly over the canal, as most of the modern nails are straight **(TECH FIG 3A,B)**. The tendon is incised in line with the fibers, avoiding the area of tendon insertion (Sharpey fibers).
- The nail entry portal is medial to the sulcus at the base of the GT. The sulcus includes the insertion of the supraspinatus and infraspinatus tendons and is to be avoided. The subchondral bone at the entry site is strong and becomes a point of fixation once the nail is inserted.
- The correct insertion site is confirmed on the lateral view as well. Access to the correct entry point is facilitated by some extension of the shoulder.
- After the guidewire is placed, the supraspinatus tendon is incised 12 to 15 mm. The edges of the tendon are tagged with no. 1 braided suture. This allows for retraction of the tendon edges while reaming and also repair of the incision after nail insertion **(TECH FIG 3C)**.

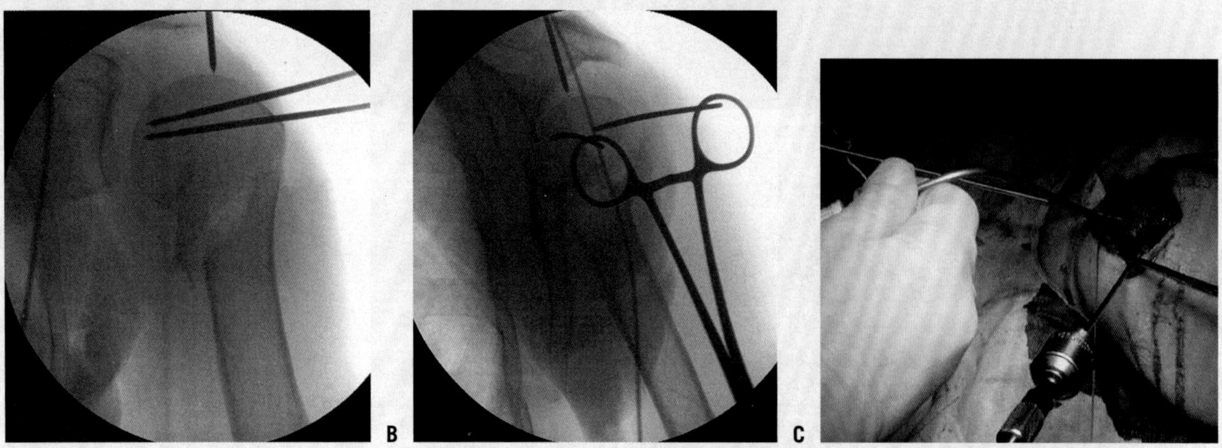

A B C

TECH FIG 3 A,B. The nail starting point is identified by using a guidewire on orthogonal views. **C.** The head fragment is controlled with a Schanz screw on a chuck, and the edges of the split in the supraspinatus are retracted with suture.

- A cannulated hollow drill is an ideal way to open the entry portal. Use of a solid cannulated drill or an awl can result in fragmentation of the head segment.
  - The cannulated hollow drill is placed deep enough to accommodate the wider proximal length of the nail. Reaming of the medullary canal is optional.

Intramedullary Nail and Interlock Screw Placement

- The nail is introduced with the jig and seated to the level of subchondral bone. The nail cannot be prominent, yet having it engage in the subchondral bone at the entry portal improves fixation. Most nail systems have a means of checking the level of the top of the nail, with a pin that goes into the insertion jig **(TECH FIG 4A–D)**.
  - If a nail is inserted too deeply, the interlocks may not be positioned appropriately and could put the axillary nerve at risk with insertion. An end cap can be added to ensure that the top of the nail engages subchondral bone, being careful not to make it prominent.
- Next, the proximal interlock screws can be placed **(TECH FIG 4E)**. The screw aiming arm allows for most interlocks to be placed through the incision, although they can be placed percutaneously if needed.
  - Regardless, it is essential that the axillary nerve be located, typically by palpation, and protected when placing screws.

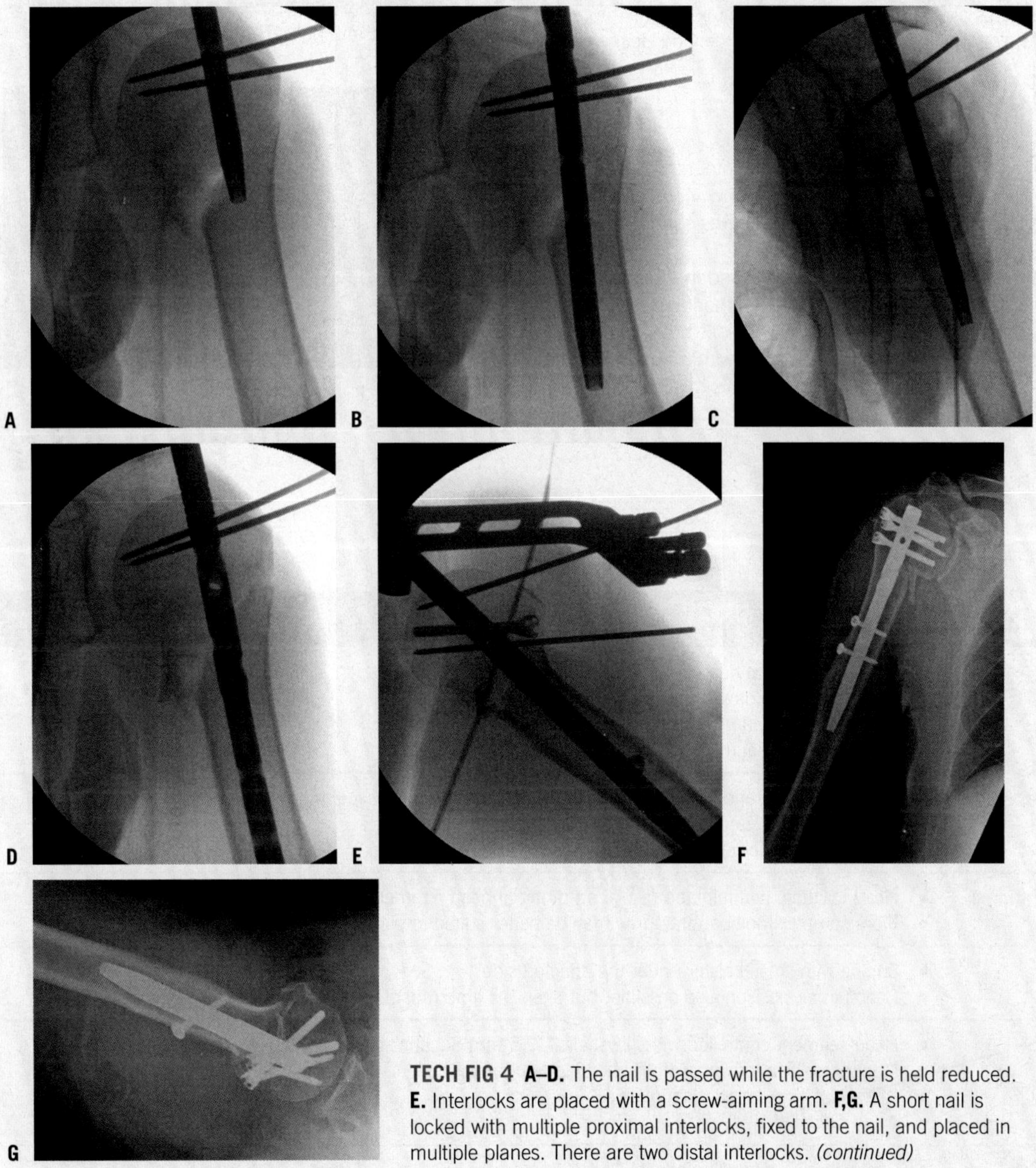

TECH FIG 4 A–D. The nail is passed while the fracture is held reduced. **E.** Interlocks are placed with a screw-aiming arm. **F,G.** A short nail is locked with multiple proximal interlocks, fixed to the nail, and placed in multiple planes. There are two distal interlocks. *(continued)*

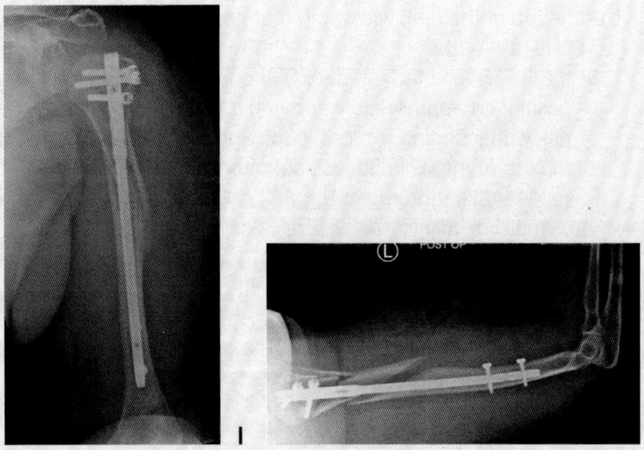

TECH FIG 4 *(continued)* **H,I.** A segmental fracture can be fixed with a long nail that also has multiple interlocks proximally, in multiple planes, and two distal interlocks placed with a "freehand" technique.

- It is important to avoid screw penetration into the shoulder joint. Multiple fluoroscopic views can help confirm screw position, but avoiding placing screws into the joint requires careful drilling technique and accurate measurement.
  - Most nails have interlocks that are placed in multiple planes, some with trajectories through the tuberosities to fix multipart fractures. In addition, many nails have a means of fixing the screw to the nail, typically with a bushing in the interlock hole through which the screw is threaded.
- The distal interlock screws are inserted to secure the nail within the IM canal. Fixation is more secure with two distal interlocks than it is with one **(TECH FIG 4F,G)**.
- For surgical neck fractures, a short nail can be used and the distal interlocks placed with the use of the screw aiming guide.
  - For bifocal neck or shaft injuries, or for fractures with extended metaphyseal/diaphyseal extension, a long nail can be used, in which case the distal interlocks are placed with a freehand technique **(TECH FIG 4H,I)**.

Completion

- Finally, the split in the rotator cuff is repaired with side-to-side sutures.
- The hole in the humeral head will be covered with fibrocartilage and will not articulate with the glenoid.
- The deltoid split is repaired with interrupted sutures and the skin closed routinely **(TECH FIG 5)**.

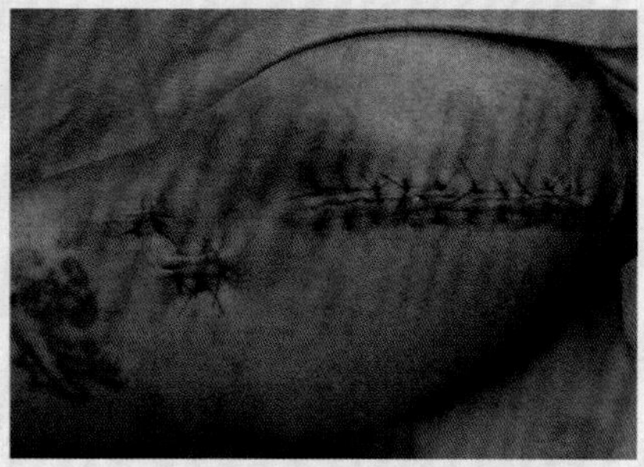

TECH FIG 5 Final closure.

TECHNIQUES

Pearls and Pitfalls

Indications	• Two-part proximal humerus fracture • Some three-part proximal humerus fractures • Bifocal injuries (surgical neck and shaft) • Extended proximal metadiaphyseal fractures
Prerequisites	• Radiolucent operating room table, image intensification, and *experienced* radiology technician • Be aware of the learning curve. • Plan B: plate/screws, arthroplasty as needed
Contraindication	• Head-splitting, comminuted displaced humeral head fragment devoid of soft tissue attachment • More complex multipart fractures may be better suited to plate/screw construct or arthroplasty.
Positioning	• Supine with small bolster under the affected side • Beach-chair position also possible, but often the limb must be moved to obtain fluoro images
Reduction Technique	• Head segment controlled with "joysticks" (2.5-mm Schanz screw); shoulder at neutral position • Manipulate arm to align with the head in neutral position. • Beware of apex anterior angulation. • Avoid malrotation.
Nail Entry Site	• Centered over medullary canal • Medial to the sulcus of GT, through the articular surface • Incision in the supraspinatus tendon in line with the fibers, avoiding the insertion site

Screw Placement	• A drill guide is used to prevent injury to the nerves and long head of the biceps. • Axillary is best identified and then avoided.
Orientation	• Neutral AP, accurate axillary view, with arm in neutral position are best ways to assess alignment.
Pitfalls	• Rotational malunion occurs when the nail is locked proximally and distally with the arm in internal rotation; this leads to decreased humeral retroversion and consequently external rotation. • Surgical neck nonunion occurs in cases of persistent distraction at the fracture site, and two-part fractures should be compressed prior to proximal locking. • Improper starting point can lead to malreduction and/or iatrogenic soft tissue damage. • Axillary nerve may be at risk from interlock placement.

POSTOPERATIVE CARE

- Sling for comfort
- Gentle pendulum shoulder exercises as well as mobilization of the elbow, wrist, and fingers are started immediately.
- Avoid weight bearing through the arm for 6 to 8 weeks.
- External rotation of the shoulder with the arm at side and internal rotation with the hand in the back by a physiotherapist are prohibited for 6 to 8 weeks postoperatively.
- Active-assisted range-of-motion exercises of the shoulder are allowed 6 to 8 weeks postoperatively.

COMPLICATIONS

- Most early complications can be avoided by attention to surgical technique, the locking nail design, and proper measurement and orientation of the screws.
- Early
  - Injury to axillary nerve
  - Joint penetration
  - Loss of reduction
  - Infection
  - Rotator cuff avulsion
- Late
  - Nonunion
  - Posttraumatic arthrosis
  - AVN of humeral head
  - Prominent hardware

SUGGESTED READINGS

Boileau P, ed. Intramedullary nail for proximal humerus fractures: an old concept revisited. In: Shoulder Concepts 2010–Arthroscopy & Arthroplasty. Montpellier, France: Sauramps, 2010:201–223.

Dilisio MF, Nowinski RJ, Hatzidakis AM, et al. Intramedullary nailing of the proximal humerus: evolution, technique, and results. J Shoulder Elbow Surg 2016;25:e130–e138.

Euler SA, Petri M, Venderley MB, et al. Biomechanical evaluation of straight antegrade nailing in proximal humeral fractures: the rationale of the "proximal anchoring point." Int Orthop 2017;41:1715–1721.

Gracitelli MEC, Malavolta EA, Assunção JH, et al. Locking intramedullary nails compared with locking plates for two- and three-part proximal humeral surgical neck fractures: a randomized controlled trial. J Shoulder Elbow Surg 2016;25:695–703.

Gradl G, Dietze A, Kääb M, et al. Is locking nailing of humeral head fractures superior to locking plate fixation? Clin Orthop Relat Res 2009;467(11):2986–2993.

Hepp P, Lill H, Bail H, et al. Where should implants be anchored in the humeral head? Clin Orthop Relat Res 2003;(415):139–147.

Konrad G, Audigé L, Lambert S, et al. Similar outcomes for nail versus plate fixation of three-part proximal humeral fractures. Clin Orthop Relat Res 2012;470:602–609.

Sheehan S, Gaviola G, Sacks A, et al. Traumatic shoulder injuries: a force mechanism analysis of complex injuries to the shoulder girdle and proximal humerus. AJR Am J Roentgenol 2013;201:W409–W424.

Südkamp NP, Audigé L, Lambert S, et al. Path analysis of factors for functional outcome at one year in 463 proximal humeral fractures. J Shoulder Elbow Surg 2011;20:1207–1216.

Zhu Y, Lu Y, Shen J, et al. Locking intramedullary nails and locking plates in the treatment of two-part proximal humeral surgical neck fractures: a prospective randomized trial with a minimum of three years of follow-up. J Bone Joint Surg Am 2011;93:159–168.

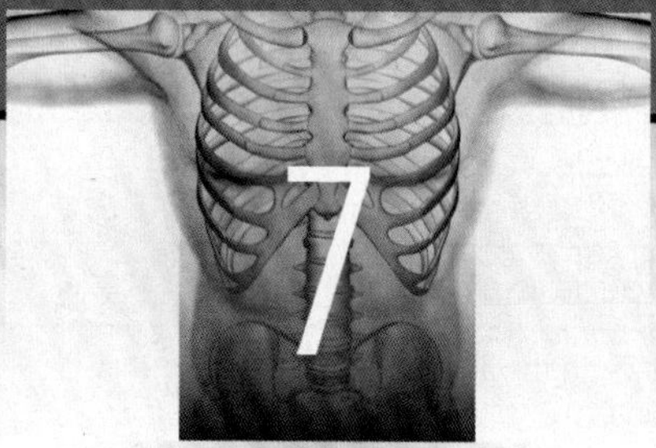

CHAPTER

Hemiarthroplasty for Proximal Humerus Fractures

Kamal I. Bohsali, Michael A. Wirth, and Steven B. Lippitt

DEFINITION

- Proximal humerus fractures involve isolated or combined injuries to the greater tuberosity, lesser tuberosity, articular segment, and proximal humeral shaft.
- Overall, proximal humerus fractures account for 4% to 5% of all fractures.[3,7,12,13]

ANATOMY

- The proximal humerus consists of four segments: the greater tuberosity, lesser tuberosity, articular segment, and humeral shaft (**FIG 1**).
- The most cephalad surface of the articular segment is, on average, 8 mm above the greater tuberosity.[20] Humeral version averages 28.8 degrees.[16,20]
- The intertubercular groove lies between the tuberosities and forms the passageway for the long head of the biceps, as it traverses from the intra-articular origin into the distal arm.
- The tuberosities attach to the articular segment at the anatomic neck. The greater tuberosity has three facets for the corresponding insertions of the supraspinatus, infraspinatus, and teres minor tendons; the lesser tuberosity has a single facet for the subscapularis.
- The deltoid, pectoralis major, and latissimus dorsi all insert on the humerus distal to the surgical neck. These soft tissue attachments contribute to the deforming forces sustained with proximal humerus fractures.
- The humeral head receives its blood supply from the anterolateral branch of the anterior humeral circumflex artery (the arcuate artery of Laing) and the posterior humeral circumflex artery. The artery of Laing courses parallel to the lateral aspect of the long head of the biceps and enters the humeral head at the interface between the intertubercular groove and the greater tuberosity.[22] More recent studies have indicated that the posterior branch plays a significant role in perfusion of the fractured humeral head, reducing the risk of osteonecrosis in this clinical setting.[11,17,18,21]

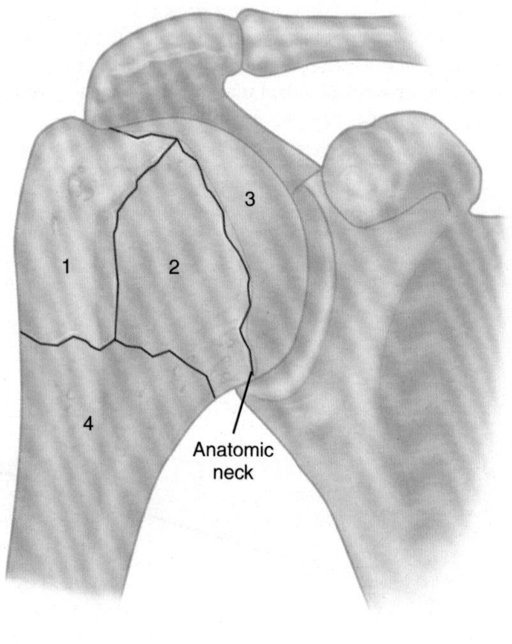

FIG 1 Neer classification of proximal humerus fractures: *1*, greater tuberosity; *2*, lesser tuberosity; *3*, articular surface; *4*, shaft.

PATHOGENESIS

- The incidence of proximal humerus fractures is increasing with an aging population and associated osteoporosis.
- The mechanism of injury may be indirect or direct and secondary to high-energy collisions in younger patients (eg, motor vehicle accidents, athletic injuries) or falls from standing height in elderly patients.
- Pathologic fractures from primary or metastatic disease should be included in the differential diagnosis.
- Risk factors for the development of proximal humerus fractures in the elderly patient population include low bone density, lack of hormone replacement therapy, previous fracture history, three or more chronic illnesses, and smoking.[19]

NATURAL HISTORY

- Neer's[25] classic study in 1970 compared the results of nonoperative treatment with hemiarthroplasty for three- and four-part displaced proximal humerus fractures. No satisfactory results were found in the nonoperative group owing to inadequate reduction, nonunion, malunion, and humeral head osteonecrosis with collapse.
- Stableforth[32] reaffirmed this in a study in which patients were randomized to nonoperative management or prosthetic replacement. The patients with displaced fractures treated nonoperatively had worse overall results for pain, range of motion, and activities of daily living.
- Olerud et al[29] most recently demonstrated significantly improved quality of life with a positive trend toward pain scores with four-part fractures treated with hemiarthroplasty versus observation.

PATIENT HISTORY AND PHYSICAL FINDINGS

- A thorough history and complete physical examination should be performed. History should include mechanism of injury, premorbid level of function, occupation, hand dominance, history of malignancy, and ability to participate in a structured rehabilitation program.[3,15]
- A review of systems should involve queries regarding loss of consciousness, paresthesias, and ipsilateral elbow or wrist pain.
- On physical examination, the orthopaedic surgeon should look for swelling, soft tissue injuries, ecchymosis, and deformity. Posterior fracture-dislocations will demonstrate flattening of the anterior aspect of the shoulder with an associated posterior prominence. Anterior fracture-dislocations present with opposite findings.[3,15]

IMAGING AND OTHER DIAGNOSTIC STUDIES

- Appropriate radiographs include biplanar views of the shoulder (**FIG 2A,B**).[3,15] If the axillary view cannot be obtained because of patient discomfort, alternate views such as the Velpeau trauma axillary view can be used to evaluate and classify the injury.[3]
  - The Neer classification is based on the four anatomic segments of the proximal humerus: the humeral head, the greater and lesser tuberosities, and the humeral shaft (see **FIG 1**).[12] Number of parts is based on 45 degrees of angulation or 1 cm of displacement from neighboring segments.
  - The AO/ASIF/OTA Comprehensive Long Bone Classification system distinguishes the valgus impacted four-part proximal humerus fracture from other four-part fractures with partial preservation of the vascular inflow to the articular segment through an intact medial capsule.[9,21,30]
  - The current fracture classification systems have fair intraobserver and interobserver reliability, even with the addition of computed tomography (CT) scans. Despite the limitations of these systems, they remain clinically useful when deciding on nonoperative versus operative treatment.[3,11,28]
- CT scans may be helpful in evaluating tuberosity displacement and articular surface involvement (**FIG 3**).[12,14,28]

DIFFERENTIAL DIAGNOSIS

- Hematoma/contusion
- Traumatic rotator cuff tear
- Simple dislocation
- Acromioclavicular separation
- Calcific tendinitis[3]

NONOPERATIVE MANAGEMENT

- Nonoperative treatment usually is reserved for minimally displaced fractures of the proximal humerus, which account for nearly 80% of these injuries.[3]
- The characteristics of the fracture (ie, bone quality, fracture orientation, concurrent soft tissue injuries), the personality of the patient (eg, compliance, expectations, mental status), and surgeon experience all affect the decision to proceed with surgical intervention.
- Moribund individuals and patients unable to cooperate with a postoperative rehabilitation program (eg, obtunded from closed head injury) are not appropriate candidates for operative intervention. In general, nonoperative management of complex, displaced proximal humerus fractures has not proven as successful.
- Initial immobilization with a sling and axillary pad may be helpful. Gentle range-of-motion exercises may be started by 7 to 10 days after the fracture event when pain has decreased and the patient is less apprehensive.[3]
- Intermittent biplanar radiographs are required to determine additional displacement and the interval stage of healing.[3]
- Active and active-assisted range-of-motion exercises are initiated with evidence of radiographic union. Educate the patient that he or she may never obtain symmetric range of motion or strength to the uninjured side.

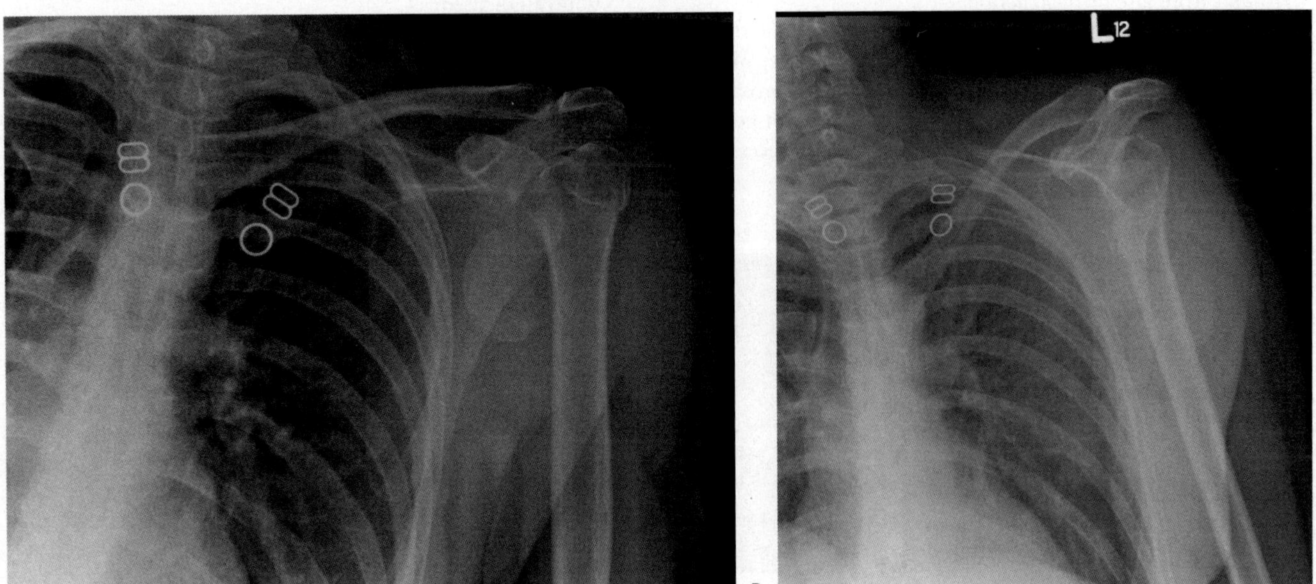

A B

FIG 2 Anteroposterior (**A**) and scapular "Y" views (**B**) of a displaced four-part proximal humerus fracture-dislocation. (Copyright Kamal I. Bohsali, MD.)

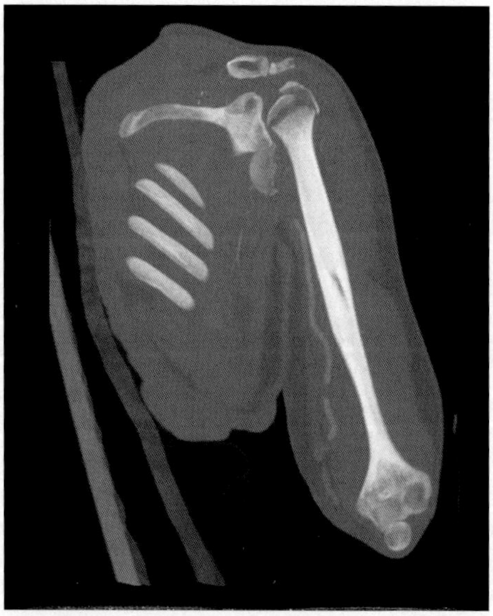

FIG 3 Coronal image from CT-angiogram indicates intact axillary vessel flow to upper extremity in the setting of a four-part proximal humerus fracture-dislocation. (Copyright Kamal I. Bohsali, MD.)

SURGICAL MANAGEMENT

- The goal of surgery is to anatomically reconstruct the glenohumeral joint with restoration of humeral height, replication of appropriate prosthetic retroversion, and establishment of secure tuberosity fixation.
- Prosthetic replacement is the preferred treatment of most four-part fractures, three-part fractures and dislocations in elderly patients with osteoporotic bone, head-splitting articular segment fractures, and chronic anterior or posterior humeral head dislocations with more than 40% of the articular surface involvement.[1,3,25]
- Studies have indicated that the outcome of primary hemiarthroplasty for acute proximal humerus fractures is superior to that from late reconstruction.[6,27]
- There are commercially available fracture-specific stems that allow for improved bone grafting and tuberosity placement, some with bone windows with reduced proximal stem diameter, and others with a suture collar with potential conversion to a reverse shoulder prosthesis if necessary.

Preoperative Planning

- Although some studies have suggested urgent intervention (eg, within <48 hours), most authors recommend preoperative planning with a careful neurovascular assessment of the injured shoulder, medical optimization of the patient, and preoperative templating with standard radiographs of the contralateral uninjured shoulder.[13]
- A CT scan may provide improved characterization of the fracture pattern such as intra-articular involvement and degree of tuberosity comminution for surgical planning.[12,14,28]
- To reduce the need for postoperative opioid consumption, we recommend an interscalene block (single shot or indwelling catheter) to supplement general anesthesia.
- Endotracheal intubation is recommended to allow for intraoperative muscle relaxation, but laryngeal mask intubation may be used.[13,15]

Positioning

- The patient is placed on an operating table in the beach-chair or semi-Fowler position with the arm positioned in a sterile articulating arm holder or draped free with a padded Mayo stand if an appropriate number of assistants are available **(FIG 4A,B)**.
- Intraoperative C-arm fluoroscopy is strongly recommended and will assist the surgeon in implant placement and tuberosity positioning.

Approach

- The surgical prep site should include the entire upper extremity and shoulder region, including the scapular and pectoral regions.
- Appropriate prophylactic intravenous antibiotics are given to the patient before skin incision.
- Antifibrinolytics may be given intravenously, topically, or both to reduce intraoperative blood loss, unless medically contraindicated.
- A standard deltopectoral incision is used. Care is taken to minimize injury (eg, surgical detachment, contusion secondary to retractors) to the deltoid and conjoint complex. The musculocutaneous and axillary nerves are identified and protected during the procedure.

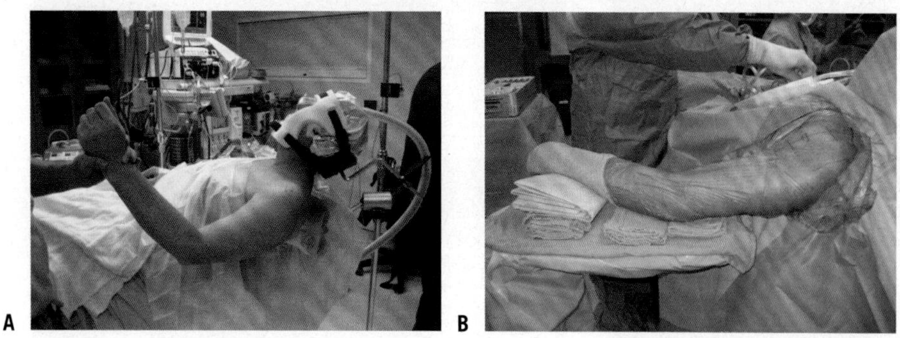

FIG 4 A,B. The patient is placed on an operating table in the beach-chair position, with the arm positioned in a sterile articulating arm holder or draped free with use of a padded Mayo stand. (Copyright Kamal I. Bohsali, MD.)

DELTOPECTORAL APPROACH

- The incision begins superior and medial to the coracoid process and extends toward the anterior aspect of the deltoid insertion **(TECH FIG 1A)**.
- The cephalic vein is identified, preserved, and retracted laterally with the deltoid muscle. The pectoralis major is mobilized medially. If additional exposure is necessary, the proximal portion (1 cm) of the pectoralis major insertion is released **(TECH FIG 1B)**.
- Fracture hematoma usually is encountered once the clavipectoral fascia is incised. At this time, fracture fragments and the rotator cuff musculature become evident.
- The axillary and musculocutaneous nerves can be identified through digital palpation of the anteroinferior aspect of the subscapularis and the posterior aspect of the coracoid muscles, respectively. External rotation of the humerus results in reduced tension on the axillary nerve.

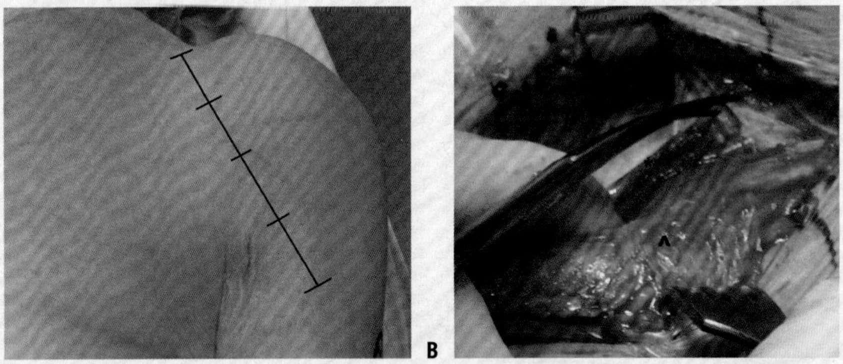

A B

TECH FIG 1 Skin incision and deltopectoral approach. **A.** The skin incision is centered over the anterior deltoid. The deltopectoral interval is developed with lateral retraction of the cephalic vein. **B.** For more exposure, the superior 1 cm of the pectoralis major (*caret*) tendon may be incised. *pound*, deltoid; *asterisk*, cephalic vein.

TUBEROSITY MOBILIZATION

- The tendon of the long head of the biceps is identified, as it courses within the bicipital groove toward the rotator cuff interval. The biceps tendon serves as a key landmark when reestablishing the anatomic relationship between the greater and lesser tuberosities.
  - The rotator cuff interval and coracohumeral ligament are both released to allow for mobilization of the tuberosities **(TECH FIG 2A,B)**.
- If the fracture does not involve the bicipital groove, an osteotome or saw may be necessary to create a cleavage plane for tuberosity mobilization. Preservation of the coracoacromial ligament is advisable to maintain the coracoacromial arch and reduce the risk of proximal humeral head migration.
- Large caliber, nonabsorbable traction sutures are placed through the rotator cuff tendon insertions in proximity to the tuberosities. Two or three sutures should be placed through the subscapularis tendon and three or four sutures through the supraspinatus. When using a suture collar system, definitive sutures may be placed after implantation of the humeral stem.
- Tuberosity fragments vary in size and may require bulk reduction for repair **(TECH FIG 2C,D)**.
- With the tuberosities retracted on their muscular insertions, the humeral head and shaft fragments are removed. In four-part fractures, the humeral head articular surface will be devoid of soft tissue attachments and easily removed.
- The native articular surface is removed and sized with a template for trial humeral head replacement **(TECH FIG 2E)**. Obtain cancellous bone from the extracted humeral head or tuberosities for later bone grafting.
- The glenoid must be examined for concomitant pathology. Hematoma and cartilaginous or bony fragments are removed and irrigated with antibiotic-impregnated saline.
- Glenoid fractures should be stabilized with internal fixation. If the glenoid exhibits significant degenerative wear or irreparable damage, a glenoid component may be necessary.

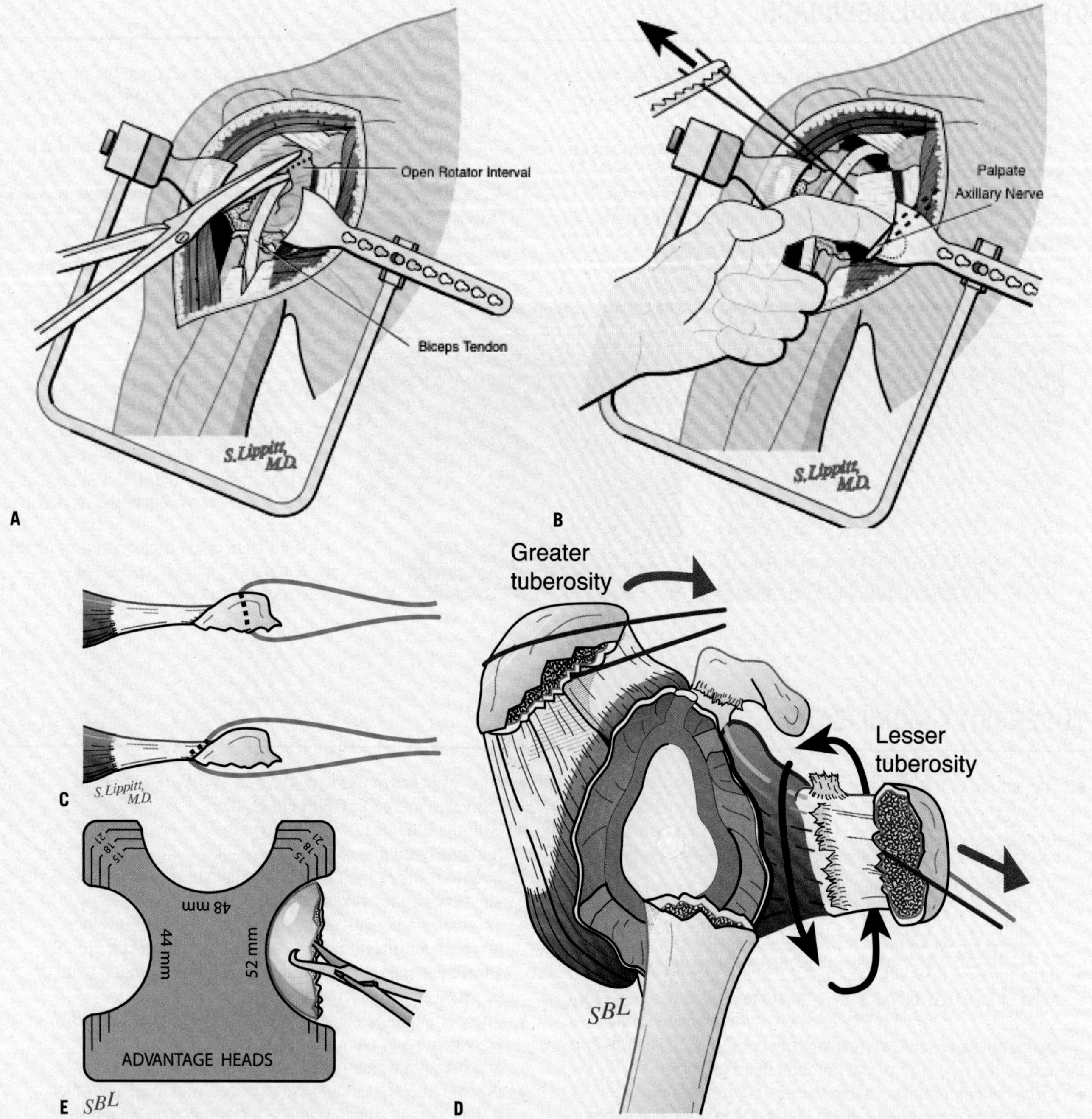

TECH FIG 2 A. The long head of the biceps is identified and traced superiorly to the rotator interval. The tendon serves as a key landmark when reestablishing the anatomic relation between the greater and lesser tuberosities. **B.** The axillary nerve is identified at the anteroinferior border of the subscapularis. **C.** Nonabsorbable sutures are placed at the junction of the tendon–tuberosity interface and not through the tuberosities. **D.** Once the native humeral head is removed, the tuberosities with their respective rotator cuff attachments are mobilized for humeral canal preparation and later repair. **E.** Humeral head sizing. The extracted native humeral head is sized with the use of a commercially available template guide. (Copyright Steven B. Lippitt, MD.)

HUMERAL SHAFT PREPARATION

- The proximal end of the humeral shaft is delivered into the incisional wound. Loose endosteal bone fragments and hematoma are removed from the canal of the humeral shaft.
- Axial reamers in 1-mm increments are used without power to prepare the humeral shaft for trial implantation. We recommend reaming at least 1 mm greater than the definitive implant when performing cement fixation.
- In systems without a suture collar, we recommend placing the trial humeral implant with the lateral fin slightly posterior to the bicipital groove and with the medial aspect of the trial head at least at the height of the medial calcar.
- A commercially available fracture jig may be used to maintain height and retroversion of the trial component through a functional range of motion during provisional reduction **(TECH FIG 3)**.[13,15] When performing press fit fixation, the trial humeral implant may be positioned with a stem inserter that allows for version and height assessment.

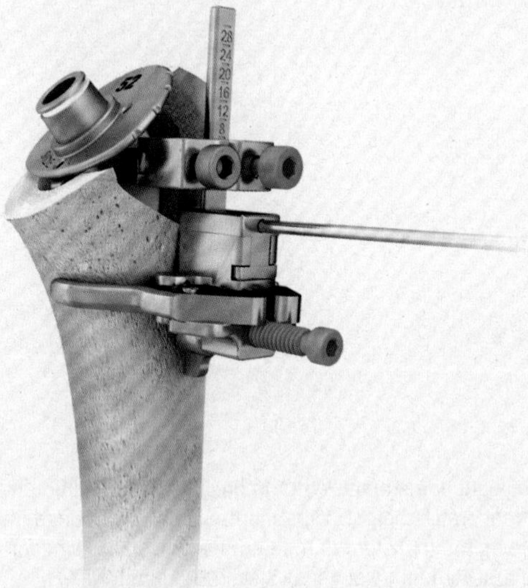

A

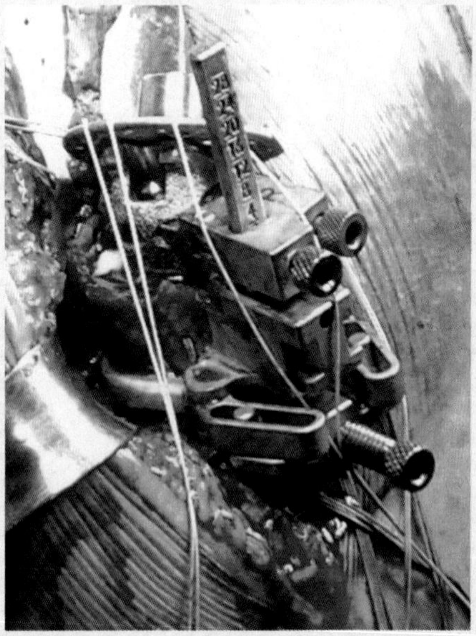

B

TECH FIG 3 A,B. A commercially available fracture jig stably positions the implant at appropriate height and retroversion. (**A:** Courtesy of DePuy Synthes. **B:** Copyright Kamal I. Bohsali, MD.)

DETERMINATION OF HUMERAL RETROVERSION

- Correct humeral retroversion is critical when recreating the glenohumeral articulation. Most techniques suggest 30 degrees as a guide during reconstruction, although native retroversion may vary from 10 to 50 degrees.[20,31]
- Several methods are employed to gauge this angle:
  - External rotation of the humerus to 30 degrees from the sagittal plane of the body with the humeral head component facing straight medially
  - An imaginary line from the distal humeral epicondylar axis that bisects the axis of the prosthesis
  - Positioning of the lateral fin of the prosthesis about 8 mm posterior to the biceps groove **(TECH FIG 4)**

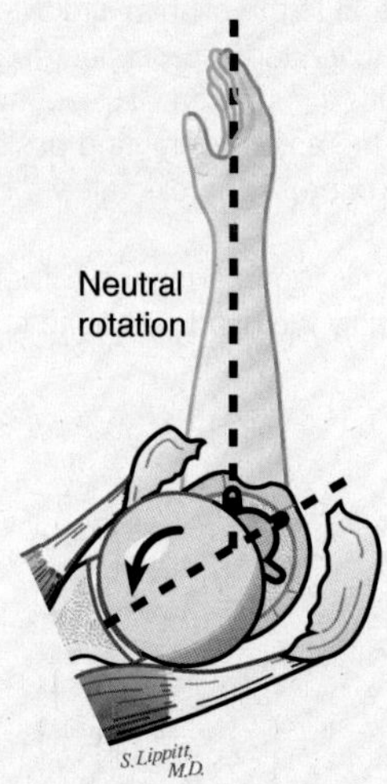

TECH FIG 4 Retroversion assessment. The anterior fin of the prosthesis is aligned with the forearm in neutral rotation, and the lateral fin is positioned about 8 mm posterior to the biceps groove, establishing a retroversion angle of about 30 degrees. (Copyright Steven B. Lippitt, MD.)

DETERMINATION OF PROSTHETIC HEIGHT

- The prosthetic height is critical in reestablishing appropriate muscle tension and shoulder mechanics.
- Preoperative templating such as x-rays of the contralateral unaffected shoulder may assist in the goal of anatomic reconstruction.
- Intraoperative examination of soft tissue tension, including the deltoid, rotator cuff, and the long head of the biceps, combined with fluoroscopic imaging aids in prosthetic height placement.
- Humeral height is established by placing the top of the prosthetic humeral head approximately 5.6 cm proximal to the superior border of the pectoralis major tendon.[24]
- Common errors involve placing the prosthesis too low, resulting in poor deltoid muscle tension and no room for the tuberosities **(TECH FIG 5)**.

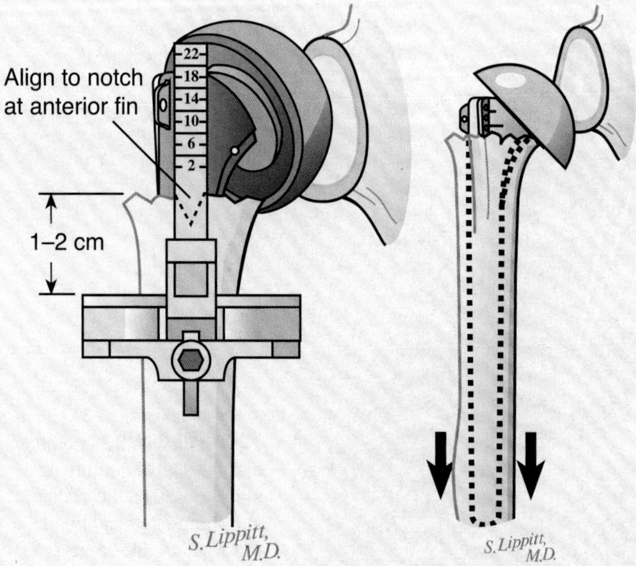

TECH FIG 5 Height adjustment. A commercially available fracture jig permits intraoperative height adjustment. Similarly, a sponge may be placed holding the trial stem at a determined level, allowing for intraoperative assessment. (Copyright Steven B. Lippitt, MD.)

TRIAL REDUCTION

- Two to four drill holes are placed in the proximal humerus medial and lateral to the bicipital groove, with no. 2 nonabsorbable sutures subsequently passed for fixation of the tuberosity to the shaft. With the suture collar technique, drill holes are made through the anterolateral and posterolateral aspects of the proximal humerus, approximately 2 cm below the fracture line **(TECH FIG 6A)**.
- A trial reduction is then performed with the mobilized tuberosities fitted below the head of the modular prosthetic head or suture collar.
- A towel clip or specially designed tuberosity clamp may be used to hold the tuberosities for fluoroscopic examination and assessment of glenohumeral stability.
- Intraoperative fluoroscopy is helpful in confirming appropriate implant height and glenohumeral stability **(TECH FIG 6B,C)**.
- To ensure adequate deltoid tensioning, the humeral head should not subluxate more than 25% to 30% of the glenoid height inferiorly.

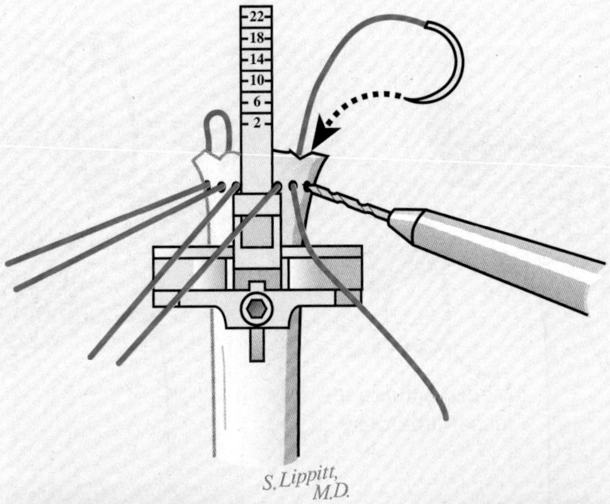

A

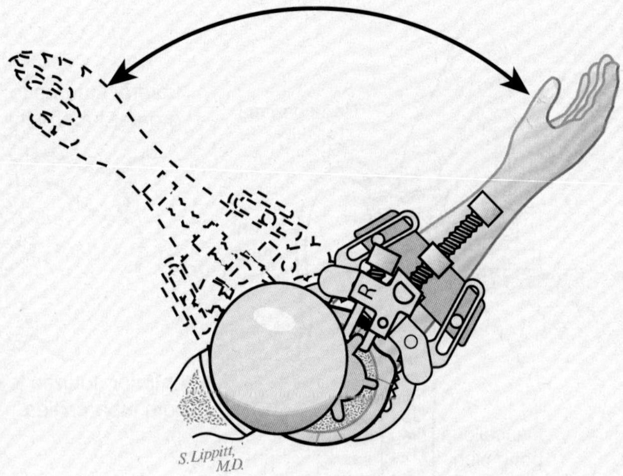

B

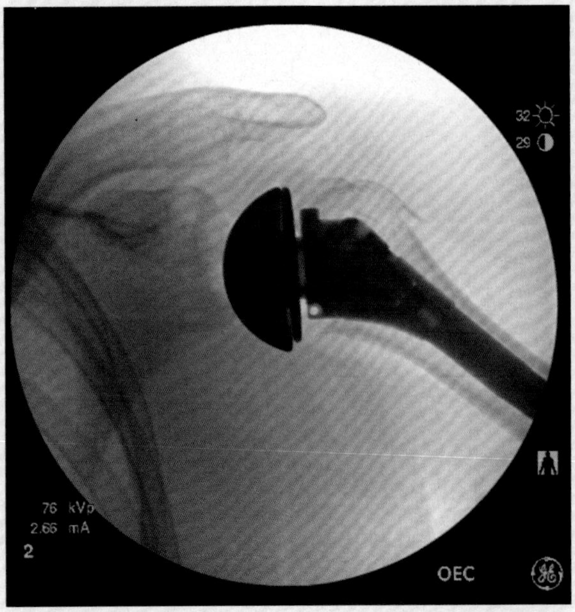

C

TECH FIG 6 **A.** Humeral shaft preparation. Drill holes are placed in the proximal humerus medial and lateral to the bicipital groove with 1-mm cottony Dacron or no. 2 nonabsorbable sutures. **B.** Trial reduction. A trial reduction may be performed with the fracture jig in place, allowing assessment of the functional range of motion. **C.** An intraoperative fluoroscopic image confirms prosthetic height and tuberosity reduction prior to placement of the final implant. (**A,B:** Copyright Steven B. Lippitt, MD; **C:** Copyright Kamal I. Bohsali, MD.)

FINAL IMPLANT PLACEMENT

- The final humeral component should be cemented in patients with osteoporotic bone and/or poor diaphyseal fixation. More recent implant designs allow for press-fit placement of the humeral component.
  - A cement restrictor is placed to prevent cement extravasation distally.
  - Pulsatile lavage and retrograde injection of cement with suction pressurization may be used **(TECH FIG 7A)**. Excess cement is removed during the curing phase. As an alternative, cement may also be applied to the humeral stem in a doughy state for proximal metadiaphyseal fixation.
- Spaces between the tuberosities, prosthesis, and shaft are packed with autogenous cancellous bone graft from the resected humeral head or debulked tuberosities **(TECH FIG 7B)**.
- A second reduction may be performed with the trial head after cement or press-fit fixation of the humeral stem.
- The final head may be impacted before stem implantation or after the repeat trial reduction. When using a suture collar, suture passage may be more facile without the final humeral head in position.
- A cerclage suture is placed circumferentially around the greater tuberosity and through the supraspinatus insertion and then medial or through the prosthesis and subscapularis insertion (lesser tuberosity). Studies have indicated superior fixation with the cerclage suture when compared to tuberosity-to-tuberosity and tuberosity-to-fin fixation alone **(TECH FIG 7D)**.[10,26]
- Overreduction of the tuberosities should be avoided to prevent limitations in external (lesser tuberosity) and internal (greater tuberosity) rotation.

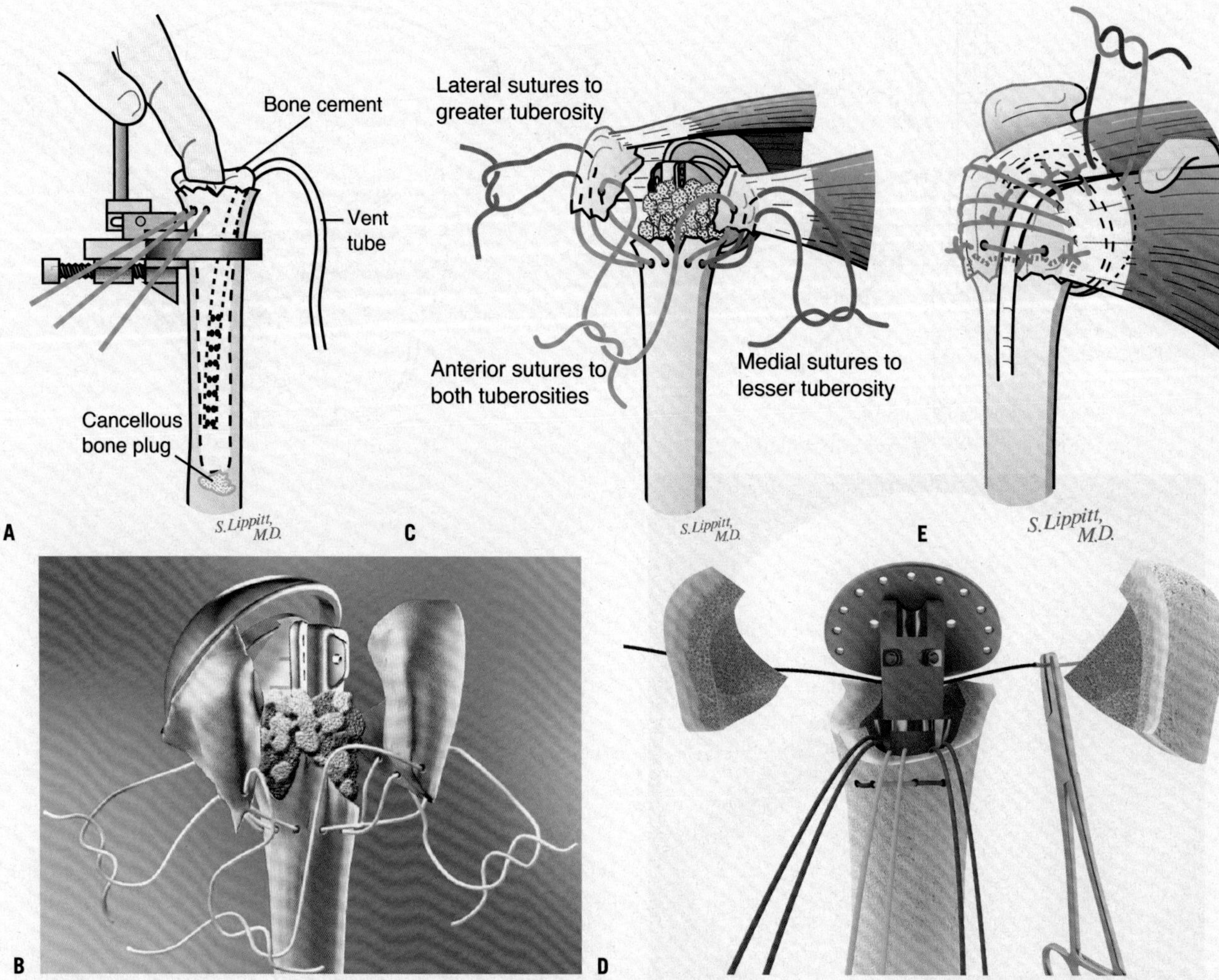

TECH FIG 7 A. If using cement, a restrictor is placed to prevent extravasation distally. Pulsatile lavage and retrograde injection of cement with suction pressurization are also used. **B.** Morselized cancellous bone graft is placed between the tuberosities and shaft. **C.** Tuberosity fixation. Previously placed suture limbs through the tuberosities and shaft are reapproximated. **D.** A medial cerclage suture is placed circumferentially around the greater tuberosity and through the supraspinatus insertion and then medial to or through the medial hole of the prosthesis and through the subscapularis insertion (lesser tuberosity) and tied. **E.** The rotator interval is closed with no. 2 nonabsorbable suture with the arm in about 30 degrees of external rotation. (**A,C,E:** Copyright Steven B. Lippitt, MD; **B,D:** Courtesy of DePuy Synthes.)

- The order and configuration of suture tying varies due to surgeon preference and implant-specific considerations. In general, sutures are tied, beginning with tuberosity-to-shaft followed by tuberosity-to-tuberosity closure using the previously placed suture limbs (**TECH FIG 7C**).
- The lateral portion of the rotator interval is closed with the arm in approximately 30 degrees of external rotation with no. 2 nonabsorbable sutures as needed (**TECH FIG 7E**).

SURGICAL WOUND CLOSURE

- The deltopectoral interval generally should not be closed. Drain suction is recommended in both acute and chronic injuries to prevent hematoma formation. Antifibrinolytics may reduce the need for drain placement, but its use is ultimately at the discretion of the surgeon.
- The subcutaneous tissues are reapproximated with 2-0 absorbable suture. Subcuticular closure is performed with 2-0 absorbable monofilament suture.
- The patient is then placed in a sling or shoulder immobilizer for comfort.

Pearls and Pitfalls

Indications	• A complete history and physical examination should be performed, with careful attention paid to the neurovascular status.
Imaging Studies	• Appropriate plain radiographs with CT scan supplementation aid in the surgical decision making. Fluoroscopy should be used for intraoperative implant and tuberosity positioning.
Tuberosity Identification	• Use the long head of the biceps to define the tuberosities for mobilization. • Tag this for later tenodesis before wound closure.
Implant Placement	• Know the specifics of the implant system including its limitations. • Place the implant in appropriate retroversion for the patient (approximately 20–30 degrees). • Use the pectoralis major insertion as a guide when restoring stem height. • Intraoperative fluoroscopy should be used to confirm trial and final implant positioning.
Tuberosity Fixation	• Avoid loss of external rotation or internal rotation with overreduction of the lesser and greater tuberosities, respectively.
Postoperative Rehabilitation	• On postoperative day 1, initiate gentle pendulum exercises, with passive forward flexion and external rotation (at 0 degrees of abduction). Always modify rehabilitation protocol based on intraoperative assessment of bone quality (tuberosity), soft tissue (rotator cuff), and patient neurologic status.

POSTOPERATIVE CARE

- Physician-directed therapy is initiated on postoperative day 1 with gentle, gravity-assisted pendulum exercises, as well as passive pulley-and-stick exercises to maintain forward flexion and external rotation (motion limits placed by surgeon based on intraoperative stability).
- After discharge, the patient's wound is reexamined and sutures removed at 10 to 14 days. Biplanar radiographs are performed to assess joint stability and tuberosity positioning. Gentle range-of-motion exercises are continued.
- At 6 weeks, repeat radiographs are obtained to evaluate tuberosity healing. When tuberosity healing is evident, phase 2 exercises are initiated with isometric rotator cuff exercises and active-assisted elevation with the pulley.
- At 3 months, strength training with graduated rubber bands (phase 3) is implemented. Functional gains may occur up to 12 months from date of intervention.

OUTCOMES

- About 90% of patients treated with hemiarthroplasty demonstrate minimal pain, despite a wide range of function, motion, and strength.[3]
- Factors that portend a poor outcome after hemiarthroplasty for fractures include tuberosity malposition, tuberosity resorption, superior migration of the humeral prosthesis, stiffness, persistent pain, poor initial positioning of the implant (excessive retroversion, decreased height), and age older than 75 years in women.[4,5]
- When comparing acute intervention versus late reconstruction, most authors report inferior outcomes with delayed surgical intervention (more than 2 weeks), particularly with functional results.[6,27,33]

COMPLICATIONS

- Complications include delays in wound healing, infection, nerve injury, humeral fracture, component malposition, instability, nonunion of the tuberosities, rotator cuff tearing, regional pain syndrome, periarticular fibrosis, heterotopic bone formation, component loosening, and glenoid arthritis.[2,8,23]
- The most common problems in acute fracture treatment involve stiffness, nonunion, malunion, or resorption of the tuberosities.[8,23]
- In patients with chronic fractures treated with hemiarthroplasty, the most common problems encountered were instability, heterotopic ossification, tuberosity malunion or nonunion, and rotator cuff tears.[23]

REFERENCES

1. Beredjiklian PK, Iannotti JP, Norris TR, et al. Operative treatment of malunion of a fracture of the proximal aspect of the humerus. J Bone Joint Surg Am 1998;80:1484–1497.
2. Bohsali KI, Bois AJ, Wirth MA. Complications of shoulder arthroplasty. J Bone Joint Surg Am 2017;99(3):256–269.
3. Bohsali KI, Wirth MA. Fractures of the proximal humerus. In: Rockwood CA Jr, Matsen FA III, Wirth WA, et al, eds. The Shoulder, ed 5. Philadelphia: Elsevier, 2016:183–242.
4. Boileau P, Krishnan SG, Tinsi L, et al. Tuberosity malposition and migration: reason for poor outcomes after hemiarthroplasty for displaced fractures of the proximal humerus. J Shoulder Elbow Surg 2002;11:401–412.
5. Boileau P, Walch G, Trojani C, et al. Surgical classification and limits of shoulder arthroplasty. In: Walch G, Boileau P, eds. Shoulder Arthroplasty. Berlin: Springer-Verlag, 1999:349–358.
6. Bosch U, Skutek M, Fremery RW, et al. Outcome after primary and secondary hemiarthroplasty in elderly patients with fractures of the proximal humerus. J Shoulder Elbow Surg 1998;7:479–484.
7. Cadet ER, Ahmad CS. Hemiarthroplasty for three- and four-part proximal humerus fractures. J Am Acad Orthop Surg 2012;20:17–27.
8. Compito CA, Self EB, Bigliani LU. Arthroplasty and acute shoulder trauma. Clin Orthop Relat Res 1994;307:27–36.
9. DeFranco MJ, Brems JJ, Williams GR Jr, et al. Evaluation and management of valgus impacted four-part proximal humerus fractures. Clin Orthop Relat Res 2006;442:109–114.
10. Frankle MA, Ondrovic LE, Markee BA, et al. Stability of tuberosity attachment in proximal humeral arthroplasty. J Shoulder Elbow Surg 2002;11:413–420.
11. Gerber C, Schneeberger A, Vinh T. The arterial vascularization of the humeral head: an anatomical study. J Bone Joint Surg Am 1990;72:1486–1494.
12. Green A. Proximal humerus fractures. In: Norris T, ed. Orthopaedic Knowledge Update: Shoulder and Elbow 2. Rosemont, IL: American Academy of Orthopaedic Surgeons, 2002:209–217.
13. Green A, Lippitt SB, Wirth MA. Humeral head replacement arthroplasty. In: Wirth MA, ed. Proximal Humerus Fractures. Rosemont, IL: American Academy of Orthopaedic Surgeons, 2005:39–48.

14. Green A, Norris T. Proximal humerus fractures and fracture-dislocations. In: Jupiter J, ed. Skeletal Trauma, ed 3. Philadelphia: WB Saunders, 2003:1532–1624.
15. Hartsock LA, Estes WJ, Murray CA, et al. Shoulder hemiarthroplasty for proximal humeral fractures. Orthop Clin North Am 1998;29(3):467–475.
16. Hernigou P, Duparc F, Hernigou A. Determining humeral retroversion with computed tomography. J Bone Joint Surg Am 2002;84(10): 1753–1762.
17. Hertel R, Stiehler M, Leunig M. Predictors of humeral head ischemia after intracapsular fracture of the proximal humerus. J Shoulder Elbow Surg 2004;13:427–433.
18. Hettrich CM, Boraiah S, Dyke JP, et al. Quantitative assessment of the vascularity of the proximal part of the humerus. J Bone Joint Surg Am 2010;92(4):943–948.
19. Huopio J, Kroger H, Honkanen R, et al. Risk factors for perimenopausal fractures: a prospective study. Osteoporos Int 2000;11:219–227.
20. Iannotti JP, Gabriel JP, Schneck SL, et al. The normal glenohumeral relationships: an anatomical study of one hundred and forty shoulders. J Bone Joint Surg Am 1992;74A:491–500.
21. Jakob R, Miniaci A, Anson P, et al. Four-part valgus impacted fractures of the proximal humerus. J Bone Joint Surg Br 1991;73B: 295–298.
22. Laing P. The arterial supply of the adult humerus. J Bone Joint Surg Am 1956;38A:1105–1116.
23. Muldoon MP, Cofield RH. Complications of humeral head replacement for proximal humerus fractures. Instr Course Lect 1997;46:15–24.
24. Murachovsky J, Ikemoto RY, Nascimento LG, et al. Pectoralis major tendon reference (PMT): a new method for accurate restoration of humeral length with hemiarthroplasty for fracture. J Shoulder Elbow Surg 2006;15(6):675–678.
25. Neer CS. Displaced proximal humeral fractures. Part II: treatment of 3-part and 4-part displacement. J Bone Joint Surg Am 1970;52A: 1090–1103.
26. Nho SJ, Brophy RH, Barker JU, et al. Innovations in the management of proximal humerus fractures. J Am Acad Orthop Surg 2007;15:12–26.
27. Norris TR, Green A, McGuigan FX. Late prosthetic shoulder arthroplasty for displaced proximal humerus fractures. J Shoulder Elbow Surg 1995;4:271–280.
28. Ohl X, Mangin P, Barbe C, et al. Analysis of four-fragment fractures of the proximal humerus: the interest of 2D and 3D imagery and inter- and intra-observer reproducibility. Eur J Orthop Surg Traumatol 2017;27(3):295–299.
29. Olerud P, Ahrengart L, Ponzer S, et al. Hemiarthroplasty versus non-operative treatment of displaced 4-part proximal humeral fractures in elderly patients: a randomized controlled trial. J Shoulder Elbow Surg 2011;20:1025–1033.
30. Orthopaedic Trauma Association Committee for Coding and Classification. Fracture and dislocation compendium. J Orthop Trauma 1996;10(suppl 1):1–155.
31. Pearl ML, Volk AG. Retroversion of the proximal humerus in relationship to the prosthetic replacement arthroplasty. J Shoulder Elbow Surg 1995;4:286–289.
32. Stableforth PG. Four part fractures of the neck of the humerus. J Bone Joint Surg Br 1984;66B:104–108.
33. Zuckerman JD, Cuomo F, Koval KJ. Proximal humeral replacement for complex fractures: indications and surgical technique. Instr Course Lect 1997;46:7–14.

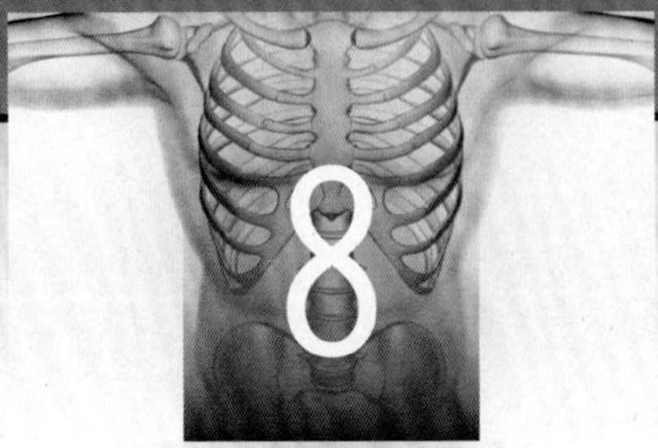

CHAPTER 8

Reverse Shoulder Arthroplasty for Proximal Humerus Fractures

Michael M. Hussey, Brandon M. Steen, and Mark A. Frankle

DEFINITION

- Fractures involving the proximal region of the humerus that provide the supporting framework for the glenohumeral articulation are termed *proximal humerus fractures*.
- These fractures typically occur along the physeal lines as described by Ernest Codman in 1934, most commonly involving the surgical neck and lesser and greater tuberosities.
- Proximal humerus fractures remain the second most common fracture of the upper extremity and the third most common fracture in patients older than age 65 years.[1]

ANATOMY

- The proximal humerus is composed of the humeral head, greater tuberosity, lesser tuberosity, and upper humeral shaft. In the normal shoulder, the head is covered with articular cartilage which allows for a smooth articulation with the glenoid. The greater and lesser tuberosities are separated by the intertubercular groove through which the long head of biceps tendon traverses.
- The superior most point of the humeral head is on average 8 mm cephalad to the greater tuberosity[11] and shown to average 30 degrees of retroversion in relation to the shaft.[19]
- The upper edge of the pectoralis major tendon is on average 56 mm inferior to the top of the humeral head.[16]
- The rotator cuff complex (subscapularis, supraspinatus, infraspinatus, teres minor) inserts onto the proximal humerus at the lesser and greater tuberosities. This complex works in concert not only to bring about intricate movements of the arm in space but also to secondarily stabilize the glenohumeral joint.
- This region consists primarily of metaphyseal bone surrounded by a vascular network of the circumflex humeral vessels.
- The humeral head receives the majority of its vascular supply from the arcuate artery, a terminal branch of the anterior circumflex humeral artery **(FIG 1A)**. Disruption of this vessel by fracture or iatrogenic causes has the potential to cause avascular necrosis and a poor outcome.
- The posterior aspect of the greater tuberosity and head are supplied by branches of the posterior circumflex humeral artery[9] **(FIG 1B)**.
- The axillary nerve courses around the lateral aspect of the proximal humerus at an average of 61 mm from the midportion of the acromion.[4]

PATHOGENESIS

- These injuries are most commonly due to a ground level fall onto the upper extremity in the elderly population with osteopenia.
- The majority of fractures are minimally displaced. However, if sufficient energy and diminished bone density exist,

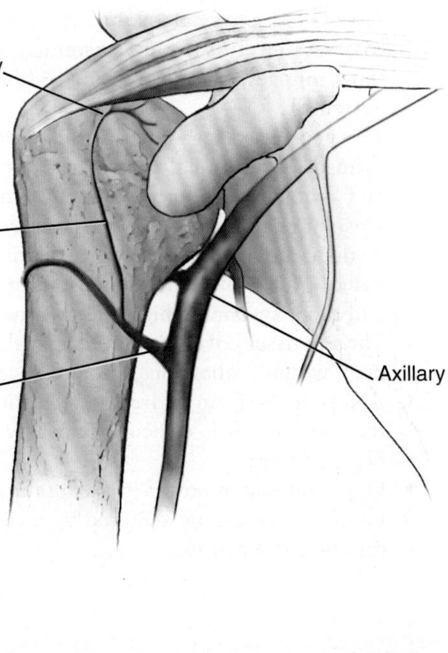

A

FIG 1 A. Anterior view. The anterior circumflex humeral artery branches off the axillary artery, giving rise to the ascending branch, which travels along the bicipital groove to supply the humeral head. *(continued)*

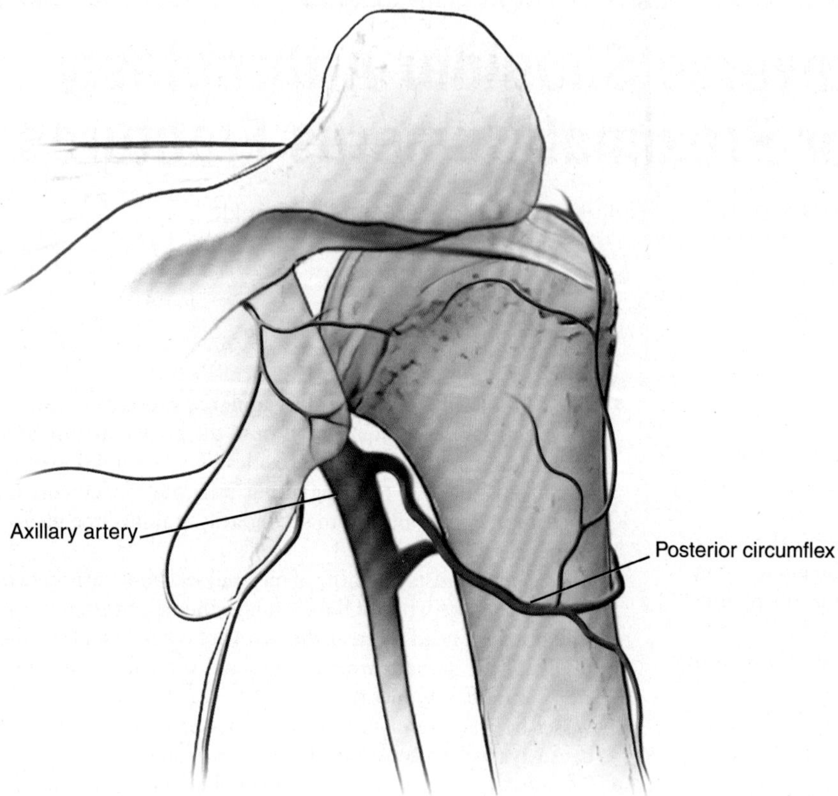

B

FIG 1 *(continued)* **B.** Posterior view. The posterior circumflex humeral artery sends many branches to supply the posterior head and greater tuberosity.

displacement can occur, which often follows characteristic fracture patterns as described by Neer.[17]

- The Neer classification is commonly used to describe these injuries and is based on displacement and/or angulation of the fracture "parts."[17] The use of this classification has led to a better understanding of the prognostic implications of treatment as well as improved therapeutic interventions.
- Due to multiple tendon attachments onto the proximal humerus, these parts undergo characteristic patterns of displacement.
- The greater tuberosity is frequently displaced posterosuperiorly by the strong external rotators of the cuff. The lesser tuberosity is pulled medially by the subscapularis, and the shaft is pulled superiorly and medially by the deltoid and pectoralis major, respectively (**FIG 2**). The head typically maintains a concentric alignment with the glenoid due to capsular attachments, except for cases of dislocation or valgus collapse.
- A valgus impacted fracture involves lateral rotation and collapse of the head onto the shaft, with displacement of the tuberosities and impaction of the underlying cancellous bone.

NATURAL HISTORY

- Significant displacement occurs in less than 15% of all proximal humerus fractures.[17]
- Left untreated, displaced three- and four-part fractures are often associated with poor patient outcomes, leading to chronic pain, loss of motion, and impairment with activities of daily living.
- Significant fracture comminution and displacement can potentially lead to avascular necrosis of the humeral head (**FIG 3**). Predictors of humeral head ischemia include posteromedial metaphyseal head extension less than 8 mm, loss of the medial hinge, four-fragment fractures, and angular displacement of the head greater than 45 degrees.[10]

PATIENT HISTORY AND PHYSICAL FINDINGS

- A thorough history should be taken from the patient to include age, mechanism of injury, arm dominance, occupation, prior history of falls, and smoking status.
- Also critical to consider in the elderly population is functional status, living situation, and medical comorbidities.
- A detailed physical examination should be performed to assess level of trauma sustained, presence of concomitant injuries, and degree of dysfunction of the injured extremity.
- The neurovascular status of the extremity should be performed. Distal radial and ulnar pulses should be palpated and compared to the uninjured arm. Distal motor and sensory examinations in the axillary, musculocutaneous, median, radial, and ulnar nerve distribution should be evaluated. This is extremely important in polytrauma patients and those sustaining high-energy trauma.
- The soft tissue envelope should be evaluated for ecchymoses, open wounds, abrasions, and presence of skin tenting.
- Ability to perform active arm elevation and assessment of the rotator cuff is difficult secondary to pain and fracture displacement.
- Of paramount importance is determination of axillary nerve injury, which can be achieved by testing sensation and deltoid motor function.

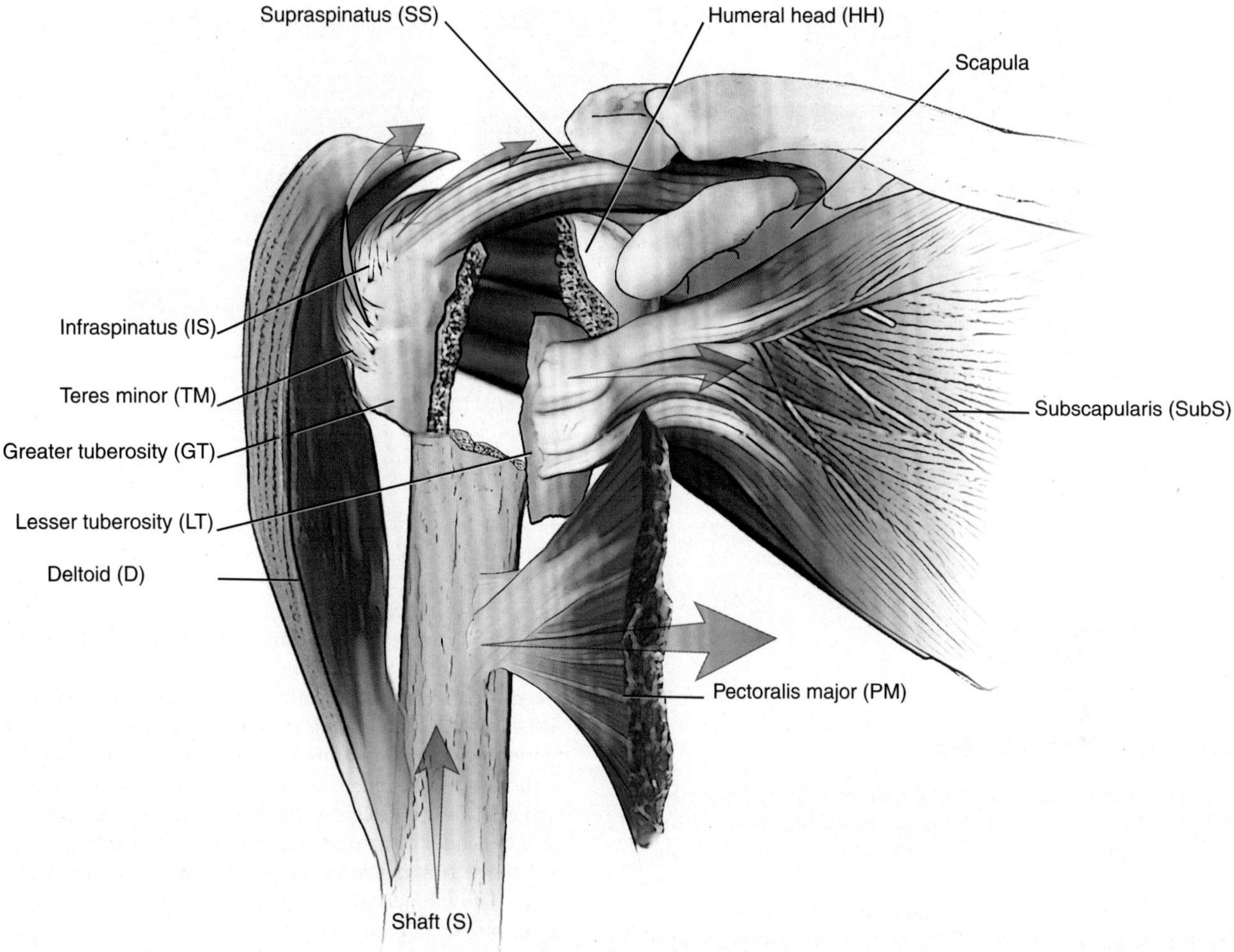

FIG 2 Illustration shows the greater tuberosity (GT) is frequently displaced posterosuperiorly by the supraspinatus (SS)/infraspinatus (IS)/teres minor (TM). The lesser tuberosity (LT) is displaced medially by the subscapularis (SubS), and the shaft (S) is pulled superiorly and medially by the deltoid (D) and pectoralis major (PM), respectively.

IMAGING AND OTHER DIAGNOSTIC STUDIES

- In fracture cases, patient discomfort often limits radiographic analysis. Typically, a true scapular anteroposterior (AP), scapular Y, and axillary lateral radiographs are obtained to evaluate details of the fracture and whether or not a dislocation is present. A Velpeau view may be helpful in situations where obtaining an axillary lateral is extremely painful (**FIG 4A,B**).
- In certain instances, computed tomography (CT) scan can be obtained to better characterize fracture pattern and aid in preoperative surgical planning. CT can be very helpful to evaluate head impaction as well as tuberosity fragmentation and displacement (**FIG 4C**).
- In cases where there is significant comminution that extends into the shaft, it is helpful to obtain bilateral humerus radiographs to measure length and assess for shortening that can aid in implant positioning.

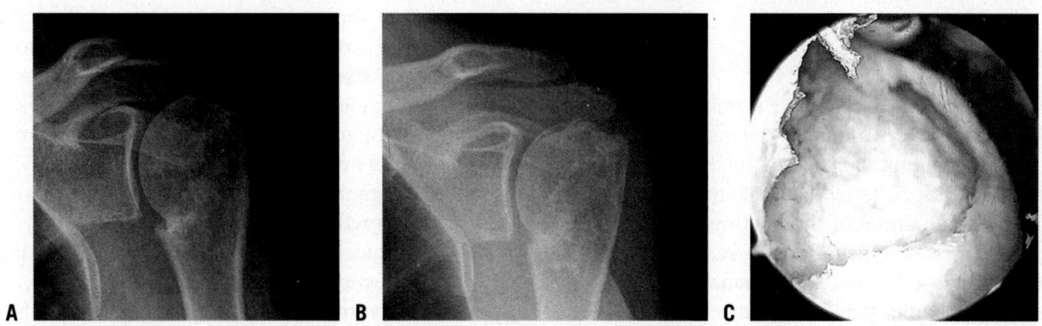

FIG 3 **A.** AP view of proximal humerus fracture healed in varus malalignment 8 months after initial injury. **B.** At 15 months, a crescent sign is visualized demonstrating avascular necrosis and collapse of the humeral head. **C.** Arthroscopic view of same patient after débridement of necrotic lesion.

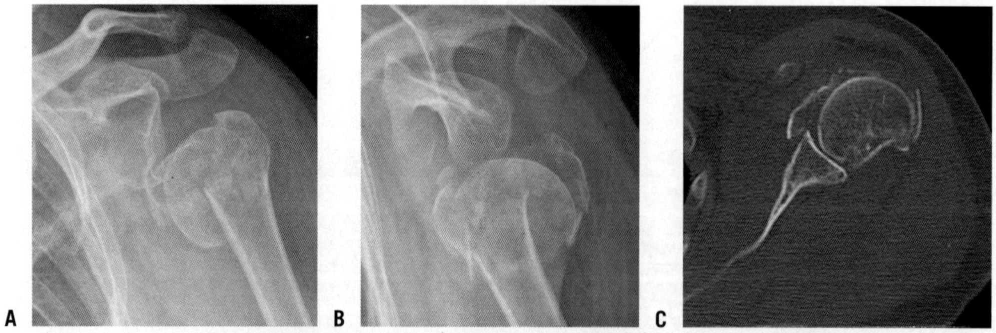

FIG 4 **A.** AP view of a comminuted displaced proximal humerus fracture. **B.** Velpeau view demonstrating collapse of the humeral head with outward displacement of the tuberosities. **C.** Axial CT scan showing medial displacement of the lesser tuberosity and extreme external rotation of the humeral head.

DIFFERENTIAL DIAGNOSIS

- Humeral shaft fracture
- Rotator cuff tear
- Scapular fracture
- Glenohumeral dislocation
- Brachial plexus injury

NONOPERATIVE MANAGEMENT

- Conservative management is the mainstay of treatment for the majority of proximal humerus fractures, as most are minimally displaced. These injuries have a very low nonunion rate.
- Most patients are able to resume normal activities once fracture healing is achieved. Some loss of motion is typically well tolerated due to the large arc of motion of the shoulder.
- Patients are placed in a sling or shoulder immobilizer for comfort during the first 10 to 14 days. They are instructed to start elbow/wrist/hand range-of-motion (ROM) exercises immediately after injury to prevent stiffness.
- Once pain subsides, patients are encouraged to perform daily gentle ROM exercises of the shoulder such as pendulums.
- When fracture consolidation is evident on follow-up radiographs (typically between 4 and 6 weeks), increased passive and active ROM exercises are added to the therapy regimen.
- By 3 or 4 months, strengthening is begun and resumption of normal daily activities usually achieved.

SURGICAL MANAGEMENT

- Proximal humerus fractures that have significant comminution and displacement are commonly managed by surgical means. In the young population and in those with good bone quality, every effort should be taken to obtain an anatomic reduction and fixation of the fracture.
- Frequently used methods include open reduction internal fixation (ORIF), closed reduction percutaneous pinning (CRPP), and intramedullary nail fixation.
- Prosthetic replacement is considered in three- and four-part fractures, particularly in the elderly with osteoporotic bone and in those with significant head involvement.
- Hemiarthroplasty has been used most commonly but has been met with mixed results. Postoperative ROM and functional outcomes as well as reduction in pain have proven unpredictable, as hemiarthroplasty relies heavily on correct tuberosity positioning and healing.[2,12,18]
- More recently, reverse shoulder arthroplasty (RSA) has been used as primary treatment for these complex injuries. RSA can be an invaluable option in the elderly, osteoporotic patient with a comminuted fracture, where tuberosity reconstruction and healing is felt to be difficult and unpredictable. Inherent in the design of the prosthesis, a good outcome is less dependent on tuberosity quality and healing, allowing for more confidence in reconstruction with varied pathology.[6] The biomechanical advantage of RSA allows the deltoid to take a greater role in arm elevation and abduction.

Preoperative Planning

- Assessment of deltoid function is paramount when deciding whether to perform RSA due to its reliance on deltoid motor function.
- Plain radiographs of the uninvolved arm can be obtained to assist in preoperative planning and templating.
- If ORIF is still being considered in the treatment plan, a CT scan can be useful to evaluate tuberosity and head displacement prior to surgery.

Positioning

- The patient is placed in the beach-chair position with all bony prominences padded appropriately. The affected extremity is draped free to allow uninterrupted access.
- Complete arm extension and adduction should be ensured prior to starting to facilitate glenoid exposure and access to the humeral canal. If a cutout is not present on the bed, then the patient should be moved as far lateral as possible to ensure impingement-free ROM.
- An assistant should be placed behind the shoulder to help with retracting.
- The surgical arm is allowed to rest on a well-padded Mayo stand throughout the case.
- C-arm fluoroscopy is positioned at the head of the bed to allow for intraoperative imaging. The C-arm can be pushed toward the contralateral shoulder to allow uninterrupted access to the surgical field when fluoroscopy is not needed **(FIG 5)**.

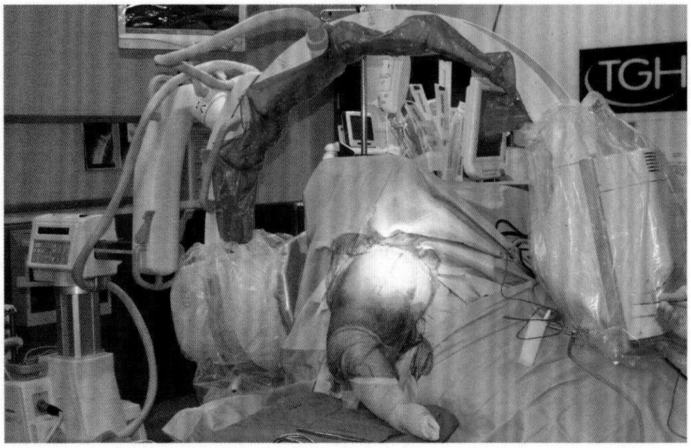

FIG 5 Prior to beginning the procedure, a fluoroscopic C-arm unit is sterilely draped and brought in from the head of the bed to ensure adequate images can be obtained. The C-arm unit is then pushed over toward the contralateral shoulder to allow the surgeon and assistant to stand beside the patient throughout the procedure.

Approach

- The standard deltopectoral approach is used and allows excellent exposure to the glenohumeral joint through an internervous plane (axillary and pectoral nerves).
- A low threshold should be maintained to further extend the incision when appropriate visualization is compromised.
- Bony prominences to include the clavicle, coracoid, and humeral shaft at the deltoid insertion should be palpated.

DELTOPECTORAL APPROACH

- A deltopectoral incision is used, starting about 5 cm medial to the acromioclavicular joint and following the anterior edge of the deltoid toward its insertion on the humerus **(TECH FIG 1A)**.
- If preserved, the cephalic vein is identified and taken medially with the pectoralis major, cauterizing lateral tributaries from the deltoid.
- The subdeltoid, subacromial, and subcoracoid spaces are developed and freed of all adhesions. A Browne deltoid retractor is placed into the subdeltoid space, facilitating exposure of the fracture. Any overlying bursa is removed to improve visualization.
- The long head of biceps tendon is identified and tenodesed to the upper edge of the pectoralis major tendon with a nonabsorbable suture **(TECH FIG 1B)**.

A

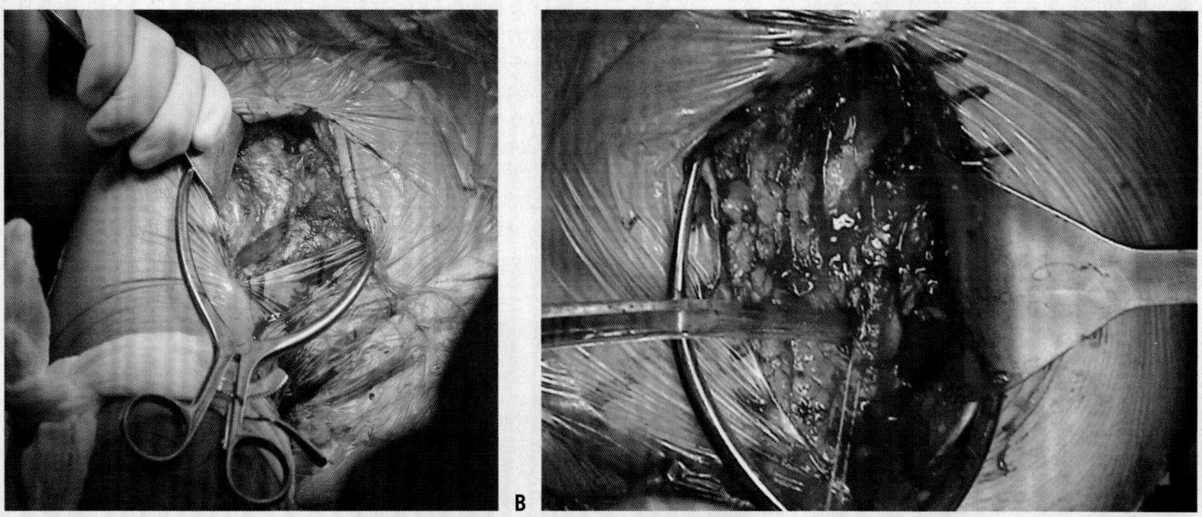

B

TECH FIG 1 **A.** Standard deltopectoral incision following the anterior edge of the deltoid. **B.** The long head of biceps tendon is identified and tenodesed to the upper edge of the pectoralis major tendon.

TUBEROSITY MOBILIZATION IN FOUR-PART FRACTURES

- The biceps tendon is divided above the tenodesis and the rotator interval is opened by following the tendon into the joint. Once exposed, the tendon stump is amputated at its origin on the supraglenoid tubercle.
- The lesser tuberosity with attached subscapularis is identified, mobilized, and a tagging suture placed at the tendon–bone interface to aid in mobilization. The greater tuberosity fragment with attached rotator cuff is identified, and another tagging suture is placed to facilitate mobilization **(TECH FIG 2A)**. Care is taken to release only adhesions that prevent adequate manipulation of the fragments.
- Through the rotator interval, the humeral head fragment and any free comminuted fragments are removed with a rongeur. The metaphyseal bone from the head is saved to be used as bone grafting later in the procedure **(TECH FIG 2B,C)**.
- With tuberosities retracted, any remaining capsule attached to the surgical neck is released using electrocautery and facilitated by progressive external rotation and extension of the adducted arm.

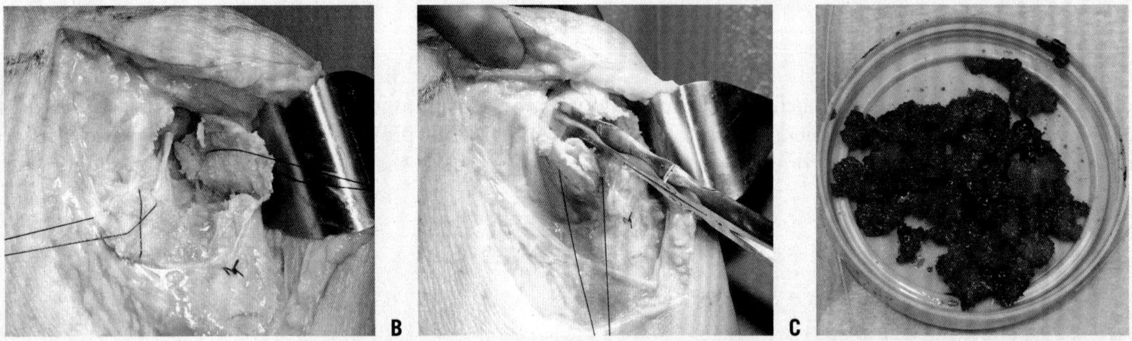

A B C

TECH FIG 2 **A.** Tagging sutures are placed around the tuberosities to aid in mobilization. **B.** The humeral head is removed through the rotator interval with a rongeur. **C.** Metaphyseal bone can be obtained from the removed humeral head and saved for grafting during tuberosity repair.

PREPARATION OF THE GLENOID

- The Browne retractor is removed and the Mayo stand elevated to bring the arm into abduction, relaxing the deltoid and allowing the humerus to retract posteriorly.
- Large, sharp Hohmann retractors are placed superiorly and posteriorly to the glenoid, whereas a Cobra retractor is placed anteriorly.
- A 360-degree release of the labrum/capsule is performed using electrocautery, with special care taken to protect the axillary nerve while resecting the inferior capsule.
- Once excellent exposure is achieved, a 2.5-mm drill bit is used to create a center hole perpendicular to the glenoid face with 10 to 15 degrees of inferior tilt, exiting the anterior scapula **(TECH FIG 3A)**. A depth gauge can be used to ensure that the depth of the drill hole is approximately 30 mm, allowing adequate purchase of the baseplate central screw.
- A 6.5-mm tap is inserted into the center hole. The tap should be firmly seated in bone and should not toggle if manually tested **(TECH FIG 3B)**.
- Sequential cannulated glenoid reamers are placed over the tap, and the glenoid is reamed until bleeding subchondral bone is evident.
- Once the tap is removed, the fixed-angle baseplate with central screw is inserted in line with the central hole. The baseplate should sit flush with the bone and secure fixation is achieved when attempted further advancement of the screw causes the entire scapula to rotate **(TECH FIG 3C)**.

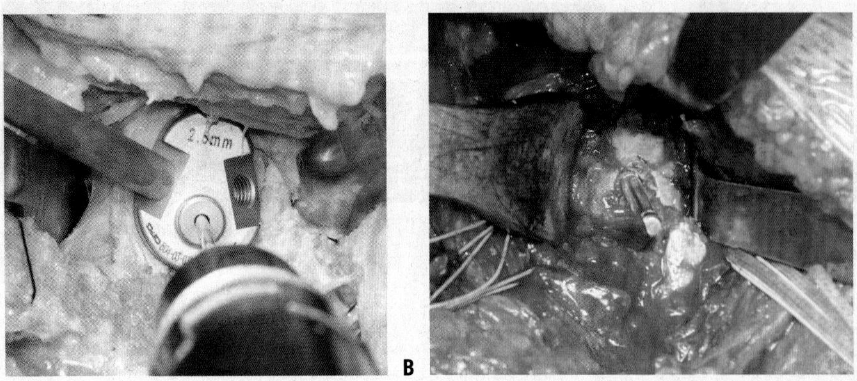

A B

TECH FIG 3 **A.** A 2.5-mm drill bit is used to create a pilot hole with the aid of a drill guide. **B.** A 6.5-mm tap is placed in line with the pilot hole. *(continued)*

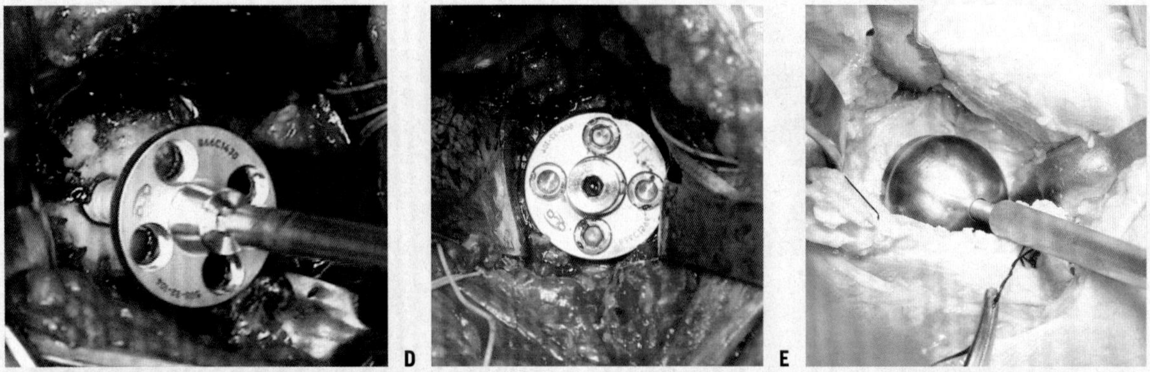

C D E

TECH FIG 3 *(continued)* **C.** The glenoid baseplate is screwed into place and appropriate seating is confirmed with rotation of the scapula. **D.** Locking or nonlocking screws can be placed into the baseplate to enhance stable fixation. **E.** A trial glenosphere is selected based on gender and size. It engages the baseplate via a Morse taper.

- Four 5.0-mm peripheral locking screws are typically placed into the baseplate for additional fixation. An option to use 3.5-mm nonlocking screws is available when inadequate bone stock prevents perpendicular locking screw placement **(TECH FIG 3D)**.
- An appropriate-sized glenosphere trial is selected based on size and quality of the glenoid, soft tissue contracture, and anticipated degree of instability. The glenosphere engages the baseplate via a Morse taper **(TECH FIG 3E)**.

HUMERAL PREPARATION

- Retractors are removed and the arm is placed into adduction and relative extension. The Browne retractor is placed back underneath the deltoid and a large Hohmann placed medially around the calcar, exposing the humerus.
- The lesser tuberosity is fully mobilized with traction sutures **(TECH FIG 4A)**.
- Three no. 5 braided nonabsorbable sutures and two 2-mm nonabsorbable tape sutures are placed at the tendon–bone interface of the greater tuberosity, evenly spaced apart and in alternating sequence **(TECH FIG 4B)**.
- The humeral canal is then sequentially reamed by hand, stopping at the reamer where good cortical chatter is obtained.

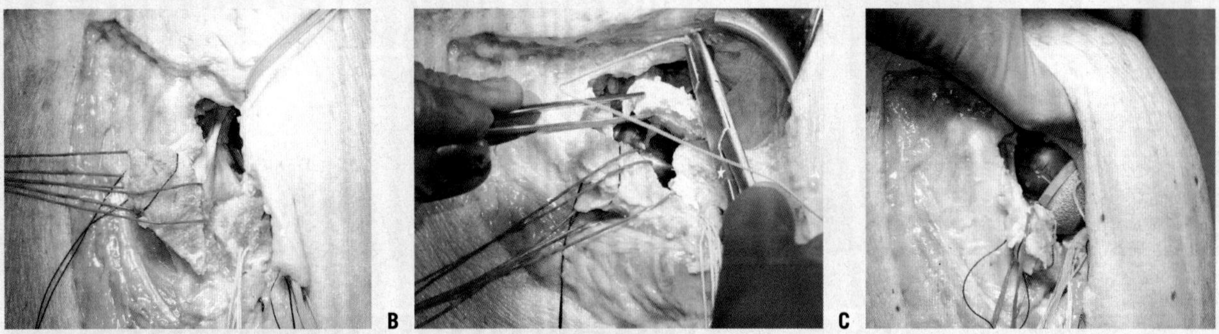

A B C

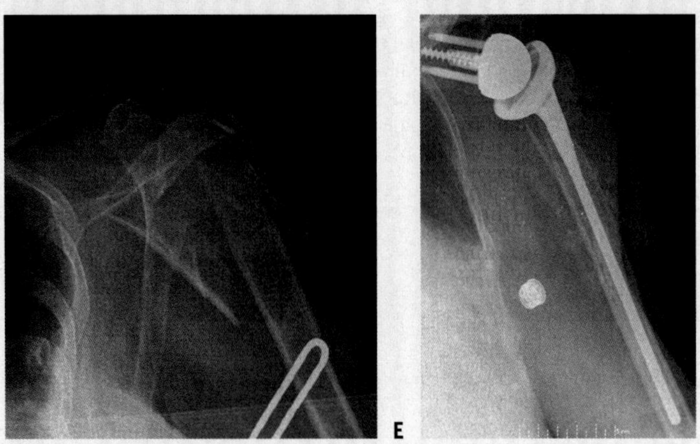

D E

TECH FIG 4 A. Traction sutures (*red*) are placed around the lesser tuberosity at the enthesis. **B.** Three no. 5 nonabsorbable sutures and two 2-mm nonabsorbable tape sutures (*green*) are placed medial to the greater tuberosity in alternating sequence. **C.** The trial glenoid and humeral components have been placed, and stability is assessed through a full ROM. **D.** Proximal humerus fracture with shaft extension and comminution. **E.** The shaft and medial calcar have been reconstructed which serves as an intraoperative template for prosthesis height assessment. *(continued)*

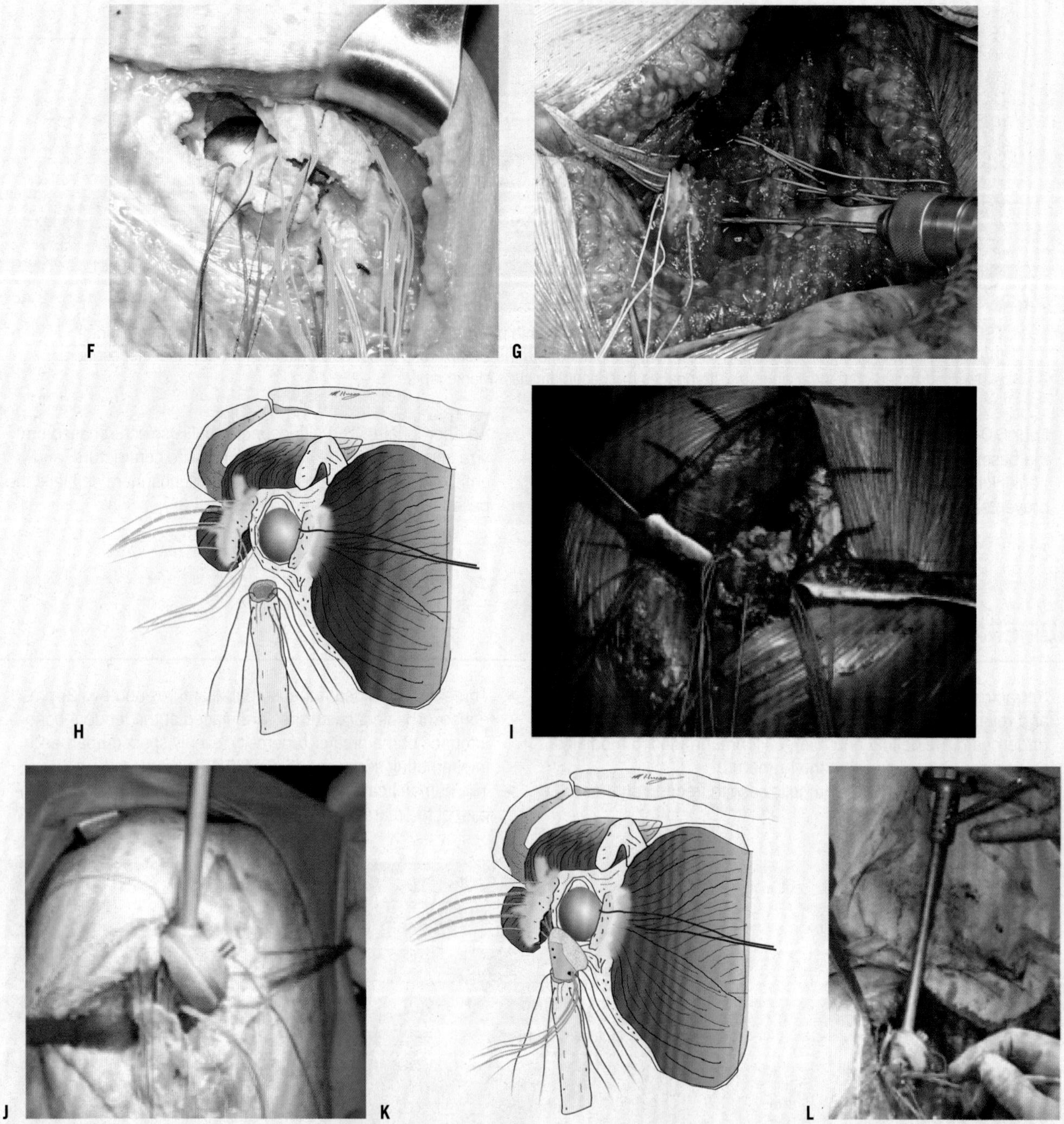
F G H I J K L

TECH FIG 4 *(continued)* **F.** The tuberosities are reapproximated to ensure that they can be reduced around the implant. **G.** Drill used to make holes for three diaphyseal sutures. **H.** Illustration shows lesser tuberosity suture (*blue*), greater tuberosity sutures (*green*), and shaft sutures (*red*) are placed appropriately. **I.** The Black-and-Tan technique for proximal humeral bone grafting is utilized, in which the upper 1 cm of the canal is packed with cancellous bone above the cement mantle. **J,K.** Intraoperative photo and illustration shows the greater tuberosity sutures (*green*) have been placed through the medial eyelet of the real humeral implant prior to cementing. **L.** The real humeral implant is inserted down the cemented canal to the height and version determined during trialing. (Panels H, I, and K copyright the Foundation for Orthopaedic Research and Education, Tampa, FL.)

The real prosthesis is typically undersized by one size to make room for an appropriately thick cement mantle. The appropriate-sized trial is placed down the canal. Alternatively, the real humeral implant can be used to perform the trial reduction with the trial socket insert prior to cementing **(TECH FIG 4C)**.

- The height of the implant can be approximated by two methods. Commonly, the fracture exits medially at the level of the surgical neck, and if the calcar is intact, the humeral socket can be allowed to sit against it, providing a close estimate of normal height. If the calcar is disrupted, then every attempt should be taken to reconstruct it to serve as a guide in height reconstruction **(TECH FIG 4D,E)**.
- Another method that can be employed when significant comminution and shaft extension is present is to obtain bilateral full length humeral radiographs with a radiographic ruler to approximate humeral length on the injured side. The uninvolved humeral length is measured from the lateral epicondyle of the distal humerus to the top of the greater tuberosity. Next, the length from the proximal shaft fracture to the lateral epicondyle is measured, and this is subtracted from the uninvolved humeral measurement. The difference is the expected length that should be restored to the proximal shaft, giving a good estimate of humeral height reconstruction.
- Humeral version is obtained using an alignment guide rod, placing the implant into 30 degrees of retroversion relative to the forearm. The humeral socket liner trial is then chosen from a variety of sizes and constraint.
- Retractors are removed and a trial reduction is performed, allowing soft tissue tension to dictate prosthesis height relative to the shaft. The tuberosities are brought around the trial implant, approximating their normal configuration **(TECH FIG 4F)**. Ideally, the trial will verify that the tuberosities can be anatomically reduced and repaired.
- The prosthesis is shucked laterally to assess the tension at the glenohumeral interface. If excessive looseness is encountered, the humeral socket liner trial can be exchanged for a thicker size or the glenosphere can be upsized. Care should be taken when increasing component size, as it may prevent anatomic tuberosity reconstruction. ROM may also be sacrificed in favor of stability; therefore, forward elevation should be checked whenever trial components are changed to ensure that there has not been significant loss of motion.
- Fluoroscopy is used to ensure that the scapulohumeral arch is restored and that the sphere and socket are well aligned. Once height is deemed appropriate, the humeral stem is marked at the proximal aspect of the fractured shaft to serve as a reference during final stem implantation.
- Next, the trial components are removed and the real glenosphere is placed onto the baseplate. The glenosphere is locked into place with a central set screw.
- The humeral canal is irrigated and prepared for cementing. A cement restrictor is inserted 1.5 cm below the estimated tip of the implant.
- Three drill holes are placed along the anterolateral proximal humeral diaphysis and three no. 5 braided nonabsorbable sutures are passed through the drill holes **(TECH FIG 4G,H)**. These sutures will be used to fix the tuberosities to the shaft once the stem is implanted.
- The deep ends of the five greater tuberosity sutures are next placed through the medial hole of the final humeral implant and set aside while the cement is prepared.
- Antibiotic-containing cement is pressurized down the canal with the use of a cement gun until cement is extruding from the proximal portion of the canal. The Black-and-Tan technique for proximal humeral bone grafting, in which the upper 1 cm of the canal is packed with cancellous bone above the cement mantle to aid in tuberosity healing, is performed **(TECH FIG 4I)**.
- The humeral stem with medial sutures already passed is then introduced into the canal to the trial determined appropriate depth marked on the prosthesis **(TECH FIG 4J,K)**.
- The version guide attached to the stem is used to ensure the implant is in 30 degrees of retroversion relative to the forearm **(TECH FIG 4L)**.
- Once the cement has appropriately cured, the prosthesis is reduced again with the trial socket liner. Stability and motion are again verified before final insertion of the real humeral socket liner.

SUTURE AND TUBEROSITY MANAGEMENT

- The three no. 5 braided nonabsorbable suture limbs of the greater tuberosity that were passed through the medial hole at the neck of the prosthesis are then passed through the bone–tendon interface at the lesser tuberosity spaced evenly apart **(TECH FIG 5A)**.
- More bone graft taken from the humeral head is packed around the shaft–implant interface. The bone graft provides an optimal environment to promote tuberosity healing once the tuberosities are reduced into place.
- The two 2-mm nonabsorable tape sutures around the greater tuberosity that were not shuttled around the lesser tuberosity are tied, to reduce the greater tuberosity to the prosthesis **(TECH FIG 5B)**. Other suture eyelets around the humeral socket are frequently used to assist in tuberosity repair around the implant.
- Next, the inner limbs of the three no. 5 shaft sutures are passed through the cuff superior to the tuberosities. Typically, the lateral two sutures are passed above the greater tuberosity through the supraspinatus and infraspinatus tendons. The medial suture is placed through the subscapularis tendon superior to the lesser tuberosity **(TECH FIG 5C)**.
- Once the greater tuberosity has been reduced, the three no. 5 greater tuberosity sutures that were shuttled around the lesser tuberosity are tied sequentially. These sutures reduce the lesser tuberosity and cerclage both tuberosities to the stem, providing strong fixation about the porous coated humeral socket **(TECH FIG 5D,E)**.
- The vertical fixation sutures are then tied, securing the tuberosities to the shaft, creating a circumferential cross-hatch construct compressing the fragments to the underlying bone graft and prosthesis **(TECH FIG 5F,G)**.
- Final intraoperative motion is assessed, followed by fluoroscopic imaging is performed to assess component positioning and tuberosity reduction **(TECH FIG 5H)**.
- The wound is closed in layers, with the subcutaneous tissue being closed with 2-0 absorbable suture. The skin is closed with a running subcuticular 3-0 monofilament suture.

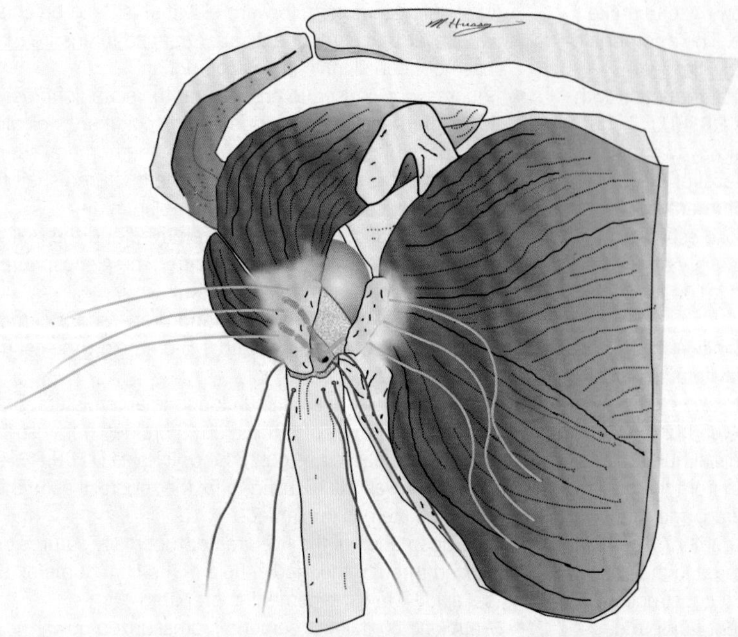

A

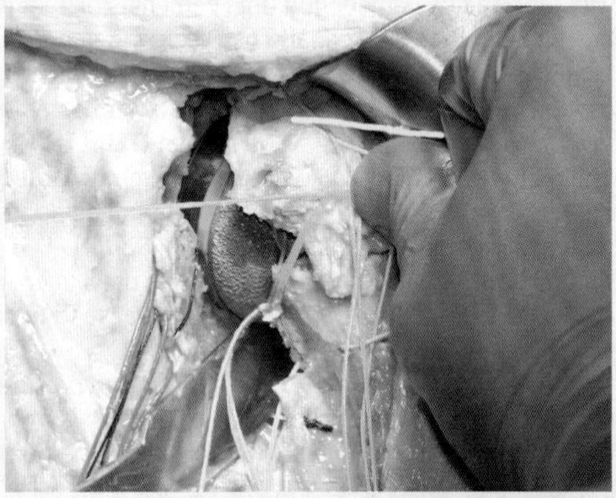

B

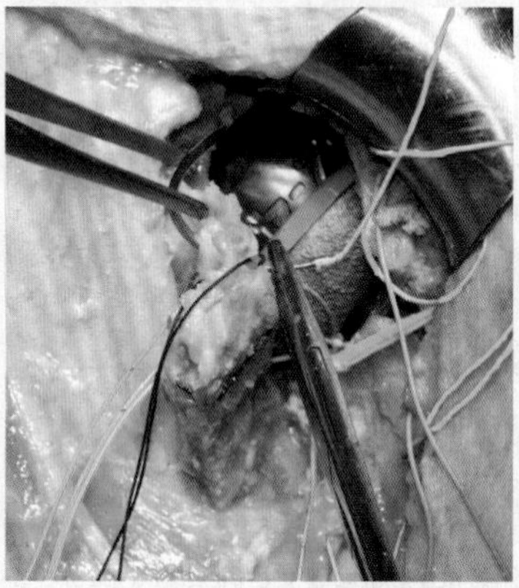

C

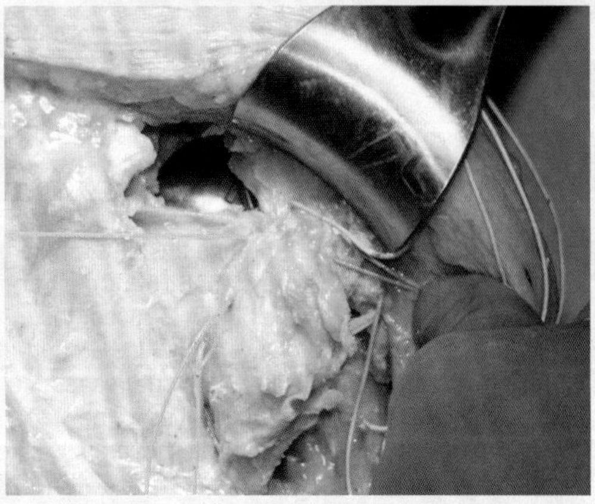

D

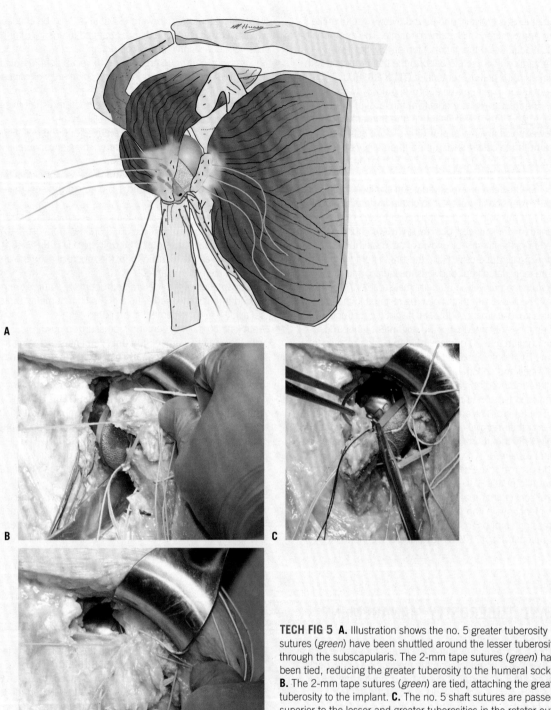

TECH FIG 5 **A.** Illustration shows the no. 5 greater tuberosity sutures (*green*) have been shuttled around the lesser tuberosity through the subscapularis. The 2-mm tape sutures (*green*) have been tied, reducing the greater tuberosity to the humeral socket. **B.** The 2-mm tape sutures (*green*) are tied, attaching the greater tuberosity to the implant. **C.** The no. 5 shaft sutures are passed superior to the lesser and greater tuberosities in the rotator cuff. **D,E.** Intraoperative photo and illustration shows the no. 5 greater tuberosity sutures (*green*) are tied, cerclaging the lesser and greater tuberosities to the implant. *(continued)*

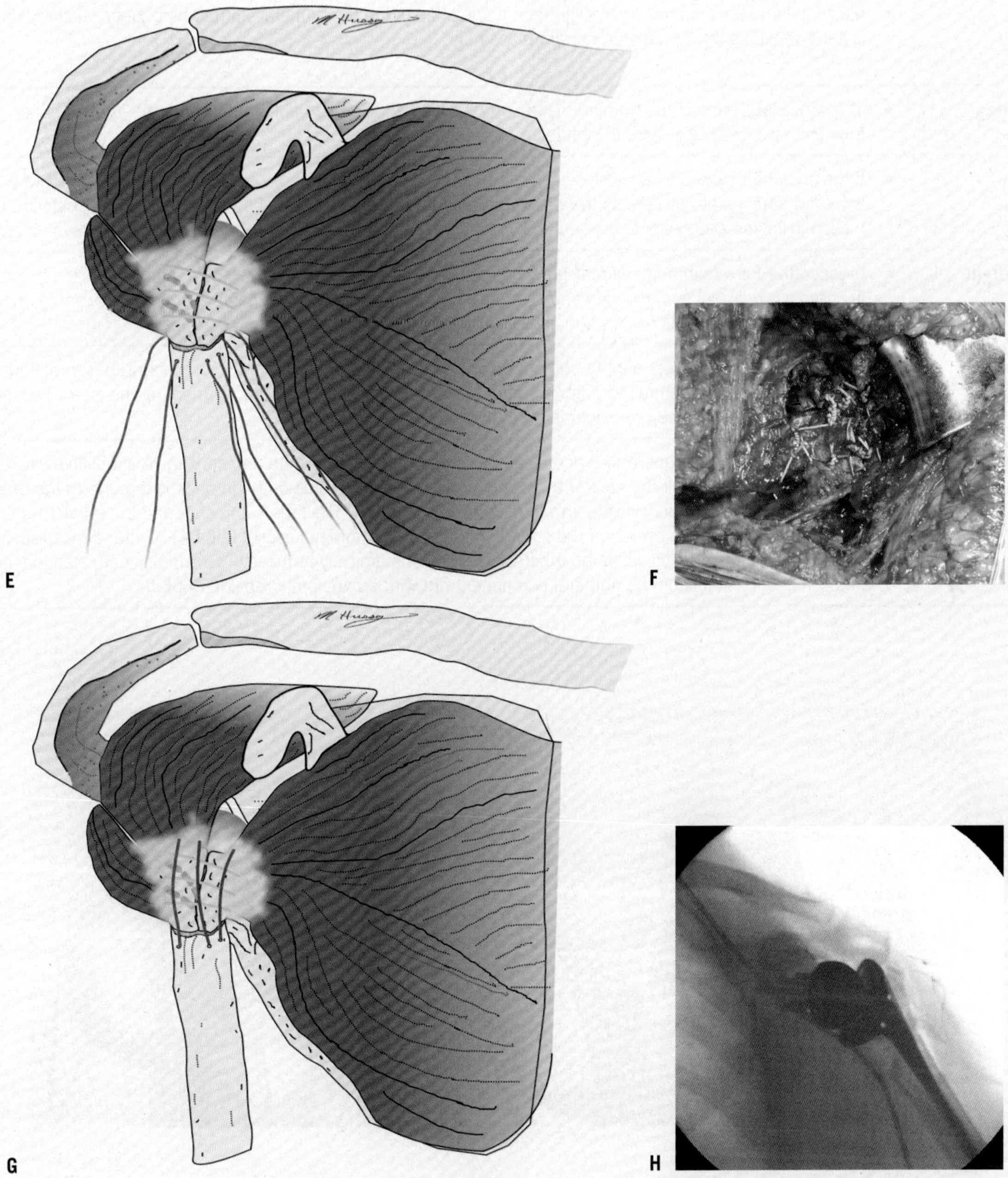

TECH FIG 5 *(continued)* **F,G.** Intraoperative photo and illustration shows final repair construct demonstrating horizontal cerclage sutures and vertical shaft sutures tied providing secure fixation of the tuberosities to the implant and shaft. **H.** Intraoperative fluoroscopic image of final repair. (Panels A, E, and G copyright the Foundation for Orthopaedic Research and Education, Tampa, FL.)

Pearls and Pitfalls

Humeral Component Version	• Most implant systems provide an alignment guide attached to the humeral stem to help judge version. The forearm is a convenient guide to assist in correct placement.
Bone Grafting	• The cancellous bone of the humeral head can be saved and used as autograft around the implant, shaft, and tuberosities, providing a more favorable environment for healing.
Soft Tissue Tensioning	• If the implant is placed in excessive tightness, ROM will be restricted postoperatively. The passive ROM that is achieved intraoperatively reflects the maximum amount of active ROM that should be expected postoperatively. If motion is limited secondary to overstuffing, consideration should be given to downsizing the humeral liner.
Implant Height	• Preoperative full-length humeral radiographs of the uninvolved side can be used as a template to restore implant height in cases of significant comminution and shaft involvement. The use of intraoperative fluoroscopy can be an invaluable aid to reconstruct the tuberosities and achieve appropriate implant height.
Suture Management	• Place all tuberosity sutures prior to cementing and implantation of the humeral component. It is important to pass the greater tuberosity sutures through the medial eyelet of the implant prior to cementing the stem. The use of large needles helps facilitate suture placement around the tuberosities.
Tuberosity Repair	• Anatomic repair of the tuberosities is critical for optimal shoulder function and stability. A simplified way to reapproximate and repair the greater tuberosity around the lateral side of the implant is to perform the repair while the humerus is dislocated with the arm in maximum adduction. The tape sutures around the greater tuberosity are shuttled through the rim eyelets at the superior aspect of the humeral socket **(FIG 6A)**. Under direct visualization, these tape sutures are tied while the tuberosity is held anatomically reduced. The supraspinatus tendon–bone junction should sit just off the humeral component rim with an anatomic repair **(FIG 6B,C)**.

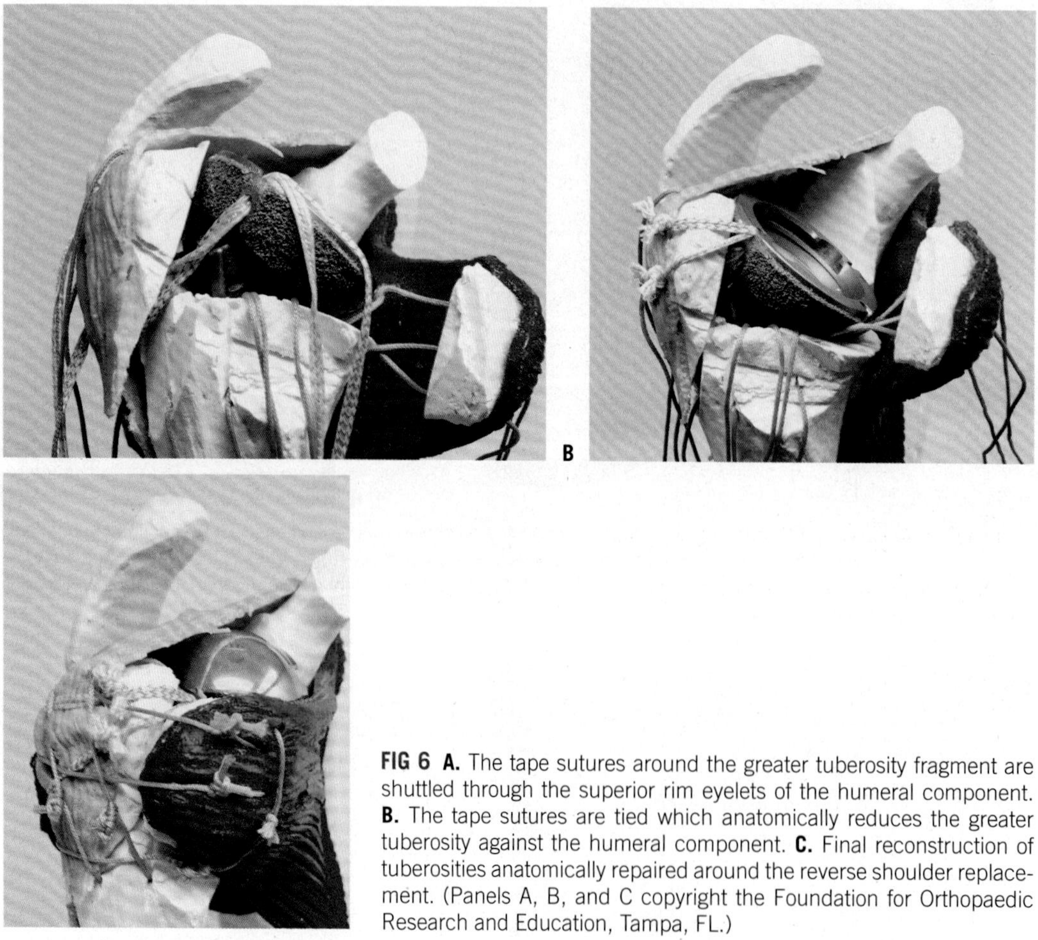

A B C

FIG 6 A. The tape sutures around the greater tuberosity fragment are shuttled through the superior rim eyelets of the humeral component. **B.** The tape sutures are tied which anatomically reduces the greater tuberosity against the humeral component. **C.** Final reconstruction of tuberosities anatomically repaired around the reverse shoulder replacement. (Panels A, B, and C copyright the Foundation for Orthopaedic Research and Education, Tampa, FL.)

POSTOPERATIVE CARE

- Regional anesthesia of the operative extremity is frequently used by the anesthesia team to assist in postoperative pain management.
- The patient wears a shoulder immobilizer during the first 6 weeks, coming out only for hygiene purposes and to perform gentle pendulum exercises. Elbow, wrist, and hand exercises are encouraged daily.
- The subcuticular suture is removed in 10 to 14 days at the first postoperative visit.
- After 6 weeks, the immobilizer is discontinued and a sling is worn in public only. Active-assisted ROM exercises are instituted, which includes supine active-assisted forward elevation. Patients are instructed not to lift anything heavier than a telephone receiver.
- At 3 months, active ROM is allowed as tolerated. Light strengthening is begun and progressively increased over several weeks.
- Radiographs of the shoulder are taken at the 2-week, 3-month, 6-month, and 1-year follow-up visits to evaluate tuberosity position and healing.
- Maximal improvement in function is typically expected about 1 year after surgery.

OUTCOMES

- Despite the lack of long-term published studies, there is increasing support for the use of RSA in management of acute fractures of the proximal humerus. Multiple recent studies have demonstrated average American Shoulder and Elbow Surgeons (ASES) scores of 70 with low reoperation and complication rates when RSA is used for management of acute proximal humerus fractures.[15,20,21]
- Levy et al[14] showed that RSA can provide a reliable salvage procedure for failed hemiarthroplasty by improving ROM, functional outcome, and patient satisfaction at short-term follow-up.
- RSA appears to reliably restore motion and function when used for acute proximal humerus fractures.[13] Importantly, restored forward elevation and abduction can be expected, regardless of tuberosity healing. However, every attempt should be taken to anatomically repair the tuberosities around the prosthesis, as shoulder rotation depends more heavily on tuberosity consolidation.
- Chun et al[5] was able to demonstrate a significant improvement in external rotation in patients who had radiographic tuberosity healing postoperatively, compared to the patients that failed to heal their tuberosities.
- Gallinet et al[7] evaluated their outcomes of RSA in patients in which an anatomic repair of the tuberosities had been performed compared to a group without repair. Their results showed that a consolidated anatomic repair led to significantly better rotation and functional outcome scores compared to nonrepair.
- RSA has also demonstrated value in maintaining independent living in the elderly population. Wolfensperger et al[21] found that 91% of patients undergoing RSA for fracture returned to their preinjury level of independence at 1 year postsurgery. Those patients also demonstrated Constant-Murley scores reaching 87% of their uninjured side.
- We evaluated our results of RSA for acute proximal humerus fractures in 18 patients with an average follow-up of 27 months and have experienced very promising outcomes with these complicated injuries. At final follow-up, the mean active forward elevation, abduction, external rotation, and internal rotation was found to be 139, 112, 37.5 degrees, and L1, respectively. The mean ASES score was 69.9, whereas the mean visual analog scale pain score was 1.7 in this patient cohort.
- Recent studies comparing RSA to hemiarthroplasty for these injuries appear to show superior short-to-midterm results for those treated with RSA.[3,6,8]
- Although short- and midterm studies appear to be favorable, long-term prospective studies are needed to fully assess the outcomes of RSA in this injury type. Currently, a multicenter randomized controlled trial, the ReSHaPE trial is underway to compare outcomes of RSA to nonoperative management in patients with three- and four-part proximal humerus fractures, who are older than the age of 70 years.[20]

COMPLICATIONS

- Infection
- Dislocation
- Neurapraxia
- Complex regional pain syndrome
- Acromial fracture
- Scapular notching with baseplate failure
- Tuberosity nonunion/malunion

REFERENCES

1. Baron JA, Barrett JA, Karagas MR. The epidemiology of peripheral fractures. Bone 1996;18(3 suppl):209S–213S.
2. Boileau P, Krishnan SG, Tinsi L, et al. Tuberosity malposition and migration: reasons for poor outcomes after hemiarthroplasty for displaced fractures of the proximal humerus. J Shoulder Elbow Surg 2002;11(5):401–412.
3. Boyle MJ, Youn SM, Frampton CM, et al. Functional outcomes of reverse shoulder arthroplasty compared with hemiarthroplasty for acute proximal humeral fractures. J Shoulder Elbow Surg 2013;22(1):32–37.
4. Burkhead WZ Jr, Scheinberg RR, Box G. Surgical anatomy of the axillary nerve. J Shoulder Elbow Surg 1992;1(1):31–36.
5. Chun YM, Kim DS, Lee DH, et al. Reverse shoulder arthroplasty for four-part proximal humerus fracture in elderly patients: can a healed tuberosity improve the functional outcomes? J Shoulder Elbow Surg 2017;26(7):1216–1221.
6. Cuff DJ, Pupello D. Comparison of hemiarthroplasty and reverse shoulder arthroplasty for the treatment of proximal humeral fractures in elderly patients. J Bone Joint Surg Am 2013;95(22):2050–2055.
7. Gallinet D, Adam A, Gasse N, et al. Improvement in shoulder rotation in complex shoulder fractures treated by reverse shoulder arthroplasty. J Shoulder Elbow Surg 2013;22(1):38–44.
8. Garrigues GE, Johnston PS, Pepe MD, et al. Hemiarthroplasty versus reverse total shoulder arthroplasty for acute proximal humerus fractures in elderly patients. Orthopedics 2012;35(5):e703–e708.
9. Gerber C, Schneeberger AG, Vinh TS. The arterial vascularization of the humeral head. An anatomical study. J Bone Joint Surg Am 1990;72(10):1486–1494.
10. Hertel R, Hempfing A, Stiehler M, et al. Predictors of humeral head ischemia after intracapsular fracture of the proximal humerus. J Shoulder Elbow Surg 2004;13(4):427–433.
11. Iannotti JP, Gabriel JP, Schneck SL, et al. The normal glenohumeral relationships. An anatomical study of one hundred and forty shoulders. J Bone Joint Surg Am 1992;74(4):491–500.

12. Kralinger F, Schwaiger R, Wambacher M, et al. Outcome after primary hemiarthroplasty for fracture of the head of the humerus. A retrospective multicentre study of 167 patients. J Bone Joint Surg Br 2004;86(2):217–219.
13. Lenarz C, Shishani Y, McCrum C, et al. Is reverse shoulder arthroplasty appropriate for the treatment of fractures in the older patient? Early observations. Clin Orthop Relat Res 2011;469(12):3324–3331.
14. Levy J, Frankle M, Mighell M, et al. The use of the reverse shoulder prosthesis for the treatment of failed hemiarthroplasty for proximal humeral fracture. J Bone Joint Surg Am 2007;89(2):292–300.
15. Longo UG, Petrillo S, Berton A, et al. Reverse total shoulder arthroplasty for the management of fractures of the proximal humerus: a systematic review. Musculoskelet Surg 2016;100(2):83–91.
16. Murachovsky J, Ikemoto RY, Nascimento LG, et al. Pectoralis major tendon reference (PMT): a new method for accurate restoration of humeral length with hemiarthroplasty for fracture. J Shoulder Elbow Surg 2006;15(6):675–678.
17. Neer CS II. Displaced proximal humeral fractures. I. Classification and evaluation. J Bone Joint Surg Am 1970;52(6):1077–1089.
18. Noyes MP, Kleinhenz B, Markert RJ, et al. Functional and radiographic long-term outcomes of hemiarthroplasty for proximal humeral fractures. J Shoulder Elbow Surg 2011;20(3):372–377.
19. Pearl ML, Volk AG. Retroversion of the proximal humerus in relationship to prosthetic replacement arthroplasty. J Shoulder Elbow Surg 1995;4(4):286–289.
20. Smith GCS, Bateman E, Cass B, et al. Reverse shoulder arthroplasty for the treatment of proximal humeral fractures in the elderly (ReShAPE trial): study protocol for a multicentre combined randomised controlled and observational trial. Trials 2017;18(1):91.
21. Wolfensperger F, Grüninger P, Dietrich M, et al. Reverse shoulder arthroplasty for complex fractures of the proximal humerus in elderly patients: impact on the level of independency, early function, and pain medication. J Shoulder Elbow Surg 2017;26(8):1462–1468.

CHAPTER 9

Plate Fixation of Humeral Shaft Fractures

Eric M. Black, Matthew J. Garberina, and Charles L. Getz

DEFINITION

- Humeral shaft fractures, which account for about 3% of adult fractures, usually result from a direct blow or indirect twisting injury to the brachium.
- These injuries are most commonly treated nonoperatively with a prefabricated fracture brace. The humerus is the most freely movable long bone, and anatomic reduction is not required.
- Patients often can tolerate up to 20 degrees of anterior angulation, 30 degrees of varus angulation, and 3 cm of shortening without significant functional loss.
- There are, however, several indications for surgical treatment of humeral shaft fractures:
  - Open fracture
  - Bilateral humeral shaft fractures or polytrauma; floating elbow
  - Segmental fracture
  - Inability to maintain acceptable alignment with closed treatment (ie, angulation >20 degrees, complete or near complete fracture displacement with lack of bony contact)—seen more commonly with transverse fractures **(FIG 1)**
  - Humeral shaft nonunion
  - Pathologic fractures
  - Arterial or brachial plexus injury
- Open reduction with internal plate fixation requires extensive dissection and operative skill. However, it offers advantages over intramedullary fixation because the rotator cuff is not violated, which leads to improved postoperative shoulder function.[3]

ANATOMY

- The humeral shaft is defined using key landmarks: the area between the upper margin of the pectoralis major tendon and the supracondylar ridge.[5]
- The blood supply of the humeral shaft comes from the posterior humeral circumflex vessels and branches of the brachial and profunda brachial arteries.
- The radial nerve and profunda brachial artery pass through the triangular interval (bordered superiorly by the teres major, medially by the medial head of the triceps, and laterally by the humeral shaft). The nerve then transverses from medial to lateral behind the humeral shaft and travels distally to a location between the brachialis and brachioradialis muscles **(FIG 2)**.
- The musculocutaneous nerve lies on the undersurface of the biceps muscle and terminates distally as the lateral antebrachial cutaneous nerve.
- The humeral shaft has anteromedial, anterolateral, and posterior surfaces. Proximal and midshaft fractures are more amenable to plating on the anterolateral surface, whereas distal fractures often require posterior plate fixation.

PATHOGENESIS

- Humeral shaft fractures occur after both direct and indirect injuries. Direct blows to the brachium can fracture the humeral shaft in a transverse pattern, often with a butterfly fragment. Injuries with high degrees of energy often result in a greater degree of fracture comminution.
- Indirect injuries, such as those that can occur with activities such as arm wrestling, often involve a twisting mechanism and result in a spiral fracture pattern. Higher energy injuries may result in muscle interposition between the fracture fragments, which can inhibit reduction and healing.
- A study of 240 humeral shaft fractures revealed radial nerve palsies in 42 patients, for an overall rate of 18% (17% in closed injuries). Fractures in the midshaft were more likely

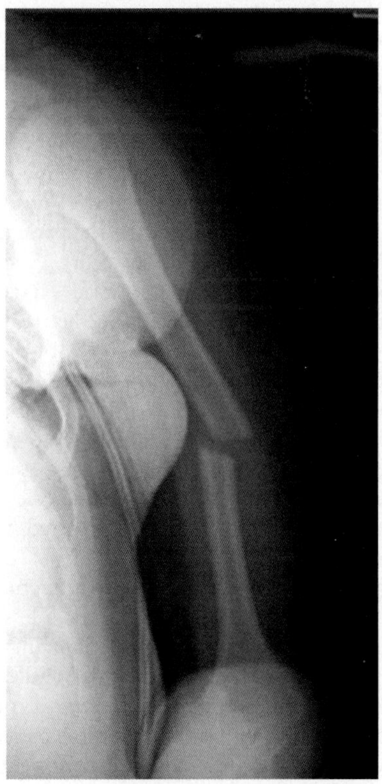

FIG 1 X-ray of an unstable transverse humeral shaft fracture.

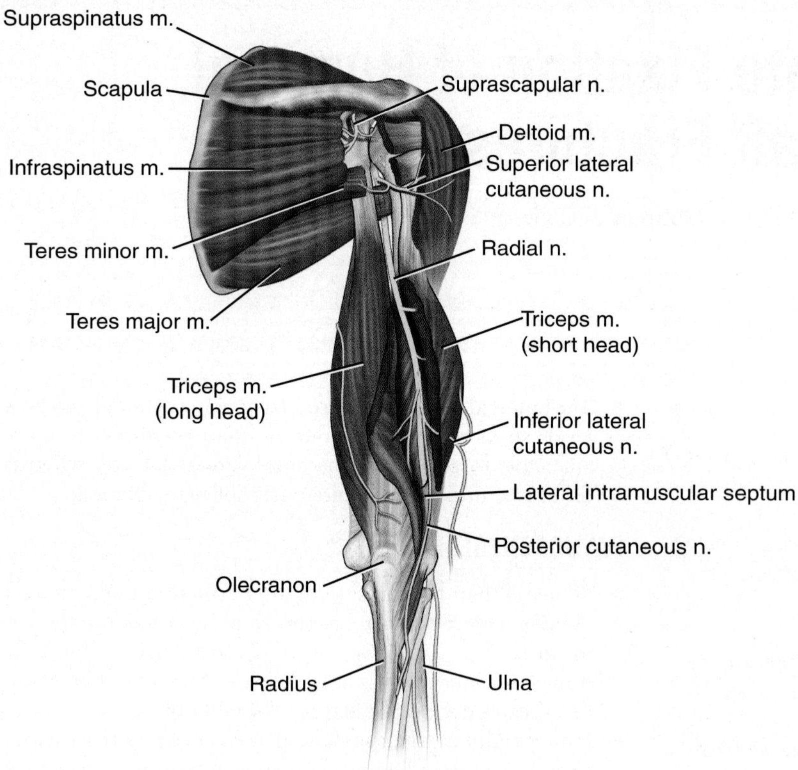

FIG 2 The course of the radial nerve along the position humerus is illustrated.

to have concomitant radial nerve palsy. Twenty five of these patients had complete recovery in a range of 1 day to 10 months. Ten patients did not have radial nerve recovery. Median and ulnar nerve palsies were seen very rarely, mostly in patients with open fractures.[7]

- Concomitant vascular injuries are present in about 3% of patients with humeral shaft fractures.

NATURAL HISTORY

- Most humeral shaft fractures heal with nonoperative management. The most common treatment method is initial splinting from shoulder to wrist, followed by application of a prefabricated fracture brace when the patient is comfortable, usually within 2 weeks of the injury.
- Studies by Sarmiento and coauthors[10,11] have shown the effectiveness of functional bracing in the treatment of humeral shaft fractures. Nonunion rates with this method of treatment are in the 4% range, lower than seen when treating with external fixators, plates, or intramedullary nails.
- Closed fractures with initial radial nerve palsy can be observed, with expected recovery over a period of 3 to 6 months. Late-developing radial nerve palsies may require surgical exploration in cases of suspected radian nerve entrapment.
- Angulation of the humeral shaft after fracture healing is expected and is well tolerated when it is less than 20 to 30 degrees. Varus deformity is most common.[10]
- Adjacent joint stiffness of the shoulder and elbow also is common. If the situation dictates treatment, physical therapy reliably restores joint motion in these patients.
- Relative contraindications to closed treatment include bilateral humeral shaft fractures or patients with polytrauma who require an intact brachium to ambulate. Transverse fractures and those with significant muscle imposition also are more amenable to operative fixation.[11] Higher level athletes and manual laborers may experience faster return to sport or work with early operative intervention, and this should be taken into account on an individualized basis.

PATIENT HISTORY AND PHYSICAL FINDINGS

- The examining physician must perform a complete examination of the affected limb to rule out concomitant injuries.
- The skin should be thoroughly evaluated for evidence of an open fracture. This includes examination of the axilla. Entry and exit wounds are sought in gunshot victims. Swelling is common, and the patient may have an obvious deformity.
- The patient often braces the affected limb to his or her side, making evaluation of shoulder and elbow range of motion difficult. Bony prominences should be gently palpated to evaluate for other injuries, such as an olecranon fracture.
- Evaluate the appearance and skeletal stability of the forearm to rule out the presence of a coexisting both-bone forearm fracture ("floating elbow"). This finding necessitates operative fixation of humeral, radial, and ulnar fractures.
- Determine the vascular status of the upper extremity by palpating the radial and ulnar pulses at the wrist. Compare these findings with the unaffected limb. Selected cases may require Doppler arterial examination.[2] If there is suspicion for arterial injury, a CT angiogram may be ordered.
- A complete neurologic assessment is necessary, with particular attention focused on the status of the radial nerve. This structure is at risk proximally, as it passes posteriorly to the humeral shaft after emerging from the triangular interval, as well as distally, as it lies adjacent to the supracondylar ridge (near the location of the Holstein-Lewis distal one-third spiral humeral shaft fracture).

- Examine sensory function in the first dorsal web space, wrist extension, and thumb interphalangeal joint hyperextension to determine the functional status of the radial nerve.

IMAGING AND OTHER DIAGNOSTIC STUDIES

- At least two plain radiographs at 90-degree angles to each other are necessary to evaluate the displacement, shortening, and comminution of the humeral shaft fracture.
- Radiographic views of the shoulder and elbow are necessary to rule out proximal extension of the shaft fracture or concomitant elbow injury (ie, olecranon fracture). This is especially important in high-energy injuries.
- If swelling or evidence of skeletal instability about the forearm is present, dedicated forearm radiographs can determine the presence of a floating elbow (ie, ipsilateral humeral shaft fracture plus both-bone forearm fractures).

DIFFERENTIAL DIAGNOSIS

- Distal humerus fracture
- Proximal humerus fracture
- Elbow dislocation
- Shoulder dislocation

NONOPERATIVE MANAGEMENT

- Most isolated humeral shaft fractures can be treated nonoperatively. Initial treatment can vary with fracture location and involves splinting in either a posterior elbow or coaptation splint. The elbow is positioned in 90 degrees of flexion. An isolated humeral shaft fracture rarely necessitates an overnight hospital stay.
- In the past, definitive nonoperative treatment involved coaptation splinting or the use of hanging arm casts. Currently, functional fracture bracing provides adequate bony alignment, whereas local muscle compression and fracture motion promote osteogenesis. These braces provide soft tissue compression and allow functional use of the extremity.[11]
- Timing of brace application depends on the degree of swelling and patient discomfort. On average, the brace is applied about 2 weeks after the injury. A collar and cuff help with initial patient comfort and should be worn during recumbency until the fracture heals.
- The brace often requires frequent retightening over the first 2 weeks as swelling subsides. Active and passive elbow and wrist range-of-motion exercises out of the sling are encouraged.
- Functional bracing requires that the patient be able to sit erect, and weight bearing on the humerus is not allowed. The level of humeral shaft fracture does not preclude the use of functional bracing, even if the fracture line extends above or below the brace.
- Anatomic alignment of the humerus rarely is achieved, with varus deformity most common. However, patients often are able to tolerate some bony angulation and still perform activities of daily living after injury. A cosmetic deformity rarely exists. Severe varus deformity may hinder the ability to reach overhead, and allow hand-to-mouth activities.
- Pendulum exercises are encouraged as soon as possible postinjury. Active shoulder elevation and abduction are avoided until bony healing has occurred to prevent fracture angulation. The surgeon obtains radiographs after brace application and again 1 week later. If alignment is acceptable, repeat radiographs are obtained at 3- to 4- week intervals until fracture healing occurs.[10,11] Initially, radiographs in brace are most helpful to determine fracture stability in the brace.

SURGICAL MANAGEMENT

- Certain humeral shaft fractures are not amenable to conservative treatment. Open fractures or high-energy injuries with significant axial distraction are treated with open reduction and internal fixation. Patients with polytrauma, bilateral humeral shaft fractures, vascular injury, or an inability to sit erect are best treated with operative fixation. Unacceptable fracture alignment requires abandonment of nonoperative treatment. Finally, humeral shaft nonunion is a clear indication for open reduction and internal fixation with bone grafting.[4,9]

Preoperative Planning

- The surgeon must review all radiographic images and must rule out ipsilateral elbow or shoulder injury.[1]
- Preoperative radiographs help the surgeon estimate the required plate length. Higher energy injuries with comminution may benefit from plating and supplemental bone grafting. The surgeon must plan for various scenarios based on these studies: Moderate comminution or bone loss can be addressed with cancellous allograft or autograft bone, whereas more extensive bone defects may require strut grafting.
- Proximal and middle-third humeral shaft fractures are addressed using an anterolateral approach. Distal-third humeral shaft fractures often are treated via a posterior approach because the distal humeral shaft is flat posteriorly, making it an ideal location for plate placement.
- Fracture patterns with extension into the proximal humerus can be exposed with a deltopectoral extension to the anterolateral humeral dissection. Often, a long, anatomic proximal humeral locking plate is helpful to ensure adequate superior fixation **(FIG 3)**.
- The surgeon notes any preexisting scars that may affect the desired surgical approach, and neurovascular status is documented, with particular attention to radial nerve function.

Positioning

- Positioning depends on the intended surgical approach. For an anterolateral or medial approach, the patient is brought to the edge of the bed in the supine position. A hand table is attached to the bed, and the patient's injured arm is placed on the hand table in slight abduction **(FIG 4A)**.
- For a posterior approach, the patient can be placed prone or in the lateral decubitus position. A stack of pillows can support the brachium during the procedure **(FIG 4B)**.

Approach

- The approach depends on fracture location and the presence of any previous surgical incisions. The anterolateral and posterior approaches to the humerus are used most commonly for proximal two-thirds and distal third fractures, respectively.
- In patients who have already undergone multiple procedures to the affected extremity, Jupiter[6] recommends consideration of a medial approach to take advantage of virgin tissue planes.

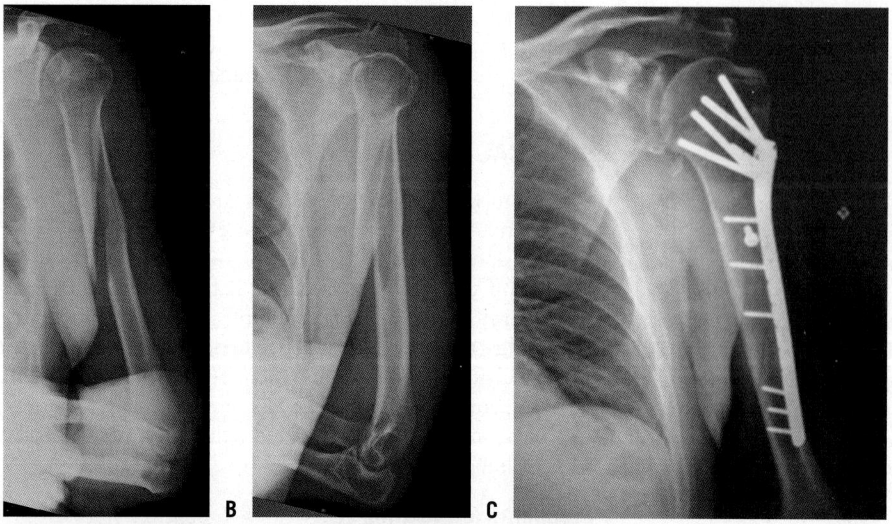

A B C

FIG 3 A. Anteroposterior (AP) and (**B**) lateral views of a humeral shaft fracture with proximal extension. **C.** A deltopectoral approach extended distally into an anterolateral approach allows proper exposure and placement of a long proximal humeral locking plate.

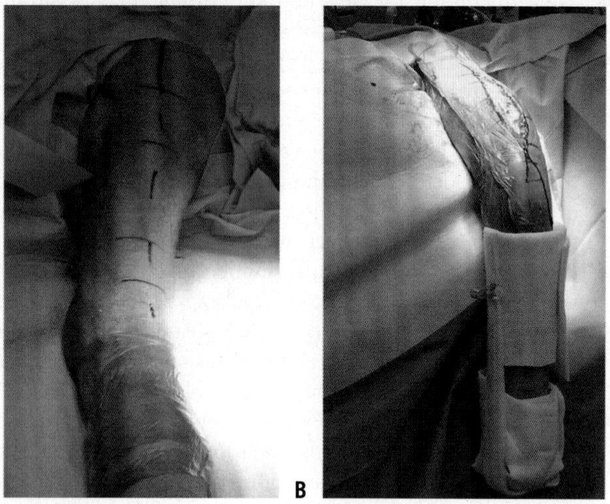

A B

FIG 4 A. Positioning for the anterolateral approach to the humeral shaft with the shoulder abducted and the arm on a hand table. **B.** Positioning for the posterior approach to the humeral shaft with the patient in the lateral decubitus position.

ANTEROLATERAL APPROACH TO THE HUMERUS

- The incision courses over the lateral aspect of the biceps, beginning proximally at the deltoid tubercle and terminating just proximal to the antecubital crease **(TECH FIG 1A)**. For more proximal fractures, the incision may extend proximally toward the coracoid to allow deltopectoral exposure.
- A tourniquet rarely is used because it often limits proximal exposure. The biceps fascia is incised in line with the incision to expose the underlying biceps muscle **(TECH FIG 1B)**.
- The lateral antebrachial cutaneous nerve lies in the distal aspect of the incision and must be protected if exposure extends far distally.
- Bluntly enter the interval between the biceps and brachialis by sweeping a finger from proximal to distal and lateral to medial.
- At the level of the midhumerus, identify the musculocutaneous nerve on the undersurface of the biceps muscle **(TECH FIG 1C)**. Trace this nerve out distally to protect its terminal branch, which forms the lateral antebrachial cutaneous nerve.

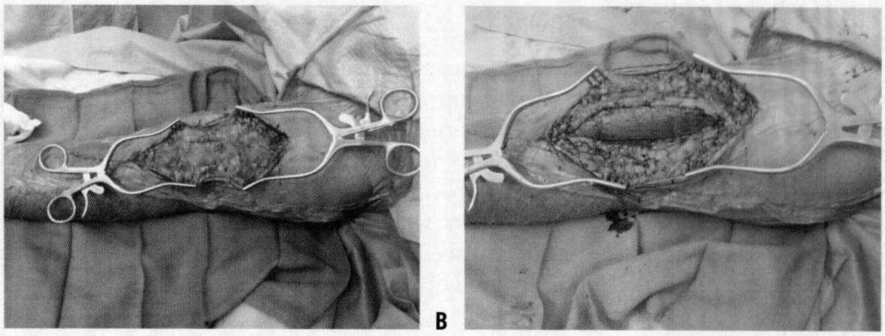

A B

TECH FIG 1 A. Initial incision along the anterolateral brachium with exposure of the biceps fascia. **B.** The biceps fascia is incised in line with the skin incision exposing the underlying biceps muscle. *(continued)*

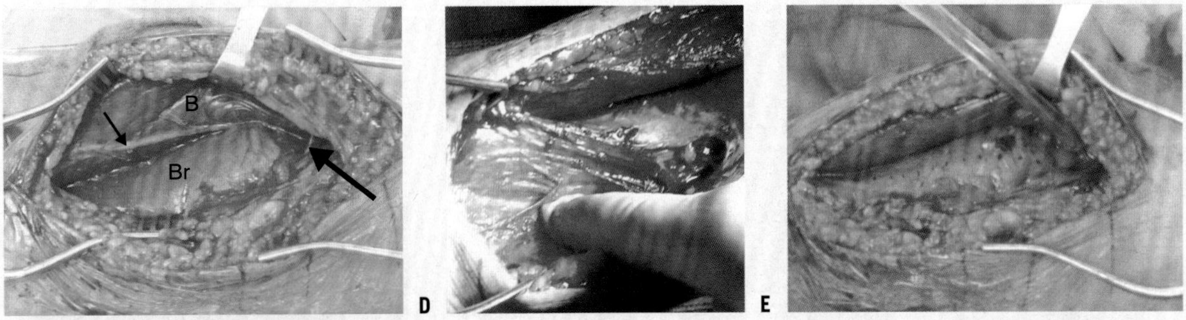

C D E

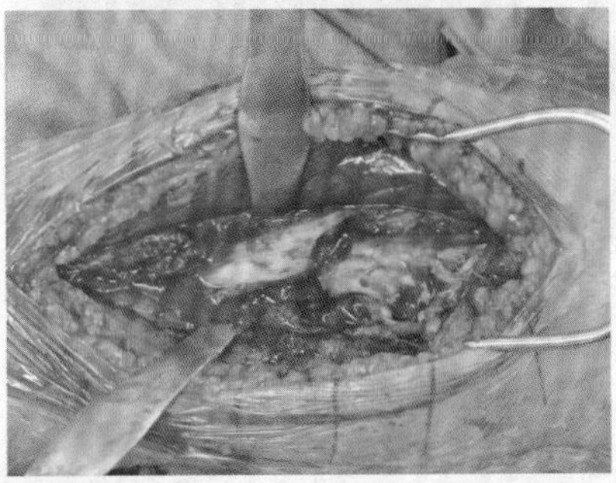

F

TECH FIG 1 *(continued)* **C.** The biceps (*B*) is bluntly lifted up exposing the underlying musculocutaneous nerve (*small arrow*), brachialis muscle (*Br*), and proximal vascular leash (*large arrow*). **D.** Radial nerve in interval between brachialis and brachioradialis. **E.** The brachialis is incised at the interval between its lateral and middle thirds. **F.** The fracture is well visualized through the brachialis split.

- Distally, the interval between the brachialis and brachioradialis is dissected to expose the radial nerve **(TECH FIG 1D)**. Protect the radial nerve with a vessel loop so that it can be identified at all times.
- The brachialis is split in line with its fibers between the medial two-thirds and lateral one-third. This is an internervous plane between the radial nerve laterally and the musculocutaneous nerve medially **(TECH FIG 1E)**.
- Identify the fracture site and remove any hematoma. Sharply remove fragments of periosteum off of the fracture ends to aid in reduction **(TECH FIG 1F)**.

EXPOSURE OF FRACTURE NONUNION

- Exposure of the radial nerve is more challenging, but it is very important in this situation. In many cases, it is best to dissect out the nerve distally in the interval between the brachialis and brachioradialis and proximally medial to the spiral groove. The nerve is then carefully dissected free from the nonunion site.
- Pinpoint the exact location of the nonunion with a no. 15 scalpel.
- The ends of the nonunion can be brought out through the wound, and all fibrous material is extracted.
- After thorough fracture débridement, the amount of bone loss becomes clear. The surgeon can now determine whether standard cancellous bone grafting or strut grafting is necessary. In cases of hypertrophic nonunion, local bone graft and rigid fixation usually facilitate healing without the need for autograft harvest from additional sites.

POSTERIOR APPROACH TO THE HUMERUS

- Make a generous incision over the midline of the posterior arm extending to the olecranon fossa **(TECH FIG 2)**.
- Identify the interval between the long and lateral heads of the triceps proximally. Bluntly dissect this interval, taking the long head medially and the lateral head laterally.
- Distally, several blood vessels cross this plane; they require coagulation before transection.
- Identify the radial nerve proximal to the medial head of the triceps in the spiral groove. Protect the radial nerve throughout the case.
- Split the medial head of the triceps in its midline from proximal to distal to expose the fracture site.
- Alternatively, the entire lateral head of the triceps can be reflected medially and dissection is carried up to the level of the radial nerve. The radial nerve is then mobilized and deep muscular tissue is split in line of the humerus proximally.
- A sterile tourniquet place high in the arm can facilitate dissection and identification of the radial nerve during initial approach, and once the radial nerve is properly identified, the tourniquet is removed and proximal extension is continued. This can allow efficient dissection, nerve identification, and minimization of bleeding from perforating vessels on the surgical approach.

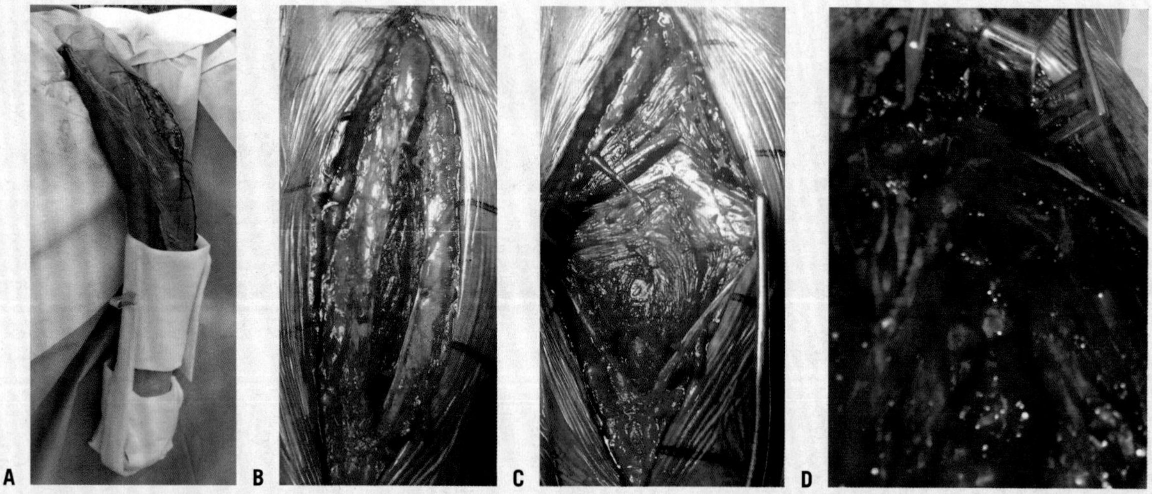

TECH FIG 2 **A.** Incision for posterior approach. **B.** Superficial triceps split. **C.** Deep triceps split. **D.** The probe points to the radial nerve as it exits the spiral groove from medial to lateral; the fracture site is seen distally.

MEDIAL APPROACH

- Positioning is similar to the anterolateral approach.
- Make an incision over the medial intermuscular septum from the axilla to 5 cm proximal to the medial epicondyle **(TECH FIG 3)**.
- Mobilize the ulnar nerve.
- Resect the medial intermuscular septum; identify and coagulate the adjacent venous plexus with bipolar electrocautery.
- Mobilize the triceps posteriorly and the biceps/brachialis anteriorly.
- Expose the fracture site.
- The axillary incision raises concern for infection; there is also concern that the ulnar nerve can scar to the plate.

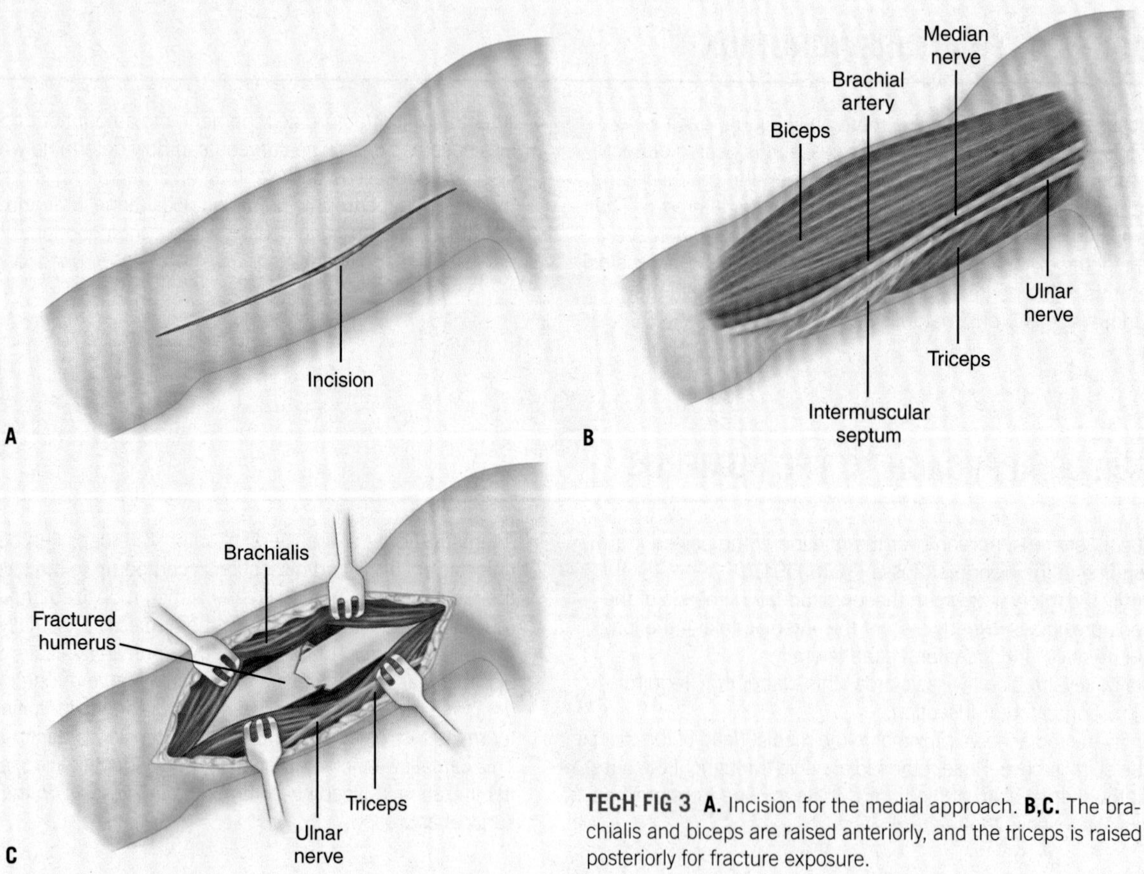

TECH FIG 3 **A.** Incision for the medial approach. **B,C.** The brachialis and biceps are raised anteriorly, and the triceps is raised posteriorly for fracture exposure.

FRACTURE REDUCTION

- Sharp periosteal dissection exposes the fracture site. Evaluate the degree, if any, of comminution.
- Limit periosteal stripping to adequately expose the fracture. Make every attempt to leave some soft tissue attached to each fragment so as not to devascularize the fragments.
- Gentle traction and rotation often can bring the fracture fragments into better alignment.
- Anatomically reduce the fracture with one or more reduction clamps. It is advisable to reduce the fracture completely before definitive fixation, and this often requires the use of multiple reduction clamps **(TECH FIG 4A)**.
- Care should be taken to ensure the radial nerve does not become entrapped underneath reduction clamps.
- After the fracture is reduced, 3.5- or 4.5-mm interfragmentary screws can be used to hold the fracture aligned until plate fixation. Temporary Kirschner wires may also be used in this capacity.
- Alternatively, fractures with minimal comminution often can be directly reduced with the plate and Verbrugge clamps **(TECH FIG 4B,C)**.

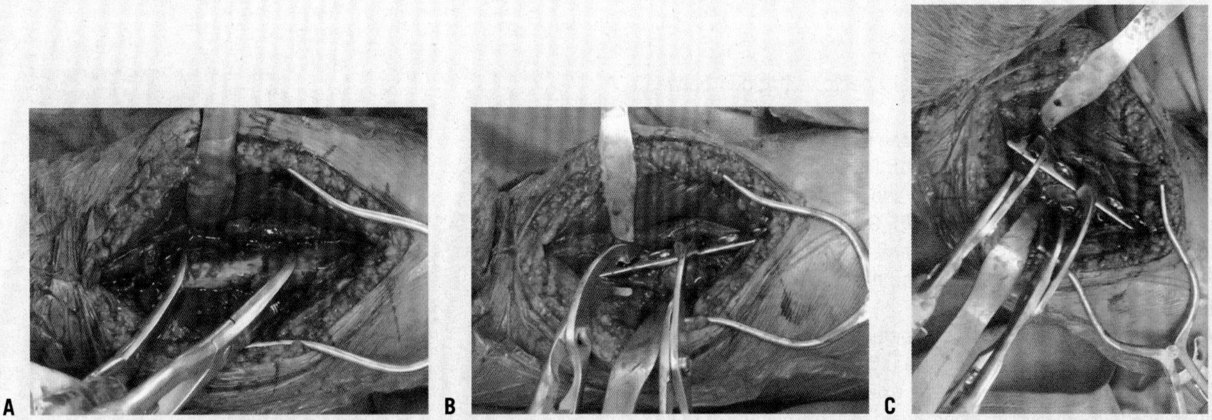

TECH FIG 4 **A.** Bone reduction clamps help realign the fracture ends. **B,C.** Verbrugge clamps can hold plate and fracture alignment intact prior to drilling and placement of cortical screws.

PLATE APPLICATION

- After fracture reduction, the plate length is determined.
- Humeral shaft fractures require at least six cortices of fixation above and below the fracture site **(TECH FIG 5A)**.
- In larger bones, a narrow 4.5-mm dynamic compression plate can provide optimal fixation. In smaller bones, a 4.5-mm limited contour dynamic compression plate often provides a better fit.
- Provisionally, place the plate on a flat surface of the humerus and hold it in place with a plate-holding clamp.
- A 4.5-mm cortical screws are placed through the plate holes proximal and distal to the fracture. Compression techniques can be used where appropriate **(TECH FIG 5B)**.

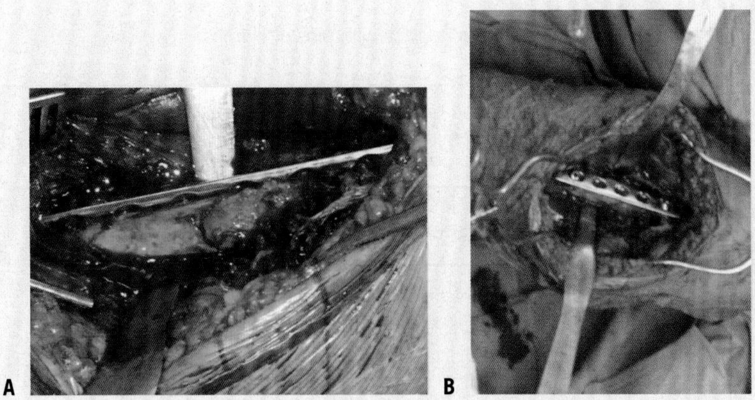

TECH FIG 5 **A.** Stable fixation requires six cortices of fixation above and below the fracture. **B.** A 4.5-mm cortical screws are placed in compression mode proximal and distal to the fracture. *(continued)*

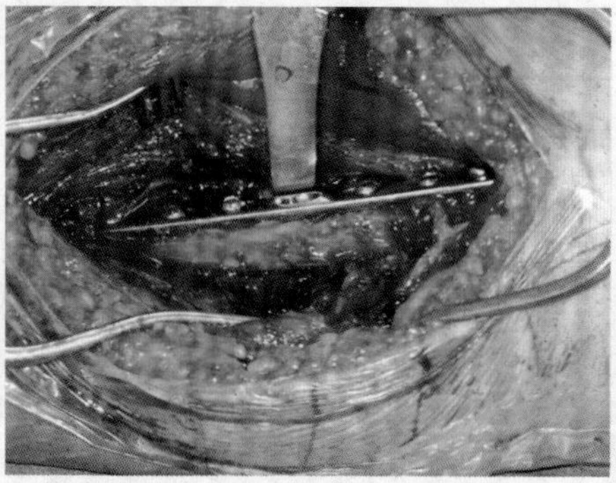

C

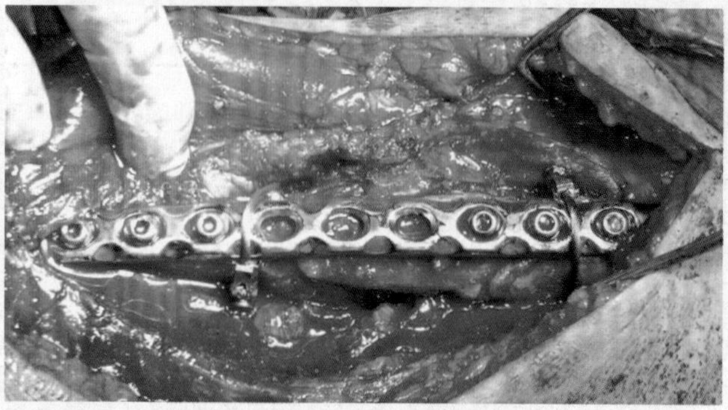

D

TECH FIG 5 *(continued)* **C.** Six cortices of fixation proximal and distal to the fracture site. **D.** Supplemental cerclage wire fixation can augment stability in weak bone.

- Ensure that no soft tissue, especially nerve, is trapped between the plate and the bone.
- Make sure to obtain screw purchase in at least six cortices above and below the fracture **(TECH FIG 5C)**.
- Cerclage wiring over the plate can add supplemental fixation, especially in weak bone **(TECH FIG 5D)**. Great care should be taken to identify and protect the radial nerve in cases of cerclage wiring.
- Rotate the arm and flex and extend the elbow to evaluate fracture stability.
- Apply cancellous bone graft into defects as needed.
- Close the brachialis over the plate **(TECH FIG 6)**.
- Distal fractures may require plate extension into the posterolateral distal humerus for appropriate fixation. The most distal screws in these constructs are often unicortical locking screws into the lateral column of the humerus.

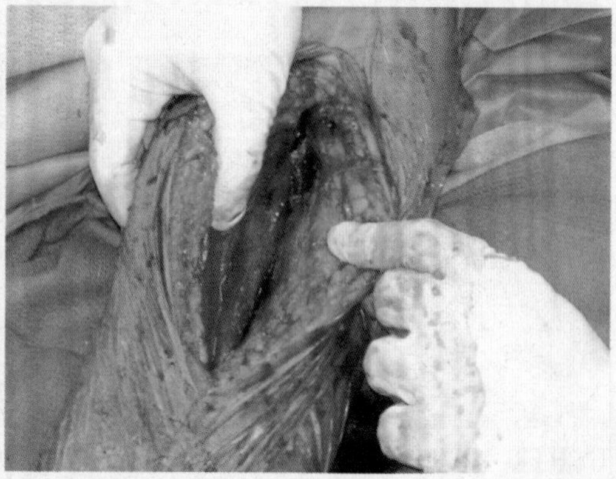

TECH FIG 6 Close the brachialis interval after definitive fracture fixation.

Pearls and Pitfalls

Indications	• Operative treatment is reserved for open fractures, patients with multiple fractures, and fractures with inadequate reduction.
Preoperative Planning	• Review all radiographs and determine the best surgical approach. • Estimate potential plate length and prepare for possible bone grafting.
Surgical Exposure	• Locate and protect the radial nerve. • Expose and reduce fracture fragments and temporarily hold them in place with pins or clamps. • Alternatively, fix larger fragments with interfragmentary screws.
Plate Fixation	• Ensure that plate length allows six cortices of fixation proximal and distal to the fracture. • Use 4.5-mm dynamic compression plates or limited contact dynamic compression plates. • Use compressive techniques when indicated.
Radial Nerve Function	• Preoperatively, document a detailed neurovascular examination. • Ensure that the radial nerve is not trapped within the plate before closure.

POSTOPERATIVE CARE

- Postoperative radiographs ensure proper fracture alignment and plate placement (**FIG 5**).
- Initially, the patient can be placed in a sling or posterior elbow splint. This is removed and range-of-motion exercises are started when patient comfort allows (usually 1 to 2 days postoperative).
- Assess radial nerve function. Debate exists regarding the role of immediate exploration in cases of intact preoperative radial nerve function, which becomes nonfunctional after surgery. In most cases, as long as there is little suspicion of radial nerve transection or compression by hardware, nerve function can be observed for up to 4 months.[13]
- Weight bearing on the affected upper extremity is allowed based on patient comfort.[12]
- Initial therapy consists of elbow range-of-motion, shoulder pendulum, and passive self-assisted exercises.
- The patient can come out of the sling after 2 weeks and start waist-level activities with the operative arm.
- At 6 weeks, elbow motion should be near normal range, and shoulder strengthening is added to the patient's physical therapy.
- At 3 months, radiographs should reveal callus formation. If no callus is evident, radiographs are repeated every 6 weeks until evidence of healing appears.

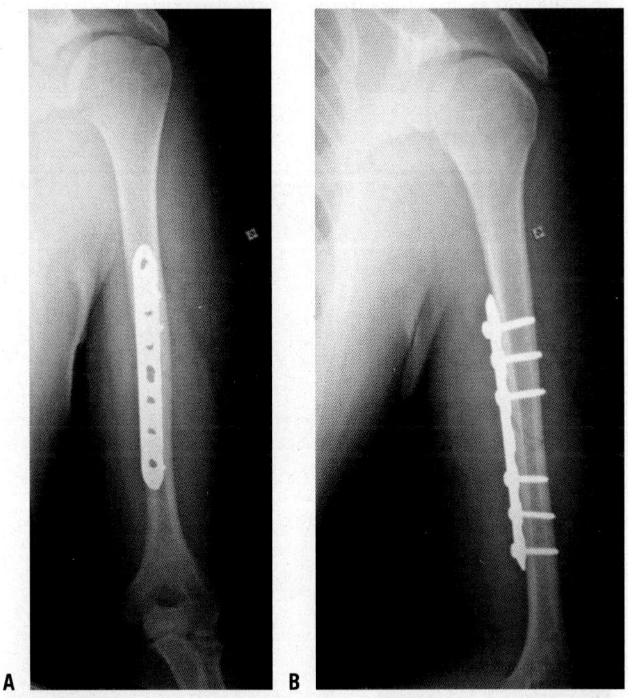

FIG 5 A,B. AP and lateral radiographs after humeral shaft fixation with a 4.5-mm dynamic and compression plate and screws.

OUTCOMES

- Plate fixation leads to union in 90% to 98% of cases.
- Plating offers decreased complication rates compared to intramedullary nailing, especially in terms of shoulder dysfunction and union rates.[8]
- Iatrogenic radial nerve palsy occurs in about 2% to 5% of cases and usually resolves in 3 to 6 months. Electromyography helps monitor return of nerve function in patients with prolonged palsy. Radial nerve exploration is indicated when no nerve function returns by 6 months.
- Elbow and shoulder range of motion usually return to normal postoperatively.

COMPLICATIONS

- Infection
- Nonunion
- Malunion
- Hardware failure
- Radial nerve palsy
- Shoulder impingement
- Elbow stiffness

REFERENCES

1. Garberina MJ, Getz CL, Beredjiklian P, et al. Open reduction and internal fixation of humeral shaft nonunions. Tech Shoulder Elbow Surg 2006;7:131–138.
2. Gregory PR. Fractures of the shaft of the humerus. In: Bucholz RW, Heckman JD, eds. Rockwood and Green's Fractures in Adults, ed 5, vol 1. Philadelphia: Lippincott Williams & Wilkins, 2001:973–996.
3. Gregory PR, Sanders RW. Compression plating versus intramedullary fixation of humeral shaft fractures. J Am Acad Orthop Surg 1997;5:215–223.
4. Healy WL, White GM, Mick CA, et al. Nonunion of the humeral shaft. Clin Orthop Relat Res 1987;(219):206–213.
5. Hoppenfeld S, deBoer P. Surgical Exposures in Orthopaedics: The Anatomic Approach. Philadelphia: Lippincott Williams & Wilkins, 1994:51–82.
6. Jupiter JB. Complex non-union of the humeral diaphysis. Treatment with a medial approach, an anterior plate, and a vascularized fibular graft. J Bone Joint Surg Am 1990;72(5):701–707.
7. Mast JW, Spiegel PG, Harvey JP Jr, et al. Fractures of the humeral shaft: a retrospective study of 240 adult fractures. Clin Orthop Relat Res 1975;(112):254–262.
8. McCormack RG, Brien D, Buckley RE, et al. Fixation of fractures of the shaft of the humerus by dynamic compression plate or intramedullary nail. A prospective, randomised trial. J Bone Joint Surg Br 2000;82(3):336–339.
9. Ring D, Perey BH, Jupiter JB. The functional outcome of operative treatment of ununited fractures of the humeral diaphysis in older patients. J Bone Joint Surg Am 1999;81(2):177–190.
10. Sarmiento A, Latta LL. Functional fracture bracing. J Am Acad Orthop Surg 1999;7:66–75.
11. Sarmiento A, Waddell JP, Latta LL. Diaphyseal humeral fractures: treatment options. J Bone Joint Surg Am 2001;83A:1566–1579.
12. Tingstad EM, Wolinsky PR, Shyr Y, et al. Effect of immediate weightbearing on plated fractures of the humeral shaft. J Trauma 2000;49:278–280.
13. Vaishya R, Kandel IS, Agarwal AK, et al. Is early exploration of secondary radial nerve injury in patients with humerus shaft fracture justified? J Clin Orthop Trauma 2019;10:534–540.

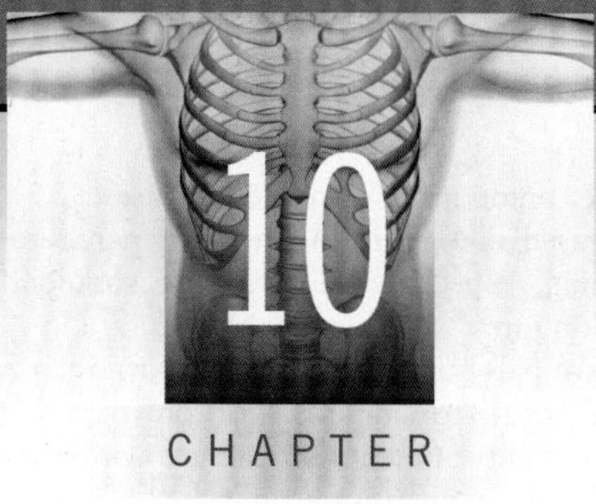

Intramedullary Fixation of Humeral Shaft Fractures

Saqib Rehman, Christopher Born, and Phillip Langer

DEFINITION

- Incidence: 3% to 5% of all fractures[12]
- The AO/ASIF classification of humeral shaft fractures is based on increasing fracture comminution and is divided into three types according to the contact between the two main fragments:
  - Type A: simple (contact >90%)
  - Type B: wedge/butterfly fragment (some contact)
  - Type C: complex/comminuted (no contact)
- Intramedullary nailing (IMN) can be used to stabilize fractures 2 cm distal to the surgical neck to 3 cm proximal to the olecranon fossa.[12]
- The precise role of IMN is not defined. Proponents offer the following benefits over formal open reduction with internal fixation (ORIF): It is minimally invasive, causing limited soft tissue damage and no periosteal stripping (preservation of vascular innervation)[15]; it is biomechanically superior; it is cosmetically advantageous (smaller incision); and it is capable of indirect diaphyseal fracture reduction and metaphyseal fracture approximation. It can be helpful in severe open fractures in which plate and screw constructs could be less ideal from an infection standpoint **(FIG 1)**.
  - Complications such as shoulder pain (with antegrade nailing), delayed union or nonunion, fracture about the implant, iatrogenic fracture comminution, and difficulty in the reconstruction of failures raise questions regarding the usefulness of IMN over ORIF.[7]
- Biomechanically, intramedullary nails are closer to the normal mechanical axis; consequently, they can act as a load-sharing device if there is cortical contact.
  - Unlike plate-and-screw fixation, a load-bearing construct, intramedullary nails are subjected to lower bending forces, making fatigue failure and cortical osteopenia secondary to stress shielding less likely.

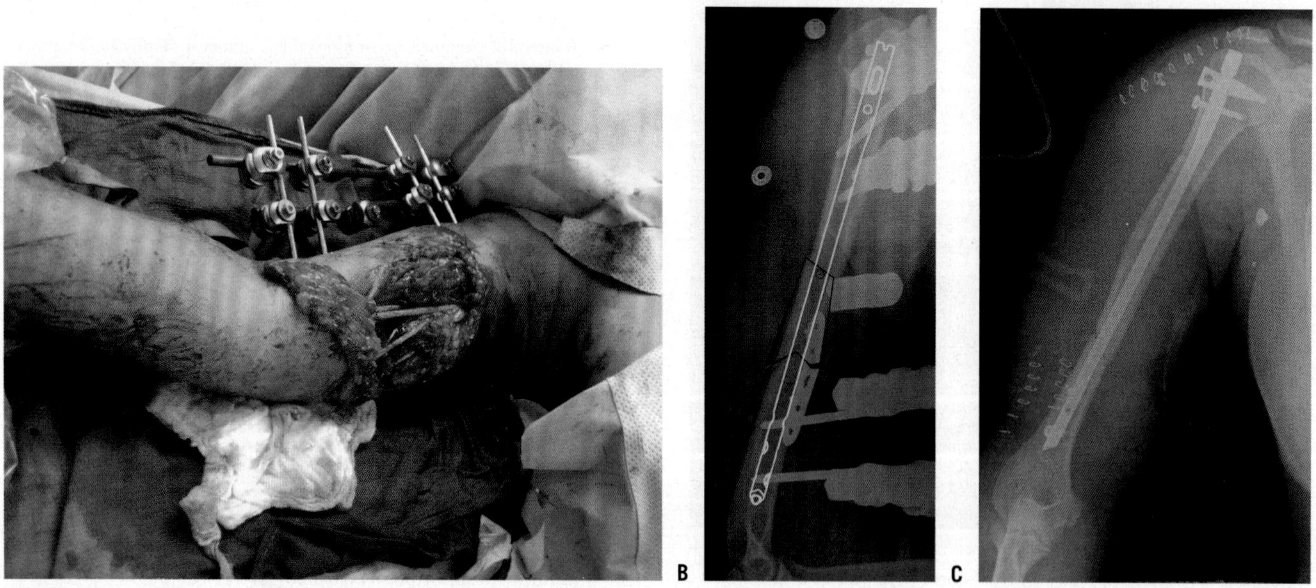

FIG 1 **A.** Intraoperative image of a type 3C open humerus fracture after undergoing vascular repair, débridement, limited internal fixation to protect the vascular repair (which was immediately adjacent to the fracture site), and external fixation. The medial and ulnar nerves as well as the vascular repair are seen here. **B.** Initial postoperative radiograph with preoperative template planning for IMN. It was felt that with her soft tissue injury and segmental fracture, extensive stripping and placement of a long plate-and-screw construct might be a higher risk for infection. If that were to occur, future treatment could be hazardous from a neurovascular standpoint in this case. So conversion to a nail was done after 2 days after discussing this with the vascular surgeon. **C.** Postoperative radiograph after removal of the external fixator and temporary plate-and-screw construct and placement of an antegrade intramedullary nail.

ANATOMY

- Comparatively, there are several anatomic differences between the long bones of the upper extremity versus the long bones of the lower extremity (femur, tibia).
  - The medullary canal terminates at the metaphysis (vs. diaphysis).
  - Isthmus: Junction is at the middle–distal third (vs. proximal–middle third).
  - Trumpet shape: The proximal two-thirds of the humeral canal is cylindrical; distally, the medullary canal rapidly tapers to a prismatic end at the diaphysis (hard cortical bone) versus the wide flare of the metaphysis (soft cancellous bone).
- Because of the funnel shape of the humeral shaft, a true interference fit is difficult to obtain; therefore, proximal and distal static locking has become the standard of care for IMN of humeral fractures.
- Neurovascular considerations include average distances of key structures from notable bony landmarks.
  - Axillary nerve to proximal humerus, 6.1 ± 0.7 cm (range 4.5 to 6.9 cm)
  - Axillary nerve to surgical neck, 1.7 ± 0.8 cm (range 0.7 to 4.0 cm)
  - Axillary nerve to greater tuberosity, 45.6 mm
  - Axillary nerve to distal edge acromion, 5 to 6 cm
  - Crossing of radial nerve at lateral intermuscular septum to proximal humerus, 17.0 ± 2.3 cm (range 13 to 22 cm)
  - Crossing of radial nerve at lateral intermuscular septum to olecranon fossa, 12.0 ± 2.3 cm (range 7.4 to 16.6 cm)
  - Crossing of radial nerve at lateral intermuscular septum to distal humerus, 16.0 ± 0.4 cm (range 9.0 to 20.5 cm)[2,5,8]

PATHOGENESIS

- Bimodal distribution[18]
  - Young, male 21 to 30 years old: high-energy trauma
  - Older, female 60 to 80 years old: simple fall/rotational injury
- 5% open[18]
- 63% AO/ASIF type A fracture patterns[18]
- Various loading modes and the characteristic fracture patterns they create
  - Tension: transverse
  - Compression: oblique
  - Torsion: spiral
  - Bending: butterfly
  - High energy: comminuted
- Red flags
  - Minimal trauma indicates a pathologic process.
  - Disconnection between history and fracture type suggests domestic abuse.

NATURAL HISTORY

- The humerus is well enveloped in muscle and soft tissue, hence its good prognosis for healing in most uncomplicated fractures.

PATIENT HISTORY AND PHYSICAL FINDINGS

- Patients with humeral shaft fractures present with arm pain, deformity, and swelling.
- Demographics, medical history, and information regarding the circumstance and mechanism of injury should be obtained.
- Particularly significant in upper extremity trauma: Hand dominance, occupation, age, and pertinent comorbidities must be solicited from the patient. All of these factors play a major role in determining whether to pursue surgical versus nonsurgical treatment.
- On physical examination, the arm is typically shortened, angulated, or grossly deformed, with motion and crepitus on manipulation.
- Document the status of the skin (open vs. closed fracture) and perform a careful neurovascular evaluation of the limb.
- If indicated, Doppler pulse and compartment pressures should be checked.
- Always examine the shoulder and elbow joint for possible associated musculoskeletal pathology.
- Examine the radial nerve for evidence of injury by testing resistance to wrist and finger extension, with care to distinguish intrinsic extension from extrinsic extension.[6]

IMAGING AND OTHER DIAGNOSTIC STUDIES

- Initial studies must always include orthogonal views (anteroposterior [AP] and lateral radiographs) of the fracture site, shoulder, and elbow **(FIG 2)**. To obtain these radiographs, move the patient rather than rotating the injured limb through the fracture site. Lateral imaging typically needs to be done with a transthoracic projection in order to prevent rotation through the fracture site with positioning.
  - Traction radiographs may be helpful with comminuted or severely displaced fractures, and comparison radiographs of the contralateral side may be helpful for determining preoperative length.
- Computed tomography (CT) scans rarely are indicated. Rare situations in which they should be obtained include significant rotational abnormality, precluding accurate orthogonal radiographs, and suspicion of possible intra-articular extension or an additional fracture or fractures at a different level.

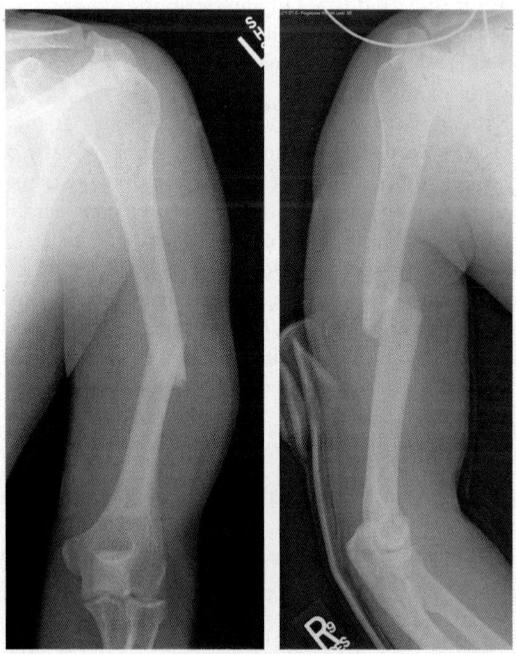

FIG 2 AP and lateral radiographs of a displaced humeral shaft fracture, shortened and in varus angulation.

- Doppler pulse and compartment pressures should be checked, if indicated, following a thorough physical examination.
- Suspicion of vascular injuries warrants an angiogram.

DIFFERENTIAL DIAGNOSIS

- Osteoporosis
- Pathologic fractures
- High- or low-energy trauma
- Open or closed fractures
- Domestic abuse

NONOPERATIVE MANAGEMENT

- Most nondisplaced or minimally displaced humeral shaft fractures can be successfully treated nonoperatively, with union rates of more than 90% often reported.[12]
- Common closed techniques include hanging arm cast, coaptation splint, Velpeau dressing, abduction humeral/shoulder spica cast, functional brace, and traction.
  - Each of these modalities has been successfully employed, but most commonly, either a hanging arm cast or coaptation splint is used for 1 to 2 weeks followed by a functional brace, tightened, as the swelling decreases.
  - Hanging arm casts are a very good option for displaced, midshaft humeral fractures with shortening, especially oblique or spiral fracture patterns, if the cast is able to extend 2 cm or more proximal to the fracture site.
- For nonoperative treatment to be effective, the patient should remain upright, either standing or sitting, and avoid leaning on the elbow for support. This allows for gravitational force to assist in fracture reduction.
  - As soon as possible, the patient should begin range-of-motion (ROM) exercises of the fingers, wrist, elbow, and shoulder to minimize dependent swelling and joint stiffness.
- Acceptable alignment of humeral shaft fractures is considered to be 3 cm of shortening, 30 degrees of varus/valgus angulation, and 20 degrees of anterior/posterior angulation.[10]
  - Varus/valgus angulation is tolerated better proximally, and more angulations may be tolerated better in patients with obesity.
  - Patients with large pendulous breasts are at increased risk for varus angulation if treated nonsurgically.
  - No set values for acceptable malrotation exist, but compensatory shoulder motion allows for considerable tolerance of rotational deformity.[10]
- Low-velocity gunshot wounds act as closed injuries after initial treatment. Following irrigation and débridement of skin at entry and exit sites, tetanus status confirmation, and prophylactic antibiotic initiation, nonoperative treatment modalities are commonly employed.[10]

SURGICAL MANAGEMENT

- Successful nonoperative management may be impossible for various reasons.
  - Fracture pattern (eg, displaced, comminuted, segmental [segmental fractures are at risk of nonunion of one or both fracture sites])
  - Prolonged recumbency
  - Morbid obesity
  - Large, pendulous breasts (in women)
  - Patient's inability to maintain a semisitting or reclined position owing to polytraumatic injuries or patient noncompliance
- Operative indications include the following:
  - Proximal humeral fractures with diaphyseal extension
  - Massive bone loss
  - Displaced transverse diaphyseal fractures
  - Segmental fractures
  - Floating elbow
  - Pathologic or impending pathologic fractures
  - Open fractures
  - Associated vascular injury
  - Intra-articular extension
  - Polytrauma
  - Spinal cord or brachial plexus injuries
  - Poor soft tissue over the fracture site(s), such as thermal burns
- The most commonly cited overall best indication for IMN from this extensive list is a pathologic or impending pathologic fracture.
- The need for operative intervention secondary to radial nerve dysfunction after closed manipulation is controversial.
  - There are advocates for both early nerve exploration and observation.
  - This condition was once thought to be an automatic indication for surgery; however, this assumption has since been called into question.[12]
- Isolated comminution is not an indication for operative treatment.[12] However, if surgical fixation is chosen over nonoperative management, antegrade IMN has been proposed by some to be favored over plate fixation for comminuted or segmental fractures.[3]
- Relative contraindications include the following:
  - Open epiphyses
  - Narrow intramedullary canal (ie, <9 mm)
  - Prefracture deformity of the humeral shaft
  - Open fractures with obvious radial nerve palsy and neurologic loss after penetrating stab injuries
    - The last two conditions require nerve exploration with subsequent plate-and-screw fixation.
- Chronically displaced fractures should be treated with ORIF rather than IMN to prevent traction-induced brachial plexus palsy and radial nerve injury.

Preoperative Planning

- When selecting implant size, consider canal diameter, fracture pattern, patient anatomy, and postoperative protocol.
  - Nail length and diameter should take into account the distal narrowing of the humerus.
- Estimations of the nail diameter, length, and necessity of reaming can be made using preoperative roentgenograms of the uninjured humerus.
- Alternatively, the length and diameter of the medullary canal can be ascertained intraoperatively using a radiopaque gauge and C-arm imaging of the intact humerus. Use of a radiolucent table top will substantially improve the quality of the image as well as the ability to obtain accurate C-arm images.
  - Position the gauge anterior to the unaffected humerus with its distal end 2.5 cm or more proximal to the superior edge of the olecranon fossa and 1 cm distal to the superior edge of the articular surface.

   - Move the C-arm to the proximal end of the humerus and read the correct length directly from the stamped measurements on the nail length gauge. The IMN should end approximately 1 to 2 cm proximal to the olecranon fossa.
- Measure the length of the IMN to allow the proximal end to be buried. This will reduce the incidence of subacromial impingement if an antegrade technique is used or encroachment on the olecranon fossa and blocked elbow extension if a retrograde approach is chosen.
   - In comminuted fractures, carefully choose the length to avoid distracting the humerus, which predisposes the patient to delayed union or nonunion.
- Measure the diameter of the medullary canal at the narrowest part that will contain the nail.
- In retrograde nailing, it is important to determine the relation between alignment of the humeral canal and the entry point of the nail by measuring the anterior deviation/distal humeral offset of the distal canal on the preoperative lateral radiograph.
   - Based on these calculations, if the deviation is small, make a distal, long entry portal that includes the superior border of the olecranon fossa.
   - If the anterior deviation is large, however, make the entry portal more proximal and shorter in length.

Positioning

- The patient's position for surgery is determined based on the method chosen for fixation.

Antegrade Intramedullary Nailing

- Place the patient in either a beach-chair or supine position on a radiolucent table with the head of the bed elevated 30 to 40 degrees (**FIG 3**).
- Put a small roll between the medial borders of the scapula and rotate the head to the contralateral side to increase exposure of the shoulder.
- Certain fracture patterns may call for skeletal traction.
   - If it is used, place an olecranon pin and apply intermittent traction to avoid brachial plexus palsy.
- Clinically assess the rotational alignment by placing the shoulder in an anatomic position and rotating the distal fragment of the fracture humerus so that the arm and hand point toward the ceiling and the elbow is flexed 90 degrees.
- Prepare the affected extremity and drape the arm free in the typical manner. The operative area should encompass the shoulder proximal to the nipple line, the midline of the chest to the nape of the neck, and the entire affected extremity to the fingertips.
- Bring the patient to the edge of the radiolucent table to improve the ability to obtain orthogonal C-arm images of the affected extremity.
   - It may be necessary to have the patient lying partially off the table on a radiolucent support.
- Cover the C-arm imager with a sterile isolation drape. Most commonly, the C-arm is brought in directly lateral on the injured side, although some surgeons favor coming in from the contralateral side.
   - Regardless of which direction the C-arm is brought into the field, it is imperative to obtain orthogonal views of the entire humerus before the first incision is made.

Retrograde Intramedullary Nailing

- Put the patient in the lateral decubitus or prone position with dorsum placed near the edge of the operating table.
   - If the patient is in the prone position, the affected arm may be supported on a radiolucent arm board or placed over a bolster or paint roller upper extremity support. The latter two options facilitate access to the olecranon fossa and prevent a traction injury to the brachial plexus. The arm should be positioned in 80 degrees of abduction with the elbow flexed at least 90 degrees.

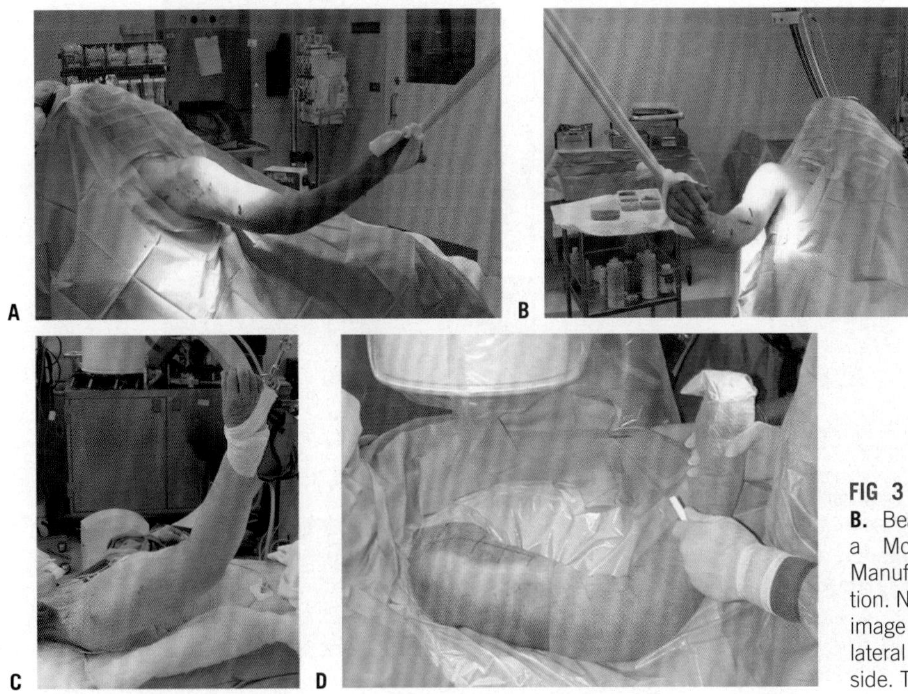

FIG 3 A. Beach-chair position for antegrade IMN. **B.** Beach-chair position for antegrade IMN using a McConnell positioner (McConnell Orthopedic Manufacturing Co., Greenville, TX). **C.** Supine position. Note the bump under the scapula and the C-arm image intensifier ready to come in from the contralateral side. **D.** C-arm imaging from the contralateral side. The patient is in the supine position.

- If the lateral decubitus position is used, suspend the fractured extremity, taking care not to distract the fracture site or cause neurovascular compromise. Suspension can be aided by an olecranon pin.
- Prepare the affected extremity and drape the arm free in the typical manner. Include the distal clavicle, the acromion, the medial scapula, and the entire arm and hand in the operative field.
- Cover the C-arm imager with a sterile isolation drape. Bring the C-arm from the ipsilateral side and make sure that adequate orthogonal C-arm images are possible before making the surgical approach.

ANTEGRADE INTRAMEDULLARY NAILING

Approach

- The antegrade approach, which has been the traditional method of IMN, typically involves a starting point at the proximal humerus—either through the rotator cuff, where the tissue is less vascular, or just lateral to the articular surface, where the blood supply is higher **(TECH FIG 1)**.
- Palpate and outline the surface anatomy of the acromion, clavicle, and humeral head.
  - Feel the anterior and posterior borders of the humeral head to locate and mark the midline.
  - Make a small longitudinal incision at the anterolateral corner of the acromion centered over the top of the greater tuberosity. Extend it 3 cm distally.
- The C-arm can be used to locate the exact entry point before performing the anterior acromial approach.
  - Place a K-wire percutaneously into the ideal entry point under C-arm imaging guidance. Confirm the location on orthogonal images.
  - Leave the K-wire intact while making an anterior acromial approach.
- Split the deltoid fibers in line with the longitudinal cutaneous incision.
  - Do not extend the incision distally more than 4 or 5 cm in the deltoid muscle to avoid damage to the axillary nerve.
  - Excise any visible subdeltoid bursae to improve your visualization of the rotator cuff.

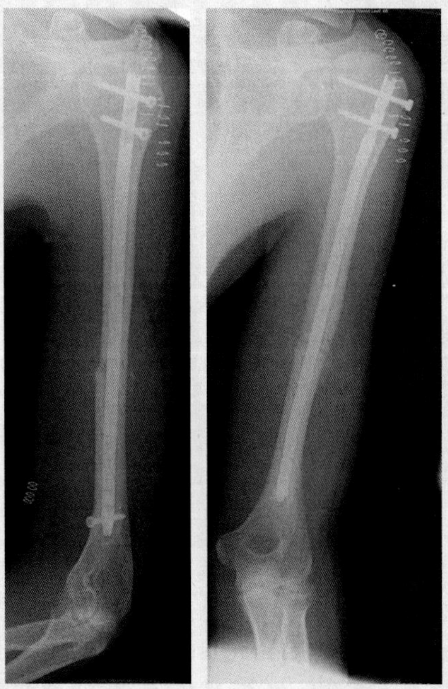

TECH FIG 1 Postoperative AP and lateral radiographs of antegrade IMN for a midshaft humerus fracture.

- Longitudinally incise the supraspinatus in line with the deltoid/cutaneous incision for 1 to 2 cm, just posterior to the bicipital tuberosity.
  - Placing suture tags at the margins of the supraspinatus will help retract its edges during the remainder of the procedure and assist in achieving an optimal rotator cuff repair during wound closure.
- There is insufficient evidence to indicate that a larger incision, in cases in which the rotator cuff is identified and purposely incised, is superior to a smaller incision made with the aid of C-arm imaging.[14]

Entry Hole

- Make the entry hole medial to the tip of the greater tuberosity, just lateral to the articular margin and approximately 0.5 cm posterior to the bicipital groove to minimize damage to the supraspinatus **(TECH FIG 2)**.
  - Linear access to the humeral medullary canal is possible only through an entry portal made in this sulcus between the greater tuberosity and the articular surface.

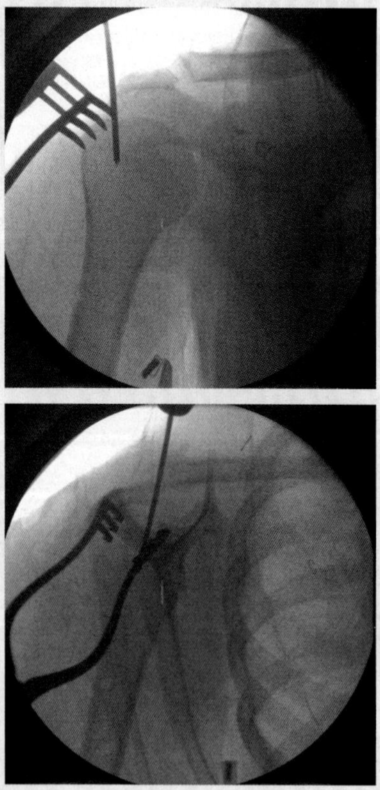

TECH FIG 2 AP and lateral intraoperative fluoroscopic images demonstrating the proper placement of a guidewire for the portal for antegrade nailing.

- Make sure the entry portal is centered on AP and lateral C-arm images to ensure the nail will be in the midplane of the humerus.
- If the entry hole is too medial, it will violate the supraspinatus; if the entry portal is too lateral, it will cause some degree of varus angulation (in proximal fractures) or substantially increase the risk of an iatrogenic fracture during nail insertion.
- Proximal third fractures may require a more medially located entry hole to avoid varus angulation at the fracture site.

Entrance into Medullary Canal

- After establishing the entry hole, insert a Kirschner wire (K-wire) through the portal into the medullary canal to the level of the lesser tuberosity.
- Next, to open the medullary canal, either use a cannulated awl or pass a cannulated drill bit over the K-wire, through a protection sleeve, and drill to the depth of the lesser tuberosity.
  - Adduct the proximal component of the fractured humerus and extend the shoulder to improve clearance of the acromion and facilitate awl or starter reamer access to the correct portal location.
- Once the medullary canal has been opened, remove the guidewire and insert a long, ball-tipped guidewire. Bending the tip of the guidewire may aid in its passage across the fracture site.

Provisional Reduction/Guidewire Passage

- Manipulate the extremity to reduce the fracture. In many cases, reduction is obtained through a combination of adduction, neutral forearm rotation, and longitudinal traction.
- While advancing the guidewire down the canal, rotate the arm about its longitudinal axis and take several C-arm images to confirm that the guidewire remains contained in the canal.
  - This is especially important if the humerus is substantially comminuted.
- Slowly and deliberately pass the guidewire across the fracture site.
  - Difficult passage may be a tip-off that soft tissue may be interposed (possibly the radial nerve).
  - An open fracture is advantageous in this situation because it provides the opportunity to directly visualize and clear the fracture site of any problematic soft tissue.
- After crossing the fracture site, advance the ball-tipped guidewire into the center of the distal fragment until the tip is 1 to 2 cm proximal to the olecranon fossa.
- Avoid shortening or distracting the fracture site while firmly securing the guidewire into the distal fragment.

Determining Nail Length

- Determine the correct nail length by one of two methods:
  - Guide rod method: With the distal end of the rod 1 to 2 cm proximal to the olecranon fossa, overlap a second guide rod extending proximally from the humeral entry portal. Subtract the length in mm of the overlapped guide rod from the total length of an identical guidewire to determine the correct nail length.
  - Nail length gauge: Position the radiopaque gauge anterior to the fractured humerus. Move the C-arm to the proximal end of the humerus and read the length from the stamped measurements on the gauge.
- The ideal length of an IMN should be measured 1 cm distal to the articular surface of the humeral head to a point 1 to 2 cm proximal to the olecranon fossa.
  - If the calculated length falls between two standardized nail lengths of the chosen implant, always choose the smaller size.
  - Excessively long nails are a risk factor for subacromial impingement and fracture site distraction.
    - Avoid the temptation to countersink an excessively long nail below the subchondral surface of the proximal humerus, as this can cause an iatrogenic split of the distal humerus or can create a supracondylar fracture when the tip of the nail is wedged too close to the olecranon fossa. In these cases, it is best to remove the nail and replace it with one which is one size shorter.

Reaming the Humeral Shaft

- Reaming the humeral shaft usually is avoided, especially in comminuted fractures, to avoid reaming injury to the radial nerve or the rotator cuff.
- If it is warranted, slowly ream the entire humerus over the ball-tipped reamer guidewire in 0.5-mm increments.
  - Exercise greater caution when reaming the humerus than when reaming the long bones of the lower extremity because the cortical thickness of the humerus is substantially less than that of the tibia or femur.
- Ream 0.5 to 1 mm larger than the selected nail diameter. Ream minimally until the sound of cortical chatter becomes audible.
- Choose a nail 1 mm smaller in diameter than the last reamer used.
- Some implant systems require that the ball-tipped guidewire be replaced with a rod that does not have a tip.
  - Use the medullary exchange tube when replacing the guidewire to maintain fracture reduction.

Inserting the Nail

- Once the correct nail length and the diameter of the selected implant have been verified, attach the nail adapter, place the nail-holding screw through the nail adapter, and then attach the radiolucent targeting device onto the nail adapter.
- Verify that this assembly is locked in the appropriate position and that its alignment is correct by inserting a drill bit through the assembled tissue protection/drill sleeve placed in the required holes of the targeting device.
- Insert the nail with sustained manual pressure.
  - Aggressive placement can result in iatrogenic fractures or displacement of the fracture fragments.
  - Use the C-arm image intensifier to identify the source of the problem if the IMN does not easily advance.
- Insert the nail at least to the first circumferential groove on the nail adapter but no deeper than the second groove.
  - Ideally, the IMN should be countersunk about 5 mm below the articular surface to avoid subacromial impingement.
  - Sinking the nail more than 1 cm below the articular surface may place the proximal interlocking screws at the level of the axillary nerve.
  - If the proximal end of the nail is properly countersunk, the incidence of shoulder pain is reportedly less than 2%.[4]

- Attach a strike plate to the targeting device and use a mallet to impact the proximal jig assembly to eliminate any fracture gap or advance the IMN.
  - Do not hit the targeting device or the nail-holding screw directly.
- The distal end of the IMN should come to lie about 2 cm proximal to the olecranon fossa.
- Remove the guidewire.

Compression

- Before proximal interlock insertion, make sure that optimal fracture site compression is present.
- Proximal compression locking can be used for transverse or short oblique fracture patterns. Severe osteopenia is a contraindication to its use.
  - Explore the radial nerve before compression locking if any possibility of radial nerve entrapment exists.
  - The nail must be overinserted by the same distance of anticipated interfragmentary travel because otherwise, during compression, the nail will back out and cause subacromial impingement.
  - Additionally, if the fracture is suitable for compression, the chosen implant should be 6 to 10 mm shorter than the calculated measurement to avoid proximal migration of the nail beyond the insertion site.
- Proximal locking screw placement
  - Oblique proximal locking screws are preferred because their insertion point is cephalad to axillary nerve.
  - It is important to make sure that these screws are inserted above the level of the humeral neck to avoid axillary nerve injury.
  - Lateral screws placed too proximal can produce subacromial impingement with terminal arm elevation.
  - Some implant systems may offer a spiral blade fixation as an option for proximal interlocking. In theory, it creates a fixed-angle construct and has a higher resistance (vs. screws) against loosening (ie, "windshield wiper" effect; **TECH FIG 3**). Other devices offer multiple screws in multiple planes in the proximal humerus for compromised bone or for proximal humeral fracture fixation.

Determining Rotation

- Confirm rotational alignment before placing distal interlock screws. Rotational alignment can be ascertained clinically and radiographically.
  - Magnified C-arm AP images of the fracture site can be used to judge the medial and lateral cortical width of the most proximal and most distal aspects of the fracture site.
  - Proper rotation is achieved when these widths are identical.

Distal Locking Screws

- Insert distal interlocking screws using a freehand technique.
  - To place AP-directed screws, advance the C-arm over the distal humerus until the distal interlocking hole is seen to be in maximal relief—that is, "perfect circle."
  - Under C-arm imaging, place a scalpel over the skin to precisely determine the location of the incision. Make every attempt to keep this incision just lateral to the biceps tendon. This will decrease the risk to brachial artery, median nerve, and musculocutaneous nerve.
- Carefully make the incision, although the skin and spread through the brachialis muscle down to the bone. This should not be a percutaneous incision, but rather, a generous enough incision so that you have adequate visualization with appropriate retractors.
- Insert a short drill bit through a soft tissue protector.
  - Center the drill bit in the locking hole and then position it perpendicular to the nail.
- Attach the drill and penetrate the near cortex. Then detach the drill bit from the drill and use a mallet to gently advance the drill bit through the nail up to the far cortex.
  - An orthogonal C-arm image may be used to verify that the position of the drill bit is satisfactory.
- Reattach the drill and penetrate the far cortex.
- A depth gauge can now be inserted to ascertain the length of the interlock screw.
- Use C-arm image intensification to confirm screw position through the nail as well as screw length.
  - Avoid articular penetration into the glenohumeral joint.
- Lateral to medial directed distal locking screws
  - Either in combination with or as an alternative to anterior to posterior screws, insert lateral to medial screws if necessary. This may be needed in cases of poor bone density and need for a second screw in an orthogonal position to the AP screw. Skin problems or anatomic issues anteriorly could also potentially obviate the placement of an AP screw, therefore requiring a lateral to medial screw.
- Make a generous 5-cm incision to decrease the risk to the radial nerve (ie, this should not be a percutaneous technique). It is due to this risk that this particular screw trajectory is less ideal compared with the anterior to posteriorly directed screws.
- Use the same technique employed when placing AP-directed screws: blunt dissection, direct visualization of the portal and the humerus, a protecting drill/screw insertion sleeve, and perfect circle freehand technique.
- Finally, confirm the IMN position, fracture reduction, and interlocking screw(s) placement with multiple orthogonal C-arm images.

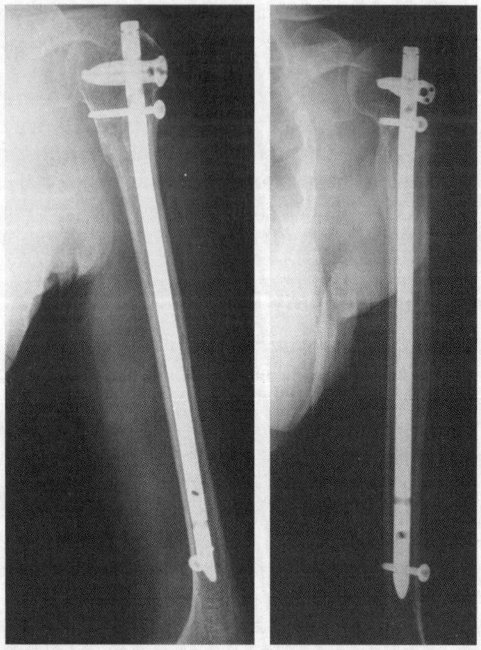

TECH FIG 3 Postoperative AP and lateral radiographs of antegrade IMN for a midshaft humerus fracture. A spiral blade has been used for proximal interlock fixation.

- After orthogonal C-arm images demonstrate satisfactory reduction and hardware implantation, remove the proximal targeting device and place an end cap (this last step is optional, depending on surgeon preference).
  - Carefully select the length of the end cap to avoid impingement.

Wound Closure

- Copiously irrigate all wounds before they are closed.
- During closure of the proximal insertion site, formally repair the surgically incised rotator cuff and deltoid raphe; side-to-side nonabsorbable sutures commonly are recommended.

RETROGRADE INTRAMEDULLARY NAILING

Approach

- Make a limited posterior approach centered over the distal humerus, starting at the olecranon tip to a point 6 cm proximal.
- Longitudinally split the triceps in line with its fibers to the cortical surface of the humerus and identify the olecranon fossa.
- Make every attempt to avoid entering the elbow joint to decrease the possibility of periarticular scarring.

Starting or Entry Portals

- As previously discussed in the Approach section, the coronal deviation of the distal humerus is variable, and, therefore, two potential starting portals exist:
  - Traditional metaphyseal entry portal: created by reaming in the midline of the distal metaphyseal triangle 2.5 cm proximal to the olecranon fossa
  - Olecranon fossa entry portal: established by reaming the proximal slope of the olecranon at the superior border of the olecranon fossa
- The more distal location of the nontraditional olecranon fossa entry portal increases the effective working length of the distal segment and provides a straighter alignment with the medullary canal.
  - However, biomechanical investigation has found that the olecranon fossa entry portal provides greater reduction in torque resistance and load to failure, which may increase the probability of an iatrogenic or postoperative fracture.[17]
- When making either entry portal, pay careful attention to the relation between the olecranon fossa and the longitudinal axis of the humerus in order to place the entry portal in line with the humeral shaft. The axis of the humerus usually is colinear with the lateral aspect of the olecranon fossa.
- Make the initial entry portal in one of two ways:
  - Open the near cortex with a 4.5-mm drill bit. Continue drilling while progressively lowering the drill toward the arm until the drill bit is in line with the medullary canal on the lateral C-arm images.
  - Drill three small pilot holes in a triangular configuration perpendicular to the cortical surface. Connect these holes with a large drill bit and small rongeur or enlarge the triangular site with a small curved awl to create a long, oval hole 1 cm wide × 2 cm long that leads directly into the medullary canal.
- Undercut the internal aspect of the posterior cortex in addition to the medial and lateral walls of the entry portal to create a distal bevel along the path of nail insertion.
  - This will facilitate easy passage of the guidewire, optional reamer, and final implant.

Provisional Reduction and Guidewire Passage

- Now, follow the same steps outlined in the antegrade IMN technique section to pass the guidewire, reduce the fracture, ream (optional), measure the desired nail length and diameter, and insert the chosen implant.
  - Reduction of the fracture usually involves gentle longitudinal traction on the distal humerus and correction of the varus–valgus displacement.

Reaming (Optional)

- If it is necessary to ream, carefully select the reamer size to avoid damage to the posterior cortex. In addition, slowly advance the reamer under C-arm image guidance to avoid excessive reaming of the anterior humeral cortex.
  - Both of these steps decrease the risk of possible iatrogenically induced fractures.

Distal Locking Screws

- Next, distally lock the nail to prevent backing out, that is, blocked elbow extension.
  - Place the distal locking screws from posterior to anterior using a guide.
  - Make an indentation with the guide, incise the cutaneous layer, and then use a blunt hemostat to spread down to the bone.
  - Follow the remaining steps unique to the chosen implant.
- After distal interlocking, gently tap the insertion bolt with a mallet to compress the fracture site. Assess the reduction with C-arm images.

Proximal Locking Screws

- Next, place a proximal interlocking screw, either anterior to posterior, posterior to anterior, or lateral to medial.
- Incise the skin and use a blunt hemostat to spread down to bone to protect the biceps tendon (anterior to posterior directed screws) or axillary nerve (posterior to anterior and lateral to medial directed screws).
- Use C-arm image intensification to confirm screw position through the nail as well as screw length.

Wound Closure

- Copiously irrigate each wound before closing it. Close triceps split with interrupted nonabsorbable sutures.

Pearls and Pitfalls

IMN Contraindications	• Antegrade nailing in patients with preexisting shoulder pathology (eg, impingement, rotator cuff) • Permanent upper extremity weight bearers (eg, para- or tetraplegics)
Antegrade IMN Entry Site	• If the entry portal is too far laterally, the lateral wall of the proximal humerus can be reamed out or fractured during nail insertion. • Pushing the reamer shaft medially may prevent this complication.
Nail Insertion	• If any resistance is met while attempting to pass the nail, either antegrade or retrograde, make a small incision to ensure that the radial nerve is not entrapped in the fracture site.
Interlocking Screws	• In most cases, soft tissues should be bluntly spread down to the bone with a hemostat before holes are drilled for any interlocking screw, to minimize neurovascular injury. • Antegrade IMN distal interlock screws: Make generous incisions rather than percutaneous incisions when placing distal locking screws. This way, proper visualization can permit safe instrumentation with regard to neurovascular structures. • Antegrade IMN: Rotate the C-arm 180 degrees, so the top can be used as a table to support the arm for placing the distal locking screws.
Nail Length	• Always err on the side of a shorter nail: Do not distract the fracture site or cause iatrogenic fractures by trying to impact a nail that is excessively long. • The retrograde IMN must be long enough to engage the cancellous part of the humeral head; the wide medullary flare of the proximal one-third of the shaft does not provide sufficient stability to the inserted nail.
Open Fractures: Reaming	• After a thorough irrigation and débridement is performed and the guidewire is successfully passed across the fracture site, close the deep muscle layer around the fracture site to keep the osteogenic reaming debris from washing away.

POSTOPERATIVE CARE

- Tailor the postoperative rehabilitation regimen to the method of nailing (antegrade vs. retrograde), stability of the fracture, overall patient health, and preinjury level of activity/workplace demands.
- Antegrade IMN
  - Place the affected arm in a sling or shoulder immobilizer at the end of surgery.
  - Postoperative day 2: Remove the dressing and begin gentle shoulder pendulum and elbow ROM exercises.
  - Postoperative days 10 to 14: Remove the sutures. Institute a structured, supervised physical therapy program. Close patient monitoring and formal therapy are key components to achieving maximum postoperative function.
  - Subsequently, schedule follow-up visits at 4- to 6-week intervals, depending on the patient's clinical and radiographic progression. Healing often takes 12 weeks or longer.
  - As union progresses, the therapist may begin supervised exercises to recover upper extremity strength. Caution the therapist against instituting programs or exercises that create large rotational stresses to the arm until radiographic healing becomes evident.
- Retrograde IMN
  - Initial postoperative management is identical to treatment following antegrade nailing, unless weight bearing is necessary for wheelchair transfers, walkers, or crutch ambulation. Use a posterior splint and platform attachment if crutches are necessary.
  - It is important to institute early elbow active ROM or gentle passive range of motion (PROM) by the patient to prevent elbow stiffness.
- Avoid the following:
  - Aggressive PROM or stretching to decrease the risk of myositis ossificans formation
  - Resisted elbow extension for the first 6 weeks after surgery to protect the repair of the triceps split

OUTCOMES

- Randomized clinical trials comparing IMN to compression plating show a higher reoperation rate and greater shoulder morbidity with the use of nails.[1,11]
- Locked antegrade IMN has resulted in loss of shoulder motion in 6% to 37% of cases.[14]
- Recent antegrade nails designed to eliminate insertion site shoulder morbidity through an extra-articular start point have been introduced, and prospective randomized trials are pending.
- Retrograde IMN union rates range from 91% to 98%, and the mean healing time is 13.7 weeks.[16]
- Retrospective reviews of retrograde IMN have found shoulder function to be excellent in 92.3% of patients and elbow function excellent in 87.2% of patients after fracture consolidation.[13,16]
  - Functional end results were excellent in 84.6% of patients, moderate in 10.3% of patients, and bad in 5.1% of patients.
- Biomechanical studies have shown that, for midshaft fractures, both antegrade and retrograde nailing showed similar initial stability and bending and torsional stiffness—20% to 30% of normal humeral shafts.[9]
  - In proximal fractures (ie, 10 cm distal to the greater tuberosity tip), antegrade nails demonstrated significantly more initial stability and higher bending and torsional stiffness, as was true for distal fractures with retrograde nailing.

COMPLICATIONS

- Nonunion
  - Nonunion of the humerus after IMN is preferentially treated with plate fixation, with or without bone grafting, depending on the biologic type of nonunion. Exchange nailing, a procedure done frequently in the tibia and femur, is not generally as successful in the humerus.
  - Antegrade IMN: 11.6%
  - Retrograde IMN: 4.5%
- Infection: 1% to 2%
- Insertion site morbidity
  - Antegrade IMN: shoulder pain, impingement, stiffness, and weakness
  - Retrograde IMN: elbow pain, stiffness, and triceps weakness
- Iatrogenic fractures
  - Antegrade IMN: 5.1%
  - Retrograde IMN: 7.1%
- Iatrogenic comminution and distraction at the fracture site[19]
- Neurovascular risk
  - Risk to the radial nerve in the spiral groove from canal preparation and nail insertion
  - Risk to the axillary nerve from proximal interlocking
  - Risk to the radial, musculocutaneous, and median nerves or brachial artery from distal interlocking
- Heat-induced segmental avascularity after reaming

REFERENCES

1. Benegas E, Ferreira Neto AA, Gracitelli MEC, et al. Shoulder function after surgical treatment of displaced fractures of the humeral shaft: a randomized trial comparing antegrade intramedullary nailing with minimally invasive plate osteosynthesis. J Shoulder Elbow Surg 2014;23(6):767–774.
2. Bono CM, Grossman MG, Hochwald N, et al. Radial and axillary nerves. Anatomic considerations for humeral fixation. Clin Orthop Relat Res 2000;373:259–264.
3. Chen AL, Joseph TN, Wolinsky PR, et al. Fixation stability of comminuted humeral shaft fractures: locked intramedullary nailing versus plate fixation. J Trauma 2002;53:733–737.
4. Crates J, Whittle AP. Antegrade interlocking nailing of acute humeral shaft fractures. Clin Orthop Relat Res 1998;350:40–50.
5. Farragos AF, Schemitsch EH, McKee MD. Complications of intramedullary nailing for fractures of the humeral shaft: a review. J Orthop Trauma 1999;13:258–267.
6. Foster RJ, Swiontowski MF, Back AW, et al. Radial nerve palsy caused by open humeral shaft fractures. J Hand Surg Am 1993;18:121–124.
7. Green AG, Reid JS, Carlson DA. Fractures of the humerus. In: Baumgaertner MR, Tornetta P, eds. Orthopaedic Knowledge Update: Trauma. Rosemont, IL: American Academy of Orthopaedic Surgeons, 2005:163–180.
8. Lin J, Hou SM, Inoue N, et al. Anatomic considerations of locked humeral nailing. Clin Orthop Relat Res 1999;368:247–254.
9. Lin J, Inoue N, Valdevit A, et al. Biomechanical comparison of antegrade and retrograde nailing of humeral shaft fracture. Clin Orthop Relat Res 1998;351:203–213.
10. Lyons RP, Lazarus MD. Shoulder and arm trauma: bone. In: Vacaro AR, ed. Orthopaedic Knowledge Update 8. Rosemont, IL: American Academy of Orthopaedic Surgeons, 2005:275–277.
11. McCormack RG, Brien D, Buckley RE, et al. Fixation of fractures of the shaft of the humerus by dynamic compression plate or intramedullary nail: a prospective randomized trial. J Bone Joint Surg Br 2000;82B:336–339.
12. McKee MD. Fractures of the shaft of the humerus. In: Bucholz RW, Heckman JD, Court-Brown C, eds. Rockwood and Green's Fractures in Adults, ed 6. Philadelphia: Lippincott Williams & Wilkins, 2006:1117–1157.
13. Patino JM. Treatment of humeral shaft fractures using antegrade nailing: functional outcome in the shoulder. J Shoulder Elbow Surg 2015;24:1302–1306.
14. Riemer BL, Foglesong ME, Burke CJ. Complications of Seidel intramedullary nailing of narrow diameter humeral diaphyseal fractures. Orthopedics 1994;17:19–29.
15. Roberts CS, Walz BM, Yerasimides JG. Humeral shaft fractures: intramedullary nailing. In: Wiss D, ed. Master Techniques in Orthopaedic Surgery: Fractures, ed 2. Philadelphia: Lippincott Williams & Wilkins, 2006:81–95.
16. Rommens PM, Verbruggen J, Broos PL. Retrograde locked nailing of humeral shaft fractures. A review of 39 patients. J Bone Joint Surg Br 1995;77B:84–89.
17. Strothman D, Templeman DC, Varecka T, et al. Retrograde nailing of humeral shaft fractures: a biomechanical study of its effects on strength of the distal humerus. J Orthop Trauma 2000;14:101.
18. Tytherleigh-Strong G, Walls N, McQueen MM. The epidemiology of humeral shaft fractures. J Bone Joint Surg Br 1998;80B:249–253.
19. Zarkadis NJ, Eisenstein ED, Kusnezov NA, et al. Open reduction–internal fixation versus intramedullary nailing for humeral shaft fractures: an expected value decision analysis. J Shoulder Elbow Surg 2018;27:204–210.

CHAPTER 11

Open Reduction and Internal Fixation of Scapular Fractures

John A. Scolaro and Alex Doermann

DEFINITION

- Scapula fractures account for approximately 0.5% of all fractures.[5]
- Nonarticular fractures account for between 62% and 98% of all scapula fractures.[12]
- Nonarticular fractures involve the glenoid neck as well as the scapular body, spine, and/or processes.
- Intra-articular fractures involve the glenoid fossa and may have extension into the earlier noted extra-articular locations.[1]
- Most fractures of the scapula can be managed nonoperatively.
- Marked fracture displacement, angulation, or resultant shoulder instability are indications for surgical intervention.[3]

ANATOMY

- The scapula is a flat, triangular bone with three processes laterally: the glenoid process, the acromial process, and the coracoid process.
- The glenoid process consists of the glenoid fossa, the glenoid rim, and the glenoid neck.
- The superior shoulder suspensory complex is a bone and soft tissue ring at the end of a superior and an inferior bony strut **(FIG 1)**. This ring is composed of the glenoid process, the coracoid process, the coracoclavicular ligament, the distal clavicle, the acromioclavicular joint, and the acromial process. The superior strut is the middle third of the clavicle, whereas the inferior strut is the junction of the most lateral portion of the scapular body and the most medial portion of the glenoid neck.[7]
- The scapula has multiple muscular and ligamentous attachments; importantly, it is the origin for all four shoulder rotator cuff muscles.

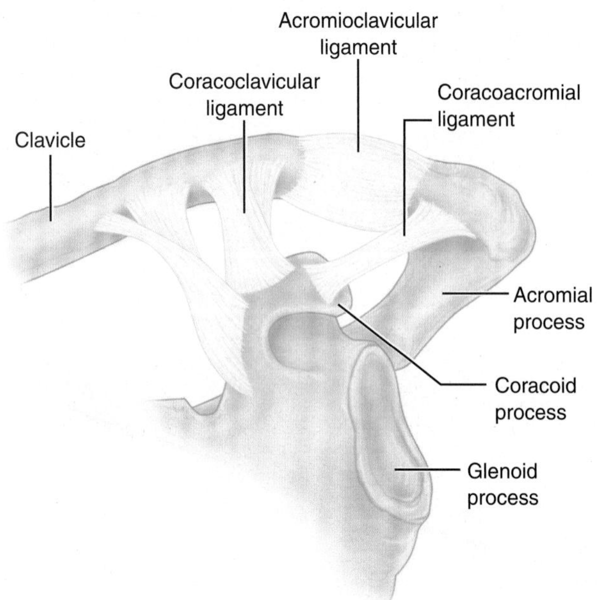

FIG 1 Superior shoulder suspensory complex.

PATHOGENESIS

- Scapula fractures commonly occur following high-energy trauma to the forequarter or upper extremity and may be associated with other musculoskeletal or thoracic injuries; low-energy injury mechanisms in older individuals can also result in scapula fractures.
- Extra-articular fractures to the body and processes commonly occur following a direct blow to the acromion process or scapular body; coracoid process fractures can also occur with sudden muscular contraction.[11]
- Glenoid neck and intra-articular glenoid fractures usually occur when the humeral head impacts the glenoid fossa or rim.

NATURAL HISTORY

- The majority of extra-articular scapula fractures are managed nonoperatively, and the functional result is very good.
- The scapula has a robust vascular and soft tissue envelope; nonunions are uncommon.
- The scapulothoracic and glenohumeral joint allow for a wide range of motion and can compensate for smaller angular deformities.
- Minimally displaced intra-articular fractures of the glenoid are also tolerated well, especially if the glenohumeral joint remains concentric.
- Displaced glenoid fractures (>5 mm) that are treated nonoperatively can result in shoulder instability, early glenohumeral posttraumatic degenerative joint disease, and functional deficits.[9]

PATIENT HISTORY AND PHYSICAL FINDINGS

- If possible, all specifics regarding mechanism of injury
- Patient factors: age, handedness, occupation, any history of previous upper extremity injury/deficits, recreational hobbies
- Soft tissue evaluation: Rashes or bruising may affect surgical timing; open lacerations or wounds may represent an open fracture.
- Complete sensory and neurovascular examination

IMAGING AND OTHER DIAGNOSTIC STUDIES

- Standard anteroposterior (AP), Grashey (true AP of the glenohumeral joint), and scapular Y view should be obtained.
- Associated glenohumeral instability should be assessed with an axillary or Velpeau view of the shoulder.
- Computed tomography (CT) scan of the shoulder, including reconstructions and three-dimensional (3-D) surface reformats, can be especially useful for evaluation, preoperative planning, and accurately measuring displacement and deformity.[14]
- Vascular abnormalities can be evaluated by CT angiography.
- Neurologic abnormalities are uncommon in these injuries, and there is a limited role for immediate electromyography evaluation.

DIFFERENTIAL DIAGNOSIS

- Extra-articular scapular fractures
- Intra-articular glenoid fractures
- Double disruptions of the superior shoulder suspensory complex including a floating shoulder (ie, glenoid neck fracture with ipsilateral middle third clavicle fracture)
- Scapulothoracic dissociation

NONOPERATIVE MANAGEMENT

- The majority of extra- and intra-articular scapula fractures can be managed nonoperatively.
- Patient is placed in a sling for 2 to 3 weeks until fracture consolidation begins and pain begins to resolve. Pendulum exercises can occur during this time.
- Therapy and range of motion begin between 3 and 4 weeks.
- At 8 weeks, gentle strengthening begins with continued focus on range-of-motion exercises.
- Goal is restriction-free activity at 3 months.

OPERATIVE INDICATIONS

- Multiple authors have proposed operative indications for scapular fractures; no clear consensus exists.[3]
- Process fractures: displaced ≥1 cm, with ≥2 concurrent disruptions to the superior shoulder suspensory complex or in the setting of ipsilateral operative scapular body/glenoid fractures
- Glenoid medialization: ≥20 mm
- Glenopolar angle: ≤22 degrees
- Sagittal angulation: ≥45 degrees
- Intra-articular step-off or displacement: ≥4 mm or 25% of glenoid surface or resultant glenohumeral instability

Preoperative Planning

- Time between injury and surgical intervention should be reviewed as this can affect surgical exposure.
- Plain radiographs of the affected extremity **(FIG 2A,B)**
- CT scan of the scapula including reconstructions and 3-D surface reformats should be reviewed to identify optimal surgical approach and anticipated surgical fixation strategy **(FIG 2C,D)**.

Positioning

- Regardless of approach and patient position, the entire shoulder, forequarter, and arm should be prepped out completely to allow unrestricted access.
- Anterior and superior (coracoid and acromion) approaches can be performed with the patient in a supine or beach-chair position **(FIG 3B)**.
- Posterior approaches can be performed with the patient in a lateral decubitus position **(FIG 3A)**.
- Concurrent access to the anterior and posterior shoulder girdle is possible in the lateral decubitus position.

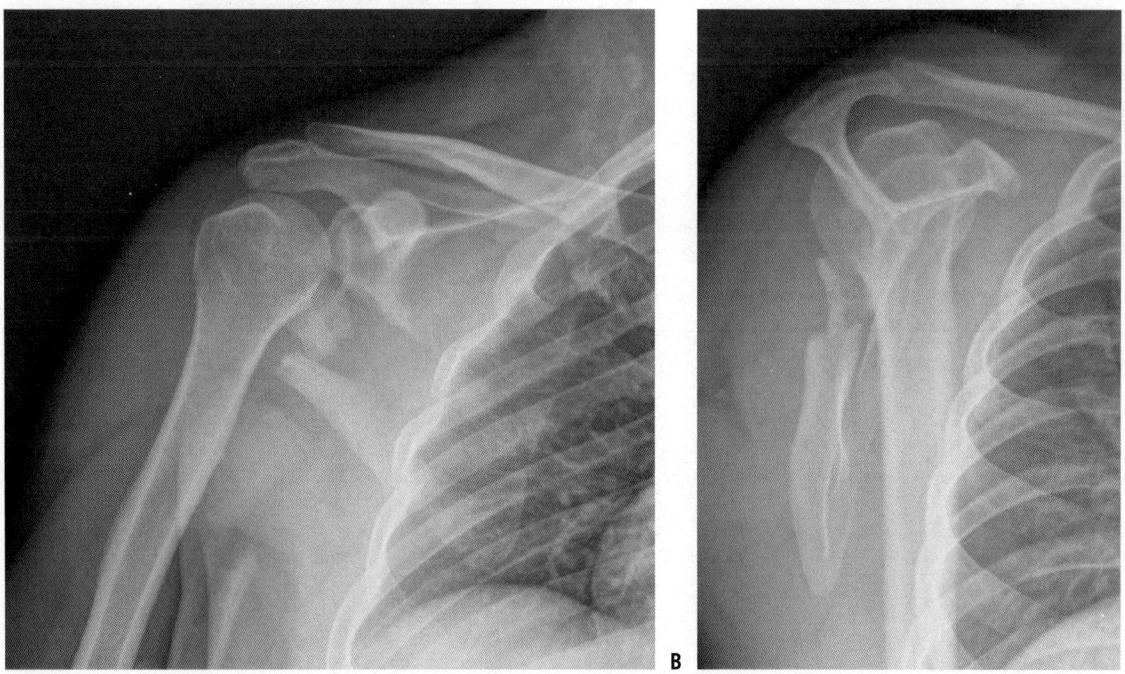

A B

FIG 2 AP (**A**) and lateral scapular Y (**B**) radiographs of a 41-year-old male with a comminuted right scapular fracture with intra-articular extension. *(continued)*

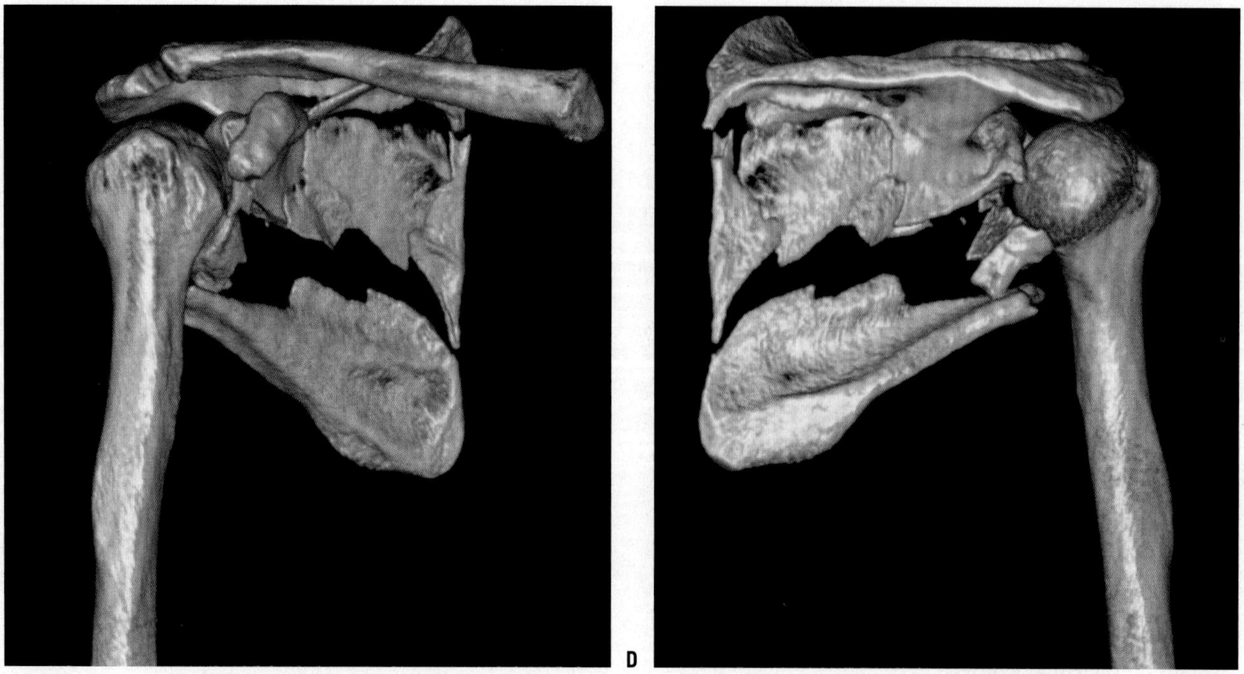

C D

FIG 2 *(continued)* Anterior (**C**) and posterior (**D**) 3-D CT surface reconstruction showing fracture morphology further injury detail.

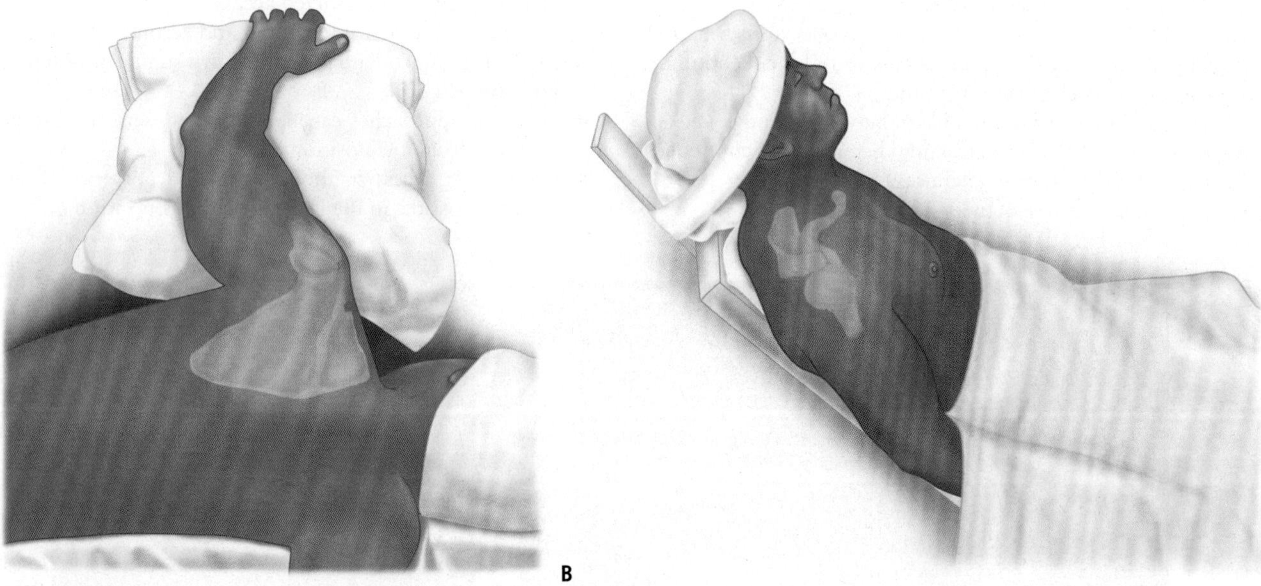

A B

FIG 3 **A.** The lateral decubitus position is used for posterior and posterosuperior approaches to the glenoid process. **B.** The beach-chair position used for anterior approaches to the scapula.

OPEN REDUCTION AND INTERNAL FIXATION OF CORACOID PROCESS FRACTURES

- Vertical incision 1 cm lateral to coracoid process **(TECH FIG 1A)**
- Development of deltopectoral interval, retract cephalic vein laterally with deltoid muscle, incise clavipectoral fascia if needed directly over coracoid and conjoint tendon
- Exposure of the fracture site (may need to open the rotator interval)
- If coracoid tip or base fracture has sufficient stock, solid or cannulated 3.5-/4.0-mm screw fixation can be performed with lag by technique or design **(TECH FIG 1B)**.
- If not, fragment excision and suture fixation of conjoint tendon to remaining coracoid is performed **(TECH FIG 1C)**.

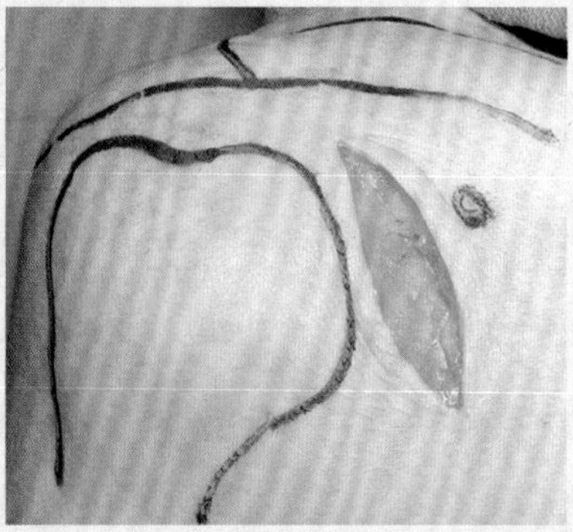

A

TECH FIG 1 A. Standard anterior incision extends from the superior to inferior margin of the humeral head, centered over the glenohumeral joint. **B,C.** Three repair techniques for coracoid fractures. **B.** Cannulated screw fixation of tip avulsion with sufficient bone to repair. **C.** Suture fixation of conjoint tendon when insufficient bone is available to repair. (**A:** Reprinted with permission from Goss TP. Open reduction and internal fixation of glenoid fractures. In: Craig EV, ed. Master Techniques in Orthopaedic Surgery: The Shoulder, ed 2. Philadelphia: Lippincott Williams & Wilkins, 2004:461–480.)

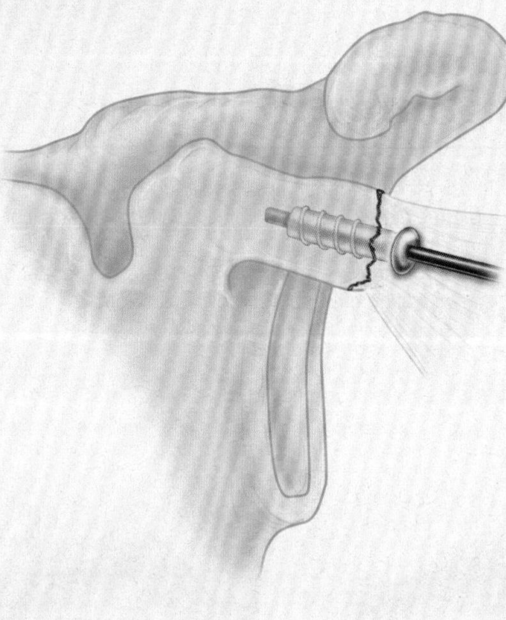

B

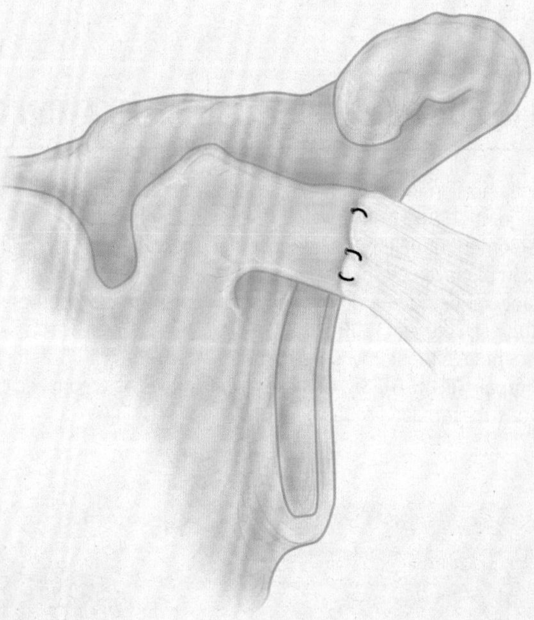

C

OPEN REDUCTION AND INTERNAL FIXATION OF ACROMIAL PROCESS FRACTURES

- Incision directly over and in line with the acromial process
- Subperiosteal dissection to expose the superior surface of the acromion
- Anatomic fracture reduction under direct visualization
- Proximal fractures: fixation with a flexible small or minifragment plate **(TECH FIG 2A)**
- Distal fractures: fixation with a tension band construct **(TECH FIG 2B)**

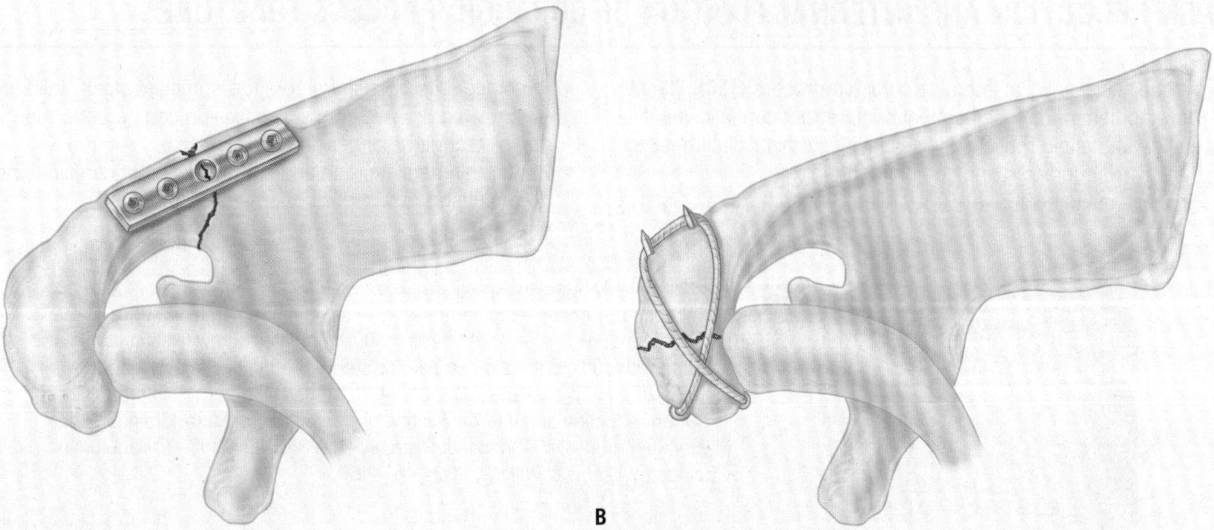

A B

TECH FIG 2 Fixation techniques for acromion process fractures. **A.** Plate-and-screw construct for a fracture of the base of the acromion. **B.** Tension band wire construct.

OPEN REDUCTION AND INTERNAL FIXATION OF ANTERIOR GLENOID FRACTURES

- Vertical incision in line with Langer lines centered over glenohumeral joint **(TECH FIG 3A)**
- Development of deltopectoral muscular interval
- Incision of clavipectoral fascia
- Retract conjoined tendon medially and protect medial neurovascular structures **(TECH FIG 3B)**.
- Subscapularis tenotomy is performed and tagged with cuff for later repair **(TECH FIG 3C)** or lesser tuberosity is osteotomized to retract subscapularis muscle.
- Incise glenohumeral capsule to expose anterior glenoid.
- Fracture is reduced anatomically with stable small or minifragment fixation.
- Subscapularis is reattached with suture, suture anchors, or screw fixation of lesser tuberosity osteotomy.

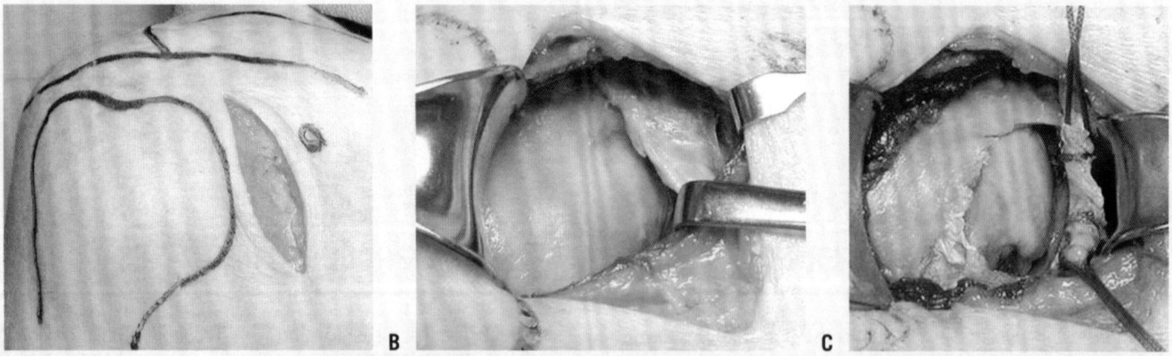

A B C

TECH FIG 3 **A.** Anterior approach using a skin incision made in Langer lines and centered over the glenohumeral joint. **B.** The conjoined tendon is retracted medially. **C.** Incise the subscapularis tendon 2 cm from its insertion on the lesser tuberosity, dissect it off the glenohumeral capsule, incise the capsule, and retract medially to gain access to the glenohumeral joint. (Reprinted with permission from Goss TP. Glenoid fractures: open reduction and internal fixation. In: Wiss DA, ed. Master Techniques in Orthopaedic Surgery: Fractures. Philadelphia: Lippincott–Raven, 1998:1–17.)

ISOLATED POSTERIOR/SUPERIOR APPROACH TO THE GLENOID NECK

- Incision is made in line with the lateral border of the scapular spine and continues anteriorly over the posterolateral deltoid **(TECH FIG 4A)**.
- The origins of the posterior and middle heads of the deltoid are split or detached from their acromion **(TECH FIG 4B)**.
- Posterior glenoid neck access is achieved by developing the interval between the infraspinatus and teres minor **(TECH FIG 4C)**.
- The glenoid fossa can be accessed with a tenotomy of the posterior infraspinatus attachment 2 cm lateral to the insertion on the humeral greater tuberosity and incision of the glenohumeral joint capsule **(TECH FIG 4D)**.
- The superior glenoid cavity is accessed by extending the posterior incision superiorly.
- The trapezius and underlying supraspinatus muscles are split in the line of their fibers **(TECH FIG 5)**.

A B C D

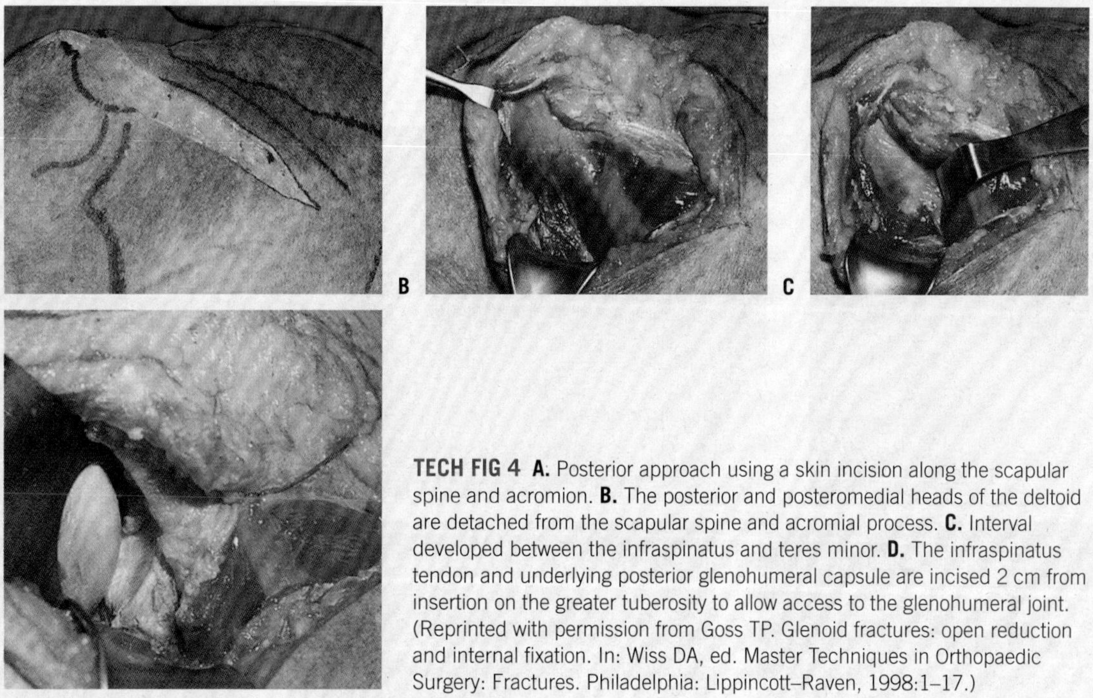

TECH FIG 4 **A.** Posterior approach using a skin incision along the scapular spine and acromion. **B.** The posterior and posteromedial heads of the deltoid are detached from the scapular spine and acromial process. **C.** Interval developed between the infraspinatus and teres minor. **D.** The infraspinatus tendon and underlying posterior glenohumeral capsule are incised 2 cm from insertion on the greater tuberosity to allow access to the glenohumeral joint. (Reprinted with permission from Goss TP. Glenoid fractures: open reduction and internal fixation. In: Wiss DA, ed. Master Techniques in Orthopaedic Surgery: Fractures. Philadelphia: Lippincott–Raven, 1998:1–17.)

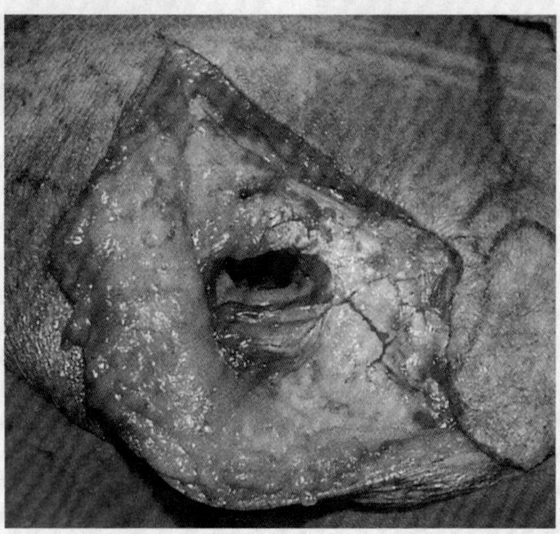

TECH FIG 5 In the interval between the clavicle and the scapular spine–acromial process, the trapezius and supraspinatus tendon have been split in line of their fibers for exposure. (Reprinted with permission from Goss TP. Glenoid fractures: open reduction and internal fixation. In Wiss DA, ed. Master Techniques in Orthopaedic Surgery: Fractures. Philadelphia: Lippincott–Raven, 1998:1–17.)

POSTERIOR APPROACH TO THE SCAPULAR BODY, POSTERIOR GLENOID NECK, GLENOID FOSSA

- Judet incision is made along the medial border of the scapula to the medial border of the scapular spine and then turns to head laterally along scapular spine **(TECH FIG 6A)**.[8]
- A full thickness skin and subcutaneous flap is then elevated above the muscular fascia **(TECH FIG 6B)**.
- The posterior deltoid musculature is then identified and the fascia between it and the infraspinatus is incised **(TECH FIG 6C)**.
- The posterior deltoid is then detached (if necessary) from the scapular spine, leaving a cuff of soft tissue for later repair; the deltoid is then retracted laterally **(TECH FIG 6D)**.
- In the modified Judet, the interval between the infraspinatus and teres minor is then identified **(TECH FIG 6E)** and developed **(TECH FIG 6F)** to expose the lateral border of the scapula, the posterior glenoid neck, and provide access to the posterior glenoid fossa.[2,10]
- Access to the medial border or scapular spine can be performed with direct exposure over these anatomic locations.
- The originally described Judet exposure provides full exposure to the scapular body and involves elevation of the infraspinatus from its origin **(TECH FIG 6G)**; this approach is typically reserved for nonunions or subacute fractures that cannot be mobilized through muscular intervals.[2]

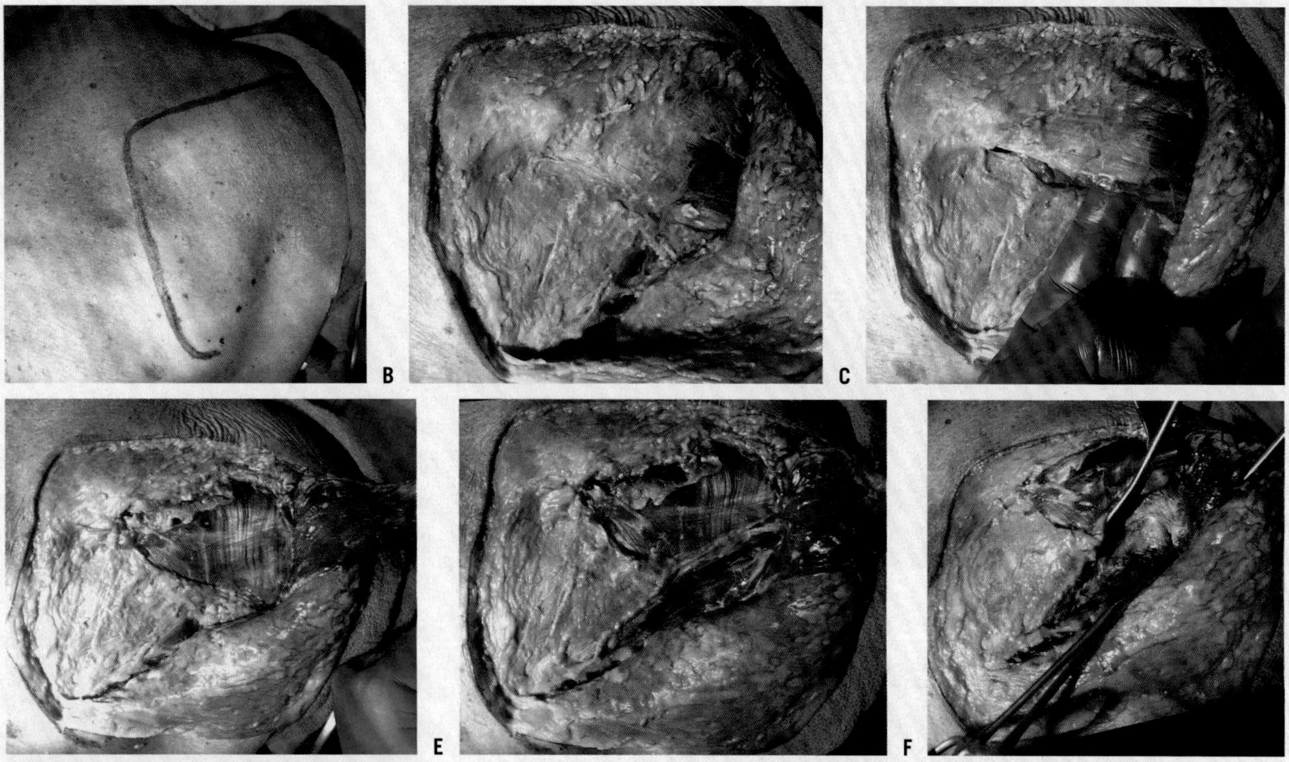

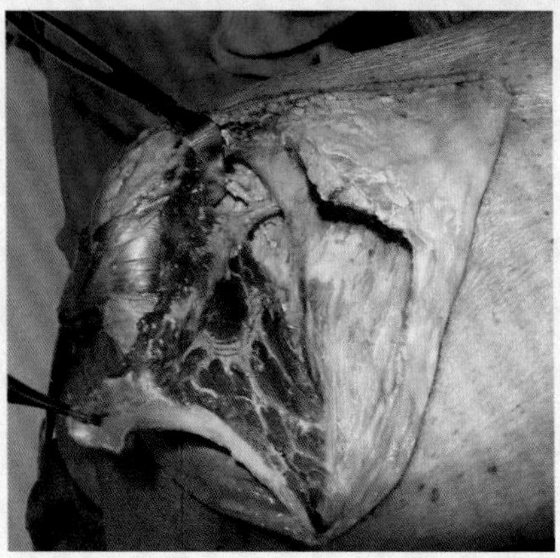

TECH FIG 6 **A.** Judet skin incision (*solid line*) with cadaveric specimen in prone position. Head is at the top of the picture and affected extremity to the right. *Dotted line* marks out the lateral border of the scapula. **B.** Full thickness skin and subcutaneous flap elevated with posterior shoulder muscle and fascia exposed. **C.** Fascia between deltoid and infraspinatus is incised and identification interval (two fingers) between these muscles. **D.** Tenotomy and retraction of medial deltoid attachment from scapular spine. **E.** Fascial incision between infraspinatus and teres minor. **F.** Surgical interval between infraspinatus and teres minor with exposure of lateral border of scapula, posterior glenoid neck and posterior glenohumeral joint. **G.** Left shoulder affected extremity at left of picture; full detachment of deltoid, infraspinatus, and teres minor exposing the full posterior surface of the scapula.

MINIMALLY INVASIVE SURGICAL APPROACH FOR OPEN REDUCTION AND INTERNAL FIXATION OF SCAPULA NECK AND BODY FRACTURES[6]

- Patient is placed in the lateral decubitus position.
- Incisions are made over the medial and lateral border of the scapula; other possible incisions are those over the scapular spine and medial inferior border.
- Lateral muscular interval is between infraspinatus and teres minor.
- Medial border of the scapula is exposed by elevation of the infraspinatus or teres minor.
- Scapular spine incision is directly over the spine.
- Pointed clamps and manipulative reduction sticks are used for reduction.
- Stable internal fixation is achieved with flexible small or minifragment implants along medial and lateral border of the scapula.

FIXATION TECHNIQUES

- Articular fractures of the glenoid require anatomic reduction and fixation; priority should be given to intra-articular locations.
- Following exposure, reduction can be aided by pointed reduction clamps **(TECH FIG 7)** and manipulative reduction pins or Kirschner wires placed in specific fragments.
- In complex fractures of the scapular body, which involve the neck and/or glenoid, reduction of the body can indirectly assist reduction of the lateral neck/glenoid.
- Fixation of scapular fractures is commonly achieved with small and minifragment implants that can be contoured to the osseous surface of the scapula. Newer minifragment implants also provide locking technology to assist in providing stable fixation in short segments **(TECH FIG 8A,B)**.
- The scapula is very thin throughout the body but has greater opportunity for fixation near the glenoid, along the lateral and medial border, and along the scapular spine.

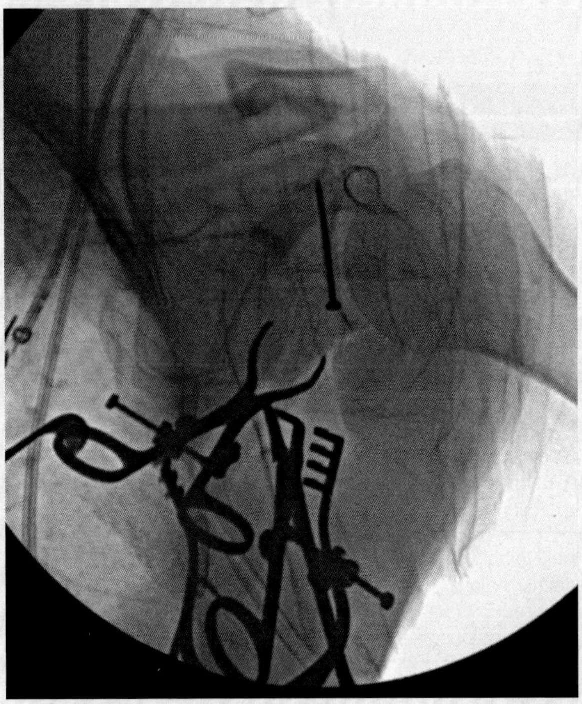

TECH FIG 7 Intra-operative fluoroscopic image showing initial minifragment screw just medial to glenoid cavity and two modified point-to-point clamps being used for provisional reduction of a displaced inferior glenoid fracture.

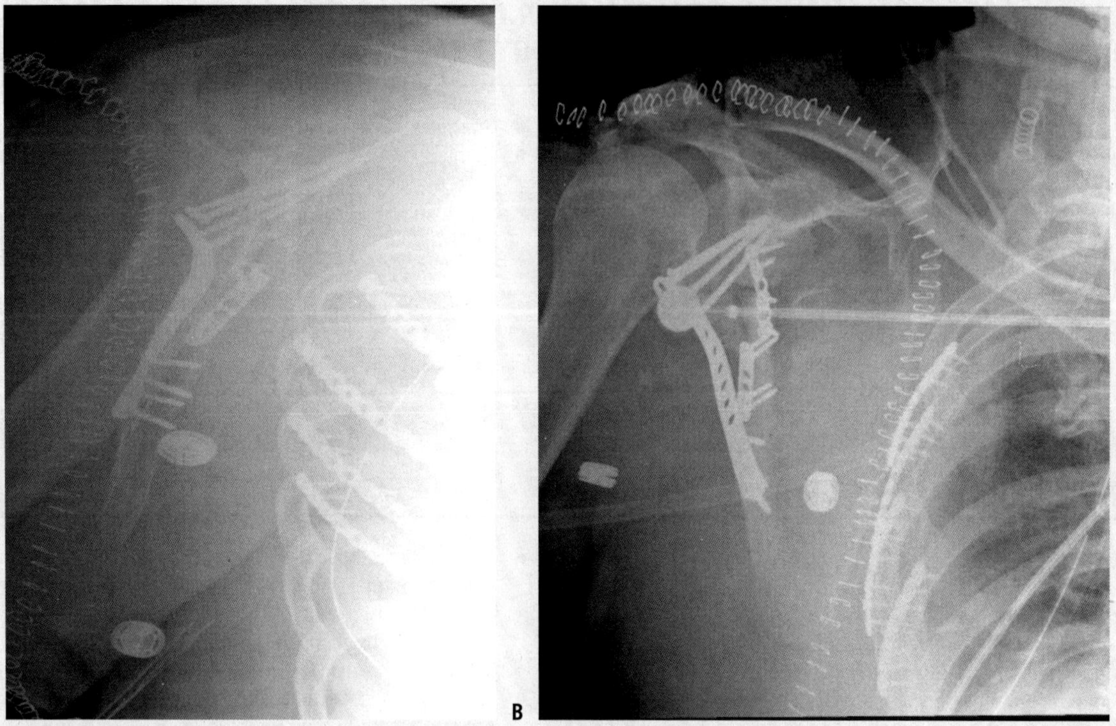

A B

TECH FIG 8 A,B. Postoperative. AP (**A**) and lateral (**B**) radiographs showing fixation of a complex scapular body and glenoid fracture with multiple minifragment plates. The lateral scapular border is an area of dense bone that is frequently used for fixation in the scapula.

TECHNIQUES

Pearls and Pitfalls

Indications	• Most scapular fractures are treated nonoperatively. • Dedicated shoulder CT and 3-D surface reconstructions can help define the fracture and intra-articular involvement. • Articular glenoid displacement ≥4 mm • Glenoid medialization ≥20 mm, glenopolar angle ≤22 degrees, sagittal angulation ≥45 degrees • Glenohumeral instability
Approach	• Identify subacute (≥3 weeks) injuries, which may not be amenable to limited exposure techniques. • Wide sterile surgical preparation; include the entire ipsilateral upper extremity. • Approach anterior glenoid fractures from the front, posterior neck, and scapular body/neck fractures from the back. • In the anterior approach to the glenoid, utilization of rotator interval or partial subscapularis tenotomy is preferred over full detachment. • Deltoid detachment provides greater scapular exposure through the posterior approach. • Avoid excessive or prolonged retraction on infraspinatus to void injury to supraspinatus nerve and artery. • Use combined or staged anterior and posterior approaches when necessary.
Reduction	• Short minifragment implants can be used effectively to hold small fragments. • Modified point-to-point clamps can help hold reductions along the medial or lateral scapular border. • Threaded Kirschner wires and Schanz pins can be used to manipulate fragments. • Reduction of the medial and/or lateral scapular border and/or spine can assist in glenoid neck/fossa reduction.
Fixation	• Small reconstruction and third/quarter tubular plates can be modified and placed on irregular scapular surfaces for fixation. • Minifragment nonlocking and locking plates are also valuable for fixation. • Treatment of complex scapula fractures requires multiple strategically placed implants to achieve stable fixation. • If severe comminution is present, an iliac crest tricortical bone graft can be used to provide a suitable glenoid rim.
Closure	• If the posterior deltoid is detached, meticulous repair of the deltoid to the scapular spine and acromion is necessary, using nonabsorbable sutures placed through drill holes. • Place a drain if necessary to avoid postoperative hematoma formation.

POSTOPERATIVE CARE

- Patients are immobilized in a sling postoperatively but are encouraged to begin gentle pendulum exercises during the first 2 weeks.
- If an anterior approach involving detachment of the subscapularis insertion is performed, shoulder external rotation past neutral is commonly prohibited until the 6-week time point.
- Progressive passive and active-assisted range-of-motion exercises are emphasized during weeks 2 through 6 postoperatively.
- Active and active-assisted range of motion is started at 6 weeks with gentle strengthening (≤10 lb) started during this period of time.
- Restrictions on weight bearing are typically lifted 3 months postoperatively with continued focus on range of motion and occupation/sport-specific rehabilitation.
- Goal is full return to all activities by 4 to 6 months.

OUTCOMES

- Limited case reports and small case series make up the majority of available literature on surgically treated acromial and coracoid process fractures; reported outcomes are generally good.
- Extra-articular fractures of the glenoid neck and scapular body that meet operative indications do very well with a low complication rate and high union rate and return of motion and function.[12]
- Operative treatment of extra-articular scapular malunions has also been shown to markedly improve patient function and ability to return to desired activity level.[4]
- Fixation of intra-articular glenoid fractures that meet operative indications (displacement ≥4 mm) has also shown to be very good with a low complication rate and high rate of retun to function.[1]
- Benefits of surgically treated intra- and extra-articular scapula fractures persist long after surgery has been performed.[15]

COMPLICATIONS

- Soft tissue complications related to surgical timing are uncommon given the robust vascular, muscular, and cutaneous soft tissue envelope around the shoulder girdle.
- Iatrogenic neurologic injury is the most common complication following scapular surgery, usually related to aggressive or prolonged retraction.[13]
  - Musculocutaneous nerve is at risk during anterior approaches to coracoid and anterior glenoid neck/fossa.
  - Supraspinatus nerve is at risk during posterior and superior approaches to the glenoid neck/fossa.
  - Axillary nerve is at risk during posterior approaches to the scapula.
- Suprascapular artery and ascending branch of circumflex scapular artery are positioned along superior and inferior border of posterior glenoid neck, respectively, and are ideally protected; if injury occurs, they should be tied off to avoid postoperative hematoma formation.
- Intraoperatively, care must be taken to avoid penetration of the thoracic cavity when instrumenting and drilling.
- Postoperative loss of fixation may be related to inadequate fixation, poor surgical technique, or patient compliance.

REFERENCES

1. Anavian J, Gauger EM, Schroder LK, et al. Surgical and functional outcomes after operative management of complex and displaced intra-articular glenoid fractures. J Bone Joint Surg Am 2012;94(7):645–653.
2. Cole PA, Dugarte AJ. Posterior scapula approaches: extensile and modified Judet. J Orthop Trauma 2018;32 suppl 1:S10–S11.
3. Cole PA, Gauger EM, Schroder LK. Management of scapular fractures. J Am Acad Orthop Surg 2012;20(3):130–141.
4. Cole PA, Talbot M, Schroder LK, et al. Extra-articular malunions of the scapula: a comparison of functional outcome before and after reconstruction. J Orthop Trauma 2011;25(11):649–656.
5. Court-Brown CM. The epidemiology of fractures. In: Court-Brown CM, Heckman JD, McQueen MM, et al, eds. Rockwood and Green's Fractures in Adults, ed 8. Philadelphia: Lippincott Williams & Wilkins, 2015:59–108.
6. Gauger EM, Cole PA. Surgical technique: a minimally invasive approach to scapula neck and body fractures. Clin Orthop Relat Res 2011;469(12):3390–3399.
7. Goss TP. Double disruptions of the superior shoulder complex. J Orthop Trauma 1993;7:99–106.
8. Judet R. Surgical treatment of scapular fractures [in French]. Acta Orthop Belg 1964;30:673–678.
9. Königshausen M, Coulibaly MO, Nicolas V, et al. Results of non-operative treatment of fractures of the glenoid fossa. Bone Joint J 2016;98-B(8):1074–1079.
10. Obremskey WT, Lyman JR. A modified Judet approach to the scapula. J Orthop Trauma 2004;18(10):696–699.
11. Ogawa K, Yoshida A, Takahashi M, et al. Fractures of the coracoid process. J Bone Joint Surg Br 1997;79(1):17–19.
12. Schroder LK, Gauger EM, Gilbertson JA, et al. Functional outcomes after operative management of extra-articular glenoid neck and scapular body fractures. J Bone Joint Surg Am 2016;98(19):1623–1630.
13. Scully WF, Wilson DJ, Parada SA, et al. Iatrogenic nerve injuries in shoulder surgery. J Am Acad Orthop Surg 2013;21(12):717–726.
14. Suter T, Henninger HB, Zhang Y, et al. Comparison of measurements of the glenopolar angle in 3D CT reconstructions of the scapula and 2D plain radiographic views. Bone Joint J 2016;98-B(11):1510–1516.
15. Tatro JM, Gilbertson JA, Schroder LK, et al. Five to ten-year outcomes of operatively treated scapular fractures. J Bone Joint Surg Am 2018;100(10):871–878.

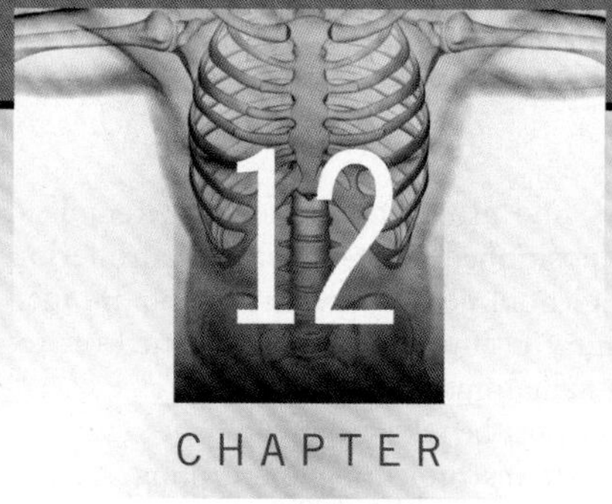

Open Reduction and Internal Fixation of Supracondylar and Intercondylar Fractures

Natalia Martínez Catalán and Joaquin Sanchez-Sotelo

PATIENT HISTORY AND PHYSICAL FINDINGS

- Fractures of the distal humerus have a trimodal age distribution[20,25]:
  - In the pediatric age, children tend to sustain supracondylar fractures or partial articular physeal injuries.
  - In middle-aged adults, high-energy distal humerus fractures are seen as a result of motor vehicle accidents or sport-related injuries.
  - In elderly patients, distal humerus fractures are typically secondary to a fall from a standing height and may be associated with complex intra-articular comminution due to age-related osteopenia.
- Distal humerus fractures are commonly classified according to the AO/ASIF/OTA classification system as A (extra-articular), B (partial articular), and C (intra-articular).[12] From a practical clinical perspective, distal humerus fractures may be divided into four major fracture patterns:
  - Supraintercondylar/column fractures: The fracture involves both the columns as well as the articular surface.
  - Articular (shear) fractures: These fractures do not extend into either column.[24]
  - Low transcondylar fractures: A single transverse extra-articular fracture line extends from the medial epicondyle to the midportion of the lateral epicondyle.
  - Partial articular fractures: Only one column is fractured, and the fracture line extends into the articular surface, typically creating a single piece.
- Articular shear fractures, low transcondylar fractures, and partial articular fractures are specific subtypes with their own nuances, and these injuries fall out of the scope of this chapter.
- These are the goals of the initial evaluation of supraintercondylar fractures:
  - Understand the fracture pattern.
  - Determine whether there was previous symptomatic elbow pathology (ie, inflammatory arthritis, previous injuries)
  - Anticipated physical demands on the elbow, especially when arthroplasty is considered
  - Determine the extent of associated soft tissue (open fractures, frail skin).
  - Identify the neurovascular status of the upper extremity.
  - Identify associated fractures (both in the same upper extremity and other locations).
  - Understand the anticipated physical demands on the elbow, especially when arthroplasty is considered.

IMAGING AND OTHER DIAGNOSTIC STUDIES

- Anteroposterior and lateral radiographs of the elbow may be difficult to interpret because of fracture displacement and comminution as well as fragment overlapping **(FIG 1A,B)**.
- Computed tomography (CT) with three-dimensional reconstruction substantially improves the identification and visualization of fracture patterns; in elderly patients with highly comminuted fractures, it may be particularly useful in deciding whether an attempt should be made at open

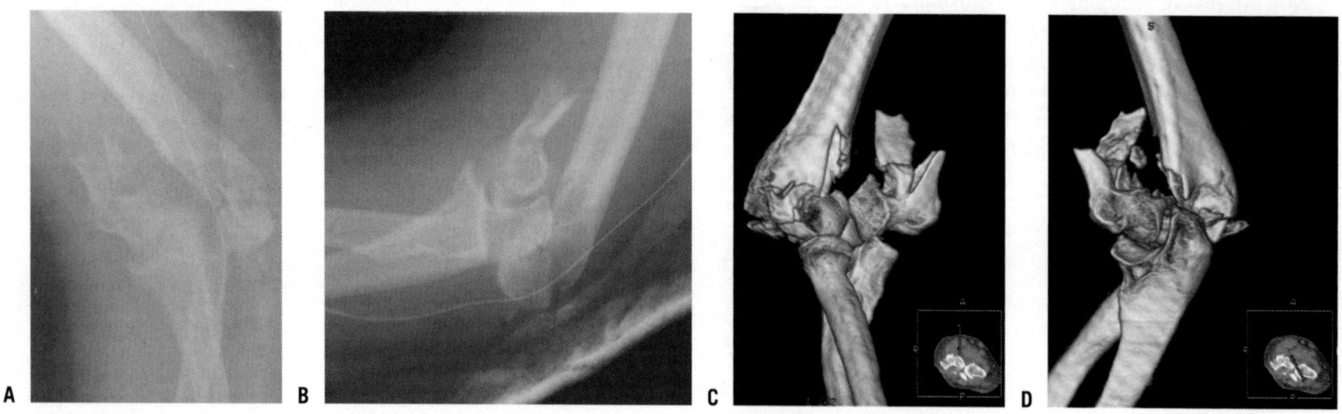

FIG 1 Anteroposterior (**A**) and lateral (**B**) radiographs showing a comminuted intra-articular supraintercondylar fracture of the distal humerus. The complexity of the fracture is difficult to appreciate fully because of the geometry of the distal humerus, fracture comminution, and fragment overlapping. **C,D.** The use of CT with three-dimensional reconstruction and surface rendering helps understand the fracture configuration and anticipate the surgical findings.

reduction and internal fixation versus proceeding directly to arthroplasty **(FIG 1C,D)**.

- Traction radiographs obtained in the operating room with the patient under anesthesia just before surgery may be useful to plan the internal fixation strategy, especially if a CT scan is not available.
- Electromyography and nerve conduction studies have been used mostly for research but demonstrate pathologic changes involving the ulnar nerve in approximately one fourth of distal humerus fractures.

SURGICAL MANAGEMENT

- Treatment of supraintercondylar fractures is challenging due to fracture comminution, poor bone quality, and difficulty in restoring the complex anatomy of the distal humerus.
- Internal fixation is selected for most patients with articular fractures of the distal humerus, whereas arthroplasty is considered for elderly patients (especially females) with osteopenia, comminution, and/or preexisting pathology.[27]
- The main goal of internal fixation is to achieve a construct stable enough to allow immediate unprotected motion without fear of redisplacement.[16]
- This can be attained in most distal humerus fractures—even the most complex—provided the following principles are adhered to **(FIG 2)**:
  - Plates used for internal fixation are applied so that fixation in the distal fragments is maximized.
  - Distal screw fixation contributes to stability at the supracondylar level, where true interfragmentary compression is achieved.

Approach

- Adequate exposure is necessary to achieve satisfactory reduction and fixation.

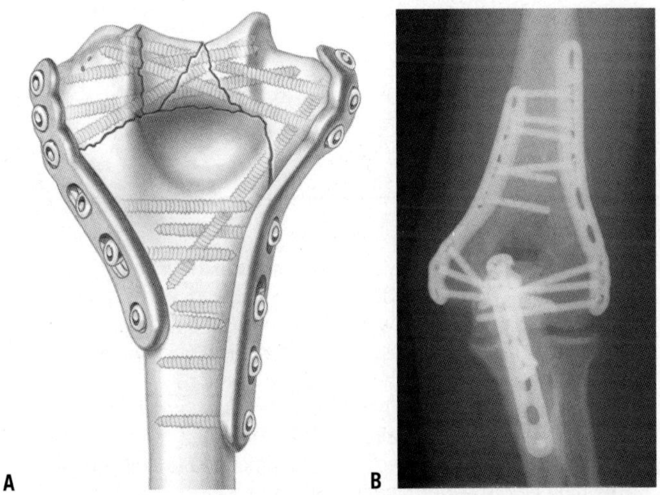

FIG 2 A. Internal fixation using two parallel medial and lateral plates allows maximal fixation of the plates in the distal fragments and increased stability at the supracondylar level. **B.** This postoperative anteroposterior radiograph shows anatomic reduction of a complex distal humerus fracture and stable fixation using the principles and technique described in this chapter. The olecranon osteotomy was fixed with a plate. (**A:** Used with permission of Mayo Foundation for Medical Education and Research. All rights reserved.)

- Although some studies have suggested that subcutaneous transposition of the ulnar nerve is associated with a decreased incidence of postoperative ulnar neuropathy,[3] the best available evidence seems to indicate no differences in ulnar nerve–related symptoms when in situ decompression versus transposition of the ulnar nerve is performed in the setting of internal fixation of a distal humerus fracture.[14]
- Approaches for distal humerus fracture fixation employ a posterior skin incision, with various strategies described to expose the distal humerus through or around the triceps to gain the access for internal fixation.
  - There is a tendency to use an Alonso-Llames bilaterotricipital approach for relatively simple fractures with minimal or no involvement of the joint surface.
  - Olecranon osteotomy seems to be the most common exposure used for the more complex fractures with intra-articular extension.
- When substantial proximal exposure of the humerus is necessary due to diaphyseal extension of the fracture or the need to use a longer lateral plate due to fracture comminution and osteopenia, the radial nerve should be formally identified and protected. The radial nerve may be identified by direct palpation at the interval between brachialis and brachioradialis. Alternatively, the posterior antebrachial cutaneous nerve (branch of the radial nerve) is identified distally and followed proximally to the main trunk of the radial nerve.
- Olecranon osteotomy is the preferred surgical approach for internal fixation for most distal humerus fractures.
  - Advantages
    - Provides excellent exposure of the articular surface and the columns[34]
    - Offers the potential of bone-to-bone healing, thereby limiting the risk of extensor mechanism insufficiency
  - Disadvantages
    - Complications: nonunion, intra-articular adhesions
    - Hardware removal may be needed.
    - Limits the ability for intraoperative conversion to elbow arthroplasty, and as such, it should be avoided in elderly patients with complex fractures when the decision to proceed with internal fixation or arthroplasty will be made after fracture exposure
    - May devitalize the anconeus muscle
    - The proximal ulna cannot be used as a template to judge reduction and motion.

Bilaterotricipital Approach (Alonso-Llames, Triceps-On, Paratricipital Approach)[1]

- Indications
  - This approach is used only for relatively simple fracture patterns, with minimal involvement of the joint surface (eg, extra-articular or simple intra-articular distal humerus fracture [AO/OTA A, C1, C2]) or when elbow arthroplasty is being considered.
  - An extension of this approach laterally through Kocher interval (between extensor carpi ulnaris and anconeus) may increase the distal exposure.
- Advantages
  - Allows visualization of the posterior aspects of both columns and the posterior aspect of the articular surface

- Leaves the extensor mechanism of the elbow completely intact by utilizing medial and lateral windows on either side of the triceps
- There is no need to protect the extensor mechanism postoperatively.
- Can be converted to an olecranon osteotomy approach to increase articular exposure and facilities conversion to a total elbow arthroplasty
- Preserves innervation and blood supply of the anconeus muscle[30]
- Disadvantage
  - Limited exposure in more complex fractures, especially in the presence of extensive articular comminution

Triceps-Reflecting, Triceps-Splitting, and Triceps-Reflecting Anconeus Pedicle

- Advantages
  - These exposures leave the proximal ulna intact, which facilitates conversion to elbow arthroplasty and facilitates use of the proximal ulna as a template for reduction of the articular surface.
  - Avoid complications related to olecranon osteotomy.
  - Allow assessment of passive extension after fracture fixation, which is especially useful in fractures requiring metaphyseal shortening.
- Disadvantages
  - Limited visualization of the anterior aspects of the articular surface
  - Risk of triceps insufficiency

Lateral Paraolecranon Approach

- Described for revision as well as primary elbow arthroplasty in an effort to maintain the triceps tendon attachment to the ulna intact but provide improved exposure in comparison to the Alonso-Llames approach
- Advantages
  - Minimal to no risk of triceps insufficiency
  - Improved visualization of the lateral aspect of the distal humerus and lateral column
  - Ease of conversion to elbow arthroplasty
- Disadvantages
  - Limited visualization of the anterior aspect of the trochlea
  - Not as triceps preserving as the bilaterotricipital exposure

Management of the Ulnar Nerve

- As mentioned, a large proportion of distal humerus fractures are associated with ulnar nerve dysfunction before surgery, and the best available evidence has failed to show differences in ulnar neuropathy rates or severity after internal fixation when in situ decompression versus subcutaneous transposition have been performed.[14]
- Authors preference is to perform a subcutaneous transposition of the ulnar nerve routinely because our impression is that it is easier to protect the nerve during surgery and also to avoid nerve to plate contact.
- The ulnar nerve is easier to identify proximally, placing a self-retaining retractor between the medial triceps and the medial skin flap. Fracture comminution leading to shortening and deformity may leave the nerve detensioned, wavy, and more difficult to identify. Longitudinal traction on the arm by an assistant may help in this part of the procedure.
- Once the nerve is dissected proximally, a vessel loop may be placed around the nerve and loosely tied, avoiding metal instruments that might constantly pull on the nerve. Some authors prefer a wider loop around the nerve, such as a Penrose drain.
- The cubital tunnel, proximal fascia of the *flexor carpi ulnaris*, and articular branch of the ulnar nerve are released, thereby mobilizing the nerve to the level of the first motor branch to the *flexor carpi ulnaris*.
- A large subcutaneous pocket is created anterior to the location of the medial epicondyle, and the ulnar nerve is mobilized and place in this pocket.

TECHNIQUES

SURGICAL EXPOSURES

Olecranon Osteotomy

- Chevron osteotomy is favored over transverse osteotomy by most because of added intrinsic stability and the potential for increased surface area for union.[21]
- The distal apex of the chevron osteotomy is centered over the "bare area" of the olecranon articular surface (the nonarticular portion of the greater sigmoid notch).
- The anconeus is divided with electrocautery in line with the lateral limb of the osteotomy.
  - In an attempt to avoid denervation of the anconeus, some authors favor elevating the anconeus off the ulna from distal to proximal without detaching it from the triceps to preserve its innervation.[17] At the end of the procedure, the anconeus is sutured back in place.
- The osteotomy is initiated with a saw and completed with an osteotome to create some irregularity at the osteotomy site, limit bone loss, and avoid inadvertent articular cartilage damage **(TECH FIG 1A)**.
- Mobilize the fragment to facilitate exposure **(TECH FIG 1B)**.
- Fixation of the olecranon osteotomy can be achieved with tension band wiring,[13] screw/tension band constructs, or compression plating **(TECH FIG 1C)**.[8]
- Plate fixation probably is the most stable, but one study reported a higher rate of soft tissue complications (wound dehiscence, infection) when plates are used.[11]
- The authors use tension-band wiring for fixation of the olecranon osteotomy for most elbows **(TECH FIG 1D,E)**.
- If screw fixation is planned, it is recommended to drill and tap the ulna before performing the osteotomy.

Bilaterotricipital Approach (Alonso-Llames, Triceps-On, Paratricipital Approach)[1]

- The triceps is elevated from the medial and lateral intermuscular septae and the posterior aspect of the humerus.
- Lateral dissection can be extended anterior to the anconeus muscle **(TECH FIG 2)**.
- The arthrotomy is performed posterior to the medial collateral ligament and lateral collateral ligament complex.

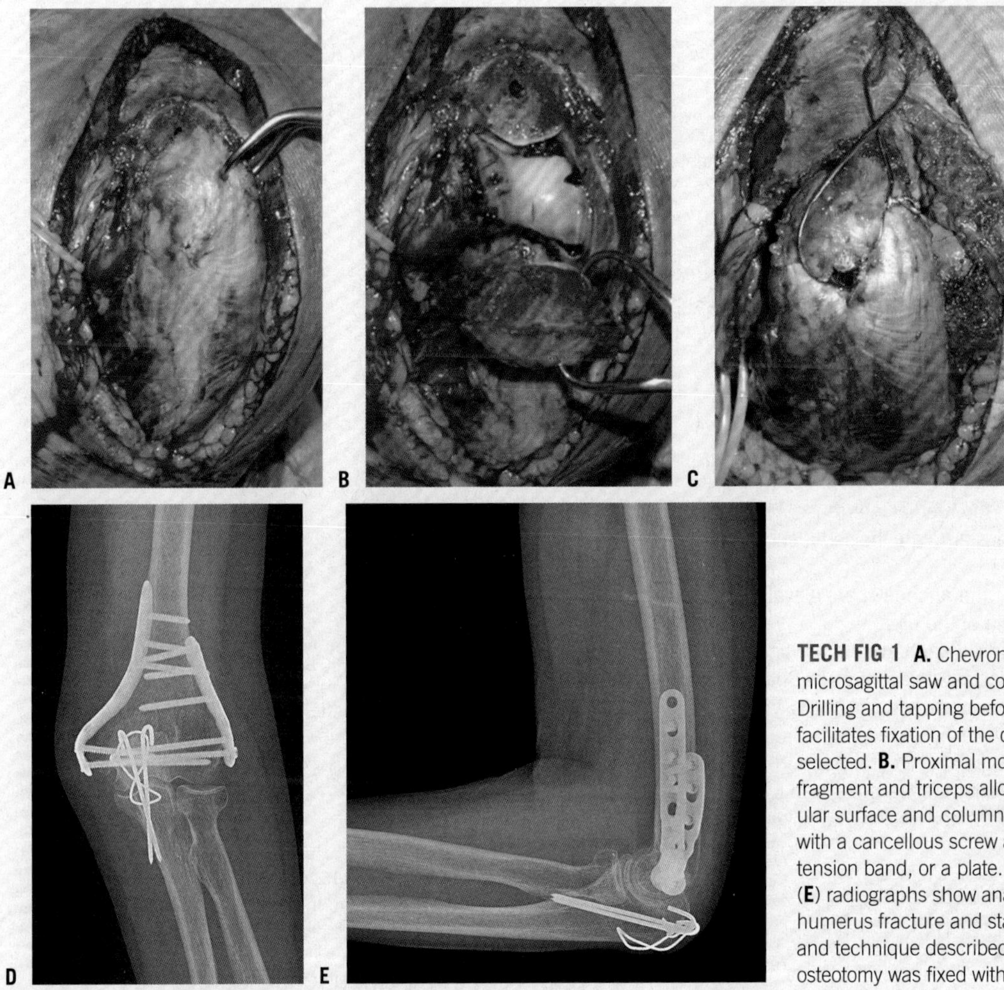

TECH FIG 1 **A.** Chevron osteotomy is initiated with a microsagittal saw and completed with an osteotome. Drilling and tapping before performing the osteotomy facilitates fixation of the osteotomy if screw fixation is selected. **B.** Proximal mobilization of the osteotomized fragment and triceps allows ample exposure of the articular surface and columns. **C.** Fixation may be performed with a cancellous screw and tension band, wires and a tension band, or a plate. Postoperative AP (**D**) and lateral (**E**) radiographs show anatomic reduction of a distal humerus fracture and stable fixation using the principles and technique described in this chapter. The olecranon osteotomy was fixed with tension band wiring.

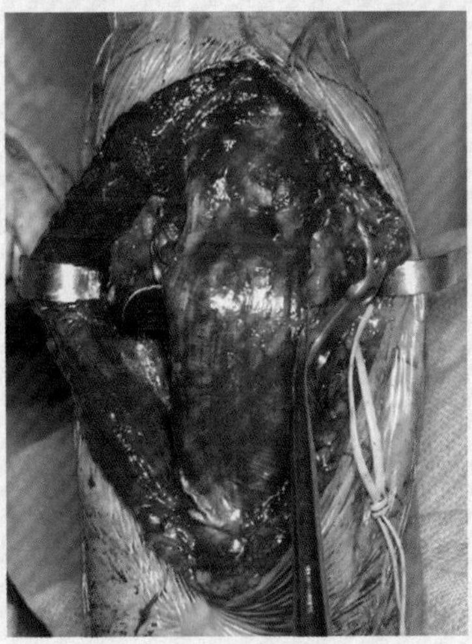

TECH FIG 2 Fractures with no or limited articular involvement may be fixed working on both sides of the triceps. As shown in this image, the extensor mechanism is left mostly undisturbed.

Lateral Paraolecranon Approach[33]

- The medial window of this exposure is identical to the paratricipital approach, elevating the medial aspect of the triceps from the medial intermuscular septum and the humerus.
- Laterally, the anconeus fascia is incised leaving a cuff of tissue on the ulna for later repair.
- The longitudinal division between the lateral portion of the triceps (not attached directly to the olecranon through Sharpey fibers) and the central portion of the triceps (attached directly to the olecranon through Sharpey fibers) is split from proximal to distal until it meets the anconeus split. This provides a lateral window with great access to the lateral distal humerus and lateral column.
- A modified triceps-splitting approach preserves most of the insertion of the triceps tendon on the olecranon while providing improved visualization of the proximal ulna relative to the paratricipital approach.

Triceps Reflection and Triceps Split

Triceps-Splitting Approach

- This approach involves a midline split through the triceps tendon. The medial and lateral columns are exposed with subperiosteal dissection starting from the midline and moving outward.
- The triceps insertion on the olecranon is split in the midline, with release of Sharpey fibers to create medial and lateral fasciocutaneuos sleeves and, at the conclusion of the procedure, the triceps tendon is repaired to the olecranon via transosseous nonabsorbable braided sutures.
- Alternatively, the medial and lateral aspects of the triceps tendon attachment are elevated with small bone chips.

Medial Triceps-Reflecting Approach (Bryan-Morrey, Medial Reflection) (TECH FIG 3)

- The triceps is elevated from the medial intermuscular septum.
- The forearm fascia and periosteum are incised just lateral to the flexor carpi ulnaris.
- The triceps, forearm fascia, and anconeus are elevated in continuity from the medial margin of the ulna.
- The triceps tendon is carefully detached from the tip of the olecranon by sharp subperiosteal detachment of Sharpey fibers.
- Finally, the extensor mechanism is reflected laterally from the margin of the lateral epicondyle.
- The anterior bundle of the medial collateral ligament and the lateral ulnar collateral ligament must be preserved to avoid postoperative instability, unless conversion to a linked elbow arthroplasty is performed.

Mayo Modified Kocher Posterolateral Triceps-Reflecting Approach[15]

- A Kocher approach is performed using the interval between the anconeus and the *extensor carpi ulnaris* and is extended proximally to separate the common extensor group anteriorly and the triceps posteriorly.
- The triceps is elevated from the lateral intermuscular septum.
- The triceps and anconeus are elevated in continuity subperiosteally off the ulna from lateral to medial.

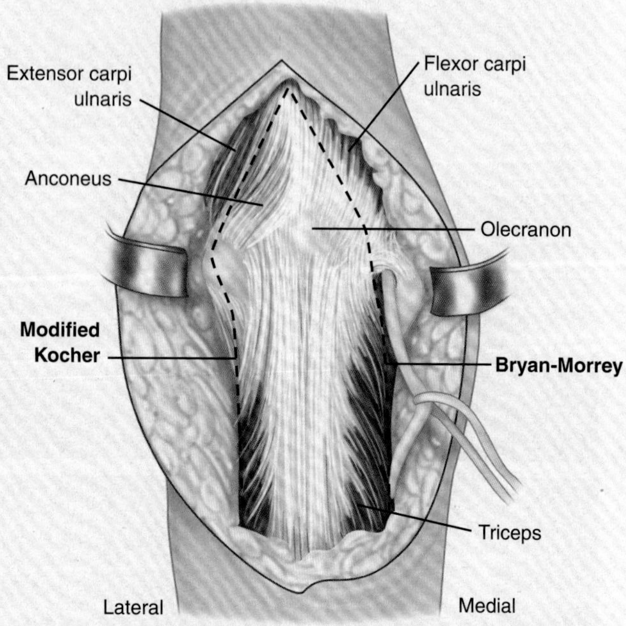

TECH FIG 3 The extensor mechanism (ie, triceps, anconeus, and forearm fascia) may be elevated off the ulna subperiosteally in continuity from medial to lateral (Bryan-Morrey approach) or from lateral to medial (Mayo modified extensile Kocher approach).

- As noted earlier, the anterior bundle of the medial collateral ligament and the lateral ulnar collateral ligament must be preserved to avoid postoperative instability, unless conversion to a linked elbow arthroplasty is performed.

Triceps-Reflecting Anconeus Pedicle Approach[17]

- This approach involves combining the Bryan-Morrey and modified Kocher approaches to reflect the triceps in continuity with the anconeus from both the medial and the lateral side.
- The triceps–anconeus complex is then reflected proximally.

INTERNAL FIXATION

- Screws in the distal fragments (articular segment) should be placed according to the following principles:
  - Every screw should pass through a plate.
  - Each screw should engage a fragment on the opposite side that also is fixed to a plate.
  - As many screws as possible should be place in the distal fragments.
  - Each screw should be as long as possible.
  - Each screw should engage as many articular fragments as possible.
  - The screws in the distal fragments should lock together by interdigitation, thereby rigidly linking the medial and lateral columns together, creating an architectural structure similar to that of an arch of dome.
- Medial and lateral plates are applied according to the following principles[29,32]:
  - Plates should be applied such that compression is achieved at the supracondylar level for both columns.
  - Plates used must be strong enough and stiff enough to resist breaking or bending before union occurs at the supracondylar level.
- All eight of these objectives are best achieved with parallel plate configuration using one plate on each column at approximately 180 degrees to each other. For relatively simple fractures with no comminution, orthogonal and parallel plating probably provide equivalent results.[29]
- Locking plates have been shown to provide improved fixation in osteoporotic bone and improved outcomes when used for

other periarticular locations,[26] but in distal humerus fractures, their utility is limited because nonpolyaxial locked screws follow a predetermined trajectory in bone, which may be difficult to fit within the complex geometry of the distal end of the humerus.
- One-third tubular plates are not strong enough for fixation of these complex fractures.

Provisional Assembly of the Articular Surface and Articular Surface Reduction

- Reduce the articular surface fragments anatomically, unless bone is missing (see in the following text). The proximal ulna and radial head may be used as templates.
- Rotational alignment should be carefully assessed.
- Used fine-threaded wires (1 to 1.5 mm) to maintain the reduction provisionally **(TECH FIG 4)**.
  - It is necessary for these wires to be placed close to the subchondral level so as not to interfere with the passage of screws from the plates into the distal fragments.
  - Occasionally, these fine-treaded wires can be cut flush with their entrance into bone and left as permanent fixation.
  - Two Steinmann pins introduced at the medial and lateral epicondyles across the distal humerus facilitate provisional placement of the plates and can be replaced by screws.

Plate Placement

- Medial and lateral plates are placed so that one of the distal holes of each plate slides over the medial and lateral Steinmann pins mentioned earlier, but no screws are placed in the distal fragments until the plates are provisionally applied proximally **(TECH FIG 5)**.
- Each plate is rotated posteriorly slightly out of the sagittal plane such that the angle between them is often in the range of 150 to 160 degrees.
- This orientation permits the insertion of at least four long screws (two from each side) through plate holes and into the distal fragments from medial to lateral and vice versa.

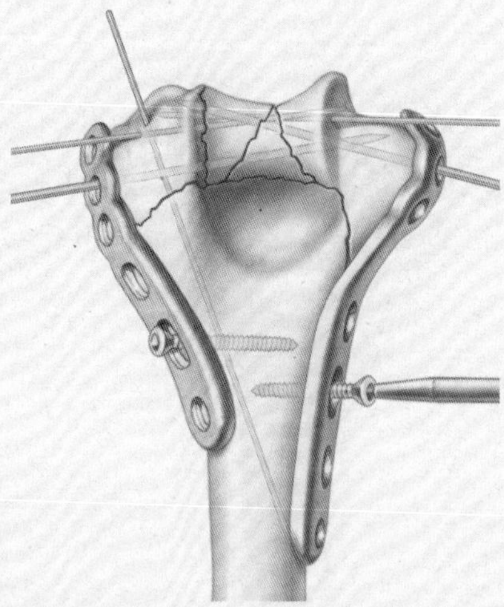

TECH FIG 5 The medial and lateral plates are held in place provisionally with two distal 2.0-mm pins (which later will be replaced by screws) and two proximal screws through an oval hole to allow small adjustments in plate positioning. (Used with permission of Mayo Foundation for Medical Education and Research. All rights reserved.)

- Plates may be contoured intraoperatively to fit the geometry of the distal part of the humerus if precontoured plates are not available. Undercontouring of the plates may be used to provide additional compression at the supracondylar level.
- The length of the plate is selected so that at least three screws can be placed in the proximal part of the humeral shaft both medially and laterally proximal to the uppermost extent of the fracture.
- Ideally, the plates should end at different levels proximally, to avoid the creation of a stress riser.
- One cortical screw is loosely introduced into an oblong hole of each plate to hold the plates in place provisionally; use of oblong holes for these screws facilitates later adjustments in plate positioning.

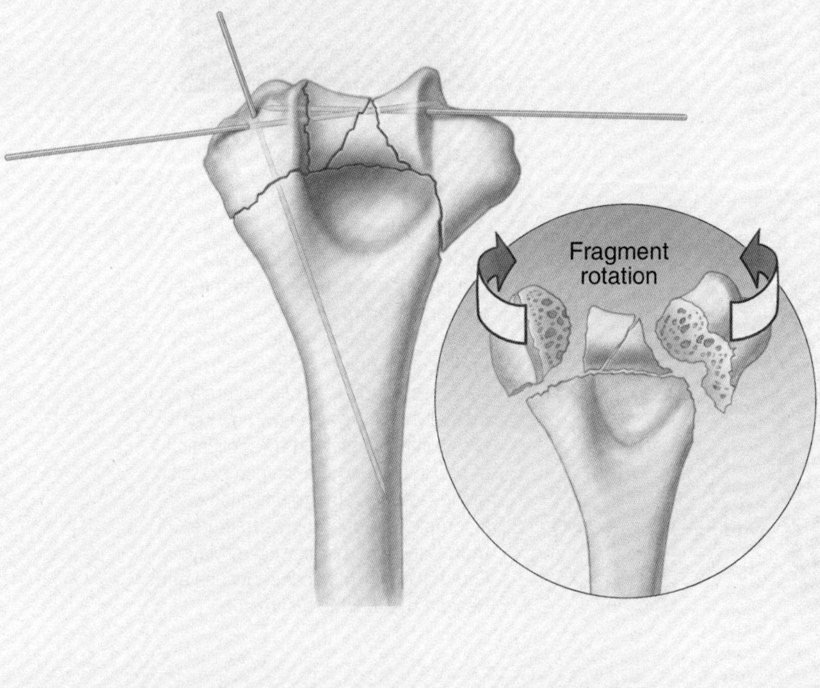

TECH FIG 4 Anatomic reduction of the articular surface is maintained provisionally with fine wires placed so that they will not interfere with plate and screw application. (Used with permission of Mayo Foundation for Medical Education and Research. All rights reserved.)

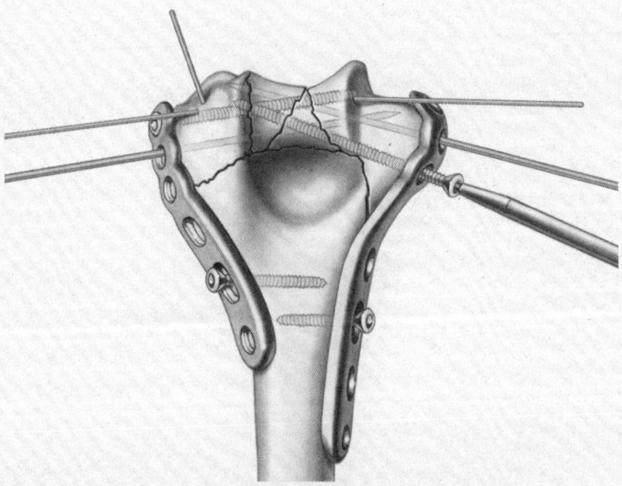

TECH FIG 6 Maximal distal plate anchorage is then achieved by insertion of multiple long screws through the plates and into the distal fragments. Usually, the screws from the medial and lateral directions will engage, creating an interlocked structure that increases fracture stability. (Used with permission of Mayo Foundation for Medical Education and Research. All rights reserved.)

Articular and Distal Fixation

- Distal fixation is achieved next by placing multiple long screws across the distal fragments, always through plate holes, and from side to side. As noted, the screws should be as long as possible and engage the opposite column.
  - Before screw application, a large bone clamp may be used to compress the articular fracture lines, unless there is comminution of the articular surface.
- The two Steinmann pins introduced earlier can be replaced with distal screws without previous drilling to avoid accidental breakage of the drill when contacting the other screws. Usually, these last screws will interdigitate with the previously applied distal screws, thereby increasing the stability of the construct **(TECH FIG 6)**.
- Care should be taken so that screws are not placed through the coronoid, radial head, or olecranon fossae, as they may lead to impingement and limit motion.

Supracondylar Compression and Proximal Plate fixation

- First, the proximal screw introduced through an oblong hole on one side is backed out, and a large bone clamp is applied distally on that side and proximally on the opposite side to apply maximum compression at the supracondylar level **(TECH FIG 7A,B)**.

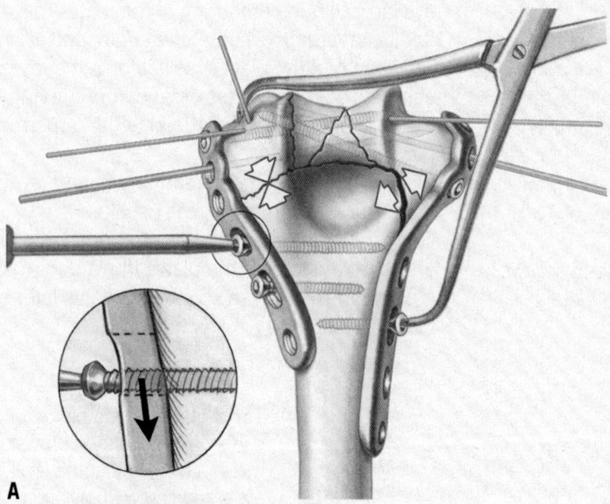

A

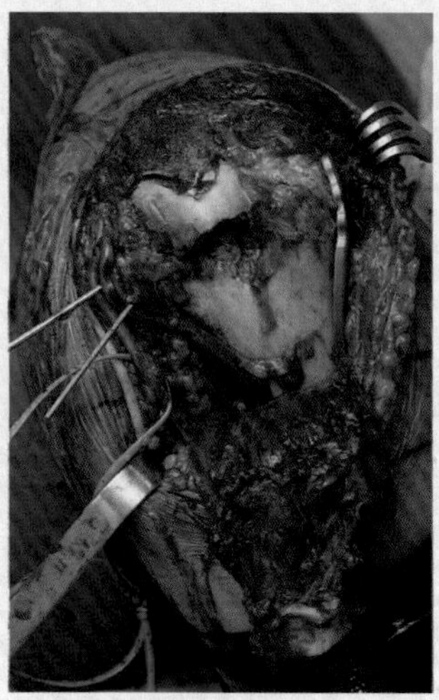

C

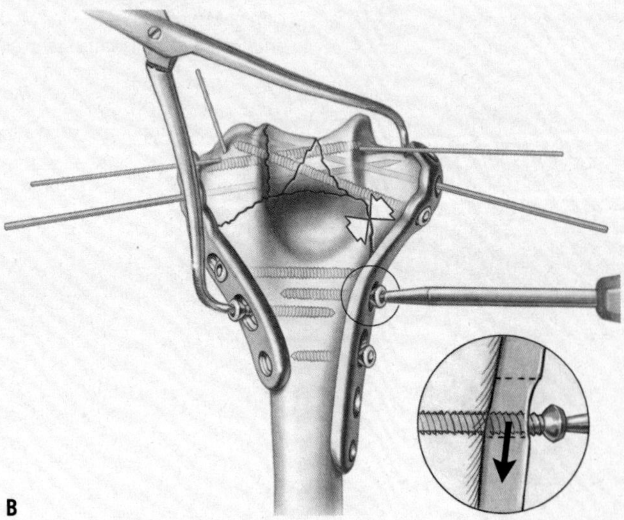

B

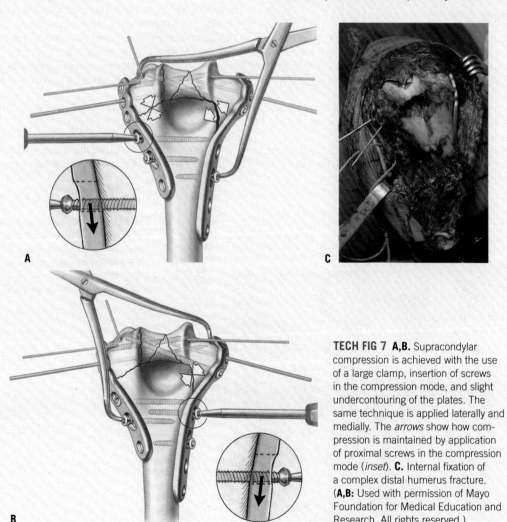

TECH FIG 7 A,B. Supracondylar compression is achieved with the use of a large clamp, insertion of screws in the compression mode, and slight undercontouring of the plates. The same technique is applied laterally and medially. The *arrows* show how compression is maintained by application of proximal screws in the compression mode (*inset*). **C.** Internal fixation of a complex distal humerus fracture. (**A,B:** Used with permission of Mayo Foundation for Medical Education and Research. All rights reserved.)

- Care must be taken not to change the varus–valgus or rotational alignment of the articular surface when the bone clamps are applied.
- Compression at the supracondylar level achieved with the bone clamp is maintained with one or more screws introduced through the plate in compression mode and selective plate undercontouring.
- The same steps are followed on the opposite side.
- The remaining diaphyseal screws are then introduced, providing additional compression as they push the undercontoured plates to gain intimate contact with the underlying bone **(TECH FIG 7C)**.
- Provisional wires are removed.
- The elbow is put through range of motion. Motion should be smooth. If extension is limited, the tip of the olecranon may be partially removed.

MANAGEMENT OF BONE LOSS

- Bone loss is common at the central aspect of the distal humerus as well as at the supracondylar region.
- Depending on the severity and location of bone loss, humeral shortening or bone grafting may be required.

Metaphyseal Shortening (Supracondylar Shortening)[19]

- The distal segment is intentionally fixed in a nonanatomic position to shorten the humerus in order to maximize contact and compression **(TECH FIG 8A,B)**.
- The distal aspect of the humeral shaft is reshaped to maximize contact; bone is never removed from the articular segment.
- The humerus may be shortened between a few millimeters and 2 cm with only minor losses in extension strength.
- Shortening leads to absence of the fossae to allow the coronoid and the radial head to fit in flexion and the olecranon in extension. As such, shortening will lead to substantial motion loss unless:
  - The articular segment is translated anteriorly to recreate anterior space for the coronoid and radial head in flexion.
  - A new space to receive the olecranon posteriorly is sculpted by removing bone from the distal aspect of the diaphysis to develop a new olecranon fossa **(TECH FIG 8C)**.
- Once the opposing bone surfaces at the metaphyseal shortening have been compressed and fixed with the plates following the principles and techniques outlined earlier, stability is satisfactory enough to permit early motion without protection.
- It is acceptable to translate the distal segment slightly medially or laterally as well as anteriorly. However, rotational and varus–valgus malalignment of the articular segment may inadvertently occur with this technique and should be avoided.

Bone Grafting

- Occasionally, the severity of metaphyseal comminution exceeds the limits of supracondylar shortening; corticocancellous iliac crest may be needed in these circumstances.
- Comminution of the central aspect of the trochlea may also be managed with bone grafting to avoid narrowing of the distal humerus with mediolateral compression during plate fixation.
- The articular cartilage of the central aspect of the trochlea is not critical, as long as the capitellum and medial trochlea are preserved.
- As such, the graft does not need to articulate with the proximal ulna and can be recessed from the articular surface.
- Allograft may be used for this particular application.

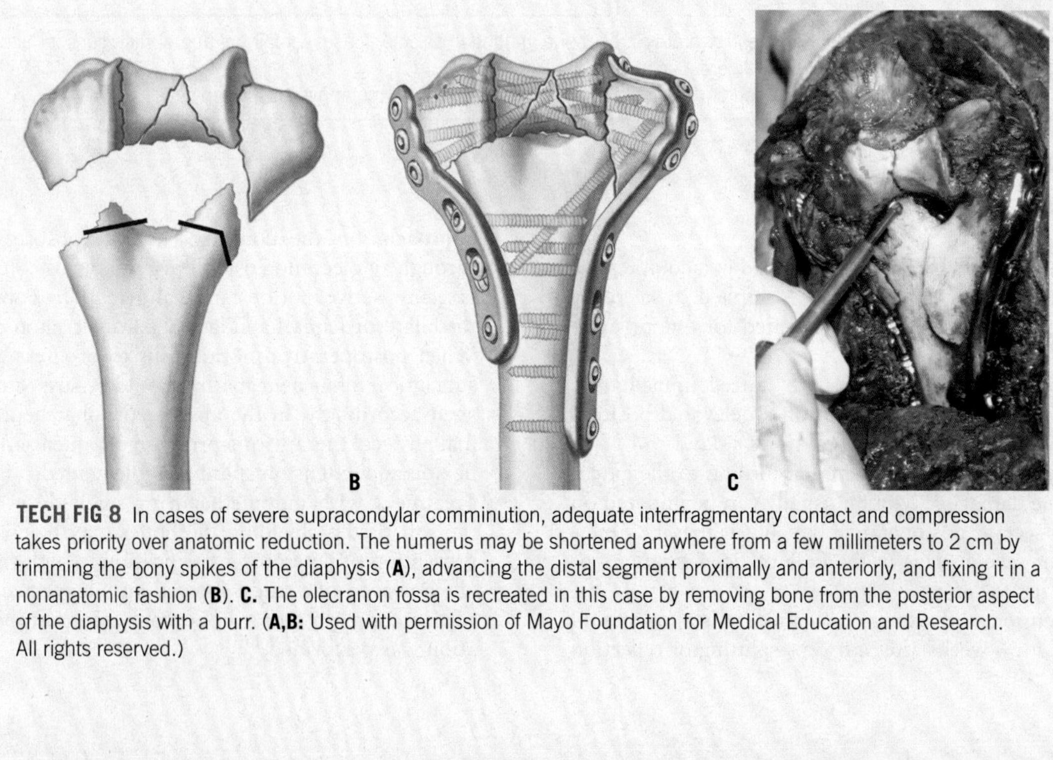

A B C

TECH FIG 8 In cases of severe supracondylar comminution, adequate interfragmentary contact and compression takes priority over anatomic reduction. The humerus may be shortened anywhere from a few millimeters to 2 cm by trimming the bony spikes of the diaphysis (**A**), advancing the distal segment proximally and anteriorly, and fixing it in a nonanatomic fashion (**B**). **C.** The olecranon fossa is recreated in this case by removing bone from the posterior aspect of the diaphysis with a burr. (**A,B:** Used with permission of Mayo Foundation for Medical Education and Research. All rights reserved.)

Pearls and Pitfalls

Exposures

Olecranon Osteotomy	• Position the apex of the osteotomy distally. • Use a thing oscillating saw to minimize bone loss. • If plate fixation is preferred, consider drilling the holes for the plate before per the osteotomy. This facilitates plate fixation of the osteotomy at the conclusion of the surgery. • Similarly, if tension band fixation with an intramedullary screw is preferred, predrill and pretap the screw hole before performing the osteotomy. • Beware of the possibility of an angled reduction of the osteotomy in the lateral plane when applying a compression plate on the dorsal aspect of the ulna.
Triceps Reflection and Triceps Split	• Meticulous subperiosteal detachment of the extensor mechanism is critical to preserve its thickness and facilitate a strong reattachment. • Reproduce anatomic reattachment of the extensor mechanism. • Use heave nonabsorbable sutures (no. 5 Ethibond [Ethicon Inc., Somerville, NJ], no. 2 FiberWire [Arthrex, Naples, FL], or equivalent). • Protect extension against resistance for 6 weeks.
Bilaterotricipital Approach	• Identify the whole width of the triceps • Resect the posterior capsule and fat pad to improve visualization.
Lateral Paraolecranon Approach	• Split the triceps from proximal to distal to avoid creating an angled split into the triceps.

Surgical Technique

Articular Surface Reduction	• Kirschner wires for provisional fixation should be placed in the subchondral region, rather than in the center of the articular segments, to avoid interference with distal screw placement. • Avoid use of distal screws not passing through the plates, so that every distal screw contributes to fixation at the supracondylar level.
Plate Placement	• Place the plates at a slight posteromedial and posterolateral angle, as opposed to exactly 180 degrees from each other. • Place the lateral plate so that it does not extend into the origin of the common extensor group and humeral origin of the lateral collateral humeral complex, to avoid late soft tissue failure by attrition. • When a longer lateral plate will be used, formal identification and protection of the radial nerve is mandatory.
Screw Placement	• Carefully check elbow range of motion for completeness and smoothness to detect inadvertent intra-articular screw placement or impingement with coronoid, radial head, or olecranon. • Once several distal screws are applied, use of a drill bit distally can easily lead to breakage.
Failure to Recognize Bone Loss	• Anticipate the potential for iliac crest bone grafting in selected cases, obtaining appropriate consent and preparing and draping the iliac crest donor site. • Understand the techniques of central trochlear grafting and metaphyseal shortening.

POSTOPERATIVE MANAGEMENT

- After closure, the elbow is lightly wrapped in a compressive dressing, an anterior plaster splint is applied to keep the elbow in extension, the elbow is elevated for one or more days, and ice may be applied.
- Hand range-of-motion exercises are started immediately, and the elbow is brought down from an elevated position to a normal resting position several times a day.
- Elbow range of motion is initiated according to the extent of soft tissue damage.[18] Motion usually can be initiated on the first or second postoperative day, but it may be necessary to wait several days in the case of open fractures or severe soft tissue damage.
- Active extension and extension against resistance should be avoided for 6 weeks after a triceps-splitting or reflection approach; on the contrary, when exposure was gained through an olecranon osteotomy and the osteotomy fixation is secure, active motion can be allowed. The same applies for the bilaterotricipital and lateral paraolecranon exposures.
- When postoperative motion fails to progress as expected, subclinical ulnar neuropathy should be suspected and managed accordingly. In the absence of ulnar neuropathy, formal physical therapy or a program of patient-adjusted static flexion and extension splint is implemented.
- Treatment with indomethacin or single-dose radiation to the soft tissues shielding the bones may be considered for prevention of heterotopic ossification in high-risk individuals; however, one study showed an unexpectedly high rate of olecranon osteotomy nonunion when postoperative radiation was performed.[10]

OUTCOMES

- The results of different studies are difficult to interpret because the severity of the injuries included sometimes varies widely, and there may be variations in the accuracy of range-of-motion measurements.[2,4–7,9,22,23,28]
- In general, reasonable outcomes can be expected when the principles of anatomic restoration of the joint surface, bicolumnar plating, and stable internal fixation to allow early motion are employed.[2,4,5,7,9,22,23]
- Improvements in fixation techniques have resulted in a decreased rate of hardware failure and nonunion; however, range of motion is not reliably restored in every patient, and other complications remain relatively common, as detailed in the following text.

COMPLICATIONS

- Infection
- Nonunion
- Stiffness, with or without heterotopic ossification
- Need for removal of the hardware used for fixation of the olecranon osteotomy
- Ulnar neuropathy
- Posttraumatic osteoarthritis
- Avascular necrosis
- Management of these complications often requires additional surgery or the occasional used of salvage procedures such as interposition arthroplasty or elbow replacement.[31]

REFERENCES

1. Alonso-Llames M. Bilaterotricipital approach to the elbow. Its application in the osteosynthesis of supracondylar fractures of the humerus in children. Acta Orthop Scand 1972;43:479–490.
2. Athwal GS, Hoxie SC, Rispoli DM, et al. Precontoured parallel plate fixation of AO/OTA type C distal humerus fractures. J Orthop Trauma 2009;23:575–580.
3. Chen RC, Harris DJ, Leduc S, et al. Is ulnar nerve transposition beneficial during open reduction internal fixation of distal humerus fractures? J Orthop Trauma 2010;24:391–394.
4. Clavert P, Ducrot G, Sirveaux F, et al. Outcomes of distal humerus fractures in patients above 65 years of age treated by plate fixation. Orthop Traumatol Surg Res 2013;99:771–777.
5. Doornberg JN, van Duijn PJ, Linzel D, et al. Surgical treatment of intra-articular fractures of the distal part of the humerus. Functional outcome after twelve to thirty years. J Bone Joint Surg Am 2007;89:1524–1532.
6. Ellwein A, Lill H, Voigt C, et al. Arthroplasty compared to internal fixation by locking plate osteosynthesis in comminuted fractures of the distal humerus. Int Orthop 2015;39:747–754.
7. Flinkkilä T, Toimela J, Sirniö K, et al. Results of parallel plate fixation of comminuted intra-articular distal humeral fractures. J Shoulder Elbow Surg 2014;23:701–707.
8. Gofton WT, Macdermid JC, Patterson SD, et al. Functional outcome of AO type C distal humeral fractures. J Hand Surg Am 2003;28:294–308.
9. Greiner S, Haas NP, Bail HJ. Outcome after open reduction and angular stable internal fixation for supra-intercondylar fractures of the distal humerus: preliminary results with the LCP distal humerus system. Arch Orthop Trauma Surg 2008;128:723–729.
10. Hamid N, Ashraf N, Bosse MJ, et al. Radiation therapy for heterotopic ossification prophylaxis acutely after elbow trauma: a prospective randomized study. J Bone Joint Surg Am 2010;92:2032–2038.
11. Lawrence TM, Ahmadi S, Morrey BF, et al. Wound complications after distal humerus fracture fixation: incidence, risk factors, and outcome. J Shoulder Elbow Surg 2014;23:258–264.
12. Marsh JL, Slongo TF, Agel J, et al. Fracture and dislocation classification compendium - 2007: Orthopaedic Trauma Association classification, database and outcomes committee. J Orthop Trauma 2007; 21(suppl 10):S1–S133.
13. McCarty LP, Ring D, Jupiter JB. Management of distal humerus fractures. Am J Orthop (Belle Mead NJ) 2005;34:430–438.
14. McKee MD, Veillette CJ, Hall JA, et al. A multicenter, prospective, randomized, controlled trial of open reduction–internal fixation versus total elbow arthroplasty for displaced intra-articular distal humeral fractures in elderly patients. J Shoulder Elbow Surg 2009;18:3–12.
15. Morrey BF. Surgical exposures of the elbow. In: Morrey BF, ed. The Elbow and Its Disorders, ed 3. Philadelphia: W.B. Saunders Co., 2000:109–134.
16. Morrey BF, Askew LJ, Chao EY. A biomechanical study of normal functional elbow motion. J Bone Joint Surg Am 1981;63:872–877.
17. O'Driscoll SW. The triceps-reflecting anconeus pedicle (TRAP) approach for distal humeral fractures and nonunions. Orthop Clin North Am 2000;31:91–101.
18. O'Driscoll SW, Giori NJ. Continuous passive motion (CPM): theory and principles of clinical application. J Rehabil Res Dev 2000;37: 179–188.
19. O'Driscoll SW, Sanchez-Sotelo J, Torchia ME. Management of the smashed distal humerus. Orthop Clin North Am 2002;33:19–33, vii.
20. Palvanen M, Kannus P, Parkkari J, et al. The injury mechanisms of osteoporotic upper extremity fractures among older adults: a controlled study of 287 consecutive patients and their 108 controls. Osteoporos Int 2000;11:822–831.
21. Patterson SD, Bain GI, Mehta JA. Surgical approaches to the elbow. Clin Orthop Relat Res 2000;(370):19–33.
22. Proust J, Oksman A, Charissoux JL, et al. Intra-articular fracture of the distal humerus: outcome after osteosynthesis in patients over 60 [in French]. Rev Chir Orthop Reparatrice Appar Mot 2007;93:798–806.
23. Reising K, Hauschild O, Strohm PC, et al. Stabilisation of articular fractures of the distal humerus: early experience with a novel perpendicular plate system. Injury 2009;40:611–617.
24. Ring D, Jupiter JB, Gulotta L. Articular fractures of the distal part of the humerus. J Bone Joint Surg Am 2003;85:232–238.
25. Robinson CM, Hill RM, Jacobs N, et al. Adult distal humeral metaphyseal fractures: epidemiology and results of treatment. J Orthop Trauma 2003;17:38–47.
26. Rozental TD, Blazar PE, Franko OI, et al. Functional outcomes for unstable distal radial fractures treated with open reduction and internal fixation or closed reduction and percutaneous fixation. A prospective randomized trial. J Bone Joint Surg Am 2009;91: 1837–1846.
27. Sanchez-Sotelo J. Distal humeral fractures: role of internal fixation and elbow arthroplasty. J Bone Joint Surg Am 2012;94:555–568.
28. Sanchez-Sotelo J, Ramsey ML, King GJ, et al. Elbow arthroplasty: lessons learned from the past and directions for the future. Instr Course Lect 2011;60:157–169.
29. Sanchez-Sotelo J, Torchia ME, O'Driscoll SW. Complex distal humeral fractures: internal fixation with a principle-based parallel-plate technique. J Bone Joint Surg Am 2007;89:961–969.
30. Schildhauer TA, Nork SE, Mills WJ, et al. Extensor mechanism-sparing paratricipital posterior approach to the distal humerus. J Orthop Trauma 2003;17:374–378.
31. Schmidt-Horlohé KH, Bonk A, Wilde P, et al. Promising results after the treatment of simple and complex distal humerus type C fractures by angular-stable double-plate osteosynthesis. Orthop Traumatol Surg Res 2013;99:531–541.
32. Shin SJ, Sohn HS, Do NH. A clinical comparison of two different double plating methods for intraarticular distal humerus fractures. J Shoulder Elbow Surg 2010;19:2–9.
33. Studer A, Athwal GS, MacDermid JC, et al. The lateral para-olecranon approach for total elbow arthroplasty. J Hand Surg Am 2013;38: 2219.e3–2226.e3.
34. Wilkinson JM, Stanley D. Posterior surgical approaches to the elbow: a comparative anatomic study. J Shoulder Elbow Surg 2001; 10:380–382.

CHAPTER 13

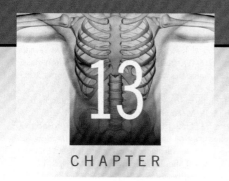

Open Reduction and Internal Fixation of Capitellum and Capitellar–Trochlear Shear Fractures

James Stenson and Luke Austin

DEFINITION

- Capitellar fractures are uncommon, accounting for less than 1% of all elbow fractures and 6% of all distal humerus fractures.[4]
- They often are associated with radial head fractures and posterior elbow dislocations.
- A classification system for capitellar fractures has been proposed by Bryan and Morrey[4] and modified by McKee et al[19]:
  - Type 1: complete fractures of the capitellum[12]
  - Type 2: superficial subchondral fractures of the capitellar articular surface[26]
  - Type 3: comminuted fractures[2]
  - Type 4: coronal shear fractures that include a portion of the trochlea as well as the capitellum as one piece (**FIG 1**)[19]
- Ring et al[23] have proposed a new classification, expanding on the growing understanding that isolated capitellum fractures are rare and often are involved as part of articular shear fractures of the distal humerus. The classification includes five anatomic components, with type 1 articular injuries encompassing the capitellum and capitellar–trochlear shear patterns (**FIG 2**):
  - Type 1: capitellum and lateral aspect of the trochlea
  - Type 2: lateral epicondyle
  - Type 3: posterior aspect of the lateral column
  - Type 4: posterior aspect of the trochlea
  - Type 5: medial epicondyle
- More recently, Dubberley and colleagues[6] introduced a classification system based on radiographic pattern of injury taking posterior comminution into account.
  - Type 1: fracture of the capitellum (with or without trochlear ridge involvement)
  - Type 2: capitellum and trochlea fracture that remain as one fragment
  - Type 3: capitellum and trochlea as separate fragments
  - Type A: no posterior condyle comminution
  - Type B: posterior condyle comminution present

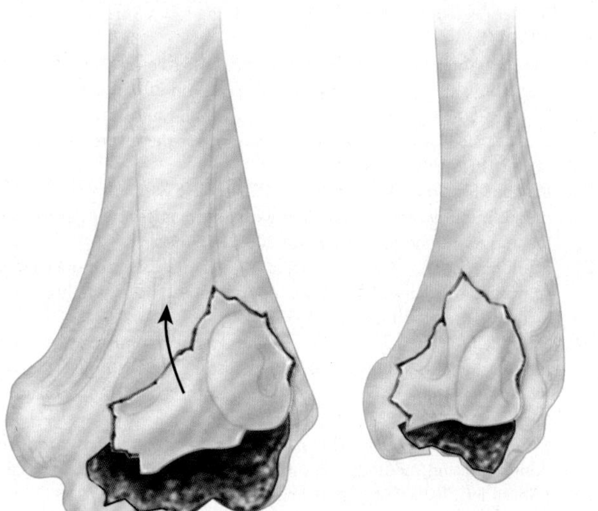

FIG 1 Type 4 coronal shear fractures of the distal humerus. Arrow indicates the direction of the shear force in the displacement of the fracture (Reprinted with permission from McKee MD, Jupiter JB, Bamberger HB, et al. Coronal shear fractures of the distal end of the humerus. J Bone Joint Surg Am 1996;78A[1]:49–54. Copyright © 1996 by The Journal of Bone and Joint Surgery, Incorporated.)

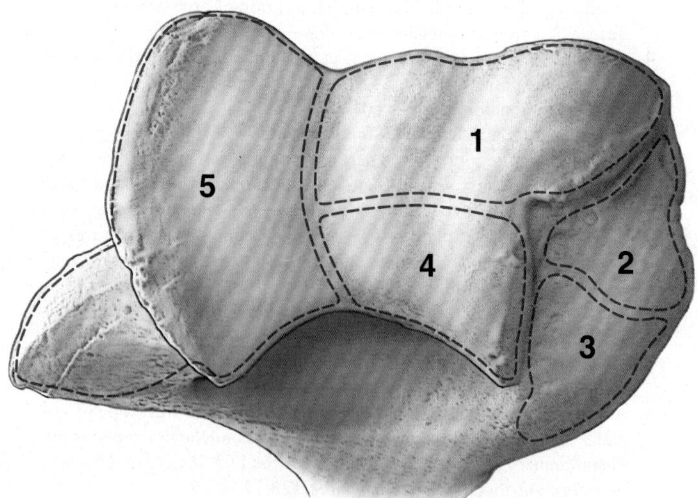

FIG 2 Articular fractures of the distal part of the humerus, including type 1 fractures that encompass capitellum and capitellar–trochlear shear fractures. (Reprinted with permission from Ring D, Jupiter JB, Gulotta L. Articular fractures of the distal part of the humerus. J Bone Joint Surg Am 2003;85-A[2]:232–238. Copyright © 2003 by The Journal of Bone and Joint Surgery, Incorporated.)

ANATOMY

- The two condyles of the distal humerus diverge from the humeral shaft to form the lateral and medial columns, which support the trochlea between them. The anterior aspect of the lateral column is covered with articular cartilage, forming the capitellum. Distally, these two condyles can be visualized as forming a triangle at the end of the humerus.
- The capitellum is the first epiphyseal center of the elbow to ossify.
- It is covered by articular surface anteriorly but devoid of it posteriorly.
- The capitellum is directed distally and anteriorly at an angle of 30 degrees to the long axis of the humerus.
- The radial head rotates on the anterior surface of the capitellum in elbow flexion and articulates with its inferior surface in elbow extension.
- The lateral collateral ligament inserts next to the lateral margin of the capitellum.
- The blood supply of the capitellum is derived posteriorly. It arises from the lateral arcade, which is the anastomosis of the radial collateral arteries of the profunda brachii and the radial recurrent artery.[27]

PATHOGENESIS

- Capitellum and capitellar–trochlear shear fractures involve impaction of the radial head against the lateral column of the distal humerus in a partially extended position, resulting in shearing of the articular cartilage of the distal humerus.
- Fracture fragments vary in size and displace superiorly and anteriorly into the radial fossa, resulting in impingement with elbow flexion.
- Associated injuries include proximal and distal radial as well as carpal fractures; ligamentous injuries include collateral ligament (lateral more common than medial) and triceps ruptures.[6]

NATURAL HISTORY

- Capitellar fractures occur almost exclusively in adults. These fractures do not occur in children because in that age group, the capitellum is largely cartilaginous, and a similar mechanism of injury would instead cause a supracondylar or lateral condyle fracture.
- Capitellar fractures are more common in females, a finding that can be attributed to the increased carrying angle of the female elbow.
- Displaced fractures that go untreated can be expected to have a poor outcome owing to the progressive loss of motion from the mechanical block to flexion, potential longitudinal instability of the forearm, and the likely development of subsequent posttraumatic arthrosis from the residual articular incongruity.
- Capitellar and trochlear fractures are prone to nonunion if multiple articular fragments are present or the posterior column is involved.[3]

PATIENT HISTORY AND PHYSICAL FINDINGS

- Capitellum fractures occur secondary to a fall onto an outstretch arm, direct blow, or after a significant high-energy traumatic event.
- Symptoms of capitellar fractures are similar to those of radial head fractures, including pain and swelling along the lateral elbow and pain with elbow motion.
- Although there may be variable loss of forearm rotation, loss of flexion and extension is most common, often accompanied by crepitus and pain.
- The association of concomitant radial head fractures and ligamentous injuries with capitellar fractures is high.[20]
- The shoulder and wrist should also be examined for concomitant injury.

IMAGING AND OTHER DIAGNOSTIC STUDIES

- Standard radiographs are often inadequate for accurate assessment of capitellar fractures.
- Lateral radiographs are best for obtaining an initial evaluation of capitellar fractures.
- Anteroposterior views do not reliably show the fracture because the outline of the distal humerus is not consistently affected.
- The radial head–capitellum view can help identify fractures of the capitellum. This view is a lateral oblique projection taken with the x-ray beam pointing 45 degrees dorsoventrally, thereby eliminating the ulno- and radiohumeral articulation shadows.[11]
  - A type 1 fracture appears as a semilunar fragment sitting superiorly with its articular surface pointing up and away from the radial head in most cases.
  - Type 2 fractures are more difficult to diagnose, depending on the amount of subchondral bone accompanying the articular fragment. They may appear as a loose body lying in the superior part of the joint.
  - Type 3 fractures display variable amounts of comminution.
  - Coronal shear fractures show a characteristic "double arc" sign on lateral radiographic views (**FIG 3A**).
- Computed tomography (CT) scans can provide excellent characterization of the fracture, and we subsequently recommend routinely obtaining a CT scan for preoperative planning.
  - CT scanning of the elbow should be done at 1- to 2-mm intervals using axial or transverse cuts.
- Three-dimensional (3-D) CT reconstructions provide the best detail and ability to appreciate the anatomic orientation of the fracture patterns and should be considered, if available (**FIG 3B,C**).

DIFFERENTIAL DIAGNOSIS

- Radial head fracture
- Distal humeral lateral condyle fracture
- Elbow dislocation

NONOPERATIVE MANAGEMENT

- We recommend operative management for capitellum and capitellar–trochlear shear fractures.
- Truly nondisplaced and isolated capitellum fractures can be splinted for 3 weeks, followed by protected motion. However, close supervision is required, as this fracture is inherently unstable and prone to displacement.
- Closed reduction techniques, which have been described in the literature, should be performed with caution, and only complete anatomic reduction should be accepted for nonoperative management.[21]

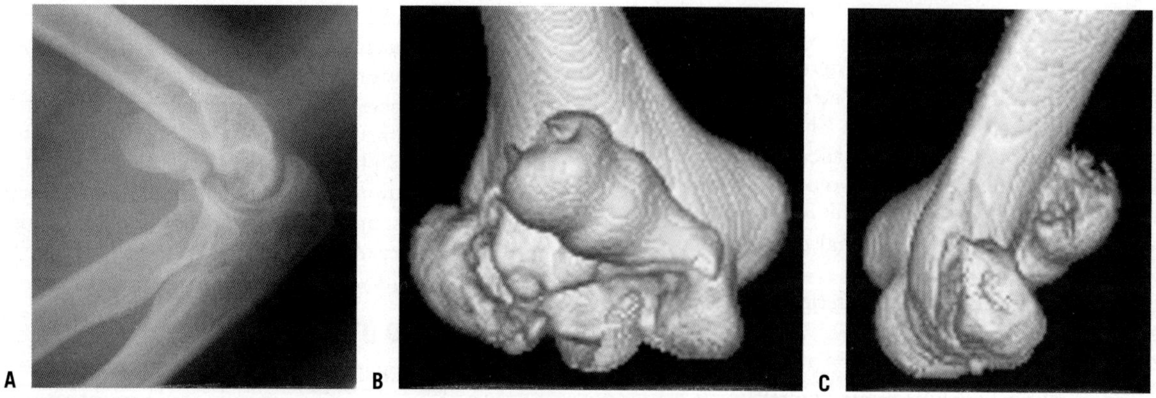

FIG 3 A. Characteristic double arc sign on lateral radiograph of coronal shear fractures. **B,C.** The 3-D CT reconstructions of a coronal shear fracture of the distal humerus.

- Capitellar–trochlear shear fractures should not be treated nonoperatively because of their inherent instability and the expectant loss of motion and posttraumatic arthrosis from residual articular incongruity.

SURGICAL MANAGEMENT

- The short-term goal of surgery is anatomic reduction and stable fixation of the fracture to allow for early motion without mechanical block.
- The long-term goals of surgery are a pain-free elbow with maximal motion, minimal stiffness, and avoidance of posttraumatic arthrosis.
- Capitellar fractures are uncommon, and the wide array of treatment options presented in the literature is based on relatively small series.
  - Treatment options include closed reduction[21] open excision,[1,8,18] open reduction and internal fixation (ORIF), hemiarthroplasty,[25] and arthroplasty.[5,9]
  - Hemiarthroplasty is not currently U.S. Food and Drug Administration approved.
- With the improvement in techniques for fixation of small fragments and management of articular surfaces, ORIF has become the mainstay of treatment.
  - Advantages of ORIF include restoration of the native anatomy and function.
  - Disadvantages include stiffness and possible failure of fixation.
- In elderly patients, we do consider total elbow arthroplasty for complex intra-articular distal humerus fractures.[14]
  - Advantages include early return to function and motion.
  - Disadvantages include functional limitations.

Preoperative Planning

- Before proceeding with surgery, a thorough understanding of the fracture and its orientation should be obtained with the help of a CT scan and, if possible, 3-D reconstructions.
- The timing of surgery is important. Fractures preferably should be approached within 2 weeks, before osseous healing sets in, but after swelling has diminished.
- Ensure that the necessary implants and hardware are available.
- Reduction and fixation of the fracture may require Kirschner wires (K-wires), articular or headless screws, and small-fragment AO screws.
- An image intensifier should be used during surgery to confirm reduction of the fracture and proper positioning of implanted hardware.

Positioning

- General anesthesia is recommended for maximum soft tissue relaxation.
- The patient usually is positioned supine on the operating table, with the arm extended onto a radiolucent hand table, facilitating the lateral approach.
- Alternatively, a lateral or prone position can be considered, with the anterior surface of the elbow supported by a padded bolster if a posterior approach is planned.

Approach

- An anterolateral, lateral, or posterior midline incision should be used.
- A lateral incision allows for direct visualization to a lateral approach to the elbow.
- A posterior incision not only allows for access to the lateral approach to the elbow but also facilitates access to the posterior and medial approaches to the elbow, if necessary.
- Multiple intervals can be used in the lateral approach to the elbow, including the Kocher, Kaplan, and Wagner approaches.
  - We advocate the Wagner approach, which uses the interval between the extensor carpi radialis longus (ECRL) and the extensor digitorum communis (EDC), as it provides ready access to the anterolateral aspect of the radiocapitellar joint while protecting the insertion of the lateral collateral ligament complex.
  - To increase exposure, the lateral collateral ligament complex can be raised posteriorly sharply with a scalpel or osteotomized with a wedge of lateral epicondyle for subsequent suture anchor repair or internal fixation, respectively.
- The Kocher approach, which uses the interval between the extensor carpi ulnaris and the anconeus, can provide access to the capitellum while affording greater protection of the posterior interosseous nerve.
- In many cases, a capsular violation has occurred. This can be exploited and used as the interval to expose the fracture, thereby avoiding the need to cause an additional soft tissue defect.

CAPITELLAR FRACTURES

Exposure

- The incision should begin 2 cm proximal to the lateral epicondyle and extend 3 to 4 cm distally toward the radial neck.
- If no large soft tissue or capsular defect is present, a direct lateral Wagner approach between the ECRL and EDC interval is recommended.
- The remaining common extensor origin is sharply raised off the lateral epicondyle and reflected anteriorly to expose the anterolateral elbow joint.
  - The capitellar fracture will most likely be found displaced anteriorly and proximally.
  - Care must be taken to avoid excessive proximal dissection and injury to the radial nerve traveling between the brachialis and brachioradialis.
  - Care must also be taken to avoid excessive distal dissection and injury to the posterior interosseous nerve by limiting dissection to only the radial neck. In addition, the forearm should be kept pronated, and no retractors should be placed anteriorly around the radial neck.
- Often, the lateral ligamentous complex will be avulsed from the distal aspect of the humerus, with or without some aspect of the lateral epicondyle.
  - This ligamentous violation can be exploited to improve exposure by hinging open the joint on the medial collateral ligament with a varus stress.
- The capitellar fracture fragment will typically be displaced anteriorly and proximally **(TECH FIG 1)**.
- The fracture fragment will also typically be devoid of any soft tissue attachments and therefore prone to displacing out of the joint with excessive manipulation. Hence, care must be taken to avoid losing the fragment off the surgical field.

Reduction and Fixation

- The fragment is reduced under direct visualization, held with reduction tenaculums, and provisionally fixed with 0.045-inch K-wires. Alternatively, the guidewires that will be used for cannulated screw fixation can be used for provisional fixation as well.
- Internal fixation options include fixation with (1) headless compression screws from either an anterior or posterior direction, (2) cancellous screws from a posterior direction, (3) posterolateral column locking plate fixation, or (4) a hybrid construct using any or all of these techniques.
- Headless compression screws allow for guidewire-directed placement, direct fracture reduction, and maximal compression of the fracture fragment. Similarly, headless compression screws may be particularly useful in cases with fragments with less subchondral bone, such as type 2 and small type 1 fracture fragments **(TECH FIG 2A)**. However, anterior screw placement can be challenging due to the thick anterior soft tissue envelope that will be present with an intact lateral collateral ligament complex. Alternatively, headless compression screws can be placed retrograde from a posterior direction to ease hardware placement **(TECH FIG 2B)**. However, this direction does not achieve maximum fracture compression and can risk fracture distraction.
- Cancellous screws are best for fracture fragments with a large subchondral component as with type 1 fracture fragments. However, extending the dissection posteriorly around the lateral column theoretically increases the risk of osteonecrosis **(TECH FIG 2C)**. We recommend using partially threaded cannulated screw to optimize fracture reduction, screw placement, and fracture compression.

A

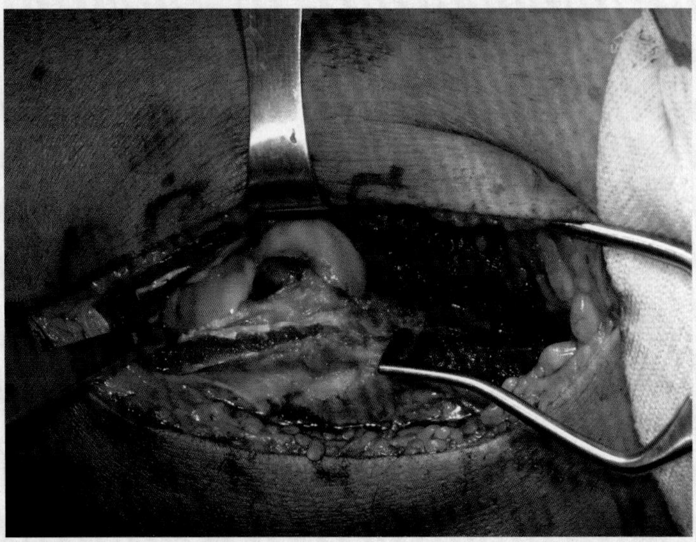

B

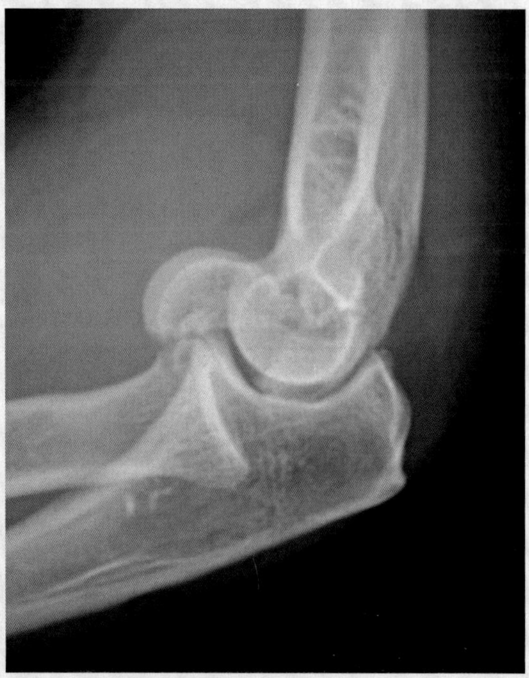

TECH FIG 1 A,B. The displaced capitellar fracture fragment will typically be displaced anteriorly and proximally and will be devoid of any soft tissue attachments.

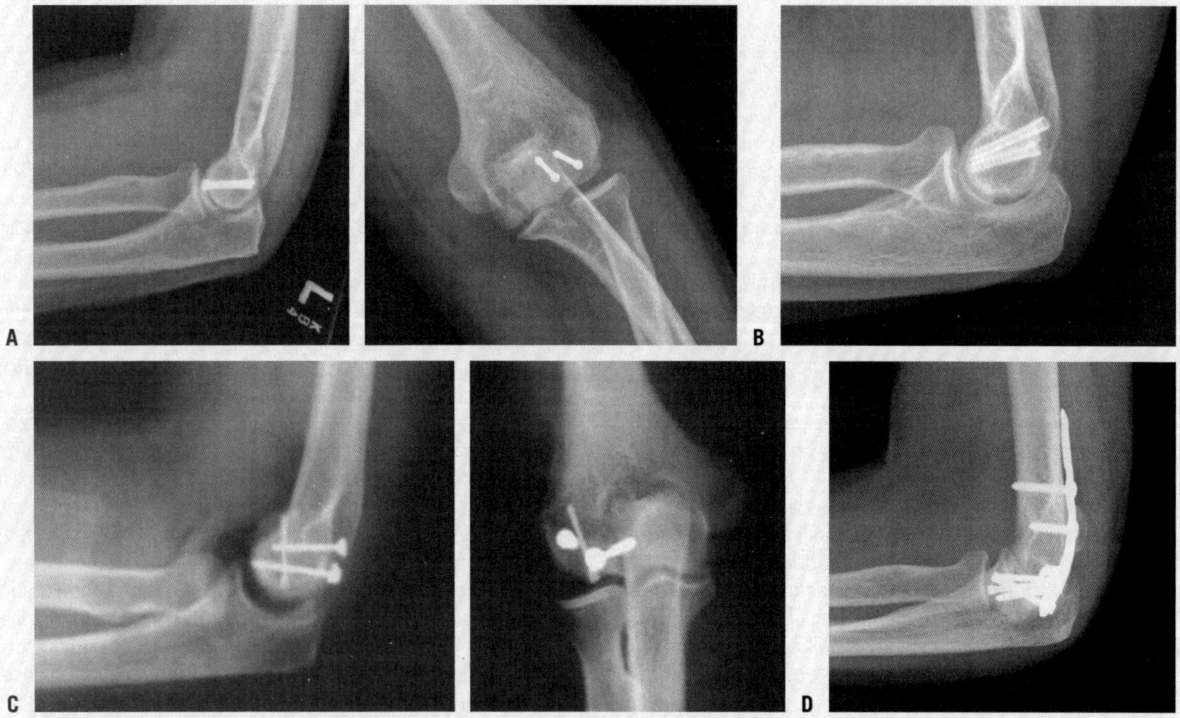

TECH FIG 2 Fixation of capitellar fractures with anteriorly placed headless compression screws (**A**), posteriorly placed headless compression screws (**B**), combination of a headless screw anteriorly and cancellous screws posteriorly (**C**), and hybrid fixation using anteriorly placed headless compression screws (**D**) followed by neutralization of the fracture with a locked periarticular plate applied posteriorly.

- Use of a periarticular locking plate alone or in a hybrid construct with headless compression screws can be of value to improve the stability of the construct **(TECH FIG 2D)**. This technique will require greater posterior dissection, therefore increasing the theoretical risk of osteonecrosis. However, application of a posterolateral plate can provide posterior stability in cases with posterior cortical extension or comminution.
- Excision of fracture fragments can be considered in type 2 fractures with small, thin articular pieces and type 3 comminuted fractures where the fragments are not amenable to internal fixation.
- Fragment reduction and hardware position should be confirmed by image intensifier.
- Unrestricted forearm rotation and elbow flexion–extension without mechanical block or catching should be confirmed intraoperatively.
- If the lateral collateral ligament complex is found to be avulsed, it should be repaired back to the lateral epicondyle with drill holes and heavy nonabsorbable sutures or suture anchors.
- The capsule should be closed.
- The retracted extensor origin should be relaxed and closed to the surrounding soft tissue.

CAPITELLAR–TROCHLEAR SHEAR FRACTURES

Exposure

- A posterior midline incision should be used, but initially, a lateral approach to the joint will be performed.
  - A posterior incision provides extensile exposure, access to both sides of the elbow, and ease of osteotomy, if necessary **(TECH FIG 3A)**.
- A direct lateral Wagner approach between the ECRL and EDC interval is recommended.
- The remaining common extensor origin is sharply raised off the lateral epicondyle and reflected anteriorly to expose the anterolateral elbow joint. Alternatively, a capsular violation may be present that can be exploited **(TECH FIG 3B)**.
- The capitellar–trochlear shear fracture will most likely be found displaced anteriorly and proximally.
  - Care must be taken to avoid excessive proximal dissection and injury to the radial nerve traveling between the brachialis and brachioradialis.
  - Care must also be taken to avoid excessive distal dissection and injury to the posterior interosseous nerve by limiting dissection to only the radial neck. In addition, the forearm should be kept pronated, and no retractors should be placed anteriorly around the radial neck.

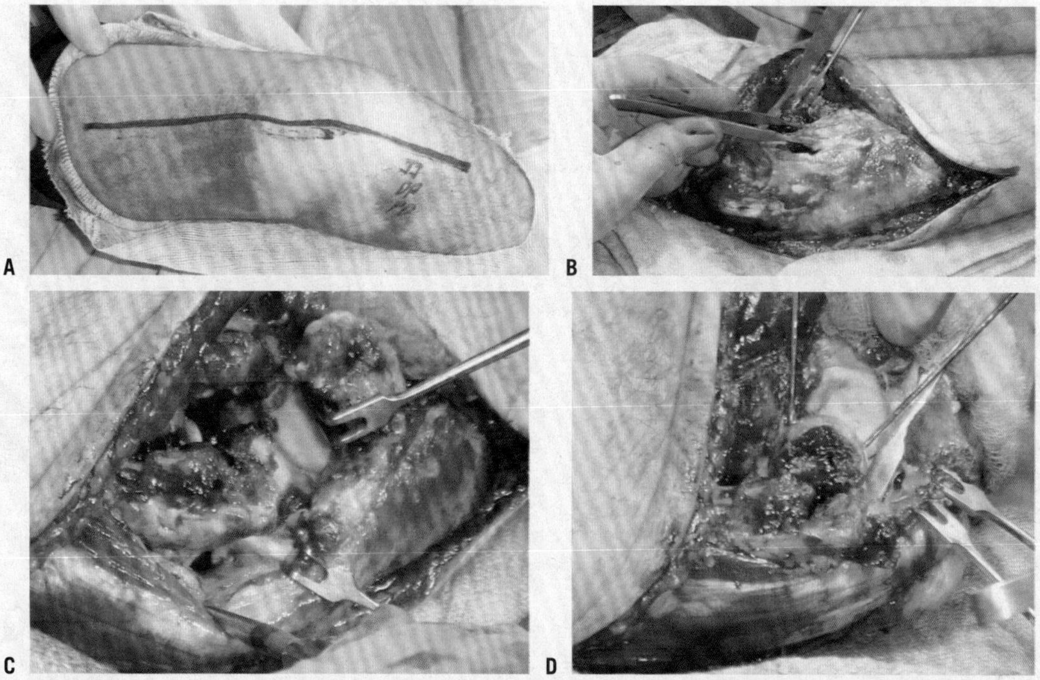

TECH FIG 3 **A.** Posterior midline incision used for capitellar–trochlear shear fractures. **B.** Deep lateral approach to the elbow using the capsular violation to enter the radiocapitellar joint. **C.** The fracture fragments tend to displace proximally and internally rotate. Note avulsion of the lateral epicondyle with subsequent retraction allowing for excellent visualization. **D.** The fracture is reduced and provisionally pinned with 0.045-inch K-wires.

- Often, the lateral ligamentous complex will be avulsed from the distal aspect of the humerus, with or without some aspect of the lateral epicondyle.
  - This ligamentous violation can be exploited to improve exposure by hinging open the joint on the medial collateral ligament with a varus stress.
  - Alternatively, a formal lateral epicondyle osteotomy can be performed to enhance visualization while maintaining the integrity of the lateral ligamentous complex.
  - Additionally, a formal olecranon osteotomy may be performed to improve visualization and fixation of fractures extending medially and posteriorly.
- The fracture fragments should now be visualized and accounted for. They are most commonly displaced proximally and internally rotated **(TECH FIG 3C)**.

Reduction and Fixation

- The fragment is reduced under direct visualization, held with reduction tenaculums, and provisionally fixed with 0.045-inch K-wires **(TECH FIG 3D)**.
- Inability to reduce the fracture anatomically may represent fracture impaction, requiring either disimpaction or bone grafting, or both.
- Internal fixation options include fixation with (1) headless compression screws from either an anterior or posterior direction, (2) cancellous screws from a posterior direction, (3) posterolateral column locking plate fixation, or (4) a hybrid construct using any or all of these techniques.
- Headless compression screws allow for guidewire-directed placement, direct fracture reduction, and maximal compression of the fracture fragment **(TECH FIG 4A)**. Similarly, headless compression screws may be particularly useful in cases with fragments with less subchondral bone, such as type 2 and small type 1 fracture fragments.
- Cancellous screws are best for fracture fragments with a large subchondral component as with type 1 fracture fragments. However, extending the dissection posteriorly around the lateral column theoretically increases the risk of osteonecrosis. We recommend using partially threaded cannulated screw to optimize fracture reduction, screw placement, and fracture compression.
- Use of a periarticular locking plate alone or in a hybrid construct with headless compression screws can be of value to improve the stability of the construct **(TECH FIG 4B)**. This technique will require greater posterior dissection, therefore increasing the theoretical risk of osteonecrosis. However, application of a posterolateral plate can provide posterior stability in cases with posterior cortical extension or comminution.
- Fragment reduction and hardware position should be confirmed by image intensifier.
- Unrestricted forearm rotation and elbow flexion–extension without mechanical block or catching should be confirmed intraoperatively.
- The lateral epicondyle, if avulsed or osteotomized, should be repaired with a tension band technique or plate and screws.
- The capsule should be closed.
- The interval and released extensor origin should be relaxed and closed to the surrounding soft tissue.

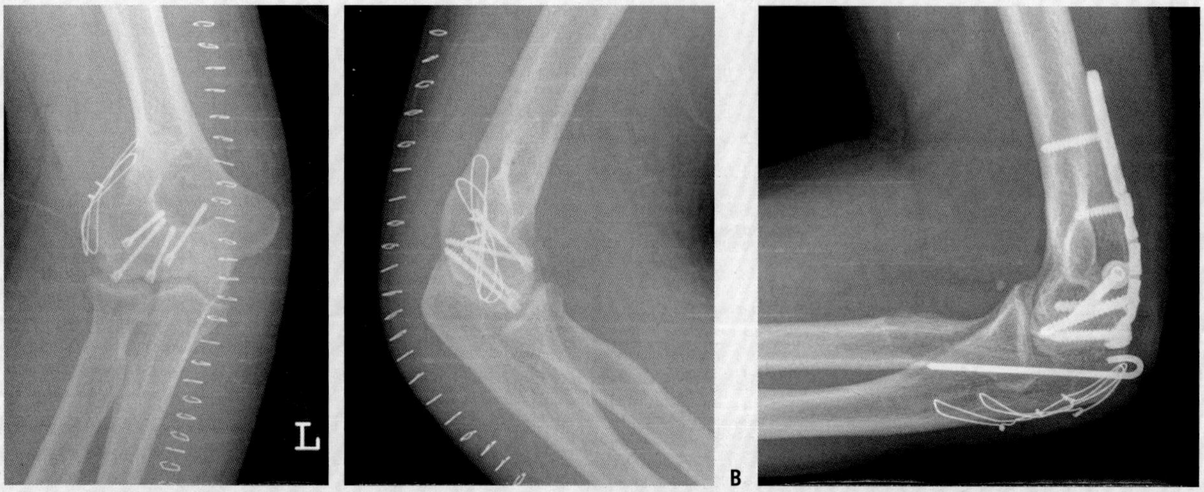

A B

TECH FIG 4 A. Postoperative radiographs illustrating repair of the lateral epicondyle and anterior fixation of a capitellar–trochlear shear fracture with multiple headless compression screws. **B.** Alternatively, note repair of a different capitellar–trochlear shear fracture using a periarticular locking plate applied to the posterolateral aspect of the distal humerus, facilitated with an olecranon osteotomy.

Pearls and Pitfalls

Diagnosis	• Diligence should be paid to identifying concomitant injuries such as elbow dislocations, radial head fractures, and ligamentous instability.
Imaging	• Plain radiographs are insufficient, and a CT scan should be considered routinely. • Order 3-D reconstructions if possible as two-dimensional CT scans are prone to positioning pitfalls.
Nonoperative Management	• Nonoperative management should be chosen cautiously. Anatomic and stable reduction of the fracture is necessary. Otherwise, a painful elbow with restricted motion may result. • We do not recommend nonoperative management of any capitellar–trochlear shear fractures.
Surgical Management	• Lateral epicondyle osteotomy can enhance exposure. • A posterior skin incision will afford access to both sides of the joint and an olecranon osteotomy, if necessary. • Inability to reduce the fracture anatomically may represent impaction of the lateral column and require disimpaction or bone grafting. • Excision of small comminuted fragments that cannot be fixed internally is preferred over nonanatomic reduction and malunion. • Concomitant fractures and ligamentous injuries should be treated simultaneously to optimize outcomes.
Postoperative Management	• Stable fixation should be sought to facilitate early motion. • Heterotopic ossification is common after elbow fractures, and prophylaxis with nonsteroidal anti-inflammatory drugs or radiation should be considered.

POSTOPERATIVE CARE

- If secure fixation has been obtained, immediate mobilization can be initiated postoperatively.
- If fixation is tenuous, splint or cast the elbow for 3 to 4 weeks, followed by active and assisted range-of-motion exercises. Some advocate the use of hinged external fixator for complex articular fractures or with severe ligamentous injuries.[10]

OUTCOMES

- Focusing initially on outcomes after ORIF of type 1 and 2 capitellar fractures, multiple small series have shown good results using Herbert screws in an anterior to posterior direction.[13,15,22]
- More recently, Mahirogullari et al[17] reported on 11 cases of type 1 capitellum fractures treated with Herbert screws, which yielded 8 excellent and 3 good results. They recommended

fixation in a posterior to anterior direction with at least two Herbert screws.

- Reported outcomes on type 4 capitellar–trochlear shear fractures are limited. McKee et al[19] originally described this pattern and reported on six cases.
  - Each case involved an extended lateral Kocher approach and fixation with Herbert screws from an anterior to posterior direction. Good or excellent results were achieved in all cases, with average elbow motion of 15 to 141 degrees, forearm rotation of 83 degrees pronation, and 84 degrees supination.
- Ring et al[23] examined 21 cases of articular fractures of the distal humerus treated with Herbert screw fixation and found 4 excellent results, 12 good results, and 5 fair results.
  - All of the fractures healed and had an average range of motion of 96 degrees. No ulnohumeral instability, arthrosis, or osteonecrosis was reported.
  - The authors stressed the importance of proper evaluation of these fractures and awareness that apparent capitellum fractures often are complex articular fractures of the distal humerus.[23]
- Lopiz et al[16] reported placement of screws in a posterior to anterior direction and patient exhibited better postoperative flexion and functional outcomes within the patient cohort.
- Dubberley et al[6] further subclassified type 4 fractures in their series of 28 cases. They achieved an average range of motion of flexion–extension of 25 degrees less than the contralateral elbow and 4 degrees of supination–pronation less than the contralateral elbow.
  - Two comminuted cases required conversion to a total elbow arthroplasty.
  - Varied fixation methods were used, including Herbert screws, cancellous screws, absorbable pins, and supplementation with K-wires.
- Ruchelsman and colleagues[24] reported a case series of 16 patients that were treated with ORIF.
  - All patients achieved full forearm rotation, and all but two had functional arc of elbow range of motion.
  - They reported 15 good to excellent results and 1 fair result.
  - The authors did not find association between concomitant radial head fracture and worse outcomes.
- Comminuted fractures (Dubberley type B) have been shown to be more prone to inferior outcomes complicated by avascular necrosis, degenerative arthritis, and heterotopic ossification.[7]

COMPLICATIONS

- The most common complication of capitellar fractures is loss of elbow motion and residual pain. The compromised motion most commonly is manifested in loss of flexion and extension.
- Ulnar neuropathy after ORIF ranges from 7.7% to 9.5%, and some recommend routine ulnar nerve decompression.[23] This is especially important in capitellar–trochlear shear fractures, as hinging of the elbow on the medial side increases the risk of ulnar nerve compression.
- Osteonecrosis may occur from the initial fracture displacement or surgical exposure. Blood is supplied to the capitellum from a posterior to anterior direction and may be compromised by surgical dissection.
  - In symptomatic cases in which revascularization after fixation has not occurred, delayed excision is indicated.
- Malunions may occur when the patient has delayed seeking treatment, when inadequate reduction or loss of closed reduction occurs, or after ORIF. Malunions result in loss of motion and may require excision of the fragment and soft tissue releases.
- Nonunions may occur, although this is uncommon. They most likely result secondary to inadequate reduction or lack of revascularization of the fragment.

REFERENCES

1. Alvarez E, Patel M, Nimberg P, et al. Fractures of the capitulum humeri. J Bone Joint Surg Am 1975;57(8):1093–1096.
2. Broberg MA, Morrey BF. Results of delayed excision of the radial head after fracture. J Bone Joint Surg Am 1986;68(5):669–674.
3. Brouwer KM, Jupiter JB, Ring D. Nonunion of operatively treated capitellum and trochlear fractures. J Hand Surg Am 2011;36(5):804–807.
4. Bryan RS, Morrey BF. Fractures of the distal humerus. In: Morrey BF, ed. The Elbow and Its Disorders. Philadelphia: WB Saunders, 1985:302–399.
5. Cobb TK, Morrey BF. Total elbow arthroplasty as primary treatment for distal humerus fractures in elderly patients. J Bone Joint Surg Am 1997;79(6):826–832.
6. Dubberley JH, Faber KJ, Macdermid JC, et al. Outcome after open reduction and internal fixation of capitellar and trochlear fractures. J Bone Joint Surg Am 2006;88(1):46–54.
7. Durakbasa MO, Gumussuyu G, Gungor M, et al. Distal humeral coronal plane fractures: management, complications and outcome. J Shoulder Elbow Surg 2013;22(4):560–566.
8. Fowles JV, Kassab MT. Fracture of the capitulum humeri. Treatment by excision. J Bone Joint Surg Am 1975;56(4):794–798.
9. Garcia JA, Mykula R, Stanley D. Complex fractures of the distal humerus in the elderly. The role of total elbow replacement as primary treatment. J Bone Joint Surg Br 2002;84(6):812–816.
10. Giannicola G, Sacchetti FM, Greco A, et al. Open reduction and internal fixation combined with hinged elbow fixator in capitellum and trochlea fractures. Acta Orthop 2010;81(2):228–233.
11. Greenspan A, Norman A. The radial head, capitellum view: useful technique in elbow trauma. AJR Am J Roentgenol 1982;138(6):1186–1188.
12. Hahn NF. Fall von einer besonderes Varietat der Frakturen des Ellenbogens. Z Wund Geburt 1853;6:185.
13. Lansinger O, Mare K. Fracture of the capitulum humeri. Acta Orthop Scand 1981;52:39–44.
14. Lee JJ, Lawton JN. Coronal shear fractures of the distal humerus. J Hand Surg Am 2012;37(11):2412–2417.
15. Liberman N, Katz T, Howard CV, et al. Fixation of capitellar fractures with Herbert screws. Arch Orthop Trauma Surg 1991;110:155–157.
16. Lopiz Y, Rodríguez-González A, García-Fernández C, et al. Open reduction and internal fixation of coronal fractures of the capitellum in patients older than 65 years. J Shoulder Elbow Surg 2016;25(3):369–375.
17. Mahirogullari M, Kiral A, Solakoglu C, et al. Treatment of fractures of the humeral capitellum using Herbert screws. J Hand Surg Br 2006;31:320–325.
18. Mazel MS. Fracture of the capitellum. J Bone Joint Surg 1935;17:483–488.
19. McKee MD, Jupiter JB, Bamberger HB. Coronal shear fractures of the distal end of the humerus. J Bone Joint Surg Am 1996;78(1):49–54.
20. Milch H. Fractures and fracture-dislocations of the humeral condyles. J Trauma 1964;4:592–607.
21. Ochner RS, Bloom H, Palumbo RC, et al. Closed reduction of coronal fractures of the capitellum. J Trauma 1996;40(2):199–203.

22. Richards RR, Khoury GW, Burke FD, et al. Internal fixation of capitellar fractures using Herbert screw: a report of four cases. Can J Surg 1987;30(3):188–191.
23. Ring D, Jupiter JB, Gulotta L. Articular fractures of the distal part of the humerus. J Bone Joint Surg Am 2003;85(2):232–238.
24. Ruchelsman DE, Tejwani NC, Kwon YW, et al. Open reduction and internal fixation of capitellar fractures with headless screws. J Bone Joint Surg Am 2009;91(suppl 2, pt 1):38–49.
25. Sabo MT, Shannon HL, Deluce S, et al. Capitellar excision and hemiarthroplasty affects elbow kinematics and stability. J Shoulder Elbow Surg 2012;21(8):1024.e4–1031.e4.
26. Steinthal D. Die isolirte Fraktur der eminentia Capetala in Ellengogelenk. Zentralk Chir 1898;15:17.
27. Yamaguchi K, Sweet FA, Bindra R, et al. The extraosseous and intraosseous arterial anatomy of the adult elbow. J Bone Joint Surg Am 1997;79(11):1653–1662.

CHAPTER 14

Open Reduction and Internal Fixation of Radial Head and Neck Fractures

Rajesh Rangarajan and John M. Itamura

DEFINITION

- Radial head and neck fractures are the most common (~33%) of all adult fractures about the elbow joint.
- They may occur in isolation or with concurrent osseous, osteochondral, and/or ligamentous injuries.
- Management (which involves nonoperative, open reduction internal fixation [ORIF], fragment excision, radial head excision, or radial head replacement) is aimed at restoring motion or both motion and stability to the elbow and forearm, depending on the pattern of injury. This chapter focuses on the decision-making principles and operative techniques for ORIF of radial head and neck fractures.

ANATOMY

- The radial head is entirely intra-articular with two articulations:
  - The *radiocapitellar joint* has a saddle-shaped articulation allowing flexion, extension, and forearm rotation.
  - The *proximal radioulnar joint* (PRUJ), constrained by the annular ligament, allows rotation of the radial head in the lesser sigmoid notch of the proximal ulna.
- To avoid creating a mechanical block to pronation and supination, implants must be limited to a 90-degree arc (the "safe zone") outside the PRUJ **(FIG 1)**.[7]
- There is considerable variability in the shape of the radial head, from nearly round to elliptical, as well as variability in the offset of the head from the neck.[16]
- Blood supply to the radial head is tenuous, with a major contribution from a single branch of the radial recurrent artery in the safe zone and minor contributions from both the radial and interosseous recurrent arteries which penetrate the capsule at its insertion into the neck **(FIG 2)**.[28]
- The anterior band of the medial collateral ligament (MCL) is the primary stabilizer to valgus stress. The radial head, a secondary stabilizer, maintains up to 30% of valgus resistance in the native elbow. Therefore, in cases where the MCL is ruptured:
  - An irreparable radial head should be replaced with a prosthesis and not excised given its biomechanical importance.
  - It may be prudent to protect a repaired radial head from high valgus stress during early range of motion.
- The radial head also functions in the transmission of axial load, transmitting 60% of the load from the wrist to the elbow.[23] This is a crucial consideration when the interosseous membrane is disrupted in the Essex-Lopresti lesion.[9] Resection of the radial head in this setting results in devastating longitudinal radioulnar instability, proximal migration of the radius, and possible ulnar–carpal impingement.

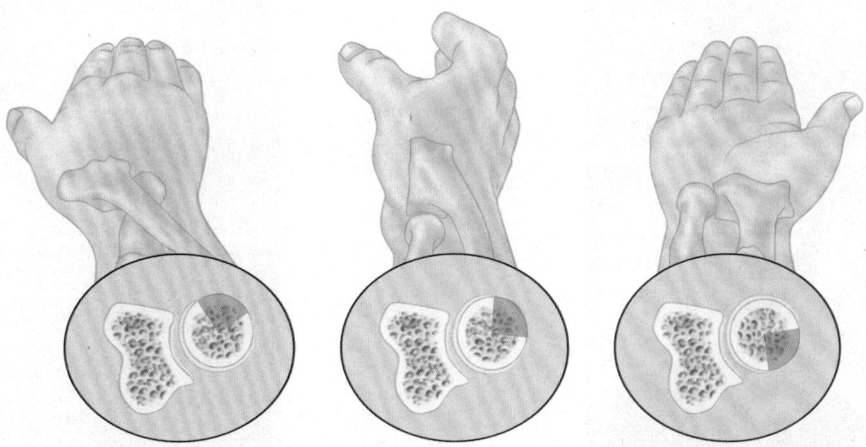

FIG 1 The safe zone is a 90-degree arc of the radial head that does not articulate with the ulna at the PRUJ during pronosupination. With the forearm in neutral rotation, the safe zone is anterolateral.

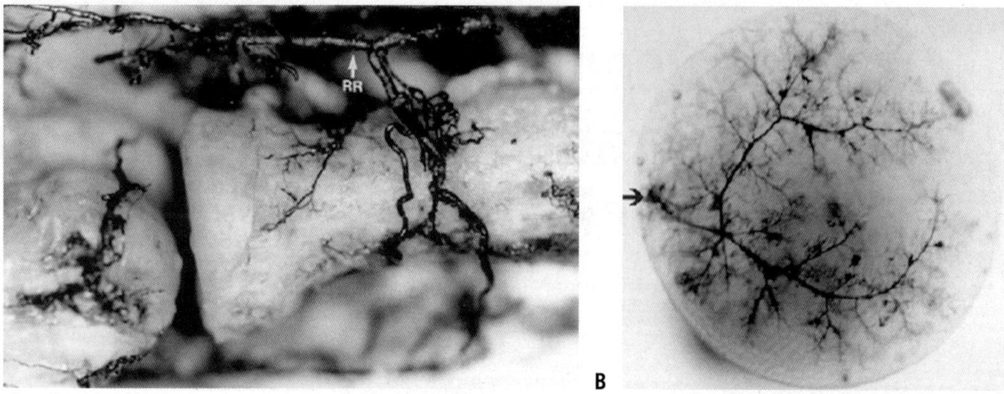

A B

FIG 2 **A.** The radial recurrent artery, a branch of the radial artery, provides the main blood supply to the radial head. **B.** In most cadaveric specimens, a branch of the radial recurrent penetrates the radial head in the safe zone. (Reprinted with permission from Yamaguchi K, Sweet FA, Bindra R, et al. The extraosseous and intraosseous arterial anatomy of the adult elbow. J Bone Joint Surg Am 1997;79A[11]:1653–1662. Copyright © 1997 by The Journal of Bone and Joint Surgery, Incorporated.)

PATHOGENESIS

- Radial head fractures result from trauma. A fall on an outstretched hand with the elbow in extension and the forearm in pronation produces an axial or valgus load (or both) driving the radial head into the capitellum, fracturing the relatively osteopenic radial head.[2]
- Nondisplaced or minimally displaced fractures typically occur as isolated injuries.
- Displaced, comminuted, or unstable fractures have a high association of soft tissue **(FIG 3)** and/or bony injuries:
  - Capitellar cartilage defects, capitellar bone bruises, and/or posterior dislocation can occur with radial head fractures.
- Axial loading may also rupture the interosseous membrane causing longitudinal radioulnar instability with dislocation of the distal radioulnar joint (DRUJ) (Essex-Lopresti fracture). An impacted radial neck or depressed radial head fracture should be highly suspicious of a concomitant interosseous membrane and DRUJ injury **(FIG 4)**.
- The "terrible triad" injury results from valgus loading of the elbow resulting in an elbow dislocation with fractures of the radial head and coronoid process.
- Radial head fractures can also occur with proximal ulnar fractures (Monteggia fracture) **(FIG 5)**.

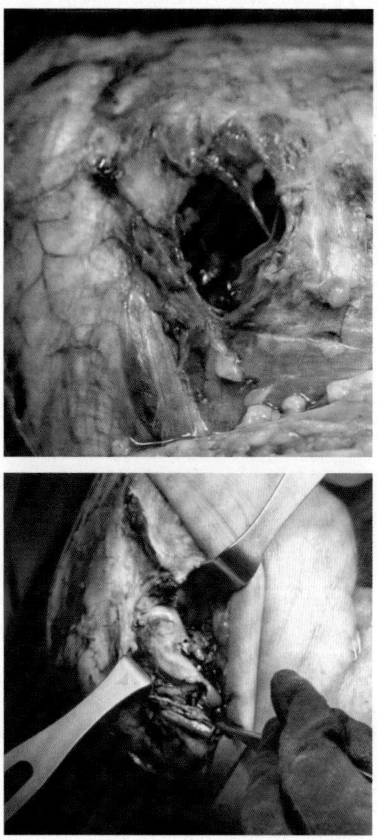

A

B

FIG 3 Soft tissue injuries may occur with unstable comminuted, displaced radial head fractures such as large capsular ruptures (**A**) and avulsions (**B**) of the lateral collateral ligament and common extensor tendons from the lateral epicondyle.

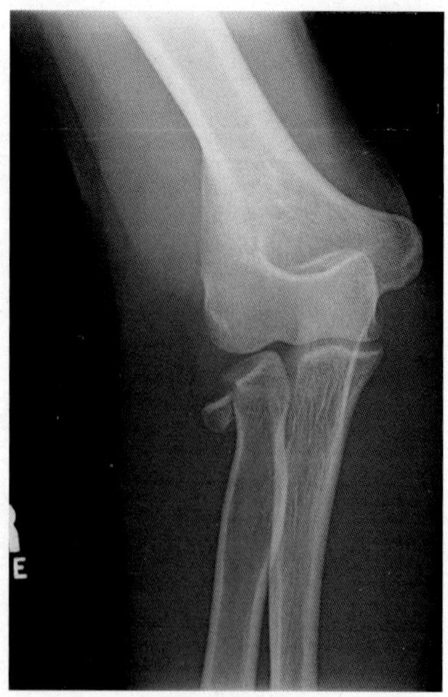

FIG 4 AP radiograph showing a depressed articular fracture with impaction at the radial neck. This fracture pattern is highly suspicious for an Essex-Lopresti fracture.

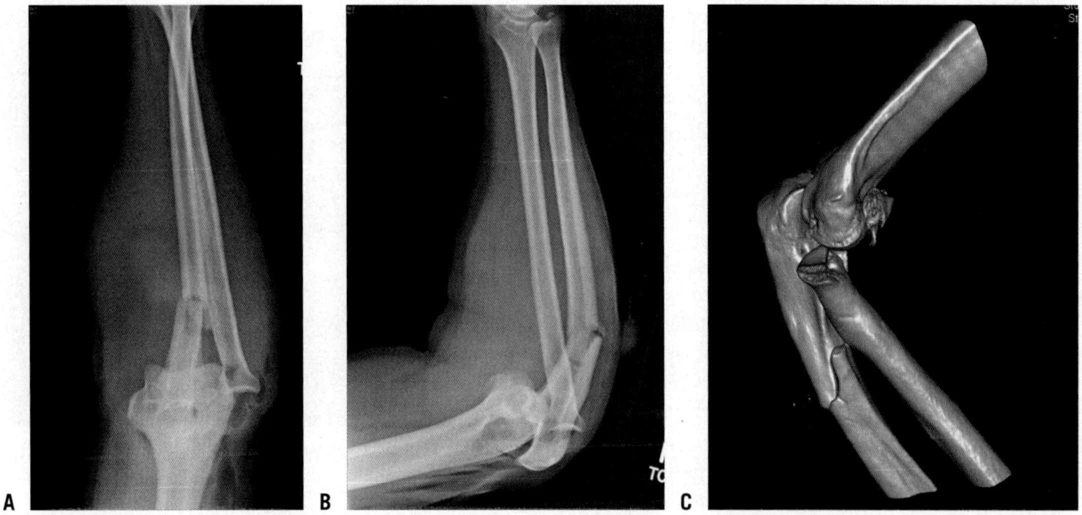

FIG 5 AP (**A**) and lateral (**B**) forearm radiographs showing a type II Monteggia fracture—posterior dislocation of radial head (or fracture) and proximal ulnar fracture with posterior angulation. CT scan (**C**) demonstrating an impaction fracture of the radial head not clearly evident on plain radiographs.

NATURAL HISTORY

- The original Mason classification was modified by Johnson and then Morrey. Hotchkiss proposed that the classification system be used to provide guidance for treatment[15]; however, interobserver reliability has been shown to be poor **(FIG 6)**.[10]

Type I Fractures

- Nondisplaced fractures with no block to pronation and supination on examination
- Represent approximately 82% of radial head fractures[20]
- Nonoperative treatment generally results in good to excellent outcomes with minimal loss of motion or resultant arthrosis.[1,3,8,13]
- Stiffness due to capsular contracture is the main reason for a poor outcome; however, it can often be managed successfully with physical therapy.

Type II Fractures

- Displaced marginal segments that can block normal forearm rotation. According to Broberg and Morrey,[6] the fragment should be at least 30% of the articular surface and be displaced 2 mm or more. We only include fractures with three or fewer articular fragments, which meet criteria for fractures that can be operatively reduced and fixed with reproducibly good results.
- Represent approximately 14% of radial head fractures[20]
- Earlier studies suggested nonoperative treatment or radial head excision as the standard treatment,[14,21,22,25] but as knowledge and technology advanced, optimal treatment has become more controversial.
- Greater than 2 mm of displacement has often been cited as an indication for ORIF, but good results have been obtained in studies treating 2 to 5 mm of displacement nonoperatively.[1,13]
- A mechanical block is the only clear indication for surgery.
- A meta-analysis[18] found successful nonoperative treatment in 80% compared to successful ORIF treatment in 93% for stable Mason type II fractures; however, the authors concluded that there was insufficient evidence to recommend optimal treatment.
- Complications from nonoperative treatment such as painful clicking, nonunion, and arthrosis can be treated with radial head excision or arthroplasty.

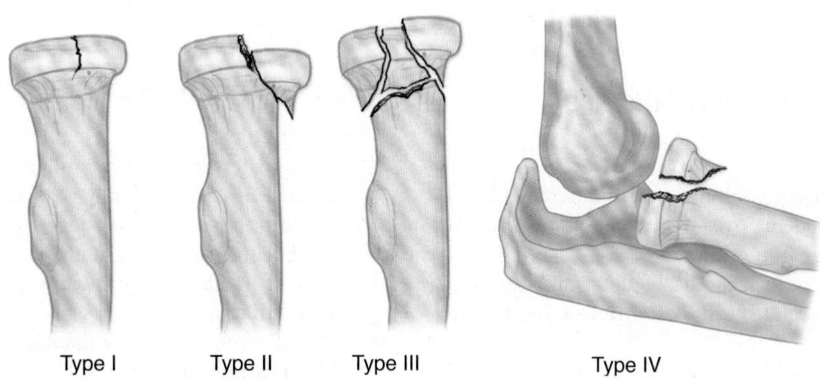

FIG 6 The modified Mason classification for radial head fractures.

- Delayed excision of the radial head after failed nonoperative management may be considered, although one study showed only modest increase in function with 23% of patients with fair or poor results at 15 years of follow-up.[5] Other studies suggested that there is no difference between delayed and primary excision.[12]

Type III Fractures

- Comminuted or impacted articular fractures (see **FIG 4**)
- Represent approximately 3% of radial head fractures[20]
- Radial head arthroplasty or excision is considered when satisfactory reduction and stable fixation is not obtained or in comminuted fractures because fixation of a radial head with more than three articular fragments is fraught with poor results.[24]
- Radial head excision should be reserved for patients with low functional demands, limited life expectancy, or in the presence of infection, and when the surgeon has excluded rotational and/or longitudinal elbow instability with a fluoroscopic examination.
- Excision is contraindicated in patients with concomitant MCL, coronoid, or interosseous membrane injury, and thus, arthroplasty should be performed in these cases.
- Radiographic, but often clinically silent, degenerative changes such as cysts, sclerosis, and osteophytes occur radiographically in about 75% of elbows after radial head excision.
- There is also a demonstrable increase in ulnar variance at the wrist and increased carrying angle, and a 10% to 20% loss of strength is expected.
- Radial head arthroplasty provides radiocapitellar contact similar to the native radial head. It restores valgus and posterior stability and resists proximal migration of the radius in response to axial loading, thereby facilitating uneventful healing of the MCL, interosseous ligaments, and the DRUJ when concomitant injuries to these structures occur.

Type IV Fractures

- Radial head fractures associated with elbow instability
- Represents approximately 1% of radial head fractures[20]
- Treatment involves immediate reduction of the elbow joint and treatment of the radial head fracture and associated bony injuries. Whether the radial head is fixed or replaced, it must be capable of bearing load immediately. If the radial head can be fixed, repair of the torn ligaments and application of a hinged fixator to protect the repaired radial head may be considered. Otherwise, satisfactory results have been obtained with radial head replacement without ligamentous repair.[11]
- The radial head should never be resected in the acute setting in these cases due to concomitant ligamentous injury.

PATIENT HISTORY AND PHYSICAL FINDINGS

History

- The history typically involves a fall on an outstretched hand followed by pain and edema over the lateral elbow, accompanied by limited range of motion.
- The mechanism of the injury should be determined to add information about associated elbow injuries or injuries to the shoulder or hand.
- The examiner should note the patient's activity level and profession.

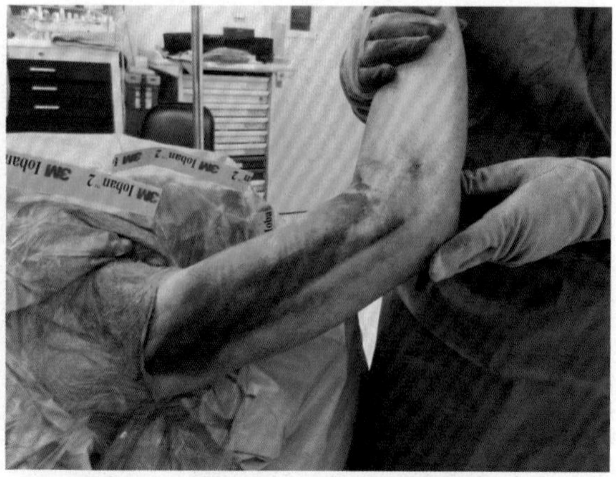

FIG 7 MCL disruption with extensive medial ecchymosis.

Physical Examination

- Physical examination should include neurovascular status, examination of the joint above (shoulder) and below (wrist), and examination of the skin to look for medial ecchymosis (**FIG 7**), which may suggest injury to the MCL.
- A detailed examination of the elbow must include bony palpation of the medial and lateral epicondyles, olecranon process, DRUJ, and radial head as well as the squeeze test of the interosseous membrane and DRUJ to screen for potential longitudinal instability.
- Varus and valgus stress testing, with or without fluoroscopy, can indicate injury to the anterior band of the MCL or to the lateral ulnar collateral ligament, respectively.
- Range-of-motion and stress examinations are vital to proper decision making and may obviate the need for advanced imaging if performed correctly with adequate anesthesia. If omitted, this will lead to undiagnosed associated injuries and may result in flawed decision making.
- In the emergency department or office, hematoma aspiration and intra-articular injection of 5 mL of local anesthetic can provide adequate anesthesia for examination under fluoroscopy. This may be performed using the "soft spot" or posterolateral approach or directly posterior into the olecranon fossa (**FIG 8**).[27] A mechanical block is an indication for operative intervention.
- If operative intervention is clearly indicated, this examination can also be performed intra-operatively under general anesthesia prior to surgery.
- Normal elbow range of motion is 0 to 145 degrees of flexion–extension, 85 degrees of supination, and 80 degrees of pronation.

IMAGING AND OTHER DIAGNOSTIC STUDIES

- Radiography
- Anteroposterior (AP), lateral, and oblique views are the standard of care, but they may underestimate or overestimate joint impaction and degree of comminution.
- A radiocapitellar view with the forearm in neutral and elbow at 45 degrees of flexion gives an improved view of the articular surfaces.
- A "sail" sign, caused by displacement of the posterior fat pad, on a lateral radiograph should prompt suspicion for an occult radial head or neck fracture.

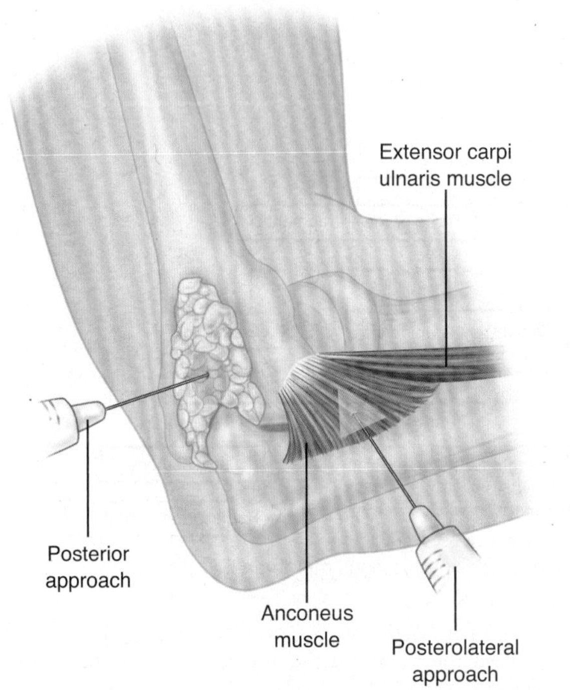

FIG 8 The elbow joint can be aspirated and injected through the posterolateral or direct posterior approaches.

- If the examination reveals wrist or forearm tenderness, the examiner should have a low threshold for obtaining bilateral wrist posteroanterior (PA) views to rule out an Essex-Lopresti lesion. Alternatively, this can be done with a one cassette view to minimize radiation exposure (**FIG 9**).
- Magnetic resonance imaging (MRI) is a useful adjunct to physical examination for evaluating associated injuries such as collateral ligament tears, chondral defects, and loose bodies.[17] It is not routinely indicated, however, as most of the associated injuries seen on MRI at the time of injury have not been found to be of clinical significance.[17,19]
- If the amount of displacement is unclear on plain radiographs or the decision has been made to proceed with operative management, we routinely obtain a computed tomography (CT) scan to better understand the fracture pattern. Three-dimensional reconstructions provide further information not always easily appreciated on routine CT scans.

DIFFERENTIAL DIAGNOSIS

- Simple elbow dislocation
- Distal humerus fracture
- Olecranon fracture
- Septic elbow
- Complex elbow instability (terrible triad)

NONOPERATIVE MANAGEMENT

- The standard protocol for treating radial head fractures is shown in **FIG 10**.
- Nonoperative management is the treatment of choice in fractures with less than 2 mm of displacement, with minor head involvement, and without a mechanical block to motion.
- A 7-day period of cast, splint, or sling immobilization is followed by aggressive motion.
- Our current practice for fractures that are more than 2 mm displaced is to determine whether there is a mechanical block to motion during fluoroscopic examination.
- If there is maintenance of at least 50 degrees of both pronation and supination, we typically recommend conservative treatment.
- If there is a blockage or instability, then fragment excision, operative fixation, or arthroplasty is recommended based on patient factors and joint stability.

FIG 9 A. The Itamura simultaneous DRUJ view is a PA radiograph of both wrists performed in 90-degree shoulder flexion, 90-degree elbow flexion, and neutral forearm rotation. **B.** Sample radiograph showing negative ulnar variance on the uninjured left side compared with neutral ulnar variance of the injured right side suggesting interosseous membrane disruption. This patient had an Essex-Lopresti injury.

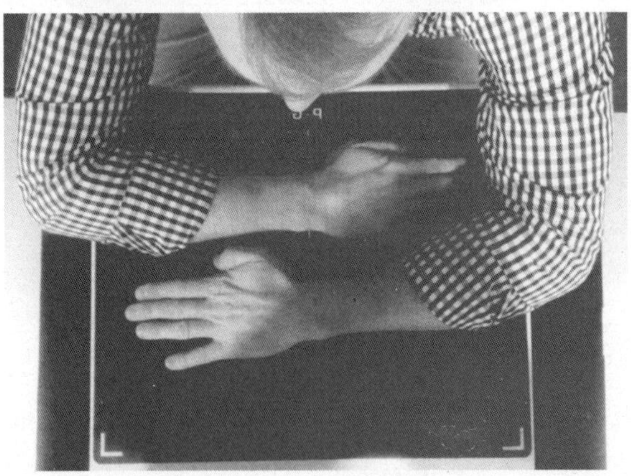
A

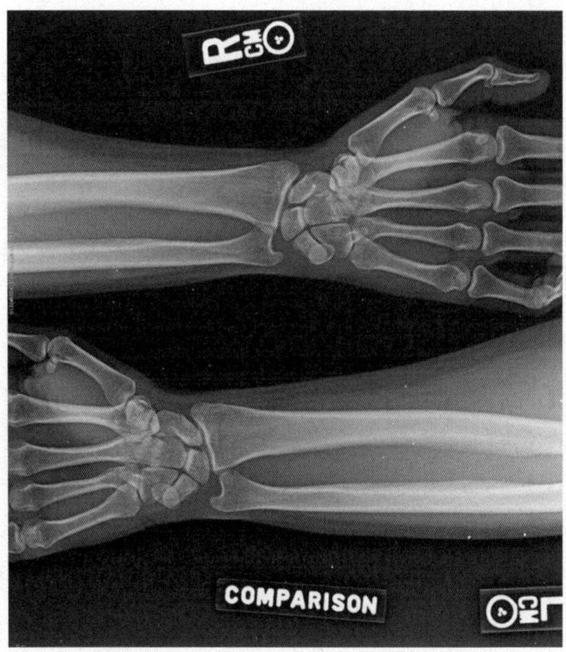

B

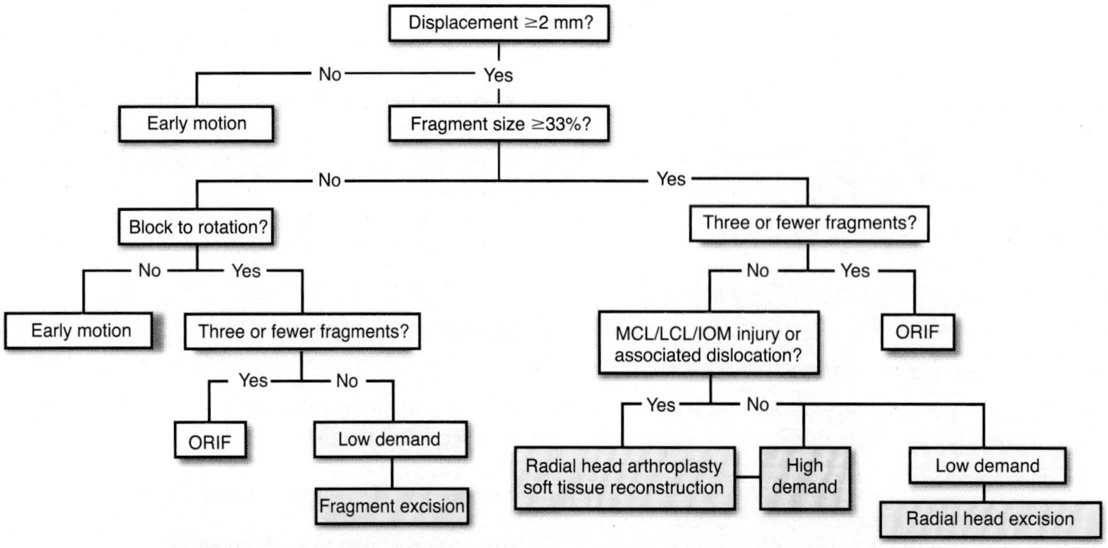

FIG 10 Treatment algorithm for radial head fractures. *IOM*, interosseous membrane.

- A recent report regarding the long-term results of nonoperative management (similar to that described) of 49 patients with radial head fractures encompassing over 30% of the joint surface and displaced 2 to 5 mm revealed that 81% of patients had no subjective complaints and minimal loss of motion versus the uninjured extremity. Only one patient had daily pain.[1]

SURGICAL MANAGEMENT

Preoperative Planning

- It is essential to review all imaging and perform thorough history, physical, and fluoroscopic examinations before making an incision.
- The presence of instability or associated fractures warrants a more extensile approach.

Positioning

- Positioning depends on the planned approach and the surgeon's preference.
- We prefer the patient supine with the affected extremity brought across the chest over a bump to allow access to the posterolateral elbow.
- A sterile tourniquet is placed high on the arm.

Approach

- The posterolateral (Kocher) approach has traditionally been presented to approach radial head fractures; however, we prefer a modified Wrightington approach,[26] which is a modified posterior (Boyd) approach[4] using the interval between the ulna and the anconeus for the following reasons (**FIG 11**):
  - It offers superior visualization of the radial head and neck which is especially critical during ORIF.
  - It is also the only approach that allows visualization of the radioulnar, radiohumeral, and ulnohumeral joint spaces, which is essential in selecting the appropriate radial head implant size if arthroplasty is warranted.
- The approach is extensile and allows concurrent management of ligamentous injuries with less risk of neuroma formation and neurologic injury.

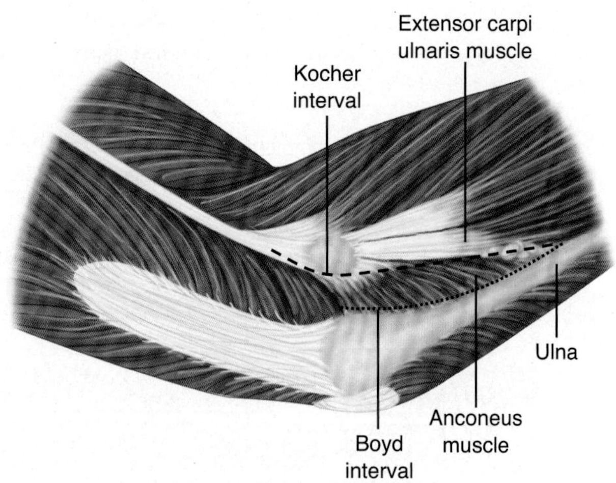

FIG 11 Surgical intervals for the Boyd approach and the Kocher approach.

KOCHER APPROACH

- The traditional posterolateral (Kocher) approach between the anconeus and extensor carpi ulnaris is cosmetic and spares the lateral ulnar collateral ligament.
- We recommend not using an Esmarch tourniquet to allow visualization of penetrating veins that help identify the interval.
- A 5-cm oblique incision is made from the posterolateral aspect of the lateral epicondyle obliquely to a point three fingerbreadths below the tip of the olecranon in line with the radial neck **(TECH FIG 1A)**.
- The radial head and epicondyle are palpated, and the fascia is divided in line with the skin incision.
- The Kocher interval is identified distally by small penetrating veins and bluntly developed, revealing the lateral ligament complex and joint capsule **(TECH FIG 1B)**.
- The anconeus is reflected posteriorly, and the extensor carpi ulnaris origin anteriorly. The capsule is incised obliquely anterior to the lateral ulnar collateral ligament **(TECH FIG 1C,D)**.
- The proximal edge of the annular ligament may also be divided and tagged, with care taken not to proceed distally and avoid injury to the posterior interosseous nerve.

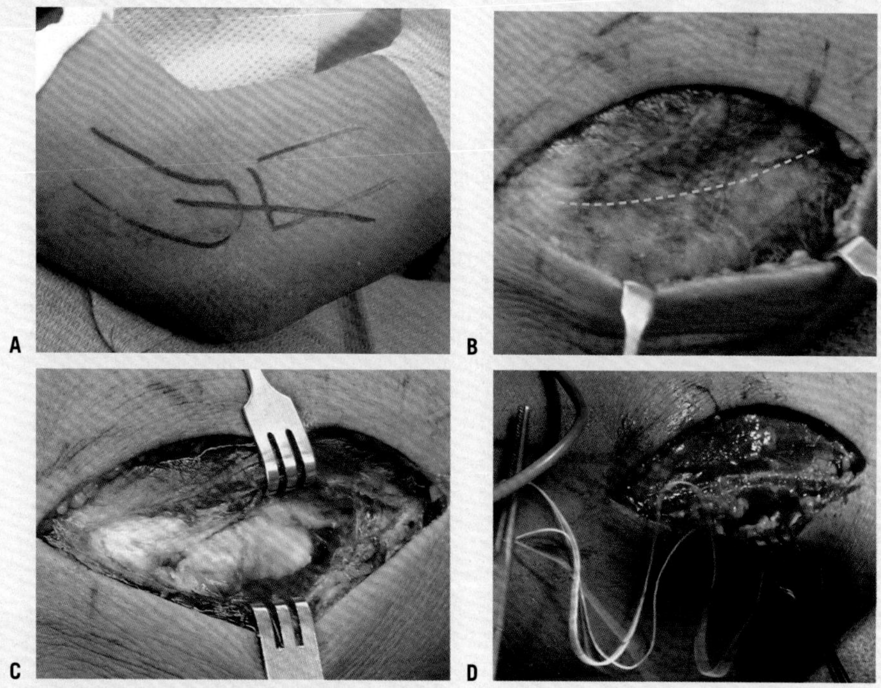

TECH FIG 1 Kocher approach. **A.** The skin incision proceeds distally from the posterolateral aspect of the lateral epicondyle to the posterior aspect of the proximal radius. **B.** Full-thickness flaps are made, and the fascial interval (*dashed yellow line*) between the extensor carpi ulnaris and anconeus muscles is identified. **C.** With longitudinal incision of the fascia and blunt division of the muscles, the joint capsule is evident. **D.** The capsule is longitudinally incised, and the fascia is tagged with figure-8 stitches for later anatomic repair.

MODIFIED WRIGHTINGTON APPROACH

- An 8-cm straight longitudinal incision is made just lateral to the olecranon **(TECH FIG 2A)**.
- Full-thickness skin flaps are developed bluntly over the fascia.
- The fascia is longitudinally incised in the interval between the anconeus and ulna and tagged with suture to facilitate repair during closure **(TECH FIG 2B)**.
- The anconeus is dissected off the ulna, elevating proximal to distal to preserve the distal vascular pedicle. Great care is taken not to violate the joint capsule or lateral ulnar collateral ligament by using a blunt elevator **(TECH FIG 2C)**.
- The lateral ulnar collateral ligament and annular ligament complex are sharply divided and tagged from their insertion on the crista supinatoris of the ulna. The radial head and its articulation with the capitellum are now evident **(TECH FIG 2D)**.
- After repair or replacement, the ligaments are repaired to their insertion with suture anchors.

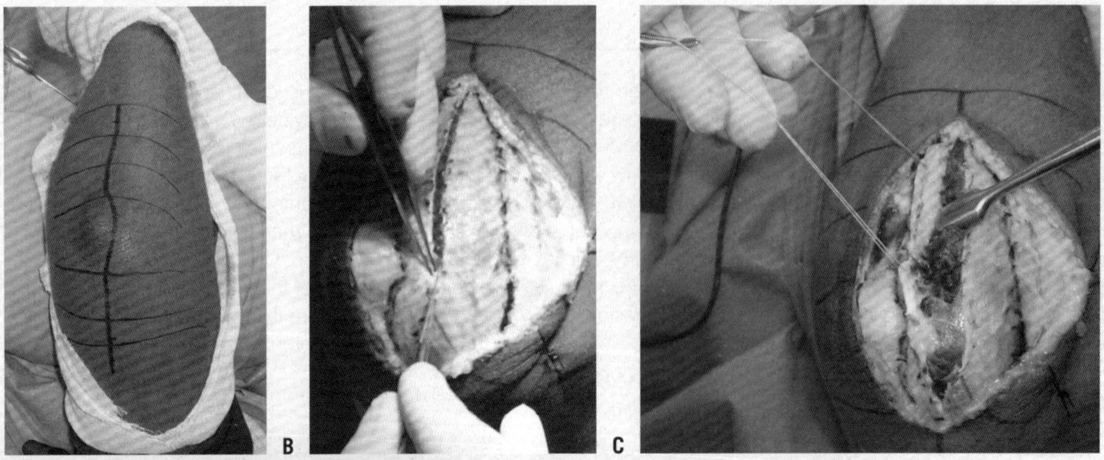

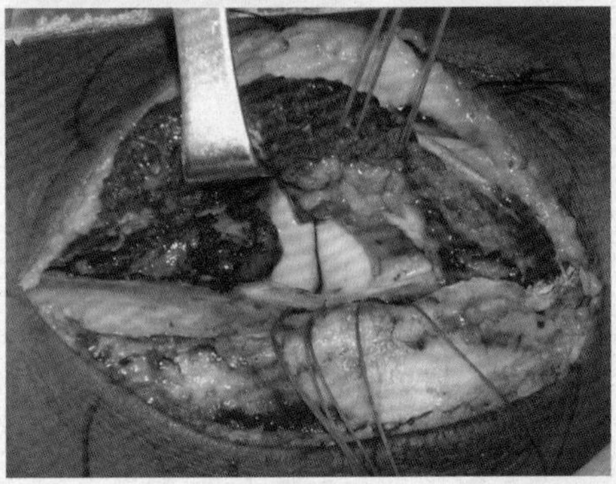

A B C D

TECH FIG 2 Modified Wrightington approach. **A.** Make an 8-cm longitudinal incision at the junction of the ulna and anconeus starting about four fingerbreadths distal to the olecranon and extending 2 cm proximal to the olecranon. **B.** The interval between the ulna and anconeus is incised sharply, with care taken not to violate the periosteum or muscle to minimize the risk of proximal radioulnar synostosis. **C.** Blunt elevation of the anconeus is crucial to avoid damaging the capsule or lateral ligament complex. **D.** The capsule and lateral ligament complex are tagged during the approach to facilitate final repair with suture anchors.

FRACTURE INSPECTION AND PREPARATION

- The fracture is now completely visible along with full visualization of the radial head by posteriorly dislocating the radial head out of the joint **(TECH FIG 3)**.
- The wound is irrigated, and loose bodies are removed.
- The forearm is rotated to obtain a circumferential view of the fracture and appreciate the safe zone for hardware placement.
- If comminution (more than three fragments) is evident at this step or significant impaction is noted with a DRUJ injury, we elect to replace the radial head.

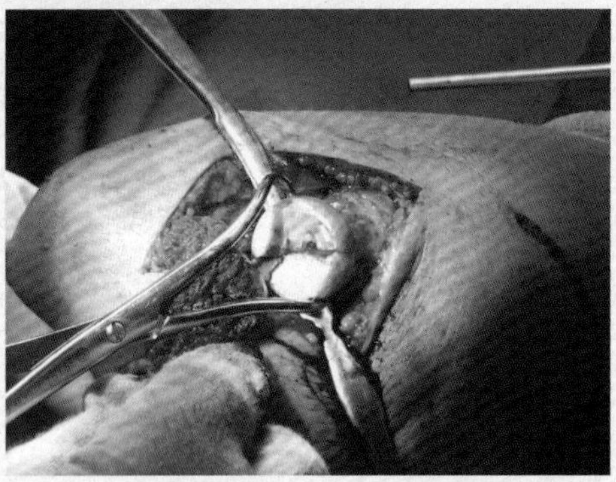

TECH FIG 3 The modified Wrightington approach provides excellent visualization of the fracture by dislocating the radial head posteriorly.

REDUCTION AND PROVISIONAL FIXATION

- Any joint impaction is elevated and the void filled with local cancellous graft from the lateral epicondyle.
- The fragments are reduced provisionally with a tenaculum and held with small Kirschner wires placed out of the zone where definitive fixation is planned.
- It is acceptable to place this temporary fixation in the safe zone.

FIXATION

- There are many options for definitive fixation[7]:
  - One or two countersunk 2.0- or 2.7-mm cortical screws perpendicular to the fracture
  - Miniplates
  - Small headless screws
  - Polyglycolide pins
  - Poly-L-lactic acid screws
  - Small threaded wires
- We prefer to use two parallel Biotrak screws (Acumed, Hillsboro, OR), which are cannulated, headless, resorbable, and variable pitched for isolated head fractures **(TECH FIG 4)**.
- For fractures with neck extension, we prefer 2.0- or 2.7-mm miniplates along the safe zone.

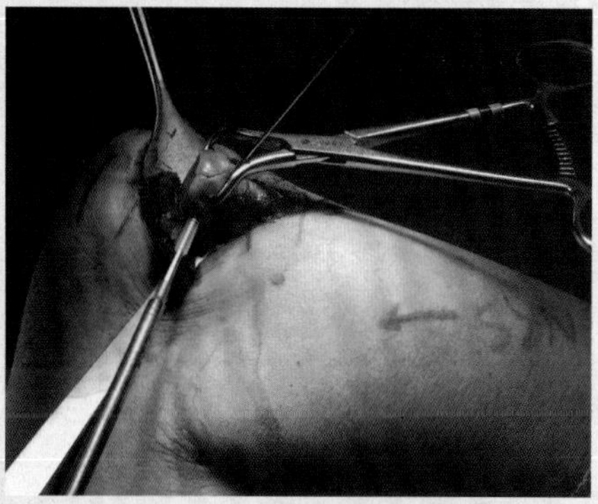

TECH FIG 4 Tenaculum clamps and 0.062-inch Kirschner wires are placed outside the safe zone for provisional fixation. Two Biotrak screws are used for definitive fixation.

CLOSURE

- Any releases or injury to the annular ligament or lateral ulnar collateral ligament must be repaired anatomically. Drill holes with transosseous sutures are a proven method, but we prefer all-suture anchors for annular ligament repair and radiopaque titanium anchors for lateral ulnar collateral ligament repair.
- Skin closure is performed in standard fashion with drain placement at the surgeon's discretion.

Pearls and Pitfalls

Protection of the Posterior Interosseous Nerve	• Pronation of the forearm moves the posterior interosseous nerve away from the operative field during posterior approaches. • Dissection should remain subperiosteally.
Comminution	• Maintain a low threshold for excision or arthroplasty in the setting of comminution.
Fluoroscopy	• Fluoroscopy should be available for examination under anesthesia before sterile preparation.
Hardware	• The possibility of radial head arthroplasty should always be discussed with the patient prior to surgery, and implants should be available in the room if needed. • A hinged external fixator should also be available for persistent instability.
Examination	• A thorough fluoroscopic examination is the most important factor in deciding what treatment is appropriate. To obtain a true lateral view, we recommend abducting the arm and externally rotating the shoulder while placing the elbow on the image intensifier.

POSTOPERATIVE CARE

- The elbow is immobilized in a splint for 7 to 10 days.
- Serial radiographs are obtained to detect any loss of reduction at the first postoperative visit and then at 4 weeks, 8 weeks, and 3 months, until adequate healing is noted **(FIG 12)**.
- Active range of motion is allowed as soon as tolerable. Formal physical therapy should begin within 2 weeks of surgery.
- Associated injuries may call for more protected range of motion.
- Light activities of daily living are allowed at 2 weeks, with increased weight bearing at 6 weeks.

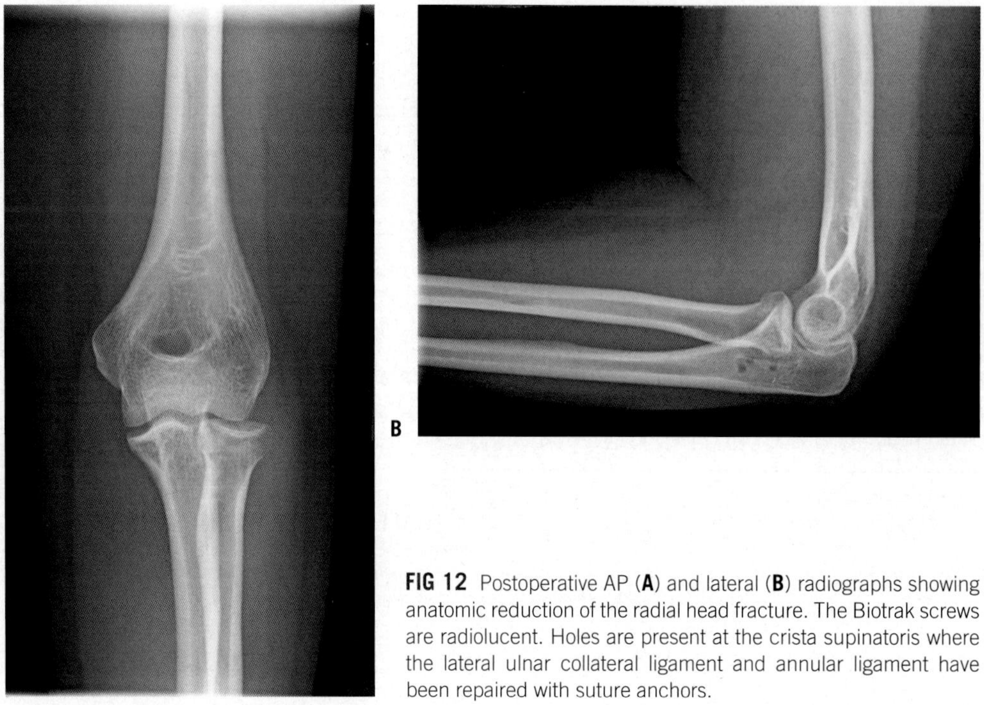

A B

FIG 12 Postoperative AP (**A**) and lateral (**B**) radiographs showing anatomic reduction of the radial head fracture. The Biotrak screws are radiolucent. Holes are present at the crista supinatoris where the lateral ulnar collateral ligament and annular ligament have been repaired with suture anchors.

OUTCOMES

- The results of ORIF depend both on host factors such as the type of fracture, smoking, compliance, level of physical demand, as well as surgical and rehabilitation protocols.
- In uncomplicated fractures, over 90% satisfactory results can be expected.
- Complications and resultant secondary procedures will be more likely in cases with undiagnosed instability or other associated injuries.

COMPLICATIONS

- Stiffness is the most common complication, with loss of terminal extension, supination, and pronation being most evident.
- Arthritis of the radiocapitellar joint or PRUJ
- Heterotopic ossification
- Nonunion **(FIG 13)**
- Infection
- Early and late instability from missed or failed treatment of associated injuries
- The rate of avascular necrosis is about 10%, significantly higher in displaced fractures. This is expected, given that the radial recurrent artery inserts in the safe zone where hardware is placed. This is generally clinically silent.
- Loss of reduction
- Symptomatic or malpositioned implants requiring secondary surgery for removal **(FIG 14)**.

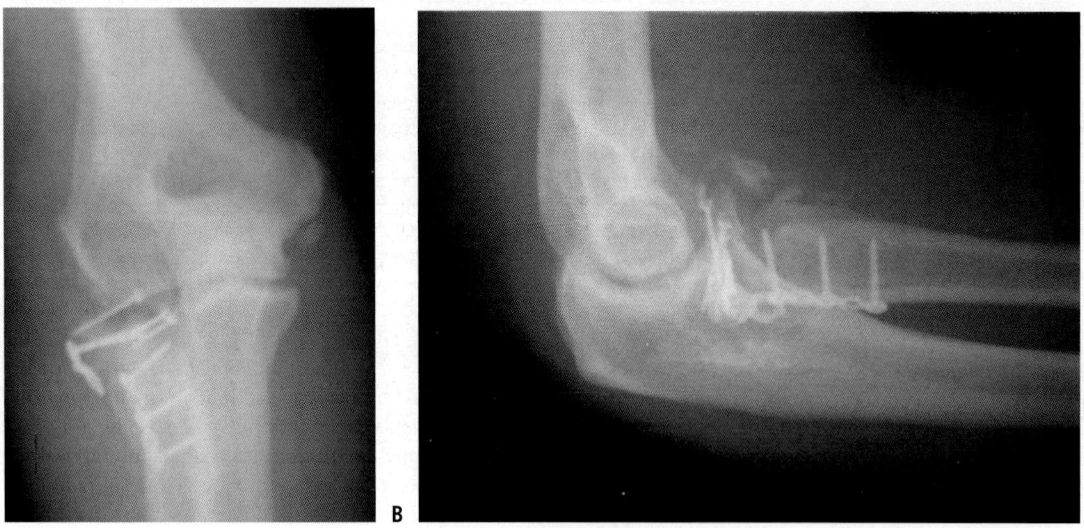

A B

FIG 13 AP (**A**) and lateral (**B**) radiographs after ORIF of a radial neck fracture that went on to nonunion and avascular necrosis.

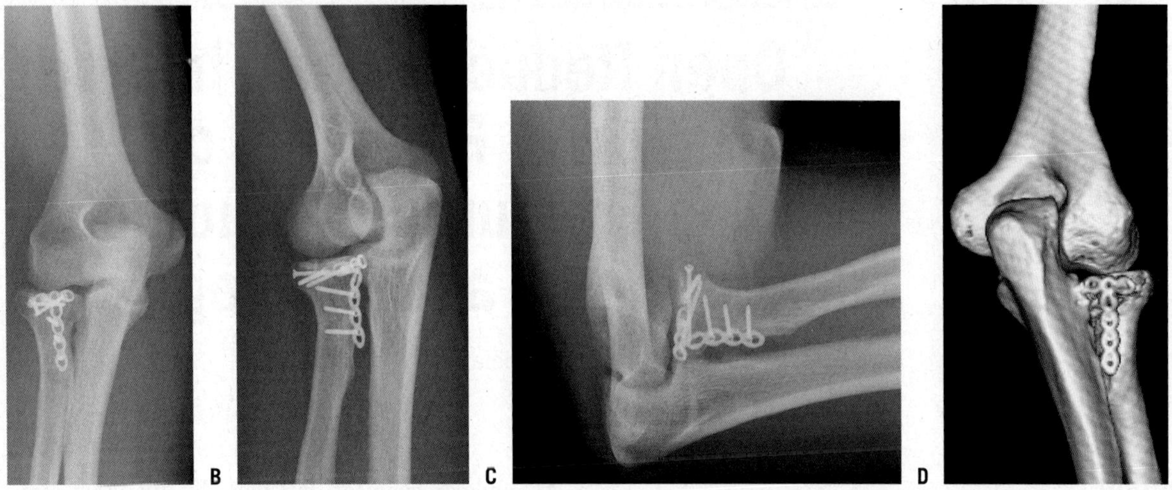

FIG 14 AP (**A**), oblique (**B**), and radiocapitellar (**C**) radiographs and three-dimensional CT rendering (**D**) of a plate placed outside of the safe zone during ORIF of a radial head fracture.

REFERENCES

1. Akesson T, Herbertsson P, Josefsson PO, et al. Primary nonoperative treatment of moderately displaced two-part fractures of the radial head. J Bone Joint Surg Am 2006;88(9):1909–1914.
2. Amis AA, Miller JH. The mechanisms of elbow fractures: an investigation using impact tests in vitro. Injury 1995;26(3):163–168.
3. Antuna SA, Sánchez-Márquez JM, Barco R. Long-term results of radial head resection following isolated radial head fractures in patients younger than forty years old. J Bone Joint Surg Am 2010;92:558–566.
4. Boyd HB. Surgical exposure of the ulna and proximal third of the radius through one incision. Surg Gynecol Obstet 1940;71:86–88.
5. Broberg MA, Morrey BF. Results of delayed excision of the radial head after fracture. J Bone Joint Surg Am 1986;68(5):669–674.
6. Broberg MA, Morrey BF. Results of treatment of fracture-elbow dislocations of the elbow and intraarticular fractures. Clin Orthop Relat Res 1989;(246):126–130.
7. Caputo AE, Mazzocca AD, Sontoro VM. The nonarticulating portion of the radial head: anatomic and clinical correlations for internal fixation. J Hand Surg Am 1998;23(6):1082–1090.
8. Esser RD, Davis S, Taavao T. Fractures of the radial head treated by internal fixation: late results in 26 cases. J Orthop Trauma 1995;9:318–323.
9. Essex-Lopresti P. Fractures of the radial head with distal radio-ulnar dislocation; report of two cases. J Bone Joint Surg Br 1951;33(2):244–247.
10. Guitton TG, Ring D; for Science of Variation Group. Interobserver reliability of radial head fracture classification: two-dimensional compared with three-dimensional CT. J Bone Joint Surg Am 2011;93(21):2015–2021.
11. Harrington IJ, Tountas AA. Replacement of the radial head in the treatment of unstable elbow fractures. Injury 1981;12(5):405–412.
12. Herbertsson P, Josefsson PO, Hasserius R, et al. Fractures of the radial head and neck treated with radial head excision. J Bone Joint Surg Am 2004;86-A(9):1925–1930.
13. Herbertsson P, Josefsson PO, Hasserius R, et al. Uncomplicated Mason type-II and III fractures of the radial head and neck in adults: a long-term follow-up study. J Bone Joint Surg Am 2004;86-A(3):569–574.
14. Hotchkiss RN. Displaced fractures of the radial head: internal fixation or excision? J Am Acad Orthop Surg 1997;5:1–10.
15. Hotchkiss RN. Fractures and dislocations of the elbow. In: Rockwood CA Jr, Green DP, eds. Fractures in Adults, ed 4. Philadelphia: Lippincott-Raven, 1996:929–1024.
16. Itamura JM, Roidis NT, Chong AK, et al. Computed tomography study of radial head morphology. J Shoulder Elbow Surg 2008;17(2):347–354.
17. Itamura J, Roidis N, Mirzayan R, et al. Radial head fractures: MRI evaluation of associated injuries. J Shoulder Elbow Surg 2005;14(4):421–424.
18. Kaas L, Struijs PA, Ring D, et al. Treatment of Mason type II radial head fractures without associated fractures or elbow dislocation: a systematic review. J Hand Surg Am 2012;37(7):1416–1421.
19. Kaas L, van Riet RP, Turkenburg JL, et al. Magnetic resonance imaging in radial head fractures: most associated injuries are not clinically relevant. J Shoulder Elbow Surg 2011;20(8):1282–1288.
20. Kovar FM, Jaindl M, Thalhammer G, et al. Incidence and analysis of radial head and neck fractures. World J Orthop 2013;4(2):80–84.
21. McKee MD, Jupiter JB. Trauma to the adult elbow and fractures of the distal humerus. In: Browner BD, Jupiter JR, Levine AM, et al, eds. Skeletal Trauma, ed 2. Philadelphia: WB Saunders, 1998:1455–1522.
22. Morrey BF. Radial head fracture. In: Morrey BF, ed. The Elbow and Its Disorders, ed 3. Philadelphia: WB Saunders, 2000:341–364.
23. Morrey BF, An KN, Stormont TJ. Force transmission through the radial head. J Bone Joint Surg Am 1988;70(2):250–256.
24. Ring D, Quintero J, Jupiter JB. Open reduction and internal fixation of fractures of the radial head. J Bone Joint Surg Am 2002;84-A(10):1811–1815.
25. Roidis NT, Papadakis SA, Rigopoulos N, et al. Current concepts and controversies in the management of radial head fractures. Orthopedics 2006;29(10):904–916.
26. Stanley JK, Penn DS, Wasseem M. Exposure of the head of the radius using the Wrightington approach. J Bone Joint Surg Br 2006;88(9):1178–1182.
27. Tang CW, Skaggs DL, Kay RM. Elbow aspiration and arthrogram: an alternative method. Am J Orthop 2001;30:256.
28. Yamaguchi K, Sweet FA, Bindra R, et al. The extraosseous and intraosseous arterial anatomy of the adult elbow. J Bone Joint Surg Am 1997;79(11):1653–1662.

CHAPTER 15

Open Reduction and Internal Fixation of Fractures of Ulna Fractures (Including Olecranon and Monteggia)

David Ring and Abed Abdelaziz

DEFINITION

- The proximal ulna is composed of the olecranon process, coronoid process, greater sigmoid notch, and the lesser sigmoid notch.
- It plays an important role in elbow stability, with the ulnohumeral joint serving as the primary static elbow stabilizer.
- Fractures of the olecranon process are common accounting for 20% of proximal forearm fractures.
- Important injury characteristics of olecranon fractures include displacement, comminution, and subluxation or dislocation of the elbow; all of which are accounted for in the Mayo classification (**FIG 1**).
- Fracture-dislocations of the olecranon can be anterior (transolecranon) or posterior in direction.[2,4,11,12]
- The "terrible triad" injury of the elbow is characterized by an elbow dislocation, radial head or neck fracture, and a coronoid fracture.
- The eponym Monteggia is best applied to metaphyseal or diaphyseal proximal ulnar fracture associated with dislocation of the radiocapitellar and/or radioulnar joints.
- The Bado classification of Monteggia fractures-dislocations with Jupiter subclassification of type II injuries is shown in **TABLE 1**.

ANATOMY

- The greater sigmoid notch of the ulna is formed by the coronoid and olecranon processes and forms a nearly 180-degree arc capturing the trochlea.
- The region between the coronoid and olecranon articular facets is the nonarticular transverse groove of the olecranon, a common location of fracture and a place where precise articular reduction is not critical.
- The triceps has a broad and thick insertion from just superior to the point of the olecranon and the tip of the olecranon process that can be used to enhance fixation of small, osteoporotic, or fragmented fractures and can be split longitudinally, if needed, when applying a plate.
- The radioulnar articulation is stabilized by the triangular fibrocartilage complex at the distal radioulnar joint, the interosseous ligament in the midforearm, and the annular ligament at the proximal radioulnar joint (PRUJ). Fracture of the ulna with dislocation of the PRUJ disrupts the annular ligament, but typically, the other structures are spared.

PATHOGENESIS

- Fractures of the olecranon and proximal ulna can result from a direct blow to the point of the elbow or indirect forces during a fall on the outstretched hand.

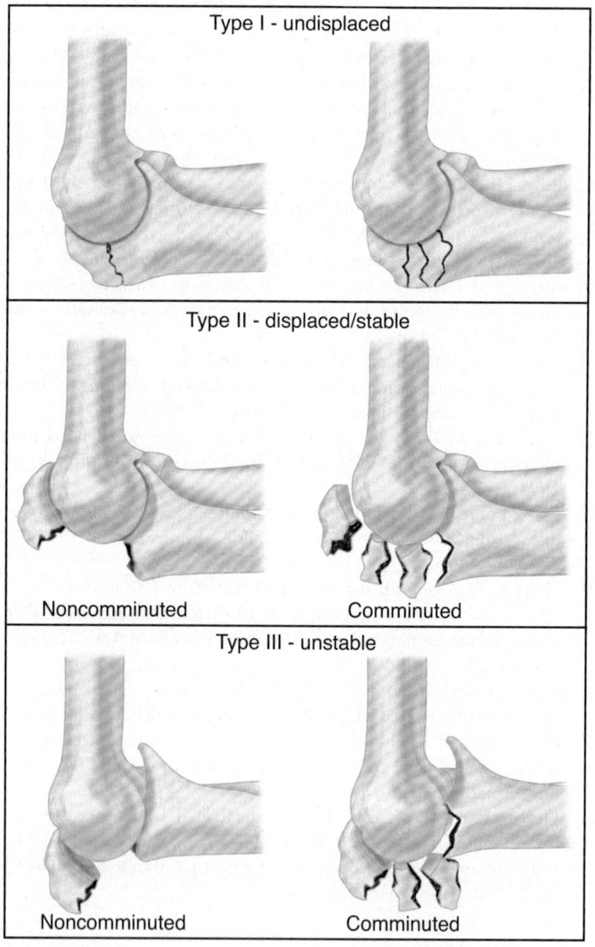

FIG 1 The Mayo classification of olecranon fractures accounts for the factors that will influence treatment decisions: displacement, comminution, and dislocation or subluxation of the articulations.

TABLE 1 Bado Classification of Monteggia Lesions with Jupiter Subclassification of Type II Fractures

Type	Description	Illustration
I	Anterior dislocation of the radial head with fracture of the diaphysis of the ulna with anterior angulation of the ulnar fracture (most common type of lesion)	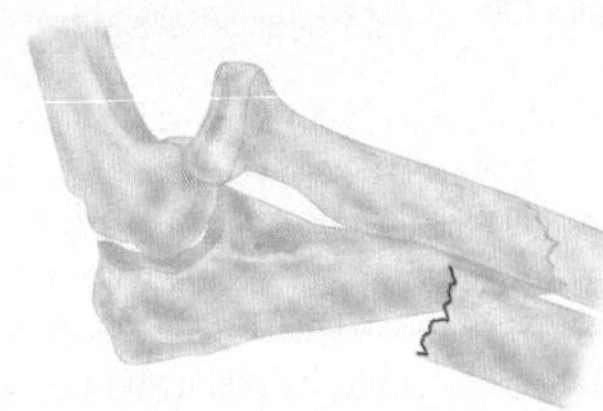
II	Posterior or posterolateral dislocation of the radial head with fracture of the ulnar diaphysis with posterior angulation of the ulnar fracture	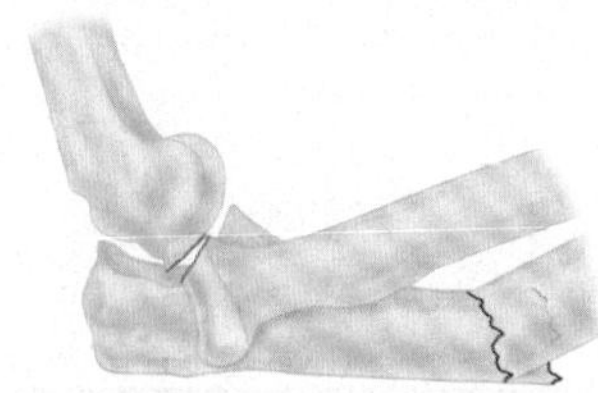
IIA	Fracture at the level of the trochlear notch (ulnar fracture involves the distal part of the olecranon and coronoid)	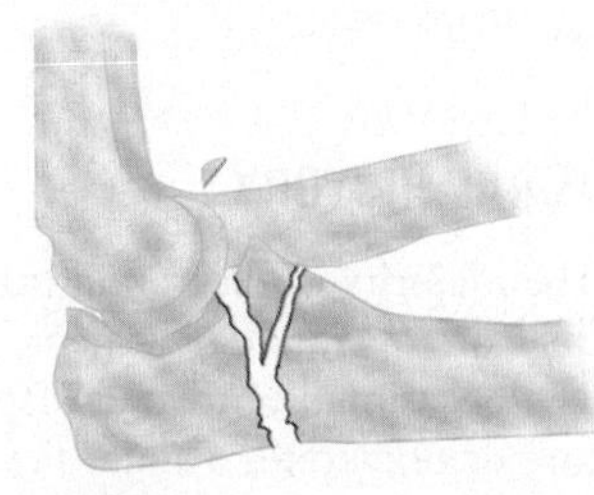
IIB	Ulnar fracture is at the metaphyseal–diaphyseal junction, distal to the coronoid.	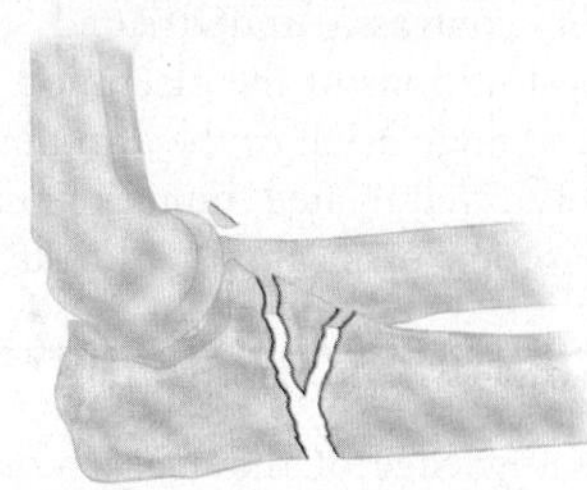
IIC	Ulnar fracture is diaphyseal.	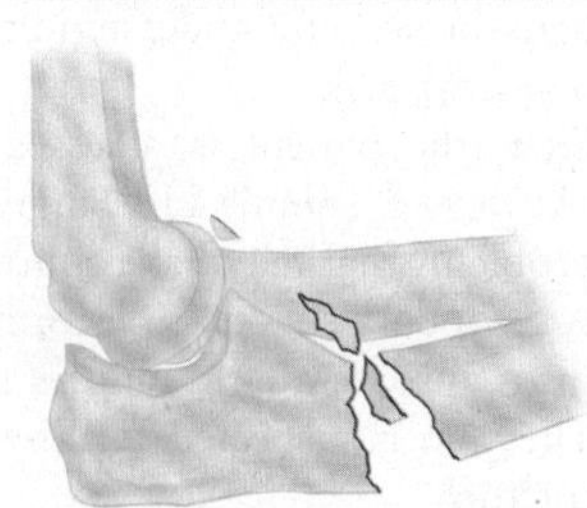
IID	Comminuted fractures involving more than one region	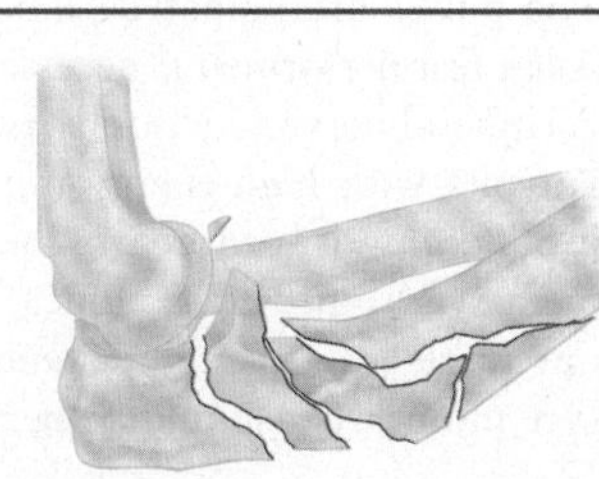

(continued)

TABLE 1 *(continued)*

Type	Description	Illustration
III	Lateral or anterolateral dislocation of the radial head with fracture of the ulnar metaphysis	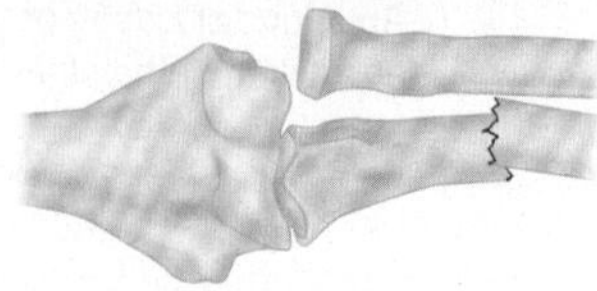
IV	Anterior dislocation of the radial head with a fracture of the proximal third of the radius and ulna at the same level	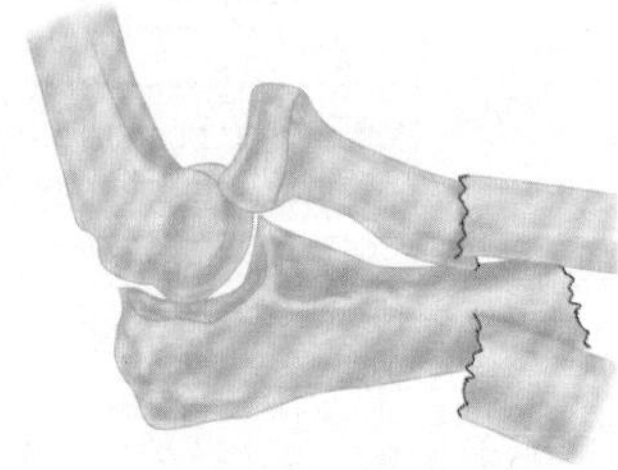

Adapted from Bado J. The Monteggia lesion. Clin Orthop Relat Res 1967;50:71–86; Jupiter JB, Leibovic SJ, Ribbans W, et al. The posterior Monteggia lesion. J Orthop Trauma 1991;5:395–402.

NATURAL HISTORY

- The majority of olecranon fractures is displaced and benefits from operative treatment.
- The occasional untreated displaced simple olecranon fracture demonstrates a slight flexion contracture, some weakness of extension, no arthrosis, and little, if any, pain.
- In contrast, undertreated or poorly treated fracture-dislocations of the olecranon often lead to severe arthrosis and angulation of the arm under the influence of gravity.
- Even well-treated complex injuries are at risk for stiffness, heterotopic ossification, arthrosis, and occasionally nonunion.

PATIENT HISTORY AND PHYSICAL FINDINGS

- Knowledge of the characteristics of the patient (age, sex, medical health) and the injury (mechanism, energy) will help the surgeon understand the injury and determine optimal treatment.
- First, the patient is assessed for life-threatening injuries (Advanced Trauma Life Support protocol) and any medical problems that may have contributed to the injury.
- A secondary survey is performed to identify any other fractures, ipsilateral arm injuries in particular.
- The skin is inspected for any wounds associated with the fracture.
- The pulses are palpated, capillary refill inspected, and an Allen test performed if necessary.
- Peripheral nerve function is assessed.
- Patients with high-energy injuries, particularly those with ipsilateral wrist or forearm injuries, are at risk for compartment syndrome. If the clinical examination is suggestive or unreliable (due to altered mental status), compartment pressure monitoring should be performed.

IMAGING AND OTHER DIAGNOSTIC STUDIES

- Anteroposterior and lateral radiographs are used for initial characterization of the injury. Oblique views may be beneficial for some fracture patterns.
- Radiographs after reduction or splinting can be useful.
- Computed tomography (CT) is useful for characterization of fracture-dislocations. In particular, three-dimensional CT reconstructions can be useful for assessment of the coronoid and radial head.

DIFFERENTIAL DIAGNOSIS

- Elbow dislocation
- Essex-Lopresti fracture-dislocation of the forearm (disruption of the interosseous ligament and or triangular fibrocartilage complex usually with fracture of the radial head)
- Fracture-dislocations of the elbow ("terrible triad" injury)
- Distal humerus fracture

NONOPERATIVE MANAGEMENT

- Nonoperative management is appropriate for fractures of the olecranon that is less than 2 mm displaced with the elbow flexed 90 degrees. Four weeks of splint immobilization followed by active-assisted mobilization of the elbow will usually result in a healed fracture and good elbow function.
- Fractures of the anteromedial coronoid facet may be treated nonoperatively when subluxation is excluded and the fracture fragment is small and minimally displaced.[15]

SURGICAL MANAGEMENT

- The vast majority of olecranon fractures are displaced and merit operative treatment.
- Transverse, noncomminuted fractures not associated with fracture-dislocation are treated with tension band wiring.[5,10]
- Comminuted fractures and fracture-dislocations are treated with dorsal contoured plate and screw fixation.[1,2,4]
- The treatment of fracture-dislocations requires attention to the coronoid, radial head, and lateral collateral ligament.[2,11,12,14]

- Debate exists as to whether coronoid fractures require fixation,[3,9,13] but increased elbow stability and alignment through coronoid fixation may reduce arthrosis.
- Fracture-dislocations of the forearm (anterolateral Monteggia injuries) are treated with anatomic realignment of the ulna and plate and screw fixation.[12]

Preoperative Planning

- The fracture characteristics that determine treatment are defined on radiographs and CT.
- Templating the surgery with tracings of the radiographs is a useful way of running through the surgery in detail before performing it, familiarizing oneself with the anatomy, anticipating problems, and ensuring that all of the implants and equipment that might be necessary are available.

Positioning

- In most patients, a lateral decubitus position with the arm over a bolster or support is best.
- Some patients with fracture-dislocations that require both medial and lateral access may be positioned supine with the arm supported on a hand table.
- A sterile pneumatic tourniquet is used.

Approach

- A dorsal longitudinal skin incision is used.

TENSION BAND WIRING

Reduction and Kirschner Wire Fixation

- Blood clot and periosteum are cleared from the fracture site to facilitate reduction.
- Limited periosteal elevation is performed at the fracture site to monitor reduction.
- One or two small pointed reduction forceps are used to secure the fracture in a reduced position **(TECH FIG 1A,B)**. A drill hole can be made in the dorsal cortex of the distal fragment to facilitate clamp application.
- Two 1.0-mm smooth Kirschner wires are drilled across the fracture site **(TECH FIG 1C)**.
- If these are drilled obliquely from dorsal-proximal to volar-distal, they will exit the anterior ulnar cortex distal to the coronoid process, providing an anchoring point of cortical bone to limit the potential for pin migration.
- In anticipation of later impaction of the proximal ends of the wires, the Kirschner wires should be retracted 5 to 10 mm after drilling through the anterior ulnar cortex.

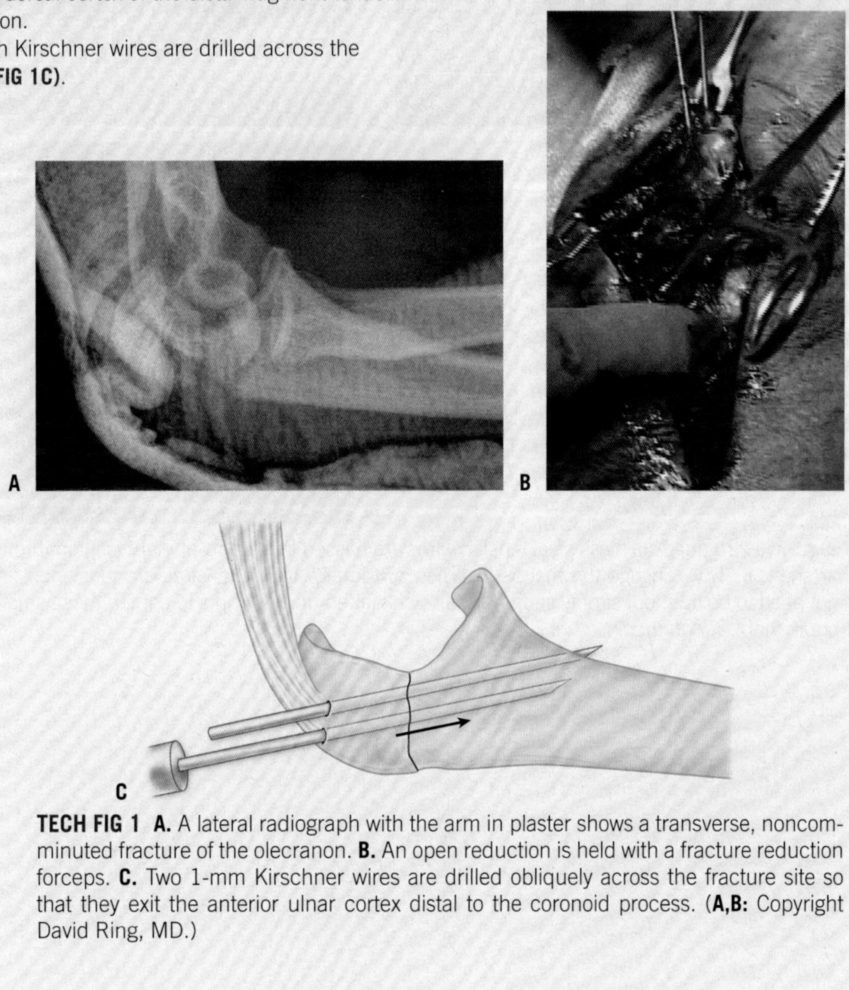

TECH FIG 1 **A.** A lateral radiograph with the arm in plaster shows a transverse, noncomminuted fracture of the olecranon. **B.** An open reduction is held with a fracture reduction forceps. **C.** Two 1-mm Kirschner wires are drilled obliquely across the fracture site so that they exit the anterior ulnar cortex distal to the coronoid process. (**A,B:** Copyright David Ring, MD.)

Wiring

- The apex of the ulnar diaphysis just distal to the flat portion of the proximal ulna is drilled with a 2.0-mm drill, with or without prior subperiosteal dissection. It is typically 4 cm distal to the fracture line.
- When two wires are used, a second drill hole is made a centimeter more distal.
- If one wire is used, it should be 18 gauge. Author preference is to use two 22-gauge stainless steel wires to limit the size of the knots, which may diminish implant prominence. The wires are passed through the drill holes. A large-bore needle can be used to facilitate passage of the wire through the drill hole **(TECH FIG 2A)**.
- The two tension wires are each passed over the dorsal ulna in a figure-of-eight fashion, then around the Kirschner wires, and underneath the insertion of the triceps tendon using a large-bore needle **(TECH FIG 2B)**.
- Each wire is tensioned both medially and laterally by twisting the wire with a needle holder **(TECH FIG 2C,D)**.
- This should be done to take up slack only. These small wires will break if they are firmly tightened, which is not necessary.
  - The tightening should be done in a place that will make the wire knots less prominent.
  - After tightening, the knots are trimmed and bent into the soft tissues to either side.
  - The proximal end of the Kirschner wires are then bent 180 degrees and trimmed, leaving a bend of about 5 to 6 mm.
- These bent ends are then impacted into the proximal olecranon, beneath the triceps insertion, using a bone tamp **(TECH FIG 2E–H)**.

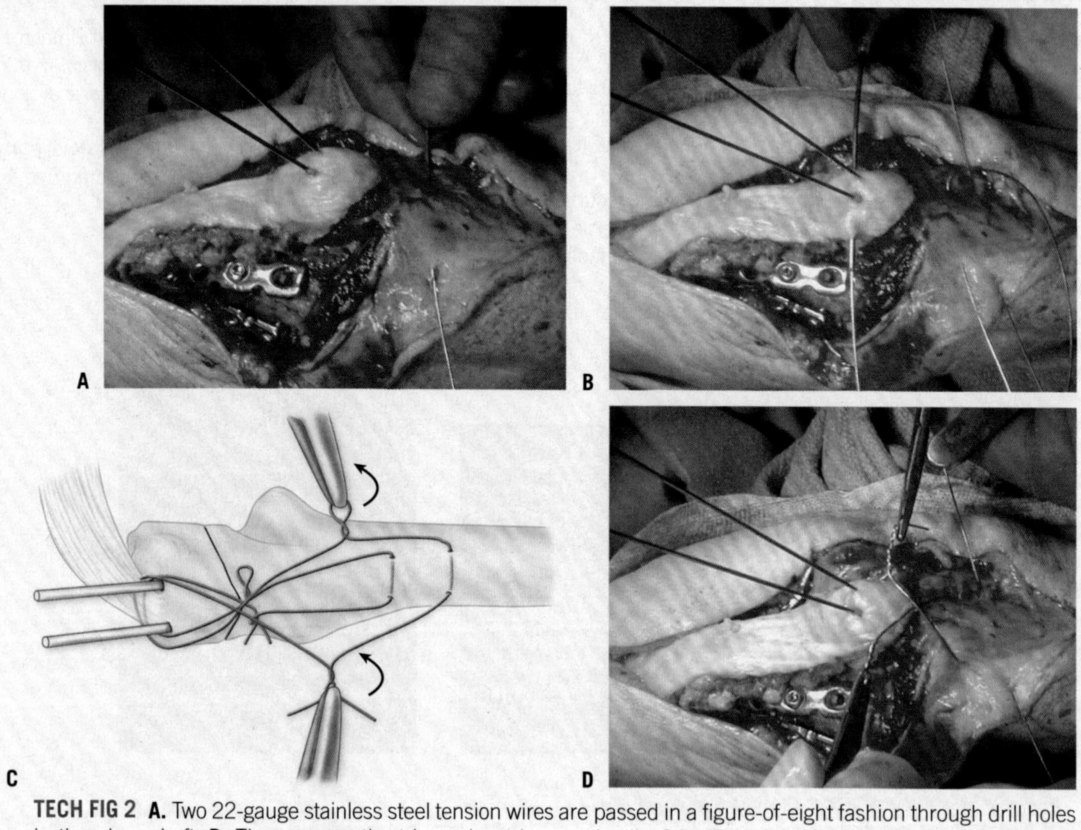

TECH FIG 2 **A.** Two 22-gauge stainless steel tension wires are passed in a figure-of-eight fashion through drill holes in the ulnar shaft. **B.** They engage the triceps insertion proximally. **C,D.** The wires are tensioned on both sides. These do not need to be tight but simply snug, with all slack taken up. Attempts to tighten these smaller 22-gauge wires will break them. *(continued)*

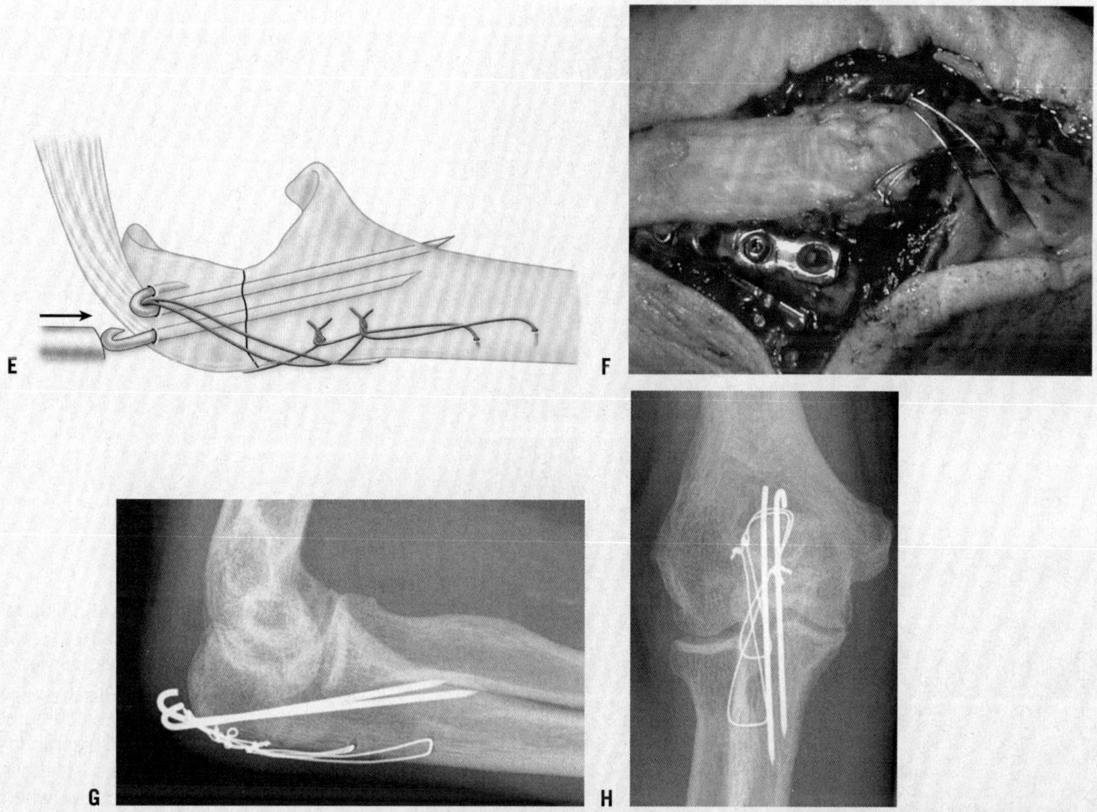

TECH FIG 2 *(continued)* **E.** The proximal ends of the Kirschner wires are bent 180 degrees and impacted into the olecranon process, beneath the triceps insertion. **F.** The resulting fixation has a relatively low profile and is unlikely to migrate. Postoperative anteroposterior (**G**) and lateral (**H**) radiographs demonstrating the final fixation construct. (**A,B,D,F–H:** Copyright David Ring, MD.)

PLATE AND SCREW FIXATION OF OLECRANON FRACTURES

- Reduce the fracture using pointed reduction forceps and Kirschner wires for provisional fixation.
- Contour the plate to wrap around the proximal aspect of the olecranon or use a precontoured plate **(TECH FIG 3A–C)**.
- A straight plate will have only two or three screws in metaphyseal bone proximal to the fracture.
- Bending the plate around the proximal aspect of the olecranon provides additional screws in the proximal fragment. The most proximal screws can be very long, crossing the fracture line into the distal fragment. In some cases, these screws can be directed to engage one of the cortices of the distal fragment, such as the anterior ulnar cortex.
- A plate contoured to wrap around the proximal ulna can be placed on top of the triceps insertion. Alternatively, the triceps insertion can be incised longitudinally and partially elevated medially and laterally sufficiently to allow direct plate contact with bone.
- Distally, a dorsal plate will lie directly on the apex of the ulnar diaphysis. The muscle need only be split sufficiently to gain access to this apex—there is no need to elevate the muscle or periosteum off either the medial or lateral flat aspect of the ulna.
- No attempt is made to precisely realign intervening fragmentation—once the relationship of the coronoid and olecranon facets is restored and the overall alignment is restored, the remaining fragments are bridged, leaving their soft tissue attachments intact.
- Bone grafts are rarely necessary if the soft tissue attachments are preserved.
- If the olecranon fragment is small, osteoporotic, or fragmented, a wire engaging the triceps insertion should be used to reinforce the fixation **(TECH FIG 3C,D)**.
- The plate and screws will serve to hold the coronoid and olecranon facets in proper alignment and bridge fragmentation, and the wire will help ensure fixation even if screw purchase is lost.

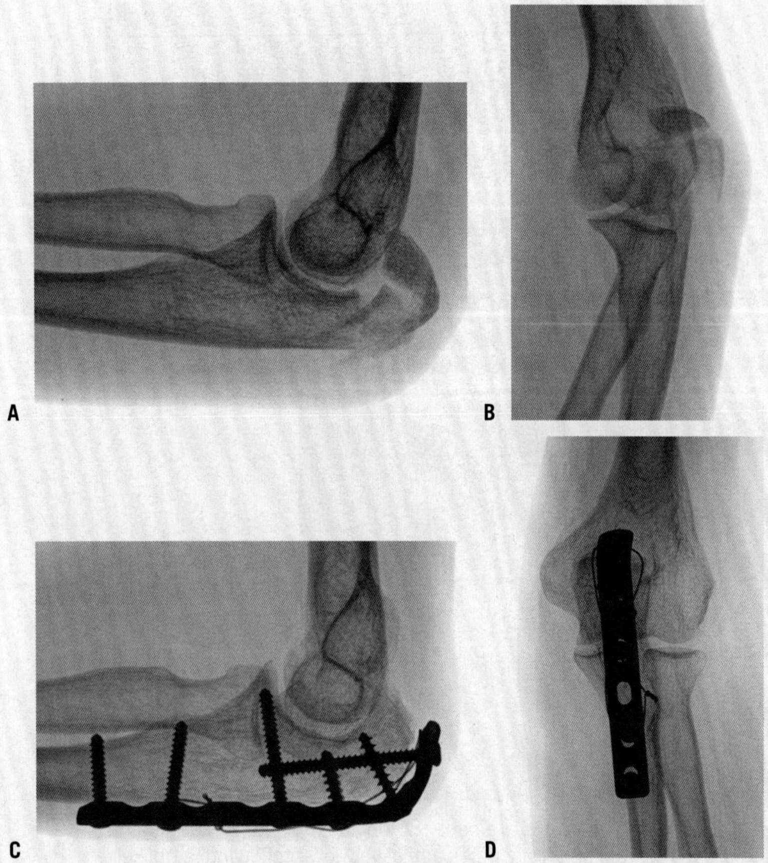

TECH FIG 3 **A.** A lateral radiograph illustrates a comminuted olecranon fracture with a small proximal olecranon fragment. **B.** An oblique view shows the fragmentation. **C.** A 3.5-mm limited-contact dynamic compression plate and screws contoured to wrap around the dorsal surface of the olecranon is used for fixation. **D.** A 22-gauge stainless steel wire engages the triceps insertion—this is useful when the olecranon fragment is small, fragmented, or osteopenic. (Copyright David Ring, MD.)

PLATE AND SCREW FIXATION OF THE FRACTURE-DISLOCATIONS OF THE OLECRANON

Exposure

- In the setting of a fracture-dislocation of the olecranon **(TECH FIG 4A)**, fractures of the radial head and coronoid process can be evaluated and often definitively treated through the exposure provided by the fracture of the olecranon process.
  - With little additional dissection, the olecranon fragment can be mobilized proximally as one would do with an olecranon osteotomy, providing exposure of the coronoid through the ulnohumeral joint.
- If the exposure of the radial head through the posterior injury is inadequate, a separate muscle interval (eg, Kocher or Kaplan intervals) accessed by the elevation of a broad lateral skin flap can be used.
- If the exposure of the coronoid is inadequate through posterior injury and olecranon fracture, a separate medial or lateral exposure can be developed.
  - A medial exposure—between the two heads of the flexor carpi ulnaris, or by splitting the flexor–pronator mass more anteriorly, or by elevating the entire flexor–pronator mass from dorsal to volar—may be needed to address a complex fracture of the coronoid, particularly one that involves the anteromedial facet of the coronoid process.[8]
  - A lateral approach to the coronoid requires moving or removing the radial head fragment. In this situation, the coronoid would be fixed first, followed by fixation of the radial head.
- When the lateral collateral ligament is injured, it is usually avulsed from the lateral epicondyle. This facilitates repair that can be performed using suture anchors or suture placed through drill holes in the bone.
- The fracture of the coronoid can often be reduced directly through the elbow joint using the limited access provided by the olecranon fracture **(TECH FIG 4B,C)**.

Fixation

- Provisional fixation can be obtained using Kirschner wires to attach the fragments either to the metaphyseal or diaphyseal fragments of the ulna or to the trochlea of the distal humerus when there is extensive fragmentation of the proximal ulna. Small or minifragment plates can also be used to provisionally or definitively fix segmental comminuted fragments to the distal diaphysis.
- An alternative to keep in mind when there is extensive fragmentation of the proximal ulna is the use of a skeletal distractor (a temporary external fixator; **TECH FIG 5A**).
  - External fixation applied between a wire driven through the olecranon fragment and up into the trochlea and a second wire in the distal ulnar diaphysis can often obtain reduction indirectly when distraction is applied between the pins.
  - Definitive fixation can usually be obtained with screws applied under image intensifier guidance.

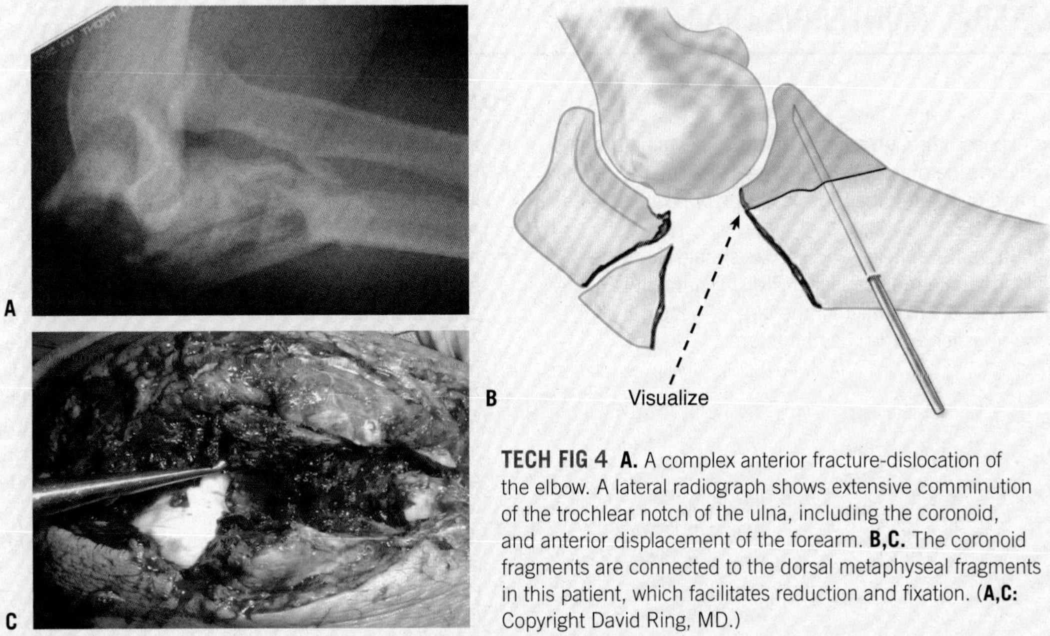

TECH FIG 4 **A.** A complex anterior fracture-dislocation of the elbow. A lateral radiograph shows extensive comminution of the trochlear notch of the ulna, including the coronoid, and anterior displacement of the forearm. **B,C.** The coronoid fragments are connected to the dorsal metaphyseal fragments in this patient, which facilitates reduction and fixation. (**A,C:** Copyright David Ring, MD.)

- The screws are placed through the plate when there is extensive fragmentation of the proximal ulna.
- For coronoid fixation, screws may be used for large fragments and sutures for small fragments.
- If the coronoid fracture is very comminuted and cannot be securely repaired, the ulnohumeral joint should be protected with temporary hinged or static external fixation or temporary pin fixation of the ulnohumeral joint, depending on the equipment and expertise available.
- A long plate is contoured to wrap around the proximal olecranon **(TECH FIG 5B)**.
  - A very long plate should be considered (between 12 and 16 holes), particularly when there is extensive fragmentation or the bone quality is poor.
- When the olecranon is fragmented or osteoporotic, a plate and screws alone may not provide reliable fixation.
  - In this situation, it can be useful to use ancillary tension wire fixation to control the olecranon fragments through the triceps insertion **(TECH FIG 5C)**.

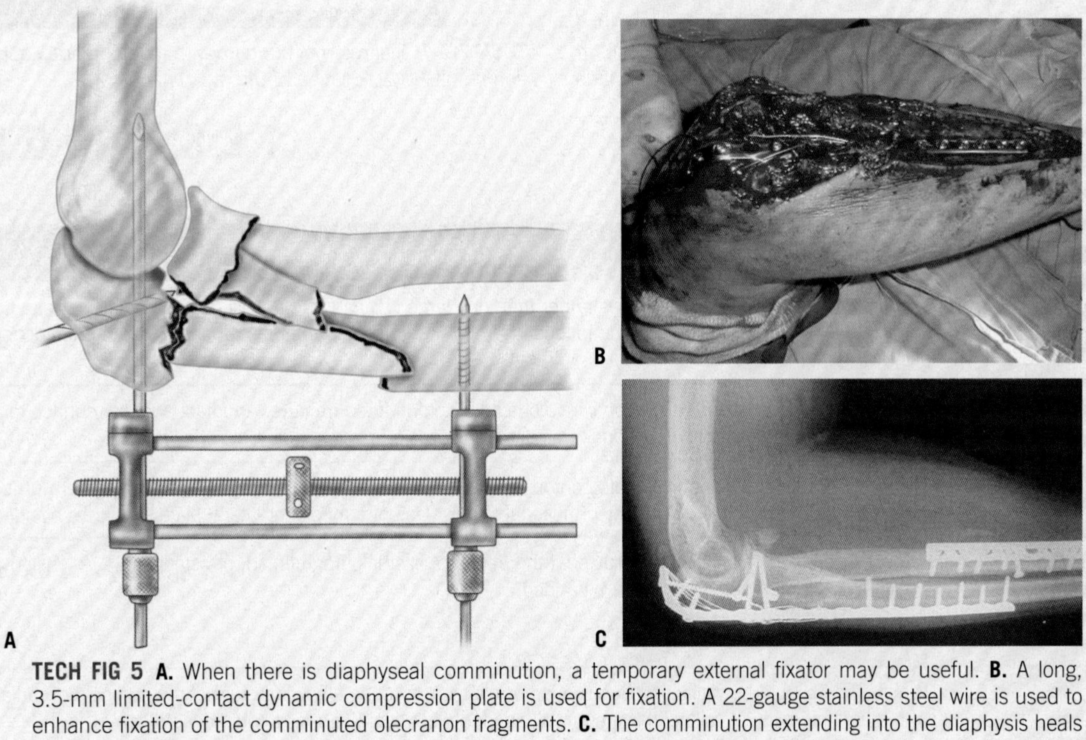

TECH FIG 5 A. When there is diaphyseal comminution, a temporary external fixator may be useful. **B.** A long, 3.5-mm limited-contact dynamic compression plate is used for fixation. A 22-gauge stainless steel wire is used to enhance fixation of the comminuted olecranon fragments. **C.** The comminution extending into the diaphysis heals with the bridging plate. The trochlear notch is restored with good elbow function. (**B,C:** Copyright David Ring, MD.)

ANTEROLATERAL MONTEGGIA FRACTURES

Exposure

- The ulna is exposed through a dorsal incision elevating the muscle from one side of the ulnar diaphysis, leaving the periosteum intact and disrupting the muscle on the opposite side as little as possible **(TECH FIG 6)**.
- Exposure of the radiocapitellar and PRUJs should rarely be necessary. Inadequate radiocapitellar/PRUJ alignment is nearly always due to residual malunion of the ulna. If necessary, expose the joint as for a radial head fracture.

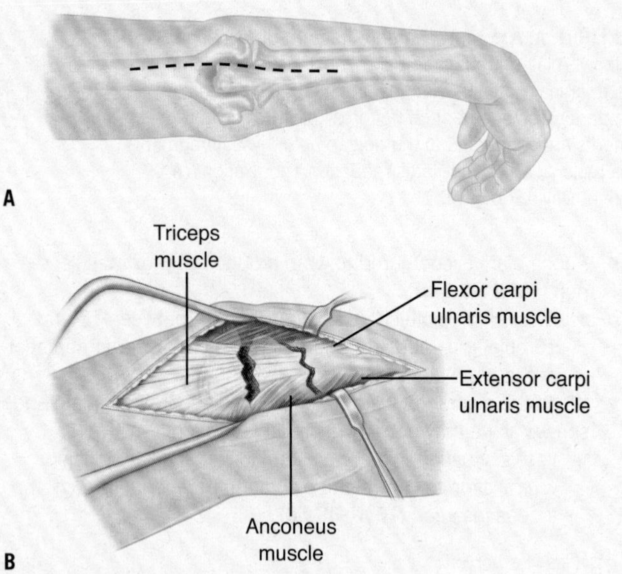

TECH FIG 6 A. Posterior midline incision positioned just off the lateral aspect of the olecranon. **B.** Deep surgical interval uses the internervous plane between the anconeus and flexor carpi ulnaris.

Fixation

- Reduce the radiocapitellar joint or PRUJ.
- Realign the ulnar fracture and provisionally apply a 3.5-mm limited contact dynamic compression plate or equivalent.
  - In osteoporotic bone, a locking plate should be used
- If there is fragmentation at the ulnar fracture site, it might be helpful to provisionally hold the reduction with a temporary external fixator (which the author has done) or temporary stabilization of the radiocapitellar articulation (which the author has not done) while getting provisional fixation of the ulna.
- Place two screws in each side of the plate proximal and distal to the fracture side and then check radiocapitellar/PRUJ alignment in several positions of elbow and forearm rotation and from several different radiographic angles under the image intensifier.
- If the alignment is inadequate, revise your fixation of the ulna accordingly.
- Failure to obtain adequate length of the ulna can lead to persistent dislocation of the radial head **(TECH FIG 7)**.
- Only enter the radiocapitellar joint if you can be 100% certain that the ulna is aligned properly. Interposition of the annular ligament is very uncommon.

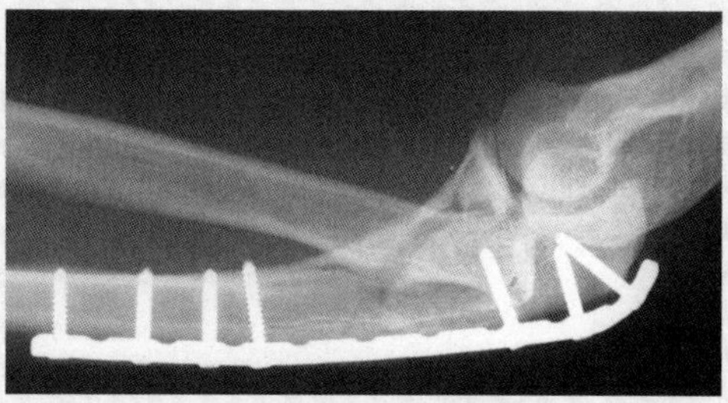

TECH FIG 7 Malunion of the ulna with resulting apex dorsal angulation results in dislocation of the radial head.

TECHNIQUES

Pearls and Pitfalls

Prominence of Olecranon Hardware	• The use of two small (22-gauge) wires rather than one large (18-gauge) wire will result in smaller knots. Care taken to place the Kirschner wires below the triceps insertion and impacting them into bone will limit prominence and the potential for migration.[6,10]
Narrowing of Trochlear Notch	• The surgeon should not use a tension wire alone on a comminuted fracture. An intact articular surface to absorb compressive forces with active motion is mandatory for tension band wiring to be effective.
Plate Loosening	• The surgeon should use a dorsal plate contoured to wrap around the olecranon, providing a greater number of screws and screws at different, nearly orthogonal angles. Use of a medial or lateral plate should be avoided.[12,14]
Loss of Fixation of the Proximal (Olecranon) Fragment	• Screw fixation alone should not be trusted if the fragment is small, fragmented, or osteoporotic. A tension wire engaging the triceps insertion should be added.
Failure to Recognize a Complex Injury	• The surgeon should be vigilant for subluxation or dislocation of the elbow, fracture of the coronoid or radial head, and injury to the lateral collateral ligament. When identified, each injury is treated accordingly.

POSTOPERATIVE CARE

- When good fixation is obtained (which occurs in most patients), active-assisted and gravity-assisted elbow and forearm exercises can be initiated immediately after surgery. A delay of several days for comfort is reasonable.
- If the lateral collateral ligament was repaired, the patient must be instructed not to abduct the shoulder for the first month, as this imparts a varus moment across the elbow and stresses the ligament repair.
- If the fixation is tenuous, it is reasonable to immobilize the arm in a splint for a month or so before beginning exercises.

OUTCOMES

- Nonunion rates for olecranon fractures are very low, reported at 1%.[7]
- Tension band wiring of simple olecranon fractures are still associated with high rates of hardware removal. The techniques described reduce incidence of hardware irritation.[10]
- Macko and Szabo[6] pointed out that it was initial implant prominence and not migration that led to implant-related problems after tension band wiring of olecranon fractures.
- In any case, a second surgery for implant removal is not unreasonable, and it may be appropriate to not consider this a complication.
- Some surgeons have considered plate-and-screw fixation of simple, noncomminuted olecranon fractures.[1] However, plates can also cause symptoms, and if only a few screws can be placed in the olecranon fragment, particularly in the setting of fragmentation or osteoporosis, it may be preferable to use the soft tissue attachments to enhance fixation rather than relying on implant–bone purchase alone.
- Medial and lateral plates have been associated with early failure, malunion, and nonunion in the treatment of complex proximal ulnar fractures.[12,14]
- Dorsal plates perform better, but the elbow is often compromised in the setting of such complex injuries.

COMPLICATIONS

- Symptomatic hardware
- Stiffness
- Heterotopic ossification
- Arthrosis
- Nonunion
- Ulnar nerve symptoms
- Loss of extension strength

REFERENCES

1. Bailey CS, MacDermid J, Patterson SD, et al. Outcome of plate fixation of olecranon fractures. J Orthop Trauma 2001;15:542–548.
2. Doornberg J, Ring D, Jupiter JB. Effective treatment of fracture-dislocations of the olecranon requires a stable trochlear notch. Clin Orthop Relat Res 2004;(429):292–300.
3. Garrigues GE, Wray WH III, Lindenhovius AL, et al. Fixation of the coronoid process in elbow fracture-dislocations. J Bone Joint Surg Am 2011;93:1873–1881.
4. Jupiter JB, Leibovic SJ, Ribbans W, et al. The posterior Monteggia lesion. J Orthop Trauma 1991;5:395–402.
5. Karlsson M, Hasserius R, Besjakov J, et al. Comparison of tension-band and figure-of-eight wiring techniques for treatment of olecranon fractures. J Shoulder Elbow Surg 2002;11:377–382.
6. Macko D, Szabo RM. Complications of tension-band wiring of olecranon fractures. J Bone Joint Surg Am 1985;67(9):1396–1401.
7. Morrey BF. Current concepts in the treatment of fractures of the radial head, the olecranon, and the coronoid. J Bone Joint Surg Am 1995;77:316–327.
8. O'Driscoll SW, Jupiter JB, Cohen M, et al. Difficult elbow fractures: pearls and pitfalls. Instr Course Lect 2003;52:113–134.
9. Pugh DMW, Wild LM, Schemitsch EH, et al. Standard surgical protocol to treat elbow dislocations with radial head and coronoid fractures. J Bone Joint Surg Am 2004;86:1122–1130.
10. Ring D, Gulotta L, Chin K, et al. Olecranon osteotomy for exposure of fractures and nonunions of the distal humerus. J Orthop Trauma 2004;18:446–449.
11. Ring D, Jupiter JB, Sanders RW, et al. Transolecranon fracture-dislocation of the elbow. J Orthop Trauma 1997;11:545–550.
12. Ring D, Jupiter JB, Simpson NS. Monteggia fractures in adults. J Bone Joint Surg Am 1998;80(12):1733–1744.
13. Ring D, Jupiter JB, Zilberfarb J. Posterior dislocation of the elbow with fractures of the radial head and coronoid. J Bone Joint Surg Am 2002;84:547–551.
14. Ring D, Tavakolian J, Kloen P, et al. Loss of alignment after surgical treatment of posterior Monteggia fractures: salvage with dorsal contoured plating. J Hand Surg Am 2004;29(4):694–702.
15. van der Werf HJ, Guitton TG, Ring D. Non-operatively treated fractures of the anteromedial facet of the coronoid process: a report of six cases. Shoulder Elbow 2010;2:40–42.

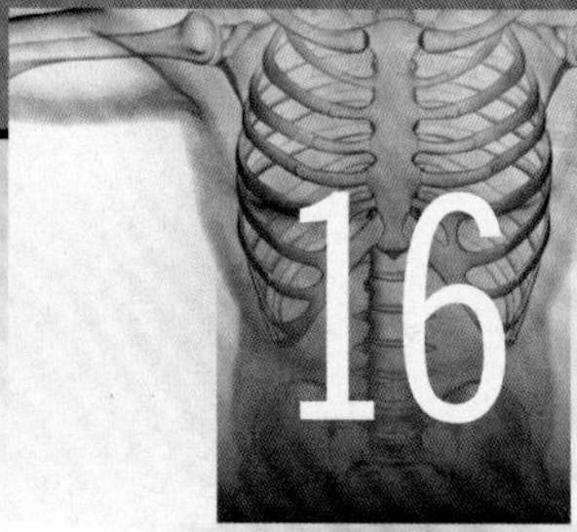

CHAPTER 16

Surgical Management of Sternoclavicular Injuries

Christina J. Hajewski and Brian R. Wolf

DEFINITION

- Sternoclavicular joint (SCJ) injuries include instability (acute and chronic), dislocation, and degenerative disease.
- Although relatively uncommon, representing 1% of all dislocations,[6] SCJ injuries with posterior displacement of the medial clavicle are potentially life-threatening due to their proximity to the great vessels and airway. For these reasons, prompt intervention is warranted for posterior sternoclavicular dislocations.
- Anterior dislocations are more common and can often be treated nonoperatively; yet, operative intervention can be considered for those that are irreducible or have recurrent instability.

ANATOMY

- The SCJ is the articulation of the medial clavicle and the manubrium. It provides the only bony attachment between the axial skeleton and the upper extremity.
- The SCJ is a diarthrodial synovial joint that is saddle shaped and reinforced with multiple ligaments: the interclavicular ligament superiorly, the costoclavicular (rhomboid) ligament inferiorly, and an anterior and posterior sternoclavicular ligament. The joint is further stabilized by its capsular ligaments and sternocleidomastoid and subclavius muscles **(FIG 1)**.[4]
- Within the joint, a fibrocartilaginous articular disc separates the manubrium and clavicle and divides the joint into two synovial articular cavities. This disc functions to absorb force transmitted through the clavicle.
- The medial clavicle epiphysis ossifies by age 25 years[7]; therefore, injuries in teenagers and young adults may represent physeal separations.

PATHOGENESIS

- Anterior SCJ dislocations are more common than posterior dislocations, which may be due to the superior strength of the posterior ligamentous structures.[8,12]

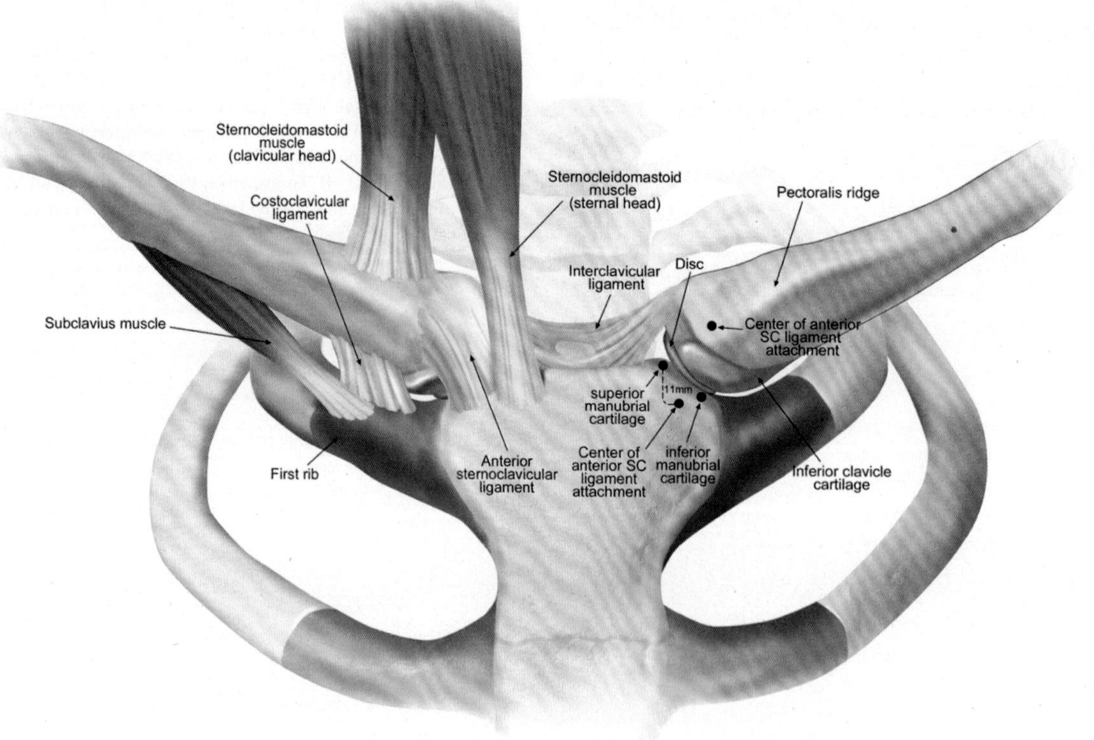

FIG 1 Anatomy of the sternoclavicular (*SC*) joint. (Reprinted with permission from Lee JT, Campbell KJ, Michalski MP, et al. Surgical anatomy of the sternoclavicular joint: a qualitative and quantitative anatomical study. J Bone Joint Surg Am 2014;96[19]:e166. Copyright © 2014 by The Journal of Bone and Joint Surgery, Incorporated.)

- Traumatic SCJ dislocations result from high energy force, either directly to the joint or indirectly with forces transmitted from the shoulder and through the clavicle.
- Common causes of traumatic injury include motor vehicle accidents, falls, and participation in contact sports.
- Direct anterior to posterior directed force applied on the medial clavicle may push the medial clavicle posteriorly behind the sternum. Examples of this scenario may occur with athletes, if a direct blow or kick is delivered to the medial clavicle, or if a person is pinned or run over by a vehicle.[12]
- Indirect forces through the shoulder more commonly cause SCJ dislocation. Posterior SCJ dislocations may occur if the shoulder rolls forward while under lateral compressive forces, whereas backward motion of the shoulder with lateral compression can produce an anterior SCJ dislocation.[12]
- If the ligamentous structures around the SCJ fail to completely heal after injury, patients may experience static subluxation or recurrent instability of the joint resulting in subluxation or dislocation.
- Degenerative changes to the SCJ may occur over time secondary to a prior traumatic injury or due to osteoarthritis or inflammatory arthritis.

NATURAL HISTORY

- Acute sprains of the SCJ are treated conservatively. More severe sprains that can result in subluxation of the SCJ may be immobilized temporarily and then protected for 4 to 6 weeks, as the capsuloligamentous structures heal.
- After reduction of acute SCJ dislocations, if the joint remains reduced, the ligamentous structures typically heal in 4 to 6 weeks following reduction.
- Acute anterior SCJ dislocations treated with closed reduction have good long-term results, although they are often more unstable than posterior dislocations.
- Chronic anterior dislocations may be managed with conservative symptomatic treatment with acceptable outcomes. However, chronic anterior dislocation can result in significant deformity to the upper chest and can cause pain and impair function.
- Chronic posterior dislocations have a risk of compromise of the mediastinal structures, including the subclavian vessels. Cases have been reported with symptoms ranging from exertional cyanosis from compression of the great vessels to complete obstruction months to years after initial injury.[5,9]

PATIENT HISTORY AND PHYSICAL FINDINGS

- Patients with acute SCJ injury usually present with a history of acute trauma and pain, yet these injuries may be easily missed, especially in the multitrauma patient; therefore, clinical suspicion is key.
- Patients with an SCJ sprain may report pain and tenderness to palpation of the SCJ and may have laxity compared to the contralateral side. Patients with SCJ dislocation usually have more severe pain and deformity of the medial clavicle and SCJ.
- Depending on the patient's body habitus or degree of swelling, deformity may or may not be grossly obvious at the SCJ on exam.
- Anterior dislocations demonstrate prominence of the medial clavicle, whereas posterior dislocations may present with a step-off or defect next to the sternum.
- Compression of mediastinal structures has been shown to occur in up to 25% of posterior SCJ dislocations.[12] Symptoms of this may include dyspnea or hoarseness from tracheal involvement or dysphagia or difficulty swallowing if the esophagus is compressed. Additionally, neurovascular symptoms may occur such as cyanosis or venous congestion of the ipsilateral upper extremity or neck from compromise of the subclavian vessels or paresthesias from compression of the brachial plexus.

IMAGING AND OTHER DIAGNOSTIC STUDIES

- Plain anteroposterior radiographs of the clavicle and chest are often difficult to interpret with many overlapping structures such as the ribs, vertebrae, clavicle, and sternum.
- A serendipity view radiograph may be obtained by tilting the radiographic beam 40 degrees cephalad, and this view shows both SCJs.[3]
- Computed tomography (CT) permits clearer evaluation of SCJ injuries and is the preferred imaging modality with its ability to differentiate medial clavicle fractures, physeal injuries, subluxations, and dislocations **(FIG 2)**. CT can also help identify degenerative changes of the SCJ.
- Magnetic resonance imaging (MRI) can be used to assess soft tissue structures including the trachea, esophagus, great vessels, and ligaments. MRI can also identify degenerative changes and effusion of the SCJ.
- Angiography can be considered if there is concern for vascular injury with a posterior SCJ dislocation.
- Ultrasound can be used to identify degenerative changes and effusion within the SCJ.

DIFFERENTIAL DIAGNOSIS

- SCJ sprain
- SCJ dislocation
- SCJ arthritis
- Clavicle fracture
- Physeal injury of the clavicle
- Rib fractures
- Pneumothorax
- Glenohumeral pathology

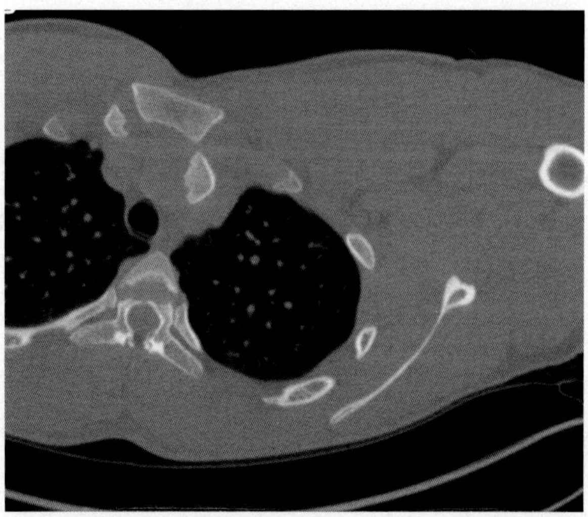

FIG 2 Axial CT scan demonstrating a left posterior SCJ dislocation. (Reprinted from Sullivan JP, Warme BA, Wolf BR. Use of an O-arm intraoperative computed tomography scanner for closed reduction of posterior sternoclavicular dislocations. J Shoulder Elbow Surg 2012; 21[3]:e17–e20. Copyright © 2012 Journal of Shoulder and Elbow Surgery Board of Trustees. With permission.)

NONOPERATIVE MANAGEMENT

- Strains and subluxations should be treated conservatively with ice, analgesics, and short-term shoulder immobilization in a sling. A figure-of-eight bandage can also be used for stability after sprain, subluxation, or dislocation.
- Anterior dislocation
  - Urgent closed reduction should be attempted under local anesthesia, sedation, or general anesthesia. This is most easily accomplished within 48 hours of injury.
  - Prior to intervention, patients should be counseled that there is a relatively high rate of recurrent subluxation or instability with anterior dislocation injuries. However, this uncommonly results in significant functional limitations.
  - The patient should be placed supine on a table with a solid pad placed posteriorly between the shoulders to retract the scapula.
  - A reduction maneuver is performed with posterior directed force on the medial end of the clavicle with abduction of the shoulder to 90 degrees and 10 to 15 degrees of extension.
  - Asymptomatic anterior SCJ subluxation should be treated with benign neglect. Physical therapy (PT), supportive taping, and patient education can be done for symptomatic anterior SCJ subluxation.
- Posterior dislocation
  - Due to the risk of complications from compression of the mediastinal structures, prompt closed reduction of posterior dislocations should be attempted in the operating room under heavy sedation or general anesthesia. We recommend alerting a cardiothoracic or vascular surgery team to be available if needed.
  - Place the patient supine on the operating room table. A 3- to 4-inch solid pad should be placed beneath the thoracic spine to extend the shoulder (**FIG 3**).

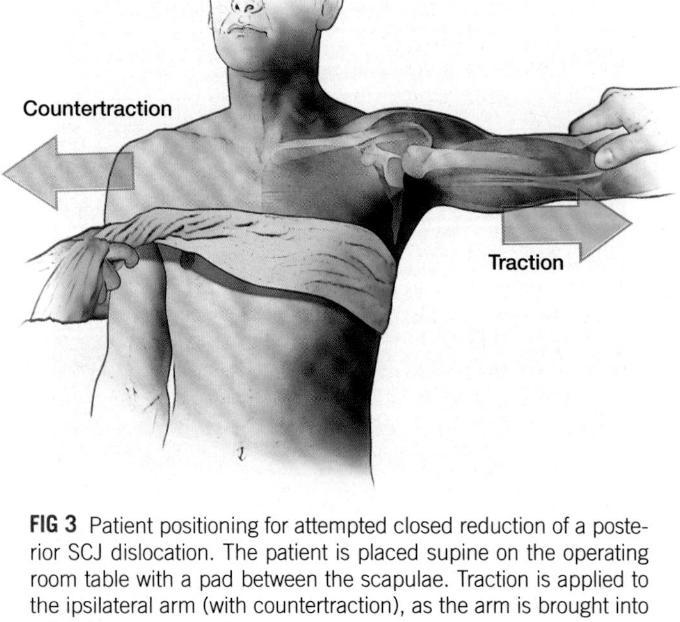

FIG 3 Patient positioning for attempted closed reduction of a posterior SCJ dislocation. The patient is placed supine on the operating room table with a pad between the scapulae. Traction is applied to the ipsilateral arm (with countertraction), as the arm is brought into extension.

  - Gentle traction is applied to the ipsilateral upper extremity with the shoulder abducted while the arm is slowly extended. Anterior traction may be applied manually to the clavicle.
  - If this is unsuccessful, a sterile towel clamp may be used to grasp the medial clavicle to provide anterior traction after the skin has been prepped.
  - Another reduction technique has been described with the shoulder adducted with traction and posterior directed pressure on the shoulder to attempt to lever the clavicle anteriorly.[1]
  - There is often a palpable or audible pop with reduction, yet this should be confirmed radiographically either with a plain radiograph or O-arm CT scan in the operating room.[10]
  - Following reduction, the patient should be admitted for observation and neurovascular checks and immobilized.
  - CT scan confirmation of joint reduction is recommended.

SURGICAL MANAGEMENT

- Irreducible and grossly displaced anterior dislocations can be surgically reduced and stabilized.
- Surgery can be performed for recurrent symptomatic anterior subluxations/dislocations that have failed conservative treatment.
- Acute posterior dislocations that are irreducible or that will not remain reduced after closed reduction should undergo operative intervention to reduce and stabilize the SCJ and prevent potential life-threatening complications.
- Surgical management of chronic posterior dislocations is controversial.
- Degenerative SCJ disease that has failed conservative management may be managed operatively with a medial clavicle resection.

Preoperative Planning

- A preoperative history and physical examination should be performed, with particular attention paid to the neurovascular status of the ipsilateral upper extremity, especially in the cases of posterior SCJ dislocation.
- The authors recommend routine case coordination with vascular or cardiothoracic surgery teams in case assistance with bleeding is needed. This would include simple coordination so that vascular or thoracic surgery is available if needed for most SCJ cases. For chronic posterior SCJ dislocation, the authors would recommend vascular or thoracic surgery assistance with surgical exposure due to risk to surrounding great vessels.
- If performing a reconstruction with soft tissue graft, then graft choices of allograft versus palmaris versus gracilis graft should be discussed with the patient preoperatively.

Positioning

- The patient is placed supine on the operating room table. In cases of posterior displacement of the clavicle, a rolled towel or pad placed between the scapulae is helpful to extend the shoulder.
- The surgical field is prepped wide to include both SCJs, the lower neck, and the majority of the chest in case bleeding is encountered and a sternotomy needs to be performed.

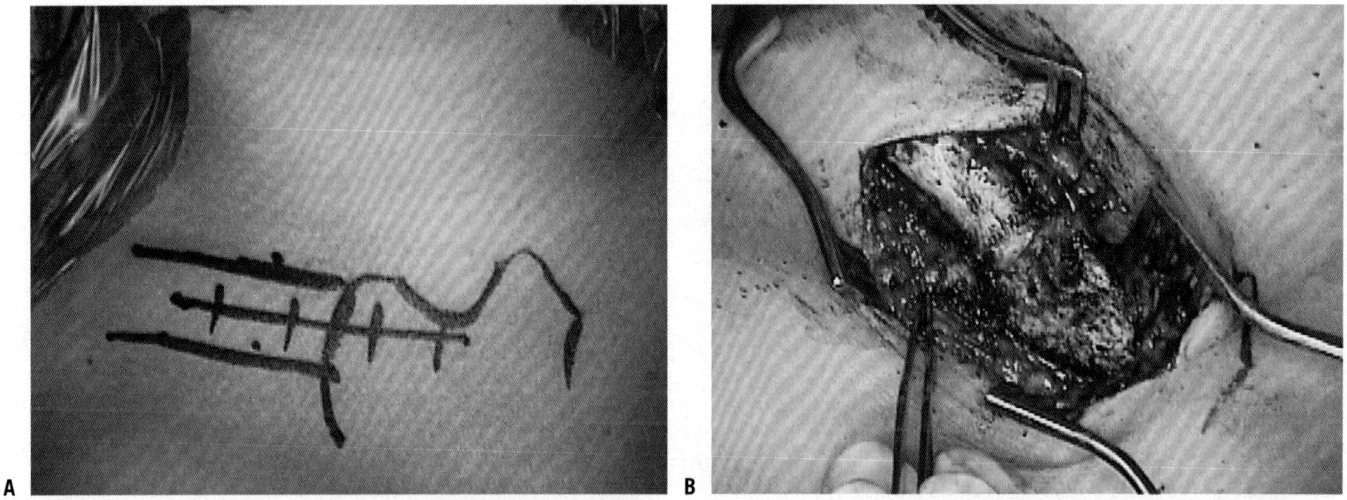

FIG 4 **A.** Skin incision with the manubrium and medial clavicle marked on the skin. Both SCJs and most of the neck and chest should be included in the prepped surgical field in case further exposure for a sternotomy would be needed. **B.** Subperiosteal exposure of the medial clavicle and sternum. (Reprinted from Guan JJ, Wolf BR. Reconstruction for anterior sternoclavicular joint dislocation and instability. J Shoulder Elbow Surg 2013;22[6]:775–781. Copyright © 2013 Elsevier. With permission.)

Approach

- A longitudinal incision is made approximately 8 to 10 cm in length from the medial fourth of the clavicle to the central upper sternum **(FIG 4A)**.
- The incision should be slightly inferior to the middle of the clavicle to produce a more cosmetic scar.
- Dissection is carried down through subcutaneous tissue.
- Incise the platysma and raise it as a separate layer in line with the incision.
- The medial end of the clavicle is further exposed by dissecting off the superior and clavicular fibers of the pectoralis major muscle.
- The periosteum is dissected from lateral to medial off the clavicle as well as the SCJ capsule.
- The intra-articular disc should remain in place and be inspected for damage.
- Periosteal dissection can continue medially off the sternum, also dissecting off the sternocleidomastoid superiorly to expose the superior sulcus of the sternum **(FIG 4B)**.

SUTURE REPAIR OF UNSTABLE POSTERIOR STERNOCLAVICULAR PHYSEAL FRACTURES

- Approach and exposure as described earlier, but it is not necessary to expose as far medial, stopping at the SCJ
- Expose the physeal fracture by dissecting off soft tissue.
- Reduce the fracture with a towel clip **(TECH FIG 1A)**.
- Drill a vertical row of three 2-mm holes on each side of the physeal fracture, only through the anterior cortex, approximately 1 cm from the fracture line.
  - Drilling through the anterior cortex only protects the mediastinal structures deep to the SCJ.
- Be cognizant to avoid the SCJ medially when drilling.
- Three no. 2 FiberWire sutures (Arthrex, Inc., Naples, FL) are passed through the drill holes and exiting out the fracture site.
- The sutures are then passed through the medial epiphyseal fragment, which is cartilaginous in nature. The sutures are passed from the fracture site to the anterior surface **(TECH FIG 1B)**.
- The fracture is reduced and the sutures are tied over the fracture and stability is assessed with gentle posterior pressure **(TECH FIG 1C)**.
- The wound is copiously irrigated and closed in a layered fashion.

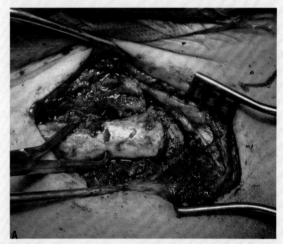

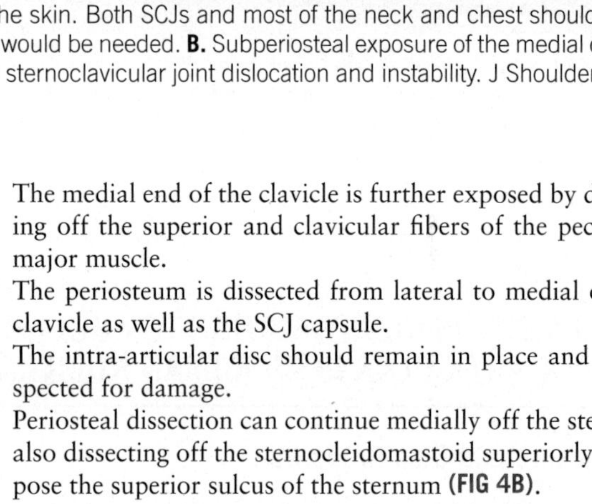

TECH FIG 1 A. Subperiosteal exposure of the medial clavicle with a physeal fracture. A towel clip is used to reduce the fracture. *(continued)*

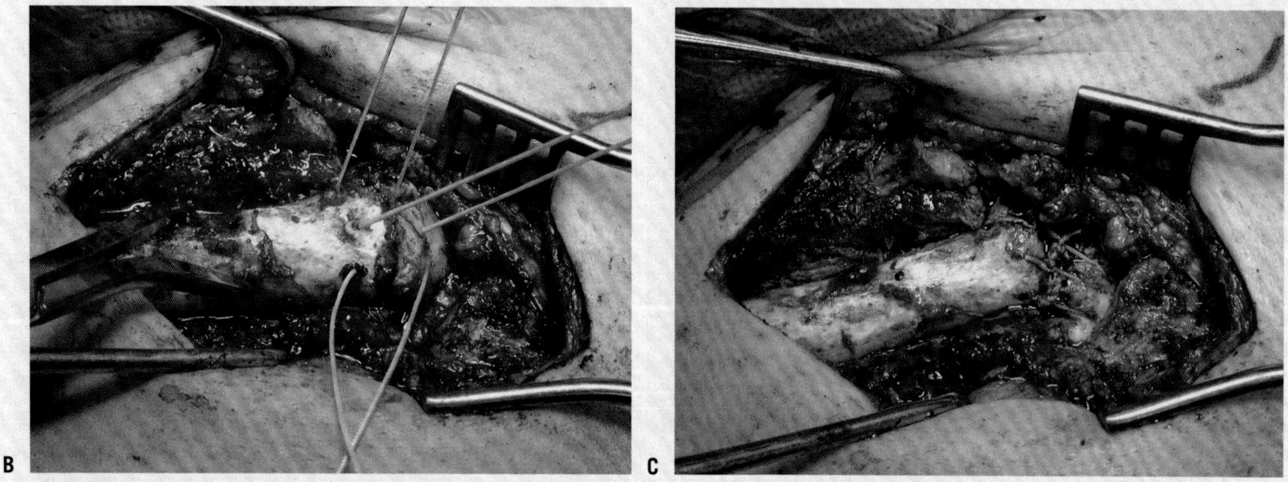

TECH FIG 1 *(continued)* **B.** Sutures are passed through drill holes prepared in the medial clavicle through the fracture site and into the medial physeal fragment horizontally from lateral to medial. **C.** Reduced physeal fracture with suture repair. (From Van Hofwegen C, Wolf B. Suture repair of posterior sternoclavicular physeal fractures: a report of two cases. Iowa Orthop J 2008;28:49–52.)

LIGAMENT RECONSTRUCTION FOR SCJ INSTABILITY WITH INTACT INTRA-ARTICULAR DISC: ROMAN NUMERAL X RECONSTRUCTION

Exposure and Disc Preparation

- Approach and exposure as described earlier. Unlike for physeal fractures, medial dissection is necessary, continuing at least 3 cm medial to the SCJ.
- The intra-articular cartilaginous disc should be closely inspected.
  - If intact, it is left in situ.
  - If the disc is significantly damaged, it can be débrided or removed (see alternative procedure modification in the following text).

Graft Preparation and Hole Placement

- A soft tissue graft is used for the reconstruction.
  - Options for an autograft include gracilis and palmaris longus tendon.
  - Soft tissue allograft can be substituted. When allograft is used, a semitendinosus allograft split longitudinally can be a good option.
- No. 0 nonabsorbable sutures are placed on each end of the graft.
- On the medial clavicle, drill two unicortical holes 15 to 20 mm lateral to the SCJ, one anterosuperior and the other anteroinferior.
  - Be sure there is an adequate cortical bridge between the holes.
  - The drill holes should be 3.5 to 4.5 mm in diameter, according to the diameter of the graft to be used and the size of the patient. A protective guide sleeve should be used to avoid the drill slipping superior or inferior off clavicle.
- Connect the drill holes with a curette subcortically, taking care to maintain the cortical bridge.
- Drill holes are placed in a similar fashion on the sternum approximately 15 to 20 mm medial to the SCJ **(TECH FIG 2)**.
  - Again, be sure to leave at least a 15-mm bone bridge and connect the drill holes subcortically with curettes.

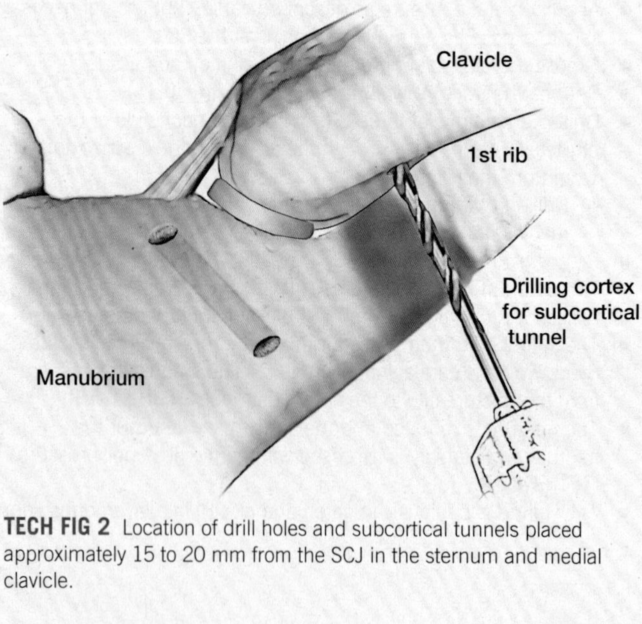

TECH FIG 2 Location of drill holes and subcortical tunnels placed approximately 15 to 20 mm from the SCJ in the sternum and medial clavicle.

Graft Passage

- One limb of the graft and a loop of suture are passed through the clavicle tunnel with a suture passer from superior to inferior.
  - The loop of suture will be used to pass the graft through the clavicle a second time when weaving the graft.
- The graft is then directed diagonally across the SCJ and passed from superior to inferior through the sternum tunnel, also with an additional loop of suture **(TECH FIG 3A)**.
- Again, the graft is taken diagonally across the SCJ toward the superior clavicle and passed from superior to inferior through the clavicle tunnel using the loop of suture previously placed **(TECH FIG 3B,C)**.
- The graft is then directed medial to the inferior sternum drill hole and passed from inferior to superior through the sternum using the suture loop **(TECH FIG 3D)**.
- Finally, the graft is crossed with the other graft end coming from the superior clavicle tunnel to create a Roman numeral X configuration.

SCJ Reduction and Completion

- If the SCJ is subluxed, reduction should be attempted.
  - Do not overreduce the SCJ, causing posterior displacement of the clavicle.
  - Judge reduction with direct visualization as the joint capsule has been elevated and compared to the opposite SCJ if possible.
  - If the SCJ cannot be reduced, the clavicle may be shortened to allow for reduction. This can be the case with subacute or chronic anterior dislocations.

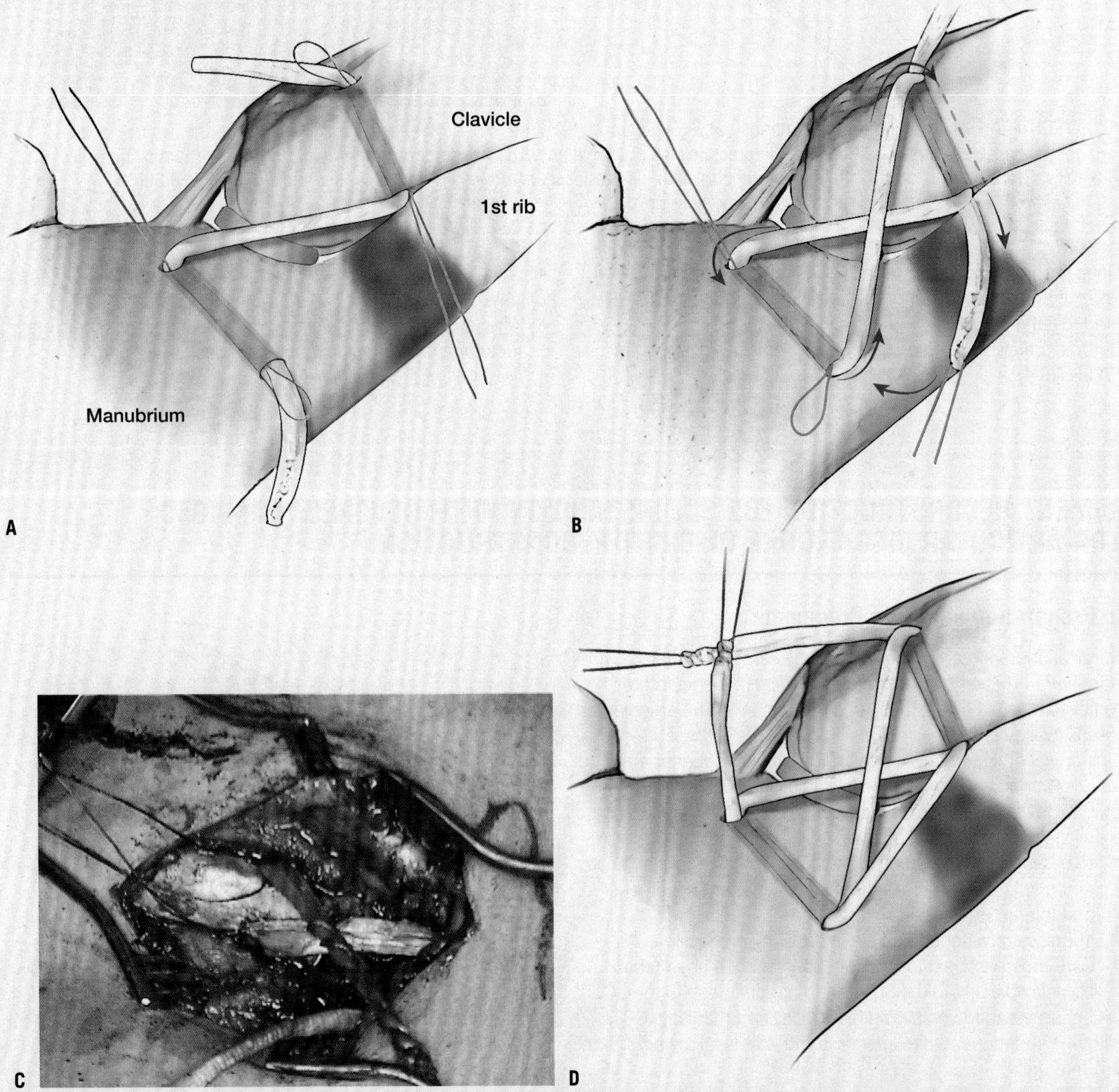

TECH FIG 3 A. The graft is passed first from superior to inferior through the medial clavicle tunnel. The suture loops through the clavicle and sternal tunnels are shown. The graft is then passed diagonally across the SCJ and again taken from superior to inferior through the sternal tunnel. **B,C.** The graft is taken again diagonally across the SCJ and passed via the suture loop from superior to inferior through the clavicle tunnel. **D.** The graft is passed horizontally to the inferior sternal hole and then passed through the sternal tunnel via the suture loop from inferior to superior. The two ends of the graft are now exiting out of the superior sternum and clavicle. (**C:** Reprinted from Guan JJ, Wolf BR. Reconstruction for anterior sternoclavicular joint dislocation and instability. J Shoulder Elbow Surg. 2013;22[6]:775–781. Copyright © 2013 Elsevier. With permission.)

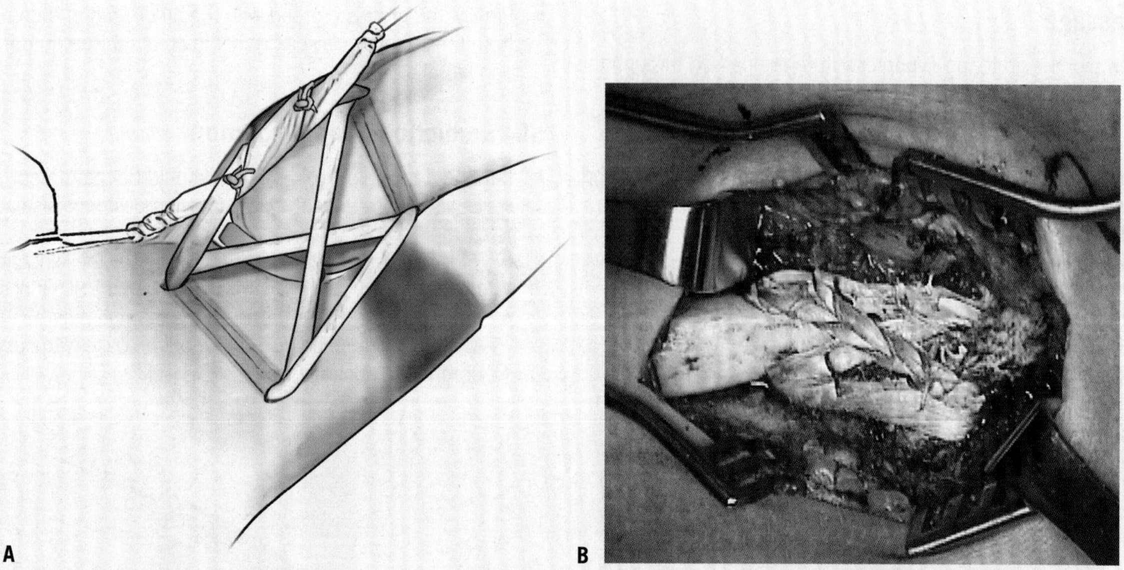

TECH FIG 4 Illustration (**A**) of and intraoperative photograph (**B**) of the roman numeral X configuration with the two free ends of the graft sewn together superiorly. Sutures are also placed at any crossing portions of the graft. (**B:** Reprinted from Guan JJ, Wolf BR. Reconstruction for anterior sternoclavicular joint dislocation and instability. J Shoulder Elbow Surg 2013;22[6]: 775–781. Copyright © 2013 Elsevier. With permission.)

- Once the SCJ is reduced, tension the graft and suture the free ends of the graft together or tie the suture from the ends of the graft together.
- Sutures are also placed at any crossing portions of the graft **(TECH FIG 4)**.
- Repair the periosteal layer and joint capsule with no. 0 absorbable suture.
- After copious fluid irrigation, the wound is closed in layers including the platysma, subcutaneous tissue, and skin.

LIGAMENT RECONSTRUCTION FOR SCJ INSTABILITY WITH SEVERELY DAMAGED INTRA-ARTICULAR DISC: FIGURE-OF-EIGHT RECONSTRUCTION

Disc Preparation and Hole Placement

- Surgical approach and exposure are the same as earlier.
- If the intra-articular disc is torn and damaged, it should be removed to avoid future mechanical symptoms. The articular disc is avascular and will not heal.
- Unicortical drill holes are made on the anterior superior and anterior inferior surface of the clavicle using a 3.5- to 4.5-mm drill, 15 to 20 mm lateral to the SCJ. It is recommended to use a drill sleeve to avoid drill slippage.
  - In cases with removed disc, the drill is directed to the center of the articular surface of the medial clavicle. The superior and inferior drill holes converge here.
  - Tunnels are widened and cleared using curettes.
  - Care must be taken to maintain cortical bone on anterior clavicle adjacent to the SCJ and to not drill deep to the SCJ.
- Drill holes are made on sternum 15 to 20 mm medial to SCJ, with one superior and one inferior to the joint level, using 3.5- to 4.5-mm drill.
  - Drill holes are directed to the articular surface of the sternum within the SCJ. The tunnels converge at the joint line and are further widened using curettes.
  - Use of a drill guide is recommended, and care must be taken to not drill deep to the SCJ. Maintain a cortical bone surface on lateral sternum over the drill tunnels **(TECH FIG 5)**.

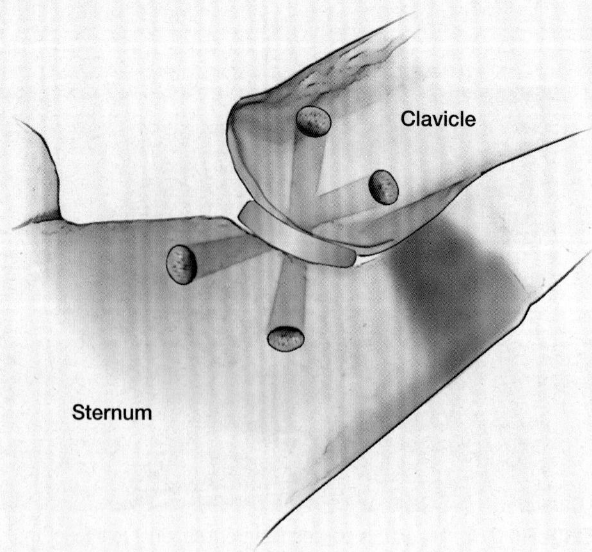

TECH FIG 5 Drill holes and subcortical tunnels are placed in the clavicle and sternum for the figure-of-eight reconstruction. The drill holes are made approximately 15 to 20 mm from the SCJ, and the subcortical tunnels converge and exit in the intra-articular space of the SCJ.

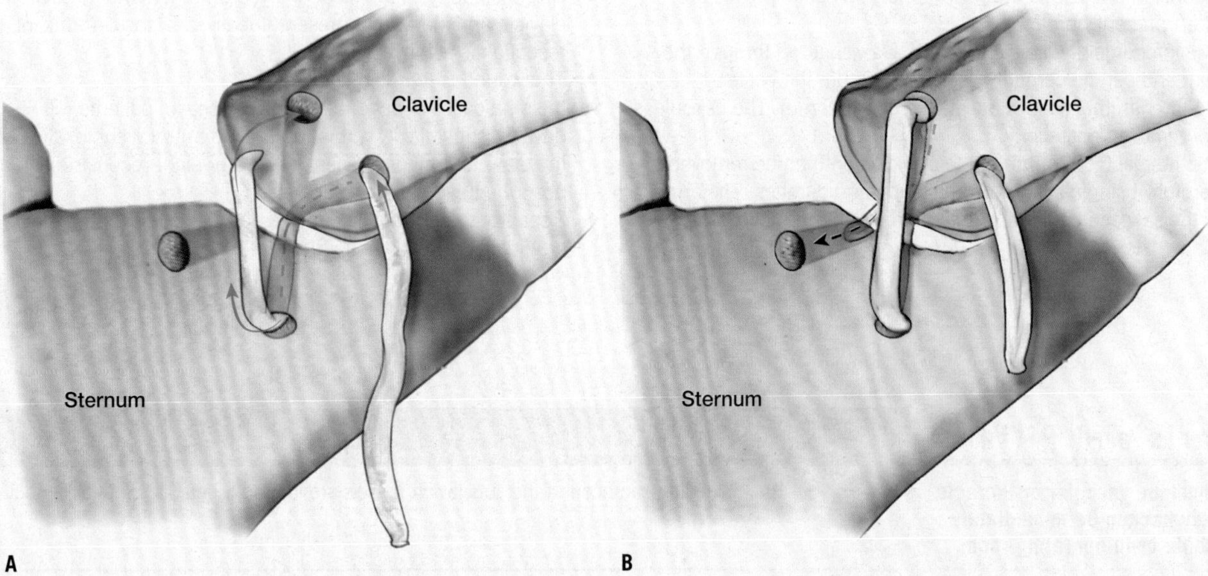

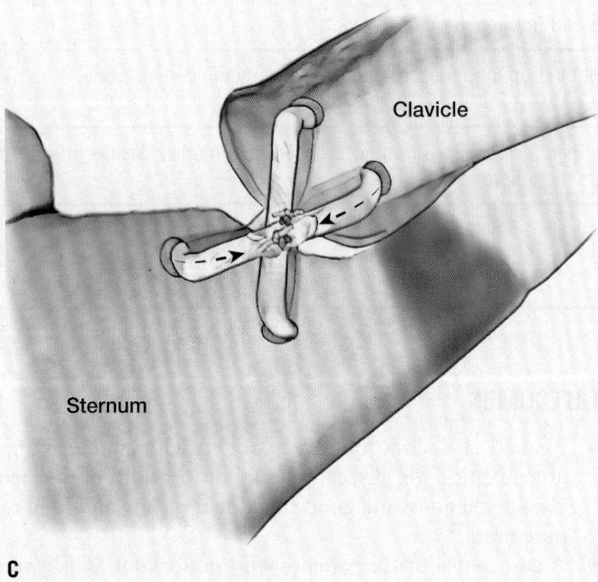

TECH FIG 6 **A.** The graft is passed from the inferior clavicle drill hole and tunnel into the SCJ intra-articular space and out of the inferior sternal tunnel and drill hole. It is then directed diagonally anterior to the SCJ toward the superior clavicle drill hole. **B.** The graft is next passed from the superior clavicle drill hole and tunnel into the SCJ intra-articular space and then passed out of the superior sternal tunnel and drill hole. **C.** The two ends of the graft are tied together with nonabsorbable suture anterior to the SCJ to complete the figure-of-eight construct.

Graft Passage

- The graft options are similar to the ligament reconstruction outlined earlier.
- The graft is passed from the inferior clavicular holes into the SCJ using a Hewson Suture passer (Smith & Nephew, Andover, MA).
  - The graft is pulled through the sternum and out the inferior sternum tunnel **(TECH FIG 6A)**.
  - It is crossed over the anterior SCJ to the superior clavicle tunnel and passed lateral to medial through the SCJ again using the superior tunnels **(TECH FIG 6B)**.
- The intra-articular graft can help substitute for the missing intra-articular cartilage disc.
- The two graft ends are then tied and/or sutured together using size 0 nonabsorbable suture **(TECH FIG 6C)**.
- Closure is similar to aforementioned.

Medial Clavicle Resection Arthroplasty for Degenerative SCJ

- The approach to the SCJ is similar to aforementioned.
- The anterior capsule of the SCJ is reflected superiorly and inferiorly.
- Remnants of the intra-articular disc are removed. Any loose bodies are removed. Synovitis is carefully removed.
- Careful subperiosteal exposure of the medial clavicle is done on the anterior superior and anterior inferior clavicle at the joint line. Careful attention should be paid to the inferior clavicle, as it is not uncommon to have inferior osteophytes and arthritis change contacting the medial first rib.
- The joint line of the sternum should be similarly exposed in a careful manner. Again, careful attention to the inferior

extension of the SCJ line is important, as osteophytes are often present here.
- The inferior joint capsule of the SCJ is visualized through the joint and can be carefully peeled away from the posterior clavicle through the joint for a distance of 5 to 8 mm. The capsule is not removed posteriorly.
- The medial 5 to 10 mm of the clavicle can then be removed carefully using a small saw, rongeurs, and curettes. The angle of the saw can be tilted so that more bone is removed anteriorly than posteriorly.
- Bony osteophytes are also removed on the inferior medial clavicle and sternum if present. Ideally, a 5- to 10-mm joint resection is achieved.
- The wound is thoroughly irrigated.
- In some cases of degenerative SCJ disease, patients will develop subtle laxity with superior and anterior subluxation of the clavicle. In these cases, a figure-of-eight reconstruction as described earlier can be done.
- Repair of the remaining capsule and periosteum is crucial if graft reconstruction is not done.

Pearls and Pitfalls

Recommend vascular or thoracic surgery backup be immediately available or in operating room.	• Brisk bleeding can occur if the subclavian vessels are injured. There is risk of air embolus.
Must maintain cortical bridges for tunnels through clavicle and sternum.	• Loss of anterior cortex over tunnels. This can usually be avoided by started tunnels far enough from joint line and from each other.
Avoid using a graft that is too big for 3.5- to 4.5-mm tunnels. Trim graft to fit tunnels.	• If graft is too big, it will bind up in tunnels or damage surrounding cortical bone.
Closely inspect intra-articular disc for pathology.	• If SCJ will not reduce, then further exposure may be needed or medial clavicle may need to be resected to facilitate reduction.
In degenerative SCJ cases, carefully inspect inferior medial clavicle and SCJ area for osteoarthritis changes.	• Residual pain can occur if complete resection arthroplasty not accomplished.

POSTOPERATIVE CARE

- Suture repair of posterior sternoclavicular physeal fractures
  - Week 0 to 3: sling immobilization coming out for pendulum exercises only
  - Week 3 to 6: Sling may be removed for passive shoulder range of motion (ROM) in addition to pendulums.
  - Week 6 to 12: active ROM as tolerated according to pain
  - Release to full activities at 12 weeks if asymptomatic
- SCJ ligament reconstruction (Roman X and figure of eight)
  - Week 0 to 8: sling immobilization with only elbow and wrist ROM
  - Week 8 to 12: shoulder ROM below 90 degrees with gradual reduction of sling use
  - Week 12: full ROM and strengthening initiated
  - Return to work and sport at 5 to 6 months
- Medial clavicle resection arthroplasty.
  - Sling for 6 weeks to allow capsule to heal
  - PT to begin gentle passive ROM; can begin at 2 weeks
  - Active ROM at 4 to 6 weeks
  - Strengthening can begin after 6 weeks if ROM appropriate

OUTCOMES

- A small case series following patients who underwent operative fixation for physeal fracture dislocations of the medial clavicle demonstrate good functional results and long-term outcomes.[11]
- A case series of six patients who underwent SCJ ligament reconstruction, as described earlier, showed improvement in pain and function and were able to return to their preinjury activities. One patient had recurrence at 4 years and was treated with revision surgery.[2]

COMPLICATIONS

- Recurrent instability
- Damage to mediastinal structures
- Infection

REFERENCES

1. Buckerfield CT, Castle ME. Acute traumatic retrosternal dislocation of the clavicle. J Bone Joint Surg Am 1984;66(3):379–385.
2. Guan JJ, Wolf BR. Reconstruction for anterior sternoclavicular joint dislocation and instability. J Shoulder Elbow Surg 2013;22(6):775–781.

3. Hobbs DW. Sternoclavicular joint: a new axial radiographic view. Radiology 1968;90(4):801.
4. Lee JT, Campbell KJ, Michalski MP, et al. Surgical anatomy of the sternoclavicular joint: a qualitative and quantitative anatomical study. J Bone Joint Surg Am 2014;96(19):e166.
5. Mehta JC, Sachdev A, Collins JJ. Retrosternal dislocation of the clavicle. Injury 1973;5(1):79–83.
6. Renfree KJ, Wright TW. Anatomy and biomechanics of the acromioclavicular and sternoclavicular joints. Clin Sports Med 2003;22(2):219–237.
7. Schulz R, Mühler M, Mutze S, et al. Studies on the time frame for ossification of the medial epiphysis of the clavicle as revealed by CT scans. Int J Legal Med 2005;119(3):142–145.
8. Spencer EE, Kuhn JE, Huston LJ, et al. Ligamentous restraints to anterior and posterior translation of the sternoclavicular joint. J Shoulder Elbow Surg 2002;11(1):43–47.
9. Stankler L. Posterior dislocation of the clavicle. A report of 2 cases. Br J Surg 1962;50:164–168.
10. Sullivan JP, Warme BA, Wolf BR. Use of an O-arm intraoperative computed tomography scanner for closed reduction of posterior sternoclavicular dislocations. J Shoulder Elbow Surg 2012;21(3):e17–e20.
11. Van Hofwegen C, Wolf B. Suture repair of posterior sternoclavicular physeal fractures: a report of two cases. Iowa Orthop J 2008;28:49–52.
12. Wirth MA, Rockwood CA Jr. Acute and chronic traumatic injuries of the sternoclavicular joint. J Am Acad Orthop Surg 1996;4(5):268–278.

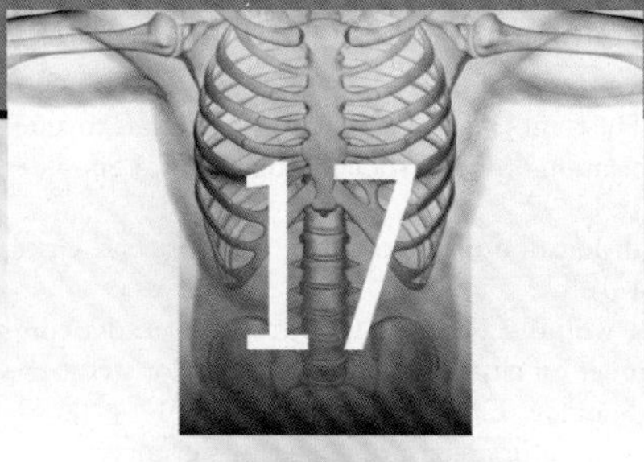

CHAPTER 17

Hand, Wrist, and Forearm
Open and Closed Techniques for Treatment of Metacarpal Fractures

R. Glenn Gaston, Casey M. Sabbag, and Jed I. Maslow

DEFINITION

- Hand metacarpals form the bony architecture of the palm and extend from the carpus to the phalanges.
- Fractures of the metacarpals can involve the head, neck, shaft, or base and can involve multiple adjacent metacarpals.
- Hand function may be compromised by fractures that involve shortening, rotation, angulation, or intra-articular extension.
- Although nonoperative treatment is effective for many metacarpal fractures, surgical treatment may be indicated based on fracture morphology or patient characteristics.[3]

ANATOMY

- The metacarpals are tubular bones. The four nonthumb metacarpals are triangular in shape and possess a cam-shaped head that is wider in both the coronal and sagittal planes palmarly, thus lending greater stability to the joint in flexion. A condyloid articulation is present with the carpus proximally and the proximal phalanx distally.
- The radial two carpometacarpal (CMC) joints are highly constrained and exhibit minimal motion, whereas in contrast, the fourth and fifth CMC joints demonstrate significant flexion and extension of nearly 30 degrees, which allows "cupping" of the hands.
- The thumb metacarpal is more round in shape, shorter, and wider than the other metacarpals. It articulates only with the trapezium proximally as a saddle joint.
- At the head of the metacarpals, the proper collateral ligaments extend from the recess to the base of the proximal phalanx at a 30-degree angle, whereas the accessory collateral ligaments run nearly perpendicular to insert on the volar plate. These provide varus and valgus stability to the metacarpophalangeal (MP) joint.
- The robust volar plate serves to resist hyperextension of the MP joint. The deep transverse intermetacarpal ligament attaches to the volar plate between each nonthumb metacarpal and provides inherent length stability in the setting of a fracture.
- Bordering the metacarpals are the interossei muscles on the volar radial and volar ulnar surfaces and the extensor tendons on the dorsal surface. The interossei and lumbricals pass volar to the MP joint contributing to MP flexion and imparting an apex-dorsal deforming force on metacarpal shaft fractures. The extensor tendons travel along the dorsal surface and are stabilized distally at the MP joint by the radial and ulnar sagittal bands that originate from the volar plate.
- Important dorsal tendon attachments to the metacarpals include the extensor carpi radialis longus and extensor carpi radialis brevis onto the second and third metacarpal base, respectively. Extensor carpi ulnaris inserts onto the base of the fifth metacarpal, and abductor pollicis longus inserts onto the base of the thumb metacarpal. Volar tendon insertions include the flexor carpi radialis and the flexor carpi ulnaris onto the base of the second metacarpal and fifth metacarpal, respectively.
- Within close proximity to the nonthumb metacarpal volar surface is the deep branch of the ulnar nerve and the deep palmar arch travelling between the two heads of the adductor pollicis on the volar aspect of the third metacarpal. Dorsal veins may be encountered during surgical fixation of metacarpal fractures through a dorsal approach and should be preserved when possible **(FIG 1)**.[4,5,19]

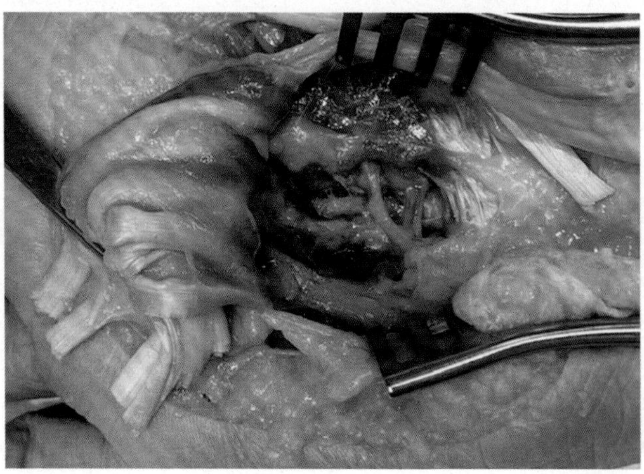

FIG 1 Volar view of the palm. The flexor tendons are reflected to reveal the deep palmar arch and deep motor branch of the ulnar nerve directly volar to the base of the third metacarpal.

PATHOGENESIS

- Axial load is the most common injury mechanism for a metacarpal fracture. Because of the normal curvature of the fifth metacarpal, such an axial load will include a bending component and lead to an apex dorsal fracture at the neck, also known as *a boxer's fracture* (**FIG 2A**).
- Axial loads may also be transmitted proximally on the metacarpal and lead to a CMC fracture-dislocation.
- Torsional injuries will lead to spiral oblique fractures (**FIG 2B**).
- Bending injuries from direct impact may lead to short oblique or transverse metacarpal fractures (**FIG 2C**). The addition of butterfly fragments and comminution is dependent on a combination of additional loads.
- Crush injuries can lead to comminuted fractures with significant soft tissue injuries and a heightened risk of compartment syndrome (**FIG 2D**).

NATURAL HISTORY

- Metacarpal fractures are mainly affected by shortening and rotation. The effect of these two components is minimized in the central metacarpals due to the stabilizing effect of the deep transverse metacarpal ligaments and the bordering intact metacarpals. This stabilizing effect is lost in cases of multiple metacarpal fractures and more severe injuries (see **FIG 2D**).
- Shaft fractures of the third and fourth metacarpals tend to do well with minimal intervention. Border metacarpals are more prone to shortening and rotation.
- Every 2 mm of shortening of the metacarpal can lead to a 7-degree lag at the MP joint.
- Fractures of the metacarpal neck typically result in apex dorsal angulation, which may lead to significant shortening. The increased mobility afforded by the ulnar CMC joints allows more tolerance of angulation in the ulnar metacarpals (fourth and fifth). Although some have accepted up to 70 degrees, most authors have recommended intervention if the angulation exceeds 30 to 40 degrees. The radial metacarpals (second to third) have stiffer CMC joints, and correspondingly, the tolerance for angulation is reduced to only 10 to 15 degrees.
- Thumb metacarpal extra-articular base and shaft fractures can easily tolerate 30 degrees of angulation due to its highly mobile CMC joint.
- Fractures of the metacarpal head with a significant gap or step-off, or fractures that involve a significant portion of the articular surface, should be considered for open reduction and stabilization.

PATIENT HISTORY AND PHYSICAL FINDINGS

- When evaluating a patient with a suspected or known metacarpal fracture, the key elements of history are mechanism of injury, patient handedness, past medical/surgical history, occupation, smoking history, any relevant previous injury or preexisting disability of the ipsilateral limb and hand, timing of the injury, and circumstances of the injury.[3]
- The mechanism of injury often results in specific fracture patterns within the metacarpal.
- Metacarpal head fractures typically result from a direct impact with the MP joint flexed and are often seen with an open wound from a human teeth impact after a direct blow (the eponymous fight bite).

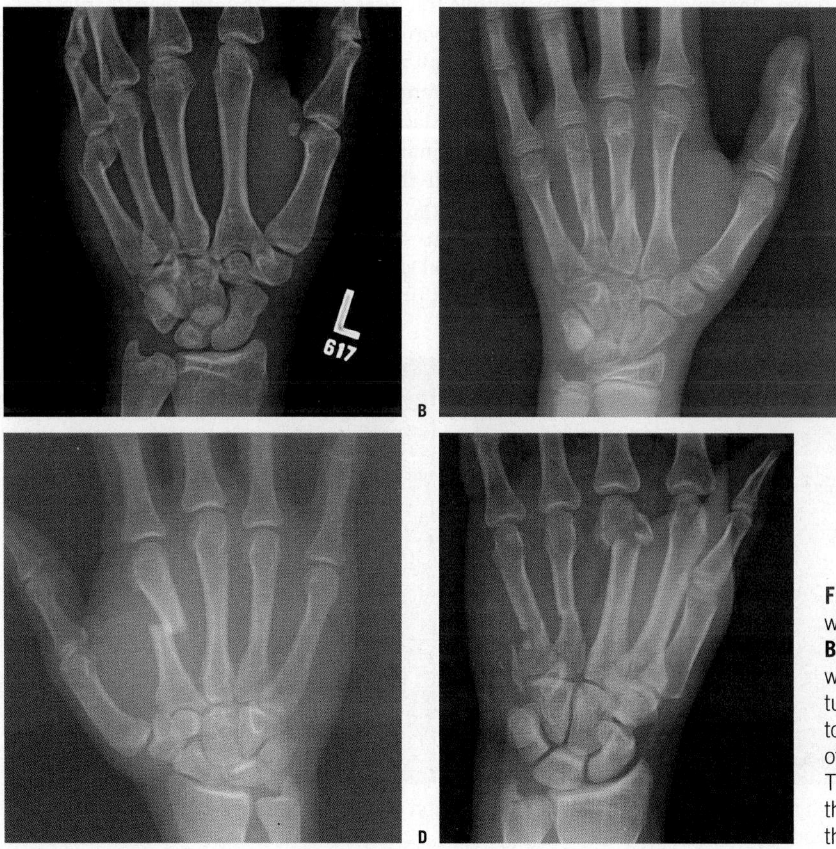

A B C D

FIG 2 A. Fracture of the neck of the fifth metacarpal with a flexed, apex dorsal angulation (boxer's fracture). **B.** Torsional injuries lead to long oblique fractures with a risk for malrotation. **C.** Short transverse fracture from a direct impact. **D.** Crush injuries can lead to a combination of injuries with an increased risk of compartment syndrome and significant stiffness. The shortened fourth metacarpal pulls the head of third metacarpal in a proximal and ulnar direction through deep transverse metacarpal ligament.

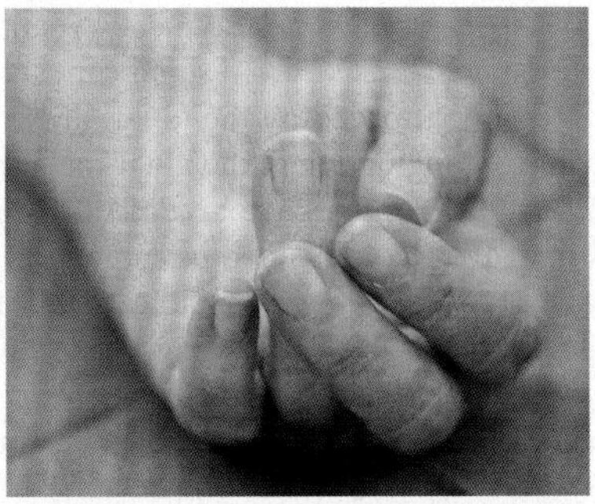

FIG 3 Malrotation in a patient with a metacarpal fracture. Clinically, this can present as digital overlap that impairs function.

- Metacarpal neck fractures typically result in a similar manner from an axial load with a flexed MP joint and are more common on the ulnar side of the hand (the eponymous boxer's fracture when involving the fifth metacarpal neck).
- Metacarpal shaft fractures can occur by various mechanisms including bending and axial compression, twisting, torque and axial load, or direct blows.
- Metacarpal base fractures more often occur from forced flexion of the wrist with simultaneous longitudinally directed force.
- Inspection should be performed in comparison to the uninjured hand and should determine the presence of any swelling, discoloration (ecchymosis, pallor, erythema), temperature changes, deformity, malrotation of the digits, shortening of the ray, joint depression of the MP joint, and presence of skin compromise or lacerations.
- To evaluate for malrotation, the hand should be inspected in with the digits in full flexion and full extension. Malrotated fingers are identified by the tip of the affected digits crossing over or under adjacent digits in full flexion compared to contralateral hand **(FIG 3)**.
- If there is an open injury, the level of contamination (ie, farm injuries, fight bite contamination) must be assessed and appropriate antibiotics given along with assessment of the patient's tetanus prophylaxis status.
- In the case of open injuries, a high degree of suspicion should be present for an open joint or extensor tendon injury. The juncturae tendinae can easily mask these injuries and provide digital extension albeit more weakly and with associated pain typically. The combination of fracture and soft tissue injury has been shown to worsen outcome with a complication rate of 17% following fractures with soft tissue injury versus 8% in those without significant soft tissue injury.[5]

IMAGING AND OTHER DIAGNOSTIC STUDIES

- Initial imaging studies in the evaluation of metacarpal fractures are posteroanterior (PA), lateral, and oblique views of the hand. Oblique views in relative pronation and supination allow for a true lateral of each metacarpal **(FIG 4)**.
- "Skyline view" of the MP joints can be obtained to determine the presence of metacarpal head impaction as a result of human tooth impaction in fight bite injuries.
- The Brewerton view offers an excellent anteroposterior view of the MP joint.
- A semipronated view is useful for assessing fourth and fifth CMC joint injuries where subtle instability may be difficult to appreciate on routine imaging.
- Computed tomography scan can be helpful if concern of intra-articular extension or associated CMC fracture-dislocations.

INDICATIONS

- The vast majority of metacarpal fractures can be effectively managed nonoperatively.
- Absolute surgical indications include open fractures, open MP or CMC joints, significant malrotation, and those fractures with associated soft tissue injuries such as tendon or nerve injuries necessitating repair.
- Relative indications include excessive shortening (>5 mm); extensor lag; and prominence of the metacarpal head in the palm, multiple fractures,[14] and intra-articular fractures.
- Malrotation is poorly tolerated as digital overlap may occur with even a small degree of malrotation. Pronation of the index and supination of the small finger can be better tolerated given the lack of overlapping with adjacent digits.
- Angulation in ulnar digits is better tolerated than the radial two digits given the increased CMC motion. Acceptable angulation for the ring and small finger metacarpal shaft fractures is 30 to 40 degrees, whereas the index and long finger metacarpal shaft fractures can generally only tolerate 15 to 20 degrees of angulation.[4,5,19]

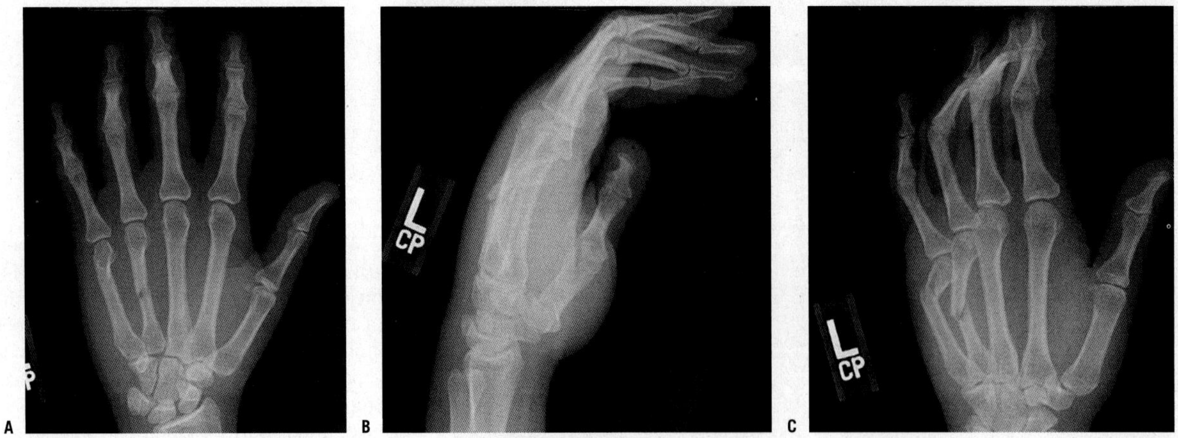

FIG 4 Standard x-ray evaluation of suspected metacarpal fractures. PA hand radiograph (**A**), lateral hand radiograph (**B**), and oblique hand radiograph (**C**) showing fourth and fifth metacarpal fractures.

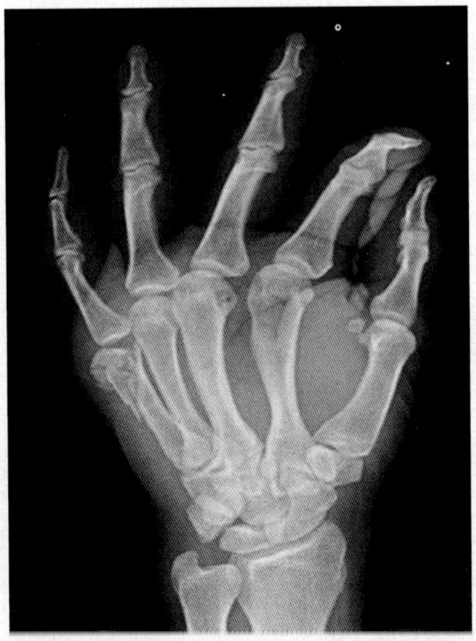

FIG 5 Intra-articular, comminuted fracture of the fifth metacarpal head with shortening and malrotation.

- Angulation up to 30 degrees is well tolerated in thumb metacarpal shaft fractures with the increased mobility of the thumb CMC joint.
- Several patient factors may contribute to a decision for or against surgery including patient age, medical comorbidities, occupation, handedness, and ability to tolerate the requisite period of immobilization for nonoperative care, especially in polytrauma patients.
- The probability of MP joint involvement when a dorsal wound is present over the knuckle (aka fight bite) must be suspected and warrants exploration in a timely fashion.[2,4,5]
- Metacarpal head fractures with intra-articular displacement of more than 1 mm or 25% of articular surface, bone loss, comminution, a block to motion, or ligamentous avulsion fractures often require surgical intervention **(FIG 5)**.

SURGICAL MANAGEMENT

- Prior to proceeding with surgery, decisions should be made about the type of anesthesia (local, regional, general, combination), the equipment needed for the planned procedure, and the postoperative dressing and immobilization.
- The degree of associated soft tissue injuries is important to consider. The reconstructive ladder can offer guidelines for the management of these combined injuries and should be considered before proceeding with surgical intervention.[13] When a fracture is associated with severe soft tissue injury, bone loss, or contamination, a staged treatment approach may be performed. Initial irrigation and debridement with antibiotic spacer placement may be followed with delayed bone grafting, tendon reconstruction, or soft tissue coverage if required.

Approach

- The overwhelming majority of metacarpal fractures are approached dorsally given the relative subcutaneous location of the bones and the ease of handling the extensor tendons and dorsal cutaneous nerves. Distally, the juncturae tendinae may require division and subsequent repair if limiting exposure. When exposing the MP joint on the border digits, the common extensor may be split from the ulnar accessory tendon (extensor indicis proprius [EIP] or extensor digiti quinti), whereas the common extensor tendon is split midline for the central two digits.
- Some coronal shear fractures of the metacarpal head or base are best approached palmarly **(FIG 6)**. A longitudinal or Bruner skin incision is made similar to the approach for a trigger finger. The A1 pulley is released and the flexor tendons retracted to either side. Care should be taken to avoid injury to the A2 pulley, which could result in unwanted pathologic bowstringing of the flexor tendons. The volar plate can then be split or longitudinally incised to expose the articular surface of the metacarpal head.

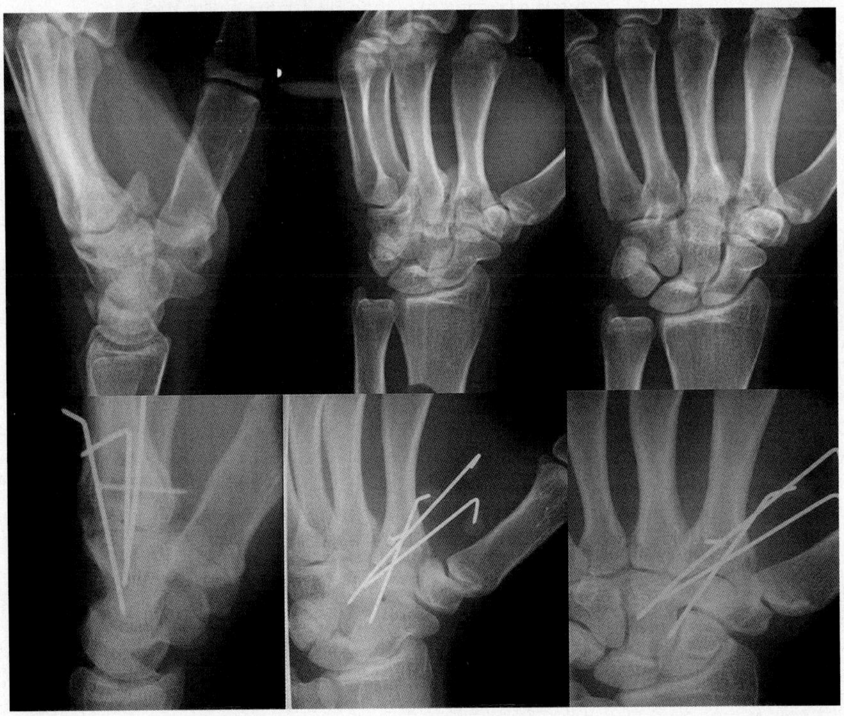

FIG 6 Fracture of the base of the second metacarpal may be one scenario when a volar approach to reduction may be used. Both volar and dorsal fixation was used to maintain reduction.

CLOSED REDUCTION

- Given the apex dorsal angulation of most metacarpal neck[16] and shaft fractures, closed reduction typically requires a dorsally directed pressure on the metacarpal head.
- One well-described technique for closed reduction is the Jahss maneuver. In this technique, the MP joint is flexed to 90 degrees to relax the pull of the intrinsic muscles and collateral ligaments.
- With the proximal interphalangeal (IP) joint flexed to 90 degrees, a dorsally directed force can then be applied through the proximal phalanx base to reduce the metacarpal head dorsally **(TECH FIG 1)**.
- Once the reduction has been achieved, immobilization should include the MP joint but the IP joints should be free to allow mobility. Studies have shown no difference in outcome if the MP joints are immobilized in flexion or extension.[8] The position of extension is often easier to allow molding of the splint or cast.

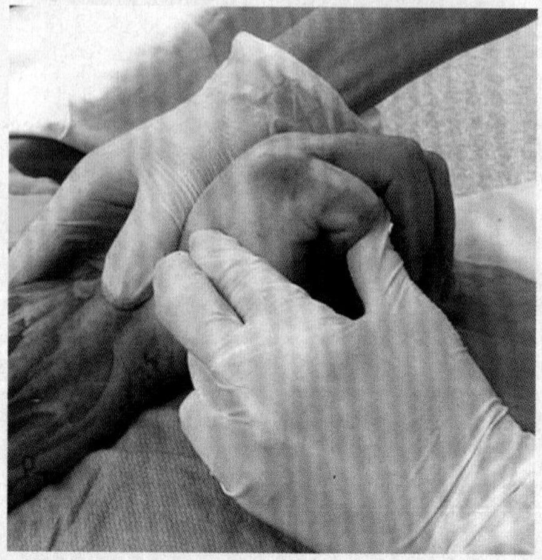

TECH FIG 1 Jahss maneuver for closed reduction of metacarpal neck fractures. The proximal IP and MP joints are flexed to 90 degrees, and a dorsally directed force can be applied.

CLOSED REDUCTION AND PERCUTANEOUS PINNING

- For fractures that can be reduced closed but are unstable, percutaneous pinning has the advantage of minimizing soft tissue injury. This may be performed retrograde, transversely, or antegrade with a limited open approach.

Retrograde Pinning

- This technique is well suited for metacarpal neck and shaft fractures. Two smooth 0.035- to 0.045-inch Kirschner wires (K-wires) are placed from distal to proximal starting in the collateral recess on the radial and ulnar aspect of the metacarpal head while the MP joint is held in flexion **(TECH FIG 2)**.
- A 14-gauge needle may be used as a guide to assist in starting point and trajectory of K-wire insertion. Pin ends may either be cut leaving a 1-cm tail out of the skin, the ends are bent to 90 degrees to aid in pin removal and prevent pin migration, or cut beneath the skin.
- Full passive motion of the MP joint and proper rotation of the digit should be ensured.

Transverse Pinning

- This technique is more commonly performed in the border digits especially in the face of comminution and requires a stable adjacent metacarpal. Longitudinal traction is applied to the digit to restore length, and the distal fragment is pinned to the adjacent metacarpal to maintain length and rotation. The trajectory is typically volar to dorsal for pin placement owing to the archlike configuration of the metacarpals **(TECH FIG 3)**.

Antegrade Intramedullary Pinning (Bouquet Pinning)

- Increased motion and decreased shortening compared to crossed K-wire fixation[10]
- A small longitudinal incision is made over the metacarpal base. The sensory nerves and extensor tendons are identified and retracted.
- A curved awl or drill[10] is then used to create a small opening in the metaphysis of the metacarpal base and ideally directed from proximal to distal.
- Three prebent 0.35-inch K-wires or two prebent 0.045-inch K-wires[10] are passed antegrade up the metacarpal diaphysis, across the fracture site and into the metacarpal head.
- Care must be taken to avoid penetrating the distal cortex. The pins may then be cut flush with the dorsal cortex and left in place permanently or subsequently removed.
- The goal is to have the tips diverge in the head as to create a "flower bouquet."

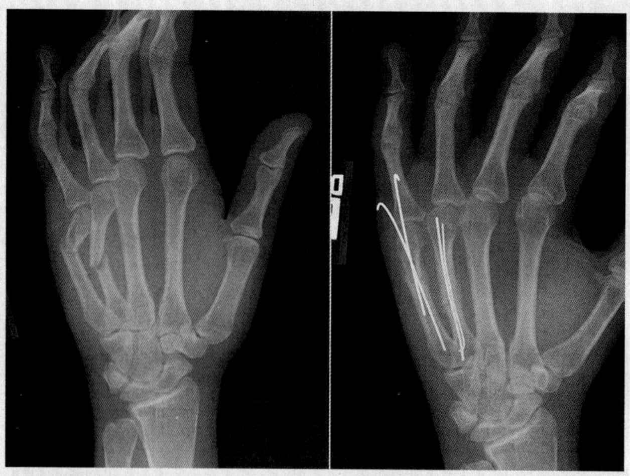

TECH FIG 2 Antegrade and retrograde IM K-wire fixation of a fourth and fifth metacarpal fracture. To aid in maintaining start point and trajectory, a 14-gauge hypodermic needle may be used as a guide.

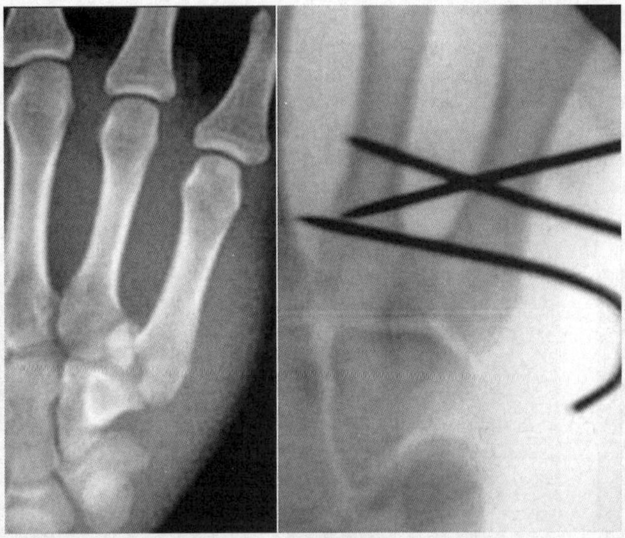

TECH FIG 3 Transverse metacarpal pin fixation for a metacarpal fracture with CMC subluxation.

OPEN REDUCTION AND LAG SCREW FIXATION

- Interfragmentary lag screw fixation is acceptable for long oblique and spiral fractures of the metacarpal shaft that are at least twice the diameter of the bone at the level of the fracture.
- Smooth K-wires can be used to hold temporary reduction if the clamp prevents adequate visualization of the fracture site.
- K-wires can also be used as "drill holes." Use 0.035-inch (0.9-mm) K-wires for 1.2-mm screws, 0.045-inch (1.1-mm) K-wires for 1.5-mm screws, and 0.062-inch (1.6-mm) K-wires for 2.0-mm screws.
- The screws are drilled to lag by technique, by overdrilling the near cortex to create a gliding hole for interfragmentary compression.[17] Typically, the first screw is placed perpendicular to the fracture for maximal compression, and the second may be placed perpendicular to the bone to resist longitudinal forces.
- A countersink is used to increase surface area of contact between the screw head and the bone, which reduces hoop stresses. This also decreases screw head prominence.
- Multiple screws should be used to increase compression across the fracture and resist the rotational torque associated with long oblique and spiral fractures **(TECH FIG 4)**.
- Intraoperative assessment of rotation alignment is tested via tenodesis effect in the operating room prior to wound closure.
- If possible, periosteum and interosseous muscle fascia should be closed with a 3-0 absorbable braided suture to prevent any hardware irritation.
- The hand is placed in an intrinsic plus splint with the IP joints free.

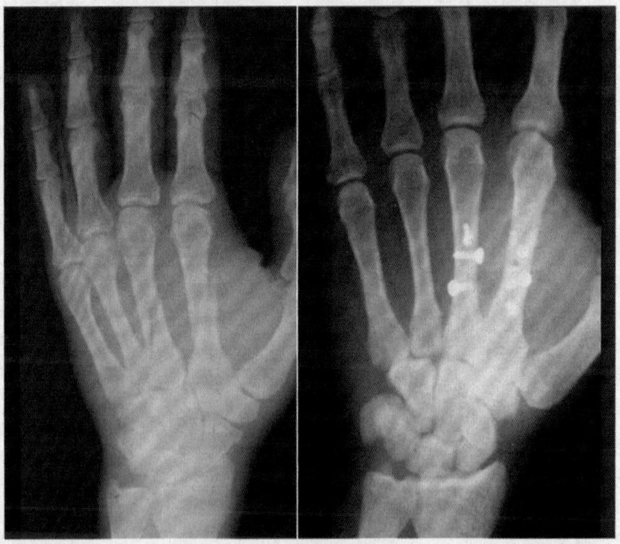

TECH FIG 4 Multiple lag screw fixation of long oblique metacarpal fractures.

OPEN REDUCTION AND PLATE FIXATION

- Transverse and short oblique fractures that are not amenable to lag screw fixation alone may undergo osteosynthesis with a plate and screw construct.
- If comminution, bone loss, or osteopenia is present, locked plating may be performed.
- A plate of length allowing four to six cortices of fixation on each side of the fracture is selected. If two-dimensional plating is performed, a 2.0-mm plate may be cut to length and positioned onto the dorsal surface of the metacarpal ideally minimizing direct contact with the overlying extensor

tendons **(TECH FIG 5A–D)**. If three-dimensional plating is performed, a 1.5- or 2.0-mm staggered or H plate may be selected **(TECH FIG 5E–H)**.

- The plate should be bent to accommodate the dorsal curvature of the metacarpal shaft to allow compression of the far cortex.[18]
- Care should be taken to avoid overdrilling the far cortex especially in the third metacarpal given the proximity of the motor branch of the ulnar nerve.
- Adequate alignment is confirmed with fluoroscopy and the wound thoroughly irrigated.
- When possible, the periosteum and interosseous muscle fascia are closed over the plate with absorbable sutures to decrease extensor irritation on the hardware.
- The skin is closed in a standard fashion and an intrinsic plus splint with the IP joints free is applied for 3 to 5 days before starting therapy and gentle motion.

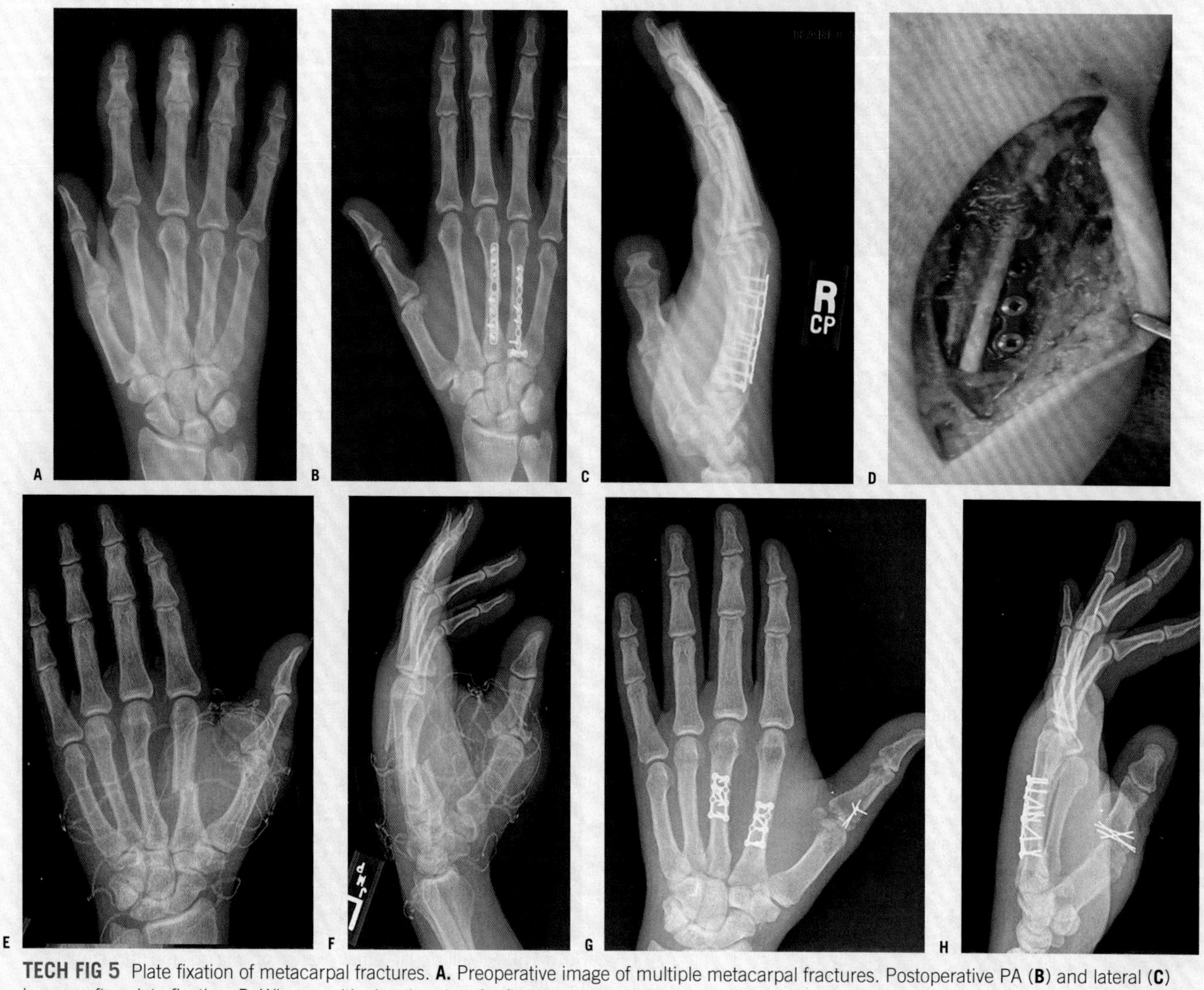

TECH FIG 5 Plate fixation of metacarpal fractures. **A.** Preoperative image of multiple metacarpal fractures. Postoperative PA (**B**) and lateral (**C**) images after plate fixation. **D.** When positioning the plate for fixation, slightly oblique or off-center positioning will avoid direct extensor tendon contact over the prominent portions of the plate. In a different patient, preoperative (**E,F**) and postoperative (**G,H**) radiographs of three-dimensional plate fixation with restoration of length, alignment, and rotation.

INTRAMEDULLARY SCREW FIXATION

- Intramedullary (IM) fixation is a treatment option that offers reliably strong fixation and limited soft tissue disruption or irritation.
- Prior to placing an IM screw, fracture reduction is performed in a closed or limited open fashion.
- With the MP joint flexed to 90 degrees, the extensor tendon is split or retracted to one side with incision through a portion of the sagittal band, followed by a small arthrotomy.
- The starting point is over the dorsal third of the metacarpal head.

- Under fluoroscopic guidance, the guidewire is passed down the medullary canal, across the fracture site, and down to the metacarpal base.
- Appropriate screw length can be measured and then the guidewire advanced across the CMC joint to avoid inadvertent removal during drilling.
- The screw is inserted in a coaxial fashion over the guidewire and countersunk 2 mm below the articular surface of the metacarpal head.
- The screw diameter should allow interference fit within the isthmus of the metacarpal shaft, whereas the screw length should traverse the length of the metacarpal if possible. In general, 3.5-mm screws fit well for ring finger metacarpals, whereas 4.0- or 4.5-mm screws are needed for the middle and small finger metacarpals **(TECH FIG 6)**.
- The hand is placed in an intrinsic plus splint with the IP joints free or soft dressing depending on the construct stability, with initiation of therapy for range of motion after 3 to 5 days.

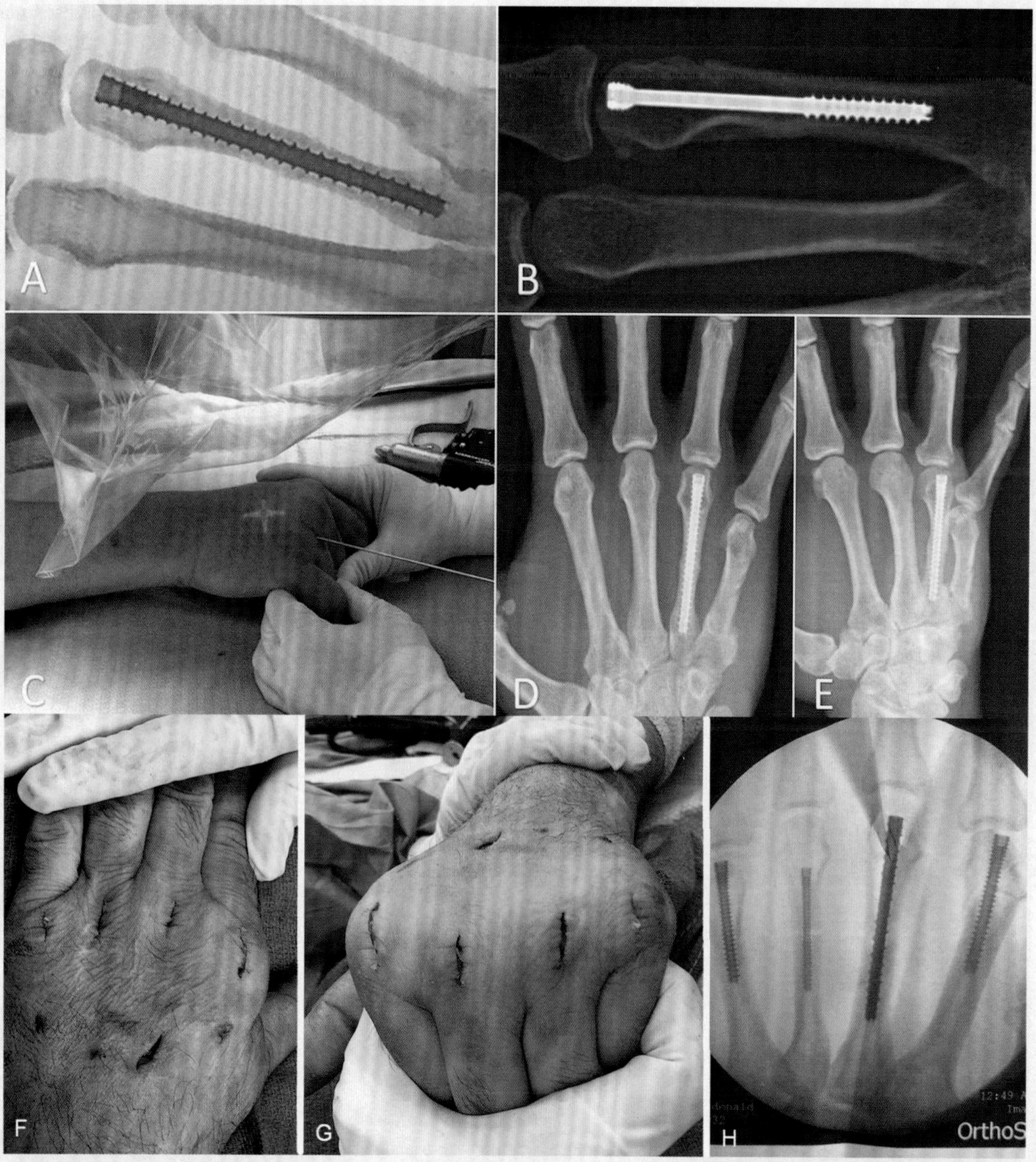

TECH FIG 6 IM screw fixation. IM screws can be fully threaded with variable pitch (**A**) or partially threaded (**B**). **C.** Intraoperative photograph of guidewire insertion is shown under fluoroscopy during IM screw fixation of a fourth metacarpal shaft fracture. **D,E.** Postoperative radiograph fixation with a fully threaded conical screw. **F–H.** Operative fixation of the index through small finger metacarpals in a different patient. The dorsal approach to the metacarpal head is performed through a longitudinal incision centered over the head with the MP joint flexed to 90 degrees. Of note, screw diameter varies by metacarpal. The smallest diameter is frequently the fourth metacarpal.

METACARPAL HEAD FRACTURE OPEN REDUCTION AND INTERNAL FIXATION

- Methods of fixation of metacarpal head fractures varies and can include headless compression screw fixation, K-wire fixation, plate fixation, or hybrid fixation.
- The dorsal approach is preferred for most fractures as it provides excellent metacarpal head exposure; however, in some coronal shear fractures, a volar approach is preferred.
- The dorsal approach can be performed through an extensor split. For the index finger, the extensor tendons of extensor digitorum communis (EDC) and EIP may be split to access the capsule. Similarly, the small finger metacarpal head may be accessed between the EDC and extensor digiti minimi tendons.
- Alternatively, the sagittal band may be incised. The ulnar sagittal band is preferred as injury to the weaker radial sagittal band can lead to postoperative subluxation.
- Care should be taken to preserve soft tissue attachments to the articular fragments when possible to minimize risk of devascularization.
- For noncomminuted fractures, reduction may be obtained with a reduction clamp followed by fixation with headless compression screws, countersunk extra-articular screws, or K-wires based on fracture size and location **(TECH FIG 7A)**.
- Screws should be advanced with special attention to not rotate the fragment and be completely countersunk beneath the articular surface.
- For volar shear coronal fractures, the volar approach may be more effective for reduction and fixation through a longitudinal or Brunner zigzag incision.
- If the comminution proves to be nonreconstructable, then volar plate interposition (aka Tupper arthroplasty), prosthetic arthroplasty, or osteochondral autograft transplantation may be considered **(TECH FIG 7B)**.[11]

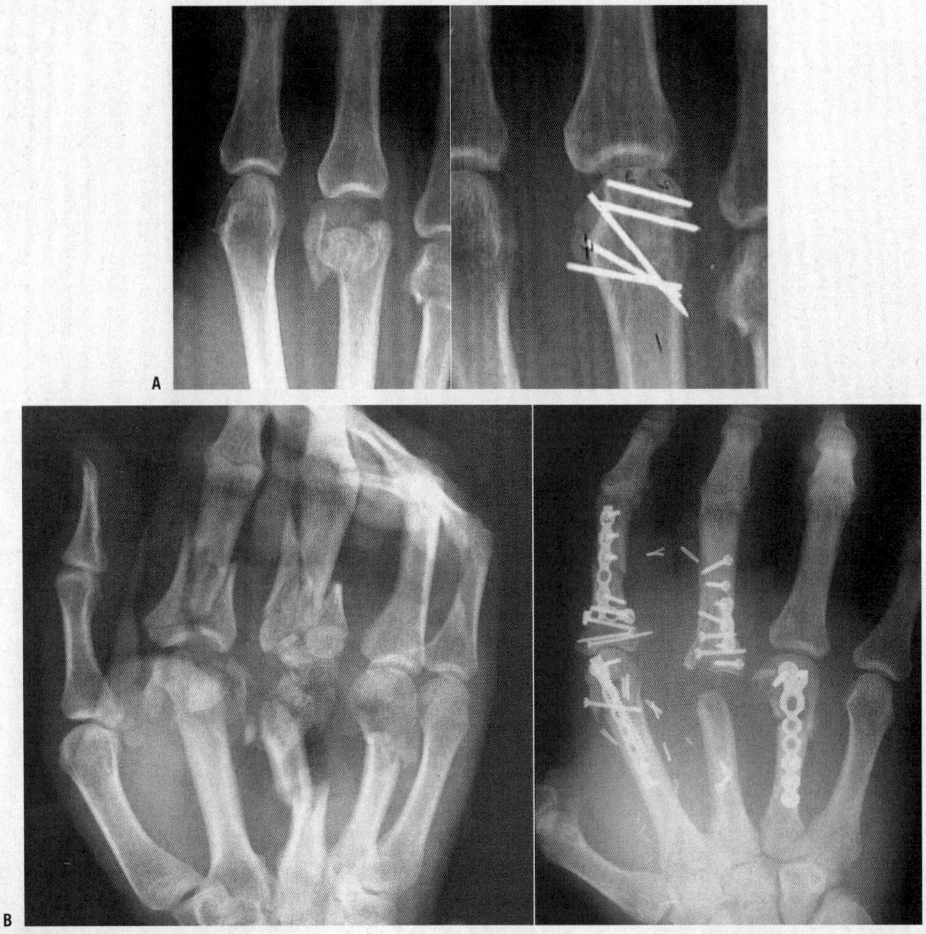

TECH FIG 7 A. Intra-articular metacarpal head fracture with fixation using multiple K-wires. **B.** Multiple metacarpal and proximal phalanx fractures with reconstruction using interfragmentary screws, plate fixation, and IM screw fixation. The long finger metacarpal head had significant comminution and bone loss that was treated with a Tupper arthroplasty.

Pearls and Pitfalls

Indications	• Malrotation is poorly tolerated in all digits. • Ring finger, small finger, and thumb metacarpals tolerate more angulation than the index finger and long finger metacarpals. • Dorsal angulation can cause extensor lag and decreased grip strength but is often well tolerated.
Surgical Approaches	• Closed reduction should be attempted first. • Use of IM K-wires (bouquet pinning) or screws allows for less soft tissue disruption. • Dorsal approach is most often preferred with the volar approach reserved for certain coronal shear metacarpal head fracture patterns.
Surgical Implants	• Lag screw fixation if long oblique or spiral fracture longer than two times the diameter of the bone • Careful periosteal elevation over the fracture site and closure of the periosteum and interosseous muscle fascia when possible to decrease risk of extensor tendon irritation and adhesions • K-wires can serve as drill bits with 0.035 inch (0.9 mm) used for 1.2-mm screws, 0.045 inch (1.1 mm) used for 1.5-mm screws, and 0.062 inch (1.6 mm) used for 2.0-mm screws. • IM fixation: Select appropriate screw diameter for interference fit (3.5 mm for ring finger metacarpal and 4.0 or 4.5 mm for middle and small finger metacarpal).

POSTOPERATIVE CARE

- Surgically treated metacarpal fractures should be immobilized in a well-padded splint in intrinsic plus position.
- Fractures stabilized with retrograde or transverse K-wires for metacarpal neck fractures should be immobilized for 4 weeks while pins are in place, with early IP motion.[7]
- Early active motion of the digits is ideal and can be initiated in fractures treated with rigid internal fixation (open reduction internal fixation with plate, IM screws, and interfragmentary lag screws).
- Weight bearing through the extremity should be delayed until bony union has been occurred.

OUTCOMES

- Most metacarpal fractures with less than 5 mm of shortening and without malrotation can be effectively managed without surgery.[15] The tolerance of malalignment may be as high as 70 degrees of angulation in small finger metacarpal neck fractures **(FIG 7)**.[9]
- When oblique fractures may be treated with lag screw fixation alone, two 2.0-mm lag screws may offer the same biomechanical strength as three 1.5-mm lag screws.[6]
- Plate fixation has consistently provided excellent restoration of range of motion and functional outcomes even with low-profile plates or in complex cases with bone loss requiring structural autograft but will at times require subsequent hardware removal.[19]
- The use of IM headless compression screws is a relatively newer technique of fixation for metacarpal fractures and in the studies reported has shown good healing on radiographs and full restoration of grip strength with acceptable range of motion.[1]
- Operative fixation of metacarpal head fractures can lead to favorable functional outcomes, although stiffness is common.[4,12]

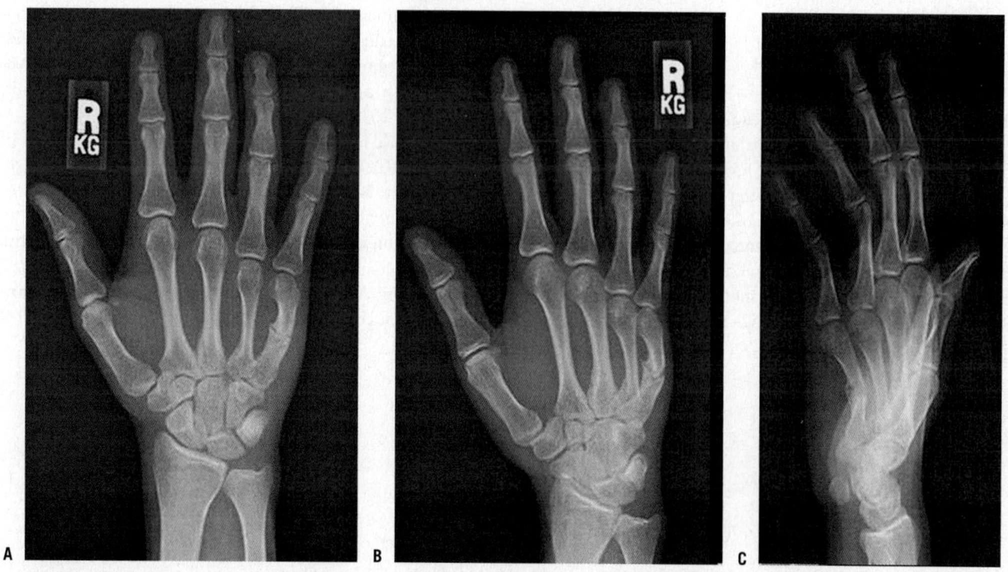

FIG 7 A–C. Malunion, specifically involving the fourth and fifth metacarpals, can be well tolerated with minimal clinical dysfunction. *(continued)*

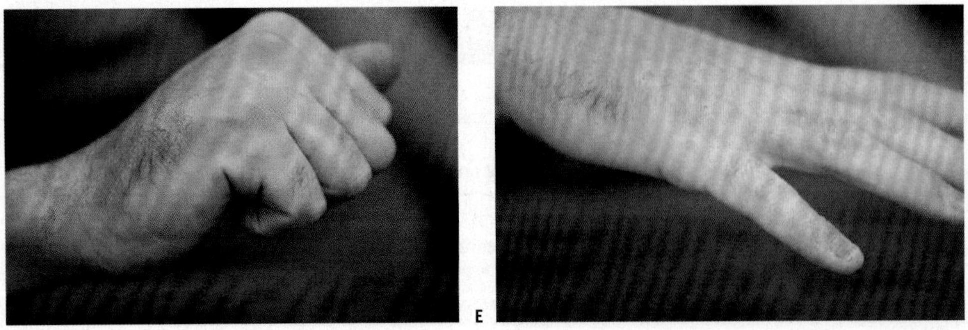

D E

FIG 7 *(continued)* **D,E.** This patient achieved full digital extension and flexion after healing a fifth metacarpal shaft fracture with residual volar angulation.

COMPLICATIONS

- Malunion with significant residual angulation can lead to weakness in grip. In addition, excessive shortening (>5 mm) can lead to extensor lag (7 degrees for every 2 mm of shortening).
- Malrotation of only 5 degrees can lead to 1.5 cm of digital overlap and impaired function.[2]
- Pin tract infections may occur in 5% to 6% of cases and can rarely lead to osteomyelitis. Burying the pins may reduce the risk of infection but complicate removal.
- Deep infection may occur with open reduction and plate osteosynthesis that may require antibiotics and hardware removal.[1]
- Nonunion is a rare occurrence in metacarpal fractures and is generally atrophic in nature due to significant soft tissue injury or bone loss. Treatment of painful nonunion or delayed union with revision fixation and autograft can be performed.
- Decreased range of motion can occur due to extensor tendon adhesions or contracture of the collateral ligaments and joint capsule. Metacarpal head fractures may result in a block to motion should the articular surface remain incongruent.[5]
- Nerve irritation or neuroma can occur as a result of operative dissection or from percutaneous pin placement and open approaches.[2]

REFERENCES

1. Avery DM III, Klinge S, Dyrna F, et al. Headless compression screw versus Kirschner wire fixation for metacarpal neck fractures: a biomechanical study. J Hand Surg Am 2017;42(5):392.e1–392.e6.
2. Balaram AJ, Bednar MS. Complications after the fractures of metacarpal and phalanges. Hand Clin 2010;26:169–177.
3. Ben-Amotz O, Sammer DM. Practical management of metacarpal fractures. Plast Reconstr Surg 2015;136(3):370e–379e.
4. Bloom JM, Hammert WC. Evidence-based medicine: metacarpal fractures. Plast Reconstr Surg 2014;133(5):1252–1260.
5. Day CS, Stern PJ. Fractures of the metacarpals and phalanges. In: Wolfe SW, Hotchkiss RN, Pederson WC, et al, eds. Green's Operative Hand Surgery, ed 6. Philadelphia: Elsevier, 2011:239–258.
6. Eu-Jin Cheah AE, Behn AW, Comer G, et al. A biomechanical analysis of 2 constructs for metacarpal spiral fracture fixation in a cadaver model: 2 large screws versus 3 small screws. J Hand Surg Am 2017;42(12): 1033.e1–1033.e6.
7. Gregory S, Lalonde DH, Fung Leung LT. Minimally invasive finger fracture management: wide-awake closed reduction, K-wire fixation, and early protected movement. Hand Clin 2014;30(1):7–15.
8. Hofmeister EP, Kim J, Shin AY. Comparison of 2 methods of immobilization of fifth metacarpal neck fractures: a prospective randomized study. J Hand Surg Am 2008;33(8):1362–1368.
9. Jardin E, Pechin C, Rey PB, et al. Functional treatment of metacarpal diaphyseal fractures by buddy taping: a prospective single-center study. Hand Surg Rehabil 2016;35(1):34–39.
10. Kim JK, Kim DJ. Antegrade intramedullary pinning versus retrograde intramedullary pinning for displaced fifth metacarpal neck fractures. Clin Orthop Relat Res 2015;473(5):1747–1754.
11. Kitay A, Waters PM, Bae DS. Osteochondral autograft transplantation surgery for metacarpal head defects. J Hand Surg Am 2016;41(3): 457–463.
12. Lee JK, Jo YG, Kim JW, et al. Open reduction and internal fixation for intraarticular fracture of metacarpal head. Orthopade 2017;46(7): 617–624.
13. Levin LS, Condit DP. Combined injuries—soft tissue management. Clin Orthop Relat Res 1996;(327):172–181.
14. Marjoua Y, Eberlin KR, Mudgal CS. Multiple displaced metacarpal fractures. J Hand Surg Am 2015;40(9):1869–1870.
15. Neumeister MW, Webb K, McKenna K. Non-surgical management of metacarpal fractures. Clin Plast Surg 2014;41(3):451–461.
16. Padegimas EM, Warrender WJ, Jones CM, et al. Metacarpal neck fractures: a review of surgical indications and techniques. Arch Trauma Res 2016;5(3):e32933.
17. Rüedi TP, Murphy WM, Colton CL. Techniques of absolute stability. In: Rüedi TP, Murphy WM, eds. AO Principles of Fracture Management. New York: Thieme, 2000:157–166.
18. Tannenbaum EP, Burns GT, Oak NR, et al. Comparison of 2-dimensional and 3-dimensional metacarpal fracture plating constructs under cyclic loading. J Hand Surg Am 2017;42(3):e159–e165.
19. Wong VW, Higgins JP. Evidence-based medicine: management of metacarpal fractures. Plast Reconstr Surg 2017;140(1):140e–151e.

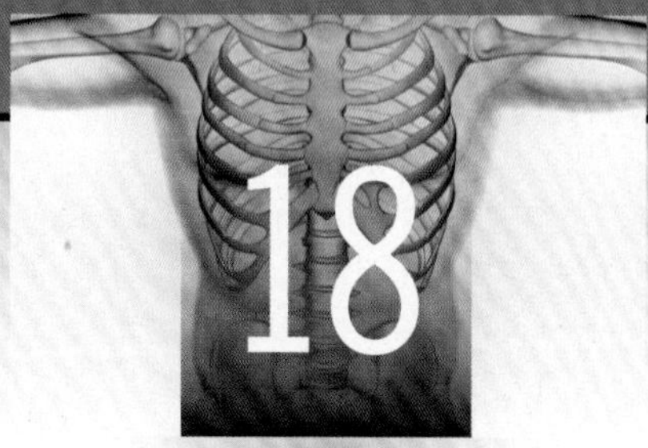

CHAPTER 18

Operative Treatment of Carpometacarpal Fracture-Dislocations Involving the Lesser Digits

Thomas J. Ergen and John J. Walsh IV

DEFINITION

- Injuries to the carpometacarpal (CMC) joints are rare. The most common CMC joints to be affected are the ring finger (RF) or the small finger (SF).[7]
- Fractures and fracture dislocations of the CMC joints of the index through SFs involve intra-articular fractures at the base of metacarpals or pure dislocations between the metacarpals and the carpus.
- The fracture can involve the base of the metacarpal, trapezoid, capitate, or hamate articular surface. These fracture dislocations can lead to joint instability and articular incongruity **(FIG 1)**.

ANATOMY

- The CMC joints connect the metacarpals to the distal carpal row.
- The shape and degree of constraint differs from finger to finger.
- The index finger (IF) and middle finger (MF) have highly constrained and stable articulations due to the shape of index finger CMC articulation and supporting soft tissues.
  - The index finger CMC joint is particularly rigid due to its bony articulation between the trapezium, the trapezoid, and the third metacarpal.[15]
  - The flexor carpi radialis tendon (IF metacarpal base) and the extensor carpi radialis longus and brevis tendons (IF metacarpal base and MF metacarpal base) allow for dynamic stability of their respective joints.
  - The strong capsular attachments aid in further joint stability.[15]
  - Due to these strong attachments and relative lack of motion of these joints, a fracture dislocation is rare **(FIG 2A)**.[3]
- The RFs and SFs have a gliding articulation on the hamate, allowing for closure of the hand around objects, crucial for power grip.
  - The mobility that occurs at the RF and SF CMC joints makes them more prone to injury.

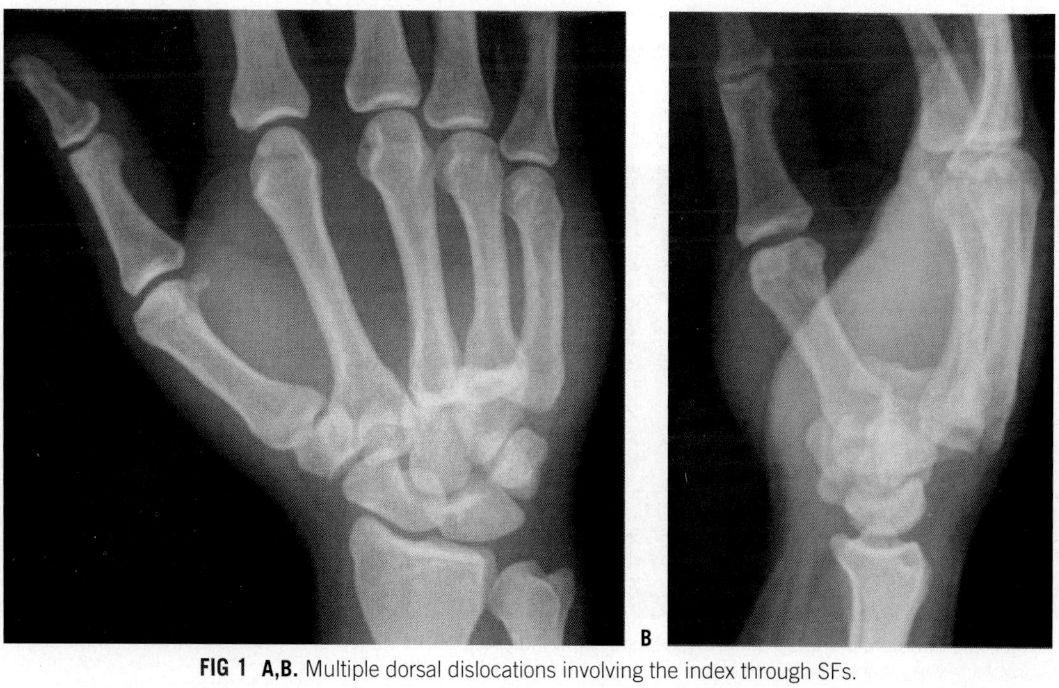

A B

FIG 1 A,B. Multiple dorsal dislocations involving the index through SFs.

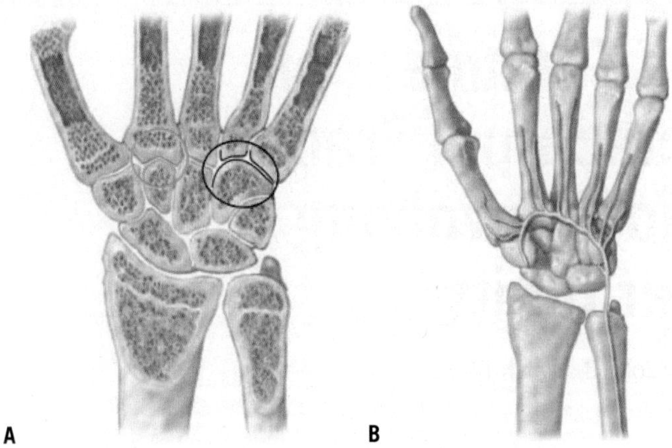

FIG 2 **A.** Variable articular congruity of the various CMC joints. *Green circle* indicating the CMC articulation of the IF, while *red circle* indicating the CMC articulation of the RF/SF. **B.** Deep motor branch of the ulnar nerve adjacent to the metacarpal bases.

- The extensor carpi ulnaris tendon attaches to the base of the SF metacarpal, which can act as a deforming force once this injury has occurred.[5]
- The deep motor branch of the ulnar nerve crosses around the base of the hamate hook from ulnar to radial and runs along the volar surface of the CMC joints. It is vulnerable at the time of injury and/or during fixation **(FIG 2B)**.
- The dorsal cutaneous branch of the radial (IF and MF) and ulnar (RF and SF) nerves are commonly encountered during the surgical approach.

PATHOGENESIS

- Injuries to the CMC joints may be divided into two broad categories, or mechanisms of injury.
  - The first is a load applied to a flexed metacarpal, which is by far the most common.
    - This occurs to the RF/SF with displacement of the metacarpals dorsally relative to the hamate.
    - It can occur as a dislocation only or a marginal fracture of the hamate.[10]
  - The second is an axially directed force that results in a comminuted fracture of the articular surface **(FIG 3A)**.
    - Severe crushing injuries can cause multiple dislocations and fractures dislocations throughout the CMC region **(FIG 3B,C)**.[1,9]

NATURAL HISTORY

- The natural history of a fracture dislocation if left untreated results in progressive arthritis of the involved CMC joint due to instability and joint incongruity.

PATIENT HISTORY AND PHYSICAL FINDINGS

- The patient's history is important to understand the mechanism of injury, which can be helpful in finding concomitant injuries of the upper extremity.
- Examine the hand for tenderness and local swelling.

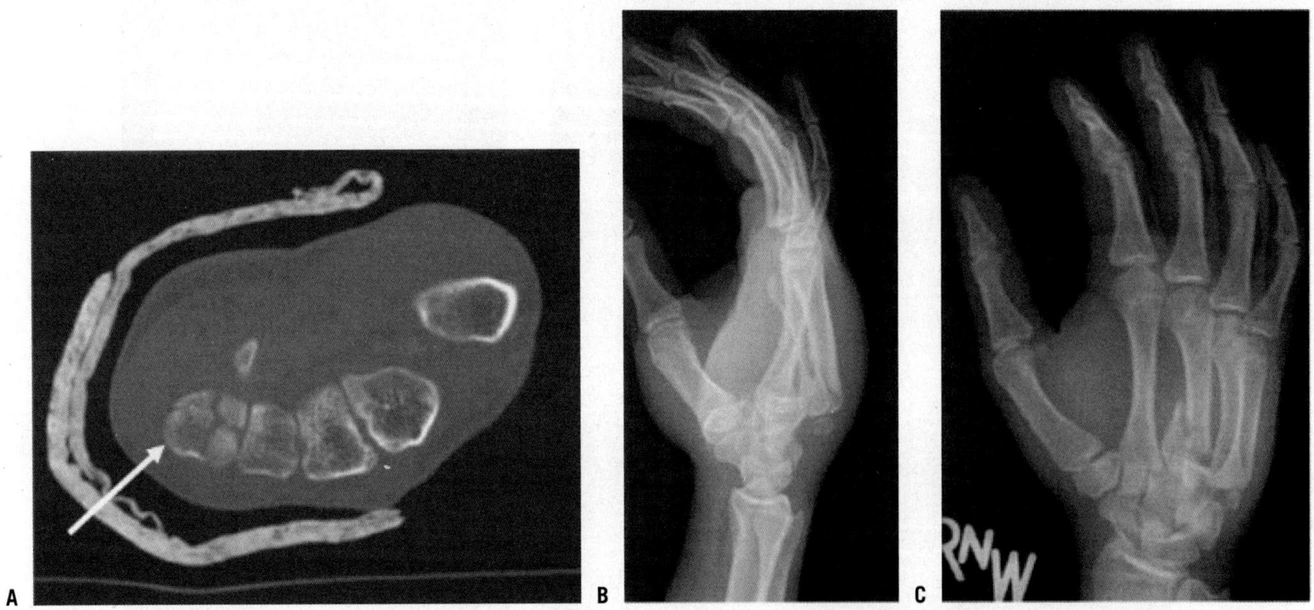

FIG 3 **A.** Comminuted fracture of the SF metacarpal base. *Arrow* indicates comminution of SF metacarpal base. **B,C.** Multiple fractures and dislocations involving the ulnar side of the hand.

- Assess the neurovascular integrity of the hand, especially the deep branch of the ulnar nerve by evaluating the intrinsic musculature (first dorsal interosseous contraction).
- Examine the limb and other extremities for concomitant injury.
- Associated injuries should be detected by physical examination and confirmed with radiographic imaging.
- Preoperative notation of nerve function is imperative when comparing function following reduction and fixation.

IMAGING AND OTHER DIAGNOSTIC STUDIES

- Radiographs of the CMC joint require careful imaging to properly assess and evaluate each joint.
- The transverse metacarpal arch causes the CMC joints of the IF and SF to appear in oblique fashion when a standard posteroanterior (PA) radiograph of the hand is obtained.
- A true frontal radiograph is most easily obtained by placing the hand in an anteroposterior (AP) projection **(FIG 4A)** with the dorsum of the hand placed flat on the cassette (or image intensifier if using fluoroscopy). The base of the affected metacarpal should lie on the cassette. This technique will result in a far more accurate portrayal of the joint trying to be visualized, essential in assessing the fracture and evaluating the hardware position after fixation.
  - Visualization of the joint surfaces at the base of the RFs and SFs differs in a typical PA projection **(FIG 4B)** when compared to the properly positioned film on the same patient **(FIG 4C)**.
- The same principle holds true for evaluating lateral radiographs of the hand.
  - A semisupinated lateral view will best visualize the base of the index and middle finger CMC joints.[7]
  - A semipronated view will best visualize the CMC joints of the RF and SF.[2]
- Due to the difficulty in evaluating the articular surface with plain radiographs, a computed tomography (CT) scan should be obtained in the majority of cases to help assess the articular involvement.
  - CT is especially helpful in evaluating the impacted articular fragments.
  - Ideally, the best visualization and determination of fracture pattern will be possible if the CT scan is obtained after a reduction of any displaced fractures or fracture dislocations has been completed **(FIG 4E)**.[12]

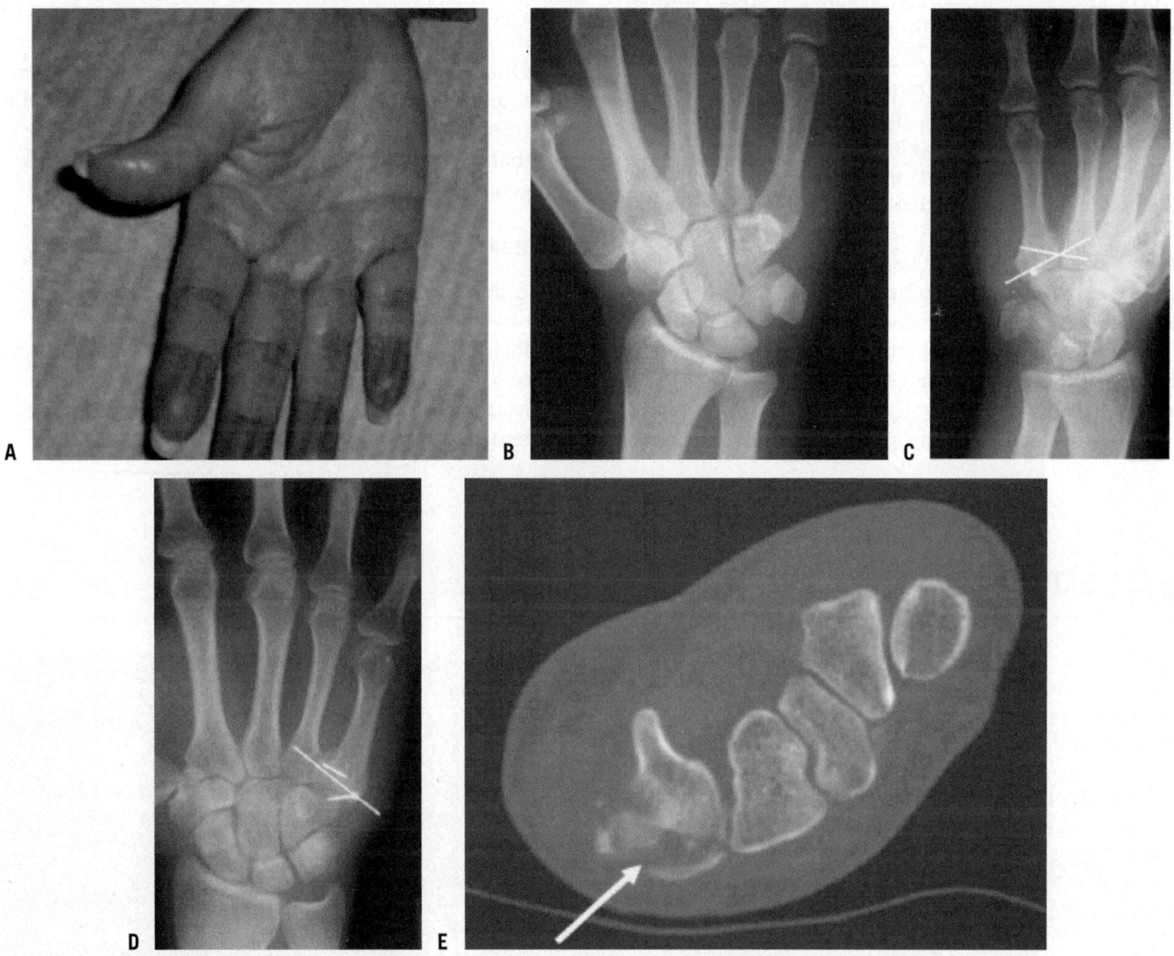

FIG 4 A. Hand properly positioned for AP view of the RF and SF CMC joints. **B.** A conventional PA view of the hand creates an oblique view of the RF and SF bases. **C.** AP projections clearly show the joint reduction in the same patient shown in **D** but with better definition of the joint surfaces. **D.** Postoperative PA film after open reduction with internal fixation of the RF and SF CMC joints. **E.** CT scan of the fracture of the dorsal lip of the hamate. *Arrow* indicates hamate comminution and displacement of dorsal lip fragment.

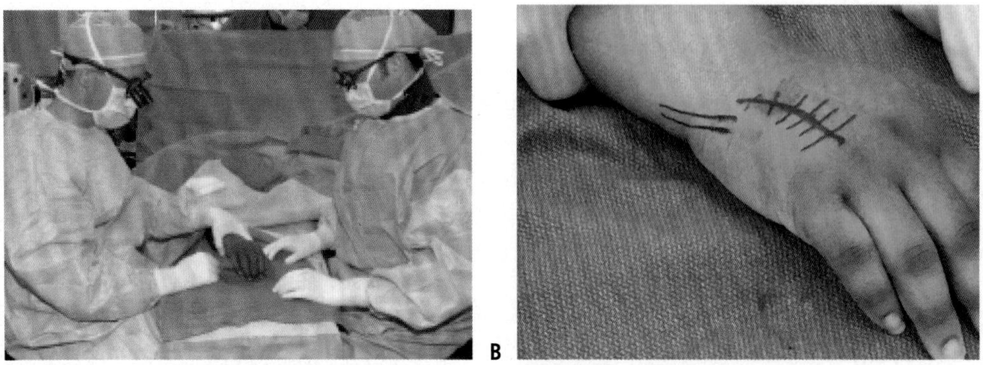

A B

FIG 5 **A.** Positioning of the surgeon (*left*) and assistant (*right*). **B.** Skin incision marked with probable course of the nerve.

DIFFERENTIAL DIAGNOSIS

- Metacarpal fracture
- Carpal bone fracture
- Fracture associated with neurovascular injury

NONOPERATIVE MANAGEMENT

- Nondisplaced injuries may be treated in a below-elbow cast that incorporates the metacarpophalangeal (MCP) joint(s) of the affected digit(s) and adjacent digit(s).[7,11]
  - Special attention should be paid to placing the MCP joints in the intrinsic-plus position. If the MCP joints are immobilized in extension, then a capsular contracture can develop relatively quickly.
- Radiographs following cast immobilization should be checked carefully to ensure that no dorsal subluxation has occurred.
  - X-rays should be repeated on a weekly basis for the first 2 weeks to monitor displacement.
- Metacarpal base fractures, especially fracture dislocations, have a propensity for recurrent dislocation following reduction. Most of these will require surgical fixation.[2,6,11] Some authors believe that nonoperative management can play a role despite shortening and intra-articular displacement.[6,14]

SURGICAL MANAGEMENT

Preoperative Planning

- Careful review of all imaging studies will facilitate planning of fracture fragment exposure and identify sites for internal fixation.

Positioning

- Place the patient supine on a regular operating table with the standard arm table.
- Often times, the surgeon is more comfortable sitting on the head side of the arm table. This helps with avoiding neck straining that may result from trying to look "over the top" that happens when the arm externally rotates while the surgeon is seating on the axilla side of the arm table **(FIG 5A)**.

Approach

- A dorsal extensile approach provides satisfactory exposure of any of the CMC joints.
- Incisions placed between metacarpals allow for access to two adjacent joints.
- Marking out the anticipated locations of nearby nerve branches can be helpful **(FIG 5B)**.

TECHNIQUES

DORSAL EXPOSURE

- Following incision of the skin, careful spreading dissection should be used to locate and protect the dorsal cutaneous nerve branches in the operative field.
- Ulnar sensory nerve branches are most commonly encountered during dorsal exposure of the CMC joints of the RF and SF **(TECH FIG 1A–C)**, and radial sensory nerves are typically encountered during exposure of the index and middle finger CMC joints.
- Extensor tendons are mobilized and retracted utilizing a no-touch technique whenever possible.

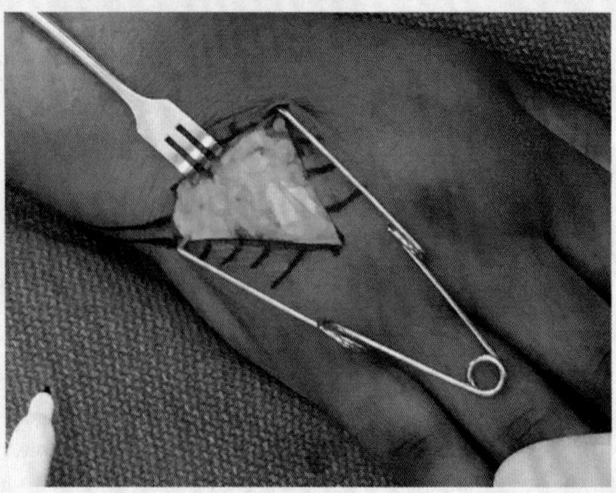

TECH FIG 1 **A.** Dorsal incision with dorsal cutaneous nerve exposed. *(continued)* A

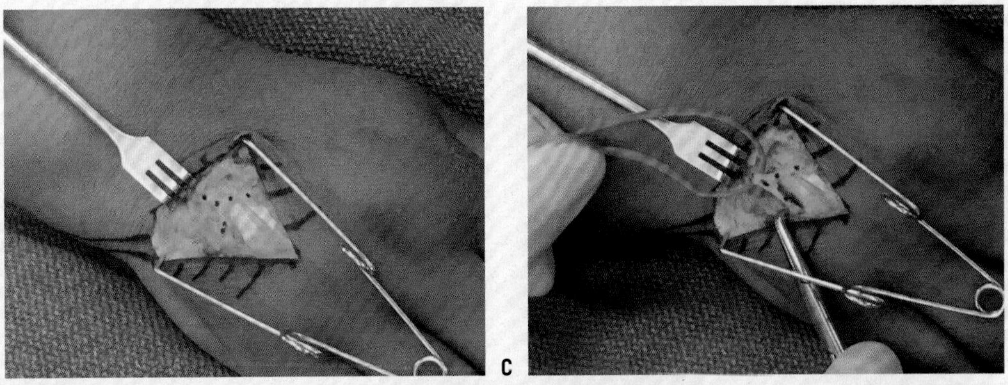

B C

TECH FIG 1 *(continued)* **B.** Dorsal cutaneous nerve drawn out with purple dots. **C.** Dorsal cutaneous nerve retracted with vessel loops.

FRACTURE EXPOSURE

- CMC capsular incisions should be planned to allow for closure following fracture and joint reduction/stabilization.
- Careful mobilization of the fracture fragments with minimal soft tissue stripping is critical.
- Exposure can be facilitated by the use of a Beaver blade, a dental pick, and a fine synovial rongeur **(TECH FIG 2A,B)**.
  - The rongeur is useful in this situation to help débride any fracture callous and hematoma.

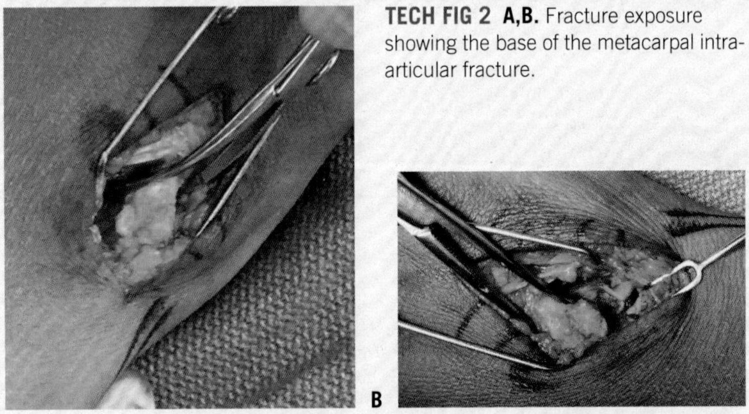

A B

TECH FIG 2 A,B. Fracture exposure showing the base of the metacarpal intra-articular fracture.

FRACTURE REDUCTION

- The fracture is then reduced and held provisionally using fine smooth Kirschner wires (K-wires) **(TECH FIG 3A)**.
  - The surgeon must be aware of the planned location for definitive hardware placement, given the limited room available.
  - K-wires temporarily driven across the base of the articular fragment into the corresponding carpal bone can be helpful in stabilizing any mobile pieces of bone (see **TECH FIG 3A**).
  - The conventional technique of first reconstructing the articular surface, followed by securing the shaft to the reassembled joint surface, is useful **(TECH FIG 3B)**.
- Confirmation of the provisional reduction should be obtained with fluoroscopy before any definitive screw placement **(TECH FIG 3C,D)**.
- The corresponding articular surface on the uninjured bone is useful as a template and also helps mold the small bone fragments into position.
  - This technique works regardless of whether the injury is in the metacarpal base, as pictured in the figures, or in a distal articular injury of one of the carpal bones.

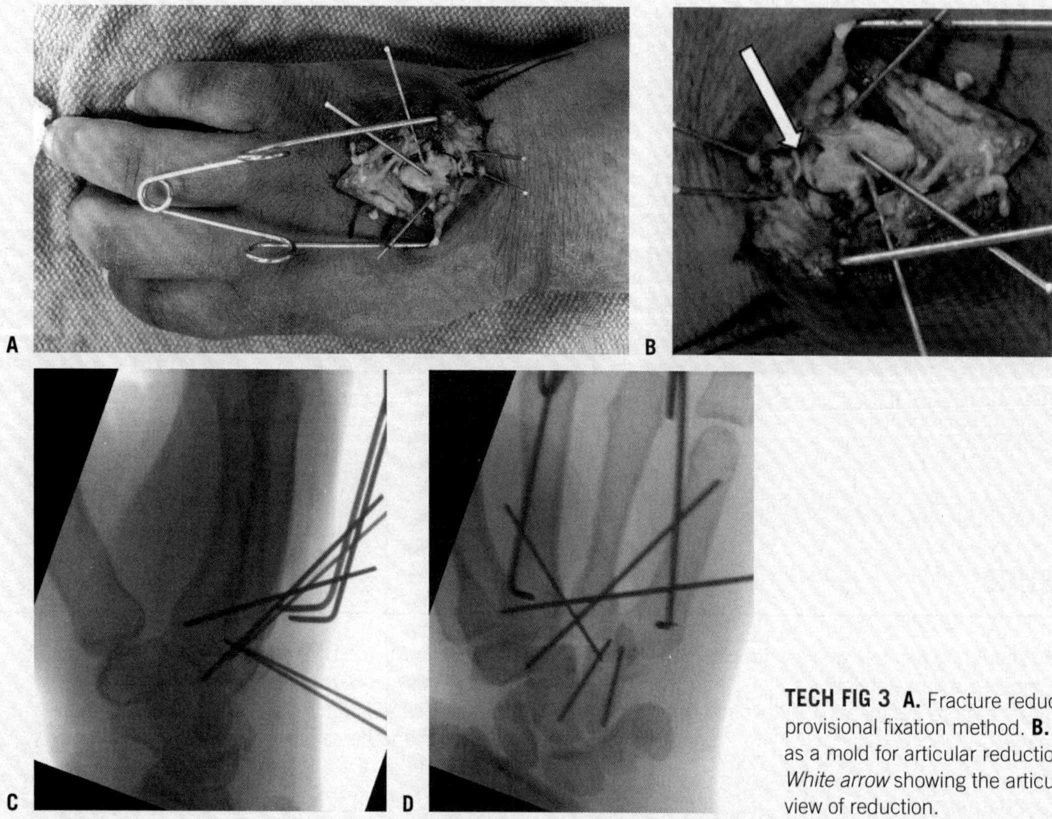

TECH FIG 3 **A.** Fracture reduction using K-wires as a provisional fixation method. **B.** Using the hamate surface as a mold for articular reduction of the metacarpal base. *White arrow* showing the articulartion. **C,D.** Fluoroscopic view of reduction.

DEFINITIVE FIXATION

- K-wires can be replaced by screws if fragment size permits **(TECH FIG 4A)**.
  - Placing the fragments under compression manually and inserting static screws sometimes is preferable to using the lag screw technique, which requires overdrilling the near side and may risk iatrogenic comminution.
- Simple K-wire fixation is satisfactory for isolated dislocations with or without fracture **(TECH FIG 4B,C)**.
  - The insertion point for a percutaneous wire often is distant from the dislocation site in a crushed and severely swollen hand.

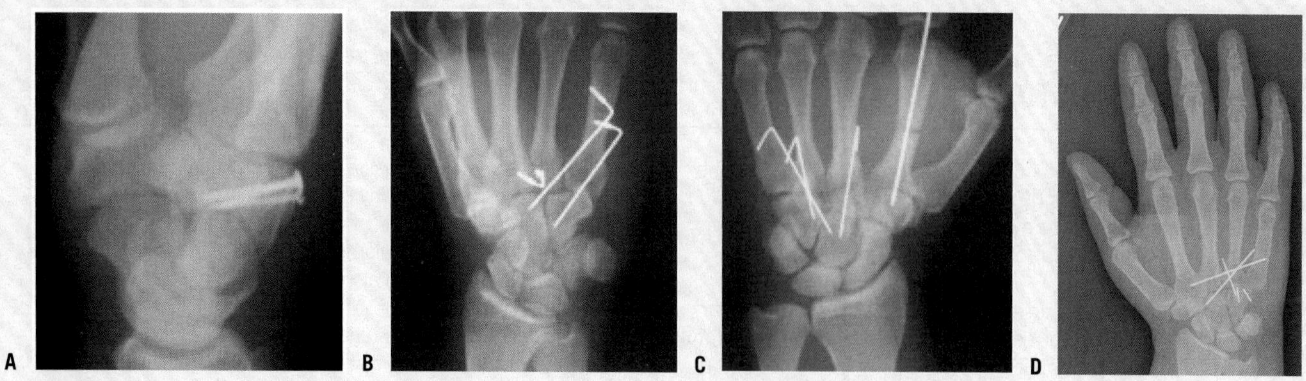

TECH FIG 4 A. Dorsal hamate lip fixation with three screws. **B.** Fracture-dislocation of the RF and SF metacarpal bases using K-wires and a screw. **C.** Percutaneous K-wire fixation of a metacarpal shaft fracture and CMC dislocation. **D.** K-wire fixation of dorsal hamate fracture and RF metacarpal shaft.

ADJUNCTIVE TECHNIQUES

- The construct can be protected by placing the affected metacarpal under slight distraction and pinning it to the adjacent metacarpal **(TECH FIG 5)**.
- Alternatively, the proximally directed deforming force of the extensor carpi ulnaris can be reduced by detaching it from the base of the SF metacarpal at the beginning of the procedure and securing it to the hamate at the close, thereby avoiding proximal pull on the base of the SF metacarpal.
  - We have never found it necessary to use this alternative approach, but it may be helpful in a delayed presentation.

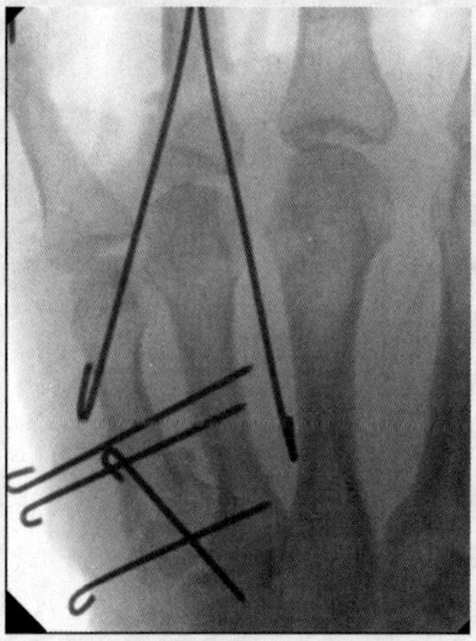

TECH FIG 5 Pinning of the fractured metacarpal to the adjacent metacarpal to allow for construct protection.

Pearls and Pitfalls

Imaging	• Ensure that adequate radiographs are available for intraoperative review. • If necessary, obtain a CT scan prior to operative fixation.
Positioning	• It is often easier for the surgeon to be seated on the outside of the hand table, instead of in the axilla between the table and patient, due to the limited internal rotation present in the shoulder, which can make visualization difficult from the usual seating position.
Exposure	• The dorsal cutaneous branch of the ulnar nerve crosses the incision obliquely and lies immediately across the operative field for exposure of the fourth and fifth CMC joints. Symptomatic neuromas are often associated with cutting the nerve. However, the sensory deficit is typically well tolerated.
Fracture Management	• Fragments can be small, and periosteal stripping can lead to devitalization. Use fracture lines for visualization of the articular surface as much as possible. A dental pick, fine K-wire joysticks, and provisional fixation before final screw placement can be helpful. Provisional fixation should be completed with careful attention to the anticipated placement of definitive fixation. Avoid malrotation of the shaft during reduction by grasping it together with one or two adjacent metacarpals when aligning it relative to the joint. A small degree of malrotation at the base of the metacarpal can lead to a substantial distal overlap of the digits.
Postoperative Protection	• Consider placing a temporary distraction K-wire between adjacent metacarpals to limit the load placed on the articular surface before it has healed.

POSTOPERATIVE CARE

- Aftercare following operative fixation falls into three general phases:
  - Acute swelling control and wound healing (10 to 14 days)
  - Fracture consolidation and maintenance of digit range of motion (4 to 6 weeks)
  - Restoration of global hand function and strength (2 to 6 months)
- Immediate measures following surgery include strict elevation and range-of-motion exercises through a full arc of motion.[6] This limits swelling, reduces pain, and prevents accumulation of protein-rich edema fluid that will slow rehabilitation.
- The relative speed at which the hand can be mobilized during the weeks after surgery depends on a number of factors, including the magnitude of the original injury, stability of fixation, reliability of the patient, and specific occupational or athletic requirements.
- The radiograph in **TECH FIG 4A** shows the hand of a physician with stable fixation of a dorsal hamate injury who was mobilized and given a 1-lb lifting restriction shortly after surgery to allow continuation of his residency training.
  - In contrast, unreliable patients require immobilization for 6 weeks in a cast (see **TECH FIG 4B,C**).
- Patients should be warned that full grip strength is the last thing that will recover and may take multiple months.[2]

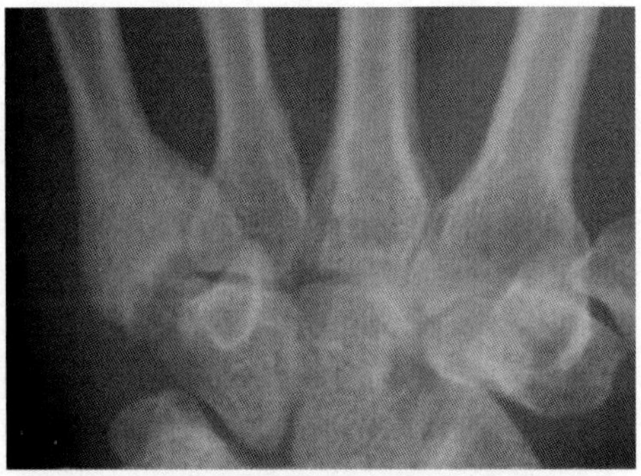

FIG 6 Radiograph taken several months following K-wire fixation of a fracture-dislocation of the fifth CMC joint. Fragments were too small for screw fixation and were resorbed.

Often times, patients will report pain even with a hand shake for an extended period of time.

OUTCOMES

- Opinions on outcomes vary with regard to overall success. A dichotomy exists between recommendation for operative and nonsurgical treatment. Kjaer-Petersen and colleagues[8] found that, regardless of treatment, long-term symptoms were present in 38% of patients at 4.3 years follow-up.
- Petrie and Lamb[14] who used unrestricted, immediate motion, reported on their results at 4.5 years and found that even with metacarpal shortening and irregularities in the articular surface, only one patient had work limitations.
- Another study found that pain was related to the degree of posttraumatic arthritis secondary to articular incongruity and advocated anatomic reduction and internal fixation.[13]
- Multiple CMC dislocations were reviewed by Lawliss and Gunther,[9] and they showed poor results in dislocations of the index and middle finger CMC dislocations (which requires higher energy for dislocation) and in those patients with an ulnar nerve injury.
- Gehrmann et al[5] showed that overall Disability of the Arm, Shoulder, and Hand (DASH) scores for SF or combined SF and RF fracture-dislocations after treatment had no significant difference, with DASH scores of 7.2 and 6.0, respectively.

COMPLICATIONS

- Complications include those common to any periarticular surgery:
  - Failure of wound healing
  - Hematoma formation
  - Neurovascular injury
  - Neuroma formation
  - Tendon adhesions
  - Posttraumatic arthritis
  - Nonunion or malunion
  - Joint stiffness
  - Weakness
- Occasionally, small fragments may resorb, leading to collapse and articular incongruity **(FIG 6)**.
- Long-term arthritis can be treated with fusion of the affected joint.[12]
- Alternatively, an interposition "anchovy" using the palmaris longus as a biologic spacer can be inserted after resection of the arthritic joint surfaces, analogous to that performed for thumb basal joint arthritis.[4]

REFERENCES

1. Bergfield TG, DuPuy TE, Aulicino PL. Fracture-dislocations of all five carpometacarpal joints: a case report. J Hand Surg Am 1985;10:76–78.
2. Bora FW Jr, Didizian NH. The treatment of injuries to the carpometacarpal joint of the little finger. J Bone Joint Surg Am 1974;56A:1459–1463.
3. Day CS, Stern PJ. Fractures of the metacarpals and phalanges. In: Wolfe SW, Hotchkiss RN, Pederson WC, et al, eds. Green's Operative Hand Surgery, ed 6. Philadelphia: Churchill Livingstone, 2011:239–290.
4. Gainor BJ, Stark HH, Ashworth CR, et al. Tendon arthroplasty of the fifth carpometacarpal joint for treatment of posttraumatic arthritis. J Hand Surg Am 1991;16:520–524.
5. Gehrmann SV, Kaufmann RA, Grassman JP, et al. Fracture-dislocations of the carpometacarpal joints of the ring and little finger. J Hand Surg Eur Vol 2015;40(1):84–87.
6. Glickel SZ, Barron OA, Catalano LW. Dislocations and ligament injuries in the digits. In: Green DP, Hotchkiss RN, Pederson WC, et al, eds. Green's Operative Hand Surgery, ed 5. Philadelphia: Churchill Livingstone, 2005:364–366.
7. Hsu JD, Curtis RM. Carpometacarpal dislocations on the ulnar side of the hand. J Bone Joint Surg Am 1970;52:927–930.
8. Kjaer-Petersen K, Jurik AG, Petersen LK. Intra-articular fractures at the base of the fifth metacarpal. A clinical and radiographical study of 64 cases. J Hand Surg Br 1992;17:144–147.
9. Lawliss JF III, Gunther SF. Carpometacarpal dislocations. Long-term follow-up. J Bone Joint Surg Am 1991;73A:52–58.
10. Lilling M, Weinberg H. The mechanism of dorsal fracture dislocation of the fifth carpometacarpal joint. J Hand Surg Am 1979;4:340–342.
11. Lundeen JM, Shin AY. Clinical results of intraarticular fractures of the base of the fifth metacarpal treated by closed reduction and cast immobilization. J Hand Surg Br 2000;25:258–261.
12. Marck KW, Klasen HJ. Fracture-dislocation of the hamatometacarpal joint: a case report. J Hand Surg Am 1986;11:128–130.
13. Papaloizos MY, Le Moine PH, Prues-Latour V, et al. Proximal fractures of the fifth metacarpal: a retrospective analysis of 25 operated cases. J Hand Surg Br 2000;25:253–257.
14. Petrie PW, Lamb DW. Fracture-subluxation of the base of the fifth metacarpal. Hand 1974;6(1):82–86.
15. Takami H, Takahashi S, Ando M. Isolated volar displaced fracture of the ulnar condyle at the base of the index metacarpal: a case report. J Hand Surg Am 1997;22(6):1064–1066.

CHAPTER 19

Surgical Treatment of Thumb Carpometacarpal Joint Fractures, Dislocations, and Instabilities

Chia H. Wu, Richard Kim, and Robert J. Strauch

DEFINITION

- The first carpometacarpal (CMC) joint comprises the thumb metacarpal base and the trapezium.
- The thumb CMC joint is vital to the function of the hand, and injuries can result in pain, weakness, and loss of grip or pinch strength. Thumb CMC joint instability can occur as a result of ligament laxity or trauma.
  - The most common instability pattern comes from injury to or incompetence of the dorsoradial ligament, resulting in dorsoradial subluxation of the thumb metacarpal.
- Two fracture-dislocation patterns commonly result from trauma to the thumb CMC joint: *Bennett* and *Rolando* fractures.
  - Bennett fractures are intra-articular fractures in which the metacarpal shaft is radially displaced by the pull of the abductor pollicis longus (APL) tendon, leaving an intact ulnar fragment at the base of the thumb metacarpal that is held reduced by the volar beak ligament **(FIG 1A)**.
  - Rolando fractures are complex intra-articular fractures involving the base of the thumb metacarpal that often have a T- or Y-type pattern. These fractures are classically described as being three-part; however, the name also applies to more comminuted fracture variants **(FIG 1B)**.

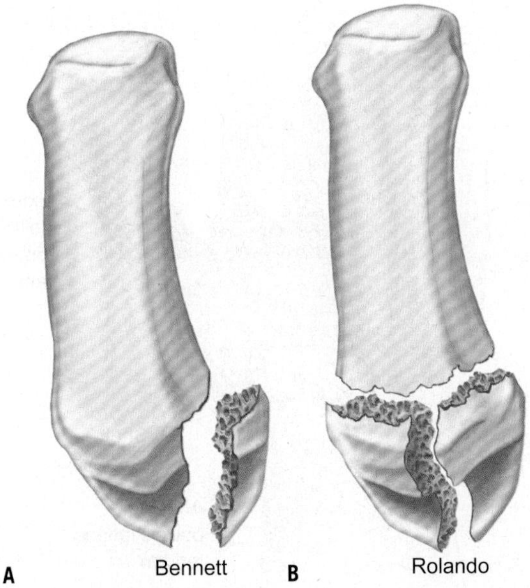

FIG 1 **A.** A typical Bennett fracture is a unicondylar fracture of the base of the first metacarpal with the fracture fragment consisting of the volar ulnar corner of the proximal metacarpal. **B.** A Rolando fracture is multifragmentary, with the entire articular base of the metacarpal being involved. By definition, no portion of the metacarpal shaft is in continuity with the CMC joint.

ANATOMY

- Understanding the deforming forces in these fracture-dislocations is important when deciding on treatment options and determining prognosis.
- The thumb metacarpal serves as the site of attachment for several tendons, including the APL at the proximal base, the adductor pollicis distally, and the thenar muscles volarly.
- The articular surfaces of the thumb metacarpal base and trapezium resemble a horseback rider's saddle and allow motion in many planes.
  - The base of the thumb metacarpal has a prominent volar styloid process (beak) that articulates with a recess in the volar trapezium when in flexion.
- Sixteen ligaments provide stability to the thumb CMC joint. The two that provide the most restraint against dorsoradial subluxation of the thumb metacarpal are the dorsoradial and volar beak ligaments **(FIG 2A,B)**.[4]
  - The dorsoradial ligament originates from the dorsoradial tubercle of the trapezium and inserts onto the dorsal base of the thumb metacarpal. It is the thickest, widest, shortest, and strongest of the CMC ligaments.
- There are three zones at the base of the thumb metacarpal **(FIG 2C)**:
  - Zone 1: volar aspect of the joint
  - Zone 2: central portion of the joint that is normally loaded
  - Zone 3: dorsal aspect of the joint
- The trapezium has several important adjacent articulations: the first metacarpal base, the radial aspect of the second metacarpal base, the scaphoid, and the trapezoid **(FIG 3)**.
  - Along with the trapezium, these last two make up the scaphotrapeziotrapezoid (STT) joint.

PATHOGENESIS

- The biconcave–convex nature of the thumb CMC joint allows for a wide range of thumb motion but is inherently unstable.
  - Pathologic instability can be a result of ligament incompetence, fracture, or both. It is worth noting that ligament incompetence can be from injury of supporting ligaments, especially the dorsoradial ligaments, or collagen disorders such as Ehlers-Danlos syndrome.

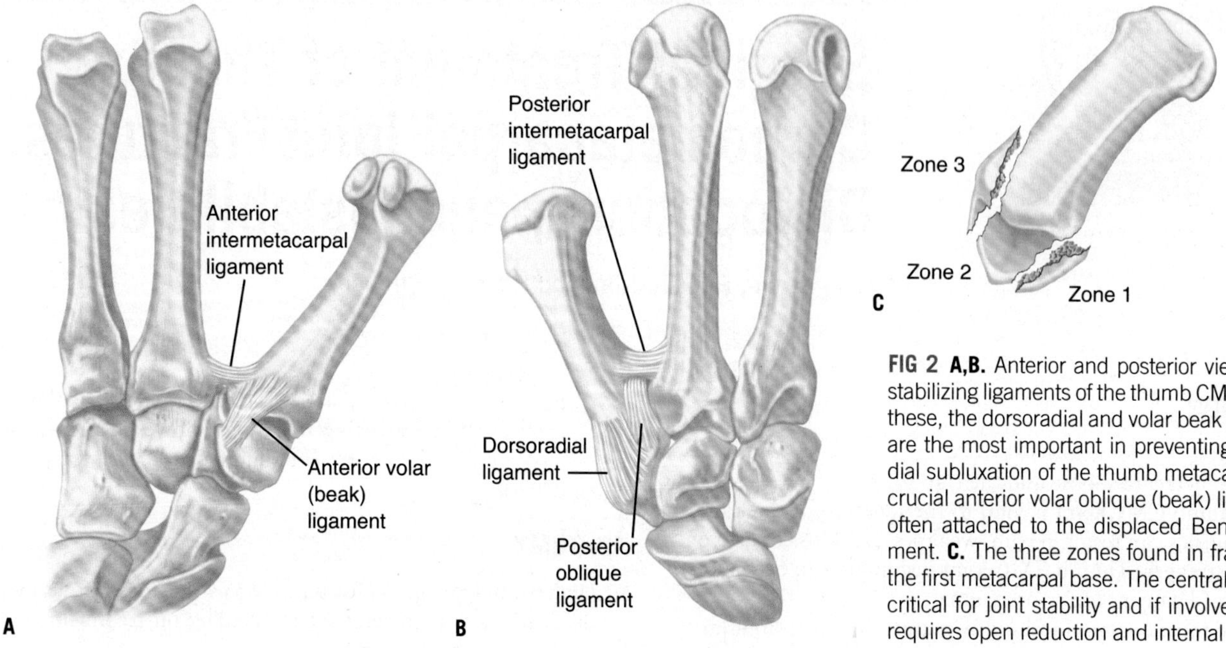

FIG 2 A,B. Anterior and posterior views of the stabilizing ligaments of the thumb CMC joint. Of these, the dorsoradial and volar beak ligaments are the most important in preventing dorsoradial subluxation of the thumb metacarpal. The crucial anterior volar oblique (beak) ligament is often attached to the displaced Bennett fragment. **C.** The three zones found in fractures of the first metacarpal base. The central zone 2 is critical for joint stability and if involved usually requires open reduction and internal fixation.

- Bennett fractures occur when the partially flexed thumb metacarpal is axially loaded, resulting in a Bennett articular fragment (the volar ulnar portion of the metacarpal base). The remainder of the metacarpal displaces dorsally, proximally, and radially.
- Rolando fractures result from a similar injury mechanism and may have a variable degree of comminution at the base of the thumb metacarpal.
- In Bennett-type fractures, the thumb metacarpal shaft is displaced dorsally and proximally by the pull of the APL at the metacarpal base, the extensor pollicis longus (EPL) which inserts more distally, and adducted and supinated by the opponens pollicis (**FIG 4**).
- Rolando-type fractures are subject to the same deforming forces, except that the APL can sometimes displace both the shaft and the dorsoradial basilar articular fragment.
- Because of the deforming forces that act on the fracture fragments, both injury patterns are usually unstable and difficult to reduce and stabilize by closed means only.

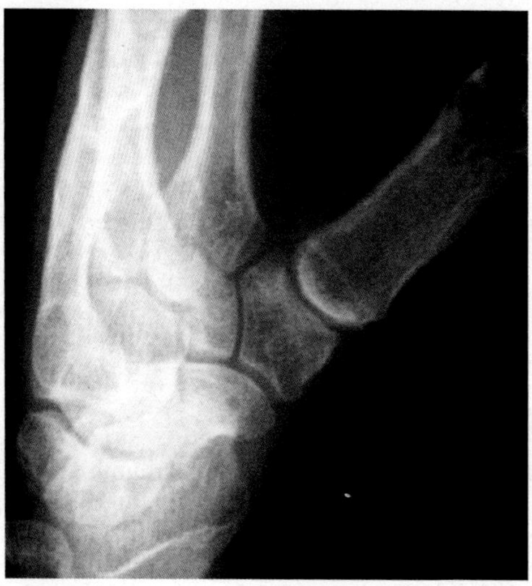

FIG 3 A radiographic view of the trapezium and its articulations including the basal joint. The view is taken with the patient's arm abducted 45 degrees with the hand pronated 45 degrees with the x-ray beam vertically oriented. This evaluates both sides of the basal joint and associated trapezial joint fractures. (Copyright Joshua Mitgang, MD.)

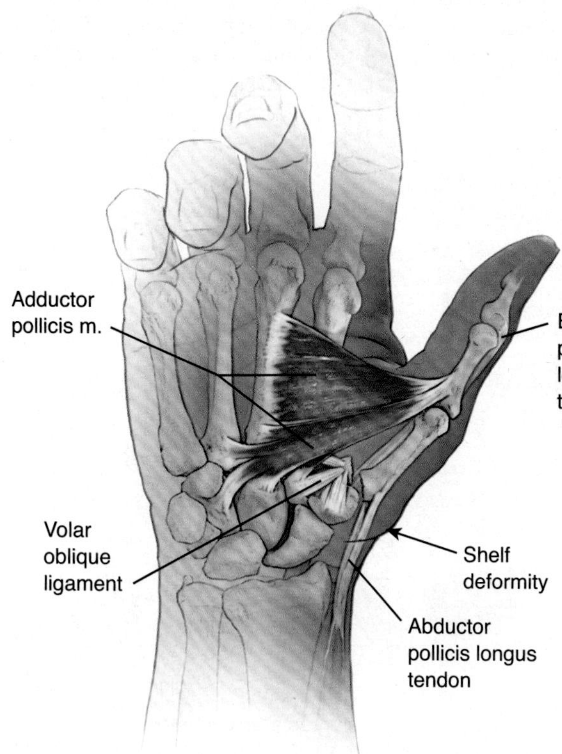

FIG 4 The typical deforming forces about a Bennett fracture. The APL and EPL serve to subluxate the main portion of the thumb metacarpal dorsally and radially, whereas the adductor pollicis rotates the fragment ulnarly. The volar oblique ligament holds the volar ulnar fragment of the thumb metacarpal in place.

NATURAL HISTORY

- Ligamentous laxity at the thumb CMC joint may cause degenerative changes to the joint cartilage and lead to arthritis, corresponding to higher stages in the Eaton-Littler staging system.
  - If the ligamentous laxity is symptomatic and causing pain, ligament reconstruction can be successful in reducing pain in over 90% of patients in the absence of preexisting arthritis. Ligament reconstruction resulting in a more stable joint has also been shown to potentially halt the progression of arthritis.[6]
- Injuries to the thumb metacarpal base represent 80% of all thumb metacarpal fractures.
- Nonoperative treatment is generally reserved for nondisplaced or minimally displaced fractures. Maintenance of reduction for displaced or comminuted fractures with a cast is unlikely.
- Residual subluxation of the metacarpal shaft leads to basal joint incongruity and the potential for developing posttraumatic arthrosis. In addition, residual intra-articular step-off greater than 1 mm may predispose the patient to the development of arthrosis.[3]

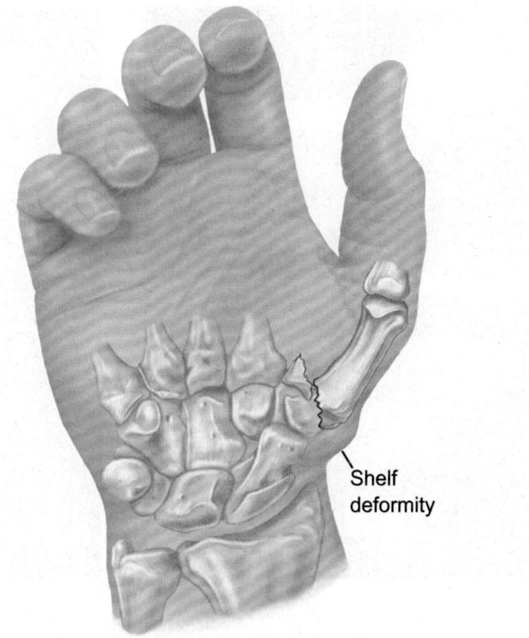

FIG 5 A typical shelf deformity is depicted in a Bennett fracture. When viewing the thumb from the lateral perspective, the thumb metacarpal shaft can be seen riding dorsally as it displaces from the unstable CMC joint.

PATIENT HISTORY AND PHYSICAL FINDINGS

- The history should include questions about general ligament laxity involving other joints as well as preexisting arthritis. Metabolic diseases such as Ehlers-Danlos syndrome are notable.
- Most of the fractures of the base of the thumb occur with direct trauma to the thumb, often from a fall or sports-related injury. The injury is most common in young males, and two-thirds occur in the dominant hand.
- Common physical examination findings include tenderness and ecchymosis surrounding the thumb CMC joint, crepitus with attempted motion, instability, and a "shelf" deformity resulting from displacement of the metacarpal shaft dorsally and radially (**FIG 5**).
- Function of the EPL, flexor pollicis longus, and extensor pollicis brevis should be confirmed.
- The thumb metacarpophalangeal (MCP) joint should also be examined for possible hyperextension laxity.
  - Range of motion is decreased and may be associated with crepitus. Adjacent joints may also have arthrosis and decreased range of motion.
- It is important to perform a complete neurovascular examination and to search for associated pathology such as wrist ligamentous injuries.
  - Neurovascular injuries are uncommon, but compartment syndrome should be suspected in higher energy injuries. A case study describing thenar compartment syndrome from a thumb metacarpal base fracture has been reported.[20]
  - The hand should also be evaluated for concomitant carpal tunnel syndrome, flexor carpi radialis tunnel syndrome, and de Quervain tenosynovitis.

IMAGING AND OTHER DIAGNOSTIC STUDIES

- Posteroanterior (PA), lateral, and oblique images of the hand should be obtained, although the oblique plane of the thumb in relation to the hand may make these images difficult to interpret.
  - A true anteroposterior (AP) view of the thumb CMC joint, known as the *Roberts view*, can be obtained with the forearm maximally pronated with the dorsum of the thumb placed on the cassette (**FIG 6A**).
  - A true lateral view is obtained with the hand pronated 20 degrees and the thumb positioned flat on the cassette. The x-ray beam is tilted 10 degrees from vertical in a distal to proximal direction (**FIG 6B**).[14]
  - A 30-degree oblique stress view of the thumb CMC joint is performed by pressing the radial side of the thumb tips together. This maneuver will subluxate the thumb metacarpal base radially, thereby demonstrating the degree of laxity in the radial direction.
  - A traction view may be helpful in Rolando-type fractures (**FIG 6C**).
- Radiographs of the contralateral, uninjured basal joint are helpful in certain cases as a template for reconstruction.
- Computed tomography may be indicated if a significant amount of articular comminution is present or when plain films inadequately demonstrate the pathology.
- Fluoroscopy alone should be used with caution when ensuring fracture and joint reduction (eg, after closed treatment), as this has recently been shown to be less accurate than plain x-rays or direct visualization.[2]

DIFFERENTIAL DIAGNOSIS

- Bennett-type fracture
- Rolando-type fracture
- Basal joint degenerative joint disease
- STT joint arthrosis
- Thumb CMC joint ligamentous injury
- Trapezial body fracture
- C6 radiculopathy
- Flexor carpi radialis tunnel syndrome
- De Quervain tenosynovitis

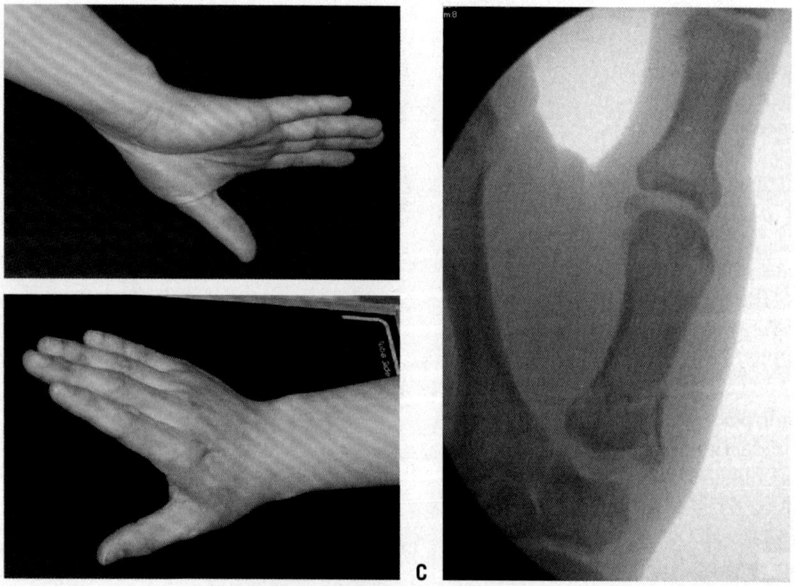

A B C

FIG 6 **A.** An ideal AP view of the thumb and CMC joint is taken with the forearm hyperpronated and the dorsum of the thumb on the cassette. **B.** A true lateral view of the CMC joint is obtained with the radial aspect of the thumb on the cassette and the other fingers clear of the x-ray beam. **C.** A fluoroscopic view of a Rolando fracture with traction applied. Distraction at the CMC joint helps to delineate the fragments at the base of the metacarpal. (Copyright John T. Capo, MD.)

NONOPERATIVE MANAGEMENT

- Instability from ligamentous laxity
  - Symptomatic ligament laxity and stage I or II basal joint disease should be treated conservatively first. This includes thumb spica splint immobilization and anti-inflammatory medications.[7]
  - If the symptoms do not improve, a steroid injection into the CMC joint can be attempted. The number of injections should be limited to a maximum of three; theoretically, more than three injections can increase joint destruction.
- Instability from thumb metacarpal base fractures
  - Nondisplaced, minimally comminuted fractures may be treated with closed reduction and thumb spica casting, but precise molding of the cast and close observation for fracture displacement are necessary.
  - In a Bennett fracture, closed treatment may be indicated if there is minimal displacement between the volar ulnar fragment and the metacarpal shaft. Most importantly, a concentric reduction of the thumb CMC joint in Bennett fractures must be maintained.[3]
- Several factors make closed treatment of these intra-articular fractures problematic:
  - Providing accurate three-point molding of the thumb metacarpal
  - Delay in treatment of 4 or more days after the initial injury
  - Assessing the adequacy of reduction with radiographs taken through the cast
- Decreased motion, grip strength, and radiographic evidence of degenerative joint disease have been seen at long-term follow-up after closed treatment.
- Development of degenerative changes may occur if there is any residual subluxation of the thumb metacarpal shaft.
  - Based on reported evidence, McCarthy and Awan[12] reiterate a useful algorithm for treatment.
  - After accurate physical and radiographic diagnosis of a thumb CMC joint dislocation, closed reduction and splint immobilization should be first attempted. If reduction without subluxation is achieved, cast treatment can be attempted.
  - If subluxation persists in the acute setting, surgical open dorsoradial ligament repair with/without suture anchors and temporary pin fixation is the author-preferred option.
  - For cases of chronic subluxation/dislocation, ligament reconstruction with tendon graft is likely the preferred option.

SURGICAL MANAGEMENT

Instability Attributed to Ligamentous Laxity

- The goal of surgery is to restore the articular congruity of the thumb CMC joint and to align the articular surfaces of the first metacarpal base and the trapezium.
  - Freedman et al[6] hypothesized that open ligament reconstruction for symptomatic thumb CMC joint laxity could potentially halt or slow the progression to degenerative arthritis.
  - In the presence of articular pathology, arthroplasty may be the treatment of choice, depending on the degree of chondromalacia.
  - If greater than 30 degrees of MCP hyperextension is present with lateral pinch, MCP capsulodesis or arthrodesis may also need to be considered, especially if the metacarpophalangeal joint collapses into hyperextension with attempted key pinch.
  - While ligament reconstruction is superior to percutaneous pinning of unstable joints in traumatic thumb CMC joint dislocations in adults; in children, reduction along with percutaneous pinning has been shown to be an effective option without the need for open ligament repair.[17]

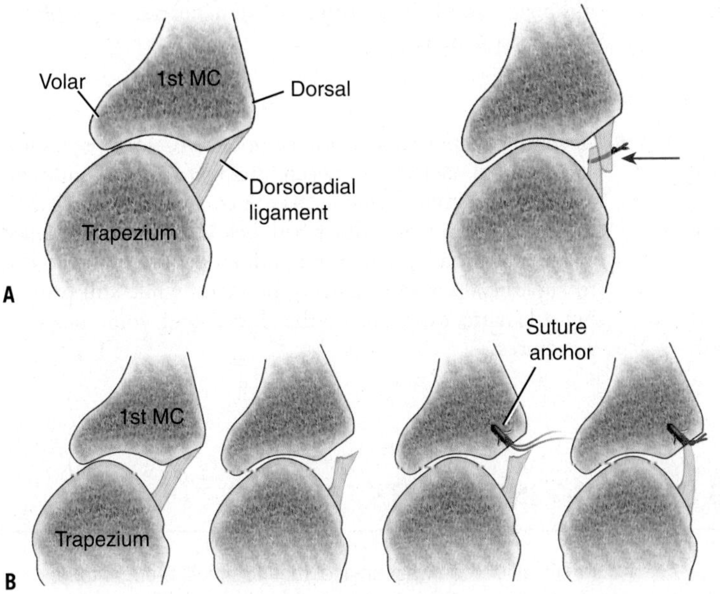

FIG 7 A. Rayan and Do's technique for thumb CMC stabilization: The dorsoradial ligament is imbricated and tightened and the CMC joint is pinned with a 0.045 K-wire for 4 weeks. **B.** The technique favored by Rosenwasser: The dorsoradial ligament is advanced into a suture anchor placed into the thumb metacarpal base in order to stabilize the CMC joint. The joint is immobilized in a thumb spica splint for 4 weeks, no pin is used. *MC*, metacarpophalangeal.

- Rayan and Do[15] described a method for capsulodesis of the important dorsoradial ligament in the setting of either traumatic CMC joint instability or early Eaton stage I disease ligament laxity **(FIG 7A)**. The technique is an imbrication of the dorsoradial ligament followed by trapeziometacarpal joint pinning.
  - An alternative technique involves advancement of the dorsoradial ligament either distally or proximally by means of a suture anchor placed into either the metacarpal insertion or the trapezial origin of the dorsoradial ligament, respectively **(FIG 7B)**.
  - The senior author (RJS) similarly tightens and advances the dorsoradial ligament by means of a suture anchor placed into its metacarpal insertion. This is a promising technique compared to open ligament reconstruction, although long-term outcomes are not yet reported.[1]
- When the injury pattern results in fracture-dislocations such as unstable Bennett and Rolando fractures, percutaneous pinning or open reduction and internal fixation should be performed in addition to repair of the dorsoradial ligament.

Instability Attributed to Fracture-Dislocation

Bennett Fractures

- In thumb metacarpal base fractures associated with trapezial body fractures, the articular surface of the trapezium should first be reduced anatomically before treating the thumb metacarpal fracture.[8,14]
- Closed reduction and percutaneous pinning is the preferred treatment for most Bennett fractures, with displaced fracture fragments representing less than 25% to 30% of the articular surface.[4,14] The metacarpal base often needs to be pinned to the second metacarpal, trapezoid, or trapezium to lessen the deforming forces on the fracture.
- Open reduction is necessary when there is residual displacement of the joint surface greater than 2 mm after attempted closed reduction and percutaneous pinning, if the fracture occupies more than 25% to 30% of the joint surface, or if there is impaction in the force-bearing aspect of the joint surface (Buchler zone 2).
  - A 2-mm or greater step-off has been significantly associated with development of posttraumatic arthritis.[10]
  - A systematic review reported that posttraumatic arthritis was present in approximately 26% and 58% of patients who underwent closed reduction with pinning and open reduction, respectively.[16]

Rolando Fractures

- Closed reduction with longitudinal traction and percutaneous pinning is indicated if successful reduction can be achieved under fluoroscopic guidance; this is rarely successful and only when large T- or Y-type fragments are present.
- If the joint cannot be reduced by closed methods, open reduction and internal fixation with a combination of smooth wires; screws; and 1.5- to 2.7-mm L, T, or blade plates are indicated.
- Significant comminution may require either external fixation or a combination of external fixation, limited internal fixation with Kirschner wires (K-wires) and small (1.3 or 1.5 mm) screws, and cancellous bone grafting.

Preoperative Planning

- A thorough history and physical examination are mandatory to choose the appropriate treatment and rule out associated injuries.
- True PA, lateral, and oblique radiographs of the thumb should be obtained in all cases along with the specific views detailed previously. Traction radiographs help assess the effects of ligamentotaxis on fracture reduction.
- A preoperative Allen test should be performed because all procedures involving the thumb CMC joint are in close proximity to the radial artery and iatrogenic injury may occur.
- Surgery may be performed acutely, but if significant soft tissue swelling is present, elevation in a well-padded thumb

spica splint for 2 to 5 days may be necessary before undergoing operative fixation.[14]

Positioning

- The patient is placed supine on the operating room table.
- A radiolucent hand table is used to allow for intraoperative fluoroscopy.
- The patient is moved toward the operative side to center the hand on the table.
- A nonsterile tourniquet is placed on the upper arm.
- General, regional (axillary or infraclavicular), or local (wrist block with local infiltration) anesthesia can be used, although muscle relaxation is often necessary to obtain proper reduction.[4,14]

Approach

- A common approach to the thumb CMC joint is a short longitudinal incision between the first and second dorsal extensor compartments, centered over the first CMC joint. The technique described below uses the modified Wagner approach, which the authors believe limit the risk to superficial cutaneous nerve branches while still providing adequate exposure of the dorsal and volar ligament structures.

LIGAMENT RECONSTRUCTION FOR THUMB CMC JOINT INSTABILITY

- The dorsal ligaments are the most important stabilizers of the thumb CMC joint.[11] The goal is to restore the stability of the CMC injury by restoring the critical anatomy.
- A number of techniques have been described for ligament reconstruction of the thumb CMC joint using a variety of different tendons, including the flexor carpi radialis, palmaris longus, extensor carpi radialis longus, extensor pollicis brevis, and APL.
  - The technique presented here is the classic volar ligament reconstruction,[5] which effectively reconstructs both the volar and dorsal ligaments using a portion of the flexor carpi radialis.

Modified Wagner Approach

- The incision is started longitudinally along the radial side of the thenar mass in the midportion of the metacarpal, at or palmar to the junction between the glabrous and nonglabrous skin **(TECH FIG 1A)**.
- Proximally, at the wrist crease, the incision is brought transversely across the wrist to the ulnar side of the flexor carpi radialis tendon.
- Once through the skin, care should be taken to avoid transection of superficial radial sensory nerve branches that may be crossing the operative field.
- The soft tissue is bluntly dissected until the thenar musculature is identified **(TECH FIG 1B)**.
  - The radial border of the thenar muscle mass is incised, and the muscles are elevated extraperiosteally to expose the CMC joint capsule.
  - The capsule is incised, and the thumb metacarpal base, the CMC joint, and the trapezium exposed **(TECH FIG 1C)**.
- Blunt dissection is continued dorsally toward the EPL and brevis tendons. The dorsal metacarpal cortex is exposed between these tendons.

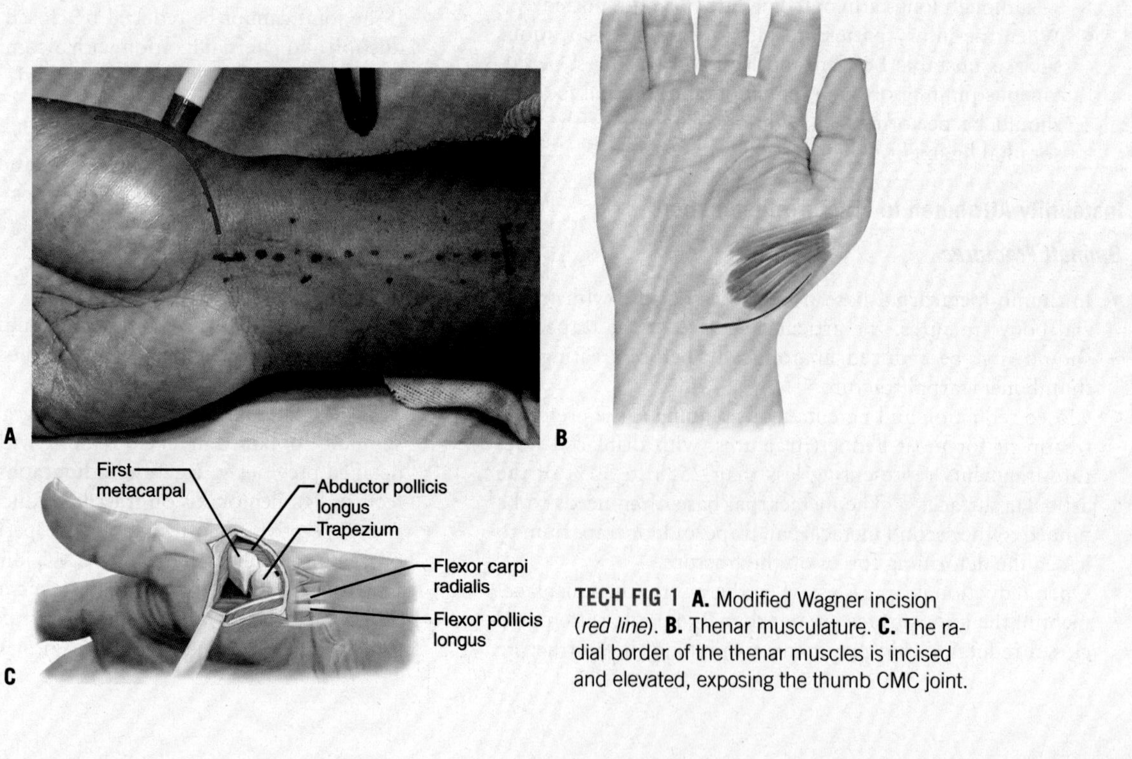

TECH FIG 1 **A.** Modified Wagner incision (*red line*). **B.** Thenar musculature. **C.** The radial border of the thenar muscles is incised and elevated, exposing the thumb CMC joint.

Flexor Carpi Radialis Graft Harvest

- The flexor carpi radialis tendon is identified just radial to the palmaris longus tendon at the wrist crease. The tendon sheath is then opened.
- A transverse incision is made proximally in the forearm overlying the flexor carpi radialis musculotendinous junction, about 8 to 10 cm proximal to the wrist crease **(TECH FIG 2A,B)**.
- The soft tissue is bluntly dissected until the tendon sheath is identified and opened. The flexor carpi radialis tendon is then exposed.
- A longitudinal split is made in the midline of the tendon just proximal to the trapezium. A 0-Prolene suture is then passed through the tendon split **(TECH FIG 2C)**.
- A pediatric feeding tube is now passed from the proximal wound into the distal wound, in the flexor carpi radialis sheath, and superficial to the flexor carpi radialis tendon fibers.
  - The tip of the feeding tube is cut off, and the two ends of the Prolene suture are passed through the end of the feeding tube from distal to proximal.
  - Once the suture is seen in the proximal wound, the feeding tube can be removed, leaving the ends of the Prolene suture in the proximal wound site **(TECH FIG 2D–F)**.
- The two suture ends in the proximal wound are now pulled so that the rest of the suture is delivered from the distal to the proximal wound. In so doing, the suture will divide the flexor carpi radialis tendon in half along its course into the proximal wound **(TECH FIG 2G)**.
- At this time, the ulnar half of the tendon is transected proximally just after the musculotendinous junction. The fibers of the flexor carpi radialis tendon spiral, so the ulnar half of the tendon will continue to become the radial half of the tendon distally at the wrist.
  - Before transection, traction should be applied to the proximal ulnar half of the tendon to ensure that it corresponds to the distal radial half of the tendon.
- The split flexor carpi radialis tendon is finally delivered into the distal wound **(TECH FIG 2H)**.

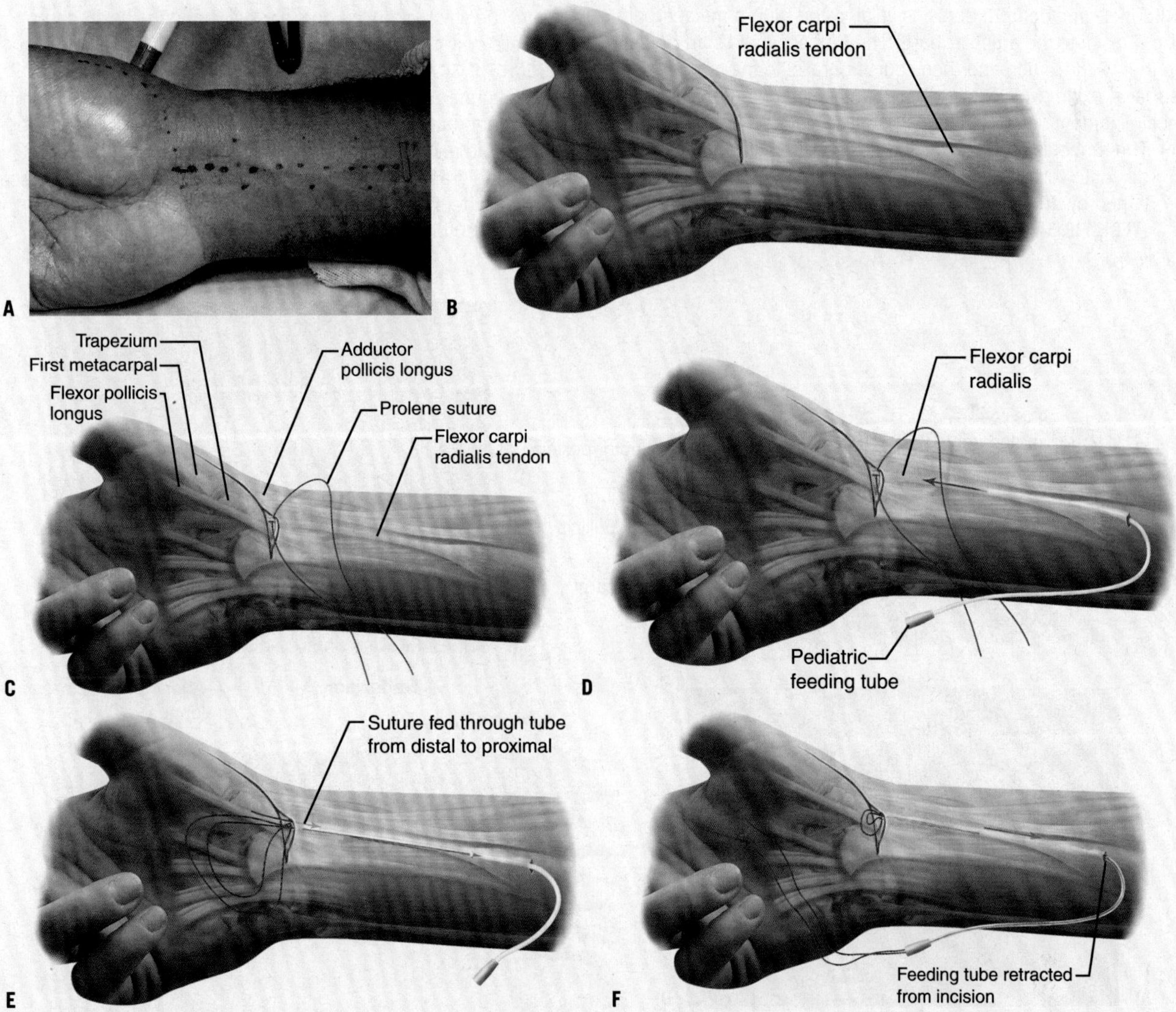

TECH FIG 2 A. Flexor carpi radialis harvest incision is made 8 to 10 cm proximal to the wrist crease (*red line*). **B.** Flexor carpi radialis musculotendinous junction. **C.** A longitudinal split is made through the flexor carpi radialis distally and a 0-Prolene suture is passed through it. **D.** A pediatric feeding tube is passed from the proximal to the distal wound. **E.** The Prolene suture is then passed through the feeding tube from distal to proximal. **F.** The feeding tube is removed, leaving the Prolene suture ends in the proximal wound. *(continued)*

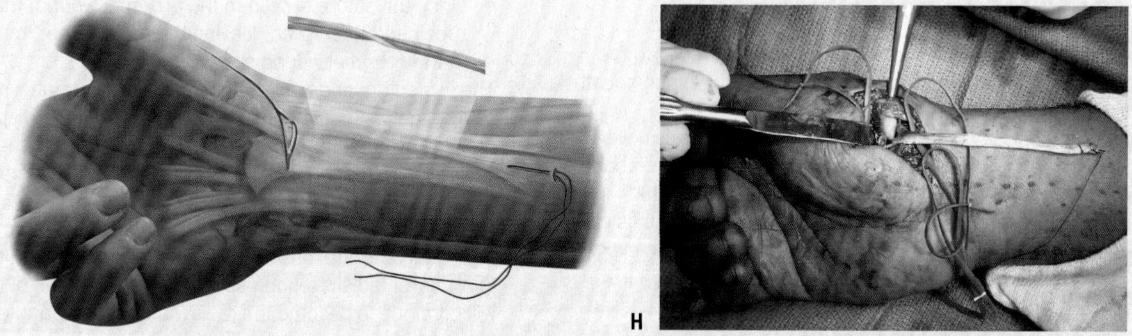

G H

TECH FIG 2 *(continued)* **G.** The two suture ends are pulled, thereby dividing the flexor carpi radialis tendon in half until the proximal wound is reached. The flexor carpi radialis tendon spirals, so the distal radial half corresponds to the proximal ulnar half of the tendon. **H.** The split flexor carpi radialis tendon is delivered into the distal wound.

Metacarpal Tunnel Placement and Flexor Carpi Radialis Graft Passage and Fixation

- A tunnel is made from dorsal to volar in the thumb metacarpal, 1 cm distal to the articular base. The tunnel should start dorsal to the APL insertion and then course parallel to the articular surface, exiting volarly just distal to the insertion of the volar beak ligament onto the metacarpal base.
  - The tunnel is started by first drilling a 0.045 K-wire from dorsal to volar in the manner described. The tunnel is enlarged by drilling a 0.062 K-wire, followed by a 3.5-mm drill **(TECH FIG 3A,B)**.
- Once completed, a nylon whipstitch is placed in the end of the flexor carpi radialis graft. The ends of the stitch are passed through the metacarpal tunnel from a volar to dorsal direction. The stitch is pulled dorsally, delivering the flexor carpi radialis graft through the metacarpal tunnel to the dorsum **(TECH FIG 3C)**.
- As the graft exits the dorsal hole in the metacarpal, the thumb is extended and abducted. The graft is pulled tightly and then allowed to relax 2 to 3 mm to set the appropriate tension.
- Once the graft tension is set, the graft is sutured to the metacarpal periosteum where it exits the dorsal hole using nonabsorbable 3-0 suture material.

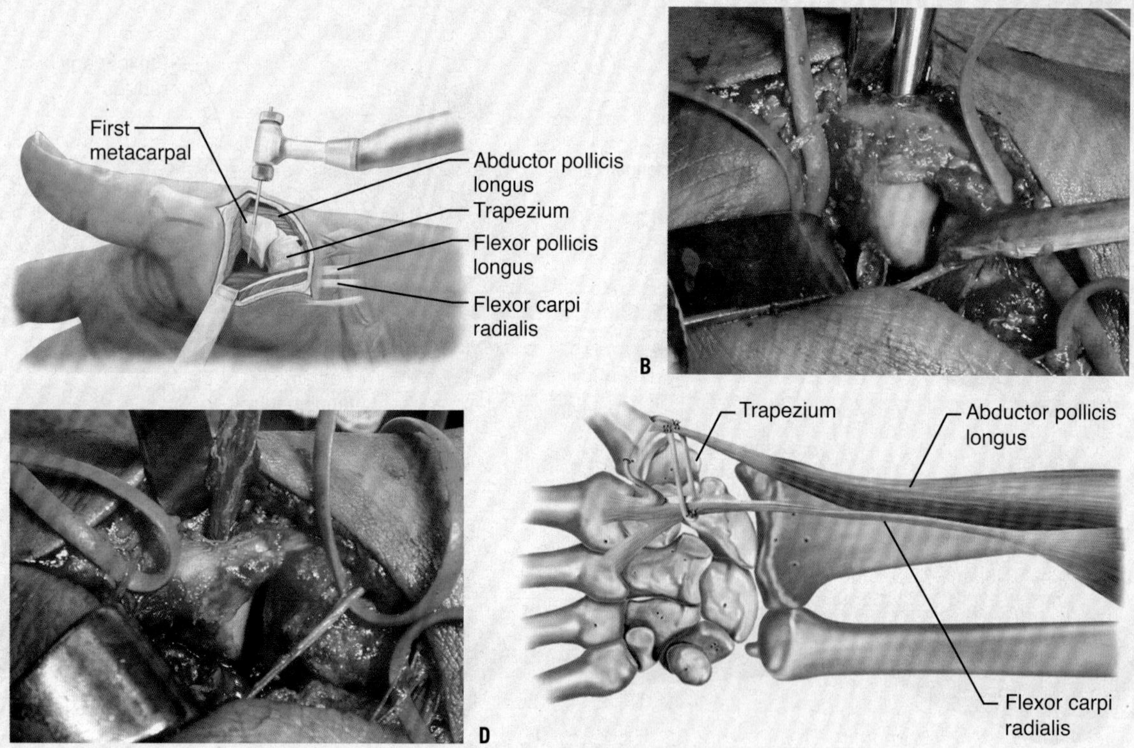

TECH FIG 3 **A.** The tunnel is drilled from dorsal to volar, staying parallel and 1 cm distal to the metacarpal articular base. **B.** A curette is shown in the metacarpal tunnel to illustrate its size and direction. **C.** The flexor carpi radialis graft is passed through the tunnel from volar to dorsal. **D.** The flexor carpi radialis graft is passed underneath and sutured to the APL, the remaining flexor carpi radialis, and back dorsally to the APL if the graft length permits. *(continued)*

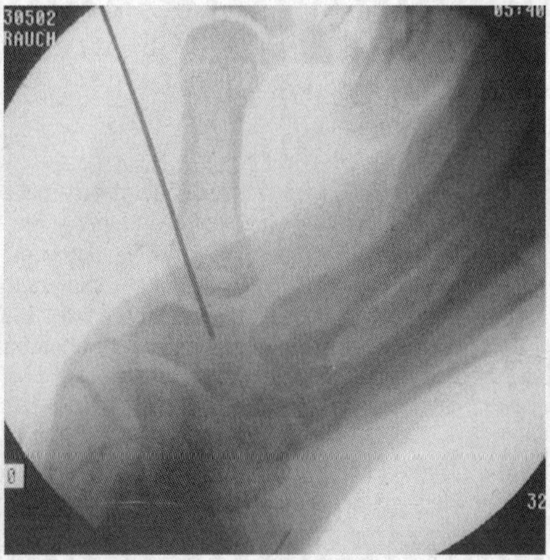

E

TECH FIG 3 *(continued)* **E.** A 0.045-inch K-wire is drilled from the thumb metacarpal into the trapezium to protect the ligament repair.

- The flexor carpi radialis graft is then passed under the APL tendon radially toward the volar side of the wrist. The graft is sutured to the APL with similar nonabsorbable 3-0 suture material as it is passed underneath it.
- The graft is then passed underneath and around the ulnar portion of the flexor carpi radialis tendon that has remained intact. The graft is also sutured to the flexor carpi radialis tendon as it is looped around it.
- If there is additional length to the graft, it is brought back dorsally and again passed underneath and sutured to the APL **(TECH FIG 3D)**.
- A 0.045-inch K-wire is drilled from the radial thumb metacarpal base into the trapezium to immobilize the CMC joint.
  - An additional K-wire can be drilled from the thumb metacarpal base to the index metacarpal base for additional support.
  - The wire is removed after 5 weeks once adequate soft tissue healing has occurred **(TECH FIG 3E)**.

Wound Closure

- If there are no fractures, the thenar muscle mass is reapproximated and sutured using synthetic absorbable 3-0 suture material.
- The proximal and distal skin incisions are closed with 5-0 nylon sutures **(TECH FIG 4)**.
- The hand is then placed in a short-arm thumb spica splint.

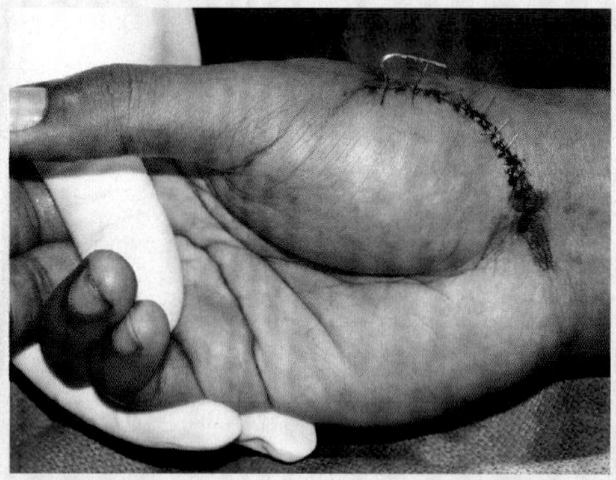

TECH FIG 4 Final wound closure with nylon sutures.

CLOSED REDUCTION AND PERCUTANEOUS PINNING OF BENNETT AND ROLANDO FRACTURES

- Longitudinal traction, abduction, and pronation of the thumb is performed while applying direct manual pressure over the metacarpal base.[14]
- Traction is maintained, and the reduction is held while fluoroscopy is used to verify acceptable fracture reduction and alignment of the articular surface **(TECH FIG 5A,B)**.
- Fine-tuning the amount of traction, abduction, and pronation can be done using fluoroscopic guidance.
- Smooth 0.045-inch K-wires are inserted from the proximal thumb metacarpal shaft into the uninjured index metacarpal base or trapezium. These wires stabilize the concentrically reduced metacarpal shaft and CMC joint. Typically, this fracture

A B

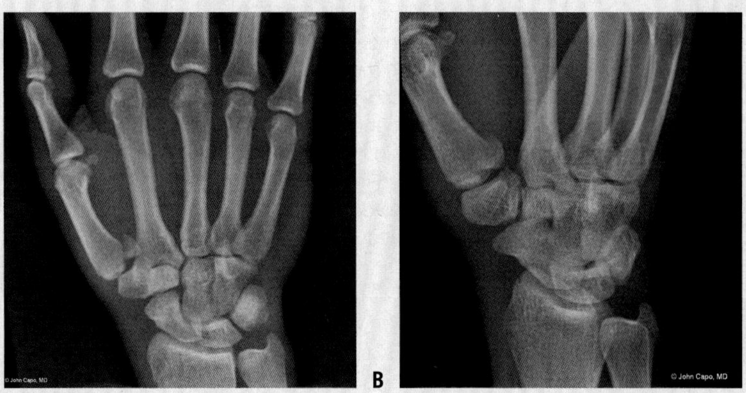

TECH FIG 5 A,B. Lateral and PA views of a Bennett fracture with intra-articular displacement. *(continued)*

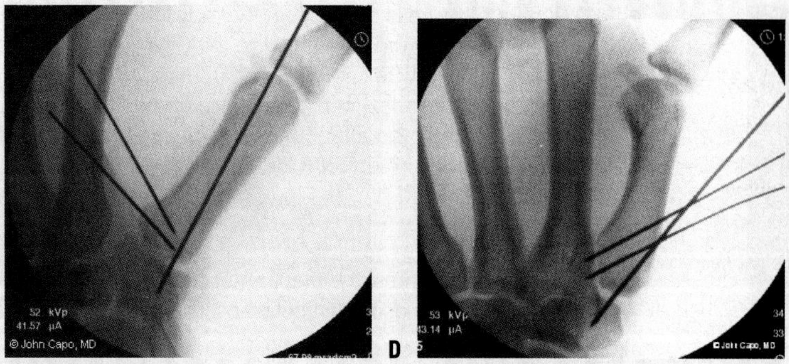

TECH FIG 5 *(continued)* **C.** The metacarpal base is first reduced to the trapezium and then a pin (0.045) is placed across the CMC joint. Two additional pins are provisionally placed and readied to stabilize the Bennett fracture fragment. **D.** The two smaller pins (0.035) are then advanced across into the Bennett fragment. (Copyright John T. Capo, MD.)

pattern requires at least two K-wires to achieve stable reduction **(TECH FIG 5C)**.

- If the Bennett fracture fragment is of ample size, fixation to the fragment may be used in addition **(TECH FIG 5D)**.
- Large fragments may be manipulated percutaneously with K-wire joysticks and then stabilized.
- The wires are bent and cut outside of the skin, followed by application of a well-padded thumb spica splint with the thumb in abduction and wrist in extension.
- If less than 2 mm of step-off cannot be obtained by closed reduction, the surgeon should consider abandoning this technique for an open reduction and internal fixation.[9]
  - Alternatively, arthroscopic-assisted reduction and pinning has been described with good outcome and could be considered.[13,18]
- In rare instances, a similar technique can be used for Rolando fractures, with large T- or Y-type fracture patterns with minimal comminution.

OPEN REDUCTION AND INTERNAL FIXATION OF BENNETT FRACTURES

Exposure

- A Wagner approach is used for open reduction of a Bennett fracture **(TECH FIG 6A)**.
- An incision is made on the dorsoradial aspect of the thumb CMC joint at the junction of the glabrous and nonglabrous skin and curved in a volar direction toward the distal wrist crease to the flexor carpi radialis tendon sheath **(TECH FIG 6B)**.
  - The palmar cutaneous branch of the median nerve, the superficial radial nerve, and distal branches of the lateral antebrachial cutaneous nerve are at risk in this approach and should be carefully protected **(TECH FIG 6C)**.
- The thenar muscles are elevated extraperiosteally from the CMC joint, and a longitudinal capsulotomy is made to expose the joint and the fracture fragments.
- An effort should be made to preserve all soft tissue attachments to the fracture fragments **(TECH FIG 6D)**.
- The fracture is exposed and cleaned of all intervening soft tissue and early fracture callous.
  - This often requires abduction, supination, and dorsal displacement of the metacarpal shaft to expose the volar Bennett fragment.

Reduction and Fixation

- The displaced thumb metacarpal shaft should be reduced with fine reduction clamps to the volar ulnar fragment under direct visualization and secured with 0.028 to 0.035 smooth K-wires placed from dorsal to palmar through the intact dorsal metacarpal and into the volar fragment **(TECH FIG 7A)**.
  - K-wires may serve as the definitive means of fixation if so desired.
- Alternatively, the wires may be exchanged for 1.3- to 2.0-mm screws to provide interfragmentary compression and therefore improved stability **(TECH FIG 7B)**.
  - One K-wire is removed at a time and replaced with a screw.
  - Generally, the path of the removed K-wire effectively guides the drill in the appropriate direction. Use of a mini-fluoroscopy unit is helpful.
  - Care should be exercised to avoid over compression, which may cause an alteration in the arc of curvature of the articular surface.
  - Screws should be precisely evaluated radiographically to be certain they are not in the CMC joint or adjacent second metacarpal base **(TECH FIG 7C,D)**.
- Anatomic reduction of the articular surface and fracture stability are verified under direct visualization.
- It is generally advisable to use one or two K-wires placed from the metacarpal into the trapezium and/or second metacarpal to protect and maintain fracture and joint reduction.
- The wound is closed in layers with absorbable sutures in the joint capsule, followed by nylon sutures in the skin. A thumb spica splint is applied.

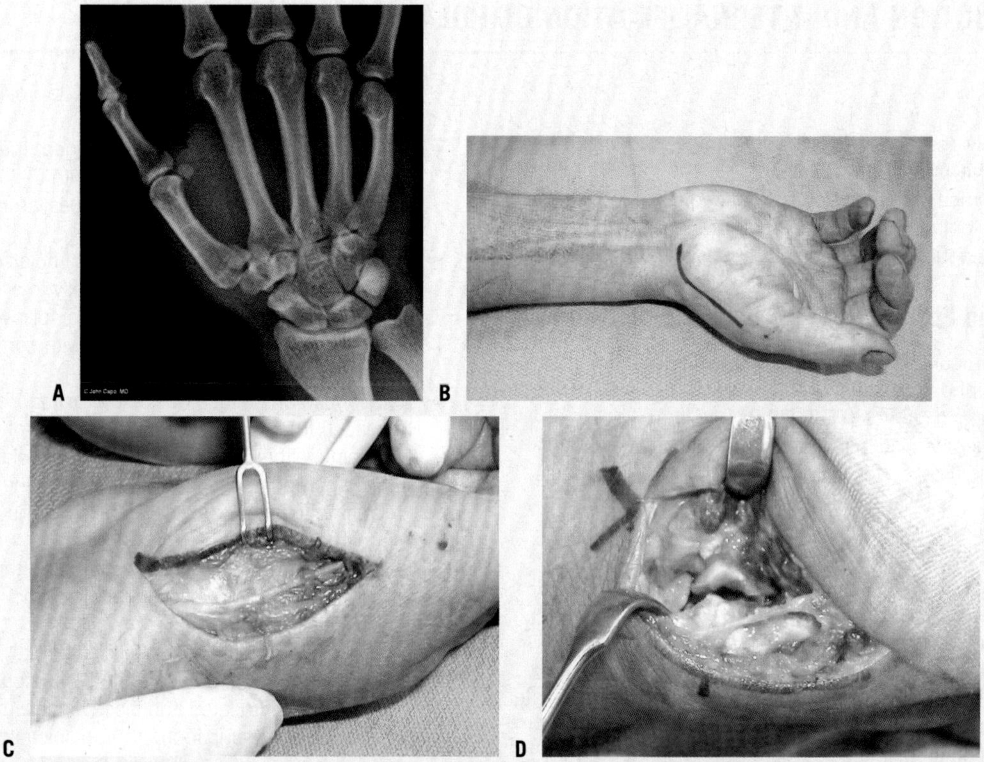

TECH FIG 6 **A.** A preoperative radiograph demonstrating a large (~40%) Bennett fracture with intra-articular displacement. **B.** The typical incision for open reduction and internal fixation of a Bennett or Rolando fracture. The proximal aspect starts at the flexor carpi radialis tendon sheath. In the case of a Rolando fracture, especially one treated by plate fixation, the distal portion of the incision should extend along the thumb metacarpal. **C.** Distal nerve branches are seen during the exposure of these fractures. The nerves can usually be retracted dorsally to allow exposure of the CMC joint. **D.** The thenar muscles are reflected volarly and the CMC joint is entered. The volar oblique fracture is now clearly visualized. Care is taken to maintain soft tissue attachments. (Copyright John T. Capo, MD.)

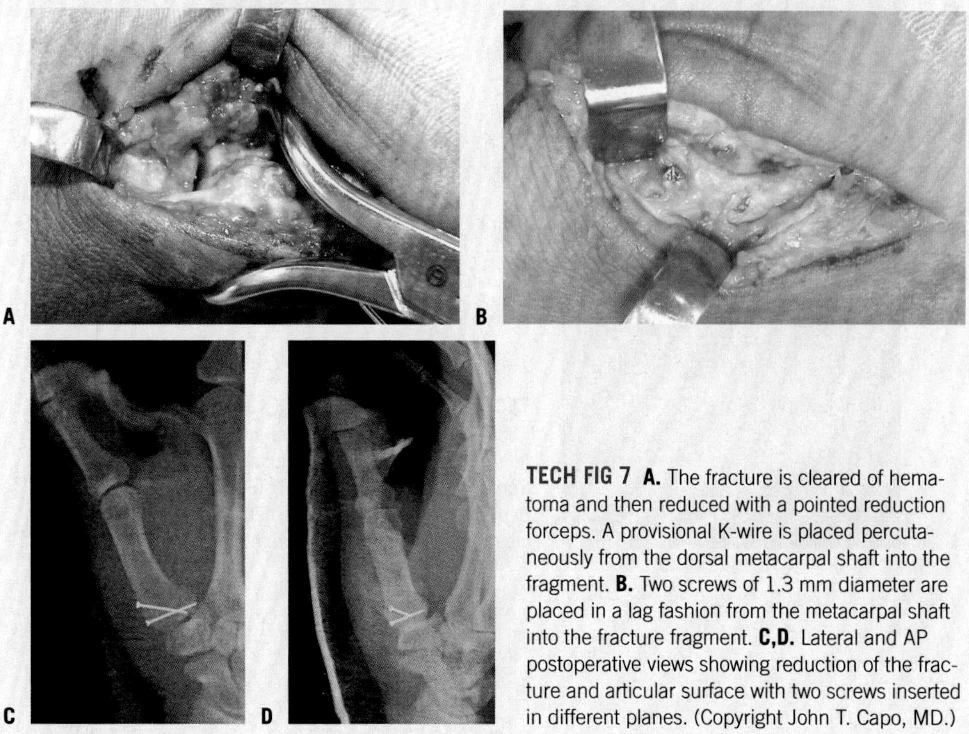

TECH FIG 7 **A.** The fracture is cleared of hematoma and then reduced with a pointed reduction forceps. A provisional K-wire is placed percutaneously from the dorsal metacarpal shaft into the fragment. **B.** Two screws of 1.3 mm diameter are placed in a lag fashion from the metacarpal shaft into the fracture fragment. **C,D.** Lateral and AP postoperative views showing reduction of the fracture and articular surface with two screws inserted in different planes. (Copyright John T. Capo, MD.)

OPEN REDUCTION AND INTERNAL FIXATION OF ROLANDO FRACTURES

Exposure

- The previously described Wagner approach is used to expose the thumb CMC joint **(TECH FIG 8A,B)**.
- The radial portion of the incision is extended distally to expose the diaphysis of the thumb metacarpal. Branches of the radial sensory nerve must be protected at this stage **(TECH FIG 8C)**.

Reduction and Fixation

- The basilar articular fragments are then reduced under direct visualization, and provisional fixation is performed with K-wires or bone reduction clamps **(TECH FIG 9A)**.
- A lag screw can be placed in a transverse direction by overdrilling the proximal cortex to compress the basilar fragments together, followed by application of a minifragment neutralization plate or by additional K-wires to stabilize the shaft **(TECH FIG 9B,C)**.[3,14]
- If greater fracture stability is desired, a small (1.5 to 2.7 mm) T, L, or blade plate can be used. If proximal fixation in the metaphysis is poor, a locking plate should be considered.
  - The palmar radial incision is extended further distally to expose the thumb metacarpal shaft to accommodate the plate.
  - Reduction is obtained using the earlier techniques, with axial traction to maintain appropriate length and bone reduction forceps or smooth K-wires to provisionally hold the articular reduction.
  - Once the fracture fragments are aligned, the plate is secured to the thumb metacarpal, with the transverse portion of the plate placed over the basilar fracture fragments.[14]
  - The most palmar and dorsal proximal holes of the T portion of the plate can be drilled eccentrically to allow for compression of the articular basilar fragments, followed by fixation of the plate to the metacarpal shaft with cortical screws **(TECH FIG 9D,E)**.
  - Additionally, an oblique (distal to proximal) lag screw can be placed from the shaft fragment to one of the basilar fragments, either within or outside of the plate.
    - An appropriate bit is used for overdrilling of the shaft fragment, followed by core drilling of the distal basilar fragment.
    - This interfragmentary screw increases the stability of the construct and may allow for earlier functional range of motion.
- The joint surface reduction is visualized directly with distal traction of the thumb and ensured to be anatomic.
- The wound is then irrigated and closed in layers, followed by immobilization in a well-padded thumb spica splint.

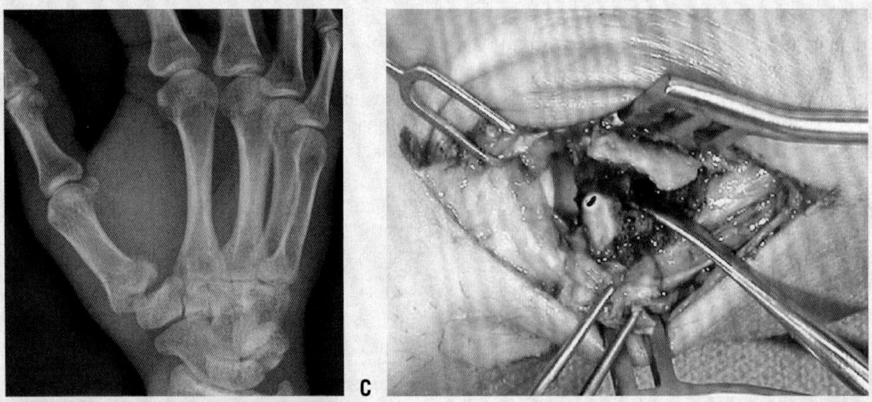

A C

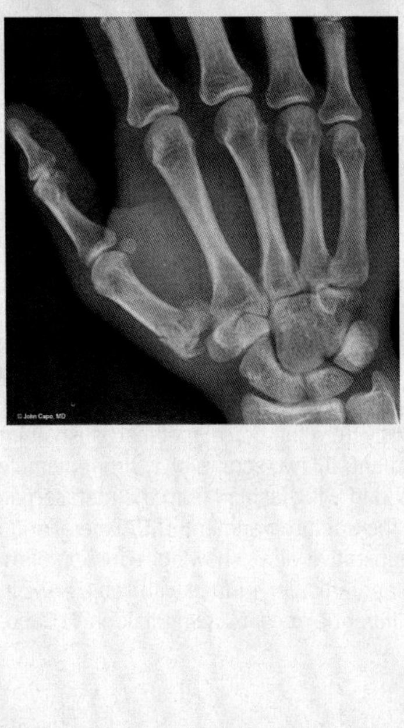

B

TECH FIG 8 A,B. Preoperative radiographs of a Rolando fracture demonstrating severe intra-articular comminution. **C.** The thumb thenar muscles have been elevated from the CMC joint and a capsulotomy has been performed. The fracture fragments are identified and cleared of hematoma. (Copyright John T. Capo, MD.)

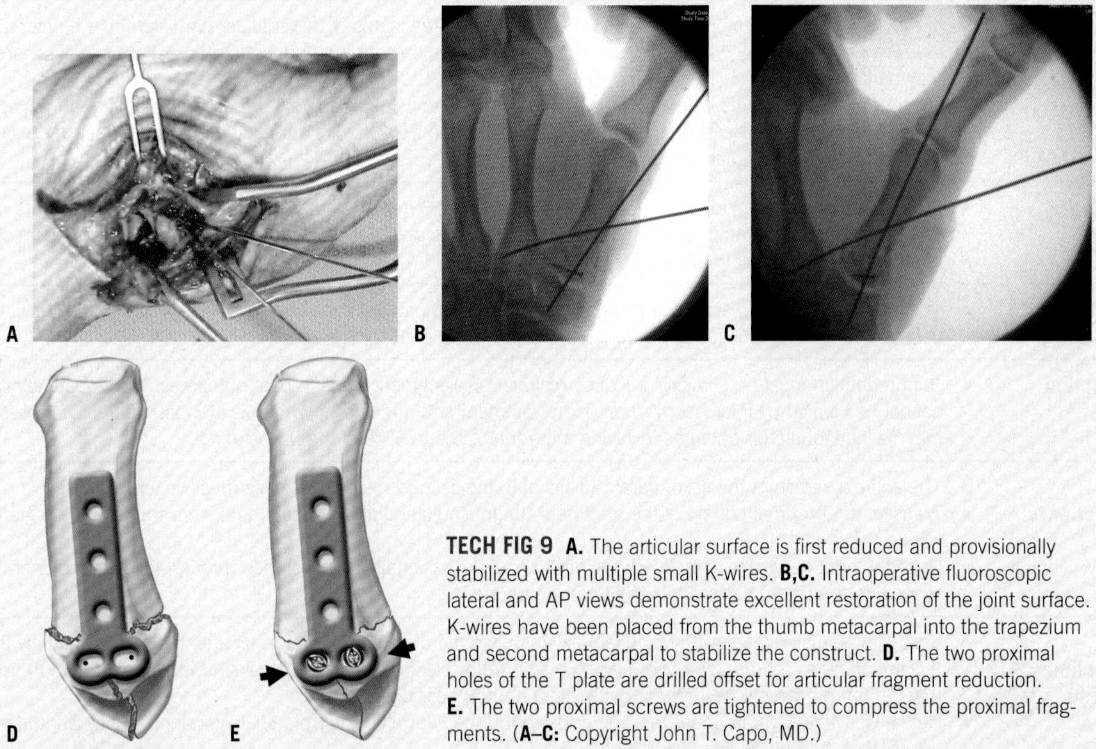

TECH FIG 9 **A.** The articular surface is first reduced and provisionally stabilized with multiple small K-wires. **B,C.** Intraoperative fluoroscopic lateral and AP views demonstrate excellent restoration of the joint surface. K-wires have been placed from the thumb metacarpal into the trapezium and second metacarpal to stabilize the construct. **D.** The two proximal holes of the T plate are drilled offset for articular fragment reduction. **E.** The two proximal screws are tightened to compress the proximal fragments. (**A–C:** Copyright John T. Capo, MD.)

APPLICATION OF AN EXTERNAL FIXATOR FOR COMMINUTED ROLANDO FRACTURES

- Before this procedure, a radiograph of the contralateral thumb CMC joint is advised for templating and to judge postreduction length.
- A mini-external fixator (2.0- to 2.5-mm pins) is applied to the thumb and index metacarpals using standard technique with a quadrilateral frame configuration.
- Exposure and open reduction are then performed as discussed previously.
- Distraction is maintained using the external fixator, and the depressed joint fragments are elevated and aligned using the preoperative radiograph of the opposite side as a guide.
  - A sharp dental pick is an excellent tool to manipulate small fragments.
- K-wires or interfragmentary screws can then be used to secure the fracture fragments.
- The external fixator is loosened to decrease the flexion deformity of the thumb metacarpal shaft and to ensure the base of the thumb is maintained in the proper position. It should be colinear with the base of the second metacarpal base.
- At the end of the procedure, the thumb should be in 45 degrees of palmar and radial abduction and about 120 degrees of pronation in relation to the plane of the hand **(TECH FIG 10)**.

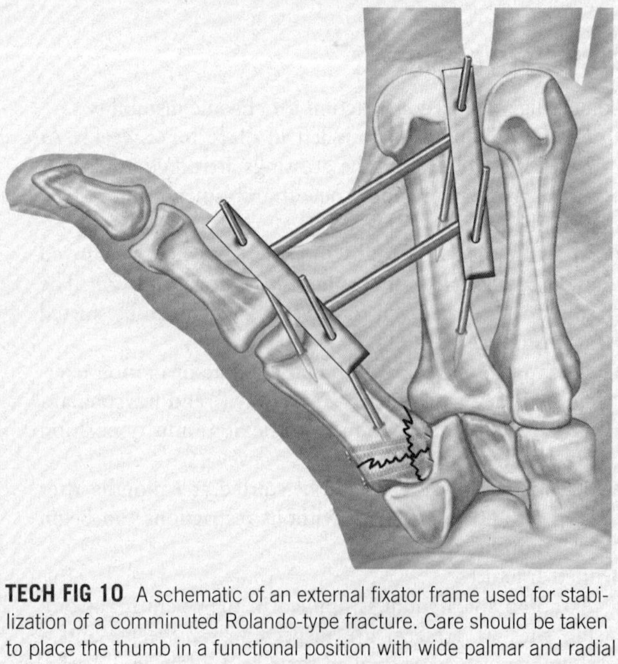

TECH FIG 10 A schematic of an external fixator frame used for stabilization of a comminuted Rolando-type fracture. Care should be taken to place the thumb in a functional position with wide palmar and radial abduction.

Pearls and Pitfalls

Indications	• In the setting of ligamentous laxity without acute trauma, the status of the articular cartilage must be carefully assessed intraoperatively. If significant cartilage damage is present, and depending on patient specifics, arthroplasty may be preferred. • For thumb base fractures, operative treatment should be considered if greater than 2 mm of step-off persists after closed reduction. Displaced Bennett fractures greater than 25% of joint surface often require open reduction and internal fixation for optimal reduction.
Preoperative Evaluation	• Proper radiographs, including a true lateral view and an AP hyperpronated view, must be obtained before operative treatment. Computed tomography scanning is usually indicated only if significant comminution is present or if plain radiographs are difficult to interpret.
Thumb Position	• The thumb should be placed in a position of function with pinning and postoperative splinting. This position is palmar and radial abduction of 45 degrees and pronation of 120 degrees.
Joint Reduction	• Joint reduction must be obtained because residual displacement leads to poor outcomes. If adequate joint reduction cannot be verified by fluoroscopy, then open treatment and direct visualization is mandatory. Percutaneous methods may be inadequate for fractures involving more than 25% to 30% of the joint surface.
Ligament Reconstruction: Harvest	• The entire insertion of the flexor carpi radialis onto the second metacarpal base must be left intact. • Transect the proximal portion of the graft near the musculotendinous junction to ensure that adequate graft length will be obtained. • Once the graft harvest is completed, the graft should occasionally be moistened through the remainder of the procedure to prevent desiccation and tenocyte injury.
Ligament Reconstruction: Passage and Fixation	• Start with a small-diameter tunnel. Gradually increase the diameter of the tunnel until the graft fits snugly through it. • It is important to set the appropriate graft tension. After placing a few periosteal sutures to hold the graft, make sure that the thumb can still be brought back into a neutral position. • Before weaving the graft under the APL and around the intact flexor carpi radialis tendons, check an image to ensure that the CMC is adequately reduced. • Braided synthetic suture such as Ethibond is soft and may be less palpable than stiffer suture such as Prolene.
Postoperative Management	• Thumb spica casting for 6 weeks is necessary if percutaneous K-wire fixation is used for fracture fixation. Premature early motion may break K-wires that span the adjacent joints. Range-of-motion exercises can be begun 2 weeks postoperatively if stable plate fixation is used. Many can expect return to pretrauma level of activity at 12 weeks after surgery.[19]

POSTOPERATIVE CARE

- Isolated ligament reconstruction for chronic instability
  - The thumb spica splint is left in place for 2 weeks. At 2 weeks of follow-up, the dressings are taken down, sutures are removed, and a new thumb spica splint or cast is applied.
  - At 5 to 6 weeks of follow-up, the K-wires are removed and a removable thumb splint is used for protection. The splint can be removed for therapy, which can be started at this time.
  - Therapy should start with active range-of-motion exercises of the wrist, thumb CMC, MCP, and interphalangeal joints. Thumb abduction, flexion, and opposition are emphasized.
  - Strengthening exercises can be started at 2 months after surgery, and full activity without restrictions can begin at 3 months.
- Bennett fractures
  - A thumb spica splint is applied in the operating room. Pin sites (if present) are inspected at 2 weeks, and a thumb spica cast is applied for 3 to 4 additional weeks, until fracture union.
  - Hand therapy is begun 2 to 3 weeks after surgery for thumb interphalangeal and index through small finger range of motion.
  - If pins were used, they are removed at 5 to 6 weeks, and therapy is advanced to the metacarpophalangeal and CMC joint along with intermittent immobilization using a removable thumb spica splint.[14]
  - Even in the setting of stable screw fixation, starting motion earlier than 5 to 6 weeks is not advisable as the dorsoradial ligament is not healed, risking subluxation of the thumb metacarpal
- Rolando fractures
  - Patients treated with closed reduction and percutaneous pinning are placed in a thumb spica splint, which is removed at 2 weeks for pin inspection. A thumb spica cast is applied for an additional 4 weeks.
  - The pins are removed 6 weeks after surgery. A removable splint may be continued for 4 additional weeks while active range-of-motion exercises are advanced.[14]
  - In patients treated with stable plate fixation, active range-of-motion exercises may be instituted at 2 weeks after surgery if the CMC joint was found to be stable without subluxation using intraoperative fluoroscopy. Patients typically wear a removable splint for 2 to 4 weeks.
  - If a severe injury dictated the use of external fixation, the pins and frame should remain in place for about 6 weeks or until fracture stability is adequate based on interval

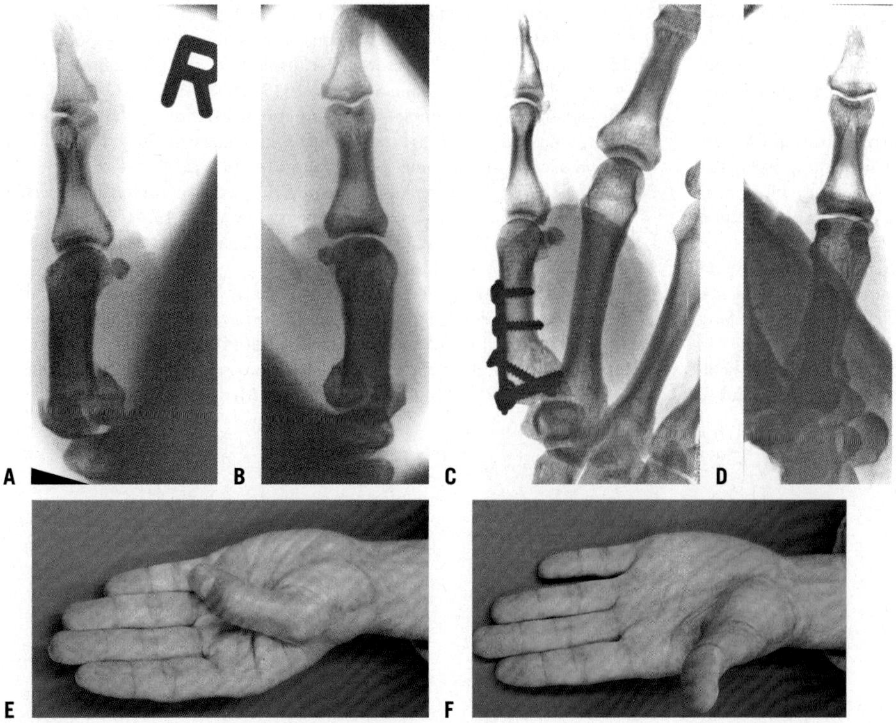

FIG 8 A,B. AP and lateral views of a comminuted, displaced Rolando fracture. **C,D.** Postoperative radiographs demonstrating excellent articular reduction using a 2-mm T plate. **E,F.** Different patient with a Rolando fracture who had undergone open reduction and internal fixation 8 months previously, demonstrating a functional range of flexion and extension. (**A–D:** Courtesy of Dominik Heim, MD. **E,F:** Copyright John T. Capo, MD.)

radiographs. A removable thumb spica splint can then be worn for an additional 4 to 6 weeks.

OUTCOMES

- Most patients can expect a successful recovery after operative treatment of Bennett or Rolando fractures (**FIG 8**).
- Superior results are seen in operatively treated fractures in which there is no residual subluxation of the thumb metacarpal shaft and less than 2 mm of intra-articular displacement.
- When ligament reconstruction is performed without preexisting basal joint arthritis, good results can be expected.
  - In a number of long-term follow-up studies of over 5 years, 87% to 100% of patients demonstrated joint stability against stress testing, 29% to 67% of patients reported no pain, and 83% to 100% reported marked improvement in pain. Interestingly, only 0% to 37% of patients progressed to a higher stage of arthritis.[6]
  - Freedman et al[6] reviewed their long-term results of 24 thumbs that underwent ligament reconstruction for stage I or II disease.
    - After a minimum of 10 years of follow-up, 29% of patients reported no pain, 54% reported pain with strenuous activity only, and 17% of patients had pain during activities of daily living.
    - When tested against stress, 87% demonstrated joint stability.

COMPLICATIONS

- Malunion and subsequent arthrosis resulting from inadequate articular reduction
- Pin tract infection
- Injury to the superficial cutaneous nerves during open dissection and percutaneous fixation
- Contracture of the first web space from immobilization or pinning of the thumb in an adducted position
- Residual joint instability
- Radial artery injury
- Superficial radial nerve or lateral antebrachial cutaneous nerve injury

ACKNOWLEDGMENT

- Drs. John T. Capo, Joshua T. Mitgang, and Colin Harris were instrumental in the creation of this chapter.

REFERENCES

1. Birman MV, Danoff JR, Yemul KS, et al. Dorsoradial ligament imbrication for thumb carpometacarpal joint instability. Tech Hand Up Extrem Surg 2014;18(2):66–71.
2. Capo JT, Kinchelow T, Orillaza NS, et al. Accuracy of fluoroscopy in closed reduction and percutaneous fixation of simulated Bennett's fracture. J Hand Surg Am 2009;34(4):637–641.
3. Cullen JP, Parentis MA, Chinchilli VM, et al. Simulated Bennett fracture treated with closed reduction and percutaneous pinning. A biomechanical analysis of residual incongruity of the joint. J Bone Joint Surg Am 1997;79:413–420.
4. Day S, Stern P. Fractures of the metacarpals and phalanges. In: Wolfe S, Hotchkiss R, Pederson W, et al, eds. Green's Operative Hand Surgery, ed 6. Philadelphia: Elsevier, 2011:283–287.
5. Eaton RG, Littler JW. Ligament reconstruction for the painful thumb carpometacarpal joint. J Bone Joint Surg Am 1973;55(8):1655–1666.
6. Freedman DM, Eaton RG, Glickel SZ. Long-term results of volar ligament reconstruction for symptomatic basal joint laxity. J Hand Surg Am 2000;25:297–304.
7. Glickel SZ, Gupta S. Ligament reconstruction. Hand Clin 2006;22:143–151.
8. Goyal T. Bennett's fracture associated with fracture of trapezium: a rare injury of first carpo-metacarpal joint. World J Orthop 2017;8(8):656–659.
9. Greeven AP, Van Groningen J, Schep N, et al. Open reduction and internal fixation versus closed reduction and percutaneous fixation

in the treatment of Bennett fractures: a systematic review. Injury 2019;50(8):1470–1477.
10. Kamphuis SJ, Greeven AP, Kleinveld S, et al. Bennett's fracture: comparative study between open and closed surgical techniques. Hand Surg Rehabil 2019;38(2):97–101.
11. Lin JD, Karl JW, Strauch RJ. Trapeziometacarpal joint stability: the evolving importance of the dorsal ligaments. Clin Orthop Relat Res 2014;472:1138–1145.
12. McCarthy CM, Awan HM. Trapeziometacarpal dislocation without fracture. J Hand Surg Am 2014;39(11):2292–2293.
13. Pomares G, Strugarek-Lecoanet C, Dap F, et al. Bennett fracture: arthroscopically assisted percutaneous screw fixation versus open surgery: functional and radiological outcomes. Orthop Traumatol Surg Res 2016;102(3):357–361.
14. Raskin K, Shin S. Surgical treatment of fractures of the thumb metacarpal base: Bennett's and Rolando's fractures. In: Strickland J, Graham T, eds. Master Techniques in Orthopaedic Surgery: The Hand. Philadelphia: Lippincott Williams & Wilkins, 2005:125–135.
15. Rayan G, Do V. Dorsoradial capsulodesis for trapeziometacarpal joint instability. J Hand Surg Am 2013;38:382–387.
16. Simonian PT, Trumble TE. Traumatic dislocation of the thumb carpometacarpal joint: early ligamentous reconstruction versus closed reduction and pinning. J Hand Surg Am 1996;21:802–806.
17. Soldado F, Mascarenhas VW, Knörr J. Paediatric trapeziometacarpal dislocation: a case report. J Hand Surg Eur Vol 2016;41(9):999–1000.
18. Solomon J, Culp R. Arthroscopic management of Bennett fracture. Hand Clin 2017;33(4):787–794.
19. Uludag S, Ataker Y, Seyahi A, et al. Early rehabilitation after stable osteosynthesis of intra-articular fractures of the metacarpal base of the thumb. J Hand Surg Eur Vol 2015;40(4):370–373.
20. Werman H, Rancour S, Nelson R. Two cases of thenar compartment syndrome from blunt trauma. J Emerg Med 2013;44(1):85–88.

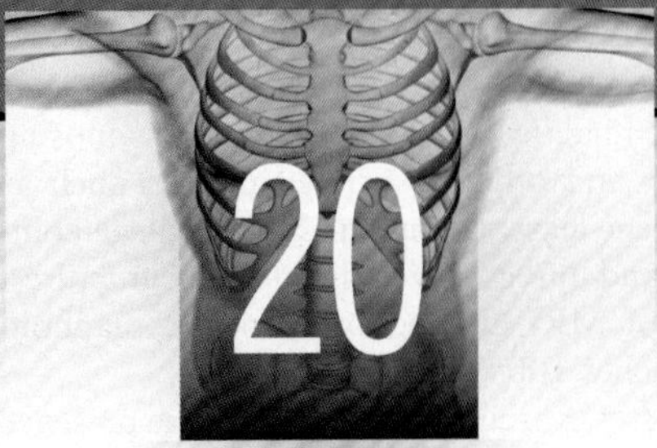

CHAPTER

Percutaneous Treatment of Scaphoid Fractures

Seth D. Dodds and Kirsten A. Sumner

DEFINITION

- Located in the proximal carpal row, the scaphoid serves as an important link between the proximal and distal carpal rows.
- Scaphoid fractures most commonly result from a fall on a hyperextended and radially deviated wrist. Less commonly, it can occur following forced palmar flexion of the wrist or axial loading of the flexed wrist.
- The scaphoid typically fractures through the waist and less frequently through the proximal pole or the distal pole.

ANATOMY

- The scaphoid has a complex three-dimensional geometry with the shape of a "twisted peanut" or cashew.
- Scaphoid dimensions vary between genders; the male scaphoid is usually longer and wider than the females. Understanding the variability of scaphoid anatomy allows for more accurate percutaneous treatment of scaphoid fractures.[14]
- The scaphoid articulates with the radius, lunate, capitate, trapezium, and trapezoid; thus, its surface is almost completely covered with hyaline cartilage. The fact that articular cartilage covers the majority of the scaphoid has several important implications:
  - Poor blood supply as there is more articular surface than periosteal surface
  - The scaphoid is nearly entirely surrounded by synovial fluid.
  - Instrumenting the scaphoid with a screw requires penetrating the articular surface.
  - Access to the scaphoid requires an arthrotomy either over the radioscaphoid joint, or the scaphotrapezio-trapezoidal joint, which can lead to stiffness and joint problems.
- The blood supply from the radial artery enters the scaphoid via two main routes[8]:
  - A dorsal branch, which enters the scaphoid via the dorsal ridge, provides the primary supply and 70% to 80% of the overall vascularity, including the entire proximal pole (via retrograde endosteal branches).
  - A volar branch, which enters through the tubercle, supplies 20% to 30% of the internal vascularity, all in the distal pole.
  - This primarily retrograde blood supply contributes to the high incidence of nonunion after a fracture at the scaphoid waist or proximal pole. It also places the proximal pole at risk for the development of avascular necrosis.
  - A central axis screw or an antegrade screw has been shown to be the least disruptive of the scaphoid vasculature.[21]

PATHOGENESIS

- A scaphoid fracture classically occurs in a young, active adult or teenager, most commonly following a fall onto an outstretched hand.
- Seventy percent to 80% of scaphoid fractures occur at the waist region, whereas 10% to 20% involve the proximal pole, and 5% occur at the distal pole or tuberosity.
- Although rare, scapholunate ligament injuries can occur in association with a scaphoid fracture.[15]

NATURAL HISTORY

- The true natural history of an untreated scaphoid fracture is unknown due to limitations in the existing literature, particularly with respect to study design. However, one retrospective study has suggested a predictable pattern of wrist arthritis develops following scaphoid nonunions, usually within 10 years of the injury.[23]
- Unrecognized, untreated, or inadequately treated scaphoid fractures have an increased likelihood of nonunion and secondary carpal instability.[18]
- A fracture through the proximal pole has the highest likelihood of nonunion, followed by a fracture of the scaphoid waist.
- If a scaphoid waist fracture does not heal, flexion forces at the distal fragment result in a flexion ("humpback") deformity of the scaphoid.
  - This deformity and loss of scaphoid support leads to a dorsal intercalated segment instability pattern with lunate extension.
  - If a proximal pole fracture does not heal, flexion deformity is not always present, potentially due to the integrity of the dorsal fibers of the scapholunate ligament, which may still be inserting on the intact waist of the scaphoid. Without bone bridging, the proximal pole frequently becomes an island as it loses its blood supply, and the articular fluid will find a way between the fragments.

HISTORY AND PHYSICAL FINDINGS

- A patient with an acute or subacute scaphoid fracture presents with radial-sided wrist pain, swelling, possibly ecchymosis, and, very characteristically, loss of wrist extension.
- Classic physical examination findings include the following:
  - Swelling over the dorsoradial aspect of the wrist
  - Tenderness to palpation at the "anatomic snuffbox" (between the abductor pollicis longus/extensor pollicis brevis and the extensor pollicis longus [EPL])

- With the wrist held in flexion, there will be tenderness over the dorsal aspect of the proximal pole, between the third and fourth extensor compartments of the wrist.
- Tenderness to palpation volarly over the distal pole of the scaphoid just proximal to the trapezium
- Pain with axial compression of the wrist (scaphoid compression test)

IMAGING AND OTHER DIAGNOSTIC STUDIES

- The following plain radiographs should routinely be ordered in the patient with a suspected scaphoid fracture: posteroanterior (PA), oblique, lateral, and a "navicular" or scaphoid view.
  - The PA view allows visualization of the proximal pole of the scaphoid.
  - The lateral view permits an assessment of fracture angulation, carpal alignment, and carpal instability.
  - The dedicated scaphoid view is a PA view with the wrist in ulnar deviation and extension. This results in scaphoid extension, allowing visualization of the scaphoid in profile. This scaphoid or "navicular" view offers the best outline of a scaphoid waist fracture and the scaphocapitate articulation **(FIG 1A)**.
  - The volar oblique or semipronated oblique view provides good visualization of the volar waist and distal pole regions **(FIG 1B)**.
  - The dorsal oblique or semisupinated oblique view provides ideal visualization of the proximal pole, dorsal waist, and dorsal ridge as well as the screw position **(FIG 1C)**.
- Computed tomography (CT) scan is helpful in identifying and characterizing an acute fracture and evaluating for a nonunion.
  - Thin 1-mm cuts along the axis of the scaphoid are particularly helpful but need to be requested at most institutions.
  - Up to 30% of scaphoid fractures seen as nondisplaced on plain films have been found to be displaced on CT scan imaging.
  - A CT scan is an ideal test to determine the indications for scaphoid fracture repair as well as the approach for scaphoid fracture fixation.[11]
- Magnetic resonance imaging (MRI) is useful for diagnosing an occult fracture[17] and other associated injuries such as scapholunate ligament tears, triangular fibrocartilage complex (TFCC) tears, and unrecognized distal radius fractures.
  - The sensitivity of MRI at diagnosing occult scaphoid fractures approaches 100% at 24 hours.
  - MRI is used to assess vascularity and determine presence of avascular necrosis.

DIFFERENTIAL DIAGNOSIS

- Wrist sprain
- Wrist contusion
- Scapholunate injury
- Fracture of other carpal bones
- Distal radius fracture

NONOPERATIVE MANAGEMENT

- Nonoperative management, specifically cast immobilization, is indicated for a nondisplaced, acute (<4 weeks from injury) fracture of the distal pole or even displaced fractures of the distal tubercle of the distal pole of the scaphoid.
- For a nondisplaced, acute waist fracture, there is debate regarding the preferred treatment approach—cast immobilization or surgical stabilization.
  - Some studies have shown more reliable healing rates after surgical repair of scaphoid fractures with quicker recovery of function.[1,2,24]
- With cast immobilization, there is no consensus regarding the preferred position of the wrist, the need to immobilize other joints besides the wrist, and the duration of immobilization.
  - Studies have demonstrated no difference in union rates with use of a long-arm versus short-arm cast; however, a small randomized prospective study by Gellman et al[9] demonstrated a shorter time to union and fewer nonunions and delayed unions with the initial use of a long-arm cast.
  - In a cadaveric study, there was no difference in scaphoid angulation or rotation when comparing use of a short-arm cast versus a thumb spica cast.[25]
  - Clinical studies have demonstrated no benefit with thumb immobilization or any influence of wrist position on the rate of union.[4]

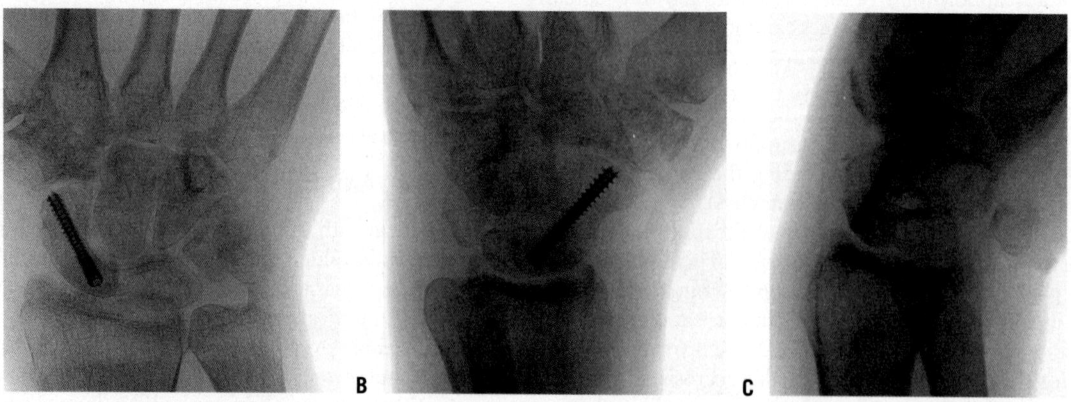

A B C

FIG 1 A–C. Fluoroscopic views of the scaphoid include the scaphoid view (**A**), the volar oblique or semipronated view (**B**) that allows good visualization of the volar aspect of the scaphoid, and the dorsal oblique or semisupinated view (**C**), which reveals the dorsal ridge of the scaphoid and dorsal aspect of the proximal pole.

- In general, cast immobilization is required for 6 weeks after a distal pole fracture and 10 to 12 weeks following a nondisplaced waist fracture.
  - Confirmation of fracture union can be performed with serial plain radiographs demonstrating progressive obliteration of the fracture line and clear trabeculation across the fracture site.[6]
- If there is any question regarding fracture union (with or without surgical repair), particularly if the patient is returning to a contact sport, a CT scan should be obtained.[5]

SURGICAL MANAGEMENT

- Percutaneous treatment of scaphoid fractures was primarily developed and advocated by Dr. Joseph Slade. In an era when scaphoid fracture fixation with the Herbert screw was intimidating, he took advantage of two important contingencies:
  - A limited dorsal approach to the scaphoid (either mini-open or percutaneous) did not disrupt the blood supply along its dorsal ridge. Excellent access to the proximal pole could be achieved leaving these capsular attachments undissected.
  - Simplification of the technique used to place a cannulated headless compression screw into five straightforward steps: fracture reduction, center–center guidewire placement, length measurement, drilling/reaming over the wire, and screw insertion.
- Although the procedure was originally developed for minimally displaced fractures that reduce with simple ulnar deviation of the wrist and a dorsally directed force on the distal pole, displaced scaphoid fractures and even select scaphoid nonunions can be treated percutaneously.
- Arthroscopy can be used not only to assess the wrist for scaphoid fracture displacement but also, and more importantly, to evaluate for associated injuries such as scapholunate and lunotriquetral ligament tears and TFCC tears. The senior author has also diagnosed a handful of distal radius fractures arthroscopically, not seen on plain films.
- The small joint arthroscope is placed in the midcarpal joint to assess the scaphoid reduction along the scaphocapitate articulation. For antegrade screw placement, the arthroscope can be inserted in the radiocarpal joint to assess the starting point of the screw.
- Displaced and unstable fractures are defined by the following criteria:
  - 1 mm of fracture displacement
  - Fracture comminution
  - More than 10 degrees of angular displacement
  - Proximal pole fractures
  - Intrascaphoid angle more than 35 degrees on the lateral radiograph
- Operative treatment is advocated for fractures that are unstable or displaced (see earlier criteria) and fractures with a significant treatment delay in adequate immobilization.[20]
- Operative indications have expanded over time to include nondisplaced scaphoid waist fractures with advantage of fasting healing and return to work.[2]
- Utilization of percutaneous fixation is reasonable for the following:
  - Nondisplaced fractures of the scaphoid waist
  - Displaced fractures of the scaphoid waist
  - Proximal pole fractures
- Percutaneous stabilization of scaphoid fractures may be performed using either a volar or dorsal approach under fluoroscopic guidance.[12,13] If desired, a dorsal arthroscopically assisted reduction and fixation (AARF) technique can be used, which allows direct visualization before and/or after fracture reduction and stabilization.[27–29]
- Regardless of the technique used, the screw should cross the length of the scaphoid and be inserted in a biomechanically advantageous position along the central axis of the scaphoid as perpendicular to the fracture as possible. Longer screws are more stable than shorter screws, but must be buried at least 2 mm beneath the chondral surface. Adhering to these biomechanical principles provides the greatest stability and stiffness and potentially decreases time to union.[7]

Preoperative Planning

- All imaging studies should be reviewed to identify the location of the fracture and the size of the scaphoid, both of which influence implant selection.
- Plain radiographs may be templated preoperatively to determine the approximate screw length.
  - The smaller size of the female scaphoid should be taken into consideration when planning internal fixation to ensure appropriate screw diameter and length.[14]
- Operative equipment
  - Portable mini-fluoroscopy unit (a standard large fluoroscopy unit may be used as well)
  - Kirschner wires (K-wires)
  - Cannulated headless compression screw system
  - Wrist arthroscopy equipment and traction tower, as desired, for AARF

Positioning

- The patient is positioned supine on the operating table, with the shoulder abducted 90 degrees and the arm on a hand table.
- A pneumatic tourniquet is applied to the upper arm, if desired.
- The portable fluoroscopy unit is positioned at the end of the hand table **(FIG 2)**.

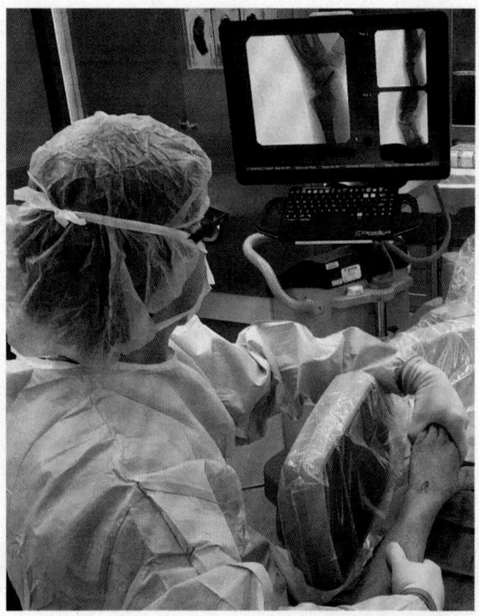

FIG 2 This photograph demonstrates simple positioning of the fluoroscopy unit at the end of the hand table with the screen in clear view of the operating surgeon.

PERCUTANEOUS SCAPHOID FRACTURE REPAIR FROM A DORSAL APPROACH (ANTEGRADE SCREW)

Minimally Displaced Fracture of the Scaphoid Waist or Proximal Pole

- Suspend the hand vertically in finger traps and apply 10 lb of traction to the upper arm to distract the radiocarpal and midcarpal articulations.
- Perform a diagnostic arthroscopy to assess for any associated injuries and to evaluate the fracture displacement and subsequent reduction.
- The 3-4 and 4-5 radiocarpal portals are used to assess the integrity of the radiocarpal and intercarpal ligaments.
- The radial midcarpal portal is used to evaluate for fracture displacement and comminution.
- Remove the hand from traction for screw insertion.
- Position the wrist and the fluoroscopy unit to obtain a PA view of the wrist.
- Under fluoroscopic guidance, gently pronate the wrist until the scaphoid appears as an oblong cylinder, indicating that the proximal and distal poles are aligned.
  - Flex the wrist about 75 degrees until the cylinder rotates into the plane of imaging, forming a "ring" sign. The center of the ring indicates the central axis of the scaphoid **(TECH FIG 1A,B)**.[27]
- Using a guidewire from a headless compression screw set, place the tip of the guidewire through the skin just proximal and ulnar from the 3-4 arthroscopy portal. This landmark can also be localized approximately 5 to 6 mm distal and 5 to 6 mm ulnar to Lister tubercle. Carefully advance the wire onto the proximal pole of the scaphoid, at the center of the scaphoid ring. Confirm correct positioning with fluoroscopy.[27,28]
- If you want to see the wire on the anteroposterior (AP) view, you must hold the wrist flexed and obtain a shoot-through fluoroscopy shot of the wrist.
- Insert the guidewire down the central axis of the scaphoid using a wire driver. Keep the wrist flexed to avoid bending the guidewire **(TECH FIG 1C–E)**.
- Once you believe your guidewire is central within the proximal and distal poles of the scaphoid, make a small surgical incision at the wire's entry to the skin. Incise only the skin.
  - Use blunt dissection with a blunt-tipped hemostat or a tenotomy scissor to dissect down to the wrist capsule.
  - Enter the wrist capsule with the small blunt-tipped hemostat to create a small capsulotomy to be able to pass the drill and the scaphoid screw.
- To obtain a true scaphoid view to see the trajectory of the guidewire, advance the guidewire distally through the distal pole of the scaphoid while holding the thumb in full adduction and extension. The wire will frequently exit through the STT joint or more distally over the thumb metacarpal.
  - The wire is further pulled out volarly until the trailing edge of the wire is just at the proximal pole of the scaphoid.
  - Now, the wrist can be fully extended for ideal radiographic assessment of its position.
- Confirm correct wire position with fluoroscopy.[19]

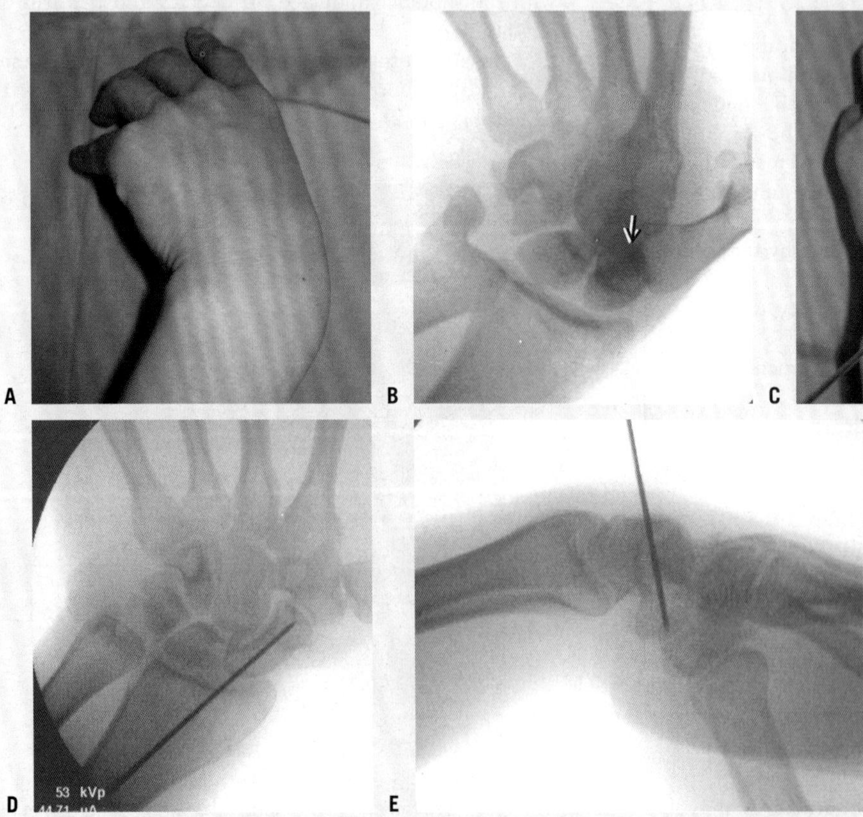

TECH FIG 1 The scaphoid ring sign targets the central axis of the scaphoid. The center of this "ring" is critical for accurate insertion of the cannulated compression screw. **A,B.** The wrist is positioned in flexion and pronation until the scaphoid appears as a ring (*arrow*) on fluoroscopic imaging. A guidewire is inserted through the center of the ring. **C–E.** Before screw insertion, the position of the K-wire must be changed from its position used for arthroscopy. The K-wire should be driven from volar to dorsal until the distal end lies just beneath the articular surface of the scaphoid. *(continued)*

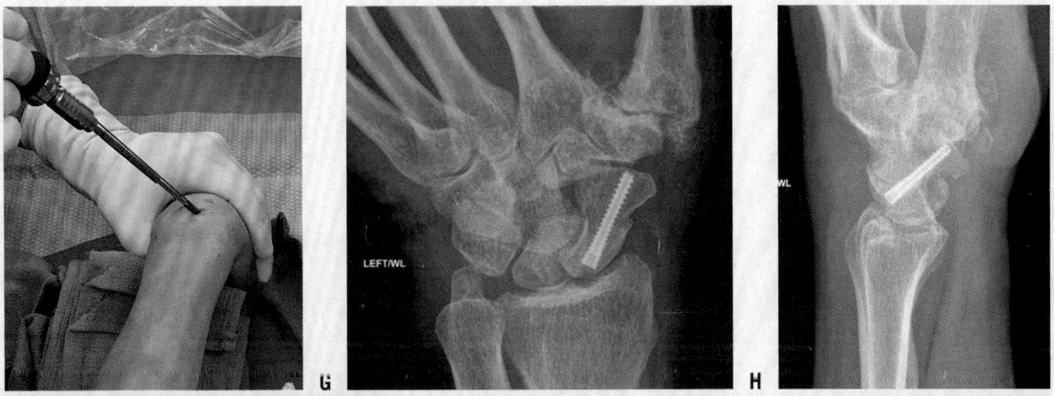

F G H

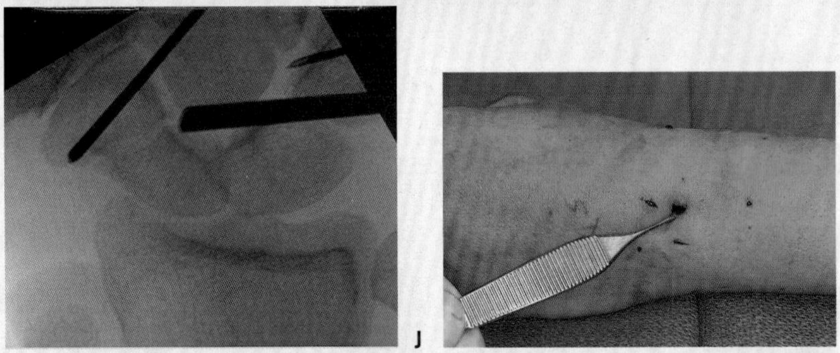

I J

TECH FIG 1 *(continued)* **F.** Using a percutaneous technique, the scaphoid screw insertion is monitored under fluoroscopic guide. **G,H.** The screw tip should rest approximately 2 mm from the distal articular surface and countersunk 2 to 3 mm from the proximal articular surface. **I.** Fluoroscopic image demonstrating insertion of the arthroscope in the radial midcarpal portal to view the scaphoid fracture site at the scapho-capitate articulation. **J.** This arthroscopic portal can be seen in relationship to the 3-4 radiocarpal portal and scaphoid screw starting point.

- Drive the guidewire back from volar to dorsal through the small, dorsal, percutaneous skin incision until the distal tip of the wire lies just within the distal pole of the scaphoid.
- Measure the guidewire length. If measurement is a challenge, you may also place a second guidewire of equal length against the tip of the proximal pole, parallel and next to the first guidewire. The difference between lengths of the protruding wires represents the length of the scaphoid.
- Subtract 4 to 6 mm from the length of the scaphoid to obtain the desired screw length.
- Use the cannulated reamer to ream the scaphoid. It is preferential to do this by hand with care and attention to the direction of the wire, as to avoid breaking the K-wire (thus, a slow reaming of the scaphoid rather than a quick drilling with the power drill).
- If you prefer to drill under power, advance the K-wire volarly again, through the volar soft tissues, and place a hemostat on the K-wire. If the K-wire breaks, both ends of the wire can then be easily retrieved.
- Insert a headless compression screw of the appropriate length **(TECH FIG 1F)**.
  - The tip of the screw should not penetrate the distal surface, and the proximal end of the screw should rest 2 to 3 mm deep to the proximal articular cartilage **(TECH FIG 1G,H)**.
- Confirm satisfactory screw position and fracture reduction with fluoroscopy including oblique imaging. The screw should be inserted down the central axis of the scaphoid. If any doubt exists, use the arthroscopic portals to confirm that the screw is buried in the scaphoid.
  - The 3-4 portal provides good visualization of the screw buried beneath the subchondral bone of the scaphoid. The radial midcarpal portal provides ideal viewing of the fracture reduction and confirmation that there is no breach of the screw at the scaphocapitate articulation **(TECH FIG 1I,J)**.

Displaced Scaphoid Fractures

- Percutaneously insert 0.062-inch K-wires dorsally into the proximal and distal poles of the scaphoid perpendicular to the long axis of the scaphoid to be used as joysticks to reduce the fracture **(TECH FIG 2A,B)**.
- It is beneficial to place these K-wires out of the way of your central guidewire.
- The distal pole tends to be flexed. One can simultaneously extend the distal fragment and flex the proximal fragment K-wires by clamping the K-wires (bringing the distal pole wire proximally and the proximal pole K-wire distally).
- Position the wrist in flexion with ulnar deviation and pronation.
- The central guidewire is then inserted from proximal to distal, starting dorsally and aiming for the central axis of the distal fragment.
  - An additional 0.045-inch K-wire is inserted parallel to the guidewire to prevent rotation of the scaphoid fragments during reaming and screw implantation.
  - Maintenance of reduction during hand reaming and screw insertion is confirmed with fluoroscopy.
  - All wires are subsequently removed after screw fixation.
- In highly unstable fractures, a second parallel screw may be placed, often through the same dorsal percutaneous incision **(TECH FIG 2C,D)**.
- Alternatively, we prefer to place a scaphocapitate screw using the same percutaneous techniques.
  - Scaphocapitate screw fixation is directed from volar radial at the distal pole of the scaphoid to dorsal ulnar in the capitate **(TECH FIG 2E,F)**.

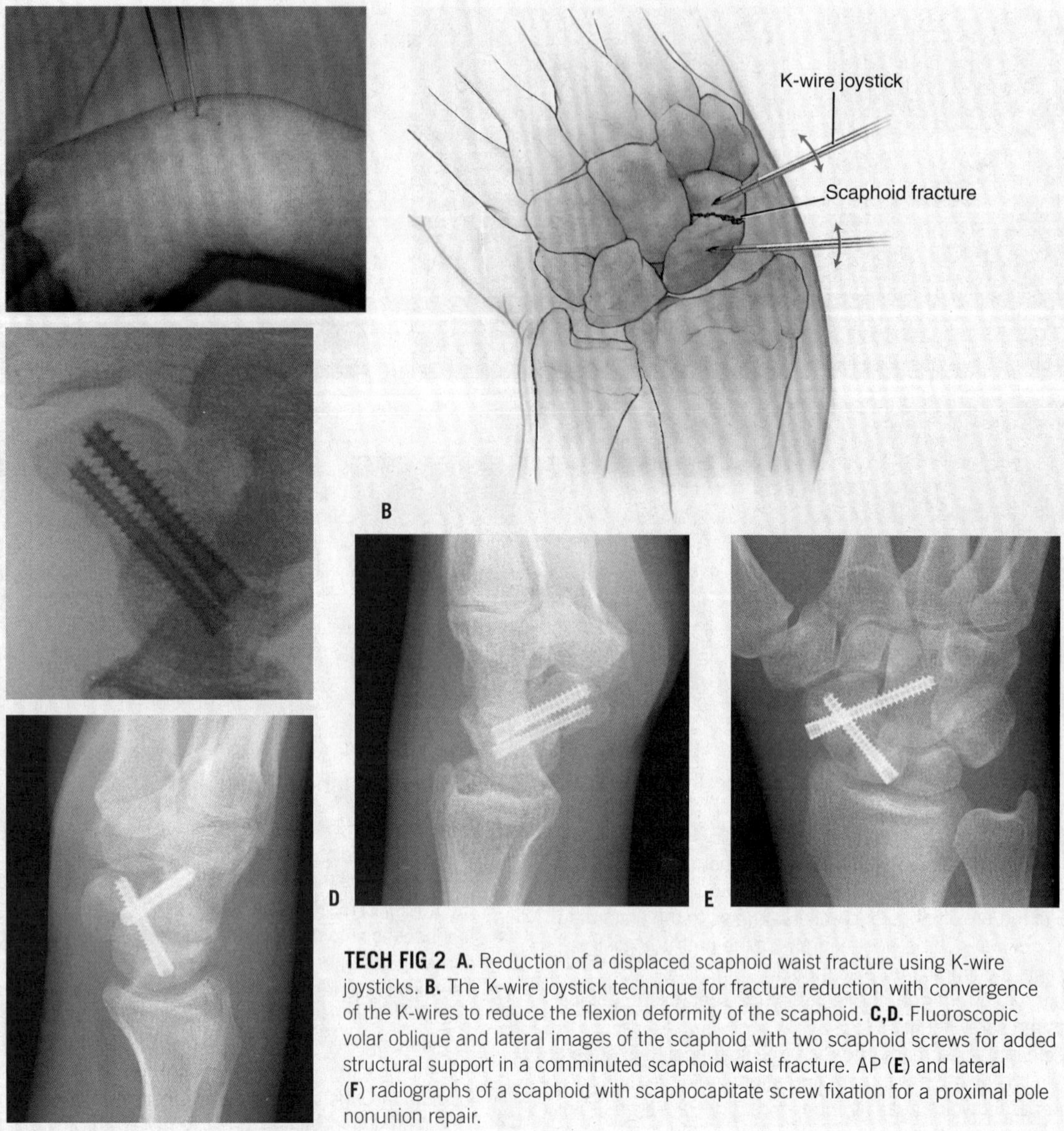

TECH FIG 2 **A.** Reduction of a displaced scaphoid waist fracture using K-wire joysticks. **B.** The K-wire joystick technique for fracture reduction with convergence of the K-wires to reduce the flexion deformity of the scaphoid. **C,D.** Fluoroscopic volar oblique and lateral images of the scaphoid with two scaphoid screws for added structural support in a comminuted scaphoid waist fracture. AP (**E**) and lateral (**F**) radiographs of a scaphoid with scaphocapitate screw fixation for a proximal pole nonunion repair.

VOLAR PERCUTANEOUS APPROACH

- Position the patient supine with the shoulder abducted and the forearm in supination. The wrist is placed into an extended and ulnarly deviated position over a rolled towel to gain access to the distal pole of the scaphoid.[13]
- Place the portable fluoroscopy unit such that AP and lateral views of the wrist can be obtained. Image intensification is used to locate the distal scaphoid tuberosity.
- A small longitudinal incision is made at this point, and the soft tissues are bluntly dissected down to the scaphotrapezial articulation, taking care to protect radial sensory nerve branches in this area.
- Introduce the guidewire on the distal scaphoid tuberosity. Under image guidance, the wire is advanced toward the center of the proximal pole, aiming for Lister tubercle **(TECH FIG 3)**.
- The volar prominence of the trapezium may be partially excised to facilitate the correct starting point and trajectory for the guidewire.
- A K-wire can also be placed into the distal pole of the scaphoid as a joystick to flex the scaphoid, to improve access to the center of the distal pole of the scaphoid.
- Alternatively, the guidewire may be placed directly through the trapezium into the scaphoid distal pole.[12] This technique requires drilling of the trapezium as well as the scaphoid and carries the risk of trapezium fracture.

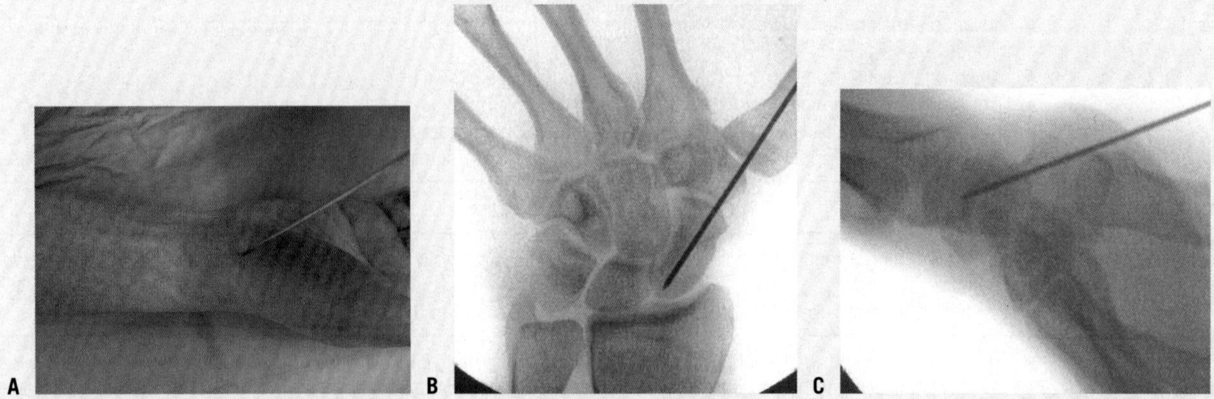

TECH FIG 3 A–C. In the percutaneous volar approach, the guidewire is inserted into the scaphoid at the scaphotrapezial joint and into the center of the proximal pole. The wire should be inserted aiming for the Lister tubercle.

- Use a depth gauge or place a second guidewire of equal length against the surface of the distal scaphoid, adjacent and parallel to the first guidewire. The difference between the lengths of the wires represents the length of the scaphoid.
- Use the cannulated reamer to ream along the guidewire for scaphoid screw placement.
- Insert an appropriate diameter screw of a length 4 to 6 mm short of the total scaphoid length measured by the central guidewire.
- Confirm satisfactory screw position and fracture reduction with fluoroscopy.

MINI-OPEN DORSAL APPROACH TO SCAPHOID SCREW FIXATION

- An alternative to the percutaneous approach is to make a 1.5-cm skin incision just ulnar and distal to Lister tubercle to allow for better visualization of the starting point of the screw and to protect the extensor tendons.
  - Although the third dorsal compartment may be opened, and the EPL transposed, a less invasive option is to create a capsular window just ulnar to the EPL and the extensor carpi radialis brevis (ECRB) without transposing the EPL **(TECH FIG 4A)**.
- Careful dissection just distal to the dorsal rim of the distal radius is used to identify the extensor digitorum communis (EDC) tendons ulnarly and the EPL and ECRB tendons radially. There is a clear area of capsule at this location.
- A 1-cm longitudinal capsulotomy is created directly over the proximal pole of the scaphoid, taking care to not only protect the dorsal capsular ridge of the scaphoid but also the underlying scapholunate ligament.
- Alternatively, a transverse arthrotomy just distal to the dorsal rim of the distal radius can be performed, which prevents dissection of the scapholunate ligament and its dorsal capsular attachments.
- Once the proximal pole is directly visualized, scaphoid screw fixation may proceed as described earlier **(TECH FIG 4B)**.

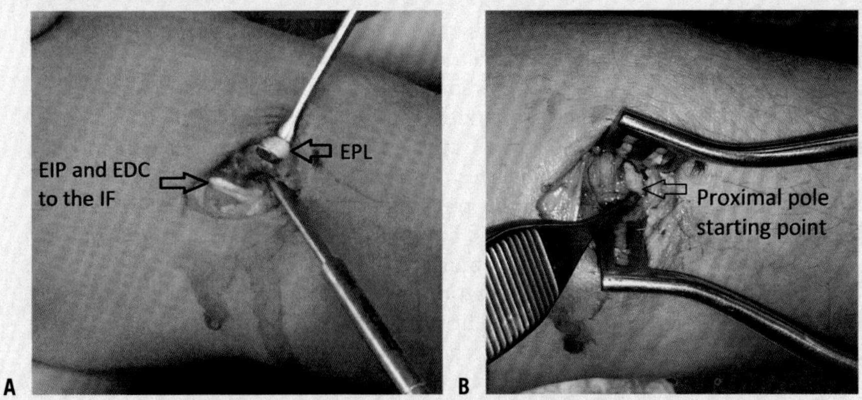

TECH FIG 4 A. This clinical photograph demonstrates the EPL tendon radial to the guidewire hand reamer and the EDC and extensor indicis proprius (*EIP*) tendons ulnar to it. These tendons can be kept safe with a small self-retaining retractor or Ragnell retractors with an assistant during instrumentation of the scaphoid. *IF*, index finger. **B.** The starting point on the proximal pole of the scaphoid can be visualized through this small arthrotomy. Care is taken while making this small capsular window to protect the scapholunate ligament and the dorsal capsular attachments of the scapholunate ligament complex.

Pearls and Pitfalls

General	• Advanced imaging for suspected scaphoid fractures in the setting of negative radiographs is cost-effective and reduces morbidity.[17] • Union rates using thumb spica cast and short-arm cast are similar.[3,4,25] • The senior author prefers the dorsal approach for all proximal pole and waist fractures. • The percutaneous volar approach is used for very distal waist fractures in my practice. • Percutaneous volar approach can work well for routine waist fractures as well and is preferred by some surgeons.
Dorsal Technique	
Approach	• Blunt dissection through the incision minimizes the risk of injury to the extensor tendons and radial sensory nerve branches. • For the arthrotomy, use a blunt-tipped hemostat to avoid injury to the articular cartilage and dorsal ligaments.
Guidewire Placement	• Pronate and flex the wrist until the ring sign is noted; the center of the ring is the insertion point for the guidewire. • Direct visualization of the proximal pole of the scaphoid following capsulotomy allows for more accurate guidewire placement and decreases risk of the guidewire bending. • It is not difficult to break a bent or malpositioned guidewire, especially if a smaller caliber screw is being used (the smaller the screw diameter, the smaller the guidewire).
Screw Placement	• Drill or ream the central guidewire by hand to decrease the chance of guidewire breakage. • Select a screw that is 4 to 6 mm shorter than the measured length. • A common mistake is to place a screw that ends up too long once the screw compresses the fragments. • Confirm central position of guidewire via fluoroscopy on each of the views (scaphoid, semipronated, semisupinated, and lateral)
Reduction of Displaced Fractures	• K-wires may be used as joysticks for reduction. • The distal fragment is typically flexed and pronated. For reduction, the distal K-wire is extended and supinated. • A derotational K-wire should be placed before reaming, and screw insertion if the fragments are unstable or if there is fracture comminution.
Extremely Small Proximal Pole Fractures	• Use a smaller size caliber screw to prevent breaking apart the proximal fracture fragment. • Noncannulated, countersunk screws with a head may also be used; a dorsal mini-open approach is recommended for visualization in this scenario.
Volar Technique	
Approach	• Blunt dissection to the scaphoid minimizes the risk of injury.
Guidewire Placement	• A central starting point on the distal scaphoid tuberosity can be hindered by the trapezium. • Part of the volar trapezium can be resected to achieve a correct starting point for trajectory of the guidewire. • Alternatively, the guidewire and the drilling can be performed through the trapezium. • Some symptoms related to partial trapezium excision may be expected.

POSTOPERATIVE CARE

- After application of sterile dressings, a volar, short-arm, wrist splint is applied. Typically, there is no need to immobilize the thumb if there is a solid scaphoid screw in place. The thumb and fingers remain free for range-of-motion exercises.
- At 2 weeks postoperatively, the sutures are removed, and the patient is transitioned to a removable wrist brace or a short-arm cast, depending on fracture stability.
  - Plain radiographs are obtained at 2, 6, and 12 weeks postoperatively.
- If there is any question regarding fracture union, a CT scan is obtained.
- Unprotected strenuous activity or contact sports are not permitted until definitive evidence of union across the fracture site is obtained, defined as at least 50% of bridging trabecular bone.
  - Players may be permitted to return to sport sooner, at their own peril, in a brace or a cast.

OUTCOMES

- Results of contemporary techniques of percutaneous fixation are excellent; it has been shown to allow for earlier mobilization and return to activity and high satisfaction rates compared to nonoperative measures.[12,13,26,27,29]
  - The surgical approach (dorsal vs. volar percutaneous) does not affect the clinical and functional outcome.[12]
  - Use of the transtrapezial approach does not lead to symptomatic scaphotrapezial arthritis at the short- to medium-term follow-up.[10]
- Earlier mobilization avoids complications such as muscle atrophy and joint stiffness.[2]
- Percutaneous techniques result in decreased soft tissue damage compared to conventional open techniques.[29]
- In a series of 27 consecutive patients treated with percutaneous internal fixation of their scaphoid fracture via an arthroscopically assisted dorsal approach, the union rate (confirmed by CT) was 100%. The average time to union

was 12 weeks, with a prolonged time to union noted in patients with a proximal pole fracture.[27]

- Although waist fractures can be treated with surgical or nonsurgical treatment depending on the fracture characteristics as well as surgeon and patient preference, surgically treated proximal pole fractures have a higher union rate and decreased time to union when compared to cast immobilization.[24]
- Treatment of nondisplaced scaphoid waist fractures
  - Similar union rates, faster return to work, and faster time to union with surgical fixation compared to cast immobilization without increased complication rate.[1,2]
  - Cost–utility analysis favors early open reduction and internal fixation (ORIF) with overall cost being higher in casting due to delayed return to work.[22]
- Volar versus dorsal approach: No significant difference in percentage or time to union.[16]

COMPLICATIONS

- The risks associated with ORIF, such as damage to the ligamentous support of the carpus and disruption of the dorsal blood supply, are minimized with percutaneous fixation.
- Possible complications include the following[28]:
  - Nonunion
  - Malunion
  - Injury to the dorsal sensory branch of the radial nerve
  - Extensor tendon injury with percutaneous dorsal approach
  - Infection
  - Technical problems: screw protrusion, screw malposition, bending or breakage of the guidewire
  - Erosion of the trapezium and discomfort from the head of the screw has been reported with the use of a percutaneous cannulated screw inserted via the volar approach.[29]

REFERENCES

1. Alnaeem H, Aldekhayel S, Kanevsky J, et al. A systematic review and meta-analysis examining the differences between nonsurgical management and percutaneous fixation of minimally and nondisplaced scaphoid fractures. J Hand Surg Am 2016;41(12):1135.e1–1144.e1.
2. Bond CD, Shin AY, McBride MT, et al. Percutaneous screw fixation or cast immobilization for nondisplaced scaphoid fractures. J Bone Joint Surg Am 2001;83:483–488.
3. Buijze GA, Goslings JC, Rhemrev SJ, et al. Cast immobilization with and without immobilization of the thumb for nondisplaced and minimally displaced scaphoid waist fractures: a multicenter, randomized, controlled trial. J Hand Surg Am 2014;39:621–627.
4. Clay NR, Dias JJ, Costigan PS, et al. Need the thumb be immobilised in scaphoid fractures? A randomised prospective trial. J Bone Joint Surg Br 1991;73:828–832.
5. Clementson M, Jørgsholm P, Besjakov J, et al. Union of scaphoid waist fractures assessed by CT scan. J Wrist Surg 2015;4:49–55.
6. Dias JJ, Taylor M, Thompson J, et al. Radiographic signs of union of scaphoid fractures: an analysis of inter-observer agreement and reproducibility. J Bone Joint Surg Br 1988;70:299–301.
7. Dodds SD, Panjabi MM, Slade JF III. Screw fixation of scaphoid fractures: a biomechanical assessment of screw length and screw augmentation. J Hand Surg Am 2006;31(3):405–413.
8. Gelberman RH, Menon J. The vascularity of the scaphoid bone. J Hand Surg Am 1980;5:508–513.
9. Gellman H, Caputo RJ, Carter V, et al. Comparison of short and long thumb-spica casts for non-displaced fractures of the carpal scaphoid. J Bone Joint Surg Am 1989;71(3):354–357.
10. Geurts G, van Riet R, Meermans G, et al. Incidence of scaphotrapezial arthritis following volar percutaneous fixation of nondisplaced scaphoid waist fractures using a transtrapezial approach. J Hand Surg Am 2011;36(11):1753–1758.
11. Gilley E, Puri SK, Hearns KA, et al. Importance of computed tomography in determining displacement in scaphoid fractures. J Wrist Surg 2018;7(1):38–42.
12. Gürbüz Y, Kayalar M, Bal E, et al. Comparison of dorsal and volar percutaneous screw fixation methods in acute type B scaphoid fractures. Acta Orthop Traumatol Turc 2012;46(5):339–345.
13. Haddad FS, Goddard NJ. Acute percutaneous scaphoid fixation. A pilot study. J Bone Joint Surg Br 1998;80(1):95–99.
14. Heinzelmann AD, Archer G, Bindra RR. Anthropometry of the human scaphoid. J Hand Surg 2007;32(7):1005–1008.
15. Jørgsholm P, Thomsen NO, Björkman A, et al. The incidence of intrinsic and extrinsic ligament injuries in scaphoid waist fractures. J Hand Surg Am 2010;35(3):368–374.
16. Kang KB, Kim HJ, Park JH, et al. Comparison of dorsal and volar percutaneous approaches in acute scaphoid fractures: a meta-analysis. PLoS One 2016;11(9):e0162779.
17. Karl JW, Swart E, Strauch RJ. Diagnosis of occult scaphoid fractures: a cost-effectiveness analysis. J Bone Joint Surg Am 2015;97(22):1860–1868.
18. Kerluke L, McCabe SJ. Nonunion of the scaphoid: a critical analysis of recent natural history studies. J Hand Surg Am 1993;18(1):1–3.
19. Kupperman A, Breighner R, Saltzman E, et al. Ideal starting point and trajectory of a screw for the dorsal approach to scaphoid fractures. J Hand Surg Am 2018;43(11):993–999.
20. Martus JE, Bedi A, Jebson PJ. Cannulated variable pitch compression screw fixation of scaphoid fractures using a limited dorsal approach. Tech Hand Upper Ext Surg 2005;9:202–206.
21. Morsy M, Sabbagh MD, van Alphen NA, et al. The vascular anatomy of the scaphoid: new discoveries using micro-computed tomography imaging. J Hand Surg Am 2019;44(11):928–938.
22. Ram AN, Chung KC. Evidence-based management of acute nondisplaced scaphoid waist fractures. J Hand Surg Am 2009;34:735–738.
23. Ruby LK, Stinson J, Belsky MR. The natural history of scaphoid non-union. A review of fifty-five cases. J Bone Joint Surg Am 1985;67(3):428–432.
24. Saltzman EB, Rancy SK, Lee SK, et al. Acute management of proximal pole scaphoid fractures. In: Buijze GA, Jupiter JB, eds. Scaphoid Fractures: Evidence-Based Management. Philadelphia: Elsevier, 2017.
25. Schramm JM, Nguyen M, Wongworawat MD, et al. Does thumb immobilization contribute to scaphoid fracture stability? Hand (N Y) 2008;3(1):41–43.
26. Slade JF III, Dodds SD. Minimally invasive management of scaphoid nonunions. Clin Orthop 2006;445:108–119.
27. Slade JF III, Gutow AP, Geissler WB. Percutaneous internal fixation of scaphoid fractures via an arthroscopically assisted dorsal approach. J Bone Joint Surg Am 2002;84:21–36.
28. Slade JF III, Jaskwhich D. Percutaneous fixation of scaphoid fractures. Hand Clin 2001;17:553–574.
29. Yip HS, Wu WC, Chang RY, et al. Percutaneous cannulated screw fixation of acute scaphoid waist fracture. J Hand Surg Br 2002;27(1):42–46.

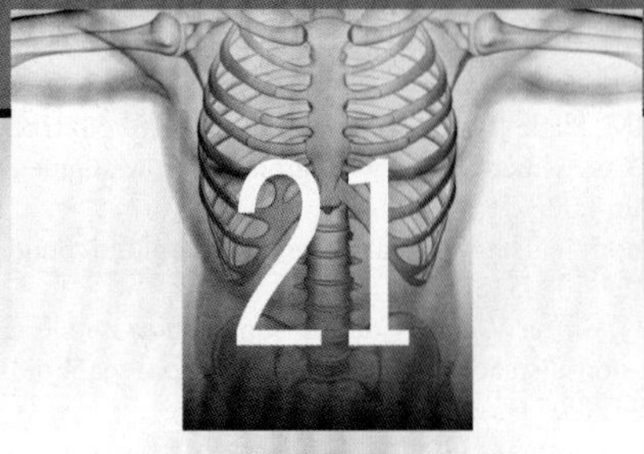

CHAPTER 21

Open Reduction and Internal Fixation of Scaphoid Fractures and Nonunions

Kevin Chan, Peter J.L. Jebson, and Levi L. Hinkelman

DEFINITION

- The scaphoid is the most commonly fractured carpal bone, accounting for 1 in every 100,000 emergency department visits.[9]
- A scaphoid nonunion is defined as a nonhealed scaphoid 6 months after injury.
- Scaphoid nonunion or proximal pole avascular necrosis (AVN) after a fracture has been associated with considerable morbidity and a predictable pattern of wrist arthritis.
- The complex anatomy and tenuous blood supply to the scaphoid make operative management of these fractures technically challenging.

ANATOMY

- The scaphoid has a complex three-dimensional geometry that has been likened to a "twisted peanut." It can be divided into three regions: proximal pole, waist, and distal pole.
- The scaphoid functions as the primary link between the forearm and the distal carpal row and therefore plays a critical role in maintaining normal carpal kinematics.
- Articulating with the scaphoid fossa of the radius, the lunate, capitate, trapezium, and trapezoid, more than 70% of the scaphoid is covered with articular cartilage.
- The main arterial supply to the scaphoid is from the radial artery; it enters the scaphoid via two main branches:
  - A dorsal branch, entering through the dorsal ridge, is the primary supply and provides 70% to 80% of the vascularity, including the entire proximal pole via retrograde endosteal branches.
  - A volar branch, entering through the tubercle, supplies the remaining 20% to 30%, predominantly the distal pole and tuberosity.
- The proximal pole is at increased risk for AVN secondary to disruption of its tenuous retrograde blood supply after a fracture of the scaphoid waist or proximal pole.
- Due to its tenuous vascular supply, the scaphoid heals almost entirely by primary bone healing, which makes anatomic reduction and bony apposition even more critical. There is usually minimal callus formation.
- The size and shape of the scaphoid demands attention to detail and accurate implantation of fixation devices during fracture fixation. Scaphoid dimensions vary between genders as the male scaphoid is usually longer and wider than the females. In addition, the diameter of many commercially available standard headless compression screws is larger than the size of the proximal pole of the female scaphoid.

PATHOGENESIS

- Scaphoid fractures are most commonly seen in young, active males.[9]
- Scaphoid fractures typically result from a fall on an outstretched hand. With the wrist dorsiflexed greater than 95 degrees, in combination with 10 degrees or more of radial deviation, the distal radius abuts the scaphoid and precipitates a fracture.[9]
- Less commonly, the scaphoid can also be fractured with forced palmar flexion of the wrist or axial loading of the flexed wrist.
- Most of these fractures occur at the waist region, although 10% to 20% occur in the proximal pole.
- Proximal pole fractures are associated with an increased risk of nonunion, delayed union, and AVN.
- In children, scaphoid fractures are less common and are most frequently seen in the distal pole.

NATURAL HISTORY

- An untreated or inadequately treated scaphoid fracture has a higher likelihood of nonunion. The overall incidence of nonunion is estimated at 5% to 10%, but the risk is significantly increased with nonoperative treatment of a displaced waist or proximal pole fracture.
- The natural history of scaphoid nonunions is controversial, but they are believed to result in a predictable pattern of progressive radiocarpal and midcarpal arthritis.
- In an established scaphoid nonunion, the distal portion of the scaphoid may flex, producing a "humpback" deformity of the scaphoid. The loss of scaphoid integrity can result in carpal instability and abnormal carpal kinematics, most frequently manifesting as a dorsal intercalated segment instability pattern.
  - The pattern of carpal instability and secondary arthrosis due to an unstable scaphoid nonunion has been termed a *SNAC wrist* (scaphoid nonunion advanced collapse pattern of wrist arthritis).
  - In the SNAC wrist, there is a loss of carpal height with proximal capitate migration, flexion and pronation of the scaphoid, and secondary midcarpal arthritis.
- Factors associated with the development of a scaphoid fracture nonunion include the following:
  - Delayed diagnosis or treatment
  - Inadequate immobilization
  - Proximal fracture
  - Initial and progressive fracture displacement
  - Fracture comminution
  - Presence of associated carpal injuries (ie, perilunate injury)

PATIENT HISTORY AND PHYSICAL FINDINGS

- Scaphoid fractures classically occur in the active, young adult population. Patients can present with radial-sided wrist pain, painful thumb movement, reduced wrist range of motion, and decreased grip strength.
- Classic physical examination findings include the following:
  - Swelling over the dorsoradial aspect of the wrist
  - Tenderness to palpation dorsoradially in the "anatomic snuffbox"
  - Tenderness volarly over the distal tubercle of the scaphoid
  - Pain with axial compression of the thumb metacarpal (scaphoid compression test)
- It is important to maintain a high index of suspicion and carefully scrutinize radiographs because not all patients with a scaphoid fracture will present with the classic physical exam findings. The diagnostic sensitivity of clinical examination is high, but the specificity ranges from 74% to 80%.[7]
- Scaphoid fractures can be part of a greater arc injury.
  - The physician should examine the entire wrist carefully for areas of tenderness and swelling.
  - Plain radiographs are scrutinized for an associated ligamentous injury or disruption of the midcarpal joint as seen in a transscaphoid perilunate fracture-dislocation.

IMAGING AND OTHER DIAGNOSTIC STUDIES

- The following plain radiographs should routinely be ordered in the patient with a suspected scaphoid fracture: posteroanterior (PA), oblique, lateral, and dedicated scaphoid views.
  - The PA view allows visualization of the proximal pole of the scaphoid.
  - The 45-degree semipronated oblique view provides the best visualization of the waist and distal pole regions.
  - The 45-degree semisupinated oblique view provides the best visualization of the dorsal ridge.
  - The lateral view permits an assessment of fracture angulation, carpal alignment, and carpal instability.
  - The dedicated scaphoid view is a PA view with the wrist in ulnar deviation. This results in scaphoid extension, allowing visualization of the scaphoid in profile **(FIG 1A)**.
- The sensitivity of radiographs for scaphoid fractures is approximately 70%.
- There is controversy surrounding the ideal method of detecting occult scaphoid fractures.
  - Approximately 20% of patients with a scaphoid fracture will initially present with normal radiographs and require additional imaging to establish a definitive diagnosis.[11] Some surgeons advocate immobilization and follow-up radiographs, whereas others recommend advanced imaging, including bone scintigraphy, magnetic resonance imaging (MRI), or computed tomography (CT).[7]
- A technetium bone scan has been shown to be up to approximately 100% sensitive in identifying an occult fracture. Unfortunately, it is associated with a lower specificity and often will not be positive immediately after the fracture (<72 hours after injury). A Cochrane systematic review[11] concluded that bone scans are statistically the best diagnostic test compared to CT and MRI, but it is more invasive, can lead to overtreatment, and may be inappropriate for use in children.
- MRI may be indicated in the evaluation of an occult scaphoid fracture as well **(FIG 1B,C)** and may be superior to

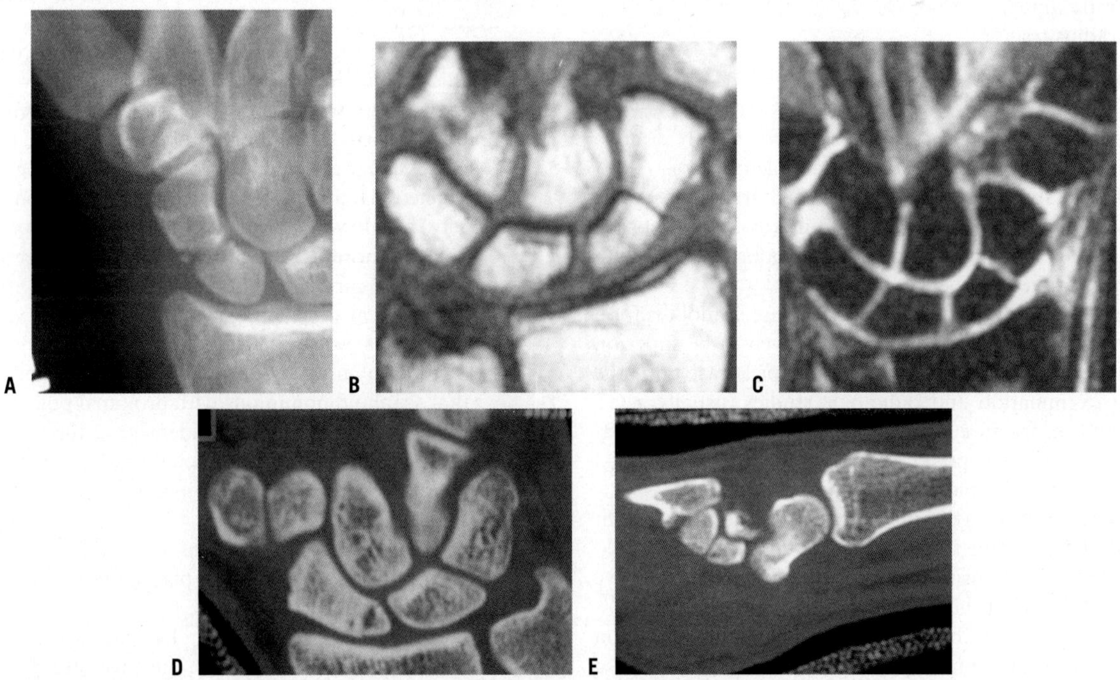

FIG 1 A. Radiograph (scaphoid view) of an acute, displaced, comminuted scaphoid waist fracture. **B,C.** T1- and T2-weighted MRI images demonstrating a nondisplaced scaphoid waist fracture. **D,E.** Axial and sagittal CT scan images demonstrating a fracture of the proximal pole of the scaphoid. (Copyright Peter J.L. Jebson, MD.)

bone scintigraphy because of improved specificity. MRI is highly sensitive with a specificity approaching 100% when performed within 48 hours of injury. Immediate testing using an MRI has also been shown to be cost-effective in establishing a diagnosis in patients with a suspected scaphoid fracture and negative radiographs.[17]
  - Bone bruising without a fracture detected on MRI can lead to an occult fracture in a small percentage of cases.
  - MRI with intravenous gadolinium contrast may be helpful in assessing the vascularity of the proximal pole, particularly in the patient with an established nonunion.
- CT with reconstruction images in multiple planes can be used to identify an acute fracture not detected on plain radiographs but is arguably most useful in evaluating an established scaphoid fracture, nonunion, or malunion.
  - CT is indicated to rule out displacement for scaphoid fractures because plain radiographs can be unreliable **(FIG 1D,E)**.
  - CT is our preferred modality for confirming union after a scaphoid fracture, particularly before permitting a return to contact sports. We use 50% bridging bone as the minimum criteria to allow patients to return to unrestricted activities.[5]
- The following criteria define a displaced or unstable fracture:
  - At least 1 mm of displacement
  - More than 10 degrees of angular displacement
  - Fracture comminution
  - Radiolunate angle of more than 15 degrees
  - Scapholunate angle of more than 60 degrees
  - Intrascaphoid angle of more than 35 degrees

DIFFERENTIAL DIAGNOSIS

- Scapholunate injury
- Wrist sprain
- Wrist contusion
- Fracture of other carpal bone
- Greater arc injury
- Distal radius fracture

NONOPERATIVE MANAGEMENT

- Nonoperative management is indicated for a truly nondisplaced, stable scaphoid waist or distal pole fracture.
  - Unstable fractures and nondisplaced fractures of the proximal pole are indications for internal fixation based on studies that have demonstrated a poor outcome with nonoperative treatment.
- The appropriate type and duration of cast immobilization remain controversial, and none has proven to be superior. Our preference is a short-arm thumb spica cast until the clinical examination and radiologic studies (usually a CT scan) confirm fracture union. If there are concerns for patient compliance, we prefer an initial period (4 to 6 weeks) of long-arm thumb spica cast immobilization.
  - Clinical studies have failed to demonstrate any benefit from including the thumb or fingers in the cast.
  - Similarly, wrist position has not been proven to improve scaphoid fracture healing.
  - Numerous studies have revealed no difference in union rates for a long-arm versus short-arm cast; however, a randomized prospective study by Gellman et al[4] documented a shorter time to union and fewer nonunions and delayed unions with initial use of a long-arm cast.
- The morbidity of a nonoperative approach, specifically cast immobilization, has become of increasing concern.
  - A prolonged duration of immobilization is often required for waist and proximal pole fractures (8 to 12 weeks), and this can be accompanied by muscle atrophy, stiffness, reduced grip strength, and residual pain. In addition, cast immobilization can cause significant inconvenience for the patient and interference with activities of daily living.
  - The prolonged duration of immobilization is of particular concern in the young laborer, athlete, or military personnel, who typically desire expedient functional recovery.

SURGICAL MANAGEMENT

- Indications for open reduction and internal fixation (ORIF) of scaphoid fractures include the following:
  - Proximal pole fracture
  - A displaced, unstable fracture of the scaphoid waist
  - Associated carpal instability or perilunate instability
  - Associated distal radius fracture
  - Delayed presentation (more than 3 to 4 weeks) with no prior treatment
  - A nondisplaced, stable scaphoid waist fracture in a patient who wishes to avoid the morbidity of cast immobilization. In this clinical scenario, operative treatment may proceed after shared decision-making and an explanation of the rationale for, and the risks and benefits of, operative treatment versus cast immobilization.
- Scaphoid nonunions are generally treated with surgical intervention to prevent scaphoid nonunion advanced collapse and secondary degenerative arthritic changes.
- Currently available surgical treatments include nonvascularized and vascularized bone grafting with and without internal fixation.
- There is controversy surrounding the ideal surgical treatment, including the use of nonvascularized versus vascularized bone graft, corticocancellous versus cancellous bone graft,[8,15,16] and the importance of proximal pole vascularity.[16]
- There is no consensus on which modality predicts proximal pole vascularity, including radiographs, MRI, intraoperative assessment of punctate bleeding, or histology.[15]
- Our preferred technique for an established nonunion with no deformity is ORIF with nonvascularized cancellous bone grafting.[3]
  - Screw fixation is superior to use of Kirschner wires with improved carpal stability and union.[14]
  - There is insufficient evidence to support vascularized bone over nonvascularized bone for scaphoid healing or time to union.[15] A growing body of evidence suggests that scaphoid nonunions with proximal pole AVN can be treated with operative débridement of the nonunion site, nonvascularized bone graft, and rigid internal fixation.[16]
- For patients with a humpback deformity, a structural bone graft should be used.
  - Intercalary corticocancellous wedge graft from the iliac crest of distal radius can be placed after correction of the humpback deformity.
  - Pure cancellous bone graft has the advantages of decreased surgical complexity, but there are concerns with mechanical stability.
  - We prefer a modified Russe technique using a single corticocancellous strut and intramedullary screw[10] or volar

plate fixation.[19] An intercalary wedge graft can be used but may be technically difficult to accurately shape the bone graft and to place a screw across three fragments.

Preoperative Planning

- All imaging studies should be reviewed to accurately define the fracture pattern.
- Required equipment are as follows:
  - Portable minifluoroscopy unit
  - Kirschner wires
  - Cannulated headless compression screw system. We prefer to use the Acutrak 2 or mini-Acutrak 2 screw system (Acumed, Beaverton, OR), but any headless cannulated screw system that permits screw insertion beneath the articular surface and generates adequate compression at the fracture site may be used.

Positioning

- General or regional anesthesia may be used. Wide-awake local anesthesia no tourniquet (WALANT) may be an alternative.
- The patient is positioned supine on the operating table with a radiolucent hand table at the shoulder level.
- The fluoroscopy unit is draped and positioned at the end of the hand table.
- A pneumatic tourniquet is carefully applied to the proximal arm, unless WALANT is used.
- An intravenous antibiotic is provided before inflation of the tourniquet as prophylaxis for infection.
- The limb is prepared and draped, followed by exsanguination of the limb with an Esmarch bandage and tourniquet inflation, usually to a pressure of 250 mm Hg.

Approach

- ORIF of scaphoid fractures can be performed through either a dorsal or volar approach.
- The specific approaches that will be described include the following:
  - Open dorsal approach (our preferred approach)[12]
  - Open volar approach
- ORIF of scaphoid nonunion is performed through a dorsal approach.

TECHNIQUES

OPEN REDUCTION AND INTERNAL FIXATION OF SCAPHOID FRACTURE: OPEN DORSAL APPROACH

Exposure

- Pronate the forearm and make a longitudinal skin incision, about 2 to 3 cm long, beginning at the proximal aspect of the tubercle of Lister and extending distally along the axis of the third metacarpal **(TECH FIG 1A)**.
  - If the fracture is nondisplaced, a smaller skin incision and limited capsulotomy may be used.
- Raise skin flaps at the level of the extensor retinaculum.
- Incise the extensor retinaculum overlying the third compartment immediately distal to the tubercle of Lister and carefully release the fascia overlying the extensor pollicis longus (EPL) tendon, permitting gentle retraction of the EPL radially. Similarly, incise the dorsal hand fascia longitudinally.
  - Gently retract the extensor digitorum communis tendons ulnarly while retracting the extensor carpi radialis brevis and extensor carpi radialis longus tendons radially with the EPL tendon, thus exposing the underlying radiocarpal joint capsule **(TECH FIG 1B)**.
- For nondisplaced fractures, make a limited transverse capsulotomy just distal to the dorsal rim of the radius.
  - Evacuate fracture hematoma.
  - Inspect the scapholunate ligament complex for associated injury.
- If the fracture is displaced, it is often helpful to create an inverted T-shaped capsulotomy with the longitudinal limb directly over the scapholunate ligament complex **(TECH FIG 1C)**. Extend the longitudinal limb of the capsulotomy to expose the scaphocapitate articulation and the radial aspect of the midcarpal joint.
  - The tubercle of Lister is helpful in locating the scapholunate articulation.

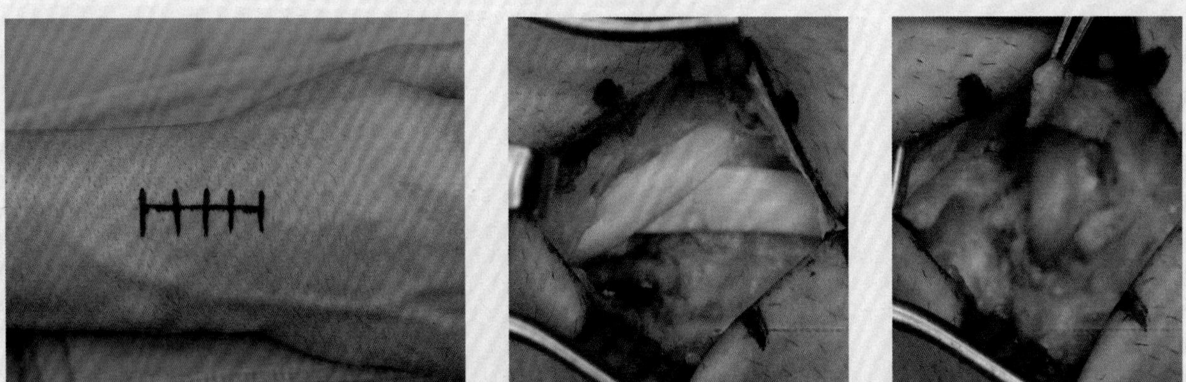

A B C

TECH FIG 1 **A.** Skin incision used for ORIF of scaphoid fractures via the dorsal approach. **B.** Retracting the thumb and wrist extensor tendons radially and the finger extensor tendons ulnarly facilitates exposure of the underlying capsule. **C.** A limited capsulotomy should be performed to expose the proximal scaphoid and scapholunate ligament. (Copyright Peter J.L. Jebson, MD.)

- Carefully elevate the capsular flaps from the proximal pole of the scaphoid and lunate. Avoid damaging the important dorsal component of the scapholunate ligament.
  - When elevating the radial flap, take care to avoid stripping the dorsal ridge vessels entering at the scaphoid waist region.

Fracture Reduction and Provisional Fixation

- Distract the carpus manually via longitudinal traction on the index and long fingers.
- If the fracture is displaced, insert 0.045-inch Kirschner wire joysticks perpendicularly into the proximal and distal scaphoid fragments to assist in the reduction **(TECH FIG 2A)**.
  - The accuracy of the reduction can be determined by visually assessing congruency of the radioscaphoid and scaphocapitate articulations.
- When a satisfactory reduction has been achieved, obtain provisional fixation with parallel derotational 0.045-inch Kirschner wires.
  - The first wire is inserted dorsal and ulnar to the central axis of the scaphoid, into the trapezium for enhanced stability.
  - The second derotational wire may be inserted volar and radial to the anticipated central axis insertion site if more fixation is needed.
  - The derotational wires must be placed such that they will not interfere with central axis guidewire placement, reaming, and screw insertion **(TECH FIG 2B)**.

Guidewire Placement

- The starting position for guidewire is at the membranous portion of the scapholunate ligament origin **(TECH FIG 3A,B)**.
  - In very proximal fractures, the starting point for the guidewire is as far proximally in the scaphoid as possible, at the midaspect of the membranous portion of the scapholunate ligament complex. This point is critical to avoid propagation of the fracture into the proximal scaphoid during insertion of the screw.
- With the wrist flexed over a bolster, insert the guidewire down the central axis of the scaphoid in line with the thumb metacarpal.
  - Be very patient with this important step; proceed with reaming and screw insertion only after central placement has been confirmed on the PA, lateral, and 30-degree pronated lateral views **(TECH FIG 3C)**.
  - Central placement of the screw is biomechanically advantageous, with greater stiffness and load to failure.
  - It is critical to insert the wire in the optimal position in all three views to avoid violating the midcarpal joint or the volar surface of the scaphoid.
  - Take care to avoid bending the guidewire.
- Advance the wire up to but not into the scaphotrapezial joint.

Screw Insertion

- Determine screw length by measuring the guidewire **(TECH FIG 4A)**.
  - In the case of minimal fragment separation, subtract 4 mm from the measured length of the wire to allow recession of the proximal screw beneath the articular surface and avoid distal violation of the scaphotrapezial articulation.
  - If fragments are more displaced, consider choosing an even shorter screw as the fracture will be compressed.
  - The common mistake is placement of a screw that is too long.
- Advance the wire into the trapezium to avoid loss of position during drilling.
- Use the cannulated drill to open up the proximal cortex **(TECH FIG 4B)** and manually insert the screw **(TECH FIG 4C,D)**.
  - We use the larger Acutrak 2 screw when feasible, but the mini-Acutrak 2 system may be necessary in patients with a small scaphoid or if the fracture is located proximally such that insertion of an Acutrak 2 screw may result in inadvertent propagation of the fracture to the insertion site with fragmentation of the proximal scaphoid. Any cannulated, headless compression screw may be used but size is critical.
  - Remove the guidewire and assess screw position via fluoroscopy using the same views.
    - If the fracture is highly unstable or the quality of fixation is less than ideal, two micro-Acutrak 2 screws (or equivalent small size screws) may be carefully inserted for enhanced stability.
    - The capsulotomy is not repaired as we have found this to lead to adhesions and a loss of wrist palmar flexion postoperatively.

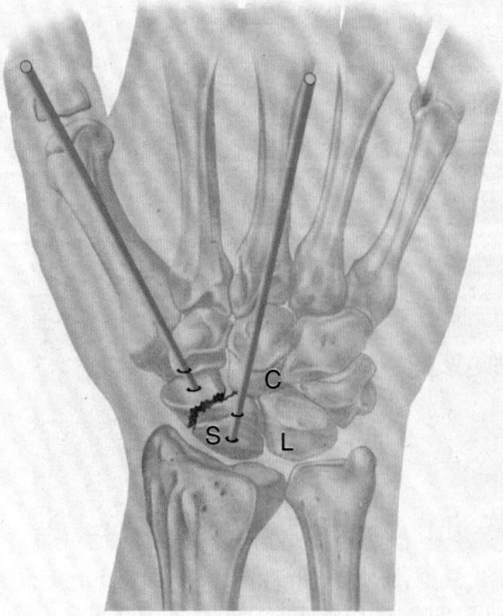

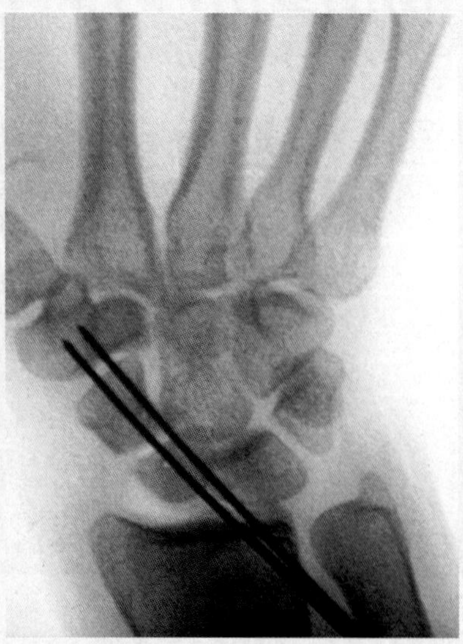

TECH FIG 2 A. Percutaneous insertion of Kirschner wires into the proximal and distal scaphoid (*S*) fragments is helpful to facilitate manual reduction of a displaced fracture. *C*, capitate; *L*, lunate. **B.** A displaced S waist fracture has been stabilized with a derotational Kirschner wire placed dorsally and ulnarly to the guidewire. The derotational Kirschner wire does not interfere with insertion of the screw in the central axis. (**B:** Copyright Peter J.L. Jebson, MD.)

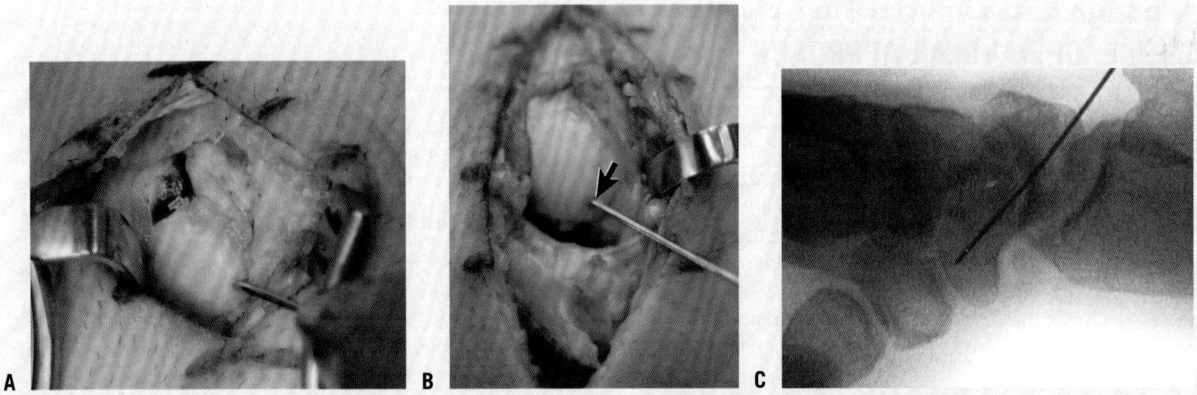

TECH FIG 3 A,B. Note the starting point at the membranous portion of the scapholunate ligament (*arrow*). (In **A**, top is distal, bottom is proximal, left is radial, and right is ulnar.) **C.** The 30-degree pronated oblique view demonstrating guidewire placement down the central axis of the scaphoid. (Copyright Peter J.L. Jebson, MD.)

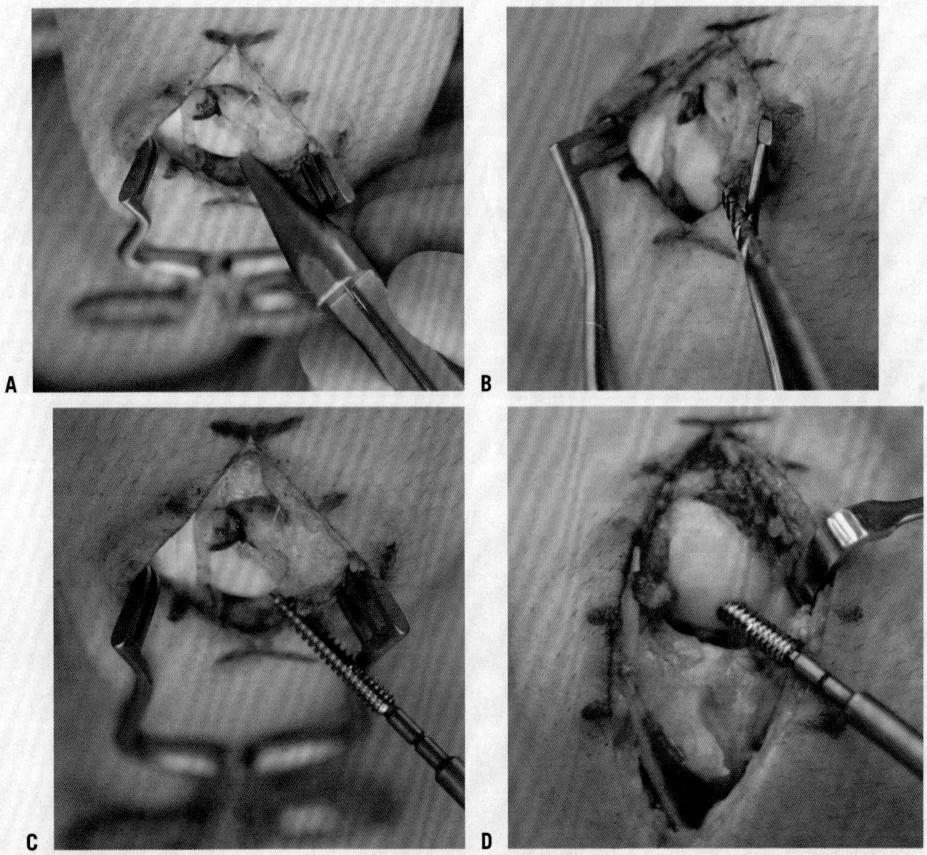

TECH FIG 4 A. Determining the appropriate screw length. **B.** Reaming with the cannulated reamer. **C,D.** Insertion of the screw. (In all, top is distal, bottom is proximal, left is radial, and right is ulnar.) (Copyright Peter J.L. Jebson, MD.)

OPEN REDUCTION AND INTERNAL FIXATION OF SCAPHOID FRACTURE: OPEN VOLAR APPROACH

Exposure

- Radially, deviate the wrist and palpate the scaphoid tubercle.
- Make a 3- to 4-cm incision centered over the scaphoid tubercle, directed distally toward the base of the thumb and proximally over the flexor carpi radialis (FCR) tendon sheath (a "hockey-stick" incision) **(TECH FIG 5A)**.
- Open the FCR sheath and retract the tendon ulnarly. If the superficial volar branch of the radial artery is encountered, cauterize it at the level of the wrist flexion crease. Open the floor of the sheath distally to expose the underlying volar wrist capsule.
- Distally, develop the interval by splitting the origin of the thenar muscles in line with their fibers over the distal scaphoid and trapezium.
- Incise the capsule longitudinally or using a nerve-sparing approach as described by Hagert et al,[6] taking care to avoid damage to the underlying articular cartilage **(TECH FIG 5B,C)**.
    - Proximally, the radioscaphocapitate ligament can be divided to allow better exposure of the proximal scaphoid pole.
    - The capsule needs to be preserved and repaired at the end of the case, as it contains the radioscaphocapitate ligament. Some surgeons prefer to tag the capsule with nonabsorbable sutures now for later repair.
- Identify the scaphotrapezial joint with a Freer elevator and bluntly expose it.
    - Dissection over the radial aspect of the scaphoid is limited to avoid injury to the dorsal ridge vessel.
- Define and clear the fracture site by irrigation, sharp excision of periosteal flaps, and curetting of debris and hematoma.
    - Assess the stability of the fracture by wrist manipulation.
    - It is critical to identify any bone loss, as compression during screw placement can result in an iatrogenic malunion.

Fracture Reduction and Fixation

- Obtain correct fracture alignment through longitudinal traction, followed by wrist manipulation.
    - An anatomic reduction may also be achieved by direct manipulation of the fragments with a dental pick, pointed reduction forceps, or joystick Kirschner wires.
- Place a provisional 0.045-inch Kirschner wire to secure the reduction. Insert the wire in a retrograde manner from volar distal to dorsal proximal, gaining fixation in the proximal pole.
    - It is critical to place this wire such that it does not interfere with subsequent screw placement in the central axis of the scaphoid.
- To gain the needed dorsal starting position in the distal scaphoid pole for central screw placement, displace the trapezium dorsally with an elevator or resect a small portion of the proximal volar trapezium with a rongeur **(TECH FIG 6)**.
    - Alternatively, a transtrapezial approach can reliably achieve central screw placement in the scaphoid as well.[15]
- The cannulated compression screw may be inserted using a freehand technique or a commercial device, which simultaneously facilitates fracture reduction and guidewire positioning.
    - Fluoroscopy is invaluable during wire and screw insertion and to confirm accurate placement and fracture reduction as described earlier.
- Precisely repair the volar wrist capsule and radiolunate and radioscaphocapitate ligaments with permanent suture.

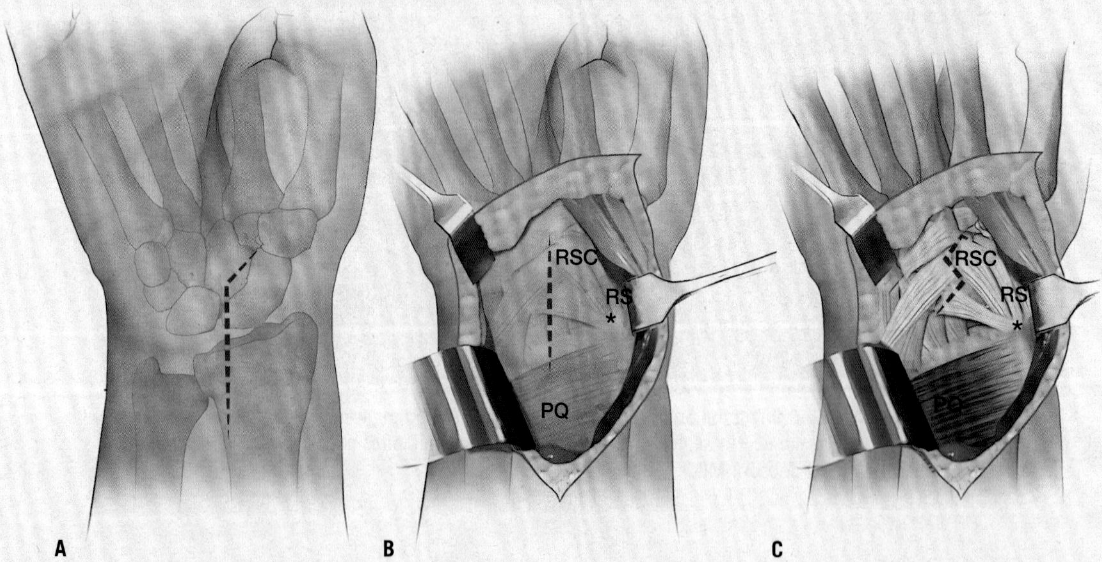

TECH FIG 5 Volar approach to the scaphoid. **A.** Orientation and location of the planned skin incision. **B,C.** Once the volar radiocarpal ligaments are exposed, either a longitudinal or nerve-sparing capsulotomy can be made to expose the entire scaphoid. *RS*, radioscaphoid ligament; *RSC*, radioscaphocapitate ligament; *PQ*, pronator quadratus; *asterisk*, radial styloid.

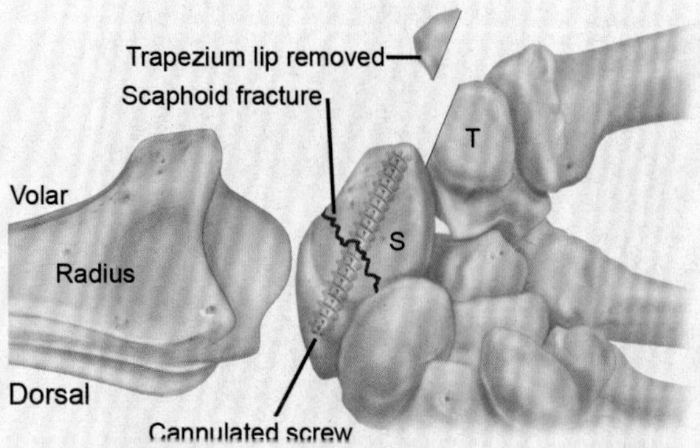

TECH FIG 6 Accurate insertion of a screw via the volar approach usually requires partial resection or dorsal displacement of the volar trapezium (*T*) to expose the distal scaphoid (*S*).

OPEN REDUCTION AND INTERNAL FIXATION OF SCAPHOID NONUNION WITH NONVASCULARIZED CANCELLOUS BONE GRAFTING

- An open dorsal approach is used as previously described.
- The nonunion site is identified. A Kirschner wire and mini C-arm can be helpful if the nonunion site is not readily visible.
- Preparations for screw placement occur next.
  - A guidewire is inserted down the central axis of the scaphoid. Unlike screw placement for acute fractures, we prefer to place this guidewire slightly volar to the central axis on a sagittal view and centrally on a coronal view **(TECH FIG 7A)**.
  - A derotational wire (0.045-inch Kirschner wire) can be inserted for stability.
  - Determine the screw length off the guidewire and subtract 4 mm to account for recession until beneath the articular surface of the proximal pole. The guidewire can then be driven into the trapezium for stability.
  - A headless compression screw is carefully inserted over the guidewire. Kirschner wires can then be removed **(TECH FIG 7B)**.
  - Insertion of the screw at this point allows for stable fixation and a thorough curetting of the nonunion site.
- A 3-mm rounded burr is used to enter and débride the nonunion site dorsally **(TECH FIG 7C)**. Care is taken to avoid violating the volar cortex and midcarpal articulation.
  - We burr down to the screw until we can visualize the threads but avoid destabilizing the screw.
  - Microcurettes can then assist with débriding the nonunion site to ensure removal of all intervening fibrous tissue.
  - We curette above the screw and across the nonunion site proximally and distally.
- Lister tubercle is débrided with a rongeur, and a curette or an osteotome is used to open the dorsal cortex of the distal radius **(TECH FIG 7D)**.
  - Angled curettes can then be used to harvest cancellous bone graft.
- The cancellous bone graft is packed tightly into the nonunion site **(TECH FIG 7E)**.
  - To achieve this, the smooth side of a microcurette can be used to apply pressure, similar to a dentist filling a cavity **(TECH FIG 7F)**.
- Capsule and skin incision can be repaired. We prefer to not repair the capsule for the reasons noted previously.

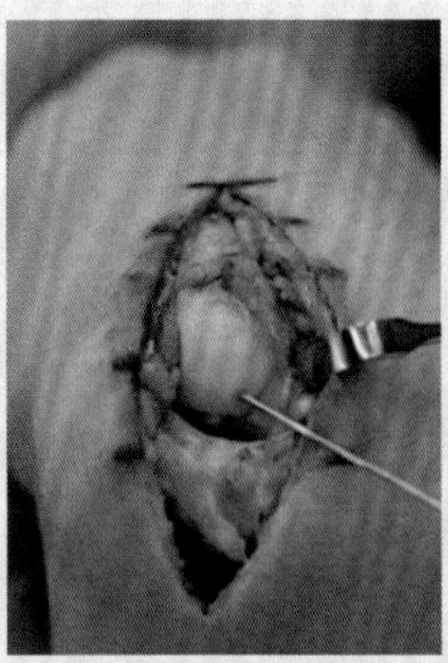
A

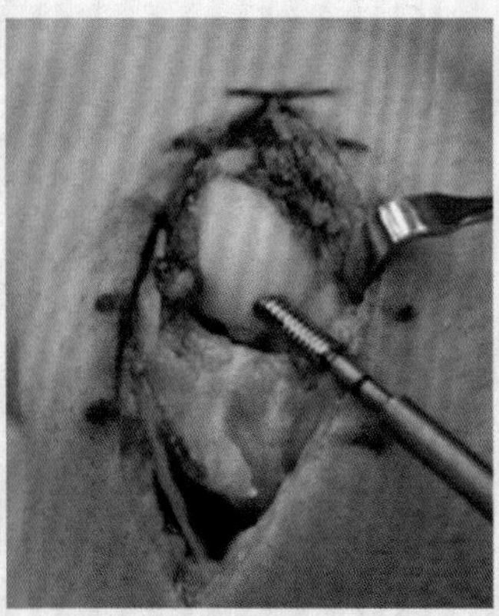
B

TECH FIG 7 ORIF of a scaphoid nonunion from a dorsal approach with nonvascularized cancellous bone graft. **A.** A guidewire is inserted down the central axis of the scaphoid on a coronal view and just volar to the central axis on the sagittal view. **B.** The cannulated headless compression screw is inserted over the guidewire. *(continued)*

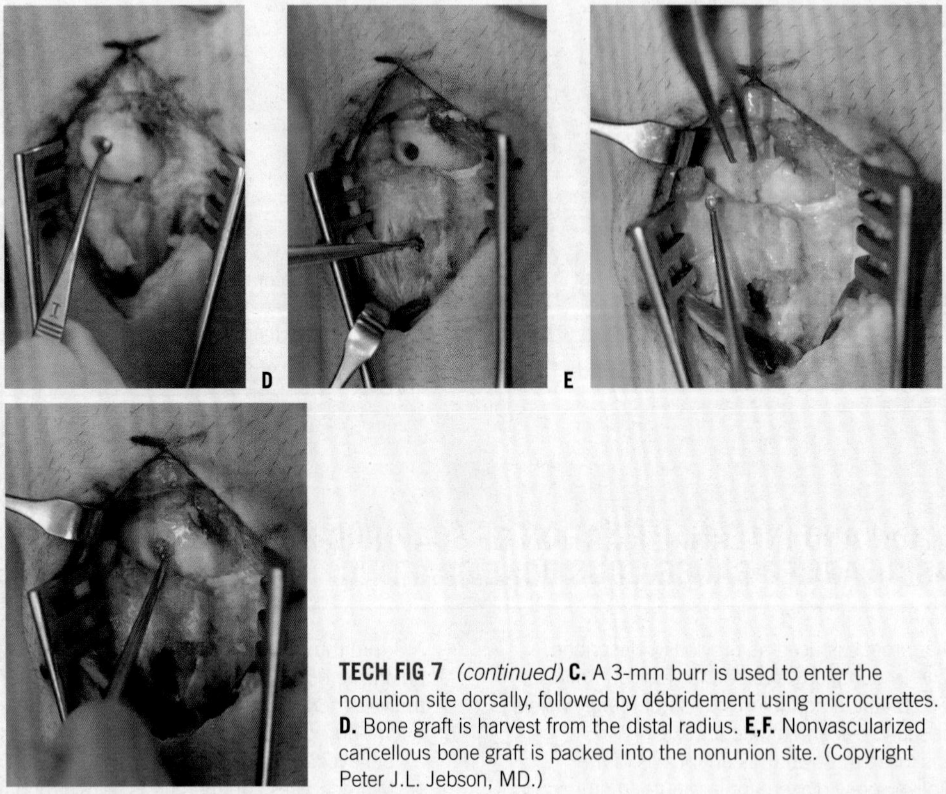

C D E F

TECH FIG 7 *(continued)* **C.** A 3-mm burr is used to enter the nonunion site dorsally, followed by débridement using microcurettes. **D.** Bone graft is harvest from the distal radius. **E,F.** Nonvascularized cancellous bone graft is packed into the nonunion site. (Copyright Peter J.L. Jebson, MD.)

TECHNIQUES

Pearls and Pitfalls

Injury to the Scaphoid Blood Supply	• Meticulous limited dissection of the capsule. Avoid any dissection on the dorsal ridge of the scaphoid.
Malpositioning of Guidewire	• Pronate and flex wrist during the dorsal approach to allow appropriate trajectory. Confirm position on multiple views to ensure insertion in the central axis of the scaphoid.
Screw Position	• Select a screw that is 4 mm shorter than measured length unless fracture fragments are separated; in that case, choose a shorter screw.
Reduction of an Unstable Fracture	• Perpendicular Kirschner wire joysticks inserted into the proximal and distal scaphoid fragments are useful to obtain a reduction. • Provisional derotational Kirschner wires placed before screw insertion can be used to stabilize fragments during screw insertion. • Recognize comminution and bone loss to avoid inadvertent shortening or malreduction with screw compression. • Consider use of two small screws for unstable fractures or revision of a scaphoid nonunion.
Small Proximal Pole Fracture	• Use of a small screw (ie, mini-Acutrak 2) may be necessary to prevent comminution of the proximal fragment. • Confirm central axis screw position, especially in the proximal pole.

POSTOPERATIVE CARE

- The patient is immobilized in a below-elbow volar plaster splint and discharged to home with instructions on strict limb elevation and frequent digital range-of-motion exercises.
- At 2 weeks, the patient returns for suture removal and transitions to a well molded short-arm fiberglass cast.
- Casting is continued until at least 50% bridging bony healing has occurred.
- After cast removal, a formal supervised therapy program is initiated to achieve satisfactory range of motion, strength, and function.
- Fracture healing is assessed at 2, 6, and 12 weeks postoperatively with plain radiography. Fracture union is defined as

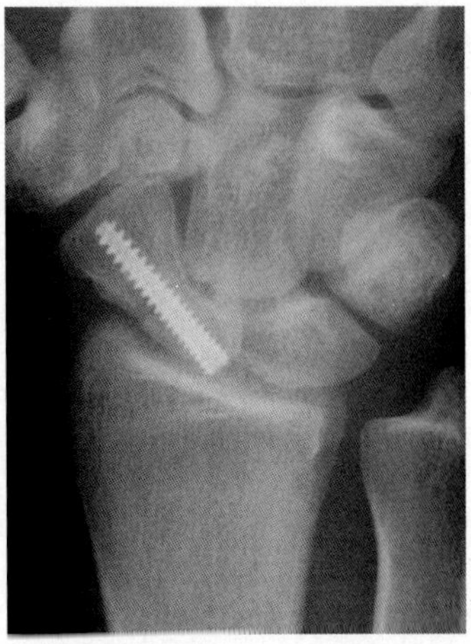

FIG 2 A healed scaphoid waist fracture after ORIF via the dorsal approach. Although the screw may appear slightly long, both the proximal scaphoid and distal scaphoid are covered with hyaline cartilage not detected on diagnostic imaging. (Copyright Peter J.L. Jebson, MD.)

progressive obliteration of the fracture and clear trabeculation across the fracture site **(FIG 2)**.

- If there is any question regarding fracture union, a CT scan is obtained at 3 months postoperatively or before the patient is allowed to return to unrestricted sporting activities.

OUTCOMES

- Surgical fixation of unstable, displaced scaphoid fractures has been increasingly advocated, given the unsatisfactory outcomes that have been reported with nonoperative management.
- Rigid internal fixation allows for early physiotherapy throughout the healing phase, a more rapid time to union, improved range of motion, and rapid functional recovery.[2,12,20] Several studies have reported a high rate of union and excellent clinical outcome with minimal morbidity using both limited open and percutaneous techniques.[1,2,18,20]
- Our preferred technique for fixation of a scaphoid proximal pole or waist region fracture involves a limited dorsal approach with compression screw fixation.[12] The technique is simple and permits visualization of a reliable starting point for screw placement within the central axis of the scaphoid, offering a significant potential advantage over the volar approach.[13] In a consecutive series of nondisplaced scaphoid waist fractures treated in this fashion, 17 out of 18 fractures healed at a mean duration of 8 weeks.[1]
- In a recent review article evaluating the current literature, overall union rate for scaphoid nonunions treated with nonvascularized or vascularized bone grafts was 87% and 85%, respectively.[15] There is insufficient evidence to support one type of bone graft over another.

COMPLICATIONS

- Postoperative wound infections are rare and can be prevented with routine preoperative antibiotic prophylaxis, thorough wound irrigation, and appropriate soft tissue management.
- Intraoperative technical problems
  - Inadvertent bending or breakage of the guidewire can occur if the wrist is dorsiflexed with the wire in position or during drilling before screw insertion.
  - Care should be taken to confirm that the screw is fully seated beneath the articular cartilage to avoid prominence and erosion of the distal radius articular surface. Similarly, failure to carefully judge accurate screw length intraoperatively can result in prominence within the scaphotrapezial articulation.
- Nonunion with or without AVN can occur despite compression screw fixation, particularly with a proximal pole or displaced waist fracture. Stripping of the dorsal ridge vasculature should be avoided. Supplemental cancellous bone graft from the distal radius may be used at the time of fixation of a displaced or comminuted fracture if desired.
- Other potential but rare complications
  - Hypertrophic scar
  - Injury to the dorsal branches of the superficial radial nerve
  - Damage to the scaphotrapezial articulation
  - Proximal pole fragment comminution

REFERENCES

1. Bedi A, Jebson PJ, Hayden RJ, et al. Internal fixation of acute, nondisplaced scaphoid waist fractures via a limited dorsal approach: an assessment of radiographic and functional outcomes. J Hand Surg Am 2007;32(3):326–333.
2. Chen AC, Chao EK, Hung SS, et al. Percutaneous screw fixation for unstable scaphoid fractures. J Trauma 2005;59(1):184–187.
3. Ernst SMC, Green DP, Saucedo JM. Screw fixation alone for scaphoid fracture nonunion. J Hand Surg Am 2018;43(9):837–843.
4. Gellman H, Caputo RJ, Carter V, et al. Comparison of short and long thumb-spica casts for non-displaced fractures of the carpal scaphoid. J Bone Joint Surg Am 1989;71(3):354–357.
5. Guss MS, Mitgang JT, Sapienza A. Scaphoid healing required for unrestricted activity: a biomechanical cadaver model. J Hand Surg Am 2018;43(2):134–138.
6. Hagert E, Ferreres A, Garcia-Elias M. Nerve-sparing dorsal and volar approaches to the radiocarpal joint. J Hand Surg Am 2010;35:1070–1074.
7. Kawamura K, Chung KC. Treatment of scaphoid fractures and nonunions. J Hand Surg Am 2008;33(6):988–997.
8. Kim JK, Yoon JO, Baek H. Corticocancellous bone graft vs cancellous bone graft for the management of unstable scaphoid nonunion. Orthop Traumatol Surg Res 2018;104(1):115–120.
9. Kozin SH. Incidence, mechanism, and natural history of scaphoid fractures. Hand Clin 2001;17(4):515–524.
10. Lee SK, Byun DJ, Roman-Deynes JL, et al. Hybrid Russe procedure for scaphoid waist fracture nonunion with deformity. J Hand Surg Am 2015;40(11):2198–2205.
11. Mallee WH, Wang J, Poolman RW, et al. Computed tomography versus magnetic resonance imaging versus bone scintigraphy for clinically suspected scaphoid fractures in patients with negative plain radiographs. Cochrane Database Syst Rev 2015;(6):CD010023.
12. Martus JE, Bedi A, Jebson PJ. Cannulated variable pitch compression screw fixation of scaphoid fractures using a limited dorsal approach. Tech Hand Up Extrem Surg 2005;9(4):202–206.
13. Meermans G, Van Glabbeek F, Braem MJ, et al. Comparison of two percutaneous volar approaches for screw fixation of scaphoid waist fractures: radiographic and biomechanical study of an osteotomy-simulated model. J Bone Joint Surg Am 2014;96(16):1369–1376.
14. Merrell GA, Wolfe SW, Slade JF III. Treatment of scaphoid nonunions: quantitative meta-analysis of the literature. J Hand Surg Am 2002;27(4):685–691.
15. Rancy SK, Schmidle G, Wolfe SW. Does anyone need a vascularized graft? Hand Clin 2019;35(3):323–344.

16. Rancy SK, Swanstrom MM, DiCarlo EF, et al. Success of scaphoid nonunion surgery is independent of proximal pole vascularity. J Hand Surg Eur Vol 2018;43(1):32–40.
17. Rua T, Malhotra B, Vijayanathan S, et al. Clinical and cost implications of using immediate MRI in the management of patients with a suspected scaphoid fracture and negative radiographs results from the SMaRT trial. Bone Joint J 2019;101-B(8):984–994.
18. Trumble TE, Gilbert M, Murray LW, et al. Displaced scaphoid fractures treated with open reduction and internal fixation with a cannulated screw. J Bone Joint Surg Am 2000;82(5):633–641.
19. Wu F, Ng CY, Hayton M. The authors' technique for volar plating of scaphoid nonunion. Hand Clin 2019;35(3):281–286.
20. Yip HS, Wu WC, Chang RY, et al. Percutaneous cannulated screw fixation of acute scaphoid waist fracture. J Hand Surg Br 2002;27(1):42–46.

CHAPTER 22

K-wire Fixation of Distal Radius Fractures with and without External Fixation

Christopher Doumas, David Lee, and David J. Bozentka

DEFINITION

- Distal radius fractures occur at the distal end of the bone, originating in the metaphyseal region and often extending to the radiocarpal and distal radioulnar joints (DRUJ).
- Distal radius fractures can be classified as stable or unstable and extra- or intra-articular to assist in treatment decisions.
- Fractures may angulate dorsally or volarly and may have significant comminution depending on the energy of the injury and the quality of the bone.
- Percutaneous pins or Kirschner wires (K-wires), typically 0.062 or 0.045 inches, can be used for treatment of simple intra-articular or extra-articular fractures with mild comminution and no osteoporosis.
- Percutaneous pins can aid reduction and stabilize the fragments in a minimally invasive manner.
- Percutaneous pins can support the subchondral area of the distal radius and maintain the articular reduction in highly comminuted fractures, which is useful when combined with other fixation methods.
- Smooth percutaneous pins may also be placed across the physis to maintain a reduction in children with minimal risk of a growth arrest.
- Highly comminuted fractures are more difficult to fix rigidly and often require external and/or internal fixation to maintain alignment during healing.
- External fixators can be hinged or static and may or may not bridge the wrist joint.
- K-wire fixation of extra-articular and simple intra-articular fractures has received more support over the last few years after several prospective randomized trials comparing K-wire fixation to volar plating has shown no difference in outcome at 1 year.

ANATOMY

- The distal radius consists of three articular surfaces: the scaphoid fossa, the lunate fossa, and the sigmoid notch.
- Ligamentotaxis aids in the reduction of intra-articular and comminuted fractures.
  - Volar extrinsic ligamentous attachments include the radioscaphocapitate, long radiolunate, and short radiolunate ligaments.
  - Dorsal extrinsic ligamentous attachments include the radiotriquetral ligament.
- Dorsal and radial to the second metacarpal lie the first dorsal interosseous muscle and the terminal branches of the radial sensory nerve.
- The distal radial sensory nerve branches lie superficial to the distal radius and should be protected during dissection and pin placement.
- The radial sensory nerve emerges between the brachioradialis and the extensor carpi radialis longus (ECRL) muscle bellies **(FIG 1)**.
- The terminal branches of the lateral antebrachial cutaneous nerve lie superficial to the forearm fascia at the radial wrist.
- There is a bare spot of bone between the first and second dorsal compartments in the region of the radial styloid.
- The brachioradialis tendon inserts onto the radial styloid deep to the first dorsal compartment.

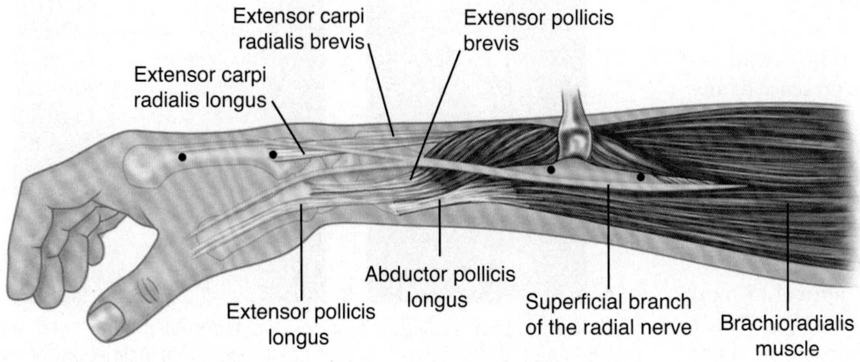

FIG 1 Anatomy surrounding the radial sensory nerve branch in the forearm.

- The ECRL and the extensor carpi radialis brevis (ECRB) lie dorsal to the brachioradialis in the second dorsal compartment.
- Lister's tubercle is dorsal, with the extensor pollicis longus (EPL) tendon on its ulnar side, in the third dorsal compartment.
- The extensor digitorum communis tendons lie over the dorsal ulnar half of the distal radius in the fourth dorsal compartment.
- The extensor digiti minimi lies over the DRUJ in the fifth dorsal compartment.

PATHOGENESIS

- Distal radius fractures are the most common fractures of the upper extremity in adults, representing about 20% of all fractures seen in the emergency room.[22]
- Mechanism of injury typically is a fall on an outstretched hand with axial loading, but other common histories include motor vehicle accidents or pathologic fractures.
- Higher energy injuries cause increased comminution, angulation, and displacement.
- Osteoporosis, tumors, and metabolic bone diseases are risk factors for sustaining pathologic distal radius fractures.
- In children, fractures typically occur along the physis due to its relative weakness compared to the surrounding ligaments.

NATURAL HISTORY

- Distal radius fractures needing no reduction and those that are stable after reduction typically recover functional range of motion with minimal long-term sequelae.
- Three parameters that affect outcome include articular congruity, angulation, and shortening.[21,26]
  - Two millimeters or more of articular surface incongruity of the distal radius can lead to degenerative changes, pain, and stiffness.
  - Dorsal angulation can lead to decreased range of motion and increased load transfer to the ulna.
  - Radial shortening can lead to decreased range of motion, pain, and ulnar impaction of the carpus.

PATIENT HISTORY AND PHYSICAL FINDINGS

- The history of a fall on an outstretched hand is the most common presentation for a patient with a distal radius fracture.
- Motor vehicle or motorcycle accidents and osteoporosis account for most comminuted fractures.
- It may be clinically indicated to implement a workup for osteoporosis.
- Pain, tenderness, swelling, crepitus, deformity, ecchymosis, and decreased range of motion at the wrist are typical symptoms and warrant radiographic evaluation.
- Physical examination should include the following:
  - Inspection: Evaluate the integrity of the skin, cascade of the digits, direction of displacement, and presence of any swelling.
  - Identify points of maximal tenderness to differentiate between distal radius injuries and carpal or ligamentous injuries.
  - Palpate specific areas of the wrist and hand to differentiate distal intra-articular, DRUJ, and carpal injuries.
  - Two-point discrimination: Higher than normal (5 mm) results in the form of progressive neurologic deficit may signify an acute carpal tunnel syndrome or ulnar neuropathy.
- Passive finger stretch test to assist with diagnosis of compartment syndrome
- EPL tendon function should be evaluated.
  - EPL assessment: Assess the resting position of the thumb interphalangeal joint and the patient's ability to lift the thumb off of a flat surface to determine the continuity of the EPL tendon.
- Palpation of forearm and elbow to assess for concomitant injury proximally
- The DRUJ must be assessed for displacement and instability.
- The bony anatomy must be carefully evaluated to avoid missing minimally displaced fractures, which may displace without treatment.
- Skin should be assessed to avoid missing an open fracture.
- Swelling should be monitored to allow for early diagnosis of compartment syndrome.
- Sensory examination should be monitored for progressive changes, which may represent acute carpal tunnel syndrome.

IMAGING AND OTHER DIAGNOSTIC STUDIES

- Radiographic evaluation should include posteroanterior (PA), lateral, and oblique views to assess displacement, angulation, comminution, and intra-articular involvement and allow for radiologic measurements.[18,22] Often, comparison x-rays of the uninjured wrist are helpful.
  - Lateral articular (volar) tilt is the angle between the radial shaft and a tangential line parallel to the articular margin as seen on the lateral view **(FIG 2A)**. The normal angle is 11 degrees.
  - Radial inclination, measured on the PA view **(FIG 2B)**, is the angle between a line perpendicular to the shaft of the radius at the ulnar articular margin and the tangential

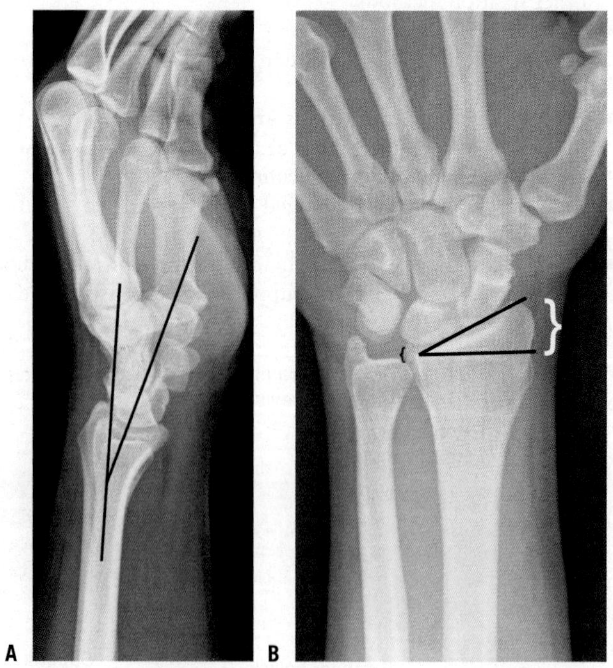

FIG 2 A. Lateral radiograph of the wrist demonstrating volar tilt (*black lines*). **B.** PA radiograph demonstrating radial inclination (*black lines*), ulnar variance (*red bracket*), and radial height (*white bracket*).

line along the radial styloid to the ulnar articular margin. The normal angle is 22 degrees.
- Ulnar variance, also measured on the PA view (see **FIG 2B**), is the distance between the radial and ulnar articular surfaces. It should be measured with the wrist in neutral forearm rotation with the elbow flexed 90 degrees and the shoulder abducted 90 degrees. Ulnar variance is compared to the contralateral side.

- Traction radiographs help assess intra-articular involvement, intercarpal ligamentous injury, and potential fracture reduction through ligamentotaxis.
- Computed tomography (CT) scans are useful in fully elucidating the anatomy of the fracture, including impaction, comminution, and size of the fragments.
  - CT scans often significantly alter the original treatment plan.[14]
- Magnetic resonance imaging is rarely performed acutely but can diagnose concomitant ligamentous injuries, triangular fibrocartilage complex injuries, and occult carpal fractures.

DIFFERENTIAL DIAGNOSIS

- Bony contusion
- Radiocarpal dislocation
- Scaphoid or other carpal fracture
- Perilunate or lunate fracture-dislocation
- Distal ulnar fracture
- Wrist ligament or triangular fibrocartilage complex injury
- DRUJ injury

NONOPERATIVE MANAGEMENT

- Nonoperative treatment consists of splinting or casting for stable fracture patterns using a three-point mold.
- Fractures amenable to nonoperative treatment include those that are stable after reduction with minimal metaphyseal comminution, shortening, angulation, and displacement.
  - Evaluation for secondary displacement weekly for 2 to 3 weeks is critical as the swelling subsides.
- Unstable patterns will displace if not surgically stabilized.
  - There is little role for nonoperative treatment in highly comminuted fractures.
- The physiologic age, medical comorbidities, and functional level of the patient should be considered in determining the need for surgical treatment.
- Early range of motion of the nonimmobilized joints is essential in the nonoperative treatment of all fractures near the wrist to prevent contracture.
  - The cast or splint must not extend past the metacarpophalangeal joints to allow digital motion.

SURGICAL MANAGEMENT

- Surgical treatments are indicated to prevent malunion and improve pain control, function, range of motion, and to decrease the time of return to function.
- Surgery is reserved for unstable fractures, including displaced, intra-articular, comminuted, or severely angulated injuries and fractures that displace following attempted closed management.
- Percutaneous pinning can assist in obtaining and maintaining reduction of displaced fractures with limited comminution in a minimally invasive manner.
- External fixators maintain radius length but cannot always control angulation and displacement; therefore, supplementation with percutaneous pins is typically performed.[2]
- Conversely, external fixators may augment percutaneous pins and plate fixation when extensive comminution is present.
  - Supplemental external fixation should be considered for fractures with comminution of over 50% of the diameter of the radius on a lateral view or when significant volar cortical comminution is present.
- External fixation may be used as a neutralization device because the distraction forces decrease soon after fracture reduction.
- External fixators also are useful for "damage control orthopaedics" to temporarily stabilize wrist fractures, especially for complex, combined, open injuries.
- For nonbridging external fixation, there must be at least 1 cm of volar cortex intact and adequate fragment sizes to allow proper pin placement.
- A relative contraindication to pin fixation with or without external fixation is a volar shear injury, which should be reduced and stabilized using a volar plate and screws.

Preoperative Planning

- All radiographs should be reviewed before surgery and brought into the operating room.
- Analysis of the pattern and presumed stability of the fracture fragments determines whether percutaneous fixation, with or without external fixation, is suitable.
- For intra-articular fractures, the specific fragments to be reduced and fixed must be identified preoperatively to avoid incomplete reduction of the joint surface.
- The surgeon must be prepared to change his or her management decision intraoperatively if the fracture behavior is different from anticipated. A variety of fixation devices should be available in the operating room.

Positioning

- The patient is positioned supine on the operating table with a radiolucent arm board.
- A tourniquet is applied near the axilla **(FIG 3)**.

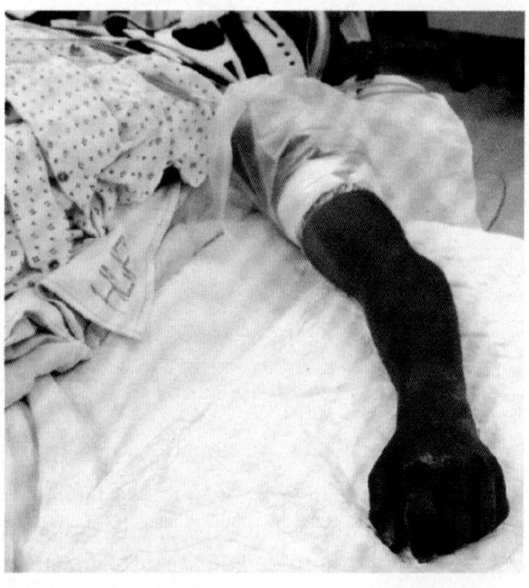

FIG 3 Positioning of patient supine on the hand table with tourniquet in place.

- Fluoroscopy should be used for confirmation of reduction and fixation throughout the procedure.
- There must be enough range of motion of the shoulder and elbow to allow standard anteroposterior, lateral, and oblique images.

Approach

- Various approaches can be used in the application of external fixators and the insertion of percutaneous pins.
- Distal external fixator half-pins may be placed directly into the second metacarpal or into other carpal bones (for injuries including the second metacarpal). Wires and half-pins from nonbridging fixators may be placed in the distal radius itself.
- Percutaneous pins can be inserted through the radial styloid between the first and second dorsal compartments, through Lister tubercle, through the interval between the fourth and fifth dorsal compartments, and across the DRUJ **(FIG 4)**.
  - Caution is taken to avoid skewering tendons and nerves and to avoid penetrating the articular surface.

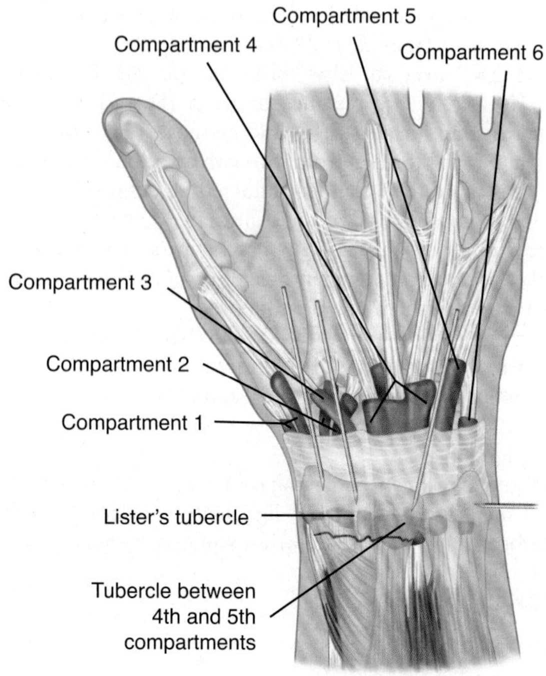

FIG 4 Areas for K-wire insertion at the distal radius.

CLOSED REDUCTION OF A DISTAL RADIUS FRACTURE

- Closed reduction should be performed before fixation using a combination of distraction and palmar translation of the distal radius fragment and carpus.[1]
- The elbow is flexed 90 degrees and manual traction is pulled upward through the hand. An assistant provides countertraction by keeping the elbow on the hand table.
- The surgeon's opposite thumb is placed on the distal fragment, and the deformity is recreated/exaggerated to disimpact the fragments.
- The reverse motion is then performed, and the thumb is used to push/reduce the fracture **(TECH FIG 1A–C)**.
- Use of a padded bump or towel roll can also aid in obtaining and maintaining reduction **(TECH FIG 1D)**.
- Overdistraction will cause increased dorsal angulation due to the intact short, stout volar ligaments.[1]
- Excessive palmar flexion of the wrist can restore volar tilt but leads to an increased incidence of stiffness and carpal tunnel syndrome.[7,8]
- Overdistraction can be assessed by measuring the carpal height index, measuring the radioscaphoid and midcarpal joint spaces, checking full finger flexion into the palm, or evaluating index finger extrinsic extensor tightness.[9]

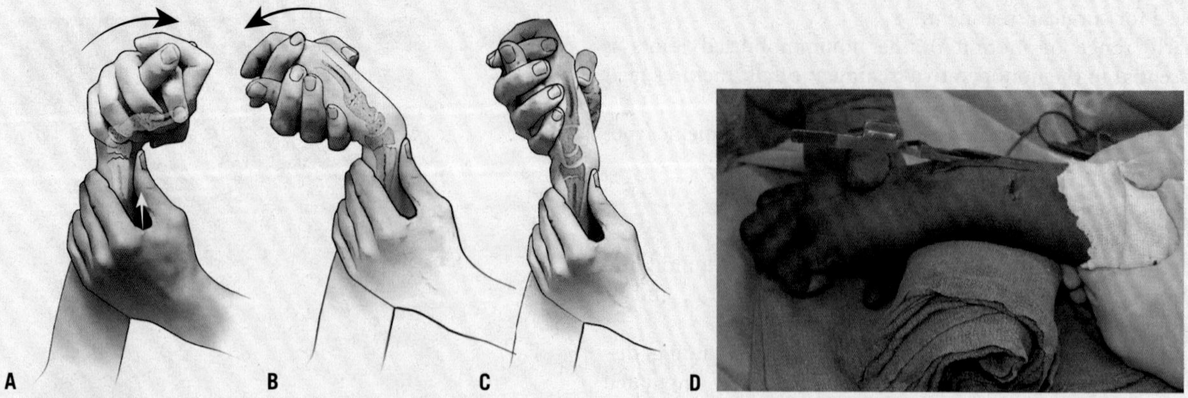

TECH FIG 1 Closed reduction of a distal radius fracture on a hand table. **A.** The elbow is flexed 90 degrees, and manual traction is pulled upward through the hand. An assistant provides countertraction by keeping the elbow on the hand table. **B.** The surgeon's opposite thumb is placed on the distal fragment and the deformity is recreated/exaggerated to disimpact the fragments. **C.** The reverse motion is then performed, and the thumb is used to push/reduce the fracture **D.** Closed reduction over a towel bump using traction and palmar translation.

KAPANDJI TECHNIQUE FOR PERCUTANEOUS PINNING

- Closed reduction is obtained using a bump, and the reduction is confirmed using fluoroscopy.
- This technique should be employed in patients younger than 55 years of age with minimal comminution. It should not be used in osteoporotic, elderly patients or those with comminution secondary to a higher risk of reduction loss. External fixation should be used to supplement pinning in these patient populations.[27]
- An incision is made radially, and a 0.062-inch pin is manually inserted into the fracture site, taking care to protect the sensory nerve branches and the first dorsal compartment tendons **(TECH FIG 2A)**.
  - The pin is angled distally, levering the bone back into its normal position and restoring the radial inclination **(TECH FIG 2B)**. The pin is advanced proximally and ulnarly through the far cortex using power. This pin act as a buttress to maintain radial inclination **(TECH FIG 2C)**.
- A second incision is placed dorsally, and a second pin is manually inserted into the fracture **(TECH FIG 2D)**.
  - The pin is angled distally, levering the bone back into its normal position and restoring the volar tilt **(TECH FIG 2E)**. This pin acts as a buttress to maintain volar tilt **(TECH FIG 2F)**.
- Using the modified technique, a third pin is inserted retrograde using power, starting at the radial styloid and proceeding into the ulnar cortex of the radius, proximal to the fracture line.
- The pins are buried and cut just below the skin, and the skin is sutured.
  - Alternatively, the pins may be bent using two needle drivers and left outside the skin.
- The pins are then cut and covered with pin caps or antibiotic gauze.
- A sterile dressing is applied, followed by a splint.

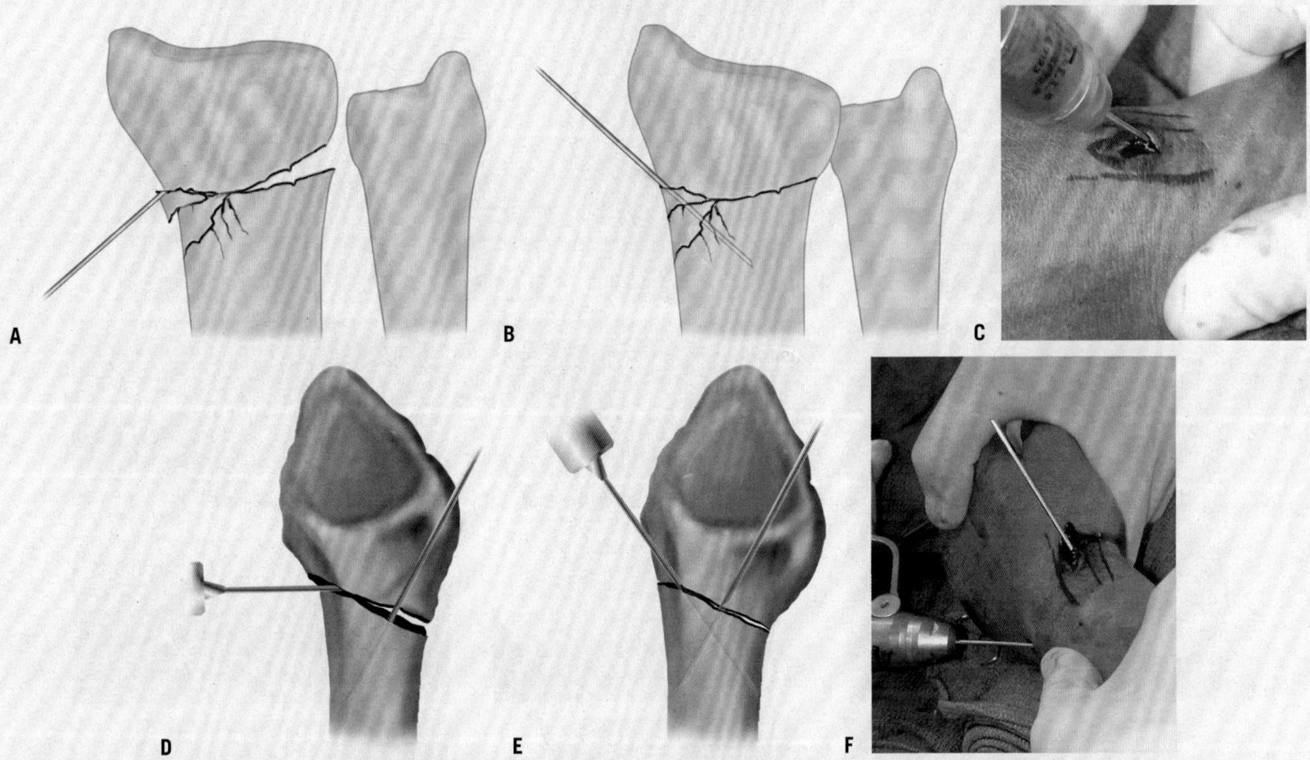

TECH FIG 2 **A.** An incision is made over the radial styloid, and a K-wire is manually inserted into the fracture site. **B.** The wire is levered distally to correct the radial inclination. **C.** The wire is advanced proximally, using power, into cortical bone. **D.** An incision is made over Lister tubercle, and a wire is inserted into the fracture site. **E,F.** The wire is levered distally to correct the dorsal angulation and advanced proximally using power into cortical bone.

AUTHORS' PREFERRED TECHNIQUE FOR PERCUTANEOUS PINNING

- Closed reduction is obtained using a bump, and the reduction is confirmed using fluoroscopy **(TECH FIG 3A,B)**.
- A small incision is placed over the bare spot on the radial styloid between the first and second dorsal compartments **(TECH FIG 3C)**.
- The radial styloid is exposed by blunt dissection, and care is taken not to injure the superficial branch of the radial nerve or the extensor tendons.
- If there is a separate, intra-articular lunate facet fragment, it can be reduced with a pointed reduction forceps and a wire can be introduced in a subchondral manner from the radial styloid across and into the fragment.
- Two 0.062-inch smooth K-wires are placed retrograde from the radial styloid across the reduced fracture, engaging the opposite cortex in a divergent fashion **(TECH FIG 3D,E)**. A small incision is placed over the interval between the fourth and fifth dorsal compartments.
- One or two K-wires are placed retrograde from the dorsoulnar corner of the distal radius across the reduced fracture, engaging the opposite cortex in a divergent fashion **(TECH FIG 3F–H)**.
- The pins are cut just beneath the skin, which is closed with a 5-0 nylon suture.
- Alternatively, the pins are bent and cut and left outside the skin **(TECH FIG 3I)**.
- A dressing and splint are then applied.

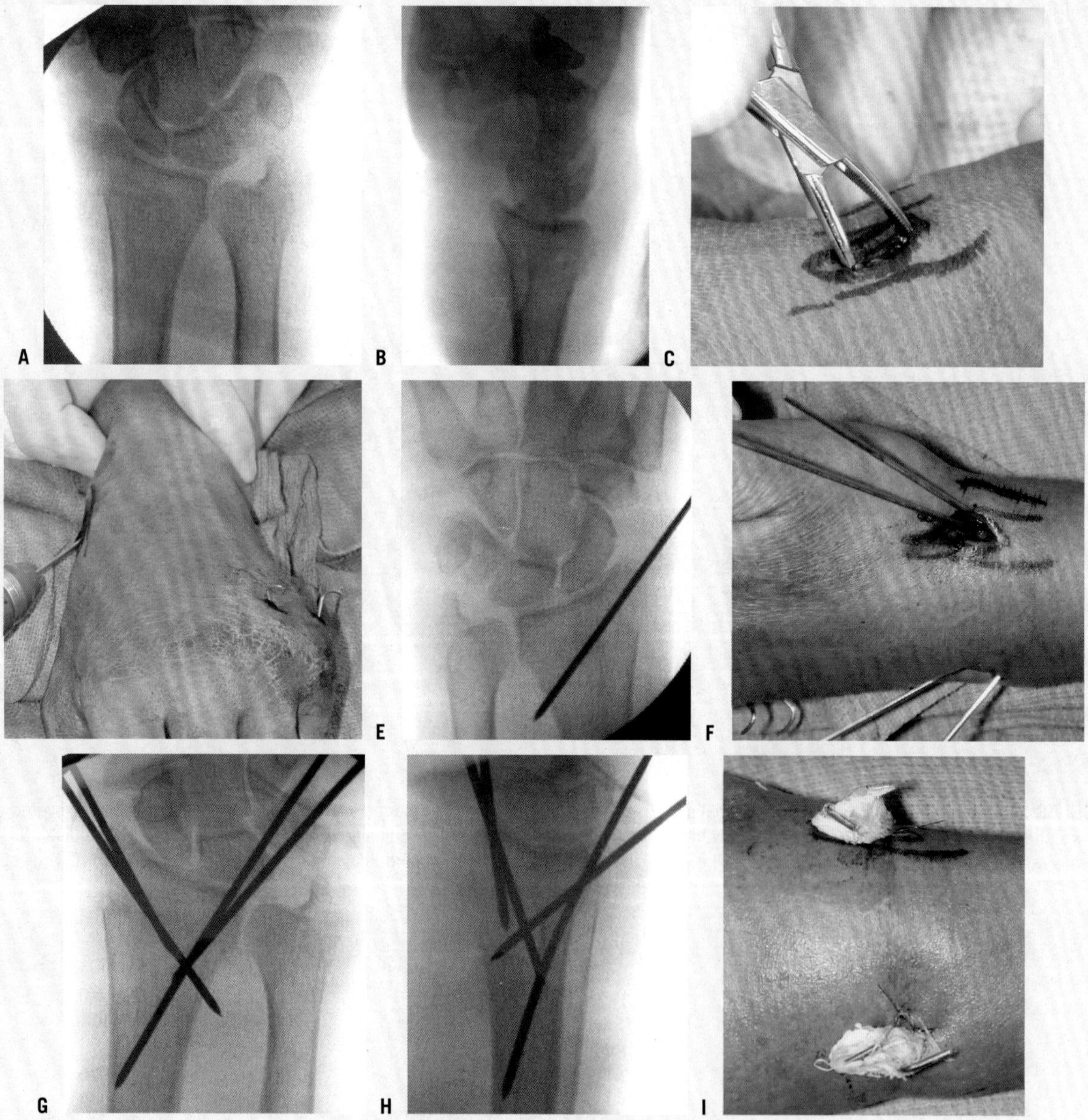

TECH FIG 3 A,B. PA and lateral views demonstrating reduction of distal radius fracture. **C.** The incision is made over the radial styloid. **D.** A pin is inserted retrograde into the radial styloid. **E.** PA radiograph demonstrating the course of the radial styloid wire. **F.** Two radial styloid wires and two dorsoulnar wires are in place. **G.** PA view showing fixation and the path of the wires. **H.** Lateral view showing fixation and path of wires. **I.** Pins are bent, cut, and covered above the skin.

BRIDGING EXTERNAL FIXATOR APPLICATION

Distal Pin Placement

- A 3-cm incision is made over the dorsal index metacarpal, exposing the proximal two-thirds.
- The distal sensory nerve branches are retracted, and the first dorsal interosseous muscle is elevated from the metacarpal to identify the insertion of the ECRL **(TECH FIG 4A)**.
- The index metacarpophalangeal joint is flexed to protect the sagittal band and first dorsal interosseous aponeurosis.
- The metacarpal drill guide is placed on the radial base of the index metacarpal at the flare of the metaphysis. Partially threaded 3- to 4-mm pins are used, with or without predrilling.
- A long-threaded pin is placed through the index and long metacarpal bases, obtaining three cortices of fixation.
- Care is taken not to enter the carpometacarpal joint.
- The double drill guide is then placed over the first pin, and the distal short-threaded pin is placed through both cortices of the index metacarpal shaft **(TECH FIG 4B,C)**.
- Fluoroscopy confirms placement and length of the pins.

Proximal Pin Placement and Frame Construction

- A 4- to 5-cm incision is made over the radial forearm, proximal to the first dorsal compartment musculature, through skin and subcutaneous tissue, avoiding the lateral antebrachial cutaneous nerve branches.
- The fascia overlying the interval between the brachioradialis and the ECRL is divided, and the radial sensory nerve is identified and retracted **(TECH FIG 5A)**.
  - The interval between the ECRL and ECRB may also be used to avoid the radial sensory branch.
- The double drill guide is placed onto the diaphysis of the radius between the brachioradialis and the radial wrist extensors or between the ECRL and ECRB **(TECH FIG 5B)**.
- Threaded 3- to 4-mm pins are placed, with or without predrilling.
  - The fracture should be reduced and the pins placed parallel to the metacarpal pins to facilitate alignment of the fracture.
  - A frame can be provisionally placed on the metacarpal pins to assist in manipulation and obtaining reduction.
  - The proximal pin should be placed bicortically, just distal to the tendon of the pronator teres.
  - The distal pin is then drilled bicortically through the double drill guide.
- Pin placement is confirmed using fluoroscopy.
- The incisions are closed using nylon suture, ensuring no tension is on the skin at the pin sites.
- Clamps and rods or adjustable fixators may then be applied to the pins to achieve and maintain final reduction **(TECH FIG 5C)**.
- Supplementary K-wire fixation is added before or after external fixation **(TECH FIG 5D)**.

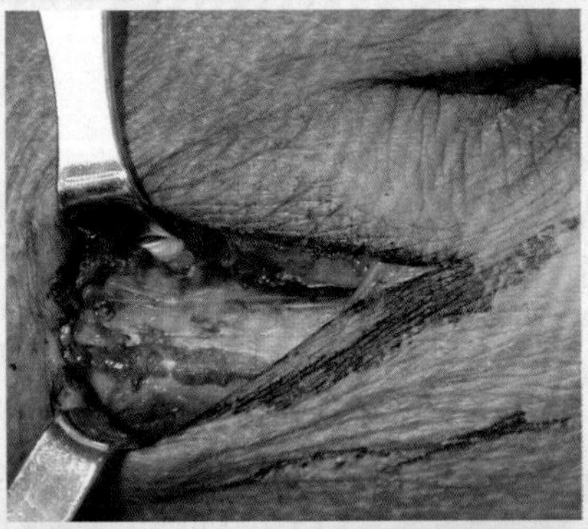
A

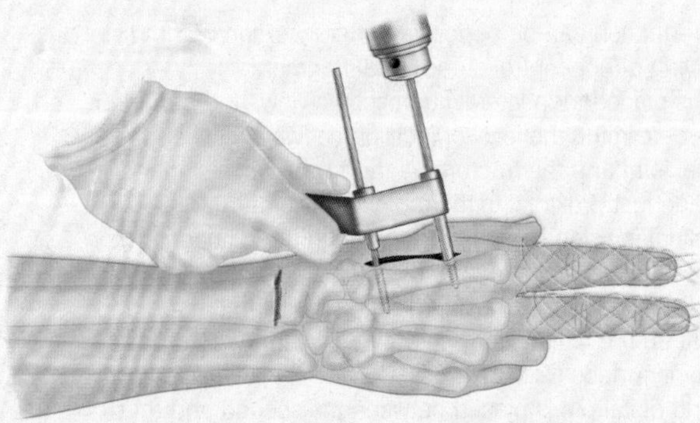
B

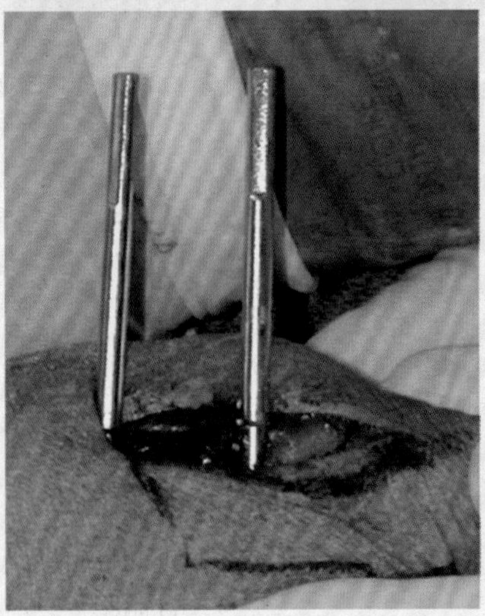
C

TECH FIG 4 **A.** An incision is made over the second metacarpal base, with reflection of the first dorsal interosseous muscle and radial sensory nerve terminal branches. (The thumb is at the top of the photograph.) **B.** Diagram showing placement of fixator pins in the shaft of the index and the base of the index and long metacarpals. **C.** Parallel placement of two metacarpal pins.

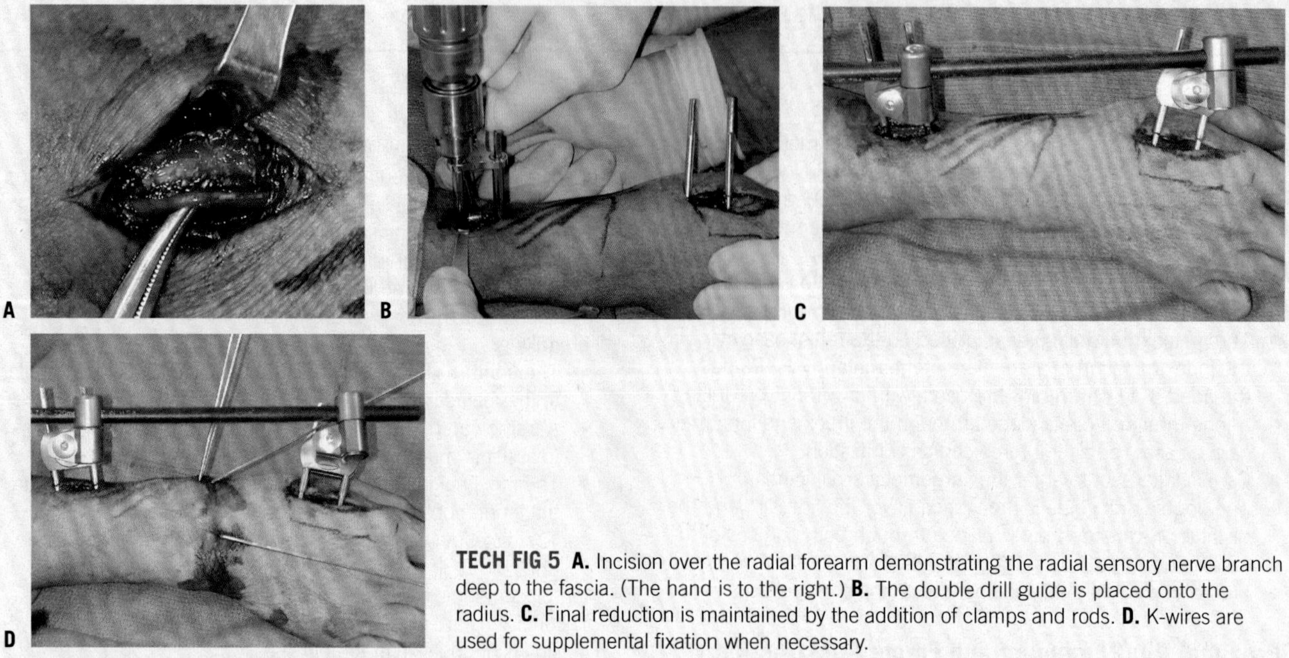

TECH FIG 5 **A.** Incision over the radial forearm demonstrating the radial sensory nerve branch deep to the fascia. (The hand is to the right.) **B.** The double drill guide is placed onto the radius. **C.** Final reduction is maintained by the addition of clamps and rods. **D.** K-wires are used for supplemental fixation when necessary.

NONBRIDGING EXTERNAL FIXATOR APPLICATION

- Fracture reduction can be performed after insertion of the distal pins, allowing direct control of the distal fragment.
- The wrist is placed for a lateral fluoroscopic view, and a marker is used to determine the level of incision halfway between the radiocarpal joint and the fracture. A short transverse skin incision is made just proximal to the radiocarpal joint.
- A longitudinal incision is then made through the retinaculum on either side of Lister tubercle, and the EPL is protected.
- The first distal pin is drilled using power, parallel to the radiocarpal joint on the lateral view, halfway between the fracture and the joint surface **(TECH FIG 6A)**.
- The second distal pin is placed between the second and third dorsal compartments, between the radial wrist extensors and the EPL tendon.
- This pin should be placed parallel to the first pin in both planes, with the starting point halfway between the radiocarpal joint and the fracture.
- The two proximal radius pins are placed using the technique described for placement of a bridging external fixator.
- The incisions are closed, after which the clamps are applied but not tightened.
- Reduction is achieved by manipulation of the distal pins and clamps.
  - Pushing the pins in the dorsal/volar plane corrects dorsal tilt.
  - Adjusting the pin clamp can correct radial inclination.
- Reduction is confirmed using fluoroscopy, and the clamps are tightened **(TECH FIG 6B)**.

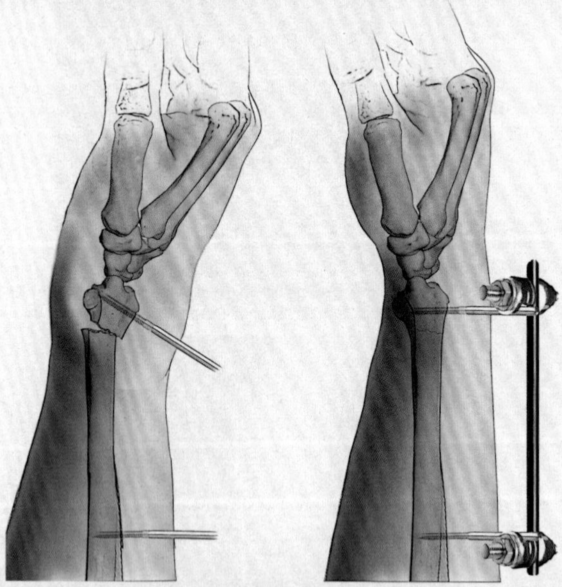

TECH FIG 6 **A.** Distal pin placement. **B.** Final reduction with nonbridged external fixator in place.

Pearls and Pitfalls

Indications	• K-wire fixation: adequate bone quality, simple articular and extra-articular fractures without significant comminution • External fixation: temporary stabilization, open injuries/soft tissue compromise, supplemental fixation to K-wires
Surgical Approach	• Make incisions and use blunt dissection for pin placement to avoid sensory nerves, tendons, and crossing veins. • Obtain adequate exposure of the radial sensory branch at forearm and hand to avoid injury.
Hardware Placement	• Choose pins of appropriate diameter. • Supplement fixation with pins using external or internal fixation as necessary. • Do not leave pins more than 1–2 mm out of the cortex and keep all pins extra-articular. • If placing the proximal metacarpal pin in metaphyseal bone, ensure that three cortices are penetrated. • Ensure that no extensor tendons are trapped by passively flexing the digits. • Do not back out conical pins because fixation will be lost. • Determine comminution and supplement fixation with external or internal fixation as necessary. • Evaluate the DRUJ after fixation to determine stability. • Subcutaneous pins are more costly to remove because that requires a second procedure, but they have a lower infection rate. Therefore, if fixation is needed for an extended period, bury the pins. • Overdistraction of the carpus must be avoided because it is associated with chronic pain–mediated syndromes and nonunion.
Postoperative Management	• Allow for adequate immobilization. • Encourage early range of motion of the fingers, elbow, and shoulder whenever possible. • Educate the patient regarding appropriate pin care. • Begin strengthening only after healing is complete and range of motion is maximized.

POSTOPERATIVE CARE

- After fixation with percutaneous pins, the wrist is immobilized alone in a short-arm splint to allow for swelling but provide stability. A cast is applied after the swelling goes down.
- Isolated radial styloid fractures fixed with pins can be placed in a volar wrist splint.
- External fixation devices typically require no additional immobilization, although a volar forearm–based Orthoplast (Johnson & Johnson, Langhorne, PA) splint may be used for support and patient comfort.
- The splint or cast is continued for 4 to 8 weeks until healing occurs, and the pins are removed.
- K-wires and half-pins should be inspected and cleaned regularly using either soap and water or half-strength hydrogen peroxide and water.
- Finger, elbow, and shoulder range of motion are begun immediately, and wrist range of motion is begun as the fracture heals.

OUTCOMES

- Multiple prospective randomized trials comparing volar plate fixation to closed reduction and percutaneous pinning have demonstrated quicker return to functional recovery with volar plate fixation but no difference in function at 1 year.[12,13,20,28]
- Functional and cost comparison of extra-articular and simple intra-articular fractures treated with volar plate fixation versus closed reduction and percutaneous fixation showed only a significant cost increase with volar plate fixation and no difference in function. This study calls into question the extra cost associated with volar plate fixation. No external fixation was used to augment the percutaneous fixation, which would increase the cost of this treatment method and may negate the cost benefit of percutaneous fixation.[5]
- A prospective randomized trial comparing percutaneous pinning and casting versus external fixation with augmentation (eg, pins, screws, bone graft) found no difference in clinical outcomes for fractures with minimal articular displacement.[10]
- In patients older than 60 years of age, percutaneous pinning has been shown to provide only marginal radiographic improvement over cast immobilization alone, with no correlation with clinical outcome.[4]
- Ebraheim et al[6] reported excellent outcomes for restoration of radiographic parameters and functional outcomes with intrafocal pinning and trans-styloid augmentation.
- An evaluation of percutaneous pinning outcomes found the best results for metaphyseal fractures. Good results were found for intra-articular fractures. The worst results were seen in fractures with associated ulnar styloid fractures and fractures in elderly persons.[19]
- A retrospective review of radiographic and clinical outcomes of open reduction internal fixation (volar and dorsal) versus external fixation revealed no significant differences, except that palmar tilt was more effectively restored with dorsal plating.[29]
- A meta-analysis found no evidence for the use of internal fixation over external fixation for unstable distal radius fractures.[16]
- Women older than 55 years of age with unstable intra-articular distal radius fractures treated with external fixation have a high rate of secondary displacement but can have acceptable functional outcomes.[11]
- Patients older than the age of 55 years have better results with external fixation and pinning than with pinning alone. Younger patients with two or more sides having comminution also have better results with supplemental external fixation.[27]
- Nonbridging external fixation has been shown to maintain volar tilt and carpal alignment better than bridging external fixation while having significantly better function during the first year.[17]
- Nonbridging external fixation was shown to have no clinical advantage in patients older than 60 years of age with moderately or severely displaced distal radius fractures.[3]
- A prospective, randomized comparison of bridging versus nonbridging external fixation revealed more complications in the nonbridging fixators and better outcomes in the bridged fixator group.[23]

- A prospective study compared unrepaired ulnar styloid fractures to those without ulnar styloid fractures and found no significant differences in clinical outcome. However, DRUJ instability was not evaluated.[24]

COMPLICATIONS

- Infection (pin tract or deep). Pin tract infections occur in 10% to 30% of patients and historically have been a major problem with this treatment method.[9,10]
- Pin tract infections can be minimized by reducing the time pins are left in place or by burying the pins beneath the skin.[15,25]
- One study showed that pin tract infections can be reduced to a 2% incidence if they are only left in place for 30 days, then removed in the office, and the wrist then casted for another 2 weeks without the pins in place.
- If K-wires are going to be left in place for longer than 30 days, they should be buried under the skin at the time of surgery to help prevent pin tract infections.
- Injury to tendons, vessels, and nerves due to percutaneous technique. Stiffness may result if tendons are inadvertently skewered, and the radial sensory branch can be injured.
- Injury to the radial sensory branch can cause a painful neuroma and should be avoided.
- Loss of range of motion
- Posttraumatic arthritis
- Weakness in grip or pinch
- Tenosynovitis and tendon rupture
- Malunion or nonunion
- Compartment syndrome
- Carpal tunnel syndrome
- Hardware failure
- Nonunion (associated with overdistraction with an external fixator)
- Complex regional pain syndrome (CRPS)[30]
- Vitamin C should be prescribed to prevent CRPS (500 mg once a day for 50 days).

REFERENCES

1. Agee JM. Distal radius fractures. Multiplanar ligamentotaxis. Hand Clin 1993;9(4):577–585.
2. Anderson JT, Lucas GL, Buhr BR. Complications of treating distal radius fractures with external fixation: a community experience. Iowa Orthop J 2004;24:53–59.
3. Atroshi I, Brogren E, Larsson GU, et al. Wrist-bridging versus non-bridging external fixation for displaced distal radius fractures: a randomized assessor-blind clinical trial of 38 patients followed for 1 year. Acta Orthop 2006;77(3):445–453.
4. Azzopardi T, Ehrendorfer S, Coulton T, et al. Unstable extra-articular fractures of the distal radius: a prospective, randomised study of immobilisation in a cast versus supplementary percutaneous pinning. J Bone Joint Surg Br 2005;87(6):837–840.
5. Dzaja I, MacDermind JC, Roth J, et al. Functional outcomes and cost estimation for extra-articular and simple intra-articular distal radius fractures treated with open reduction and internal fixation versus closed reduction and percutaneous Kirschner wire fixation. Can J Surg 2013;56(6):378–384.
6. Ebraheim NA, Ali SS, Gove NK. Fixation of unstable distal radius fractures with intrafocal pins and trans-styloid augmentation: a retrospective review and radiographic analysis. Am J Orthop (Belle Mead NJ) 2006;35(8):362–368.
7. Gupta A. The treatment of Colles' fracture. Immobilisation with the wrist dorsiflexed. J Bone Joint Surg Br 1991;73(2):312–315.
8. Gupta R, Bozentka DJ, Bora FW. The evaluation of tension in an experimental model of external fixation of distal radius fractures. J Hand Surg Am 1999;24:108–112.
9. Hargreaves DG, Drew SJ, Eckersley R. Kirschner wire pin tract infection rates: a randomized controlled trial between percutaneous and buried wires. J Hand Surg Br 2004;29(4):374–376.
10. Harley BJ, Scharfenberger A, Beaupre LA, et al. Augmented external fixation versus percutaneous pinning and casting for unstable fractures of the distal radius—a prospective randomized trial. J Hand Surg Am 2004;29(5):815–824.
11. Hegeman JH, Oskam J, Vierhout PA, et al. External fixation for unstable intra-articular distal radial fractures in women older than 55 years. Acceptable functional end results in the majority of the patients despite significant secondary displacement. Injury 2005;36(2):339–344.
12. Jeudy J, Steiger V, Boyer P, et al. Treatment of complex fractures of the distal radius: a prospective randomised comparison of external fixation 'versus' locked volar plating. Injury 2012;43(2):174–179.
13. Karantana A, Downing ND, Forward DP, et al. Surgical treatment of distal radial fractures with a volar locking plate versus conventional percutaneous methods: a randomized controlled trial. J Bone Joint Surg Am 2013;95(19):1737–1744.
14. Katz MA, Beredjiklian PK, Bozentka DJ, et al. Computed tomography scanning of intra-articular distal radius fractures: does it influence treatment? J Hand Surg Am 2001;26(3):415–421.
15. Lakshmanan P, Dixit V, Reed MR, et al. Infection rate of percutaneous Kirschner wire fixation for distal radius fractures. J Orthop Surg (Hong Kong) 2010;18:85–86.
16. Margaliot Z, Haase SC, Kotsis SV, et al. A meta-analysis of outcomes of external fixation versus plate osteosynthesis for unstable distal radius fractures. J Hand Surg Am 2005;30(6):1185–1199.
17. McQueen MM. Redisplaced unstable fractures of the distal radius. A randomised, prospective study of bridging versus non-bridging external fixation. J Bone Joint Surg Br 1998;80(4):665–669.
18. Nana AD, Joshi A, Lichtman DM. Plating of the distal radius. J Am Acad Orthop Surg 2005;13(3):159–171.
19. Rosati M, Bertagnini S, Digrandi G, et al. Percutaneous pinning for fractures of the distal radius. Acta Orthop Belg 2006;72(2):138–146.
20. Rozental TD, Blazar PE, Franko OI, et al. Functional outcomes for unstable distal radial fractures treated with open reduction and internal fixation or closed reduction and percutaneous fixation. A prospective randomized trial. J Bone Joint Surg Am 2009;91(8):1837–1846.
21. Short WH, Palmer AK, Werner FW, et al. A biomechanical study of distal radial fractures. J Hand Surg Am 1987;12(4):529–534.
22. Simic PM, Weiland AJ. Fractures of the distal aspect of the radius: changes in treatment over the past two decades. Instr Course Lect 2003;52:185–195.
23. Sommerkamp TG, Seeman M, Silliman J, et al. Dynamic external fixation of unstable fractures of the distal part of the radius. A prospective, randomized comparison with static external fixation. J Bone Joint Surg Am 1994;76(8):1149–1161.
24. Souer JS, Ring D, Matschke S, et al. Effect of an unrepaired fracture of the ulnar styloid base on outcome after plate-and-screw fixation of a distal radial fracture. J Bone Joint Surg Am 2009;91(4):830–838.
25. Subramanian P, Kantharuban S, Shilston S, et al. Complications of Kirschner-wire fixation in distal radius fractures. Tech Hand Up Extrem Surg 2012;16(3):120–123.
26. Trumble TE, Schmitt SR, Vedder NB. Factors affecting functional outcome of displaced intra-articular distal radius fractures. J Hand Surg Am 1994;19(2):325–340.
27. Trumble TE, Wagner W, Hanel DP, et al. Intrafocal (Kapandji) pinning of distal radius fractures with and without external fixation. J Hand Surg Am 1998;23(3):381–394.
28. Wei DH, Raizman NM, Bottino CJ, et al. Unstable distal radial fractures treated with external fixation, a radial column plate, or a volar plate. A prospective randomized trial. J Bone Joint Surg Am 2009;91(7):1568–1577.
29. Westphal T, Piatek S, Schubert S, et al. Outcome after surgery of distal radius fractures: no differences between external fixation and ORIF. Arch Orthop Trauma Surg 2005;125(8):507–514.
30. Zollinger PE, Tuinebreijer WE, Breederveld RS, et al. Can vitamin C prevent complex regional pain syndrome in patients with wrist fractures? A randomized, controlled, multicenter dose-response study. J Bone Joint Surg Am 2007;89(7):1424–1431.

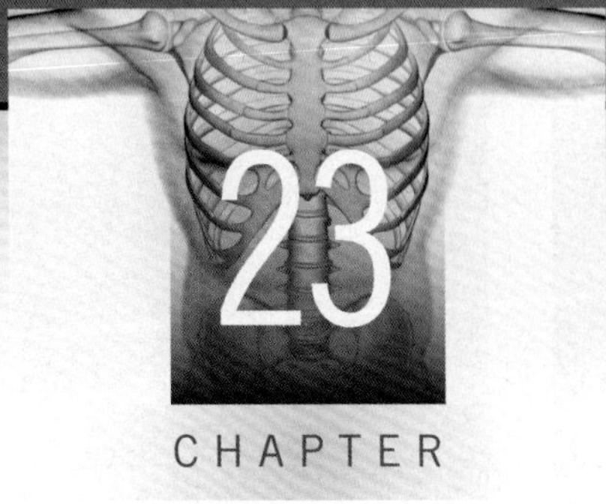

Volar Plating of Distal Radius Fractures

John J. Fernandez and David J. Wilson

DEFINITION

- Distal radius fractures are defined by their involvement of the metaphysis of the distal radius.
- They are assessed on the basis of fracture pattern, alignment, and stability:
  - Articular versus nonarticular
  - Reducible versus irreducible
  - Stable versus unstable
- Irreducible or unstable fractures require surgical reduction and stable fixation.
- Volar plating historically has been the method of choice for volar shear–type fractures.
  - Fixed-angle plates remain the preferred method of fixation for most types of distal radius fractures.

ANATOMY

- The distal radius serves as a buttress for the proximal carpus, transmitting 75% to 80% of its forces into the forearm.
  - The remaining 20% to 25% of force is transmitted through the distal ulna and the triangular fibrocartilage complex (TFCC).
- Thickness of distal radius articular cartilage is 1 mm or less.[18]
- Dorsally
  - The distal radius is the origin for the dorsal radiocarpal (DRC) ligament (**FIG 1A**).
  - It is the floor of the fibro-osseous extensor tendon compartments and includes Lister tubercle, assisting in extensor pollicis longus function (**FIG 1B**).
  - The extensor tendons are in immediate contact with the dorsal surface of the distal radius.
- Volarly
  - The distal radius is the origin for volar extrinsic ligaments of the wrist, including the radioscaphocapitate (RSC) ligament and long and short radiolunate ligaments (see **FIG 1A**).
  - It is also the origin of the pronator quadratus.
  - The flexor tendons are separated from the volar surface of the distal radius by the pronator quadratus.
- Ulnarly
  - The distal radius is the origin for the triangular fibrocartilage (see **FIG 1A**).
  - It also contains the sigmoid notch, which articulates with the head of the distal ulnar, allowing forearm rotation through the distal radioulnar joint (DRUJ).
- Distally
  - The surface is divided into a triangular scaphoid fossa and a square lunate fossa articulating with each respective carpal bone (see **FIG 1A**).
- The distal articular surface is inclined approximately 22 degrees ulnarly in the coronal plane and 11 degrees volarly in the sagittal plane (**FIG 1C,D**).
- The metaphysis is defined as the length of the distal radius, proximal to the articular surface, equivalent to the widest portion of the entire wrist.
- The dorsal cortical bone is less substantial than the volar cortical bone, contributing to the characteristic dorsal bending fracture pattern of distal radius fractures.

PATHOGENESIS

- The mechanism of injury in a distal radius fracture is an axial force across the wrist, with the pattern of injury determined by bone density, the position of the wrist, and the magnitude and direction of force.
- Most distal radius fractures result from falls with the wrist extended and pronated, which places a dorsal bending moment across the distal radius.
  - Relatively weaker, thinner dorsal bone collapses under compression, whereas stronger volar bone fails under tension, resulting in a characteristic "triangle" of comminution with the apex volar and greater comminution dorsal.
- Other possible mechanisms form a basis for some fracture classifications such as the one proposed by Jupiter and Fernandez.[8]
  - Bending
  - Axial compression
  - Shear
  - Avulsion
  - Combinations
- Articular involvement and its severity are the basis of some fracture classifications, such as the AO Foundation and Orthopaedic Trauma Association (AO/OTA)[12] and Melone[14] classifications.
- Articular involvement splits the distal radius into distinct fragments separate from the radius shaft (**FIG 2**):
  - Scaphoid fossa fragment
  - Lunate fossa fragment. Comminution of this fragment may result in two impacted articular fragments, involving the dorsal ulnar corner and the volar ulnar rim.[13]

NATURAL HISTORY

- Clinical outcome usually, but not always, correlates with deformity.
  - Variable residual deformity can be tolerated best by individuals with fewer functional demands.

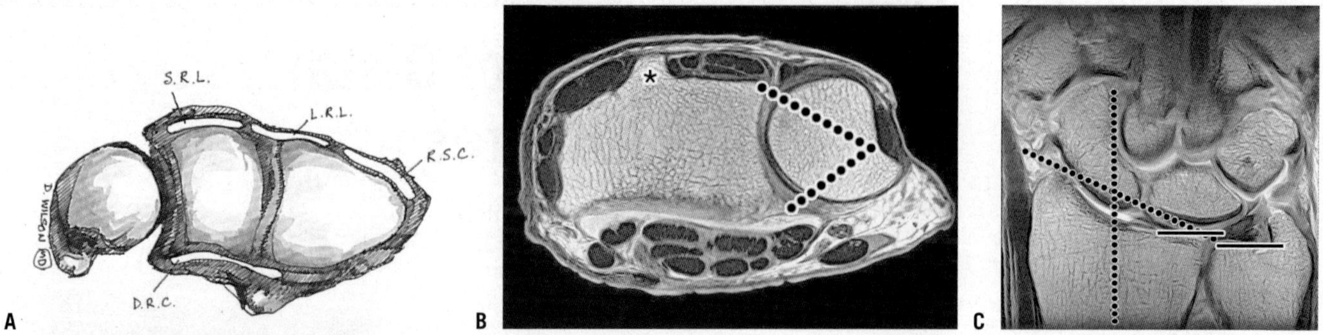

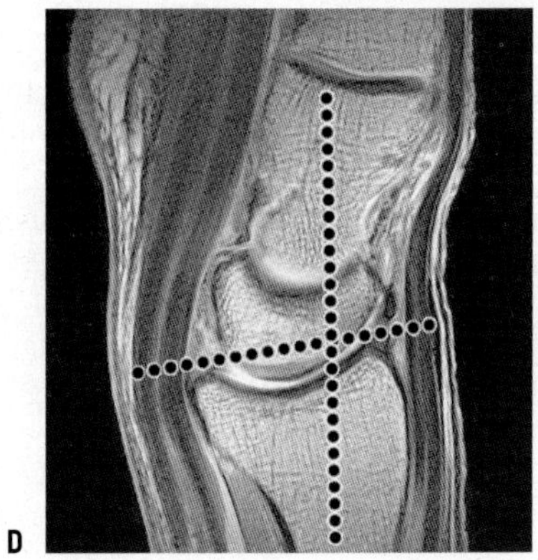

FIG 1 **A.** The distal articular surface of the radius is divided into a triangularly shaped scaphoid fossa and a square-shaped lunate fossa. The distal ulna and the TFCC act as ulnar buttresses for the wrist. The origins of the DRC ligament, RSC ligament, long and short radiolunate ligaments are shown. **B.** Axial magnetic resonance (MR) image of the wrist at the level of the distal radius. Lister tubercle is marked with an *asterisk*. *Dotted lines* represent dorsal and volar borders of the triangular fibrocartilage that helps stabilize the DRUJ. The dorsal distal radius acts as an attachment for dorsal extensor compartment sheaths. **C.** MR coronal cut of the distal radius. The articular surface of the distal radius is inclined about 22 degrees relative to the forearm axis (*dotted lines*). The ulnar aspect of the distal radius (ie, the lunate fossa) usually is distal to the end of the distal ulna (ie, negative ulnar variance). Note the *solid lines* marking ulnar variance. **D.** MR sagittal cut of the distal radius. The articular surface of the distal radius is inclined approximately 11-degree palmar relative to the forearm axis (*dotted lines*). Proximally, there exists relatively thinner dorsal cortical bone versus the thicker volar bone.

- As wrist deformity increases, physiologic function is progressively altered.
  - Intra-articular displacement of 1 to 2 mm results in an increased risk of osteoarthritis.[5,9]
  - Radial shortening of 3 to 5 mm or more results in increased loading of the ulnar complex.[1,17]
  - Dorsal angulation greater than 10 degrees shifts contact forces to the dorsal scaphoid fossa and the ulnar complex, causing increased disability.[20,23]
- The incidence of associated intracarpal injuries increases with fracture severity. Such injuries can account for poor outcomes. These injuries often are not recognized at first, leading to delayed treatment.[6,21]
  - TFCC tears
  - Scapholunate and lunotriquetral ligament tears

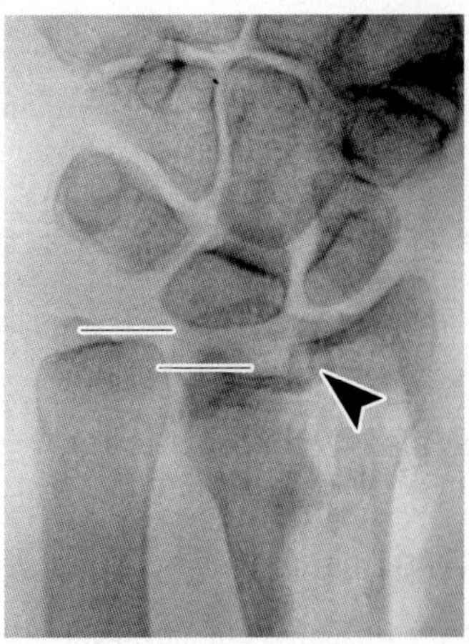

FIG 2 The *arrowhead* points to the articular split. Articular displacement of the scaphoid fossa fragment radially and the lunate fossa fragment ulnarly is apparent, as is significant shortening (ulnar positive variance) as outlined by the *lines*.

  - Chondral injuries involving the articulating surfaces
  - Distal radioulnar joint injury
  - Distal ulnar fractures
- By predicting the stability of a distal radius fracture, deformity and its complications can be minimized. Several risk factors have been suggested by Lafontaine et al[10] and others. The presence of three or more of the following indicates instability:
  - Dorsal (or volar apex) angulation greater than 20 degrees
  - Dorsal comminution
  - Intra-articular extension
  - Associated ulnar fracture
  - Patient age older than 60 years

PATIENT HISTORY AND PHYSICAL FINDINGS

- The mechanism of injury should be sought to assist in assessing the energy and level of the trauma.
- Associated injuries are not uncommon and should be carefully ruled out.
  - Injuries to the hand, carpus, and proximal arm, including other fractures or dislocations
  - Injuries to other extremities or the head, neck, and torso
- Establish the patient's functional and occupational demands.
- Document coexisting medical conditions that may affect healing such as smoking or diabetes.
- Determine possible risk factors for anesthesia and surgery, such as cardiac disease.
- The physical examination should document the following:
  - Condition of surrounding soft tissues (ie, skin and subcutaneous tissues)
  - Quality of vascular perfusion and pulses
  - Integrity of nerve function
  - Sensory two-point discrimination or threshold sensory testing
  - Motor function of intrinsic muscles, including thenar and hypothenar muscles, of the hand

- Examination of the distal ulna, TFCC, and DRUJ should rule out disruption and instability.
  - Detailed evaluation of DRUJ stability is typically only possible intraoperatively, after distal radius fracture reduction and stabilization.
- Reliable physical examination of the carpus often is difficult, making radiographic review even more critical and follow-up examinations important.

IMAGING AND OTHER DIAGNOSTIC STUDIES

- Imaging establishes fracture severity, helps determine stability, and guides the operative approach and choice of fixation.
- Plain radiographs should be obtained before and after reduction: posteroanterior (with the forearm in neutral rotation), lateral, and two separate oblique views.
  - Oblique views, in particular, help evaluate articular involvement, particularly the lunate fossa fragment **(FIG 3A,B)**.
  - The lateral view should be modified with the forearm inclined 15 to 20 degrees to best visualize the articular surface **(FIG 3C**; see **TECH FIG 5B,C)**.
- Fluoroscopic evaluation can be useful because it gives a complete circumferential view of the wrist and, with traction applied, can help evaluate injuries of the ligaments and carpus.
- Computed tomography (CT) helps define carpal subluxation from intra-articular involvement and helps detect small or impacted fragments, which may not be apparent on plain radiographs, particularly those involving the central portion of the distal radius **(FIG 3D,E)**.

DIFFERENTIAL DIAGNOSIS

- Diagnosis is directly confirmed by radiographs.
- Associated and contributory injuries should always be considered.
  - Pathologic fracture (eg, related to tumor, infection)
  - Associated injuries to the carpus (eg, scaphoid fracture, scapholunate ligament injury)

NONOPERATIVE MANAGEMENT

- Nonoperative treatment is reserved for distal radius fractures that are reducible and stable based on the criteria previously discussed.
- The goal of nonoperative treatment is to immobilize the wrist while maintaining acceptable alignment until the fracture is healed.
- Goals for treatment[11]
  - Radial inclination greater than 10 degrees
  - Ulnar variance less than 3-mm positive
  - Palmar tilt less than 10 degrees dorsal or 20 degrees volar
  - Articular congruity with less than a 2-mm gap or step-off
- Patients are immobilized in a short-arm cast for approximately 6 weeks. Radiographic follow-up is performed on a weekly basis for the first 2 to 3 weeks to identify fracture displacement that may warrant operative treatment.

SURGICAL MANAGEMENT

- The goal of operative treatment is to achieve acceptable alignment and stable fixation.

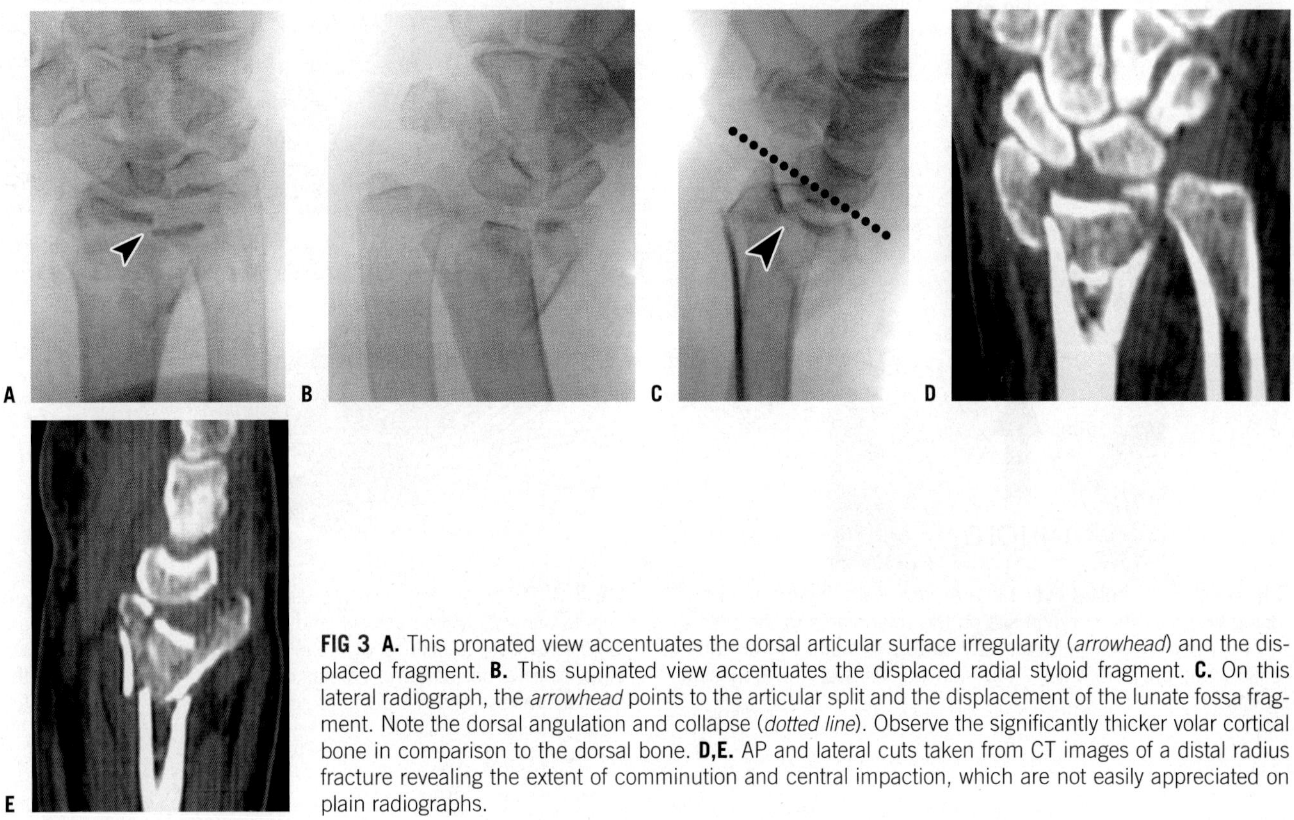

FIG 3 A. This pronated view accentuates the dorsal articular surface irregularity (*arrowhead*) and the displaced fragment. **B.** This supinated view accentuates the displaced radial styloid fragment. **C.** On this lateral radiograph, the *arrowhead* points to the articular split and the displacement of the lunate fossa fragment. Note the dorsal angulation and collapse (*dotted line*). Observe the significantly thicker volar cortical bone in comparison to the dorsal bone. **D,E.** AP and lateral cuts taken from CT images of a distal radius fracture revealing the extent of comminution and central impaction, which are not easily appreciated on plain radiographs.

- Various methods of fixation are available: pins, external fixators, intramedullary devices, and plates (volar, dorsal, fragment specific).

Preoperative Planning

- Preoperative medical and anesthesia evaluation are performed as required.
- Discontinue blood-thinning medications (anticoagulants and nonsteroidal anti-inflammatory drugs, especially acetylsalicylic acid).
- Request necessary equipment, including fluoroscopic, power equipment, and implants.
- Look for and document the presence of median nerve paresthesias, signifying acute compartment syndrome. If noted, consider a carpal tunnel release along with fracture stabilization.
- Confirm the plate fixation system to be used, and check the equipment before beginning surgery for completeness (ie, all appropriate drills, plates, and screws).
- Have a contingency plan or additional fixation (external fixator, bone graft, or bone graft substitute).
- Review and have previous radiographic studies available.
  - Consider having radiographs of the uninjured wrist to use as a template.
- Consider use of a regional anesthetic for postoperative pain control.

Positioning

- Place the patient in the supine position with the affected extremity on an arm table.
- Apply an upper arm tourniquet, preferably within the sterile field.
- Incorporate weights or a traction system to apply distraction across the fracture **(FIG 4)**.
- The surgeon is seated so that the elbow is pointing toward the patient's torso and the dominant hand works toward the fingers of the patients.
- The assistant is seated opposite the surgeon.
- The fluoroscopy unit is brought in from the end or corner of the table.

Approach

- Dorsal exposure allows for direct visualization of the articular surface when necessary.
- Fracture comminution is more severe dorsally, making overall alignment more difficult to judge.
- The thicker volar cortex is less comminuted, allowing for more precise reduction and buttressing of bone fragments.
- Sometimes, both dorsal and volar exposures may be necessary to achieve articular congruency and volar reduction and fixation, respectively.
- An extended volar ulnar exposure may be necessary to manage isolated volar ulnar fractures of the lunate facet or to perform a simultaneous carpal tunnel release if indicated.
- The techniques described in this chapter use the volar approach to distal radius, as described by Henry **(FIG 5)**.

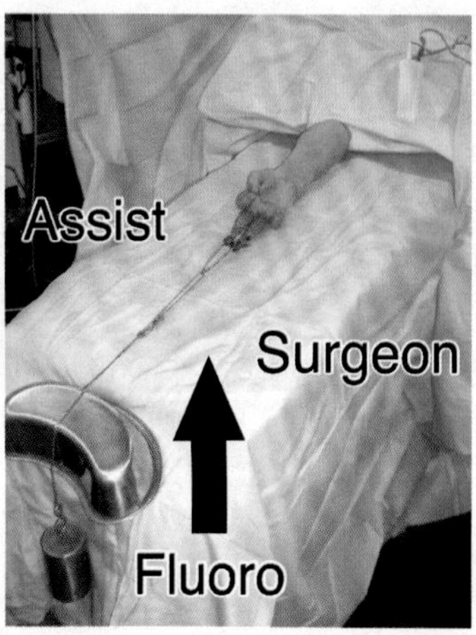

FIG 4 Traction is applied over the arm table with finger traps and hanging weights. The surgeon sits on the volar side and the assistant on the dorsal side. Fluoroscopy can be brought in from any direction but preferably from the side adjacent or the opposite surgeon.

A

B

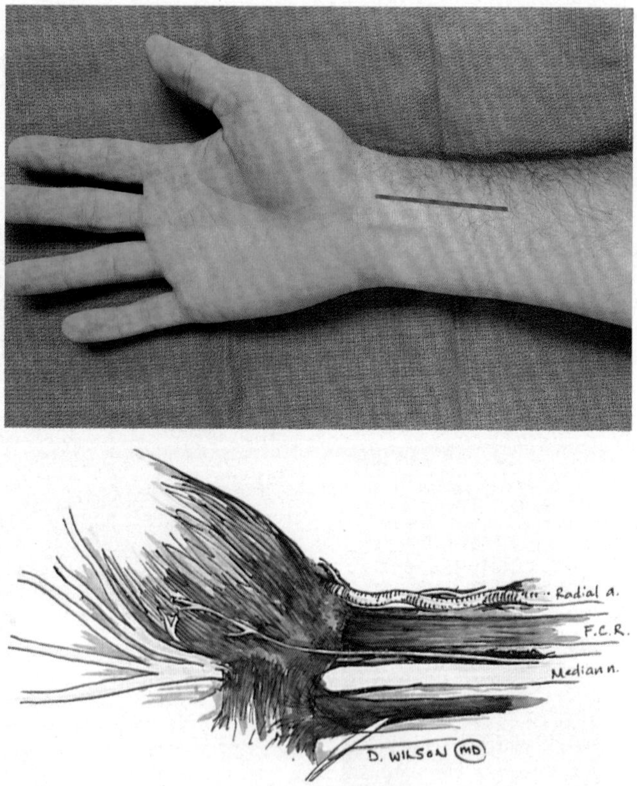

FIG 5 **A.** The volar incision is represented by the *solid line* just proximal to the wrist flexion creases and radial to the flexor carpi radialis longus. **B.** Care is exercised to avoid dissection ulnar to the flexor carpi radialis because the palmar cutaneous nerve branch of the median nerve is at risk.

VOLAR FIXED-ANGLE PLATE FIXATION OF THE DISTAL RADIUS

Incision and Dissection

- Make a 4- to 8-cm longitudinal incision from the proximal wrist flexion crease proximally, along the radial border of the flexor carpi radialis tendon.
  - Use a zigzag incision to cross the wrist flexion creases if required.
  - If performing a concurrent carpal tunnel release, consider performing this after stable fixation of an anatomic reduction, as traumatic deformity can distort the anatomy.
- Carefully avoid the palmar cutaneous branch of the median nerve, which arises within 10 cm proximal to the wrist flexion crease and travels along the ulnar side of the flexor carpi radialis tendon distally.
  - Branches of the dorsal radial sensory nerve and lateral antebrachial cutaneous nerve may appear along the path of the incision and also need to be protected.
- At the distal end of the incision, protect the palmar branch of the radial artery to the deep palmar arch.
  - It usually is not necessary to dissect out the radial artery **(TECH FIG 1A)**.
- Incise the anterior sheath of the flexor carpi radialis tendon and retract the tendon ulnarly to help protect the median nerve **(TECH FIG 1B)**.
- Incise the posterior sheath of the flexor carpi radialis tendon.
  - The deep tissues likely will bulge out from the pressure of swelling and fracture hematoma.
  - The median nerve is at risk lying within the subcutaneous tissues along the ulnar portion of the wound **(TECH FIG 1C,D)**.
  - The flexor pollicis longus tendon sits along the radial margin of the wound.
- Using blunt dissection with a gauze-covered finger, sweep the flexor tendons and the median nerve ulnarly.
  - A self-retaining retractor is carefully placed just deep to the radial artery radially and the tendons and median nerve ulnarly.
  - The pronator quadratus is now visualized on the floor of the wound.
- Incise the pronator quadratus at its radial insertion. Leaving fascial tissue on either side facilitates later repair if desired. Determine the proximal and distal extent of the muscle, and make horizontal incisions at both of those points creating an ulnarly based muscle flap **(TECH FIG 1E)**.
  - The distal margin of the pronator quadratus attaches along the distal volar lip of the distal radius, along the "teardrop" and the watershed line.
  - The radial margin is in proximity to the tendons of the first dorsal compartment and the brachioradialis.

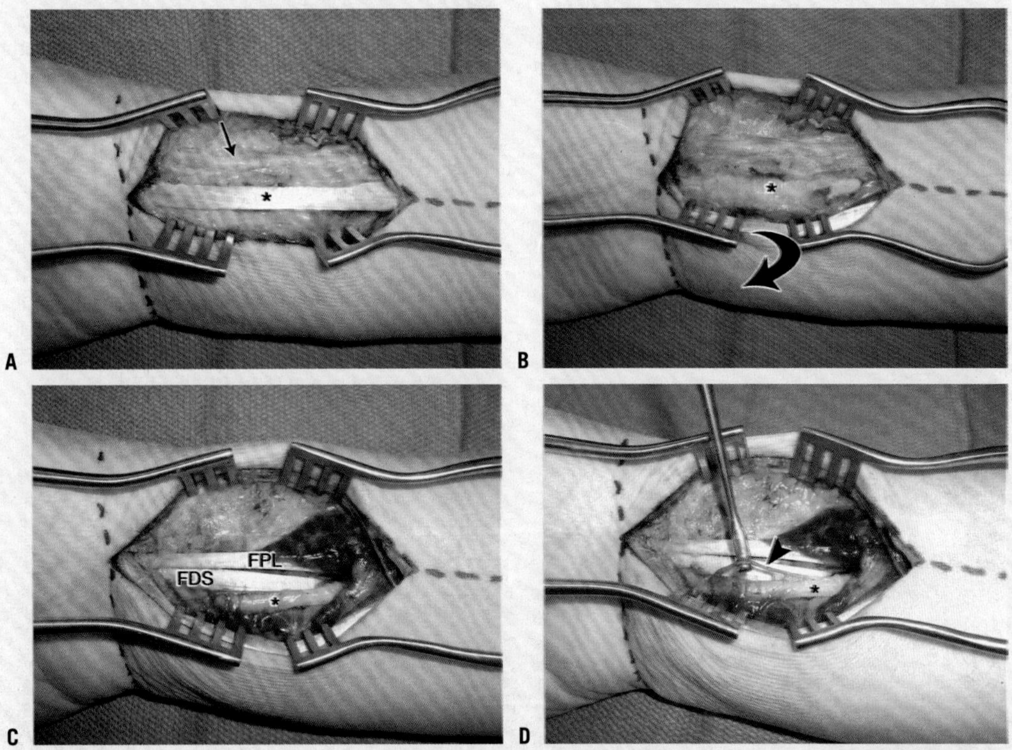

TECH FIG 1 **A.** The interval between the radial artery (*arrow*) and the flexor carpi radialis tendon (*asterisk*) is seen. **B.** The posterior sheath (*asterisk*) of the flexor carpi radialis is visible after retracting the flexor carpi radialis ulnarly (*curved arrow*). Be careful during deeper dissection because swelling and hematoma may distort the position of the median nerve beneath the sheath. **C.** Following incision in the flexor carpi radialis posterior sheath, the deep tendons are visible, including the flexor pollicis longus (*FPL*) and the flexor digitorum superficialis (*FDS*) of the index finger. The median nerve also is visible (*asterisk*). **D.** The palmar cutaneous nerve branches of the median nerve (*arrowhead*) and median nerve (*asterisk*) are both at risk for injury during this approach. Be careful regarding placement of retractors and during dissection and plate placement. *(continued)*

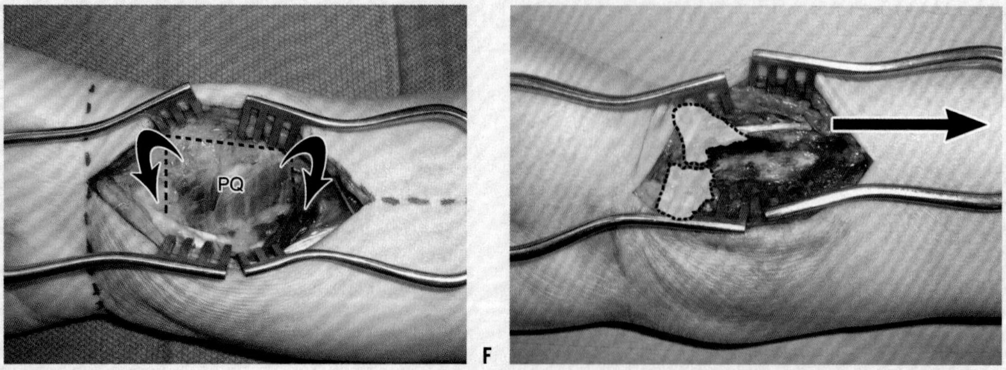

TECH FIG 1 *(continued)* **E.** The pronator quadratus (*PQ*) is incised distally, radially, and proximally and then reflected ulnarly after dissection off the volar distal radius (*curved arrows* and *broken lines*). **F.** The brachioradialis (*arrow*) can be a deforming force, especially in comminuted fractures and in those for which treatment has been delayed. This tendon can be released if necessary (*broken lines*).

- Subperiosteally, dissect the pronator quadratus off the volar surface of the distal radius as an ulnarly based flap with a knife or elevator.
- Retract the pronator ulnarly with the flexor tendons and median nerve.
- Particularly, if significant shortening of radial-sided fracture fragments has occurred, incise the broad insertion of the brachioradialis to eliminate the deforming force **(TECH FIG 1F)**.
  - Release the first dorsal compartment and retract the tendons before releasing the brachioradialis.
  - Alternatively, Z-lengthen the brachioradialis tendon to allow for repair at the completion of the case.

Fracture Reduction and Provisional Fixation

- Apply a lobster claw clamp around the radius shaft at a perpendicular angle to the volar surface at the most proximal portion of the wound **(TECH FIG 2A)**.
  - This allows for excellent control of the proximal shaft for rotation and translation, providing counterforce when correcting the dorsal angulation collapse.
  - It also aids in soft tissue retraction.
- With the fracture now exposed, apply traction distally to distract and disimpact the fragments.
- Carefully clean the fracture of any interposed muscle, fascia, hematoma, or callus while maintaining the bony contours.
- In the case of significant volar comminution, reduce and provisionally stabilize the fragments with Kirschner wires (K-wires).
  - Take plate positioning into account when placing these K-wires.
- The articular surface is first reduced, if necessary.
- Under fluoroscopic guidance, manipulate the articular fragments through the fracture with a periosteal elevator, osteotome, or K-wires **(TECH FIG 2B,C)**.
  - Longitudinal traction is important during this reduction phase. It can be performed by an assistant or using cross-table weights and finger traps.
  - A dorsal exposure may be performed at this stage if there is significant articular impaction, particularly centrally, that cannot be corrected using the extra-articular technique described here.
- Place K-wires from the radial styloid fragment into the lunate fossa fragment to maintain the articular reduction **(TECH FIG 2D)**.
  - The K-wires should be placed as close as possible to subchondral bone **(TECH FIG 2E,F)**.

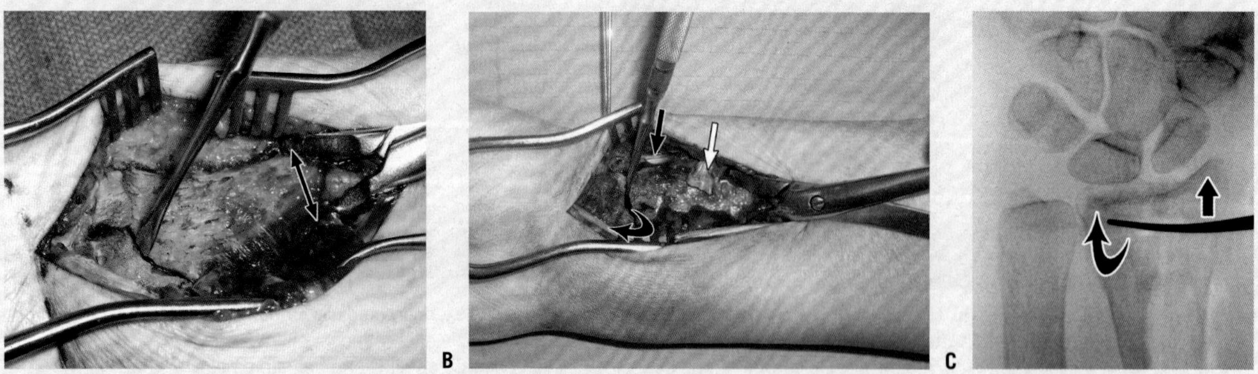

TECH FIG 2 **A.** A lobster claw clamp (*double arrow*) is applied to the radius shaft well proximal to the fracture. This instrument helps the surgeon control the radius during reduction and defines the lateral margins of the radius. A Freer elevator is inserted into the fracture to help disimpact the fragments and assist in their reduction. **B.** The brachioradialis (*white arrow*) is released, and the first compartment extensor tendons are visible in the background (*black arrow*). An instrument can now be placed to assist in the reduction (*curved arrow*). **C.** The Freer elevator is used to reduce the fragments. In this case, the intra-articular step-off is being corrected, and the radial length and inclination are being restored (*arrows*). *(continued)*

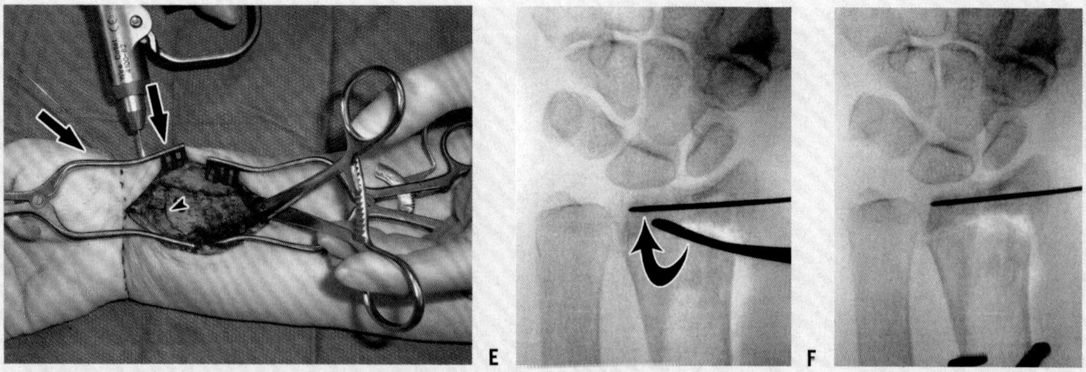

D E F

TECH FIG 2 *(continued)* **D.** K-wires are placed across the radial styloid into the reduced ulna fossa fragment. An assistant usually applies traction, and the lobster claw clamp can be used for powerful leverage. If there is no articular involvement, this K-wire can be placed into the radius metaphysis or diaphysis proximally (*arrows* and *arrowhead*). **E.** The K-wire should be placed as close as possible to the subchondral bone, avoiding areas of comminution (*curved arrow*). **F.** The K-wire should maintain the articular reduction without any support.

- Once the distal articular reduction is complete, reduce the distal radius as a single unit to the radius shaft.
- Insert K-wires as required to maintain the provisional reduction between the distal fragments and the proximal shaft fragment.
  - If radial collapse and translation are prominent, a large K-wire can be introduced into the radial portion of the fracture. By advancing it proximally and ulnarly, it behaves like an intrafocal pin, providing a radial buttress by pushing the distal fragment ulnarly.
  - A similar technique can be applied through the dorsal fracture to assist in maintaining palmar tilt correction.

Plate Application

- Apply a fixed-angle volar plate to the volar surface of the distal radius and shaft. Position the plate to accommodate for the unique design characteristics of the plating system as well as the location of the fracture fragments.
  - Each plating system has unique characteristics that determine its optimal placement.
  - Ideally, the plate should be placed so that subchondral screw purchase is maximized, without the distal locking pegs or screws penetrating the joint.
  - If the fracture has not yet been fully reduced, this must be taken into account when placing the device.
  - Plate placement distal to the watershed line should be avoided as this increases the risk for flexor tendon rupture.
- Clamp the previously applied lobster claw to the proximal portion of the plate to keep the plate centralized on the radius shaft.
- Place provisional K-wires through the plate to maintain position **(TECH FIG 3)**. Then, fluoroscopically confirm proper plate position in both the distal proximal and radioulnar directions.
  - Proper alignment of the plate can be determined only using a true anteroposterior (AP) image in which the DRUJ is well visualized.
  - The K-wires allow for fine adjustment in plate position before committing to insertion of a screw.
- Drill and insert a provisional screw in the oblong hole in the plate.
  - If the bone is osteopenic, a screw longer than the initial measurement should be placed to ensure that both cortices are engaged. Otherwise, the plate may not be held securely, and reduction will be compromised. After the remaining screws have been secured, this screw must be replaced with one of appropriate length.
- Insert at least one additional proximal screw and remove the provisional K-wires holding the plate in place.

Distal Fragment Reduction

- Once the plate has been secured proximally, execute any additionally needed reduction.
  - A well-designed plate serves as an excellent buttress for correction of palmar tilt **(TECH FIG 4A)**.
- Apply counterforce through the lobster claw clamp in a dorsal direction while the distal hand and wrist are translated palmarly and flexed **(TECH FIG 4B)**.
  - This maneuver reduces the distal radius to the plate, effectively restoring volar tilt by pushing the lunate against the volar lip of the distal radius **(TECH FIG 4C,D)**.
- Additional distraction and ulnar deviation correct radial collapse and loss of radial inclination.

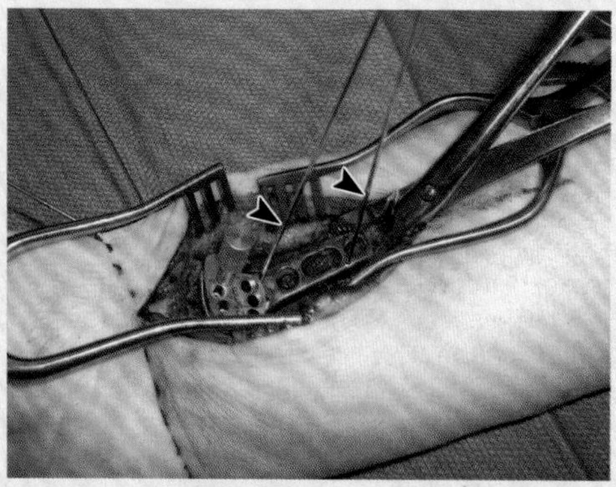

TECH FIG 3 Keep the plate centered on the radius and as distal as possible. The lobster claw clamp helps keep the plate centered. K-wires (*arrowheads*) are helpful as provision fixation until alignment can be confirmed radiographically and screws placed.

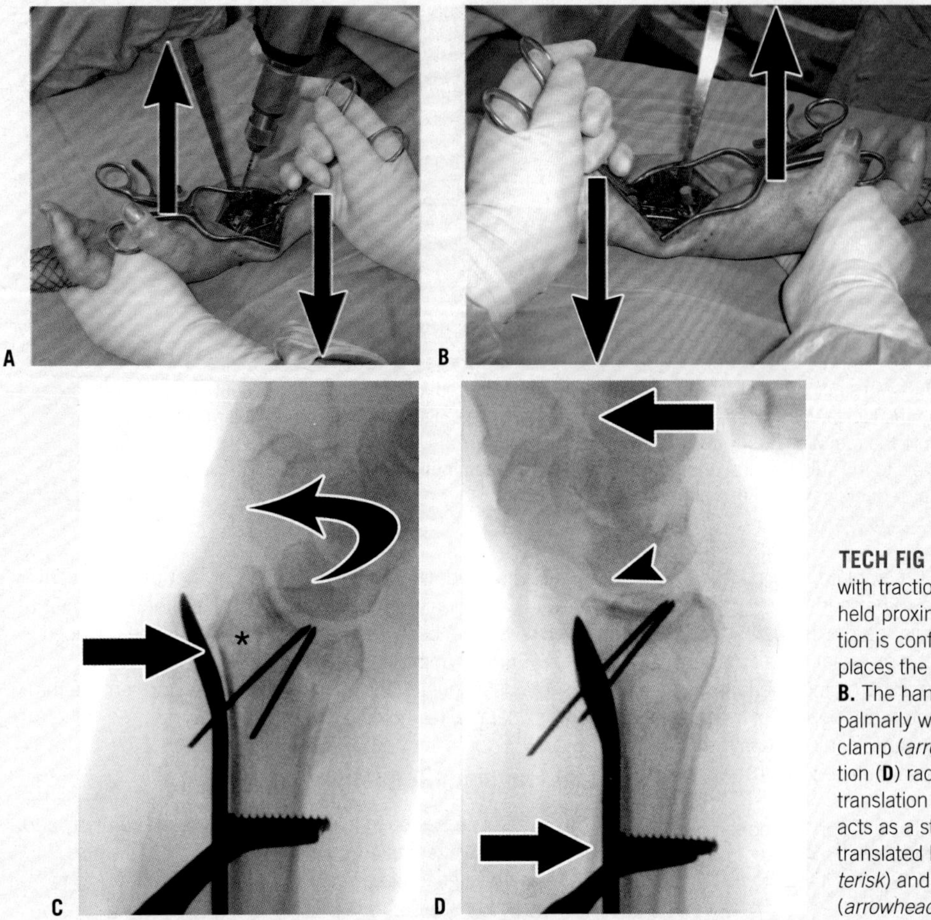

TECH FIG 4 A. The final reduction is performed with traction on the hand and with the radius held proximally with a clamp. Once the reduction is confirmed radiographically, the assistant places the distal screws or K-wires (*arrows*). **B.** The hand is translated (not appreciably flexed) palmarly while the radius shaft is held with the clamp (*arrows*). Prereduction (**C**) and postreduction (**D**) radiographs demonstrating the palmar translation reduction maneuver. The volar plate acts as a strong buttress (*arrows*), allowing the translated lunate to push on the volar radius (*asterisk*) and correct the dorsal angulation deformity (*arrowhead*).

Plate Fixation

- While the reduction is held, drill the holes in the distal plate segment **(TECH FIG 5A)**.
  - Some plate systems allow for provisional fixation using K-wires placed through the distal plate segment.
  - Penetrating the dorsal distal radius with the drill risks injury to the dorsal extensor tendons.
- Consider drilling and placing the distal ulnar screws first and then proceed radially and proximally.
- Accurate screw placement using the same inclination of the drill is required to avoid cross-threading into the plate and lessening stability.
- Judge the placement of all distal screws or pegs precisely using fluoroscopic imaging in multiple planes.
  - In order to confirm extra-articular placement of distal screws, perform a "true" lateral view of the wrist with the x-ray beam at a 20-degree angle to the radius shaft **(TECH FIG 5B,C)**. This is facilitated by lifting the wrist off the table with the elbow maintained on the table and the forearm at a 20-degree angle to the table **(TECH FIG 5D,E)**.
  - The extensor pollicis longus is at greatest risk of injury from a protruding screw.
  - Because of the prominence of Lister tubercle and the triangular configuration of the distal radius, the lateral view of the wrist may not accurately rule out dorsal screw protrusion.
  - The dorsal tangential (also known as *Horizon*) view can aid in assessing adequate screw length dorsally. It is obtained by wrist hyperflexion and aiming the beam of the image intensifier along the long axis of the radius.[7]
- Sequentially insert the remaining distal screws or pegs, followed by the remaining proximal plate screws **(TECH FIG 5F)**.
- If necessary, add bone graft or bone graft substitute around the plate into the fracture site or through a small dorsal incision.
- Precisely assess the stability of the construct after the plate has been applied. If appropriate, remove the provisional K-wires.
  - If the K-wires are deemed critical for fracture stability, they can be left in place and removed 4 to 8 weeks later.
  - If residual instability exists, add additional fixation with K-wires, an external fixator, a dorsal plate, or a combination.

Closure

- If desired, repair the pronator quadratus to its insertion site with a series of 3-0 absorbable horizontal mattress sutures **(TECH FIG 6A)**.
  - In many cases, it is impossible to repair the pronator quadratus because the muscle and fascia are extremely thin or the muscle is damaged. In this situation, the muscle can be débrided or simply left in place.
- Before skin closure, obtain final radiographs and assess the stability of the DRUJ.

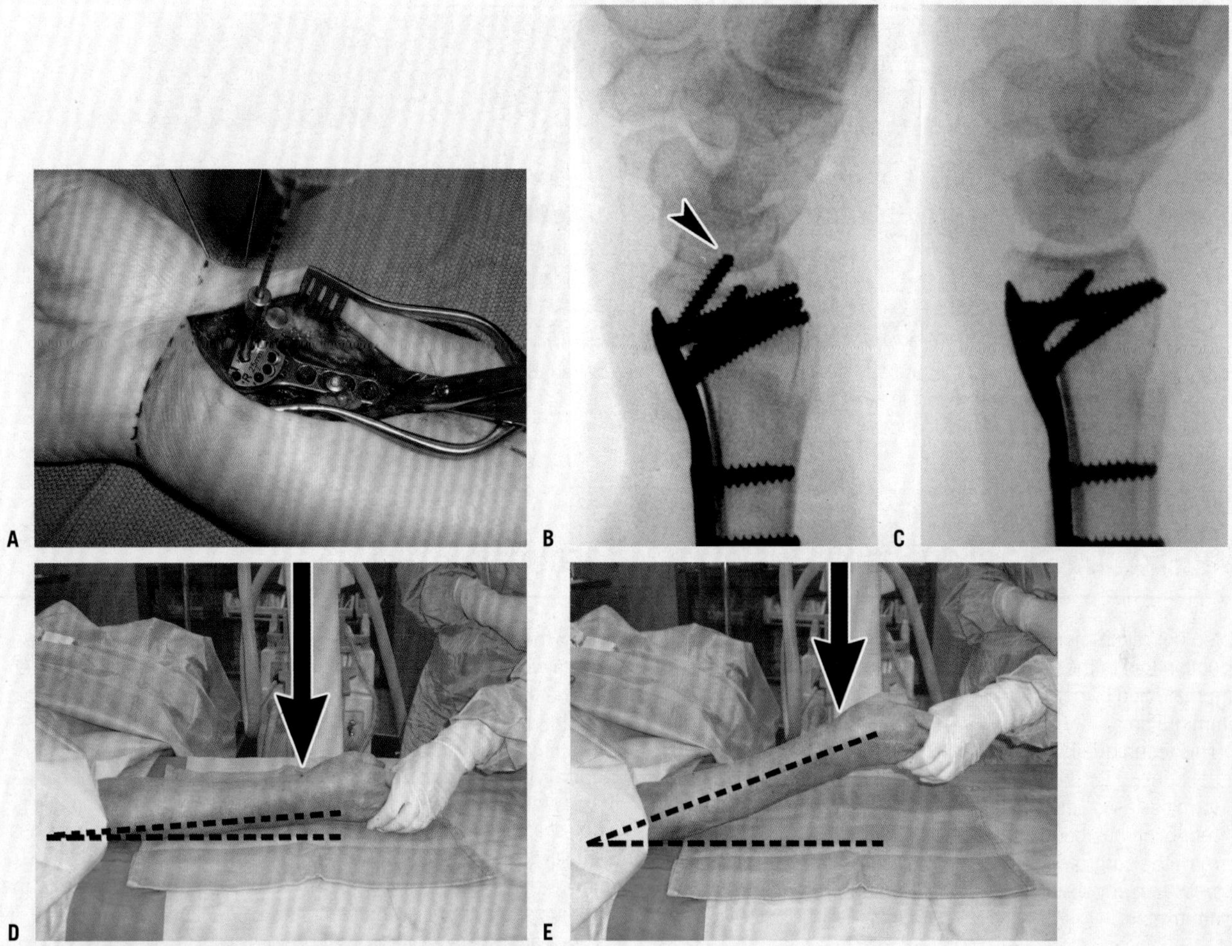

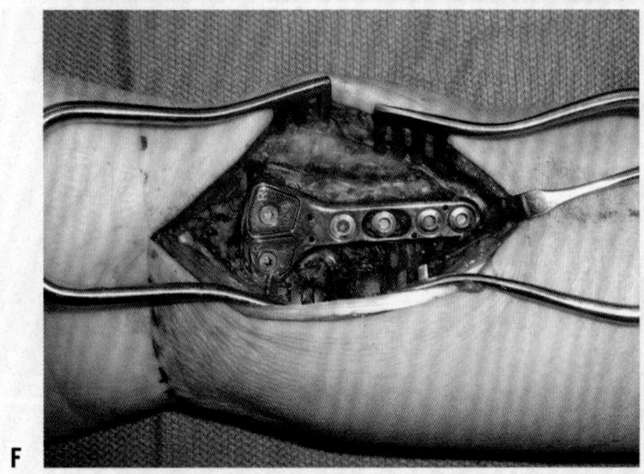

TECH FIG 5 **A.** The remaining holes can now be drilled and screws placed where needed. **B.** This radial styloid screw (*arrowhead*) looks as though it has penetrated the joint, when in reality, it is simply the angle of the radiographic beam that throws its projection into the joint. **C.** A true lateral view of the distal radius is necessary to judge placement of the radial screws. In this lateral view, and perhaps in the previous lateral x-ray image, the screws may be penetrating the dorsal cortex, endangering the extensor tendons. A dorsal tangential "horizon" view would be beneficial to assess screw length. In most instances, the screws would be removed and shorter screws inserted. **D.** A radiograph is being taken with the wrist perpendicular to the x-ray beam (*arrow*). This is not a true lateral image because the distal surface of the radius is inclined 20 degrees radially (*broken lines*). **E.** By lifting the hand and wrist 20 degrees off the table, a true lateral image can be achieved. The x-ray beam is now perpendicular to the joint (*arrow* and *broken lines*). **F.** The remaining screws have been placed.

- Place a drain only if excessive bleeding is anticipated.
- Consider methods to minimize postoperative pain if indicated.
  - Percutaneous placement of a pain pump catheter
  - Injection of a long-acting local anesthetic
- Close the subcutaneous tissues with a 4-0 or 5-0 braided absorbable suture and reapproximate the skin with interrupted 4-0 or 5-0 nylon sutures or a running subcuticular stitch.
- Place two layers of gauze and a nonadherent gauze over the wound, wrap the wrist and forearm with thick Webril (Kendall, Mansfield, MA), and apply a below-elbow splint in a neutral wrist position, leaving the metacarpophalangeal joints free for range of motion (ROM) **(TECH FIG 6B)**.
- If there is injury to the ulnar wrist (eg, ulnar styloid fracture, DRUJ injury):
  - Evaluate stability of the DRUJ and compare with the uninjured wrist. If needed, proceed with repair or fracture stabilization.
  - If additional surgery is not deemed necessary, immobilize the forearm in slight supination with an above-elbow or sugar-tong (Muenster) splint.

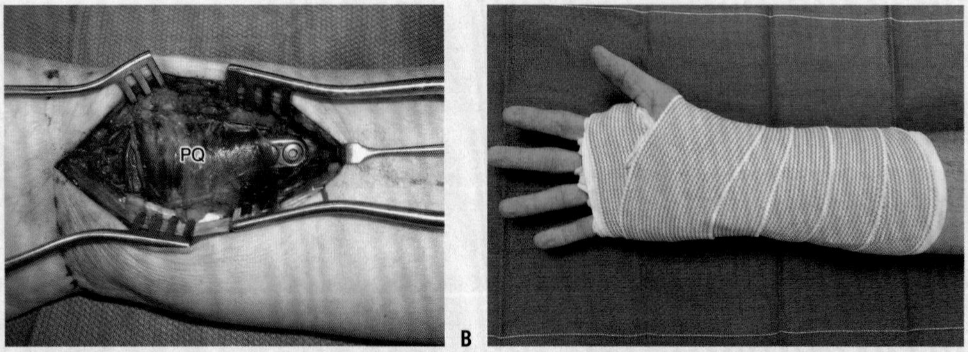

A B

TECH FIG 6 **A.** The pronator quadratus (*PQ*) has been repaired. **B.** A bulky dressing is applied with a volar splint holding the wrist in a neutral position.

VOLAR FIXED-ANGLE PLATE USING THE PLATE AS REDUCTION TOOL

- We do not recommend use of the volar fixed-angle plate as a reduction tool in the acute setting. It is best employed (if at all) for a malunion or perhaps for a fracture with minimal articular comminution.
  - This technique is difficult because the plate must be applied accounting for the coronal, sagittal, and translational deformities associated with the fracture fragments before the reduction has been achieved.
- Perform the surgical approach as previously described.
- Address first any distal articular involvement with reduction and K-wire fixation.
- Affix the plate to the distal fragment, accounting for where the plate will sit on the radius shaft once the reduction is completed.
- Place the screws so that they are parallel to the articular surface on the lateral x-ray view **(TECH FIG 7A,B)**.
- On the AP radiograph, align the plate 20 degrees off parallel to the radially inclined articular surface of the distal radius. Proper position of the plate on the distal segment allows proper position along the shaft segment, once anatomic restoration of radial inclination is achieved. (20 degrees;**TECH FIG 7C,D**).
- Once distal fixation is complete, secure the proximal plate to the radius shaft, thereby completing the reduction.
- Close and splint as described previously.

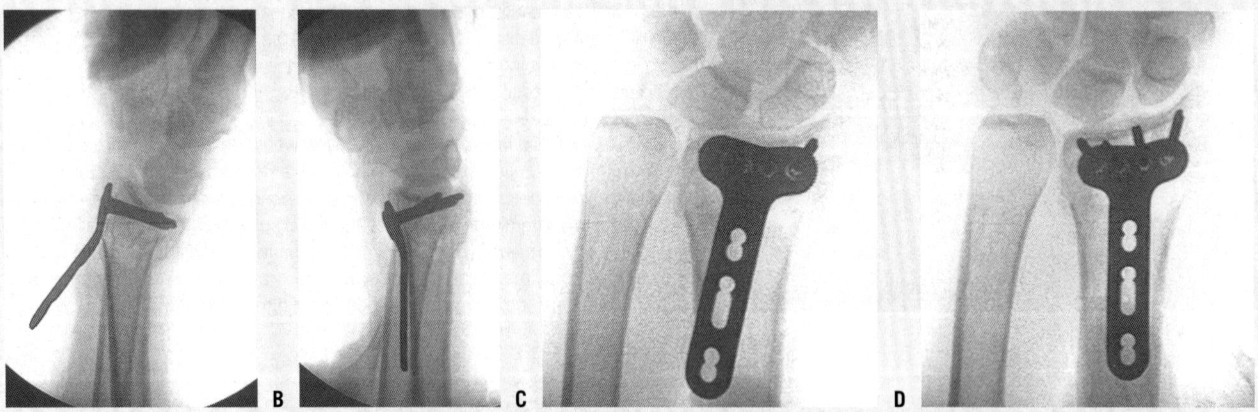

A B C D

TECH FIG 7 **A.** The volar plate is applied with the distal screws placed first (parallel to distal articular surface). **B.** Reducing the plate to the diaphysis proximally accomplishes the reduction. **C.** The plate is applied at approximately a 20-degree angle relative to the distal articular surface or to the amount of angulation that is estimated. **D.** By reducing the plate to the diaphysis, the distal angulation is corrected.

Pearls and Pitfalls

Preoperative Planning	• Obtain multiple radiographs in different positions (eg, several oblique views), especially in the setting of comminution or articular involvement. • Obtain a CT scan if assessing the pattern of fracture when radiographs alone are difficult or uncertain.
Surgical Approach	• Avoid crossing the distal flexion creases of the wrist. • Avoid ulnar exposure to the midline of the flexor carpi radialis. • Use extra care with deep dissection in the presence of hematoma or significant swelling.
Fracture Reduction	• Employ traction across the wrist with a device or weights. • Use a lobster claw clamp on the proximal radius shaft for control of the forearm and as a reference for the lateral margins. • Use instruments to disimpact and reduce articular fragments through the fracture itself, either volarly, dorsally, or both. • Employ a temporary K-wire to stabilize the reduction before placement of the plate.
Plate Alignment	• Confirm appropriate radial–ulnar positioning of the proximal plate using a true AP radiograph (ie, forearm in supination with open view of the DRUJ). • Confirm proper distal plate position on a true lateral view (ie, forearm 20 degrees off the table). • Place the plate as distal as possible, up to the volar teardrop (watershed line) of the distal radius, if possible. • Evaluate the screws for possible joint penetration using 360-degree fluoroscopic images.
Plate Fixation	• Use K-wires to fix the plate provisionally to the proximal radius. • The initial "oblong hole" screw should be slightly longer than the measured length to ensure better initial fixation.
Postoperative	• Closure of the pronator quadratus is not critical and should be reserved for more substantial muscles with limited trauma. • Begin immediate ROM to digits with edema.

POSTOPERATIVE CARE

- The wrist is splinted in a neutral position, leaving the digits free.
  - If the fracture is particularly tenuous or there is injury to the ulnar wrist, a long-arm or sugar-tong (Muenster) splint is applied.
- Vitamin C 500 to 1500 mg per day for 6 weeks has been recommended to reduce the incidence of complex regional pain syndrome; however, newer data calls the efficacy of this practice into question.[3,4,25]
- The patient is instructed to perform active ROM exercises for the digits every hour and to engage in strict elevation for at least 3 days.
  - It is critical to emphasize edema prevention and immediate ROM of the digits.
- At 1 week postoperatively, the splint is removed and the wound is examined.
- If fracture stability and swelling permit, the therapist fabricates a molded Orthoplast splint (Johnson & Johnson Orthopedics, New Brunswick, NJ) to be worn at all times.
  - Active ROM exercises of the wrist are implemented 1 week postoperatively.
- At 4 to 6 weeks, putty and grip exercises are added.
- At 6 to 8 weeks, the splint is discontinued, and progressive strengthening exercises are advanced.
- If necessary, progressive passive ROM can begin, including use of dynamic splints.
- At 10 to 12 weeks, the patient usually can be discharged to all activities as tolerated.
- Elderly patients with distal radius fractures are at increased risk of sustaining other osteoporosis-related fractures. A referral to an osteoporosis clinic is advised.

OUTCOMES

- Overall good to excellent results can be expected in over 80% of patients with ROM, strength, and outcomes scoring.[15,16,22,24]
- Studies comparing volar fixation to other forms of fixation (eg, external fixators, pins, and dorsal plating) have revealed similar if not superior results.
  - Results appear to be superior in the early recovery period, with the final outcome yielding equivalent results among all fixation groups.
  - Some studies suggest better maintenance in overall reduction compared to other forms of fixation.

COMPLICATIONS

- Complication rates as high as 27% have been reported.
- Complications can be categorized into those involving hardware, fracture, soft tissues, nerves, and tendons.[2]
- Failures of hardware, such as plate or screw breakage, can occur but are rare. Usually, such failures are an indication of other problems, such as nonunion.
- The hardware becomes unacceptably prominent in a minority of patients.
  - This complication may become evident only after some time has elapsed, as swelling of fibrous tissue subsides and bone remodels.
  - The most common sites include the dorsal wrist, when screws have been inserted, and the radial wrist, when a plate has been used.
  - It can be avoided with careful screw and plate placement and radiographic verification of their position.
- Nonunion and delayed union are unusual. Consider a diagnosis of osteomyelitis or other risk factors such as smoking.

- Loss of fracture reduction and fixation can occur and is most common in patients with osteopenic bone or comminuted and articular fractures.
  - This can be avoided with frequent and early follow-up with repeat radiographs.
  - If instability is suspected, the fracture can be casted.
  - In the operating room, if instability is suspected, additional fixation should be considered (eg, external fixator, pins, bone graft).
- Soft tissue complications are proportional to the energy of the initial injury.
- Open wounds usually can be addressed with local measures.
- Significant swelling must be addressed with early and aggressive modalities. Swelling can lead to other complications, such as joint stiffness and tendon adhesions.
- Nerve injuries can be the result of initial trauma or subsequent surgical trauma.
  - Assess and document neurologic status before surgery.
  - Avoid further injury to nerves with careful placement of retractors.
  - The palmar cutaneous branch of the median nerve can be injured during incision and exposure.
  - Avoid the nerve with a well-placed incision radial to the flexor carpi radialis and careful deep dissection.
- Postoperative neuromas can cause pain and sensitivity along scar. Carpal tunnel syndrome (CTS) can occur with distal radius fractures. Acute CTS occurs with a reported incidence of 5.4% to 8.6% and develops in hours to days after the fracture and should be addressed with an expeditious release.[19]
- Complex regional pain syndrome is reported with incidence as high as 10% in all distal radius fractures. Despite early evidence of protective benefit, recent data suggests no difference in patients prophylactically treated with vitamin C versus placebo.[3,4]
- Tendon complications include adhesions and ruptures.
- Most tendon adhesions involve the dorsal extensor tendons resulting in extrinsic extensor tightness.
- Flexor tendon adhesions are uncommon and involve primarily the flexor pollicis longus.
- Tendon ruptures have been described, especially involving the flexor pollicis longus and the extensor pollicis longus, as a result of plate and screw prominence, respectively.
  - The distal screws must not be left prominent, and caution must be applied when drilling.
  - The sagittal and coronal profiles of the plate being used must be taken into consideration—some plates are very prominent and extend far radially.

REFERENCES

1. Aro HT, Koivunen T. Minor axial shortening of the radius affects outcome of Colles' fracture treatment. J Hand Surg Am 1991;16(3): 392–398.
2. Arora R, Lutz M, Hennerbichler A, et al. Complications following internal fixation of unstable distal radius fracture with a palmar locking-plate. J Orthop Trauma 2007;21(5):316–322.
3. Ekrol I, Duckworth AD, Ralston SH, et al. The influence of vitamin C on the outcome of distal radius fractures: a double-blind, randomized controlled trial. J Bone Joint Surg Am 2014;96(17):1451–1459.
4. Evaniew N, McCarthy C, Kleinlugtenbelt YV, et al. Vitamin C to prevent complex regional pain syndrome in patients with distal radius fractures: a meta-analysis of randomized controlled trials. J Orthop Trauma 2015;29(8):e235–e241.
5. Fernandez JJ, Gruen GS, Herndon JH. Outcome of distal radius fractures using the short form 36 health survey. Clin Orthop Relat Res 1997;(341):36–41.
6. Geissler WB, Freeland AE, Savoie FH, et al. Intracarpal soft-tissue lesions associated with an intra-articular fracture of the distal end of the radius. J Bone Joint Surg Am 1996;78(3):357–365.
7. Joseph SJ, Harvey JN. The dorsal horizon view: detecting screw protrusion at the distal radius. J Hand Surg Am 2011;36(10):1691–1693.
8. Jupiter JB, Fernandez DL. Comparative classification for fractures of the distal end of the radius. J Hand Surg Am 1997;22(4):563–571.
9. Knirk JL, Jupiter JB. Intra-articular fractures of the distal end of the radius in young adults. J Bone Joint Surg Am 1986;68(5):647–659.
10. Lafontaine M, Hardy D, Delince P. Stability assessment of distal radius fractures. Injury 1989;20(4):208–210.
11. Lichtman DM, Bindra RR, Boyer MI, et al. American Academy of Orthopaedic Surgeons clinical practice guideline on: the treatment of distal radius fractures. J Bone Joint Surg Am 2011;93(8):775–778.
12. Marsh JL, Slongo TF, Agel J, et al. Fracture and dislocation classification compendium - 2007: Orthopaedic Trauma Association classification, database and outcomes committee. J Orthop Trauma 2007; 21(10 suppl):S1–S133.
13. Medoff RJ. Essential radiographic evaluation for distal radius fractures. Hand Clin 2005;21(3):279–288.
14. Melone CP Jr. Articular fractures of the distal radius. Orthop Clin North Am 1984;15(2):217–236.
15. Musgrave DS, Idler RS. Volar fixation of dorsally displaced distal radius fractures using the 2.4-mm locking compression plates. J Hand Surg Am 2005;30(4):743–749.
16. Orbay JL, Fernandez DL. Volar fixed-angle plate fixation for unstable distal radius fractures in the elderly patient. J Hand Surg Am 2004;29(1):96–102.
17. Pogue DJ, Viegas SF, Patterson RM, et al. Effects of distal radius fracture malunion on wrist joint mechanics. J Hand Surg Am 1990;15(5):721–727.
18. Pollock J, O'Toole RV, Nowicki SD, et al. Articular cartilage thickness at the distal radius: a cadaveric study. J Hand Surg Am 2013;38(8):1477–1481.
19. Pope D, Tang P. Carpal tunnel release and distal radius fractures. Hand Clin 2018;34:27–32.
20. Porter M, Stockley I. Fractures of the distal radius. Intermediate and end results in relation to radiologic parameters. Clin Orthop Relat Res 1987;(220):241–252.
21. Richards RS, Bennett JD, Roth JH, et al. Arthroscopic diagnosis of intra-articular soft tissue injuries associated with distal radial fractures. J Hand Surg Am 1997;22(5):772–776.
22. Rozental TD, Blazar PE, Franko OI, et al. Functional outcomes for unstable distal radial fractures treated with open reduction and internal fixation or closed reduction and percutaneous fixation. A prospective randomized trial. J Bone Joint Surg Am 2009;91(8):1837–1846.
23. Short WH, Palmer AK, Werner FW, et al. A biomechanical study of distal radial fractures. J Hand Surg Am 1987;12(4):529–534.
24. Wright TW, Horodyski M, Smith DW. Functional outcome of unstable distal radius fractures: ORIF with a volar fixed-angle tine plate versus external fixation. J Hand Surg Am 2005;30(2):289–299.
25. Zollinger PE, Tuinebreijer WE, Breederveld RS, et al. Can vitamin C prevent complex regional pain syndrome in patients with wrist fractures? A randomized, controlled, multicenter dose-response study. J Bone Joint Surg Am 2007;89(7):1424–1431.

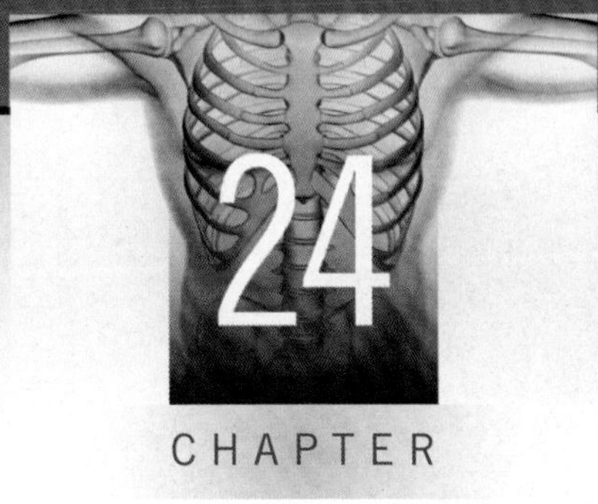

Fragment-Specific Fixation of Distal Radius Fractures

Robert J. Medoff

DEFINITION

- Fragment-specific fixation of complex periarticular fracture patterns follows four basic core principles:
  - Identification of primary fracture components
  - Independent fixation with specific implants for each fracture component
  - Use of semielastic fixation mechanisms, which avoid dependence on thread purchase
  - Creation of a load sharing construct **(FIG 1)**
- Fragment-specific implants are low profile and have a "spring-like" elasticity; this characteristic, combined with independent fixation of multiple fragments in different planes, creates a load sharing construct that restores articular anatomy while avoiding limitations and potential complications caused by ineffective thread purchase in small periarticular fragments **(FIG 2)**.
- Surgical planning is essential to determine whether a single approach or a combination of surgical approaches is needed to visualize and fix each of the main fracture components that make up a particular injury.
  - For distal radius fixation, a complete set of implants should be available to address any of the five primary fracture elements: the radial column, ulnar corner, volar rim, dorsal wall, and/or impacted articular fragments.
  - Identification and treatment of distal radioulnar joint (DRUJ) disruption and injuries of the ulnar column should also be included.
- Fragment-specific fixation avoids creation of large holes in small distal fragments, with fixation based and often triangulated to the stable ipsilateral cortex of the proximal fragment.
- The goal of fragment-specific fixation is creation of a multiplanar, load-sharing construct that restores an anatomic articular surface with sufficient stability to allow motion to be initiated in the early postoperative period.[2,7,11]

ANATOMY

Essential Basic Anatomy

- The palmar cutaneous branch of the median nerve typically lies in the subcutaneous tissue between the flexor carpi radialis (FCR) and palmaris longus tendons; radial-based incisions should *not* extend distally into a carpal tunnel approach in order to avoid injury to this nerve.
- The terminal branches of the lateral antebrachial cutaneous nerve and dorsal sensory branch of the radial nerve run in the subcutaneous tissue radial to the course of the radial artery. Exposure of the radial column by elevating a thick radial skin and subcutaneous flap using blunt dissection from a proximal to distal direction along the surface of the first dorsal compartment tendons helps avoid injury to these structures.
- The pronator quadratus inserts along the ridge at the distal flare of the radius volarly; dissection distally should be limited to no more than 1 to 2 mm distal to the ridge to avoid compromise of the important volar carpal ligaments.
- Because the position of the radial artery deep to the tendons of the first dorsal compartment limits soft tissue exposure to either side, exposure of the volar surface of the radius should be done in a plane ulnar to the radial artery, and exposure of the radial column should be done in a plane radial to the radial artery.

Essential Osseous Anatomy

- Structurally, the wrist can be thought of in terms of three basic support columns: a radial column that includes the radial border of the distal radius and scaphoid facet, a middle column consisting of the central and ulnar part of the radial shaft and lunate facet, and an ulnar column that includes the DRUJ, the triangular fibrocartilage complex (TFCC), and the ulnar head.

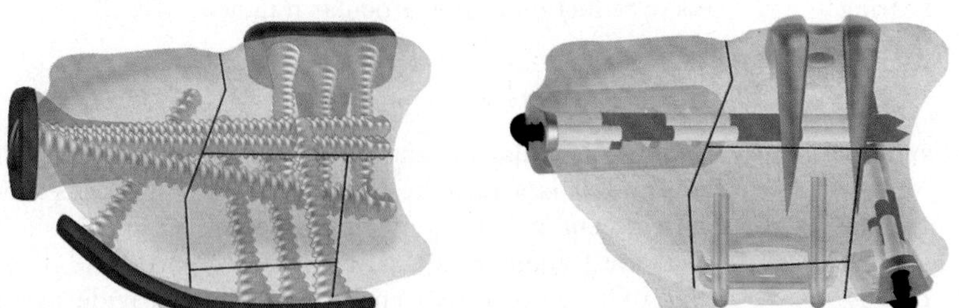

A B

FIG 1 Comparison of standard fixation with multiple plates/screws to fragment-specific fixation. **A.** Plates are applied to multiple surfaces but rely on thread purchase in bone and thicker, more rigid interface for locking screws; fixation is not load sharing. **B.** Fragment-specific implants control the position of each of the major fracture components without the need for thread purchase; implants are semielastic, resulting in interfragmentary compression and creating a load sharing fixation construct.

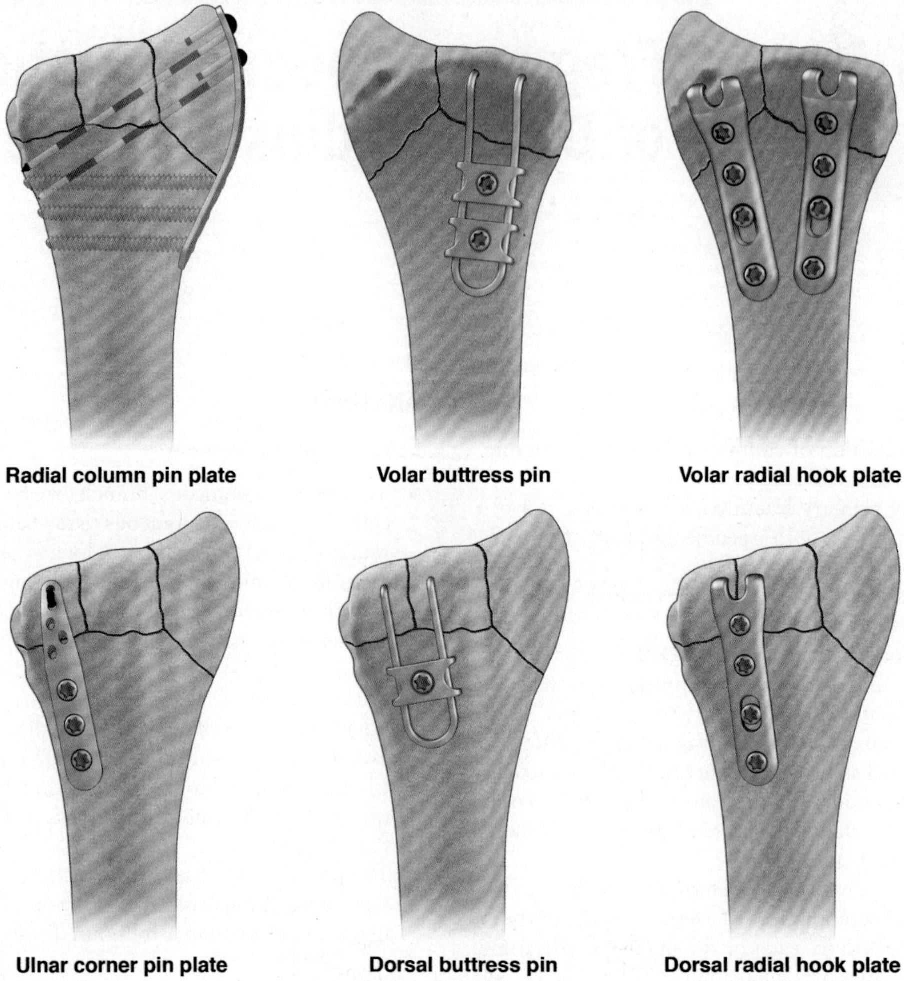

FIG 2 Fragment-specific implants.

- The radial column fragment involves the pillar of bone along the radial border of the distal radius. Restoration of radial length is important to correct the axial position of the carpus, unloading deforming compressive forces that can interfere with reduction of middle column injuries. Typically, the terminal portion of the brachioradialis inserts on the base of the radial column fragment and may be a deforming force that contributes to proximal displacement of the fragment. Metaphyseal comminution along the base of the radial column fragment may also contribute to radial column instability. Although not common, radial column injuries with secondary coronal fracture or segmental comminution into the shaft proximally can be particularly unstable fracture patterns.
- The volar rim of the lunate facet is a primary load-bearing structure of the articular surface. Instability of the volar rim occurs in two patterns:
  - In the volar instability pattern, the volar rim migrates in a proximal and volar direction resulting in secondary palmar translation of the carpus.
  - In the axial instability pattern, axial impaction of the carpus drives the volar rim into dorsiflexion, resulting in secondary axial and dorsal subluxation of the carpus.
- The ulnar corner fragment involves the dorsal half of the sigmoid notch and may include part of the articular surface of either the sigmoid notch and/or lunate facet. This fracture component is the result of impaction of the lunate into the articular surface and may be associated with dorsal and proximal migration of this fragment. Residual displacement of the ulnar corner may result in instability of the DRUJ as well as restriction of forearm rotation.
- Dorsal wall fragmentation is a common finding with either dorsal bending or axial loading injuries. If displaced, this fracture component is often associated with dorsal subluxation of the carpus in addition to the typical dorsal angulation of the articular surface.
- Free articular fragments may be impacted within the metaphyseal cavity and result in incongruity of the articular surface. Elevation of dorsal wall fragments allows direct access to reduction of free articular fragments **(FIG 3)**.

PATHOGENESIS

- Complex articular injuries of the distal radius are not all the same; it is a mistake to expect that a single method of treatment will be uniformly effective. Careful analysis of the fragmentation pattern and the principle directions of fracture displacement can often provide useful information about the mechanism of injury and type of instability.[4]

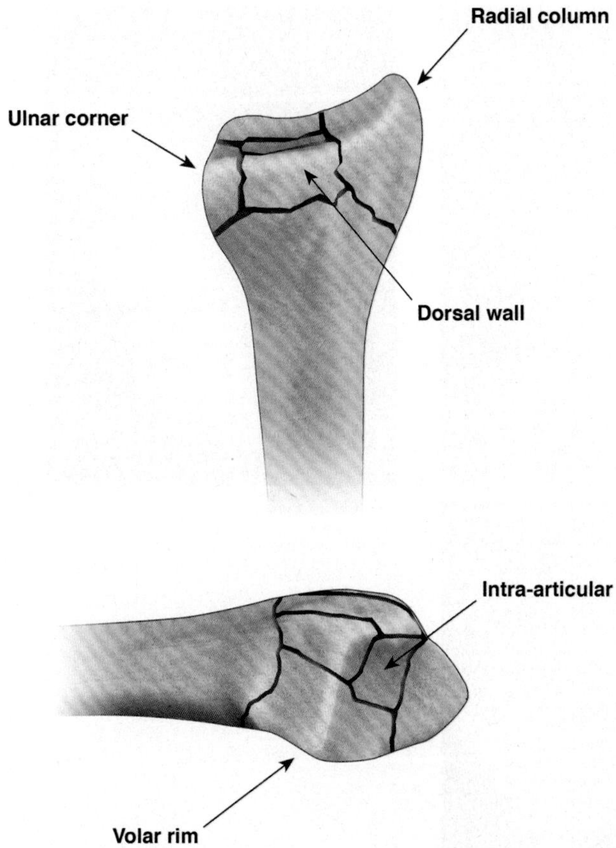

FIG 3 Articular fracture components.

- Dorsal bending injuries result in extra-articular fractures with dorsal displacement **(FIG 4A)**. Comminution of the dorsal wall and compression into metaphyseal cavity can result in dorsal instability.
- Volar bending injuries result in extra-articular fractures with volar displacement **(FIG 4B)**. Fractures with significant volar displacement are nearly always unstable and require some type of intervention to obtain and hold a reduction until union.
- Dorsal shearing injuries present as fractures of the dorsal rim and are often associated with dorsal instability of the carpus **(FIG 4C)**. These injuries often have a depressed articular fragment and may have additional radial column involvement.
- Volar shearing injuries present as displaced fractures of the volar rim and result in volar instability of the carpus **(FIG 4D)**. This pattern often has multiple articular fragments and is highly unstable. It is not usually amenable to closed methods of treatment.
- Radial shearing fractures (chauffeur's fracture) are identified by a characteristic transverse fracture line across the radial styloid that extends into the radiocarpal joint. These injuries often have more extensive chondral disruption than may be appreciated from the radiographic findings **(FIG 4E)**.
- Simple three-part fractures are usually the result of low-energy injuries that combine a dorsal bending mechanism with some axial loading across the carpus **(FIG 4F)**. This pattern is characterized by the presence of an ulnar corner fragment involving the dorsal portion of the sigmoid notch, a main articular fragment, and a proximal shaft fragment.
- Complex articular fractures are usually the result of axial loading injuries from moderate to high-energy trauma. In addition to articular comminution, this pattern may often generate a significant defect in the metaphyseal cavity or complete disruption of the DRUJ **(FIG 4G)**.
- The avulsion/carpal instability pattern is primarily a ligamentous injury of the carpus with associated osseous avulsions of the distal radius. Bone fragments are typically small and very distal **(FIG 4H)**.
- Injuries from a high-energy mechanism present as complex comminuted fractures of the articular surface with extension into the radial/ulnar shaft **(FIG 4I)**.

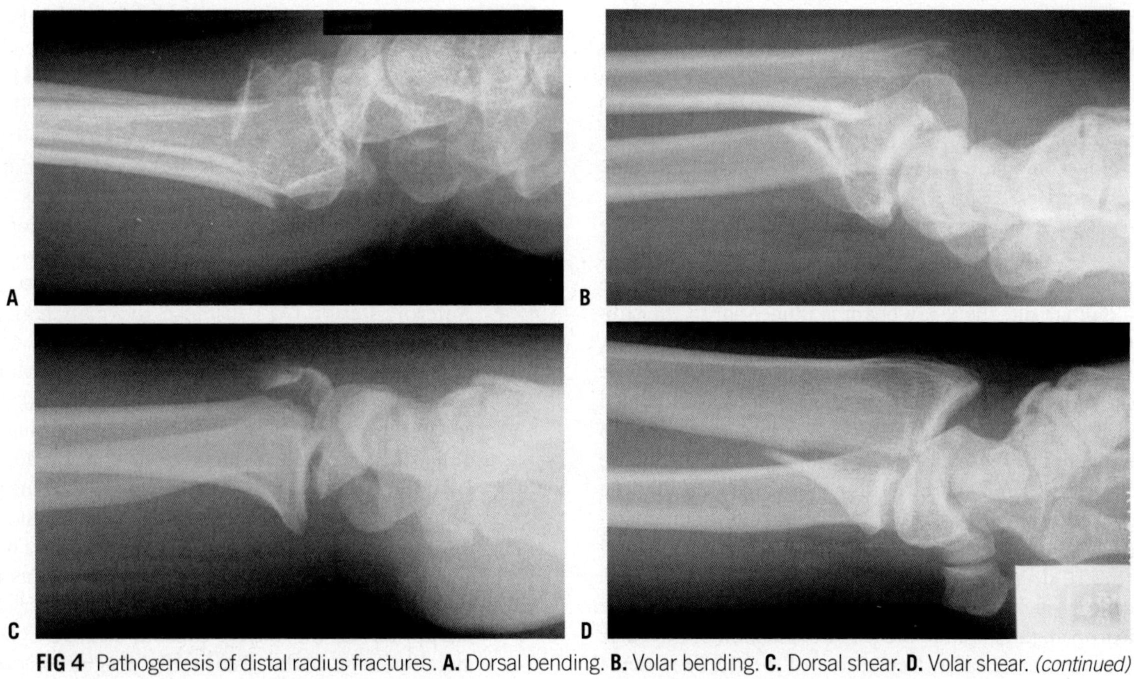

FIG 4 Pathogenesis of distal radius fractures. **A.** Dorsal bending. **B.** Volar bending. **C.** Dorsal shear. **D.** Volar shear. *(continued)*

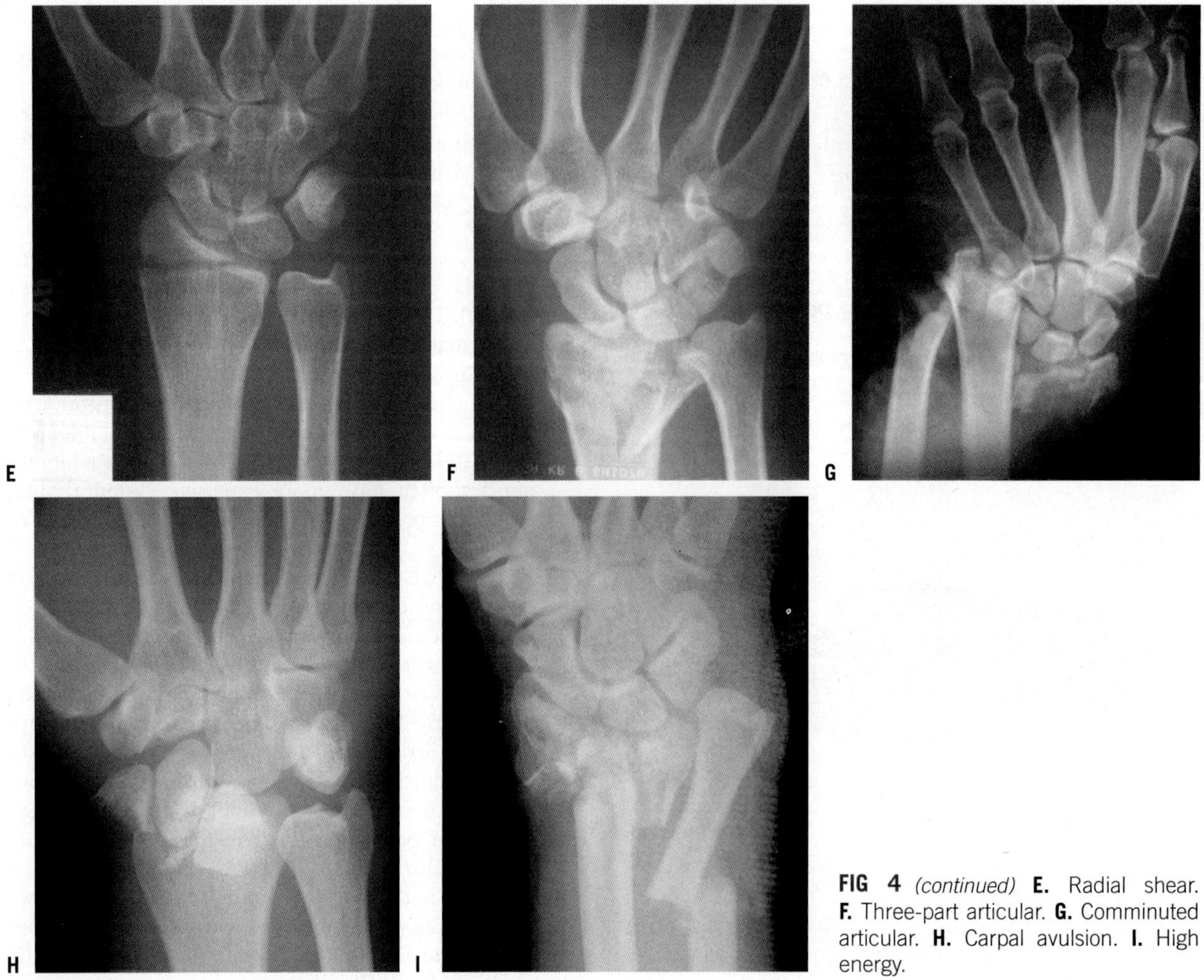

FIG 4 *(continued)* **E.** Radial shear. **F.** Three-part articular. **G.** Comminuted articular. **H.** Carpal avulsion. **I.** High energy.

IMAGING AND OTHER DIAGNOSTIC STUDIES

- Posteroanterior (PA), standard lateral **(FIG 5A,B)**, and 10-degree lateral views are routine views for radiographic evaluation of the distal radius. The 10-degree lateral view **(FIG 5C,D)** clearly visualizes the ulnar two-thirds of the articular surface from the base of the scaphoid facet through the entire lunate facet. Oblique views may also be helpful for evaluating the injury.
- The radiographic features of distal radius fractures include the following[8]:
  - Carpal facet horizon **(FIG 6A,B)**. This is the radiodense horizontal landmark that is used to identify the volar and dorsal rim on the PA view. If the articular surface has palmar tilt, the x-ray beam is tangential to the subchondral bone of the volar portion of the lunate facet, with the result that the carpal facet horizon identifies the volar rim. However, if the articular surface has displaced into dorsal tilt, the x-ray beam becomes tangential to the subchondral bone of the dorsal portion of the lunate facet instead, and the carpal facet horizon identifies the dorsal rim (not shown). The carpal facet horizon corresponds to the portion of the articular surface visualized on the 10-degree lateral x-ray projection.
  - Teardrop angle (normal 70 ± 5 degrees; **FIG 6C,D**). The teardrop angle is used to identify dorsiflexion of the volar rim of the lunate facet. Depression of the teardrop angle to a value less than 45 degrees indicates that the volar rim of the lunate facet has rotated dorsally and impacted into the metaphyseal cavity (axial instability pattern of the volar rim). This may be associated with axial and dorsal subluxation of the carpus. Restoration of the teardrop angle is necessary to correct this type of malreduction.
  - Congruency of the articular surface **(FIG 6E,F)**. The subchondral outline of the articular surface of the distal radius is normally both congruent and concentric with the subchondral outline of the base of the lunate; a uniform joint interval should be present between the radius and lunate along the entire articular surface. When the joint interval between these articular surfaces is not uniform, discontinuity and disruption of the lunate facet has occurred.
  - Anteroposterior (AP) distance (normal: females 18 ± 1 mm, males 20 ± 1 mm; **FIG 6G**). The AP distance is the point-to-point distance from the dorsal to palmar rim of the lunate facet. It is best evaluated on the 10-degree lateral view. Widening of the AP distance implies discontinuity of the volar and dorsal portion of the lunate facet.
  - DRUJ interval **(FIG 6H)**. The DRUJ interval measures the degree of apposition between the head of the ulna and the sigmoid notch (normal: 2 mm or less). This parameter is best measured with the forearm in neutral rotation. Significant widening of the DRUJ interval implies disruption of the DRUJ capsule and TFCC. Coronal malalignment of the distal radial fragment is often suggested by widening of the DRUJ interval.

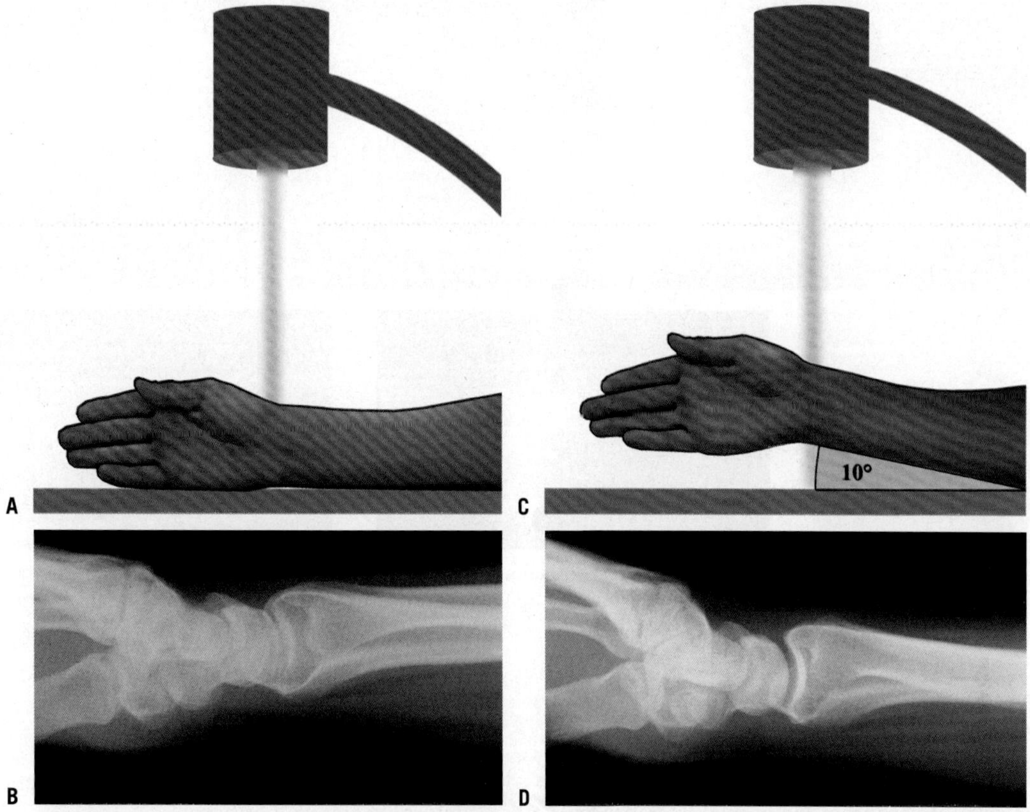

FIG 5 A. Positioning for standard lateral radiography. **B.** Standard lateral radiograph. **C.** Positioning for 10-degree lateral radiography. **D.** Ten-degree lateral radiograph. Note the improved visualization of the articular surface of the base of the scaphoid facet and the entire lunate facet.

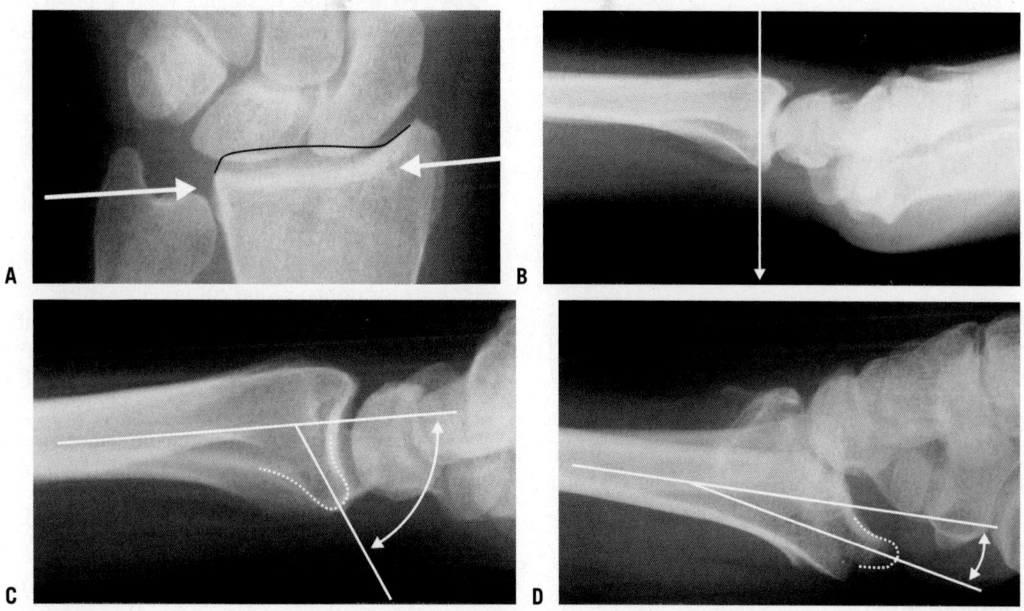

FIG 6 A. Carpal facet horizon (*arrows*). Used to differentiate between the volar and dorsal rim on the PA projection. **B.** Origin of carpal facet horizon. The carpal facet horizon is formed by that part of the articular surface that is parallel to the x-ray beam and depends on whether the articular surface is in volar or dorsal tilt. **C.** Normal teardrop angle. **D.** Depressed teardrop angle in this case is caused by axial instability of the volar rim. *(continued)*

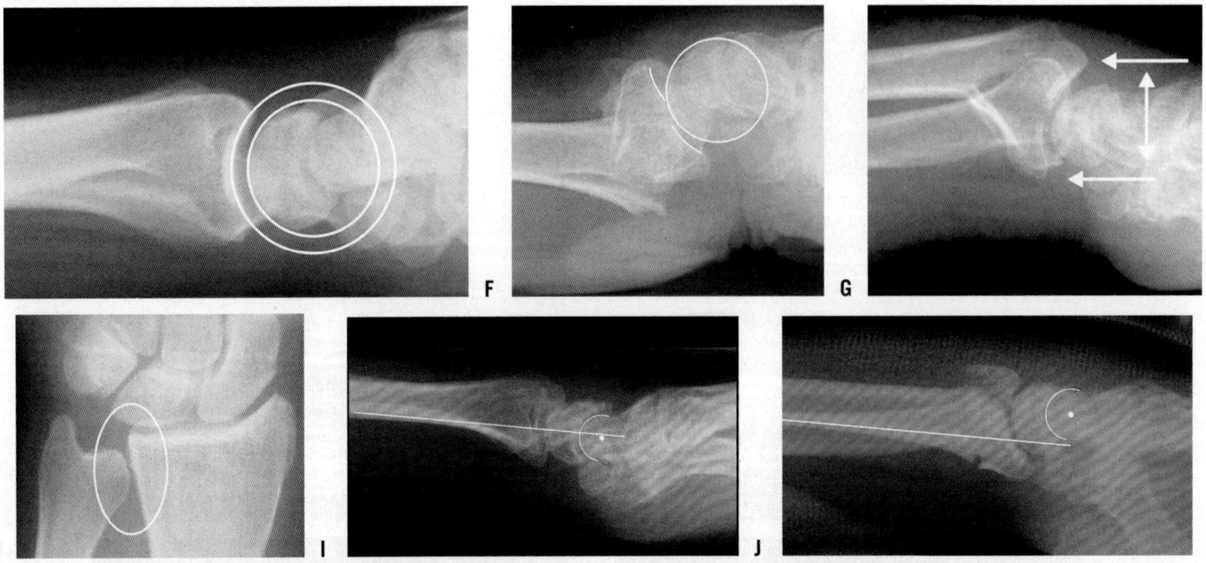

E F G H I J

FIG 6 *(continued)* **E.** Normal articular congruency. **F.** Abnormal articular congruency, indicating disruption across the volar and dorsal surfaces of the lunate facet. **G.** AP interval is the point-to-point distance between the corners of the dorsal and volar rim. **H.** DRUJ interval. **I.** Normal lateral carpal alignment. **J.** Dorsal subluxation of the carpus.

- Lateral carpal alignment **(FIG 6I,J)**. On the 10-degree lateral view and with the wrist in neutral position, the rotational center of the capitate normally aligns with a line extended from the volar surface of the radial shaft. Significant displacement from the normal lateral carpal alignment can adversely affect grip strength by placing the tendons at a mechanical disadvantage as well as disrupting normal carpal kinematics. Dorsal rotation of the volar rim results in a dorsal shift of lateral carpal alignment as the carpus subluxes dorsally. Palmar rotation or displacement of the articular surface such as observed with volar bending injuries and shear fractures results in palmar shift of lateral carpal alignment.
- In addition to injury films, reassessing radiographs after reduction can be very helpful in determining the personality and specific components of a particular fracture.
- Computed tomography (CT) scans allow higher resolution and definition of fracture characteristics, particularly for highly comminuted fractures. Preferably, an attempt at closed reduction before obtaining a CT scan will help limit distortion of the image. CT scans are particularly helpful for visualizing intra-articular fragments as well as DRUJ disruption and incongruity of the sigmoid notch.
- Clinical evaluation of the carpus, interosseous membrane, and elbow, combined with radiographic studies when needed, should be included to identify the presence of other injuries that may affect the decision for a particular treatment approach.

SURGICAL MANAGEMENT

Operative Indications

- General parameters
  - Shortening of more than 5 mm
  - Radial inclination of less than 15 degrees
  - Dorsal angulation of more than 10 degrees
  - Articular step-off of more than 1 to 2 mm
  - Depression of teardrop angle to less than 45 degrees
  - Volar instability
  - DRUJ instability
  - Displaced articular fractures
  - Young, active patients are generally less tolerant of residual deformity and malposition.

Preoperative Planning

- Extra-articular fractures: multiple options
  - Volar plating through a volar approach
  - Dorsal plating through a dorsal approach
  - Fragment-specific fixation
    - Radial pin plate (TriMed, Inc., Valencia, CA) and volar buttress pin (TriMed, Inc.) fixation through a limited incision volar or standard volar approach
    - Radial pin plate and either an ulnar pin plate dorsally or a dorsal buttress pin through a dorsal or combined approach
    - Fixed-angle radial column plate using either a volar or dorsal radial column exposure
    - Volar hook plates with or without radial column plate using a volar approach
- Intra-articular fractures: Surgical approach is based on the fragmentation pattern.
  - Unstable volar rim fragments require a standard volar or occasionally an ulnar-based volar approach for adequate visualization.
  - Fixation of the radial column can be done either through a limited-incision volar radial approach (Henry), a volar approach with radial extension combined with pronation of the forearm, or a dorsal approach with radial extension combined with supination of the forearm.
  - Fixation of dorsal, ulnar corner, and free intra-articular fragments can be done through a dorsal approach.

Positioning

- The patient is supine.
- The affected arm is placed on an arm board out to the side.

- C-arm
  - If the arm board is radiolucent, the C-arm can be brought in from the end of the arm board and images taken directly with the wrist on the arm board.
  - If the arm board is not radiolucent, the C-arm is brought in along the side of the table from the foot, and the arm is brought off the arm board for each image.

Operative Sequence

- Initial restoration of radial column length with traction and provisional trans-styloid pin fixation can be helpful to hold the carpus out to length and unload the lunate facet.
- The volar rim is anatomically reduced to restore length and a normal teardrop angle and fixed. For complex injuries, this is often the keystone for building stable fixation.
- The ulnar corner dorsally is reduced, taking care to restore the anatomy of both the sigmoid notch and radiocarpal joint as well as fully correct lateral carpal alignment; it is then secured with an appropriate implant.
- Free intra-articular fragments and the dorsal wall fragments are reduced and stabilized as necessary to restore a congruent joint surface, correct the AP interval, and correct lateral carpal alignment.
- Bone graft is applied if the metaphyseal defect is large.
- Fixation is completed with a radial column plate. Rigid fixation of the radial column is performed last to ensure the radial column fixation does to prevent anatomic reduction of the lunate facet fragments.
- Depending on the nature of the fracture, fixation may be a subset of these steps.
- If adequate stability is not obtained, fixation is supplemented with additional protection such as a spanning bridge plate.
- Fragment-specific fixation techniques may be used to supplement other types of fixation, such as a volar plate.

Approach

- The repair is undertaken by means of one of the following approaches:
  - Limited-incision volar approach (distal limb of Henry approach)
  - Dorsal approach
  - Extensile volar approach (FCR approach)
  - Volar ulnar approach

TECHNIQUES

LIMITED-INCISION (HENRY) VOLAR APPROACH

- A limited incision using the distal segment of a Henry volar approach allows wide exposure of the radial column, but only provides limited exposure of the volar surface.
- Make a longitudinal incision along the radial side of the radial artery.
- Proximally, insert the tip of a tenotomy scissors superficial to the surface of the first dorsal compartment sheath and sweep distally to elevate a radial skin flap.
- Pronate the forearm and sharply expose the bare area of bone over the radial styloid situated in the interval between the first and second dorsal compartments **(TECH FIG 1A)**.
- Leaving the distal 1 cm of sheath intact, open the first dorsal compartment proximally and mobilize the tendons. Reflect the insertion of brachioradialis to complete exposure of the radial column **(TECH FIG 1B)**.
- If needed, the dissection can be continued through the floor of the incision to expose the volar surface. Detach the insertion of the pronator quadratus radially and distally and reflect to the ulnar side. Alternatively, create an ulnar skin flap superficial to the artery and continue the exposure through a standard volar approach.
- Exposure of the ulnar side of the volar rim may be difficult with this approach, particularly with large patients or in the presence of significant swelling.

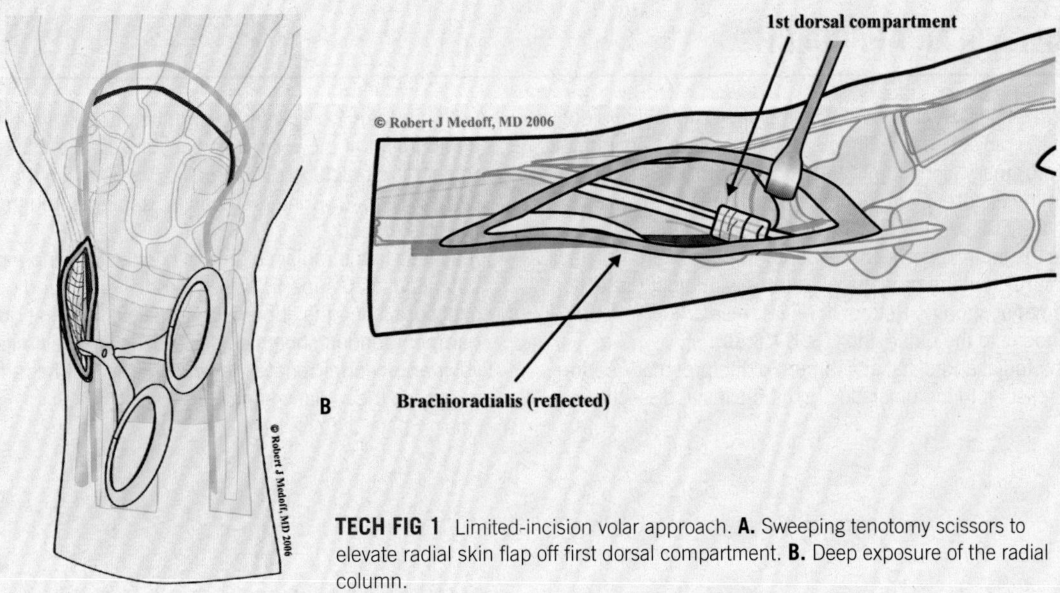

A B

TECH FIG 1 Limited-incision volar approach. **A.** Sweeping tenotomy scissors to elevate radial skin flap off first dorsal compartment. **B.** Deep exposure of the radial column.

DORSAL APPROACH

- Make a longitudinal skin incision dorsally along the ulnar side of the tubercle of Lister **(TECH FIG 2A)**.
- Identify the extensor digitorum communis tendons visible proximally through the translucent extensor sheath. Incise the dorsal retinacular sheath.
- Develop the interval between the third and fourth compartment tendons for access to dorsal wall and free, impacted articular fragments. Resect a segment of the terminal branch of the posterior interosseous nerve **(TECH FIG 2B)**.
- Transpose the extensor pollicis longus from the tubercle of Lister if required for additional exposure.
- Develop the interval between the fourth and fifth extensor compartments to gain access to the ulnar corner fragment.
- A dorsal capsulotomy can be done by incising the capsule from the scaphoid facet to the center of origin of the dorsal radiocarpal ligament as needed to visualize the articular surface and carpus.
- The radial column can be accessed through a dorsal exposure by extending the incision and elevating a radial subcutaneous flap. Supinate the forearm to visualize the radial column and release the proximal sheath of the first dorsal compartment.
- To gain access to the distal ulna, extend the incision as needed and elevate an ulnar subcutaneous flap.

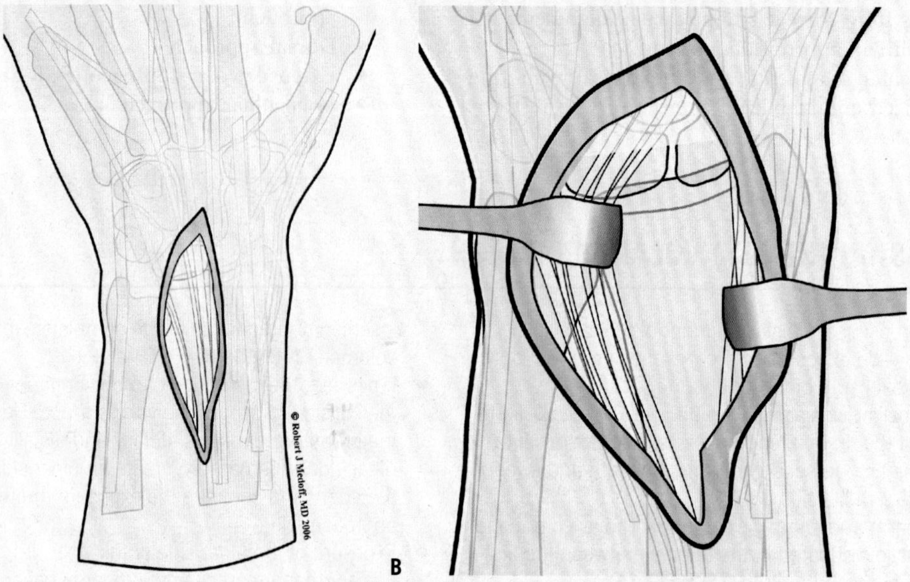

TECH FIG 2 Dorsal approach. **A.** Initial incision. **B.** Deep exposure.

EXTENSILE VOLAR APPROACH

- Start the skin incision at the distal pole of the scaphoid and angle it toward the radial border of the flexor wrist crease. Continue the incision proximally along the FCR tendon **(TECH FIG 3A)**.
- Continue the exposure with deeper dissection in the plane between the FCR tendon and the radial artery.
- Separate the interval between the contents of the carpal tunnel and the surface of the pronator quadratus with blunt dissection with a finger or sponge. Retract the FCR, median nerve, and flexor tendons to the ulnar side **(TECH FIG 3B)**.
- Divide the radial and distal attachment of the pronator quadratus and reflect it to the ulnar side. Limit the distal dissection to no more than 1 or 2 mm beyond the distal radial ridge to avoid detachment of the volar wrist capsular ligaments **(TECH FIG 3C)**.
- Reflect the brachioradialis from its insertion on the distal fragment if needed. Bone graft can be applied through the radial fracture defect.
- If access to the radial column is needed, elevate a radial subcutaneous flap superficial to the radial artery and continue the exposure along the superficial surface of the first dorsal compartment tendon sheath as described with the limited incision volar approach. Pronate the wrist, retracting the radial skin flap to expose the radial column.

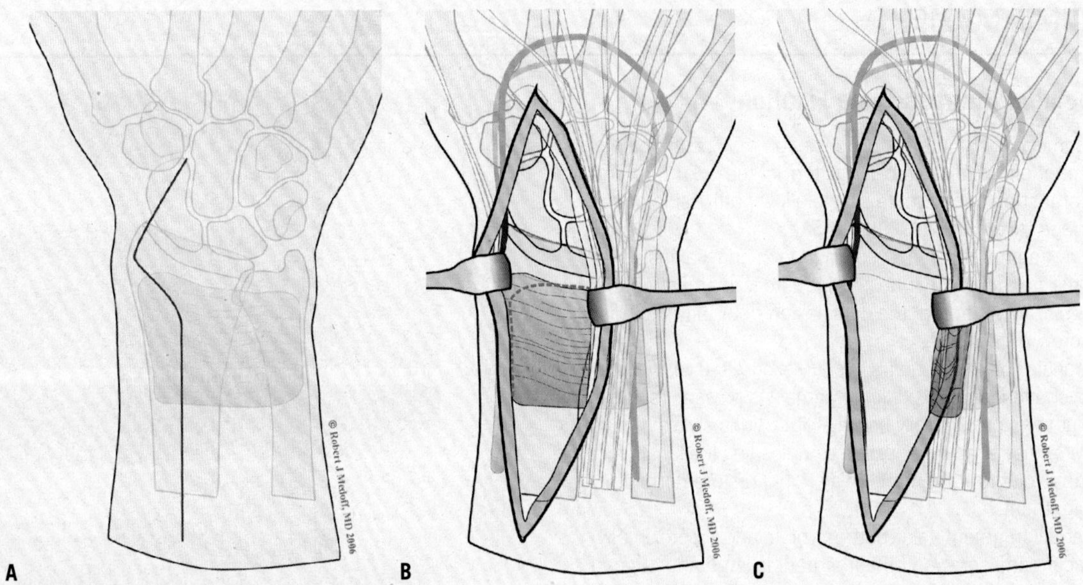

TECH FIG 3 Extensile volar approach. **A.** Initial incision. **B.** Line of incision in pronator quadratus. **C.** Deep exposure.

VOLAR ULNAR APPROACH

- Make a longitudinal skin incision along the radial border of the flexor carpi ulnaris (FCU) tendon **(TECH FIG 4A)**.
- Reflect the FCU tendon and the ulnar artery and nerve to the ulnar side **(TECH FIG 4B)**.
- With blunt finger or sponge dissection, develop the plane along the superficial surface of the pronator quadratus.
- Retract the contents of the carpal tunnel to the radial side **(TECH FIG 4C)**.
- Reflect the pronator quadratus from its ulnar and distal attachment. Do not dissect more than 1 to 2 mm beyond the distal radial ridge to avoid detachment of the volar wrist capsule.

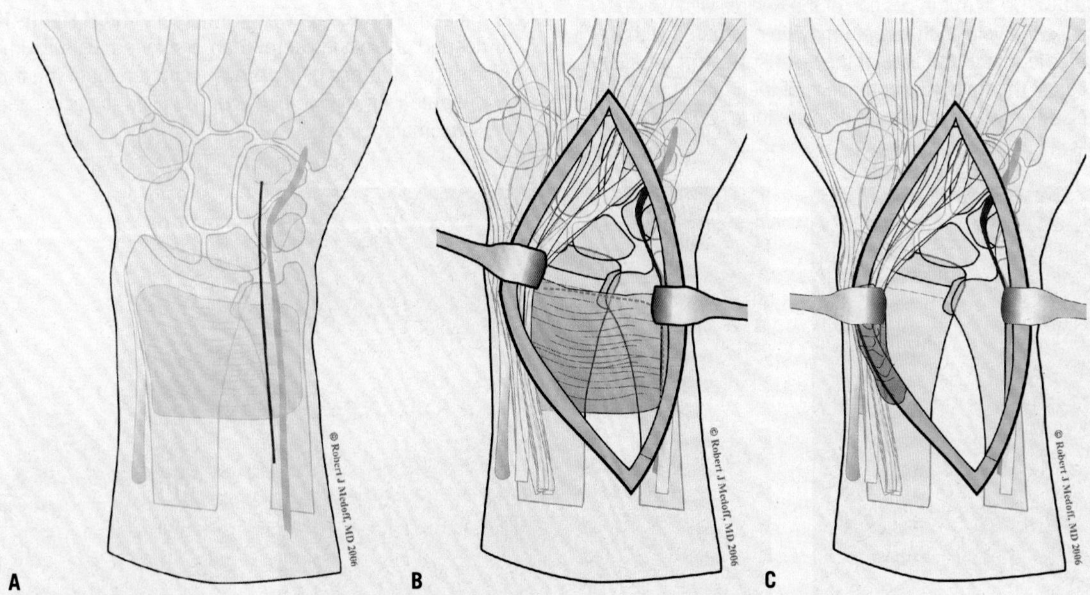

TECH FIG 4 Volar ulnar approach. **A.** Incision. **B.** Initial exposure. **C.** Completed exposure.

VOLAR RIM FRAGMENT

Small Fragment Buttress Plate Fixation

- Small fragment volar buttress plate fixation may be indicated for treatment of a volar instability pattern of the volar rim. The fragment must be of adequate size to allow buttressing on the volar surface by the plate **(TECH FIG 5A)**.
- If volar rim fragmentation is associated with an axial instability pattern, the fragment must be of adequate size and strength to allow angular correction of the dorsiflexion deformity with distal locked screw purchase.
- An appropriate volar approach is used to expose the volar rim fragment. If a shortened radial column fragment is present, restoring radial length and provisionally holding with a trans-styloid Kirschner wire (K-wire) may simplify reduction by unloading the lunate facet.
- Reduce the volar rim fragment; this should restore normal carpal alignment.
- Apply a small fragment volar buttress plate and fix proximally with cortical bone screws. If the fragment is large and of good quality, standard or locking bone screws distally may be added **(TECH FIG 5B)**.

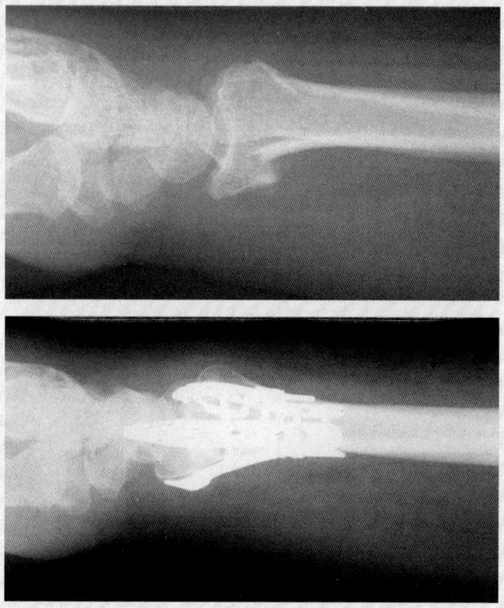

A B

TECH FIG 5 Volar rim fixation with small fragment plate. **A.** Shear fracture of volar rim with volar instability pattern. **B.** Fixation with small fragment plate.

Volar Buttress Pin Fixation

- Volar buttress pin fixation is indicated for unstable volar rim fragments and can be a particularly effective technique when faced with small distal fragments or axial instability patterns of the volar rim (depressed teardrop angle; **TECH FIG 6A,B**).
- Use an appropriate volar approach to expose the volar rim fragment. If necessary, restore radial length and provisionally hold it with a trans-styloid K-wire to unload the lunate facet.
- Continue exposure for up to 1 to 2 mm beyond the distal radial ridge. Reduce the volar rim fragment as much as possible and note the orientation of the teardrop on the 10-degree lateral view.
- Insert two 0.045-inch K-wires transverse to one another starting at an entry site 1 to 2 mm beyond the distal radial ridge. They should be placed within the center of the teardrop on the lateral view **(TECH FIG 6C)**. Confirm the position of the K-wires with C-arm.
- If necessary, the volar buttress pin may be contoured with a wire bender to match the flare of the volar surface of the distal radius. Adjust the trajectory of the legs of the implant to make a 70-degree angle with the base of the wire form. Cut the legs to appropriate length, leaving the ulnar leg 2 to 3 mm longer than the radial leg **(TECH FIG 6D)**.
- While controlling exposure of the entry site by using a forceps to prevent soft tissue from obstructing the hole, place the longer leg of the buttress pin adjacent to the entry site of the ulnar K-wire, remove the ulnar K-wire, and immediately engage the longer leg of the volar buttress pin into the hole. Repeat the procedure with the radial leg. Impact and seat the implant into the volar rim fragment. Apply to the proximal shaft fragment to correct any dorsiflexion of the volar rim **(TECH FIG 6E)**.
- Fine-tune the reduction and fix the implant proximally with a minimum of two screws and washers **(TECH FIG 6F–H)**. If needed, a blocking screw can be placed just proximal to the end of the buttress pin to prevent shortening of the fragment.
  - Alternatively, a wire plate can be used to secure the implant proximally.

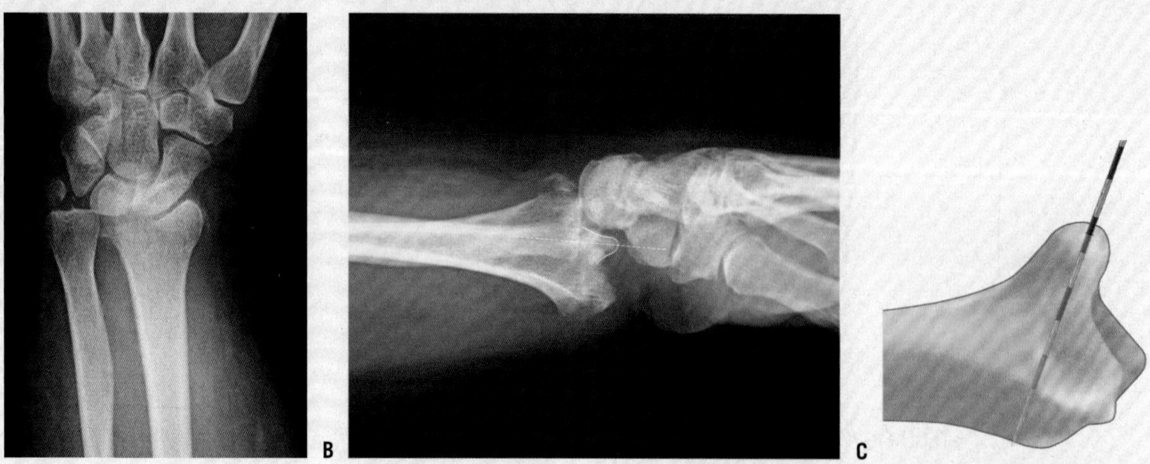

A B C

TECH FIG 6 Volar rim fixation with a volar buttress pin. **A,B.** Articular fracture with axial instability pattern of volar rim. **C.** Insertion of K-wires. *(continued)*

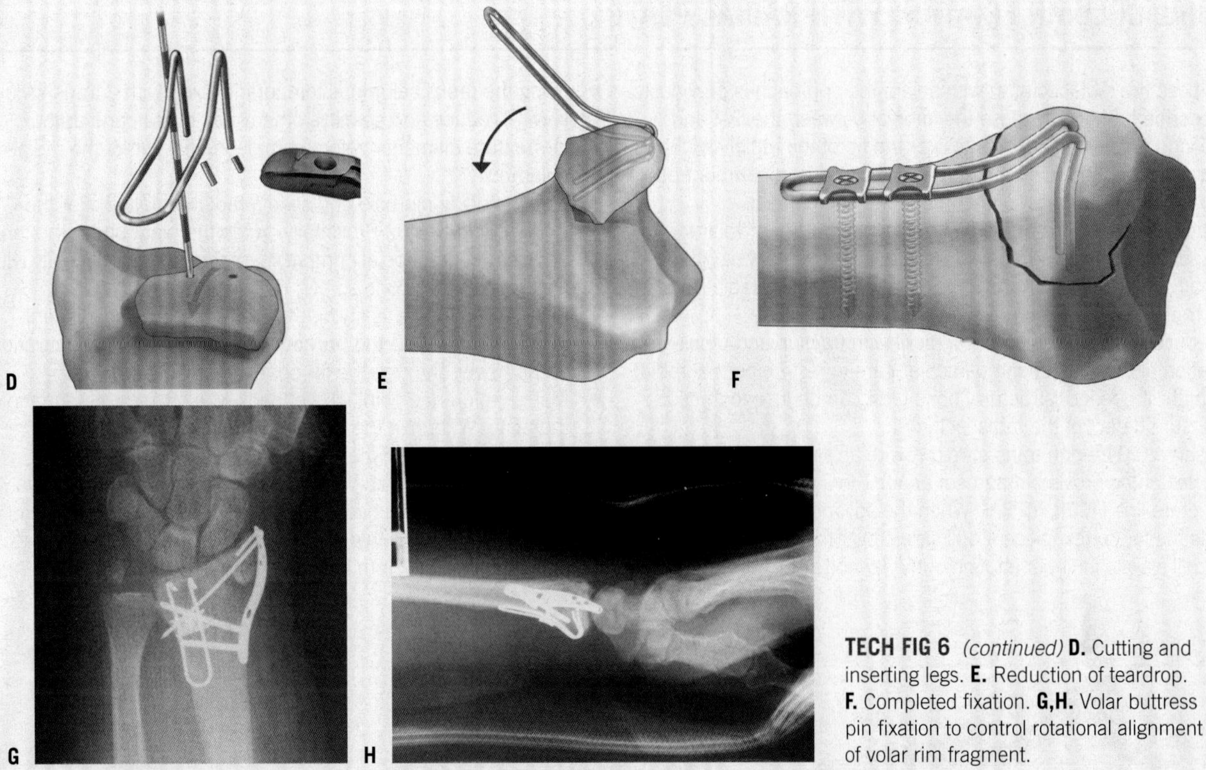

TECH FIG 6 *(continued)* **D.** Cutting and inserting legs. **E.** Reduction of teardrop. **F.** Completed fixation. **G,H.** Volar buttress pin fixation to control rotational alignment of volar rim fragment.

Volar Hook Plate Fixation

- Volar hook plates are useful alternative to volar buttress pins for fixation of unstable volar rim fragments, particularly for small distal fragments associated with axial instability patterns of the volar rim or volar instability patterns associated with volar shear fractures.
- Expose and reduce the volar rim fragment according to the technique described for the volar buttress pin. If possible, provisionally hold the reduction with a K-wire in the radial and ulnar border.
- Contour the plate if needed to match the morphology of the bone. Orientation of the hooks at an angle of 70 degrees to the long axis of the plate is typical to help restore the normal teardrop angle.
- Position and insert a 0.045-inch K-wire distally down the center of the teardrop along the intended path of the hooks of the plate. Confirm the position with the C-arm.
- Place a volar hook plate drill guide over the guidewire and predrill the cortex for insertion of the hooks.
- Insert the volar hook plate over the guide pin and seat into the distal fragment **(TECH FIG 7)**. Place a distal locking peg of appropriate length after predrilling with a fixed-angle peg guide. Fix the plate proximally with standard bone screws.

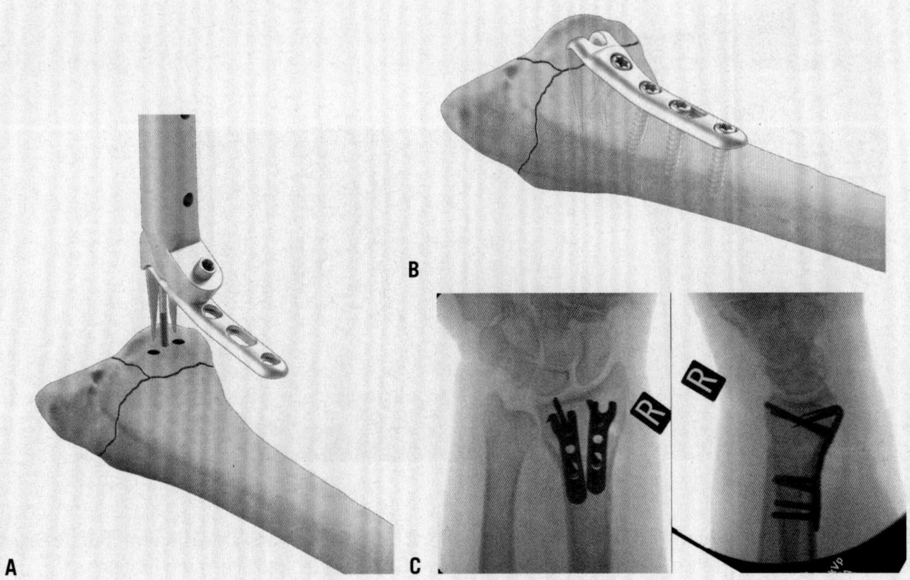

TECH FIG 7 Volar rim fixation with a volar hook plate. **A.** Insertion of volar hook plate over guide pin through predrilled holes. **B.** Completed fixation. **C.** Final intraoperative x-ray showing placement of two volar hook plates into separate distal rim fragments.

RADIAL COLUMN FIXATION WITH RADIAL PLATE

- Expose the radial column with any of the approaches previously described. Sharply expose the interval between the first and second dorsal compartments over the tip of the radial styloid. Release the tendon sheath of the first dorsal compartment proximally, leaving the last 1 cm of tendon sheath intact.
- Retract the tendons of the first dorsal compartment volar for exposure distally and dorsal for exposure proximally along the shaft. Release the terminal insertion of the brachioradialis to complete wide exposure of the radial column.
- Reduce the radial column fragment with traction and ulnar deviation of the wrist taking particular care to restore normal radial length. If needed, structural bone graft can be inserted into the fracture defect of the radial column.
- Insert a 0.045-inch trans-styloid K-wire angled to engage the far cortex of the proximal fragment about 1 to 2 cm proximal to the fracture line **(TECH FIG 8A)**. When the advancing tip of the K-wire hits the far cortex, place a drill sleeve over the K-wire and use as a drill stop to limit penetration of the far cortex to 1 to 2 mm.
- Once the radial column is temporarily fixed with a trans-styloid K-wire, reduce and stabilize other volar, dorsal, and articular fracture elements before completing fixation of the radial column.
- Select a distal pin hole and slide a radial pin plate over the trans-styloid K-wire. Proximally, guide the plate under the tendons of the first dorsal compartment and secure it initially with a single 2.3-mm bone screw.
- Insert a second trans-styloid K-wire through a nonadjacent distal pin hole. Use the previous technique to limit penetration of the K-wire through the far cortex to 1 to 2 mm.
- Mark a reference point where the K-wire crosses the surface of the plate. Withdraw the K-wire 1 cm and cut it 1 cm or more above the reference mark **(TECH FIG 8B)**.
- Position the reference mark between the lower two posts of a wire bender and create a hook **(TECH FIG 8C)**. By starting the bend at the reference mark, this ensures that a K-wire of proper length that extends 1 to 2 mm beyond the far cortex is created.

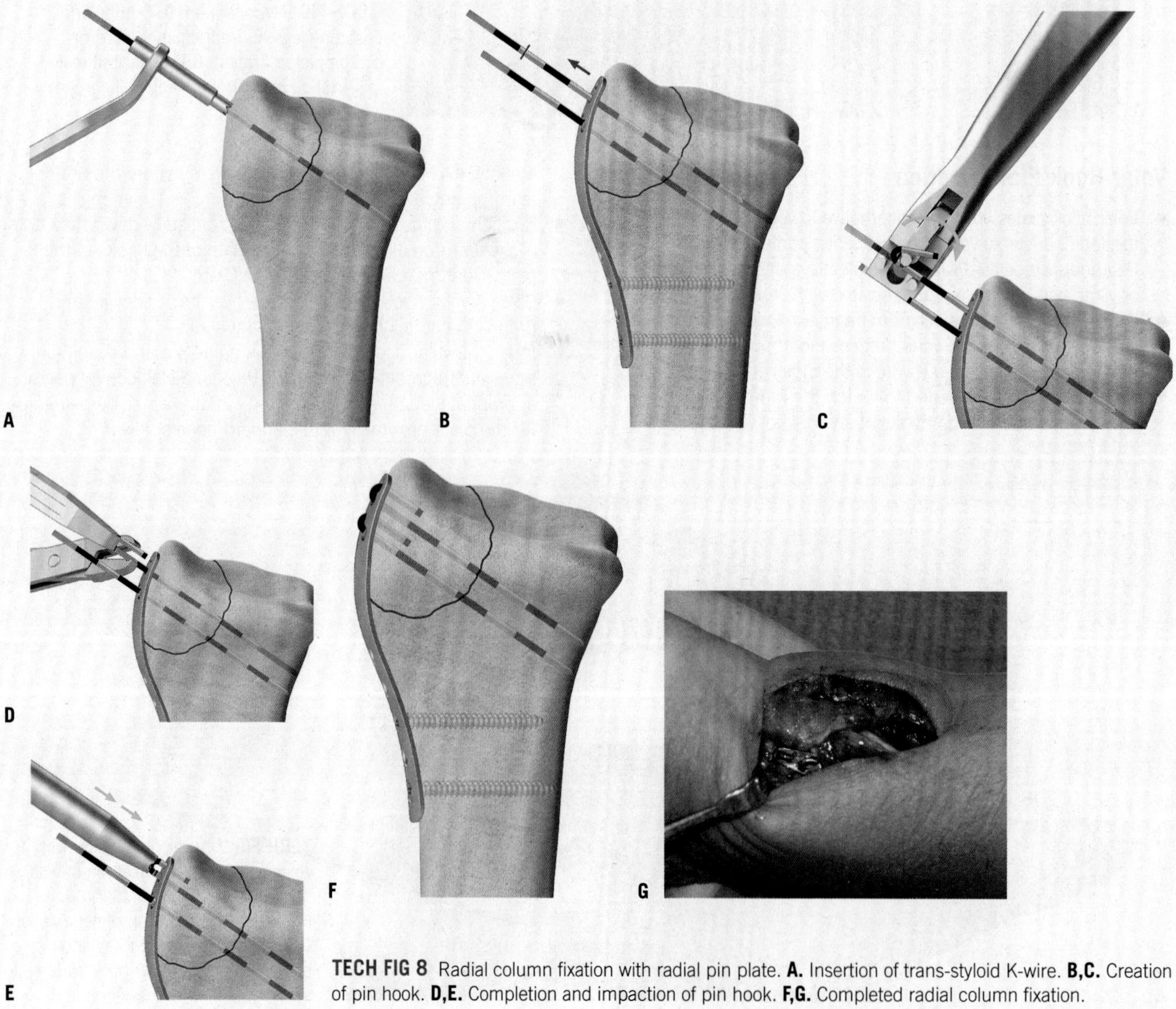

TECH FIG 8 Radial column fixation with radial pin plate. **A.** Insertion of trans-styloid K-wire. **B,C.** Creation of pin hook. **D,E.** Completion and impaction of pin hook. **F,G.** Completed radial column fixation.

- Complete the bend with a pin clamp, overbending slightly to allow the hook to snap into an adjacent pin hole or over the edge of the plate **(TECH FIG 8D)**. With a free 0.045-inch K-wire, predrill a hole to accept the end of the hook.
- Impact the K-wire with a pin impactor and fully seat the hook **(TECH FIG 8E)**. Repeat the procedure with the second K-wire.
- Complete proximal fixation with 2.3-mm cortical bone screws **(TECH FIG 8F,G)**.

RADIAL COLUMN FIXATION WITH FIXED-ANGLE RADIAL COLUMN PLATE

- Although small fixed-angle plates are not technically considered fragment-specific implants, they can be useful as adjunctive fixation particularly if additional resistance to axial settling is needed. In this context, a hybrid of fragment-specific fixation and fixed-angle devices is used.
- Expose and reduce the radial column with the technique described previously.
- Position the fixed-angle radial column plate and temporarily fix with a K-wire both proximally and distally **(TECH FIG 9A)**. Confirm reduction of the radial column and plate position with the C-arm.
- Using fixed-angle drill guides, drill, measure, and insert locking fixation pegs of appropriate length into the distal fixed-angle holes in the plate and standard bone screws proximally into the shaft **(TECH FIG 9B–E)**.

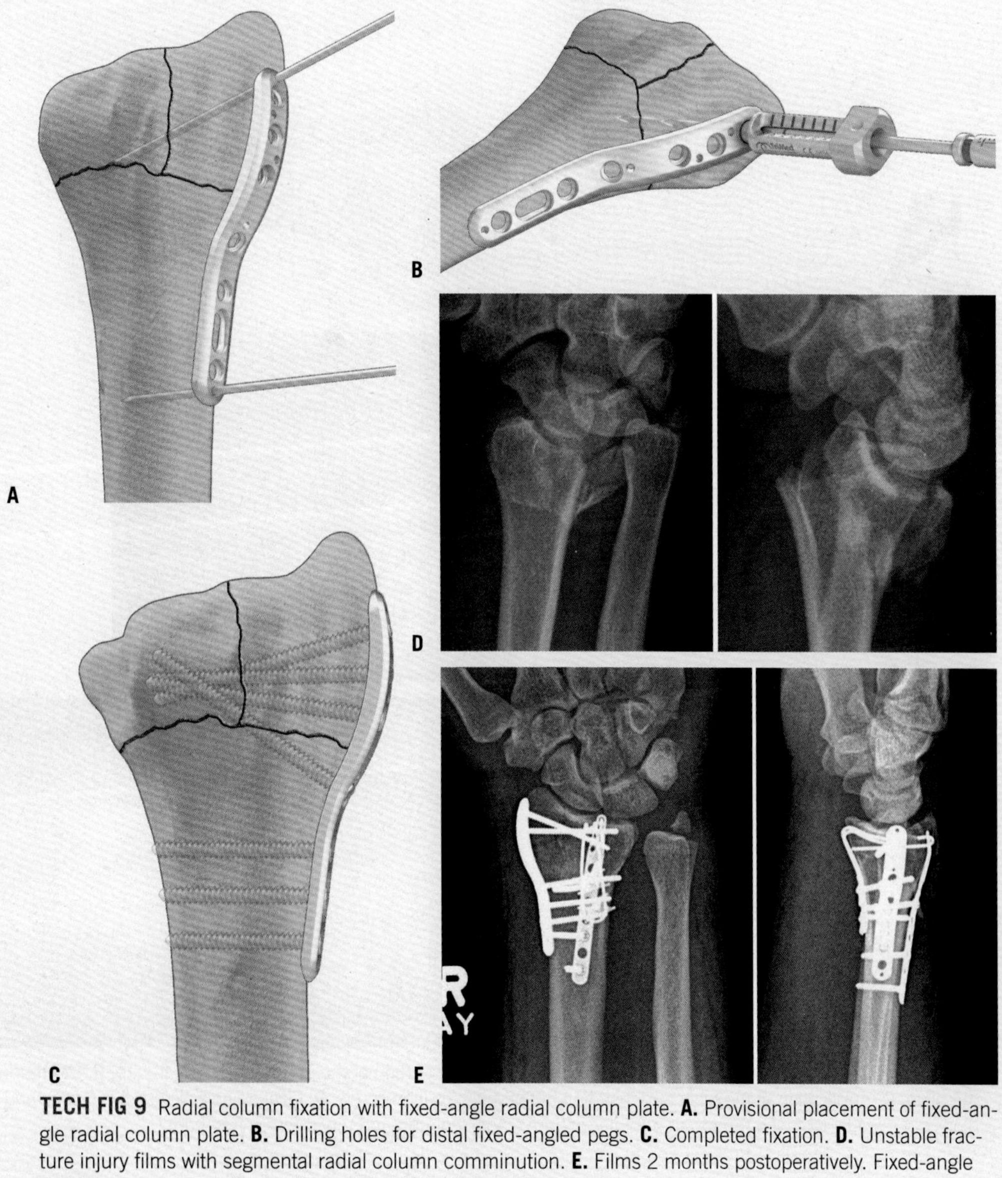

TECH FIG 9 Radial column fixation with fixed-angle radial column plate. **A.** Provisional placement of fixed-angle radial column plate. **B.** Drilling holes for distal fixed-angled pegs. **C.** Completed fixation. **D.** Unstable fracture injury films with segmental radial column comminution. **E.** Films 2 months postoperatively. Fixed-angle radial column support is used to avoid radial column shortening.

ULNAR CORNER AND DORSAL WALL FIXATION

Ulnar Pin Plate

- Through a dorsal approach, expose and reduce the dorsal ulnar corner fragment, dorsal wall fragment, or both.
- Insert a 0.045-inch K-wire through the fragment **(TECH FIG 10A)**, angled proximally and slightly radially to purchase the far cortex of the proximal fragment.
- Insert structural bone graft into the metaphyseal defect as needed to support the subarticular surface.
- If alignment of the plate along the ulnar border of the shaft is desired, add a 15-degree torsional bend to the plate (twist the proximal end of the plate into slight supination) to avoid supination of the distal end of the plate as the bone screws are secured. Often, contouring the plate with slight extension at the distal end produces a better fit **(TECH FIG 10B)**.
- Slide the plate over the K-wire and fix it proximally with a 2.3-mm bone screw **(TECH FIG 10C)**.
- Insert a second K-wire if the fragment is large enough. Create and impact hooks as described for the radial pin plate **(TECH FIG 10D–F)**.
- If the K-wire tips protrude beyond the volar cortex, they can be cut flush to the bone surface through a volar incision.

Dorsal Buttress Pin

- Through a dorsal approach, expose and reduce the dorsal ulnar corner fragment, dorsal wall fragment, or both.
- Insert structural bone graft into the metaphyseal defect if present to support the subarticular surface.
- Insert two 0.045-inch K-wires through the dorsal cortex and behind the subchondral bone; check the position with the C-arm **(TECH FIG 11A)**.
  - The K-wires should be separated by about 1 cm and should be transverse to the longitudinal axis of the shaft; on the

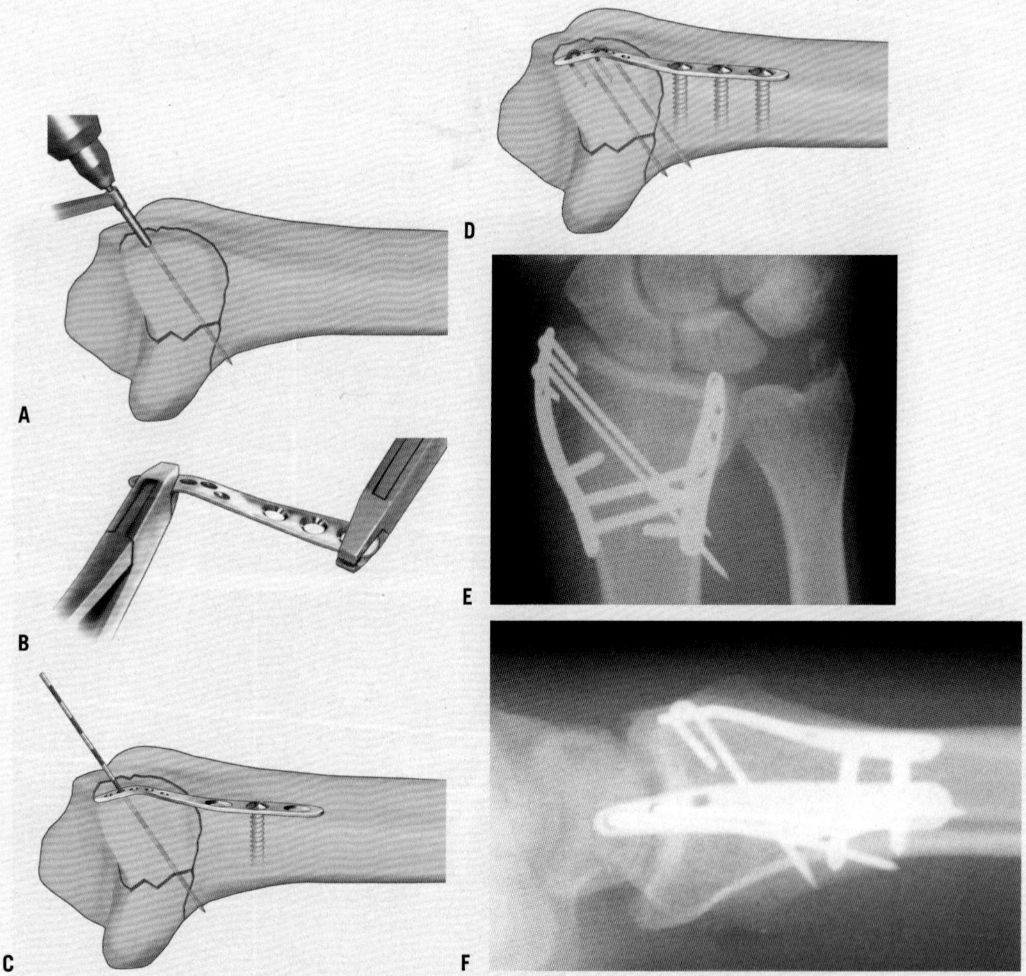

TECH FIG 10 Ulnar corner fixation with an ulnar pin plate. **A.** Insertion of the interfragmentary K-wire. **B.** Contouring the plate. **C.** Application of the plate and insertion of the initial fixation screw. **D.** Fixation completed. **E,F.** Radial and ulnar pin plate fixation of a three-part articular pattern (radial column and ulnar corner fragment).

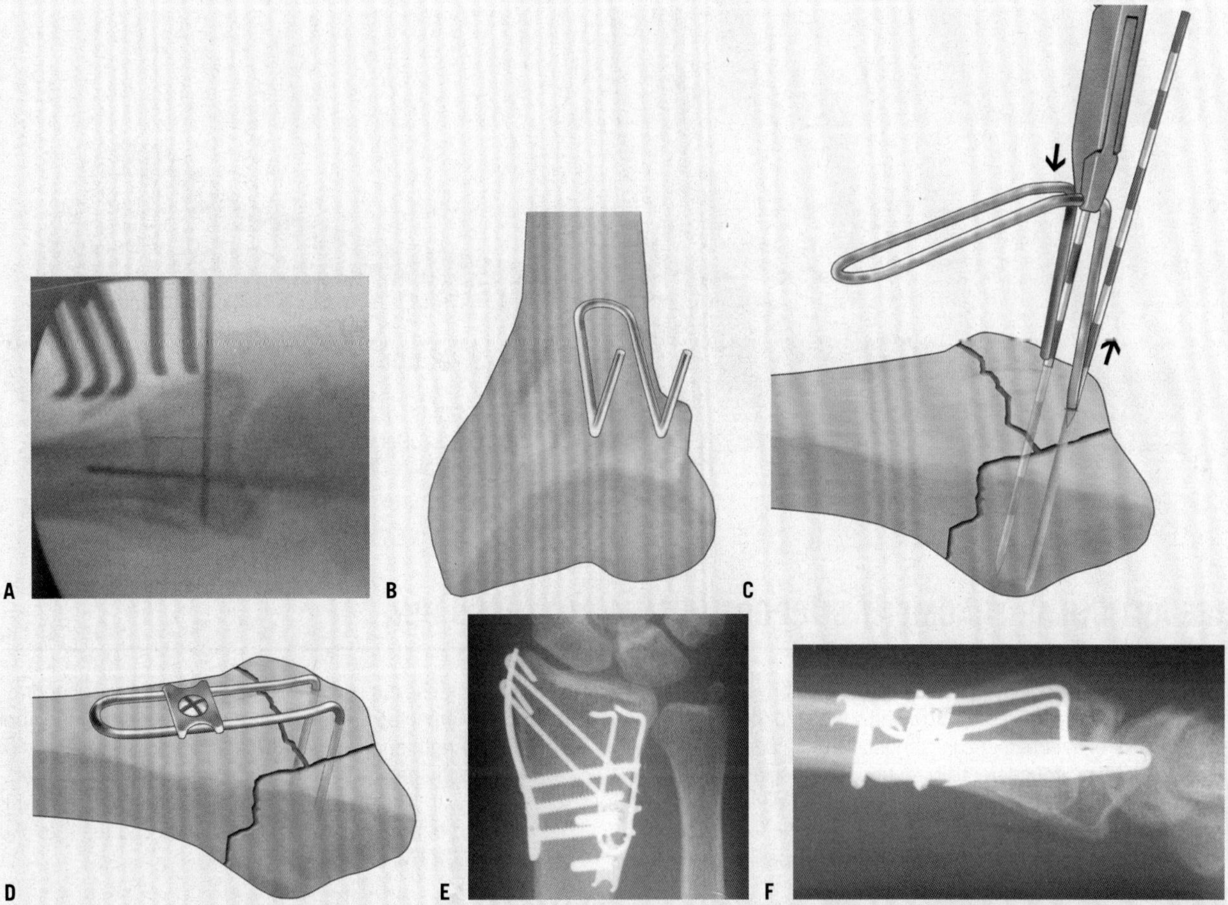

TECH FIG 11 Dorsal buttress pin fixation. **A.** The position of the K-wires is checked with a C-arm before inserting the implant. **B.** Placing an implant upside down on bone to template the trajectory of the K-wires. **C.** Inserting the dorsal buttress pin. **D.** Buttress pin fixation completed. **E,F.** Fixation of a three-part articular fracture with radial column and ulnar corner fragment with radial column plate and dorsal buttress pin.

lateral view, it may be necessary to angle the K-wires proximally to avoid penetration into the joint if the entry site is near the dorsal rim.

- Initially applying the dorsal buttress pin upside down on the bone as a template can be helpful to aid in visualization of the proper position and insertion angle of the K-wires; this helps determine the relative amount of pronation or supination of the pin trajectory that is needed for the site of application **(TECH FIG 11B)**.
- Ensure that the leading tips of the legs of the dorsal buttress pin are straight and cut to the required length. Leave the ulnar leg 2 to 3 mm longer than the radial leg, so one leg can be engaged at a time. Direct the legs proximally if needed to match the insertion angle of the K-wires.
- Place the ulnar leg of the buttress pin adjacent to the insertion site of the ulnar K-wire and then withdraw the K-wire and immediately engage the leg in the hole **(TECH FIG 11C)**. Repeat with the radial K-wire to engage the radial leg of the buttress pin. Impact and seat the buttress pin **(TECH FIG 11D)**.
- Fine-tune the reduction and complete the fixation proximally with one or two 2.3-mm cortical bone screws and washers **(TECH FIG 11E,F)**. If needed, a blocking screw can be placed just proximal to the end of the buttress pin to prevent shortening of the fragment.

Dorsal Hook Plate Fixation

- Dorsal hook plates are another alternative for fixation of dorsal fragments.
- Expose and reduce ulnar corner and/or dorsal wall fragments according to the technique described previously.
- Position and insert a 0.045-inch K-wire distally along the intended path of the hooks of the plate. Confirm the position with the C-arm.
- If needed, predrill the holes for insertion of the hooks. In osteoporotic bone, the hooks can be simply pushed into the fragment **(TECH FIG 12A)**.
- Verify the position and reduction with C-arm and complete fixation with proximal bone screws **(TECH FIG 12B)**.

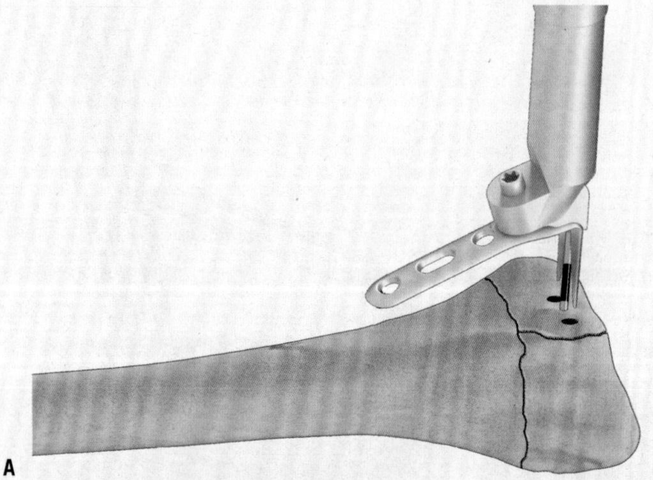

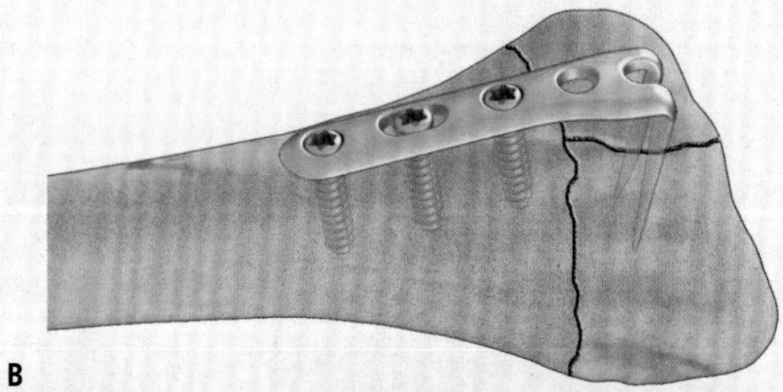

TECH FIG 12 Dorsal hook plate fixation. **A.** Placement of dorsal hook plate. **B.** Completed fixation.

FREE ARTICULAR FRAGMENT SUPPORT WITH A BUTTRESS PIN

- Free articular fragments impacted into the metaphyseal cavity can be reduced and stabilized by providing support to the subchondral surface of the fragment, in combination with peripheral cortical stabilization circumferentially around the articular fragment.
- Structural bone graft may be used to support free articular fragments in combination with fragment-specific fixation of the surrounding cortical shell, resulting in containment of the graft within the metaphysis.
- A dorsal buttress pin is useful to provide direct subchondral support of impacted articular fragments. The legs of the implant are cut to length and inserted through the dorsal defect, slid distally directly behind the articular fragment and then fixed proximally with a screw and washer. The articular fragment is sandwiched between the base of the lunate and the legs of the implant **(TECH FIG 13)**.

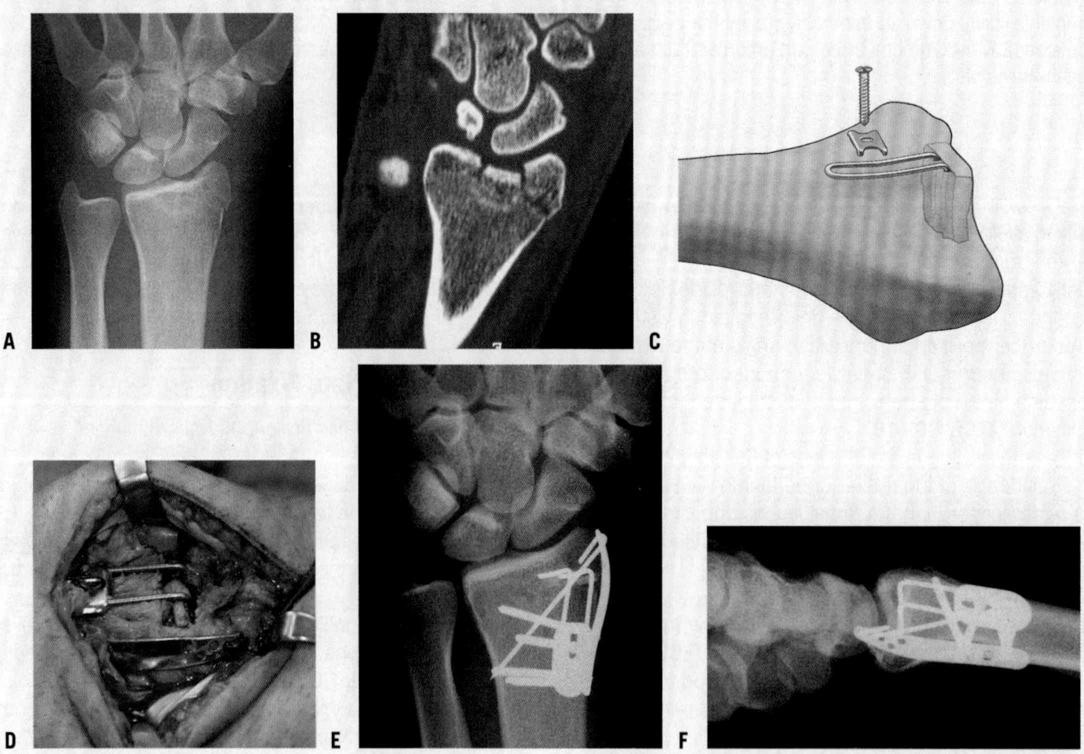

TECH FIG 13 **A,B.** Dorsal shear fracture with depressed articular fragment. **C,D.** Support of free articular fragment with a buttress pin and bone graft. **E,F.** Final x-rays.

Pearls and Pitfalls

Determining whether a Fragment Is on the Volar or Dorsal Side of the Distal Radius on the PA View	• Correlation of the carpal facet horizon with the lateral view allows identification whether a fragment is dorsal or volar. • If the articular surface is positioned in dorsal tilt, the carpal facet horizon identifies the dorsal rim. • If the articular surface is positioned in volar tilt, the carpal facet horizon identifies the volar rim.
Reduction of Unstable Fracture Pattern	• Identify and initiate reduction with the fragment that best stabilizes the carpus to its normal spatial relationship. • Initial reduction of the radial column with a provisional trans-styloid K-wire can help restore carpal length and unload impaction along the lunate facet. • Reduction of the volar rim of the lunate facet, paying particular attention to restoration of length and correction of the teardrop angle, is often the keystone to management of complex articular injuries. • The addition of structural bone graft, either through the fracture line at the base of the radial column or through a dorsal defect, can help stabilize the reduction during operative fixation.
Coronal Malalignment of the Distal Fragment with Widening of the DRUJ	• Correction of coronal malalignment by reducing radial translation of distal fragments before completing volar fixation both proximally and distally • An elastic, slightly overcontoured radial column plate such as a radial pin plate can help close sagittal fracture gaps and seat the sigmoid notch against the ulnar head. • Assess the clinical stability of the DRUJ and consider TFCC repair or ulnar styloid fixation as needed.
Loss of Fixation of Small or Dorsally Rotated Volar Ulnar Fragment	• Ensure adequate fixation of volar ulnar corner fragment. • Consider volar buttress pin or volar hook plate fixation for extremely distal or dorsally rotated volar rim fragments. • Avoid release of the volar wrist capsule. When necessary, the legs of an implant can be inserted through the capsule. • Larger fragments may have adequate support with a standard volar plate.
Unrecognized Intercarpal Ligament Injury	• Maintain a high index of suspicion for ligamentous injuries of the carpus. Consider arthroscopic evaluation, particularly in the context of radial or dorsal shear fractures, carpal avulsion/instability patterns, or articular fractures associated with a significant longitudinal step-off between the scaphoid and lunate facets.
Missed Stabilization of a Major Articular Fragment or Fracture Displacement after Surgery	• Careful analysis of radiographic features both before and during reduction; CT scan when needed. • Preoperative planning to select approaches that allow complete visualization of all major fragments • Availability of complete set of implants and instruments available before surgery including fragment-specific plates and possible spanning bridge plate • Evaluate stability of fixation with range of motion under observation before closing operative incision.
Loss of Radial Length: Proximal Migration of Articular Surface	• Graft the metaphyseal defect when needed with structural bone graft in cases of depression of articular fragments. • Use implants that buttress the subchondral bone.
DRUJ Dysfunction: Pain, Instability, or Limitation of Forearm Rotation	• Assess clinical stability of DRUJ at the end of procedure. • Ensure restoration of lateral carpal alignment. • Ensure correction of coronal alignment. • Use radial column plate to push distal fragment against ulna to seat sigmoid notch against ulnar head. • Evaluate and repair TFCC and capsular tears when necessary. • Reduce and fix ulnar corner and volar rim fragments to restore congruity of sigmoid notch. • Ensure that radial length is restored. • Mild, uncomplicated postoperative ulnar-sided wrist pain from ulnar styloid fracture without DRUJ instability often spontaneously resolves over 6–12 months.
Stiffness: Slow, Restricted Return of Movement of Wrist, Forearm, and Fingers; Associated with Pain	• Early range of motion and mobilization of soft tissues • Avoidance of constricting bandages • Strict elevation to decrease postoperative swelling • Consider occupational therapy when needed.
Tendinitis or Rupture: Pain with Resisted Motion, Loss of Tendon Function, Clicking, and Pain	• Use implants that have a low distal profile. • For small distal fragments, consider use of buttress pins. • Avoid placing sharp, bulky edges of hardware in proximity to tendons. • Cover dorsal plates distally with retinacular flap when possible. • Remove any pins or hardware that back out or become prominent postoperatively. • Ensure that volar plates do not extend up beyond distal volar ridge (watershed line) into soft tissues. • Avoid long screws or pins, particularly when placed from volar to dorsal. Distal screws should normally be 2–4 mm shy of the dorsal cortical margin to minimize risk of injury to the extensor tendons.

POSTOPERATIVE CARE

- At the end of the surgical procedure, confirm the stability of fixation as well as the stability of the DRUJ.
- If stable, apply a removable wrist brace and instruct the patient to initiate gentle range-of-motion exercises of the fingers, wrist, and forearm twice or more daily as tolerated. For noncompliant patients or injuries with tenuous fixation, use a cast for 2 to 3 weeks postoperatively or until radiographic evidence of healing is identified.
- Avoid resistive loading across the wrist until signs of radiographic healing are present; typically, this occurs by 4 weeks postoperatively. Specifically instruct older patients not to push up out of a chair or lift heavy objects after surgery.
- If there is persistent stiffness after 4 weeks, initiate physical and occupational therapy.

OUTCOMES

- Konrath and Bahler[5] reported 27 patients with at least 2 years of follow-up:
  - One fracture lost reduction.
  - Patient satisfaction was high (average Disabilities of the Arm, Shoulder, and Hand [DASH] scores 17 and Patient-Rated Wrist Evaluation [PRWE] scores 19 at follow-up).
  - In only three cases was hardware removed; no tendon ruptures occurred.
- Schnall et al[10] reported on two groups of patients: Group I had sustained high-energy trauma, and group II had lower energy injuries.
  - Group I patients averaged return to work in 6 weeks, with all fractures uniting without loss of position or deformity.
  - Two patients in group I required removal of painful hardware.
  - Group II patients averaged 2 degrees of loss of volar tilt, a 0.3-mm change in ulnar variance, and no loss of joint congruity at follow-up.
  - Grip strength in group II patients was 67% of the contralateral side.
- Benson et al[3] reported on 85 intra-articular fractures in 81 patients with a mean follow-up of 32 months.
  - There were 64 excellent and 24 good results, with an average DASH score of 9 at final follow-up.
  - Flexion and extension motion was 85% and 91% of the opposite side at final follow-up.
  - Grip strength was 92% of the opposite side at final follow-up.
  - Sixty-two percent of patients had a 100-degree arc of flexion–extension and normal forearm rotation by 6 weeks postoperatively.
  - Postoperative radiographic alignment was maintained at follow-up.
  - There were no cases of symptomatic posttraumatic arthritis.
- Abramo et al[1] reported a randomized, prospective study on 50 unstable fractures randomized to either external fixation or fragment-specific fixation and with follow-up at 1 year[1] and 5 years.[6]
  - At 1 year, internal fixation resulted in better grip strength and range of motion.
  - No difference in subjective outcome was observed at 5 years.
  - There were five malunions in the external fixation group, compared to only one malunion in the fragment-specific group.
  - Differences in grip strength tended to equalize at 5-year follow-up.
- Saw et al[9] reported on 22 unstable C2 and C3 fractures of the distal radius treated with fragment-specific fixation with a minimum of 6 months follow-up.
  - At follow-up, radial inclination was restored to an average of 25 degrees and volar tilt to 8 degrees.
  - Twenty of 22 fractures had restoration of articular congruity to less than 2 mm.
  - Mean wrist flexion/extension was 50 to 63 degrees and mean pronation/supination arc of 149 degrees.
  - Mean subjective PRWE score at follow-up was 20.
  - Treatment approach was felt to be a powerful tool for difficult fractures, but acknowledge a significant learning curve.

COMPLICATIONS

- Stiffness: common early, uncommon at follow-up
  - Recovery can be accelerated by anatomic fixation that is stable enough to start motion immediately after surgery. The relative degree of trauma to the bone and soft tissues, combined with underlying physiologic factors, is also a critical factor that can lead to slow recovery of motion or residual stiffness.
- Malunion or nonunion: rare
  - Loss of reduction may occur, particularly if a major fracture component is missed and left untreated. In addition, osteoporosis, failure to graft the metaphyseal defect, and associated DRUJ injuries may contribute to loss of reduction or malunion.
  - Pin plates are able to resist translational displacements but are less effective for preventing loss of length; they require osseous contact between the proximal and distal fragments or additional support by bone graft or a secondary implant that will buttress the subchondral surface.
  - Nonunions are extremely rare.
- Tendinitis or tendon rupture: uncommon
  - If pins are noted postoperatively to back out, they should be removed. Leaving the distal 1 cm of tendon sheath of the first dorsal compartment intact helps avoid tendon contact with hardware.
  - Using low-profile implants dorsally, covering the distal ends with a strip of retinacular sheath or both, is also helpful.
  - The surgeon should avoid leaving screws or pins protruding from the dorsal or volar surfaces of the bone.
- Painful hardware: rare
  - Painful hardware can be related to migration of a pin or settling of the fracture proximally. Overbending pin hooks and using bone graft or buttressing implants can help avoid this problem.
  - Remove hardware when painful.
- Late arthritis is uncommon and related to the articular damage at the time of injury as well as the quality of the articular restoration.

- Infections, bleeding, carpal tunnel syndrome, and other nerve injuries are uncommon and often related to the primary injury.
- Complex regional pain syndrome is uncommon.

REFERENCES

1. Abramo A, Kopylov P, Geijer M, et al. Open reduction and internal fixation compared to closed reduction and external fixation in distal radial fractures: a randomized study of 50 patients. Acta Orthop 2009;80(4):478–485.
2. Barrie K, Wolfe S. Internal fixation for intraarticular distal radius fractures. Tech Hand Up Extrem Surg 2002;6:10–20.
3. Benson LS, Minihane KP, Stern LD, et al. The outcome of intraarticular distal radius fractures treated with fragment-specific fixation. J Hand Surg Am 2006;31(8):1333–1339.
4. Fernandez DL, Jupiter JB. Fractures of the Distal Radius, ed 2. New York: Springer, 2002:42–50.
5. Konrath G, Bahler S. Open reduction and internal fixation of unstable distal radius fractures: results using the TriMed fixation system. J Orthop Trauma 2002;16:578–585.
6. Landgren M, Jerrhag D, Tägil M, et al. External or internal fixation in the treatment of non-reducible distal radial fractures? Acta Orthop 2011;82(5):610–613.
7. Leslie BM, Medoff RJ. Fracture specific fixation of distal radius fractures. Tech Orthop 2000;15:336–352.
8. Medoff R. Essential radiographic evaluation for distal radius fractures. Hand Clin 2005;21:279–288.
9. Saw N, Roberts C, Cutbush K, et al. Early experience with the TriMed fragment-specific fracture fixation system in intraarticular distal radius fractures. J Hand Surg Eur Vol 2008;33(1):53–58.
10. Schnall SB, Kim BJ, Abramo A, et al. Fixation of distal radius fractures using a fragment-specific system. Clin Orthop Relat Res 2006;445:51–57.
11. Swigart C, Wolfe S. Limited incision open techniques for distal radius fracture management. Orthop Clin North Am 2001;32:317–327.

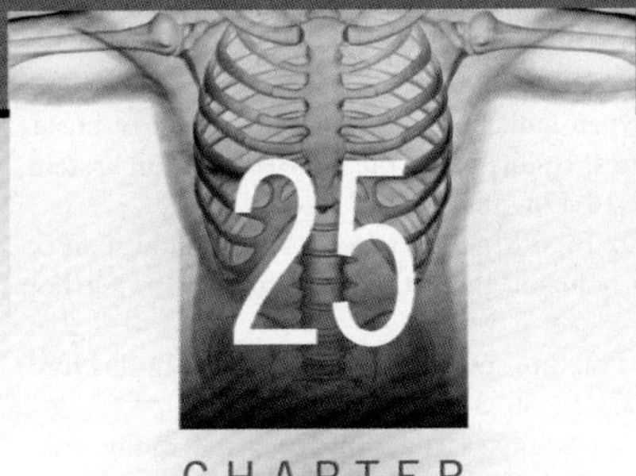

CHAPTER 25

Bridge Plating and External Fixation of Distal Radius Fractures

Venus Vakhshori, Ram K. Alluri, and Alidad Ghiassi

DEFINITION

- High-energy fractures of the distal aspect of the radius with extensive articular comminution and diaphyseal extension represent a major treatment challenge. Standard plates and techniques may be inadequate for the management of such fractures.
- These highly comminuted fractures are often amenable to relative stability techniques, which rely on radiocarpal joint distraction and ligamentotaxis to restore length, alignment, and rotation. This can be achieved with external fixation or internal radiocarpal distraction plating (dorsal spanning plates).

ANATOMY

- On average, the articular surface of the distal radius has a volar tilt of 11 degrees, radial inclination of 22 degrees, and radial height of 12 mm.
- The dorsal cortex surface of the distal radius thickens to form Lister tubercle.
- A central ridge divides the articular surface of the radius into a scaphoid facet and a lunate facet.
- Because of the different areas of bone thickness and density, fractures tend to occur in the relatively weaker metaphyseal bone and propagate into the joint between the scaphoid and lunate facets.
- The degree, direction, and magnitude of applied load may cause coronal or sagittal splits within the lunate or scaphoid facets.
- The distal forearm may be conceptualized by a three-column model. The radial column is composed of the radial styloid and scaphoid facet; the intermediate column includes the lunate facet and the sigmoid notch; and the ulnar column is made up of the ulnar head, distal radioulnar joint (DRUJ), the ulnar styloid, and the triangular fibrocartilage. The intermediate column may be split into volar ulnar and dorsoulnar fragments. The volar ulnar corner, or the "critical corner," is especially challenging to treat and may lead to volar subluxation of the carpus if not properly stabilized.[23]

PATHOGENESIS

- Three subsets of patients with distal radius fractures continue to represent unique treatment challenges.
  - Patients with high-energy wrist injuries with significant comminution and fracture extension into the radial diaphysis. These patients may also have multiple injuries including abdominal, pelvic, and lower extremity injuries making early postoperative mobilization very challenging.
  - Radiocarpal dislocations and fracture-dislocations. These may include volar or dorsal shearing injuries and periarticular dislocations with and without bony avulsion.
  - Elderly patients with low bone density and periarticular fractures with gross instability and severe displacement

NATURAL HISTORY

- In comminuted distal radius fractures treated by closed methods, the final radiographic results resembled the prereduction radiographs more than any other radiographs during treatment, even when the initial reduction successfully restored wrist anatomy.
- Restoration of normal bony anatomy of a distal radius fracture can lead to improved function. Functional outcome scores in patients without anatomic reduction may be poor in the short-term; however, multiple factors contribute to patient's long-term functional outcome.[6]
- Malunions of the distal radius have been associated with pain, stiffness, weak grip strength, and carpal instability in a substantial percentage of patients. Long-term consequences include degenerative arthrosis, especially with intra-articular fractures and malunions.[18]
- Surgical treatment ensures more consistent correction of fracture fragment displacement and maintenance of reduction. Over the last two decades, there has been a trend toward operative treatment with internal fixation in both the elderly and the young population.[21]

PATIENT HISTORY AND PHYSICAL FINDINGS

- In the management of high-energy distal radius fractures, a complete history should include the mechanism of injury, degree of initial displacement, any attempts at reduction (on the field or in outside facilities), and other concomitant injuries.
- Examination of the soft tissue envelope of the wrist should be performed to rule out open fractures and plan potential surgical incisions for open reduction and internal fixation.
- Patients with high-energy injuries are at increased risk for neurovascular compromise and tendon injury.[10] Careful examination for signs of median and ulnar nerve dysfunction from an acute nerve compression should be clearly documented. Surgeons should be suspicious of compartment syndrome in high-energy injuries, especially in polytrauma patients with altered mental status. If the postreduction splint and dressings are excessively constrictive, the bandage should be released and loosened to ensure space for adequate soft tissue swelling.

IMAGING AND OTHER DIAGNOSTIC STUDIES

- Adequate quality pre- and postreduction wrist radiographs should be obtained preoperatively to assess the fracture pattern and rule out associated injuries to the carpus or DRUJ.
- Although there is no consensus regarding the use of preoperative computed tomography scans, they may be helpful for surgical planning of complex intra-articular distal radius fractures.[2]

NONOPERATIVE MANAGEMENT

- For extra-articular fractures, even with acceptable reduction, open reduction and internal fixation with volar locking plates led to better functional outcomes at all time points.[22] In addition, there is a high risk of redisplacement necessitating surgical fixation at a later time point as well as future symptomatic malunion.
- For high-energy comminuted intra-articular distal radius fractures, nonoperative management is usually unacceptable.
- Patients and their family members should be included in the shared decision-making process as it relates to the risks and benefits of nonoperative treatment.

SURGICAL MANAGEMENT

- Displaced, highly comminuted distal radius fracture patterns are prone to shortening/collapse with resultant displacement and malalignment of the radiocarpal joint. If standard volar locking plate fixation or fragment-specific fixation is not sufficient for fracture stabilization due to the fracture pattern, external fixation or bridge plating may be indicated **(TABLE 1)**.

TABLE 1 Indications for Bridge Plating or External Fixation of Distal Radius Fractures

Indication	Explanation
Metadiaphyseal comminution of the radius	Extensive comminution in metadiaphyseal region is difficult to treat with standard implants used for distal radius fractures.
Need for early weight bearing through the upper extremity	Patients with associated lower limb injuries may require the need for early weight bearing through the upper extremities.
Polytrauma	Nursing care of the multiply injured patient may be easier with spanning internal fixation than with external fixation. However, in an unstable patient, external fixation may require less surgical time and may be preferred.
Augmented fixation	In osteoporotic bone with multiple small articular fragments, bridge plating can be used to augment tenuous fixation to provide axial stability.
Radiocarpal dislocation	Radiocarpal dislocations or fracture-dislocations may be held in a reduced position with the help of spanning internal fixation.

- External fixation allows for indirect reduction through ligamentotaxis and prevention of shortening by spanning the radiocarpal joint. This can restore length, alignment, and rotation. However, external fixators may be complicated by pin site infections, malreduction, overdistraction of the radiocarpal joint, hand stiffness, and increased risk of chronic regional pain syndrome.[20] The rate of external fixation in the treatment of distal radius fractures has been steadily declining, with only 4.9% of distal radius fractures were treated with external fixators in 2014.[27]
- For patients with large dorsal soft tissue loss or degloving injuries, external fixation can be used until definitive fixation and soft tissue coverage.
- The rigidity of an external fixator construct is inversely proportional to the distance between the longitudinal fixator and the bone. Bridge plating creates a bar to bone distance of 0, increasing the rigidity of an external fixation construct, allowing it to act as an "internal fixator."[30] Bridge plate fixation has increased mean stiffness compared to external fixation.[30]
- Both external fixation and bridge plating offer relative stability and an indirect reduction of the distal radius fracture. These techniques can be combined with a limited articular fixation approach for fracture patterns with intra-articular extension.
- Distal fixation to the third metacarpal results in greater stiffness in flexion, compared to second metacarpal fixation; however, there is a theoretical increased risk of tendon entrapment with use of the middle metacarpal.[1,17]

Preoperative Planning

- Bridge plates allow the placement of smaller screws in the metacarpal and larger screws in the radial shaft. Locking screw options are available for use in osteoporotic bone. Some manufacturer plates allow for articular surface fixation through the plate with center holes.
- Compared to wrist arthrodesis plates, bridge plates are longer, providing increased stability for fractures with proximal extension. These plates are produced by multiple manufacturers and are available in 2.4-, 2.7-, 3.2-, and 3.5-mm sizes.[15]
- A small external fixation device with 2.5-mm threaded Kirschner wires (K-wires) or 3.0- to 4.0-mm Schanz pins may be used with corresponding bars, as available by several different manufacturers. Larger pin size confers increased stability; however, in the metacarpal, an excessively large pin has a high risk of metacarpal fracture and may not be able to be placed bicortically. Therefore, smaller diameter pins (generally 2.5 to 3.2 mm) are used in the metacarpal, and larger diameter pins (generally 4.0 mm) are used in the radius.
- In extra-articular or simple articular distal radius fractures, nonspanning external fixators may be used to allow radiocarpal motion, but this is often not possible in highly comminuted intra-articular distal radius fractures.[19]

Positioning

- With the patient anesthetized and supine on the operating table, a nonsterile tourniquet is placed on the upper arm, and the involved extremity is draped free and centered on a radiolucent hand table.

- A C-arm is used, positioned such that the operating surgeon can easily view the fluoroscopy screen. The C-arm can be flipped 180 degrees, with the large image intensifier placed under the table, and the smaller x-ray tube above the table to increase working space in the surgical field. The surgeon may also use the foot pedal to better control image acquisition.
- In polytrauma patients with lower extremity injuries, concomitant surgery can be performed in a highly coordinated team effort between orthopaedic traumatologists and hand surgeons.
- Finger traps can be applied to the index and middle fingers with 4.5 kg of longitudinal traction applied at the edge of the table through a rope and pulley system.

CLOSED REDUCTION MANEUVER OF AGEE

- Longitudinal traction is first used to restore length and to assess the benefit of ligamentotaxis for the restoration of articular step-off **(TECH FIG 1A,B)**.
- Next, the hand is translated palmarly relative to the forearm to restore sagittal tilt and to assess the integrity of the volar lip of the radius **(TECH FIG 1C–F)**.
- Finally, pronation of the hand relative to the forearm is performed to correct the supination deformity.
- Once the initial reduction maneuver is completed, K-wire fixation may be used to hold the reduction before the application of the bridge plate or external fixator.
- The Kapandji intrafocal pinning technique can be used to help support articular fragments and restore anatomic alignment.[29]
- Additionally, fragment-specific fixation may be used to stabilize key articular fragments prior to the application of the spanning plates.
- We only recommend limited internal fixation of important articular fragments when there is underlying instability or displacement.

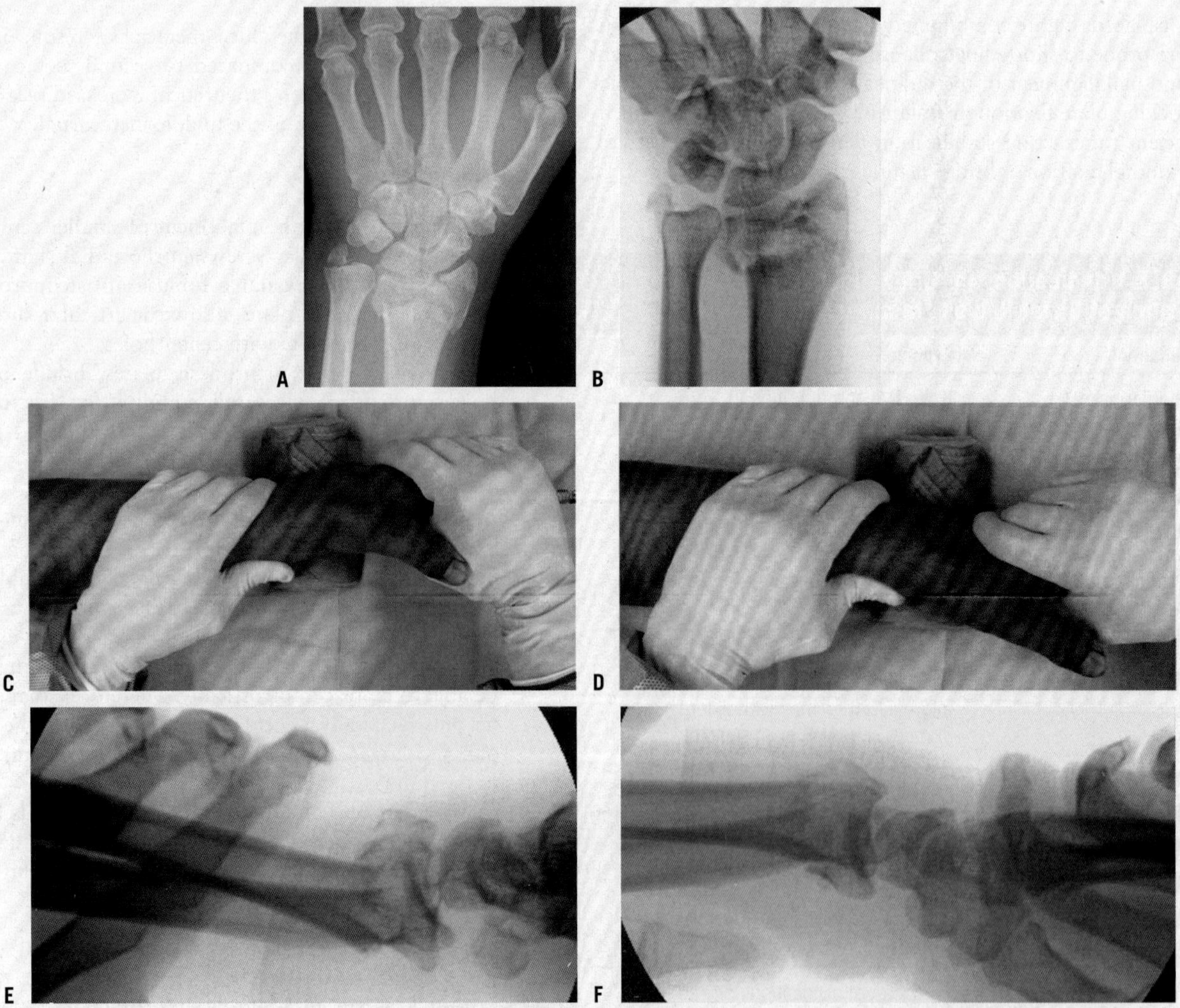

TECH FIG 1 Radiographs show an anteroposterior (AP) projection of the wrist injury before (**A**) and after (**B**) distraction is applied. Clinical pictures show the wrist deformity before (**C**) and after (**D**) application of the Agee reduction maneuver, which is a combination of longitudinal traction and volar translation of the carpus. Radiographs show the wrist deformity before (**E**) and after (**F**) application of the Agee reduction maneuver.

EXTERNAL FIXATOR PLACEMENT

Proximal Fixator Pins

- The radial shaft is palpated 10 cm proximal to the radial styloid, ideally at least 5 cm outside the zone of injury. The bare area of the radius is identified in the palpable interval between the brachioradialis and the extensor carpi radialis longus (ECRL) muscles.
- Generous incisions are made at the pin sites on the dorsal surface of the forearm, with careful attention to protect the branches of the superficial radial and lateral antebrachial cutaneous nerves. The incisions should allow for adequate visualization of passing nerve branches.
- Holes are predrilled.
- Proximal pins are placed from the dorsal–radial aspect of the radius to the volar ulnar side at a 45-degree angle.
- After the first pin is placed, a fixator clamp can be used to determine the placement of the second pin.
- Unicortical pin placement should be avoided to prevent creation of a stress riser **(TECH FIG 2)**.
- Fluoroscopy is used to confirm Schanz pin placement and length. The threads of the pin should be in the far cortex.

Distal Fixator Pins

- The bare area between the first dorsal interosseous muscle and the extensor tendon complex to the index finger is identified, and incisions are made at the pin sites on the dorsal surface of the index metacarpal.
- Holes are predrilled.
- Pins are placed from the dorsal surface volarly in the center of the metacarpal shaft. Careful attention should be paid to avoid eccentric placement of the pins resulting in unicortical pins or metacarpal fracture.
- A clamp can be used after placement of the first pin to guide the second pin placement. Fluoroscopy is used to confirm placement.
- In case of an iatrogenic metacarpal fracture, we recommend open reduction and internal fixation of the metacarpal bone, followed by application of pins to the adjacent metacarpal.

Assembly

- Pin to bar connectors are used.
- Ideally, rods should be 1 to 2 cm dorsal to the skin to avoid contact between the bar and the skin, which can occur due to postoperative swelling.
  - A second rod can be used to increase stiffness of the overall construct.
  - Rods are connected proximally first, then distally.
- Distraction is used to achieve ligamentotaxis and reduction. This is confirmed fluoroscopically.
- Overdistraction should be avoided to prevent hand stiffness and intrinsic contracture. The amount of distraction of the radiocarpal and midcarpal joints should be checked fluoroscopically.
- Intra-articular reduction can be further adjusted by using limited periarticular incisions to allow for direct manipulation of articular fragments, placement of subchondral bone grafts, repair of intercarpal ligament injuries, and augmentation of fracture fixation with K-wires and periarticular plates.
- Displaced volar medial fracture fragments that are not reduced with this technique require a separate volar incision and appropriate buttress support.
- Pin sites are dressed using occlusive gauze and dry dressings.

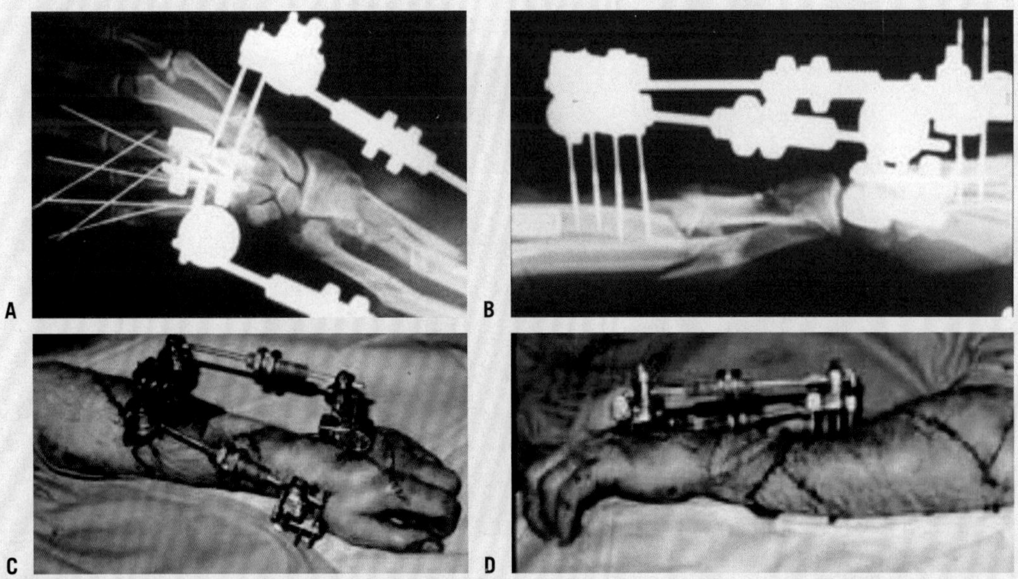

TECH FIG 2 AP (**A**) and lateral (**B**) radiographs of the external fixator construct, demonstrating restored distal radius fracture alignment. **C,D.** Pin and bar placement. *(continued)*

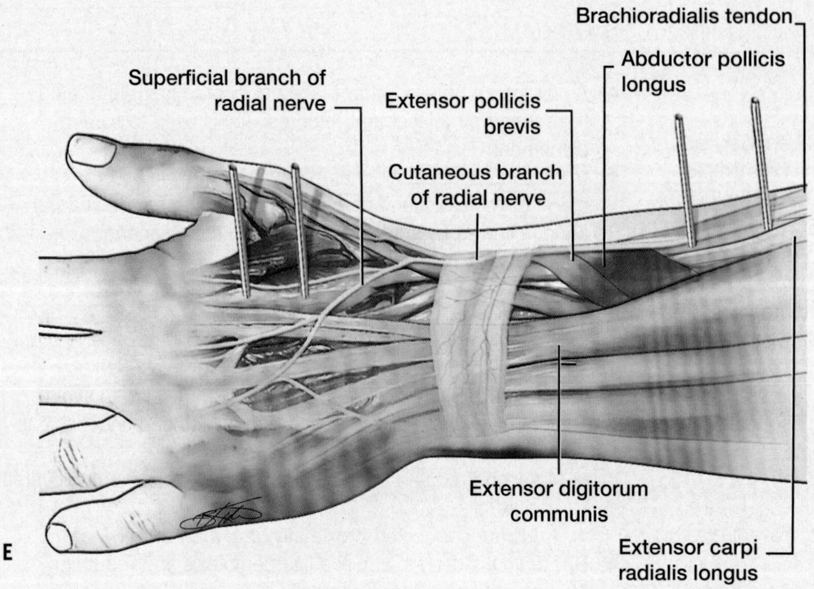

TECH FIG 2 *(continued)* **E.** Pin positioning between the brachioradialis and ECRL tendons proximally and on the index metacarpal distally. (**C,D:** Courtesy of Roy Meals, MD.)

BRIDGE PLATE APPLICATION

- The closed reduction maneuver of Agee can again be performed as described earlier.

Approach

- The bridge plate is superimposed on the skin from the radial diaphysis to the distal metadiaphysis of the second or third metacarpal. The position of the plate is verified with image intensification, and markings are placed on the skin at the level of the proximal and distal four screw holes of the plate **(TECH FIG 3A–C)**.
- We recommend fixation to the third metacarpal for radiocarpal dislocations and to the second metacarpal for distal radius fractures.[3]
- A 5-cm incision is made at the base of the second or third metacarpal and continued along the metacarpal shaft. In the depths of this incision, the insertions of the ECRL and extensor carpi radialis brevis (ECRB) are identified as they pass beneath the distal edge of the second dorsal wrist compartment to insert on the second and third metacarpal bases, respectively.
- A second incision is made just proximal to the outcropper muscle bellies (abductor pollicis longus and extensor pollicis

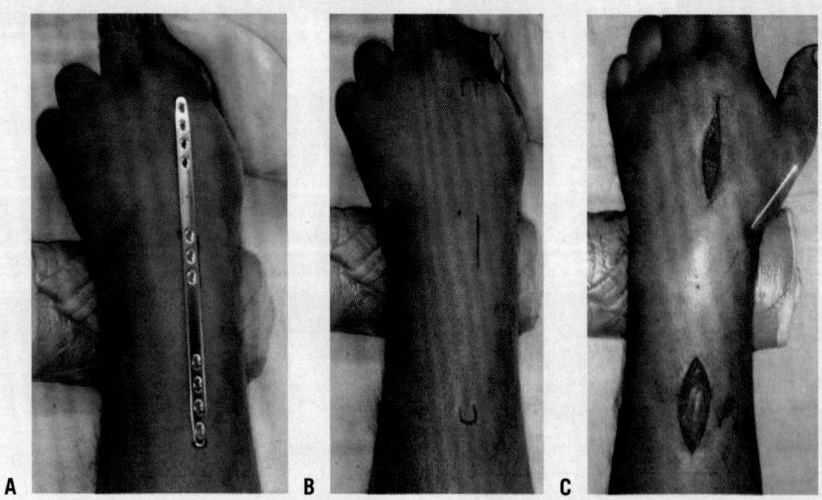

TECH FIG 3 **A.** The plate is placed over the forearm and hand. Radiographs can be taken to confirm the position of the plate. The plate should be centered over the second metacarpal distally and the radius proximally. This will be along the course of the extensor carpi radialis longus (*ECRL*). **B.** Outline of the plate. **C.** Incisions are made over the second metacarpal and the radius. *(continued)*

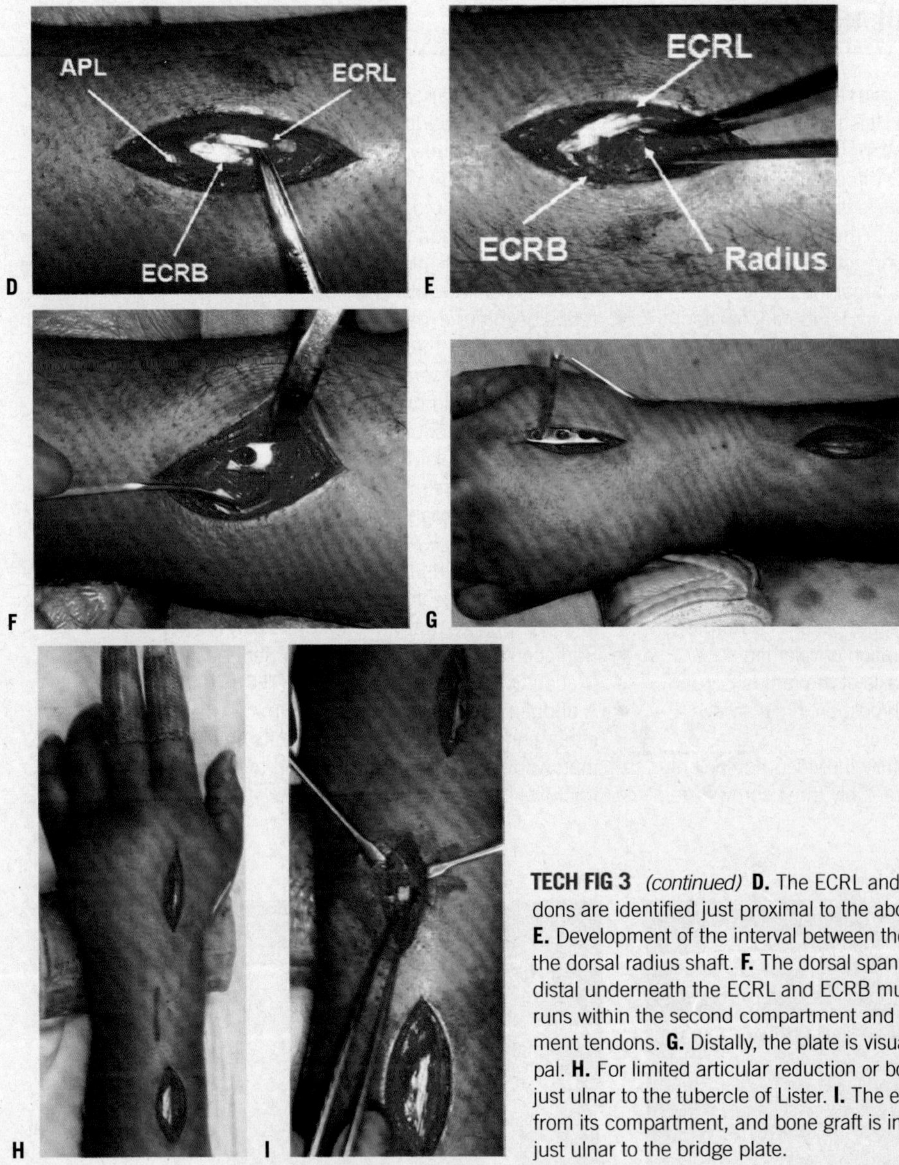

TECH FIG 3 *(continued)* **D.** The ECRL and extensor carpi radialis brevis (*ECRB*) tendons are identified just proximal to the abductor pollicis longus (*APL*) in the forearm. **E.** Development of the interval between the ECRL and ECRB tendons to gain access to the dorsal radius shaft. **F.** The dorsal spanning bridge plate is passed from proximal to distal underneath the ECRL and ECRB muscles. It is important to ensure that the plate runs within the second compartment and not superficial to the first and third compartment tendons. **G.** Distally, the plate is visualized, emerging over the second metacarpal. **H.** For limited articular reduction or bone grafting, a third incision is marked out just ulnar to the tubercle of Lister. **I.** The extensor pollicis longus tendon is released from its compartment, and bone graft is inserted through the dorsal fracture fragment just ulnar to the bridge plate.

brevis), in line with ECRL and ECRB tendons. The interval between the ECRL and ECRB is developed and the diaphysis of the radius exposed **(TECH FIG 3D,E)**.

- We prefer passing the plate from a distal to proximal direction in order to avoid passing the plate into the fracture site, which can occur if the plate is passed from the proximal to distal direction. With direct visualization of the ECRL tendon insertion on the base of the index metacarpal, the plate can be passed just deep to this.
- Alternatively, the plate can be introduced beneath the muscle bellies of the outcroppers extraperiosteally and advanced from proximal to distal between the ECRL and ECRB tendons **(TECH FIG 3F)**.
- Some resistance may be encountered as the plate emerges distally but can usually be easily overcome with gentle manipulation of the plate **(TECH FIG 3G)**.
- Occasionally, the plate will not pass through the compartment. In these cases, a blunt surgical instrument, such as a Freer elevator, may be used to create a path for the plate. Alternatively, a guidewire or stout suture retriever is passed along the compartment from distal to proximal. The plate is secured to the distal end of the wire and delivered into the hand.
  - In the rare instance that these measures fail, a third incision is made directly over the metaphysis of the radius. The retinaculum over the proximal half of the second compartment is incised, and the plate is passed under direct vision.
- For fixation to the third metacarpal, the plate passes under the fourth dorsal compartment under the finger extensors. A third incision should be made to facilitate passing of the plate under the extensor digitorum communis (EDC) tendons deep to the extensor retinaculum. Otherwise, there is risk of compression of the EDC tendons under the bridge plate.
- The third, or periarticular, incision may also be used to assess the articular surface, reduce die-punch fragments, and introduce bone graft in the metaphyseal region **(TECH FIG 3H,I)**.

PLATE FIXATION AND ARTICULAR FIXATION

- After the bridge plate is passed, it is confirmed fluoroscopically to be on bone rather than in soft tissue. It is then secured to the metacarpal (index or middle) by placing a nonlocking fully threaded 2.4- or 2.7-mm cortical screw through the most distal plate hole. The proximal end of the plate is then identified in the forearm. The distal aspect of the plate must be centered in the metacarpal diaphysis to avoid placing eccentric unicortical screws that may cause iatrogenic metacarpal fractures.
- If the plate design includes K-wire holes for temporary fixation, these can be used to maintain the plate position prior to final fixation.
- Additionally, if the plate design includes an oval sliding hole, we recommend this as the first point of fixation in the proximal aspect of the radius. This allows for further adjustment of length prior to final stabilization.
- If the radial length has not been restored, then the plate, secured to the second metacarpal, is pushed distally until the length is re-established and a fully threaded 2.4-, 2.7-, or 3.2-mm nonlocking screw is placed in the most proximal plate hole across the radial shaft. By using nonlocking screws, the plate is compressed onto the intact bone, aiding in the restoration of volar tilt.
- Plate alignment along the longitudinal axis of the radius is guaranteed by securing the most distal and most proximal screw holes first.
- The remaining holes are secured with fully threaded nonlocking screws inserted with bicortical purchase. Only three screws are required proximally and distally, with no biomechanical difference seen with addition of a fourth screw.[30]
- Locking screws may be used in cases of osteoporosis for increased stability. The initial cortical screws placed can also be exchanged for locking screws after the remaining holes have been filled. The ideal modulation of stiffness by varying the combination of nonlocking screws, locking screws, and working length is not known.
- It has been our experience that as the plate is passed along the radial diaphysis, through the second compartment and along the second metacarpal, extra-articular alignment, radial inclination, volar tilt, and radial length are restored.
- Intra-articular reduction may be further adjusted by using limited periarticular incisions to allow for direct manipulation of articular fragments, placement of subchondral bone grafts, repair of intercarpal ligament injuries, and augmentation of fracture fixation with K-wires and periarticular plates.
- Displaced volar lunate facet fracture fragments that are not reduced with this technique may require a separate volar incision and appropriate buttress support **(TECH FIG 4)**.
- Radiocarpal dislocations are often better aligned with distal fixation to the middle metacarpal **(TECH FIG 5)**.
- A bridge plate fixed with a minimum of three screws at either end of the plate confers significantly more stability than would an external fixator used to stabilize a comparable fracture.[30]

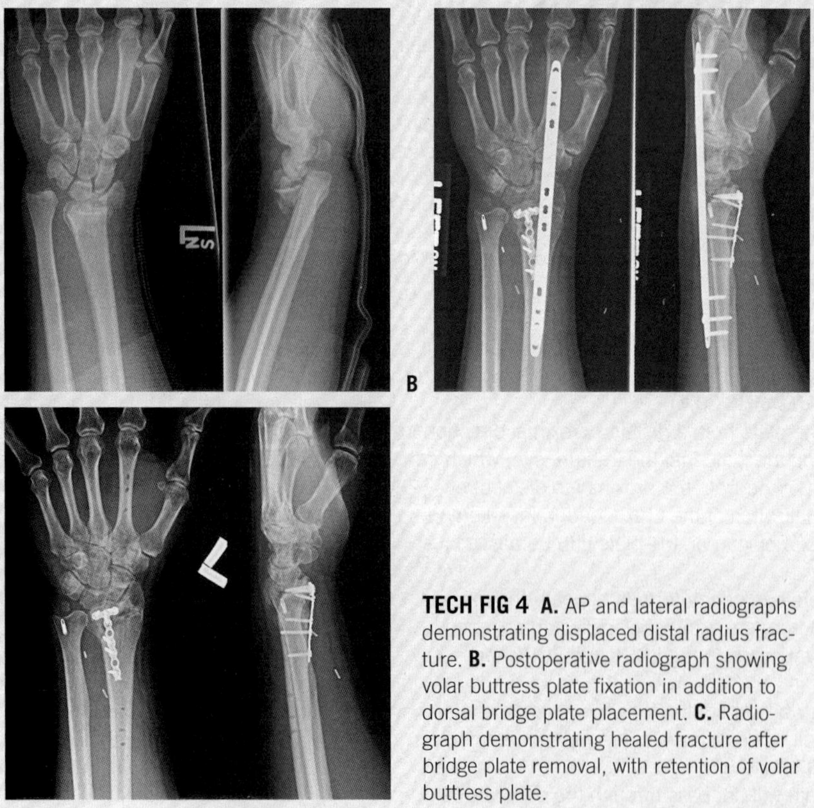

TECH FIG 4 A. AP and lateral radiographs demonstrating displaced distal radius fracture. **B.** Postoperative radiograph showing volar buttress plate fixation in addition to dorsal bridge plate placement. **C.** Radiograph demonstrating healed fracture after bridge plate removal, with retention of volar buttress plate.

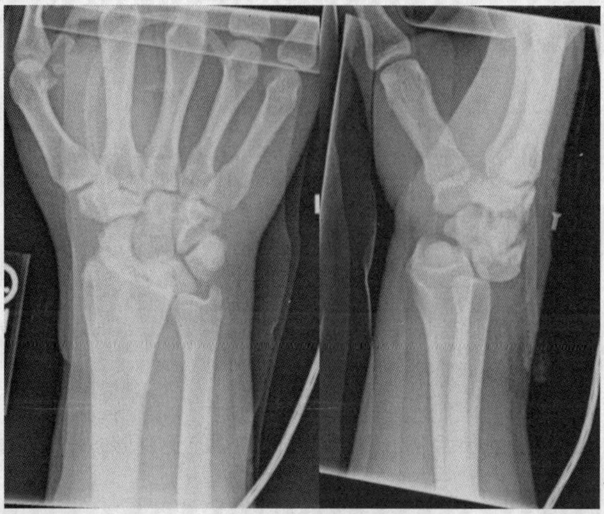

A

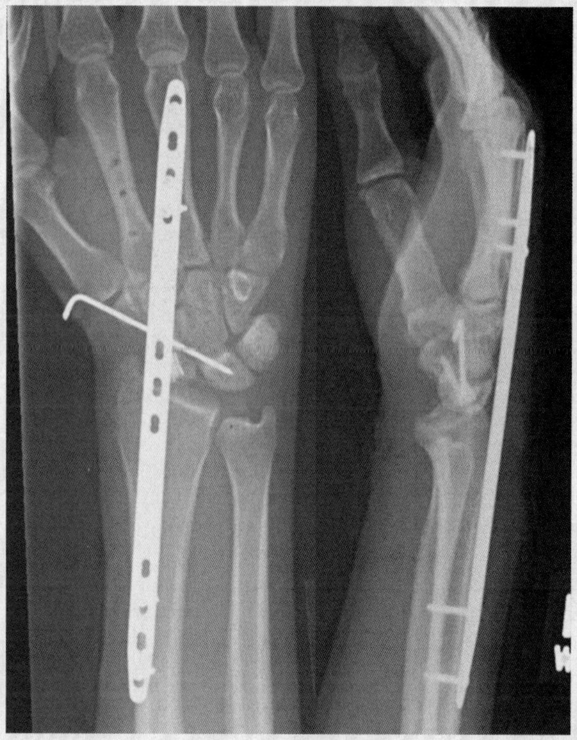

B

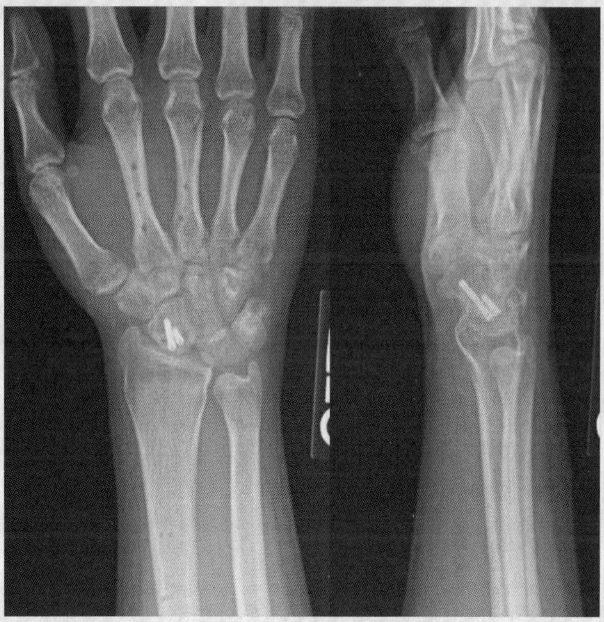

C

TECH FIG 5 **A.** AP and lateral radiographs demonstrating a radiocarpal dislocation with associated transscaphoid perilunate fracture-dislocation. **B.** Postoperative radiograph showing reduction of the radiocarpal dislocation with spanning bridge plate fixation with screw fixation of the scaphoid fracture and K-wire fixation across the scapholunate joint. Initially, fixation to the second metacarpal was performed, but intraoperatively, carpal malalignment was noted. Distal fixation was then placed on the third metacarpal with some improvement. **C.** Radiographs demonstrating healed radiocarpal dislocation with concentrically reduced joint, as well as healed scaphoid fracture, after removal of bridge plate and K-wire.

DISTAL RADIOULNAR JOINT MANAGEMENT

- DRUJ stability is assessed after radius reconstruction. If the DRUJ is stable, the limb is immobilized in a long-arm splint with the forearm in supination for the first 10 to 14 days postoperatively.
- If the DRUJ is unstable, and there are no contraindications to prolonging the operation, repair or reconstruction of the triangular fibrocartilage complex is undertaken.
- If, however, the patient's condition does not allow the operation to be prolonged, the ulnar head is reduced manually into the sigmoid notch, and the ulna is transfixed to the radius with two 1.6-mm K-wires passed proximal to the DRUJ. Radioulnar transfixation is performed with the forearm in neutral position.

Pearls and Pitfalls

Hardware Removal	• Bridge plates require a second surgery for hardware removal, whereas external fixators can generally be removed without anesthesia. At the time of hardware extraction, the prior incisions are used, the screws are removed, and the plate is removed through one of the prior incisions. • A removable short-arm splint is worn for 2–3 weeks after plate removal. Hand therapy at this point is directed at regaining motion and strength.
Index versus Middle Metacarpal Fixation	• We prefer distal fixation to the index metacarpal to avoid traumatizing the finger extensors and risk of compression of the tendons under the bridge plate. • For radiocarpal dislocations, fixation to the middle metacarpal allows for more anatomic reduction.
Overdistraction	• Distraction of greater than 5 mm may lead to digital stiffness and complex regional pain syndrome (CRPS). • Increased midcarpal joint space compared to the radiocarpal joint space is indicative of overdistraction of the wrist.

POSTOPERATIVE CARE

- Digit range-of-motion and forearm rotational exercises start immediately after surgery. Load bearing through the forearm and elbow is allowed immediately as well as the use of a platform crutch when the patient is physiologically stable. Lifting, pushing, pulling, and carrying are restricted until fracture healing. However, light activities of daily living are allowed for self-care, including driving.
- Supplemental K-wires for articular fixation are removed 6 weeks postoperatively.
- The bridge plate and screws or external fixator is removed traditionally not earlier than 12 weeks after injury once radiographic healing is confirmed. However, the plates may be removed as soon as both clinical and radiographic signs of fracture healing are observed.

OUTCOMES

- Compared to plaster immobilization, external fixation shows improved radiographic and clinical outcomes in those patients with comminuted distal radius fractures.[11] However, some studies demonstrate a high complication rate, and recent evidence has illustrated a decrease in external fixator use with a corresponding increase in bridge plate utilization.[4]
- Three studies assessing second metacarpal fixation with a total of 105 patients included[7,8,14] 1 ECRL tendon rupture, 4 hardware failures, 19 cases of stiffness requiring tenolysis, and 2 cases of wrist pain were reported. Range of motion and grip strength returned to functional levels after healing.
- Third metacarpal fixation has been reported in three studies of 43 total patients.[5,13,26] In this cohort, there were 2 delayed unions, 8 cases of stiffness or extensor tendon lag, and 1 case of CRPS. Range of motion and grip strength also returned to functional levels.
- In two studies evaluating fixation to either metacarpal without stratifying results based on which metacarpal was used, 177 patients were assessed.[9,25] Range of motion and grip strength improved, but 4 patients had wound healing complications, there were 5 hardware failures, 2 malunions, 2 nonunions, 2 deep infections, 12 cases of stiffness, 1 EPL rupture, 1 transient superficial radial neuritis, and 1 case of CRPS.
- The authors of each of these studies propose that bridge plating allows fracture reduction and fixation over a broad metadiaphyseal area while effectively diverting compression forces away from the fracture site.
- The use of bridge plating in the treatment of distal radius fractures avoids some of the complications of external fixation. A bridge plate can remain implanted for extended periods without the potential for increased risks of infection. Plate or screw failure with an extended duration of plate retention is possible, but most hardware failures occur after fracture healing, at an average of 10 months after surgery.[9] In patients with multiple traumatic injuries, bridge plating may allow earlier postoperative load bearing across the affected wrist, especially with a stout plate that does not contain central holes.[12] Forearm weight bearing with a modified crutch or walker may also be used. This may enable independent transfers and the use of ambulatory aids. Application of bridge plates is simple, and surgical time is likely comparable with the application of an external fixator.
- It is important to educate patients on the need for hardware removal when spanning plates are used, as retained plates may break and lead to tendon injury.[16]

COMPLICATIONS

- The use of external fixation is often limited by pin site complications. Infection and loosening may necessitate earlier pin removal. There is a reported 50% to 62% complication rate associated with external fixation, most commonly loose pins, pin tract infection, digital stiffness, and malreduction.[28] Generally, the external fixator may be removed at the bedside without anesthesia or sedation.
- Bridge plate removal requires a second operative procedure and cannot be done in clinic. However, they can be removed easily with local anesthesia, with or without light sedation.
- Stiffness is commonly reported after external fixation and bridge plate fixation, often requiring tenolysis, particularly if excessive distraction is used.[9,28]
- Tendon entrapment, rupture, or adhesions are possible with bridge plate fixation (**FIG 1**).[17] There is a higher risk of tendon entrapment with fixation to the third metacarpal, with the finger extensors at risk at the level of the extensor retinaculum. For index finger metacarpal fixation, branches of the superficial radial nerve must be identified and protected distally.
- Fracture may result from using excessively large screws or external fixator pins, particularly in the metacarpal.
- Excessive distraction may lead to CRPS, especially if distraction exceeds 5 mm.[24]

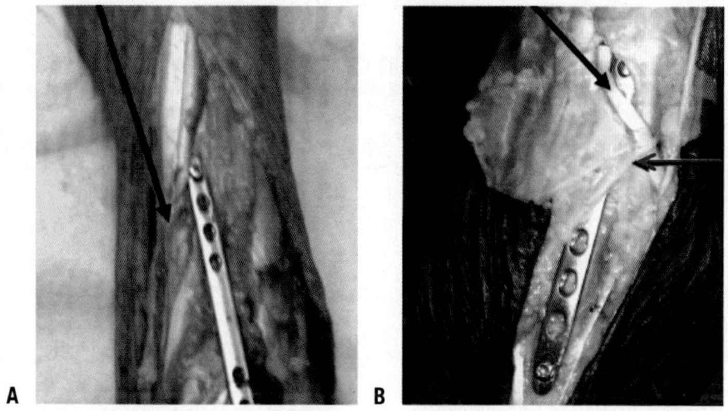

FIG 1 A. Plate to the third metacarpal demonstrating its position on top of the tendons of the first dorsal compartment (*arrow*). **B.** Plate to the second metacarpal demonstrating its position under the EPL (*black arrow*) and proximity to the terminal branches of the superficial radial nerve (*red arrow*).

REFERENCES

1. Alluri RK, Bougioukli S, Stevanovic M, et al. A biomechanical comparison of distal fixation for bridge plating in a distal radius fracture model. J Hand Surg Am 2017;42(9):748.e1–748.e8.
2. Alluri RK, Hill JR, Ghiassi A. Distal radius fractures: approaches, indications, and techniques. J Hand Surg Am 2016;41:845–854.
3. Azad A, Choi JT, Fisch R, et al. Wrist-spanning fixation of radiocarpal dislocation: a cadaveric assessment of ulnar translation [published online ahead of print September 13, 2019]. Hand (N Y). doi:10.1177/1558944719873148.
4. Brogan DM, Richard MJ, Ruch D, et al. Management of severely comminuted distal radius fractures. J Hand Surg Am 2015;40:1905–1914.
5. Burke EF, Singer RM. Treatment of comminuted distal radius with the use of an internal distraction plate. Tech Hand Up Extrem Surg 1998;2:248–252.
6. Chung KC, Kotsis SV, Kim HM. Predictors of functional outcomes after surgical treatment of distal radius fractures. J Hand Surg Am 2007;32:76–83.
7. Dodds SD, Save AV, Yacob A. Dorsal spanning plate fixation for distal radius fractures. Tech Hand Up Extrem Surg 2013;17:192–198.
8. Hanel DP, Lu TS, Weil WM. Bridge plating of distal radius fractures: the Harborview method. Clin Orthop Relat Res 2006;445:91–99.
9. Hanel DP, Ruhlman SD, Katolik LI, et al. Complications associated with distraction plate fixation of wrist fractures. Hand Clin 2010;26:237–243.
10. Hill JR, Alluri RK, Ghiassi A. Acute isolated flexor tendon laceration associated with a distal radius fracture. Hand (N Y) 2017;12:NP39–NP42.
11. Howard PW, Stewart HD, Hind RE, et al. External fixation or plaster for severely displaced comminuted Colles' fractures? A prospective study of anatomical and functional results. J Bone Joint Surg Br 1989;71:68–73.
12. Huang JI, Peterson B, Bellevue K, et al. Biomechanical assessment of the dorsal spanning bridge plate in distal radius fracture fixation: implications for immediate weight-bearing. Hand (N Y) 2018;13(3):336–340.
13. Jain MJ, Mavani KJ. A comprehensive study of internal distraction plating, an alternative method for distal radius fractures. J Clin Diagn Res 2016;10:RC14–RC17.
14. Lauder A, Agnew S, Bakri K, et al. Functional outcomes following bridge plate fixation for distal radius fractures. J Hand Surg Am 2015;40:1554–1562.
15. Lauder A, Hanel DP. Spanning bridge plate fixation of distal radius fractures. JBJS Rev 2017;5(2):01874474-201702000-00002.
16. Lefebvre R, Intravia J, Cao L, et al. Bridge plate failure with extensor tendon injury: a case report and literature review. Case Rep Orthop 2018;2018:3256891.
17. Lewis S, Mostofi A, Stevanovic M. Risk of tendon entrapment under a dorsal bridge plate in a distal radius fracture model. J Hand Surg Am 2015;40:500–504.
18. Lutz M, Arora R, Krappinger D, et al. Arthritis predicting factors in distal intraarticular radius fractures. Arch Orthop Trauma Surg 2011;131:1121–1126.
19. McQueen MM. Non-spanning external fixation of the distal radius. Hand Clin 2005;21:375–380.
20. Mellstrand-Navarro C, Ahrengart L, Törnqvist H, et al. Volar locking plate or external fixation with optional addition of K-wires for dorsally displaced distal radius fractures: a randomized controlled study. J Orthop Trauma 2016;30:217–224.
21. Mellstrand-Navarro C, Pettersson HJ, Tornqvist H, et al. The operative treatment of fractures of the distal radius is increasing: results from a nationwide Swedish study. Bone Joint J 2014;96-B:963–969.
22. Mulders MAM, Walenkamp MMJ, van Dieren S, et al. Volar plate fixation versus plaster immobilization in acceptably reduced extra-articular distal radial fractures: a multicenter randomized controlled trial. J Bone Joint Surg Am 2019;101:787–796.
23. O'Shaughnessy MA, Shin AY, Kakar S. Stabilization of volar ulnar rim fractures of the distal radius: current techniques and review of the literature. J Wrist Surg 2016;5:113–119.
24. Papadonikolakis A, Shen J, Garrett JP, et al. The effect of increasing distraction on digital motion after external fixation of the wrist. J Hand Surg Am 2005;30:773–779.
25. Richard MJ, Katolik LI, Hanel DP, et al. Distraction plating for the treatment of highly comminuted distal radius fractures in elderly patients. J Hand Surg Am 2012;37:948–956.
26. Ruch DS, Ginn TA, Yang CC, et al. Use of a distraction plate for distal radial fractures with metaphyseal and diaphyseal comminution. J Bone Joint Surg Am 2005;87:945–954.
27. Vakhshori V, Rounds AD, Heckmann N, et al. The declining use of wrist-spanning external fixators. Hand (N Y) 2020;15(2):255–263.
28. Weber SC, Szabo RM. Severely comminuted distal radial fracture as an unsolved problem: complications associated with external fixation and pins and plaster techniques. J Hand Surg Am 1986;11:157–165.
29. Weil WM, Trumble TE. Treatment of distal radius fractures with intrafocal (Kapandji) pinning and supplemental skeletal stabilization. Hand Clin 2005;21:317–328.
30. Wolf JC, Weil WM, Hanel DP, et al. A biomechanic comparison of an internal radiocarpal-spanning 2.4-mm locking plate and external fixation in a model of distal radius fractures. J Hand Surg Am 2006;31:1578–1586.

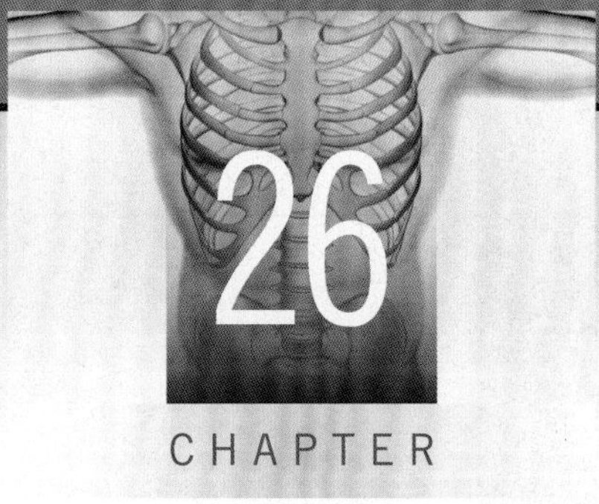

Open Treatment of Radiocarpal Fracture-Dislocations

Michael U. Okoli and Asif M. Ilyas

DEFINITION

- The radiocarpal joint's stability is provided by the carpal articulation at the scaphoid and lunate fossae as well as the soft tissue restraints of the capsule and extrinsic radiocarpal ligaments.
- Radiocarpal dislocations occur through a traumatic separation of the proximal carpal row from the articular surface of the distal radius.
- Radiocarpal dislocations can occur in either a volar or dorsal direction, with the most common direction being dorsal.
- Radiocarpal dislocations can occur with only soft tissue disruption or, more commonly, in association with marginal rim fractures of the distal radius or ulnar styloid.
- Radiocarpal dislocations are often confused with distal radius fractures of the marginal rim or volar/dorsal shear fractures (ie, "Barton" fractures) **(FIG 1)**.
  - Radiocarpal dislocations represent a shear or avulsion injury of the wrist that may or may not be associated with an avulsion fracture of the distal radius or ulna **(FIG 1A)**.
  - Barton fractures of the distal radius represent compression and/or shear fractures **(FIG 1B)**.

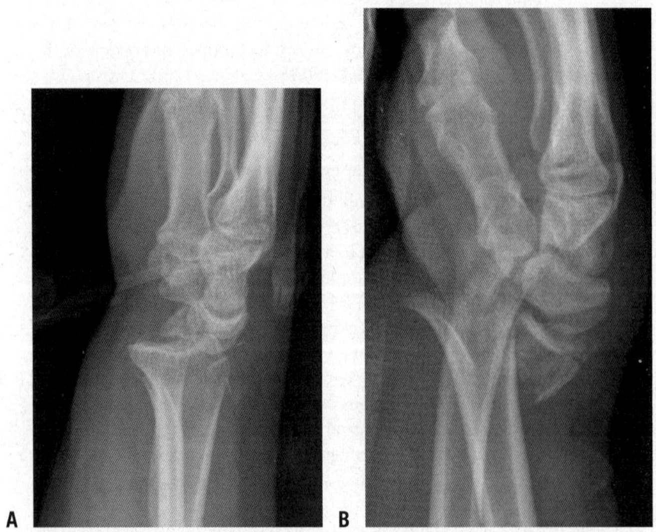

FIG 1 Radiocarpal dislocations can be confused with shear fractures of the distal radius. **A.** Note the disruption of the carpus from the distal radius in this lateral view of a radiocarpal fracture-dislocation. **B.** In contrast, note in this lateral view of this distal radius fracture that the relationship between the carpus and distal radial articular surface is maintained.

- Two classification systems are typically used to describe radiocarpal dislocations.
  - Moneim et al[12] classified radiocarpal dislocations based on the presence or absence of an intercarpal ligament injury.
    - Type 1 dislocations do not have an associated intercarpal injury.
    - Type 2 injuries are associated with a concomitant scapholunate ligament.[12]
  - Dumontier et al[4] classified radiocarpal dislocations based on the presence or absence of an associated avulsion fracture off the radial styloid.
    - Type 1 injuries are considered purely ligamentous with minimal cortical avulsion off the radial styloid.
    - Type 2 injuries are associated with a large radial styloid fracture compromising of at least one-third of the scaphoid fossa.[4]

ANATOMY

- The average arc of motion in a normal wrist ranges from 68 degrees of flexion to 50 degrees of extension.[9]
- Radiocarpal joint stability is provided by both the osseous joint articulation between the scaphoid and lunate bones and their corresponding fossae of the distal radius, along with the extrinsic radiocarpal ligaments and the wrist capsule **(FIG 2)**.
- Among the various volar radiocarpal ligaments, the primary ligaments important to radiocarpal stability are the short radiolunate and the radioscaphocapitate ligaments.
  - The short radiolunate ligament originates from the stout margin of the lunate facet of the volar distal radius and serves as the primary restraint against volar translation of the carpus.
  - The stout radioscaphocapitate ligament originates from the radial styloid and resists ulnar translation of the carpus.
- The ulnocarpal ligaments, including the ulnolunate and the ulnotriquetral ligaments, take their origin from the ulnar styloid. Along with the triangular fibrocartilage complex (TFCC), they assist in providing radiocarpal and ulnocarpal joint stability.
- The dorsal radiocarpal ligaments are highly variable[11] and also assist in imparting stability to the radiocarpal joint, although to a much lesser extent than the volar radiocarpal ligaments.

PATHOGENESIS

- Radiocarpal dislocations can occur in either a volar or dorsal direction, with dorsal being far more common (~85%).[4]
- The injury requires pronation and hyperextension of the wrist with a shear force across the joint. With increasing amounts of supination, the risk of a perilunate dislocation rather than a radiocarpal dislocation increases.[10]

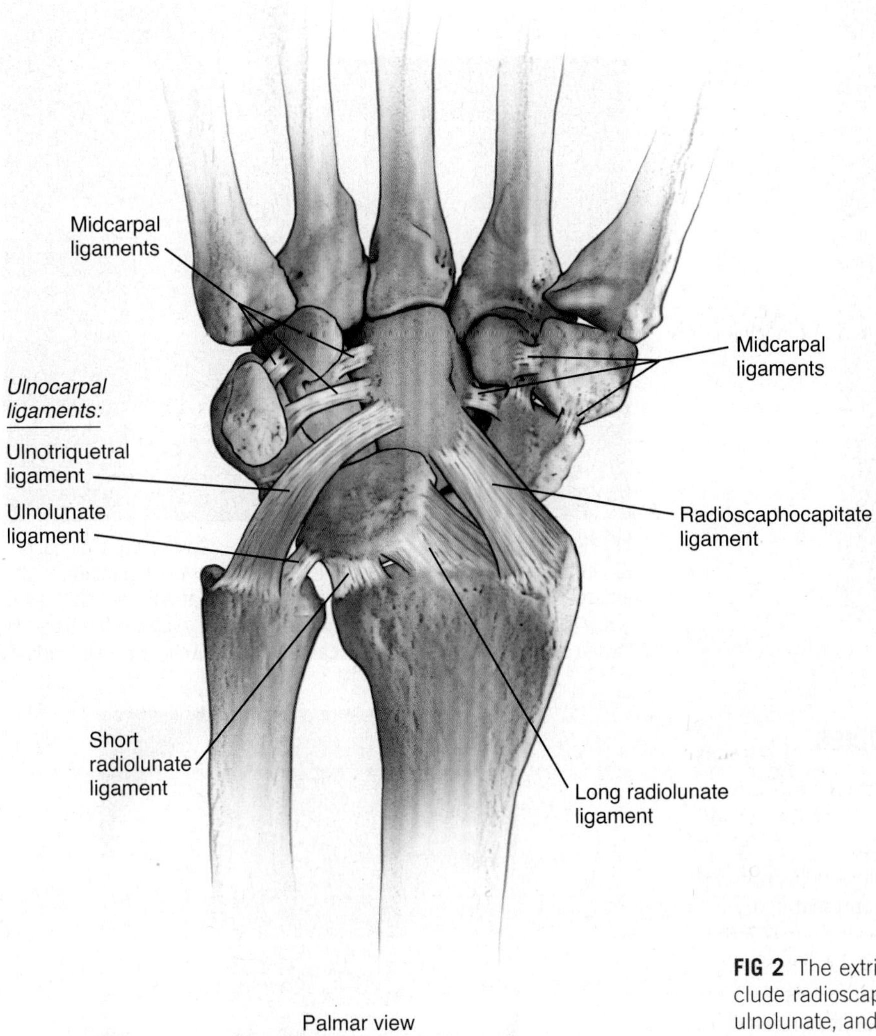

FIG 2 The extrinsic volar radiocarpal ligaments of the wrist include radioscaphocapitate, long radiolunate, short radiolunate, ulnolunate, and ulnotriquetral ligaments.

- Disruption of the radiocarpal ligaments, the most critical of which are the radioscaphocapitate and the short radiolunate, is necessary to dislocate the radiocarpal joint.
- A pure dislocation without a bony injury is less common. More often, a fracture of the radial styloid, volar marginal rim, or ulnar styloid is identified representing an avulsion of the origin of the radioscaphocapitate, short radiolunate, or ulnocarpal ligaments, respectively.

NATURAL HISTORY

- Radiocarpal dislocations are high-energy injuries most often seen in males aged 20 to 40 years.[4,8]
- Mechanisms of injury are typically falls from a height, industrial injuries, and motor vehicle accidents.
- The incidence of radiocarpal dislocations has been published to be as low as 0.2% of all hand and wrist dislocations.[5] More recent studies have found incidence of radiocarpal dislocations to be as high as 2.7% of all distal radius fractures and wrist dislocations.[8]
- Due to the high-energy nature of these injuries, there is a high association of associated injuries including neurologic injuries, vascular injuries, and open wounds.[1,4,12]
- Residual radiocarpal instability and posttraumatic wrist degeneration is common, particularly with purely ligamentous injuries (Dumontier type 1).[4]

PATIENT HISTORY AND PHYSICAL FINDINGS

- Radiocarpal dislocations typically present with a very swollen and painful wrist, with likely deformity **(FIG 3)**.
- Physical examination should include a thorough neurologic, vascular, and tendon examination.
  - Neurologic deficits, particularly of the median nerve, are common with displaced radiocarpal dislocations.
  - Vascular embarrassment to the hand may occur with prolonged displacement and swelling.
  - Incarceration of the dorsal extensor tendons can occur pre- and postreduction.
- Close inspection of the skin should also be performed, as open wounds can also be present possibly signifying an open arthrotomy of the wrist or an associated open fracture.[15]
- A full secondary survey is mandatory, as these injuries are typically high-energy and may be associated with concomitant fractures of other limbs and visceral injuries,[13] which have been reported to occur in 58% and 37% of cases, respectively.[4]

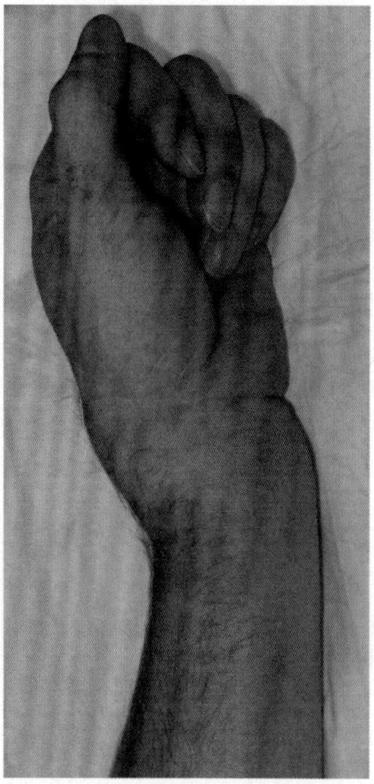

FIG 3 Typical deformity following a dorsally displaced radiocarpal dislocation.

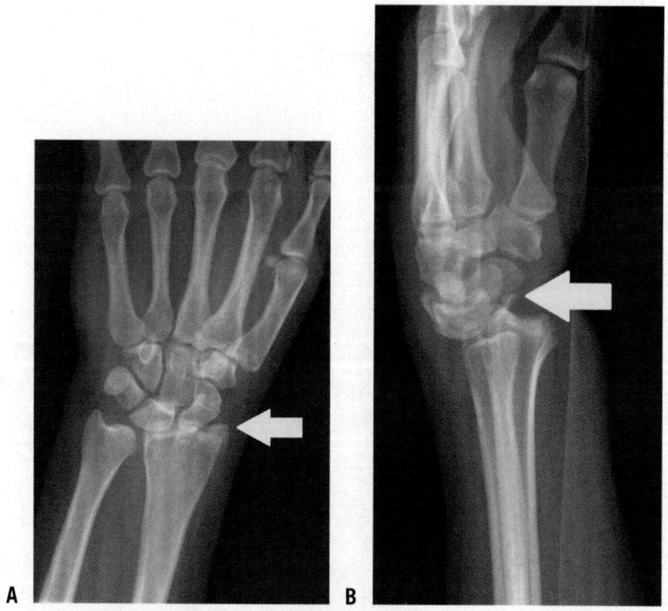

FIG 4 Anteroposterior and lateral views of a radiocarpal dislocation. **A.** On the anteroposterior view, note the *yellow arrow* is pointing to the avulsed fracture of the radial styloid. **B.** On the lateral view, the *yellow arrow* is pointing to a volar radiocarpal ligament avulsion fracture following disruption of the proximal carpal row relative to the distal radius.

IMAGING AND OTHER DIAGNOSTIC STUDIES

- Evaluation should begin with plain radiographs including a posteroanterior and lateral views of the wrist **(FIG 4)**. Additional oblique views can help in assessment.
  - On the lateral view, the radiograph should be scrutinized for the alignment of the arcs of Gilula, representing the relationship between the midcarpal and radiocarpal joints. Disruption between the lunate and the distal radius signifies a radiocarpal disruption, whereas disruption between the capitate and lunate may represent a perilunate injury **(FIG 5)**.
  - On the posteroanterior view, the radiograph should be scrutinized for associated avulsion fractures of the distal radius or ulna, ulnar translation of the carpus relative to the distal radius, and intercarpal diastasis.
- Computed tomography (CT) may be helpful in identifying marginal rim fractures and to further evaluate intra-articular fracture patterns **(FIG 6)**.
- Magnetic resonance imaging (MRI) is useful in evaluating the soft tissue stabilizers of the radiocarpal joint. In addition, MRI can provide better evaluation of associated injuries such as to the intercarpal ligaments and TFCC.

DIFFERENTIAL DIAGNOSIS

- Colles fracture
- Smith fracture
- Barton fracture
- Perilunate dislocation

NONOPERATIVE MANAGEMENT

- Surgical repair is indicated for all displaced radiocarpal dislocations. Uniformly poor outcomes have been shown with nonoperative management and minimal repair techniques due to the high risk of persistent radiocarpal instability and resulting posttraumatic degeneration.[2]

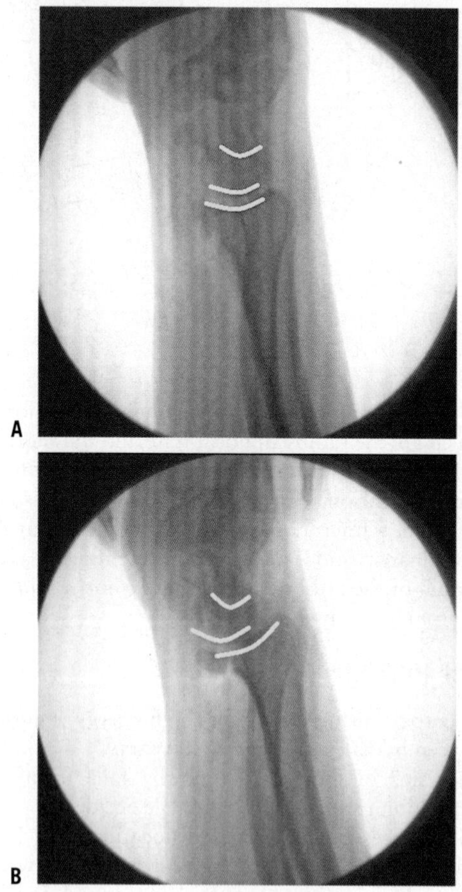

FIG 5 The arcs of Gilula represent the "cup-shaped" (*yellow lines*) alignment of the capitates, lunate, and distal radial articular surfaces on the lateral view. **A.** When the wrist is reduced, the "cups" stack up symmetrically. **B.** When the radiocarpal joint is subluxated or dislocated, as is the case with this radiocarpal dislocation with an associated volar marginal rim fracture, the cups will not be aligned.

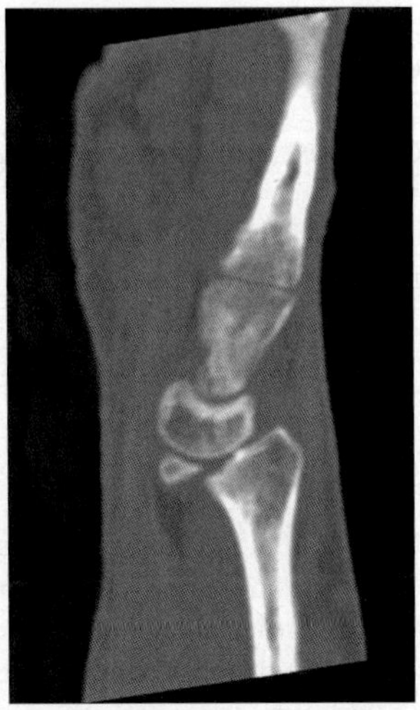

FIG 6 CT image provide detailed characterization of a marginal rim fracture and subluxated radiocarpal joint.

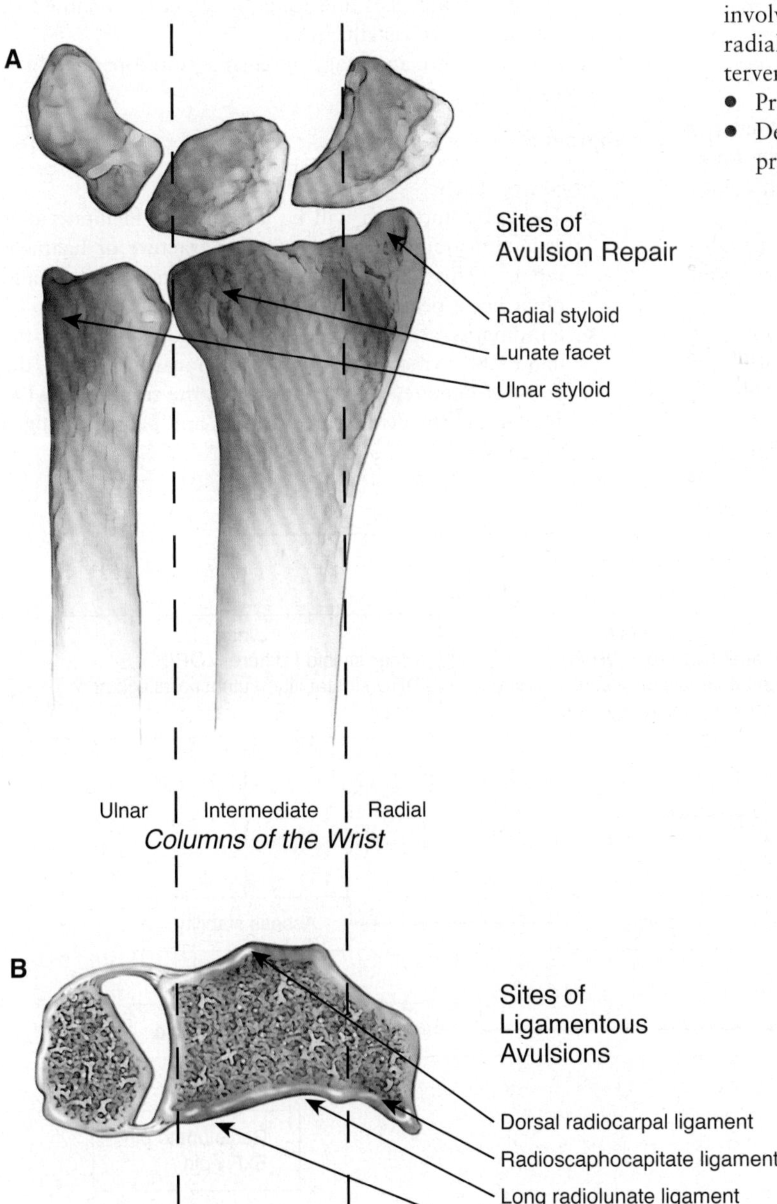

FIG 7 A,B. The three columns of the wrist including the radial, intermediate, and ulnar columns. Each column consists of respective bone, joint, and ligaments.

SURGICAL MANAGEMENT

- Successful management of radiocarpal dislocations is dependent on achieving concentric joint reduction and ligament or fracture repair to restore stability.
- Although we recommend routine operative treatment for all cases of radiocarpal dislocations due to their inherent instability, the following are absolute indications for surgery:
  - Open injuries
  - Injuries with neurovascular compromise
  - Irreducible dislocations
- Timing of surgery depends on the ability to achieve a provisional closed radiocarpal reduction, soft tissue status, and neurovascular function.
- Successful management of radiocarpal dislocations requires adherence to three treatment principles:
  - Concentric, stable reduction of the radiocarpal joint
  - Repair of intercarpal ligament injuries, if present
  - Repair of extrinsic ligament avulsion injuries
- Preoperative planning should take into account the presence of any intercarpal ligament injuries and the extent of involvement of the three columns of the wrist including the radial, intermediate, and ulnar columns **(FIG 7)**. Surgical intervention should then follow a stepwise approach:
  - Provisional reduction of the radiocarpal joint
  - Decompression of the median nerve, if paresthesias are present

- Joint exposure and débridement
- Repair of intercarpal ligament injury, if present
- Repair or fracture fixation of extrinsic ligamentous avulsion injuries
- Confirmation of reduction and stability of the three columns of the wrist
- Neutralization of the wrist with a temporary external fixator or bridge plate

- When approaching step 5, repair or fracture fixation of extrinsic ligamentous injuries, the three columns of the wrist should be approached in a stepwise order and associated fractures and ligamentous injuries repaired to restore radiocarpal stability **(FIG 8)**.
  - Radial column
    - Radial styloid fracture
    - Radioscaphocapitate ligament injury
  - Intermediate column
    - Lunate facet fracture
    - Short radiolunate ligament injury
  - Ulnar column
    - Ulnar styloid fracture
    - Ulnocarpal ligament injury

Preoperative Planning

- As these are typically young individuals with a high-energy injuries, patients should be counseled regarding the long-term risk of developing posttraumatic arthritis. Those with intercarpal ligament injuries are at higher risk.
- Standard and traction radiographs may be useful in evaluating for radiocarpal alignment, associated fractures, and intercarpal ligament injuries.
- Consider advanced imaging in the form of CT scanning for better fracture characterization or MRI scanning for better intercarpal and extrinsic ligament injury visualization.
- Necessary equipment to have available include suture anchors, Kirschner wires, small fragment or modular hand set, distal radius plating system, external fixator set, tension band materials, arthroscopy equipment, and bone graft/substitutes.
- Arthroscopy can assist in evaluating the extent of ligament and cartilage injury.
  - Use arthroscopy with caution, as excessive extravasation of fluid may occur due to the underlying capsular injury.
- Surgical repair may require use of several approaches to the wrist, including volar extensile and radial and dorsal approaches **(FIG 9)**.

Positioning

- Axillary or interscalene block anesthesia is helpful for muscle relaxation as well as postoperative pain control. General anesthesia is recommended over monitored anesthesia care.
- The patient is positioned supine on the operating table with the operative extremity extended on a radiolucent hand table. This allows for adequate pronation/supination in order to access both the dorsal and volar surfaces of the wrist.
- Tourniquet hemostasis and loupe magnification should be used to maximize visualization.
- Ready access to an image intensifier intraoperatively is necessary.

Approach

- Volar approach[7]
  - The volar approach will be indicated to facilitate joint reduction, joint débridement, and fracture or ligament repairs. This approach will also facilitate median and ulnar nerve decompression, if necessary.
  - Landmarks are identified on the volar surface of the hand and wrist, including Kaplan cardinal line, the hook of hamate, the thenar crease, the transverse wrist crease, and the flexor carpi radialis and palmaris longus tendons.

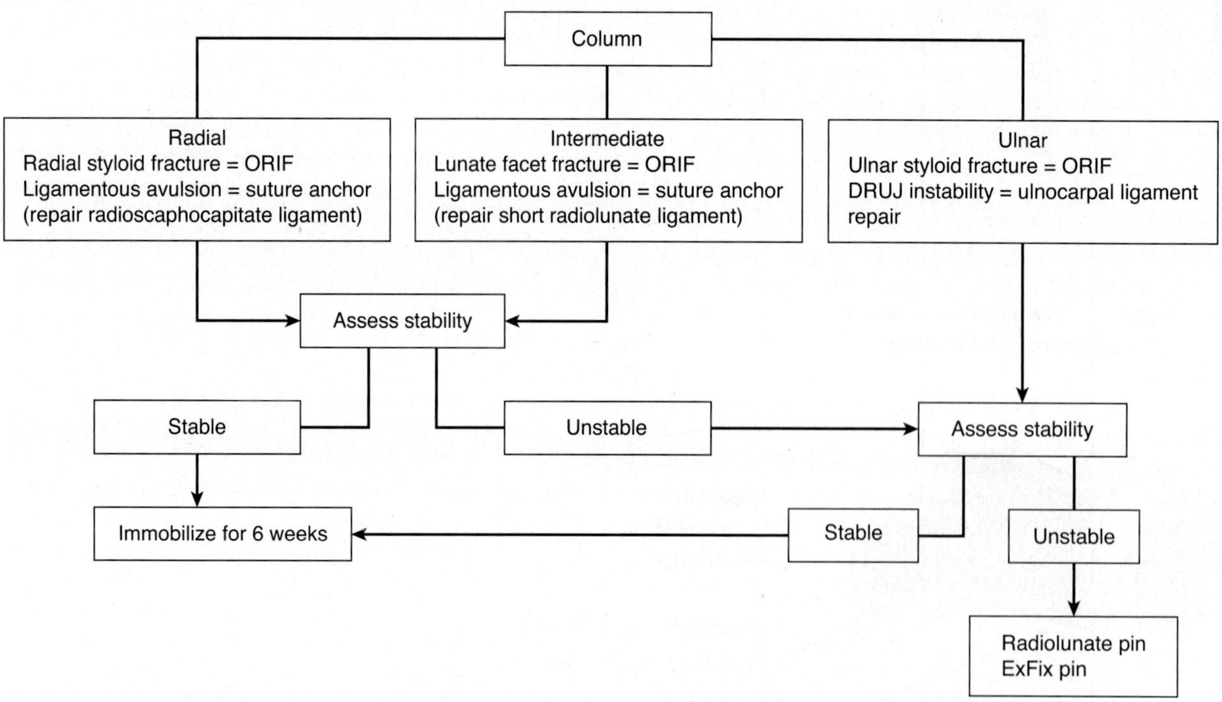

FIG 8 Algorithm for repair of the columns of the wrist. *ORIF*, open reduction internal fixation; *DRUJ*, distal radioulnar joint; *ExFix*, external fixator.

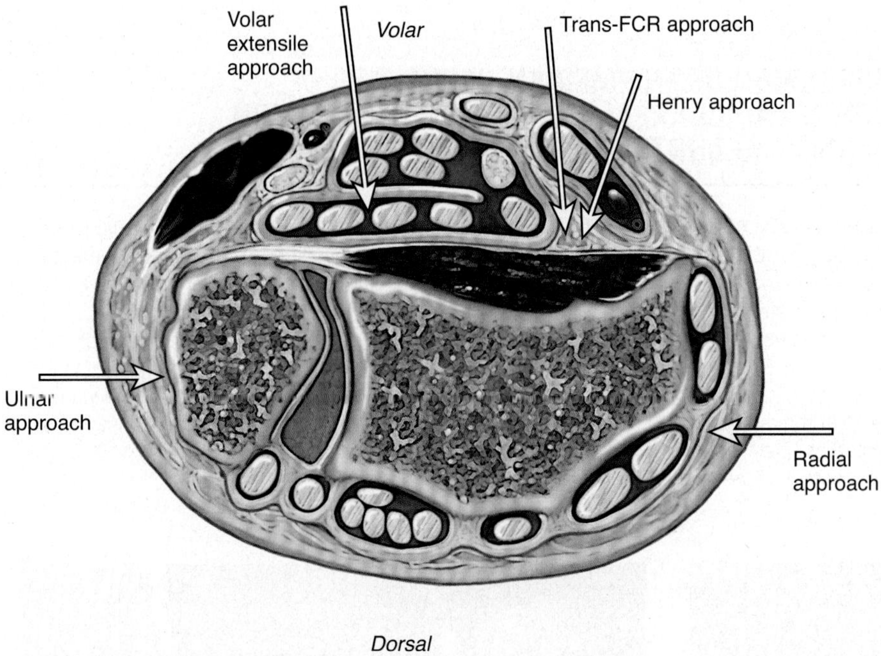

FIG 9 Multiple approaches to the wrist are possible including ulnar, between the extensor and flexor carpi ulnaris tendons; radial, between the extensor pollicis brevis and extensor carpi radialis longus tendons; the distal extent of the approach of Henry, between the flexor carpi radialis (*FCR*) tendon and radial artery; the trans-FCR approach; and the volar extensile approach, that is developed between the palmaris longus and flexor carpi ulnaris tendons. In the extensile approach, the median nerve and finger flexor tendons are taken radially and the ulnar neurovascular structures are taken ulnarly.

- The standard volar approach can be performed through the floor of the flexor carpi radialis tendon or through the distal extent of Henry approach between the radial artery and the brachioradialis tendon (see **FIG 9**). Elevation of the distal extent of the pronator quadratus may be necessary to maximize exposure of the avulsed radiocarpal ligaments or fractures.
- An extensile volar approach to the wrist may be used beginning ulnar to the thenar eminence and extending proximally ulnar to the contents of the carpal tunnel (see **FIG 9**). This allows for access and decompression to both Guyon canal and the carpal tunnel. To expose the volar capsule, the median nerve and flexor tendons are retracted radially, and the ulnar neurovascular structures are retracted ulnarly.

- Radial approach[7]
  - The radial approach is indicated for radial-sided fracture and ligament repairs.
  - Landmark is the radial styloid.
  - A longitudinal incision is made directly over the radial styloid. Great care must be taken to avoid injury to branches of the radial sensory nerve. The radial styloid and origin of the radioscaphocapitate ligament can be found deep to and between the first and second dorsal compartments.
- Dorsal approach[7]
  - The dorsal approach is indicated for intercarpal ligament injury repair and to facilitate joint reduction and débridement.
  - Landmarks include the radial and ulnar styloids and Lister tubercle.
  - A longitudinal incision is made just ulnar to Lister tubercle, crossing the dorsal wrist crease. The extensor retinaculum is identified, and the capsule is exposed between the third and fourth compartments. The extensor pollicis longus tendon in the third compartment is left in place unless more exposure is necessary, and then the tendon may be fully released from its compartment and retracted radially to expose the dorsal cortex of the distal radius.
  - Joint arthrotomy should be done with care as to not cause an iatrogenic intercarpal ligament injury.
- Ulnar approach[7]
  - The ulnar approach is indicated for repair of the ulnar styloid, TFCC, or ulnocarpal ligaments.
  - Landmark is the ulnar styloid.
  - A longitudinal incision is made over the ulnar styloid. Care is taken not to injure any branches of the dorsal ulnar sensory nerve. The ulnar styloid can be found deep or volar to the extensor carpi ulnaris tendon.

VOLAR EXPOSURE FOR DECOMPRESSION OF THE MEDIAN NERVE, IDENTIFICATION OF THE DISRUPTED RADIOCARPAL LIGAMENTS OR AVULSION FRACTURES, AND PROVISIONAL JOINT REDUCTION AND DÉBRIDEMENT

- If decompression of the median nerve is deemed necessary, an extensile volar approach to the wrist may be used that will facilitate both complete decompression of the median nerve as well as access to the radial and intermediate columns of the wrist. Alternatively, a standard volar approach can be used **(TECH FIG 1)**.
- Following exposure of the volar wrist, soft tissue avulsion and/or marginal rim fractures will be encountered at the radiocarpal joint level **(TECH FIG 1B)**. Their elevation will allow direct visualization of the joint and identification of impaction injury and/or articular defects.
- The joint should be provisionally reduced and thoroughly irrigated and débrided of any loose bone or cartilage fragments.
  - Displaced and incarcerated intra-articular fragments can potentially block concentric reduction.
- Stay sutures are placed in the ends of the disrupted radiocarpal ligaments and wrist capsule but not initially sewn down. Once the intercarpal ligament injuries have been addressed via the dorsal side, as indicated, the volar capsular avulsions will be repaired last via direct repair or suture anchors.

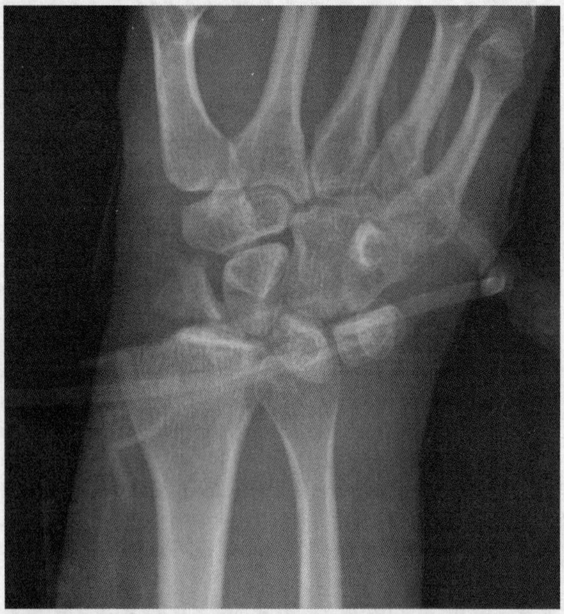

A

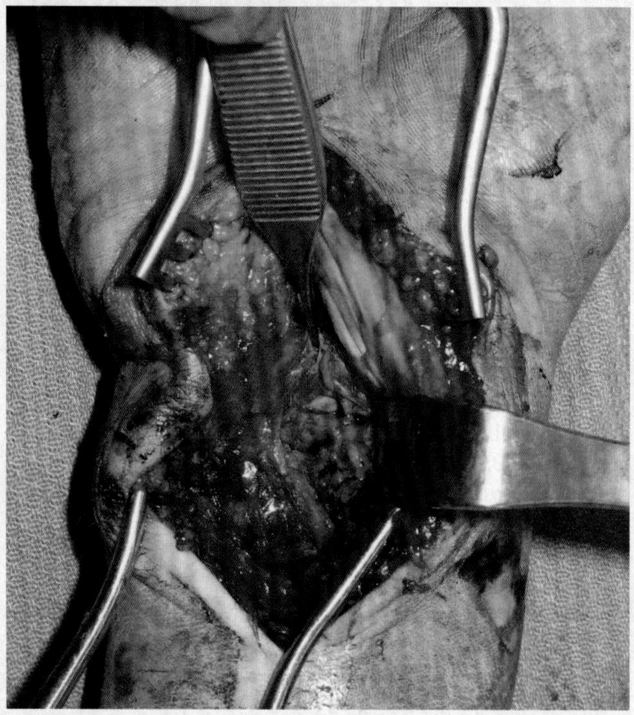

B

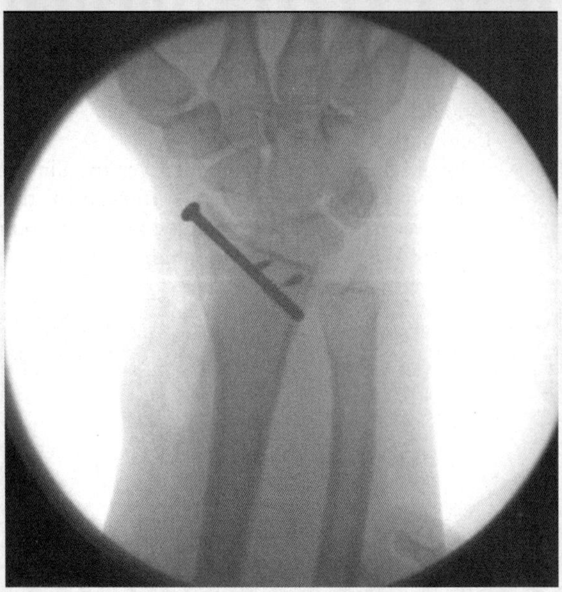

C

TECH FIG 1 **A.** Radiocarpal dislocation, displaced dorsally with a radial styloid avulsion fracture. **B.** Exposure through a volar extensile approach demonstrating the avulsed radiocarpal ligaments. **C.** Repair consisted of radial styloid internal fixation to stabilize the radial column and suture anchor repair of the intermediate column's avulsed volar radiocarpal ligaments.

DORSAL EXPOSURE AND INTERCARPAL LIGAMENT STABILIZATION

- If intercarpal ligament injuries are present requiring repair, they should be approached through a separate dorsal incision and repaired definitively prior to returning volar.
- In addition, the dorsal approach to the wrist can facilitate joint exposure, débridement, and reduction.
- If necessary, the dorsal approach can also allow for repair of the avulsed dorsal capsule. Stay sutures can be placed in the avulsed capsule and repaired to the dorsal cortex of the distal radius with suture anchors. Alternatively, if large dorsal marginal rim avulsion fractures are present, they can similarly be repaired with any internal fixation of choice.

RADIAL COLUMN

- Fractures of the radial styloid are common and require diligent anatomic reduction and stable fixation.
  - Smaller styloid fragments can be stabilized with suture anchors.
  - Screw fixation is preferable when the fragments are of adequate size.
  - Larger radial styloid fragments may be amenable to radial plate fixation.
  - Volar plating can also be used to repair a radial styloid fracture. However, volar plate fixation of the styloid may be tenuous, as it is at a mechanical disadvantage to counter the shear stress that a radiocarpal dislocation will place on the radial styloid fragment. Therefore, compression fixation with a screw or radial plate is preferable **(TECH FIG 1C)**.
- When a radial styloid fracture fragment is not present, avulsion of the radioscaphocapitate ligament must be suspected and repaired to its footprint on the radial styloid with suture anchors.

CENTRAL COLUMN

- Fractures of the lunate facet are common and must be precisely repaired if amenable. Fixation options include screws, tension band,[3] or hook plates. Alternatively, a volar plate may be applied to serve as a buttress but must be used with care and placed adequately distal to fully buttress and reduce the lunate facet fracture **(TECH FIG 2)**.
- Lunate facet fracture reduction may be facilitated with provisional pinning of the radiolunate articulation. The pin, however, should be removed at the end of the procedure.
- In cases of small lunate facet avulsion fractures or exclusively soft tissue avulsion of the volar wrist capsule, repair of the capsule and short radiolunate with suture anchors placed in the volar distal radius should be performed to recreate the volar capsular buttress.

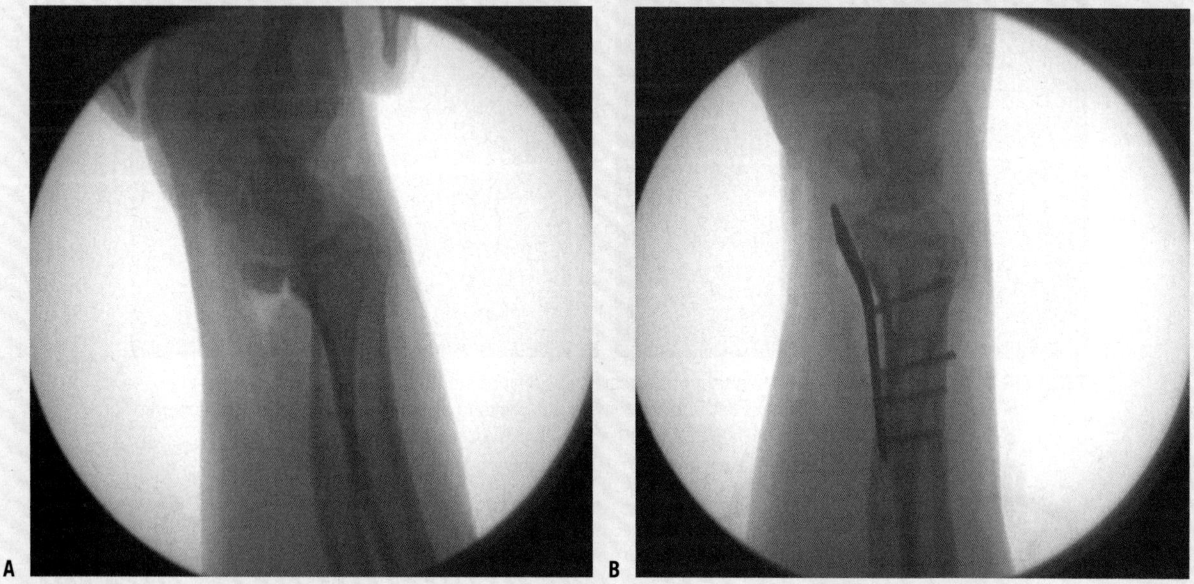

TECH FIG 2 A,B. Buttress plate fixation of a radiocarpal dislocation with an associated volar rim marginal rim fracture.

ULNAR COLUMN

- Indicators of potential ulnar column instability include an associated large ulnar styloid base fracture, distal radioulnar joint instability on examination, or MRI findings consistent with peripheral tear of the TFCC and/or injury to the ulnolunate or ulnotriquetral ligaments.
- We recommend routine repair of large ulnar styloid fragments using either a screw or tension band construct.
- If the ulnar column remains unstable after styloid fixation, repair of the ulnocarpal ligaments should also be considered.

EVALUATION OF WRIST STABILITY

- Upon repair of the columns of the wrist and intercarpal ligament injuries, the operative wrist should be gently taken through a full range of motion under fluoroscopy. Any residual wrist instability should be addressed to avoid poor long-term outcomes.
- If additional stabilization is deemed necessary, consider temporary use of an external fixator or an internal bridge plate **(TECH FIG 3)**.

A B

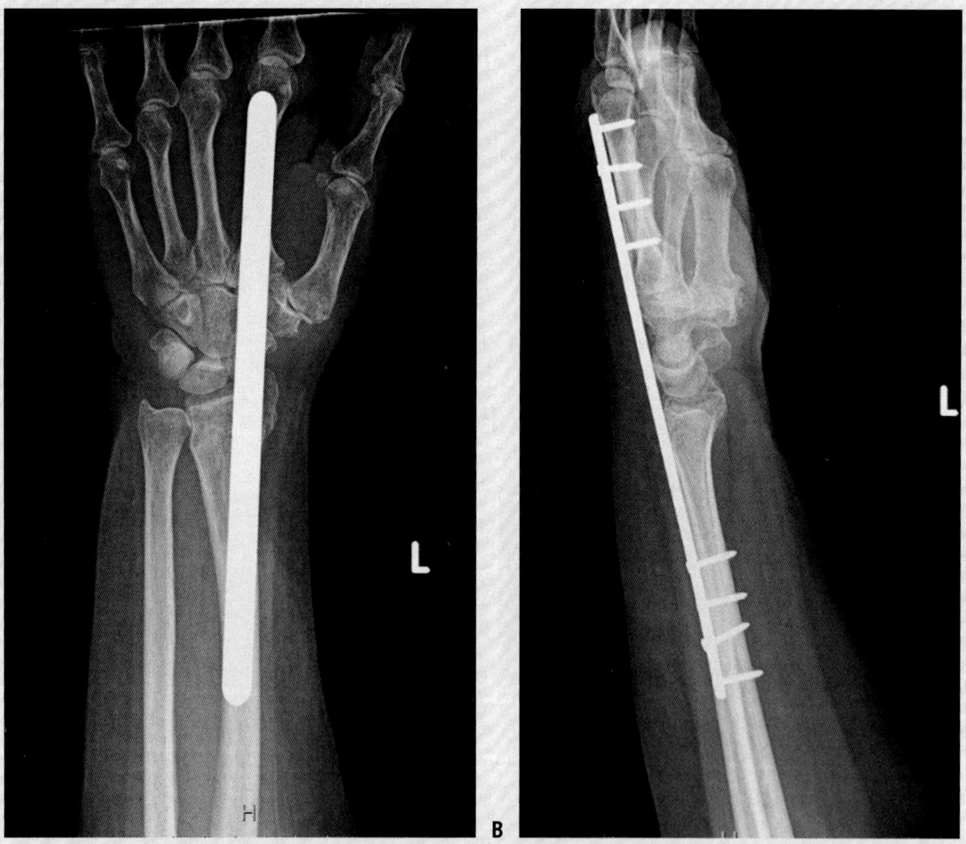

TECH FIG 3 A,B. Neutralization of a soft tissue radiocarpal dislocation neutralized with a temporary bridge plate after soft tissue repair. The plate is left in place for 8 to 12 weeks to allow the soft tissue to heal, followed by staged removal.

Pearls and Pitfalls

Diagnosis	• These are high-energy injuries with other extremity fractures or head and visceral organ injuries. • In the setting of a prolonged unreduced dorsal radiocarpal dislocation, the risk of median neuropathy and acute carpal tunnel syndrome increases.
Imaging	• These injuries can be missed on radiographs when not associated with a fracture or confused with a distal radius fracture if the radiographic alignment of the radiocarpal joint is not scrutinized. • CT scan may be helpful in assessing marginal rim and articular fractures. • MRI scan may be helpful in assessing concomitant intercarpal ligament and TFCC injuries.
Surgical Management	• Use a stepwise approach: • Provisional reduction of the radiocarpal joint • Decompression of the median nerve, if paresthesias are present • Joint exposure and débridement • Repair of intercarpal ligament injury, if present • Repair or fracture fixation of extrinsic ligamentous avulsion injuries of all three columns of the wrist • Confirmation of reduction and stability of the three columns of the wrist

POSTOPERATIVE CARE

- Unlike with standard distal radius fractures, where postoperative motion is often initiated early, secure immobilization for a minimum of 6 weeks following radiocarpal dislocation repair is recommended to allow sufficient soft tissue healing.
- Once satisfied with maintenance of concentric radiocarpal joint reduction, protected range of motion can be initiated after 6 weeks under the supervision of a therapist.
- It is highly recommended to inform the patient early that some permanent loss of motion in the flexion–extension arc is to be anticipated.
  - Expect a 30% to 50% loss of total wrist motion.

OUTCOMES

- Limited long-term data exists in the literature specific to radiocarpal dislocations.
- A number of small retrospective series have reported a range of outcomes generally consisting of decreased range of motion and mild pain at short-term follow-up.[4] Range of motion in the flexion–extension arc generally decreases by 30% to 40%.[8] Secondary radiocarpal instability, including late volar and ulnar translation, was seen with inadequate soft tissue or fracture repairs.[4]
- Marginal rim fractures and intercarpal injuries are indicative of poor outcome,[12,16] as are open injuries and those with neurovascular complications.[15]
- Pure ligamentous injuries demonstrated inferior outcomes relative to fracture-dislocation variants.[4]
- Posttraumatic arthritis was seen in 11% to 25% of cases at final follow-up.[4,6,14] The presence of late arthritic changes was generally attributed to residual radiocarpal instability or the presence of concomitant intercarpal ligament injury. Reconstruction of concomitant intercarpal instability has shown to have improved patient reported outcomes.[17]

COMPLICATIONS

- Complications can be separated into preoperative, early postoperative, and late postoperative.
- In the preoperative setting, sources of complication include open wounds, infection, and neurovascular embarrassment including acute carpal tunnel syndrome. These can be minimized with aggressive management of open wounds and early provisional joint reduction.
- In the early postoperative setting, complications can arise from persistent radiocarpal instability or frank dislocation due to inadequate repair and possibly associated persistent median neuropathy **(FIG 10)**.
- In the late postoperative setting, complications can include stiffness, decreased range of motion, decreased strength, posttraumatic degeneration, and hardware-related soft tissue irritation.

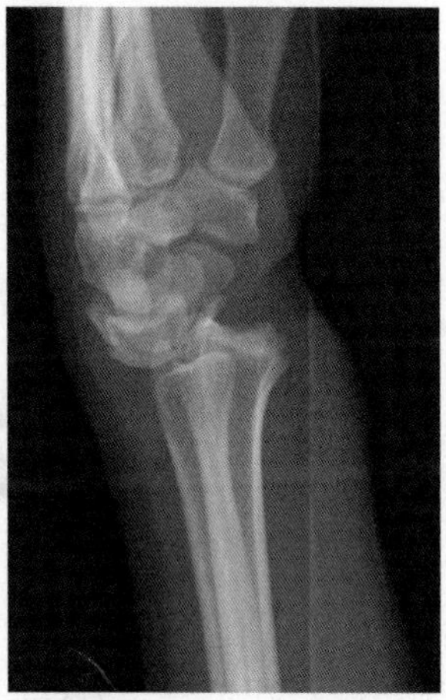

A

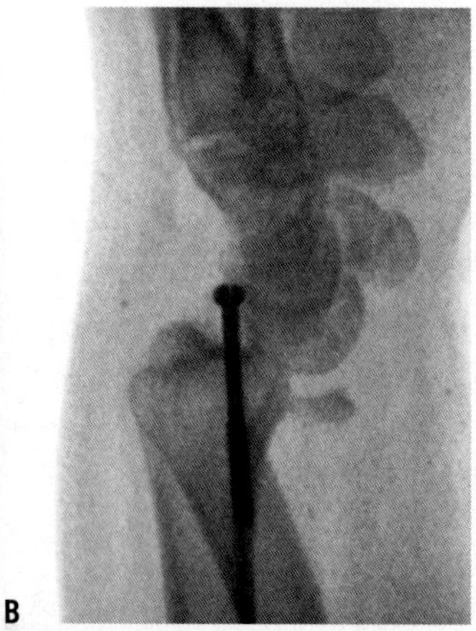

B

FIG 10 A,B. This is a case of a radiocarpal dislocation treated by repair of the radial column alone with radial styloid fixation but without repair of the intermediate and ulnar columns and resultant failure.

REFERENCES

1. Bilos ZJ, Pankovich AM, Yelda S. Fracture-dislocation of the radiocarpal joint. J Bone Joint Surg Am 1977;59(2):198–203.
2. Brown D, Mulligan MT, Uhl RL. Volar ligament repair for radiocarpal fracture-dislocation. Orthopedics 2013;36(6):463–468.
3. Chin KR, Jupiter JB. Wire-loop fixation of volar displaced osteochondral fractures of the distal radius. J Hand Surg Am 1999;24(3):525–533.
4. Dumontier C, Meyer zu Reckendorf G, Sautet A, et al. Radiocarpal dislocations: classification and proposal for treatment. A review of twenty-seven cases. J Bone Joint Surg Am 2001;83(2):212–218.
5. Dunn AW. Fractures and dislocations of the carpus. Surg Clin North Am 1972;52(6):1513–1538.

6. Girard J, Cassagnaud X, Maynou C, et al. Radiocarpal dislocation: twelve cases and a review of the literature [in French]. Rev Chir Orthop Reparatrice Appar Mot 2004;90(5):426–433.
7. Ilyas AM. Surgical approaches to the distal radius. Hand (N Y) 2011;6(1):8–17.
8. Ilyas AM, Williamson C, Mudgal CS. Radiocarpal dislocation: is it a rare injury? J Hand Surg Eur Vol 2011;36(2):164–165.
9. Kaufmann RA, Pfaeffle HJ, Blankenhorn BD, et al. Kinematics of the midcarpal and radiocarpal joint in flexion and extension: an in vitro study. J Hand Surg Am 2006;31(7):1142–1148.
10. Mayfield JK, Johnson RP, Kilcoyne RK. Carpal dislocations: pathomechanics and progressive perilunar instability. J Hand Surg Am 1980;5(3):226–241.
11. Mizuseki T, Ikuta Y. The dorsal carpal ligaments: their anatomy and function. J Hand Surg Br 1989;14(1):91–98.
12. Moneim MS, Bolger JT, Omer GE. Radiocarpal dislocation—classification and rationale for management. Clin Orthop Relat Res 1985;(192):199–209.
13. Mourikis A, Rebello G, Villafuerte J, et al. Radiocarpal dislocations: review of the literature with case presentations and a proposed treatment algorithm. Orthopedics 2008;31(4):386–392.
14. Mudgal CS, Psenica J, Jupiter JB. Radiocarpal fracture-dislocation. J Hand Surg Br 1999;24(1):92–98.
15. Nyquist SR, Stern PJ. Open radiocarpal fracture-dislocations. J Hand Surg Am 1984;9(5):707–710.
16. Spiry C, Bacle G, Marteau E, et al. Radiocarpal dislocations and fracture-dislocations: injury types and long-term outcomes. Orthop Traumatol Surg Res 2018;104(2):261–266.
17. Yuan BJ, Dennison DG, Elhassan BT, et al. Outcomes after radiocarpal dislocation: a retrospective review. Hand (N Y) 2015;10(3):367–373.

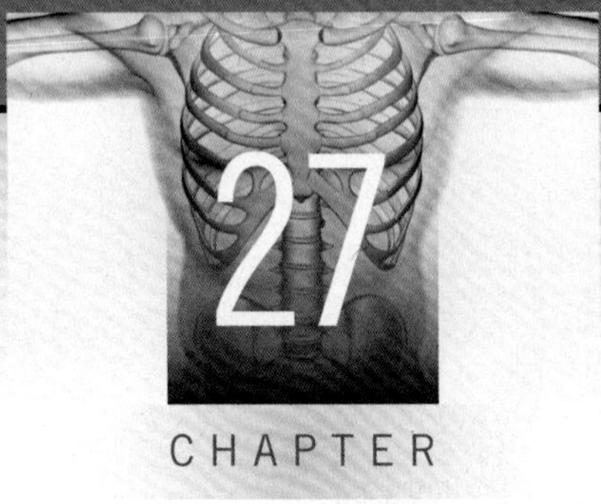

Open Reduction Internal Fixation of Radius and Ulna Shaft Fractures (Volar and Dorsal Approaches)

Joseph T. Labrum IV and Mihir J. Desai

BACKGROUND

- The forearm plays a pivotal role in upper extremity function.
- Hand position and use in space is largely reliant on flexion and extension at the wrist and elbow as well as supination and pronation of the forearm, movements that are intimately associated with the radius and ulna, their biomechanical integrity, and their linking articulations.
- The diaphysis of the radius encompasses the radial shaft distal to the bicipital tuberosity to the region just proximal to the distal radius metaphyseal flare (**FIG 1**).[5]
- The diaphysis of the ulna begins distal to the coronoid and extends to the diametaphyseal junction of the distal ulna.[1]
- Diaphyseal shaft fractures of the forearm do not involve dislocation or disruption of the proximal or distal radioulnar joints as can be observed in Galeazzi fractures, Monteggia fractures, or Essex-Lopresti injuries, which are considered distinct entities.[6]
- The synergic relationship of the radius and ulna is often disrupted in the setting of diaphyseal shaft fractures, which can lead to a significant loss of upper extremity function.
- These injuries often require operative intervention by an orthopaedist, as slight angular or rotation deformities can lead to significant deficits in forearm rotation and upper extremity function.

ANATOMY

- The forearm is made up of the radius and ulna, which are intricately linked via a triarticular complex.[6]
  - The triarticular complex of the forearm is made up of the proximal and distal radioulnar joints as well as the interosseous membrane and its associated structures, referred to as the *middle radioulnar joint*.[7]
- The radius and ulna lie parallel to one another when the forearm is supinated.
- The convex shape of the radius, referred to as *radial bow*, allows the radius to rotate over the longitudinal axis of the ulna during pronation. Loss of radial length or alterations in native radial bow will result in significant loss of forearm rotation as well as loss of grip strength.
- Detailed knowledge of the muscular and neurovascular anatomy of the volar and dorsal forearm is needed when carrying out plate osteosynthesis of diaphyseal radius and ulnar shaft fractures (**FIG 2**).
- The forearm is composed of four muscular compartments: superficial volar compartment, deep volar compartment, dorsal compartment, and mobile wad (see **FIG 2**).
  - The interval between the mobile wad and superficial volar compartments is used in the volar approach to the radius.
  - The interval between the dorsal compartment and the mobile wad is used in the dorsal approach to the radius.

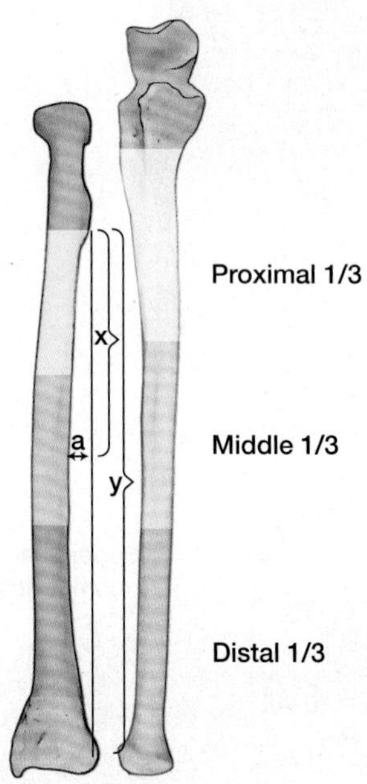

FIG 1 The diaphysis of the radius encompasses the radial shaft distal to the bicipital tuberosity to the region just proximal to the distal radius metaphyseal flare. The diaphysis of the ulna begins distal to the coronoid and extends to the diametaphyseal junction of the distal ulna. Diaphyseal radial and ulnar shaft fractures are also referred as *2R2* and *2U2* fractures, respectively, within the AO Foundation/Orthopaedic Trauma Association (AO/OTA) fracture classification system. Measurement of radial bow can assist in restoration of anatomic reduction of the radius in cases of radial shaft fractures with significant comminution or segmental bone defects. To evaluate radial bow, a line (*y*) is drawn from the bicipital tuberosity to the ulnar-most aspect of the distal radius in line with the longitudinal axis of the radius. The point of maximum radial bow as measured in millimeters with a perpendicular line (*a*) is determined. The distance from the bicipital tuberosity to maximum radial bow (*x*) is divided by the overall length (*y*) and multiplied by 100.

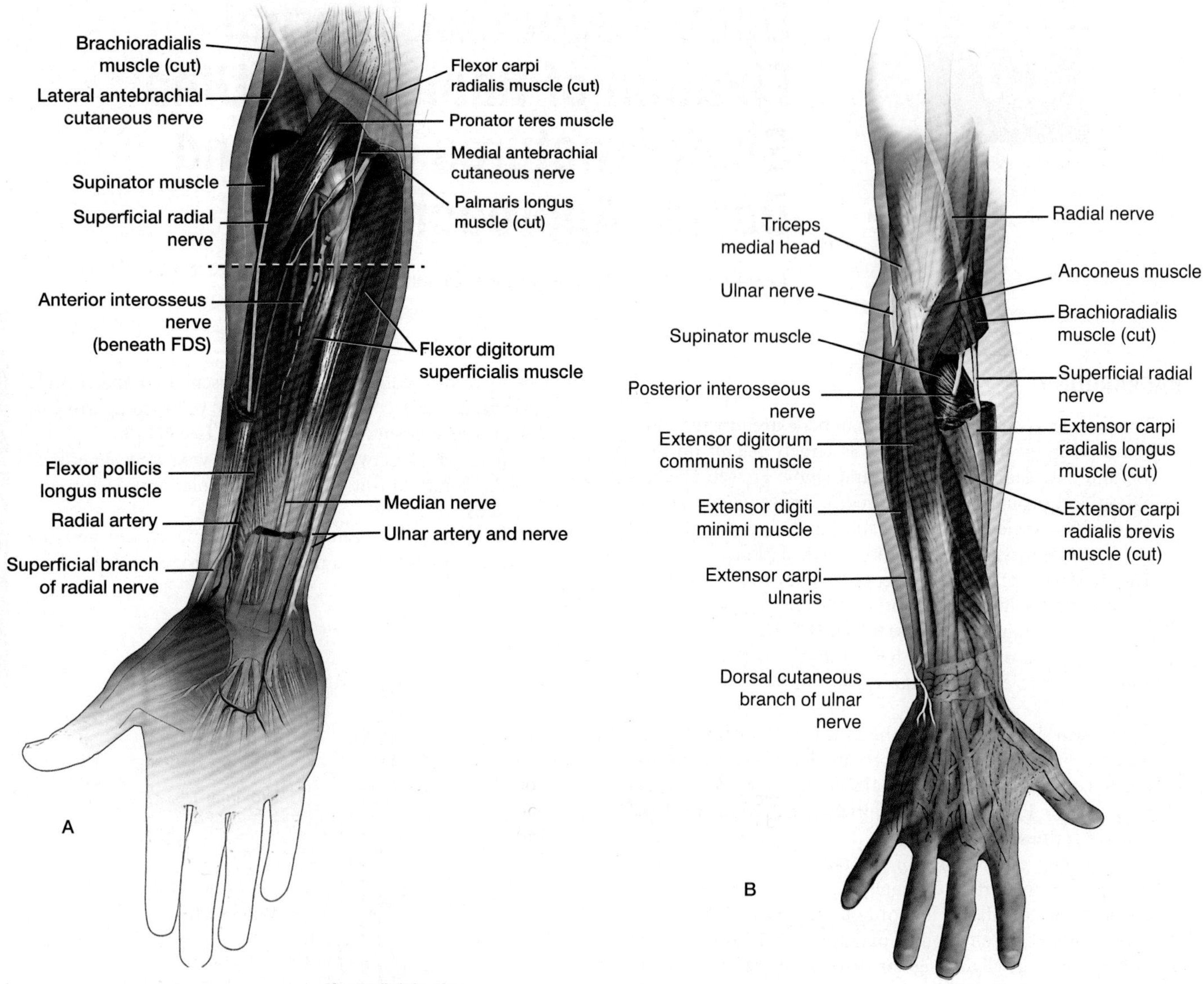

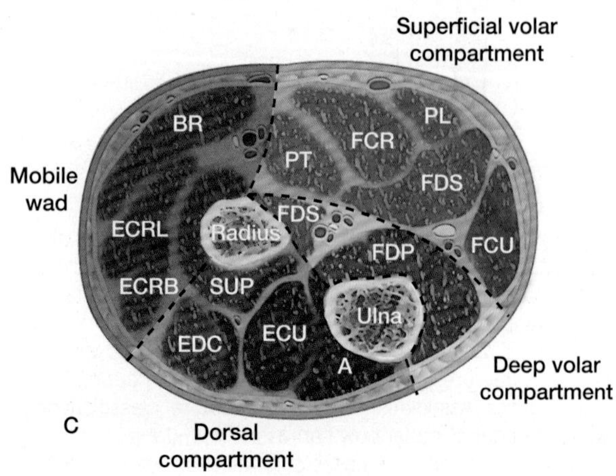

FIG 2 Muscular and neurovascular anatomy of the forearm. **A.** During a volar approach to the forearm, the radial artery, superficial radial nerve, anterior interosseous neurovascular structures, and PIN may all be encountered. Detailed knowledge of their location and ability to visually identify these structures are critical to avoiding injury when their anatomic location is disrupted by injury. **B.** Dorsal approaches must demand identification of the PIN proximally and superficial radial nerve branches distally. During distal third ulnar approaches, the dorsal cutaneous branch of the ulnar nerve may be encountered, notably when anatomy is aberrant. **C.** Axial view at the level of the *dashed line* in **A**. The interval between the mobile wad and superficial volar compartment is used in the volar approach to the radius. The interval between the dorsal compartment and the mobile wad is used in the dorsal approach to the radius. These four compartments must be released in the setting of a forearm fasciotomy through a volar and dorsal incision.

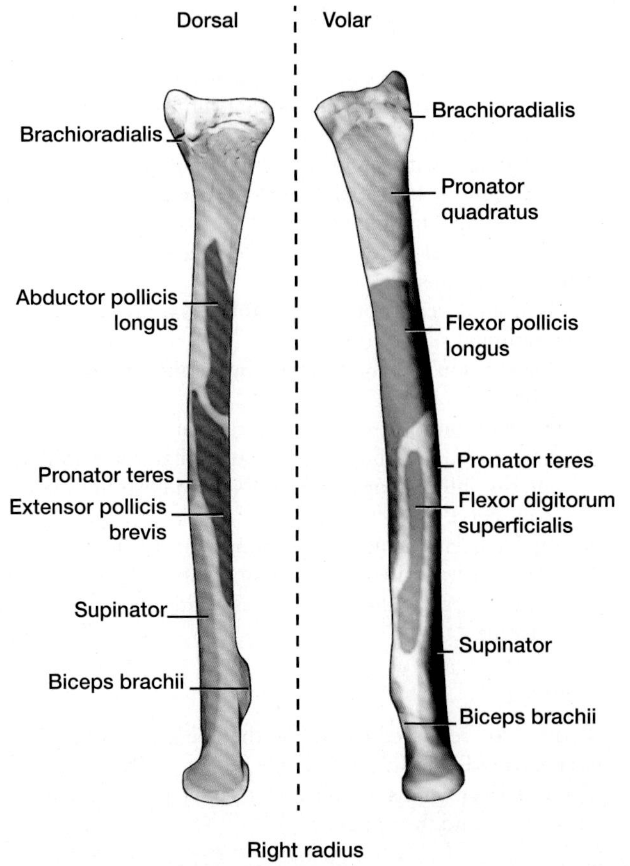

FIG 3 The diaphysis of the radius is covered by five muscles volarly and four dorsally. The volar radius is covered by the supinator, flexor digitorum superficialis, PT, flexor pollicis longus, and pronator quadratus from proximal to distal. The dorsal radius is covered by the supinator, abductor pollicis longus, and PT proximally and extensor pollicis brevis distally. The "bare area" of the radius is found dorsally in the mid-shaft.

- These four compartments must be released in the setting of a forearm fasciotomy through a volar and dorsal incision. Epimysiotomy of individual muscle bellies can also be carried out in addition if they appear tense or pale following fascial release.
- The diaphysis of the radius is covered by five muscles volarly and four dorsally **(FIG 3)**. These muscles will be encountered in approaches to the radial diaphysis. These muscles can undergo significant damage from the initial injury, and identification can be challenging. Therefore, a thorough understanding of the anatomy is needed.

PATHOGENESIS

- Diaphyseal shaft fractures typically result from indirect axial force that is applied through the hand into the forearm or a direct trauma to the forearm itself, as in the case of "nightstick" ulna fractures. These injuries commonly occur secondary to high-energy trauma but can also be seen following low-energy mechanisms in patients with poor bone quality.[6]
- Diaphyseal forearm fractures typically result in significant bony displacement and forearm deformity with secondary loss of function.
- Patients presenting with radius and ulna shaft fractures often present with other traumatic injuries and therefore should undergo a thorough initial evaluation.

PATIENT HISTORY AND PHYSICAL FINDINGS

- Both operative and nonoperative management of forearm fractures require a thorough patient history and physical exam.
- Patient history should include mechanism of injury, handedness, occupation, and baseline activity level in addition to the classic history gathered in all evaluations. A thorough social history is also advised.
- Physical examination of the injured extremity should include the following:
  - Close examination for open fracture, neurologic deficit, or vascular injury. Preoperative nerve assessment is best performed via measurement of static two-point discrimination of the injured and uninjured extremity. Motor examination is equally important but can be difficult to obtain acutely in some cases secondary to pain.
  - Examination of forearm compartments to evaluate for active or impending compartment syndrome both on presentation and perioperatively
  - In instances of isolated radial or ulnar shaft fractures, the treating surgeon should closely evaluate the elbow, wrist, proximal and distal radioulnar joints on x-ray, and physical exam to avoid misdiagnosis of occult Monteggia or Galeazzi injuries.

IMAGING AND OTHER STAGING STUDIES

- Orthogonal radiographs of the forearm, wrist, and elbow of the injured extremity should be carried out during initial evaluation.
- In forearm fractures with segmental bone loss or significant comminution, orthogonal radiographs of the contralateral forearm can be obtained for intraoperative comparison of radial bow (see **FIG 1**).
  - This provides a useful tool for intraoperative assessment and restoration of radial length and rotation.
- If nonoperative management is planned, repeat anteroposterior (AP) and lateral radiographs of the affected forearm should be carried out following immobilization to confirm adequate alignment.
- Advanced imaging is typically not necessary for diaphyseal fractures of the radius or ulna.
  - Computed tomography scans can be obtained in instances where there is concern for radial or ulnar shaft fractures with proximal or distal, intra-articular extension, or complex dislocation.
  - Magnetic resonance imaging can be carried out when abnormal bony or soft tissue lesions or pathologic fractures are suspected.

NONOPERATIVE MANAGEMENT

- Open injuries should be irrigated upon initial presentation with subsequent sterile dressing application. Intravenous antibiotics as well as tetanus immunization, when indicated, should be administered as soon as possible.
- The injured extremity should be immobilized in a splint that prohibits wrist flexion/extension, forearm pronation/supination, and elbow flexion/extension.
- Nonoperative management of diaphyseal forearm fractures is typically reserved only for patients with significant medical comorbidities that cannot undergo anesthesia or surgical intervention safely.

- Nonoperative management can be successfully employed in minimally displaced ulnar shaft fractures with good overall alignment.
  - Patients should be immobilized in an above-elbow splint or cast for at least 2 weeks prior to allowing active range of motion (AROM).
  - Patients should be monitored with close follow-up and repeat radiographs to confirm maintenance of acceptable alignment and forearm rotation.
- Rarely, nonoperative management of isolated, nondisplaced radial shaft fractures can be carried out with immobilization in a cast until resolution of pain.
- Radiographic union can be expected between 8 and 10 weeks.

SURGICAL MANAGEMENT

- Operative fixation typically represents the treatment of choice in the management of diaphyseal radius and ulna fractures.
- Both preoperative and postoperative peripheral nerve blocks should never be used in multimodal pain regimens employed for these injuries in order to avoid masking compartment syndrome.
- Partial exsanguination of the operative extremity can aid in visualization of forearm vasculature.
- When treating diaphyseal both-bone forearm fractures, it is recommended that each fracture is approached through an independent surgical incision to decrease the rate of posttraumatic radioulnar synostosis.
- In both-bone forearm fractures, the surgeon should first select the fracture that has the simpler fracture pattern or superior cortical read in order to best restore length, alignment, and rotation.
- Forearm fascia should be left open in all cases to mitigate risk of postoperative compartment syndrome.
- If skin closure cannot be obtained acutely, the volar incision is left open with plans for delayed closure within 72 hours.

Preoperative Planning

- Operative timing, fixation construct, goals of treatment, and surgical approach should be carefully considered prior to any surgical intervention.
- Timing
  - Closed forearm fractures with normal neurovascular examinations and acceptable soft tissue swelling represent a nonurgent injury that can be treated either acutely or on a delayed, outpatient basis depending on surgeon and patient preference.
  - Open forearm fractures should be taken to the operating room urgently after management and stabilization of life-threatening injuries and when a capable operative team is available.[6]
  - Any forearm fracture with concurrent or impending compartment syndrome or vascular injury, threatening limb viability, should be taken to the operating room emergently.
    - Forearm crush injuries and AO/OTA type C forearm fractures have a significantly increased association with the development of compartment syndrome and should therefore be monitored closely.[1]
- Fixation construct
  - Standard fixation constructs include 3.5-mm compression plating with fixation in six cortices both proximal and distal to the fracture site.
  - Anatomically contoured plates or prebent plates aid in restoration of radial bow.
  - In patients with poor bone quality, significant comminution, or fracture patterns that limit fixation, locking constructs should be used.
  - In patients with significant comminution or segmental bone defects, bridge plating technique is useful in restoring and maintaining length.
  - Stainless steel plates can provide added rigidity.
- Goals of treatment
  - Anatomic reduction and stable fixation of forearm fracture(s)
  - Preservation of blood supply by minimizing soft tissue exposure
  - Preservation of at-risk structures, which include the radial artery, superficial branch of radial nerve (SBRN), anterior interosseous nerve (AIN), and posterior interosseous nerve (PIN)[2]
  - Avoiding iatrogenic complications, including neurovascular injury, malreduction, postoperative infection, posttraumatic radioulnar synostosis, and poor functional outcome

Positioning

- Patient can be placed supine on the operating table with a standard radiolucent arm table.
- A nonsterile pneumatic tourniquet can be placed circumferentially around the upper arm.

Approach

- Radial shaft approaches include the volar Henry approach and the dorsal Thompson approach.
- The classically described volar Henry approach uses the plane between the pronator teres (PT) (median nerve) and brachioradialis (radial nerve) proximally and the radial artery and flexor carpi radialis (FCR) tendon distally.
  - SBRN can also be found deep to brachioradialis proximally and should be visualized and protected during deep dissection.
  - The radial artery should be visualized and protected during the entirety of the procedure.
  - This approach can be used for all radial shaft fractures. It is the standard of care for midshaft and distal third radial shaft fractures. Volar dissection of the proximal third of the radius is attainable but can be challenging.
- Alternatively, the modified volar Henry approach, which uses the FCR tendon sheath interval superficially to gain access to the distal radius, can be used for access to distal radial shaft fractures based on surgeon preference.
- The dorsal Thompson approach can be used for access to fractures in the proximal third and middle third of the radial diaphysis.
  - Superficially, this approach uses an interval between extensor carpi radialis brevis (ECRB) and extensor digitorum communis (EDC).
  - The abductor pollicis longus and extensor pollicis brevis, also known as the *outcropper muscles*, define the interval between the wrist and finger extensors and can be used as a point of reference in this approach.[2]
  - Deep dissection to expose the radial shaft proximally requires elevating supinator ulnarly.

- The forearm should be pronated during mobilization of the supinator and exposure of the proximal radius in order to move PIN distally and radially.[1]
- For all ulnar shaft fractures, a direct approach along the subcutaneous border of the ulna can be used.
  - Internervous plane between flexor carpi ulnaris (ulnar nerve) volarly and extensor carpi ulnaris (PIN) dorsally is used.[2]
  - Distally, the dorsal cutaneous branch of the ulnar nerve crosses the subcutaneous approach to the ulna at or just proximal to the ulnar styloid.
  - Proximally, care must be taken to protect the ulnar nerve medially and the lateral ulnar collateral ligament insertion along the supinator crest laterally.[2]

Intraoperative Imaging

- Anatomic analysis of the forearm has shown that the radial styloid and radial tuberosity and the coronoid and ulnar styloid are oriented on average 158 and 185 degrees, respectively, from one another with significant variability, not 180 degrees as classically described.[9]
- Weinberg et al[9] observed that 20 degrees of supination following visualization of the maximal bicipital tuberosity profile on AP fluoroscopy should yield the largest profile of the radial styloid.
  - This provides a useful radiographic landmark for restoration of rotation alignment during the treatment of radial shaft fractures with significant comminution or segmental bone loss.

ANTERIOR (VOLAR) APPROACH TO THE RADIUS

- Light exsanguination is performed by elevation or loose circumferential wrapping with a sterile elastic wrap, and the tourniquet is inflated.
- The incision is drawn centered on the fracture from the lateral edge of the biceps tendon to the radial styloid.
  - Length depends on the degree of fracture comminution but in general will encompass roughly one-third of the forearm length **(TECH FIG 1A)**.
- An incision is made through the skin followed by blunt dissection down to fascia.
  - The lateral antebrachial cutaneous nerve at risk during superficial dissection and should be visualized and protected **(TECH FIG 1B)**.
  - A sponge can be used to bluntly sweep away deep fat from the underlying fascia if necessary.
- The fascia is incised and released with scissors.
- The radial artery and venae comitantes must be identified and mobilized. In the proximal third of the forearm, the radial artery lies deep to the brachioradialis muscle belly, which at this level nears the midline of the anterior forearm.
- Bipolar cauterization of brachioradialis perforators allows ulnar (medial) mobilization of the radial artery.
- In the mid-forearm, the radial artery is more superficial as it exits the interval between brachioradialis and FCR **(TECH FIG 1C)**. The artery is mobilized ulnarly (medially) in this region.
- In the distal third of the forearm, it is often safer to mobilize the radial artery radially (laterally).
  - In the modified Henry approach through the floor of the FCR tendon sheath, the radial artery will not be visualized but will be retracted radially.
- The superficial radial nerve is identified, and care is taken to avoid injury with retractor placement.
- Distally, flexor pollicis longus and pronator quadratus can be reflected from the radius from radial (lateral) to ulnar (medial).
- In the middle third of the radius, flexor digitorum profundus and PT can be sharply released from the radius from radial (lateral) to ulnar (medial).
- PT can be Z-lengthened or taken off the bone in a subperiosteal fashion. If release of PT is required, it can be repaired by suturing down the plate **(TECH FIG 1D–F)**.

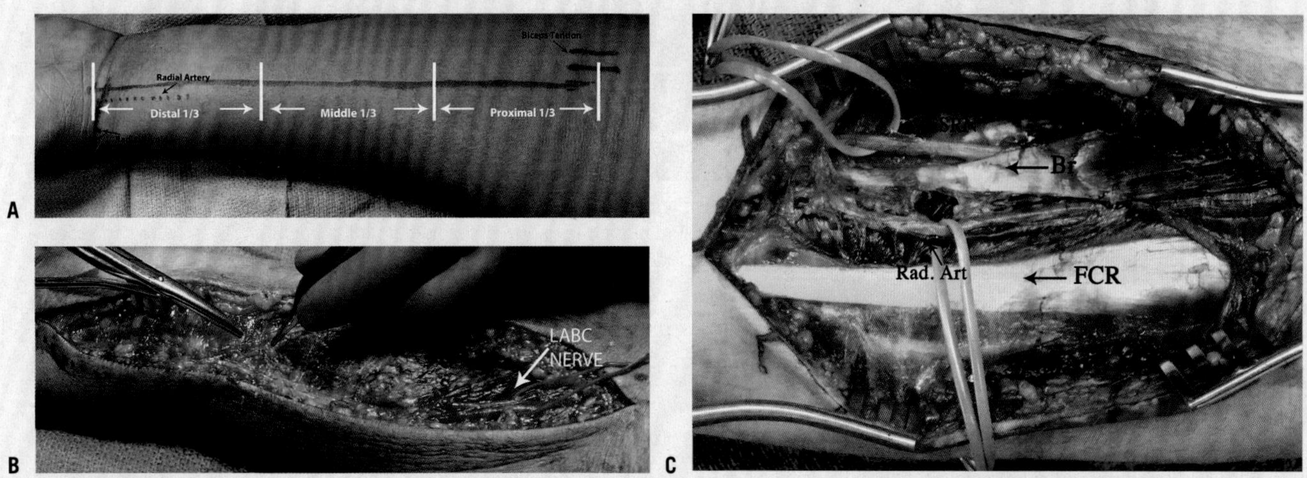

TECH FIG 1 Anterior approach to the radius. **A.** The forearm is mentally divided in thirds. Each third has unique anatomic structures that must be recognized during the approach. Extensile exposure extends from the biceps tendon to the radial styloid. Distal third fractures can alternatively be approached through the floor of the FCR tendon. **B.** Blunt dissection is performed superficially, and the main trunk of the lateral antebrachial cutaneous (*LABC*) nerve is identified and protected. **C.** In the middle third, the radial artery (*Rad. Art.*) and venae comitantes are identified exiting between brachioradialis (*Br*) and FCR. Light exsanguination assists in identifying vascular structures. The superficial radial nerve (*SRN*) is seen coursing between Br and FCR. *(continued)*

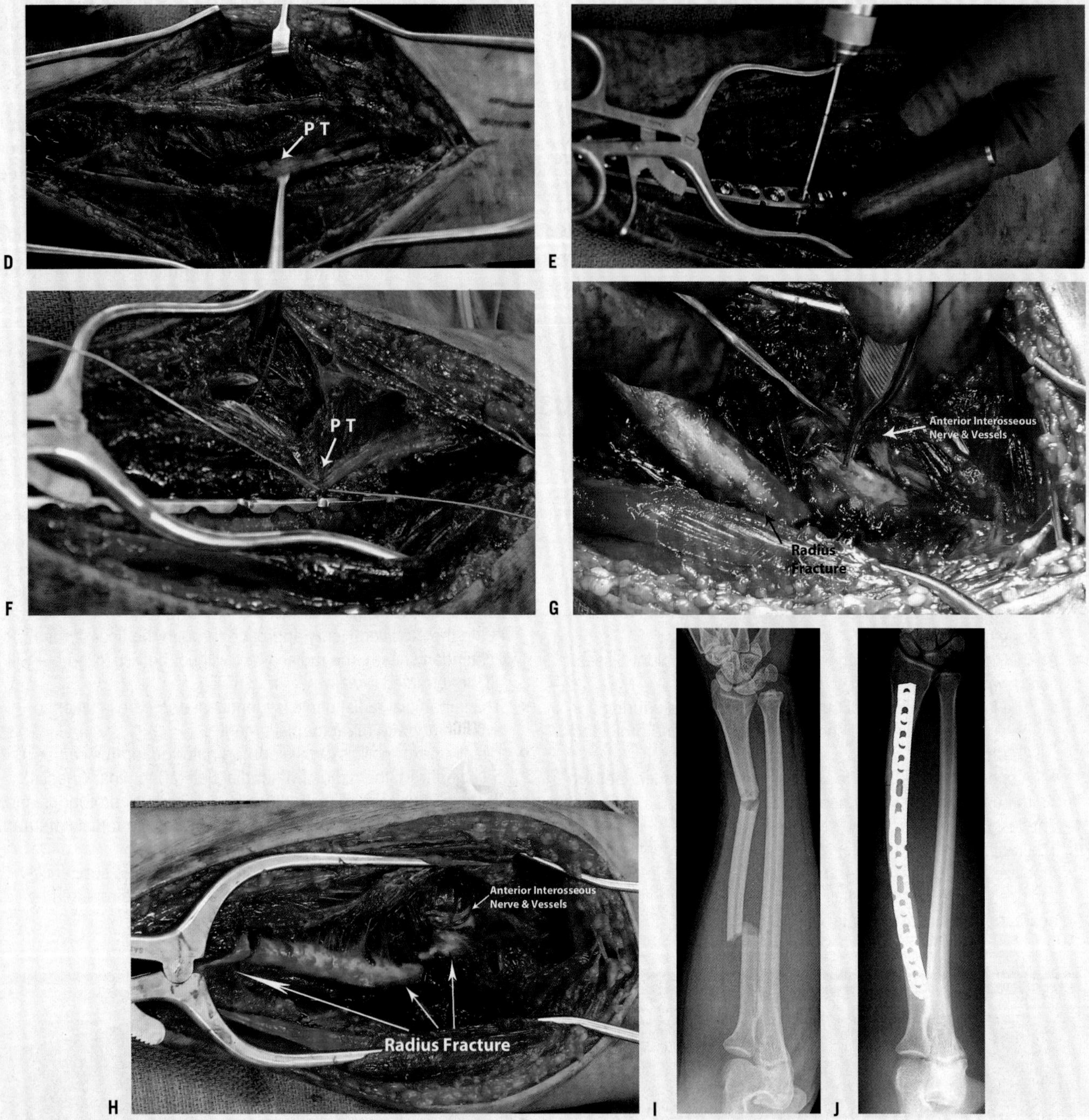

TECH FIG 1 *(continued)* **D.** The PT insertion on the radius. Drill holes are placed through the plate and radius (**E**) for reattachment of PT (**F**). Retraction of neurovascular bundle with a Freer elevator, allowing exposure of the radius (**G**). A segmental radius fracture with the AIN and vessel in close proximity to the proximal fragment (**H**). Pre- and post-operative radiographs of the segmental radius fracture (**I**) treated via anatomic plate fixation with restoration of the radial bow (**J**).

- In the proximal forearm, the soft tissue envelope is deep. Dissection proceeds along the ulnar border of the brachioradialis.
- The supinator can be identified by its obliquely orientated muscle fibers.
- The PIN runs from medial to lateral as it courses distally and enters between the two heads of the supinator at right angle with respect to the supinator muscle fiber orientation.
- The forearm should be supinated when dissecting proximally in order to protect the PIN as this allows the nerve to migrate laterally away from the surgical field. Dissection should be carried out on the ulnar (medial) border of the radius to avoid PIN injury.
  - When the radius is broken **(TECH FIG 1G)** and adequate supination cannot be achieved, a reduction forceps can be placed on the proximal radius distal to the supinator insertion to ensure adequate supination and PIN mobilization and protection.

- When dissection is carried proximally near the biceps tuberosity, the surgeon will often encounter a small amount of clear, thick fluid originating from the biceps bursa. This can aid in orientation. Just proximal to the bursa, there are multiple crossing vessels that can be mobilized en masse with blunt retraction if necessary.
- Following reduction and fixation of the forearm **(TECH FIG 1H–J)**, the tourniquet should be taken down and meticulous hemostasis should be obtained.
- Forearm fascia is left open in all cases. Subcutaneous tissues can be approximated with Vicryl or Monocryl sutures (3-0 or 4-0). Nylon sutures can be used for superficial skin closure.

POSTERIOR (THOMPSON) APPROACH TO THE RADIUS

- Light exsanguination is performed by elevation or loose, circumferential wrapping with a sterile Ace wrap, and the tourniquet is inflated.
- Skin incision is centered over the fracture and drawn in line with the lateral epicondyle of the humerus to Lister tubercle on the distal radius **(TECH FIG 2A)**.
  - Skin incision length roughly equal to one-third the length of the radius will provide sufficient exposure.
- Blunt dissection is carried out to the level of the forearm fascia where the extensor mass can be visualized.
- In the middle third of the radius, the abductor pollicis longus and extensor pollicis brevis are identified and elevated off the radius sharply for exposure.
- Proximally, the interval lies between the thick tendinous band of EDC tendon ulnarly (medially) and the ECRB muscle belly, which lies dorsal and radial (lateral) **(TECH FIG 2B)**.
- The radial portion of the lateral collateral ligament complex of the elbow lies directly deep to the tendinous origin of EDC. Care should be taken to identify the EDC origin and avoid iatrogenic injury to the lateral elbow stabilizers.
- Fascia is incised just anterior to the white tendinous band of EDC, and a Freer elevator is used to elevate the muscle fibers off the septum, exposing the deep fascia.
- The deep fascia layer is carefully opened with scissors from distal to proximal, exposing the underlying supinator muscle, which can be readily identified by its obliquely oriented muscle fibers **(TECH FIG 2C)**.
- Blunt retraction of the radial wrist extensors and brachioradialis from the supinator often allows PIN visualization.
  - The PIN can be identified running from medial to lateral as it courses distally and enters between the two heads of the supinator at right angle with respect to the supinator muscle fiber orientation (see **TECH FIG 2C**).
  - If PIN cannot be visualized, the surgeon can identify PIN distally and traced proximally through the supinator **(TECH FIG 2D–G)**.

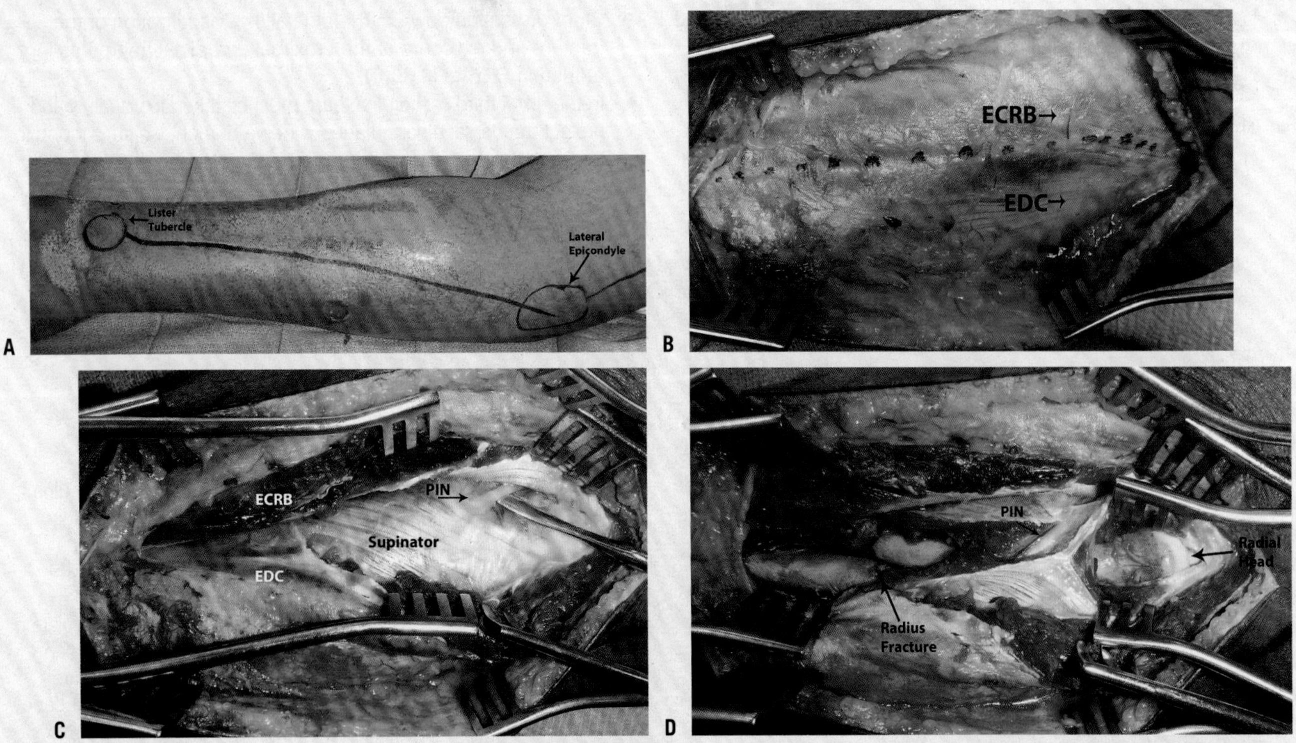

TECH FIG 2 Posterior approach to the radius. **A.** Extensile exposure (lateral humeral epicondyle to Lister tubercle). **B.** Proximal interval is located between EDC and ECRB. **C.** The deep fascia of ECRB and EDC has been divided, and the oblique fibers of the supinator are now visualized. The PIN can be seen entering supinator perpendicular to its fibers. **D.** The supinator has been partially divided to reveal the PIN coursing through its substance. The radial head is seen proximally and the radius fracture is seen distally. *(continued)*

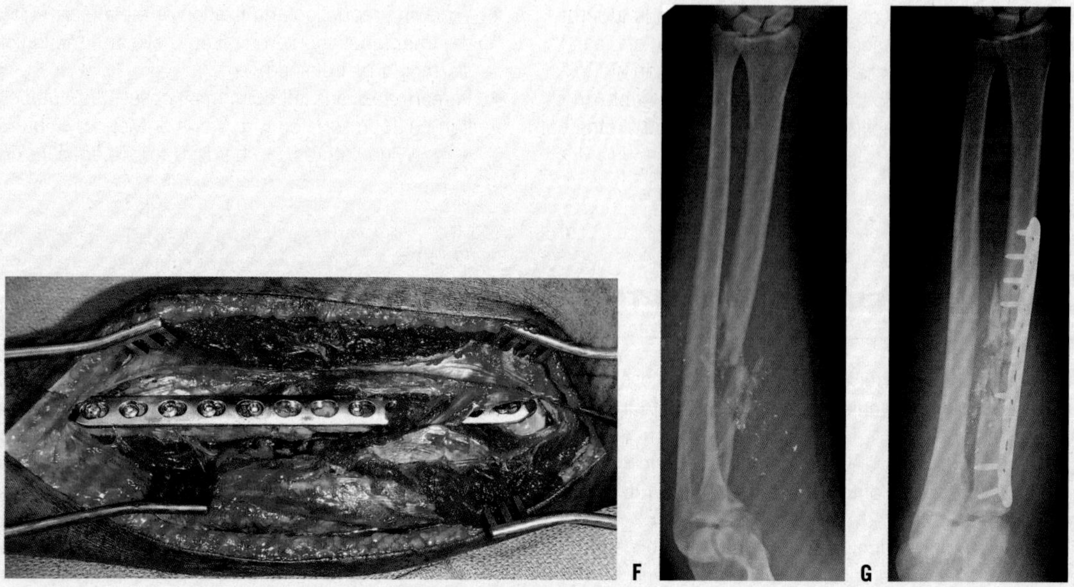

E F G

TECH FIG 2 *(continued)* **E.** A 3.5-mm locking compression plate has been applied to the proximal radius. In this case, only two screws of proximal fixation were available; therefore, locking screws were used. **F,G.** Preoperative and postoperative radiographs demonstrating bridge plating of this comminuted proximal radius fracture. A 3.5-mm locking plate was used. Proximally, the plate placement must be scrutinized to avoid impingement during forearm pronosupination. In our experience, this fracture is at significant risk for infection and nonunion. Acute bone grafting was not performed secondary to concern for infection.

SUBCUTANEOUS APPROACH TO THE ULNA

- Light exsanguination is performed and the tourniquet is inflated.
  - In cases where radial reduction and fixation may be challenging, this approach can be carried out in the absence of tourniquet.
- The incision is drawn from the olecranon to the ulnar styloid centered over the fracture site **(TECH FIG 3A)**.
- Blunt dissection down to the ulna allows visualization of the fracture and exposure of the proximal and distal fragments for reduction **(TECH FIG 3B,C)**.
- In the distal third of the ulna, care must be taken to visualize and protect the dorsal ulnar cutaneous nerve branch, which is found in the subcutaneous tissues just distal to the ulnar styloid.

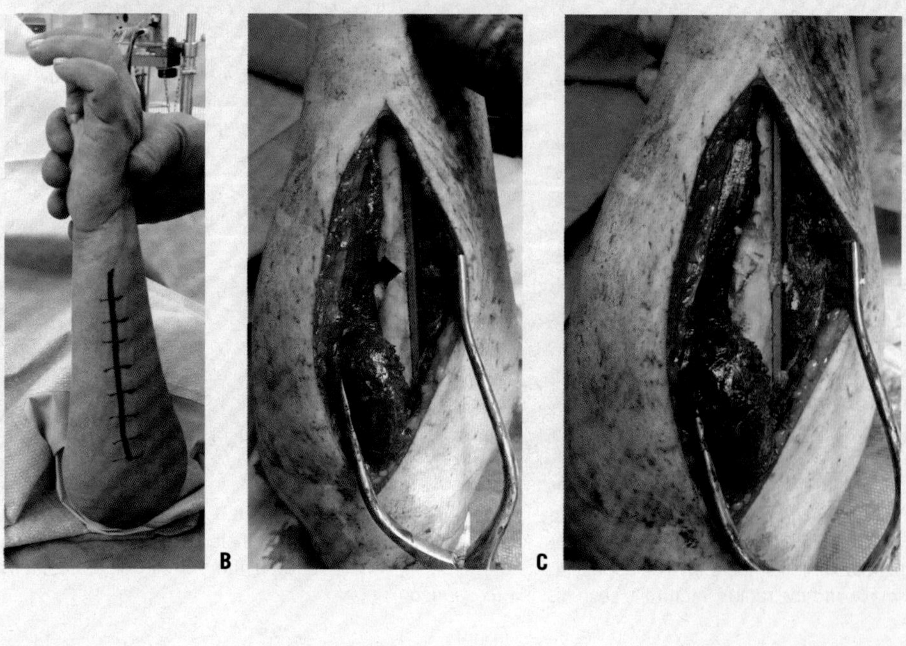

A B C

TECH FIG 3 Approach to the ulna. **A.** Incision drawn along the ulnar subcutaneous border. **B.** Open reduction internal fixation (ORIF) of the ulna with comminuted butterfly fragment with dorsal plate. **C.** Comminuted butterfly fragment and supplemental allograft bone graft fills the defect. (Autograft bone grafting for this type of defect may be preferred. This can be performed acutely in closed fractures if necessary.)

Pearls and Pitfalls

Compartment Syndrome	• Both preoperative and postoperative peripheral nerve blocks should never be used in order to avoid the potential masking of compartment syndrome. • Forearm crush injuries and AO/OTA type C forearm fractures are noted to have a significantly increased association with the development of compartment syndrome and should therefore be monitored closely. • Forearm fascia should never be closed following fixation of radial and/or ulna fractures. • If significant swelling precludes primary wound closure, close the ulnar wound and leave the radial approach open for up to 72 hours.
Preoperative Planning	• To best restore length, alignment, and rotation, the fracture that has the simpler fracture pattern or superior cortical read should be addressed initially.
Transverse Fractures	• Prebending of the plate to create a 1- to 2-mm gap between the plate and the fracture site can prevent gapping at the far cortex following fracture compression. • Reduction technique: Blunt reduction forceps ("lobster claws") can be used to clamp one side of the fracture to plate with subsequent reduction of the other fracture fragment to the plate.
Oblique Fractures	• When reducing oblique fractures, it is best to fix the plate to the bone fragment that creates an axilla. This facilitates fracture compression and maintenance of reduction by using the plate to neutralize shear force at the fracture site during compression.
Butterfly Fragments	• Use interfragmentary 2.4-mm lag screws to fix the butterfly fragment to one side of the fracture in order to create a two-part fracture. If necessary, this interfragmentary screw can be placed through the plate.
Comminution/ Segmental Bone Defect	• Bridge plating with anatomic precontoured plates should be used for increased construct rigidity. If a significant bone defect is present, Masquelet technique can be carried out with methylene blue–dyed cement for subsequent identification and removal.[8]
Restoring Radial Bow	• Use radial bow from the contralateral extremity as well as the 20-degree supination view of maximal radial styloid profile to ensure restoration of length, alignment, and rotation. • Anatomic precontoured plates can assist in recreating radial bow.
Osteoporotic Fractures	• In patients with poor bone quality, locking constructs should be used. If possible, fracture site compression should be achieved prior to locking.

POSTOPERATIVE CARE

- Orthogonal forearm radiographs should be obtained following surgery.
- Soft dressing versus splint immobilization for 1 to 2 weeks following surgery is recommended.
- Postoperative neurovascular and compartment pressure check should be carried out following surgery.
- Encourage immediate AROM of the injured extremity.
- Encourage smoking cessation and metabolic optimization when necessary to mitigate postoperative complications.
- 2 weeks
  - Remove soft dressing or splint, evaluate wound for complications, and remove sutures.
  - Continue AROM/passive range of motion of the forearm, encouraging pronation, supination, and grip strength exercises.
- 6 to 8 weeks and after
  - Progressive weight bearing following radiographic evidence of union with clearance to normal activity

OUTCOMES

- Outcomes following ORIF of diaphyseal radius and/or ulna fractures are very favorable.
- Although outcomes following plate osteosynthesis of forearm fractures are favorable, patients can be counseled that a slight decrease in grip strength and forearm rotation should be expected following the procedure.[3,4] This loss of function is more pronounced in cases of malreduction.

COMPLICATIONS

- Infection
- Symptomatic hardware or hardware failure
- Iatrogenic nerve injury
- Refracture
- Radioulnar synostosis

REFERENCES

1. Auld TS, Hwang JS, Stekas N, et al. The correlation between the OTA/AO classification system and compartment syndrome in both bone forearm fractures. J Orthop Trauma 2017;31(11):606–609.
2. Catalano LW III, Zlotolow DA, Hitchcock PB, et al. Surgical exposures of the radius and ulna. J Am Acad Orthop Surg 2011;19(7):430–438.
3. Droll KP, Perna P, Potter J, et al. Outcomes following plate fixation of fractures of both bones of the forearm in adults. J Bone Joint Surg Am 2007;89(12):2619–2624.
4. Goldfarb CA, Ricci WM, Tull F, et al. Functional outcome after fracture of both bones of the forearm. J Bone Joint Surg Br 2005;87(3):374–379.
5. Meinberg EG, Agel J, Roberts CS, et al. Fracture and dislocation classification compendium—2018. J Orthop Trauma 2018:32(suppl 1):S1–S170.
6. Schulte LM, Meals CG, Neviaser RJ. Management of adult diaphyseal both-bone forearm fractures. J Am Acad Orthop Surg 2014;22(7):437–446.
7. Soubeyrand M, Wassermann V, Hirsch C, et al. The middle radioulnar joint and triarticular forearm complex. J Hand Surg Eur Vol 2011;36(6):447–454.
8. Walker M, Sharareh B, Mitchell SA. Masquelet reconstruction for posttraumatic segmental bone defects in the forearm. J Hand Surg Am 2019;44(4):342.e1–342.e8.
9. Weinberg DS, Park PJ, Boden KA, et al. Anatomic investigation of commonly used landmarks for evaluating rotation during forearm fracture reduction. J Bone Joint Surg Am 2016;98(13):1103–1112.

CHAPTER 28

Surgical Decompression of the Forearm, Hand, and Digits for Compartment Syndrome

Dipak B. Ramkumar, Niveditta Ramkumar, Marci D. Jones, and Lance G. Warhold

"Dedicated to the memory of our friend and colleague, Rodrigo Santamarina, MD (1969-2017)"

DEFINITION

- Acute compartment syndrome is a condition in which increased tissue pressure compromises the circulation within the enclosed space of fascial compartments. As a result of this elevated interstitial pressure, the blood supply to the soft tissues is impaired. If left untreated, elevated pressures can cause irreversible soft tissue necrosis resulting in fibrosis and contracture.

ANATOMY

- Compartment syndrome is most common in the forearm and hand but can occur in the arm and in the finger as well.
- The arm is divided into two fascial compartments, the forearm into three compartments, the hand into 10 compartments, and the finger into two compartments.
- The two arm compartments are the anterior and posterior, separated by the medial and lateral intermuscular septa **(FIG 1A)**.
  - The anterior arm compartment contains the biceps brachii, brachialis, and coracobrachialis.
  - The posterior arm compartment contains the triceps brachii.
- The forearm consists of four compartments: superficial volar, deep volar, dorsal, and mobile wad of three **(FIG 1B)**.
  - The contents of the volar compartment include the flexor muscles and can be subdivided into superficial and deep components.
    - The superficial muscles are the flexor carpi ulnaris, palmaris longus, pronator teres, and flexor carpi radialis.
    - The deep muscles are the flexor digitorum superficialis and profundus, the flexor pollicis longus, and distally, the pronator quadratus.
  - The dorsal compartment of the forearm contains the extensor muscles.
    - The superficial extensors include the extensor digitorum communis, extensor digiti minimi, and extensor carpi ulnaris.
    - The deep layer includes the supinator, abductor pollicis longus, extensor pollicis longus, extensor pollicis brevis, and extensor indicis.
  - The mobile wad of three is a distinct muscle compartment that contains the brachioradialis, extensor carpi radialis longus, and extensor carpi radialis brevis.
- The wrist has one significant closed space, the carpal tunnel. Although not a compartment in the strictest sense, increased pressure in the carpal tunnel can cause damage to the median nerve.
- The hand contains 10 distinct compartments **(FIG 1C)**.
  - There are seven compartments for the interossei.
    - Each of the four dorsal and three palmar interossei has a separate compartment.
  - The adductor compartment contains the adductor pollicis.
  - The thenar compartment contains the abductor pollicis brevis, the opponens pollicis, and the flexor pollicis brevis.
  - The hypothenar compartment contains the abductor digiti minimi, flexor digiti minimi, and opponens digiti minimi.
- Compartment syndrome can also occur in the finger due to the limited skin compliance from the multiple fascial attachments.

PATHOGENESIS

- The blood flow to a compartment is determined by several factors: venous or "outflow" pressure, arterial or "inflow" pressure, and local interstitial pressure.
  - Increased pressure within a compartment decreases the blood supply to the soft tissues and can result in tissue ischemia and ultimately tissue necrosis.
  - Increased capillary permeability results from muscle ischemia. This increased permeability leads to intramuscular edema, which further increases the tissue pressure, thereby decreasing blood flow and oxygen transport. This in turn results in further tissue necrosis.

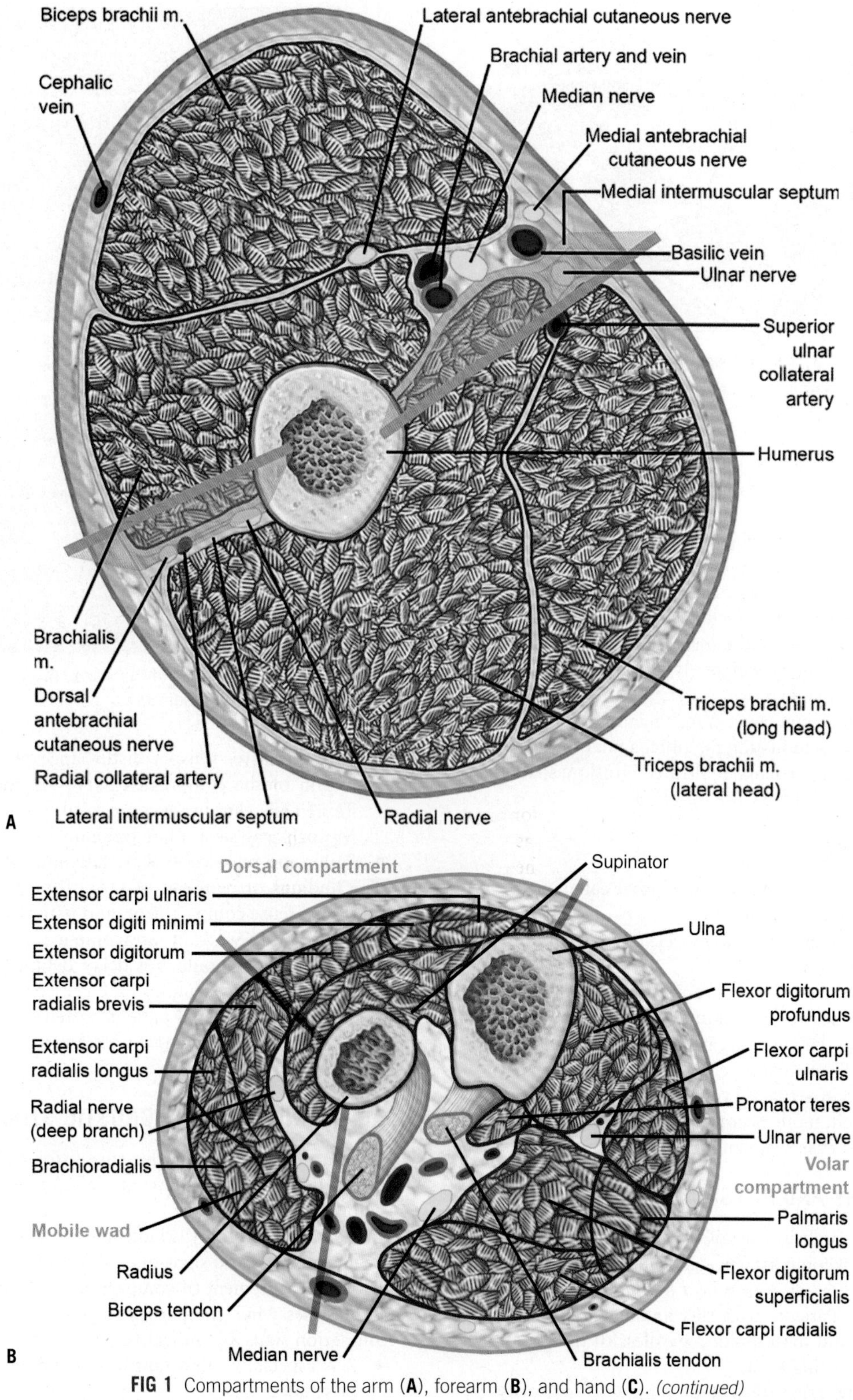

FIG 1 Compartments of the arm (**A**), forearm (**B**), and hand (**C**). *(continued)*

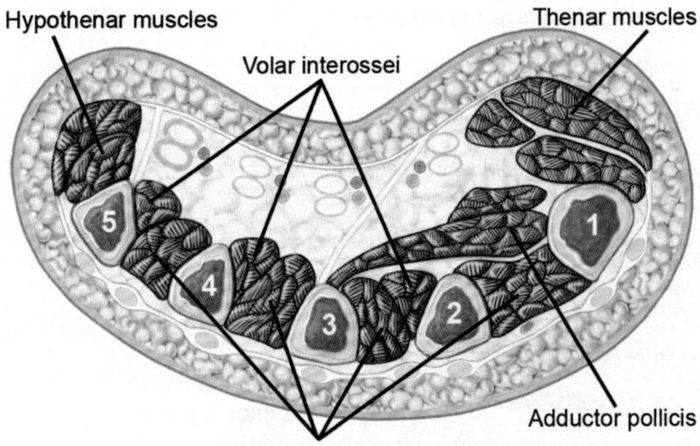

C

FIG 1 *(continued)*

- It is easy to appreciate the vicious, feed-forward cycle that escalates the pathophysiology of compartment syndrome.
- Many conditions are associated with compartment syndrome. These can be divided into two major categories[6]:
  - Conditions that decrease compartment volume: tight casts or dressings, burn eschar, limb lengthening or application of traction, and increased external pressure on limb from prolonged weight (lying on limb or entrapment under a weight)
  - Conditions that increase compartment contents: bleeding (arterial or venous injury, anticoagulation, trauma), reperfusion injury, edema, infiltrated infusion, snakebite, infection, and high-pressure injection

NATURAL HISTORY

- Compartment syndrome results in hypoxic cell damage and ultimately anoxic cell death.
  - Functional changes occur in muscle after 2 to 4 hours of total ischemia time.
  - Hypoxia to nerves causes paresthesias, dysesthesias, and hypoesthesia within 30 minutes of ischemia, but irreversible nerve damage may not occur until 12 hours or more of total ischemia time.
- An untreated compartment syndrome can result in permanent neural deficit, tissue necrosis, growth arrest, Volkmann contracture, and even wet gangrene.

PATIENT HISTORY AND PHYSICAL FINDINGS

- It is important to elicit a detailed history and evaluate the possible causes of compartment syndrome (discussed earlier).
- *Pain out of proportion to physical findings is the most important finding.* Patients with this finding should be carefully evaluated and monitored, regardless of the presumed severity of the inciting event.
- Most commonly, patients will present with a history of trauma or a crushing injury; however, other causes must not be overlooked.
- Compartment syndrome may involve single or multiple compartments in the extremity.
- Physical examination findings include the following:
  - A tense, swollen, and tender compartment (**FIG 2**)
  - Pain with passive stretch of the muscles within the compartment

A

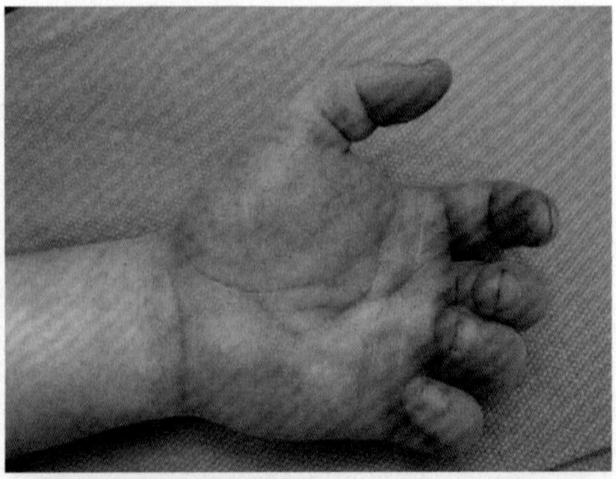

B

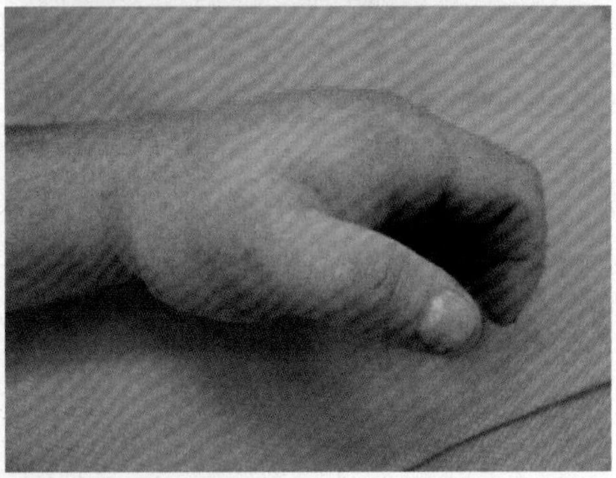

FIG 2 Diffuse, tense swelling of the hand. **A.** Palmar view with loss of palmar concavity. **B.** Radial view.

  - Paresthesias or sensory disturbances in the nerve distribution of the compressed nerve are intermediate findings. This can be accompanied by motor weakness. Motor paralysis is a late finding.
  - Pallor and pulselessness are late findings.
- The findings of pain out of proportion to physical examination, a tense compartment, and pain with passive stretch are sufficient to warrant intracompartmental pressure measurements. One should not delay definitive diagnosis and treatment until later findings are present.
- In obtunded or sedated patients, a tense, swollen compartment is sufficient to warrant intracompartmental pressure measurements.

IMAGING AND OTHER DIAGNOSTIC STUDIES

- Clinical examination is the cornerstone of the diagnosis, and it is important to have a high degree of suspicion for compartment syndrome.
- Immediate fasciotomy is indicated in patients with unequivocal symptoms and signs of compartment syndrome.
- Direct measurement of compartment pressures is indicated in all cases when the patient's symptoms and physical examination signs are indicative of compartment syndrome.
  - It is especially important in patients who are obtunded or sedated.
- Diagnosis of compartment syndrome of the finger is made clinically and not through the use of pressure measurement.
- Pressure measurement in the arm is obtained for both anterior and posterior compartments. Anteriorly, the pressure is measured over the biceps muscle and posteriorly over the triceps muscle.
  - The physician must be careful not to injure the radial nerve when measuring the arm compartment pressure.

The nerve courses deep to the triceps in the spiral groove of the humerus. Ten centimeters proximal to the lateral epicondyle, it passes through the lateral intermuscular septum to the anterior compartment.

- In the forearm, the pressure is measured within the volar, mobile wad, and dorsal compartments.
  - The median and ulnar nerves are at risk during measurement of the volar compartment. The ulnar nerve courses deep to the flexor carpi ulnaris in the ulnar forearm; the median nerve is between the flexor digitorum superficialis and profundus muscles.
  - When measuring the mobile wad, the superficial branch of the radial nerve is deep to the brachioradialis in the forearm but emerges between the brachioradialis and extensor carpi radialis longus tendons about 8 cm proximal to the radial styloid.
    - The posterior interosseous nerve courses around the radial neck in the proximal radial forearm and should be avoided when measuring the mobile wad and dorsal compartments.
- In the hand, pressure measurements should be made in the affected compartments; measurements are generally made in the area of the planned incisions.
- There is no absolute increased compartment pressure that warrants fasciotomy. When the pressure approaches 30 to 45 mm Hg, or 30 mm Hg less than the diastolic pressure (ie, the "ΔP"), with concordant physical examination findings, decompressive fasciotomy should be performed.[5] In the hand, lower pressures (15 to 20 mm Hg) may indicate compartment syndrome.
  - Of note, it is important to remember that many anesthetic agents and sedatives can lower the diastolic blood pressure. Thus, when measuring the ΔP between the compartment and the diastolic pressure, it is advisable to use the diastolic pressure prior to administration of any sedatives or anesthetics.[3]
- Plain radiographs should be performed to evaluate any underlying bony abnormality. Fractures and dislocations should be reduced in order to minimize further soft tissue injury and swelling.
- Arterial injury can lead to ischemia and can present similarly. Arteriography is indicated if the history may be significant for arterial injury (fracture, avulsion, or laceration).

DIFFERENTIAL DIAGNOSIS

- Arterial injury
- Nerve injury

NONOPERATIVE MANAGEMENT

- There is no role for nonoperative management of an acute compartment syndrome. In acute cases of compartment syndrome with elevated compartment pressure, prompt decompressive fasciotomies are required to relieve tissue ischemia.
- In patients with early symptoms and signs of compartment syndrome, but without elevated compartment pressures, removal of all compressive/circumferential dressings and casts and elevation of the affected extremity to the level of the heart is indicated.
  - Frequent close monitoring by physical examination and repeated compartment pressure measurements as necessary are critical.[6]
- In patients presenting late with aseptic muscle necrosis, acute fasciotomy and débridement may not be indicated.

SURGICAL MANAGEMENT

Preoperative Planning

- The surgeon should review radiographs and plan for surgical stabilization of any underlying fractures or dislocations, as necessary.

Positioning

- The patient is positioned supine on the operating table with the upper extremity on an arm board.
- Tourniquets are frequently applied but not routinely used during decompressive fasciotomy.
- If the arm is affected, the shoulder and axilla are included in the sterile field to allow for exposure of the entire extremity.

Approach

- Skin is considered a significant compressive structure, and it is important to create a skin incision of sufficient length to allow complete decompression of a compartment.
  - Cosmesis should not be of concern.
- Incisions are planned to afford complete and rapid decompression of the compartments while maintaining coverage of vital structures and avoiding joint contractures due to scarring.
- The viability of muscles is determined by muscle tone and color, contractility, and bleeding.
  - If the viability is still unclear, the muscle should be left alone and reinspected in 24 to 48 hours, to allow for declaration.
- The skin is left open, and the wounds are copiously irrigated and covered with wet saline dressings, or more commonly, a wound vacuum dressing. The latter can reduce edema and pain associated with frequent dressing changes.[4,7]
  - Negative-pressure wound therapy (NPWT) using a vacuum-assisted closure (VAC) system has become common place in the management of fasciotomy wounds.[4,7]
  - In this technique, the forearm wound is first filled with a porous material. This can include foam sponges (ie, black polyurethane ether, V.A.C. GranuFoam [KCI, San Antonio, TX] or white polyvinyl alcohol, V.A.C. WhiteFoam [KCI, San Antonio, TX]) or gauze-based systems (**FIG 3A,B**).
  - The porous material facilitates pressure transmission within the wound. A drainage port is then attached above the porous material, which is secured onto the wound with adhesive films. The drainage port is usually connected to vacuum pump, which maintains the negative pressure anywhere from 50 to 150 mm Hg, depending on the clinical situation. The pressure can be applied in three different modes: continuous, intermittent, or variable mode.
  - NWPT is thought to promote wound healing by four different mechanisms (**FIG 3C**):
    - Macrodeformation: refers to induced wound shrinkage, which occurs when suction is applied to the foam, causing collapse. This results in force exertion on the wound edge, which draws them closer together.
    - Microdeformation: describes the mechanical changes that occur on the microscopic scale when suction is applied to the wound bed. Negative pressure causes

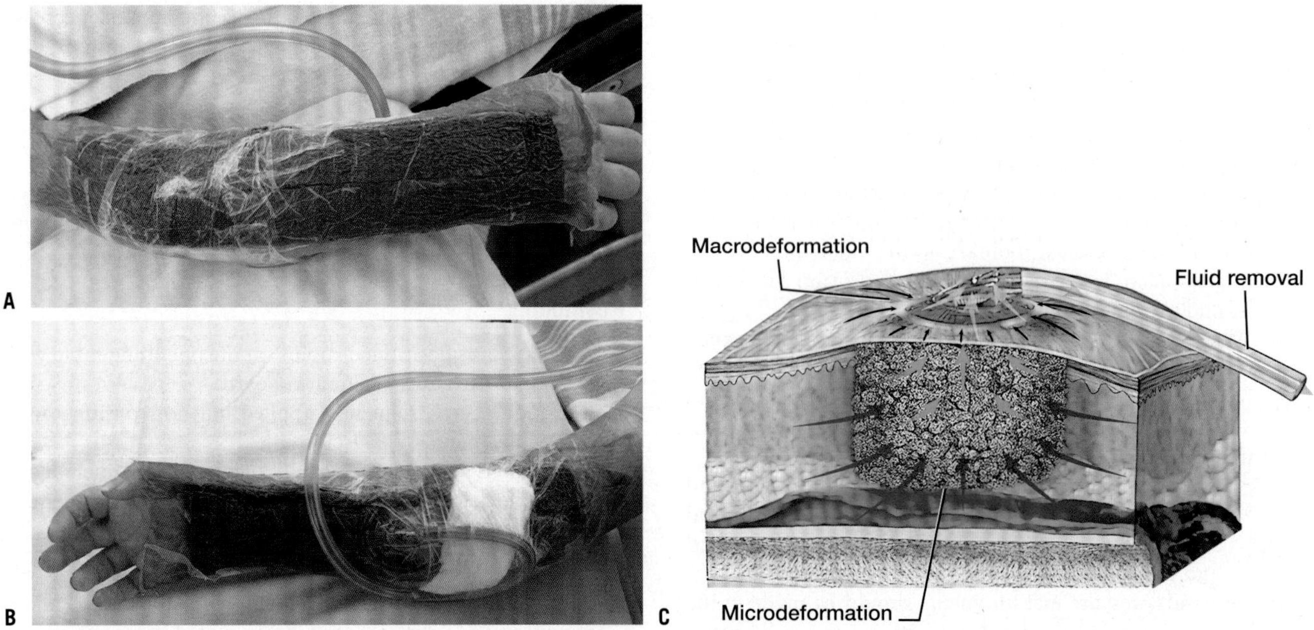

FIG 3 NPWT applied to dorsal (**A**) and volar (**B**) forearm fasciotomy sites. **C.** The four primary mechanisms for promoting wound healing in NPWT. (**A,B:** From Lee G, Murray PC, Hasegawa IG. Closed incision negative pressure wound therapy in the management of a complex fasciotomy wound in a pediatric patient. Cureus 2020;12[3]:e7413. https://creativecommons.org/licenses/by/4.0/.)

undulation of the wound surface. These forces result in shear forces that affect the cytoskeletal structures, leading to the activation of various signaling cascades that upregulates granulation tissue formation, and thus, wound healing.

- Fluid removal: Fluid accumulation in the extracellular space inhibits wound healing by elevating interstitial pressure, compressing cells and tissues, and inhibiting cellular proliferation by decreasing the building of intrinsic tension. Furthermore, removing fluid also decreases hydrostatic compression of the microvasculature, allowing for increased blood flow and perfusion of the tissue.
- Alteration of the wound environment: When fluid is evacuated, electrolytes and proteins are removed, allowing for stabilization of osmotic and oncotic gradients at the wound surface. Furthermore, the foam and adhesive help maintain temperature and a warm wound environment. These factors can also potentiate wound healing.

- Once the wound is considered to be stable and clean, the skin can be closed if under no tension. If minimal tension is present, tension dissipation suture ladders (**FIG 4**), including many commercially available products, can be used. If significant tension is present, split-thickness skin grafts are usually applied.

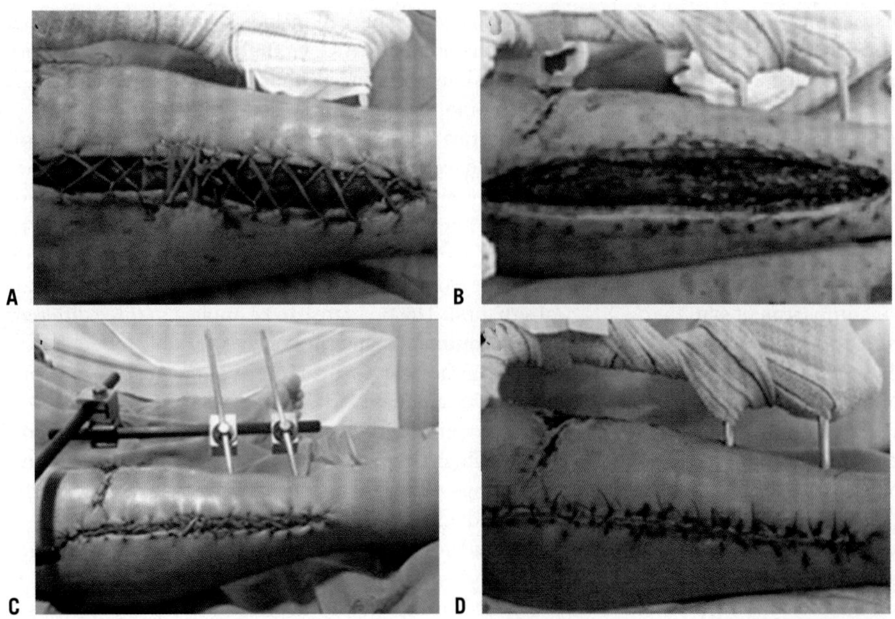

FIG 4 Tension-dissipating elastic suture technique at initial application (**A**), after 48 hours (**B**), after removal in 7 days (**C**), and after secondary suture application (**D**). (Reprinted from Branco PS, Cardoso M Jr, Rotbande I, et al. Elastic suture [shoelace technique] for fasciotomy closure after treatment of compartmental syndrome associated to tibial fracture. Rev Bras Ortop 2016;52[1]:103–106. Copyright © 2016 Elsevier. With permission.)

DECOMPRESSION OF THE ARM

- Compartment syndrome of the arm is rare. It can be approached from the lateral, posterior, or anteromedial approach.
  - The choice of incision may be based on the need for fracture fixation.[1,2]
- The lateral approach begins at the deltoid insertion and extends to the lateral epicondyle. The fascia overlying the biceps anteriorly and triceps posteriorly is split through the incision **(TECH FIG 1A)**.
- The anteromedial approach extends from the medial epicondyle toward the axilla, and the fascia overlying the biceps and triceps is split **(TECH FIG 1B)**. This incision can be continued from the forearm skin incisions.
  - The ulnar nerve must be protected in this approach.
- For isolated posterior compartment syndrome, a posterior incision can be made from 8 cm distal to the acromion to the olecranon **(TECH FIG 1C)**. The triceps fascia is directly exposed and incised.[2]
  - The radial nerve runs between the long and lateral heads of the triceps and is at risk during muscle débridement.

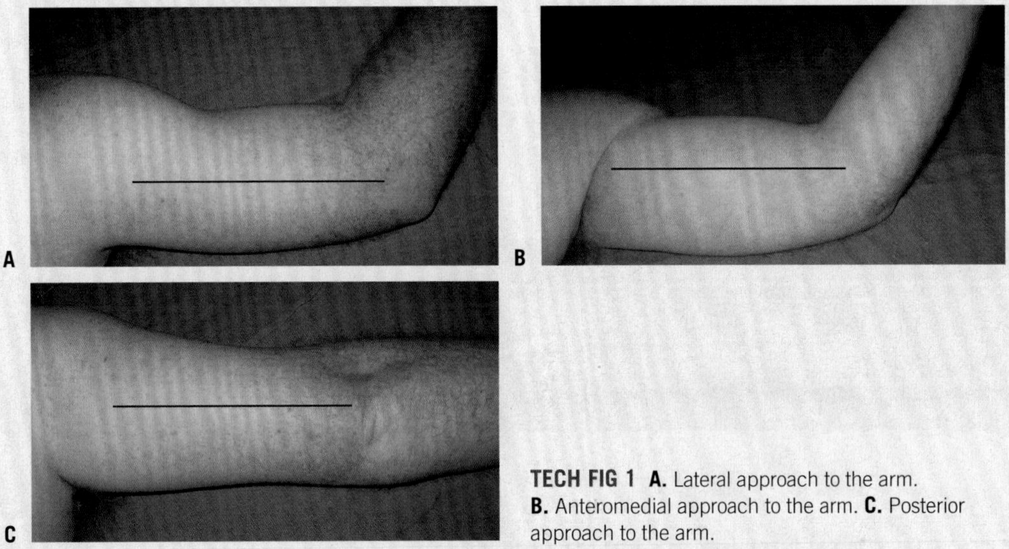

TECH FIG 1 A. Lateral approach to the arm. **B.** Anteromedial approach to the arm. **C.** Posterior approach to the arm.

DECOMPRESSION OF THE VOLAR FOREARM

- Design a curvilinear incision from the carpal tunnel to the antecubital fossa. A complete carpal tunnel release is indicated if symptoms of median nerve compression are present **(TECH FIG 2)**.
- Start the incision distally between the thenar and hypothenar eminences in line with the radial border of the ring finger. Release the skin, palmar fascia, and transverse carpal ligament.
- Continue the incision proximally to the distal wrist crease, then curve it ulnarly to the pisiform, and extend it proximally along the ulnar side of the distal forearm.
  - This prevents exposure of the flexor tendons and median nerve and protects the palmar cutaneous branch of the median nerve.
- Curve the incision radially in the midforearm and then just anterior to the medial epicondyle at the elbow.
  - Creation of this flap provides coverage of the median nerve.
- At the antecubital fossa, curve the incision slightly anteriorly to meet the incision of the arm, if necessary.
  - This prevents a linear incision at the level of the elbow and provides coverage for the brachial artery.
- Release the fascia covering the superficial and deep compartment of the forearm, as well as the mobile wad, through this incision. Release the lacertus fibrosus at the elbow. Release individual muscle fascia if release of the compartment fascia does not relieve the pressure within each muscle.

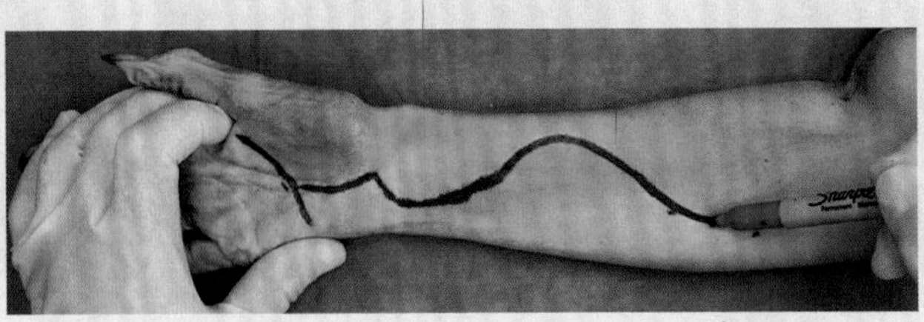

TECH FIG 2 Incision for volar forearm decompression.

- Loosely close the wound over the carpal tunnel; it is generally left open over the forearm.
  - If the swelling is mild, the fascia may be left open, and the skin closed or the skin edges may be approximated with a vessel loop-stapling technique.
  - If the wound is left open, it is covered with a sterile nonocclusive dressing. Alternatively, a VAC dressing may be applied.
- An alternative incision uses the Henry approach between the brachioradialis and the flexor carpi radialis, connecting to the carpal tunnel distally and proximally, crossing the antecubital fossa obliquely from radial to ulnar.
  - If this approach is used, take care not to injure the palmar cutaneous branch of the median nerve at the wrist.

DECOMPRESSION OF THE DORSAL FOREARM

- In the forearm, release of the volar compartment and mobile wad may decrease the pressure in the dorsal compartment. Once the palmar fasciotomy has been performed, the dorsal compartment should be reevaluated for the need for fasciotomy.
- Make a longitudinal dorsal incision just ulnar to the tubercle of Lister and extending proximally toward the lateral epicondyle. Release the fascia over the dorsal compartment **(TECH FIG 3)**.
- Release individual muscle fascia if necessary.
- If posterior interosseous nerve involvement is suspected, separate the extensor carpi ulnaris and extensor digitorum communis muscles to expose and release the fascia overlying the supinator.
- The wound is managed in a similar way to that described for the volar forearm fasciotomy.

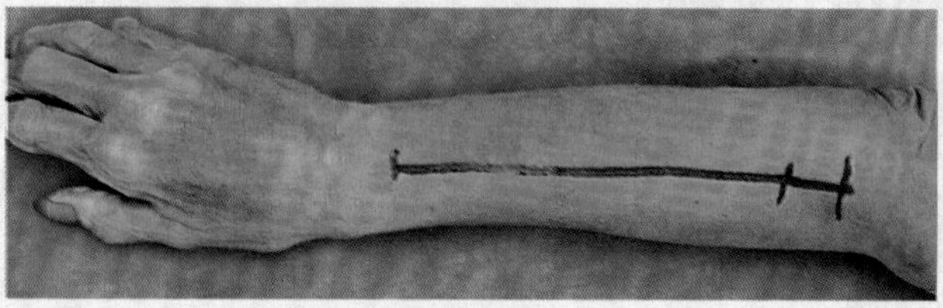

TECH FIG 3 Incision for dorsal forearm decompression.

DECOMPRESSION OF THE HAND COMPARTMENTS

- To release the four dorsal and three palmar interosseous compartments and the adductor compartment, make two dorsal longitudinal incisions over the second and fourth metacarpals **(TECH FIG 4A)**.
- Take the incisions to the level of the extensor tendons. Avoid the sensory branches of the radial and ulnar nerves and preserve dorsal veins to minimize postoperative edema.
- Retract the extensor tendons and expose the dorsal surface of the metacarpal. Release the dorsal compartments on each side of the metacarpal (the first and second dorsal compartments are reached on either side of the second metacarpal, and the third and fourth dorsal compartments are found on either side of the fourth metacarpal). Continue blunt dissection palmarly through the dorsal interossei to release the three palmar interosseous compartments.
- Release the adductor compartment through the incision over the second metacarpal.
- Release the thenar compartment through a longitudinal incision along the radial border of the thumb metacarpal and release the hypothenar compartment through an incision along the ulnar border of the fifth metacarpal **(TECH FIG 4B)**. Split the underlying fascia longitudinally.
- The wounds are left open **(TECH FIG 4C)**, and the hand is placed in a bulky splint in intrinsic-plus position (metacarpophalangeal joints flexed 70 degrees and interphalangeal joints extended).

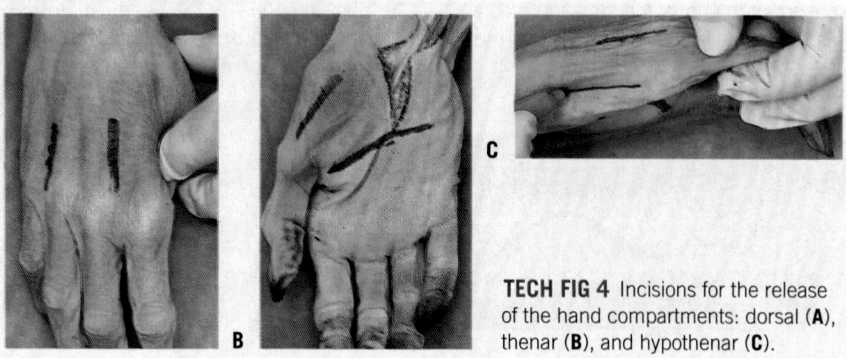

A B C

TECH FIG 4 Incisions for the release of the hand compartments: dorsal (**A**), thenar (**B**), and hypothenar (**C**).

DECOMPRESSION OF THE FINGER

- Make longitudinal midaxial incisions along the finger. These incisions are made by connecting the most dorsal portions of the joint flexion creases **(TECH FIG 5A)**. These are more easily seen with the finger in flexion.
- Avoid making a more palmar, midlateral incision to prevent postoperative flexion contracture.
- Carefully divide the transverse retinacular ligament and Cleland ligament to release the neurovascular bundles on both radial and ulnar sides **(TECH FIG 5B)**.
- If possible, loosely approximate the skin.

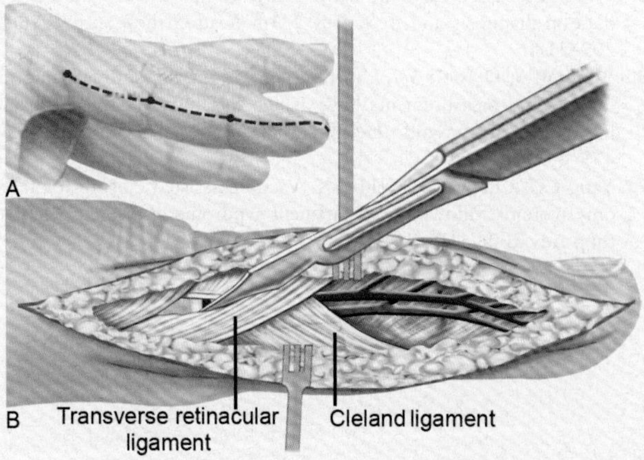

TECH FIG 5 A. Incision for the release of the finger. *Dots* are placed at the apex of each flexion crease and connecting the dots provides the midaxial line. **B.** Division of the transverse retinacular ligament and Cleland ligament.

TECHNIQUES

Pearls and Pitfalls

Indications	• Have a low threshold for measurement of compartment pressures. Perform pressure measurements if clinical examination findings are equivocal.
Surgical Management	• Take care to completely decompress the skin and fascia. • Do not injure superficial nerves. • Débride any devitalized muscle. • Do not close the fascia. • Close the skin loosely or leave it open at the initial procedure.
Postoperative Management	• Return to the operating room for a second look if there is muscle of questionable viability. • Base closure of the wounds on the skin tension and viability. Choose delayed primary closure, split-thickness skin grafting, or flaps as appropriate.

POSTOPERATIVE CARE

- A second look is planned 48 to 72 hours after the index procedure.
  - Additional débridement of devitalized tissue is performed. Serial débridements are performed until no devitalized tissue remains.
  - Delayed primary closure of the skin (not fascia) may be possible. More frequently, split-thickness skin grafting is performed to cover the wounds **(FIG 5)**. If significant soft tissue has been lost with exposed tendon, nerve, or bone, flap coverage is planned.
- Wound coverage should be performed as soon as possible to minimize complications such as infection, desiccation, and amputation.
- The upper extremity should be elevated and splinted in an intrinsic-plus position. Gentle active and active-assisted range of motion of the hand, wrist, and elbow should be initiated as soon as swelling begins to subside, generally within 2 to 3 days after wound closure. Placement of a flap or skin graft may preclude motion at certain joints, but unaffected joints should be ranged.

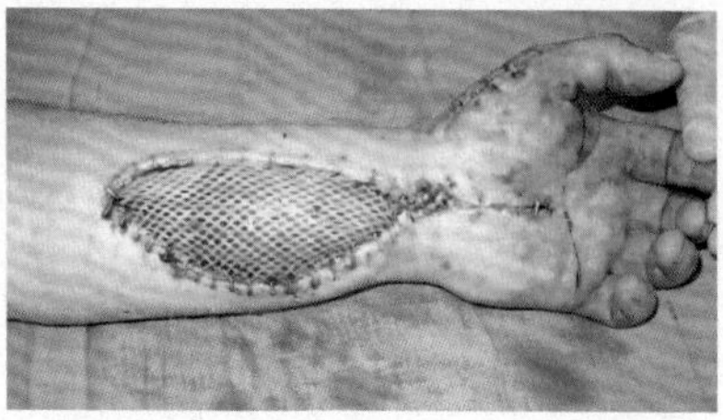

FIG 5 Wound coverage after second look with delayed primary closure and split-thickness skin grafting.

OUTCOMES

- The outcome after compartment release depends both on the severity of the initial injury and the time elapsed before release.
- Patients with prompt diagnosis and treatment and limited devitalized tissues generally have favorable outcomes.
- Patients with severe initial injuries, delayed treatment, or extensive tissue necrosis have a more guarded prognosis for functional recovery of the upper extremity.

COMPLICATIONS

- Volkmann ischemic contracture is the result of untreated acute compartment syndrome.
- Necrosis and fibrosis of the muscle occur, with a resultant claw hand deformity. This deformity is due to extrinsic flexor and extensor contracture with concomitant intrinsic muscle dysfunction.
- Nerve dysfunction results either from the initial ischemic injury or from subsequent compressive neuropathy due to the dense scarring of the tissues surrounding the nerves.
- The deeper compartments are more severely compromised, with the flexor digitorum profundus alone affected in milder cases, and fibrosis of all muscles in the most severe.

REFERENCES

1. Antebi A, Herscovici D Jr. Acute compartment syndrome of the upper arm: a report of 2 cases. Am J Orthop (Belle Mead NJ) 2005;34(10):498–500.
2. Diminick M, Shapiro G, Cornell C. Acute compartment syndrome of the triceps and deltoid. J Orthop Trauma 1999;13(3):225–227.
3. Kakar S, Firoozabadi R, McKean J, et al. Diastolic blood pressure in patients with tibia fractures under anaesthesia: implications for the diagnosis of compartment syndrome. J Orthop Trauma 2007;21(2): 99–103.
4. Tarkin IS. The versatility of negative pressure wound therapy with reticulated open cell foam for soft tissue management after severe musculoskeletal trauma. J Orthop Trauma 2008;22(10 suppl):S146–S151.
5. Whitesides TE, Heckman MM. Acute compartment syndrome: update on diagnosis and treatment. J Am Acad Orthop Surg 1996;4(4): 209–218.
6. Whitney A, O'Toole RV, Hui E, et al. Do one-time intracompartmental pressure measurements have a high false-positive rate in diagnosing compartment syndrome? J Trauma Acute Care Surg 2014;76(2): 479–483.
7. Yang CC, Chang DS, Webb LX. Vacuum-assisted closure for fasciotomy wounds following compartment syndrome of the leg. J Surg Orthop Adv 2006;15(1):19–23.

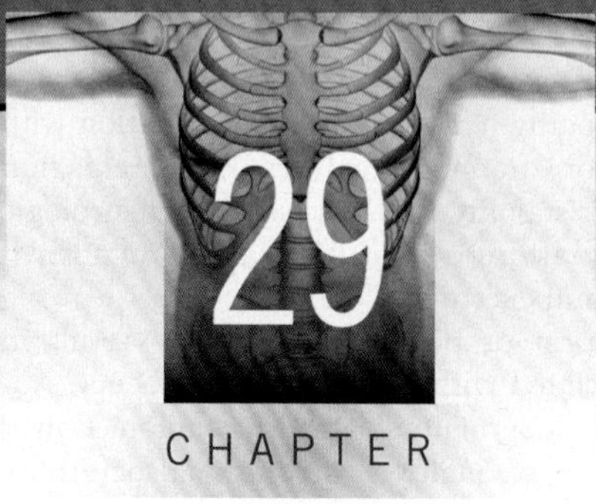

Pelvis and Hip
External Fixation and "Infix" of the Pelvis

Robert D. Wojahn, Stephen A. Kottmeier, and Reza Firoozabadi

DEFINITION

- Pelvic ring fractures represent a diverse group of injury patterns ranging from stable fractures suitable for immediate weight bearing to rotationally and vertically unstable injuries with significant morbidity and mortality.
- Acute management of severe pelvic ring injuries seeks to control intrapelvic hemorrhage, whereas the goal of definitive treatment is to provide structural stability to facilitate easier patient mobilization, minimize deformity, and prevent long-term disability.[14]
- Historic nonoperative treatment of pelvic ring injuries with traction, spica casts, or overhead slings associated with significant patient discomfort and complications[37]
- External fixation first proposed as definitive treatment for pelvic fractures in 1973 with improved reduction, fewer complications, and more rapid patient mobilization.[37]
- Modern role of external fixation has decreased with availability of commercially available pelvic binders and sheeting as well as increasing use of percutaneous fixation techniques.
- Pelvic external fixation remains useful in acute stabilization when the situation precludes use of a binder or sheet and in definitive fixation when the injury prohibits safe internal fixation or necessitates augmentation of other fixation methods.

ANATOMY

- Pelvis composed of two innominate: bones and the sacrum
- Serves as structural continuity between the axial skeleton and lower extremities
- Affords protection and passage for genitourinary, gastrointestinal, and neurovascular structures
- Pelvic stability defined as the ability of the pelvis to assume physiologic loads without displacement or functional compromise
- Stability afforded by ligamentous, rather than osseous, structures
  - Anterior sacroiliac and sacrospinous ligaments resist rotational deformity of the hemipelvis.
  - Interosseous ligaments provide stability against anteroposterior (AP) translation.
  - Posterior sacroiliac and sacrotuberous ligaments resist shear and flexion of the hemipelvis.
  - Iliolumbar ligaments confer additional stability against vertical translation and rotation.
- Anterior portion of the pelvic ring assumes minimal weight-bearing function and affords little pelvic ring stability.
- Life-threatening massive hemorrhage, a potential complication of pelvic ring injury, can be of arterial (branches of the internal iliac system), venous plexus, or fracture surface origins.
- Additional concerns when treating pelvic ring trauma include injury to the lumbosacral plexus and male urethra.

PATHOGENESIS

- Pelvic injury patterns determined by the direction, point of application, and magnitude of applied forces
- Applied forces can be simplified into anteroposterior compression (APC), lateral compression (LC), vertical shear (VS), and combined mechanisms according to the Young-Burgess classification.[40]
- Resultant instability patterns may be categorized as rotationally and vertically stable (Tile A), rotationally unstable and vertically stable (Tile B), and both rotationally and vertically unstable (Tile C) according to the Tile classification.[32]
- Disruption of the ischiosacral (sacrospinous and sacrotuberous) ligaments in the presence of intact posterior sacroiliac ligaments will render a pelvis rotationally unstable. Further disruption of the posterior sacroiliac ligaments will result in both rotational and vertical instability.
- Hemipelvic rotational forces in the APC2 injury cause disruption of the "anterior ligamentous" complex (symphysis pubis, ischiosacral ligaments, anterior sacroiliac ligament) with resulting rotational instability, but the posterior sacroiliac ligaments maintain vertical stability **(FIG 1A)**.
- LC injuries result in internal collapse of the pelvis. Ligaments both anteriorly and posteriorly generally remain intact. Osseous injuries are often stable impaction variants, but internal rotatory instability is occasionally sufficient to warrant surgical stabilization.
- VS injuries imply complete disruption of the posterior tension band of the pelvic ring. This may be of osseous, ligamentous, or combined origin. The involved hemipelvis is unstable in the axial, sagittal, and coronal planes **(FIG 1B)**.
- Any injury mechanism (APC, LC, VS, or combined) may result in complete (vertical and rotational) instability if the force magnitude is sufficient.

NATURAL HISTORY

- Hemorrhage associated with pelvic fractures may be intrapelvic or extrapelvic. In the absence of extrapelvic or intraperitoneal sources, external compression of the pelvis may prevent life-threatening exsanguination.
  - Early sheeting or binder placement may offer an initial beneficial hemodynamic response. Suspected sustained

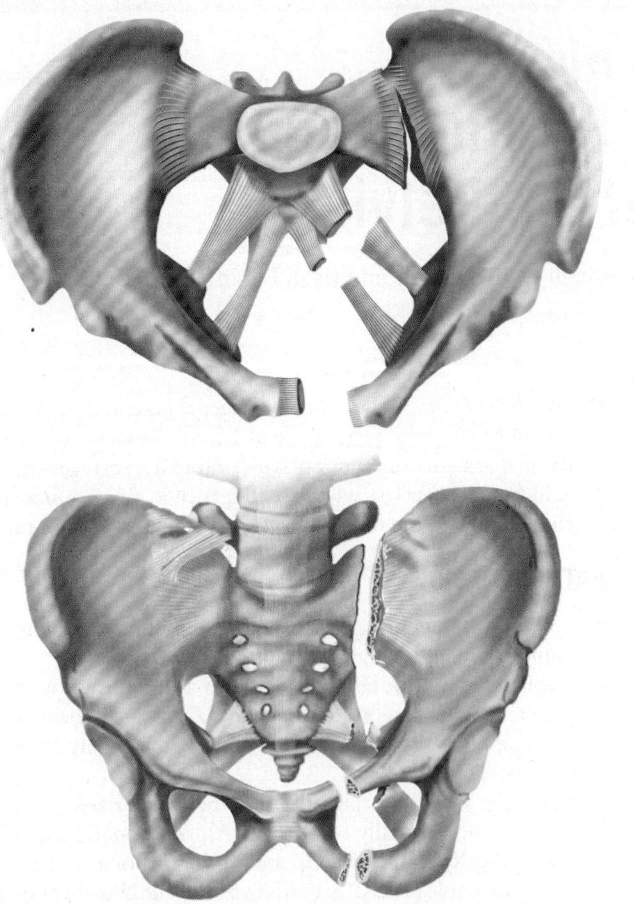

A

B

FIG 1 **A.** An external rotation injury (APC) resulting in "anterior ligamentous complex injury." Instability is rotational in character and demonstrated in the axial plane. The posterior tension band is intact, and vertical stability is preserved. **B.** A VS injury. In addition to compromise to the "anterior ligamentous complex," the integrity of the posterior tension band is disrupted. The involved hemipelvis is unstable in all planes. (Modified from Buckle R, Browner B, Morandi M. Emergency reduction for pelvic ring disruptions and control of associated hemorrhage using the pelvic stabilizer. Tech Orthop 1995;9:258–266.)

hemorrhage of indeterminate source may be intrapelvic arterial in origin, which may respond favorably to angiographic transcatheter embolization.[2]
- Role and timing of exploratory laparotomy remains controversial.
- Imaging findings, results of diagnostic peritoneal lavage (if indicated), and response to aggressive fluid resuscitation must be considered before exposing the unstable trauma victim to the potential negative effects of abdominal exploration (decompression of intrapelvic tamponade, among others).

- Pelvic fractures associated with violation of the perineal, rectal, or vaginal regions must be identified immediately, and early measures directed toward preventing regional and systemic sepsis must be implemented.
  - Appropriate soft tissue management requires early aggressive débridement and restoration of pelvic stability to facilitate wound care. External fixation is of paramount importance in many such cases, as is diverting colostomy.
- Lumbosacral plexopathy may present in combination with sacral spinal canal or foraminal fractures. Pelvic reduction with restoration of stability and occasionally neurologic decompression may afford a more favorable prognosis if properly indicated and executed.[26]
- Insufficient restoration of pelvic stability may result in complications associated with prolonged recumbency. Additional concerns include malunion and nonunion. Lower extremity limb length inequality and rotational deformity may result in functional deficits.
- Anterior ring injuries with significant displacement such as tilt fragments can result in sexual dysfunction, particularly in females.

PATIENT HISTORY AND EXAMINATION

- Patient age is associated with physiologic reserve, which can impact the hemodynamic response. It also impacts bone quality, which can determine tolerance of the bone to various forms of fixation.
- Preexisting medical comorbidities may have considerable impact on survivability and complications associated with operative or nonoperative management of pelvic ring injuries.
- Details of the mechanism of injury offer insight into the energy imparted, which may help determine pelvic injury, instability patterns, and associated intrapelvic or extrapelvic injuries.[5]
- Resuscitative principles of Advanced Trauma Life Support (ATLS) program form the cornerstone for initial treatment of patients with pelvic ring injuries.
  - Evaluation should be undertaken for other potentially life-threatening injuries in the thorax, abdomen, or head.
- Clinical evaluation of pelvis includes inspection for abrasions, contusions, swelling, or fluctuance, which may suggest an underlying Morel-Lavallée lesion. Abnormal rotation of the lower extremities or limb length discrepancy may indicate rotational or vertical pelvic instability.
- A thorough inspection for open fracture must be performed including a vaginal or rectal examination as mortality rates in the presence of such lesions are considerable.[3] Regional hemorrhage in the genitourinary area may also imply urethral injury **(FIG 2)**.
- Neurologic assessment to identify deficits in voluntary sphincter control or perianal sensation is important as lumbosacral plexopathy implies pelvic instability.
- Palpation and manual testing for stability may be pursued with caution.
- Associated lower limb fractures or dislocations must also be assessed as these can impact the method or timing of treatment for the pelvic ring injury.

IMAGING AND OTHER DIAGNOSTIC STUDIES

- The initial AP pelvis radiograph, performed as part of the ATLS protocol, is often sufficient to reveal the injury pattern and initiate emergent treatment **(FIG 3A)**.
- In combination with the pelvic inlet and outlet views, this constitutes the pelvic trauma radiographic triad.
  - Inlet view **(FIG 3B)** depicts AP and rotational displacement, whereas the outlet view **(FIG 3C)** best demonstrates vertical displacement.

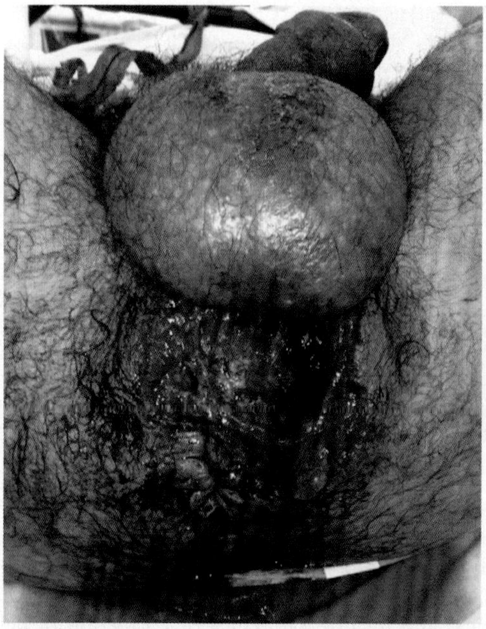

FIG 2 Open pelvis fracture with a large perineal wound in communication with a left inferior ramus fracture and associated rectal injury. Proper treatment of this patient necessitates urgent débridement with temporizing external fixation and diverting colostomy. (Reprinted from Govaert G, Siriwardhane M, Hatzifotis M, et al. Prevention of pelvis sepsis in major open pelviperineal injury. Injury 2012;43[4]:533–536. Copyright © 2011 Elsevier. With permission.)

- Posterior pelvic displacement greater than 1 cm or ramus fracture displacement greater than 2 cm may suggest pelvic instability
- Other radiographic clues of instability include the following:
  - Sacrospinous ligament avulsions (ischial spine or sacral border fractures)
  - Iliolumbar ligament avulsions (L4–L5 transverse process fractures)
  - Symphyseal diastasis of more than 2.5 mm suggests disruption of the anterior ligament complex.
- Imaging studies offer only a static view of the pelvis and may underestimate the amount of deformity at the time of injury.[9] Consequently, they may imply but do not confirm stability of the pelvic ring.
- Stress radiographs under anesthesia (internal/external rotation and "push–pull" studies) may offer a dynamic view of pelvic stability **(FIG 4)**.[30]
  - Such maneuvers are contraindicated in the presence of lumbosacral plexopathy, hemodynamic instability, or ipsilateral lower extremity fractures.
- Computed tomography serves as a valuable adjunctive study to better characterize the injury and, in particular, the posterior injury characteristics.
  - Complete sacral fractures, sacral fracture gap (instead of impaction), and posterior ilium fractures may suggest instability.
  - Sacral foraminal and central spinal canal involvement is also evaluated.

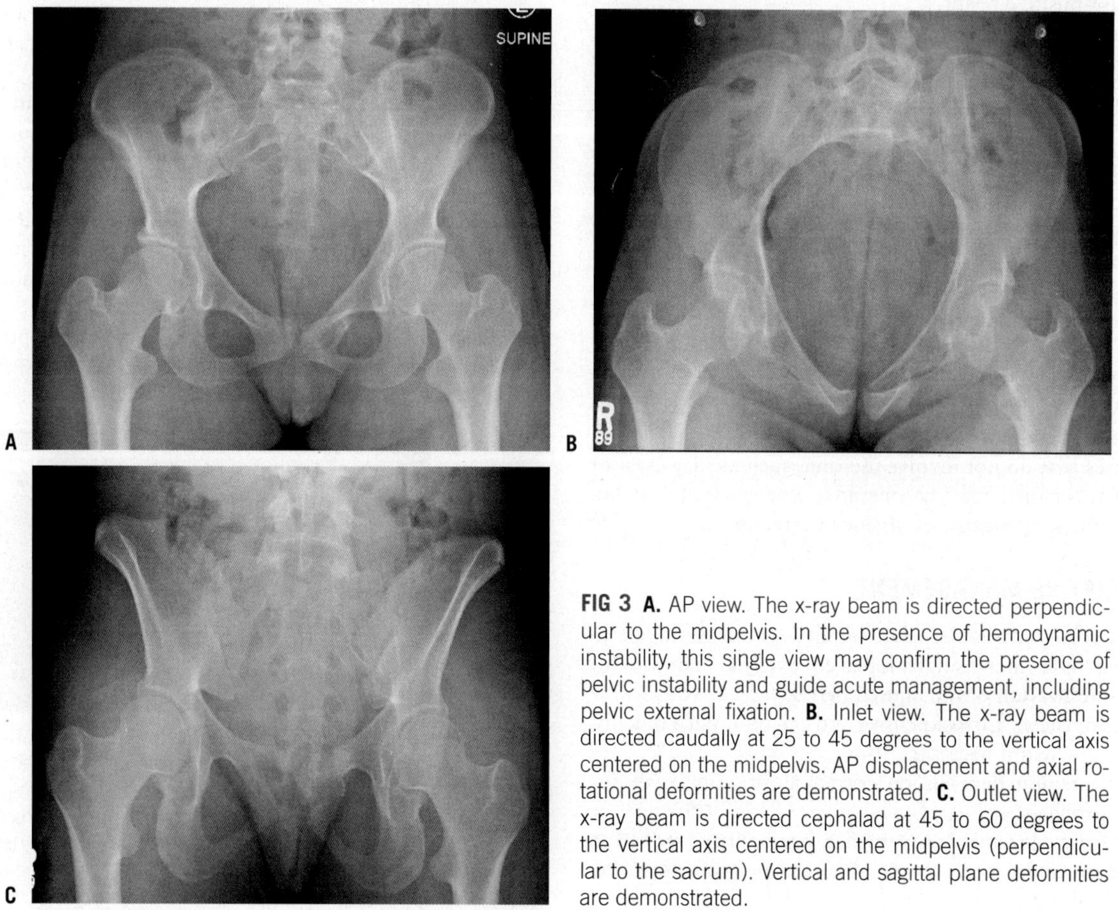

FIG 3 A. AP view. The x-ray beam is directed perpendicular to the midpelvis. In the presence of hemodynamic instability, this single view may confirm the presence of pelvic instability and guide acute management, including pelvic external fixation. **B.** Inlet view. The x-ray beam is directed caudally at 25 to 45 degrees to the vertical axis centered on the midpelvis. AP displacement and axial rotational deformities are demonstrated. **C.** Outlet view. The x-ray beam is directed cephalad at 45 to 60 degrees to the vertical axis centered on the midpelvis (perpendicular to the sacrum). Vertical and sagittal plane deformities are demonstrated.

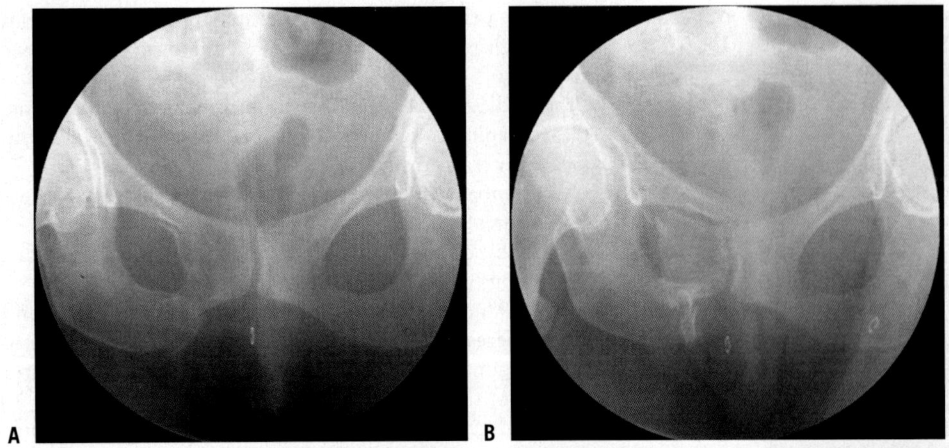

FIG 4 Stress examination under anesthesia may elucidate occult instability not appreciated on the static injury films. **A.** Unstressed AP pelvis radiograph demonstrates minimally displaced right superior and inferior pubic rami fractures. **B.** Internal rotation stress radiograph with a compressive force on the iliac crests shows significant rotatory instability of the pelvic ring with displacement of the fracture across the midline.

- Role of diagnostic and therapeutic angiography remains controversial within management pathways.[16] Ninety percent of intrapelvic hemorrhage is venous or osseous, which may be effectively arrested with a binder, sheet, or external fixation. However, sustained hemodynamic instability may suggest arterial blood loss. In such cases, angiography may be considered and therapeutic arterial embolization performed as necessary. Furthermore, arterial embolization can result in decreased downstream venous bleeding.
- Diagnostic peritoneal tap and lavage, first described in 1965, has a poorly defined contemporary role.[22] Procedure indications, performance, and result criteria remain ambiguous. The presence of a pelvic fracture may also contribute to a false-positive result.
  - Current imaging technology may prove a more reliable tool to determine the likelihood of abdominal injury and the need for laparotomy.

DIFFERENTIAL DIAGNOSIS

- Correct diagnosis of the fracture pattern, severity, soft tissue injury, and patient physiologic status is crucial for treatment planning.
- Recognition of the deforming force in turn dictates temporization and ultimate reduction maneuvers in the operating room.
- Low-energy fractures in senescent bone versus high-energy injuries in younger patients imply markedly different force magnitudes and potential associated injuries.
- Fractures that do not involve the ring, such as iliac crest or ischial tuberosity, may be operative but generally do not require the same degree of urgency in treatment.

NONOPERATIVE MANAGEMENT

- Commercially available pelvic binders and circumferential sheeting have increasingly replaced external fixation for acute stabilization of the injured pelvis.[27]
- Binders or sheets are inexpensive and can be applied quickly, even in the field if necessary.
- Proper function depends on correct positioning over the greater trochanters.
  - Incorrect placement may impact the quality of reduction and preclude access to the abdomen or groin for other procedures.
- Definitive nonsurgical management is appropriate for pelvic ring injuries determined to be clinically and radiographically stable.
  - Goals of surgical and nonsurgical management are identical and include avoidance or correction of deformity, maintenance of stability, and pain-free function.

SURGICAL MANAGEMENT

- Role remains for external fixation in acute management for those patients expected to have a prolonged medical stabilization period prior to undergoing definitive fixation.
  - May be applied at the time of exploratory laparotomy or other urgent procedure
  - By decreasing pelvic volume, it offers intrapelvic tamponade. It also diminishes fracture motion, encouraging hemostasis, and improving patient comfort.
- Temporizing external fixation most successful for pelvic ring injuries with only rotational instability (Tile B)
- Attempts to stabilize vertically unstable patterns (Tile C) with anteriorly based external fixation alone are inadequate and may even accentuate the posterior deformity **(FIG 5)**.[4]
  - These injuries may be better temporized with a binder/sheet, distal femoral traction, or with the addition of a posterior pelvic C-clamp.
- Definitive external fixation remains a viable option for patients with open perineal wounds, rectal injury, suprapubic

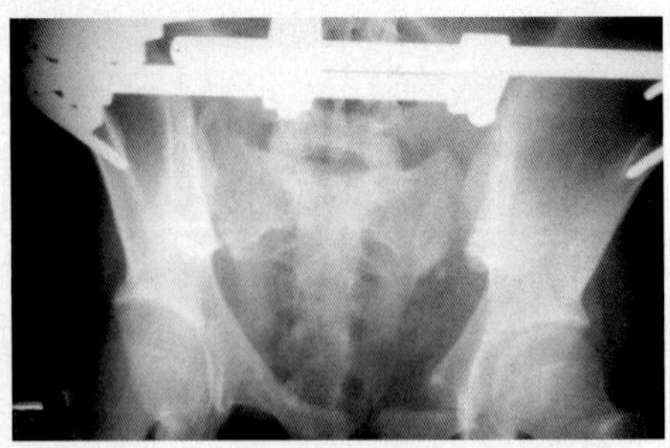

FIG 5 Anterior external fixation of the pelvis does not confer posterior stability. In this example, left posterior sacroiliac diastasis is unresolved. In such cases, anterior external fixation may effectively manage hemodynamic instability but does not offer structural posterior stability. (Reprinted with permission from Peters P, Bucholz RW. The assessment of pelvic stability following pelvic ring disruptions. Tech Orthop 1990;4:52–59.)

catheters, or those expected to undergo multiple abdominal washouts in whom internal fixation would have a high risk for infection.[20]

- Also helpful in stabilizing comminuted or segmental rami fractures and to augment other fixation options in the setting of poor bone quality
- Finally, external fixation may be considered in young male patients with parasymphyseal fractures in whom percutaneous retrograde ramus screws could injure the contralateral spermatic cord.[7]

- Certain LC1 or APC2 patterns, such as those with considerable symphyseal comminution unreceptive to plating, may be amenable to isolated anterior pelvic external fixation for definitive stabilization provided the posterior tension band remains intact.[1]
- Vertically unstable patterns require supplemental posterior fixation.

Preoperative Planning

- Associated intrapelvic, vascular, urologic, and gynecologic comorbidities must be identified.
- Patient's neurologic status should be assessed and any deficits documented. Soft tissues are inspected thoroughly and circumferentially.
- Presence and type of pelvic instability is characterized, assigning the injury pattern to a classification scheme if possible.
- The intended purpose of external fixator must be defined (resuscitative or definitive stabilization).
- If for purposes of initial resuscitation, the surgeon should determine the anticipated timing, sequence, and method of subsequent definitive stabilization.
- Frame design and pin location are selected (iliac crest, supra-acetabular, posterior pelvic C-clamp) based on the pelvic injury pattern, patient's hemodynamic status, associated soft tissue injury, available imaging, and surgeon familiarity.

Positioning

- The patient is placed supine on a fully radiolucent table, so unobstructed fluoroscopy views can be obtained.
- Midline bump is positioned beneath the sacrum to improve access to the starting point for iliosacral screws or the pelvic C-clamp (**FIG 6**).
- Provisional reduction of an APC injury is advisable prior to prepping to avoid skin tenting around pin sites as the deformity is reduced.
  - May be accomplished with a pelvic binder or sheet moved distally to the proximal thighs
  - Alternatively, working portals can be cut in a sheet to allow for a variety of percutaneous procedures while maintaining the compressive effect of the device.[12]
  - The reduction of a binder or sheet can also be augmented by internal rotation and taping of the lower extremities at the feet or anterior thigh.[13]
- Intraoperative traction through a distal femur skeletal traction pin may be a useful reduction tool for cases with vertical instability.
- Full chemical paralysis will also assist in reduction of the hemipelvis.
- Adequacy of imaging and efficacy of closed reduction maneuvers are confirmed prior to prepping.
  - Objects that may block full motion of the C-arm or obstruct the beam are removed.

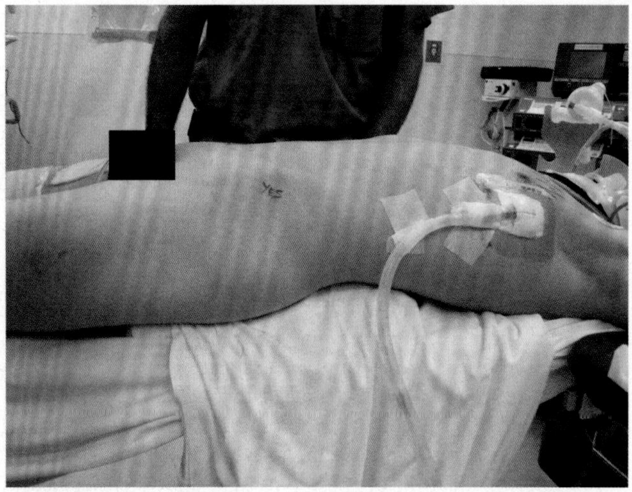

FIG 6 Patient positioning for pelvic fixation. A central bump in place beneath the sacrum to elevate the pelvis off the table. Urinary catheters, chest tubes, and venous or arterial lines are positioned so as not to obstruct the x-ray beam.

- Preparation is then done from the xiphoid to the proximal thighs with isolation of the perineum.
- One or both lower extremities are included circumferentially as required to effect rehearsed closed reduction maneuvers.

Approach

- Proper pin placement and adequate reduction and are the principal requirements for restoring pelvic stability when applying an external fixator.
- Pins may be placed in either the iliac crest or the supra-acetabular region (**FIG 7**).

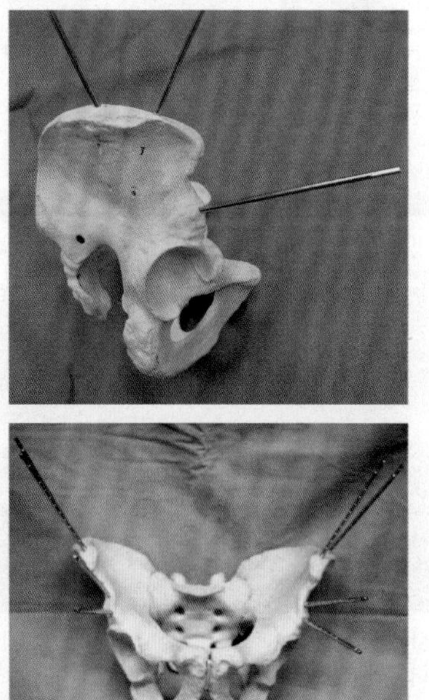

A

B

FIG 7 The anterior hemipelvis offers two sites for pin insertion: the iliac crest (superiorly) and the supra-acetabular region (more inferiorly). **A.** Profile view. **B.** Frontal view.

- Iliac crest pins are placed in the gluteal pillar, a thickening of the ilium extending inferiorly from the crest to the superior acetabulum.
  - Can by placed quickly, even without fluoroscopy if necessary, making them ideal for an emergent resuscitation frame
  - No significant regional anatomic hazards but higher rate of pin misplacement and cutout as the corridor of bone is quite narrow[31]
  - Consider two to three pins in each side for definitive frames to decrease the force seen by each pin and increase the overall stability of the construct.[31]
  - On occasion, this area may be compromised by soft tissue concerns or proximity to fracture planes.
- Supra-acetabular pins are placed through a larger column of dense bone running from the anterior to posterior aspect of the pelvis, resulting in superior stability.[11]
  - Inferior location of these pins also allows easier access to the abdomen for cases of intra-abdominal injury and is less irritating to anterolateral abdominal soft tissues.
  - Supra-acetabular pins are better tolerated in obese patients and less prone to loosening or infection.
  - Major disadvantage is that placement of these pins is more time-consuming and requires fluoroscopic guidance to avoid intra-articular penetration or damage to neurovascular structures of the greater sciatic notch.[31] Resuscitative role is therefore limited.
- Pelvic antishock C-clamp is a posteriorly applied device that offers greater stability to vertically unstable fractures than anteriorly based frames (**FIG 8**).[17]
  - Able to provide a translational force to the posterior pelvis to close down a disrupted sacroiliac joint or displaced sacral fracture

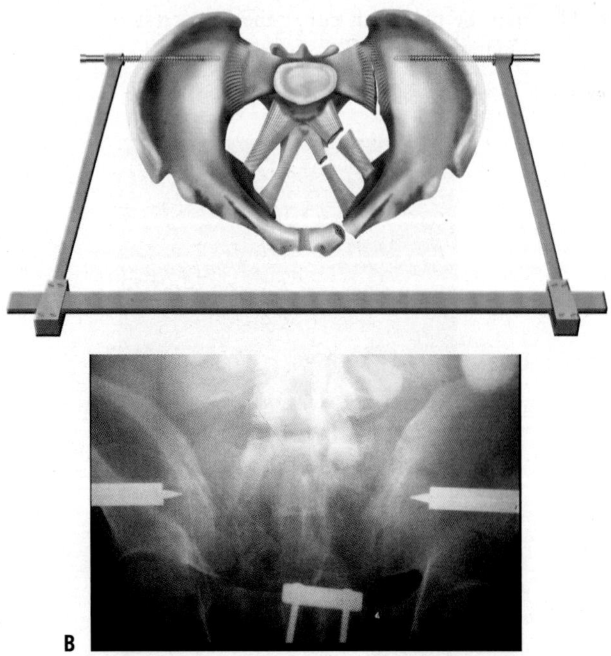

A

B

FIG 8 "Antishock" clamp. This device, applied posteriorly, may offer more stability to vertically unstable injury patterns than anteriorly applied frames. **A.** Schematic. **B.** Case AP radiograph. (**A:** Modified with permission from Simonian PT, Routt ML Jr, Harrington RM, et al. Anterior versus posterior provisional fixation in the unstable pelvis: a biomechanical comparison. Clin Orthop Relat Res 1995;[310]:245–251.)

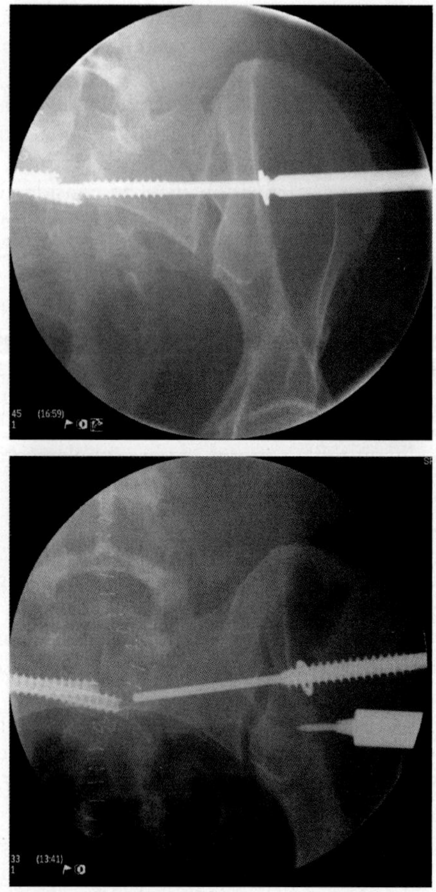

A

B

FIG 9 Use of the pelvic C-clamp as an intraoperative reduction tool. **A.** A partially threaded iliosacral screw was unsuccessful in reducing the joint diastasis for this complete sacroiliac joint injury. **B.** After removal of the screw, a C-clamp was applied with reduction of the joint, avoiding an open reduction.

  - Particularly helpful to tamponade venous bleeding from the presacral plexus but its use has been supplanted in many centers by circumferential sheets or binders, which do have some ability to generate posterior compression
  - The device is indicated for both the acute management of a hemorrhaging patient or as an intraoperative reduction tool when other methods of closed reduction of the posterior ring are insufficient (**FIG 9**)[39]; no role in definitive fixation
  - Contraindicated in cases with comminution of the sacral neural foramina where compression can cause iatrogenic nerve root compression and with comminution of the posterior ilium in which the bolts may fall into fracture lines and risk injury to internal pelvic contents[38]
- Subcutaneous anterior internal fixation has been described to overcome issues associated with transcutaneous pins such as pin tract sepsis, loosening, soft tissue impingement, and impaired patient mobilization (**FIG 10**).
  - Technique employs a precontoured rod or plate introduced via small incisions into a subcutaneous tunnel overlying the external oblique fascia and anchored by screws into the dense supra-acetabular bone.

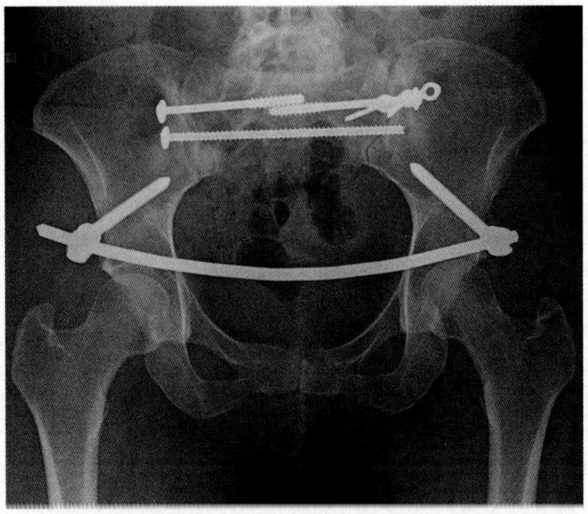

FIG 10 The subcutaneous internal fixator consists of bilateral supra-acetabular pedicle screws connected by a subcutaneously tunneled connecting rod. (Reprinted with permission from Gardner MJ, Mehta S, Mirza A, et al. Anterior pelvic reduction and fixation using a subcutaneous internal fixator. J Orthop Trauma 2012;26[5]: 314–321.)

- Shorter working distance between bone and connecting rod imparts improved stability compared to traditional external fixation.[34]
- Allows unencumbered access to the lower abdomen for surgical procedures, permits easier hip flexion, and allows patients to lie in the prone or lateral position
- Particularly advantageous in obese patients who are at higher risk for complications with traditional external fixation[34]
- Internalized, subcutaneous fixators show lower rates of infection and loosening, but heterotopic ossification is a concern, and lateral femoral cutaneous nerve (LFCN) irritation is somewhat common.[35]
- Close proximity to underlying intrapelvic and neurovascular structures demands an understanding of regional anatomy and proper surgical technique.[23]
- Not applicable for resuscitative purposes due to insertion time and need for fluoroscopy
- Obligatory removal in an operating room setting 3 to 6 months later remains a relative disadvantage.

TECHNIQUES

CIRCUMFERENTIAL PELVIC ANTISHOCK SHEETING

- Several techniques of noninvasive external pelvic ring stabilization have been described. Among them are the use of inflatable antishock trousers and spica casts. These do not permit abdominal access, require skill and familiarity, and conceal the abdomen.
- The simple application of a circumferential bed sheet may be considered during the resuscitation of the hemodynamically unstable patient.[27]
  - Uses materials that are inexpensive, easy to apply, and readily available. No incisions that may jeopardize subsequent operative procedures are required.
  - Sheet is centered at the level of the greater trochanters to allow access to the abdomen and lower extremities.
  - Sheet is folded without wrinkles, pulled tight anteriorly, and the ends secured with clamps **(TECH FIG 1)**.
- Long-term pelvic sheeting is discouraged as soft tissue compromise is a concern. It is contraindicated in the presence of unstable LC injuries where its use may aggravate deformity, resulting in internal visceral injury or posterior neurologic compression.
- Other circumferential pelvic compression devices may offer the simplicity and effectiveness of sheeting with the benefit of feedback-controlled force. This may prevent inadequate or excessive compression.

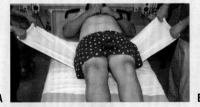

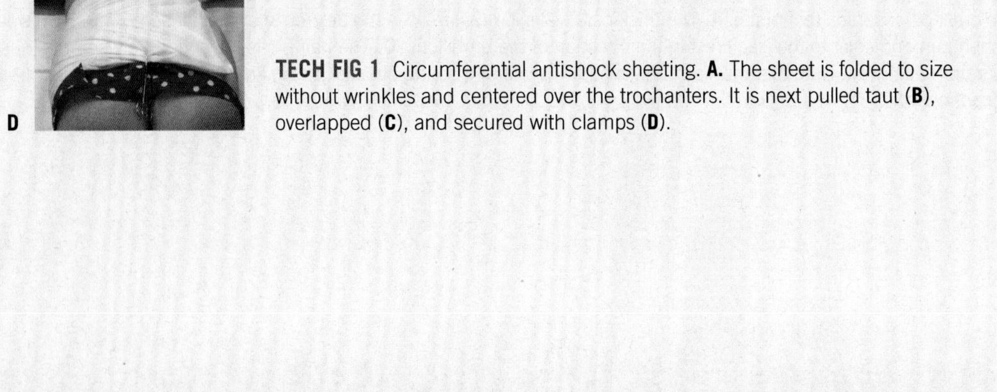

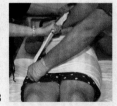

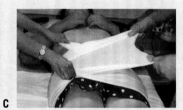

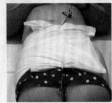

TECH FIG 1 Circumferential antishock sheeting. **A.** The sheet is folded to size without wrinkles and centered over the trochanters. It is next pulled taut (**B**), overlapped (**C**), and secured with clamps (**D**).

ILIAC CREST PIN TECHNIQUE

- Iliac crest pins can be placed with or without fluoroscopy, but it is advisable to use imaging if available to decrease the chance of pin misplacement that could lead to cutout or instability of the construct.
- A provisional reduction is recommended before establishing site of the skin incision to minimize the need for subsequent skin relief incisions after reduction. Failure to account for this can result in excessive skin tension around the pin and contribute to pin site infections or skin necrosis.
- Gluteal pillar begins 2 to 3 cm posterior to the anterior superior iliac spine (ASIS) and extends posteriorly 6 to 8 cm along the crest **(TECH FIG 2A)**. The thickness of bone in this region ranges from 8 mm at the isthmus to 4 cm in the supra-acetabular region.[28]
- Obturator outlet view is obtained as this best visualizes the inner and outer tables of the ilium.
  - View adjusted until the inner table is seen as a single cortical line without any double density
- Starting point for the anterior-most pin is 3 to 4 cm posterior to the ASIS along the crest and just medial to the midpoint between the inner and outer rims because the crest overhands laterally.
- A small incision is made perpendicular from the anterior iliac crest toward the umbilicus as this diminishes undesirable soft tissue tension around the pin on pelvic reduction **(TECH FIG 2B)**.
- Alternatively, a smooth Kirschner wire can be placed percutaneously along the inner table of the ilium to provide a visual reference for the inclination of the iliac wing. A small incision is made just lateral to the wire and the triple drill sleeve advanced to bone.
- Cortex penetrated with 3.5-mm drill and exchanged for a 5.0-mm half pin
  - Medial-lateral trajectory of the pin between the two tables of the ilium is guided by the obturator outlet view or the wire along the inner table **(TECH FIG 2C)**.
  - AP trajectory is directed toward the acetabular dome on the iliac oblique view or approximated using the greater trochanter as a guide for aiming **(TECH FIG 2D)**.[28]
- Pin length is maximized to increase pullout resistance but left at least 2 cm short of the acetabular dome to prevent inadvertent joint penetration.
  - Pin advancement beyond 5 cm without fluoroscopy is associated with an increased chance of cortical penetration, and acetabular penetration is likely to occur with pins advanced further than 10.5 cm.[28]
- Intercortical pins are preferred to transcortical pins due to increased pullout strength.
- Additional pins, if applicable, are placed posterior to the first pin in similar fashion with a 2- to 3-cm interval between each pin.
- Pins should converge slightly as the gluteal pillar narrows as it nears the supra-acetabular region **(TECH FIG 2E)**.
- Two to three pins should be placed in each side if not using fluoroscopy due to the higher risk for pin malposition and failure.

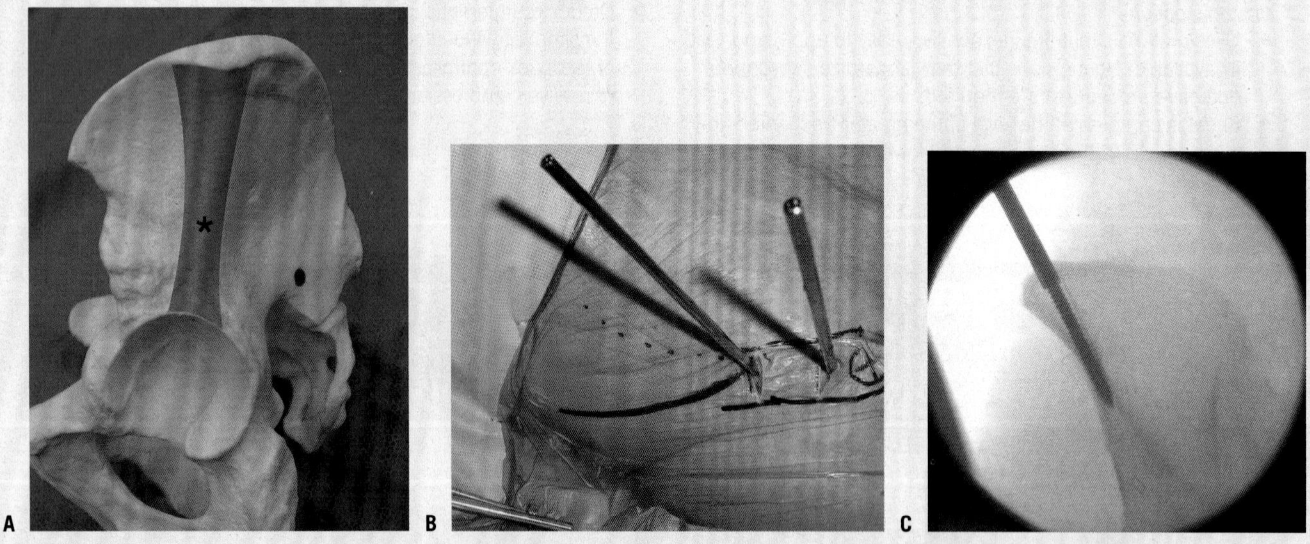

TECH FIG 2 Iliac crest pin insertion technique. **A.** The thick osseous pillar (*asterisk*) is the desired site of pin insertion. **B.** Stab wounds (1 to 2 cm long) are established perpendicular to the iliac crest in the direction of the umbilicus. **C.** The half pin is advanced between the inner and outer tables on the obturator outlet view. Note that the iliac crest overhangs laterally, so the pin start site is kept medial to the midpoint between the inner and outer rims. *(continued)*

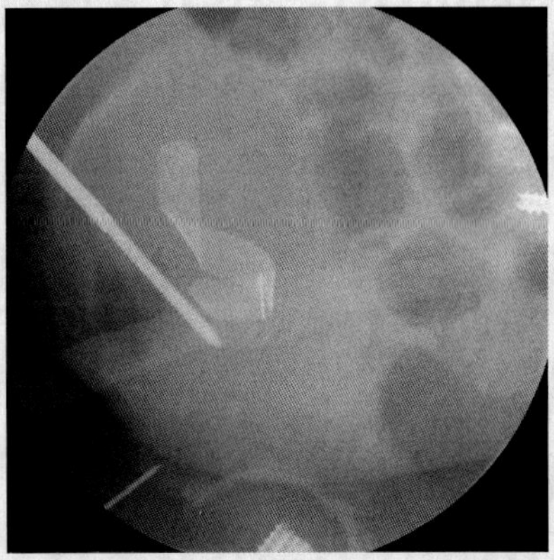
D

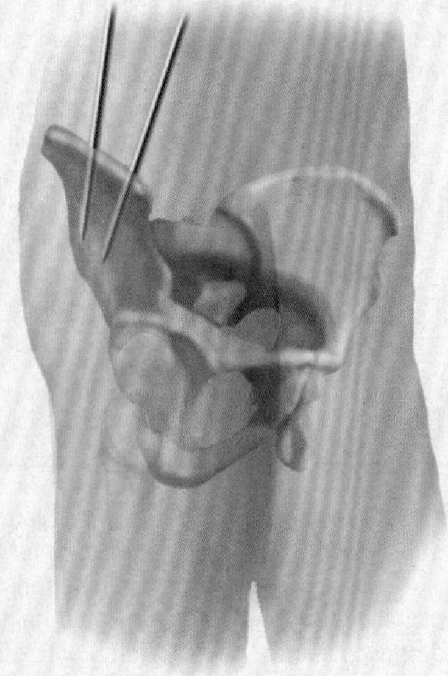
E

TECH FIG 2 *(continued)* **D.** The pin is directed toward the acetabulum on the iliac oblique view to keep it within the gluteal pillar. **E.** Pins should converge on the supra-acetabular region while remaining within the gluteal pillar. (**E:** Modified with permission from Poka A, Libby EP. Indications and techniques for external fixation of the pelvis. Clin Orthop Relat Res 1996;[329]:54–59.)

SUPRA-ACETABULAR PIN TECHNIQUE

- Safe placement and proper positioning of supra-acetabular pins require fluoroscopic guidance.
- Bone corridor is visualized on the obturator outlet view, also called the *teardrop view* in this application.
  - View should be optimized until the inferior border of the teardrop lies just above the acetabular dome, the inner table appears as a single linear density, and the corridor of bone is as narrow as possible **(TECH FIG 3A)**.[11]
- Pin starting point is in the center of the teardrop and should be at least 2 cm superior to the acetabular dome to prevent intracapsular placement and possible septic joint in the setting of pin site infection.[15]
- Skin entry site is marked using a radiopaque object and a 1-cm vertical incision made.
- Blunt dissection is carried to the bone to minimize risk to the LFCN.
  - LFCN is a mean distance of 10 mm from the pin entry site but ranges from 2 to 25 mm.[15]
- Triple drill sleeve is introduced to the cranial aspect of the anterior inferior iliac spine (AIIS) and its position confirmed fluoroscopically.[11]
- Cortex penetrated with a 3.5-mm drill and then exchanged for a 5.0-mm half pin
  - Iliac oblique view is used to assess insertion depth and direct the pin 1 to 2 cm cranial to the greater sciatic notch **(TECH FIG 3B)**.
    - Alternatively, the pin can be directed more caudally toward the notch to engage the dense bone of the sciatic buttress and allow increased hip flexion before the thigh impinges on the clamps and bar.

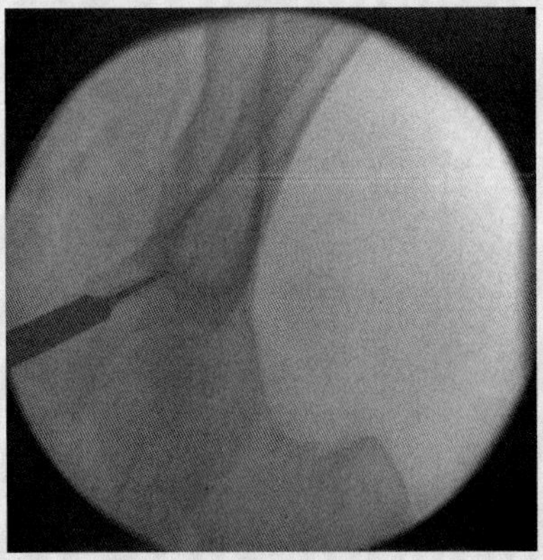
A

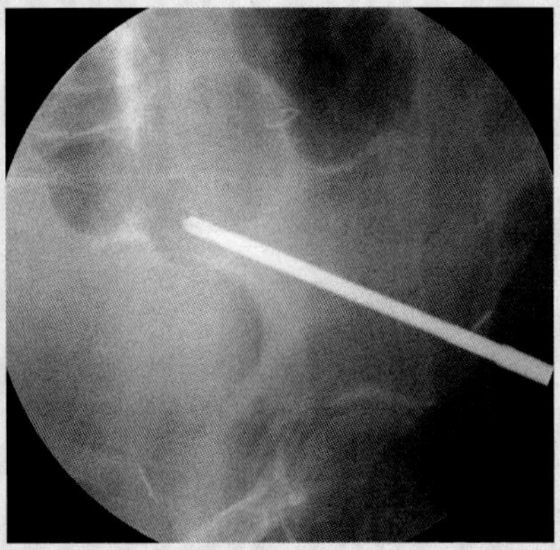
B

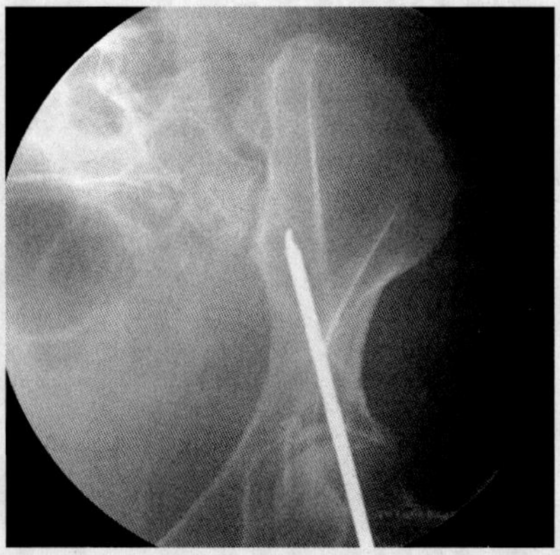
C

TECH FIG 3 Supra-acetabular pin insertion technique. **A.** The corridor of bone for pin placement is visualized on the obturator outlet or "teardrop" view. The scalpel blade marks the starting point in the center of the teardrop, at least 2 cm superior to the acetabulum. **B.** The pin is directed 1 to 2 cm superior to the greater sciatic notch on the iliac oblique view to avoid injury to the sciatic nerve or gluteal vessels. **C.** The pin is directed between the inner and outer tables of the ilium on the obturator inlet view.

- Obturator inlet view provides an orthogonal view of the column of bone running from the AIIS to posterior superior iliac spine (PSIS) and can permits visualization of the entire length of the pin between the inner and outer tables **(TECH FIG 3C)**.
- Pins have similar posterior stability whether they are advanced halfway to the PSIS or to within 1 cm of the PSIS.[8]
- A second pin is inserted in the contralateral hemipelvis using similar technique.
- Alternatively, a 0.062 Kirschner wire can be used to optimize the start site and inserted 1 to 2 cm into bone. A 4.5-mm cannulated drill is then placed over this wire and appropriate trajectory obtained using the drill within 3 to 4 cm of the cortex. This is then exchanged for a 5.0-mm Schanz pin through the outer cannula of a triple sleeve.

FRAME APPLICATION AND REDUCTION

- Simple frame constructs are preferred to permit patient mobilization, abdominal access, and performance of subsequent diagnostic and therapeutic procedures.
- Provisional construct is assembled but the clamps initially left loose, so reduction maneuvers can be performed prior to clamp tightening.
- A 3-4 bar construct is most often used for iliac crest-based frames with a bar on each side to link the pins in each crest and 1-2 bars anteriorly connecting the two lateral bars **(TECH FIG 4A)**.
- Supra-acetabular pins may instead be secured with two bars attached anteriorly with a single-bar bar clamp or with a single anterior curved bar **(TECH FIG 4B)**.
- Clamps should remain three fingerbreadths above the skin surface to avoid soft tissue impingement and allow adequate pin site care.
- Care must also be taken to allow adequate room for hip flexion and abdominal expansion.
- Pelvic deformity is reduced using the pins as levers to manipulate the affected hemipelvis.
  - Rotational deformity is corrected with internal rotation of the hemipelvis for APC injuries or external rotation for LC injuries.[1]
  - Sagittal plane deformity can be reduced with flexion or extension of the pin.
  - Cranial translation of the hemipelvis can be corrected with longitudinal traction either manually or through a distal femoral traction pin.[11]
- Oblique distraction external fixation uses a hybrid frame used for reduction and stabilization of combined flexion/internal rotation hemipelvic deformities **(TECH FIG 4C)**.[6]
  - Ipsilateral supra-acetabular pin and contralateral iliac crest pin bridged by either a femoral distractor or an external fixation bar
  - Can be used as provisional reduction for subsequent internal fixation or left in place as definitive fixation
- Anteriorly based external fixators are unable to maintain reduction of vertically unstable patterns and may even accentuate deformity in these injuries.[4]
- Use of a femoral distractor as a fixed angle compressor has been described to achieve some posterior reduction of a vertically unstable pattern **(TECH FIG 4D)**.[11]

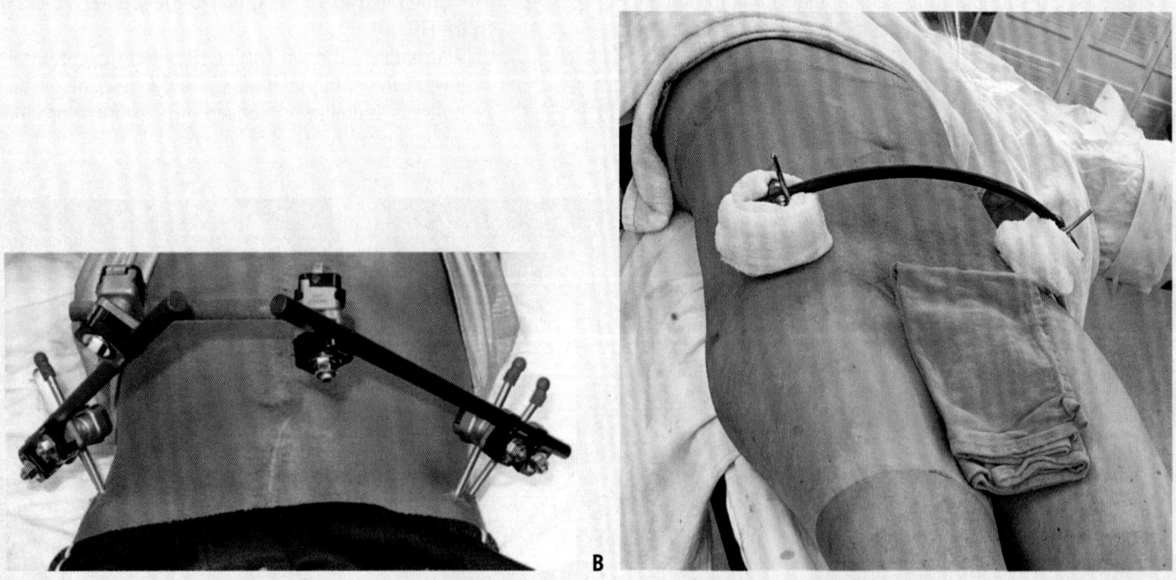

A B

TECH FIG 4 **A.** Frame configuration utilizing iliac crest pins. The two side bars are linked by a single anterior bar. Note that two pins are used in each iliac crest due to the less favorable biomechanical properties of these pins. **B.** Frame configuration utilizing supra-acetabular pins. A pin-bar clamp is applied to each pin and the two linked anteriorly with a single curved bar. Care is taken to allow adequate room for hip flexion and abdominal expansion. *(continued)*

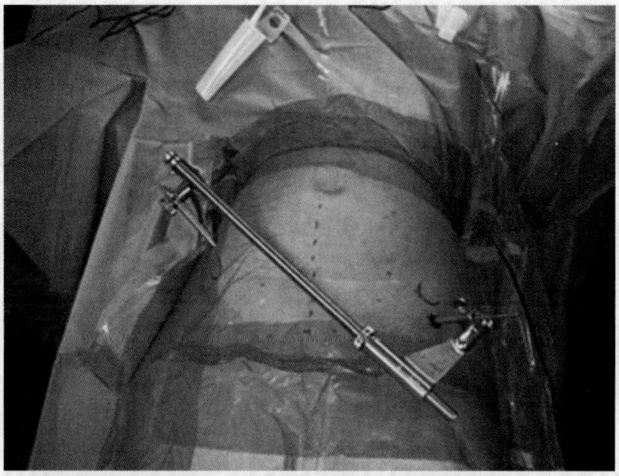

C

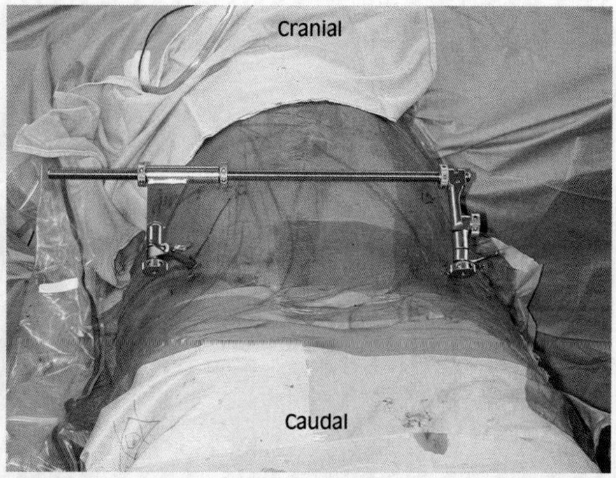

D

TECH FIG 4 *(continued)* **C.** This oblique distraction fixator configuration uses an iliac crest pin in the right hemipelvis and a supra-acetabular pin in the left hemipelvis to create an oblique reduction force vector. **D.** Use of a femoral distractor as a fixed-angle compressor to generate posterior pelvic compression utilizing supra-acetabular pins. (**A:** Reprinted with permission from Kanlic EM, Abdelgawad AA. Pelvic fractures: external fixation. In: Wiss DA, ed. Master Techniques in Orthopaedic Surgery: Fractures, ed 3. Philadelphia: Lippincott Williams & Wilkins, 2013:745–770. **C:** Reprinted with permission from Evans AR, Routt ML Jr, Nork SE, et al. Oblique distraction external pelvic fixation. J Orthop Trauma 2012;26[5]:322–326. **D:** Reprinted with permission from Gardner MJ, Nork SE. Stabilization of unstable pelvic fractures with supraacetabular compression external fixation. J Orthop Trauma. 2007;21[4]:269–273).

PELVIC ANTISHOCK C-CLAMP

- The C-clamp can be applied with or without fluoroscopy, but imaging is advised if possible to avoid risk of bolt misplacement.
- Surgeon can choose between two coronally oriented pin placement positions (posterior or anterior).[25]
  - Posterior pin placement allows for compression of the posterior pelvic ring.
  - Anterior pins are placed in the supra-acetabular region, which may provide more symmetric compression of both the anterior and pelvic ring.
- Optimal site for posterior pin placement is at the intersection of a line connecting the ASIS and PSIS (roughly a vertical line down from the ASIS) and a line along the posterior border of the femur with the leg in neutral rotation **(TECH FIG 5A)**.
  - Two- to 3-cm incision is made at this location and blunt dissection with hemostat or scissors carried down to the lateral surface of the posterior ilium.
  - In the absence of fluoroscopy, the tip of this instrument can then be used to palpate the correct insertion point as a "groove" where the orientation of the iliac wing changes at the level of the pelvic brim.[25]
  - Correct insertion point can also be localized using fluoroscopy at the anterior aspect of the sacroiliac joint on the inlet view and at the S1 or S2 level on the outlet view. This is very near the start point for a transiliac-transsacral screw, so care should be taken not to obstruct placement of definitive posterior fixation.
  - Steinman pin is then introduced to this location and driven or impacted 1 cm into the ilium. This process is repeated for the contralateral side.
- Optimal site for anterior pin placement lies along the gluteal pillar midway between the iliac crest and the greater trochanter **(TECH FIG 5B)**. The proximal extent of the gluteal pillar can be approximated as three fingerbreadths posterior to the ASIS.
  - Surgeon must ensure the leg is not externally rotated as this will place the pins too far posterior.
  - Pin site should be approximately 5 to 6 cm from the top of the iliac wing.[25]
- Contralateral pins are adjusted to be coaxial, which allows rotation of the C-clamp, permitting abdominal access.
- The threaded compression bolts with attached sidearms are then inserted over the two pins and advanced down to bone **(TECH FIG 5C)**.
- Reduction of any vertical displacement is now completed with traction or manipulation of the hemipelvis using Schanz pins prior to compressing the C-clamp.

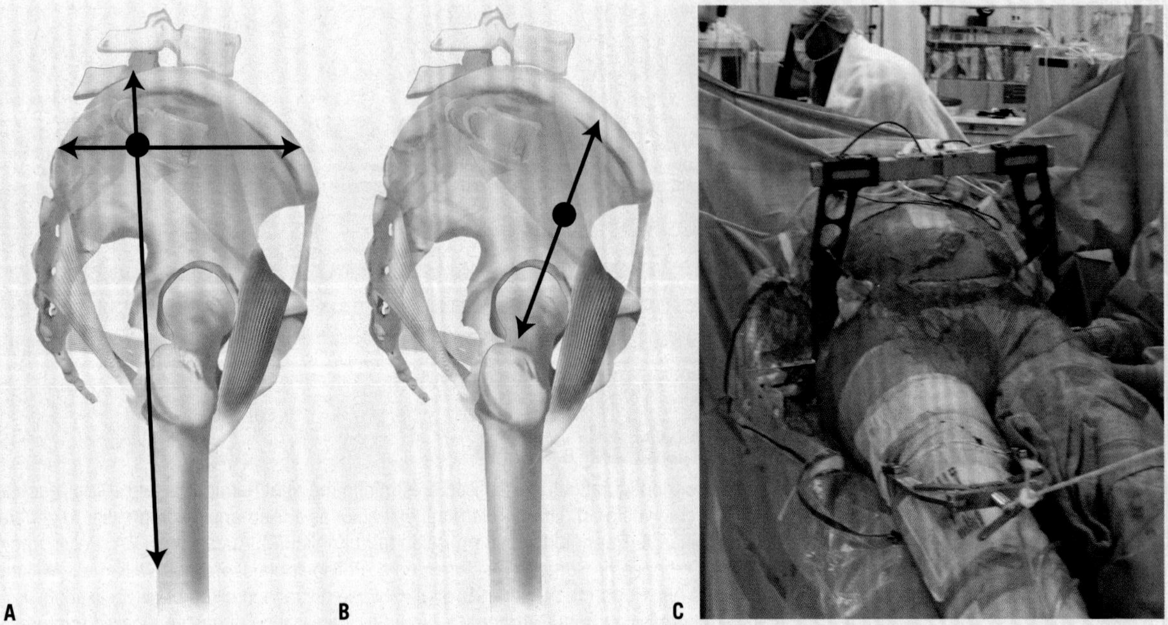

TECH FIG 5 **A.** Posterior pin location for C-clamp application at the intersection of a vertical line down from the ASIS and a line along the posterior border of the femur. **B.** Anterior pin location for C-clamp application along the gluteal pillar midway between the iliac crest and greater trochanter. **C.** Clinical photograph of the C-clamp after placement on a polytraumatized patient. Note that the clamp permits unencumbered access to the abdomen and perineum. (**A,B:** Modified from Buckle R, Browner B, Morandi M. Emergency reduction for pelvic ring disruptions and control of associated hemorrhage using the pelvic stabilizer. Tech Orthop 1995;9:258–266.)

SUBCUTANEOUS ANTERIOR PELVIC INTERNAL FIXATION

- Several different techniques have evolved using plates, screws, pins, or alternative devices. Technique depicted in this text employs cannulated instruments and implants commonly used for posterior spinal fixation.
- No commercially available subcutaneous internal fixator system is available, so any spine pedicle screw set can be used in this off-label application.
- Ideal starting point is localized at the center of the "tear drop" on an obturator outlet view similar to a supra-acetabular external fixator.
- Three-cm longitudinal skin incision is made and blunt dissection carried down to the sartorius fascia to minimize the risk of injury to the LFCN.[34]
- A Jamshidi needle is advanced between the cortices of the ilium, directed toward the PSIS, monitoring its progress on the iliac oblique and obturator inlet views **(TECH FIG 6A,B)**.
- The guidewire of the pedicle screw system is then positioned and advanced through the needle and appropriate length measured. A tap can be employed if desired **(TECH FIG 6C–E)**.
- Appropriate length 7.0- to 8.5-mm cannulated pedicle screw is placed over the guidewire using the screw assembly **(TECH FIG 6F,G)**.
  - Screw head should be left just superficial to the sartorius fascia, 15 to 40 mm off bone, to prevent compression of neurovascular structures by the connecting rod **(TECH FIG 6H)**.
  - Screw lengths are typically 75 to 110 mm with approximately 60 mm in bone.[23,34]
- Same procedure is repeated for the contralateral hemipelvis **(TECH FIG 6I)**.
- A 5.0- to 6.5-mm titanium connecting rod is then cut to size and precontoured with an anterior bow to match the patient's anatomy at the level of the lower abdominal fold.
  - Optimal contour avoids compression of abdominal contents or neurovascular structures but is also not prominent under the skin.
  - External iliac vessels are, on average, only 2.2 cm posterior to the rod when done correctly.[23]
- Rod is inserted above the abdominal fascia via a subcutaneous tunnel using the rod holder assembly to meet the contralateral screw **(TECH FIG 6J,K)**.
- Once the rod is captured and locked by an end cap on one side, powerful rotational reduction forces can be effected with use of a system-specific compression or distraction tool prior to tightening the set screws.
- The fixator is removed in the operating room after healing of fractures (typically between 3 and 6 months).

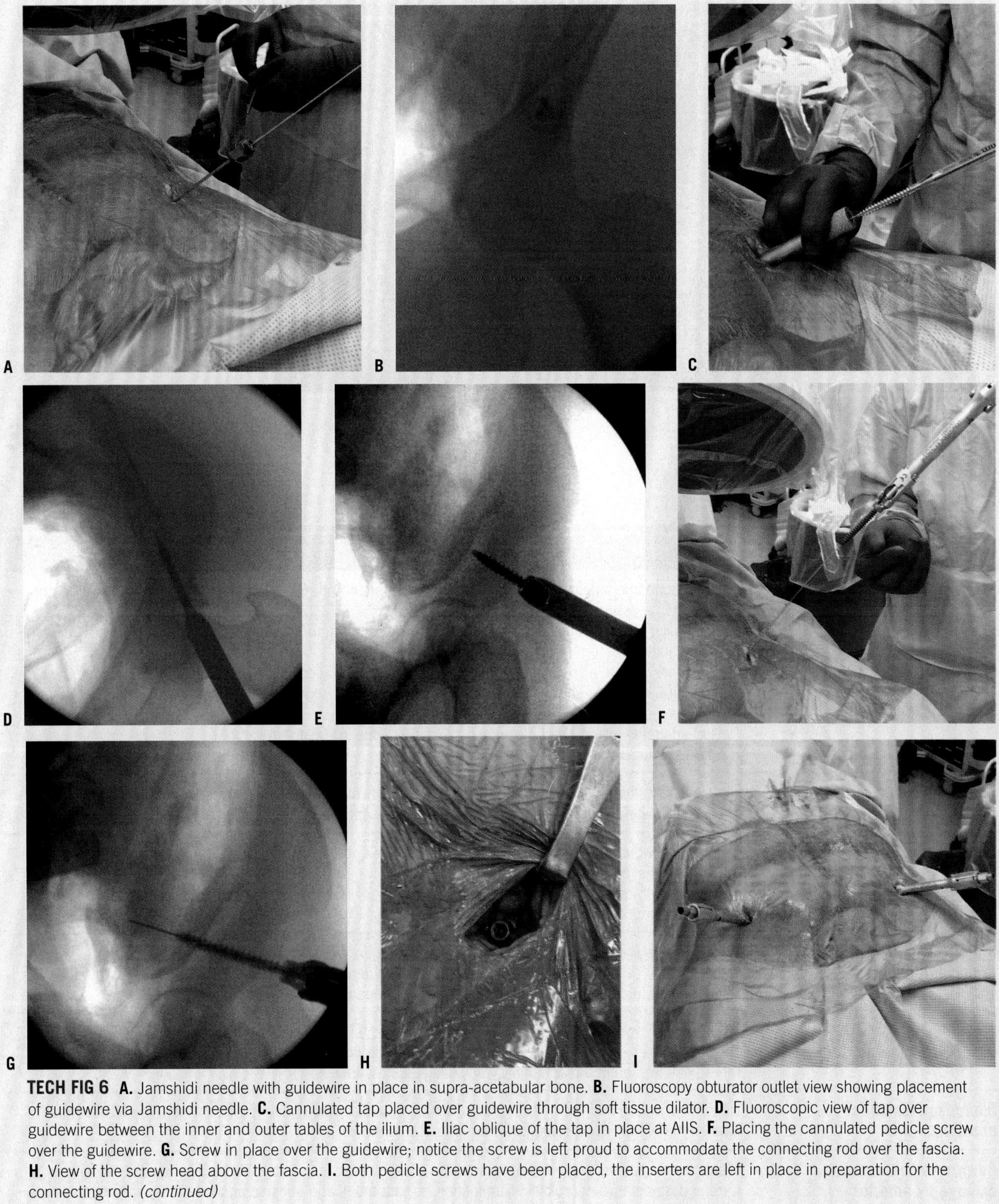

TECH FIG 6 A. Jamshidi needle with guidewire in place in supra-acetabular bone. **B.** Fluoroscopy obturator outlet view showing placement of guidewire via Jamshidi needle. **C.** Cannulated tap placed over guidewire through soft tissue dilator. **D.** Fluoroscopic view of tap over guidewire between the inner and outer tables of the ilium. **E.** Iliac oblique of the tap in place at AIIS. **F.** Placing the cannulated pedicle screw over the guidewire. **G.** Screw in place over the guidewire; notice the screw is left proud to accommodate the connecting rod over the fascia. **H.** View of the screw head above the fascia. **I.** Both pedicle screws have been placed, the inserters are left in place in preparation for the connecting rod. *(continued)*

J
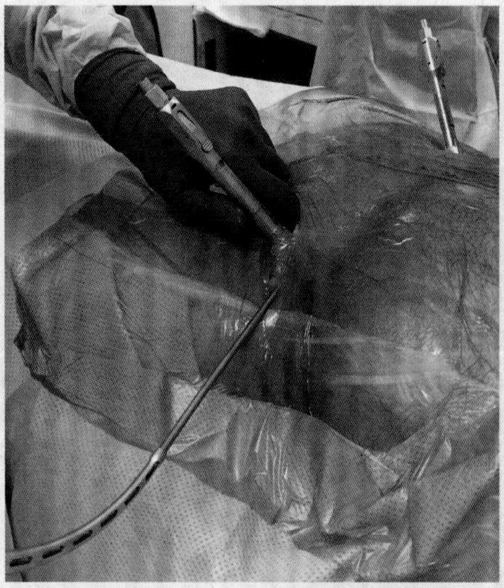

K
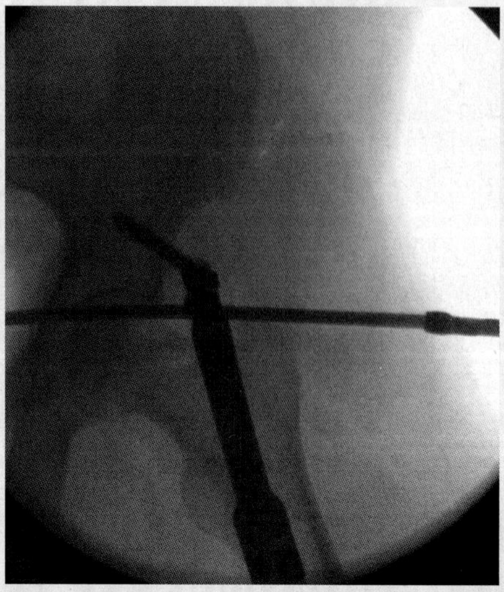

TECH FIG 6 *(continued)* **J.** The connecting rod is placed percutaneously. **K.** Fluoroscopic view confirming rod capture by the pedicle screw.

TECHNIQUES

Pearls and Pitfalls

Enhancing Pin Fixation	• The pin–bone interface has maximal stress concentration and represents the weakest component of the external frame assembly. • Bone quality, frame rigidity, pin number, and pin placement and diameter can all affect the strength of the pin–bone interface. • The insertion length, also referred to as the *intercortical distance*, greatly influences pullout forces. • As a general rule, pins should be maintained within the two cortices as long as possible. Distal cortical penetration is technically undesirable and should be avoided. • Pins of adequate intercortical distance consistently appear to outperform those with transcortical purchase (undesired extracortical exit).
Avoiding Conflicting Surgical Exposures	• Pin location in the supra-acetabular region is less likely to compromise future anticipated surgical wounds. This is particularly important if anterior access to the sacroiliac joint is anticipated and pursued later.
Anterior Iliac Crest Wound	• The surgical wound anteriorly should be placed in the anticipated region of the hemipelvis after reduction. This minimizes tension on soft tissues. • Percutaneous wounds may be made adjacent to the open exposure to allow pin introduction. • The wound is closed before frame application.
Anticipating Pin Trajectory in the Unreduced Pelvis	• Pin inclination in the unreduced pelvis does not reflect normal parameters. • Depending on deformity, pin inclination may be more vertical (LC) or horizontal (externally rotated, APC). • Provisional reduction should be achieved by closed means prior to pin placement.
Avoiding Extrapelvic Misguided Pins	• "Preferential errors" do exist! • For APC injuries, an internal exit is preferred. For LC injuries, an external exit is preferred. This maintains three-point fixation in a mechanically advantageous manner.
Overcompression is possible.	• Depending on the method of application, reduction, and fracture pattern, compression with an anteriorly applied frame may accentuate posterior displacement.
Beware of neurovascular damage by anterior subcutaneous rod.	• Compression of traversing femoral vessels and femoral nerve is to be avoided with adequate rod contouring. Careful postoperative neurologic examination is mandatory, and consideration should be given to Doppler ultrasound of femoral vessels. • LFCN irritation rates approach 30%.

POSTOPERATIVE CARE

- After frame application, individual pin sites should be scrutinized and soft tissues released as necessary to prevent tension-induced skin necrosis or subsequent infection.[20]
- A compressive dressing may be left on the pin sites for 3 to 7 days to permit soft tissue healing. Pin site care is then begun and may consist of twice daily cleansing of the pin bases with half-strength hydrogen peroxide solution or saline.[6,11,29]
- Mild serous drainage is common regardless of the thoroughness of cleansing and does not in itself indicate infection.
- Patients with signs of infection such as erythema, swelling, tenderness, or purulent drainage may be treated with a 7- to 10-day course of an oral antibiotic with adequate coverage of skin organisms. Rarely, deep infection may require operative débridement, pin removal, and intravenous antibiotics.[24,29]
- Mobilization is generally initiated on the day after surgery with weight bearing dictated by the injury pattern and designated stability classification.
- Weight-bearing restrictions are continued for 6 to 8 weeks at which time radiographs are reviewed for signs of healing and the patient's clinical healing status assessed. Weight bearing may then be progressed with a goal of full weight bearing at 3 months after surgery.
- Definitive pelvic external fixators may typically be removed 6 to 8 weeks postoperatively prior to advancing weight bearing.[6]
  - Pin removal can be accomplished in the clinic setting, but fixator removal in the operating room is still preferred by some surgeons.[24,29]
- Careful examination of femoral nerve function is advisable after internal fixator placement as dysfunction may necessitate revision.[18]

OUTCOMES

- Severe hemodynamic instability on arrival is a useful predictor of mortality and transfusion demands. Death within the first 24 hours is often due to acute blood loss, but after this time, it is usually secondary to multisystem organ failure.
- Reported mortality rates of open pelvic fractures range from 10% to 45% as these injuries are often associated with other injuries of prognostic significance.
- Vertically unstable fractures continue to have significant neurologic and associated injuries with long-term disability despite modern treatment approaches.
- Rotationally unstable injuries have a more favorable prognosis.
- Satisfactory functional outcomes have been reported in 75% of cases treated with definitive external fixation independent of injury pattern or final radiographic position, despite a malunion rate of 30.5%.[33]
- In his original series of patients treated with the C-clamp, Ganz reported good reduction of the pelvic ring in 66% of cases and 33% mortality rate, half of which occurred in the first hours after admission due to hemorrhagic shock.[17]
- Early results of the subcutaneous internal fixator show appropriate healing permitting weight bearing at 12 weeks in all patients with good to excellent Majeed functional outcome measures.[36]

COMPLICATIONS

- Historically, complication rates for external fixation were as high as 62% for definitive fixators and 21% for temporary fixators.[21]
  - Pin site infection rates as high as 50%, loss of reduction in up to 57%, and aseptic loosening in 11% of definitive frames.
- Loss of reduction was even more common in obese patients were the soft tissues place increased stress on the pin–bone interface.[19]
- More recent studies with supplemental posterior iliosacral screw fixation reported a much lower complication rate with superficial infection rate of 10%, deep infection requiring operative débridement in 5%, and maintained reduction in all patients at final follow-up.[24]
- Other potential complications include inadequate or aggravated posterior alignment, LFCN irritation, intra-articular penetration, or greater sciatic notch neurovascular injury.
- Ganz reported a 13% rate of loss of reduction in his initial series of patients treated with the C-clamp.[17]
- Subsequent studies have also reported cases of intrapelvic pin penetration, neurovascular injury, and pin site infection.[38]
- Early series on the subcutaneous internal fixator showed no delayed or nonunions, loss of reduction in 0% to 3%, and infections in 0% to 3%.[10,34,35]
- Despite careful blunt dissection, irritation of the LFCN has been reported in 8% to 30% of patients.
- Heterotopic ossification at the screw heads is also common, occurring in 25% to 35% of patients, but nearly all remain asymptomatic.[10,35]
- Placement of the connecting rod too deep may cause compression of the femoral neurovascular bundle, particularly as the patient becomes more ambulatory.[18]
  - Treatment is implant removal, but neurologic recovery is variable.

REFERENCES

1. Bellabarba C, Ricci WM, Bolhofner BR. Distraction external fixation in lateral compression pelvic fractures. J Orthop Trauma 2006; 20(1 suppl):S7–S14.
2. Blackmore CC, Cummings P, Jurkovich GJ, et al. Predicting major hemorrhage in patients with pelvic fracture. J Trauma 2006;61(2): 346–352.
3. Dente CJ, Feliciano DV, Rozycki GS, et al. The outcome of open pelvic fractures in the modern era. Am J Surg 2005;190(6):830–835.
4. Dickson KF, Matta JM. Skeletal deformity after anterior external fixation of the pelvis. J Orthop Trauma 2009;23(5):327–332.
5. Eastridge BJ, Starr A, Minei JP, et al. The importance of fracture pattern in guiding therapeutic decision-making in patients with hemorrhagic shock and pelvic ring disruptions. J Trauma 2002;53(3):446–450.
6. Evans AR, Routt ML Jr, Nork SE, et al. Oblique distraction external pelvic fixation. J Orthop Trauma 2012;26(5):322–326.
7. Firoozabadi R, Stafford P, Routt ML. Risk of spermatic cord injury during anterior pelvic ring and acetabular surgery: an anatomical study. Arch Bone Jt Surg 2015;3(4):269–273.
8. Gardner MJ, Kendoff D, Ostermeier S, et al. Sacroiliac joint compression using an anterior pelvic compressor: a mechanical study in synthetic bone. J Orthop Trauma 2007;21(7):435–441.
9. Gardner MJ, Krieg JC, Simpson TS, et al. Displacement after simulated pelvic ring injuries: a cadaveric model of recoil. J Trauma 2010;68(1):159–165.
10. Gardner MJ, Mehta S, Mirza A, et al. Anterior pelvic reduction and fixation using a subcutaneous internal fixator. J Orthop Trauma 2012;26(5):314–321.

11. Gardner MJ, Nork SE. Stabilization of unstable pelvic fractures with supraacetabular compression external fixation. J Orthop Trauma 2007;21(4):269–273.
12. Gardner MJ, Osgood G, Molnar R, et al. Percutaneous pelvic fixation using working portals in a circumferential pelvic antishock sheet. J Orthop Trauma 2009;23(9):668–674.
13. Gardner MJ, Parada S, Routt ML Jr. Internal rotation and taping of the lower extremities for closed pelvic reduction. J Orthop Trauma 2009;23(5):361–364.
14. Giannoudis PV, Pape HC. Damage control orthopaedics in unstable pelvic ring injuries. Injury 2004;35(7):671–677.
15. Haidukewych GJ, Kumar S, Prpa B. Placement of half-pins for supra-acetabular external fixation: an anatomic study. Clin Orthop Relat Res 2003(411):269–273.
16. Hak DJ. The role of pelvic angiography in evaluation and management of pelvic trauma. Orthop Clin North Am 2004;35(4):439–443.
17. Heini PF, Witt J, Ganz R. The pelvic C-clamp for the emergency treatment of unstable pelvic ring injuries. A report on clinical experience of 30 cases. Injury 1996;27(suppl 1):S-A38–S-A45.
18. Hesse D, Kandmir U, Solberg B, et al. Femoral nerve palsy after pelvic fracture treated with INFIX: a case series. J Orthop Trauma 2015;29(3):138–143.
19. Hupel TM, McKee MD, Waddell JP, et al. Primary external fixation of rotationally unstable pelvic fractures in obese patients. J Trauma 1998;45(1):111–115.
20. Lee C, Sciadini M. The use of external fixation for the management of the unstable anterior pelvic ring. J Orthop Trauma 2018;32 suppl 6:S14–S17.
21. Mason WT, Khan SN, James CL, et al. Complications of temporary and definitive external fixation of pelvic ring injuries. Injury 2005;36(5):599–604.
22. Mendez C, Gubler KD, Maier RV. Diagnostic accuracy of peritoneal lavage in patients with pelvic fractures. Arch Surg 1994;129(5):477–481.
23. Merriman DJ, Ricci WM, McAndrew CM, et al. Is application of an internal anterior pelvic fixator anatomically feasible? Clin Orthop Relat Res 2012;470(8):2111–2115.
24. Mitchell PM, Corrigan CM, Patel NA, et al. 13-Year experience in external fixation of the pelvis: complications, reduction and removal. Eur J Trauma Emerg Surg 2016;42(1):91–96.
25. Pohlemann T, Braune C, Gänsslen A, et al. Pelvic emergency clamps: anatomic landmarks for a safe primary application. J Orthop Trauma 2004;18:102–105.
26. Reilly MC, Zinar DM, Matta JM. Neurologic injuries in pelvic ring fractures. Clin Orthop Relat Res 1996(329):28–36.
27. Routt ML Jr, Falicov A, Woodhouse E, et al. Circumferential pelvic antishock sheeting: a temporary resuscitation aid. J Orthop Trauma 2006;20(1 suppl):S3–S6.
28. Rupp RE, Ebraheim NA, Jackson WT. Anatomic and radiographic considerations in the placement of anterior pelvic external fixator pins. Clin Orthop Relat Res 1994(302):213–218.
29. Ryder S, Gorczyca JT. Routine removal of external fixators without anesthesia. J Orthop Trauma 2007;21(8):571–573.
30. Sagi HC, Coniglione FM, Stanford JH. Examination under anesthetic for occult pelvic ring instability. J Orthop Trauma 2011;25(9):529–536.
31. Stahel PF, Mauffrey C, Smith WR, et al. External fixation for acute pelvic ring injuries: decision making and technical options. J Trauma Acute Care Surg 2013;75(5):882–887.
32. Tile M. Pelvic ring fractures: should they be fixed? J Bone Joint Surg Br 1988;70(1):1–12.
33. Tosounidis TH, Sheikh HQ, Kanakaris NK, et al. The use of external fixators in the definitive stabilisation of the pelvis in polytrauma patients: safety, efficacy and clinical outcomes. Injury 2017;48(6):1139–1146.
34. Vaidya R, Colen R, Vigdorchik J, et al. Treatment of unstable pelvic ring injuries with an internal anterior fixator and posterior fixation: initial clinical series. J Orthop Trauma 2012;26(1):1–8.
35. Vaidya R, Kubiak EN, Bergin PF, et al. Complications of anterior subcutaneous internal fixation for unstable pelvis fractures: a multicenter study. Clin Orthop Relat Res 2012;470(8):2124–2131.
36. Vaidya R, Martin AJ, Roth M, et al. Midterm radiographic and functional outcomes of the anterior subcutaneous internal pelvic fixator (INFIX) for pelvic ring injuries. J Orthop Trauma 2017;31(5):252–259.
37. Wild JJ Jr, Hanson GW, Tullos HS. Unstable fractures of the pelvis treated by external fixation. J Bone Joint Surg Am 1982;64(7):1010–1020.
38. Wollgarten M, Keel MJB, Pape H-C. Editorial: emergency fixation of the pelvic ring using the pelvic C clamp—has anything changed? Injury 2015;46(suppl):S1–S2.
39. Wright RD, Glueck DA, Selby JB, et al. Intraoperative use of the pelvic C-clamp as an aid in reduction for posterior sacroiliac fixation. J Orthop Trauma 2006;20:576–579.
40. Young JWR, Burgess AR, Brumback RJ, et al. Pelvic fractures: value of plain radiography in early assessment and management. Radiology 1986;160(2):445–451.

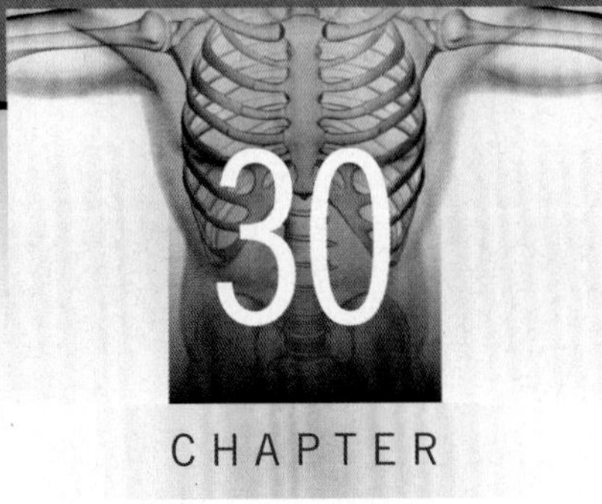

Open Reduction and Internal Fixation of the Symphysis

Jodi Siegel, Michael S.H. Kain, and Paul Tornetta III

DEFINITION

- The pubic symphysis comprises a fibrocartilaginous disc between the bodies of the two pubic bones.
- A diastasis of the pubic symphysis indicates a disruption of the pelvic ring and an unstable pelvis.
- The symphysis is disrupted in anterior–posterior compression (APC) injuries as classified by Young and Burgess[22] and occasionally in lateral compression fractures.

ANATOMY

- The symphysis is an amphiarthrodial joint, consisting of a fibrocartilaginous disc, and stabilized by the superior and inferior arcuate ligaments **(FIG 1A)**.
- The corona mortis is a vessel that represents the anastomosis between the obturator artery and the external iliac artery. It is located about 6 cm laterally on either side of the symphysis **(FIG 1B)**.[17]
- Lateral to the symphysis on the superior rami is the pubic tubercle, a prominence representing the attachment of the inguinal ligament.
  - This bony landmark must be accounted for when contouring a plate that is going to span the symphysis.
- Anatomic variation exists between the sexes, with females having a wider and more rounded pelvis, making their anterior pelvic ring more concave than males **(FIG 2)**.
  - The pelvic arch formed by the convergence of the inferior rami tends to be more rounded in females because their pubic bodies are shallower than males.
  - The cartilaginous disc of the female pelvis is several millimeters thicker with 2 to 3 mm more mobility (which increases with pregnancy) than the male pelvis.
- The arcuate ligaments are the main soft tissue stabilizers of the anterior pelvis.
  - These ligaments arc both superiorly and inferiorly and are firmly attached to the pubic rami.
- The sacrospinous and sacrotuberous ligaments play an important role in the stability of pelvic fractures. These ligaments connect the sacrum to the ilium via the ischial spine and the ischial tuberosity. The sacrospinous ligament resists the rotational forces of the hemipelvis, and the sacrotuberous ligament prevents rotation as well as translation of the hemipelvis.[15]
  - If these ligaments and the pelvic floor are torn in conjunction with a pelvic fracture, symphyseal widening is more significant (see Chap. 29).[7]

PATHOGENESIS

- The Young and Burgess classification describes the injury by the type of force acting on the pelvis. Symphyseal diastasis is most commonly seen in APC injuries or open-book pelvis injuries.

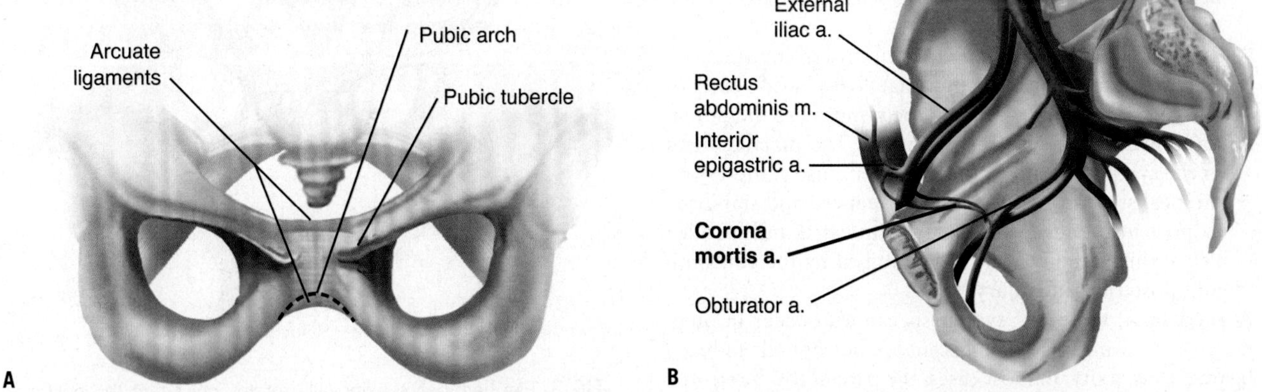

FIG 1 **A.** View of the anterior pelvis demonstrating the fibrocartilaginous disc between the pubic bodies, the superior and inferior arcuate ligaments, and the relationship between the symphysis and the pubic tubercles. **B.** The corona mortis is demonstrated on the superior pubic rami about 6 cm from the symphysis. It represents the anastomosis of the obturator artery and the external iliac artery.

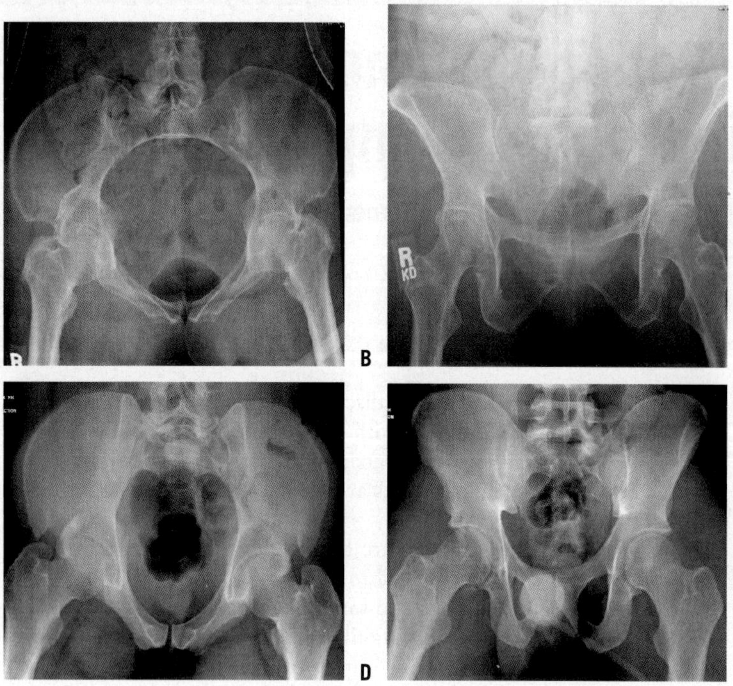

FIG 2 Examples of the anatomic variants between genders. The female pelvis has a more concave shape to the ring, and the pubic arch has less of an acute angle because of the broader pubic body, as demonstrated in the inlet (**A**) and outlet (**B**) views of a female pelvis. The male pelvic ring is more oval, with a much more acute angle anteriorly because of the thinner pubic body, as seen the corresponding inlet (**C**) and outlet (**D**) views.

- In APC injuries, minor widening of the symphysis may not involve disruption of the pelvic floor, including the sacrospinous ligaments.
- In cadaver pelvis, where the symphysis and sacrospinous ligaments were sectioned, more than 2.5 cm of symphyseal widening was observed, thus defining a rotationally unstable pelvis.[14] It should be remembered that any radiograph of the pelvis is but a moment in time and that the anatomically based cutoff of 2.5 cm is a good reference for instability when displacement is greater but not always accurate when it is less, especially if external stabilization like a sheet or binder is in place.
  - If the pelvic floor and the sacrospinous ligaments are torn, the hemipelvis is unstable and can externally rotate on the intact posterior sacroiliac (SI) ligaments **(FIG 3)**.[7]
- Occasionally, lateral compression injuries can cause symphyseal disruption.
  - Locked symphysis occurs when one pubic bone becomes lodged behind the contralateral pubic bone, or entrapped in the contralateral obturator foramen, after a lateral compression injury.
  - Tilt fractures occur as lateral compression injuries with fracture of the superior ramus that is displaced posterior and inferior, rotating through the symphysis, and potentially protruding into the perineum. The malalignment of the symphysis and/or the rami can cause compression on local structures and should be reduced and stabilized to prevent impingement of the birth canal and bladder. Pelvic ring stability will be determined by the concomitant posterior ring injury.[15]
- A diastasis of the pubic symphysis can also occur in pregnancy and during childbirth because of hormonally induced ligamentous laxity. In most cases, the patient can be treated symptomatically with a binder for comfort and the pain and instability resolves. Occasionally, chronic instability and pain results and stabilization (typically fusion) of the symphysis has been shown to relieve pain.[18]

NATURAL HISTORY

- Persistent low back pain; anterior pain; sitting imbalance; and an impaired, painful gait are common sequelae after pelvic fractures.
- Early studies looking at pelvic fractures without surgical treatment demonstrated that almost a third of these patients had disabling pain and impaired gait. Only a third were asymptomatic if the posterior ring was involved.[18]

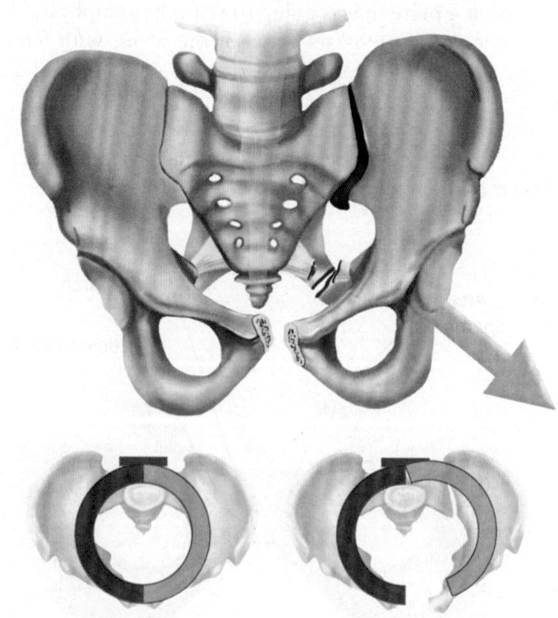

FIG 3 The hemipelvis externally rotates out when the posterior SI ligaments remain intact, as in an APC type II injury. The posterior ligaments act as a hinge, and with sacrospinous ligaments torn, the involved hemipelvis will rotate down and out, so the pubic body on the injured side will be below the intact pubic body.

- APC type I injuries are Tile type A stable pelvic injuries, which do well with nonoperative treatment. These injuries tend to occur in younger patients involved in motor vehicle trauma or in elderly patients as a result of a direct injury such as a fall.
- APC types II and III injuries are unstable injuries. Nonoperative treatment results in late pain. In a retrospective study by Tile,[15] APC type II injuries treated nonoperatively had a 13% incidence of late pain, with the majority of patients reporting persistent moderate pain. The patients with APC type III injuries reported a 16% incidence of late pain, with most pain being reported as moderate or severe.
- Patients with pelvic trauma tend to have other organ systems involved, and these associated injuries contribute to long-term disability. The more severe injuries associated with pelvic fractures are urologic and neurologic injuries.[18]
- Whitbeck et al[20] demonstrated higher morbidity and mortality rates as well as an increased incidence of arterial injuries in APC type III injuries compared to other pelvic fractures.
- Disruption of the pubic symphysis is associated with urologic injuries. Bladder ruptures and urethral tears occur about 15% of the time in association with pelvic trauma and can lead to late complications such as strictures and incontinence. These associated injuries potentially lead to a higher infection rate when open reduction and internal fixation is performed.[11] An increased incidence of incontinence has also been seen in women with APC injuries.
- Associated neurologic injuries are typically due to the posterior pathology. However, they are more common with sacral fractures and with vertically unstable fracture patterns.
- Dyspareunia and sexual dysfunction are also described as complications after pelvic fractures.[10] These can occur due to the original injury or as a result of ectopic bone formation during healing.
- Symphyseal pelvic dysfunction, a relatively common condition, presents as anterior pelvic pain secondary to the laxity in the symphysis. This condition typically resolves spontaneously and can take some time but needs to be differentiated from traumatic symphyseal diastasis as a result of childbirth. Traumatic diastasis occurs in about 1 in 2000 births to 1 in 30,000 births, and the diastases from pregnancy can be as great as 12 cm.[4]
  - Most patients with postpartum displacement recover with no residual pain or instability after treatment with pelvic binders, girdles, and the recommendation to lie in the lateral decubitus position.
  - There are a limited number of studies looking at symphyseal disruption secondary to pregnancy. The exact incidence of persistent long-term pain is unknown, but chronic pelvic instability can occur.[12]
  - In the few series reporting operative treatment, the indication was persistent pain for *at least* 4 to 6 months postpartum.[5,12]

PATIENT HISTORY AND PHYSICAL FINDINGS

- Pelvic injuries usually occur as a result of any high-energy trauma, such as high-speed motor vehicle accidents, motorcycle accidents, or falls from heights. Patients should be evaluated following the Advanced Trauma Life Support guidelines.
- Patients with pelvic fractures may become hemodynamically unstable, and close monitoring of blood pressure and fluid requirements is needed.
  - Typically, if a patient requires more than 4 units of blood to maintain hemodynamic stability, an angiogram should be obtained to identify and possibly embolize any arterial injuries. Clotting factors and platelets should also be administered.
- Patients may have tenderness to palpation in the area of the symphysis. If motion of the pelvis is detected, manipulation of the pelvis should cease, as unnecessary manipulation may disturb any clot formation (see Part 2 Pelvis and Lower Extremity Trauma Exam Table at the end of the book).
- If there is no radiographic demonstration of displacement, the iliac wings can be compressed to test for stability of the pelvic ring and each hemipelvis.
- A careful examination of the skin to identify areas of ecchymosis and hematoma formation, particularly in the flanks, groin, and abdominal regions, also needs to be performed.
  - The presence of a Morel-Lavallée lesion indicates that high-energy trauma has occurred in the pelvic region (**FIG 4**). Recognition of this lesion is important to prevent infection and may need to surgically débrided prior to proceeding with definitive fixation of the symphysis.
- A good pelvic examination and evaluation of the perineum are essential. Swelling or open wounds in the perineal area may indicate a high-energy mechanism of injury. Open injuries require emergent management. This includes an examination of the vaginal vault in women, particularly in a lateral compression injury.
- Evaluation of other organ systems, looking for associated injuries, is essential.
  - In males, a high-riding prostate on the rectal examination or blood at the meatus may indicate injury to the urethra or bladder, and placement of a Foley catheter should be delayed until a retrograde urethrogram is performed, unless the patient is in extremis.
  - Urethral injuries are less common in females because the urethra is shorter.
- A thorough neurologic examination of the lower extremities also needs to be performed as injuries to the L4 and L5 nerve roots can occur in pelvic fractures. It is essential to test the sensation and motor functions of specific roots, identifying any neurologic injury that can differentiate between a nerve root lesion or a more central lesion.
- A limb length discrepancy or a rotational deformity of the lower extremities should prompt radiographic evaluation of the pelvis.

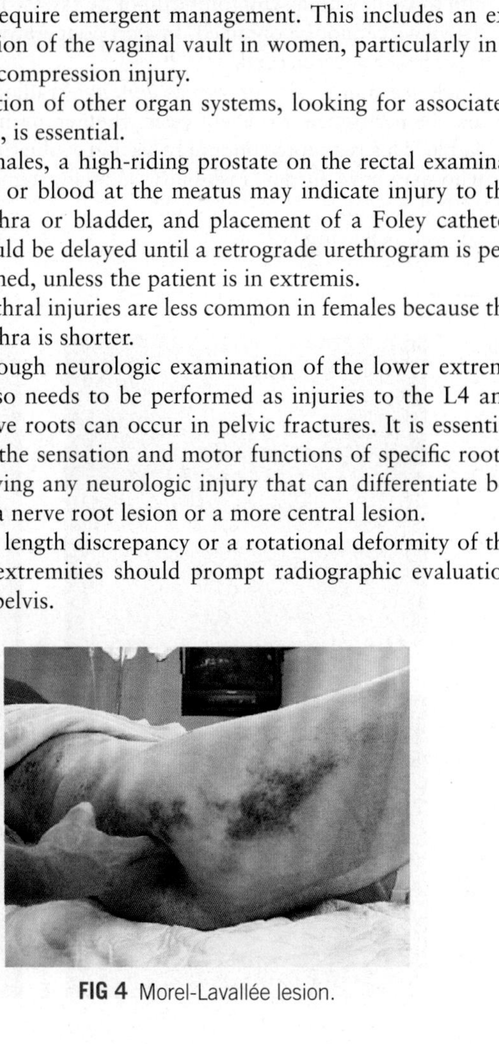

FIG 4 Morel-Lavallée lesion.

- Substantial debate exists as to whether to remove a binder placed in the field by emergency medical services. In most centers, if the patient is hemodynamically stable, then removing the binder prior to computed tomography (CT) scan will be helpful to identify the injury.

IMAGING AND OTHER DIAGNOSTIC STUDIES

- Radiographic evaluation of the pelvis consists of anteroposterior (AP), inlet, outlet, and Judet plain radiographs (**FIG 5**).
- A retrograde urethrogram and a cystogram should be performed to rule out an injury to the genitourinary system in men. A cystogram (direct or CT) is sufficient for women.
- A CT scan of the pelvis is also indicated to help evaluate intra-articular injuries to the SI joints and further delineate the fracture pattern.
- A CT angiogram can also be used at the time of the trauma scan to help identify if arterial bleed is present and requires further treatment with angiography and embolization.[13]
- Angiography may be used to treat patients who are hemodynamically unstable and do not respond to standard resuscitation, particularly if a CT angiogram indicates arterial bleeding.
- A stress examination in the operating room can be performed under fluoroscopy to assess stability if there is a question of an unstable pelvis not reliably diagnosed on the static images. This may be helpful in intubated patients and those in whom symptoms cannot be assessed and single leg views cannot be obtained. In alert cooperative patients, it is almost never needed.
- Single-leg stance (also known as *flamingo*) radiographs can also be performed if it is not clear whether an injury is unstable. This is a more commonly used in evaluating patients who may have chronic instability, such as a female patient with ligamentous laxity secondary to pregnancy or unrecognized pelvic injury.[12,17]

DIFFERENTIAL DIAGNOSIS

- Rami fractures
- Symphyseal strain
- Hip fracture
- Muscle strain or avulsion
- Lumbar fracture

ACUTE MANAGEMENT

- The patients should be hemodynamically stabilized.
- Internally rotating the lower extremities, padding the feet and ankles, and binding the ankles together with elastic wraps can reduce the acute increase in pelvic volume associated with APC injuries. The padding on the heels and ankles should be generous to prevent skin breakdown.
- Placing a sheet or binder at the level of the greater trochanters can also be used to reduce the symphysis diastasis and pelvic volume while temporarily stabilizing the pelvis. The sheet should be applied over a wide surface area and should be held with towel clips rather than tying a knot to avoid skin breakdown (see Chap. 29). Holes can be cut in the sheet to allow for access to the abdomen as needed.

NONOPERATIVE MANAGEMENT

- If minimal separation of the symphysis is present, the patient can be mobilized full weight bearing with crutches as needed for comfort and reassessed.
- Close radiographic monitoring and physical examination is needed for a few weeks to confirm the pelvic ring remains reduced and that patient's pain is improving. Single-leg stance views can be used to help identify late instability, although there is no strict cutoff that has been identified as requiring surgery to prevent late symptoms.

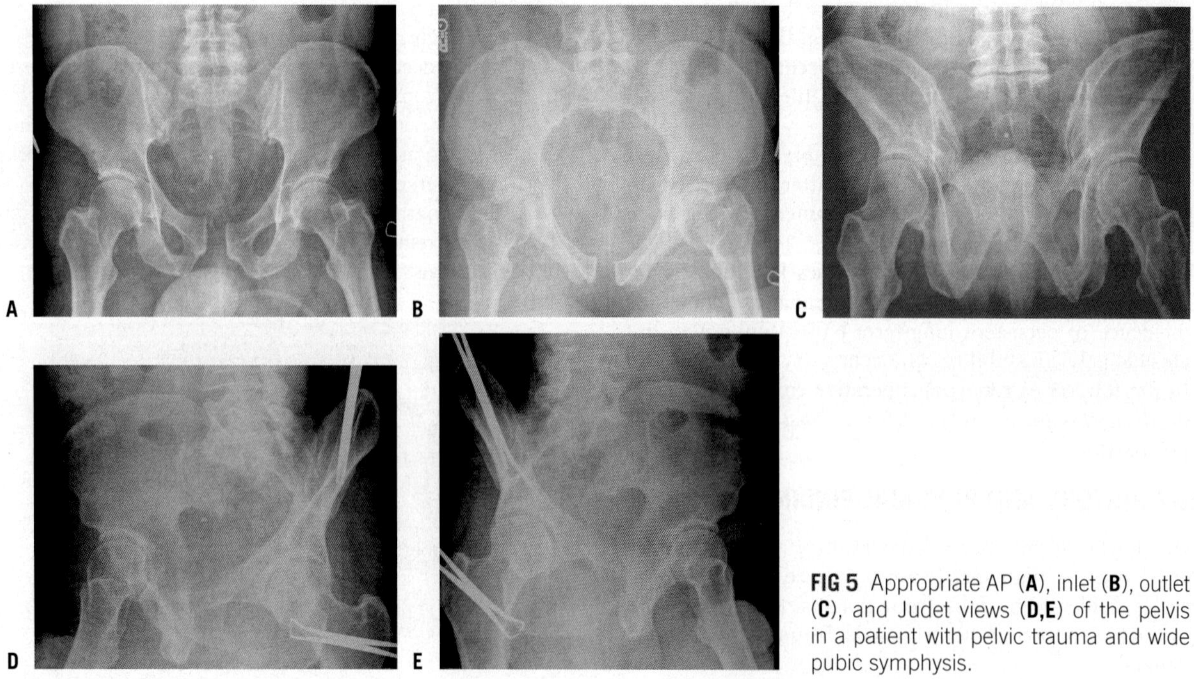

FIG 5 Appropriate AP (**A**), inlet (**B**), outlet (**C**), and Judet views (**D,E**) of the pelvis in a patient with pelvic trauma and wide pubic symphysis.

SURGICAL MANAGEMENT

- A diastasis greater than 2.5 mm indicates a disruption of the sacrospinous ligaments and thus an unstable pelvis. Anterior SI joint widening will also be present. Open treatment of the symphysis diastasis with reduction and stabilization will restore stability to the pelvic ring.[4]
- Open injuries that are highly contaminated can be stabilized with external fixation using iliac wing pins or Hanover pins placed at the level of the anterior inferior iliac spine. Refer to Chapter 29 for more details.
- Additionally, the technique of INFIX using pedicle screws at the anterior inferior iliac spine and a subcutaneously placed bar can also be used for obese patients.[19]
- In APC type II injuries with intact posterior SI joint ligaments, no posterior fixation is needed after the symphysis is reduced and stabilized.
- For APC type III injuries, the symphysis is typically addressed first. Depending on the posterior injury, simultaneous control of both the front and the back of the pelvic ring is necessary to obtain an anatomic reduction with provisional reduction and fixation with clamps in the front assisting with the reduction of the posterior structures.
- Additional symphyseal disruptions indicated for surgical treatment include in the setting of a laparotomy, when associated with rami fractures protruding into the perineum (ie, a tilt fracture), or in association with an acetabular fracture requiring open reduction.[15]

Preoperative Planning

- The surgeon should review appropriate radiographic studies (AP, inlet, and outlet views and CT scan).
  - Identifying all rami fractures and the presence of any pubic body fractures is essential as this will identify any potential obstacles to a simple reduction. Additionally, longer plates may be required to span nearby fractures.
- Presence of a bladder rupture or urethral tear must be identified preoperatively. If present, repair or protection of the field should be performed during the same exposure as internal fixation of the symphysis to avoid a more complex late reconstruction and decrease infection risk.
- Any history of previous abdominal surgery or the presence of prior incisions should be identified before going to the operating room to arrange for assistance from a general surgeon if necessary.
- Necessary equipment that should be available includes C-arm, radiolucent table, large bone clamps, pelvic external fixation equipment, pelvic internal fixation equipment, and a possibly a C-clamp or a Ganz clamp.

Positioning

- The patient is placed on a radiolucent flat-top table with feet padded and strapped together to facilitate reduction of the symphysis.
- Preincision fluoroscopic images confirming the ability to obtain adequate inlet and outlet views with the C-arm are obtained before draping the patient.
- Right-handed surgeons may prefer to have the C-arm on the patient's right and the instruments on the patient's left for easier access to the symphysis and surgeon comfort and vice versa.
- Placement of a Foley catheter is vital to decompress and protect the bladder; palpation of the Foley balloon intraoperatively can help identify the bladder.
- Sequential compression devises are placed on both legs if possible for deep vein thrombosis prophylaxis during the case.

Approach

- Open reduction of the symphysis is performed with an anterior Pfannenstiel approach.
  - Alternatively, if done in concert with the general surgeons, the midline laparotomy can be extended distally to allow access to the space of Retzius.

PFANNENSTIEL APPROACH

- The entire lower abdomen is prepared, including the proximal quarter of the thighs, the lateral hemipelves, the iliac crests, and the umbilicus. The external genitalia is draped out of the field unless necessary for the urology team.
  - Access to the anterior superior iliac spine is important if an external fixator is to be placed to assist in reduction or for additional fixation.
  - The entire posterior pelvis should be prepped into the field if there is any chance that posterior fixation will be employed.
- A transverse incision is made 2 cm above the symphysis **(TECH FIG 1A)**.
- Once through the skin, a large rake is placed distally and then proximally to help raise full thickness flaps and to open the tissue plan above the rectus fascia.
- A vertical incision is then made through the fascia of the linea alba. Take care not to cut into the bladder. The incision is carried distally past the symphysis. The proximal extent is determined by the amount of soft tissue excursion needed to safely work in the field. The rectus muscle insertion is not surgically taken down, although it is common to see an avulsion of one of the heads of the rectus muscles off the rami from the initial injury **(TECH FIG 1B)**.
- Blunt dissection is continued longitudinally to spread the rectus muscle and protect the underlying peritoneum and bladder.
  - Electric cautery can be used to divide the remaining fibers of the rectus while protecting the underlying structures.
  - If unsure of where the bladder is, split the linea alba more distally over the symphysis as this will decrease the likelihood of injuring the bladder.
- Once the retroperitoneum (space of Retzius) is opened, inspect the bladder and bladder neck for any injury. Confirm with the anesthesia team the color of the urine and ask them to alert you

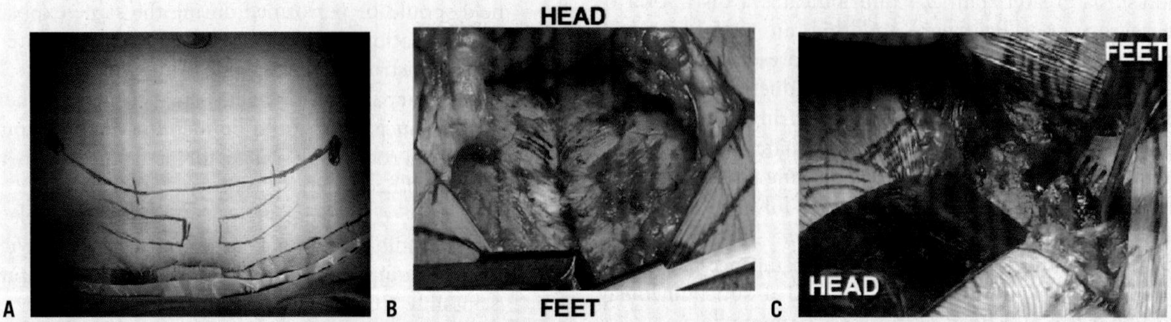

TECH FIG 1 A. The skin is marked for the incision. The entire lower abdomen is prepared to include the umbilicus and both anterior superior iliac spine as well as the anterior inferior iliac spine bilaterally. An incision is marked about two fingerbreadths superiorly to the pubic bones. **B.** The linea alba is clearly identified once the subcutaneous fat has been dissected away from the fascia. An incision along the linea alba, between the two rectus muscles, is made to allow exposure of the space of Retzius. **C.** Once the space of Retzius is exposed, a Dever or malleable blunt retractor is used to retract the bladder and two Hohmann retractors are placed on the outside of each superior rami to expose the superior aspect and to allow reduction and plating.

for any indications of new blood in the Foley catheter collection chamber.

- At this point, a blunt malleable retractor can be placed into the space of Retzius to protect the bladder **(TECH FIG 1C)**.
- Next, care should be taken to inspect the areas lateral to the symphysis for any large blood vessels running perpendicular to the superior rami. This vessel is known as the *corona mortis* and tends to be about 6 cm lateral to the symphysis.
  - The corona mortis is an anastomosis of the obturator and external iliac arteries (see **FIG 1B**).[17] If present, it should be ligated and cut to prevent injury and subsequent retraction with uncontrolled bleeding.
- A Hohmann retractor is then placed through the periosteum over the superior pubic rami on one side to retract the rectus muscle laterally to expose the superior ramus and the body of the symphysis.
  - Although placed deep to the external iliac vessels, care should be taken when passing the Hohmann retractors to be directly onto bone to avoid injury.
- The periosteum on the superior aspect of the rami is then cut with electrocautery and elevated distally. The Hohmann retractor is then repositioned to effectively retract all soft tissues away from the expose parasymphyseal area.
- These same steps are then repeated for the contralateral superior ramus. It may be helpful for the surgeon to switch sides of the table to improve visualization.
- Typically, a large hematoma is encountered within the space of Retzius. Copious irrigation will assist with removing this and improve visualization.
- At this point, the symphyseal disruption should be easily visualized.
- The authors prefer to remove the symphyseal cartilaginous disc as it allows for more compression of the pelvic ring, which imparts more stability. This technique has been shown to result to fewer hardware failures than when the cartilage is left in place.
  - To remove the cartilage, a curved osteotome is used to remove the majority by gently tapping it along the medial aspect of the symphyseal body. A large curved curette is then used to remove the rest.
  - Take care to ensure that all of the cartilage is removed to maximize bony contact.

WEBER CLAMP REDUCTION

- Once the superior aspect of the symphyseal bodies is exposed, the Weber clamp is placed anteriorly to avoid removing the insertion of the rectus **(TECH FIG 2A)**.
- The goal in using this technique is to have the tips of the Weber clamp at the same level on each symphyseal body. It is *not* placed in the obturator foramen.
- If anterior displacement is present on either side, the tip of the clamp is placed slightly anterior on that side, so at the time of reduction, the tips are at the same level.[7]
- The clamp is tilted distally to engage the tines **(TECH FIG 2B)**.
- The clamp is placed anterior to the rectus insertions.

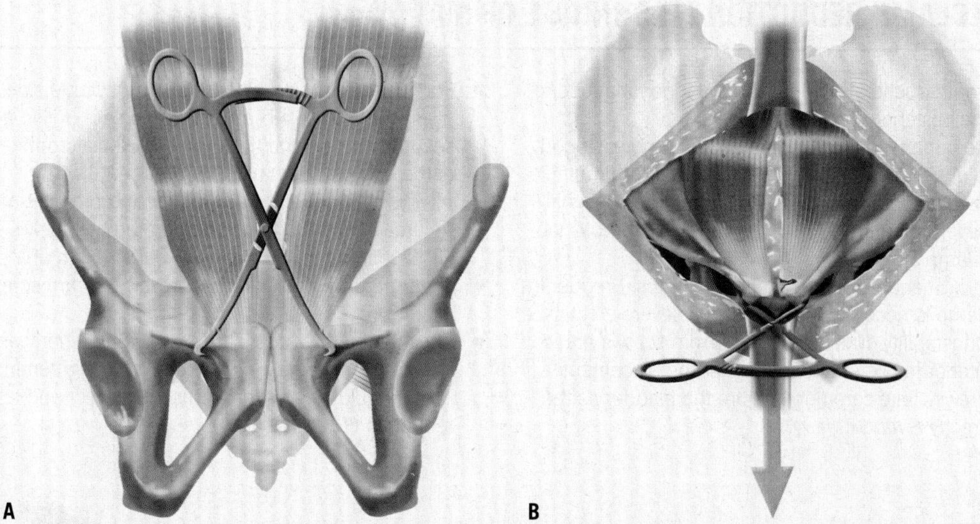

TECH FIG 2 **A.** Weber clamp or large bone tenaculum is used to reduce the symphysis with the tines at the same level on each pubic body anterior to the rectus muscle. **B.** Tilting the clamp distally will help engage the tines.

USE OF A C-CLAMP TO AID IN REDUCTION

- The C-clamp (Ace DePuy) has been described for use in unstable APC pelvic fracture patients requiring an exploratory laparotomy or for temporary pelvic fixation if a patient cannot go to the operating room. It can also be used to assist in the open reduction of the symphysis if conventional clamps alone cannot achieve or maintain the reduction.
- This is a similar concept to the one described by Wright et al[21] for assisting in the reduction of the posterior pelvic ring.
- To apply the C-clamp, the pins are placed two fingerbreadths directly posterior to the anterior superior iliac spine. This places the pins in the gluteus pillar, a thickened portion of the lateral ilium above the acetabulum **(TECH FIG 3A)**.
- Once the pins are in place, the clamp can be fitted onto the pins. The clamp is then used to compress the pelvis and reduce the rotationally unstable hemipelvis **(TECH FIG 3B,C)**. Once reduced, the clamp is tightened and locked. Fluoroscopy is used to confirm reduction of the symphysis as well as any posterior pathology. (See Chap. 29 for further description of the C-clamp.)
- Care should be taken not to overreduce rami fractures if they are present.
- The goal of this technique is to obtain most of the reduction with the C-clamp and then fine-tune any remaining malreduction with the Weber clamp once the symphysis is exposed.

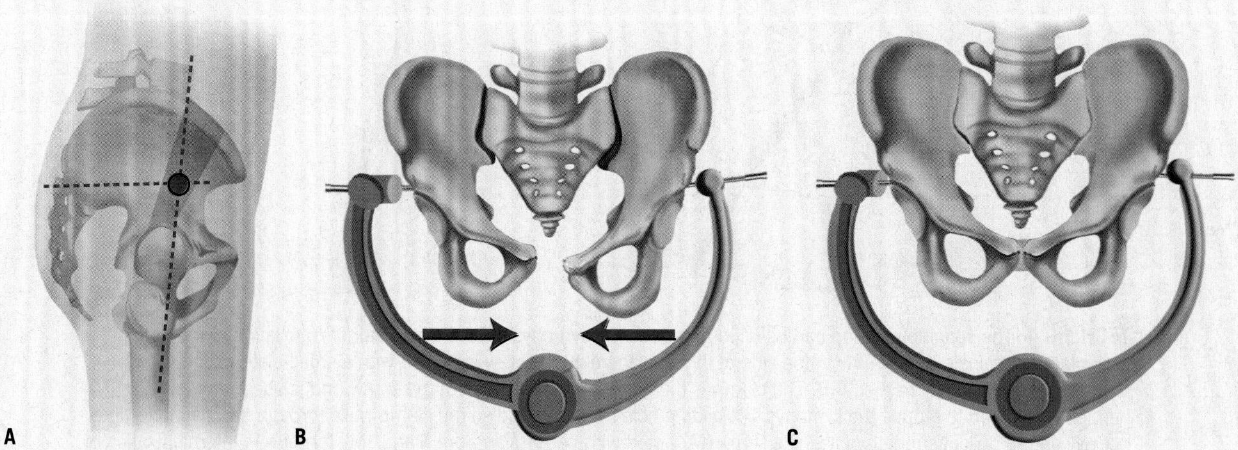

TECH FIG 3 Placement of pins for the C-clamp (**A**) and how it is applied to obtain a reduction of the symphysis (**B,C**).

JUNGBLUTH CLAMP REDUCTION (TECHNIQUE OF MATTA)

- Jungbluth clamp reduction is used when the innominate bone is intact and the posterior ring is unstable.
- The innominate bone tends to be externally rotated, posteriorly displaced, and superiorly translated. With instability in multiple planes, mobilizing the entire innominate bone requires significant force in several direction, which cannot be accomplished with a Weber clamp alone.
- There are both 3.5- and 4.5-mm Jungbluth clamps. Frequently, the 4.5-mm clamp is necessary in the case of severe soft tissue disruption and instability. Drill holes for 4.5-mm screws are made in an anterior to posterior direction for the placement for 4.5-mm screws. Take care not to injure the bladder as the trajectory is directly toward it.
- For the screw being placed on the unstable side (with posterior displacement), a 4.5-mm gliding hole is drilled and the screw is secured to the bone through a small plate on the posterior side of the pubis using a nut **(TECH FIG 4A,B)**.
  - The plate will act as a washer and provides a larger surface area of force to be exerted on the hemipelvis so one does not have to rely only on the pullout strength of a single screw.
- A standard drill hole is used for the 4.5-mm screw on the intact side.
- The Jungbluth clamp is then placed anteriorly and secured to the 4.5-mm screws. The screws are tightened to the clamp. The Jungbluth can then be used to affect and to hold the reduction **(TECH FIG 4C,D)**.[8]

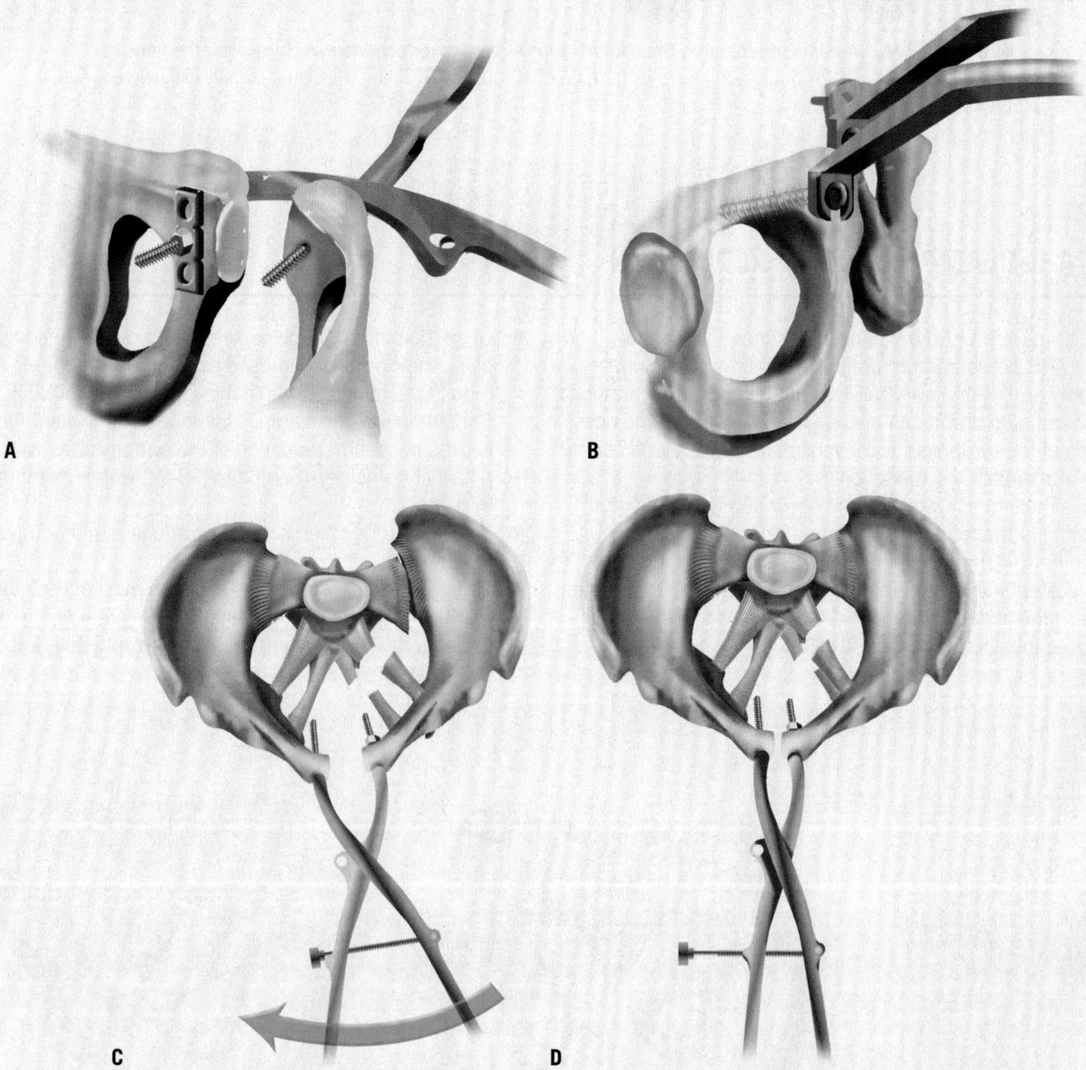

TECH FIG 4 The Jungbluth clamp can be used to reduce the symphysis if there is posterior translation of the hemipelvis and intact innominate bone. **A,B.** On the side of the displacement, a screw is placed with a small plate attached with a nut so the plate acts a washer. **C,D.** The clamp is then attached to the head of the screw and is used to pull the hemipelvis forward to reduce the symphysis. A gliding hole must be used so the clamp pulls through the plate and does not rely on the pullout strength of a single screw. (Adapted with permission from Matta JM, Tornetta P. Internal fixation of pelvic fractures. Clin Orthop Relat Res 1996;329:129–140.)

PLATE PLACEMENT

- Before placing fixation, the reduction should be confirmed by direct visualization, palpation, and fluoroscopically on AP, inlet, and outlet views.
- With the symphysis reduced, a six-hole, curved 3.5-mm reconstruction plate, or a precontoured symphyseal plate is placed across the symphysis. The authors prefer to place the plate superior-posterior to allow for drilling away from the bladder and into the long corridor of bone available there for excellent screw purchase.
- A Kirschner wire can be placed between the symphyseal bodies to aid in centering the plate.
- Before the plate is placed, it is contoured to fit the curve of the superior surface of the symphysis and rami. The ends are contoured if a six-hole plate is used to allow for anatomic contact to the ramus **(TECH FIG 5A)**. Alternatively, precontoured plates can be used.
  - In a six-hole plate, the two medial screws on each side go into the symphyseal body and the most lateral screw goes into the rami.
- Careful planning of screw placement must be considered if the Jungbluth clamp is used so that screws are placed through the plate without losing the reduction.
- The first screws placed are adjacent to the symphysis on either side **(TECH FIG 5B)**.
  - The authors prefer to drill eccentrically, along the lateral aspect of the holes, to generate compression.
  - The proper angle for drilling can be determined by placing a finger deep into the space of Retzius, along the symphysis, to feel the inner surface of the pubic body. Drilling parallel

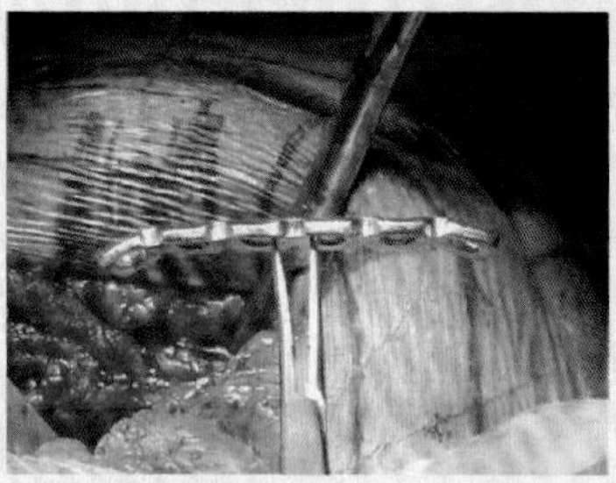

A

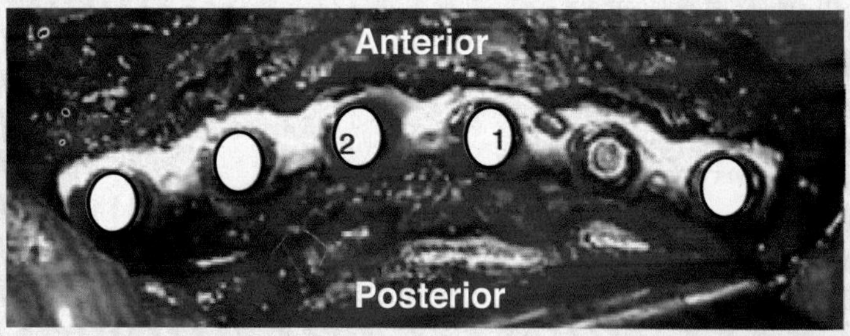

B

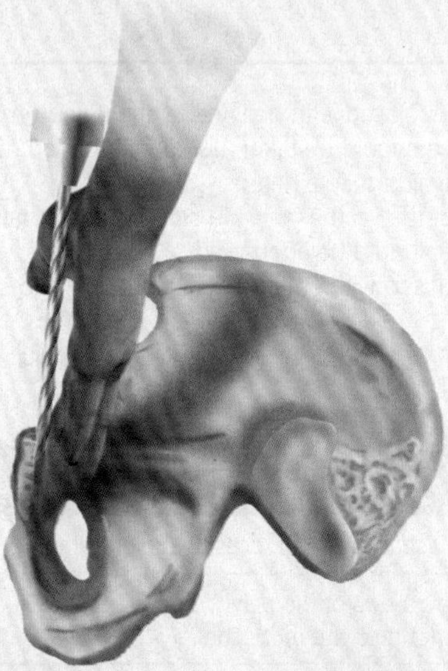

C

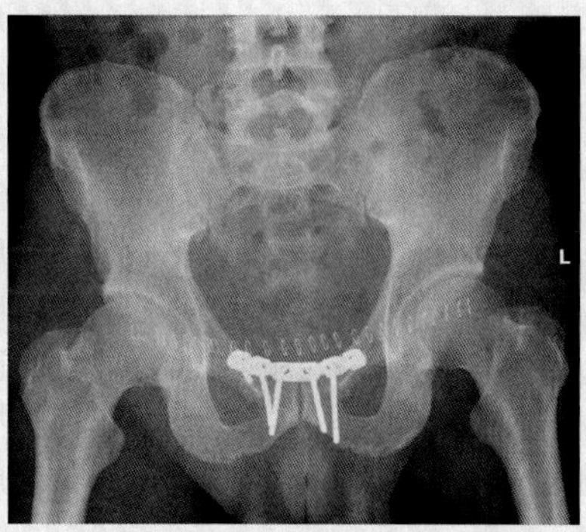

D

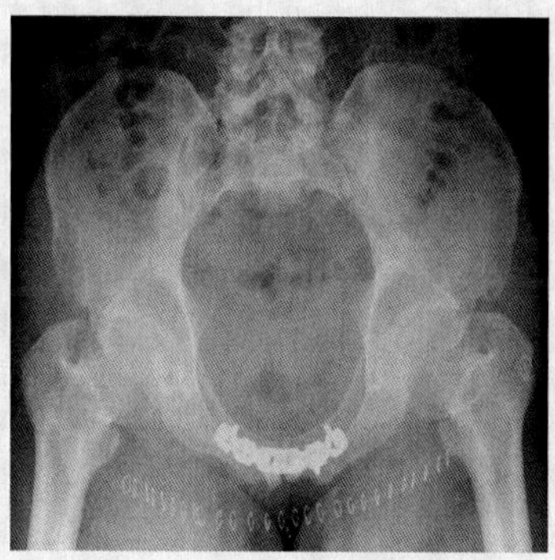

E

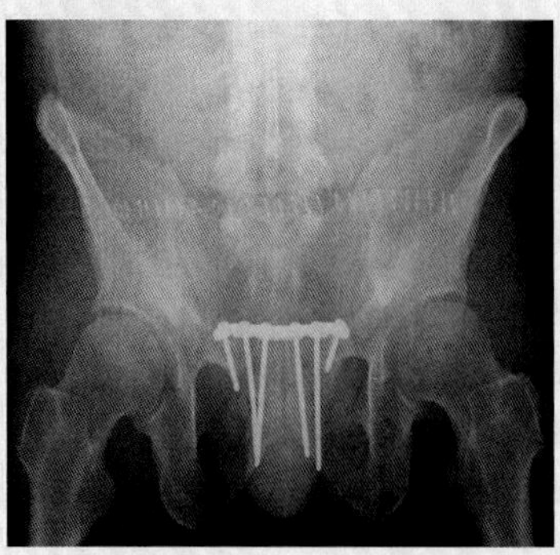

F

TECH FIG 5 **A.** Example of how the plate needs to be contoured to accommodate the pubic tubercle on either side of the symphysis. The concavity of the plate also has to be contoured, and this can vary between genders (see **FIG 2**). **B.** Clinical photograph of plate after all screws are placed. Numbering indicates the order of screw placement, with the screws closest to the symphysis being placed first. After screws *1* and *2* are placed, any order may follow for the remaining screws. **C.** Drilling the proper angle is imperative to ensure the screw will stay in bone. To gauge the angle, one may place a finger on the posterior aspect of the pubic body and then drill parallel to that finger to ensure the drill is held at the proper angle. **D–F.** Postoperative AP, inlet, and outlet view radiographs of a precontoured plate and a reduced symphysis.

to one's finger in this area will allow for long, safe screws **(TECH FIG 5C)**.
- These initial screws should be angled slightly anteriorly and laterally in the pubic body so that they stay in bone and achieve the best bite.
  - These screws can be placed all the way into the ischium if necessary.
- The two most medial screws on each side of the symphysis can be placed either parallel to each other or in a crossing pattern within the symphyseal body **(TECH FIG 5D–F)**.
- The lateral screws in the plate are placed last and will be shorter than the other screws as they will be at the level of the obturator foramen.
  - When drilling for these screws, care should be taken to avoid the nearby obturator neurovascular structures.
- Symphyseal locking plates do not offer any advantage and are not necessary.[1]

DOUBLE-PLATING TECHNIQUE

- Tile[15] described placing a second plate anteriorly if extra stability is needed in vertically unstable patterns **(TECH FIG 6)**.
- This technique can also be used if insufficient stabilization is achieved with initial plate placement.
- In placing the anterior plate, care must be taken to avoid the screws in the first plate.
- Take care to protect the bladder during drilling.
- The same sequence of screw placement should be followed, with the medial screws placed first and subsequent screws placed laterally.

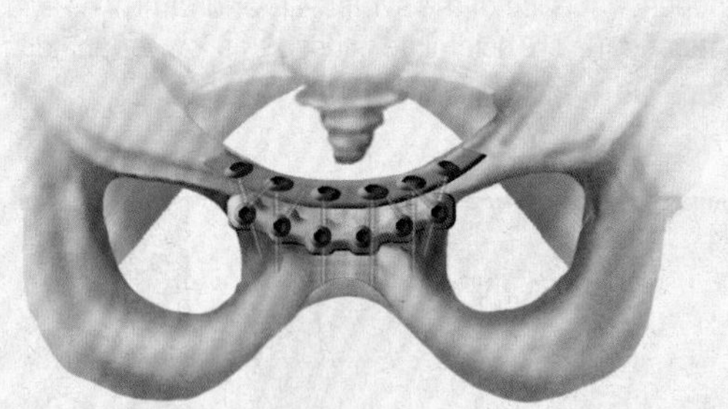

TECH FIG 6 Example of double plating described by Tile.[15]

WOUND CLOSURE

- Once the symphysis is reduced, the plate is in place, and the reduction is confirmed, the bladder is reevaluated. The urine in the Foley collection chamber is examined. The wound is thoroughly irrigated. A hemovac drain is placed in the space of Retzius, between the bladder and the symphysis, and is passed to the skin through the rectus fascia.
- The rectus fascia is closed with heavy absorbable suture in the linea alba. Care should be taken not to include too many muscle fibers to avoid muscle necrosis.
- At the distal end of the rectus fascia, a side-to-side repair of any avulsed tissue should be attempted.
- The skin is then closed with subcutaneous sutures and staples.

Pearls and Pitfalls

Setup	• It is important to be sure adequate fluoroscopic AP, inlet, and outlet visualization are possible before draping.
Reduction	• Reduction is confirmed under direct vision, palpation, and fluoroscopic views of the pelvis. The C-clamp can also be used to maintain reduction before plating if conventional clamps cannot hold the reduction.
Reduction Aids	• A second clamp or a ball spike can be used to assist in reduction if there is difficulty obtaining reduction or holding the symphysis reduced. For instance, in tilt fractures, a ball spike can be used to push against the intact rami while pulling up the pubic body on the fractured side. Again, the C-clamp or an external fixator can be placed to help approximate the pubic bodies to facilitate reduction with a Weber clamp.
Backup	• If fixation is tenuous or if the patient becomes too sick to continue with plating, an external fixator can always be added.
Screw Placement	• C-arm is used to confirm placement of screws and confirm that they are not too long. Prominent screws distal to the ischial tuberosity can cause sitting discomfort and patient complaints.
Poor Fixation with One Plate	• Double plating can be used to improve fixation by creating a 90-90 construct.
Two-Hole Plate	• A two-hole plate should not be used. It allows for rotational instability and has a high failure rate.

POSTOPERATIVE CARE

- Deep vein thrombosis prophylaxis is imperative as 35% to 60% of patients with a pelvic fracture are at risk. Of these, proximal thrombosis can occur 2% to 10% of the time; these clots pose a higher risk of leading to a pulmonary embolism.[9]
- With such a high risk of deep vein thrombosis, prophylaxis should combine mechanical and chemical means. Sequential compression devices are essential.
- Chemical modalities consist of unfractionated heparin, low-molecular-weight heparin, vitamin K antagonists, and factor Xa indirect inhibitors.
- If patients have a contraindication for chemical prophylaxis secondary to another injury such as a head bleed or spine injury, an inferior vena cava filter should be considered.
- The authors use sequential compression devices throughout the hospital course and chemical prophylaxis preoperatively as soon as permissible based on associated injuries. Postoperatively, patients are restarted on chemical prophylaxis as soon as possible as guided by intra-operative bleeding concerns. Chemical prophylaxis is continued for at least 6 weeks depending on mobility.
- Early mobilization is imperative to prevent comorbid conditions from arising.
  - Once stable fixation is in place, patients should be out of bed to a chair within 24 hours of surgery if their overall condition allows.
- The patient's weight-bearing status is dependent on the injury pattern and the overall injury pattern of the pelvic ring.
  - If anterior fixation is used alone, such as for an APC type II injury, patients are made partial weight bearing on the injured side for 6 weeks.
  - For type III injuries, which require posterior pelvic fixation, stricter weight bearing limitations are continued for up to 12 weeks.
- Patients should be followed routinely with radiographs. On postoperative day 1, before the patient gets upright, AP, inlet, and outlet radiographs are obtained to assess the reduction and more importantly to be used for comparison for future follow-up radiographs taken at 6 and 12 weeks.

OUTCOMES

- Stabilizing the anterior pelvis improves outcomes, and anatomic alignment allows for more reliable ligamentous healing.
- Kellam[3] defined an adequate reduction of anterior symphyseal widening as less than 2 cm and reported that when this was obtained in rotationally unstable fractures, 100% of patients returned to normal function. Patients with posterior pathology had poor outcomes, with only 31% reporting normal function.
- Pohlemann et al[10] reported no residual posterior displacement in 95 patients with type B fractures treated with anterior plating. This was associated with an 11% incidence of late pain that occurred after exercise. No patients had pelvic pain at rest.
- Tornetta et al[16,18] also reported that APC type II injuries, when treated with anatomic open reduction and internal fixation, have a 96% rate of good to excellent outcomes.
- Pohlemann et al[10] demonstrated that type C injuries had more residual radiographic posterior displacement than type B injuries. Only 33% of these type C patients were pain-free after combined anterior and posterior fixation.
- Lybrand et al[6] looked at the position of the anterior ring at the time of union in patients with APC II and III fractures and found that small amounts of displacement at the time of union did not affect outcome or pain. Displacement of more than 15 mm and injury severity score did result in worse outcomes.
- Implant loosening or breakage does not affect outcomes and may restore some physiology motion at the pubic symphysis.[2,6]
- In general, functional outcomes correlate with the initial displacement of the injury.
- Associated injuries also affect outcome. Patients with associated urologic injuries are at risk for urethral strictures, urinary tract infections, and late infections.
- There is a greater than 90% chance of a good outcome in patients with near-anatomic fixation of the symphysis in APC type II pelvic fractures, and 96% will be able to return to work within a year of injury.[16]

COMPLICATIONS

- Proximal deep vein thrombosis occurs in 25% to 35% of pelvic fracture patients, so it is imperative to provide proper prophylaxis both mechanically and chemically.[9]
- Plate and screw constructs can fracture or loosen secondary to fatigue due to the physiologic motion between the two pubic bodies. This tends to occur after 8 weeks and generally does not affect healing.
  - If it occurs earlier and a loss of reduction occurs, then revision osteosynthesis should be considered.[7,8,18]
- Loss of reduction can also occur with widening of the symphysis both with and without the plate breaking. Although no data exist, the quality of the initial reduction appears to be the best predictor. Therefore, if a perfect reduction cannot be maintained, additional fixation should be added or activity modification should be implemented postoperatively.[8,16]
- In most series of pelvic fracture, which report on the use of anterior fixation, there is a low incidence of anterior wounds developing deep infections.
  - Most resolve with irrigation and débridement and go on to union.[4,7,8]
- Urologic injuries occur in about 15% of pelvic fractures. Urologic complications include late urethral strictures, incontinence, and erectile dysfunction.
  - Early repair of bladder and/or urethral injuries at the same time of fixation avoids more complex reconstructions; however, the rate of late urologic complications is still relatively high.[11]

REFERENCES

1. Daily BC, Chong AC, Buhr BR, et al. Locking and nonlocking plate fixation pubic symphysis diastasis management. Am J Ortho (Belle Mead NJ) 2012;41(12):540–545.
2. Frietman B, Verbeek J, Biert J, et al. The effect of implant failure after symphyseal plating on functional outcome and general health. J Orthop Trauma 2016;30:336–339.

3. Kellam JF. The role of external fixation in pelvic disruptions. Clin Orthop Relat Res 1989;(241):66–82.
4. Lange R, Hansen ST Jr. Pelvic ring disruptions with symphysis pubis diastasis. Indications, technique, and limitations of anterior internal fixation. Clin Orthop Relat Res 1985;(201):130–137.
5. Lindsey RW, Leggon RE, Wright DG, et al. Separation of the symphysis pubis in association with childbearing. A case report. J Bone Joint Surg Am 1988;70:289–292.
6. Lybrand K, Bell A, Rodericks D, et al. APC injuries with symphyseal fixation: what affects outcome? J Orthop Trauma 2017;31: 27–30.
7. Matta JM. Indications for anterior fixation of pelvic fractures. Clin Orthop Relat Res 1996;(329):88–96.
8. Matta JM, Tornetta P III. Internal fixation of unstable pelvic ring injuries. Clin Orthop Relat Res 1996;(329):129–140.
9. Montgomery KD, Geertz WH, Potter HG, et al. Thromboembolic complications in patients with pelvic trauma. Clin Orthop Relat Res 1996;(329):68–87.
10. Pohlemann T, Bosch U, Gänsslen A, et al. The Hannover experience in management of pelvic fractures. Clin Orthop Relat Res 1994;(305):69–80.
11. Routt ML, Simonian PT, Defalco AJ, et al. Internal fixation in pelvic fractures and primary repairs of associated genitourinary disruptions: a team approach. J Trauma 1996;40:784–790.
12. Siegel J, Templeman DC, Tornetta P III. Single-leg-stance radiographs in the diagnosis of pelvic instability. J Bone Joint Surg Am 2008;90(10): 2119–2125.
13. Siegel J, Tornetta P, Burke P, et al. CT angiography for pelvic trauma predicts angiographically treatable arterial bleeding. Paper presented at: Orthopaedic Trauma Association Annual Meeting; October 2007; Boston, MA.
14. Tile M. Fracture of the Pelvis and Acetabulum. Baltimore: Williams & Wilkins, 1984.
15. Tile M. Pelvic ring fractures: should they be fixed? J Bone Joint Surg Br 1988;70:1–12.
16. Tornetta P III, Dickson K, Matta JM. Outcome of rotationally unstable pelvic ring injuries treated operatively. Clin Orthop Relat Res 1996;(329):147–151.
17. Tornetta P III, Hochwald N, Levine R. Corona mortis. Incidence and location. Clin Orthop Relat Res 1996;(329):97–101.
18. Tornetta P III, Templeman D. Expected outcomes after pelvic ring injury. Instr Course Lect 2005;54:401–407.
19. Vaidya R, Colen R, Vigdorchik J, et al. Treatment of unstable pelvic ring injuries with an internal anterior fixator and posterior fixation: initial clinical series. J Orthop Trauma 2012;26(1):1–8.
20. Whitbeck MG Jr, Zwally HJ II, Burgess AR. Innominosacral dissociation: mechanism of injury as a predictor of resuscitation requirements, morbidity, and mortality. J Orthop Trauma 1997;11:82–88.
21. Wright RD, Glueck DA, Selby JB, et al. Intraoperative use of the pelvic C-clamp as an aid in reduction for posterior sacroiliac fixation. J Orthop Trauma 2006;20:576–579.
22. Young J, Burgess A, Brumback R, et al. Pelvic fractures: value of plain radiography in early assessment and management. Radiology 1986;160(2):445–451.

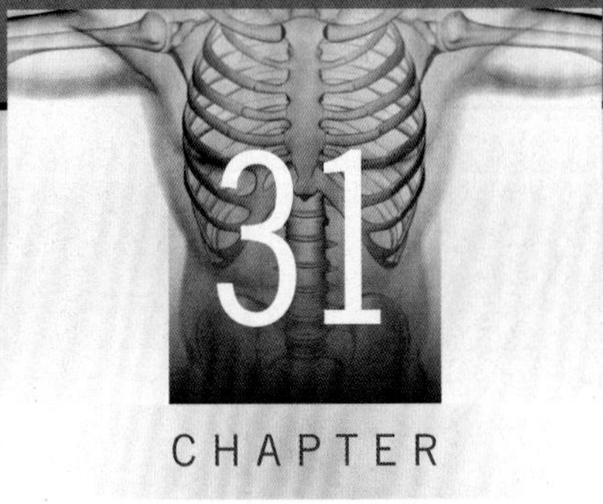

Open Reduction Internal Fixation of the Sacroiliac Joint and Sacrum

David Donohue and Henry Claude Sagi

DEFINITION

- Pelvic fractures are serious injuries associated with a diverse assortment of morbidities and mortality rates as high as 50%.
- Fractures and dislocations of the pelvis involve, in broad terms, injuries to the anterior and posterior structures of the pelvic ring.
  - Injuries to the anterior pelvic ring include symphyseal disruption and/or pubic body or rami fractures.
  - Injuries to the posterior pelvic ring involve iliac wing fractures, sacroiliac (SI) joint dislocations and fracture-dislocations, and sacral fractures.
- Treatment options vary widely based on the degree of displacement, instability, and associated injuries.
- This chapter focuses specifically on the treatment of displaced sacral fractures and SI joint dislocations.

ANATOMY

- The pelvis is a ring structure composed of the two hemipelves (innominate bones) and the sacrum. Each hemipelvis is the culmination and fusion of the three embryonic bony elements: the ilium, the pubis, and the ischium (**FIG 1**).
- The two hemipelves are joined anteriorly at the pubic symphysis (a symphyseal joint), and posteriorly, they articulate with the wings, or alae, of the sacrum via the SI joints to complete the pelvic ring (**FIG 2A,B**).
- The sacrum represents the terminal structural segment of the spinal column that connects the pelvis and extremities to the trunk and spine.
- The sacrum is the caudal segment of the axial skeleton. It is, therefore, a spinal element and subject to segmentation abnormalities and dysmorphism.
  - Most commonly, segmentation anomalies such as a lumbarized S1 or a sacralized L5 will be present (**FIG 2C,D**). The only way to be sure which defect, if any, is present, is to count down from the first thoracic vertebrae, which is the first vertebra to have transverse processes that are inclined cephalad.
  - As a general rule of thumb, however, the top of the iliac crest is usually at the same level as the L4 or L5 disc space. This rule can be used to judge the presence of dysmorphism or other segmentation anomalies at the lumbosacral junction such as sacralization of L5 (see **FIG 2C**).
  - These issues are pertinent to interpretation of the radiographic landmarks required to safely place iliosacral screws (see discussion later).
- Being wedge-shaped, the sacrum forms a keystone articulation with the innominate bones.
  - By virtue of this shape and their orientation, the SI joints are inherently unstable with respect to the bony constraints, and the maintenance of posterior pelvic ring integrity is wholly dependent on the support provided by the ligamentous structures, which include the pelvic floor (see **FIG 2A**).
  - The pelvic ligaments are structured and positioned to resist these deformations as static stabilizers of the pelvis. There are no specific dynamic stabilizers of the pelvic ring.
- With axial loading, the natural tendency is for each hemipelvis to externally rotate and translate in a cephalad and posterior direction. During two-legged stance, the symphysis is under tension, and the SI joints experience compression superiorly and tension inferiorly. During single-leg stance, the symphysis is under compression and shear, whereas the SI joints are under tension superiorly and compression inferiorly.

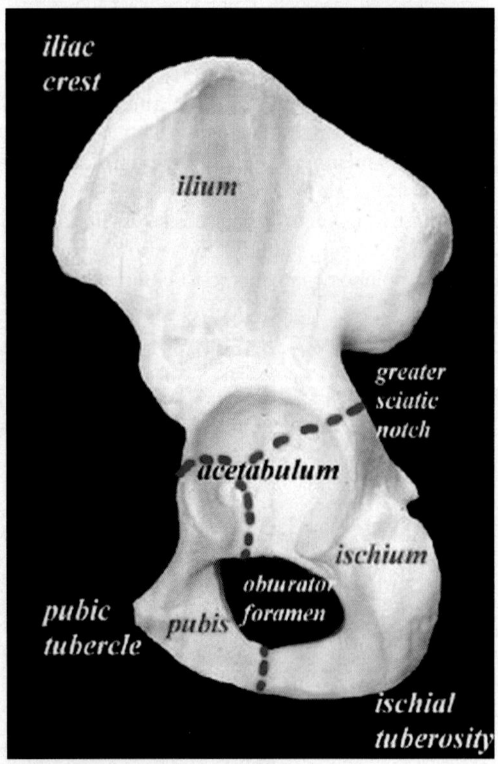

FIG 1 The three embryonic bones (pubis, ischium, ilium) fusing to form the innominate bone or hemipelvis.

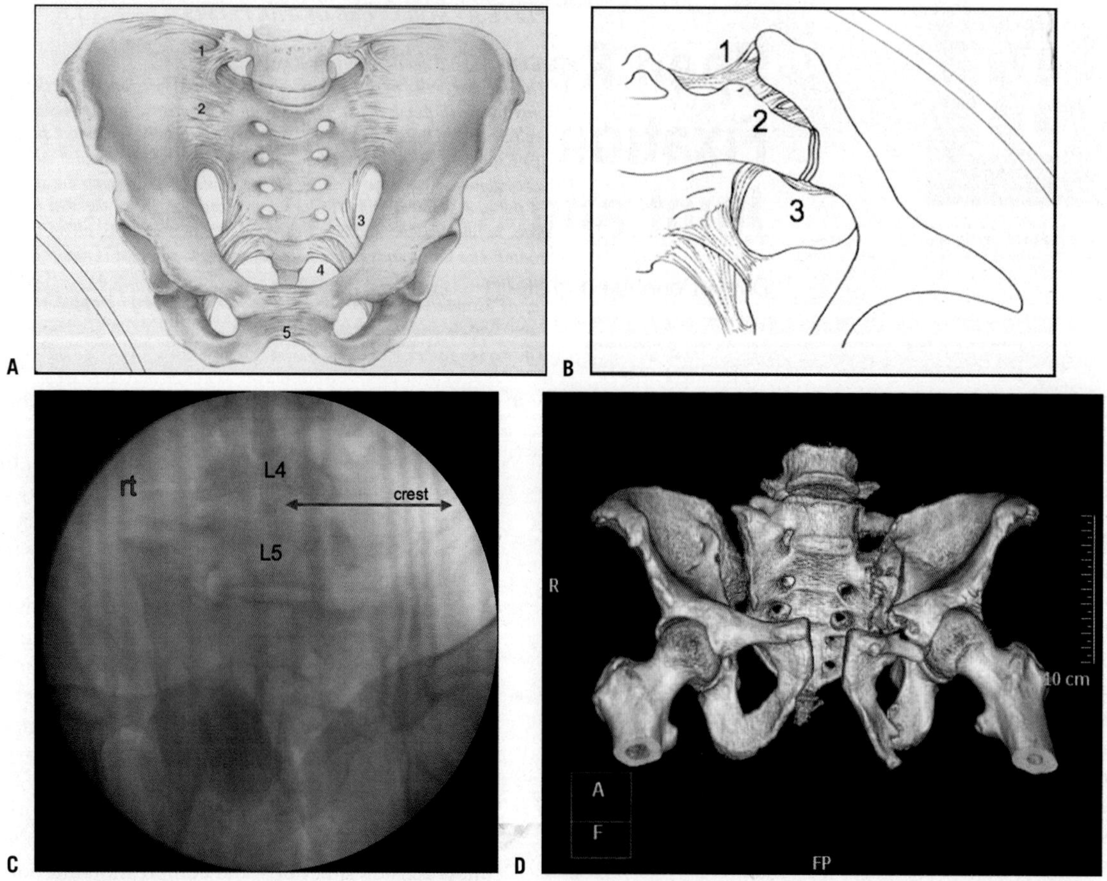

FIG 2 A. The two innominate bones and sacrum forming the pelvic ring with supporting ligaments. *1,* iliolumbar; *2,* SI; *3,* sacrospinous; *4,* sacrotuberous; and *5,* symphyseal ligaments. **B.** SI joint ligaments. *1,* posterior; *2,* intra-articular; *3,* anterior SI ligaments. **C.** Intraoperative fluoroscopy showing unilateral segmentation anomaly with partial sacralization of L5 and the level of the crest still at L4–L5. *rt,* right. **D.** Three-dimensional CT reconstruction showing segmentation anomaly.

- The SI ligaments (anterior, posterior, and intra-articular ligaments) are the strongest ligaments in the body, with the posterior SI ligaments being the most important in resisting posterior and cephalad displacement (see **FIG 2B**).
- The symphyseal ligaments (themselves contributing no more than 15% to pelvic ring stability), the sacrotuberous ligaments, and the sacrospinous ligaments resist external rotation.[13,32]
- The bladder is immediately posterior to the pubic bodies and symphysis, separated only by a thin layer of fat and the potential space of Retzius.
- The relationship of the L5 nerve root to the superior aspect of the sacral ala as it courses to join the lumbosacral plexus is a key anatomic feature that must be kept in mind during reduction and stabilization of posterior pelvic ring injuries **(FIG 3A,B)**.

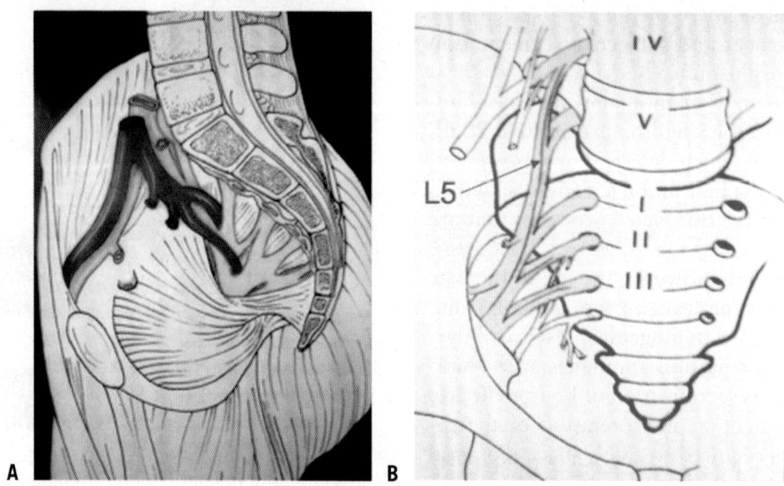

FIG 3 A,B. Neurovascular structures around the posterior pelvic ring. Note intimate relationship of L5 nerve root to sacral ala.

- The sacral nerve roots course from posterior to anterior, medial to lateral, and proximal to distal as they traverse the upper sacral nerve root tunnels. As they exit the sacrum, the nerve roots lay on the inferior and lateral aspect of the foramina.
- The superior gluteal artery is immediately lateral to the inferior aspect of the SI joint as it arises from the internal iliac artery to exit the greater sciatic notch with the superior gluteal nerve.

PATHOGENESIS

- The SI ligaments are the most resilient in the human body and therefore must be subject to substantial forces and energy transmission to result in disruption.
  - Anteroposterior (AP) compression (APC) of the pelvis or forces on the leg(s) that cause external rotation of the innominate bone(s) (which may or may not be coupled with a vertical shearing force) is the most common cause of SI joint dislocation.
- Sacral fractures, however, can occur in three distinctly different situations.
  - Insufficiency fractures of the sacrum arise secondary to failure through excessively osteoporotic or osteopenic bone.
  - Stress fractures of the sacrum resulting from fatigue and cyclic failure of normal bone in high-level athletes or military recruits
  - Traumatic disruptions resulting from high-energy lateral or APC and/or vertical shear injuries such as (in order of decreasing frequency) motorcycle crashes, autopedestrian collisions, falls from height, motor vehicle accidents, or crush injuries.[13,32]

NATURAL HISTORY

- Pelvic fractures occur in at least 20% of blunt trauma admissions, most frequently in young males.
  - They can result in small insignificant fractures of the pubic rami with no compromise of pelvic ring stability or major injuries and disruptions that can be associated with life-threatening bleeding and/or visceral injury.
- The pelvic ring encloses the true pelvis (organs contained below the pelvic brim, extraperitoneal) and the false pelvis (organs contained above the pelvic brim, both peritoneal and retroperitoneal).
  - The most commonly associated injuries to structures contained within the true pelvis are the internal iliac arterial and venous systems and branches, the bladder (20%) and urethra (14%), the lumbosacral plexus, and the rectum and vaginal vault (open pelvic fractures).
- Injuries to structures within the false pelvis as a direct result of the pelvic fracture are uncommon, but severe iliac wing fractures with abdominal wall disruption can result in intestinal injury and even entrapment **(FIG 4A–C)**.

A

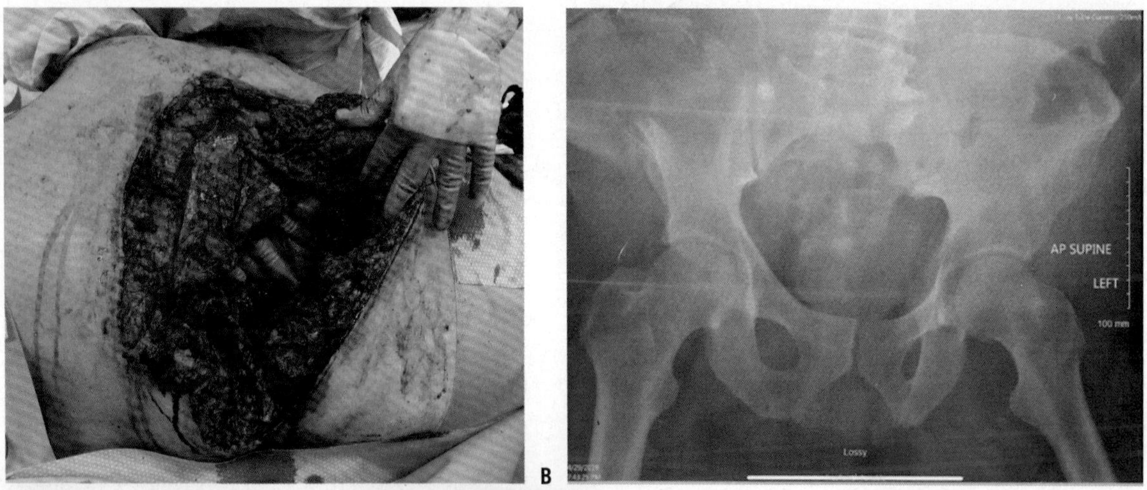

B

C

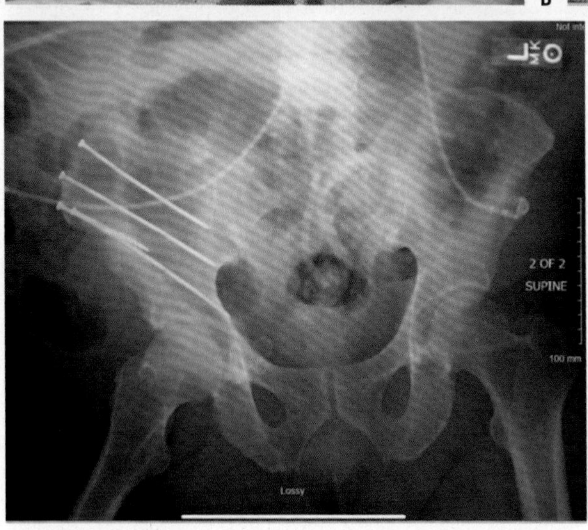

FIG 4 A. Clinical image demonstrating open iliac wing fracture with evisceration. **B.** Radiograph demonstrating comminuted right iliac wing fracture. **C.** Subsequent stabilization of the iliac wing for repair of abdominal wall musculature.

- Morbidity and mortality from pelvic fractures can be quite high and is most commonly secondary to pelvic hemorrhage.
  - The mortality rate associated with pelvic fracture with an associated bladder rupture approaches 35% in some series.
  - The mortality rate of open pelvic fractures involving the perineum used to be as high as 50%, but this has decreased to approximately 2% to 10% with the liberal use of diverting colostomies and more advanced stabilization techniques.
- Neurologic injury to the lumbosacral plexus can lead to significant sensorimotor dysfunction involving the extremities, bowel, bladder, and sexual organs.
- Because of these associated neurovascular and visceral injuries, pelvic fractures often result in prolonged recovery periods, significant chronic pain, permanent disability, and loss of psychological and socioeconomic structure.[5,7,9,19–21]

PATIENT HISTORY AND PHYSICAL FINDINGS

- Any patient presenting with a history of trauma or satisfying criteria for a trauma alert in the emergency department should be suspected of having a pelvic fracture until otherwise ruled out by radiologic and physical examination.
- The physical examination should follow the primary and secondary survey of the advanced trauma life support protocol.[1]
- Examination of a patient suspected of having a pelvic fracture should be divided into the examination of the abdomen, pelvic ring, perineum, rectum, vagina, and lower extremities.
- The abdominal examination should elucidate the following:
  - Tenderness, fullness, or rigidity
  - Abdominal wall disruptions, defects, or open wounds
  - Flank ecchymosis
  - Presence of internal degloving or a Morel-Lavallée lesion (separation of the subcutaneous tissues from the underlying muscular fascia). This can be recognized by subcutaneous fluctuance or a fluid wave and, later, extensive ecchymosis.
- The rectal and vaginal examination should consider the following:
  - The position of the prostate (A high-riding prostate may be a sign of urethral injury.)
  - Palpable bony fragments perforating the rectal or vaginal mucosa
  - Defects or tears in the wall of the rectum or vagina indicating possible bony penetration
  - Rectal or vaginal bleeding indicating possible tears or bony penetration
  - Urethral bleeding at the meatus indicating possible urethral or bladder disruption
  - Scrotal or labial swelling and ecchymosis indicating pelvic hemorrhage **(FIG 5)**
  - Rectal tone, perianal sensation, voluntary sphincter control, and bulbocavernosus reflex to assess for the presence of cauda equina syndrome, spinal shock, or lower sacral nerve root injury
- Examination of the pelvic ring and extremities should focus on the following key factors:
  - Palpable internal or external rotation instability of the pelvic ring with manually applied AP and lateral compressive forces on the iliac wings/crests. However, in an awake patient or with hemodynamic instability, multiple forceful attempts at manipulating the pelvis is not recommended, as this will be very uncomfortable to the patient and may exacerbate ongoing pelvic hemorrhage. Some surgeons recommend no examination of the stability of the pelvis and favor an initial urgent AP radiographic evaluation to avoid causing more bleeding or other injury.
  - Leg length discrepancy with asymmetric internal or external rotation

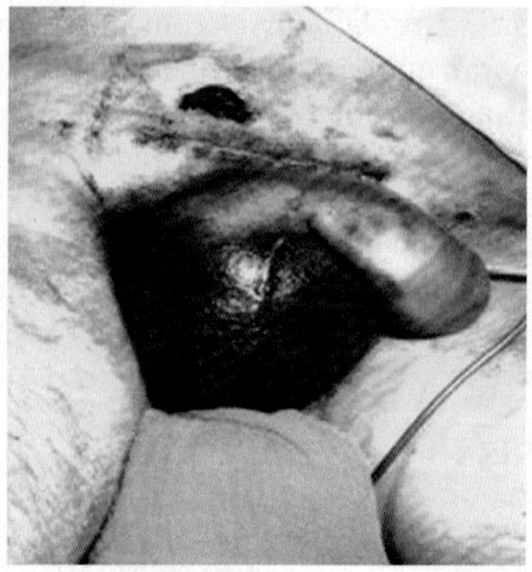

FIG 5 Scrotal ecchymosis from internal pelvic hemorrhage.

- Neurologic status in patients able to comply can be assessed as follows:
  - L1–L2: iliopsoas (hip flexors) and upper anterior thigh sensation
  - L3–L4: quadriceps (knee extensors) and lower anterior thigh/medial calf sensation
  - L5: extensor hallucis longus, digitorum longus (toe dorsiflexion), peroneal eversion (although this can have a strong L4 component), and lateral calf/dorsum of foot sensation
  - S1: gastrocsoleus complex (ankle plantar flexion) and posterior calf sensation
  - S2–S3: flexor hallucis and digitorum longus (toe plantar flexion) and sole of foot sensation

IMAGING AND OTHER DIAGNOSTIC STUDIES

Plain Radiographs

- The standard AP (pelvis) view should be part of the initial trauma series screening. With enough experience, many of the injuries to the posterior pelvic ring can be diagnosed with this single projection **(FIG 6A)**.
  - A good AP radiograph should have the pubic symphysis colinear with the sacral spinous processes, but if a displaced injury exists, this reference is lost and the quality of the film is based on the position of the lower lumbar spine using the spinous process and pedicle positions.
    - This allows side-to-side comparison of bony landmarks to aid in diagnosis of subtle displacements of the sacrum or SI joint.
  - The cortical density of the pelvic brim and iliopectineal line should be traced back to its intersection with the lateral margin of the sacral ala.
    - This intersection should be at the same level (usually the superior margin of the S2 foramen) bilaterally.

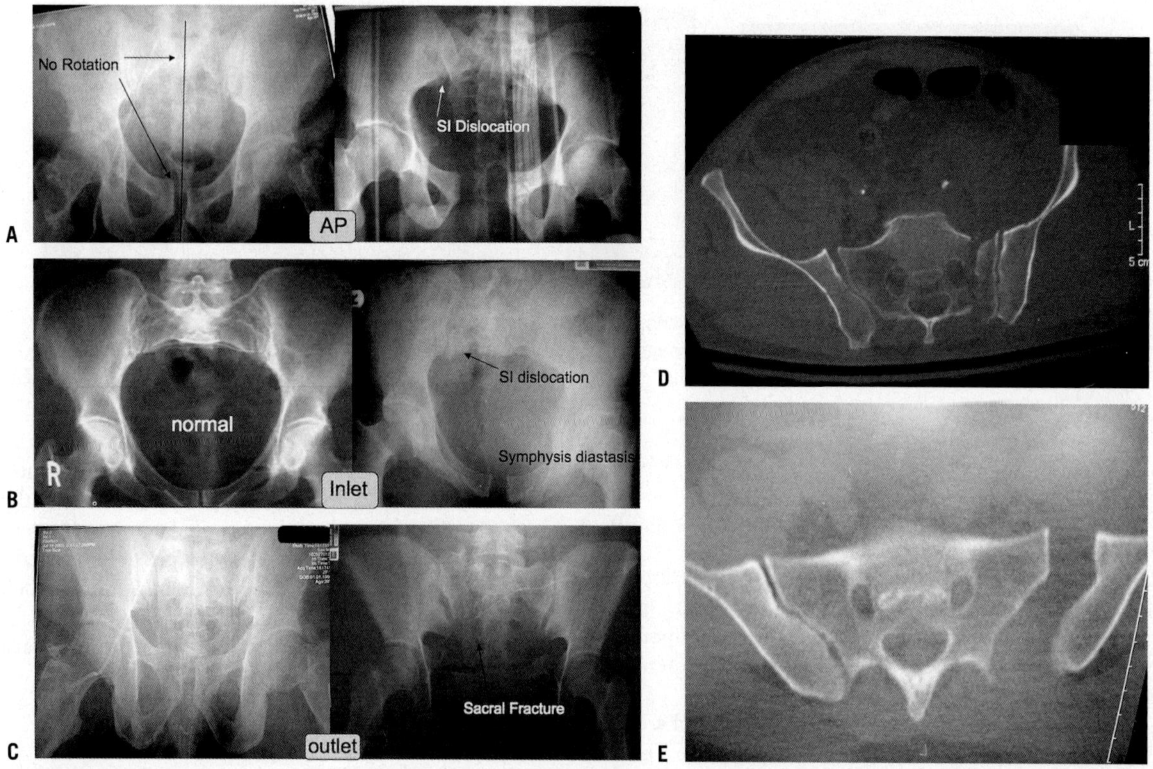

FIG 6 A. AP pelvis radiograph. Ideal film should have symphysis aligned with sacral spinous processes. **B.** Inlet pelvic radiograph. Note sacral promontory and alar regions. **C.** Outlet pelvic radiograph. Note sacral foramina and sacroiliac (*SI*) joints. Ideal image should have top of symphysis–rami at the S2–S3 level. **D.** Axial CT scan of transforaminal (Denis zone 2) sacral fracture. **E.** Axial CT scan of SI joint dislocation. Note diastasis of anterior and posterior joint.

- Asymmetry in the SI joint space and the appearance of the sacral foramina should alert the surgeon to the possibility of an SI joint dislocation or sacral fracture.
  - Fractures of the L5 transverse process may be a clue to a vertical shear or severe open book pelvic injury that has avulsed the transverse process via the iliolumbar ligament.
- Symphyseal diastasis or displaced rami fractures should alert the examiner to additional injuries in the posterior ring even though they may not be readily apparent on the initial radiographic evaluation.

- The inlet projection is taken with the x-ray beam directed caudally approximately 45 degrees to the radiographic film.
  - A true inlet view of the pelvis, however, may require variations on this degree of angulation because of the variations pelvic obliquity, sacral inclination, and dysmorphism. A perfect inlet view will show the anterior cortices of the S1 and S2 sacral bodies superimposed with the undulating promontory of the S1 body slightly anterior to the more linear S2 body.
  - This view simulates a direct view into the pelvis from above along its longitudinal axis (see **FIG 6B**).
  - The inlet view is helpful in imaging the following:
    - External or internal rotation of the hemipelvis
    - Opening of the SI joint or an impaction fracture of the sacrum
    - "AP" displacement or translation of the hemipelvis (see the following text)
- The outlet projection of the pelvis is obtained by directing the x-ray beam approximately 45 to 60 degrees cephalad to the radiographic film.
  - A true outlet view of the sacrum, however, may require variations in this degree of angulation because of the variations in pelvic obliquity, sacral inclination, and dysmorphism. A perfect outlet view will show the anterior sacral foramina as full circles.
  - This view simulates looking at the sacrum and SI joints directly en face **(FIG 6C)**.
  - The outlet view is helpful in imaging the following:
    - Cephalad or "vertical" shift of the hemipelvis
    - Sacral fractures relative to the foramina
    - Flexion–extension deformity of the hemipelvis via ischial height evaluation
- It is important to remember that these radiographs are taken at about 45 degrees to the long axis of the patient's body.
  - Therefore, a given amount of translation or displacement seen on the inlet or outlet view is in fact the sum of displacement vectors in both the coronal and axial planes. For example, "posterior" shift seen on the inlet projection is in fact a combination of both posterior and cephalad translation relative to the long axis of the body.

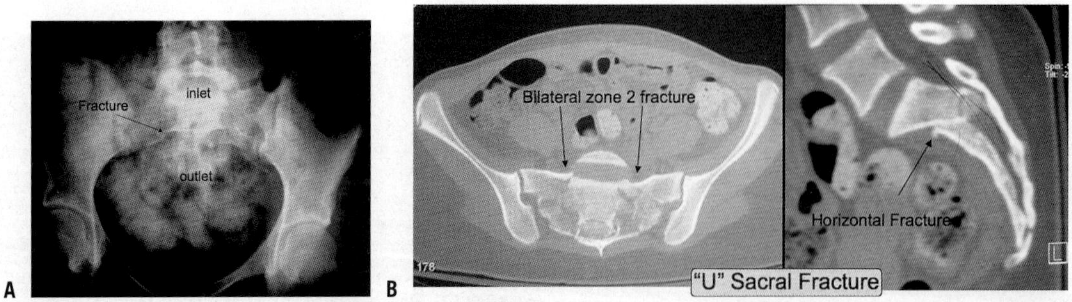

FIG 7 A. AP radiograph of patient with a U-shaped sacral fracture. Note inlet view of proximal sacrum but outlet appearance of caudal sacrum. **B.** Axial and sagittal CT scan reconstructions of the same patient with a U-shaped sacral fracture.

Computed Tomography

- Computed tomography (CT) scanning is imperative in any suspected pelvic ring injury.
  - As the pelvis is a ring structure, any disruption in one location (no matter how seemingly insignificant) must (by virtue of ring structure mechanics) be accompanied by disruption in another location (pathologic fractures excluded).
- Three-millimeter axial sections (or 3 mm of vertical travel per 360-degree rotation of the gantry in a spiral CT) are recommended to disclose the majority of significant injuries **(FIG 6D,E)**. Most standard trauma series acquire the needed resolution in current spiral scanners.
- Another important point to bear in mind is the appearance of the sacrum on the AP projection.
  - If one sees a paradoxical inlet view of the upper sacrum and outlet view of the distal sacrum, a lateral x-ray and CT scan with sagittal reconstructions must be performed to rule out an occult sacral fracture-dislocation (U-shaped sacral fracture otherwise known as *spinal–pelvic dissociation*) **(FIG 7A,B)**. This will be easily seen on the sagittal reconstructions.
  - Bilateral sacral alar fractures noted on an axial CT image of the sacrum should alert the surgeon to a U-shaped sacral fracture dislocation or spinal–pelvic dissociation.
- Computed tomography angiogram: If there is any concern for hemodynamic instability or bleeding from the pelvis based on the initial AP radiograph, adding dye to the CT is helpful as the absence of extravasation has a high negative predictive value for pelvic arterial bleeding, and a positive finding can inform the location of bleeding to be managed. However, the lack of a "blush" does not exclude arterial bleeding.

Retrograde Urethrography and Cystography

- Retrograde urethrography (in male patients) and cystography (in all patients) are mandatory in pelvic fractures with ring disruption to rule out urethral/bladder injury.
- The Foley catheter is partially inserted into the urethra, and the balloon is inflated with 2 to 3 mL of sterile saline to occlude the urethra. Ten to 15 mL of water-soluble contrast is then injected into the urethra, and the outlet view of the pelvis is repeated.
- If no extravasation is seen, the catheter is advanced into the bladder with injection of a further 300 mL of water-soluble contrast to rule out a bladder rupture. If no contrast extravasation is noted, the bladder is drained with the catheter, and any residual dye is noted.
- If passage of the catheter is not possible or there is a tear of the urethra or bladder neck, suprapubic catheterization should be performed well above the umbilicus if possible (to avoid contamination of potential future anterior pelvic operations).

Pelvic Angiography

- Angiography is indicated in those patients exhibiting persistent hemodynamic instability despite[10]
  - Adequate volume resuscitation
  - Other sources of hemorrhage being ruled out (abdomen, thorax, and long bone fractures)
  - Attempts to "close" the pelvic ring (see the following text) have failed to stop pelvic hemorrhage
- Most cases of pelvic hemorrhage (85%) arise from venous bleeding and are not amenable to angiographic embolization.
  - Arterial bleeding is usually from branches of the internal iliac system and approximately half of patients with arterial bleeding have more than one source (median sacral, superior gluteal, pudendal, or obturator arteries) **(FIG 8)**.
  - Arterial hemorrhage is more common in patients older than 65 years.
- If diagnostic peritoneal lavage is being performed to rule out abdominal hemorrhage, then it must be performed above the umbilicus and arcuate line to avoid false-positive results from pelvic hemorrhage.

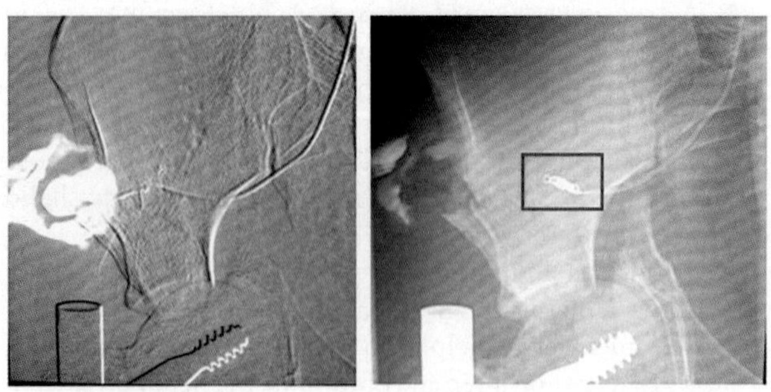

FIG 8 Angiogram showing extravasation (*left*) and coiling (*red box, right*) of superior gluteal artery. (Courtesy of Johannes Reuger, MD, with permission.)

NONOPERATIVE MANAGEMENT

- As a general rule, traumatic complete SI dislocations should not be managed nonoperatively as the ligamentous healing results in an unstable joint and chronic pain.
- Progressive cephalad displacement of the hemipelvis may occur and result in pelvic malunion. Leg length inequality, chronic mechanical low back and buttock pain, pelvic obliquity with sitting imbalance, and dyspareunia are common complaints when the hemipelvis and ischial tuberosities are malpositioned.
- For patients in extremis, sepsis, or critical medical comorbidity, nonoperative therapy may be required until the patient can tolerate pelvic reconstruction procedures. This helps to reduce the pelvic deformity, stabilize the pelvic hemorrhage and clot, and improve patient comfort in the acute resuscitative period. In such cases, the pattern of deformity dictates the maneuvers to be used to minimize deformity.
  - Patients with vertical instability should be placed into balanced longitudinal skeletal traction in an attempt to reduce and/or prevent further cephalad displacement. Traction is also an effective adjunct for hemostasis during resuscitation. Distal femoral skeletal traction is preferable.
  - Patients with external rotation deformity of the pelvic ring (ie, an open book pelvis) should be treated with circumferential wrapping with either a sheet or commercially available pelvic binder placed over the greater trochanters. Frequent skin checks are mandatory to prevent full-thickness pressure ulceration and as such, they are rarely, if ever, indicated for definitive treatment (**FIG 9**).
- Anterior pelvic external fixators can be applied either in the trauma bay or the intensive care unit (ICU) for patients in extremis.
  - Anterior pelvic external fixators are good for controlling external and internal rotation of the anterior pelvic ring. Thus, the surgeon may elect to use them definitively in situations where the SI joint is only disrupted through the anterior SI ligaments (a type 2 injury with no vertical or sagittal plane instability) or with certain lateral compression injuries where the sacral fracture is stable by virtue of its impaction.
  - By themselves, however, anterior external fixators are not effective in controlling the posterior pelvic ring and, if applied incorrectly, can make some pelvic deformities worse.[16,30]

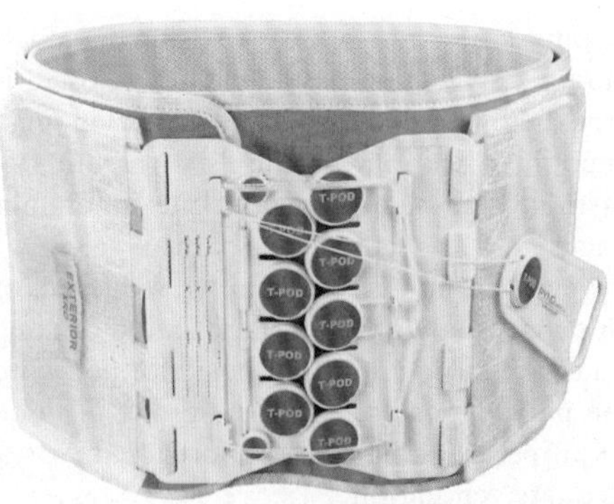

FIG 9 T-POD pelvic binder. (Image courtesy of Teleflex Incorporated. Copyright © 2020 Teleflex Incorporated. All rights reserved.)

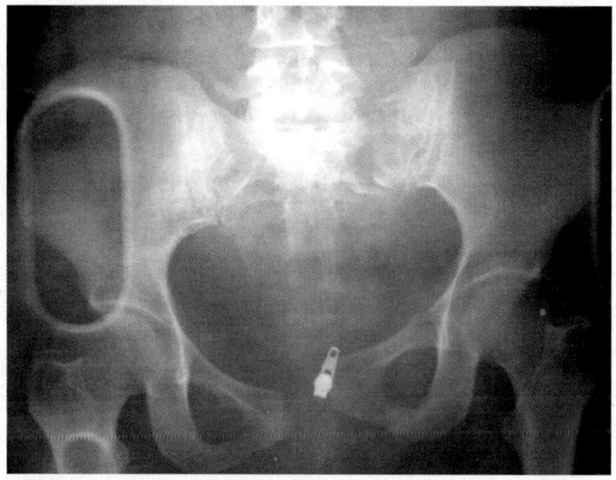

FIG 10 Nonoperative treatment of vertical shear sacral fracture with resultant malunion and leg length inequality.

  - Pelvic C-clamps can also be applied anteriorly in the gluteal pillars with excellent resultant compression. This technique also helps to compress the posterior ring.
- External fixation of the posterior pelvic ring with various commercially available pelvic clamps (Pelvic C-clamp, DePuy Synthes, Paoli, PA) are used on occasion, but expertise is required to prevent serious complications from misplacement, and contaminated pin sites from their use may mitigate options for posterior fixation.[8,18]
- In contrast to SI joint dislocations, many traumatic sacral fractures can be treated successfully with nonoperative care.
  - Although vertical shear sacral fractures represent the far end of the spectrum of unstable sacral fractures needing operative stabilization (**FIG 10**), impacted sacral fractures resulting from lateral compression mechanisms can be relatively stable injuries.
- If the radiographic and CT scanning evaluation reveals an impacted sacral alar fracture without significant displacement in other planes, a trial of nonoperative therapy is warranted if it is thought that the patient will be compliant with mobilization restrictions and appropriate radiographic follow-up to prevent late displacement and healing with a malunion (**FIG 11**).
- Often, the presentation of the patient in bed can help to predict success with nonoperative treatment of impacted sacral fractures.
  - Those patients that are able to roll in bed on their own and help with hygienic care with only minimal or moderate discomfort often have a relatively stable pelvis and will be able to mobilize with physical therapy.

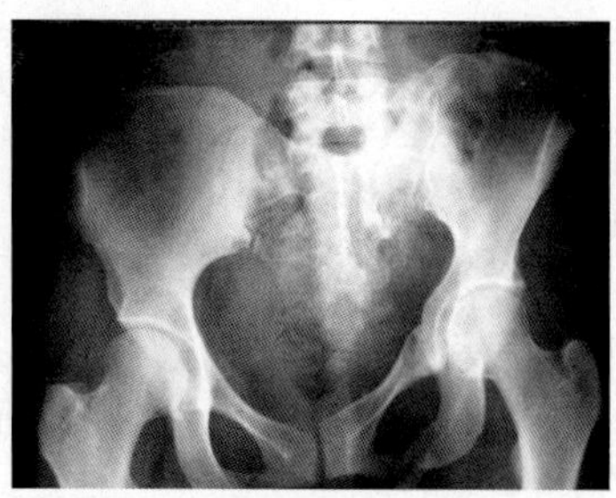

FIG 11 Impacted sacral fracture from lateral compression mechanism with internal rotation.

- Some patients, however, will not be able to tolerate even logrolling in the bed with nursing care.
  - They may be found on examination under anesthetic to have an unstable pelvis despite innocuous-appearing imaging studies.
- There is controversy related to the imaging characteristics that predict lateral compression pelvic ring injuries that might shift over time.
  - Complete sacral fractures with bilateral ramus fractures have the highest chance of displacement over time and require close monitoring.[2]
- If a patient with an impacted sacral fracture is deemed to be a candidate for nonoperative treatment, they can be mobilized with physical therapy as soon as other injuries permit.
  - The patient is instructed to be touchdown weight bearing (TDWB) on the affected extremity for 6 weeks. However, there is considerable variation with respect to weight bearing for lateral compression fractures, and many surgeons will permit immediate full weight bearing allowing the patient to self-regulate. In some cases, the presence of an incomplete or complete sacral fracture may dictate the weight-bearing status for a particular patient.
  - If they are able to successfully mobilize, then repeat clinical examination and AP, inlet, and outlet radiographs are performed within 1 to 2 weeks to assess for any further displacement and increasing leg length inequality.

SURGICAL MANAGEMENT

- In general, all complete SI joint dislocations and unstable displaced nonimpacted sacral fractures should be treated with operative stabilization. The choice of fixation in most instances for both SI joint dislocations and sacral fractures will be with iliosacral screws (SI screws).
  - Biomechanical studies have validated the strength of this technique in comparison to more traditional anterior SI plating and transsacral bars and plates.[11,27]
  - SI screws can be applied with the patient in either the prone or supine position and in either an open or closed percutaneous fashion.
  - SI screw placement requires an exacting knowledge of the radiographic correlates to anatomic landmarks to prevent serious neurologic and vascular injury.[3,6,15,22,31,34]
- Transforaminal sacral fractures with comminution and vertical instability treated with standard SI screw fixation alone may be suboptimal in some instances and have a higher failure rate.
  - In these instances, the surgeon may elect to place alternate forms of fixation to augment the SI screw (transiliac screws, transiliac plates, or some form of spinal pelvic construct) and resist the tendency for vertical displacement. This is discussed in further detail in the following text.[12,26,28]

Preoperative Planning

- Proper preparation and preoperative planning for any major pelvic surgery is mandatory.
  - Pelvic reconstructive procedures can be associated with prolonged anesthetics, lengthy prone positioning, extensive blood loss, and complex reduction maneuvers that can pose serious risk to a patient with other medical or traumatic comorbidities.
  - Having a detailed understanding of the deformity and the reduction and fixation strategy can help to significantly decrease operative time and blood loss.
- We recommend chemical anticoagulation and/or sequential compression devices within 24 hours of admission.
  - If there are contraindications to anticoagulation, inferior vena caval filter placement should be considered in consultation with the other consulting services such as neurosurgery and critical surgeons.[29]
- If an open pelvic reduction is anticipated, then an acute immediate reduction that is easier to perform but potentially associated with greater blood loss needs to be weighed against waiting for a few days to decrease potential blood loss but having a more difficult reduction and increasing patient morbidity.
  - Patients should have at least 3 units of typed and crossmatched blood on hold.
  - If large blood loss is anticipated, then cell saver can be used to avoid allogenic blood products.
  - The surgery should be performed with a surgical team that is familiar with complex pelvic surgery.

Positioning

- Patients should be positioned on a radiolucent table for intraoperative fluoroscopy and be compatible with the ability to apply traction in some fashion.
- Adequate caudal translation of an unstable hemipelvis is not possible if a perineal post is in place because the ischial tuberosity and pubis tend to abut the post, preventing any movement in a caudal direction.
  - This problem can be overcome by stabilizing the contralateral extremity in a traction boot and tightening the traction arm without applying traction to provide vertical support for the contralateral side while traction is applied to the affected extremity.
  - Another alternative in cases with severe vertical displacement is to rigidly fix the contralateral stable pelvis to the operating table with Schanz pins and an external fixator using a pelvic stabilization frame (eg, Mizuho OSI, Union City, CA).
- Patient positioning will be in either the prone or supine position, depending on the injury pattern and the surgeon's assessment of the ability to achieve reduction via closed or open means.
  - In some cases, an initial provisional reduction of the anterior pelvic ring may facilitate a closed, indirect, or percutaneous reduction of the posterior ring. The most common indication for this is if the anterior injury is a symphyseal disruption and the innominate bone is intact.
  - However, an imperfect definitive reduction of the anterior pelvic ring with rigid stabilization can impair reduction of the more important posterior pelvic injury.
- For the patient positioned in the prone position **(FIG 12)**, ensure proper padding and support for the chest to allow for adequate ventilation.
- It is preferable to use longitudinal chest rolls that come short of the pelvis, allowing the lower trunk and pelvis to

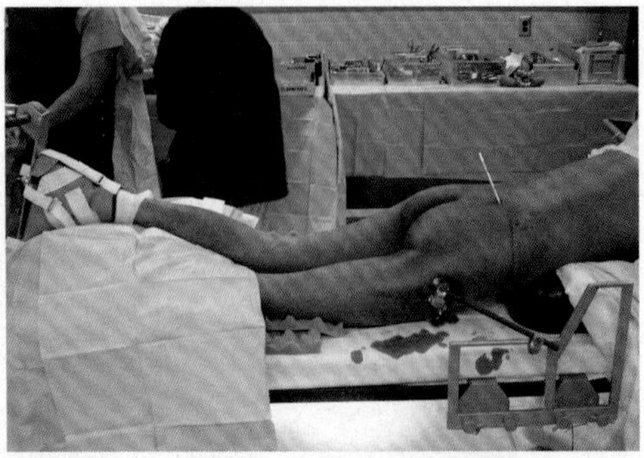

FIG 12 Positioning and setup of patient for posterior approach and reduction of sacral fracture or SI joint dislocation. Note the pelvis hanging freely, traction setup, and rigid stabilization frame on contralateral stable hemipelvis.

hang freely and not rest on the anterior superior iliac spine (ASIS).
  - If the pelvis is permitted to rest on the ASIS, posterior translation of the unstable hemipelvis may result and/or impair reduction.
- The extremity ipsilateral to the unstable hemipelvis should be draped free to allow for longitudinal traction and internal–external rotation.
  - It should be placed in either boot or skeletal (distal femoral or proximal tibial) traction that allows for rotation and abduction–adduction.
  - The hip should be extended and the knee flexed to relax the sciatic nerve and lumbosacral plexus (see **TECH FIG 4B**).
  - Extension of the hip and lumbosacral junction and longitudinal traction will help to indirectly reduce any flexion deformity that exists.
- Draping of the operative field should include the entire flank on the affected side.
  - The field should continue to include the buttock and upper thigh, with free draping of the affected extremity.
  - The natal cleft and contralateral buttock are excluded from the field.
- For the patient positioned in the supine position, have a small folded sheet or pad placed under the sacrum or buttock on the affected side to lift the pelvis away from the table. Again, the affected extremity should be placed into traction to aid in reduction, as detailed earlier.
  - If there is posterior displacement of the hemipelvis, placing the bump under the buttock will help to anteriorly translate the pelvis when traction is applied.
  - If there is anterior translation of the hemipelvis, then placing the bump directly midline will help to lift the pelvis away from the table and also let the affected hemipelvis hang freely to allow posterior translation during reduction maneuvers.

Examination Under Anesthesia[24]

- Accurate assessment of the injury AP pelvis performed in the trauma bay helps determine the mechanism of injury, necessary reduction maneuvers, and fixation constructs.
- Degree of initial displacement often underappreciated due to recoil of the pelvis following injury, manipulation by emergency medical services personnel, and application of pelvic sheets or binders.
- Allows surgeon to confirm operative indication and properly treat unstable injuries not evident on injury films or CT scans.
- We use a series of 15 images, but others have different protocols if they use stress examinations.
  - We use static, internal rotation stress, external rotation stress, and push-pull on each extremity (**TABLE 1**). Each of these is performed in on AP, inlet and outlet fluoroscopic images.
- We define instability as displacement greater than 1 cm, although all displacements are not equally important. For example, vertical displacement of the sacrum would be a more universal operative indication than a small amount of internal rotation.
- Negative stress examination performed in this fashion reliably predicts union without late displacement even in the face of pain as patients without displacement and without pain would not undergo stress examination.[33]
- Sequential intraoperative examination under anesthesia identifies occult, unstable injuries following initial fixation (ie, ongoing instability in the anterior ring following fixation of the posterior ring, injury to the contralateral SI joint in the setting of lateral compression pelvic ring injury).

Surgical Approach

- Exposure of the SI joint can be accomplished from either anterior or posterior.
- If significant displacement exists and a difficult open reduction is predicted, we prefer a posterior approach, but this varies based on individual surgeon experience.[17]

Posterior Approach to the Sacroiliac Joint

- For the posterior approach to the SI joint, the incision is vertical and paramedian, centered directly over the involved SI joint. Do not carry the incision directly over the bony prominence of the posterior superior iliac spine (PSIS); rather, place it just medial to the PSIS (**FIG 13**).
- The tissues that bridge the SI joint posteriorly in the intact state include the lumbodorsal fascia (LDF), the transverse fibers of the gluteus maximus, the erector spinae muscles, and the multifidus—in addition to the posterior SI ligaments (**FIG 14**).
- With SI joint dislocations, some or all of these fascial, muscular, and ligamentous layers may be completely disrupted, and no further dissection is needed.
  - Often, however, to visualize the inferior aspect of the SI joint posteriorly, the transverse gluteus maximus (TGM) needs to be mobilized. The TGM attachment to the sacral spinous processes and thoracolumbar fascia is released, and the TGM is reflected laterally and inferiorly to expose the inferior aspect of the SI joint. In preventing wound complications, it is imperative to preserve the attachment and origin of the TGM.
- Occasionally, some of the LDF will need to be released from the posterior iliac crest, and the piriformis can also be released and reflected posteriorly.
  - This allows dissection up over the superior aspect of the SI joint and sacral ala to permit digital palpation as an assessment of reduction of the anterior SI joint or a less cluttered access through the greater sciatic notch, respectively.

TABLE 1 Examination Under Anesthesia

Examination	Technique	Illustration
External rotation pelvic instability	Legs are positioned flexed, abducted, and externally rotated. Hands are placed on the medial knee, and an AP force is applied.	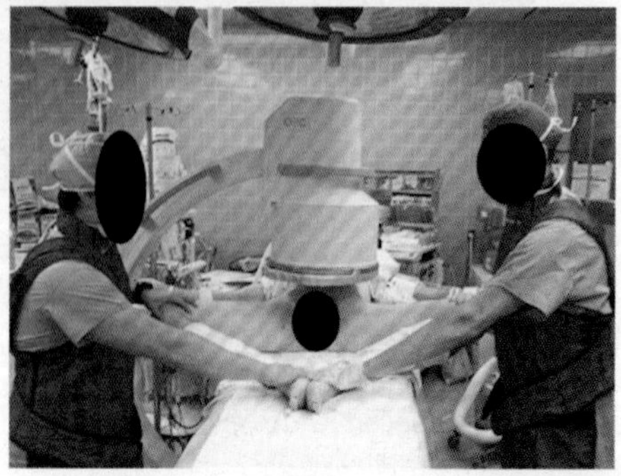
Internal rotation pelvic instability	Legs are positioned extended, adducted, and internally rotated. Hands are positioned over the greater trochanters, and a lateral to medial compressive force is applied.	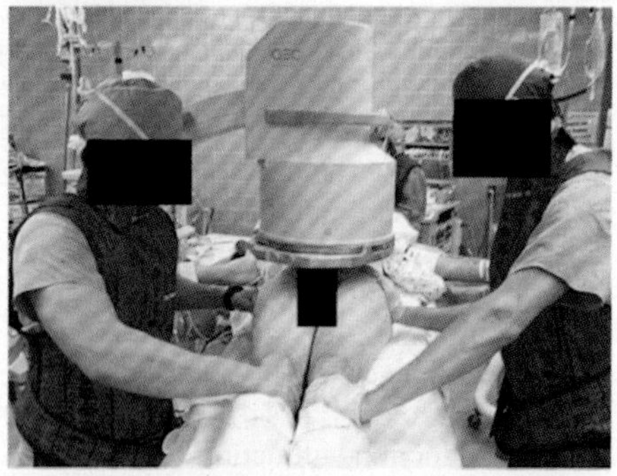
Vertical instability	Legs are positioned extended. While one extremity is supported at the heel, traction is applied to the other.	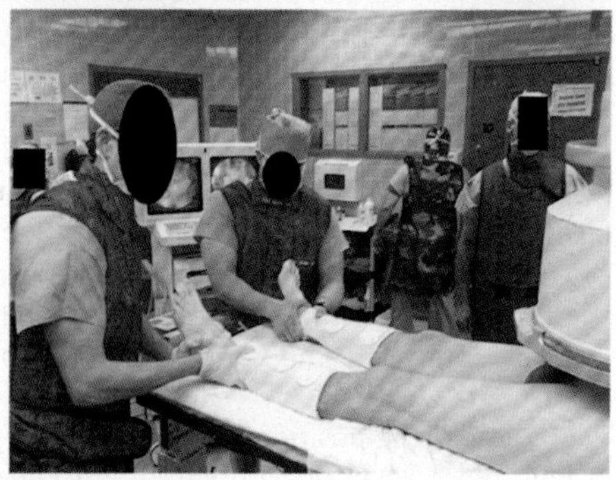

AP, anteroposterior.

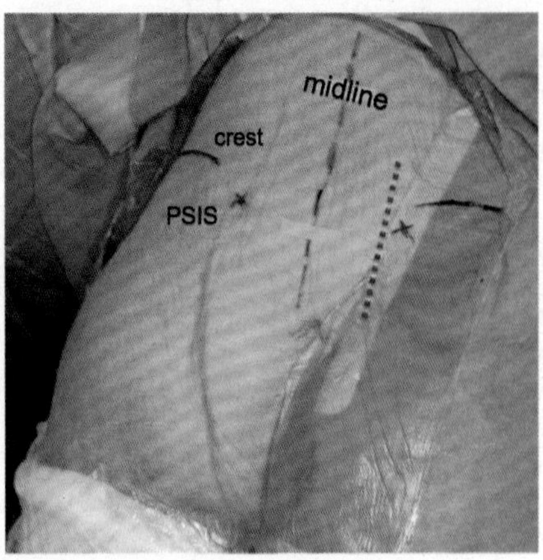

FIG 13 Skin incision for posterior approach to sacrum and SI joint. *PSIS*, posterior superior iliac spine.

- Once exposure is complete, it is usually necessary to evacuate a significant amount of blood clot and hematoma from the joint.
  - On occasion, loose fragments of denuded articular cartilage are present and should be removed.
  - Routine removal of articular surfaces for a primary SI joint fusion is not routinely performed.
- While removing blood clot and debris, specific attention must be paid to the superior gluteal vessels and the internal iliac vascular system.
  - Removal of clot may restart arterial bleeding that was initially controlled by tamponade and spasm, or direct iatrogenic injury may occur with dissection through the fracture hematoma and clot. Should significant bleeding occur, the surgeon should resist the temptation to blindly clip or ligate vessels that are not clearly visualized, as this may cause inadvertent injury to the superior gluteal

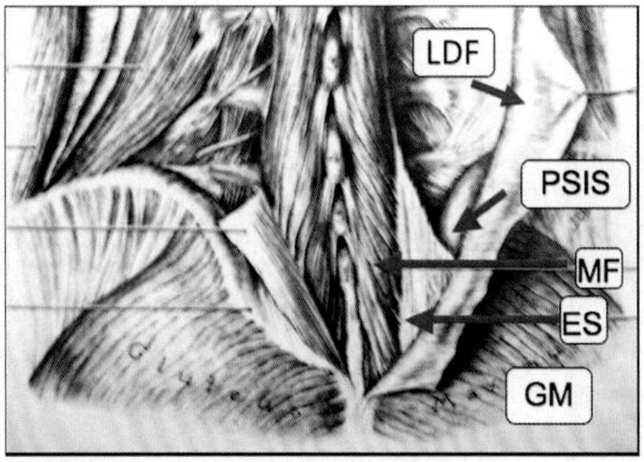

A

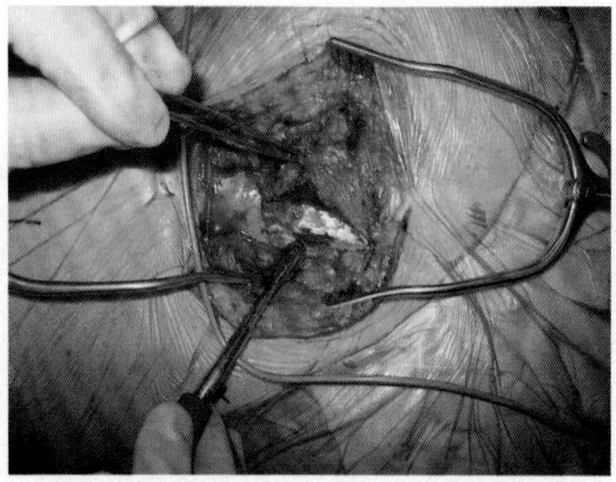

B

FIG 14 A. Diagram of fascial fibers and muscular layers for posterior approach to sacrum and SI joint. *LDF*, lumbodorsal fascia; *PSIS*, posterior superior iliac spine; *MF*, multifidus; *ES*, erector spinae; *GM*, gluteus maximus. **B.** Intraoperative surgical exposure of SI joint from posterior approach demonstrating the TGM.

nerve and continued blood loss. Unless the bleeding vessel is clearly visualized and separated from the nerve, it is best to pack the bleeding with various topical hemostatic agents such as thrombin and gel foam. If this does not control the bleeding, and/or the patient is hypotensive, maintain the packing, close the wound, and proceed with interventional radiology and embolization/coiling.

- All sacral fractures that necessitate an open reduction require a posterior approach.
  - Anterior approaches are not recommended because it is not possible to dissect onto the anterior aspect of the sacrum without posing excessive risk to the lumbosacral nerve roots and iliac vessels through a traditional anterior approach to the posterior pelvic ring.
- The posterior approach for sacral fracture reduction varies depending on the fracture location and the need for sacral nerve root decompression.
- In general, however, most sacral fractures and foraminal decompressions can be performed through the same paramedian approach as described earlier for SI joint dislocations. The only alterations in technique would be as follows:
  - Subperiosteal elevation of the paraspinal muscles from the dorsal aspect of the sacrum to the spinous processes is required to expose the whole posterior surface of the sacrum **(FIG 15)**. Keep in mind that with a sacral fracture, the posterior SI ligaments are (usually) intact, so careful elevation of the paraspinal muscles without disruption of the posterior SI ligaments must be undertaken.
  - Proximal extension along the intermuscular plane between the multifidus and erector spine is performed to expose the L4–L5 facet joint..

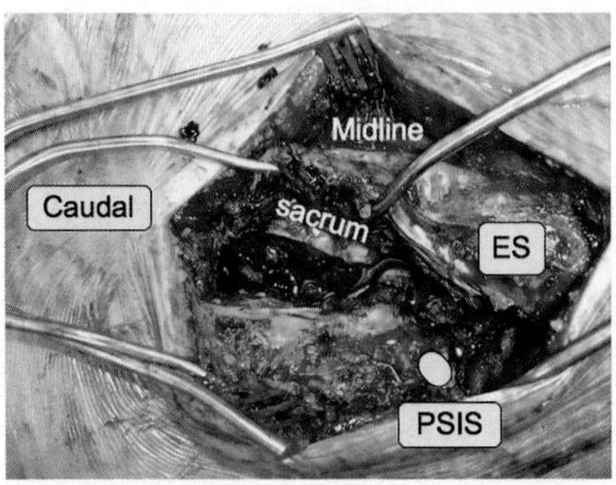

FIG 15 Posterior exposure for sacral fracture reduction demonstrating the lateral reflection of the paraspinal muscles. *ES*, erector spinae; *PSIS*, posterior superior iliac spine.

Anterior Approach to the Sacroiliac Joint

- The anterior approach provides good visualization of the superior aspect of the SI joint and is advocated in the following situations:
  - The soft tissues do not permit the posterior approach.
  - The patient will not tolerate prone positioning because of poor pulmonary status or associated spinal injuries.
  - A close-to-anatomic closed reduction of the SI joint can be obtained with traction, manipulation, or provisional anterior ring reduction with only minor adjustments needing to be made.
- The anterior approach to the SI joint uses the proximal portion of the Smith-Petersen approach by releasing the external oblique fibers from the iliac crest and elevating the iliacus muscle subperiosteally from the inner table of the ilium.
  - Remember to use the intermuscular plane between the abductors and the external oblique muscles to access the crest. The external oblique muscle tends to hang over the crest, and direct dissection down to bone through the muscle results in a weaker repair and increased postoperative pain.
- When the SI joint is encountered, careful mobilization of the tissue on the sacral ala using a blunt periosteal elevator and finger dissection helps to move the L5 nerve root medially out of harm's way.
- Once this tissue is mobilized, and the sacral ala is seen under direct vision, a sharp Hohmann retractor is driven into the alar cortex and used to protect the L5 nerve root, which lies medially **(FIG 16A)**.
  - To improve exposure and visualization of the sacrum and SI joint anteriorly, the surgeon may elect to perform an osteotomy of the ASIS, leaving the sartorius and external oblique attached to it **(FIG 16B,C)**.

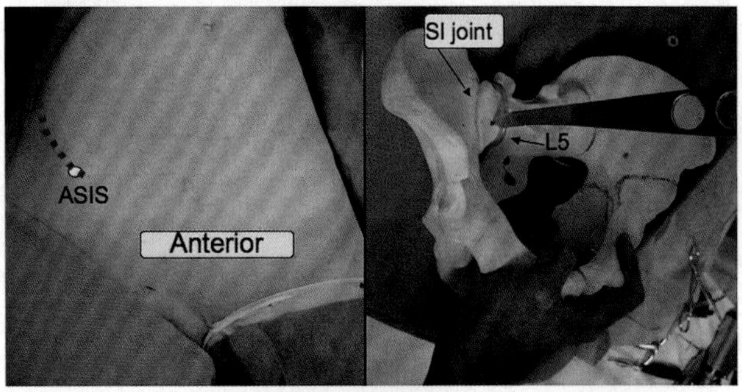

A

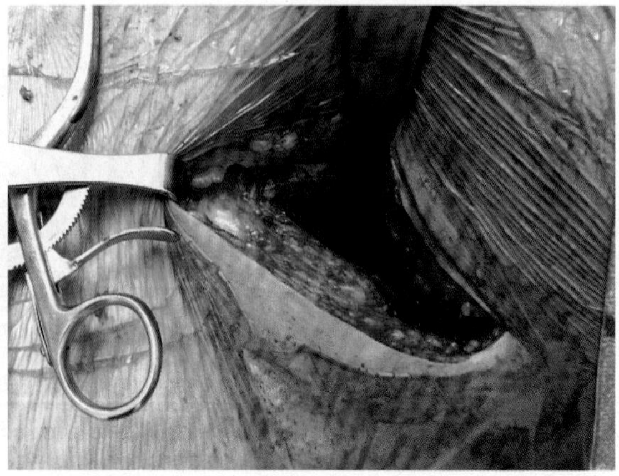

B

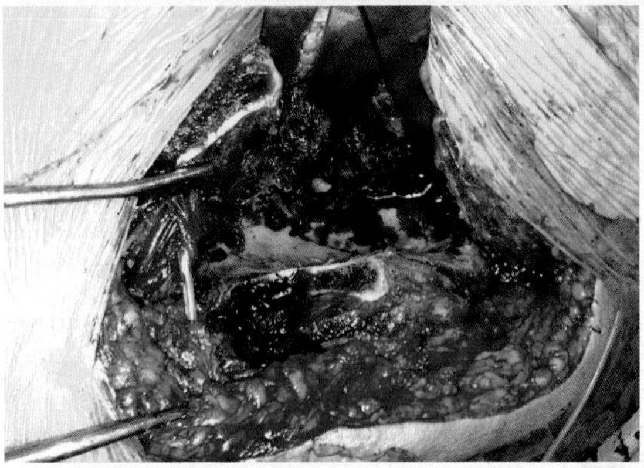

C

FIG 16 A. Diagram of incision and view of sacroiliac (*SI*) joint from the anterior approach. Note position of sharp Hohmann retractor in ala to protect the L5 nerve root. **B.** Visualization prior to osteotomy of the anterior superior iliac spine (*ASIS*) to improve anterior exposure of the posterior pelvic ring and SI joint. **C.** Visualization after osteotomy of the ASIS to improve anterior exposure of the posterior pelvic ring and SI joint.

TECHNIQUES

OPEN REDUCTION OF THE SACROILIAC JOINT VIA THE POSTERIOR APPROACH

- Reduction of the dislocated SI joint is complex and requires a good knowledge of the three-dimensional anatomy of the sacrum, ilium, and SI joint.
- Although some AP translation and lateral–medial translation may be necessary to reduce the SI joint, longitudinal traction is the single most important indirect maneuver to perform. Adequate longitudinal traction can be assessed intraoperatively with direct visualization, digital palpation, and the image intensifier.
- Reduction of the superior aspect of the SI joint can be assessed with digital palpation, ensuring that the superior–anterior aspect of the SI joint is flush.
- Final confirmation with inlet, outlet, and AP radiographs will help disclose subtle rotational deformities not appreciated by direct visualization or palpation.
- Only when adequate length has been restored can the need for additional AP or medial to lateral translation be assessed.
- Fine-tuning of the SI joint reduction will require the placement of one or two reduction clamps to medially translate and internally rotate the hemipelvis. Large pointed reduction clamps (such as the Weber clamp or angled jaw clamps) are used.
- Posteriorly, a clamp can be placed over the sacral spinous process or into the posterior cortex of the sacrum inferiorly and into the cortical bone of the medial aspect of the greater sciatic notch. This can help close the inferior aspect of the SI joint **(TECH FIG 1A)**.
- A second clamp can be used superiorly, with one tine placed carefully over the top of the joint onto the sacral ala anteriorly and the second tine placed just lateral to the PSIS. The tine on the ala should be placed laterally to avoid the L5 nerve root **(TECH FIG 1B)**.
- Alternatively, the second clamp can be placed through the greater notch, with one tine on the sacral ala lateral to the sacral nerve roots and foramina and the other tine on the posterior cortex of the ilium **(TECH FIG 1C)**.
- While these clamps are being closed to reduce the superior SI joint, internal rotation of the extremity or pushing on the anterior iliac wing with a ball spike pusher (picador) can help to close down the anterior aspect of the SI joint.

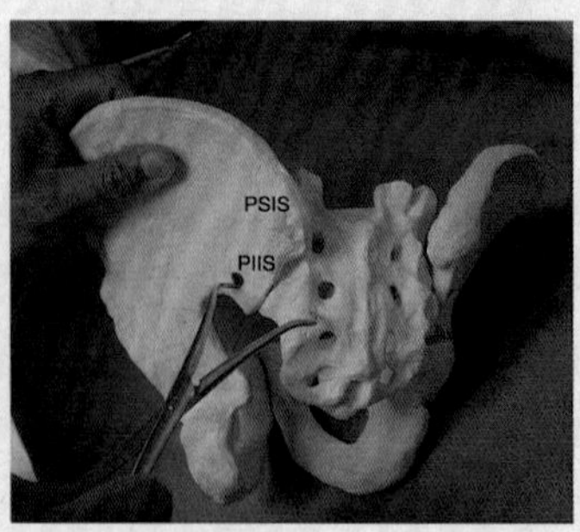

A

TECH FIG 1 A. Weber reduction clamp positioned to reduce inferior aspect of sacroiliac (*SI*) joint, from posterior approach. *PSIS*, posterior superior iliac spine; *PIIS*, posterior inferior iliac spine. *(continued)*

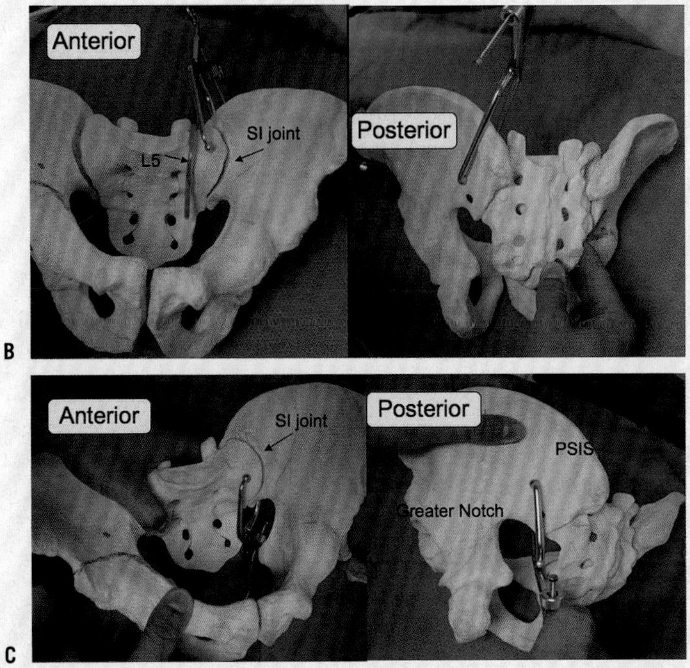

TECH FIG 1 *(continued)* **B.** Angled jaw clamp reducing superior and anterior aspect of SI. Clamp is positioned from over the top between iliac crest and L5 transverse process. **C.** Angled jaw clamp reducing anterior aspect of SI joint. Clamp is positioned through the greater notch onto lateral aspect of the ala, lateral to the L5 nerve root and sacral foramina.

OPEN REDUCTION OF THE SACRUM VIA THE POSTERIOR APPROACH

- The patient setup and surgical exposure are the same as for SI dislocations.
- Indirect reduction maneuvers are also the same as for SI dislocations, but clamp placement for reduction of the sacral fractures differs because the surgeon no longer has the ability to place clamps on the anterior aspect of the sacral ala.
- Instead, two sharp-pointed reduction clamps can be used.
  - One clamp is placed posteriorly from the PSIS to the inferior aspect of the sacrum by the sacral cornu (to correct residual cephalad displacement), and the second clamp is placed from a sacral spinous process to the outer table of the ilium to correct lateral displacement **(TECH FIG 2A,B)**. Craniocaudal displacement must be corrected prior to medial–lateral displacement.
- Residual anterior opening of the fracture can be corrected with the iliosacral or transsacral lag screw if the posterior cortex is uncomminuted.

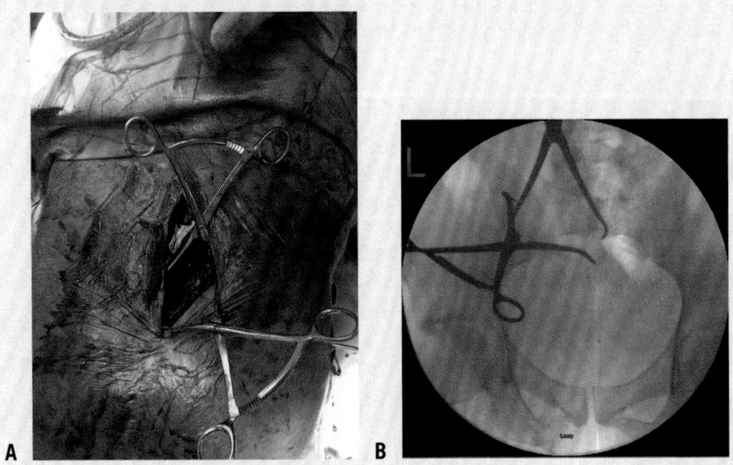

TECH FIG 2 **A.** Intraoperative photograph showing clamp placement for sacral fracture reduction. **B.** Intraoperative fluoroscopic image showing clamp placement for sacral fracture reduction.

OPEN REDUCTION OF THE SACROILIAC JOINT VIA THE ANTERIOR APPROACH

- Once the SI joint and sacral ala have been exposed for an anterior approach as outlined earlier, reduction can be carried out.
  - Similar to the posterior approach, longitudinal traction is applied with internal rotation of the extremity.
- If there is wide diastasis of the SI joint and symphysis, the surgeon may elect at this stage to expose the symphysis and temporarily reduce it with a clamp to aid in internal rotation and reduction.
- It is important to keep in mind, however, that permanent fixation of the symphysis at this time is not indicated as it may impede anatomic reduction of the SI joint by limiting motion of the unstable hemipelvis.
  - If open reduction of the symphysis is performed, hold it temporarily with a clamp so that it can be removed or adjusted if the SI joint does not reduce satisfactorily.
- Should persistent diastasis of the SI joint exist despite these indirect maneuvers, a Jungbluth or Farabeuf reduction clamp can be used to complete the reduction.
  - A single cortical screw is placed on either side of the SI joint into the ilium and sacral ala, respectively.
  - The heads of the screws are left proud off the cortex, allowing the reduction clamp to engage the screw heads.
  - The clamps can be rotated and twisted in any direction while closing the gap to achieve reduction of the joint **(TECH FIG 3A,B)**.
  - The reduction is verified by direct visualization and intraoperative fluoroscopy with AP, inlet, and outlet projections.
  - As a temporary measure until definitive SI screw fixation, an anterior SI plate can be placed to help with reduction of the SI joint by placing a two- or three-hole plates with one screw in the sacral ala and another into the ilium directed back toward the posterior inferior iliac spine (PIIS) **(TECH FIG 3C)**.

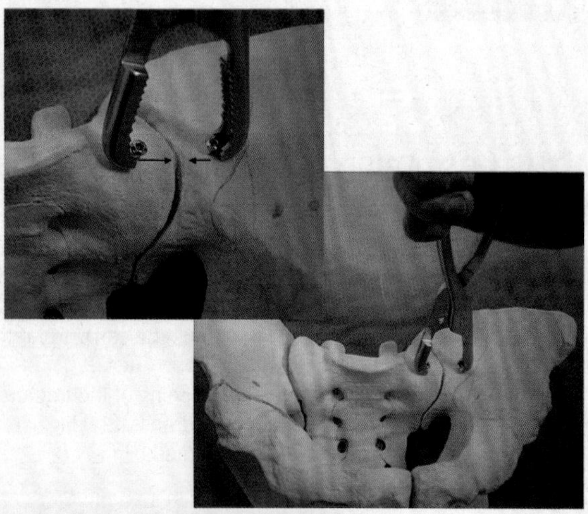
A

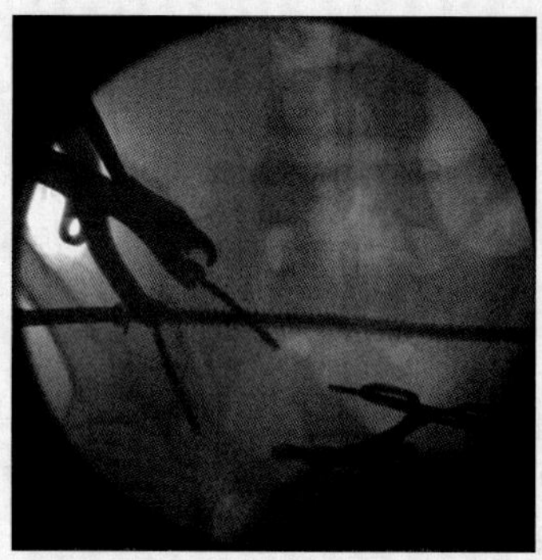
B

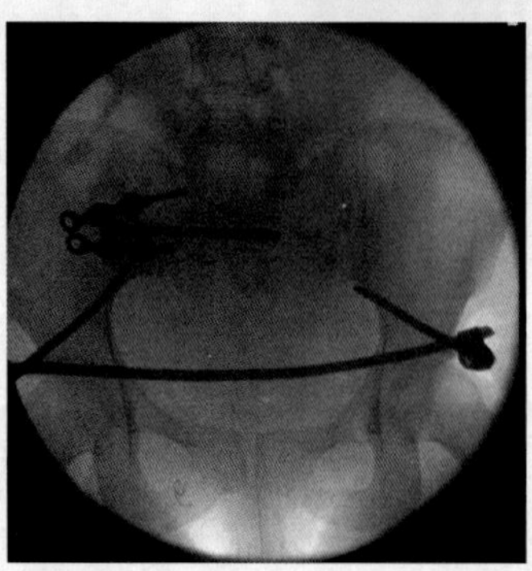
C

TECH FIG 3 A. Farabeuf pelvic reduction clamp reducing the SI joint from the anterior approach using the two-screw technique. **B.** Intraoperative fluoroscopic image demonstrating the Jungbluth reduction clamp on the anterior aspect of the SI joint with a Hohmann retractor medially protecting the L5 nerve root. **C.** Anterior SI plates place to aid with reduction of the anterior SI joint and augment the SI screw for an SI dislocation.

PLACEMENT OF ILIOSACRAL SCREWS

- Large cannulated, partially threaded lag screws are used (6.5, 7.3, or 8.0 mm) so that compression can be applied to achieve maximal stability.
- The entry point on the external surface of the ilium is typically 10 to 20 mm anterior to the crista glutea, two-thirds of the way from the iliac crest (PSIS) to the greater sciatic notch or 2 cm up and 2 cm posterior to the notch **(TECH FIG 4A)**.
- Percutaneously, the external landmark for choosing the correct entry site is the point of intersection between a line extending proximally from the greater trochanter along the axis of the femoral shaft and a horizontal line extending laterally from the PSIS **(TECH FIG 4B)**.
- Percutaneously applied SI screws (particularly into the S2 segment) must be wary of injury to the superior gluteal neurovascular bundle because the entry point is in close proximity to the superior gluteal neurovascular bundle as it exits the greater sciatic notch.[4,23]
- "Safe" placement is maximized by careful attention to radiographic bony landmarks.[3,6,22,34]
- The three critical projections for placing an SI screw are as follows:
  - The lateral projection to center the guidewire on the sacral body anterior to the canal and upper sacral nerve root tunnel and below the iliac cortical density (L5 nerve root). **(TECH FIG 4C)**. The use of the lateral projection is particularly useful when placing screws into the second sacral segment when there is substantial overlap between the anterior cortices of S1 and S2 on the inlet projection.
  - The outlet projection to ensure that the guidewire passes above or between the sacral foramina **(TECH FIG 4D)**
  - The inlet projection to ensure that the guidewire is at the proper trajectory and coming to rest all the way across in the anterior aspect of the sacral body–promontory for maximal purchase **(TECH FIG 4E)**.
- A few points merit mentioning at this point:
  - The trajectory—and therefore starting point—varies for transsacral screws and iliosacral screws. In general terms, transsacral screws are placed in the true transverse axis across the sacral body, whereas iliosacral screws are placed perpendicular to the plane of the SI joint.
  - On the lateral projection, therefore, transsacral screws will be centered more on the sacral body, whereas iliosacral screws will be placed more inferior and posterior (closer to the upper sacral nerve root tunnel).
  - Keep in mind that a safely placed screw is only verified by combining the information gleaned from at least the inlet and outlet projections. A screw that looks completely safe on the inlet may be too low on the outlet and in danger of penetrating the neural foramen. Conversely, a screw that looks completely safe on the outlet may be too anterior or posterior on the inlet and in danger of nerve root injury. In general, the safe place to target is high and anterior in the sacral body.
  - Whenever there is any question of whether a screw has been placed safely within the sacral body, the lateral projection will always be the one view that will give you the most information about a safely placed screw being within all the confines of the safe corridor (upper sacral nerve tunnel, sacral spinal canal, anterior sacral cortex, and iliac cortical density).
- Be attentive to sacral dysmorphism and segmentation defects that give rise to altered anatomy, such as lumbarized S1 or sacralized L5 vertebral bodies **(TECH FIG 4E,F)** and result in atypical safe trajectories and corridors for SI screws.
  - The case shown in **FIG 2C,D** demonstrates a unilateral sacralized L5 on the right. The left side is normal. Note that iliac crest is in line with the L4–L5 disc space.
  - The safe corridor for the SI screw is between the valley of the ala anteriorly (L5 nerve root), the sacral canal posteriorly (cauda equina), and the sacral foramen inferiorly (S1 nerve root) (see **TECH FIG 4F**).
  - Note that in the normal situation (no segmentation abnormality), the corridor is well defined (see **TECH FIG 4F**), but in the case of a sacralized L5, the safe corridor is either exceedingly narrow or nonexistent **(TECH FIG 4G,H)**. If this abnormality is not recognized, and an SI screw is placed into L5 assuming it is S1, the L5 nerve root is likely to be injured. If the surgeon is unsure, the lateral projection with the iliac cortical densities is key in determining the correct level to place the screw because they are constant with their relationship to S1 even in segmentation abnormalities **(TECH FIG 4I)**.
- For SI joint dislocations, the screw trajectory should be from inferior to superior on the outlet view and from posterior to anterior on the inlet view (perpendicular to the plane of the SI joint). Placement of the screw outside of this trajectory may result in shear rather than compression of the SI joint and therefore potentially displace or malreduce the SI joint (see **TECH FIG 4D,E**). However, if the anterior ring has been reduced, and the SI joint is situated perfectly congruent but just laterally translated, then a purely transverse trajectory may be selected in that scenario. Similarly, if only the anterior aspect of the SI joint is open, then a purely transverse trajectory for an anteriorly placed screw may be optimal.
- For sacral fractures, the screw trajectory should be straight across from lateral to medial on the inlet and outlet view (perpendicular to the fracture plane; see **TECH FIG 4J–L**).
- The tip of the SI screw should come to rest in the contralateral side of the S1 body and promontory. Carrying the screw into the contralateral ala provides weaker purchase secondary to poor bone quality and increased risk to the contralateral L5 nerve root.
- In situations of comminuted transforaminal sacral fractures, the theoretical risk of overcompression and iatrogenic L5 or sacral nerve root injury exists. To gain stability with the construct and avoid a nonunion, some compression is, however, necessary.
  - If the sacral fracture is comminuted, and fragments of bone are noted to be in the foramen, then sacral nerve root decompression can be readily performed through the fracture to mitigate the risk of iatrogenic nerve injury during the reduction and compression of the fracture.
  - If inadequate compression secondary to extensive comminution exists, then supplemental forms of fixation such as transsacral screws, transiliac plates, or spinal pelvic fixation should be considered **(TECH FIG 5)**.

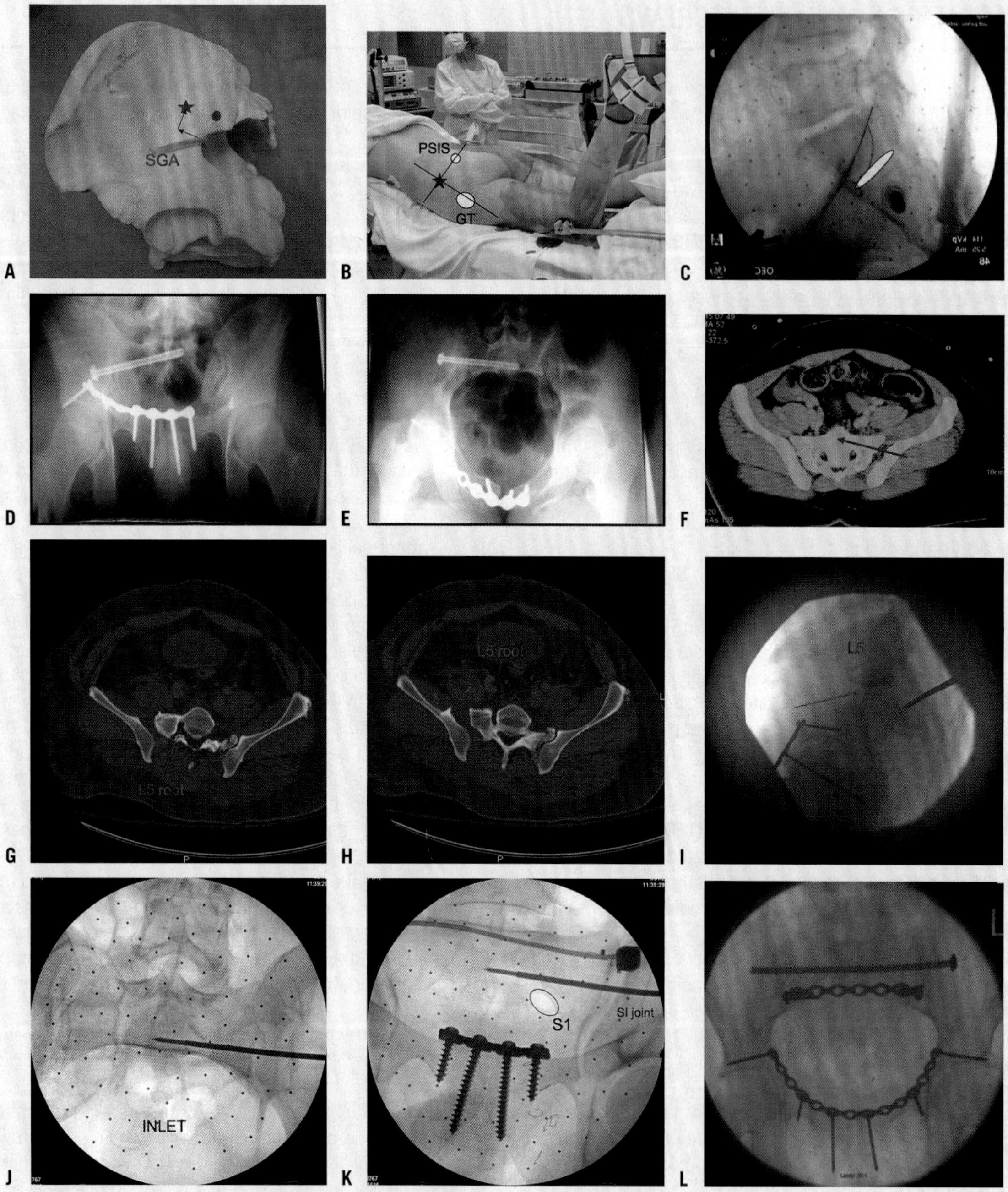

TECH FIG 4 A. Entry point for SI screw on outer table of the ilium. Note proximity to the superior gluteal neurovascular bundle. *SGA*, superior gluteal artery. **B.** Superficial landmarks for percutaneous SI screw placement. *PSIS*, posterior superior iliac spine; *GT*, greater trochanter. **C.** Lateral projection of pelvis showing the very narrow safe corridor in S1 as bordered by the iliac cortical density (L5 nerve root), the upper sacral nerve root tunnel, and the vestigial disc space at S1–S2. The iliosacral screw is in S2. **D.** Outlet projection showing path of iliosacral screw for SI joint dislocation. **E.** Inlet projection showing path of iliosacral screw for SI joint dislocation. **F.** Axial CT scan showing correct trajectory through safe corridor in S1 to perform lag technique in reducing the SI joint dislocation. **G,H.** Axial CT scan showing dysmorphic sacrum with compromised safe corridor. **I.** Lateral intraoperative fluoroscopic image demonstrating an S1 iliosacral screw below the two lilac cortical densities (*red arrow*). **J.** Intraoperative inlet projection demonstrating the correct trajectory for an iliosacral screw for a sacral fracture now perpendicular to the fracture plane, not the SI joint. **K.** Intraoperative outlet projection demonstrating the correct trajectory for an iliosacral screw for a sacral fracture now perpendicular to the fracture plane, not the SI joint. **L.** Intraoperative fluoroscopic AP projection demonstrating the use of a transiliac plate and transsacral screw for fixation of a sacral fracture.

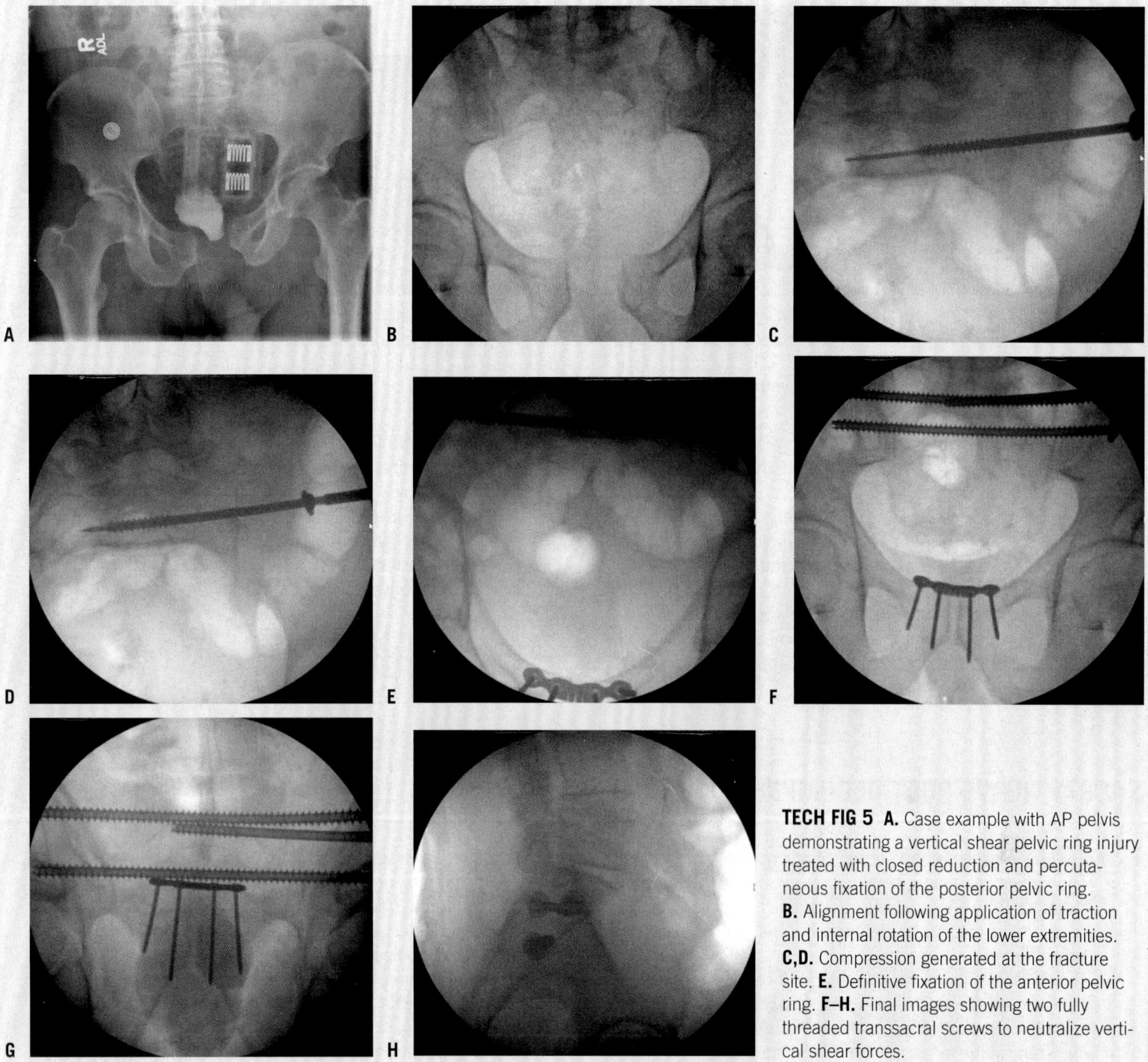

TECH FIG 5 A. Case example with AP pelvis demonstrating a vertical shear pelvic ring injury treated with closed reduction and percutaneous fixation of the posterior pelvic ring. **B.** Alignment following application of traction and internal rotation of the lower extremities. **C,D.** Compression generated at the fracture site. **E.** Definitive fixation of the anterior pelvic ring. **F–H.** Final images showing two fully threaded transsacral screws to neutralize vertical shear forces.

SPINAL PELVIC FIXATION

- This technique is also known by the terms *lumbopelvic fixation* and *triangular ostesynthesis.*[14,25]
- The purpose of this technique is to augment SI screw fixation for a very unstable posterior ring injury that has been reduced and temporarily stabilized but at risk for failure of fixation and subsequent displacement—usually in the case of extensively comminuted transforaminal sacral fractures.
- Through the posterior approach as described earlier, the L4–L5 facet joint is exposed, taking care not to disrupt the capsule.
- A Schanz screw (USS thoracolumbar fracture system, DePuy Synthes USA, Paoli, PA) or any other pedicle screw system is placed into the L5 pedicle, with the entry point being at the junction of the transverse process and the lateral border of the facet joint.
- A second Schanz screw or pedicle screw is placed into the ilium at the PSIS and then directed between the inner and outer tables of the ilium along the sciatic buttress toward the anterior inferior iliac spine.
  - The trajectory should be aiming for the ipsilateral greater trochanter as an external landmark. The screw should be directed to pass through the region of the sciatic buttress above the greater sciatic notch as seen on the iliac oblique view.

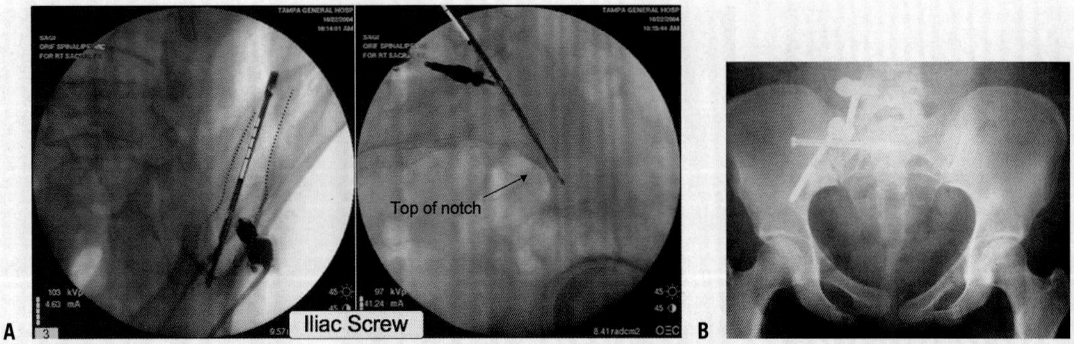

TECH FIG 6 **A.** Obturator outlet (*left*) and iliac (*right*) oblique views to show the path of the iliac screw for triangular osteosynthesis; note that path is between the inner and outer tables (outlined in *red hashmarks*) on the obturator oblique view and just above the sciatic buttress on the iliac oblique view. **B.** AP radiograph of the pelvis after spinal pelvic fixation (triangular osteosynthesis).

- Safe placement out of the SI joint and within the confines of the inner and outer tables can be confirmed on the obturator–outlet oblique view **(TECH FIG 6A)**.
- The pedicle and iliac screws are then connected with fixed angle clamps and a 5.0-mm rod, thus supplementing the SI screw to resist vertical displacement and rotation around the SI screw **(TECH FIG 6B)**.
- It is important to keep in mind that sacral fracture reduction and fixation with an SI screw as described earlier should be performed prior to placement of any spinal pelvic construct.
  - This avoids rigid fixation with residual sacral gap and subsequent nonunion or delayed union. At times, the SI or transsacral screw may interfere with the iliac screw from PSIS to the ASIS. However, there is considerably more room and leeway for placement of the iliac screw. For that reason, place the sacral screw first and adjust the trajectory of the iliac screw afterward to accommodate the position of the sacral screw.

SACRAL NERVE ROOT DECOMPRESSION

- This will be indicated in one of two situations:
  - The patient has a peripheral neurologic deficit (radiculitis or radiculopathy) attributable to a sacral nerve root injury, and preoperative imaging shows fracture fragments within the sacral foramen.
  - The patient is neurologically intact, but preoperative imaging studies disclose a large bone fragment within the foramen that during reduction will further compress the nerve root and stenose the foramen, resulting in iatrogenic nerve root injury **(TECH FIG 7A)**.
- In most cases of transforaminal fractures, the incriminating fragment of bone can be found and removed by working directly through the fracture in the sacrum **(TECH FIG 7B)**.
- A laminar spreader can be placed into the fracture to spread the respective portions of the fracture.
- After the clot is removed, careful dissection along the exposed surface of the medial sacral fragment will disclose some portion of the foramen.
- Tracing the nerve root anteriorly will usually lead to the bone fragment.

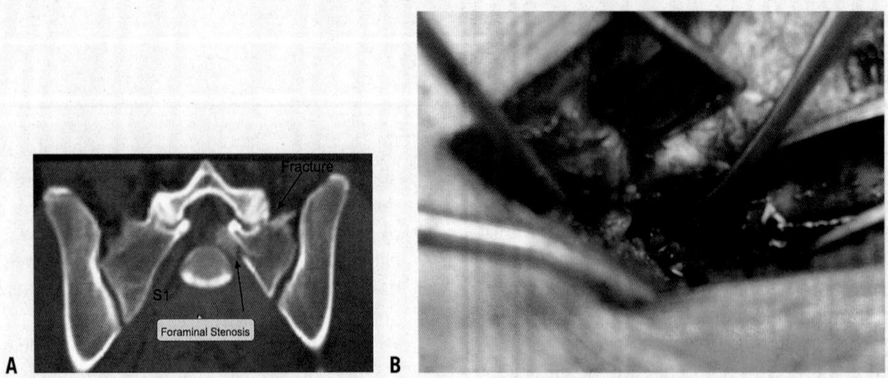

TECH FIG 7 **A.** Axial CT scan of a sacral fracture showing large intraforaminal bony fragment. **B.** Intraoperative photograph demonstrating decompression the sacral nerve root directly through the sacral fracture.

- Occasionally, a Kerrison and pituitary rongeur will be needed to remove some portion of the sacral lamina to find the nerve root, so these instruments should always be readily available.

Zone 3 Sacral Fractures

- Vertically oriented zone 3 sacral fractures are usually the result of wide APC forces and are associated with anterior ring disruption.
- Generally, they can be treated with internal rotation and anterior ring fixation alone.
- If residual sacral gapping persists, however, an SI screw with short threads can be placed into the contralateral S1 body to close the residual gap.

U-Shaped Sacral Fractures

- Otherwise known as *spinal–pelvic dissociation*, this fracture is essentially a sacral fracture-dislocation.
  - It tends to occur through the vestigial disc space and result in kyphosis.
  - These fractures can be easily missed on the standard AP pelvis radiograph and axial CT scans, making the sagittal CT reconstruction of paramount importance in diagnosing this injury (see **FIG 7A,B**).
- These injuries generally do not result in pelvic ring instability as the SI joints and distal surrounding sacrum are intact. They are more commonly associated with spinal instability.
- These injuries can be associated with cauda equina syndrome and significant spinal instability and should be treated by a surgeon experienced in treating injuries to the distal axial skeleton.
- Fractures with minimal kyphotic deformity, impaction, and no sacral canal compromise or neurologic deficit can be managed with percutaneous bilateral SI screw or transsacral screw fixation alone.
- Fractures with severe kyphosis and neurologic deficit require open reduction, decompression, and some form of bilateral posterior lumbopelvic fixation to restore the posterior tension band and control sagittal deformity **(TECH FIG 8)**.

A
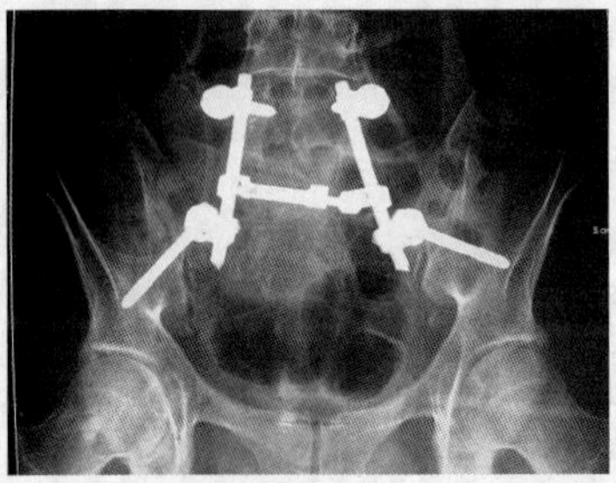
B
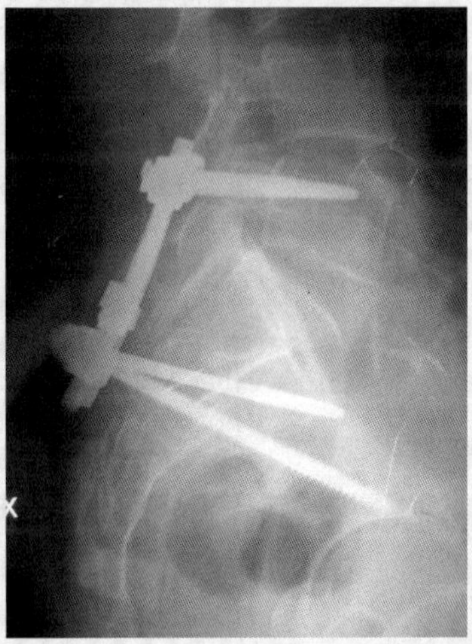

TECH FIG 8 A. AP radiograph showing a patient with a U-shaped sacral fracture with spinal–pelvic dissociation treated with a spinal pelvic construct to restore the posterior tension band and stabilize the fracture. **B.** Lateral radiograph showing a patient with a U-shaped sacral fracture with spinal–pelvic dissociation treated with a spinal pelvic construct to restore the posterior tension band and stabilize the fracture.

TECHNIQUES

Pearls and Pitfalls

Pitfall	Salvage or Bailout
Poor SI Screw Purchase	• Placement of a second SI screw into S2 • Ensure appropriate length into anterior aspect of sacral vertebral body and promontory. Alar purchase is poor secondary to low bone density here. • Placement of a transsacral SI screw into contralateral SI joint • Placement of transiliac plates
Fixation of Sacral Fracture with Residual Gap	• Use clamps and SI screw to close the fracture gap under fluoroscopic control, without overcompressing. • Do not use spinal pelvic fixation construct prior to manipulative reduction and placement of SI screw as it will lock down the fracture, preventing reduction and gap closure.
SI Screw Malpositioning	• If any symptoms or signs of radiculitis or radiculopathy exist, then postoperative CT scan and screw removal is indicated. If patient is asymptomatic from a misplaced screw, then observation is warranted. However, if symptoms develop at a later date, then the nerve root may scar or become adherent to the screw, making removal more difficult.

Sacral Dysmorphism	• Close scrutiny of the preoperative CT scan is important to plan out the safest trajectories and measure the diameter of the potential corridors. • Unilateral segmentation defects are also common. • Three-dimensional reconstructions are often helpful in diagnosing sacral dysmorphism and assessing the region of the sacral ala relative to the first sacral foramen.
Wound Dehiscence/ Infection	• These should be treated early and aggressively to avoid deep-seated pelvic abscesses and infections. • Prolonged drainage after 4–5 days (whether the patient is febrile or not and whether the white cell count is elevated or not) should be considered for a return to the operating room for open irrigation and débridement and drainage. Incisional negative pressure dressings may help to seal the wound, control drainage, and prevent wound dehiscence.

Patient wakes up with new neurologic deficit (iatrogenic nerve injury, most commonly L5).	• First, preoperatively, the patient should be informed of the risk of neurologic injury that can occur with reduction.
	• CT scan is ordered to assess for possible causes for nerve root injury:
	  • Malpositioned screw: remove
	  • Bone fragment (usually from sacral fracture): decompress, usually anteriorly on top of ala
	• However, postoperative CT scan may not disclose any offending etiology, in which case, observation and emotional support are indicated.

Inability to Reduce the SI Joint or Sacral Fracture	• First, ensure that adequate longitudinal traction is applied, as that is the key to reduction. • Do not use a standard fracture table with a perineal post as this will impede caudal translation of the hemipelvis.

POSTOPERATIVE CARE

- Provided that all other injuries permit, the patient is mobilized the first postoperative day.
  - The patient is instructed to be TDWB on the ipsilateral extremity for 10 to 12 weeks for SI dislocations and sacral alar fractures stabilized with SI screws.
  - Patients with spinal pelvic fixation can be allowed to full weight bear within 4 to 6 weeks.
  - All patients are given a regimen of pelvic, core trunk, hip, and knee range-of-motion exercises.
- Common early postoperative problems in patients with severe pelvic fractures include ileus and urinary retention, and these need to be addressed early.
  - The urinary catheter is usually not removed until the patient can mobilize well with physical therapy.
  - Diet is not advanced until flatus and normal bowel sounds have returned.
- Anticoagulation is administered in all patients for 6 weeks with low-molecular-weight heparin or Coumadin for deep venous thrombosis and pulmonary embolism prophylaxis.

OUTCOMES

- Outcome studies after fixation of pelvic fracture-dislocations are difficult to interpret because of poor follow-up, heterogeneity of the injury pattern, associated visceral and neurologic injury, and the lack of a reliable outcome measures for pelvic ring injuries.
- Improved short-term patient outcome with early stabilization and mobilization of the patient with a pelvic fracture as well as numerous reports citing improved outcome with anatomic reduction of the posterior ring continued to provide the impetus to develop more rigid and stable posterior fixation constructs.
- Earlier outcome studies support the position that the long-term functional results are improved if reduction with less than 1 cm of combined displacement of the posterior ring is obtained, especially with pure dislocations of the SI complex.
- Fractures of the posterior ring, as opposed to pure SI dislocations (ligamentous injuries), tend to display superior functional outcomes—presumably because of bony healing that restores preinjury strength and stability to the pelvic ring. Conversely, SI dislocations rely on ligamentous healing and scar formation—as a result, these patients tend to have worse functional outcomes in the short term and long term with pain and ambulation when compared to patients with other injury patterns.
- More recent detailed clinical outcome studies have shown that with current fixation techniques, a substantial proportion of patients continue to have poor outcomes with chronic posterior pelvic pain despite seemingly anatomic reductions and healing, with less than 50% returning to previous level of function and work status.
- This disparity in results is likely related to multiple confounding factors, such as
  - Poor financial and psychosocial and emotional status of trauma patients
  - The extensive soft tissue damage and associated long bone and extremity fractures
  - Associated neurologic, visceral, and urogenital injuries resulting in dyspareunia, sexual dysfunction, and incontinence
  - Prolonged recovery and rehabilitation time with loss of job, home, and family and dog.

COMPLICATIONS

- Blood loss and the need for transfusion are common with any open procedure on the posterior pelvic ring, particularly with open reduction of the SI joint and sacral fracture, where injury to the superior gluteal artery is always a danger.
- Wound infection occurs surprisingly infrequently given the medical condition of these patients, prolonged ICU and hospital admission, and associated soft tissue injury.
  - Infection and wound complications occur in approximately 3% of operative cases.

- Patients with internal degloving injuries (a Morel-Lavallée lesion), where the skin and subcutaneous fatty layer are sheared and separated from the underlying musculofascial layers, are particularly prone to severe wound complications with dehiscence, necrosis, and slough.
  - Patients identified as having an internal degloving lesion in the area of operative approach should first have drainage and débridement of the lesion, and the reduction and placement of fixation should be performed through an alternate approach.
- Similarly, patients who have undergone angioembolization during resuscitation for pelvic hemorrhage may be at higher risk for wound complications during extensive open posterior reconstructions—particularly if nonselective bilateral embolization techniques were used.
- Neurologic injury from manipulation of fracture fragments or placement of SI screws is a possibility.
  - Careful attention to the radiologic landmarks and clear appropriate imaging should allow the surgeon to avoid these iatrogenic complications, although even smooth gentle reductions of widely displaced fractures and dislocations can result in neurapraxic injury to the nerve roots and postoperative deficits.
    - Patients need to be informed of this risk preoperatively.
  - The risk of misplaced SI screws varies widely with surgeon and individual experience.
- Loss of reduction and failure of fixation can occur in very comminuted and unstable fracture-dislocations, particularly in patients with poor bone quality.
  - These situations should be recognized intraoperatively and the appropriate supplemental fixation (additional SI screws transsacral screws, transiliac plates, or spinal pelvic fixation constructs) should be applied.
- Nonunion of sacral fractures and SI dislocations is a rare occurrence and not reported specifically in the literature.
  - Rigidly stabilizing a sacral fracture with a residual gap predisposes to malunion and nonunion.
  - Some patients with SI dislocations continue to have chronic SI joint pain, requiring SI joint fusion.

REFERENCES

1. American College of Surgeons Committee on Trauma. Advanced Trauma Life Support for Doctors, ed 7. Chicago: American College of Surgeons Committee on Trauma, 2004.
2. Bruce B, Reilly M, Sims S. OTA highlight paper predicting future displacement of nonoperatively managed lateral compression sacral fractures: can it be done? J Orthop Trauma 2011;25(9):523–527.
3. Carlson DA, Scheid DK, Maar DC, et al. Safe placement of S1 and S2 iliosacral screws: the "vestibule" concept. J Orthop Trauma 2000;14(4):264–269.
4. Collinge C, Coons D, Aschenbrenner J. Risks to the superior gluteal neurovascular bundle during percutaneous iliosacral screw insertion: an anatomical cadaver study. J Orthop Trauma 2005;19(2):96–101.
5. Dalal SA, Burgess AR, Siegel JH, et al. Pelvic fracture in multiple trauma: classification by mechanism is key to pattern of organ injury, resuscitative requirements, and outcome. J Trauma 1989;29(7): 981–1002.
6. Day CS, Prayson MJ, Shuler TE, et al. Transsacral versus modified pelvic landmarks for percutaneous iliosacral screw placement—a computed tomographic analysis and cadaveric study. Am J Orthop (Belle Mead NJ) 2000;29(9 suppl):16–21.
7. Demetriades D, Karaiskakis M, Toutouzas K, et al. Pelvic fractures: epidemiology and predictors of associated abdominal injuries and outcomes. J Am Coll Surg 2002;195(1):1–10.
8. Ertel W, Keel M, Eid K, et al. Control of severe hemorrhage using C-clamp and pelvic packing in multiply injured patients with pelvic ring disruption. J Orthop Trauma 2001;15(7):468–474.
9. Flancbaum L, Morgan AS, Fleisher M, et al. Blunt bladder trauma: manifestation of severe injury. Urology 1988;31(3):220–222.
10. Gänsslen A, Giannoudis P, Pape HC. Hemorrhage in pelvic fracture: who needs angiography? Curr Opin Crit Care 2003;9(6):515–523.
11. Gorczyca JT, Varga E, Woodside T, et al. The strength of iliosacral lag screws and transiliac bars in the fixation of vertically unstable pelvic injuries with sacral fractures. Injury 1996;27(8):561–564.
12. Griffin DR, Starr AJ, Reinert CM, et al. Vertically unstable pelvic fractures fixed with percutaneous iliosacral screws: does posterior injury pattern predict fixation failure? J Orthop Trauma 2003;17(6):399–405.
13. Hearn T, Tile M. The effects of ligament sectioning and internal fixation of bending stiffness of the pelvic ring. In: Proceedings of the 13th International Conference on Biomechanics; December 9 13, 1991; Perth, Australia.
14. Käch K, Trentz O. Distraction spondylodesis of the sacrum in "vertical shear lesions" of the pelvis. Unfallchirurg 1994;97(1):28–38.
15. Keating JF, Werier J, Blachut P, et al. Early fixation of the vertically unstable pelvis: the role of iliosacral screw fixation of the posterior lesion. J Orthop Trauma 1999;13(2):107–113.
16. Kellam JF. The role of external fixation in pelvic disruptions. Clin Orthop Relat Res 1989;(241):66–82.
17. Moed BR, Karges DE. Techniques for reduction and fixation of pelvic ring disruptions through the posterior approach. Clin Orthop Relat Res 1996;(329):102–114.
18. Pohlemann T. Pelvic emergency clamps: anatomic landmarks for a safe primary application. J Orthop Trauma 2004;18(2):102–105.
19. Raffa J, Christensen NM. Compound fractures of the pelvis. Am J Surg 1976;132(2):282–286.
20. Richardson JD, Harty J, Amin M, et al. Open pelvic fractures. J Trauma 1982;22(7):533–538.
21. Rothenberger D, Velasco R, Strate F, et al. Open pelvic fracture: a lethal injury. J Trauma 1978;8(3):184–187.
22. Routt ML Jr, Simonian PT, Agnew SG, et al. Radiographic recognition of the sacral alar slope for optimal placement of iliosacral screws: a cadaveric and clinical study. J Orthop Trauma 1996;10(3):171–177.
23. Routt ML Jr, Simonian PT, Mills WJ. Iliosacral screw fixation: early complications of the percutaneous technique. J Orthop Trauma 1997;11(8):584–589.
24. Sagi HC, Coniglione FM, Stanford JH. Examination under anesthetic for occult pelvic ring instability. J Orthop Trauma 2011;25(9):529–536.
25. Schildhauer TA, Josten C, Muhr G. Triangular osteosynthesis of vertically unstable sacrum fractures: a new concept allowing early weight-bearing. J Orthop Trauma 1998;12(5):307–314.
26. Schildhauer TA, Ledoux WR, Chapman JR, et al. Triangular osteosynthesis and iliosacral screw fixation for unstable sacral fractures: a cadaveric and biomechanical evaluation under cyclic loads. J Orthop Trauma 2003;17(1):22–31.
27. Simonian PT, Routt ML Jr. Biomechanics of pelvic fixation. Orthop Clin North Am 1997;28(3):351–367.
28. Simonain PT, Routt ML Jr, Harrington RM, et al. Internal fixation for the transforaminal sacral fracture. Clin Orthop Relat Res 1996;(323):202–209.
29. Steele N, Dodenhoff RM, Ward AJ, et al. Thromboprophylaxis in pelvic and acetabular trauma surgery. The role of early treatment with low-molecular-weight heparin. J Bone Joint Surg Br 2005;87(2):209–212.
30. Stocks GW, Gabel GT, Noble PC, et al. Anterior and posterior internal fixation of vertical shear fractures of the pelvis. J Orthop Res 1991;9(2):237–245.
31. Templeman D, Schmidt A, Freese J, et al. Proximity of iliosacral screws to neurovascular structures after internal fixation. Clin Orthop Relat Res 1996;(329):194–198.
32. Vrahas M, Hearn TC, Diangelo D, et al. Ligamentous contributions to pelvic stability. Orthopedics 1995;18(3):271–274.
33. Whiting PS, Auston D, Avilucea FR, et al. Negative stress examination under anesthesia reliably predicts pelvic ring union without displacement. J Orthop Trauma 2017;31(4):189–193.
34. Xu R, Ebraheim NA, Robke J, et al. Radiologic evaluation of iliosacral screw placement. Spine (Phila Pa 1976) 1996;21(5):582–588.

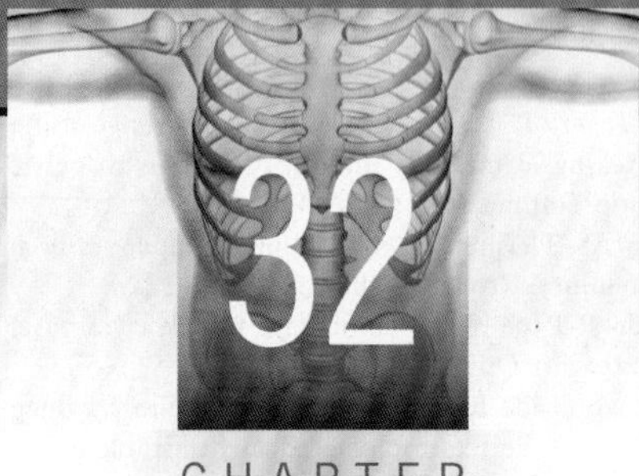

CHAPTER 32

Open Reduction and Internal Fixation of the Posterior Wall of the Acetabulum

Jodi Siegel and David C. Templeman

DEFINITION

- A posterior wall fracture is one of the elementary fracture types as described by Letournel and Judet.[6] It is a fracture of the posterior rim of the socket portion of the ball-and-socket joint of the hip (**FIG 1**).
- The disruption separates a segment of articular surface that involves varying amounts of the bony posterior wall of the acetabulum. It can exist as one single fragment or as several comminuted pieces.
- The wall fracture can exist alone or as part of an associated acetabular fracture.
- By definition, the posterior column, and therefore the ilioischial line, remains intact despite varying amounts of retroacetabular surface disruption.

ANATOMY

- The hip is a constrained ball-and-socket joint composed of the femoral head as the ball and the acetabulum as the socket.
- The capsule surrounding the joint extends from the bony acetabular rim to the intertrochanteric line anteriorly and to the femoral neck posteriorly. It is thickened in specific areas, creating ligaments.
  - Anteriorly, the iliofemoral Y ligament exists as two bands. The inferior capsule is supported by the pubofemoral ligament, and the posterior capsule is strengthened by the ischiofemoral ligament.
- The acetabular labrum is a fibrocartilaginous structure attached to the bony rim, deepening the socket and making

A B C

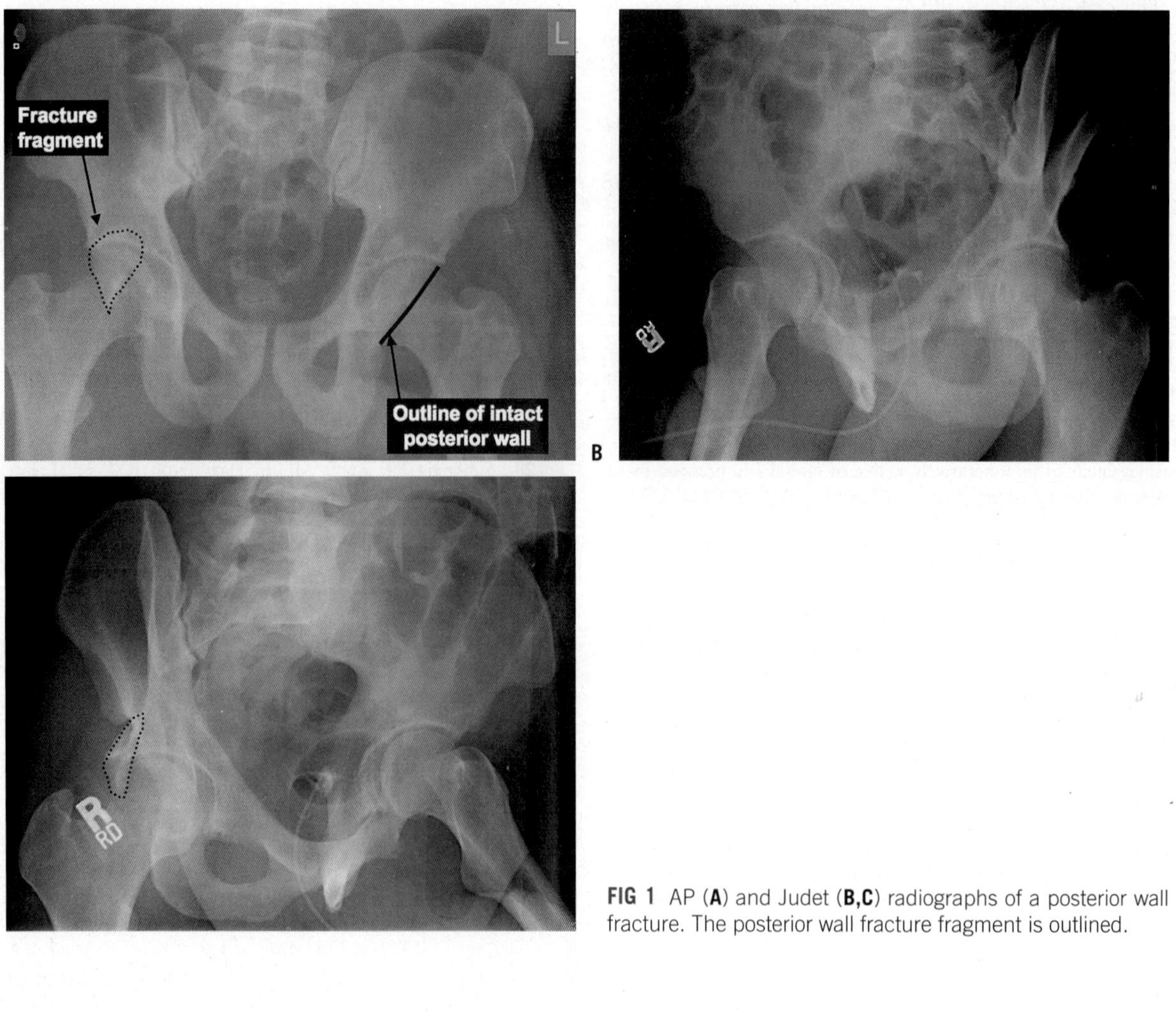

FIG 1 AP (**A**) and Judet (**B,C**) radiographs of a posterior wall fracture. The posterior wall fracture fragment is outlined.

the joint more stable. It adds an additional 10% of coverage to the femoral head.

- The acetabulum is composed of two columns, two walls, and the roof within the pelvis. The anterior and posterior columns form an inverted Y and are attached to the sacrum via the sacral buttress. The articular surface of the joint sits on the anterior and posterior walls and the roof, which is located within the arms of the Y.
  - The anatomic roof is located between the anterior inferior iliac spine and the ilioischial notch of the acetabular margin.[6]
    - The weight-bearing dome, as determined by 45-degree roof arc measurements on anteroposterior and Judet radiographs, is the most important articular portion of the acetabulum. This functional aspect of the acetabulum includes the excursions of all resultant force vectors during normal daily activities.[9]
  - Two additional segments should also be considered separately.
    - The posterosuperior segment is the bridge between the roof and the posterior wall.
    - The posteroinferior segment is the lower part of the posterior wall and the posterior horn of the cartilage.[6]
- Due to the large area of muscular attachments, the blood supply to the acetabulum is vast.[6] Small arteries start peripherally and flow centrally, parallel to each other.
  - The largest nutrient foramina on the internal aspect of the ilium is reliably located 1 cm lateral to the sacroiliac joint and 1 cm above the iliopectineal line. It is fed by a branch of the iliolumbar artery.
  - A branch of the superior gluteal artery feeds the largest nutrient foramina on the external surface in the center of the iliac wing, just anterior to the anterior gluteal line.
  - The obturator artery supplies foramina in front of the sciatic notch just below the iliopectineal line and in the roof of the obturator canal. The body of the pubis is also supplied by the obturator artery. A branch of this artery, the acetabular branch, feeds the cotyloid fossa via a number of small perforators.
  - A complete vascular circle supplies multiple nutrient vessels around the periphery of the acetabulum. The artery of the roof of the acetabulum (from the superior gluteal artery), the obturator artery, and the inferior gluteal artery are main contributors.
  - The iliac crest, from the anterior inferior iliac spine posteriorly to the auricular articular surface of the sacroiliac joint, is supplied by branches of the external anterior iliac artery, branches of the fourth lumbar artery, and branches of the iliolumbar artery.
  - The sciatic buttress receives its blood supply from multiple branches of the superior gluteal artery.

PATHOGENESIS

- Acetabular fractures occur when a force is transmitted from the femur, through the femoral head, to the acetabulum. The specific pattern of the fracture is determined by the position of the hip at the time of injury and the magnitude of the force of the trauma.
  - A common mechanism of injury of posterior wall fractures and fracture-dislocations is a motor vehicle crash in which the unrestrained patient is sitting with a flexed knee and the knee strikes the dashboard, creating an axial load along the length of the femur, loading the posterior aspect of the acetabulum.
- Posterior wall fractures of the acetabulum occur when the hip is flexed to 90 degrees and is in neutral coronal and axial plane orientation. In this position, when an axial load is applied to the femur, the posterior articular surface of the joint is stressed. The amount of comminution, displacement, and articular impaction will depend on the quality of the bone and the magnitude of the force.
  - A typical posterior wall fracture is completely below the roof of the acetabulum.
  - With less hip flexion and a force applied along the axis of the femoral shaft, a superior posterior wall variant will result, which includes part of the adjacent roof.
  - A posterior inferior fracture includes the inferior horn of the articular surface, the subcotyloid groove, and often the superior ischium.
  - Extended fractures, massive posterior wall fractures, and transitional forms are mentioned for completeness but are outside the scope of this chapter.
- A variation of a posterior wall fracture is a fracture-dislocation, which involves single or multifragmented pieces of the posterior wall separated by the dislocating femoral head. This pattern is often associated with impaction of the articular surface of either the head or the wall (**FIG 2**).
  - With a posterior wall fracture or fracture-dislocation, one of two possibilities exists for the capsule.
    - The capsule can rupture and allow the head to dislocate. In this scenario, varying sizes of wall fragments and labral injury can exist.
    - Alternatively, the capsule can remain intact to the wall fragment and to the femur, with all of the displacement (or even the dislocation) occurring through the fracture site.
    - The size of the posterior wall fragment and the integrity of the capsule and the labrum play a role in hip stability. Despite attempts to quantitate fragment size to define operative indications,[2,5,7,16] stress examination remains the only method to predict instability.[15]

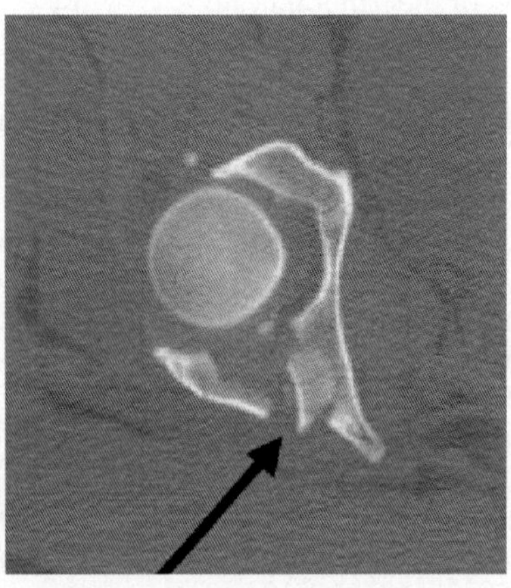

FIG 2 Axial CT cut showing impaction. The impacted fragment (*arrow*) is rotated with the articular cartilage now facing laterally.

- When the capsule remains intact and the head dislocates, the fracture edges often fragment. This creates osteochondral fragments, which can lead to impaction or incarceration of the pieces upon reduction of the femoral head.

NATURAL HISTORY

- The goal of the treatment of acetabular fractures is to achieve a stable, congruent hip joint with an anatomically reduced articular surface. Anatomic reduction and stabilization will decrease the incidence of posttraumatic arthritis.[8]
- Although fractures of the posterior wall are common, representing 24% of Letournel and Judet[6] initial series, they are frequently reported as having poor results, with 10% to 30% of patients developing posttraumatic arthritis within 1 year.
- Nonoperative treatment is unsuccessful, and Epstein[3] has documented that 88% of patients treated with closed reduction alone had unsatisfactory long-term results.
  - Roof arc and subchondral arc measurements do not apply to typical posterior wall fractures; however, the size of the posterior wall fragment may play a role.
  - Multiple authors have attempted to define the size of the fragment that will predict instability.
    - In cadaveric studies, fragments that include greater than 50% of the wall were always unstable, whereas those less than 20% were stable.[5,16]
    - A clinical study revealed that acetabuli with less than 34% of the posterior wall intact were unstable, and those with greater than 55% intact were stable.[2]
- Dynamic stress examination that uses fluoroscopy to assist with the detection of subtle subluxation can define a stable or unstable joint without depending on fragment size measurements.[15]

PATIENT HISTORY AND PHYSICAL FINDINGS

- Acetabular fractures are often the result of high-energy trauma; therefore, other associated injuries must be sought.
- Hemorrhage and hemodynamic instability are rarely associated with isolated fractures of the posterior wall; however, the superior gluteal artery and vein may be lacerated when fractures extend to the greater sciatic notch.
- Patients will frequently present with hip or groin pain and a shortened lower extremity due to the posterior, superior dislocation of the femoral head.
- Soft tissue injuries around the pelvis are uncommon because the mechanism of injury is indirect. Nonetheless, the skin overlying the hip and pelvis of any pelvic or acetabular fracture should be carefully evaluated for any subcutaneous fluctuance, ecchymosis, or cutaneous anesthesia.
  - The Morel-Lavallée lesion, a subcutaneous degloving injury, although a closed injury, is culture positive in up to 40% of cases.[4] Initial débridement of these lesions as well as a delay in internal fixation is recommended by some authors.
- Soft tissue injuries at the knee are more common and often missed. Ligamentous or chondral injuries are often discovered on secondary survey, but only if they are considered and a careful and thorough examination is performed.
- The incidence of damage to the femoral head is unknown as the head is not routinely dislocated during fixation of the acetabular fracture for complete evaluation. However, it is not surprising when associated femoral head fractures or chondral lesions are noted as the large amount of force needed to cause the acetabular fracture is transmitted via the femoral head.
- Careful neurologic examination at the time of injury reveals deficits in up to 30% of cases. The peroneal division of the sciatic nerve is the most commonly seen nerve injury, especially when the femoral head is dislocated posteriorly.
- Other ipsilateral extremity injuries often discovered include fractures of the femur, tibia, and foot.

IMAGING AND OTHER DIAGNOSTIC STUDIES

- The diagnosis and classification of an acetabular fracture is made from the initial trauma AP radiograph.
  - Two 45-degree oblique radiographs (Judet views) must be obtained also to aid in classification and treatment planning.
  - Completing the five views of the pelvis series with pelvic inlet and outlet views allows potential injuries to the pelvic ring to be evaluated.
- A computed tomography (CT) scan of the pelvis will assist in defining displacement, intra-articular fragments, marginal articular impaction, and associated femoral head injuries.
  - The size of the posterior wall fragment can also be determined more accurately using a CT scan, which is optimally obtained after the initial reduction.
  - The size and number of incarcerated fragments can be more precisely determined with a CT scan. Preoperative planning allows determination of the size and number of free fragments that must be removed from the joint as well as the location of any impaction that must be elevated.

DIFFERENTIAL DIAGNOSIS

- Posterior hip dislocation
- Associated acetabular fracture
  - Associated transverse and posterior wall fracture
  - Associated posterior column and posterior wall fracture
  - Associated T-shaped fracture
  - Associated both-column fracture
- Pelvic fracture
- Femoral head fracture
- Proximal femur fracture

NONOPERATIVE MANAGEMENT

- Nondisplaced, stable fractures with a congruent joint can be treated with protected, foot-flat weight-bearing restrictions if no instability is evident on fluoroscopic-assisted stress examination.[15]
- Posterior wall fractures that present dislocated should be considered a surgical emergency.
  - A prompt closed reduction with satisfactory general anesthesia is recommended.
  - The surgeon should check the femoral neck before reduction.
  - Once reduced, the joint should be evaluated fluoroscopically in both the AP and obturator oblique views for stability: The joint should be axially loaded with the hip in flexion and in flexion plus adduction.[15] Only if the joint is stable (nonsubluxated) is nonoperative management sufficient.

SURGICAL MANAGEMENT

- Surgical management of acetabular fractures is technically demanding. The goal of surgery is to obtain an anatomic reduction of the joint surface and to create a congruent and stable hip joint while avoiding complications.
- Other factors that play a role in surgical management include surgeon experience and the timing of operative intervention.
  - Letournel and Judet[6] described their learning curve in 4-year intervals.
  - They also reported reduced ability to achieve anatomic reduction when fractures are operated on more than 21 days after injury.
- Unlike most conditions in orthopaedic surgery, all displaced fractures of the acetabulum, which include marginal impaction, are indicated for surgery unless specific criteria for nonoperative management are met.[14] These include the following:
  - A congruent hip joint on AP and Judet radiographs and on CT scan
  - An intact weight-bearing surface, as defined by roof arc measurements and subchondral arc measurements on CT scan
    - At least 50% of the posterior wall intact on CT scan
  - A stable joint, including on a dynamic stress examination
  - Patient factors must also be considered.
    - Age, bone quality, comorbidities, preinjury functional status, type of employment, and personal expectations all must factor into the decision-making process.

Preoperative Planning

- Open reduction and internal fixation of a posterior wall fracture is based on evaluation of the AP pelvic and Judet view radiographs and the CT scan.
- The surgeon should closely evaluate the films for a transverse component, which may be overlooked on initial viewing.
- The identification of marginal impaction necessitates elevating the articular cartilage and packing behind it with some form of bone graft or bone void filler to reconstruct the joint surface successfully (see **FIG 2**).
- Careful review of the CT scan will allow identification and quantification of the number of intra-articular fragments that exist to ensure that all foreign bodies are removed from the joint upon exploration.

Positioning

- Most acetabular surgeons position the patient prone on a fracture table **(FIG 3)**.
  - The affected side is suspended using a distal femoral traction pin.
  - The peroneal post must be appropriately padded to prevent pudendal nerve palsy.
  - The affected leg is placed in traction, with the hip in extension and the knee flexed to at least 80 degrees; the foot is well padded and secured in a fracture table boot in the resting position. Sequential compression devices are applied to both lower extremities.
  - Traction is positioned to pull in line, neutral abduction–adduction, neutral internal and external rotation, with the table's arm holding the foot free enough to allow internal and external rotation intraoperatively.

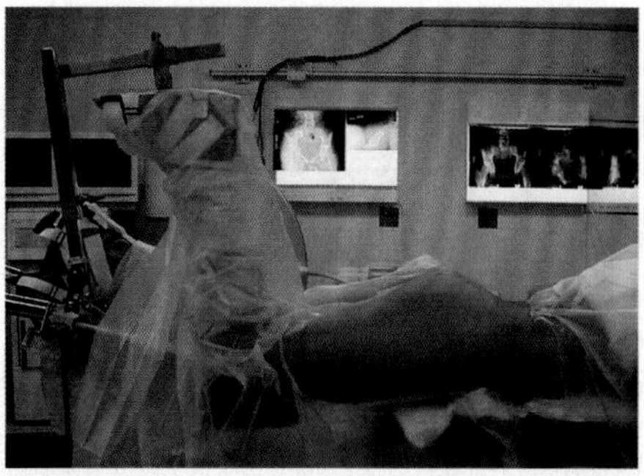

FIG 3 Prone positioning on a fracture table with the affected leg in distal femoral skeletal traction, the hip extended, and the knee flexed to at least 80 degrees. Sequential compression devices are in place on both lower extremities.

  - The contralateral leg is in extension in a fracture table boot with the foot well padded and in neutral position.
  - Pads are placed to support both thighs.
  - Chest pads are positioned to allow adequate room for the abdomen and breasts and for chest excursion.
  - Arms are abducted to 90 degrees at the shoulders and 90 degrees at the elbows.
- Once positioning is completed, posteroanterior and oblique views are obtained with the C-arm before draping or preparation to ensure that the hip is reduced and that the necessary images can be obtained.
  - The obturator oblique view can be obtained by rotating the C-arm 45 degrees toward a lateral view.
  - Pushing upward on the anterior superior iliac spine can assist with the last 15 degrees of rotation to obtain an iliac oblique view, an image that most C-arms cannot otherwise obtain.
- In certain circumstances, such as presence of a free fragment in the joint that may be difficult to access, lateral positioning may be necessary.
  - The patient is turned lateral on a radiolucent table with appropriate padding, including an axillary roll and protection of the peroneal nerve at the fibular head on the down leg.
  - The authors prefer a beanbag with a large gel pad, although Stulberg hip positioners or a peg board are also adequate if limited concerns for a lengthy procedure.
  - The affected extremity is draped free, so the leg can be moved intraoperatively to allow for subluxation or redislocation of the femoral head through the fracture as needed to access the fragment.
- Care must be taken throughout the procedure to ensure knee flexion and hip extension to decrease risk to the sciatic nerve.
- Once positioning is complete and prior to draping, C-arm images are obtained to ensure adequate radiograph visualization is obtainable.

Approach

- The posterior wall of the acetabulum is accessed via the Kocher-Langenbeck approach.

KOCHER-LANGENBECK APPROACH

Incision and Dissection

- The incision is based on two limbs **(TECH FIG 1A)**.
  - One starts at the posterior tip of the greater trochanter and extends distally along the posterior aspect of the femoral shaft, distal to the trochanter and the gluteal crease, which serves as an external landmark for the gluteus maximus tendon.
  - The proximal limb extends about 45 degrees toward a spot 1 cm cephalad to the posterior superior iliac spine. The length of this limb depends on the amount of posterior column that must be accessed.
- The skin and subcutaneous tissue are divided down to the fascia lata and the gluteal aponeurotic fascia.
- Once identified, the tensor fascia lata and iliotibial band are sharply divided longitudinally in line with the underlying femoral shaft **(TECH FIG 1B)**.
  - To open the proximal limb, the surgeon sharply divides the gluteal aponeurosis and then gently splits the gluteus maximus muscle via finger dissection.
  - The surgeon must watch for crossing vessels and cauterize them before they are torn.
  - The nerves that innervate the proximal third of the gluteus maximus will cross in this area, about halfway between the greater trochanter and the posterior superior iliac spine. The surgeon should stop splitting at the first nerve trunk to prevent postoperative palsy.
- The Charnley retractor is helpful for holding the fascia away from the operative field. The surgeon must take care not to insert too deeply to prevent iatrogenic injury to the sciatic nerve.
- The bursa over the trochanter is often hemorrhagic from the injury and can be resected at this time if it is large and hindering visualization **(TECH FIG 1C)**.

Protecting the Sciatic Nerve

- The sciatic nerve is identified. This can be difficult owing to the conditions of the traumatized tissues; often, it will be easiest to identify the nerve in an area of healthy tissue, such as at the level of the quadratus femoris.
- If overall visualization is inadequate at this point, the gluteus maximus tendon can be divided at its insertion on the femur. A cuff of tissue is left on the femur, so an adequate repair can later be performed.
- With the posterior aspect of the gluteus medius tendon retracted anteriorly, the piriformis tendon can be identified **(TECH FIG 2A)**.
  - It can be helpful to internally rotate the leg to put the short external rotators and the piriformis on stretch to assist with identification.
  - In some cases, the short external rotators have been avulsed by the dislocation.
  - It is easier to palpate the edges of the piriformis tendon with a finger and then pass a finger behind the tendon to better isolate it.
  - The surgeon confirms that the correct muscle has been identified by following its path backward and toward the greater sciatic notch.
  - Once isolated, the tendon is tagged and divided at its attachment to the femur **(TECH FIG 2B)**. This tag suture is used to retract the muscle posteriorly **(TECH FIG 2C)**.
- With the piriformis retracted, the sciatic nerve should now be easily visible, lying over the short external rotators. The surgeon visually examines the sciatic nerve for any contusion or laceration.
- Next, the surgeon identifies the tendon composed of the superior and inferior gemelli and the obturator internus.
  - Another tag suture is passed through this tendon, and it is released from the femur.
  - Because the piriformis lies superficial to the sciatic nerve, it will not retract or protect the nerve.

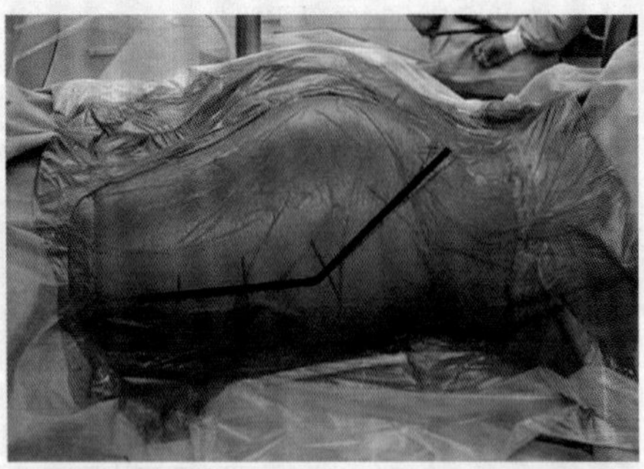

A

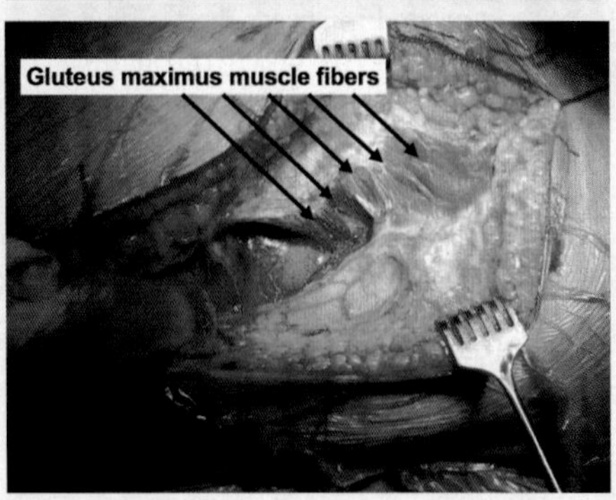

B

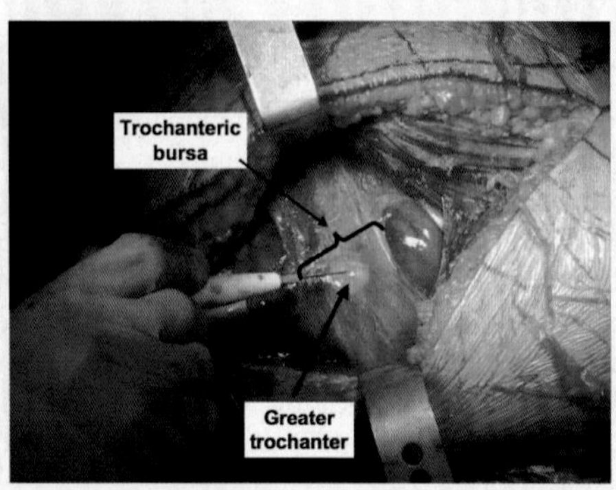

C

TECH FIG 1 **A.** Kocher-Langenbeck incision. **B.** The surgeon divides the fascia and then splits the gluteus maximus muscle. **C.** With the Charnley retractor in place, the surgeon excises the bursa if it obstructs visualization.

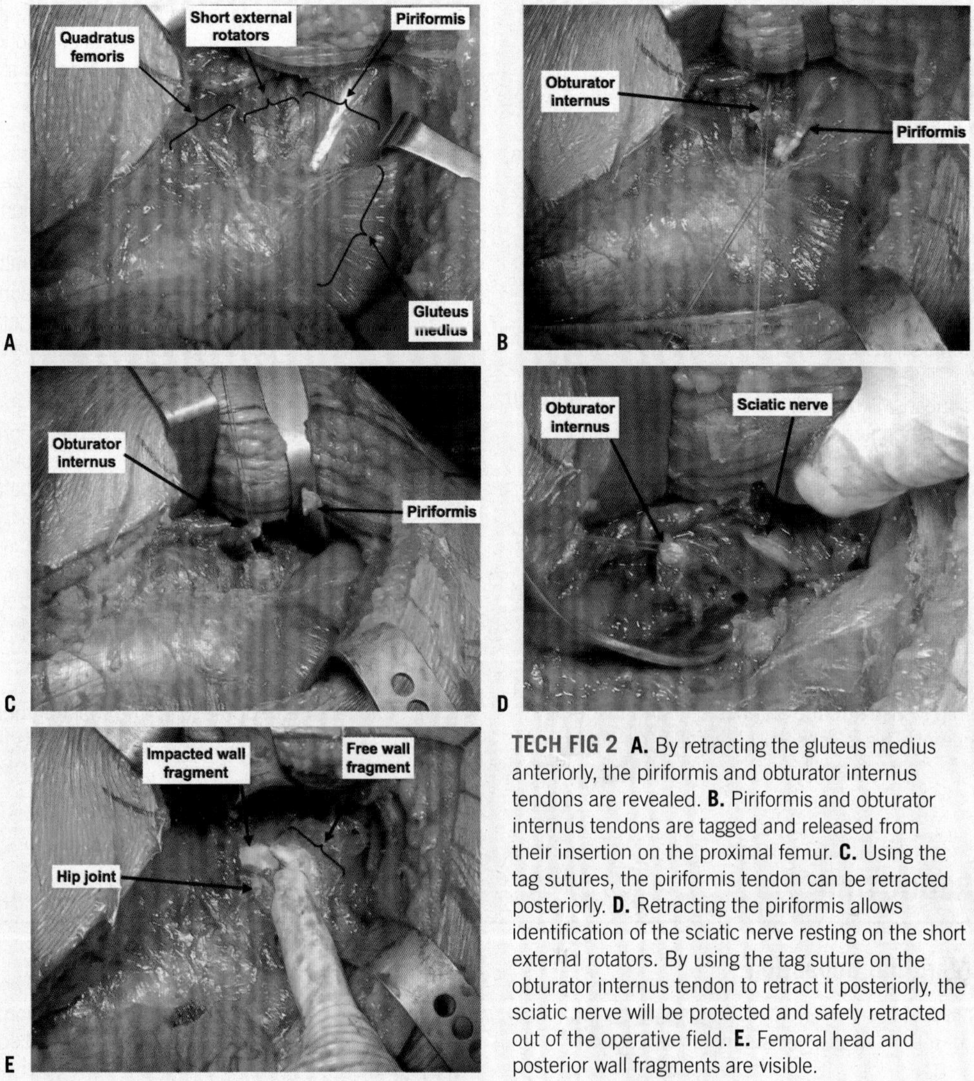

TECH FIG 2 **A.** By retracting the gluteus medius anteriorly, the piriformis and obturator internus tendons are revealed. **B.** Piriformis and obturator internus tendons are tagged and released from their insertion on the proximal femur. **C.** Using the tag sutures, the piriformis tendon can be retracted posteriorly. **D.** Retracting the piriformis allows identification of the sciatic nerve resting on the short external rotators. By using the tag suture on the obturator internus tendon to retract it posteriorly, the sciatic nerve will be protected and safely retracted out of the operative field. **E.** Femoral head and posterior wall fragments are visible.

- In contrast, the gemelli and the obturator internus can be used to effectively protect and retract the sciatic nerve posteriorly **(TECH FIG 2D)**.
- By pulling upward on this tag stitch–tendon, the surgeon can pass a finger into both the greater and lesser sciatic notches, beneath the muscle, and therefore the nerve, making a path.
  - A sciatic nerve retractor can then be placed along this path, into either notch. (Care should be exercised if a retractor must be placed into the greater sciatic notch due to the presence of the superior gluteal neurovascular bundle.)
  - By continuously checking that the external rotators are above the retractor, the surgeon can ensure that the sciatic nerve is protected. In addition to protecting the nerve, this helps to retract the soft tissues and provides excellent visualization of the retroacetabular surface.
- The posterior hip capsule, the fracture line, and the posterior wall fragment are now within the surgical field **(TECH FIG 2E)**.

FRACTURE SITE EXPOSURE AND DÉBRIDEMENT

- With the retroacetabular surface now exposed, the fracture site and the joint must be débrided and prepared.
  - By removing any residual hematoma from the field, the posterior wall fragment and the posterior column will become easily visible.
- The posterior column is inspected carefully for any nondisplaced transverse fracture line. It is better to recognize this early than to displace it later.

- The surgeon "books open" the fracture site by flipping the wall piece out into the wound.
  - The posterior wall piece will typically remain attached by the capsule and some periosteum. The surgeon strips away from the wall any periosteum that may be preventing its mobilization, taking care not to injure the labral attachments. The surgeon must be sure to peel all the periosteum off the fracture edges. Direct visualization of interdigitation at the fracture site is vital in judging anatomic reduction, and the rate of nonunion is low after reduction and fixation of acetabular fractures.[8]
  - It is often necessary to sharply dissect the overlying gluteus minimus muscle from the posterior wall to allow mobilization.
  - The femoral head will be easily visualized once the wall is mobilized, and the interior of the hip joint is inspected.
  - Any damage to the femoral head is noted.
  - Intra-articular fragments can be removed, and the joint can be irrigated to remove any other debris.
  - With the fracture table used to pull traction, the joint can be distracted, which will assist with joint débridement. If the fracture table allows such movement, the hip can be flexed to assist with fragment removal.
    - If there is concern that a fragment remains in the joint, a 70-degree arthroscope can be used while distracting the hip to visualize the anterior joint and to identify the fragment. This is especially helpful if you are in the prone position and on a table without hip flexion capabilities. Useful instruments to reach around the head to secure a fragment include a curved Kocher and a Cooley vascular clamp.
    - Alternatively, if in the lateral position, a formal surgical dislocation with a trochanteric osteotomy can be performed (see Chap. 33). This will allow easy access to any fragments in the joint and evaluation of the entire articular surface directly.
- The intact segment must be prepared in a similar fashion.
  - The surgeon strips any additional periosteum and soft tissue that remains attached to the intact retroacetabular surface at the fracture edge. Again, this area will later be inspected for fracture line interdigitation.
  - Any soft tissue is elevated from the top of the ischium. This will prepare the ischium to receive the reconstruction plate.
  - The soft tissues superolateral to the acetabulum, on the outer table of the ilium, must be elevated in preparation to receive the proximal aspect of the plate. In this area, it is often necessary to elevate the overlying gluteus minimus muscle.
    - It is safe to pass an elevator under the abductor muscles, staying on bone, down toward the iliac crest at the level of the anterior superior iliac spine. A spiked Hohmann retractor inserted in this path can also assist with retraction and visualization.
- With the fracture bed, the joint, the wall fragment, and the intact segment débrided, fracture reduction is the next step.

FRACTURE REDUCTION

Reduction of Marginal Impaction

- Careful dissection of the posterior wall fragments and the intact portion of the pelvis are necessary for an accurate reduction.
- Preoperative review of all the radiographic images will normally identify any marginal impaction, which must be reduced.
- When the femoral head is sitting in the acetabulum, the areas of impaction can be reduced to the head.
- An osteotome is placed deep to the depressed subchondral bone. Gentle malleting allows the osteotome beneath the impacted bone. By manipulating the bone and its overlying cartilage, the articular surface is reduced to the femoral head with its intact cartilage.
- Once reduced, there will be an empty space deep to the subchondral bone where the osteotome entered and the original bone collapsed. This area is packed with an osteoconductive bone void filler that can provide structure and prevent recollapse. Options include autogenous cancellous bone, allograft cancellous bone chips, and calcium sulfate bone graft substitute.
  - As in other areas of the body, overreduction is better than underreduction, as often there is settling.
- Once the fracture bed has been meticulously débrided of fracture hematoma and soft tissue, interdigitation of the posterior wall to the remaining intact retroacetabular surface can be visualized.

Reducing the Posterior Wall Fragment

- With the marginal impaction reduced, attention is turned to reducing the posterior wall fragment into its bed in the intact acetabulum.
- The wall fragment is flipped into its bed.
  - Using a ball spike pusher, the surgeon gently manipulates the piece until a smooth, convex retroacetabular surface with no external step-offs is obtained. If this cannot be produced, the wall piece is flipped out of its bed again, and the surgeon looks for a cause of the malreduction. If the fragment does not reduce perfectly at the retroacetabular surface, it will not be reduced perfectly at the joint.
  - Once reinspection is complete, the wall is reintroduced to its bed. The piece is manipulated into place. Gentle persuasion with a mallet can help the fragment find its home, especially if marginal impaction reduction required grafting.
  - Provisional fixation is placed next. This can hold the fragment in place while the surgeon evaluates the reduction and places the definitive internal fixation.
- If multiple wall fragments exist, careful planning of the order of reduction is vital. Often, certain pieces must be reduced first, as the cortical shell of other fragments may need to rest outside of the cancellous bone attached to its neighboring fragment. Without attention to this detail, an anatomic reduction may be impossible.
  - Provisionally holding a multifragmented posterior wall can be difficult. Multiple Kirschner wires or spring plates may be needed. Sometimes, only the definitive fixation can be used.

INTERNAL FIXATION

Provisional Fixation

- Once the posterior wall pieces are reduced, provisional fixation to hold the fragment in place can make the overall procedure easier.
- Options for provisional fixation include either interfragmentary lag screws (2.7 or 3.5 mm) or Kirschner wires.
- By using a ball spike pusher, the fracture fragment is stabilized within its bed, and a Kirschner wire or a lag screw can be placed to hold the reduction.
  - We prefer to use 2.7-mm lag screws. With these screws, the heads sit flush with the bony cortex and do not interfere with the subsequent placement of the definitive fixation.
  - An alternative to a lag screw is the use of one or multiple Kirschner wires. If Kirschner wires are used, the reconstruction plate can be placed around the wires without difficulty, and subsequent removal is easy.
- Occasionally, when the posterior wall piece is small or comminuted, lag screws and Kirschner wires may not be possible. A spring plate can be used (similar to when preventing medial wall "kick-up").
  - The end hole of a one-third tubular plate is cut into a V, creating tines. The plate is bent, so the tines can effect a reduction. This plate can be used as provisional fixation to hold a small wall fragment in place or as a spring plate to prevent the medial aspect of a large wall fragment from kicking up.
  - The tines and a portion of the plate are placed over the wall fragment. The fracture edge is spanned with the remaining plate. Either of the remaining holes of the plate can be used for screw placement, depending on the size of the wall being stabilized.
  - The plate is positioned, so it is possible to drill outside of the joint. Once secured, this spring plate will prevent the wall piece (if small) or the medial fracture edge (if the wall piece is large) from kicking up or displacing.

Reconstruction Plate Stabilization

- Now that the wall piece is reduced, it is definitively stabilized with a 3.5-mm pelvic reconstruction plate **(TECH FIG 3)**.
- Most commonly, a slightly underbent, contoured eight-hole plate is used. It is fashioned to sit at the edge of the posterior wall, from the top of the ischial tuberosity to the bone posterior to the anterior inferior iliac spine.

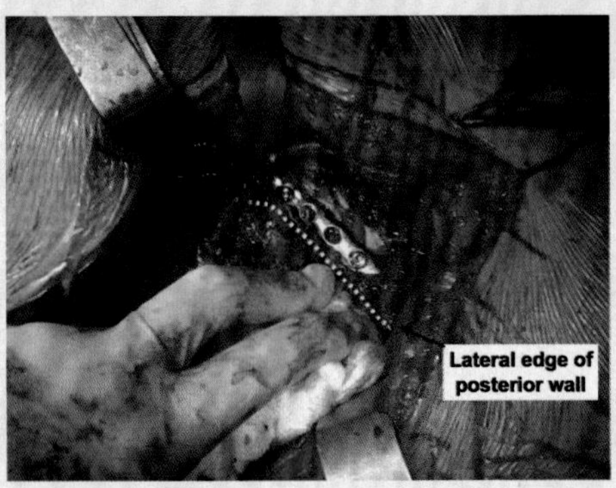

TECH FIG 3 The surgeon reduces the posterior wall piece in the fracture bed and fixes it with a buttress plate placed along the edge of the wall.

- By using a finger or a Kirschner wire to feel the edge of the wall and the labrum, the surgeon can ensure that there is no portion of the plate resting on the labrum or in the joint. Placement in this location provides the greatest biomechanical advantage in buttressing the wall.
- It is not unusual for the reconstruction plate to sit on top of the heads of the lag screws or rest over the tines of the spring plate.
- With the plate adequately contoured and positioned, it is initially fixed to the pelvis at the level of the ischial tuberosity.
  - The surgeon drills into screw hole no. 2 from the distal aspect of the plate, which should be resting within the recess at the top of the ischial tuberosity. The surgeon aims distally and medially into the proximal portion of the ischium. There will be good bone in this location.
  - Next, the plate position is checked again, at the edge of the wall but not impinging on the labrum, and then a ball spike pusher is placed into screw hole no. 8.
  - Because the plate is underbent, use of a ball spike pusher and the first proximal screw, placed in screw hole no. 7, will compress the plate to the posterior wall, further enhancing reduction, fixation, and stability of the posterior wall fragment.
    - The surgeon must take care not to violate the joint or the femoral head while drilling. In most patients, screw holes no. 7 and no. 8 are proximal to the joint even when drilling "straight" across.
- The plate will now be holding the reduction, so if any Kirschner wires were used, they can be removed.
  - The surgeon should note whether the medial aspect of the fracture fragment springs up with removal of the Kirschner wire. If it does, further fixation will be required in addition to the primary reconstruction plate.
- This is an excellent time to obtain C-arm images to evaluate the reduction and to ensure that the screws have been placed extra-articularly.
- One or two additional screws should be placed in the proximal end of the plate, and at least one more screw needs to be inserted into the distal part of the plate, at the most distal hole.
  - The most distal screw can be placed into the ischium, toward the tuberosity, where one should find great bony purchase.

Checking the Fixation

- Once the final screws are placed, the surgeon evaluates the retroacetabular surface, ensuring that the medial aspect of the fracture piece has not kicked up.
  - If the medial wall kicks up, it must be further stabilized.
    - A lag screw can be used in the same way as previously described.
    - A three-hole one-third tubular plate spring plate is another option, as described.
  - Once the medial aspect of the wall is reduced and stabilized, the smooth convexity of the retroacetabular surface should once again be restored.
- Any traction that has been applied to the extremity is removed.
- Final C-arm images are obtained to be sure that the joint is reduced and congruent and that all screws are out of the joint.
  - The proximal screws are best seen with an obturator oblique view.
  - The distal screws are best confirmed as extra-articular with the iliac oblique view.

WOUND CLOSURE

- The wound is copiously irrigated.
- The surgeon checks the integrity and condition of the sciatic nerve one final time.
- A Hemovac drain is placed on the bone, along the posterior aspect of the posterior wall. A long path will help prevent inadvertent pullout of the drain and will allow hematoma to drain over a long distance.
- The first stage of closure is to reattach the piriformis and the external rotators. This can be accomplished in several different ways, including drill holes into the greater trochanter or suturing to the gluteus medius tendon. The authors prefer to suture to the tendon, a site shorter than the original insertion site, to decrease the risk of pullout or failure of the repair.
- If the gluteus maximus tendon was released, it is repaired next. Typically, the tendon edges are easily visualized and sutured to each other.
- Any injured or devitalized muscle should be further débrided to decrease the risk of heterotopic ossification.
- Next, the fascia lata is identified and closed watertight.
- Routine soft tissue closure is performed. We prefer to decrease dead space, and therefore areas for hematoma to collect, with a layered closure, when possible, between the fascia lata and the skin.
- We prefer to obtain an AP pelvis radiograph with the patient supine on the regular hospital bed to inspect the reduction, the fixation, and the joint before extubation **(TECH FIG 4)**. Another example is seen in **TECH FIG 5**.

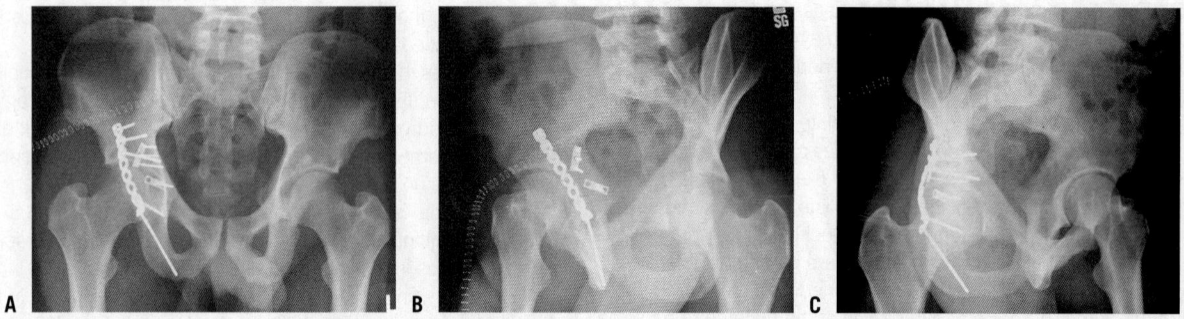

TECH FIG 4 Postoperative AP (**A**) and Judet (**B,C**) radiographs.

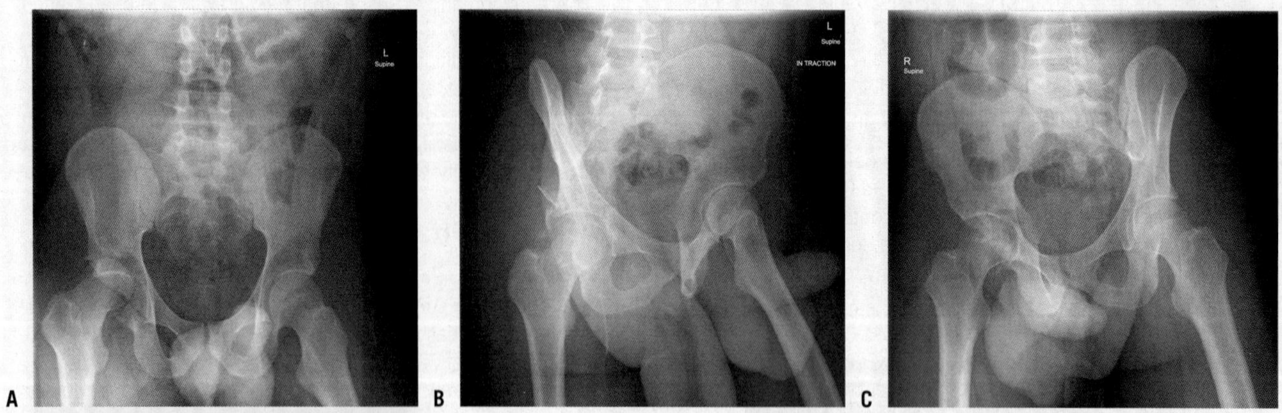

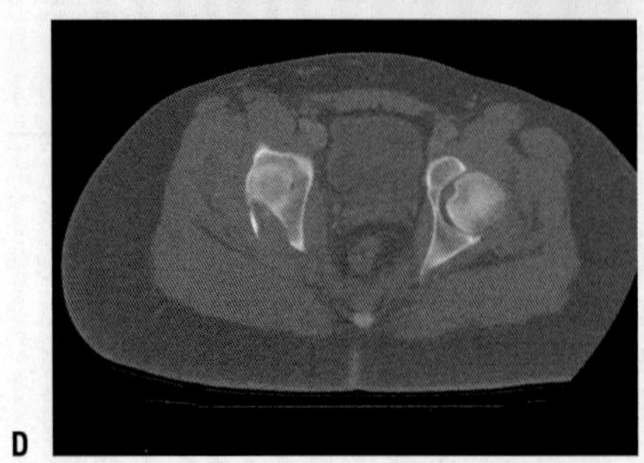

TECH FIG 5 **A.** Anteroposterior radiograph. The right femoral head is dislocated, and multiple fragments of the posterior wall are evident. **B.** Obturator oblique radiograph shows comminution of the posterior wall. **C.** Iliac oblique radiograph. There is no disruption of the sciatic notch, which indicates the fracture is confined to the posterior wall and the posterior column is not involved. **D.** CT scan at the level of the acetabular roof reveals the cranial extent of the posterior wall fracture. *(continued)*

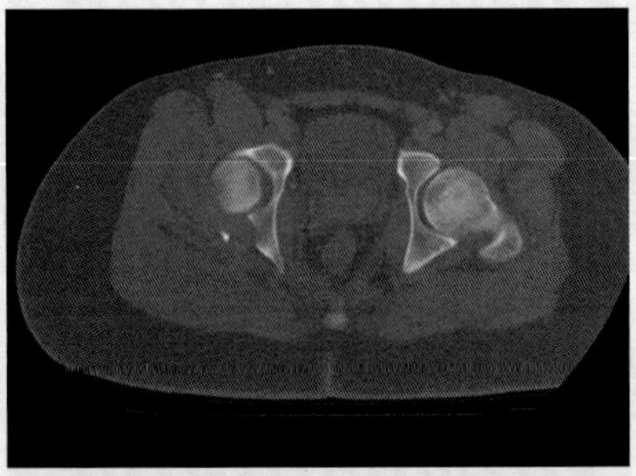

E

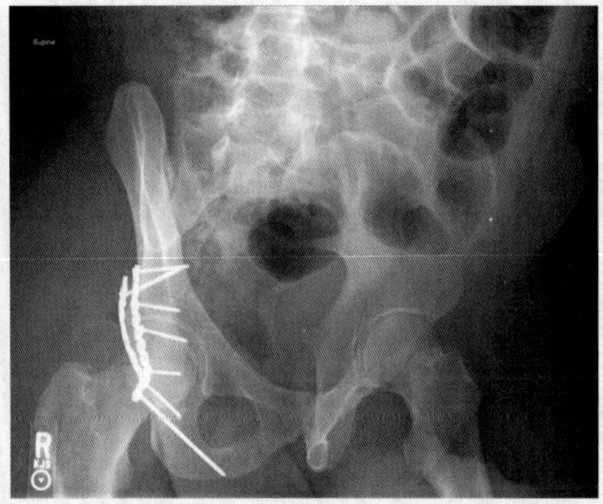

F

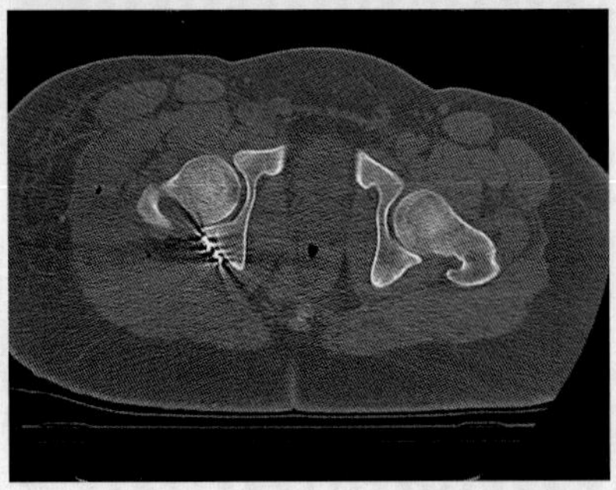

G

TECH FIG 5 *(continued)* **E.** CT scan at the level of the cotyloid fossa shows that 50% of the posterior wall is fractured. **F.** Postoperative fixation seen on the obturator oblique view. Two plates were used due to the extensive comminution. **G.** Postoperative CT.

Pearls and Pitfalls

Table and Positioning	• Using a fracture table, prone positioning, and distal femoral skeletal traction reduce the risk of injuring the sciatic nerve. The hip is extended and the knee flexed to at least 80 degrees in the prone position on the table at all times, allowing the surgeon to concentrate on the procedure. Freedom is allowed in the internal–external rotation plane during the procedure to aid in soft tissue identification and manipulation and to allow differentiation between the femoral head and the edge of the posterior wall.
Internal Fixation	• The reconstruction plate is placed at the lateral edge of the posterior wall to gain maximum buttressing capability. A Kirschner wire is used to feel the edge of the wall and the beginning of the labrum to clearly define location if unable to visualize with certainty. The plate is underbent to assist with the reduction.
Superior Posterior Buttress	• These fractures should be stabilized with a superior antiglide plate in addition to the traditional wall fractures plate.
Imaging	• Intraoperative C-arms often rotate to only 30 degrees "over the top." To obtain an adequate iliac oblique image, the surgeon can push up on the anterior superior iliac spine, which will further rotate the pelvis and provide a more familiar radiographic image. The surgeon must be certain that all screws are out of the joint. With a convex joint, if the screw is completely out on one image, it is located outside of the joint.
Transverse Fracture	• The surgeon must look for it.
Medial Wall Kick-up	• Often, the medial aspect of the posterior wall piece will kick up when the plate along the edge of the wall is secured. To prevent this, the surgeon must first look for it and recognize it. Then, a three-hole one-third tubular plate, with one distal hole cut into a V to act as a hook (or a tubular 2.7-mm minifragment plate), can be placed along this medial aspect of the fracture. One or two screws can secure this plate, which will function as a spring plate and prevent the medial wall from kicking up. This will help restore the smooth convexity of the retroacetabular surface.

POSTOPERATIVE CARE

- A drain is maintained until drainage measures less than 30 mL in a 24-hour period.
  - Antibiotics are prophylactically used until 24 hours after the drain is discontinued or until the wound is completely free of any drainage.
  - Often, hip wounds will have serous drainage for several days postoperatively. It is the authors' opinion that this signifies that the wound is not sealed, and therefore, the patient should continue to receive prophylactic antibiotics.
- Indomethacin 25 mg is given orally three times a day to prevent heterotopic ossification.
  - Chemical deep venous thrombosis prophylaxis is given at the surgeon's discretion, plus sequential compression boots for mechanical prophylaxis.
- Physical therapy restrictions
  - No active range of motion at the hip
  - Passive range of motion only; this is easily accomplished with use of a continuous passive motion machine.
  - Any necessary flexion limit will be determined by intraoperative evaluation.
- Foot-flat weight bearing for 3 months is instituted immediately, and patients are allowed to get out of bed the next day, once they understand their limitations.
  - This weight-bearing restriction (about 30 lb) unloads the weight of the extremity from the hip joint.
  - By choosing foot-flat weight bearing and no active muscle contraction, the joint reaction forces of the hip joint are decreased to attempt to further protect the internal fixation and cartilage during the reparative and healing process.
- At the 3-month mark, with evidence of callus on the radiographs, weight bearing will be advanced to partial weight bearing, with the patient and the physical therapist advancing further as tolerated.
  - Strengthening and gait training will begin at this time, with special concentration on the hip abductors.

OUTCOMES

- The outcome of an acetabular fracture after surgical intervention correlates with the quality of reduction and avoidance of complications.
- Although regarded as the simplest type of acetabular fracture, most posterior wall fractures are either comminuted or have marginal impaction, making anatomic reduction difficult and clinical outcomes worse than for most more complex, associated types of acetabular fractures.[1,13]
- Letournel and Judet[6] reported only a 93.7% perfect reduction rate for posterior wall fractures and an 82% good to excellent clinical outcome.
- Matta[8] reported 100% anatomic reduction of posterior wall fractures in his series but only 68% good to excellent clinical outcome. Similarly, Moed et al[12] had 97% perfect reductions and 89% good to excellent clinical outcomes for their series.

COMPLICATIONS

- Posttraumatic osteoarthritis was reported in 17% (97 of 569) of Letournel and Judet's[6] patients operated on within 3 weeks of injury with at least 1 year of follow-up. It occurred in 10.2% (43 of 418) of hips after perfect reductions and in 35.7% (54 of 151) of hips after imperfect reductions. The incidence of osteoarthritis for posterior wall fractures was 22.7% (22 of 97). It occurred in 16% (19 of 119) of patients with perfect reductions. The rate after perfect reductions is higher compared to perfect reductions for all types of acetabular fractures (16% vs. 10.2%, respectively).
  - Matta[8] reported a 32% (7 of 22) clinical failure rate despite perfect reduction of posterior wall fractures, which was higher than for any other fracture pattern in his series.
- Infection after acetabular surgery is reported in about 2% to 5% of patients.[6,8,9] It can be intra-articular or extra-articular, depending on the approach used. The presence of a soft tissue injury, such as a Morel-Lavallée, can increase the risk of infection.[4,6]
- Heterotopic ossification occurs after use of the extended iliofemoral approach, the Kocher-Langenbeck approach or the ilioinguinal approach when it is combined with elevation of the external fossa. Letournel and Judet[6] reported it in 20% (41 of 208) of operatively treated posterior wall fractures. They also reported a decrease from 24.6% (123 of 499) in all cases via all approaches before treatment to prevent formation to 10.2% (5 of 49) in patients receiving indomethacin for prophylaxis to 0% (0 of 29) in patients receiving both indomethacin and radiation therapy.
  - Indomethacin is generally considered safe and effective, although a randomized trial has questioned its use in prevention.[10]
  - The unknown long-term complications associated with radiation therapy, however, make it generally not recommended for isolated posterior wall fractures in young, healthy patients.
- Avascular necrosis of the femoral head must not be confused with rapid mechanical wear or deterioration due to osteochondral injury. Epstein[3] reported a rate of 5.3% in operatively treated posterior wall fractures. Letournel and Judet[6] reported a 7.5% incidence after posterior dislocation (17 of 227) and a total of 22 of 569 (3.1%) fractures operated on within the first 3 weeks after injury.
- The rate of iatrogenic nerve injury, typically the sciatic nerve, is reported to be about 2% (range 2% to 18%) in the hands of experienced surgeons.[6,9,11]

REFERENCES

1. Baumgaertner M. Fractures of the posterior wall of the acetabulum. J Am Acad Orthop Surg 1999;7:54–65.
2. Calkins M, Zych G, Latta L, et al. Computed tomography evaluation of stability in posterior fracture dislocation of the hip. Clin Orthop Relat Res 1988;227:152–163.
3. Epstein H. Posterior fracture-dislocations of the hip: long-term follow-up. J Bone Joint Surg Am 1974;56:1103–1127.
4. Hak D, Olson S, Matta J. Diagnosis and management of closed internal degloving injuries associated with pelvic and acetabular fractures: the Morel-Lavallée lesion. J Trauma 1997;42:1046–1051.
5. Keith JE Jr, Brashear HR, Guilford WB. Stability of posterior fracture-dislocations of the hip. Quantitative assessment using computed tomography. J Bone Joint Surg Am 1988;70:711–714.
6. Letournel E, Judet R. Fractures of the Acetabulum. Berlin: Springer-Verlag, 1993.
7. Lieberman J, Altchek D, Salvati E. Recurrent dislocation of a hip with a labral lesion: treatment with a modified Bankart-type repair. J Bone Joint Surg Am 1993;75:1524–1527.
8. Matta J. Fractures of the acetabulum: accuracy of reduction and clinical results in patients managed operatively within three weeks after the injury. J Bone Joint Surg Am 1996;78:1632–1645.

9. Matta J, Anderson L, Epstein H, et al. Fractures of the acetabulum. A retrospective analysis. Clin Orthop Relat Res 1986;(205):230–240.
10. Matta J, Siebenrock K. Does indomethacin reduce heterotopic bone formation after operations for acetabular fractures? A prospective randomised study. J Bone Joint Surg Br 1997;79:959–963.
11. Middlebrooks E, Sims S, Kellam J, et al. Incidence of sciatic nerve injury in operatively treated acetabular fractures without somatosensory evoked potential monitoring. J Orthop Trauma 1997;11:327–329.
12. Moed B, WillsonCarr S, Watson J. Results of operative treatment of fractures of the posterior wall of the acetabulum. J Bone Joint Surg Am 2002;84:752–758.
13. Saterbak A, Marsh L, Nepola J, et al. Clinical failure after posterior wall acetabular fractures: the influence of initial fracture patterns. J Orthop Trauma 2000;14:230–237.
14. Tornetta P III. Displaced acetabular fractures: indications for operative and nonoperative management. J Am Acad Orthop Surg 2001;9:18–28.
15. Tornetta P III. Non-operative management of acetabular fractures. The use of dynamic stress views. J Bone Joint Surg Br 1999;81:67–70.
16. Vailas J, Hurwitz S, Wiesel S. Posterior acetabular fracture-dislocations: fragment size, joint capsule, and stability. J Trauma 1989;29(11):1494–1496.

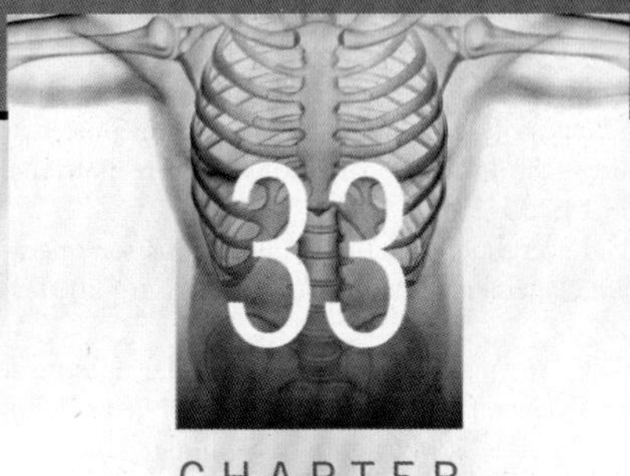

CHAPTER 33

Open Reduction and Internal Fixation of Femoral Head Fractures

Michael S.H. Kain

DEFINITION

- Fractures of the femoral head are rare and occur almost exclusively in association with high-energy hip dislocations. Femoral head fractures occur approximately in 5% to 15% of posteriorly dislocated hips.[1]
- Associated injuries to the femur, acetabulum, or acetabular labrum can affect treatment options.

ANATOMY

- The spherical femoral head is almost completely covered by articular cartilage, which often is damaged during the hip dislocation.
- Blood is primarily supplied to the superior dome of the femoral head by the medial femoral circumflex artery, which travels around the posterior aspect of the proximal femur, traveling deep to the quadratus femoris and penetrating the joint capsule just inferior to the piriformis tendon **(FIG 1)**.
  - The ligament of Weitbrecht, or the medial synovial fold, runs along the inferior calcar and has another branch of the medial femoral circumflex artery, which supplies the inferior femoral head.[4,6]
  - Additional vascular support is supplied by the foveal artery within the ligamentum teres.
  - The anterior half of the femoral neck is devoid of vascular structures. Therefore, anterior surgical approaches to the hip joint do not compromise the vascular supply of the femoral head.

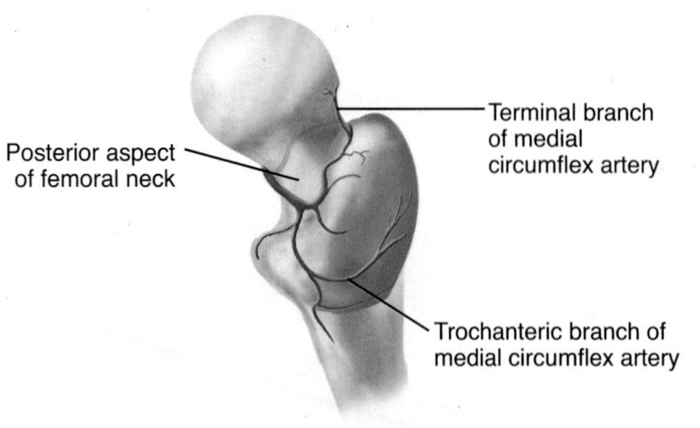

FIG 1 The blood supply to the superior dome of the femoral head is primarily supplied by the medial femoral circumflex artery. It travels around the posterior aspect of the proximal femur, traveling deep to the quadratus femoris, and penetrates the joint capsule just inferior to the piriformis tendon.

- The acetabular labrum acts as a secondary stabilizer of the hip by increasing the coverage of the femoral head and maintaining the suction seal. The labrum may be damaged during hip dislocation in particular posterior dislocations.

PATHOGENESIS

- Fractures of the femoral head are a result of a shearing injury. In posterior fracture-dislocation, the femoral head strikes the acetabular rim and is driven posteriorly with the posterior wall levering on the femoral head shearing off a piece of the femoral head as it dislocates. These injuries are articular injuries, and it is common to see impaction on both sides of the fracture edges.
- Posterior wall fractures and avulsions of the labrum are commonly associated with these fractures.
- Both the position of the leg at the time of impact and the patient's hip anatomy have been shown to play a role in the etiology of fracture-dislocations of the hip.
- Posterior dislocations, the most common type, occur when the hip is in a flexed, adducted, and internally rotated position. Decreased femoral anteversion leads to reduced femoral head coverage by the acetabulum and increases the risk of hip dislocation.
- Anterior dislocations are less common. They occur when the hip is in an abducted and externally rotated position, which results in an impaction injury to the anterolateral femoral head **(FIG 2)**.

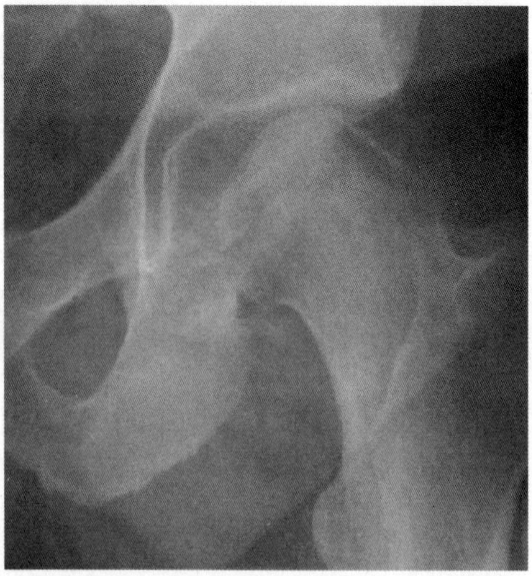

FIG 2 Anterolateral femoral head impaction injury following anterior hip dislocation.

NATURAL HISTORY

- In an intermediate-term follow-up study by Jacob et al,[5] despite open or closed treatment, only 40% of patients had satisfactory results after hip dislocation at an average of 4.5 years after injury. More than half of the patients had posttraumatic arthrosis.
- Osteonecrosis of the femoral head may develop in 20% of patients with femoral head fractures despite anatomic reduction.

PATIENT HISTORY AND PHYSICAL FINDINGS

- Because of the high energy required to induce a fracture-dislocation of the hip, all patients should undergo a thorough trauma evaluation for associated injuries.
  - Airway, cardiovascular, head, and spine injuries should be stabilized emergently.
  - Narcotic pain medication usually is required.
- Careful evaluation of the affected extremity is essential.
  - The leg often appears shortened and internally rotated after a posterior hip dislocation.
  - The leg is shortened and externally rotated in an anterior/inferior dislocation
  - Suspicion for associated injuries, particularly around the knee, should remain high, such injuries can be recognized on physical examination.
  - Injury to the knee ligaments or extensor mechanism is associated with traumatic hip dislocation and should be assessed with a knee stability examination, the presence of instability is known as a dashboard injury.
- Because sciatic nerve injuries are common, motor and sensory examination of the affected extremity is critical, with particular attention paid to strength grades (1 to 5) and sensation in the peroneal and tibial nerve distribution.

IMAGING AND OTHER DIAGNOSTIC STUDIES

- In the traumatic anteroposterior (AP) pelvis radiograph **(FIG 3A)**, both hips should be evaluated for fracture-dislocation. The goal should be to emergently reduce the hip, and further imaging should not excessively delay reduction of the dislocated hip.

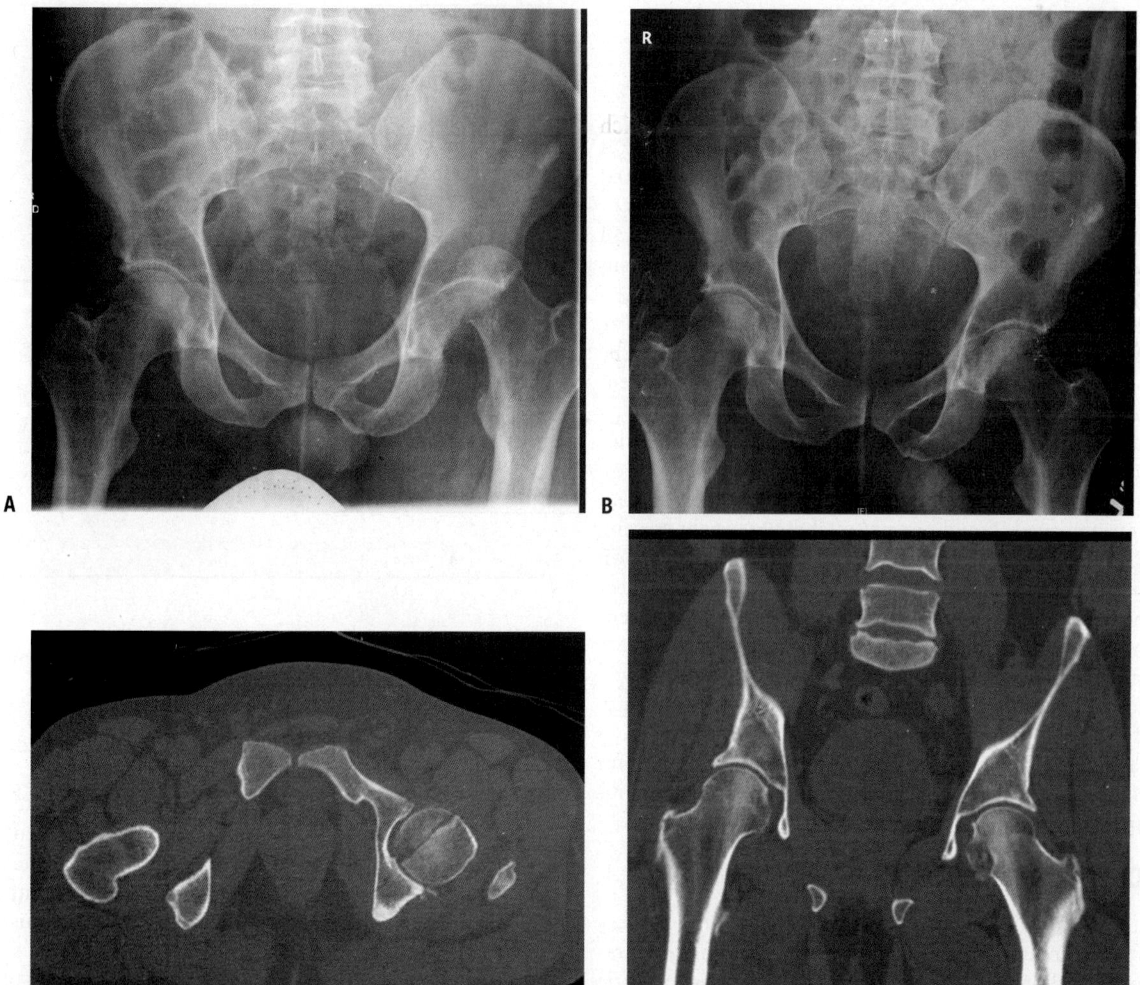

FIG 3 **A.** Prereduction AP pelvis radiograph in the trauma bay demonstrating hip dislocation and femoral head fracture. **B.** Postreduction AP pelvis taken after closed reduction in the operating room. **C,D.** Postreduction fine-cut CT scan images demonstrating femoral head fracture and assessment of the femoral neck in multiple planes.

- Associated injuries such as femoral neck fractures, acetabular fractures, or pelvis fractures may require additional dedicated hip, Judet views, or pelvic inlet and outlet radiographs **(FIG 3B)**.
- A postreduction fine-cut computed tomography (CT) scan of the pelvis and femoral neck with coronal and sagittal reconstructions will further define the anatomy of the femoral head fracture and associated injuries **(FIG 3C,D)**.
  - Although a prereduction CT scan of the hip is not often indicated, it is often obtained in the trauma workup and helps to assess the femoral neck for any nondisplaced fractures. If there is any concern for femoral neck fracture, then a CT with reconstructions should be obtained.
- Although magnetic resonance imaging can be used to evaluate femoral head osteonecrosis in follow-up care, acute imaging has not been demonstrated to be prognostic of this complication. Although, there is some suggestion thought that rupture of the obturator externus tendon may be an indicator that the femoral head blood supply has been disrupted.[10]

DIFFERENTIAL DIAGNOSIS

- Femoral head fractures are classified according to Pipkin **(TABLE 1)**.
- An isolated posterior wall fragment may be confused with a femoral head fracture.

TABLE 1 Pipkin Classification of Femoral Head Fractures

Type	Description	Illustration
I	Fracture inferior to the femoral head fovea	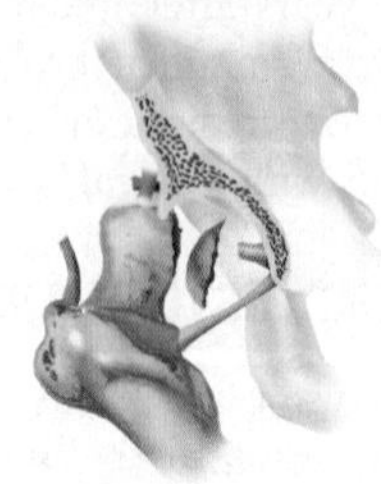
II	Fracture superior to the femoral head fovea	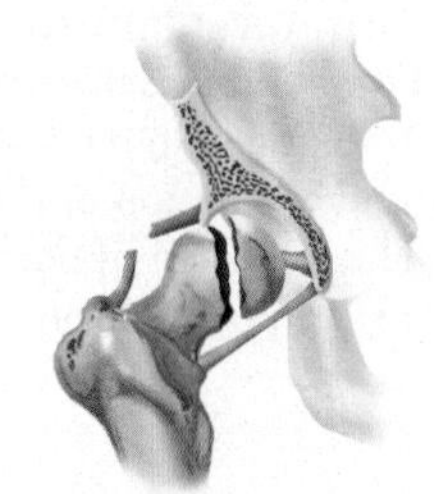
III	Femoral head fracture plus femoral neck fracture	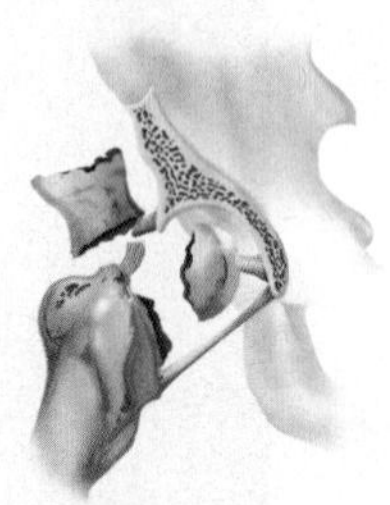
IV	Femoral head fracture plus acetabular fracture	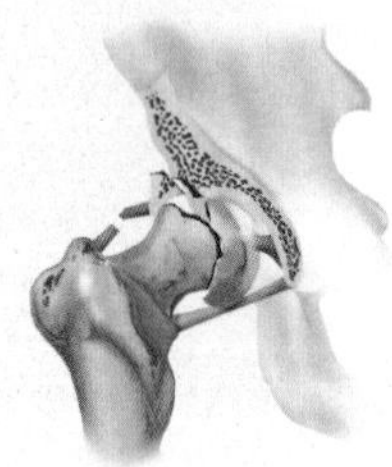

NONOPERATIVE MANAGEMENT

- The goal of treatment is to restore stability and congruency to the hip joint. In more proximal head fractures and if there is any incongruence, surgical management is required to reconstruct the femoral head.
- Nonoperative management is reserved for Pipkin type I fractures with small articular fragments if there is a concentric reduction of the hip.
  - No quality clinical studies are available to define the size of the fragment or amount of displacement that can be tolerated. The accepted guideline is that the fragment should be congruent with the intact femoral head.
  - Small impaction injuries associated with anterior dislocation also may be treated nonoperatively in many cases.
- Nonoperative and postoperative management is very similar. Patients managed should remain touchdown weight bearing for 8 to 12 weeks. For posterior dislocations, hip flexion beyond 90 degrees should be avoided for 6 weeks to protect the posterior capsule and to prevent the fracture from engaging the weakened femoral head and displacement.
  - Patients managed nonoperatively need to be followed closely to ensure no loss of reduction, loss of incongruity of the joint, or loss of motion.
  - Early range of motion with a continuous passive motion Machine or a stationary bike can be used to help maintain motion.

SURGICAL MANAGEMENT

- Most patients with femoral head fractures require surgery to provide an anatomic reduction of the femoral head, remove osteochondral loose bodies, or obtain a concentric reduction of the hip joint. Loose body removal can delay the onset of arthrosis.
- Large, displaced fragments should be anatomically fixed. Smaller fragments inferior to the fovea can be excised if a stable reduction of the fracture fragment cannot be obtained and the hip remains stable.
- Although their significance is unknown, labral tears often can be evaluated and treated surgically depending on the approach.
- Hip arthroplasty is another treatment option in elderly patients, especially with large head fragments. Femoral head fractures in this age group tend to have a large amount of articular cartilage damage and impaction of the bone at the fracture line, which compromises the patient's outcome.
- Recommendations for surgical management of isolated femoral head fractures
  - Nondisplaced fracture or small impaction injury
    - Nonoperative treatment with stable and concentric reduction

- Displaced/unstable fragment
  - Small: surgical excision, anterior approach
  - Large: surgical fixation
    - Pipkin I and II if no fragment in the joint, fragment anterior: Hueter approach
    - Pipkin II with significant displacement or comminution: surgical dislocation
    - Pipkin III or IV: surgical dislocation
    - Irreducible fracture-dislocations: surgical dislocation
  - Elderly patient
    - Small fragment without evidence of femoral head impaction: surgical excision
    - Large fragment or significant femoral head impaction: hip arthroplasty

Preoperative Planning

- If the hip is dislocated, it should be emergently reduced under general anesthesia with muscle paralysis if possible.
  - Inadequate anesthesia during hip reduction can lead to further damage to the femoral head, femoral neck, or acetabulum as the hip is relocated.
- If there is an associated fracture of the femoral neck even if nondisplaced, an open reduction of fixation of the femoral neck should be considered.
- If the hip is reduced, the patient should be placed in 30 lb of longitudinal skeletal traction until formal open reduction and internal fixation of the femoral head occurs. Traction will unload the femoral head and prevent ongoing third-body wear within the hip joint.
  - Repeat radiographs and a postreduction CT scan should be obtained to confirm reduction of the hip and evaluate for loose bodies or fracture morphology.
  - It is reasonable at this point to delay definitive surgery until the appropriate surgeon, anesthesiologist, and equipment are available.
- If the hip is irreducible, or there is an associated femoral neck fracture, emergent open reduction and internal fixation is required.

Approach

- The most difficult decision is determination of the best operative approach.

Posterior Approach (Kocher-Langenbeck)

- Epstein et al[2] originally argued that all femoral head fractures should be approached posteriorly because the posterior blood supply to the femoral head had already been damaged during hip dislocation. This left the anterior capsular blood supply intact.
  - However, the anterior capsule and anterior femoral neck provide very little vascular supply to the femoral head. In addition, visualization of the anteriorly located femoral head fracture is often inadequate.
  - This approach is best when large femoral head fragments remain dislocated posteriorly after reduction of the hip or with an associated posterior column or posterior wall fracture.
    - However, visualization of the anterior head fragment is difficult through a posterior approach and such a fracture may be better treated with a Ganz surgical dislocation.

Anterior Approach (Smith-Petersen or Hueter Interval)

- Swiontkowski et al[9] effectively demonstrated that better visualization of the femoral head was obtained for most Pipkin I and II femoral head fractures by using the distal limb of an anterior Smith-Petersen approach.
  - Lower rates of osteonecrosis were seen, although a slightly higher risk of heterotopic ossification was observed.
  - A Smith-Petersen approach is an excellent approach for the treatment of most Pipkin types I and II fractures and is the preferred approach for excision of the fragment, as long as there is a stable and concentric hip joint.
  - The distal portion of the Smith-Petersen approach is referred to as a *Hueter interval* or *direct anterior approach*.

Surgical Hip Dislocation

- Alternatively, better visualization of both the femoral head and the fracture fragment can be obtained through a surgical hip dislocation, as described by Ganz et al.[3]
  - This approach safely preserves the medial circumflex arterial supply to the femoral head.
  - It also allows the best access to associated injuries such as posterior acetabular fractures, labral tears, osteochondral debris, or posteriorly dislocated femoral head fragments.
  - Surgical dislocation also provides improved access to angulate lag screw fixation perpendicular to the femoral head fracture line and addresses any areas of articular impaction in the femoral head.

Positioning

- For an anterior Smith-Petersen approach, the patient is positioned supine on a radiolucent table with a hip bump, and the affected leg draped free or on a fracture table that allows for flexion and extension of the hip.
- For a posterior Kocher-Langenbeck approach, the patient is placed lateral on a radiolucent fracture table with the knee flexed to 90 degrees to relieve sciatic nerve tension. Prone positioning is not advised unless the surgeon feels a dual approach is necessary, as the prone position limits the ability to access the anterior femoral head. Additionally, if in the lateral position, this can be converted to a surgical hip dislocation with a trochanteric osteotomy.
- For a surgical hip dislocation approach, the patient is placed on a radiolucent table with a beanbag in the lateral decubitus position and the affected leg draped free.

SMITH-PETERSEN ANTERIOR APPROACH (HUETER INTERVAL)

Incision and Dissection

- The patient is positioned supine on a fracture table that allows for the hip to be flexed and extended.
- A vertical incision is made from the anterior superior iliac spine (ASIS) extending distally toward the lateral border of the patella **(TECH FIG 1A)**.
- The sartorius and tensor fascia lata are identified **(TECH FIG 1B)**. The fascia is incised over the medial aspect of the tensor muscle, and the medial border of the tensor muscle is followed to develop the interval between the tensor and sartorius muscles **(TECH FIG 1C)**.
- The tensor muscle is retracted laterally and the sartorius muscle medially.
- Find the lateral femoral circumflex vessel traversing the inferior part of the wound as this marks the distal aspect of the incision. This can be ligated, tied off, or cauterized.
- The direct and indirect heads of the rectus femoris muscle are identified and are retracted medially **(TECH FIG 1D)**. There is an overlying fascial layer that must be divided to be able to see this muscle. If excision if being performed, the direct head can remain intact to the anterior inferior iliac spine.
- In most patients, a residual muscle belly, the iliocapsularis muscle, is deep to the rectus muscle. This muscle is swept medially, exposing the capsule.
- Place a retractor over the anterior wall of the acetabulum to improve visualization.
- If additional exposure is necessary, a portion of the direct head of the rectus muscle may be released and repaired at the end of the case.

Capsulotomy

- A longitudinal incision is made from the base of the femoral neck along the axis of the femoral neck and extended until reaching the intact acetabular labrum. Medially, a capsular incision is made along both the acetabular rim and the base of the femoral neck **(TECH FIG 2A)**. Laterally, only a capsular incision along the articular rim is made to protect the femoral head blood supply at the posterior base of the femoral neck.

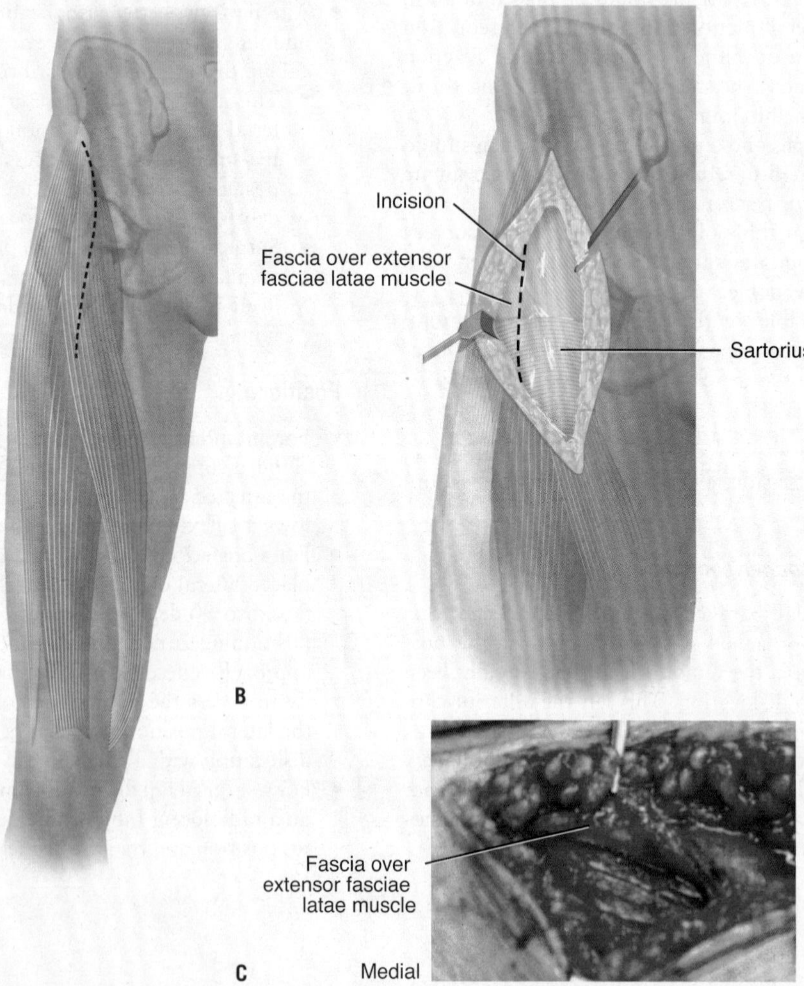

TECH FIG 1 Smith-Petersen anterior approach. **A.** Incision starts at ASIS or just lateral and extends distally toward the lateral border of the patella. **B.** The fascia is incised over the medial border of the tensor muscle. **C.** The medial border of the tensor muscle is followed to develop the interval between the tensor muscle and the sartorius muscle. *(continued)*

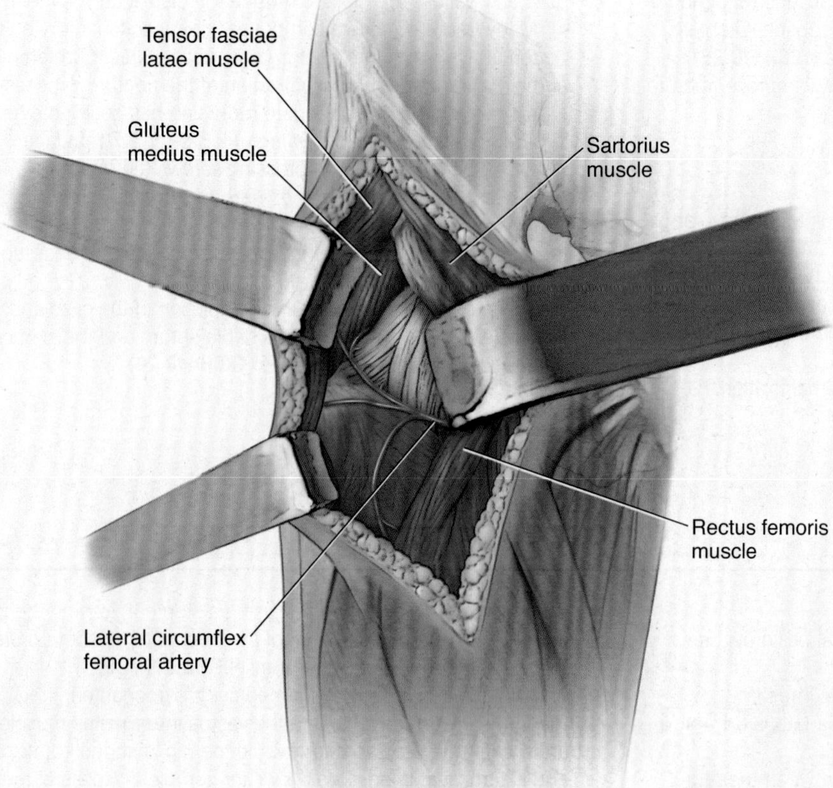

D

TECH FIG 1 *(continued)* **D.** The direct and indirect heads of the rectus femoris muscle are identified and retracted medially.

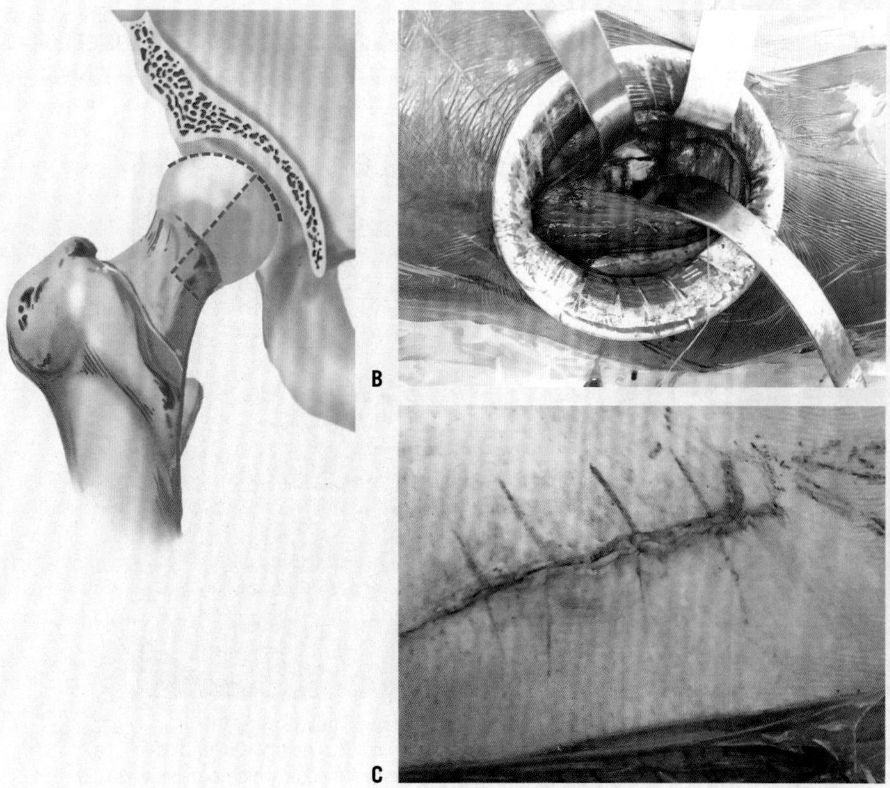

A B C

TECH FIG 2 Smith-Petersen anterior approach. **A.** A capsulotomy is performed by making a longitudinal incision from the base of the femoral neck to the articular rim along the axis of the femoral neck. Medially, a capsular incision is made along both the acetabular rim and the base of the femoral neck. Laterally, only a capsular incision is made along the articular rim. **B.** View of a Pipkin II through a Smith-Petersen approach prior to fixation. **C.** Final wound closure of a Hueter interval approach starting slightly lateral to ASIS.

- Tag sutures are placed at the corners of the "T" in the capsule near the acetabular labrum to assist with capsular retraction.
- Blunt retractors are placed within the joint capsule to obtain good exposure of the femoral head fracture **(TECH FIG 2B)**.
- External rotation of the leg and hip flexion will improve fracture visualization.

Fracture Reduction and Fixation

- Distract, lavage, and carefully inspect the joint to remove any loose bodies.
  - Visualization may be improved by cutting the ligamentum teres.
  - In some cases, complete anterior dislocation of the femoral head will facilitate fracture reduction and insertion of definitive fixation.
- The fragment is excised if too small for internal fixation.
- A pointed reduction clamp, a dental pick, or Kirschner wires used as joysticks are used to reduce the displaced fragment.
  - Many fractures have a component of impaction injury on the femoral head, so the fracture may not key in circumferentially. Circumferential visualization of the fracture is necessary to confirm that adequate reduction has been obtained.
- The fracture is fixed with countersunk 3.5- or 2.7-mm lag screws or headless self-compressing screws (eg, Acutrak [Acumed LLC, Hillsboro, OR] or Herbert-Whipple screws [Zimmer Inc., Warsaw, IN]).
- It is important to ascertain that the screw heads are recessed within the bone.
- Loosely repair the capsule at the completion of the case and
- the skin can be closed with absorbable suture and the skin can be closed with absorbable suture **(TECH FIG 2C)**.

SURGICAL HIP DISLOCATION

- The patient is in the lateral position.
- Either a direct lateral incision or a traditional posterolateral approach is used **(TECH FIG 3A)**.
- Anterior to the trochanter, the gluteus maximus is retracted posteriorly, and the tensor fascia lata is retracted anteriorly.
- Posterior to the trochanter, the interval between the gluteus minimus and the piriformis is identified. The gluteus minimus is sharply elevated anteriorly, and the piriformis is left intact.
  - The dissection is kept superior to the piriformis muscle because the medial femoral circumflex vessel penetrates the hip capsule at the inferior margin of the piriformis.
  - The vastus lateralis is elevated just distal to the insertion of the gluteus maximus tendon.
- The trochanter is osteotomized using a step cut, leaving the piriformis and a portion of the tip of the trochanter intact to protect the medial femoral circumflex vessel **(TECH FIG 3B)**.
- The gluteus minimus, gluteus medius, the trochanteric fragment, the vastus lateralis, and the vastus intermedius muscles are sharply elevated anteriorly while the hip is abducted, flexed, and externally rotated. This allows for complete expose of the hip capsule.
  - Placing the leg in the figure-4 position with the operative-side foot on the table improves exposure of the anterior capsule. This helps keep the hip abducted, flexed, and externally rotated.
- A Z-shaped capsulotomy is performed with the cephalad limb posteriorly and the caudal limb anteriorly **(TECH FIG 3C)**. Place tag sutures at the corners of the capsulotomy to improve visualization and for later repair.

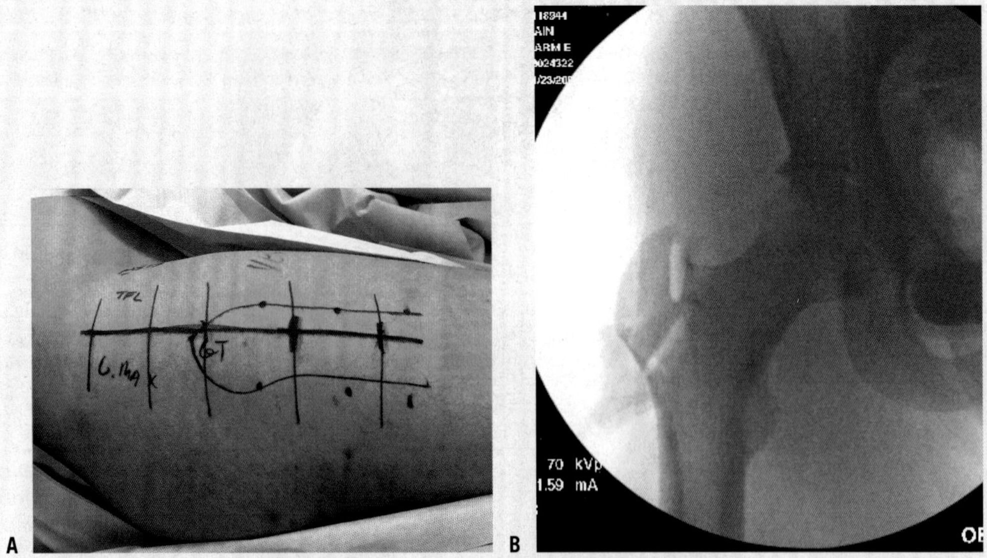

TECH FIG 3 Ganz surgical dislocation. **A.** A straight lateral Gibson incision is marked out allowing the surgeon to find the interval between the gluteus maximus and the tensor fascia lata. **B.** The trochanteric osteotomy can be made as a straight osteotomy or as shown in the C-arm image as a step cut, which provides more stability. *(continued)*

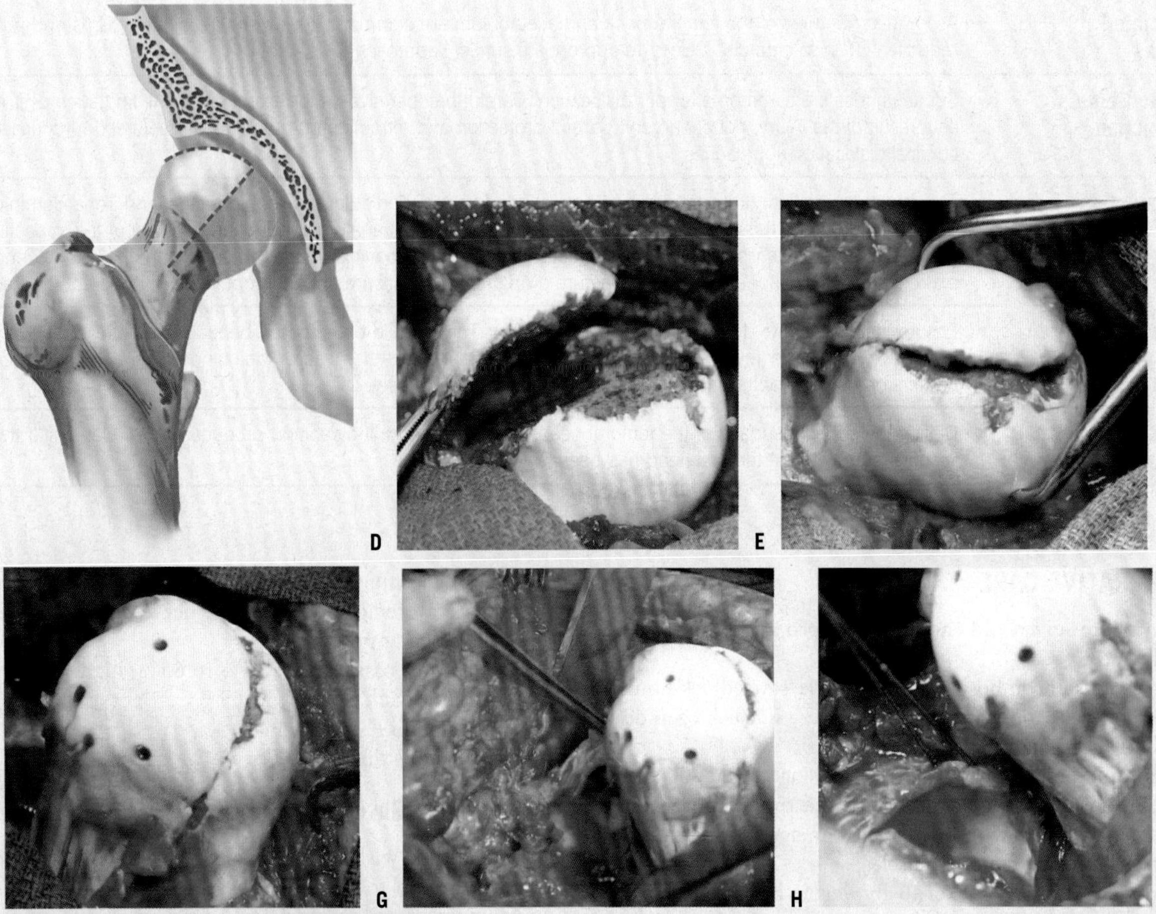

C D E F G H

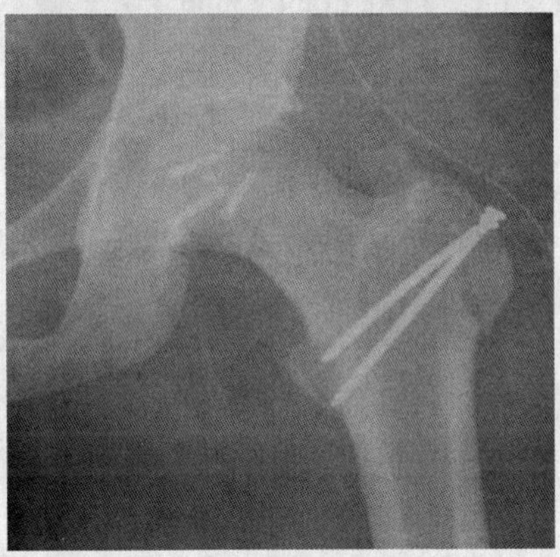

I

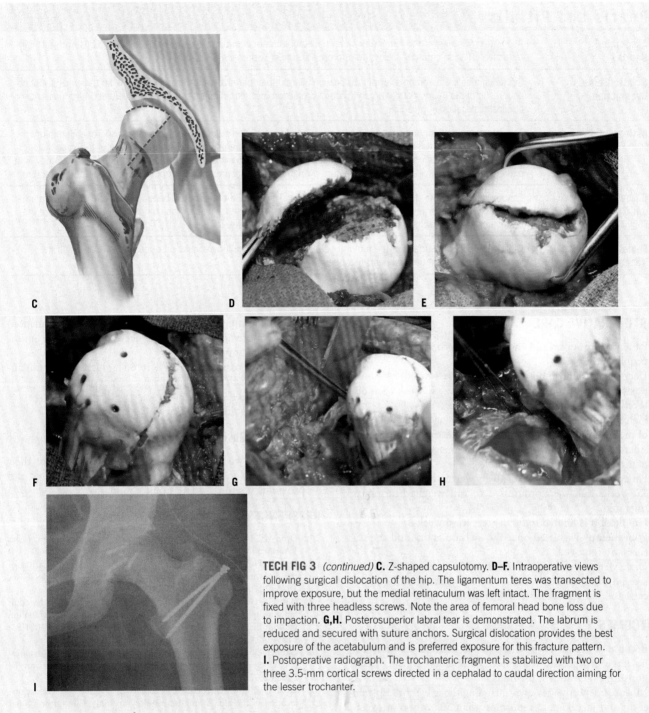

TECH FIG 3 *(continued)* **C.** Z-shaped capsulotomy. **D–F.** Intraoperative views following surgical dislocation of the hip. The ligamentum teres was transected to improve exposure, but the medial retinaculum was left intact. The fragment is fixed with three headless screws. Note the area of femoral head bone loss due to impaction. **G,H.** Posterosuperior labral tear is demonstrated. The labrum is reduced and secured with suture anchors. Surgical dislocation provides the best exposure of the acetabulum and is preferred exposure for this fracture pattern. **I.** Postoperative radiograph. The trochanteric fragment is stabilized with two or three 3.5-mm cortical screws directed in a cephalad to caudal direction aiming for the lesser trochanter.

- The femoral head is dislocated and the foot is placed into a sterile bag anteriorly. The ligamentum teres is cut to free the Pipkin fragment, but care is taken to keep the ligament of Weitbrecht intact, as this has the blood supply to this inferior fragment.
  - The femoral head fragment is reduced or excised.
  - Impacted areas are elevated and packed with bone graft if necessary **(TECH FIG 3D–F)**.
- The labrum is assessed and is fixed with suture anchors if it is torn **(TECH FIG 3H)**.
- If an associated posterior wall fragment is present, the hip is reduced and the wall fragment repaired in standard fashion.
- The capsule is loosely repaired, and the trochanter is reattached with two or three 3.5-mm cortical screws **(TECH FIG 3I)**.

Pearls and Pitfalls

Associated Injuries	• Associated fractures of the femoral neck and acetabulum are common. Review the initial injury films and post–hip reduction CT scan carefully. Select an appropriate surgical approach.
Sciatic Nerve Dysfunction	• Subtle injuries are common after hip dislocation. Careful preoperative motor examination will find such dysfunction as a result of the injury, not of surgery. Careful protection and retraction of the nerve is essential during posterior or surgical dislocation approaches.
Malreduction	• This is a shearing injury that results in a femoral head fracture, articular cartilage damage, and impaction injury to the femoral head. It can be difficult to obtain a circumferential anatomic reduction because of the impaction injury. Circumferential visualization of the fracture is necessary to avoid a large articular step-off. The tendency is to malreduce the posterior aspect of the fracture owing to poor exposure and incomplete visualization of the fracture.
Screw Length and Type	• Ensure that the screws do not penetrate into the joint. They should be recessed beneath the cortex of the femoral head. Use headless screws rather than standard screws because the head of the standard screw will displace the borders of the thin fracture fragment as the head engages the bone.
Femoral Head Vascular Supply	• Drilling the superior surface of the femoral head with a 2.0-mm drill bit should produce arterial bleeding if the vascular supply to the femoral head has been maintained.

POSTOPERATIVE CARE

- Patients are given 24 hours of appropriate antibiotic prophylaxis.
- Deep venous thrombosis prophylaxis is started 24 hours postoperatively and is used before surgery if it has been delayed for more than 24 hours after injury.
- Heterotopic ossification prophylaxis using either 700 cGy of radiation or indomethacin 25 mg three times daily is considered in patients with significant damage to the gluteus minimus or rectus femoris muscles.
- Patients are allowed 30 to 40 lb weight bearing for 8 to 12 weeks and then progressed to full weight bearing as tolerated.
- Hip flexion is limited to 90 degrees for 6 weeks.
- Pool therapy is started once the incision is dry and the sutures are removed.
- Once weight bearing is initiated at 12 weeks, more aggressive physical therapy focusing on gait training and quadriceps and hip abductor strengthening is started.

OUTCOMES

- Because of the rarity of femoral head fracture-dislocations, no large prospective trials have compared surgical versus nonsurgical treatment methods.
- Most retrospective reviews, including those by both Epstein et al[2] and Jacob et al,[5] report less than 50% good or excellent results at 5 to 10 years of follow-up.
- Scolaro et al[7] had demonstrated good outcomes for Pipkin I and II with the anterior approach.
- Using a surgical dislocation approach has been shown to improve outcomes for Pipkin IV injuries.[8]
- Posttraumatic arthrosis is common following a femoral head fracture, and patients should be warned early of the poor prognosis.

COMPLICATIONS

- Posttraumatic arthrosis: greater than 50%
- Femoral head osteonecrosis: 20%
- Neurologic injury: 10% (60% of these recover some function)
  - Lateral femoral cutaneous nerve injury after Smith-Petersen approaches
- Heterotopic ossification: 25% to 65%; higher risk with anterior approach
- Hip instability
- Deep venous thrombosis

ACKNOWLEDGMENTS

- The author wishes to thank Drs. Friess and Ellis for their contribution to the previous edition for this chapter and providing a strong foundation to build on.

REFERENCES

1. Droll KP, Broekhuyse H, O'Brien P. Fracture of the femoral head. J Am Acad Orthop Surg 2007;15:716–727.
2. Epstein HC, Wiss DA, Cozen L. Posterior fracture dislocation of the hip with fractures of the femoral head. Clin Orthop Relat Res 1985;(201):9–17.
3. Ganz R, Gill TJ, Gautier E, et al. Surgical dislocation of the adult hip a technique with full access to the femoral head and acetabulum without the risk of avascular necrosis. J Bone Joint Surg Br 2001;83: 1119–1124.
4. Gautier E, Ganz K, Krügel N, et al. Anatomy of the medial femoral circumflex artery and its surgical implications. J Bone Joint Surg Br 2000;82:679–683.
5. Jacob JR, Rao JP, Ciccarelli C. Traumatic dislocation and fracture dislocation of the hip. A long-term follow-up study. Clin Orthop Relat Res 1987;(214):249–263.
6. Kalhor M, Horowitz K, Gharehdaghi J, et al. Anatomic variations in femoral head circulation. Hip Int 2012;22:307–312.
7. Scolaro JA, Marecek G, Firoozabadi R, et al. Management and radiographic outcomes of femoral head fractures. J Orthop Traumatol 2017;18:235–241.
8. Solberg BD, Moon CN, Franco DP. Use of a trochanteric flip osteotomy improves outcomes in Pipkin IV fractures. Clin Orthop Relat Res 2009;467:929–933.
9. Swiontkowski MF, Thorpe M, Seiler JG, et al. Operative management of displaced femoral head fractures: case-matched comparison of anterior versus posterior approaches for Pipkin I and Pipkin II fractures. J Orthop Trauma 1992;6:437–442.
10. Tannast M, Pleus F, Bonel H, et al. Magnetic resonance imaging in traumatic posterior hip dislocation. J Orthop Trauma 2010;24:723–731.

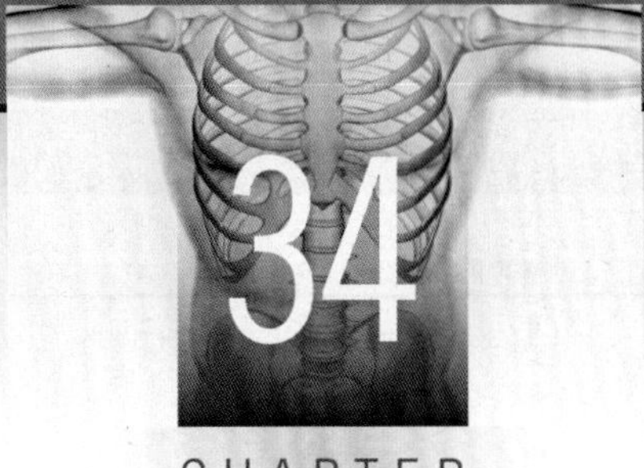

CHAPTER 34

Open Reduction and Internal Fixation and Closed Reduction and Percutaneous Fixation of Femoral Neck Fractures

Raveesh D. Richard, Brian Mullis, and Jeff Anglen

DEFINITION

- Femoral neck fractures occur in two patient populations.
  - Most commonly, they happen in older osteopenic patients after low-energy trauma, such as falls.
  - When they occur in younger patients with normal bone, they are usually the result of high-energy trauma, such as a motor vehicle collision.
- Femoral neck fractures can be classified by several characteristics. The most important distinguishing feature in regard to treatment decisions is the degree of displacement.
  - Fractures that are nondisplaced or impacted into valgus can often be treated with in situ fixation using percutaneous methods.
  - Displaced fractures require reduction and fixation or replacement.
- The location of the fracture in the femoral neck can be described as subcapital, transcervical, or basicervical (**FIG 1**).
- Transcervical femoral neck fractures can be further characterized by the angle of the fracture line with respect to the perpendicular of the femoral shaft axis. This is the Pauwels classification (**TABLE 1**).
  - The importance of this feature is to recognize high-angle fractures (more vertical), which have the greater risk of displacement when treated with screws along the neck axis due to shear stress at the fracture site.

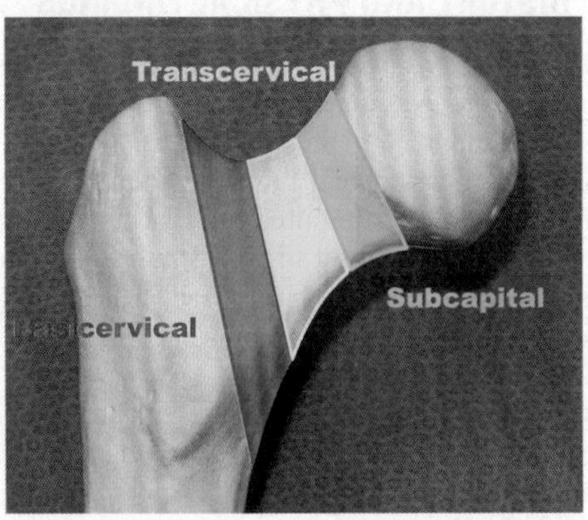

FIG 1 Definition of location for femoral neck fractures. Fractures through the *red zone* are described as basicervical; in the *yellow zone*, they are transcervical; and in the *green area*, they are designated subcapital.

ANATOMY

- The femoral neck axis forms an angle of approximately 140 degrees to the femoral shaft axis in the coronal plane. In addition, it is anteverted approximately 15 degrees with reference to the plane of the posterior condyles of the distal femur.
- When viewed in both anteroposterior (AP) and lateral radiographic views, the normal contour of the femoral head and neck forms a gentle "S" shape (**FIG 2A,B**).
- Additionally, the femoral neck is aligned with the anterior one-half of the proximal femur shaft when viewed laterally (**FIG 2C**).
- The vascular supply of the proximal femur relies on the medial femoral circumflex artery, particularly the posterior branch, which feeds the retinacula of Weitbrecht. Minor and variable contributions come from the artery of the ligamentum teres (**FIG 2D,E**).
- The strongest bone in the femoral head is in the center-center position, at the confluence of trabeculae (primary compressive group and primary tensile group).

PATHOGENESIS

- Low-energy femoral neck fractures generally are a result of a fall from standing height in an osteoporotic individual.
  - This is an increasing public health problem, with projections of 512,000 hip fractures of all types in the United States by the year 2040.[2]
- High-energy femoral neck fractures generally result from high-speed motor vehicle collision or falls from greater than 10 feet.
  - These fractures are often comminuted and significantly displaced.
  - These patients frequently have multiple injuries, which can complicate treatment.

NATURAL HISTORY

- Nondisplaced or minimally displaced fractures that are not surgically stabilized may further displace owing to the high mechanical forces associated with hip motion and the instability that comes from comminution of the cortical bone.
- Even valgus impacted fractures treated without surgery will displace approximately 40% of the time.
- Valgus impacted fractures with posterior tilt seen on the lateral view are more likely to fail.[8]

TABLE 1 Pauwels Classification of Transcervical Femoral Neck Fractures

Classification	Fracture Plane Angle[a]	Example	Effect of Vertical Forces on Fracture Site	Fixation
Pauwels 1	Low, ≤30 degrees	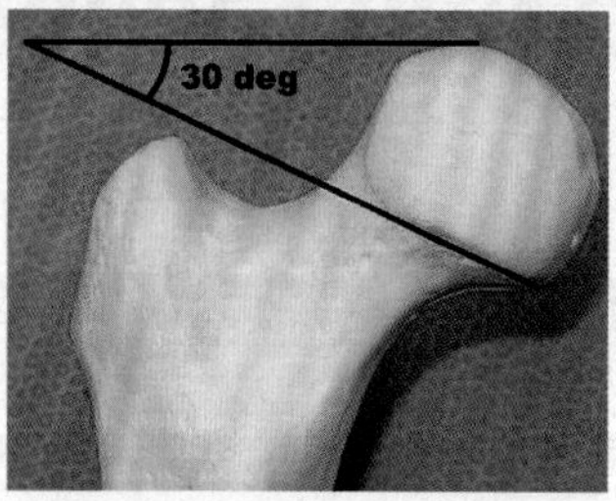	Compression, stable	Lag screws in axis of femoral neck
Pauwels 2	30–50 degrees	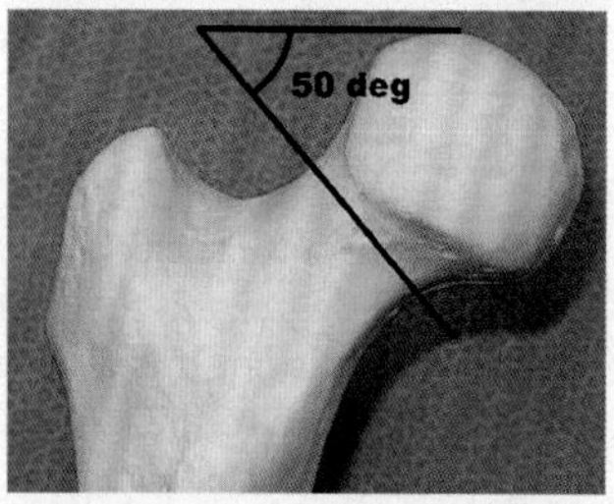	Variable	Lag screws in axis of femoral neck
Pauwels 3	High, ≥50 degrees	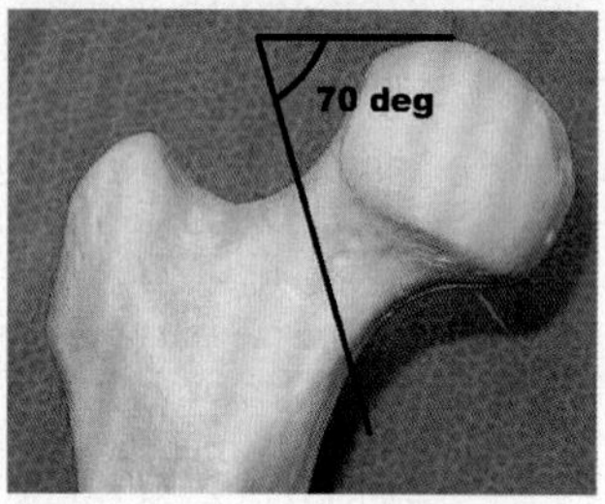	Shear, unstable; tends to displace into shortened, varus position	At least one lag screw perpendicular to fracture plane or fixed angle device

[a]Fracture plane angle is relative to a line perpendicular to the femoral axis on AP radiograph.

- Garden 2 femoral neck fractures are more likely to shorten (63%) than Garden 1 (42%) when treated with in situ cannulated screws.[1]
- The intra-articular location of the femoral neck means that there is not a well-vascularized soft tissue envelope, and the fracture is exposed to synovial fluid, which contains enzymes that lyse blood clot, the required first stage in bone healing. As a result, femoral neck fracture healing is slowed.
- In addition, the blood supply comes from tenuous retrograde blood flow.
  - Nonunion rate for untreated displaced fractures approaches 100%.
- Nonunion of the femoral neck leads to a shortened limb, variable restriction in motion, and pain with weight bearing.
- Fracture of the femoral neck can lead to interruption of the blood supply to the femoral head due to kinking or disruption of vessels or tamponade from hemarthrosis.
  - This results in avascular necrosis (AVN) in about 15% of cases.[5]
  - Many surgeons believe that time to treatment is an important factor, with delay increasing the incidence, although this remains controversial. The time imperative probably varies from patient to patient, but in general, an effort is made to fix these fractures within 24 hours of injury. A delay of internal fixation greater than 24 hours increases the odds of developing a nonunion.[9]
- About 50% of patients return to their previous level of function after surgery.[7]
- Femoral neck fractures in the elderly are associated with 20% 1-year mortality.[11]

PATIENT HISTORY AND PHYSICAL FINDINGS

- In most patients with femoral neck fracture, the history will contain a distinct traumatic episode, after which the patient could not ambulate.
  - Physical findings reveal limb shortening, external rotation, and pain on attempted hip motion.
- In some patients, the onset of pain is more insidious.
  - It is usually associated with weight bearing, and it is located in the groin rather than in the buttock or trochanteric area.
  - In the case of a stress fracture, the history of increased activity over a short period of time is suggestive.
  - Night or rest pain suggests pathologic fracture or impending fracture.
- In highly osteopenic patients with minor trauma, a history of groin pain with weight bearing may be a symptom of occult femoral neck fracture, which is a nondisplaced fracture not visible on plain radiographs.

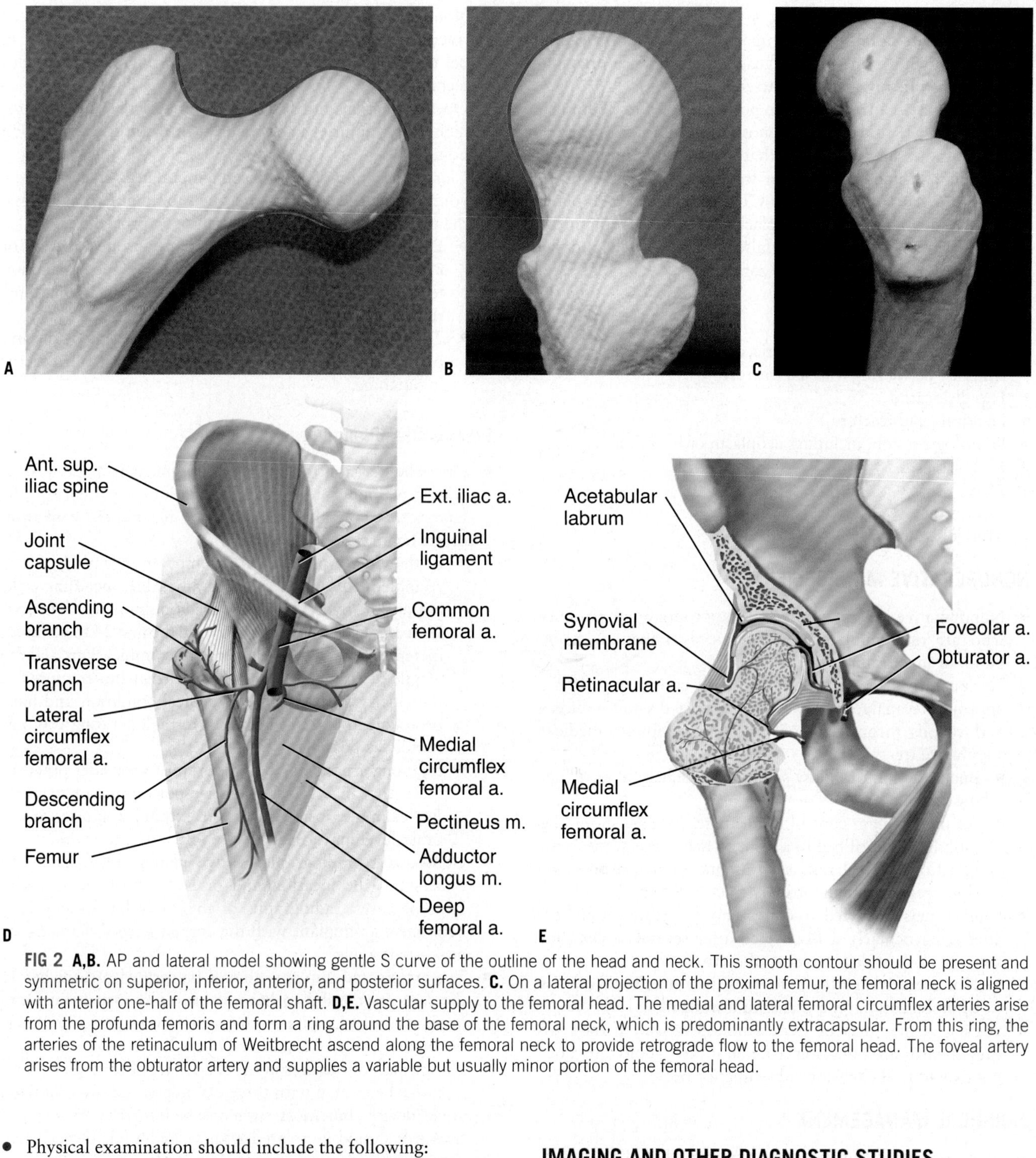

FIG 2 A,B. AP and lateral model showing gentle S curve of the outline of the head and neck. This smooth contour should be present and symmetric on superior, inferior, anterior, and posterior surfaces. **C.** On a lateral projection of the proximal femur, the femoral neck is aligned with anterior one-half of the femoral shaft. **D,E.** Vascular supply to the femoral head. The medial and lateral femoral circumflex arteries arise from the profunda femoris and form a ring around the base of the femoral neck, which is predominantly extracapsular. From this ring, the arteries of the retinaculum of Weitbrecht ascend along the femoral neck to provide retrograde flow to the femoral head. The foveal artery arises from the obturator artery and supplies a variable but usually minor portion of the femoral head.

- Physical examination should include the following:
  - Observation of the lower extremities with comparison of foot position in the supine patient. A shortened, externally rotated limb is consistent with a fracture.
  - Gait observation. Groin pain on attempted weight bearing or an antalgic gait suggests occult femoral neck fracture.
  - Internal and external rotation. Pain in the groin is concerning for femoral neck fracture but may also be caused by fractures of the anterior pelvic ring.
  - Impaction of the heel of the injured leg. Groin pain that did not exist at rest implies hip fracture.
  - A focal neurovascular exam of the involved lower extremity should be performed.

IMAGING AND OTHER DIAGNOSTIC STUDIES

- Standard plain radiographs consist of an AP view of the pelvis and AP and lateral films of the hip.
  - Lateral films may be obtained via a frog-leg technique, cross-table, or the Lowenstein method.
- An AP traction film with internal rotation can be helpful if initial films are difficult to interpret in terms of the location of injury, the fracture pattern, and the reduction obtained as a predictor of what will occur in the operating room.
- An alternative to a traction film with internal rotation view is a computed tomography (CT) scan to further delineate the fracture pattern.

- If clinical suspicion is high (eg, an elderly patient who cannot ambulate because of groin pain) but plain radiographs are negative, a bone scan or magnetic resonance imaging (MRI) may be obtained for low-energy injuries.
  - The bone scan will not turn positive for 24 to 72 hours, but the MRI should be diagnostic within hours of injury.
- Some studies have suggested that any multiply injured patient with a high-energy femur fracture should have imaging of the femoral neck with a CT scan in addition to plain films to identify minimally displaced femoral neck fractures. However, the CT scan may be false negative as well, and the routine use of this modality is controversial.

DIFFERENTIAL DIAGNOSIS

- Intertrochanteric, pertrochanteric, or subtrochanteric fracture
- Anterior pelvic ring (ramus) fracture
- Hip dislocation
- Femoral head fracture
- Pathologic lesion, including neoplasm or infection
- Arthritis
- AVN
- Contusion
- Muscle strain

NONOPERATIVE MANAGEMENT

- Nonoperative treatment may be appropriate in patients who are nonambulators, neurologically impaired, moribund, or in extremis.
- Nonoperative treatment should initially consist of bed rest, appropriate analgesia, protection against decubitus ulcers and venous thromboembolism, and appropriate medical supportive treatment.
  - Buck traction or pillow splints may be helpful in reducing pain.
  - As soon as pain control is adequate, patients should be mobilized out of bed to a chair to help prevent the complications of bed rest, such as pneumonia, aspiration, skin breakdown, and urinary tract infection.
- Some valgus impacted fractures may be treated nonoperatively, particularly if discovered after several weeks, but there is a risk of displacement of up to 46%.
  - Nonoperative treatment for these patients should consist of mobilization on crutches or a walker.[13]
- Stress fractures may be treated nonoperatively if they are caught early, are nondisplaced, and if the fracture line does not extend to the tension side (superior neck).

SURGICAL MANAGEMENT

- Most patients with femoral neck fracture should be considered for surgical treatment.
- Displaced femoral neck fractures in some patient populations may be better served by hemiarthroplasty or total hip arthroplasty, the details of which are beyond the scope of this chapter.
- This includes elderly patients, osteoporotic patients, those with neurologic disease, patients with preexisting hip arthritis, and those with medical illnesses impairing bone healing or longevity (eg, renal failure, diabetes, malignancy, or anticonvulsant treatment).
- Nondisplaced fractures, valgus impacted femoral neck fractures in the elderly, or stress fractures in athletes can be treated with fixation in situ through percutaneous techniques.
- Open reduction and internal fixation is the standard for high-energy injuries in younger healthy patients with good bone.
- Closed reduction of a displaced femoral neck fracture in the young patient is difficult, and one should not accept a less-than-perfect reduction to avoid an open procedure.
  - Evidence demonstrates no difference in rates of AVN or nonunion when comparing closed and open reduction techniques for femoral neck fractures when an anatomic reduction is achieved.[4,12]
  - The quality of the reduction and placement of the implants are the most important surgeon-controlled factor in outcome.

Preoperative Planning

- Once the decision for operative treatment is made, preoperative planning begins with evaluation of patient-specific factors that may alter the timing or technique for fixation of the femoral neck fracture.
  - In the elderly population, prompt optimization of correctable medical conditions is advisable, including evaluation of hydration and cardiopulmonary function. However, delay of surgery beyond the first 24 to 48 hours increases the risk of perioperative complications and the length of stay. Many institutions treat hip fractures in the elderly as an emergent medical condition and have protocols in place to get them to the operating room as rapidly as possible.
  - In younger patients, it is important to consider other injuries that may affect operative positioning or fixation. For example, ipsilateral lower extremity injuries at another level may affect the use of the fracture table.
- Good-quality radiographs in two planes are necessary to understand the location and orientation of the fracture. In some cases, radiographs of the contralateral side may help select an implant with the correct length, diameter, or neck–shaft angle.
- The anticipated implants should be verified present before the case. It is useful to have arthroplasty instruments and implants in the hospital in the event of unexpected findings. Fortunately, this will rarely be needed.
- Nondisplaced fractures in the subcapital or transcervical region can be treated with three cannulated screws or a fixed angle device, but most surgeons believe that basicervical fractures should be treated with a fixed-angle device, such as a sliding hip screw or cephalomedullary nail.

Positioning

- The patient is positioned on a fracture table with the operative hip flexed and contralateral hip extended, or "scissored" **(FIG 3A)**.
  - Owing to the risk of compartment syndrome, the surgeon should avoid using the "well-leg holder," which puts the contralateral leg in a hemilithotomy position (hip and knee flexed, elevating the leg).

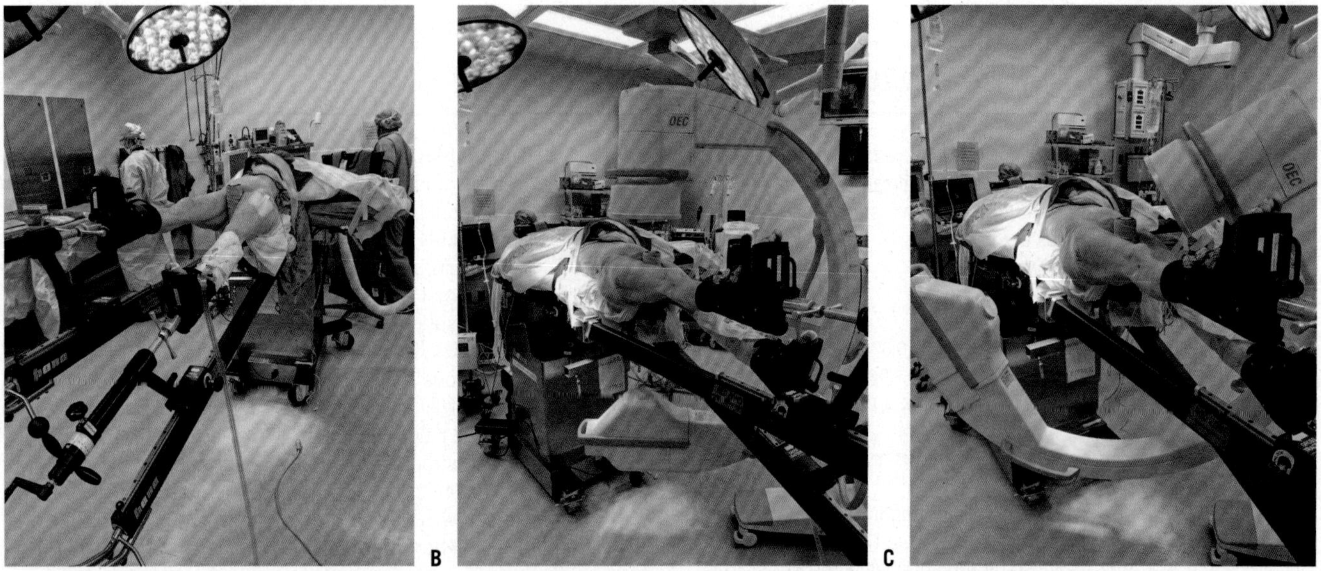

FIG 3 A. Patient setup with the operative leg parallel to the floor and with the contralateral well leg flexed or scissored on a fracture table. The injured leg may be internally rotated to assist with reduction. **B.** AP imaging, the C-arm is brought in from the contralateral side of the table. Typically, the C-arm is rotated approximately 5 to 10 degrees toward the surgeon to obtain a true AP image of the proximal femur. **C.** Lateral image, with the C-arm positioned from the contralateral side of the table.

- Intraoperative fluoroscopy is used, and good visualization of the hip and the fracture reduction in both AP (**FIG 3B**) and lateral projections (**FIG 3C**) should be verified before preparing the leg.
- A closed reduction may sometimes be obtained by applying gentle traction and internal rotation under fluoroscopic control. Vigorous, repeated, and complicated reduction maneuvers are unlikely to be effective and should be avoided. Percutaneous reduction aids such as Steinman pins, a ball-spike pusher, and blocking drill bits/screws can also be used to help facilitate a closed reduction (**FIG 4**). If simple, gentle positioning is not successful in achieving acceptable position, open reduction should be strongly considered. The patient should have full muscle relaxation by the anesthesia providers.
- Reduction is anatomic when the normal contours of the femoral neck are reestablished in both the AP and lateral projections (see **FIG 2A,B**), the normal neck–shaft angle and neck length are restored (as judged from a film of the contralateral hip, or AP pelvis), the relative heights of the femoral head and trochanter are symmetric to the contralateral side, and no gaps are seen in the fracture.
  - If the C-arm images are of poor quality because of patient obesity or other factors, the surgeon must not assume or hope it will be better intraoperatively. If adequate visualization to assess reduction or implant position is not achievable, open reduction under direct visualization is the prudent course.

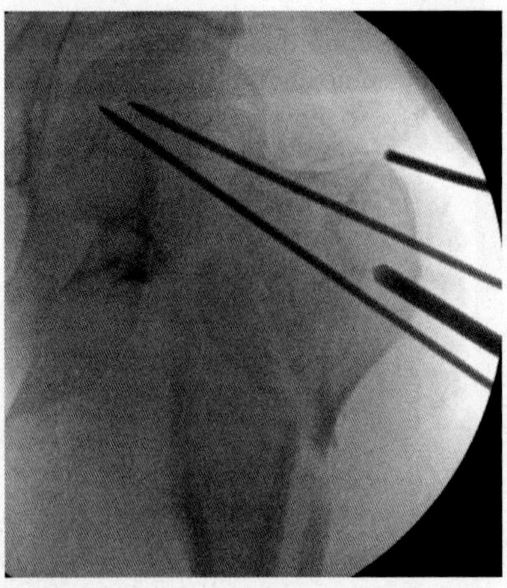

FIG 4 Percutaneous reduction techniques such as the use of a Steinman pin or K-wires can be used to facilitate a closed reduction.

Approach

- A standard lateral approach is used for percutaneous fixation of undisplaced or valgus impacted fractures.
- If an open reduction is planned, a Smith-Petersen or Watson-Jones approach may be used according to surgeon preference to afford visualization of the anterior femoral neck.
  - The Watson-Jones approach is the senior author's preference in most patients. The advantage of this approach is that the same interval can be used for reduction and fixation. However, it is more difficult to visualize the medial femoral neck, especially in morbidly obese or muscular patients.
  - The Smith-Petersen approach is used as an alternative approach in obese or muscular patients. Both are described in the following sections.

CLOSED REDUCTION AND PERCUTANEOUS FIXATION

- The patient is positioned on the fracture table and reduction is obtained as noted earlier, C-arm visualization is verified, and the leg and hip is prepared and draped in a sterile fashion.
- Preoperative antibiotics are given.

Guidewire and Screw Placement

- Guidewires for cannulated screws are placed in line with the femoral neck axis through poke holes or a single 1- to 2-cm incision.
  - The wires are placed parallel using a parallel drill guide or free hand.
  - The standard screw arrangement is an inverted triangle of three screws.
  - They should be positioned peripherally in the femoral neck with good cortical buttress, particularly against the inferior and posterior neck. Starting points below the lesser trochanter should be avoided owing to risk of subtrochanteric fracture postoperatively **(TECH FIG 1A–C)**.
- Once the position of the wires is verified in two planes by fluoroscopy, small (1 cm), full-depth incisions are made at each guide pin, and the soft tissues are spread to the bone.
- The lateral cortex may be drilled in patients with dense bone.
- Self-drilling, self-tapping cannulated screws are placed by power over the guidewires.
  - Washers should be used in the more proximal, metaphyseal locations **(TECH FIG 1D,E)**.
  - Screws should be long enough so that all screw threads are on the proximal (head) side of the fracture and end within 5 mm from subchondral bone. The screws should ideally have a good spread **(TECH FIG 2)**.
  - Some surgeons prefer fully threaded screws to prevent collapse especially in valgus impacted fractures, but this may increase the risk of nonunion or fixation failure.
  - In displaced fractures, the inferior screw shaft should be as close to the calcar as possible to resist varus collapse. If the inferior screw is greater than 3 to 5 mm from the calcar, there is a higher risk of failure.

Arthrotomy

- Many surgeons believe that an arthrotomy should be performed to relieve pressure on the blood supply to the femoral head due to intracapsular bleeding. Some consider this to be mostly important in younger patients with minimally displaced

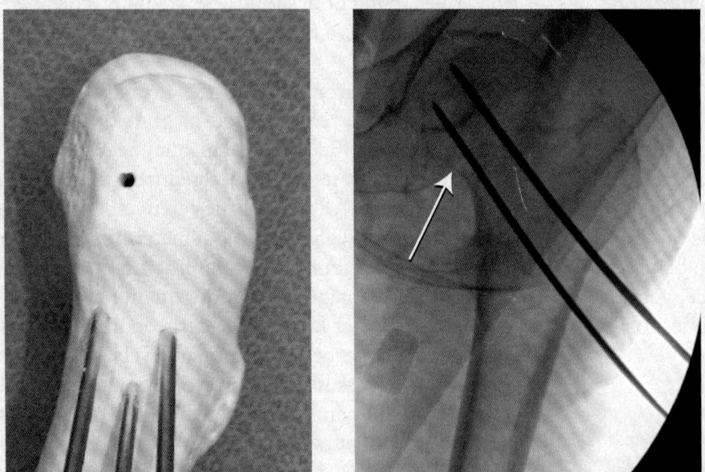

A B

TECH FIG 1 **A.** Sawbones lateral view of the proximal femur showing configuration for three parallel guidewires before placement of cannulated screws. The wire starting points form an inverted triangle. **B.** Intraoperative AP fluoroscopic view showing position and depth of the guidewires. The inferior wire runs right along the inferior cortex of the femoral neck—the "calcar" (*arrow*). **C.** Intraoperative lateral fluoroscopic view showing guidewire position. The posterior wire is directly adjacent to and supported by the posterior cortex of the neck (*arrow*). Care is necessary to ensure that the guidewire does not go outside of the neck and then reenter the femoral head. **D,E.** Intraoperative fluoroscopic views demonstrating cannulated screw insertion over guidewires. **D.** AP view showing use of washers in this metaphyseal location. **E.** Lateral view showing parallel insertion and appropriate depth.

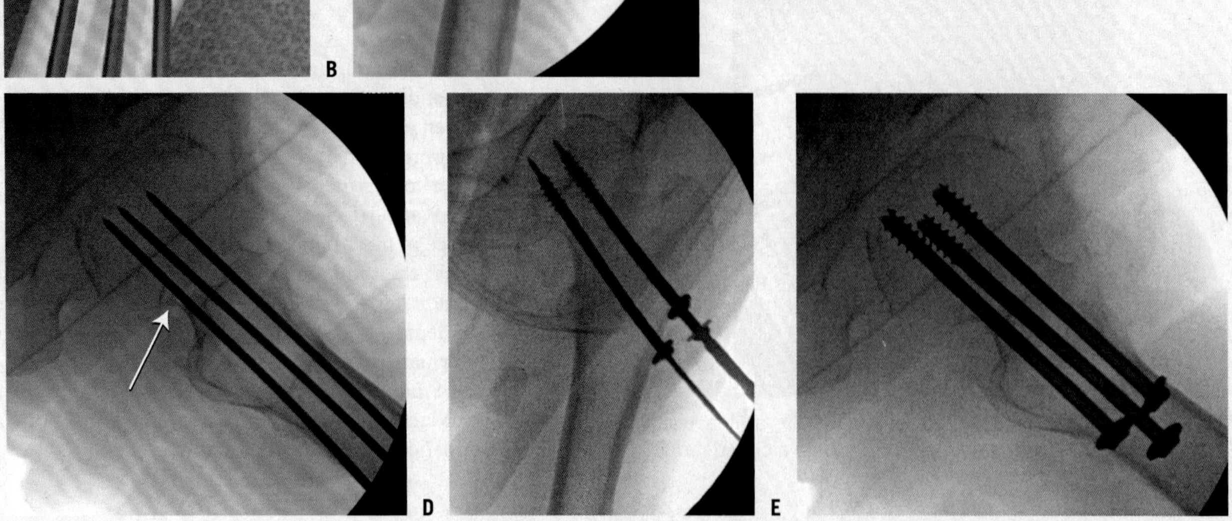

C D E

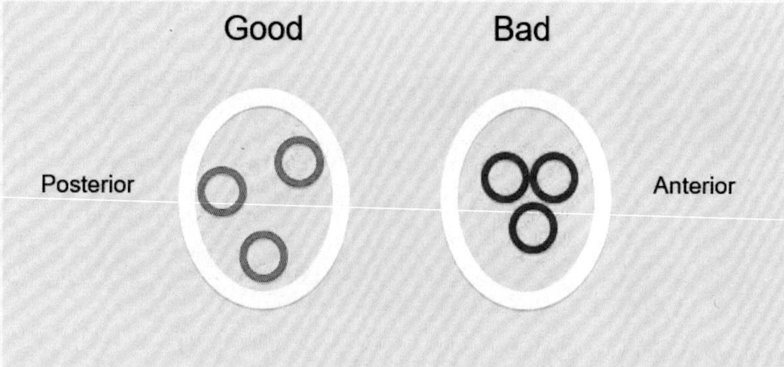

TECH FIG 2 Cannulated screws should ideally have a good spread. The posterior and inferior screws are the most important and should "hug" the cortical surface without penetrating it.

fractures because they reason that more widely displaced fractures have had decompression of the intracapsular hematoma by virtue of the injury. This is controversial, however, as increased capsular pressure has not been clinically associated with AVN.[6]

- A no. 15 blade on a long handle is positioned at the inferior margin of the base of the femoral neck on the AP fluoroscopic image.
- A small skin incision is made at this level, and the soft tissues are spread down to the joint capsule.
- With fluoroscopic verification of position, a small capsulotomy is performed to allow drainage of the hematoma from the capsule.
- A blunt sucker tip can be inserted through this small incision to evacuate any remaining hematoma.

OPEN REDUCTION AND INTERNAL FIXATION THROUGH THE WATSON-JONES APPROACH

- The patient is positioned on the fracture table as described earlier, fluoroscopic visualization is confirmed, and the leg and hip are prepared and draped in a sterile fashion.
  - Circumferential proximal thigh preparation is important.
- Preoperative antibiotics are given.

Soft Tissue Dissection

- The incision is located laterally over the anterior portion of the greater trochanter.
  - It curves slightly anteriorly as it extends proximal from the trochanter toward the crest for about 8 to 10 cm.
  - It extends straight distally about 10 cm from the trochanter **(TECH FIG 3A)**.
- The fascia lata is identified and incised just posterior to the tensor fascia lata muscle.
  - This incision through the fascia extends the length of the skin incision **(TECH FIG 3B)**.
- The anterior inferior edge of the gluteus minimus is identified.
  - The interval between the minimus and the joint capsule is developed.
  - A portion of the minimus insertion on the trochanter can be gently released to facilitate retraction with a curved, blunt Hohmann retractor.
- The reflected head of the rectus femoris is identified **(TECH FIG 3C)** and divided **(TECH FIG 3D)**, leaving a stump to repair.
  - A Cobb elevator can be used to clean muscle fibers off the anterior capsule.
- The capsule is incised in line with the femoral neck axis **(TECH FIG 3E)** and then released in a T shape along the acetabular edge **(TECH FIG 3F)**.
  - Blunt Hohmann retractors can be moved inside the capsule. The surgeon must take care to be very gentle against the posterior femoral neck **(TECH FIG 3G)**.
- The fracture should be clearly exposed.
  - If necessary, the distal part of the capsule, where it inserts anteriorly at the base of the neck, can be released, converting the T arthrotomy to a lazy H (or an I).
- This should be done gently and sparingly, and only if necessary for visualization, as it entails a risk of injury to the ring of vasculature at the base of the femoral neck.

Fracture Reduction

- A 4.5-mm Schanz pin should be placed in the proximal femoral shaft at the subtrochanteric level to facilitate reduction. The use of a T-handle chuck will allow easier manipulation of this pin.
  - A 2.5-mm terminally threaded Kirschner wire (K-wire) is placed in the femoral head at the articular margin to serve as a joystick in the proximal (head) fragment. Sometimes, it is necessary to use two such joysticks to accurately position the head, which, because of its spherical nature, may be difficult to position along three axes simultaneously.
- Reduction is performed under direct visualization using the K-wire and Schanz pin to manipulate the fragments.
  - Internal rotation of the shaft, along with external rotation and adduction of the head fragment, is usually required.
  - Occasionally, a bone hook under the medial inferior portion of the neck will help.
  - When there is significant posteromedial calcar comminution, the previous reduction techniques alone may be insufficient. Often, a Weber, Jungbluth, or other reduction clamp can be used to assist with holding reduction before placement of K-wires **(TECH FIG 4A)**.
  - The reduction is verified by keying the opposing cortical surfaces on the anterior, superior, and inferior neck together under direct visualization. A finger can be gently used to feel the surfaces and verify a smooth reduction without gaps or translation.

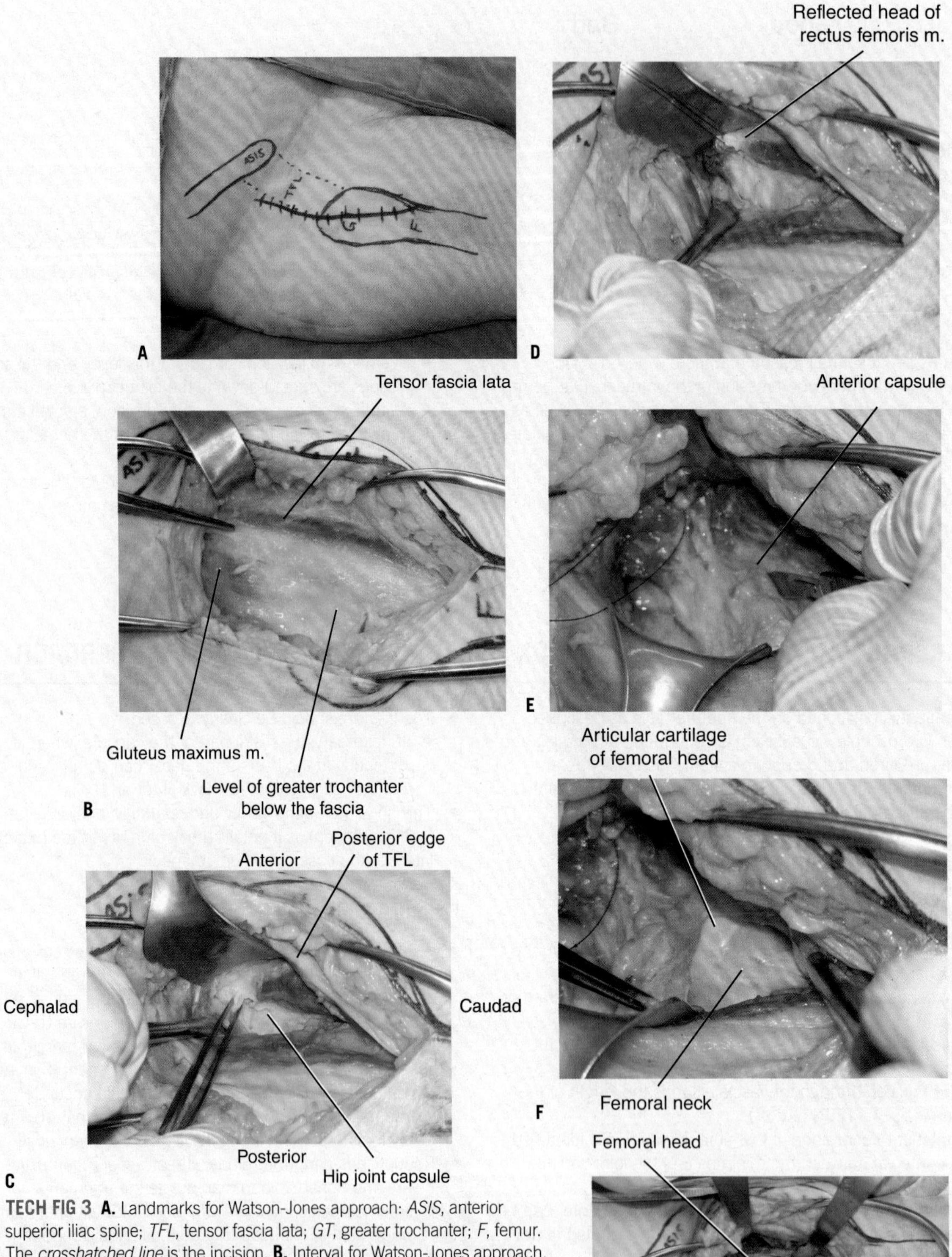

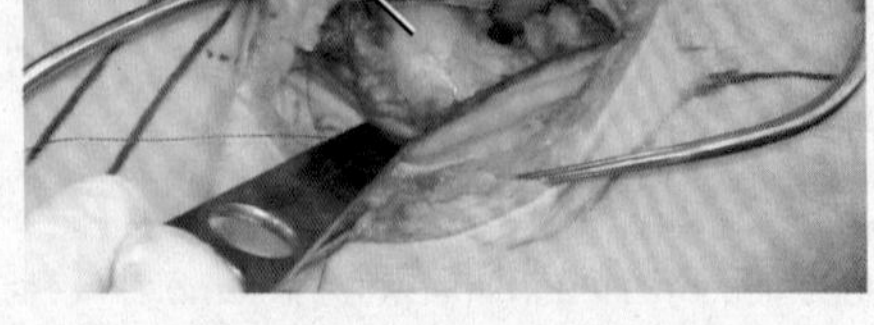

TECH FIG 3 **A.** Landmarks for Watson-Jones approach: *ASIS*, anterior superior iliac spine; *TFL*, tensor fascia lata; *GT*, greater trochanter; *F*, femur. The *crosshatched line* is the incision. **B.** Interval for Watson-Jones approach, shown here between tensor fascia lata anteriorly and gluteus maximus posteriorly, is indicated by the position of the forceps. **C.** The anterior surface of the hip joint capsule has been cleared off. The retractor at the *top* of the picture (anterior on the patient) is under the tensor fascia lata, and the retractor to the *left side* of the picture (cephalad) is under the leading edge of the gluteus minimus. The reflected head of the rectus femoris, attaching on the top of the joint capsule, is grasped by the forceps. **D.** The reflected head of the rectus femoris has been divided and tagged with suture. **E.** The scalpel is in position to perform arthrotomy of the anterior capsule in line with femoral neck. The sutures are in the proximal stump of the reflected head of the rectus. **F.** A T-capsulotomy has been performed, with the transverse arm toward the acetabulum (proximal). **G.** The femoral neck is exposed with the gentle use of Hohmann retractors inside the capsule.

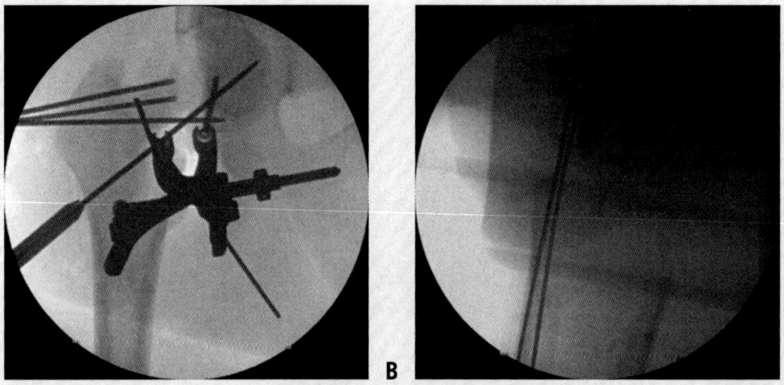

TECH FIG 4 A. When there is significant posteromedial calcar comminution, open clamping may assist with fracture reduction. Here, a Jungbluth clamp is used to assist with holding reduction before placement of K-wires in a highly comminuted femoral neck fracture. **B.** When a sliding hip screw or cephalomedullary nail is used for fixation, reduction K-wires should be kept anterior to facilitate passage of the nail and/or the lag screw into a center-center position of the head.

- The reduction is temporarily stabilized with at least two terminally threaded 2.5-mm K-wires placed from the lateral femoral cortex. In particularly unstable fracture patterns with a tenuous reduction, long K-wires can be directed across the fracture and into the acetabulum for temporary stabilization.
  - It is verified by fluoroscopy in two planes.
  - When a sliding hip screw or cephalomedullary nail is used for fixation, these K-wires should be kept anterior to facilitate passage of the nail and/or the lag screw into a center-center position of the head **(TECH FIG 4B)**.
- Additionally, a medial buttress plate can be placed along the inferomedial calcar to hold reduction. When viewing the femoral head as a clock face on the lateral view, the safe zone for this buttress plate has been described as slightly anterior between 5 o'clock and 6 o'clock.[10]
- When the reduction is anatomic and temporarily stabilized, definitive fixation devices (cannulated screw guidewires, sliding hip screw, or cephalomedullary nail guide) are positioned.

Screw Placement

- Screw fixation is performed as described earlier for percutaneous stabilization.
- For high-angle transcervical fractures (Pauwels 3), one of the lag screws should be positioned in a more horizontal orientation, perpendicular to the fracture plane, to provide compression, which will resist the tendency for shear forces to displace the fracture.
- Alternatively, a fixed-angle implant such as a sliding hip screw or cephalomedullary nail could be used and may give better mechanical fixation in a comminuted fracture or Pauwels 3 fracture pattern.
- Reduction and implant position should be verified with the C-arm.

Wound Closure

- Wound closure includes repair of the capsule, restoration of the reflected head of the rectus, and closure of the fascia lata.
  - Layered closure of the skin and sterile dressings complete the job.
- Portable radiographs in the operating room with the patient still asleep, and the back table still sterile, are useful to avoid surprises in the recovery room.

ALTERNATIVE APPROACH: OPEN REDUCTION AND INTERNAL FIXATION THROUGH THE SMITH-PETERSEN APPROACH

- The patient is positioned on the fracture table as described earlier, fluoroscopic visualization is confirmed, and the leg and hip are prepared and draped in a sterile fashion.
  - Circumferential proximal thigh preparation is important.
- Preoperative antibiotics are given.

Soft Tissue Dissection

- The incision is started approximately 1 to 2 cm distal to the anterior superior iliac spine (ASIS) and runs toward the lateral patella.
  - The incision extends toward the lateral patella approximately 8 to 10 cm. As this alternative approach is typically used in the obese or muscular patient, the incision is frequently larger to achieve adequate exposure.
  - The incision can be carried proximally along the iliac crest or distally toward the lateral border of the patella.
- The interval between the tensor fascia lata and sartorius is identified **(TECH FIG 5A)** and dissected, taking care not to violate the lateral femoral cutaneous nerve, which can typically be found as it exits the fascia 4 to 5 cm distal to the ASIS.
- As this plane is developed, the ascending branch of the lateral femoral circumflex artery crosses between the two muscles and is routinely ligated to allow adequate exposure.
- Deep dissection beyond the sartorius and tensor fascia develops the plane between the gluteus medius and rectus femoris.
  - The gluteus medius is easily retracted.
  - The rectus femoris consists of two heads: a direct head from the anterior inferior iliac spine and an indirect (or reflected) head from the superior lip of the acetabulum and anterior joint capsule.
- The indirect (or reflected) head is routinely elevated with the joint capsule. The direct head can also be detached if needed to improve exposure.

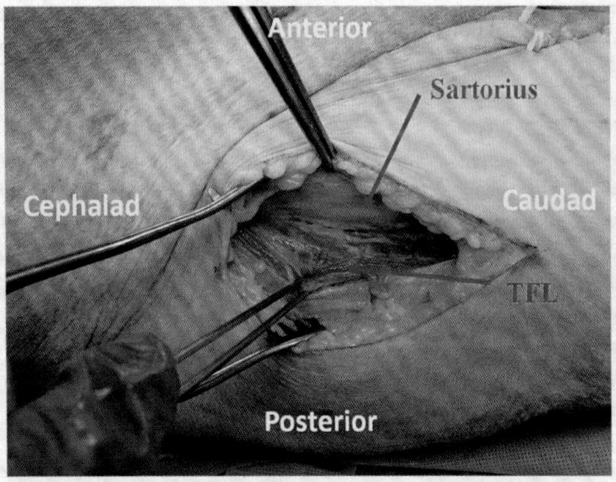

A

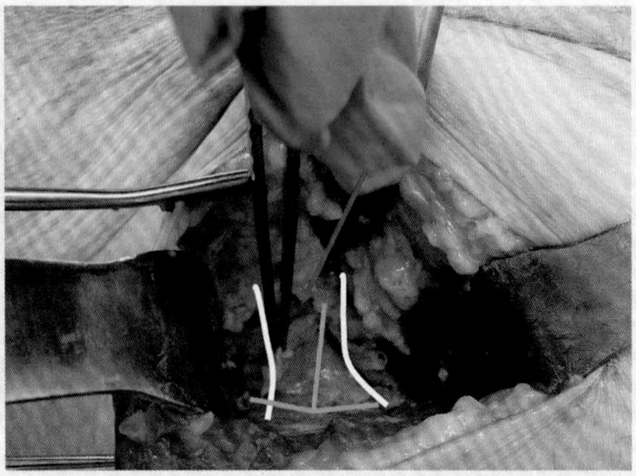

B

TECH FIG 5 **A.** Interval for Smith-Petersen approach, shown here between the sartorius and tensor fascia lata. *TFL*, tensor fascia lata. **B.** A T-capsulotomy has been performed (*green*), with the *arrow* indicating the location of the femoral head and the anterior femoral neck exposed. (Photos courtesy of Drs. Robert V. O'Toole and Ted Manson.)

- Capsulotomy is performed at the lateral neck and carried toward the femoral head **(TECH FIG 5B)**.
  - Hohmann retractors can be moved inside the capsule. The surgeon must take care to be very gentle against the posterior femoral neck.
- The fracture should be clearly exposed.
  - If necessary, the distal part of the capsule, where it inserts anteriorly at the base of the neck, can be released, converting the T arthrotomy to a lazy H (or an I).
- This should be done gently and sparingly, and only if necessary for visualization, as it entails a risk of injury to the ring of vasculature at the base of the femoral neck.
- A separate, direct lateral approach will be needed for placement of lateral hardware or a separate percutaneous approach will be needed for cephalomedullary nail fixation (see the following section).
- A small mini-frag plate can be used along the inferior neck or buttress along the calcar to both hold the reduction in comminuted fractures before placing larger implants and increase the stability especially if cannulated screws are being considered as definitive fixation.

CEPHALOMEDULLARY NAIL FIXATION

- The patient is positioned on the fracture table as described earlier, fluoroscopic visualization is confirmed, and the leg and hip are prepared and draped in a sterile fashion.
  - Circumferential proximal thigh preparation is important.
- Preoperative antibiotics are given.

Incision and Dissection

- A small incision, usually 3 to 4 cm long, is made several centimeters proximal to the tip of the greater trochanter to allow passage of the nail **(TECH FIG 6)**.
- A periosteal elevator can be used to spread the gluteus medius fibers in line with the incision.
- Blunt dissection with an elevator or a finger provides access to the starting point. The tip of the greater trochanter is palpated. The tendon of the gluteus medius attaching to the trochanter can be felt and is protected.

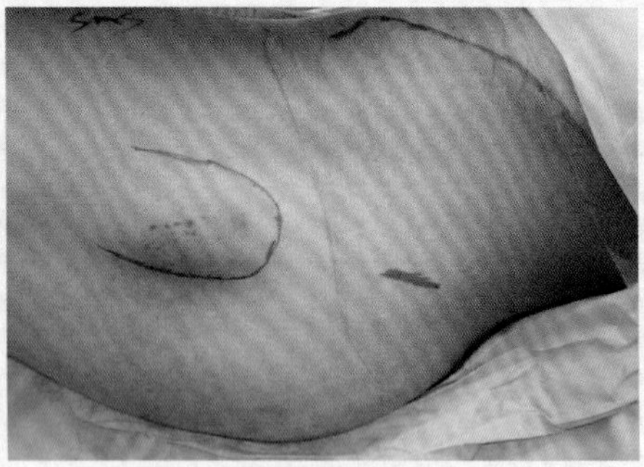

TECH FIG 6 Landmarks for cephalomedullary nail placement. The iliac crest is marked and the trochanter is outlined. The incision is in line with the femoral shaft and several centimeters proximal to the tip of the trochanter.

Starting Point and Reaming

- Using fluoroscopy, a starting point is obtained for the nail at the medial edge of the greater trochanter for a trochanteric-starting cephalomedullary nail.
  - The starting point should be just lateral to the piriformis fossa **(TECH FIG 7A)**.
  - Alternatively, an awl can also be used to obtain the proper starting point; this can be especially useful in obese patients.
- An anatomic reduction of the femoral neck must be achieved before reaming.
  - If an anatomic reduction cannot be achieved by closed means, an open reduction must be performed.
    - This can be done by a Smith-Petersen or Watson-Jones approach, as described earlier.
    - An antirotational pin may be used to maintain reduction **(TECH FIG 7B,C)**.

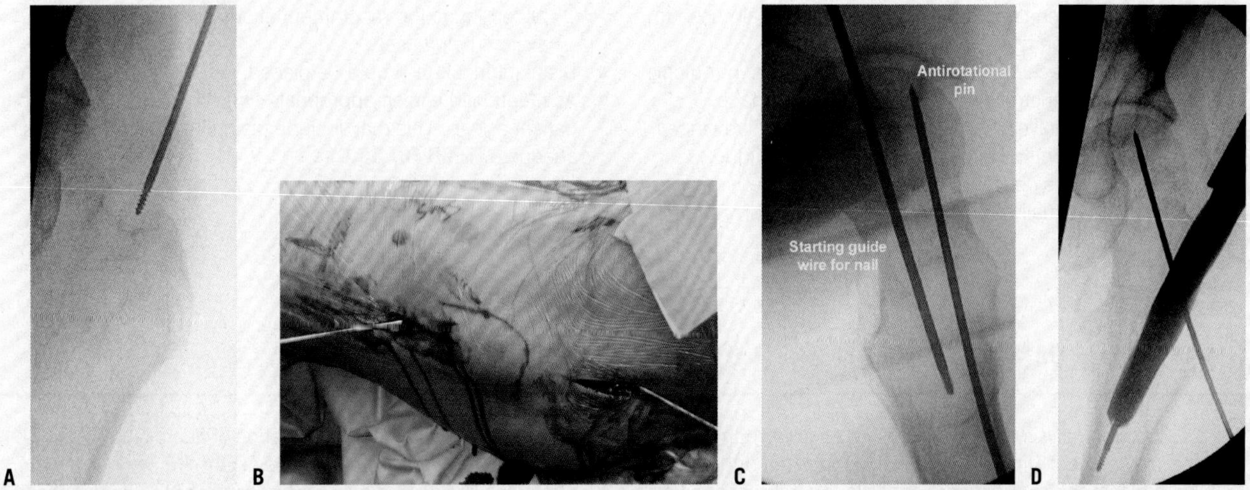

TECH FIG 7 **A.** Intraoperative AP fluoroscopic view showing starting point at medial edge of greater trochanter, in line with the mid-axis of the intramedullary canal. **B.** Intraoperative photograph showing longer incision distally used to obtain anatomic reduction with temporary stabilization pin placed to maintain reduction. **C.** Intraoperative lateral fluoroscopic view showing position of the temporary stabilization pin and the guidewire. **D.** Intraoperative AP fluoroscopic view showing the entry reamer with antirotational pin maintaining reduction of fracture.

- Once reduction has been obtained, the entry reamer is introduced **(TECH FIG 7D)**.
  - For a short cephalomedullary nail, the entry reamer is all that is needed before nail passage.
  - If a long cephalomedullary nail is being placed, serial reaming can be performed to 1 to 1.5 cm over the desired nail diameter.

Proximal and Distal Interlocking

- After the nail is positioned at the correct depth, the guidewire into the femoral head is placed.
  - Multiple fluoroscopic images are needed to make sure the tip of the guidewire is placed within the center of the femoral head for nails with a single screw going into the head.
  - Newer nails with more than one screw going into the head may necessitate adjustments to this technique to allow passage of both screws (such as placing the first lag screw slightly superior to center to allow passage of the second screw inferior to center). Each device has its own recommendations.
- A depth gauge is used to check the length of the guidewire.
- For rotationally unstable femoral neck fractures, an antirotational guidewire or screw can be placed to prevent rotation of the fracture with tapping **(TECH FIG 8A)**.
  - Many nail systems allow a pin to be placed through a sheath attached to the jig or have an antirotational bar to prevent rotational displacement during reaming and screw placement.
- A reamer is then used to open the outer cortex of the femur and is continued into the head under fluoroscopic guidance.
  - The reamer should be checked during passage to ensure the guidewire is not being driven into the pelvis and the reduction is not lost during reaming.

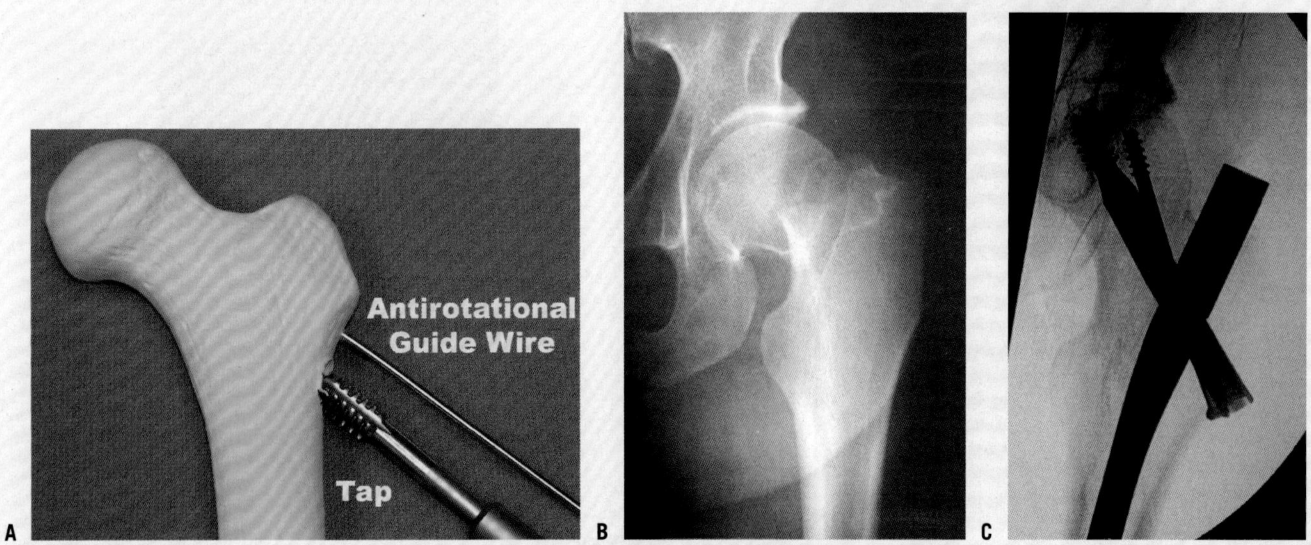

TECH FIG 8 **A.** Antirotational screw is placed in addition to guidewire before tapping when using a sliding hip screw or cephalomedullary nail. **B.** Preoperative radiograph showing a displaced femoral neck fracture. **C.** Final intraoperative AP fluoroscopic view showing anatomic reduction with antirotational screw with cephalomedullary nail.

- The lag screw is then tapped, and fluoroscopy is again used to ensure the reduction is not lost.
- The lag screw is placed and fluoroscopy undertaken in multiple views to rule out penetration of the subchondral surface.
- Most nail systems have a set screw that needs to be advanced to give rotational control for a single lag screw technique.
  - If compression is desired, the set screw then needs to be loosened, usually a quarter-turn of the screwdriver, according to the recommendations of the individual nail system being used.
- Distal interlock(s) should be placed.
- As mentioned earlier, appropriate films should be taken with the patient asleep. This may include plain films if fluoroscopy is not adequate **(TECH FIG 8B,C)**.

MINIMALLY INVASIVE FIXATION WITH A SLIDING HIP SCREW

- In a subgroup analysis, the Fixation using Alternative Implants for the Treatment of Hip Fractures trial demonstrated that sliding hip screws are superior to cancellous screws in smokers and basicervical fractures, although there does appear to be higher rate of radiographic AVN associated with their use.[3]

Positioning, Reduction, and Guidewire Placement

- The patient is positioned on the fracture table as described earlier. Fluoroscopic visualization is performed, and reduction is confirmed to be acceptable in all planes.
- In femoral neck fractures, as opposed to intertrochanteric or pertrochanteric fractures, the reduction must be verified as anatomic if one is to expect stability and healing.
- In this approach, as opposed to the technique described in Chapter 48, the guidewire is inserted percutaneously by poking through the skin under the guidance of fluoroscopy and with use of an appropriate angle guide **(TECH FIG 9A)**.
- The guidewire is positioned at the center of the femoral head as described in Chapter 48 **(TECH FIG 9B)**.
- If the fracture is rotationally unstable (transcervical, comminuted, widely displaced before reduction), an antirotational wire or screw should be placed up the neck across the fracture to prevent loss of reduction (see **TECH FIG 8A**).

Incision and Preparation of Bone

- An incision is made beginning at the guidewire and extending distally for 4 to 5 cm **(TECH FIG 10A)**.
  - A full-thickness skin-to-bone incision is made.
  - Soft tissues are gently spread with a clamp, and an elevator is used to clear tissue from the lateral cortex distal to the pin entry site for the length of a two-hole plate.
- The guidewire is measured.
- The reamer is then set to this depth **(TECH FIG 10B)**.
  - Fluoroscopy should be checked intermittently during reaming because the guidewire can migrate into the pelvis if bound by the reamer.

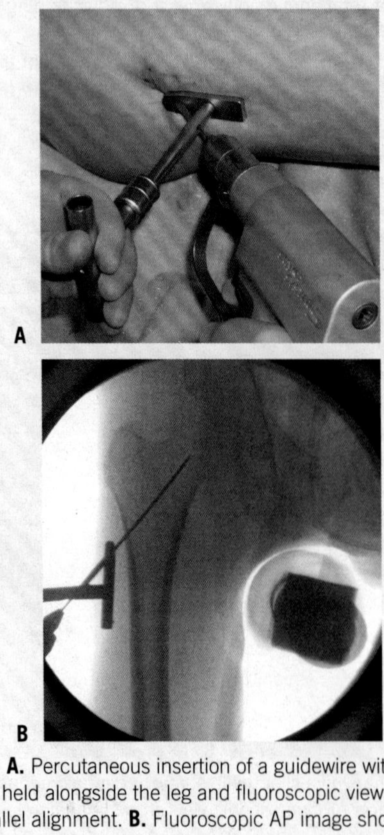

TECH FIG 9 **A.** Percutaneous insertion of a guidewire with angle guide. The guide is held alongside the leg and fluoroscopic views are obtained to verify parallel alignment. **B.** Fluoroscopic AP image showing insertion of guidewire, which has been stabbed through the skin.

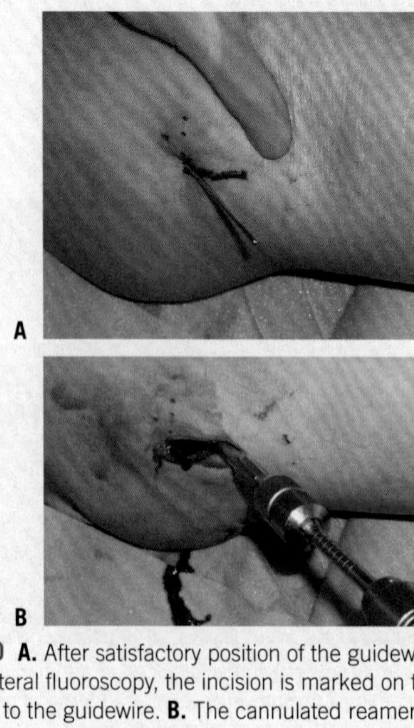

TECH FIG 10 **A.** After satisfactory position of the guidewire is verified on AP and lateral fluoroscopy, the incision is marked on the skin 4 to 5 cm inferior to the guidewire. **B.** The cannulated reamer is used to prepare the bone for the lag screw.

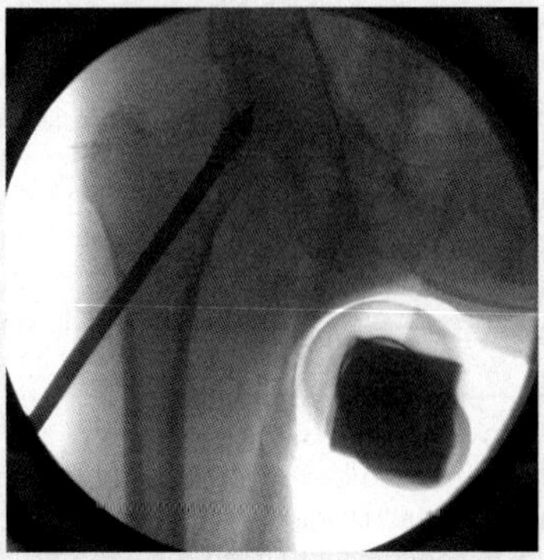

TECH FIG 11 The lag screw is placed over the guidewire after reaming and position is verified with fluoroscopy. Once the lag screw is positioned, the two-hole side plate can be placed through the same incision.

Implant Placement

- The lag screw is then placed over the guidewire in standard fashion **(TECH FIG 11)**.
- The femoral neck–shaft angle has been set by placement of the guide pin, but it can be measured intraoperatively with a guide to select the appropriate implant.
  - This is usually a 135-degree side plate if placed correctly.
- The side plate is then placed over the lag screw and gently worked through the soft tissues until it is placed into contact with the lateral cortex. The skin is quite mobile and elastic, and with a little stretching, the plate can be positioned easily.
  - Final seating can be done with light blows of a mallet with the aid of a "candlestick" impaction device.
  - A two-hole plate is sufficient.
- If the lag screw was not placed with the key parallel to the femoral shaft, most systems allow this to be corrected by simply reapplying the T-handle screwdriver to the lag screw and turning the plate and screw as one unit until the plate fits appropriately.
- Usually, only two bicortical screws are needed through the side plate into the shaft.
- Most systems allow the insertion of a compression screw to further compress the fracture site. Care must be taken in compressing high-energy, comminuted fracture patterns **(TECH FIG 12)**.
- As mentioned earlier, appropriate films should be taken with the patient asleep. This may include plain films if fluoroscopy is not adequate.

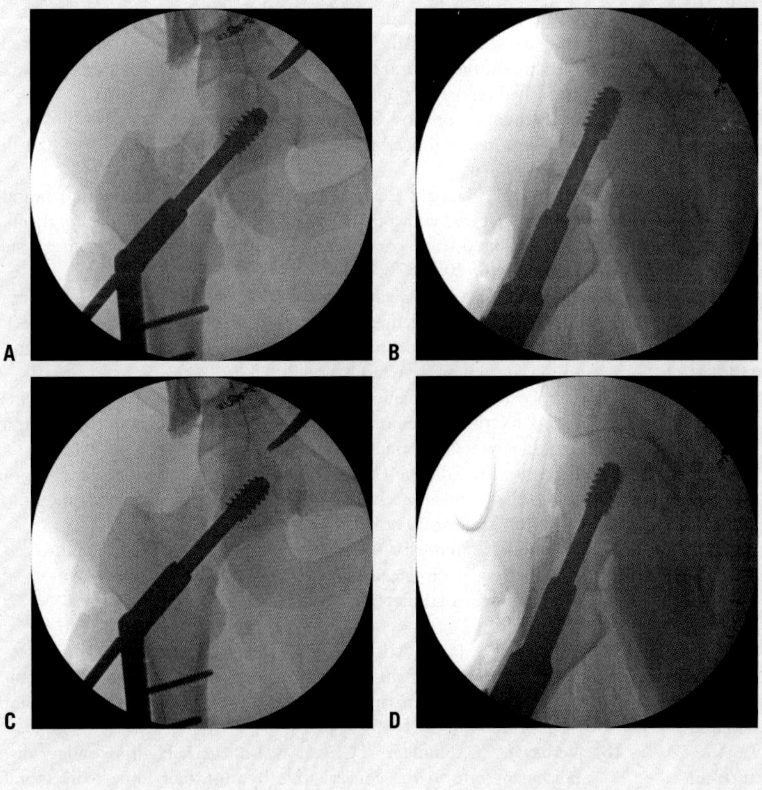

TECH FIG 12 AP (**A**) and lateral (**B**) of a right femoral neck fracture with sliding hip lag screw placed prior to compression. AP (**C**) and lateral (**D**) of the same femoral neck fracture after insertion of a compression screw to close the fracture gap.

Pearls and Pitfalls

Imaging	• The pattern of injury must be recognized preoperatively. A traction film with internal rotation can help with this as initial plain films are usually externally rotated and may be difficult to interpret. • If the clinical examination is suspicious despite negative plain films, a screening MRI is indicated to rule out an occult femoral neck fracture. • Although controversial, a CT scan of the femoral neck should be considered in all trauma patients with femur fractures.
Positioning	• Pelvic rotation: Either scissor legs with the fracture table or the torso is leaned away from the affected side to prevent pelvic tilt. • The patients should be draped wide, from the lower ribs to below the knee, to allow complete access to the femur if problems arise.
Reduction	• Internal rotation of the fractured-side leg holder will reduce anterior neck diastasis. • Guidewire joysticks using 2.5-mm terminally threaded K-wires and Schanz pins can be used to help obtain reduction (usually used when an open reduction is necessary). These should be kept anterior in the neck to facilitate passage of a nail or lag screw. • Temporarily pinning the reduced fracture to the pelvis may be helpful in very unstable fracture patterns. • Reduction is facilitated by complete muscle relaxation. • An anatomic reduction is necessary. An open approach should be used if there is any question that the reduction is not perfect.
Fixation	• The surgeon should avoid starting cannulated screws inferior to the lesser trochanter to minimize the risk of subtrochanteric femur fracture. • Screws are positioned against the femoral neck cortex, especially inferiorly and posteriorly. • For high-angle fractures (Pauwels 3), the surgeon should consider using an additional horizontal screw, sliding hip screw, or cephalomedullary nail. • If the fracture is comminuted or rotationally unstable, the surgeon should consider placing a sliding hip screw or cephalomedullary nail. • If using a sliding hip screw or cephalomedullary nail, the tip–apex distance should be 25 mm or less, calculated by adding the distance from the center of the femoral head at the level of the subchondral bone to the tip of the screw on both the AP and lateral radiographs.

POSTOPERATIVE CARE

- In the elderly, mentally competent patient with stable fixation, weight bearing is allowed as tolerated.
- Younger patients are typically made non–weight bearing or touchdown weight bearing to the affected extremity for approximately 6 to 12 weeks postoperatively, usually due to higher energy and comminution.
- For deep vein thrombosis prophylaxis, the length and type of treatment are controversial, but some form of prophylaxis should be given at least during the patient's hospital stay.
- A first-generation cephalosporin is given for 24 hours postoperatively.

OUTCOMES

- The 1-year mortality rate is about 20% in the elderly.[11]
- About 50% of elderly patients return to their previous level of function.[7]

COMPLICATIONS

- There is approximately 16% rate of AVN with displaced femoral neck fractures.[5]
- There is approximately 33% rate of nonunion with displaced femoral neck fractures.[5]

REFERENCES

1. Cronin PK, Freccero DM, Kain MS, et al. Garden 1 and 2 femoral neck fractures collapse more than expected after closed reduction and percutaneous pinning. J Orthop Trauma 2019;33(3):116–119.
2. Cummings SR, Rubin SM, Black D. The future of hip fractures in the United States. Numbers, costs, and potential effects of postmenopausal estrogen. Clin Orthop Relat Res 1990;(252):163–166.
3. Fixation using Alternative Implants for the Treatment of Hip fractures (FAITH) Investigators. Fracture fixation in the operative management of hip fractures (FAITH): an international, multicentre, randomised controlled trial. Lancet 2017;389:1519–1527.
4. Ghayoumi P, Kandemir U, Morshed S. Evidence based update: open versus closed reduction. Injury 2015;46(3):467–473.
5. Lu-Yao GL, Keller RB, Littenberg B, et al. Outcomes after displaced fractures of the femoral neck. A meta-analysis of one hundred and six published reports. J Bone Joint Surg Am 1994;76A:15–25.
6. Maruenda JI, Barrios C, Gomar-Sancho F. Intracapsular hip pressure after femoral neck fracture. Clin Orthop Relat Res 1997;(340):172–180.
7. Pajarinen J, Lindahl J, Michelsson O, et al. Pertrochanteric femoral fractures treated with a dynamic hip screw or a proximal femoral nail. A randomised study comparing post-operative rehabilitation. J Bone Joint Surg Br 2005;87B:76–81.
8. Palm H, Gosvig K, Krasheninnikoff M, et al. A new measurement for posterior tilt predicts reoperation in undisplaced femoral neck fractures. 113 consecutive patients treated by internal fixation and followed for 1 year. Acta Orthop 2009;80(3):303–307.
9. Papakostidis C, Panagiotopoulos A, Piccioli A, et al. Timing of internal fixation of femoral neck fractures. A systematic review and meta-analysis of the final outcome. Injury 2015;46(3):459–466.
10. Putnam SM, Collinge CA, Gardner MJ, et al. Vascular anatomy of the medial femoral neck and implications for surface plate fixation. J Orthop Trauma 2019;33(3):111–115.
11. Rogmark C, Johnell O. Primary arthroplasty is better than internal fixation of displaced femoral neck fractures: a meta-analysis of 14 randomized studies with 2,289 patients. Acta Orthop 2006;77:359–367.
12. Upadhyay A, Jain P, Mishra P, et al. Delayed internal fixation of fractures of the neck of the femur in young adults. A prospective, randomised study comparing closed and open reduction. J Bone Joint Surg Br 2004;86(7):1035–1040.
13. Verheyen CC, Smulders TC, van Walsum AD. High secondary displacement rate in the conservative treatment of impacted femoral neck fractures in 105 patients. Arch Orthop Trauma Surg 2005;125:166–168.

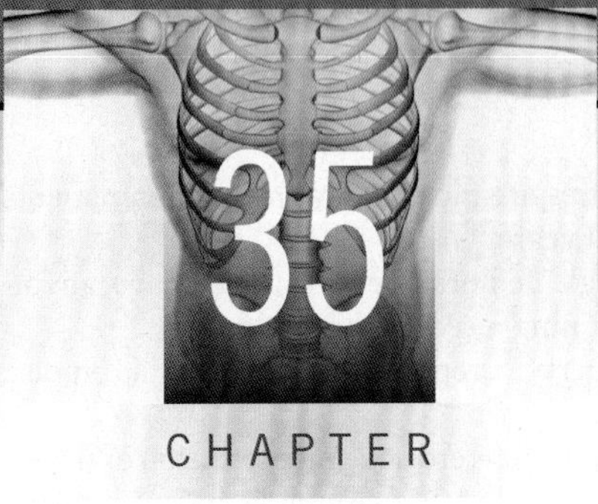

Hemiarthroplasty of the Hip

Hari P. Bezwada and Brian M. Culp

DEFINITION

- Femoral neck fractures are classified according to the Garden classification **(TABLE 1)**.[10]
  - This classification divides these fractures into displaced or nondisplaced fractures. Guidelines for treatment of nondisplaced femoral neck fractures are beyond the scope of this chapter. There are some recent reports however that suggest hemiarthroplasty may be indicated even in the setting of a nondisplaced fracture in decreasing the rate of reoperation.[19]
- The generally accepted indications for a hemiarthroplasty of the hip include displaced femoral neck fractures or other proximal femoral fractures that do not lend themselves to internal fixation and salvage for massive acetabular osteolytic defects in revision total hip arthroplasty (THA). Ideally, hemiarthroplasty should be reserved for elderly patients with low functional demands. Younger, more active patients may have improved outcomes with THA.[22]
- Published reports suggest that hemiarthroplasty has poor outcomes when used as a primary prosthesis for failures with degenerative joint disease, and this technique currently is not recommended. Similarly, poor results have been noted for hemiarthroplasty in the treatment of osteonecrosis of the femoral head.[14]
- The two types of hemiarthroplasty implants are the unipolar type (ie, Austin Moore; **FIG 1A**) and the bipolar type **(FIG 1B)**.
  - The bipolar prosthesis has been favored because of its theoretical reduction of wear on the acetabular side. Motion between the inner and outer heads of the prosthesis leads to less motion at the acetabulum–implant interface.[18] There also has been suggested slightly superior resistance to prosthetic hip dislocation with bipolar design when compared to a unipolar design but that has not born out in the literature.[15] Furthermore, there is some concern over the polyethylene wear characteristics, which may act as a source of osteolysis. Added costs associated with bipolar heads also may prove to have greater relevance especially with cost containment strategies and alternative payment models.

TABLE 1 Garden's Classification of Femoral Neck Fractures

Grade	Description
I	Incomplete fracture with valgus impaction
II	Nondisplaced fracture through femoral neck
III	Incompletely displaced fracture through femoral neck
IV	Completely displaced fracture with no engagement of fragments

ANATOMY

- The neck–shaft angle is about 130 ± 7 degrees in adults and does not vary significantly between genders.
- The femoral neck is anteverted 10.4 ± 6.7 degrees with respect to the femoral shaft in Caucasians.
  - Some ethnic groups (eg, Asians) have a propensity for higher degrees of anteversion, up to 30%.
- Native femoral head diameters range from 40 to 60 mm.
- Femoral neck length and shape vary considerably.
  - In cross-section, the femoral neck is cam-shaped, with a shorter anteroposterior (AP) than mediolateral diameter.
- The calcar femorale is a condensed, vertically oriented area of bone that originates superiorly and fuses with the cortex at the posterior aspect of the femoral neck.
- The major vascular supply of the femoral head comes from the lateral epiphyseal branch of the medial femoral circumflex artery.
  - Other contributing vessels include the inferior metaphyseal artery, arising from the lateral femoral circumflex artery, and the medial epiphyseal artery through the ligamentum teres, arising from the obturator artery.[12]

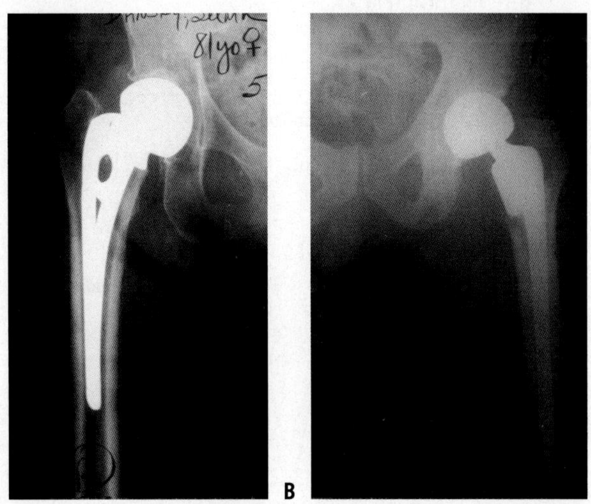

A B

FIG 1 **A.** Austin Moore prosthesis. **B.** Cemented bipolar prosthesis.

PATHOGENESIS

- In elderly persons, a femoral neck fracture is usually the result of a fall.
- Several mechanisms have been proposed:
  - A direct blow to the lateral aspect of the greater trochanter from a fall
  - A sudden increase in load with the head fixed in the acetabulum along with a lateral, rotatory force. This causes impaction of the posterior neck on the acetabulum.
  - A fatigue fracture that precedes and causes a fall
  - The incidence of femoral neck fractures increases as bone density falls to osteoporotic levels.
- Femoral neck fractures in young patients typically are the result of high-energy mechanisms.
  - The mechanical explanation is axial loading of the distal femur or the foot if the knee is extended.
  - The amount of bony displacement and associated soft tissue injury can be much higher and demonstrate more vertical fracture patterns.
- Displacement of a femoral neck fracture can lead to disruption of the vascular supply of the femoral neck.
  - This vascular compromise may contribute to the high incidence of avascular necrosis (AVN) with this injury.
- If femoral neck fracture occurs, the intraosseous cervical vessels are disrupted.
  - The risk of AVN generally corresponds to the degree of displacement of the fracture of the femoral neck on initial radiographs.
  - In displaced fractures, most of the retinacular vessels are disrupted. Femoral head blood supply is then dependent on remaining retinacular vessels and those functioning vessels in the ligamentum teres.
  - The role of early fixation and joint capsulotomy in prevention of AVN remains controversial.
- The incidence of nonunion following a displaced fracture is as high as 60% with nonoperative treatment in some reports.
- Femoral neck fractures can be divided into subcapital, transcervical, and basicervical types, based on the location of the injury.
  - Basicervical fractures can often be treated in a manner similar to intertrochanteric fractures with regard to fracture fixation (**FIG 2**).

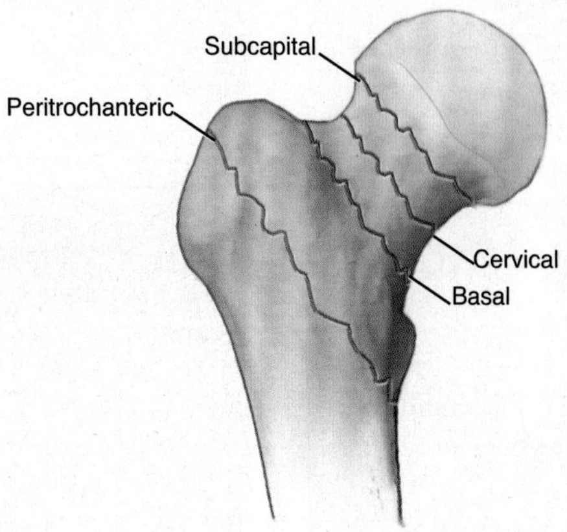

FIG 2 Geography of proximal femoral fractures.

NATURAL HISTORY

- Femoral neck fractures are most commonly seen in patients older than age of 50 years.[20]
- Patients with a single femoral neck fracture have an increased risk of sustaining a second hip fracture.
- Bateman[2] and Gilberty[11] reported the use of a bipolar prosthesis.
  - The rationale was that less erosion and protrusion of the acetabulum would occur because motion is present between the metal head and polyethylene socket's inner bearing.
  - Acetabular wear is diminished by reduction of the total amount of motion that occurs between the acetabular cartilage and metallic outer shell with interposition of the second low-friction inner bearing within the implant.
  - Overall hip motion also may be greater because of the compound bearing surface.
- Barnes et al[1] showed that mortality in the first month postoperatively was substantial, as high as 13.3% in men and 7.4% in women.
  - More importantly, delaying surgery beyond 72 hours led to a substantial increase in the mortality rate.
- Factors influencing mortality in hemiarthroplasty include cardiac history, residence in a nursing home, chronic pulmonary disease, elevated serum creatinine, pneumonia, history of myocardial infarction, duration of surgery, and gender.[8] The time from injury to surgery has also been associated with greater postoperative morbidity and amount of time spent optimizing the patient for surgery should be minimized.[17]
- Associated injuries may include subdural or epidural hematoma and ipsilateral upper extremity injury for low-energy fractures.
  - High-energy fracture patterns have a higher incidence of associated injury, including closed head injury, pneumo- or hemothorax, spinal fracture, visceral injury, and ipsilateral lower extremity bony injury.[5]

PATIENT HISTORY AND PHYSICAL FINDINGS

- A complaint of groin, proximal thigh, or, rarely, lateral hip pain following a fall in an elderly patient should raise suspicion for a low-energy femoral neck fracture.
- If a patient has fallen on the floor and is unable to bear weight, this should also raise suspicion for a femoral neck fracture.
- The patient's preinjury ambulatory status must be ascertained when the history is taken. His or her preoperative activity level can help determine the most appropriate type of surgical management.
- Care must be taken to evaluate other possible sources of injury about the hip as well as associated ipsilateral injury.
  - Pelvic fracture: Associated injury to the pelvic rami is common. Radiographs are useful in diagnosing these associated injuries.
  - Acetabular fracture: In a low-energy injury, acetabular fracture is an uncommon association with a femoral neck fracture. However, this is not the case in high-energy injury patterns. Thin-slice computed tomography (CT) may be useful for diagnosing this injury.
  - Inter- and subtrochanteric fracture: Injury to the intertrochanteric area is commonly seen about the hip in elderly patients. Subtrochanteric fractures are less common. Usually, the limb is held in extension, not in a flexed, externally

rotated position. Radiographs again are useful for establishing the diagnosis.

- A thorough physical examination should include the following:
  - Observation of the lower extremity. If it is shortened, externally rotated, and painful to move, a joint effusion secondary to fracture hematoma is most likely responsible. Flexion and external rotation of the hip is often seen as this physiologic position increases the available space within the joint capsule.
  - Logroll maneuver, which is a very sensitive physical finding. A positive result elicits pain at the groin due to the side-to-side movement of the lower extremity, which creates shear forces across a femoral neck fracture, leading to exquisite pain.
  - Axial load test, which is positive if the maneuver elicits pain at the groin. This test is less specific than the logroll test.
  - Range-of-motion tests. Pain at the end points of the range of motion may be the only clue to detect a nondisplaced occult fracture.
  - Straight leg raise should also be attempted and associated pain may also aid in diagnosis.

IMAGING AND OTHER DIAGNOSTIC STUDIES

- Plain radiographs of the AP pelvis and injured hip should be obtained.
  - If possible, the legs should be immobilized in 15 degrees of internal rotation for the film.
  - A shoot-through lateral radiograph is useful for determining the degree of displacement of the fracture fragment, especially for fractures that appear minimally displaced on an AP view.
- A radiograph taken while applying axial traction is helpful to determine location of the fracture along the femoral neck if displacement of the fracture fragments obscures a view of the fracture pattern. This may also help to differentiate between low femoral neck fractures and peritrochanteric pattern fractures amenable to fixation.
- CT scanning is useful for identifying nondisplaced fractures when clinically suspected as well as associated injuries. However, it usually is not routinely employed for an isolated, low-energy femoral neck fracture.
- Radionucleotide uptake bone scans are helpful in identifying occult femoral neck fractures but may take up to 72 hours to be apparent on film.
- Magnetic resonance imaging is more sensitive in identifying occult femoral neck fractures than CT scan or bone scan within the first 72 hours and is more commonly recommended as a diagnostic modality when the patient is able to tolerate this study.
  - It also is highly sensitive to identifying occult fractures at the ipsilateral intertrochanteric area.

DIFFERENTIAL DIAGNOSIS

- Intertrochanteric fracture
- Subtrochanteric fracture
- Pelvic fracture
- Acetabular fracture
- Hip contusion or traumatic trochanteric bursitis

NONOPERATIVE MANAGEMENT

- Acute femoral neck fractures are rarely managed nonoperatively. Both nondisplaced and displaced fracture patterns have better functional and overall outcomes when treated surgically.
  - Nonoperative management may be relatively indicated in the patient with severe medical comorbidities who is unable to tolerate anesthesia for surgical intervention.
  - Because nondisplaced fractures can be internally fixed with percutaneous techniques under local anesthetic and monitored sedation, nonoperative treatment is usually not indicated for this fracture type.
- In most cases, nonoperative treatment should be limited to initial management of the injury before surgical stabilization.
  - A soft pillow may be placed under the patient's knee and leg to keep them in a comfortable position.
- All patients with femoral neck fractures should be placed on strict bed rest with a Foley catheter and intravenous fluids on admission.
- Axial traction of the injured lower extremity is contraindicated for femoral neck fractures because it can increase displacement of the fracture fragments.

SURGICAL MANAGEMENT

- The best method of surgical fixation of femoral neck fractures is controversial.[9] The debate between internal fixation versus arthroplasty continues and is beyond the scope of this chapter.
- General indications for surgical management using hemiarthroplasty include the elderly patient with low functional demands or poor bone quality not amenable to internal fixation.
- Hemiarthroplasty is indicated for patients with displaced femoral neck fractures who meet the following criteria:
  - Reasonable general health
  - Pathologic hip fractures
  - Neurologic diseases including Parkinson disease, previous stroke, or hemiplegia
  - Physiologic age older than 75 to 80 years
  - Severe osteoporosis with loss of primary trabeculae in the femoral head
  - Inadequate closed reduction
  - Displaced fracture
  - Preexisting hip disease on the femoral side, namely osteonecrosis, without any acetabular disease
- Contraindications include the following:
  - Preexisting sepsis
  - Young age
  - Failure of internal fixation devices, mainly because of acetabular damage that often occurs in that situation
  - Preexisting acetabular disease. Even patients with normal preoperative cartilaginous space may become symptomatic after about 5 years due to degradation caused by friction between the metal and the acetabular cartilage.
- Indications for cementing a femoral stem vary from surgeon to surgeon and institution to institution.
  - Primary candidates for this approach are patients with poor bone quality, such as those with a stovepipe femur or Dorr type C femur.[6] These patients can be difficult to manage with uncemented implants because they require either massive, canal-filling, uncemented implants that

often produce significant stress shielding of the femur or have proximally filled implants that can make accurate adjustment of limb lengths very difficult.

- Antibiotic-impregnated cement may be advisable for certain high-risk groups of patients. Some patients, such as those on dialysis, may be more prone to sepsis, and use of antibiotic-impregnated cement may be considered appropriate.
  - Appropriate antibiotics include tobramycin, vancomycin, cefazolin, and erythromycin.
- Cemented stems also should be considered for patients with pathologic fractures. For these patients, the use of cement with a bone-replacing prosthesis may be the preferred treatment, regardless of age or bone quality.
- The first-generation cementing technique involved finger-packing without the use of pressurization and a reduction of porosity. Modern cementing techniques use a medullary brush, cement restrictor, medullary pulsatile lavage, the insertion of epinephrine-soaked sponges, reduction of cement porosity (ie, vacuum mixing), cement centralizers, and a cement gun for retrograde cement insertion, after which pressurization can be performed with a surgeon's gloved finger or, alternatively, with a wedge-shaped pressurization device.
- Because of the embolic load secondary to pressurization, surgeons may avoid cemented components in patients with a history of cardiopulmonary disease.
- Some data suggests a higher incidence of periprosthetic femur fracture for noncemented arthroplasty, and this may influence the choice of fixation technique in patients with poor quality bone.[13]

Preoperative Planning

- It is important that the preoperative x-rays are reviewed and templated for appropriate size and for fixation.
- Appropriate implant selection should be undertaken, whether to proceed with a tapered stem, a diaphyseal engaging stem, or a cemented stem.
- The patient should undergo an appropriate preoperative workup including medical and anesthesia evaluations.
  - Banked blood should also be available.
  - Important preoperative laboratory studies include complete blood counts, electrolytes, and coagulation studies.
  - Additional blood tests could include total protein, albumin, and appropriate liver studies to evaluate the patient's overall nutritional status. Other studies that may be helpful include vitamin D and thyroid function testing as these may point to opportunities to intervene on bone quality and future fracture prevention.
- Electrocardiogram, chest radiograph, and possibly, further cardiac studies, including echocardiogram, may be appropriate preoperatively.
- The femoral head size must be evaluated to establish the correct component size. This can be assessed with templating or with various surgical instruments at the time of surgery.
  - If the component is too large, equatorial contact occurs, which can result in a tight joint with decreased motion and pain.
  - If the component is too small, polar contact occurs, leading to increased contact stresses and, therefore, to greater erosion and possible superomedial migration.
- It is also important to template neck length and offset.
  - If the neck length is too long, reduction can be difficult, and the increased soft tissue tension could lead to increased pressure on the acetabular cartilage.
  - The offset should be reproduced postoperatively. It can be created by evaluating the distance between the center of the femoral head and the greater trochanter, thereby restoring the length of the abductor mechanism and decreasing postoperative limp.
- These procedures can be performed under neuraxial or general anesthesia. Spinal or epidural anesthesia may show some benefit because neuraxial anesthesia may have the benefit of reducing blood loss and postoperative confusion.
- Prophylactic antibiotics are administered before the surgery.
- The procedure must be performed in a clean operating room with laminar flow. Vertical laminar airflow in conjunction with operating suite and body exhaust systems is helpful.
- Associated injuries should be addressed concurrently if possible.
- Application of tranexamic acid via intravascular or topically administration may have value in blood loss prevention. Several ongoing studies are currently assessing the safety and value of this treatment.

Positioning

- Patient positioning is important and should be done very carefully.
- General positioning principles include padding all bony prominences, positioning the patient in a stable position for implant placement, and creating a range-of-motion arc so that implant position and stability can be tested intraoperatively.

Supine Position for Direct Approach (Smith-Petersen) Approach

- Once the patient is adequately anesthetized, he or she is placed in a supine position, which allows for direct measurement of leg length.
- This can be performed on a standard flat table or a specialized bed.
- When utilizing a specialized table, a well-padded post should be used, and traction should be used judiciously given the patient's risk of further fractures.
- When on a standard table, the patient is brought down the table so the leg break is at the level of the midthigh. In order to facilitate this positioning, the headpiece is often placed at the foot of the bed.
- A bump may be placed beneath the sacrum. This sacral pad is constructed of folded sheets or a gel bump approximately 1.5 to 2 inches in height and rectangular with an approximate dimension of 12 × 10 inches (**FIG 3**).
  - The modest elevation of the sacrum allows the femur to drop posteriorly when sizing and inspecting the acetabulum. This also allows space for mobilization of the femur.
  - It also allows hip stability to be evaluated in extension.
- Both arms are placed on arm boards secured at 90 degrees of abduction or secured across the body.
- Fluoroscopy may be used as an adjunct for component positioning if needed.

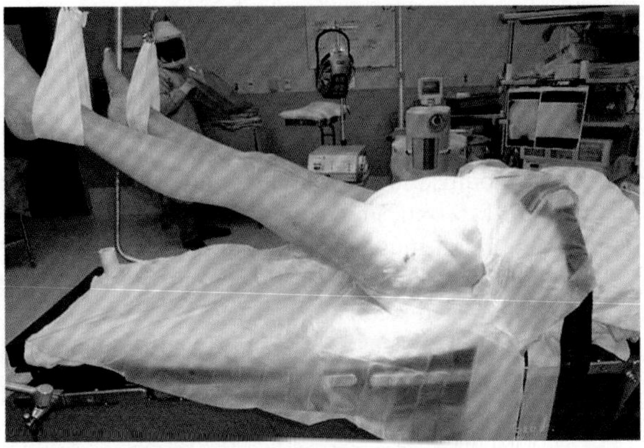

FIG 3 Positioning with sacral bump.

Supine Position for Direct Lateral (Modified Hardinge) Approach

- Once the patient is adequately anesthetized, he or she is placed in a supine position, which allows for direct measurement of leg length.
- The operating table is placed in a flat position.
- The patient is brought to the edge of the table so that the operative hip slightly overhangs the edge of the table.
- A bump is placed beneath the sacrum. This sacral pad is constructed of folded sheets or a gel bump approximately 1.5 to 2 inches in height and rectangular with an approximate dimension of 12 × 10 inches.
- The modest elevation of the sacrum allows the fat and soft tissues from above the trochanter to fall posteriorly away from the incision, thereby minimizing the amount of tissue that must be dissected in a lateral approach.
  - It also allows hip stability to be evaluated in extension.
- A footrest is fixed to the operating table so that the surgical hip is flexed 40 degrees.
- Both arms are placed on arm boards secured at 90 degrees of abduction.
- The operating room table is inclined 5 degrees away from the operating surgeon to improve visualization of the acetabulum.

Lateral Position

- The lateral position is used for a posterolateral approach to the hip and can also be used for an anterolateral approach.
- Once the patient is adequately anesthetized, he or she is placed in the lateral decubitus position in a gentle fashion.
  - The anesthesiologist controls the patient's head and neck to allow for neutral positioning.
  - One surgical team member controls the patient's hands and shoulders, and another controls the patient's hips.
- The ipsilateral arm is positioned in no more than 90 degrees of forward flexion and slight adduction.
- An axillary pad is placed by lifting the patient's chest and positioning the pad distal to the contralateral axilla.
- The contralateral arm must be kept in no greater than 90 degrees of forward flexion.
- Extremities are padded over all bony protuberances.

A

B

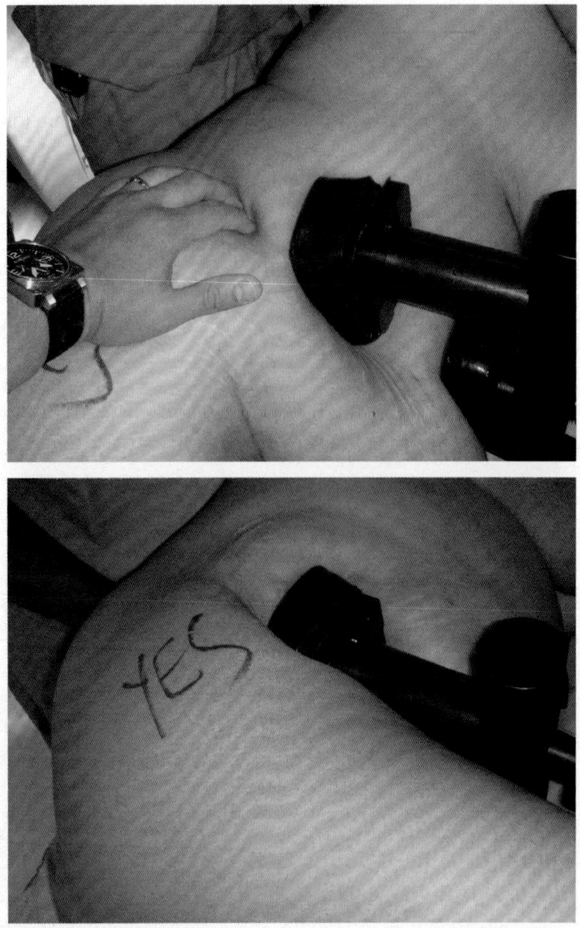

FIG 4 A. Palpation of ASIS for lateral position. **B.** Adequate range of motion must be ensured after positioning.

- The operating room table must be kept in an absolute horizontal position, parallel to the floor.
- A number of holders can be used to hold the patient in a lateral decubitus position.
  - A beanbag can be used, although it is not as rigid as a variety of other types of holders. The pubis and sacrum must be secured in the holder.
  - Placement of the pubic clamp must be done cautiously, with the pad directly against the pubic symphysis.
    - Placement of the pad more inferiorly causes occlusion or compromise of the femoral vessels in the opposite limb, which may go unrecognized.
    - Placement of the pad superiorly may compromise ipsilateral femoral vessels and may prevent adequate flexion and adduction of the operated hip.
- A sacral pad is placed over the midsacrum. It should be at least 3 to 5 inches away from the most posterior end of the skin incision **(FIG 4A)**.
- When the patient is securely positioned in lateral decubitus, the position of the pelvis is checked to make sure that it is not tilted in the AP direction **(FIG 4B)**.
- A chest positioner and pillows between the arms are helpful in preventing anterior displacement of the torso.
- The perineum is isolated using an adhesive U-shaped plastic drape.

Approach

- Hemiarthroplasty can be performed through a number of different approaches.
- There are four commonly employed approaches to the hip joint:
  - Anterior (Smith-Petersen)
    - This approach uses the interval between the sartorius and the tensor fascia superficially and between the rectus femoris and tensor fascia deeply.
    - Risks include injury to the lateral femoral cutaneous nerve.
    - Allows the surgeon direct access to the anterior hip capsule
    - Femoral preparation may be more challenging and require traction, hip extension, and the use of a hook to deliver the femur anteriorly for preparation.
  - Anterolateral (Watson-Jones)
  - Lateral (modified Hardinge)
  - Posterior (Southern)
- Choice of approach is highly dependent on surgeon preference.
  - I use a modification of the direct anterior as described by Smith-Petersen, Hueter, and Judet. Previously, I preferred a lateral muscle-splitting approach to the hip, as originally described by Hardinge and the use of a cementless tapered stem.[3]
- A variety of stem designs can be implanted through each of these surgical exposures. Similarly, cementation of implants can be performed with each.

TECHNIQUES

ANTERIOR APPROACH (MODIFIED SMITH-PETERSEN) WITHOUT A SPECIALIZED TABLE

Preparation of the Surgical Site

- Both lower extremities are prepped into the surgical field. Plastic adhesive drapes are used to isolate the operative field from the perineum and adjacent skin.
  - A large U-drape is placed, isolating the perineum and abdomen from the hip and repeated for the opposite side.
  - A second drape is placed transversely above the level of the iliac crest, completing the isolation of the wound area from the abdomen and thorax. This is also done for the nonoperative side but to a lesser degree.
  - The excess drapes are debulked down the center (perineum) with silk tape.
- Both lower extremities are scrubbed with a chlorhexidine brush, followed by a preparation with chlorhexidine and alcohol **(TECH FIG 1A)**.
- The incision area is dried to allow better adherence of Ioban drapes (3M, St. Paul, MN).
- A down sheet is placed, and a surgical towel is placed over the crotch and perineum. Both limbs are removed from the leg holders and the surgeon grasps the foot with a double-thickness stockinette.
  - Impermeable drape is placed across of the bottom of the operating table up to the level of the patient's buttock. This U-drape is placed bilaterally. A second U-drape is placed only on the operative side. A bar drape seals the upper portion of the surgical site **(TECH FIG 1B)**.
  - The stockinette is unrolled to the level of the upper thigh and higher on the nonoperative side. A bilateral extremity drape is placed over both legs, not to exceed the stockinettes. The stockinettes are secured with a Coban dressing (3M) **(TECH FIG 1C)**.
- A rectangular window is cut off the drape over the surgical site, and the sides are secured with staples. The surgical site is additionally prepped with a chlorhexidine and alcohol or Betadine and alcohol solution **(TECH FIG 1D)**.

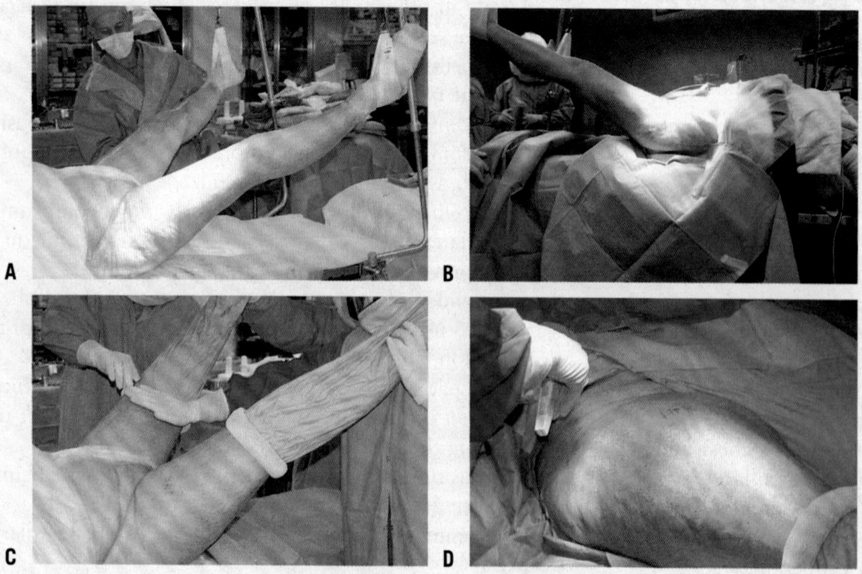

TECH FIG 1 A. Both legs prepped. **B.** First sterile U-drape. **C.** Bilateral stockinettes. **D.** Operative side isolated.

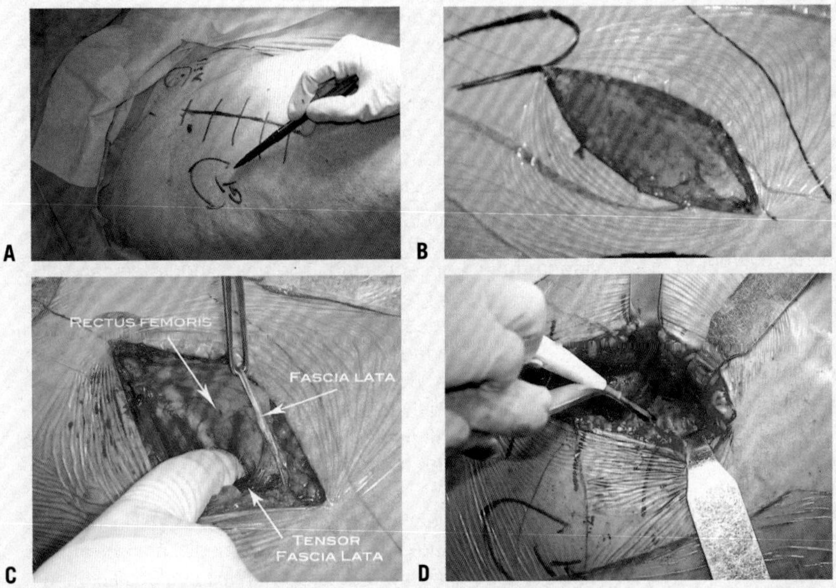

TECH FIG 2 **A.** Skin markings of ASIS, greater trochanter, and skin incision. **B.** Fascia overlying tensor muscle belly. **C.** Elevating fascia off the tensor and blunt finger dissection into the Smith-Petersen interval between tensor and rectus. **D.** Identifying the ascending branches of the lateral femoral circumflex vessels. (**B,D:** Courtesy of Jonathan Yerasamides, MD.)

Skin Incision

- The anterior superior iliac spine (ASIS) and greater trochanter are marked and an oblique skin incision approximately 3 to 4 inches in length and starting a finger's breadth distal and lateral to the ASIS is outlined. This window is then sealed with Ioban drapes **(TECH FIG 2A)**.
- The skin incision is taken down through subcutaneous tissue to the tensor fascia. The fascia over the muscle is identified. The fascial incision is directly over the tensor muscle not directly in the interval. Too medial is over the interval and too lateral is over the fascia lata **(TECH FIG 2B)**.
- The fascia is incised and elevated bluntly medially with a pickup and finger dissection. The finger must wrap around the tensor medially, dropping into the interval between the tensor and rectus. This should be done bluntly **(TECH FIG 2C)**.
- A blunt Hohmann retractor is placed around the lateral side of the femoral neck and a second double-angled Hohmann retractor is placed around the lateral femur (greater trochanter). Hibbs retractors are placed medially retracting the rectus. Ascending branches of the lateral femoral circumflex vessels are identified and coagulated or tied **(TECH FIG 2D)**.
- The distal fascia between the rectus and tensor is released; allowing the rectus to slide medially and allowing a second blunt Hohmann retractor to be placed around the medial side of the femoral neck. The rectus is then dissected from the anterior hip capsule with a Cobb elevator and a final blunt cobra retractor is placed on the anterior column.

Acetabular Preparation

- The anterior hip capsule is fully exposed. Perforating vessels are coagulated. The capsule is opened in an H fashion and excised. Both blunt Hohmann retractors are placed intracapsularly. The femoral neck fracture is identified. A femoral neck osteotomy is performed distal to the fracture, using the saddle as reference at a 45-degree angle. Typically, a blunt osteotome can be used at both the osteotomy and fracture site to remove the fractured neck segment. A more proximal osteotomy may be performed as well in the subcapital area, if necessary, to remove that segment. The femoral head is removed with a power corkscrew.
- The leg is then placed in a figure-4 position with a pointed Hohmann retractor below the lesser trochanter in order to assess the osteotomy level and perform medial capsular release (capsule above the lesser trochanter is released from the calcar). Once the level is determined to be satisfactory, the leg is placed back in a neutral position. Additional neck resection is performed if necessary.
- Three retractors are placed around the acetabulum. A blunt cobra retractor is placed on the anterior column above the labrum and beneath the capsule and rectus. A double-angled Hohmann retractor is placed at the level of the transverse acetabular ligament. A pointed Aufranc retractor is placed along the posterior acetabulum **(TECH FIG 3)**.
- The acetabulum should be inspected to remove any bony fragments and debris and then should be sized. The acetabulum should be sized with a trial bipolar or unipolar component to ensure that there will be good fit without overfilling the acetabulum.
- This can be achieved with a good suction-tight feel with placement of the trial component.

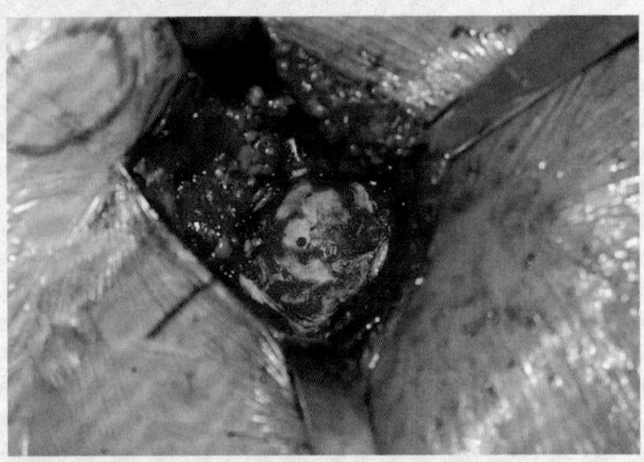

TECH FIG 3 Acetabular exposure with three retractors.

Femoral Preparation

- Attention is then placed to the femur.
  - The leg of the table is then extended 30 degrees. The nonoperative leg is placed on a padded Mayo stand. The operative leg is placed in a figure-4 position under the nonoperative leg **(TECH FIG 4A)**.
  - The second assistant places a hand on the knee, pushing down and adducting the leg, thereby creating external rotation, extension, and adduction of the operative femur. A double-footed retractor is placed along the posterior femoral neck, and a double-angled retractor is placed along the anterior femoral neck **(TECH FIG 4B)**.
- The next step is to perform the femoral releases in order to prepare the femur. The releases include the superior or lateral capsule, which is draped in front of the inside of the greater trochanter when the leg is in externally rotated position. The medial aspect of the greater trochanter should be exposed. Additionally, the conjoint tendon, which consists of the inferior gemellus, obturator internus, and superior gemellus, may need to be released. Occasionally, the piriformis tendon may need to be released in a contracted hip **(TECH FIG 4C)**.
  - Once the proximal femur is adequately exposed, the proximal femur is sometimes opened with an offset box osteotome. More commonly, it is opened with a curved canal finder, a curved rasp, and a rongeur to further open the canal. A curette can be used to clear the medial side of the trochanter and the rongeur again in this area. The curved rasp should be used to open the canal as well as feel the cortices and appreciate the orientation of the femur **(TECH FIG 4D–F)**.
  - The canal is sequentially broached until there is a tight feel. The broach should be stable to rotation.
    - The femoral broach is introduced in a neutral position, and neutral version of the rotation is judged in relation to the position of the knee and the calcar as well as the posterior femoral neck **(TECH FIG 4G)**.
- Broaching is begun with the smallest broach and then increased until appropriate fit and fill is achieved. This can be gauged by preoperative templating and tactile feedback.
- The broach is introduced each time to its full depth.
  - If significant resistance is met, broaching should continue with a series of small inward and then outward taps.
  - Broaching is continued until full cortical seating has been accomplished. This is indicated by an upward change in pitch as the broach is being seated.
- Final seating and sizing is determined by pitch, tactile feedback, and lack of progression.
- Trial reduction is performed with a minus neck trial and a standard neck offset to start. The head should be carefully reduced. This will require flexion, traction, and internal rotation. The surgeon must carefully turn the bipolar head so that it may be reduced under the rectus and anterior soft tissue sleeve. If it is a difficult reduction, then the trial construct is typically too long and a smaller broach needs to be countersunk and the femoral neck recut. If it reduces too easily, then the trial construct may be too short or have inadequate offset.
- Once a reasonable trial construct has been established, leg lengths are measured directly near the medial malleoli and heels. Anterior stability is checked with external rotation and extension in a neutral and adducted position. Posterior stability is checked with flexion and internal rotation. Once satisfactory stability is achieved, the final components are placed **(TECH FIG 4H–J)**.
  - The final stem is placed by hand and impacted until final seating. The final bipolar hemiarthroplasty is assembled on the back table and impacted onto a clean trunnion **(TECH FIG 4K,L)**.
  - The final prosthesis is reduced with flexion, traction, and internal rotation. The table is placed in a level position with a new down sheet. The wound is thoroughly irrigated and a medium Hemovac drain may be placed with a distal exit site.
- Wound closure begins with interrupted absorbable sutures in the tensor fascia. Interrupted absorbable sutures are used for the subcutaneous tissues. Skin staples are applied to the skin, sealed with Dermabond and a final sealed hydrofiber dressing **(TECH FIG 4M–O)**.

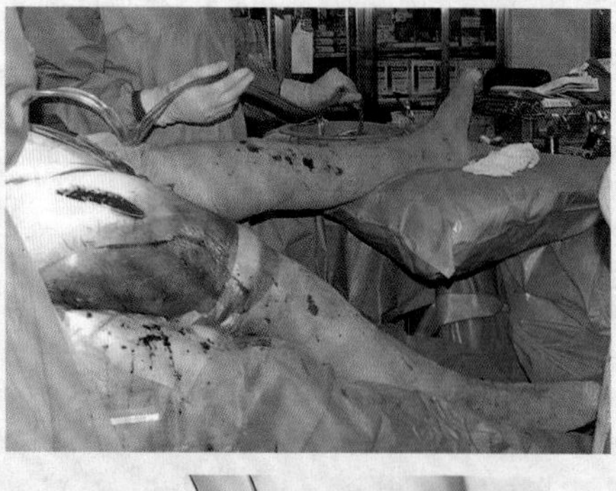
A

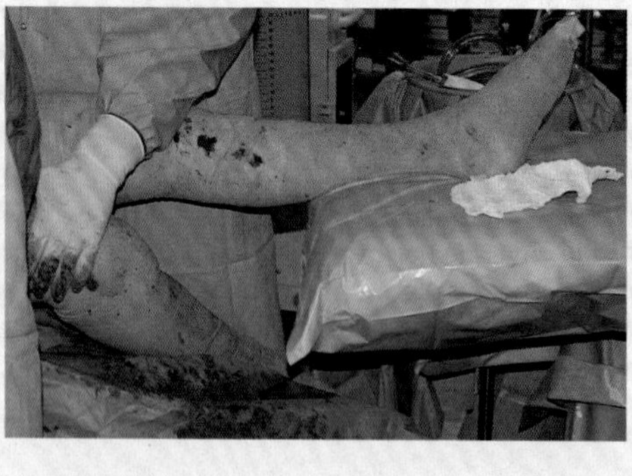
B

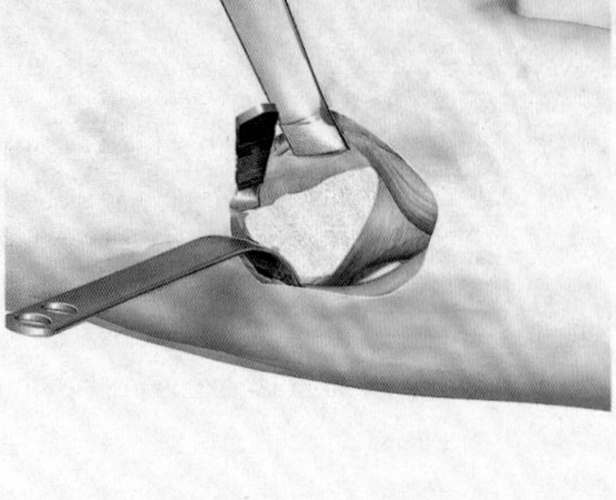
C

TECH FIG 4 A. Table position for femoral preparation. **B.** Position of nonoperative leg and second assistant maneuvering operative leg. **C.** Diagram representing superior capsular release for a right hip. *(continued)*

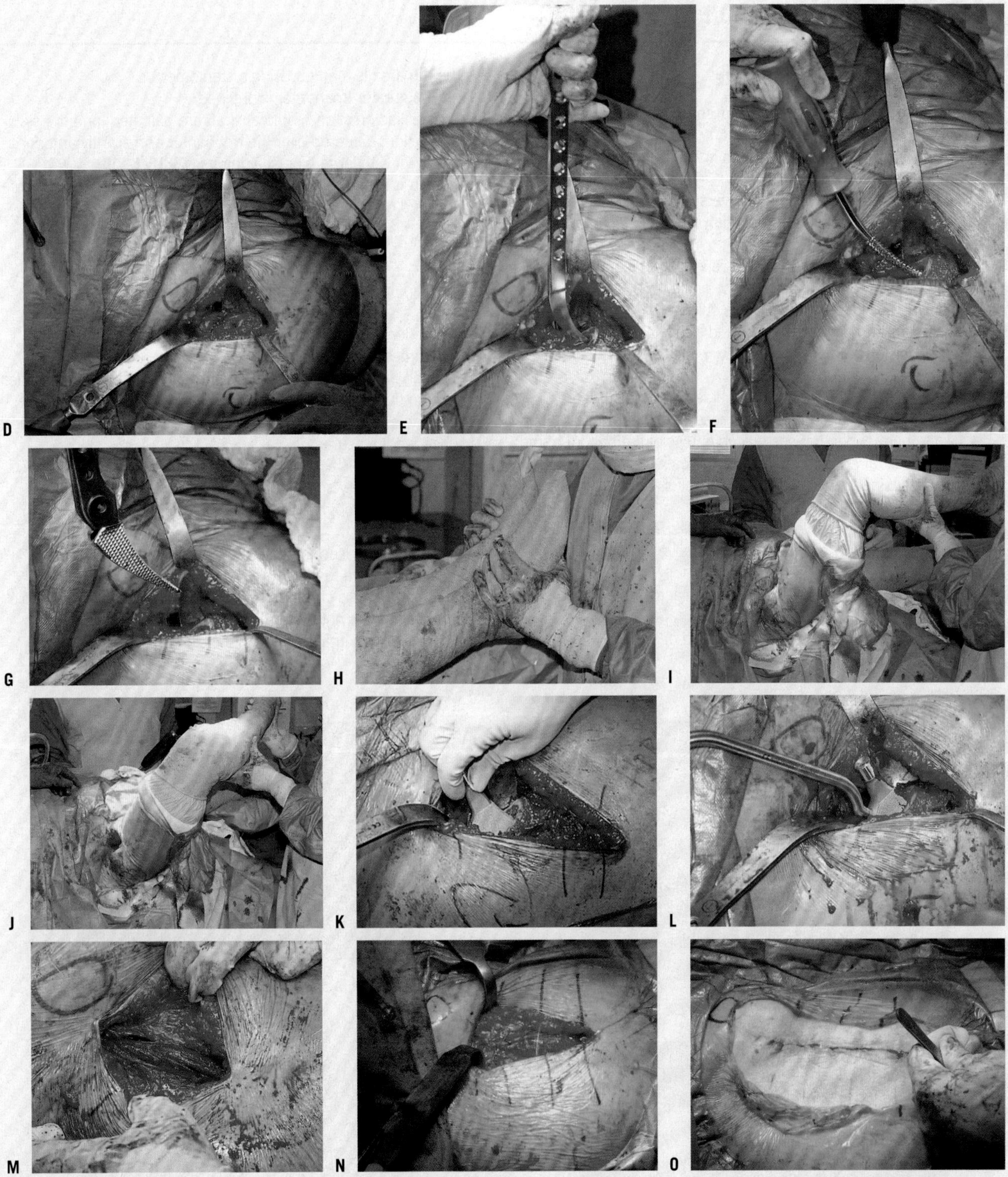

TECH FIG 4 *(continued)* **D.** Exposure of proximal femur after releases. **E.** Curved canal finder. **F.** Curved rasp. **G.** Trial broach insertion. **H.** Direct leg length evaluation. **I,J.** Stability evaluation. **K.** Final stem placement by hand. **L.** Offset impactor. **M.** Tensor muscle and fascia. **N.** Fascial closure. **O.** Subcutaneous closure.

LATERAL APPROACH (MODIFIED HARDINGE)

Preparation of the Surgical Site

- Plastic adhesive drapes are used to isolate the operative field from the perineum and adjacent skin.
  - A large U-drape is placed, isolating the perineum and abdomen from the hip.
  - A second drape is placed transversely above the level of the iliac crest, completing the isolation of the wound area from the abdomen and thorax.
  - The foot also is sealed with a plastic 10 × 10 drape, isolating the foot above the level of the ankle.
- The operative field is scrubbed with a chlorhexidine brush, followed by a preparation with chlorhexidine and alcohol **(TECH FIG 5A)**.
  - The incision area is dried to allow better adherence of Ioban drapes.
- The limb is removed from the leg holder, and the surgeon grasps the foot with a double-thickness stockinette.
  - An impermeable drape is placed across of the bottom of the operating table up to the level of the patient's buttock.
  - The stockinette is unrolled to the level of the midthigh and secured with a Coban dressing.
- The limb is draped sterilely using two full-sized sheets brought beneath the leg and buttock and held above the level of the iliac crest.
  - A double sheet is placed transversely across the abdomen above the level of the iliac crest.
  - A clean air room is sealed at the head of the operating table with sterile adhesive drape.
- The hip area is marked using a sterile pen.
  - The greater trochanter is outlined.
  - The iliac crest and femoral shaft are palpated, and the skin incision, centered over the trochanter and slightly anterior, is drawn with large cross-hatchings **(TECH FIG 5B)**.
- The hip is flexed to 40 degrees and slightly adducted. The foot is placed on the footrest.

Incision

- The skin incision is approximately 5 inches in length.
  - It is slightly anterior to the apex of the vastus ridge.
  - The length of the incision also depends on the patient's degree of obesity.
- The skin incision is taken sharply through subcutaneous tissues down to the tensor fascia lata (TFL) **(TECH FIG 6A)**.
- The fascia is exposed to a small degree to allow the incision and subsequent closure.
  - Hemostasis is achieved in the subcutaneous tissue with electrocautery and bayonet forceps.
- The incision through the fascia lata is in line with the skin incision.
  - A scalpel is used to penetrate the fascia lata and allow a safe entrance to the compartments.
  - The incision is continued with the use of heavy Mayo-Noble scissors. It is not undermined beyond the skin incision or distal or proximal to the skin incision **(TECH FIG 6B)**.

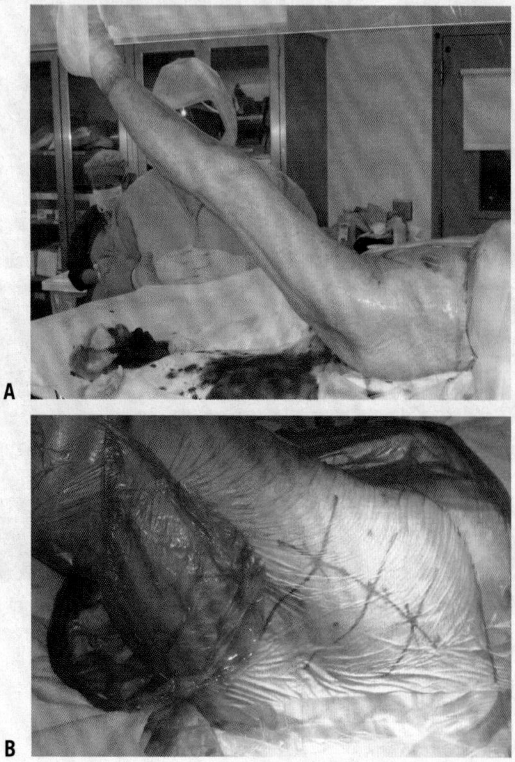

TECH FIG 5 **A.** Skin preparation for lateral (Hardinge) approach to the hip. **B.** Lateral skin incision.

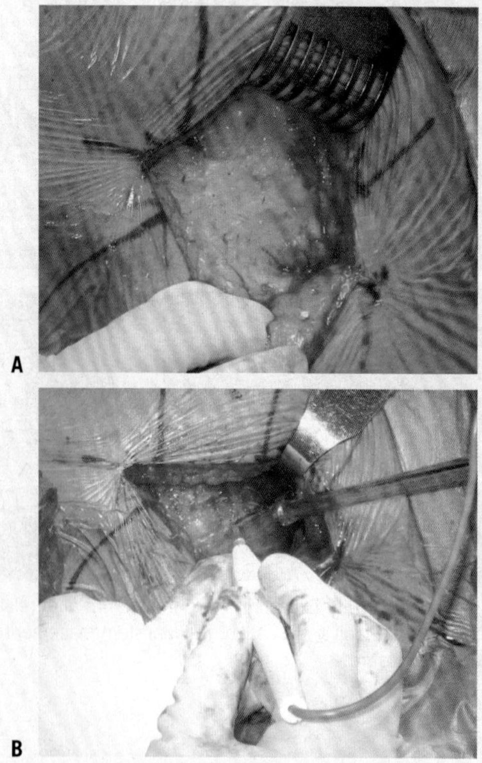

TECH FIG 6 **A.** The TFL exposed. **B.** An incision is made into the tensor fascia.

Proximal Dissection

- More proximally, the fibers of the gluteus maximus muscle are split using firm thumb dissection.
  - A Hibbs retractor is used to retract the anterior flap of the fascia lata.
  - Once that is done, the gluteus medius, greater trochanter, and vastus lateralis are clearly visualized.
- The abductor mass is split.
  - The basic premise of the modified Hardinge approach is to develop an anterior flap, composed of the anterior portion of the vastus lateralis, anterior capsule, anterior third of the gluteus medius muscle, and most of the gluteus minimus muscle to allow exposure of the hip joint.
  - The muscle split is usually located in the anterior third of the gluteus medius.
  - The muscle split is made using electrocautery through the gluteus medius **(TECH FIG 7A,B)**.
- Once the gluteus medius is penetrated, the surgeon encounters a fatty layer, beneath which is found the gluteus minimus.
  - The gluteus minimus is isolated and a more posterior incision is made with the electrocautery through the gluteus minimus and the capsule onto the acetabulum **(TECH FIG 7C)**.
- A blunt Hohmann retractor is placed posteriorly to expose the gluteus minimus and capsule. The blunt end of the Hibbs retractor is used to retract the anterior aspect of the gluteus medius.
- The capsule then is visualized in the depths of the wound.
  - The capsule is incised parallel to the superior aspect of the femoral neck, and the incision is extended to the bony rim of the acetabulum with care not to damage the labrum.
  - This area is then packed with an E-tape sponge **(TECH FIG 7D)**.

Distal Dissection

- Attention is turned to the more distal aspect of the wound and the vastus lateralis.
- The anterior third of the vastus lateralis is incised longitudinally using electrocautery, beginning at the trochanteric ridge and extending 2 to 3 cm beyond.
- Once this is dissected subperiosteally in the anterior direction, a blunt Hohmann retractor is placed around the femur medially to reflect the vastus lateralis anteriorly.
- An anterior bridge of soft tissue remains along the greater trochanter between the incision in the vastus lateralis and the incision in the gluteus medius and superior capsule. This bridge consists of the anterior fibers of the gluteus medius, minimus, and capsule.
  - This bridge is incised through the tendon in a gentle arc along the anterior aspect of the greater trochanter, connecting the incisions.
  - Healthy soft tissue must be present on both sides of this arc to allow effective repair during closure.
- The bridge is dissected using electrocautery in the anterior aspect of the greater trochanter to develop a flap in continuity consisting of the anterior portion of the gluteus minimus and going around the gluteus medius, anterior hip capsule, and gluteus minimus. This exposes the femoral neck and head.
  - The dissection is carried medially until the medial aspect of the neck is exposed **(TECH FIG 8)**.
- Exposure is usually adequate to allow for dislocation of the hip, femoral neck, or proximal femur.
  - A bone hook is placed around the neck of the femur anteriorly, and the leg is externally rotated to allow for dislocation of the hip (ie, the hip is placed in the figure-4 position).
- At this point, with a femoral neck fracture, the proximal femur will often dissociate from the femoral neck.

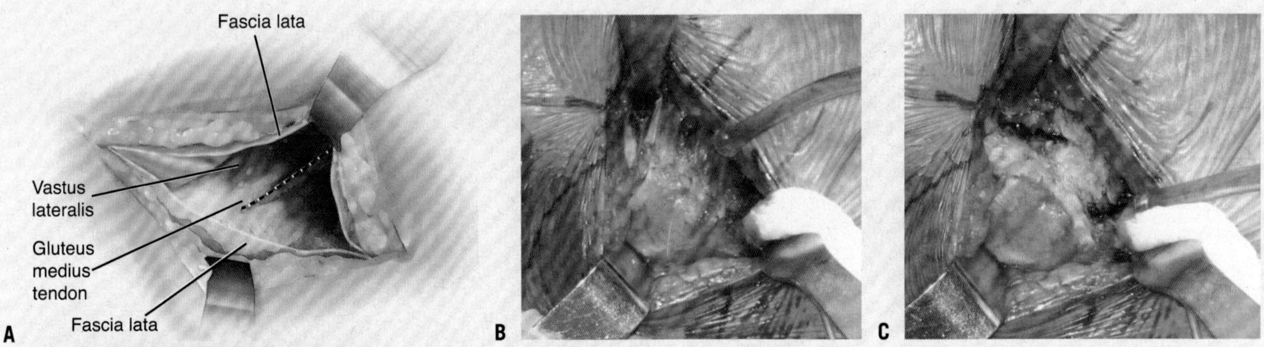

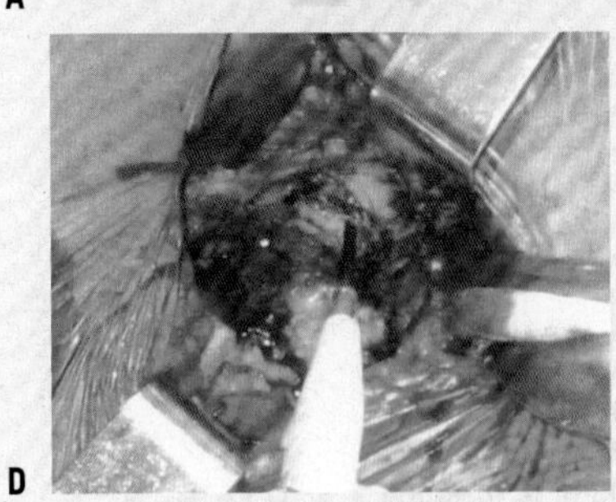

TECH FIG 7 **A.** Diagram of the splitting of the abductor mass. **B.** The abductor mass exposed. **C.** Detachment of the abductor mass. **D.** Exposure of the femoral neck.

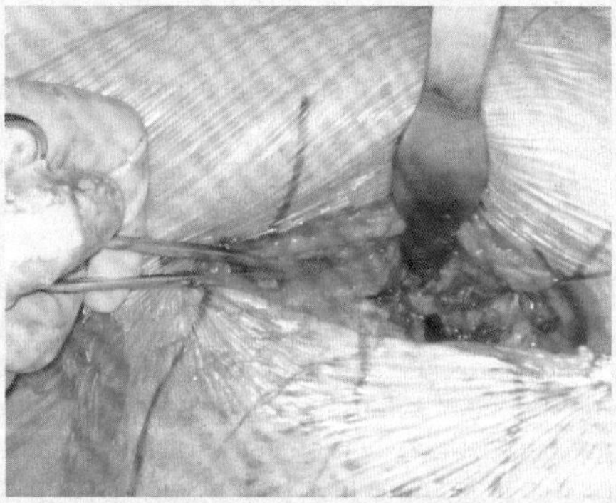

TECH FIG 8 More proximal femoral exposure.

- An initial rough cut of the femoral neck can be performed in line with appropriate preoperative templating.
  - Two blunt-tip retractors are placed around the femoral neck to protect the soft tissues.
  - Electrocautery is used to mark the femoral neck, and an initial cut of the femoral neck is made with an oscillating saw.

Placement of Acetabular Retractors

- Attention is turned to the acetabulum.
  - The first retractor is placed in the anterior acetabulum.
  - A small plane is created between the anterior wall of the acetabulum and the anterior capsule using a Cobb elevator.
- A blunt-tip Hohmann retractor is placed in the 12 o'clock position anterior to the acetabulum beneath the capsule.
  - An assistant can then easily retract the anterior soft tissues.
- The second spiked Mueller acetabular retractor is placed in the superior aspect of the acetabulum, retracting the superior capsule in the cranial direction.
  - The retractor is placed at 10 o'clock position for the right hip and 2 o'clock position for the left hip.
  - The exact placement of the retractor is outside the labrum and inside the capsule.
- Using the impactor mallet, the surgeon drives this retractor into the ilium in a slightly cranial direction.
  - The tip is not driven perpendicular to the axis of the body because it may perforate the dome of the acetabulum.
- To facilitate appropriate exposure prior to placement of the third retractor and to allow posterior mobilization of the proximal femur, a medial capsular release must be performed.
  - A curved hemostat is placed between the iliopsoas and capsule, anterior and in line with the pubofemoral ligament.
  - The capsule is incised medial to lateral, thereby increasing the mobilization of the femur in a posterior direction.
- A third, double-angled acetabular retractor is placed inferiorly in the ischium.
  - It is placed with the blade of the retractor resting on the neck of the femur rather than on the cut surface.

Femoral Head Removal and Implant Sizing

- At this point, the femoral head and neck are clearly visualized in the acetabulum.
- The femoral head and neck fracture can be removed using a corkscrew in combination with a Cobb elevator or a tenaculum.
  - This should be done carefully so as not to damage the acetabular cartilage or the labrum **(TECH FIG 9A,B)**.
- Once the femoral head is removed, it should be measured to enable the surgeon to estimate the size of the acetabulum.
- The acetabulum should be sized with a trial bipolar or unipolar component to ensure that there will be good fit without overfilling the acetabulum.
  - This can be achieved with a good suction-tight feel with placement of the trial component.
  - It should move freely without resistance.
  - If it floats freely in the acetabulum, the trial component is undersized **(TECH FIG 9C)**.

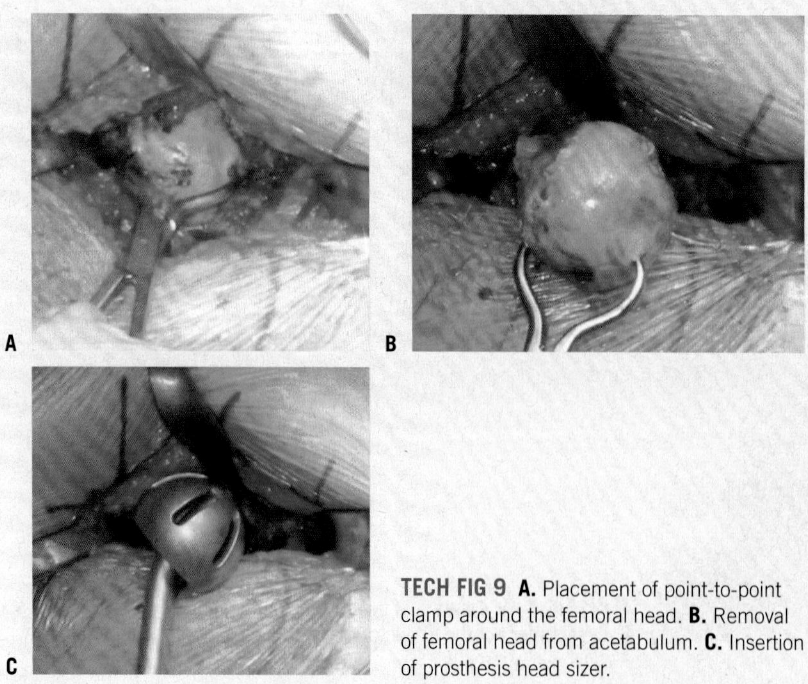

TECH FIG 9 **A.** Placement of point-to-point clamp around the femoral head. **B.** Removal of femoral head from acetabulum. **C.** Insertion of prosthesis head sizer.

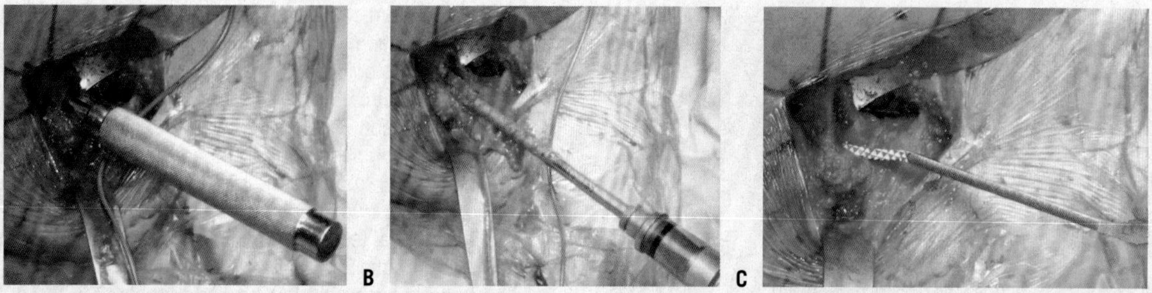

A B C

TECH FIG 10 **A.** Use of a curette for femoral orientation. **B.** Reaming of the femoral canal. **C.** Lateralization of the femoral canal with a lateral rasp.

Femoral Reaming

- The femur is exposed with the use of two double-footed retractors, one beneath the greater trochanter and a second retractor medially in the area of the calcar.
- The leg is placed in a figure-4 position, crossed over the opposite thigh.
  - The femur should be easily exposed.
  - If there is difficulty in this exposure, the leg should be placed in a greater degree of figure 4 and rotation.
- Excess soft tissue is removed from the tip of the greater trochanter to allow for reaming and broaching. This will prevent varus positioning of the component.
- A large rongeur is used to open the femoral canal slightly.
- A small, straight curette is introduced into the femoral canal in neutral orientation.
  - The second assistant should use his or her hand to create a target at the distal femur in line with the femur.
  - As the surgeon places the small curette, he or she can place his or her opposite hand on the patient's knee to help direct the small metal curette in the appropriate orientation **(TECH FIG 10A)**.
- An entry reamer is then introduced into the femoral canal, pushed into valgus, and worked into the trochanter to ensure appropriate component positioning **(TECH FIG 10B)**.
- The bone within the area of the greater trochanter in the lateral aspect of the femoral canal is removed using a lateral rasp or a curette **(TECH FIG 10C)**.

Femoral Broaching

- The femoral broach is introduced in neutral position, and neutral version of the rotation is judged in relation to the position of the knee.
- Broaching is begun with the smallest broach and then increased until appropriate fit and fill is achieved. This can be gauged by preoperative templating and tactile feedback.
- The broach is introduced each time to its full depth.
  - If significant resistance is met, broaching should continue with a series of small inward and then outward taps.
  - Broaching is continued until full cortical seating has been accomplished. This is indicated by an upward change in pitch as the broach is seated.
  - Final seating and sizing is determined by pitch, tactile feedback, and lack of progression **(TECH FIG 11A)**.
- Once the final seating of the femoral broach is accomplished, an initial reduction with the appropriate-sized hemiarthroplasty bipolar or unipolar trial component is performed **(TECH FIG 11B)**.

Evaluation of Trial Prosthesis

- The hip is reduced for evaluation.
  - Hip stability is evaluated in full flexion and in internal and external rotation.
  - One finger is kept in the joint to evaluate for anterior impingement.
  - Anterior stability is evaluated with external rotation, adduction, and extension.
  - Leg lengths are measured directly.
  - The position of the pelvis, shoulders, and knees must be evaluated as the assistants help with orientation **(TECH FIG 12)**.
- Stability also is evaluated with a longitudinal shuck test, with a goal of 1 or 2 mm of shuck.
  - Excessively tight soft tissues about the hip cause difficult or incomplete extension of the hip; excessive laxity leads to increased shuck.
  - For inadequate soft tissue tension and appropriate leg length restoration, a lateral offset can also be used.
  - It is important to achieve stability, which takes precedence over leg length.

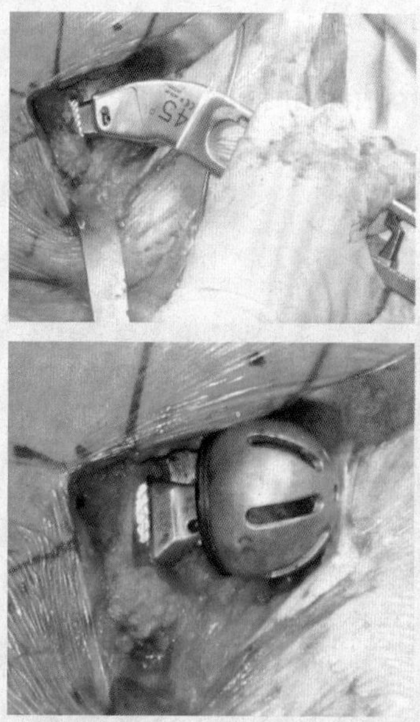

A B

TECH FIG 11 **A.** Broaching of the femoral canal. **B.** Placement of trial head onto trial femoral prosthesis.

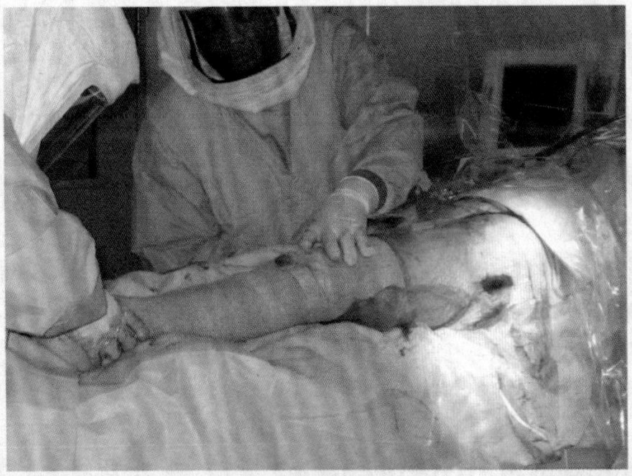

TECH FIG 12 Intraoperative evaluation of trial prosthesis leg length.

Placement of the Femoral Stem

- Once stability is satisfactory, the trial components are removed.
- The wound and the femur are irrigated with pulsatile lavage.
  - Excessive debris is removed.
  - The femur is prepared again with the curette only, to clear any soft tissue debris from the lateral aspect of the femur.
  - The femoral canal must be copiously irrigated.
  - The surgeon and assistant change outer gloves.
- The appropriately sized femoral component is placed in the femoral canal with the use of an impactor.
  - Varus positioning must be avoided. It can be prevented with appropriate valgus positioning of the stem on insertion, with attention paid to maintaining the appropriate version.
  - The femoral component is seated into position using firm taps with a mallet.
  - A pause between taps may allow some plastic deformation of the femur.
  - Final seating is determined in relation to the last broach, tactile feedback, pitch change, and lack of progression **(TECH FIG 13)**.

Completion of Implant Placement

- Once the stem is placed, a second trial reduction can be performed with the trial next segment and trial bipolar shell, or a final component can be placed if the broach and stem achieve the same position.
  - If the trial bipolar shell is desired, trial reduction is performed again.
  - The reduction is performed with the patient held in position by the second assistant and the first assistant.
  - The surgeon reduces the hip with distraction, internal rotation, and adduction.
  - The surgical technician can assist the reduction with longitudinal traction.
- The head is assembled on the back table with the outer acetabular bipolar shell impacted on the appropriately sized head.
  - This can be a 22-, 28-, or 32-mm head, depending on the implant system, with a polyethylene insert and bipolar shell that sits over it **(TECH FIG 14A)**.
- Once that is assembled on the back table, the trunnion is cleaned and dried and the bipolar shell is impacted on to the trunnion of the neck of femoral prosthesis.
- The acetabulum is checked one last time before final reduction for any debris or any soft tissue **(TECH FIG 14B)**.
- Once it is checked and cleared, the hip is reduced, and the bipolar shell is reduced and checked for appropriate position, after which the wound is thoroughly irrigated and copiously irrigated with pulsatile lavage **(TECH FIG 14C)**.
- At this point, drains can be used according to the preference of the surgeon. I prefer not to use drains.

Wound Repair and Closure

- The abductor mass is repaired.
- The vastus lateralis is repaired to the remaining tissue sleeve with interrupted absorbable sutures in figure-8 fashion with no. 1 Vicryl.
- The gluteus medius tendon and capsule are repaired to the tissue sleeve on the bridge of the trochanter.
  - This is done with heavy absorbable sutures in figure-8 fashion.
  - The repair is done at the corner of the gluteus medius tendon and then extended into the proximal split with simple sutures **(TECH FIG 15A)**.
- Once the hip abductor is adequately repaired, the TFL is approximated with absorbable sutures in figure-8 fashion.
  - This must be done to both the proximal and distal extents of the fascia lata.

A

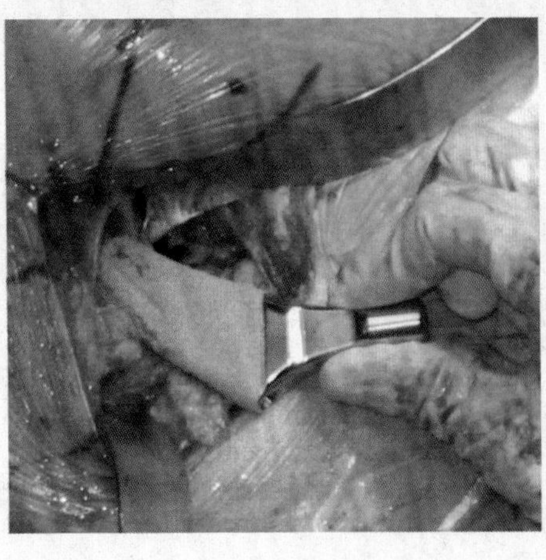

B

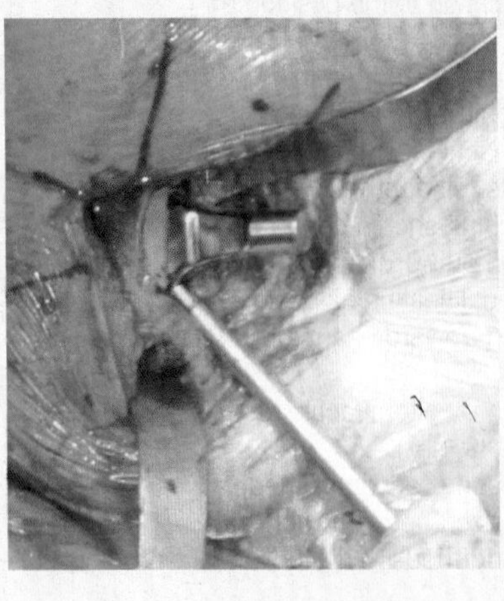

TECH FIG 13 **A.** Placement of final femoral stem. **B.** Impaction of femoral stem.

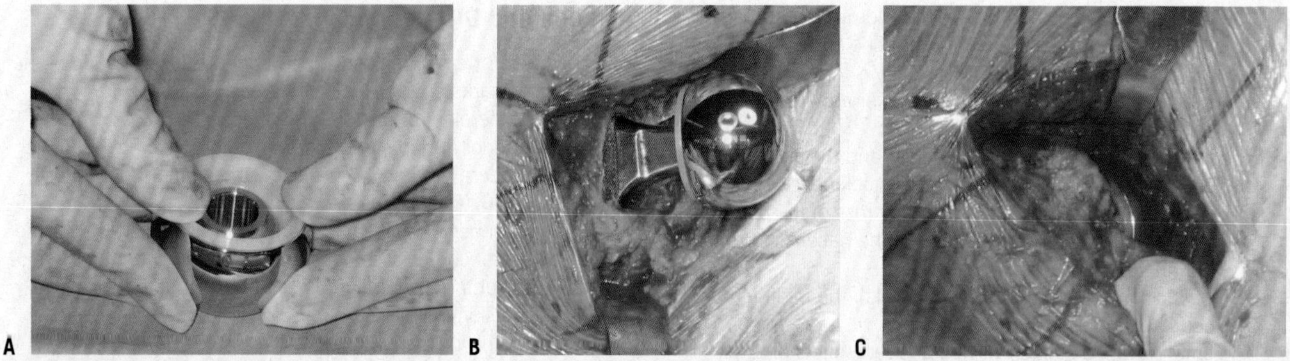

TECH FIG 14 A. Assembly of bipolar head. **B.** Placement of bipolar head onto femoral stem. **C.** Relocation of the prosthetic hip into the native acetabulum.

- The potential dead space is closed with heavy absorbable sutures, and smaller absorbable 2-0 sutures are placed in subcutaneous tissue **(TECH FIG 15B)**.
- Skin staples are applied.
- Sterile dressing is applied with Microfoam surgical tape (3M).
- An abduction pillow is placed between the legs and loosely secured.
- The patient is awakened from anesthesia and brought to the recovery room if, or as soon as, his or her condition is stable.
- Postoperative radiographs are taken in the recovery room **(TECH FIG 15C)**.

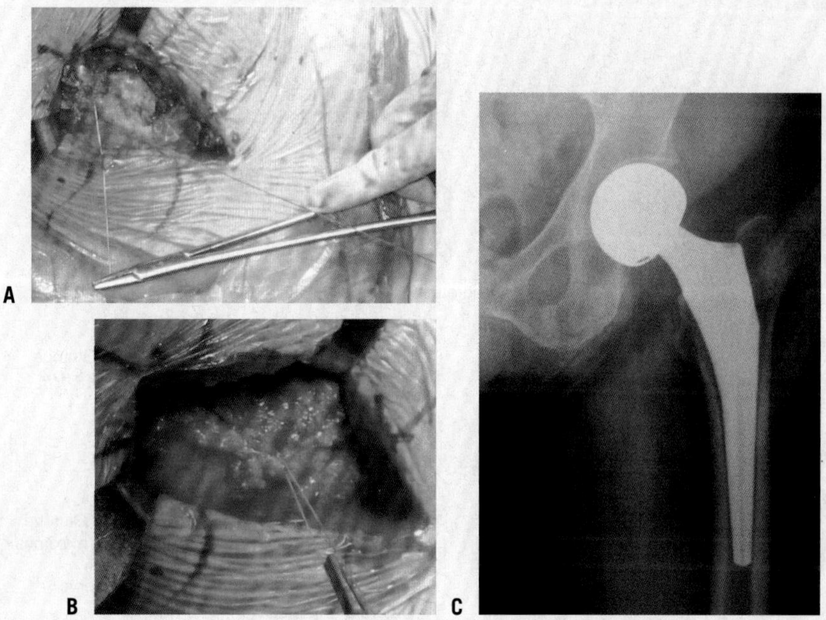

TECH FIG 15 A. Repair of the abductor mass. **B.** Repair of the TFL. **C.** AP radiograph of an implanted bipolar prosthesis.

POSTERIOR APPROACH (SOUTHERN)

Preparation of the Surgical Site

- Patient is secured in the lateral decubitus position with a holding device.
- Anatomic prominences are padded including an axillary roll on the chest wall.
- Plastic adhesive drapes are used to isolate the operative field from the perineum and adjacent skin.
  - A large U-drape is placed, isolating the perineum and abdomen from the hip.
  - A second drape is placed transversely above the level of the iliac crest, completing the isolation of the wound area from the abdomen and thorax.

- The operative field is scrubbed with a chlorhexidine brush, followed by a preparation with chlorhexidine and alcohol (see **TECH FIG 5A**).
  - The incision area is dried to allow better adherence of Ioban drapes.
- The limb is removed from the leg holder and the surgeon grasps the foot with a double-thickness stockinette.
  - An impermeable U-drape is placed across of the bottom of the operating table up to the level of the patient's buttock following the positioners.
  - The stockinette is unrolled to the level of the midthigh and secured with a Coban dressing.
- The limb is draped sterilely using full-sized sheets brought beneath the leg and buttock and held above the level of the iliac crest.
- A large extremity drape with side pockets is placed.
- The exposed skin is isolated with an adhesive drape such as Ioban.
- The hip area is marked using a sterile pen.
  - The greater trochanter is outlined.

Incision and Dissection

- Exposure of the hip begins with appropriate identification of the bony landmarks.
  - The posterolateral corner of the greater trochanter and the anterior and posterior borders of the proximal femoral shaft are marked 10 cm below the greater trochanter **(TECH FIG 16A,B)**.
- The incision begins at this point and extends obliquely over the posterolateral corner of the greater trochanter, continuing proximally, so that the acetabulum is centered in the incision.
  - The incision usually is 15 to 20 cm, although this will vary depending on the patient's body habitus **(TECH FIG 16C)**.
- Once the subcutaneous tissue is divided, the fascia lata is identified and incised in line with the incision.
  - The fibers of the gluteus maximus belly are bluntly separated with firm finger pressure **(TECH FIG 16D,E)**.
- A Charnley self-retaining retractor is placed to retract the gluteus maximus and tensor fascia. The gluteus maximus tendon may be released from the femur although this is not typically needed.

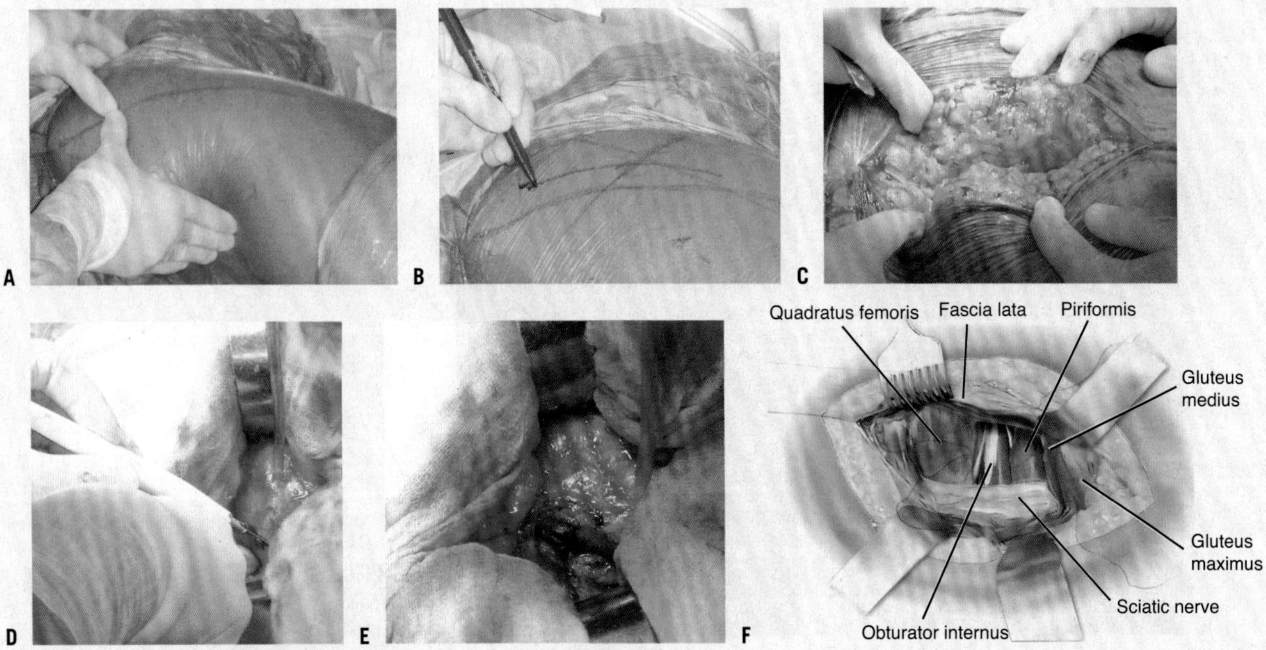

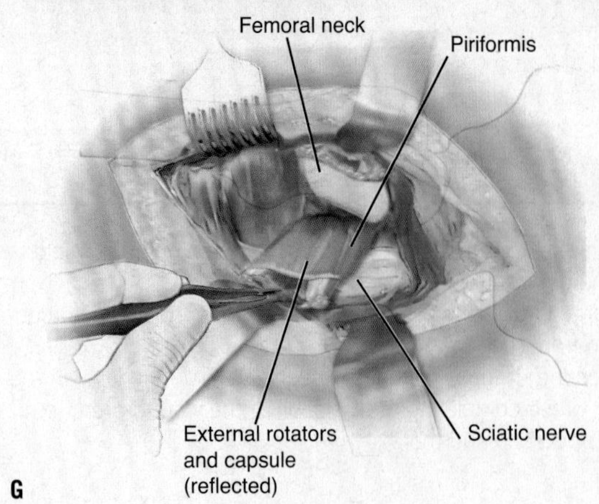

TECH FIG 16 **A.** Palpation of bony landmarks for posterior approach. This is created by the midpoint of the ASIS and the ischial tuberosity. **B.** Incisional line. Note its placement with respect to the axis of the femur, the proximal extent of the greater trochanter, and the previous line created by bony palpation. **C.** Skin incision. **D.** Identification and incision of the TFL. **E.** Exposure of the deep posterior structures of the hip after blunt separation of the gluteus maximus. **F.** Deep posterior structures of the hip. **G.** Reflection of the short external rotators. (**A–E:** Courtesy of Norman A. Johanson, MD.)

- The hip is internally rotated to offer exposure to the posterior structures.
- The piriformis tendon is identified by palpation, and a curved retractor is placed deep into the abductors just superior to the piriformis **(TECH FIG 16F)**.
  - A cobra retractor is placed inferior to the femoral neck.
- The short external rotators and piriformis may be released separately from the capsule and tagged.
  - The piriformis and conjoint tendons should be divided as close to their insertions as possible.
  - Alternatively, the external rotators and capsule can be taken down as one continuous sleeve off the trochanter and femoral neck **(TECH FIG 16G)**.
- Following the reflection of the short external rotators, the capsule is isolated by repositioning the superior and inferior retractors.
  - The curved superior retractor is placed deep to the gluteus minimus just over the superior femoral neck and capsule.

Site Preparation

- A capsulotomy is performed from this posterosuperior acetabulum and continued to the piriformis fossa in line with the posterior border of the abductors. In the setting of a hemiarthroplasty, the labrum can be preserved by cautiously performing the capsulotomy at the level of the acetabulum.
- It is continued inferiorly along the bone of the trochanter and neck reflecting this capsule as continuous sleeve to the level of the lesser trochanter **(TECH FIG 17)**.
- The quadratus femoris can be released along with the capsule, leaving a small muscular cuff with later reattachment. The capsule can be tagged with a suture.
- The hip is gently dislocated using a combination of flexion, internal rotation, and adduction.
- The leg is held at 90 degrees of internal rotation so that the femoral neck is parallel to the ground.

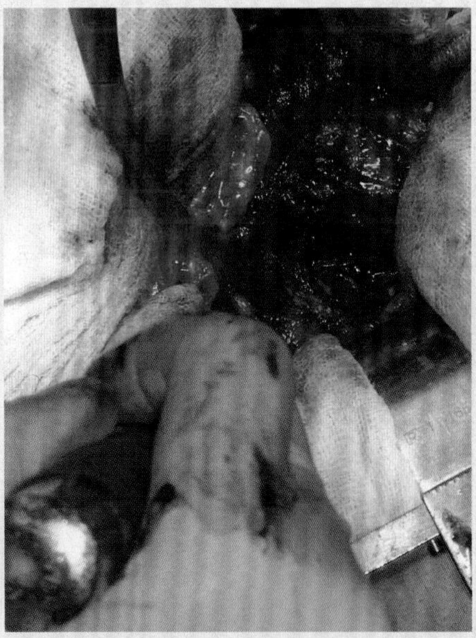

TECH FIG 17 Exposure of the hip capsule. (Courtesy of Norman A. Johanson, MD.)

- At this point, the proximal femur usually dissociates from the femoral neck and head, which often remain in the acetabulum.
  - Two retractors can be placed around the proximal femur and a fresh cut of the femoral neck can be performed with an oscillating saw.
  - Alternatively, if this is a low femoral neck fracture, this area can be smoothed with a rongeur and attention turned to the acetabulum.
- At this point, the retractors are placed around the acetabulum. Initially, a curved retractor is placed anteriorly, retracting the proximal femur out of the view of the acetabulum.
  - The operated extremity is placed in slight flexion and internal rotation, which aids in exposure.
  - Occasionally, the reflected head of the rectus femoris must be released.
- A Steinmann pin can be placed in the ilium to reflect the abductors, and a small capsulotomy can be made inferiorly to allow for placement of a cobra retractor deep to the transverse acetabular ligament.
  - A bent Hohmann retractor can be placed posteriorly, taking care to first palpate the sciatic nerve to ensure that it is out of harm's way.
- At this point, the acetabulum is exposed and the femoral head can be removed again with a corkscrew and a Cobb elevator.
  - This step should be done very carefully to avoid damaging the acetabular cartilage.
  - The acetabulum can then be inspected for bone debris or fragments.

Component Placement

- The femoral head is measured. A trial unipolar or bipolar head can be placed in the acetabulum for appropriate sizing, which is performed as described for the modified Hardinge approach.
- Once an appropriate size has been determined, the leg is flexed and internally rotated to expose the proximal femur.
  - The leg is held at approximately 90 degrees of internal rotation and 70 degrees of flexion, bringing the osteotomized neck into the surgeon's view.
  - A trochanteric elevator is placed with the teeth under the anterior aspect of the femoral neck, lifting it out of the wound. This allows for unencumbered preparation of the femoral neck **(TECH FIG 18A)**.
- The femur is then prepared in a fashion similar to that described for the modified Hardinge approach **(TECH FIG 18B–F)**.
- In cases where cemented femurs are preferred, a trial of reduction for leg lengths can be performed and a final component can be cemented into place.
  - The component must be cemented in the appropriate version and the neck of the prosthesis must sit on the femoral neck, which can be additionally prepared with a calcar planer.

Completion of the Procedure

- Once the final components are placed and the hip is reduced, two drill holes can be made in the posterior aspect of the greater trochanter for repair of the capsular and short external rotators. Alternatively, the capsule may be closed to a remaining sleeve of capsule or abductor insertion on the trochanter.

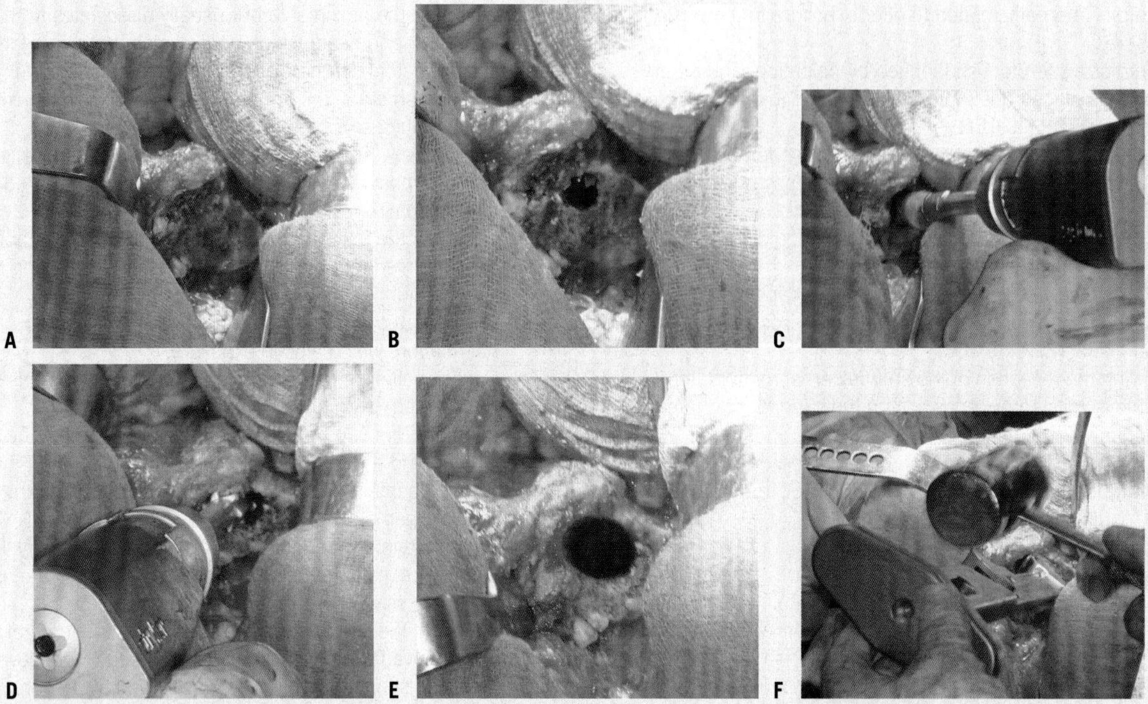

TECH FIG 18 **A.** Presentation of the proximal femur. **B.** Pilot hole for femoral preparation. **C.** Reaming of the femoral shaft. **D.** Lateralization of the femoral shaft using a reamer. **E.** Reamed femoral shaft. Note the lateralization of the canal. **F.** Broaching of the femoral shaft. (Courtesy of Norman A. Johanson, MD.)

- Two nonabsorbable sutures are placed in the capsular flap.
  - The capsular and external rotator tagging sutures are brought through the drill holes and the greater trochanter tied in layers.
  - The quadratus femoris and gluteus maximus tendon also can be repaired if that is the surgeon's preference **(TECH FIG 19)**.
- Subsequently, the Charnley retractor is removed, and the TFL and gluteus maximus fascia are reapproximated.
- Dead space is closed with absorbable sutures in the subcutaneous fat and absorbable sutures are placed in the subcutaneous tissue.
- Skin staples and a sterile compressive dressing are applied at the skin level.
- The hip must be held in an abducted position. An abduction pillow may be placed, and the patient is moved from the lateral position to the supine position at the end of the operation.

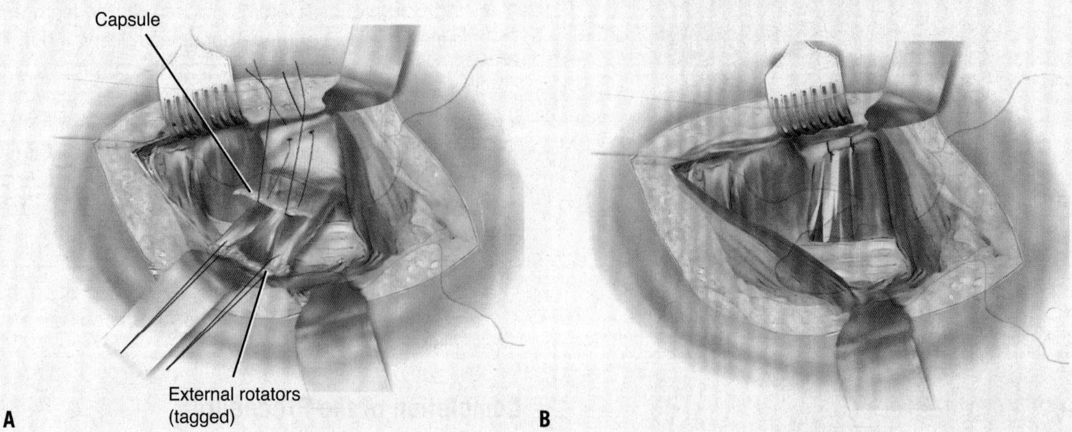

TECH FIG 19 **A,B.** Approximation and repair of the short external rotators.

CEMENTED TECHNIQUE

- The trochanteric fossa is cleared of soft tissue, and a pilot hole is made in it with a small metal curette.
  - An entry reamer is inserted along this pilot hole to seek the long access of the femoral canal.
- The residual femoral neck is cleared with a rongeur or box osteotome. Sometimes, a lateralizing reamer is used to ensure direct access to the femoral canal and minimize the possibility of varus implantation.
- Broaches often are oversized relative to the final implant size, thereby ensuring a minimum cement mantle all around the implant.
  - The final broach is determined when it adequately fills the proximal femur; it also serves as a trial component for reduction.
- Once the stability, limb length, and offset are satisfactory, cementation can be performed. The canal is gently curetted to remove any loose cancellous bone.
- The canal is irrigated with a long, pulsating, irrigating tip.
  - High-quality cancellous bone remains in the femoral canal following this preparation.
  - It is important to centralize the prosthesis to ensure an uninterrupted cement mantle around the implant.
- A plug is placed after the canal is irrigated.
  - I prefer to allow 1 to 2 cm of cement below the tip of the implant so that the plug may be placed at that level.
  - It must be secure enough to withstand pressurization.
  - Three 40-g packs of cement are typically mixed with a vacuum system.
- The canal is packed with sponges to keep it dry during the cementation. Alternatively, continuous suction may be used.
- The viscosity of the cement is an important consideration. The cement should be somewhat doughy and delivered through a cement gun.
  - Appropriate cement viscosity has been reached when the cement no longer sticks to the surgical gloves.
- Once the cement reaches the appropriate viscosity, the packing sponges are removed and the canal is suctioned. Cement is delivered in a retrograde fashion into the canal.
- Once the canal is filled with cement, a pressurizing unit can be placed over the proximal femur, or pressurization can be achieved with a gloved finger.
- The prosthesis is inserted into the doughy mass of cement with the centralizer attached to the tip.
- The leg is placed in a secure position, and the prosthesis is inserted.
  - The prosthesis must be inserted with the appropriate anteversion from insertion all the way down.
  - It is preferable not to rotate the femoral component within the canal because this will create undesirable cement voids.
  - The prosthesis must be inserted with great care to avoid varus malpositioning.
- All the excess cement is removed and the stem is held in place until the cement has fully hardened. The femoral trunnion should be cleaned at this point, and the hemiarthroplasty component should be inserted onto the stem.
- The hip is then reduced and the appropriate closure is performed.

ANTEROLATERAL (WATSON-JONES) TECHNIQUE

- One major difficulty with the Watson-Jones technique is dealing with the gluteus medius and minimus.
  - The hip abductors lie over anterior hip capsule and could be damaged in an effort to obtain adequate exposure.
  - The original approach used by Charnley placed the patient in a supine position and required a trochanteric osteotomy. This approach is used less commonly now because of problems associated with trochanteric reattachment.
- The skin incision is made 2.5 cm behind the ASIS to the tip of the greater trochanter and extended vertically along the anterior margin of the trochanter.
- The intraneural interval is between the TFL and gluteus medius. An incision is made in the underlying iliotibial band, after which the TFL is retracted medially and the gluteus medius is retracted laterally.
- Deep dissection may require release of the anterior parts of the gluteus medius and minimus, which are raised from the femur and retracted posteriorly.
  - The upper part of the capsule at the hip joint is seen with a reflected head of the rectus femoris attached to the upper part of the acetabular rim.
  - It can then be detached with greater exposure of the capsule, which may be incised.
- The ascending branch of the lateral femoral circumflex artery and the accompanying veins run deep to the muscles and must be ligated.
- A longitudinal incision is made in the joint capsule along the femoral neck and transversely from the proximal femur.
- A bone hook can be used to apply a direct lateral force to disimpact the femoral neck fracture. The femoral head can be carefully removed from the acetabulum.
- The acetabulum is then sized as previously described.
- After the femur is externally rotated, adducted, and extended, it can be prepared.
  - Femoral preparation in this approach may require specialized instruments.
- Consider detaching or splitting along the anterior third of the gluteus medius to eliminate the risk of damage to the superior gluteal nerve, which passes 4.5 cm above and 2 cm behind the tip of the greater trochanter.

Pearls and Pitfalls

Acetabular Reaming	• Not recommended for hemiarthroplasty because it leads to poor results. Appropriate femoral head size should be chosen intraoperatively to avoid reaming.
Varus Malalignment	• Care should be taken to broach the lateral cortex of the proximal femur adequately to prevent varus malalignment of the implant.
Implant Orientation (Anteversion)	• Ideally, the patient's hip should be reoriented to its native position. Ideal anteversion of the hip in adults is 10–30 degrees, depending on multiple patient-specific factors. If the patient has pathology that affects hip orientation (eg, developmental displacement of the hip), a modular THA implant could be considered.
Cement Technique	• I recommend the use of uncemented, proximal-fit, porous-coated implants in most patients, if possible. The presence of poor bone quality, stovepipe proximal femoral metaphysis and shaft, and angular/rotational deformities of the proximal femur argue for use of a cemented implant. Proper cement technique includes vacuum mixing of cement, pressurized cement delivery, proper canal preparation, placement of a cement restrictor plug, finger pressurization of cement, and stable implant pressurization of the cement. An ideal cement mantle is 2 mm circumferentially around the implant.
Posterior Approach	• Careful retractor placement is essential to avoid errant sciatic or femoral nerve injury. Enhanced posterior capsular repair is important to reduce the risk of dislocation.

POSTOPERATIVE CARE

- All patients are placed into an appropriate bed with consideration of ulcer prevention. Bilateral thromboembolic stockings or sequential venous compression devices should be used as a mechanical means to prevent thromboembolic events.
- Early ambulation and progression to full weight bearing when possible is encouraged as this minimizes the risk of postoperative complications. Furthermore, older patients are often incapable of partial weight bearing and therefore are more likely to succeed when full weight bearing can be initiated.
- Antiembolic prophylaxis is started according to the surgeon's preference. Appropriate anticoagulation choice is beyond the scope of this chapter but may range from mechanical prophylaxis alone, augmentation with aspirin, heparin, unfractionated heparin, warfarin, or novel anticoagulant medications.
  - Extended prophylaxis may be considered for these patients who are immobile.

OUTCOMES

- Bipolar hemiarthroplasty was introduced in the 1970s in an effort to prevent or retard acetabular wear.
  - These femoral prostheses have a 22- to 32-mm head that articulates with a polyethylene liner.
  - The liner is covered with a polished metal outer shell that articulates with the acetabular cartilage.
  - Depending on implant design, about 45 degrees of angular motion is achieved before the prosthetic neck impinges on the liner and axial rotation is restricted.
- Theoretically, hip motion occurs primarily at the prosthetic joint and only secondarily at the metal-cartilage interface.
  - The polyethylene liner may help to protect the native acetabular cartilage by cushioning the high-contact pressures that occur across the bearing.
- LaBelle et al[18] reported no acetabular protrusio or articular cartilage wear greater than 2 mm in 49 femoral neck fractures treated with cemented bipolar hemiarthroplasties at 5- to 10-year follow-up.
- Wetherell and Hinves[21] reported a 50% reduction in acetabular erosion for patients treated with a cemented bipolar prosthesis when compared to those treated with a unipolar prosthesis.
- Research attempting to demonstrate that motion occurs within a bipolar prosthesis has yielded conflicting results.
  - Drinker and Murray[7] fluoroscopically evaluated 13 hips in 10 young patients following bipolar reconstruction for AVN and noted that only a minor amount of motion occurred at the inner bearing and that motion tended to decrease over time.
  - They further demonstrated that in this group, most implants functioned as a unipolar prosthesis and concluded that motion will occur at the interface where there is the least frictional resistance. They found that this location is not the same in arthritic hips as in fractured hips.
  - In patients with acute hip fractures with normal articular cartilage, primary intraoperative or intraprosthetic motion occurred in only 25% and most implants functioned as unipolar.
- Brueton et al[4] whose radiographic analysis of 75 bipolar prostheses compared 32- and 22-mm heads, showed that the smaller head was associated with more motion.

COMPLICATIONS

- Thromboembolism (eg, deep vein thrombosis or pulmonary embolism)
- Kenzora et al[16] reported a mortality rate of 14% during the first year following hip fracture.
  - When compared to 9% mortality in a population of similar age, the mortality after hemiarthroplasty is 10% to 40%.
- The incidence of intraoperative femur fracture is 4.5%. Most are nondisplaced and involve either the trochanter or calcar. Recent data suggests that press-fit fixation choice has a higher incidence of periprosthetic fracture than cemented

fixation and should be considered based on bone quality, patient risk factors, and surgeon comfort level.[13]

- When an intraoperative femur fracture occurs, the full extent of the fracture should be exposed. Assessment of the fracture will dictate treatment. Choices include observation and claw plate fixation for isolated trochanteric lesions. If there is concern about component stability with the fracture, treatment options may include utilizing polymethylmethacrylate fixated stems combined with long-stem prosthesis or, alternatively, a diaphyseal engaging stem and cables.

- The rate of dislocation is less than 10%. Dislocation is more common with incorrect version, posterior capsulectomy without repair, and excessive postoperative flexion or rotation with the hip adducted. Recurrent dislocation may be treated with closed reduction, conversion to a total hip arthroplasty if constraint is desired, or alternatively resection arthroplasty (Girdlestone).
- Postoperative sepsis has been reported to range from 2% to 20%. Infections may be superficial or deep. These can be managed with either antibiotics alone, open débridement combined with antibiotics, or component removal or exchange depending on the depth of infection, chronicity, and host factors.
- Stem loosening or failure of fixation may be suspected with the presence of a radiolucent line around the prosthesis. This may manifest as thigh pain, start-up pain, or difficulty with ambulation.
  - If clinical signs and symptoms are present, or loosening or migration is present with serial imaging, a revision arthroplasty may be considered.
- Cementation presents some hazards, and, in some cases, the application of pressurized cement is associated with an embolization phenomenon with cement elements (ie, monomer, polymethylmethacrylate elements, or fat). Embolization of these materials may result in hypoxia, cardiac arrest, or death.
  - The risk factors include older age or patent foramen ovale.
  - The use of pulsatile lavage can reduce that risk by removing fat and marrow from the femoral canal.
  - In older patients with substantial medical comorbidities, it may be wise to avoid pressurization of the cement within the canal because the risk of acute embolization may be high.
  - Alternatively, the anesthesia team should be notified at the time of cementation and may consider raising the blood pressure to accommodate potential risks.
- Progressive wear may occur years later as the native acetabulum has not been resurfaced and may still develop osteoarthritis. This is more commonly seen in younger and active patients, which highlights the need for appropriate identification of patient preinjury function to allow for the correct procedure to be performed. This may be diagnosed clinically with groin pain, or with radiographic loss of articular cartilage between the prosthetic head and acetabular bone. Diagnosis may be augmented with diagnostic lidocaine injections to assess for pain relief. This progressive osteoarthritis may be treated with conservative measures as with standard hip osteoarthritis or alternatively with conversion to a total hip replacement by placing an acetabular component.

REFERENCES

1. Barnes JT, Brown JT, Garden RS, et al. Subcapital fractures of the femur: a prospective review. J Bone Joint Surg Br 1976;58:2–24.
2. Bateman JE. Single-assembly total hip prosthesis. Preliminary report. Orthop Dig 1974;2:15.
3. Bezwada HP, Shah AR, Harding SH, et al. Cementless bipolar hemiarthroplasty for displaced femoral neck fractures in the elderly. J Arthroplasty 2004;19(7 suppl 2):73–77.
4. Brueton RN, Craig JS, Hinves BL, et al. Effect of femoral component head size on movement of the two-component hemi-arthroplasty. Injury 1993;24:231–235.
5. Dedrick DK, Mackenzie JR, Burney RE. Complications of femoral neck fracture in young adults. J Trauma 1986;26:932–937.
6. Dorr LD, Faugere MC, Mackel AM, et al. Structural and cellular assessment of bone quality of proximal femur. Bone 1993;14:231–242.
7. Drinker H, Murray WR. The universal proximal femoral endoprosthesis. A short-term comparison with conventional hemiarthroplasty. J Bone Joint Surg Am 1979;61:1167–1174.
8. Eiskjaer S, Ostgård SE. Risk factors influencing mortality after bipolar hemiarthroplasty in the treatment of fracture of the femoral neck. Clin Orthop Relat Res 1991;(270):295–300.
9. Fixation using Alternative Implants for the Treatment of Hip fractures (FAITH) Investigators. Fracture fixation in the operative management of hip fractures (FAITH): an international, multicentre, randomised controlled trial. Lancet 2017;389(10078):1519–1527.
10. Garden RS. Stability and union in subcapital fractures of the femur. J Bone Joint Surg Br 1964;46-B:630–647.
11. Gilberty RP. Bipolar endoprosthesis minimizes protrusio acetabuli, loose stems. Orthop Rev 1985;14:27.
12. Grose AW, Gardner MJ, Sussmann PS, et al. The surgical anatomy of the blood supply to the femoral head: description of the anastomosis between the medial femoral circumflex and inferior gluteal arteries at the hip. J Bone Joint Surg Br 2008;90(10):1298–1303.
13. Grosso MJ, Danoff JR, Murtaugh TS, et al. Hemiarthroplasty for displaced femoral neck fractures in the elderly has a low conversion rate. J Arthroplasty 2017;32(1):150–154.
14. Ito H, Matsuno T, Kaneda K. Bipolar hemiarthroplasty for osteonecrosis of the femoral head. A 7- to 18-year followup. Clin Orthop Relat Res 2000;(374):201–211.
15. Jia, Z, Ding F, Wu Y, et al. Unipolar versus bipolar hemiarthroplasty for displaced femoral neck fractures: a systematic review and meta-analysis of randomized controlled trials. J Orthop Surg Res 2015;10:8.
16. Kenzora JE, McCarthy RE, Lowell JD, et al. Hip fracture mortality. Relation to age, treatment, preoperative illness, time of surgery, and complications. Clin Orthop Relat Res 1984;(186):45–56.
17. Klestil T, Röder C, Stotter C, et al. Impact of timing of surgery in elderly hip fracture patients: a systematic review and meta-analysis. Sci Rep 2018;8:13933.
18. LaBelle LW, Colwill JC, Swanson AB. Bateman bipolar hip arthroplasty for femoral neck fractures. A five- to ten-year follow-up study. Clin Orthop Relat Res 1990;(251):20–25.
19. Lin JCF, Liang WM. Outcomes after fixation for undisplaced femoral neck fracture compared to hemiarthroplasty compared to displaced femoral neck fracture among the elderly. BMC Musculoskeletal Dis 2015;16:199.
20. Robinson CM, Court-Brown CM, McQueen MM, et al. Hip fractures in adults younger than 50 years of age. Epidemiology and results. Clin Orthop Relat Res 1995;(312):238–246.
21. Wetherell RG, Hinves BL. The Hastings bipolar hemiarthroplasty for subcapital fractures of the femoral neck. A 10-year prospective study. J Bone Joint Surg Br 1990;72:788–793.
22. Yu L, Wang Y, Chen J. Total hip arthroplasty versus hemiarthroplasty for displaced femoral neck fractures: meta-analysis of randomized trials. Clin Orthop Relat Res 2012;470:2235–2243.

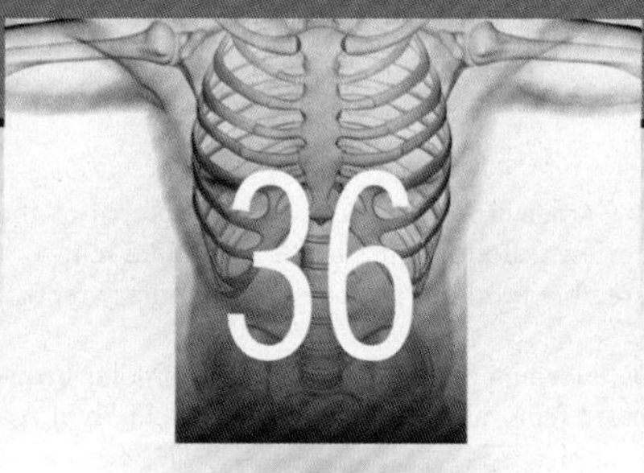

CHAPTER

Femur and Knee
Cephalomedullary Nailing of the Proximal Femur

Hassan R. Mir

DEFINITION

- Fractures of the proximal femur are usually grouped into four major types reflecting differences in the anatomic and physiologic character of these regions:
  - Femoral head fractures
  - Intracapsular femoral neck fractures
  - Pertrochanteric fractures (also referred to as *intertrochanteric* and *peritrochanteric*), which include proximal extracapsular fractures from the femoral neck region to the region along the lesser trochanter before the development of the medullary canal
  - Subtrochanteric fractures
- Cephalomedullary nailing is the surgical stabilization of the fracture with an intramedullary device usually inserted through the piriformis fossa or the greater trochanter and includes fixation into the femoral head.
- Cephalomedullary nails are most commonly indicated in extracapsular peritrochanteric and subtrochanteric fractures. Although there is occasional overlap of these regions, the personality of the fracture will be predominantly one of these major types.

ANATOMY

- The transitional anatomy from the femoral head to the subtrochanteric region affords very different fracture pathogeneses, affecting the surgical opportunity for repair **(FIG 1A)**.
  - Intracapsular fractures of the femoral neck are critically dependent on the vascular supply from the medial femoral circumflex artery for fracture repair and maintenance of vascularity of the femoral head to avoid avascular necrosis.
  - Conversely, the well-vascularized pertrochanteric region is dependent on the structural integrity of an essentially solid cancellous bone block (calcar or Adam's arch) extending from the femoral head inferiorly along Ward triangle to the lesser trochanter, where the solid nature of the structure changes to a tubular construct with the origin of the femoral medullary canal **(FIG 1C)**.[3,10]

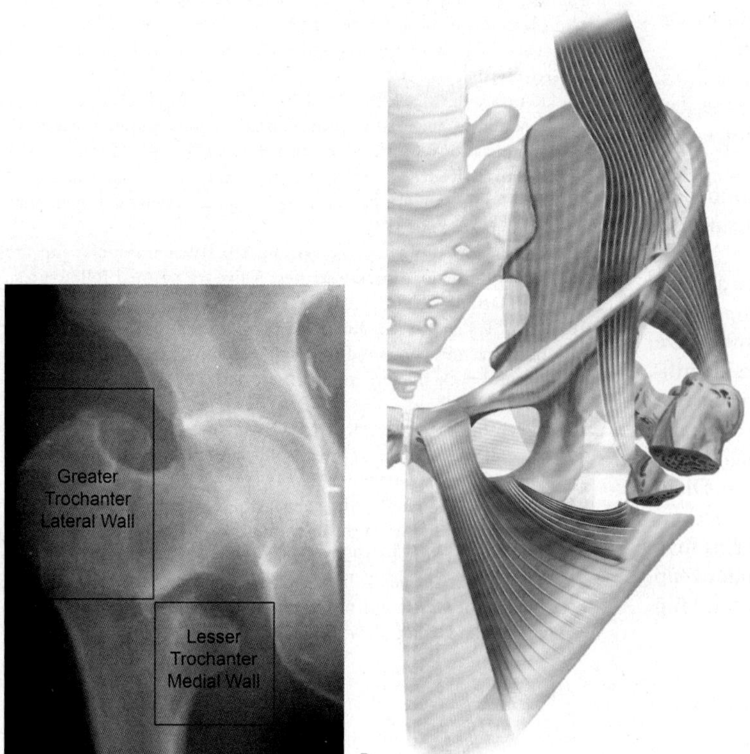

FIG 1 **A.** Radiographic anatomy of the proximal femoral fracture zones. Note greater trochanter and lateral wall and lesser trochanter and medial wall. **B.** Muscle attachments in subtrochanteric fractures accounting for the subsequent deformity of the fracture. *(continued)*

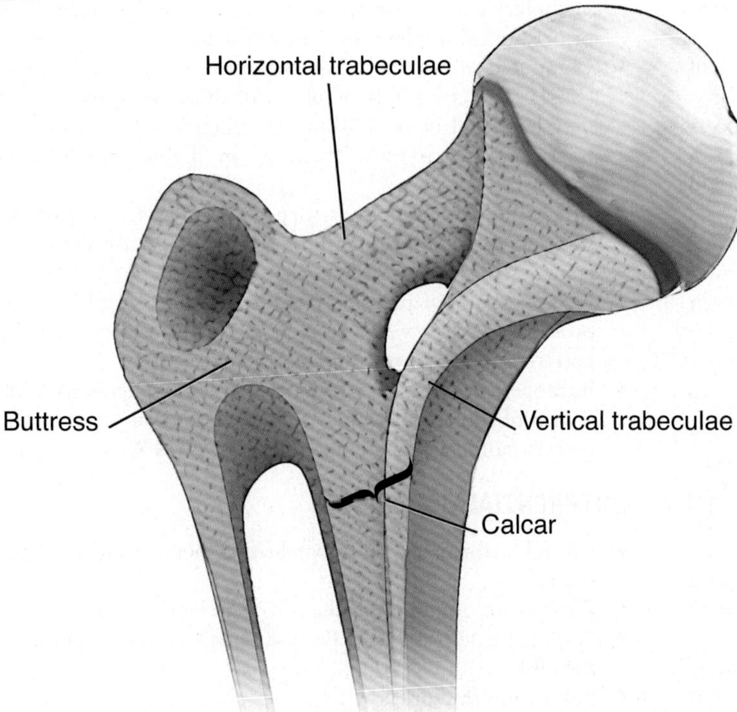

C

FIG 1 *(continued)* **C.** Drawing of Hammer model femoral head–neck trabecular patterns.

- Subtrochanteric fractures incur the highest stresses in the proximal femur owing to their tubular anatomy and the moment arm generated from the short proximal femoral region and associated musculotendinous insertions, which place high degrees of stress on the implants used for their fixation.
- The muscular attachments of the gluteus medius in the lateral aspect of the greater trochanter and the iliopsoas insertion in the lesser trochanter are key determinants in the deforming forces associated with fracture displacement and functional recovery after injury **(FIG 1B)**.

PATHOGENESIS

- Fractures of the proximal femur fall into three mechanistic categories:
  - Low-energy, same-level falls, predominantly in the physiologically senior population, often associated with osteoporosis and muscular atrophy
  - High-energy trauma in younger and healthier patients from motor vehicle collisions and falls from greater heights, typically resulting in fractures with marked displacement and comminution
  - Pathologic fractures, often the first indication of a neoplastic process

NATURAL HISTORY

- To obtain any real hope of ambulatory recovery, surgical treatment is necessary for complete fractures, as the resulting deformity of a nonoperatively treated hip invariably results in significant shortening and varus deformity.
- Functional recovery is actually very poor despite surgical treatment of these fractures with conventional techniques in the elderly age group.[2]

PATIENT HISTORY AND PHYSICAL FINDINGS

- Pertinent history for a hip fracture patient focuses on the mechanism of injury for insight into the potential quality of bone available for repair and associated injuries in high-energy trauma.
- Associated injuries or premorbid diseases may coexist with the fracture diagnosis. Syncopal episodes resulting in a fall may bring attention to cardiovascular and neurologic disease states.
- A history of any tumor or malignant disease, including the last mammogram and breast examination in women older than 45 years and the last prostate examination in men older than 40 years, may suggest an underlying pathologic etiology for the fracture.
- Drug use, either illicit or prescribed, is a confounding and contributing factor affecting anesthesia and postoperative pain and rehabilitation management.
- Preinjury ambulatory status including the use of walking aids (eg, cane, walker) is important to determine in order to counsel patients and families on postoperative expectations.
- Patients with preexisting symptomatic osteoarthritis may be considered for treatment with calcar replacing arthroplasty instead of fracture fixation.
- Unfortunately, nursing home and institutionalized patients must be examined for potential neglect and abuse.
- The physical findings of a displaced hip fracture are shortening of the extremity, deformity of rotation compared to the contralateral extremity, and pain or crepitus with motion at the hip.
  - Shortening and rotational deformity may be the result of varus deformity at the hip from associated muscular pull or telescoping of 100% displaced fragments.
- Examination may also include the Lippmann test (auscultation). Decreased tone or pitch implies fracture. Sound conduction through the pelvis and hip from the pelvis is

interrupted by any discontinuity from the patella, femur, or pelvis articulations.

- Swelling and discoloration with hematoma are signs of injury but are usually not acutely present.
- Lacerations, Morel-Lavallée lesions, and decubitus ulcers may complicate the surgical approach.
- Extracapsular proximal femur fractures extravasate blood into the surrounding tissues.
- A complete neurovascular examination must be performed as with any extremity injury. This is particularly important in elderly patients who may have vascular insufficiency even without injury.

IMAGING AND OTHER DIAGNOSTIC STUDIES

- Plain radiographs, including an anteroposterior (AP) view of the pelvis, AP, and cross-table lateral views of the affected hip are required for diagnosis and preoperative planning. Frog-leg lateral views should be avoided as they cause unnecessary pain to the patient.
- A traction view of the hip in mild internal rotation may add valuable information about the pattern and the reducibility of the fracture.
- AP and lateral radiographs of the affected femur to the knee are required, with special attention to femoral bow and medullary canal diameter, and to assess for the presence of prior surgical implants at the distal femur.
- Computed tomography or magnetic resonance imaging (MRI) scans are rarely required for displaced fractures but may be useful in establishing the diagnosis in nonobvious fractures and atypical fractures in high-energy trauma patients.
- If a pathologic etiology is suspected, however, an MRI or positron emission tomography scan of the body should be considered as part of the initial workup.
- Intraoperative or preoperative traction radiography or fluoroscopic C-arm views may be helpful in delineating the pattern and extent of complex fractures.
- Intraoperative length and rotational measurements with the C-arm of the normal femur may be helpful in selecting the correct nail length in complex fractures **(FIG 2)**.

DIFFERENTIAL DIAGNOSIS

- Painful arthropathy (osteoarthritis, rheumatoid arthritis, septic)
- Established nonunion of the proximal femur
- Pathologic deformity (ie, Paget disease, fibrous dysplasia of the hip)
- Pubic rami fracture

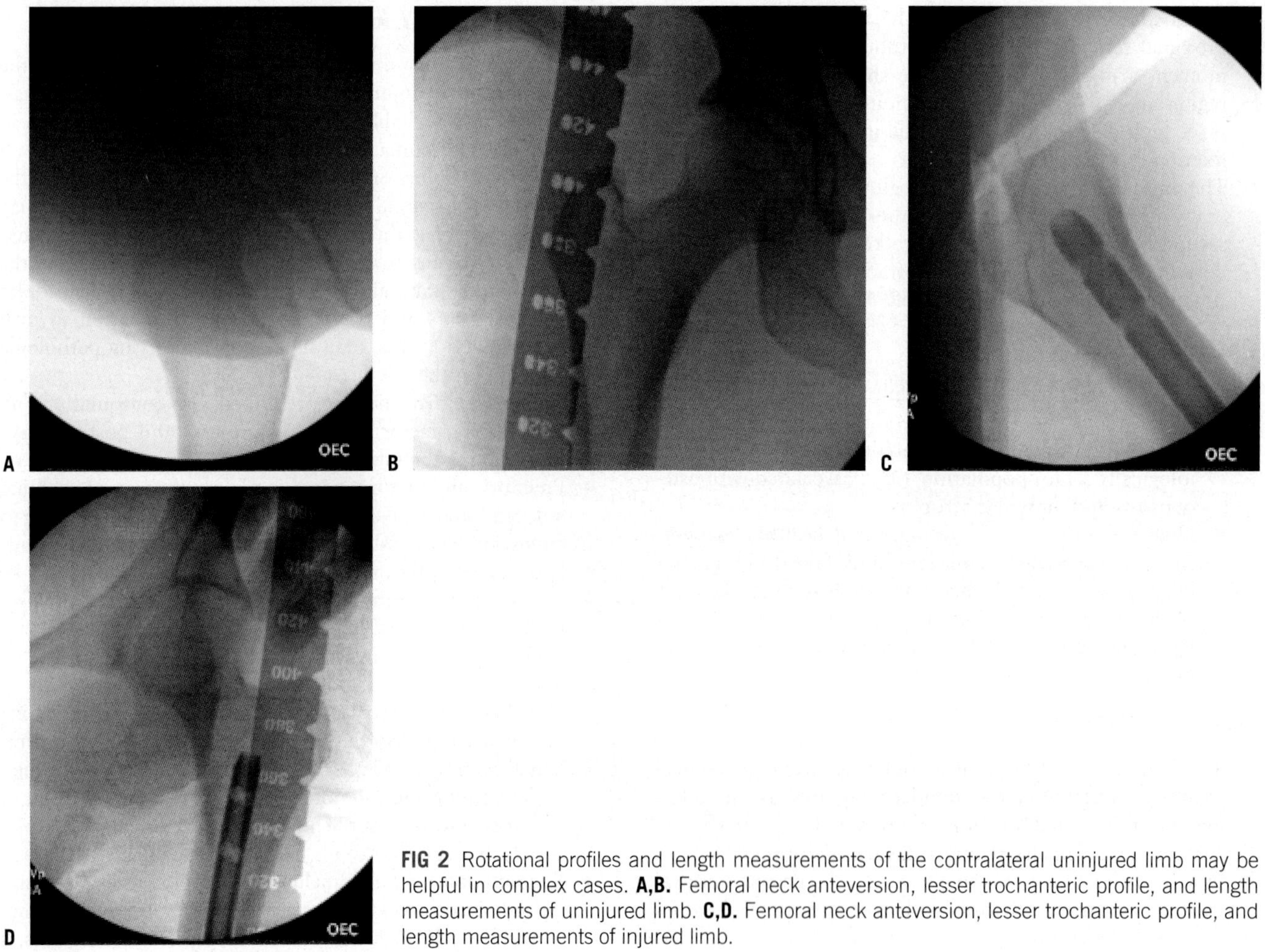

FIG 2 Rotational profiles and length measurements of the contralateral uninjured limb may be helpful in complex cases. **A,B.** Femoral neck anteversion, lesser trochanteric profile, and length measurements of uninjured limb. **C,D.** Femoral neck anteversion, lesser trochanteric profile, and length measurements of injured limb.

- Acetabular fracture
- Contiguous femoral fracture
- Hip fracture-dislocation (rare)

NONOPERATIVE MANAGEMENT

- Nonoperative treatment may be the best option in nonambulatory or chronic dementia patients with pain controllable with analgesics and rest, patients with terminal disease with less than 6 weeks of life expected, patients with irresolvable medical comorbidities that preclude surgical treatment, and patients with active infectious diseases that preclude insertion of a surgical implant.
  - An exception is incomplete pertrochanteric fractures diagnosed by MRI, which have been shown to heal with nonoperative measures in selective patients.[1]
- Nonoperative management must include attentive nursing care with frequent positioning to avoid decubiti, attention to nutrition and fluid homeostasis, and adequate analgesia. Patients may be mobilized from bed to chair as tolerated, usually after 7 to 14 days, with careful support and elevation of the affected extremity. Inadequate pain control is a contributing factor to dementia and increased complications.
- Fracture callus at 3 weeks markedly decreases motion-related pain, and by 6 weeks, most patients can be lifted into a wheelchair or reclining chair.
- Ambulatory ability may be possible after nonoperative treatment of displaced fractures.[20]

SURGICAL MANAGEMENT

- Surgical management, once selected, should be performed as soon as any correctable metabolic, hematologic, or organ system instabilities have been rectified. This is within the first 24 to 48 hours for most patients.
  - The literature shows increased mortality after this time.[26]
  - Patients with subtrochanteric fractures may benefit from skeletal traction while awaiting surgery.

Preoperative Planning

- Standard AP pelvis and AP hip radiographs are usually obtained. Cross-table lateral and films in traction are useful if the hip fracture pattern is complex. Hip fractures are three-dimensional entities, and these are apparent in high-energy trauma cases. Full-length femur radiographs of good quality are required before surgery to evaluate the full extent of damage to the femur, to estimate the length and diameter of implant selections, to assess for the presence of prior surgical implants at the distal femur, and to avoid neglect of skip lesions or segmental damage to the femur. Most importantly, the full length lateral radiograph will allow for an assessment of the femoral bow, such that the proper implant can be chosen. Substantial deformity in either plane may preclude the ability to nail the fracture with a long implant, or require bending the nail intraoperatively.
- Classifications for peritrochanteric and subtrochanteric hip fractures have not been particularly helpful in clinical situations, although increased surgical complexity is associated with unstable fracture patterns.[11]
  - Unstable characteristics include posteromedial large separate fragmentation, basicervical patterns, reverse obliquity patterns, and displaced greater trochanteric or lateral wall fractures. These findings, however, were described as creating an unstable fracture when plating is chosen and do not portend the same problems with stability if nailed with an appropriate reduction.
  - The Evans, Kyle, AO Orthopaedic Trauma Association, and Russell-Taylor classifications are commonly referred to in the literature.
- The Russell-Taylor classification assists in implant selection when nailing the proximal femur by drawing attention to the high-risk attributes of the proximal femoral anatomy, particularly the absence or presence of fracture extension into the piriformis fossa, referred to as *group I* (intact greater trochanteric region) and *group II* (fracture extension), and secondly the absence or presence of medial cortical stability in the lesser trochanteric region, referred to as *type A* (stable contact possible) and *type B* (fracture instability) **(FIG 3)**.[25] This classification was devised for nails that entered the piriformis fossa and therefore does not directly apply as directly to the current generation of trochanteric entry nails.
  - Russell-Taylor type IA fractures are in reality high diaphyseal femoral fractures within 5 cm of the lesser

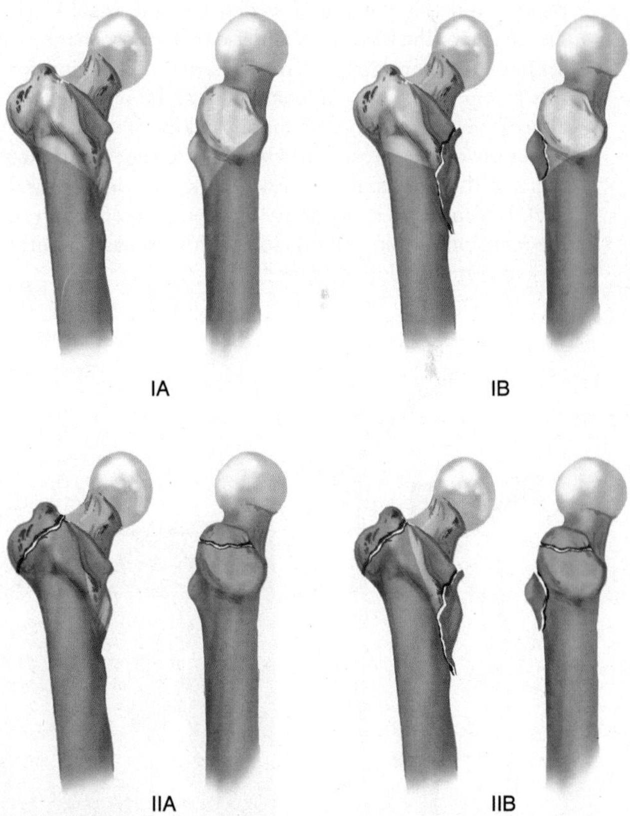

FIG 3 Russell-Taylor classification. Type IA fractures are in reality high diaphyseal femoral fractures within 5 cm of the lesser trochanter. Type IB fractures are fractures at the diaphyseal–metaphyseal junction of the proximal femur with medial instability due to fracture comminution in the lesser trochanteric region. Type IIA fractures extend into the piriformis region but have the possibility of restoration of medial cortical stability. Type IIB fractures are the most unstable fractures, with fracture extension into the greater trochanteric piriformis region and have lost medial cortical stability.

trochanter and may be treated with conventional interlocking nails, with the surgeon's choice of trochanteric, piriformis, or retrograde entry devices and without the need for cephalomedullary nails.

- Russell-Taylor type IB fractures are fractures at the diaphyseal–metaphyseal junction of the proximal femur with medial instability due to fracture comminution of the medial calcar and lesser trochanter. The greater trochanter and lateral wall are intact, and cephalomedullary nails, either of the reconstruction nail class or hip fracture nails, are indicated, with either a trochanteric or piriformis entry type of device with the respective portal.
- Russell-Taylor type IIA fractures are fractures involving the greater trochanter and piriformis region but have the possibility of restoration of medial cortical stability. If the greater trochanter is displaced, open reduction and stabilization are required. Trochanteric portal cephalomedullary nails are recommended if a nail technique is preferred. Piriformis nails are relatively contraindicated. Open plate and screw reduction with an indirect reduction technique and trochanteric buttress plating may be preferred in this group of patients especially if the greater trochanter is displaced cephalad.[14]
- Russell-Taylor type IIB fractures are the most unstable fractures, with fracture extension into the piriformis region, and they have lost medial cortical stability by disruption of the lesser trochanteric region. Trochanteric cephalomedullary nails are the preferred nail option for this group if a stable nail construct can be obtained, or alternatively, a proximal femoral locking plate if comminution of the greater trochanter precludes nail stability in the proximal fragment. If the anterior femoral neck is comminuted, accessory fixation and reduction of the anterior wall in conjunction with proximal femoral locked plate fixation is advised.[6]
    - Reverse obliquity patterns and lateral wall fractures occurring in the perioperative period have been identified as high-risk patterns for sliding compression hip screw-type implants. Failure by excessive collapse of femoral neck length and medialization of the shaft is a form of dynamic failure of the implant, and although the implant may survive, the resultant deformity will compromise the patient's functional recovery. The ability to differentiate stable from unstable pertrochanteric fractures has been shown to be the result of unstable malreductions and unappreciated osteopenia in the shaft and femoral head fixation with implant bone interface failure as the etiology of failure.[9,19]
- Determination of the preoperative neck–shaft angle and medullary canal diameter is paramount to selection of the correct nail device, as different manufacturers have different neck–shaft angle and diameter nails. Another important consideration is nail curvature for long nails. Curved nails with a 1.5- to 2-m radius are applicable to most situations, but the surgeon must beware of patients with excessive curvature or tertiary curves in the distal third of the femur, as distal penetration of long nails has been reported.[17]
- Cephalomedullary nailing involves fixation of the femoral head coupled with an intramedullary shaft implant **(FIG 4)**. These implants are designed to have a piriformis portal for insertion, usually with the shaft component straight in the AP plane or a trochanteric portal with the shaft component laterally angulated proximally.
    - Modern trochanteric designs have moved to a 4- to 6-degree proximal bend positioned above the lesser trochanteric region, which seems to be most compatible with anatomic restoration of the fracture.[18]
- Reconstruction design nails (two smaller screws into the head) have the usual advantage of a smaller head diameter (average 13 to 15 mm) and may be of a piriformis or trochanteric portal design, whereas the traditional

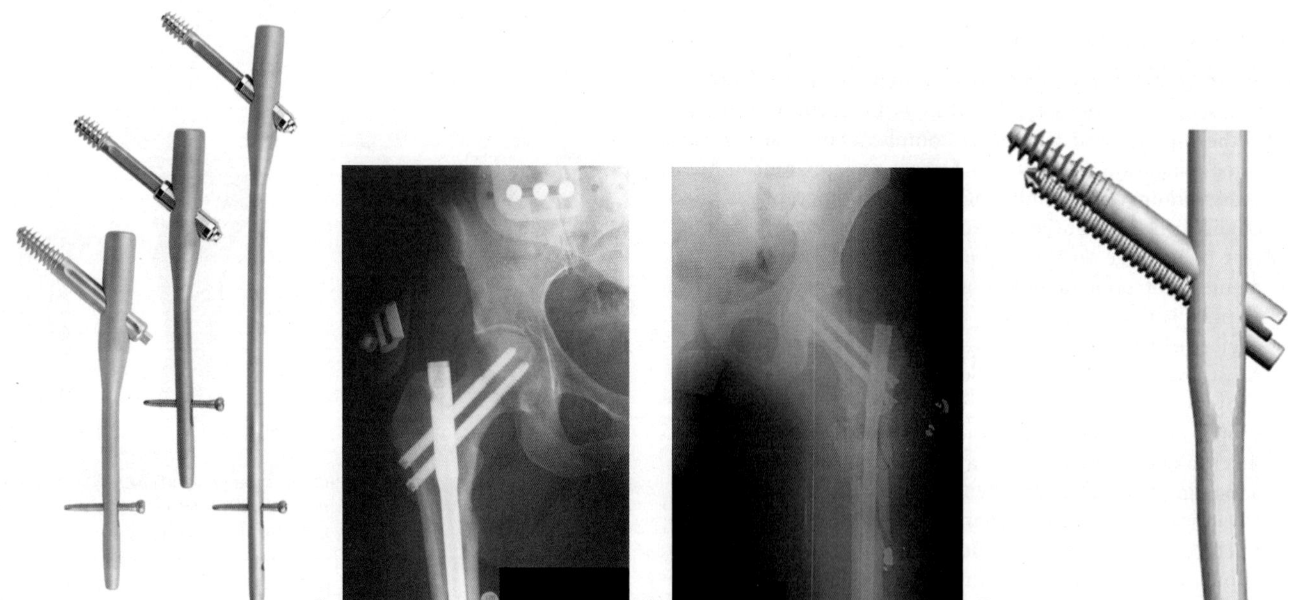

FIG 4 Cephalomedullary nail types from Smith & Nephew, Inc. **A.** Gamma class intramedullary hip screw. **B.** Piriformis TriGen reconstruction nail. **C.** Trochanteric TriGen reconstruction nail. **D.** Integrated interlocking InterTAN nail. **(A,D:** Courtesy of Smith & Nephew, Inc., Memphis, TN.)

trochanteric portal intramedullary hip fracture nails have a single large-diameter femoral head fixation screw or blade and have proximal shaft diameters around 16 to 18 mm.

- New-generation cephalomedullary nails are moving to smaller geometries of 12 to 15.5 mm of the head to maximize bone conservation in the proximal femur and avoid excessive bone removal from the lateral wall.
- New designs in femoral head fixation are also in use with constraint in the reconstruction-type two-screw design to minimize Z-effect and integrated interlocking two-screw fixation with the design goal of improving fracture construct rotational and translational stability.

Positioning

- Intramedullary techniques for the proximal femur are best managed with a modern fracture table with image intensification (C-arm) capabilities.
- Although the lateral decubitus approach may be helpful for reverse obliquity patterns, the supine position is usually preferred because of the ease of setup and radiographic visualization in a familiar frame of reference.
- The author prefers use of the fracture table with the legs in a scissored position, although attachment to the fracture table via skeletal traction through the distal femur or proximal tibia can be used if there are other injuries about the knee, leg, or foot.
  - The operative leg is raised to about 20 to 30 degrees of flexion, and the nonoperative extremity is extended 20 to 30 degrees.
  - The uninjured limb can be secured to the central bar of the fracture table with a pillow sling and Coban bandage or tape **(FIG 5)**.[5] Alternately, it can be placed in traction on most tables through a well-padded boot.
  - The injured leg is pulled in line with the body to avoid varus positioning of the hip.

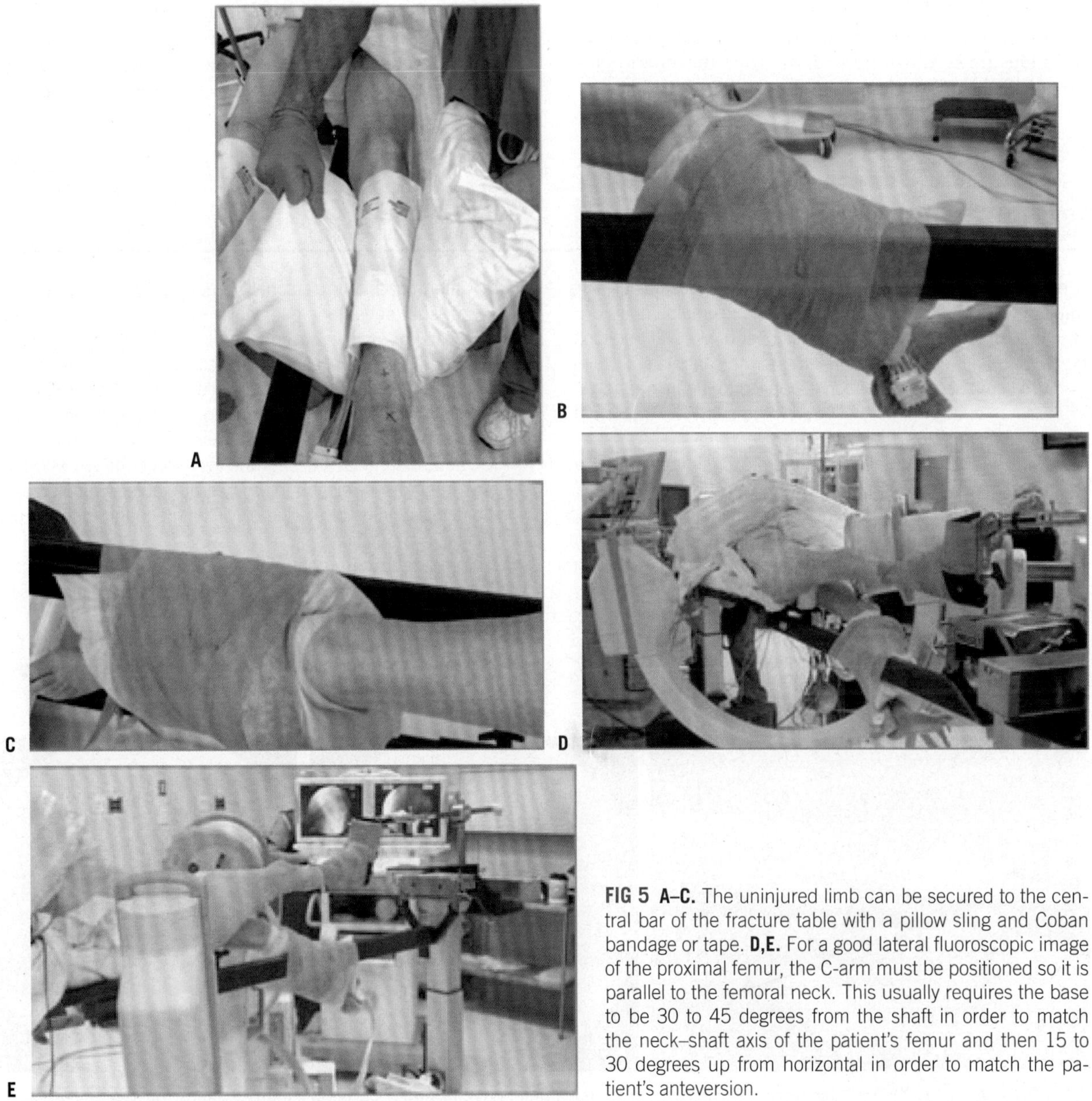

FIG 5 A–C. The uninjured limb can be secured to the central bar of the fracture table with a pillow sling and Coban bandage or tape. **D,E.** For a good lateral fluoroscopic image of the proximal femur, the C-arm must be positioned so it is parallel to the femoral neck. This usually requires the base to be 30 to 45 degrees from the shaft in order to match the neck–shaft axis of the patient's femur and then 15 to 30 degrees up from horizontal in order to match the patient's anteversion.

- The C-arm is brought in from the opposite side with the base as perpendicular to the operative femoral neck as possible to get the best view of this region.
- With this type of setup, the true AP of the hip is usually obtained with 5 to 15 degrees of rotation of the C-arm over the top.
- In order to obtain a good lateral fluoroscopic image of the proximal femur, the C-arm must be positioned so it is parallel to the femoral neck. This usually requires the base to be 30 to 45 degrees from the shaft in order to match the neck–shaft axis of the patient's femur and then 15 to 30 degrees up from horizontal in order to match the patient's anteversion (see **FIG 5**).

Approach

- The surgical approach for the entry is common for all antegrade proximal femoral nailing.
- The incision is usually 3 cm long and is about 4 cm proximal to the greater trochanter, centered over the extrapolated middle third of the trochanter.
  - In obese or muscular individuals, this can be referenced by a line drawn down transversely from the anterior superior iliac spine and the lateral position of the incision determined by the C-arm true lateral with a radiographic marker on the skin (**FIG 6**).
- This approach should not damage the gluteus medius muscle, so aggressive traction or manipulation through the muscle should be avoided. The surgeon should always instrument and ream the femur with soft tissue protection in mind.

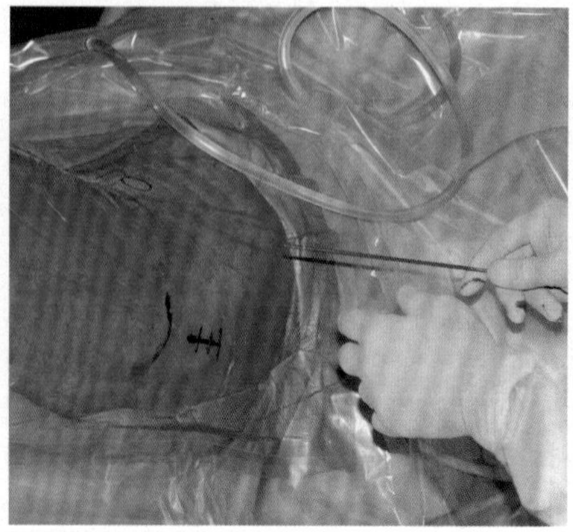

FIG 6 Skin incision position referencing the anterior superior iliac spine.

FRACTURE REDUCTION

- Reduction of the fracture is tantamount to success. There are multiple techniques for reduction of the proximal femur.
  - After attachment to the foot positioner or skeletal traction with the perineal post attached and the contralateral uninjured limb secured, traction is applied to the injured leg in order to restore length in line with the body. It is important to avoid a varus reduction.
  - The leg is rotated to align with the proximal fragment, 5 to 15 degrees of external rotation for most subtrochanteric personality fractures, and intertrochanteric personality fractures may be externally rotated 10 degrees or placed in up to 15 degrees of internal rotation as the variability of femoral neck anteversion is larger than previously recognized.[6]
  - Posterior sag is corrected at the fracture with a force directed from posterior to anterior and maintained. The leg is flexed through the foot holder 20 to 30 degrees from neutral for intertrochanteric personality fractures and 30 to 40 degrees for subtrochanteric personality fractures, maintaining the posterior to anterior reduction force at the hip. This can be aided in certain cases when necessary with a crutch, or with commercially available table attachments (**TECH FIG 1A–C**).[13]
- Acceptable alignment is confirmed with the C-arm in both views. The surgeon ensures there is adequate room in the pelvic and abdominal areas for the insertion of the wires, reamers, and implants in relation to the fracture table. A small bump may be necessary to elevate the pelvis high enough to allow room for the instrumentation.
- The reduction can then be fine-tuned with closed methods, intramedullary instruments, or by percutaneous joysticks or pushers (**TECH FIG 1D–U**).
- If the reduction is not acceptable at this point, the surgeon should stop and reevaluate the position of the C-arm and the

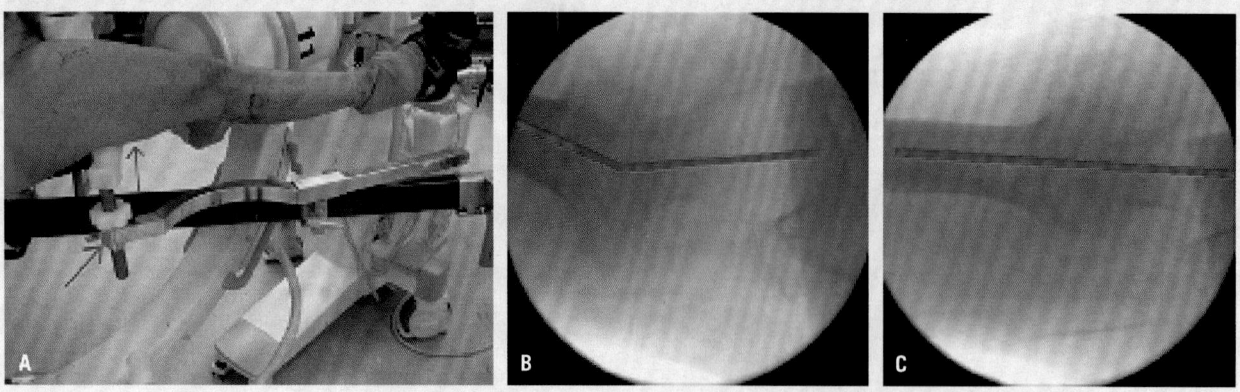

TECH FIG 1 **A.** PORD (Orthofix, McKinney, TX) attached to the fracture table. **B.** Posterior sag of an intertrochanteric fracture prereduction. **C.** Sag corrected with lift from table attachment device. *(continued)*

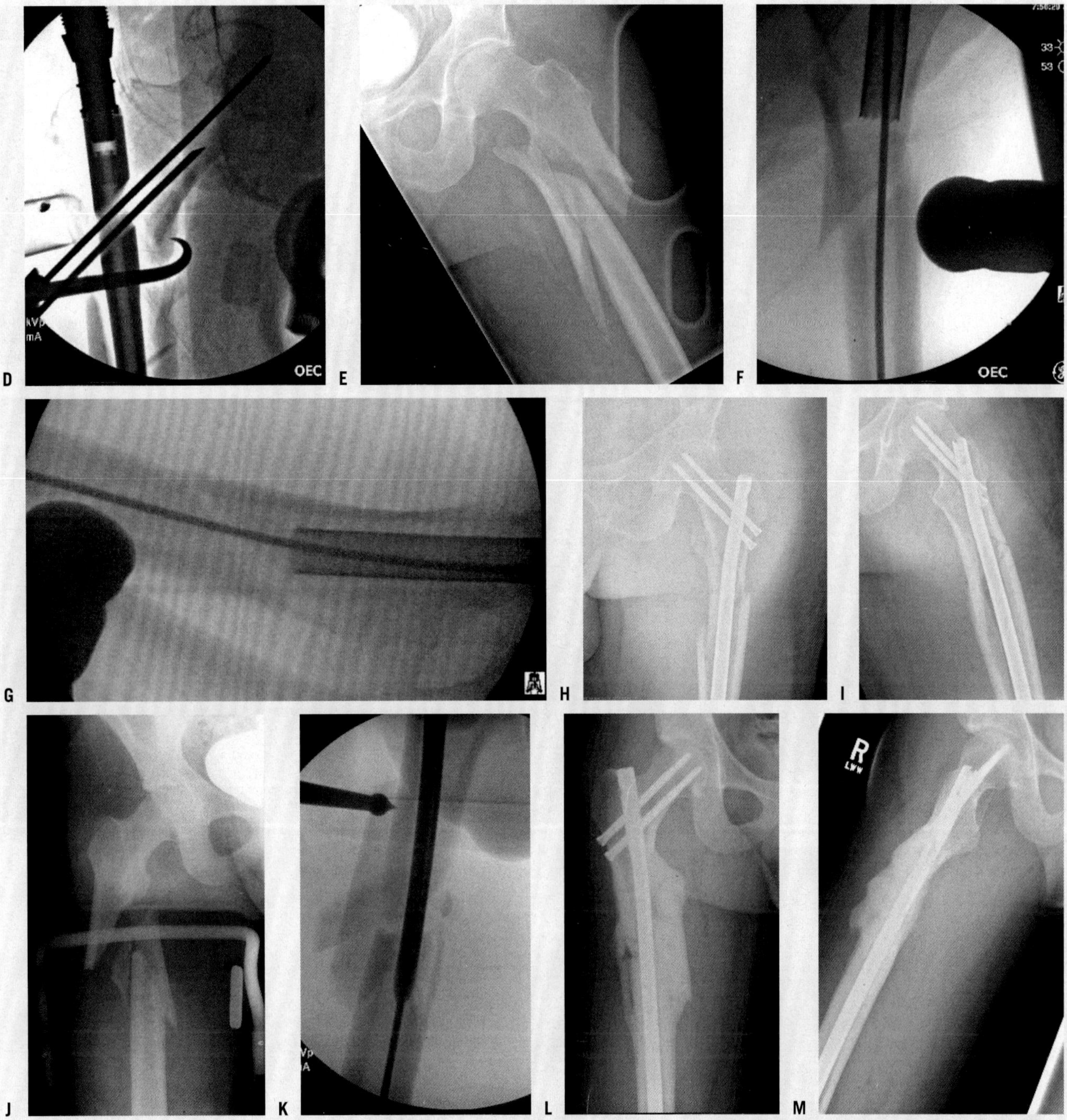

TECH FIG 1 *(continued)* **D.** Use of a bone hook to prevent calcar gapping. **E–I.** Use of closed force methods to obtain alignment (mallet, F-tool). **J–M.** Use of a percutaneous ball spike pusher to obtain alignment. *(continued)*

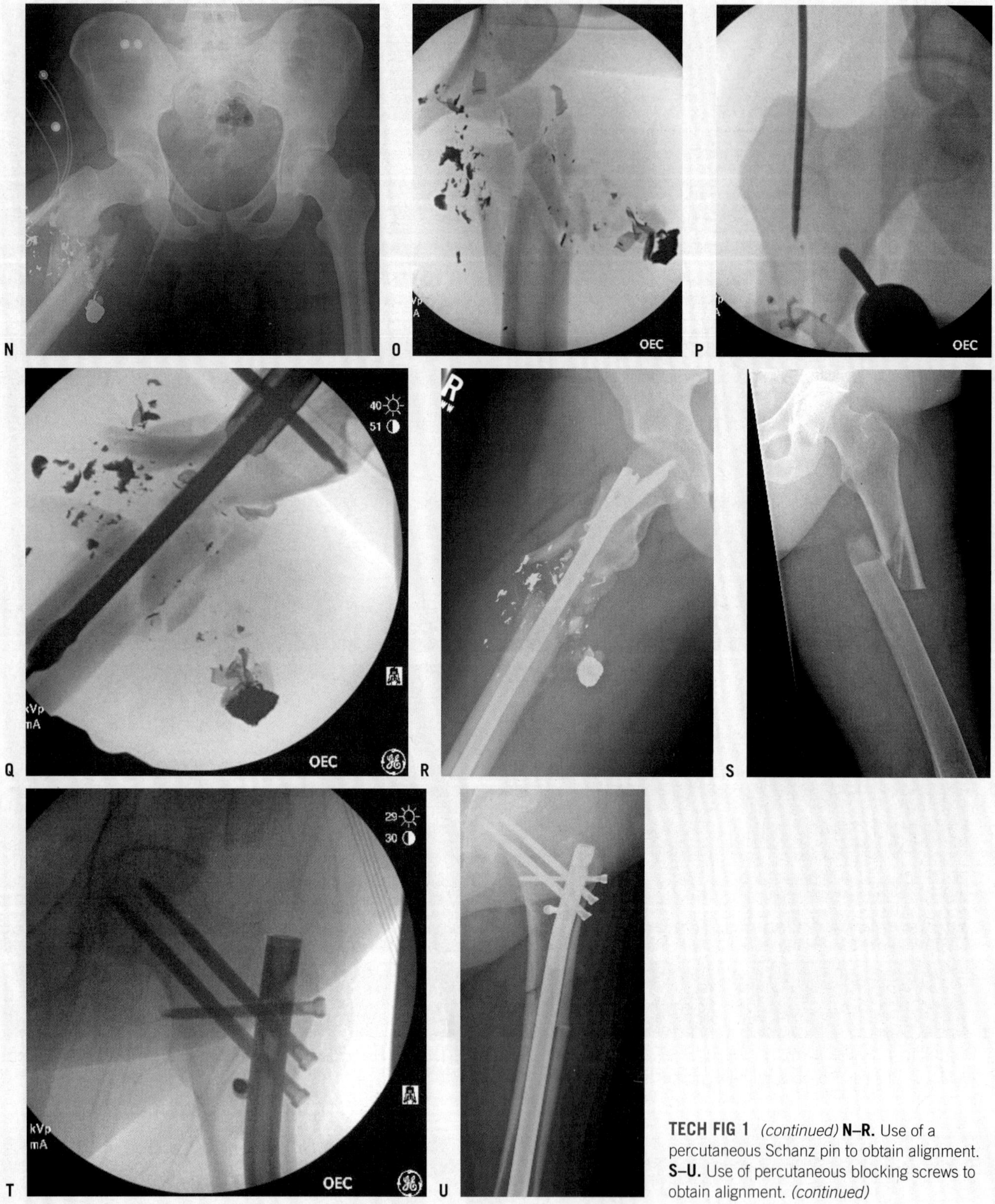

TECH FIG 1 *(continued)* **N–R.** Use of a percutaneous Schanz pin to obtain alignment. **S–U.** Use of percutaneous blocking screws to obtain alignment. *(continued)*

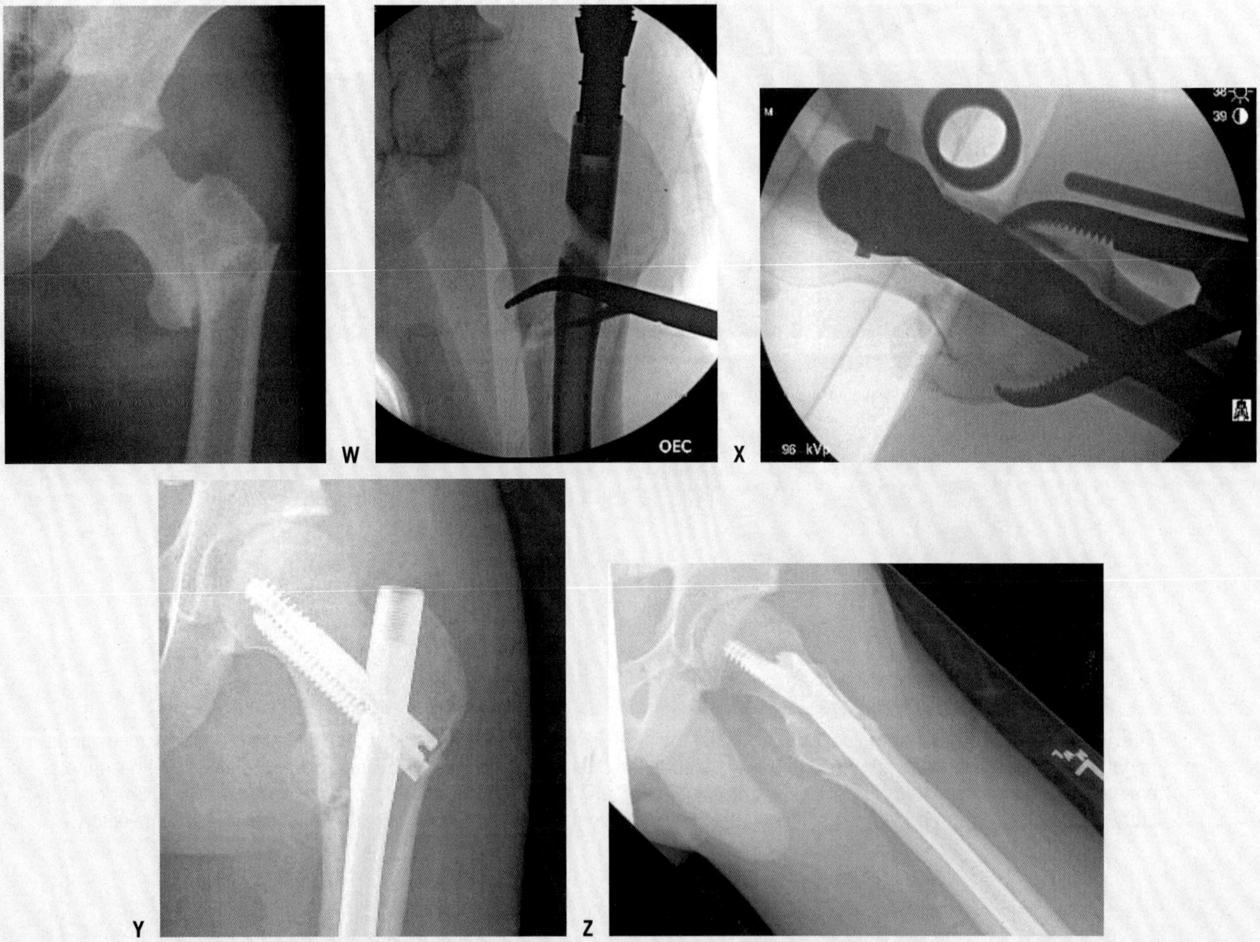

V W X Y Z

TECH FIG 1 *(continued)* **V–Z.** Use of open clamping to obtain alignment.

amount of traction (too little or too much). The surgeon should not ream across the proximal femur fracture site until reduction control is demonstrated.

- If reduction cannot be obtained by closed or percutaneous bone methods, the surgeon should proceed to open reduction using the lower portion of a Watson-Jones–type approach to the hip **(TECH FIG 1V–Z)**.
- The surgeon should avoid dissecting the medial soft tissue envelope, where the vascularity is located. A single cerclage wire will be most helpful if there is a coronal split of the proximal fragment. Use of multiple cables or wires is avoided. The clamps and reduction tools are maintained as the implant is inserted.

PRECISION PORTAL PLACEMENT AND TRAJECTORY CONTROL

- The rationale for the minimally invasive cephalomedullary surgical technique is based on three concepts to maximize bone and soft tissue conservation during nail implantation and to minimize the potential for malalignment[24]:
  - Precision portal placement
  - Trajectory control
  - Portal preservation
- A precise starting point is the first criterion in ensuring an accurate reduction of proximal fractures, whether the entry portal is a modified trochanteric entry portal or a piriformis portal as defined by the selected nail geometry **(TECH FIG 2A,B)**.
- The proximal femur is filled with a solid cancellous bone architecture from the femoral head region until the level just below the lesser trochanter, where the medullary canal begins.
- Trajectory control is the development of a precise path for the nail through this solid cancellous bone, which will restore the proximal alignment in the AP and lateral planes.
  - This correct trajectory parallels the anterior lateral cortex of the proximal femur and allows nail juxtaposition against a solid cortical structure **(TECH FIG 2C)**.
  - An incorrect trajectory will induce malalignment with nail insertion and result in an unstable juxtaposition against cancellous bone only, forcing the nail to migrate to the posterior cortex and resulting in a flexion deformity of the proximal fragment **(TECH FIG 2D,E)**.

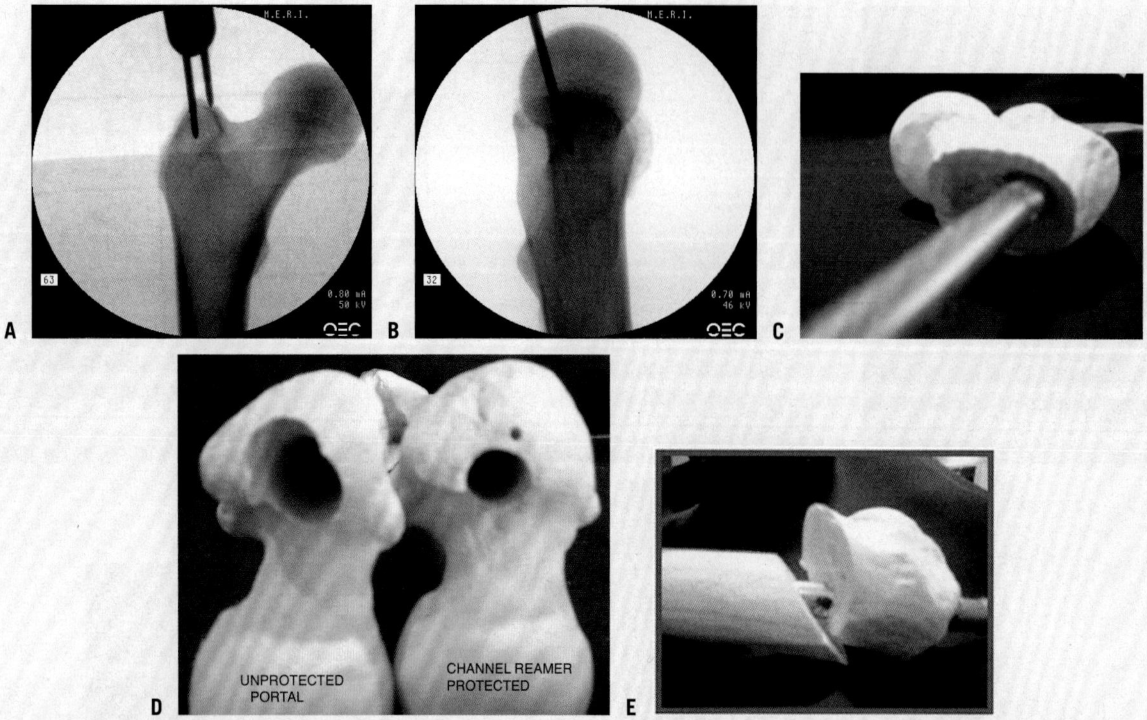

TECH FIG 2 **A.** Radiographic position of entry portal. Medial pin is medial trochanteric portal and lateral pin is lateral trochanteric portal. **B.** Lateral radiographic projection of piriformis portal; trochanteric portals will be aligned to bisect the femoral head more anteriorly. **C.** Anterolateral trajectory for nail in proximal femur. **D,E.** Incorrect nail trajectory in proximal fragment. **D.** Erosion of entry portal versus controlled reamed entry portal. **E.** Flexion deformity from posteriorly directed proximal fragment trajectory.

PORTAL ACQUISITION AND PROTECTION

- Once the correct trajectory is established, the portal and the lateral wall of the trochanter must be protected from erosion and fragmentation by the subsequent instruments for fracture reduction and canal preparation.
  - Typically, with the patient in a supine position, this erosion takes place in a posterolateral direction during reaming of the proximal femoral component, further contributing to a flexed and varus position of the proximal fragment when nail insertion occurs.
- A stepwise approach to canal preparation will simplify the nail insertion technique **(TECH FIG 3A–C)**.
- There are three currently published options for portal placement[21]:
  - Lateral trochanteric for nails with a proximal lateral angulation of more than 6 to 10 degrees. This portal is falling out of

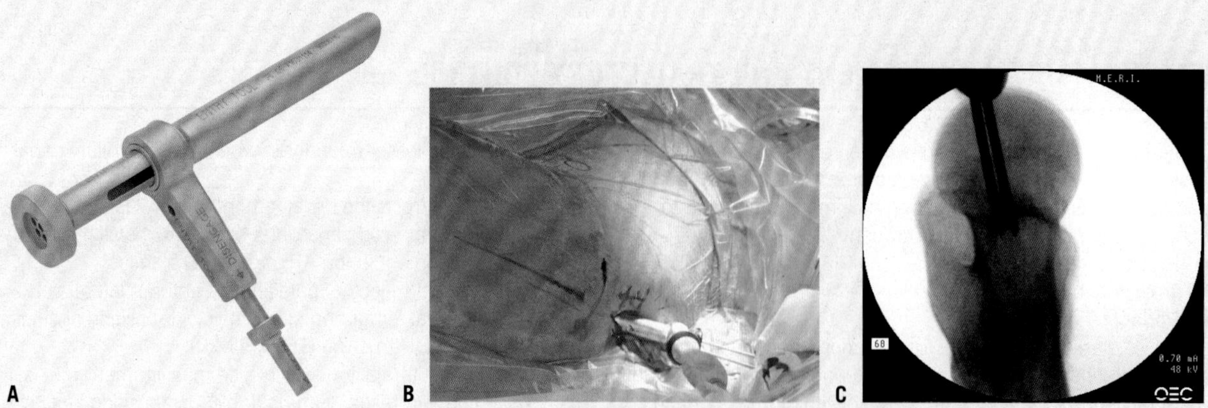

TECH FIG 3 **A.** Entry portal tool with honeycomb design targeter for pin placement (TriGen). **B.** Insertion of entry portal tool through incision. **C.** Two-pin technique through honeycomb targeter to precisely acquire entry site of pin. *(continued)*

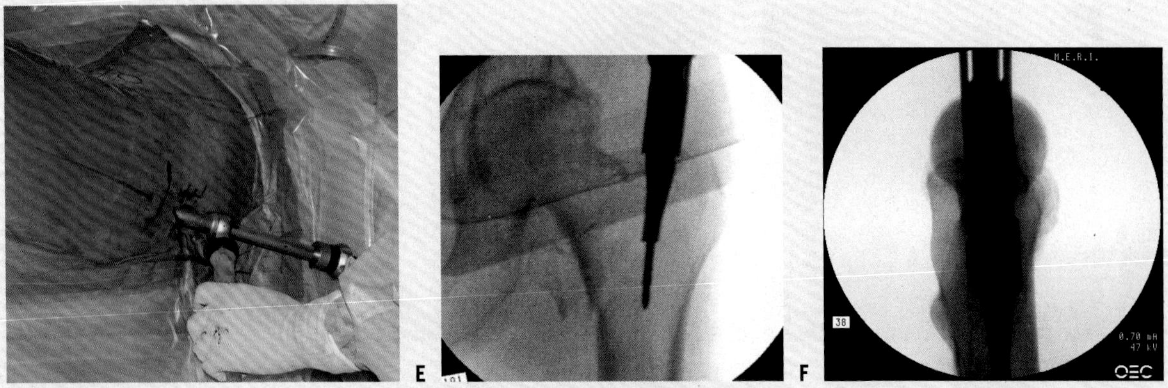

D E F

TECH FIG 3 *(continued)* **D.** Channel reamer insertion through entry portal tool for soft tissue protection. **E.** AP radiograph of trajectory for medial trochanteric portal. **F.** Lateral radiograph of correct anterolateral portal with channel reamer. (**A:** Courtesy of Smith & Nephew, Inc., Memphis, TN.)

favor as it is associated with more complications of fracture of the entry portal and reamer erosion with varus position of the hip and abductor damage. This has also been associated with trochanteric attachment complications if the nail is converted to a total hip arthroplasty.[19]

- Tip to medial trochanteric portal for nails with a proximal lateral angulation of 4 to 6 degrees. This is the preferred portal for peritrochanteric fractures currently.
- Piriformis portal for straight proximal segment nails, usually for subtrochanteric fracture patterns

- The guidewire drill system is inserted with soft tissue protection to the region of the greater trochanter. A 3.2-cm guidewire is inserted about 5 to 10 mm into bone in the lateral aspect of the greater trochanter.
  - This is a pivot pin about which a honeycomb type of targeter can be adjusted to precisely place the definitive guidewire pin at the tip of the greater trochanter.
- The definitive guidewire should be just lateral to the tip of the greater trochanter for the lateral trochanteric portal, medial to the tip of the greater trochanter for the medial trochanteric portal (see **TECH FIG 2A**), and medial to the trochanter on the nadir of the superior femoral neck for the piriformis portal on the AP C-arm view, and all portals should be centered in the femoral neck on the lateral C-arm view.
  - The definitive guidewire should be inserted 10 to 15 mm into the trochanter and does not have to be in correct canal alignment as the definitive trajectory will be obtained in the next step.
  - Insertion of the guidewire too deeply will constrain the reamer usually into a varus fracture reduction position. This is because the flexibility of the wire and the lateral approach vector of the hip will always place the wire in a varus position when nailing in a supine position. One of the real advantages of the lateral position is allowing a more direct vector approach for the guidewire.
- A cannulated rigid reamer, preferably with modular end-cutting capability (TriGen), approximating the proximal nail geometry diameter, is introduced over the guidewire through the protective sleeve **(TECH FIG 3D)**.
  - The rigid reamer or channel reamer is directed toward a point projected in the center of the medullary canal just distal to the region of the lesser trochanter **(TECH FIG 3E).**
  - The reamer is advanced in stepwise fashion while confirming maintenance of trajectory and the reduction.
- After the reamer has been inserted about 20 mm, its trajectory is confirmed with a lateral C-arm view.
  - The reamer should be directed along the anterior cortex of the proximal femur. The insertion of the reamer can be adjusted during reaming to approximate the position described and is most helpful in avoiding a varus position of the proximal femur.
- Once the canal is reamed in such a fashion, the distal femur is adjusted with the fracture table to allow correct neck–shaft angulation.
- The reamer is inserted until it reaches the medullary canal just below the region of the lesser trochanter **(TECH FIG 3F)**.
- The inner reamer is removed and the outer reamer is maintained for protection of the proximal reamer during the next step.

FRACTURE REDUCTION AND CANAL PREPARATION

- A fracture reducer (TriGen) or similar curved cannulated device is inserted through the retained channel reamer to the fracture site and threaded through the fracture site into the distal fragment intramedullary canal, with manipulation in appropriate planes to align the fracture **(TECH FIG 4A)**.
- A long guide rod is inserted to the knee if a long nail is desired, confirming that the wire does not impinge on the anterior cortex distally.
  - Preferably, the guide rod should be inserted to the old physeal scar and centered on AP and lateral C-arm views **(TECH FIG 4B)**.

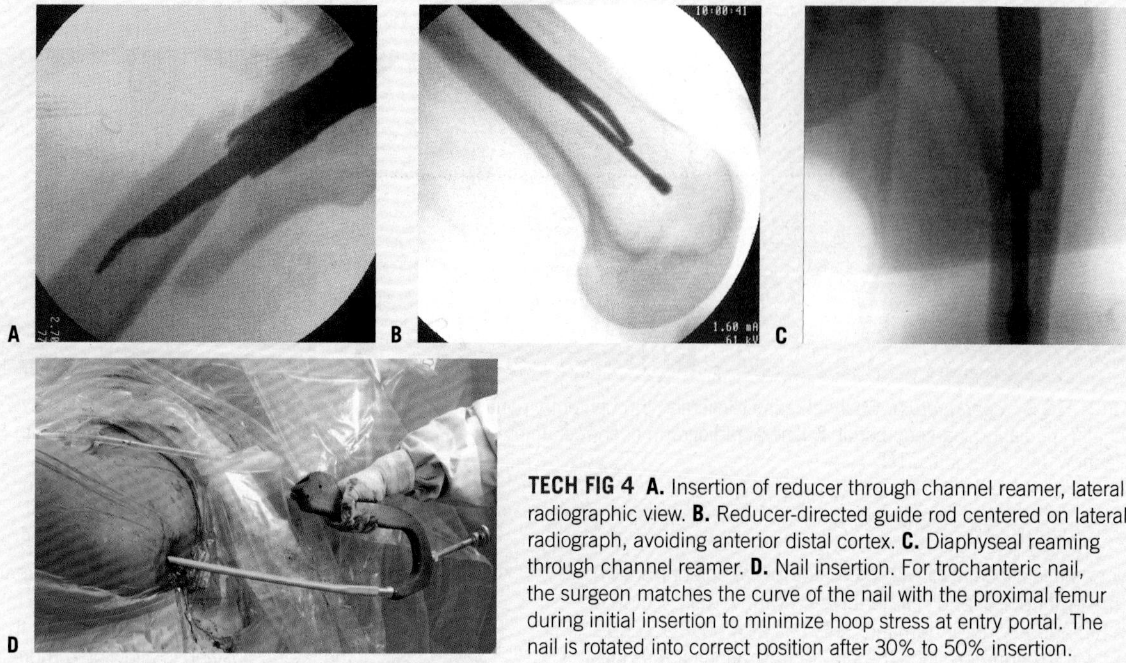

TECH FIG 4 **A.** Insertion of reducer through channel reamer, lateral radiographic view. **B.** Reducer-directed guide rod centered on lateral radiograph, avoiding anterior distal cortex. **C.** Diaphyseal reaming through channel reamer. **D.** Nail insertion. For trochanteric nail, the surgeon matches the curve of the nail with the proximal femur during initial insertion to minimize hoop stress at entry portal. The nail is rotated into correct position after 30% to 50% insertion.

- The reducer is removed and the guidewire position is maintained with an obturator proximally.
- Length is checked with an appropriate ruler, allowing for fracture distraction and nail final position.
- The diaphyseal region is reamed up to at least 1 mm over the desired nail size (up to 2.5 mm for excessive anterior bows) **(TECH FIG 4C)**.
  - The proximal expansion of the nail should have already been reamed with the entry portal reamer, but the surgeon should always confirm diameters.
- The channel reamer is removed, and the selected nail is inserted **(TECH FIG 4D)**.
  - For long trochanteric nails, it is helpful to rotate the nail 90 degrees anteriorly during the first half of the nail insertion to minimize hoop stresses in the proximal femur. After partial insertion, the nail is rotated to the anticipated anteversion required for femoral head fixation.
  - The last 5 cm of the nail is inserted after releasing distraction sufficient for fracture apposition, maintaining correct rotational alignment.
  - Most commercial guides use reference marks to align with the femoral head on the lateral C-arm view. These same guides may be used for C-arm verification of correct depth of insertion to allow optimal femoral head fixation.
  - The long guide rod is removed to proceed with interlocking.
- Proximal interlocking will depend on the type of implant selected, but most designs recommend that the screw be placed as close to center–center position as possible.
  - If a secondary screw is included in the nail design constructs (ie, reconstruction or InterTAN), there is usually sufficient room for the second screw inferiorly, but care should be exercised in small patients.

SINGLE-SCREW OR SINGLE-DEVICE DESIGNS (GAMMA, STRYKER; IMHS, SMITH & NEPHEW; TFN, DEPUY SYNTHES)

- The center–center wire is inserted to within 5 mm of subchondral bone. Fracture reduction is confirmed, and the length to lateral cortex is measured.
- If compression is desired (usually 5 mm), the surgeon reams for the screw and selects a screw 5 mm shorter than measured. For the TFN, the head is not reamed.
- The surgeon inserts the head fixation screw or nail to the desired depth; position is confirmed on AP and lateral C-arm views **(TECH FIG 5A)**.
- The option of compression and locking of the lag screw with a set screw within the nail is available on selected systems **(TECH FIG 5B)**.

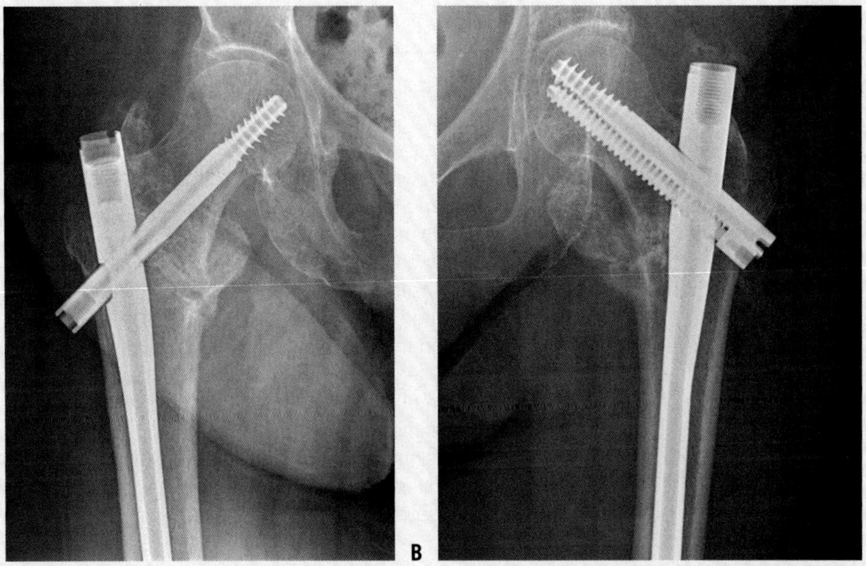

A B

TECH FIG 5 **A.** Gamma nail AP view with lateral trochanteric portal and center–center head screw position. **B.** Russell-Taylor IIB fracture with an InterTAN nail AP.

TWO-SCREW RECONSTRUCTION (TRIGEN)

- Using the proximal targeting guide attached to the nail, the surgeon inserts the most distal proximal guidewire along the femoral calcar within 5 mm of the inferior femoral neck, centered on the lateral C-arm view, to within 5 mm of subchondral bone **(TECH FIG 6A)**.
- Through the proximal targeting guide attached to the nail, the surgeon inserts the most proximal guide pin, which will be close to the center position of the femoral head parallel to the first guide pin. Its position is confirmed with the C-arm.
- The surgeon removes the inferior guidewire, drills, and reams for the selected lag screw for the system and inserts the inferior screw **(TECH FIG 6B)**.
- The same steps are repeated for the proximal screw, and final fixation is confirmed on AP and lateral radiographs **(TECH FIG 6C)**.
- Traction is released before final tightening of the lag screws to allow fracture compression.

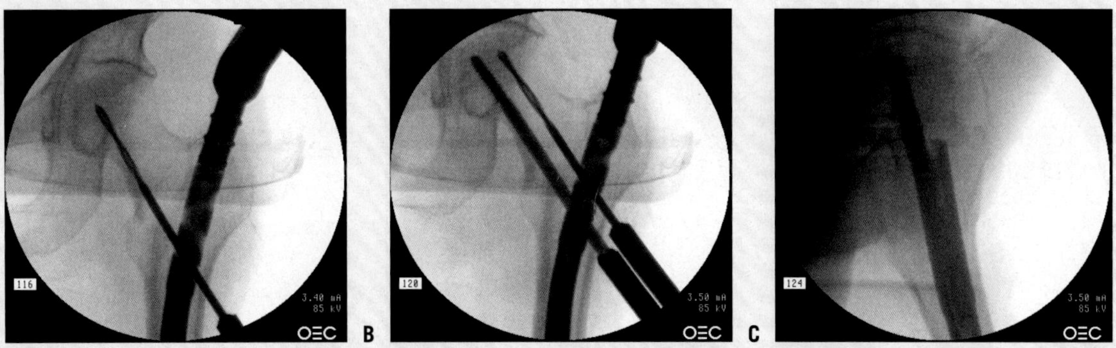

A B C

TECH FIG 6 **A.** Trochanteric reconstruction nail with inferior drill placed first along medial neck. **B.** Inferior lag screw placed first. **C.** Lateral radiographic view of head screw position.

INTEGRATED SCREW CEPHALOMEDULLARY NAIL (INTERTAN)

- Whereas the previous techniques for femoral head fixation used devices that gain compression by impaction or compression against the lateral cortex, this device uses a gear drive mechanism that compresses the nail against the endosteal surface of the medial cortex and simultaneously compresses the proximal femoral head and neck to the medial surface of the nail (see **TECH FIG 5B**).
  - This design conceptually improves rotational and translational stability to the proximal femoral construct.
- The 3.2-mm guidewire is inserted through the proximal targeting guide and advanced in a center position of the femoral head to within 5 mm of subchondral bone, after confirming correct depth and anteversion **(TECH FIG 7A–C)**.
- The inferior lateral cortex is drilled through the targeting guide with a step drill to clear away bone from the nail attachment site for the gear drive **(TECH FIG 7D)**.
- The antirotation bar is inserted into the inferior hole to augment femoral head and neck stability during large lag screw reaming **(TECH FIG 7E,F)**.
- The surgeon confirms the length for the lag screw, subtracting 5 to 10 mm from the measured length for compression if desired.
  - The 3.2-mm wire is overdrilled with the 10.5-mm cannulated drill, and the selected lag screw is inserted to within 5 mm of subchondral bone **(TECH FIG 7G)**.
- The antirotation bar is removed, and the compression gear drive screw is inserted through the guide. Traction is released from the leg, and compression is started **(TECH FIG 7H–K)**.
  - Compression through the gear drive does not begin until the head of the gear drive screw contacts the nail.
  - Visualization of compression can be confirmed by C-arm and calibrations on the guide.
- Once compression is achieved, the screwdrivers are disassembled. Static locking of the screw assembly can be achieved with the integrated set screw within the nail.

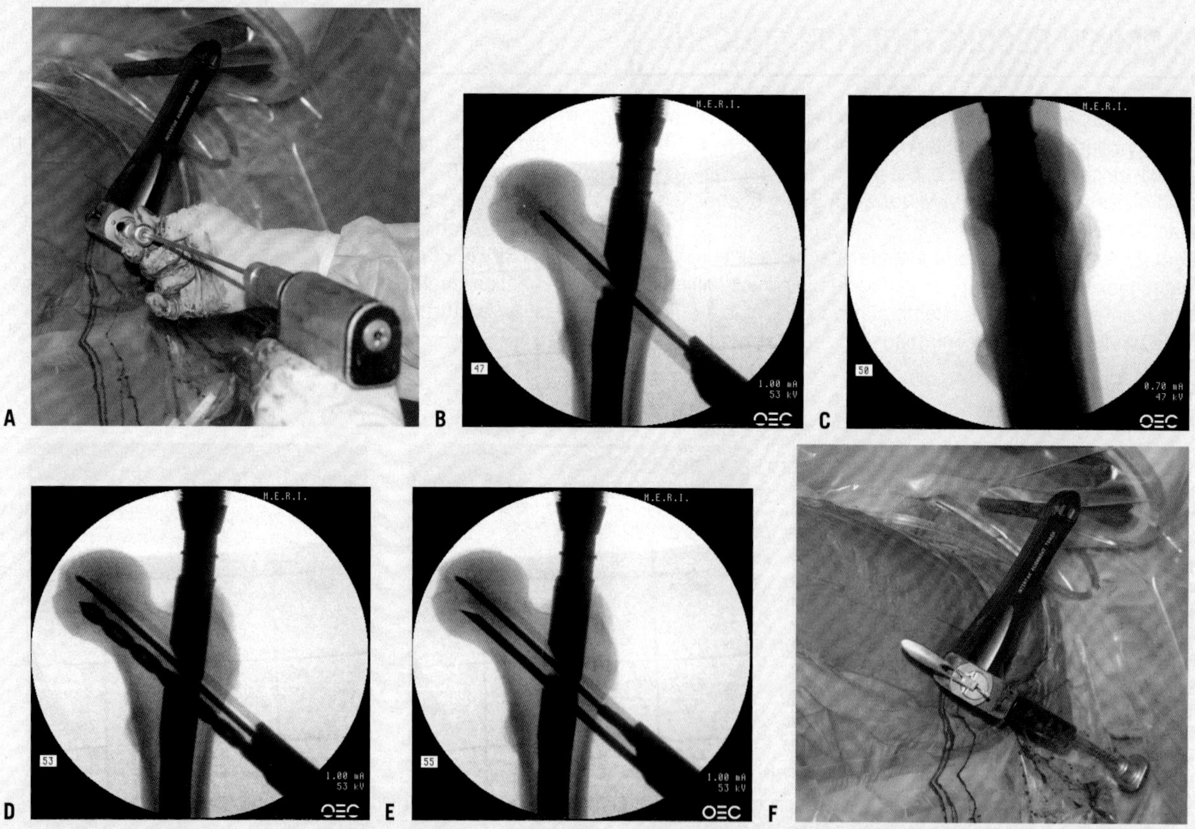

TECH FIG 7 Integrated screw cephalomedullary nail (InterTAN). **A.** Pilot drill hole for 3.2-mm wire for center–center position. **B.** AP radiograph with radiolucent alignment tower. **C.** Lateral radiograph with radiolucent guide centered over femoral head. **D.** Inferior screw hole for antirotation bar and compression screw. **E,F.** Antirotation bar inserted. *(continued)*

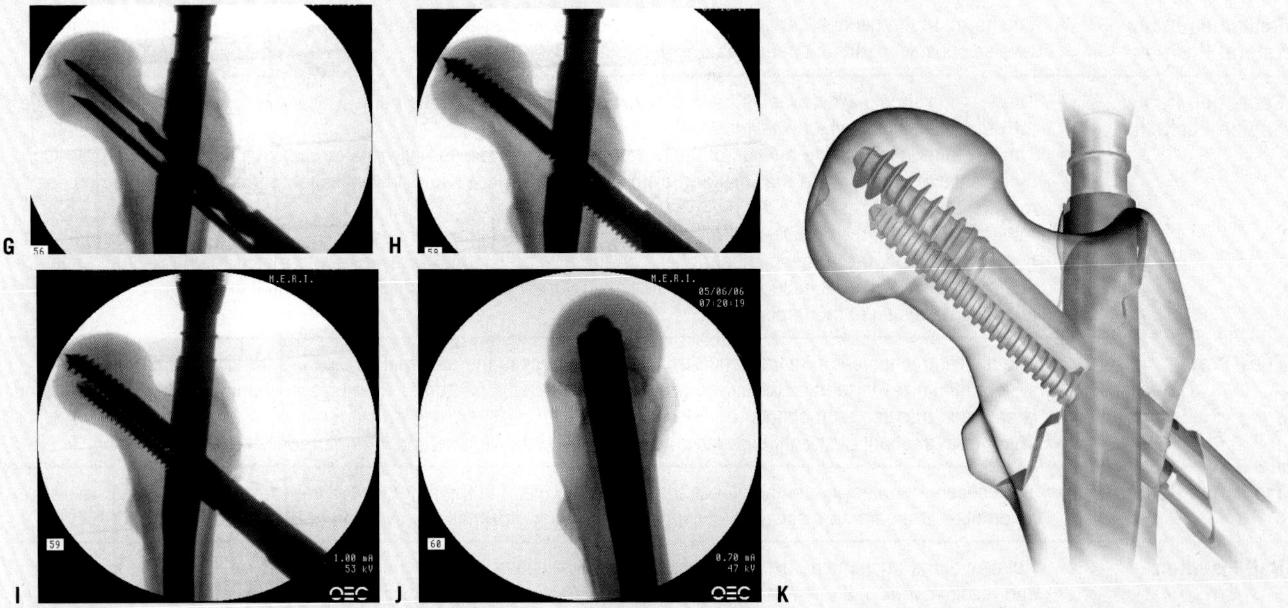

TECH FIG 7 *(continued)* **G.** Drill for cannulated center lag screw. **H–J.** Insertion of inferior compression screw and final AP and lateral views of integrated screws engaged. **K.** Schematic of integrated screws and nail in fracture. (**K:** Courtesy of Smith & Nephew, Inc., Memphis, TN.)

DISTAL INTERLOCKING TECHNIQUE

- Length, alignment, and rotation should be confirmed prior to distal interlocking. The surgeon should check on the AP and lateral C-arm views and match the neck–shaft angle and rotation. Alternatives include using cortical thickness, rotational profiles of the contralateral limb, or utilizing the built-in anteversion of the femoral nail.[7]
- Short nails have distal locking capability, usually in a static or dynamic mode with most modern designs. I prefer dynamic locking.
  - Most systems have this hole targeted through the proximal nail guide, and a single bicortical screw is usually sufficient.
- Long nails have distal locking capability with either static holes or a combination of static and dynamic.
  - For length-stable proximal fractures, one bicortical screw is sufficient in a dynamic mode.
  - Conversely, for segmental fractures or extensive comminution, two screws may be preferred.
  - Distal interlocking is most commonly done using the same freehand technique used in the conventional femoral interlocking nail technique **(TECH FIG 8)**.

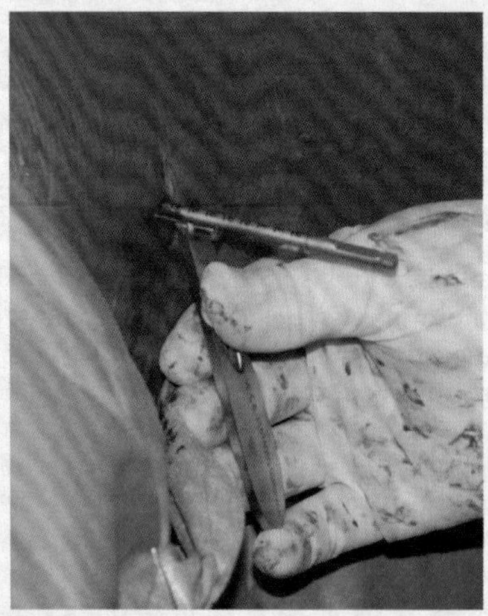

TECH FIG 8 Distal freehand technique for long nails.

WOUND CLOSURE FOR ALL NAILS

- With attention to detail, minimal damage to the muscle and skin is incurred with nail techniques, so wound irrigation and standard layered closure are performed.

Pearls and Pitfalls

Reduction in the Lateral Position	• The height of the perineal post is adjusted to effect medial displacement of the shaft. This is especially helpful with reverse obliquity pertrochanteric patterns (Russell-Taylor IIA).[22]
Reduction in the Supine Position	• The surgeon should avoid placing the hip in varus to gain entry into the bone. This leads to a varus trajectory in the proximal bone stock, which will recur with nail insertion. • The key to reduction is the rotation of the distal fragment to the externally rotated proximal fragment and apposition of the anterior cortex of the proximal and distal fragments. These two points will allow correction of the flexion and malrotation deformities. • After nail insertion, the coronal and rotational alignment of the proximal femur may change, so before proximal and distal interlocking, the surgeon should check on the AP and lateral C-arm views and match the neck–shaft angle and rotation. Alternatives include using cortical thickness, rotational profiles of the contralateral limb, or utilizing the built-in anteversion of the femoral nail.
Entry Portal	• The medial trochanteric portal greatly simplifies the access to the proximal femur, and the use of a rigid reamer system minimizes false trajectories and trochanteric iatrogenic fractures. The surgeon should avoid letting the reamer lateralize in the greater trochanter at any time. • The medial trochanteric portal uses less radiation and operative time and is preferred in the supine position.[23]
Trajectory Control	• The concept of trajectory control places the nail in apposition to the anterolateral cortex, minimizing flexion deformities at the fracture site, and conserves bone stock proximally by avoiding cutout of the reamer posteriorly.
Nail Insertion	• Rotation of the trochanteric design nails during the first half of insertion minimizes stress on the greater trochanter and medial cortex of the femur below the lesser trochanteric region in long nail designs. • The surgeon should remember to let off traction before final seating of the nail to avoid nailing the femur in distraction. • Nails must have stability by cortical contact in the proximal and distal femur. Disruption of the lateral wall places more stress on the construct and should be reconstructed separately from the nail if displaced or a locking proximal plate may be required. Special care is required for Russell-Taylor IIA and IIB fracture patterns.
Proximal Screw Targeting	• Guidewire insertion and drilling should always be performed with a high-speed rate and a *slow* feed rate. This means that the guidewires and reamers bend and can be misdirected with excessive axial force during drilling. • For single-device and integrated screw femoral head fixation, the surgeon should use a center–center position for the large lag screw. • For two-device femoral head fixation (reconstruction), the inferior screw is placed first along the medial calcar of the femoral neck; this will ensure room for the proximal screw.
Distal Locking	• Distal locking is usually recommended with a dynamic single screw for short and long nails. Two distal interlocking screws are recommended for comminuted or segmental fractures.

POSTOPERATIVE CARE

- AP and lateral radiographs of the final construct should be obtained in the surgical suite before recovering the patient to assess the construct and ensure stability.
  - If there are adjustments to be made, these are best made while the patient is still under anesthesia.
  - Radiographs should reveal the entire fracture region, including the entire implant construct.
- Patients are mobilized to a chair upright position the day after the operative procedure.
- Ambulation with supervision is allowed, with weight bearing as tolerated with a walker or crutches and emphasis on heel-strike and upright balance exercises.[12]
  - Polytrauma or patients with other comorbidities may have delayed ambulation, but it should begin as soon as possible to minimize secondary complications.
- Patients are reevaluated with an examination and radiographs at 2 weeks and then monthly thereafter until fracture healing is documented and the patients have maximized ambulatory capabilities, usually by 6 months after the injury.
- The surgeon should emphasize good nutrition and hip abductor exercises bilaterally.
- Patients must be counseled to report any increased swelling or respiratory distress as an emergency because of the high risk of thromboembolic disease.

OUTCOMES

- Union of these fractures is high (>95%) with cephalomedullary nail techniques.
- Functional recovery is poor in many patients, however, with more than 60% of patients failing to recover their preinjury level of function.[15]
- Mortality within the first year in patients older than 55 years is 20% to 30%.
- Many patients sustain progressive collapse of the hip into varus and shortening of the leg with the current generation of sliding hip screw fixation.[16]

COMPLICATIONS

- Loss of construct stability is one of the most common complications. It is manifested by collapse of the screw and varus migration of the femoral head construct, with final cutout failure in the worst cases.
  - This occurs to a small degree in all cases, as the sliding impaction was designed to minimize catastrophic cutout.

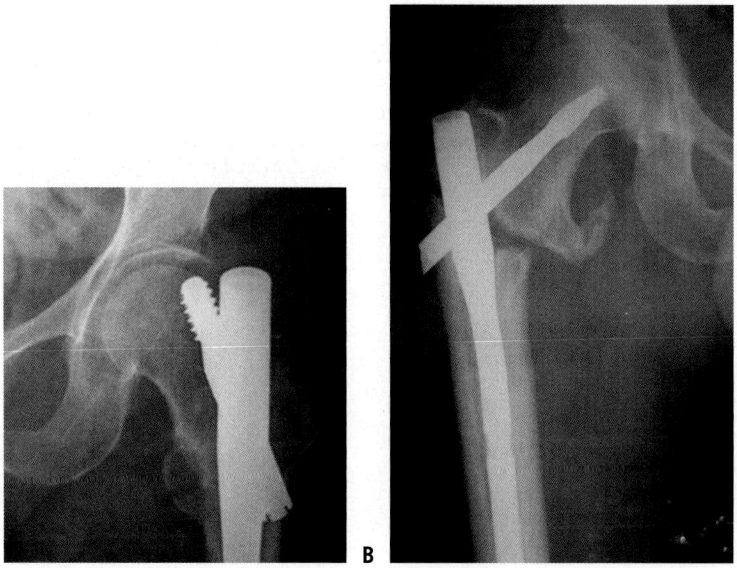

A B

FIG 7 Nail failures. **A.** Proximal screw cutout. **B.** Distraction nonunion with spiral blade nail construct.

- A center–center position of single-screw devices minimizes cutout.[4]
- Nail cutout is a much more serious complication, involving loss of fixation of the nail component in the proximal femur or periprosthetic femoral fracture with short nails; this will result in reoperation with locking construct plates or 95-degree blade plates, exchange for longer nails, or even prosthetic replacement in severe cases (**FIG 7A**). If a lateral trochanteric portal was used, prepare for trochanteric accessory fixation if arthroplasty is required.[8]
- Nonunion, although rare (1% in older patients), is usually treated with total hip replacement in older patients and revision fixation in young patients (**FIG 7B**).
- Infection occurs in 1% to 2% of postoperative cases and is minimized by preoperative antibiotics, usually a cephalosporin class of antibiotic.
  - In immunocompromised and malnourished patients, standard care involves isolation and sensitivity testing of the causative bacteria and appropriate intravenous antibiotics, in consultation with an infectious disease specialist, and standard débridement and irrigation for wound care.
  - If the implant is stable, it should be retained. Rarely will a resection arthroplasty be required.

REFERENCES

1. Alam A, Willett K, Ostlere S. The MRI diagnosis and management of incomplete intertrochanteric fractures of the femur. J Bone Joint Surg Br 2005;87(9):1253–1255.
2. American Academy of Orthopaedic Surgery. Hip fracture. AAOS Web site. Available at: http://orthoinfo.aaos.org/topic.cfm?topic=A00392. Accessed December 24, 2014.
3. Bartonícek J. Internal architecture of the proximal femur—Adam's or Adams' arch? Historical mystery. Arch Orthop Trauma Surg 2002;122:551–553.
4. Baumgaertner MR, Curtin SL, Lindskog DM, et al. The value of the tip-apex distance in predicting failure of fixation of peritrochanteric fractures of the hip. J Bone Joint Surg Am 1995;77(7):1058–1064.
5. Bible JE, Mir HR. Well-leg positioning on a fracture table: using a pillow sling. Am J Orthop (Belle Mead NJ) 2014;43(12):571–573.
6. Connelly CL, Archdeacon M. The lateral decubitus approach for complex proximal femur fractures: anatomic reduction and locking plate neutralization: a technical trick. J Orthop Trauma 2012;26: 252–257.
7. Espinoza C, Sathy AK, Moore DS, et al. Use of inherent anteversion of an intramedullary nail to avoid malrotation in femur fractures. J Orthop Trauma 2014;28(2):e34–e38.
8. Exaltacion JJ, Incavo SJ, Mathews V, et al. Hip arthroplasty after intramedullary hip screw fixation: a perioperative evaluation. J Orthop Trauma 2012;26(3):141–147.
9. Gotfried Y. The lateral trochanteric wall: a key element in the reconstruction of unstable pertrochanteric hip fractures. Clin Orthop Relat Res 2004;(425):82–86.
10. Hammer A. The structure of the femoral neck: a physical dissection with emphasis on the internal trabecular system. Ann Anat 2010;192:168–177.
11. Jin WJ, Dai LY, Cui YM, et al. Reliability of classification systems for intertrochanteric fractures of the proximal femur in experienced orthopaedic surgeons. Injury 2005;36:858–861.
12. Koval KJ, Sala DA, Kummer FJ, et al. Postoperative weight-bearing after a fracture of the femoral neck or an intertrochanteric fracture. J Bone Joint Surg Am 1998;80(3):352–356.
13. Langford J, Burgess A. Nailing of proximal and distal fractures of the femur: limitations and techniques. J Orthop Trauma 2009;23(5 suppl): S22–S25.
14. Matre K, Vinje T, Havelin LI, et al. TRIGEN INTERTAN intramedullary nail versus sliding hip screw: a prospective, randomized multicenter study on pain, function, and complications in 684 patients with an intertrochanteric or subtrochanteric fracture and one year of follow-up. J Bone Joint Surg Am 2013;95:200–208.
15. Miller CW. Survival and ambulation following hip fracture. J Bone Joint Surg Am 1978;60(7):930–934.
16. Moroni A, Faldini C, Pegreffi F, et al. Dynamic hip screw compared with external fixation for treatment of osteoporotic pertrochanteric fractures. A prospective, randomized study. J Bone Joint Surg Am 2005;87(4):753–759.
17. Ostrum RF, Levy MS. Penetration of the distal femoral anterior cortex during intramedullary nailing for subtrochanteric fractures: a report of three cases. J Orthop Trauma 2005;19:656–660.
18. Ostrum RF, Marcantonio A, Marburger R. A critical analysis of the eccentric starting point for trochanteric intramedullary femoral nailing. J Orthop Trauma 2005;19:681–686.
19. Palm H, Jacobsen S, Sonne-Holm S, et al. Integrity of the lateral femoral wall in intertrochanteric hip fractures: an important predictor of a reoperation. J Bone Joint Surg Am 2007;89(3):470–475.
20. Parker MJ, Handoll HH, Bhargara A. Conservative versus operative treatment for hip fractures. Cochrane Database Syst Rev 2000;(4):CD000337.

21. Perez EA, Jahangir AA, Mashru RP, et al. Is there a gluteus medius tendon injury during reaming through a modified medial trochanteric portal? A cadaver study. J Orthop Trauma 2007;21:617–620.
22. Prasarn ML, Cattaneo MD, Achor T, et al. The effect of entry point on malalignment and iatrogenic fracture with the Synthes lateral entry femoral nail. J Orthop Trauma 2010;24(4):224–229.
23. Ricci WM, Schwappach J, Tucker M, et al. Trochanteric versus piriformis entry portal for the treatment of femoral shaft fractures. J Orthop Trauma 2006;20:663–667.
24. Russell TA, Mir HR, Stoneback J, et al. Avoidance of malreduction of proximal femoral shaft fractures with the use of a minimally invasive nail insertion technique (MINIT). J Orthop Trauma 2008;22:391–398.
25. Russell TA, Taylor JC. Subtrochanteric fractures. In: Browner B, ed. Skeletal Trauma. Philadelphia: WB Saunders, 1993.
26. Sheehan KJ, Sobolev B, Guy P. Mortality by timing of hip fracture surgery: factors and relationships at play. J Bone Joint Surg Am 2017;99(20):e106.

CHAPTER 37

Open Reduction and Internal Fixation of Peritrochanteric Hip Fractures

Clifford B. Jones

DEFINITION

- Peritrochanteric hip fractures are defined as extracapsular hip fractures, always involving the trochanter and frequently with extension into the subtrochanteric region.
- Medicare data indicates that as management of osteoporosis has improved, individual risk of sustaining a hip fracture has declined.[7] However, with an aging population, the total number of hip fractures increases each year. According to a Medicare database, 786,717 hip fractures were reported between 1986 and 2005. These fractures account for approximately 20% of Medicare claims.
- These fractures require operative intervention to achieve stable, anatomic, fracture fixation to allow immediate patient mobilization, restoration of anatomic relationships, successful fracture healing, and return of limb function.

ANATOMY

- The intertrochanteric region of the hip is notable for the anatomic transition from the femoral neck to the femoral shaft.
  - The angles subtended by the femoral neck and long axis of the femoral shaft in the coronal plane (the neck–shaft angle) and in the sagittal plane (anteversion) are approximately 132 and 10 degrees, respectively.[29]
  - Studies have shown that this angle tends to decrease slightly with age and osteoporosis.[11]
- The peritrochanteric region of the femur is composed of multiple thickenings of trabecular bone distributed in compressive and tensile groups.[12]
  - The thickest and most structural are the primary compressive trabeculae located along the posterior medial aspect of the femoral neck and shaft, also known as the *calcar*.
- Multiple muscle groups attach to this region of the femur and can create deformity **(FIG 1)**[1]:
  - Iliopsoas: attaches to the lesser trochanter and exerts a flexion and external rotation (ER) force to the hip
  - Abductors and short external rotators: attach to the greater trochanter
  - Adductors: attach to the femoral shaft distal to the peritrochanteric region
- The blood supply to the peritrochanteric region of the femur is rich and abundant. The medial and lateral femoral circumflex arteries supply the cancellous bone of the trochanteric region through muscle attachments at the vastus origin and the insertion of the gluteus medius.

PATHOGENESIS

- In the elderly population, most peritrochanteric fractures are caused by a low-energy fall onto the lateral aspect of the hip.
- Numerous factors, such as structurally weak bone, lack of subcutaneous padding, and slowed protective reflexes lead to increased risk of hip fracture in the elderly population.
- Pathologic lesions in the peritrochanteric region are not uncommon and may lead to fractures after relatively minor trauma.
- Young patients who sustain peritrochanteric fractures are typically victims of high-energy trauma. In these cases, the fracture must be approached differently, with an attitude toward a timed surgical restoration anatomy to restore joint mechanics.

NATURAL HISTORY

- Almost all peritrochanteric hip fractures will heal without intervention. However, owing to the pull of the musculature in this region,[1] the fracture will heal in gross malalignment, leading to subsequent functional limitations.[11]

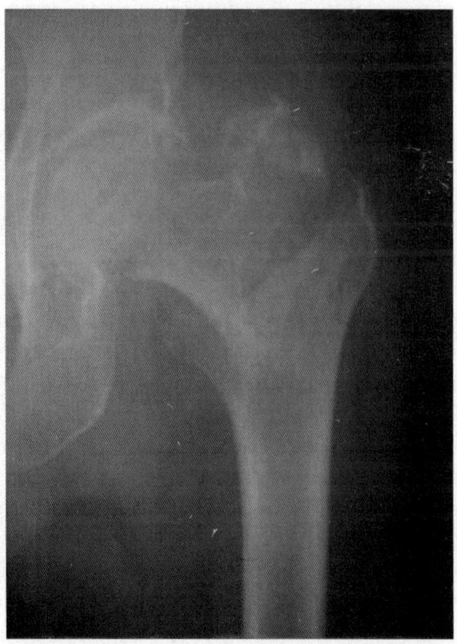

FIG 1 Injury AP hip x-ray demonstrating shortening, abduction (external rotators), and shaft ER (iliopsoas).

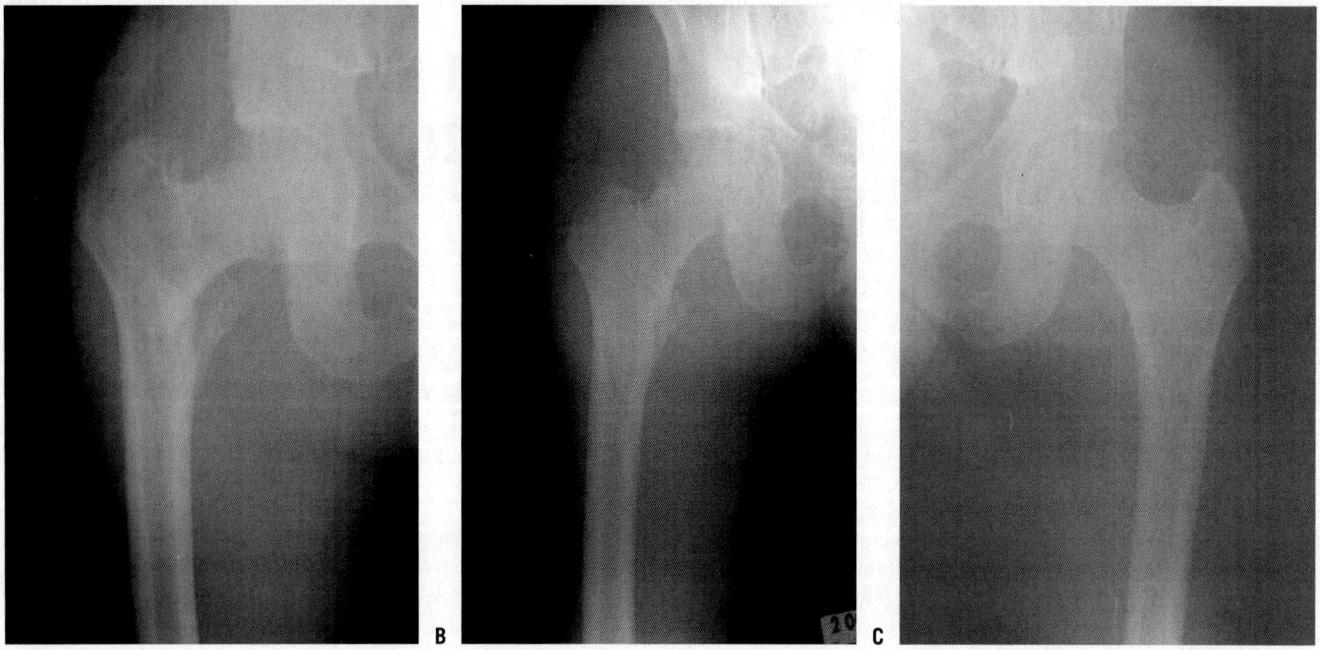

A B C

FIG 2 Injury AP hip x-ray (**A**) demonstrating displacement. Traction x-ray (**B**) demonstrates excellent indirect reduction and restoration of anatomy in comparison to normal contralateral x-ray (**C**).

- Early operative intervention of these fractures is undertaken to restore anatomic alignment, lessen blood loss, reduce pain, and enhance patient mobilization. Early fixation has been demonstrated to decrease incidence of pressure sores, pneumonia, and 30-day mortality.

PATIENT HISTORY AND PHYSICAL FINDINGS

- It is important to elicit the cause of the patient's fall, as many falls in the elderly population that result in hip fractures are due to medical comorbidities.
- Elderly patients should be carefully evaluated and treated for rhabdomyolysis, dehydration, urinary tract infection, and malnutrition. In cases of preexisting poor mobility, consider deep vein thrombosis, and in anticoagulated patients, it may be appropriate to obtain brain imaging.
- Complaints of hip pain (prodromal symptoms) before falling may indicate a preexisting pathologic process that requires further evaluation.
- A thorough whole-body musculoskeletal examination of the patient is necessary because of the high incidence of associated fractures (especially of the wrist and proximal humerus) in the elderly population sustaining hip fractures from simple falls. In cases of visible head trauma, cervical spine imaging can obviate prolonged cervical collar immobilization.
- Examination of the soft tissue overlying the lateral hip, sacrum, and heels is necessary to ensure that no pressure ulcers or abrasions have occurred in these areas.
- The classic physical finding in a patient with a peritrochanteric hip fracture is a shortened, externally rotated lower extremity.
- Passive logrolling or axial loading of the leg will elicit pain. This may be an especially helpful finding in occult hip fractures with no obvious fracture line or deformity.

IMAGING AND OTHER DIAGNOSTIC STUDIES

- Plain radiographic anteroposterior (AP) pelvis and cross-table lateral images of the injured hip should be obtained initially.
- AP and lateral views of the femur, including the knee joint, should be obtained both to assess the femoral bow as well as to evaluate the femoral canal in the event that an intramedullary device is required.
- A traction radiograph (radiograph taken with firm manual traction and internal rotation [IR] of the leg) will provide more information on the fracture pattern and will allow a better comparison to the uninjured hip **(FIG 2)**. Alternatively, an obturator oblique view of the pelvis can allow for this comparison without requiring additional analgesic medication.
- A fine-cut (2 mm) computed tomography (CT) scan with reconstruction images (sagittal, coronal, and three-dimensional [3-D]) set to bone windows may help assess the fracture when ipsilateral femoral neck or other fractures are suspected **(FIG 3)**.
- Magnetic resonance imaging (MRI) is the modality of choice to assess for the presence of an occult peritrochanteric hip fracture in the setting of significant hip pain and normal radiographs **(FIG 4)**.

DIFFERENTIAL DIAGNOSIS

- Femoral head or neck fracture
- Acetabular fracture or hip dislocation
- Femoral shaft fracture
- Greater trochanter fracture
- Septic hip
- Pelvic ring injury

NONOPERATIVE MANAGEMENT

- Early operative management of peritrochanteric fractures is associated with decreased patient morbidity and improved patient function compared to nonoperative management.
- Relative indications for nonoperative management include nonambulatory patients with little pain, patients with active sepsis, patients with soft tissue compromise at the intended

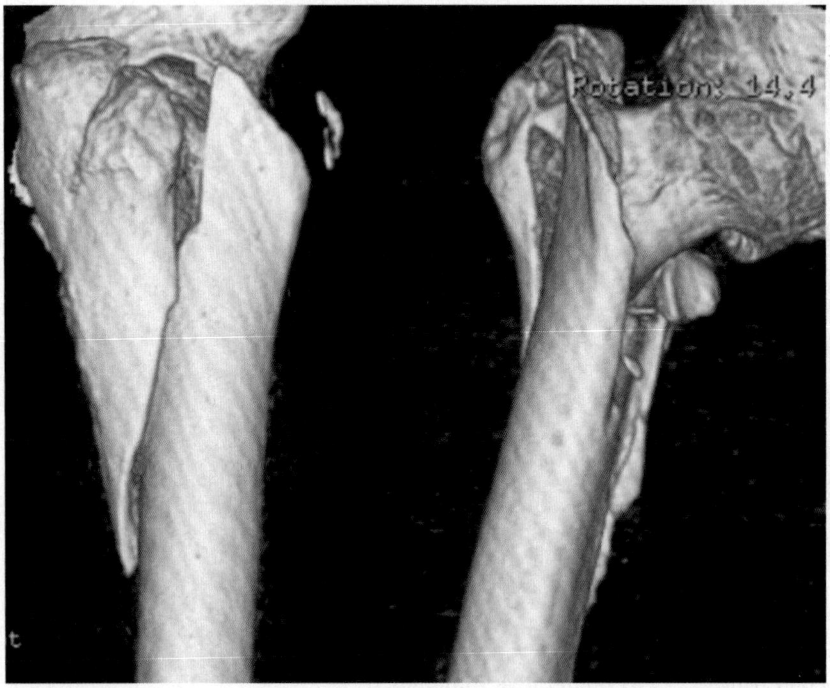

FIG 3 Injury 3-D CT of AP and lateral images demonstrates fracture planes, greater trochanteric extension, and diaphyseal coronal extension.

surgical site, and patients with severe and irreversible medical comorbidities precluding operative intervention.

- Nonoperative management consists of two regimens:
  - Early mobilization
    - No attempt at axial realignment (Can the patient sit up in pain comfortably?)
    - Used for nonambulatory patients if contraindications to surgical management exist and consists of pain control and mobilization out of bed to chair as tolerated to avoid systemic complications of prolonged bed rest
  - Traction
    - Attempted realignment with nonoperative management for ambulatory patients
    - Balanced traction for 8 to 12 weeks, with serial radiographs to assess healing
    - Progressive weight bearing as the fracture shows signs of healing and pain lessens
    - Skeletal traction is associated with fewer complications than skin traction. Skeletal traction with a tensioned bow through the distal femur is less likely to lead to knee stiffness and pain than traction placed through the proximal tibia.

SURGICAL MANAGEMENT

- Once surgical management is chosen, the timing of intervention becomes important.
  - The balance between medical optimization and early operative management in this mostly elderly or younger polytrauma patient population is delicate and coordinated.

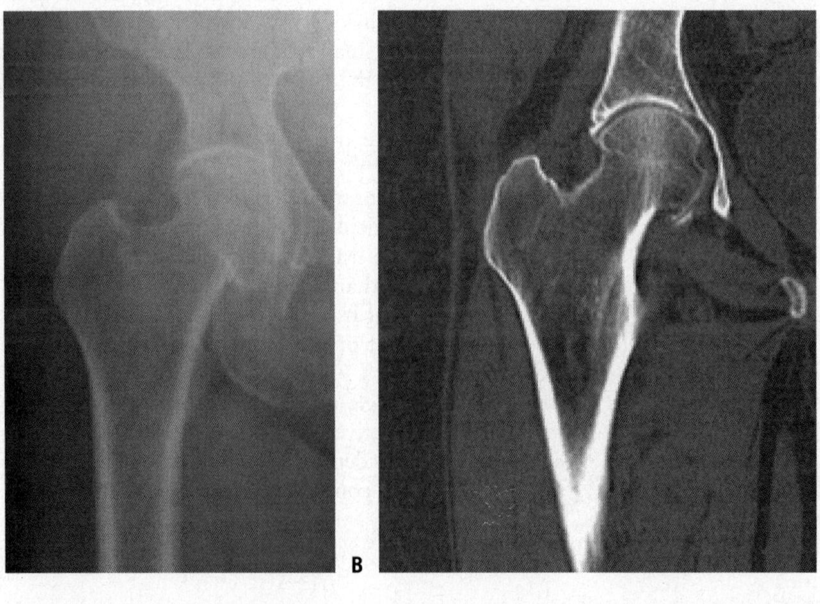

FIG 4 **A.** Injury AP hip of 77-year-old female complaining of hip pain after low-energy fall. **B.** A CT was obtained demonstrating a minimally displaced greater trochanteric fracture but no intertrochanteric extension. *(continued)*

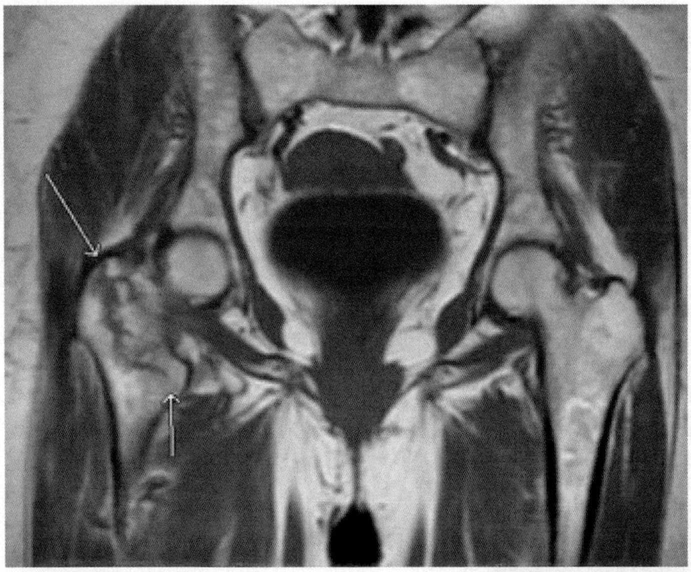

C

FIG 4 *(continued)* **C.** Because she continued to have pain and was unable to weight bear, an MRI demonstrated a complete pertrochanteric hip (*white arrows*) fracture. She was treated with operative fixation.

- Although a retrospective study of more than 2600 patients found that a surgical delay of up to 4 days did not increase patient mortality up to 1 year postoperatively, most studies suggest that delays of more than 2 days may increase patient mortality postoperatively.[26,33] Another National Surgical Quality Improvement Program (NSQIP) study of 17,459 patients demonstrated that surgical delays did not change 30-day readmissions but did prolong hospital stays.[25]

Implant Selection

- Implant selection for fracture fixation should be guided based on fracture pattern, goals of surgery, surgeon skill/expertise, and patient age.
- Implants that may be used include side plates with sliding hip screw (SHS) with or without a trochanteric stabilizing plate (TSP), intramedullary devices (intramedullary nail [IMN], discussed in another chapter), angled blade plate (ABP), proximal femoral locking plate (PFLP), and sometimes IMN/plate combination.
- All implants discussed are angular stable devices, in that they are designed to preserve the neck–shaft angle. SHS and many intramedullary devices allow for sliding of the bone along the axis of the screw, which allows fracture compression and shortening with weight bearing. With these devices, early weight bearing is allowed and encouraged. With stable fracture patterns, some shortening is expected, but with unstable fracture patterns, extensive shortening affecting leg lengths and abductor function can occur.[21]
- ABP and PFLP are fixed length and preserve proximal femoral bone stock. These implants do not allow further compression or shortening across the fracture site, and patients often have restricted weight bearing following surgery.
- Length-stable devices are generally indicated in younger patients with better bone quality or older patients with complex comminuted proximal and/or distal extension to maintain proximal femoral anatomy to facilitate preservation of the abductor lever arm allows and leg length for preserved joint mechanics return to normal ambulation.

Preoperative Planning

- Radiographs are reviewed to determine the fracture pattern.
- The Orthopaedic Trauma Association/AO (OTA/AO) fracture classification system[22] is beneficial and reliable for peritrochanteric fractures (type 31-A). It is divided into groups based on fracture geometry **(FIG 5)**:
  - Group 1 has a single fracture line extending to the medial cortex.
  - Group 2 has more than one fracture line extending to the medial cortex.
  - Group 3 has a fracture geometry that runs in a more transverse or reverse oblique pattern, with the fracture line exiting the lateral cortex below the vastus ridge.
- Implant selection for peritrochanteric fractures in elderly, low-demand patients may be guided by an understanding of this fracture classification.
- Group 1 fractures are fixed reliably with good results using either an SHS or IMN device.
- Group 2 fractures have been shown to be amenable to treatment with either SHS and screw devices or IMN devices. Recent studies have shown improved patient outcomes and better maintenance of fracture alignment and leg lengths with the use of IMN devices in this type of fracture.[5,27,31]
- Group 3 fractures are treated best with IMN devices or angular stable plates.[13,20]
  - SHS devices are contraindicated in these fractures because of the high incidence of implant failure.[18,21]
  - In a meta-analysis, IMN implants were found to have a lower failure rate than angular stable plates when used to treat this type of fracture pattern and should be considered the implant of choice for most surgeons for the elderly patient.[18]
  - The neck–shaft angle of the nonfractured femur can be measured preoperatively to estimate the reduction to be achieved but ≥130 degrees should be desired to improve implant insertion, controlled collapse, and lessen fixation failure.

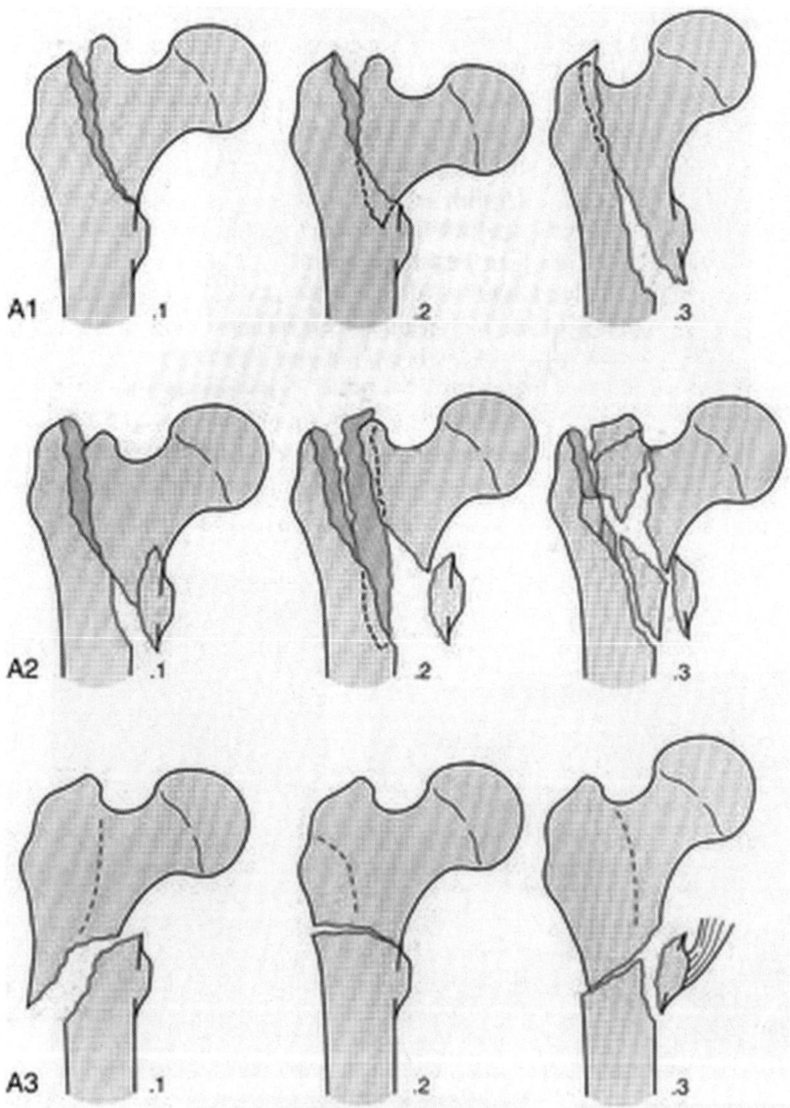

FIG 5 OTA/AO proximal femoral classification demonstrating simple (A1), comminuted (A2), and transverse (A3) or reverse oblique oriented fractures.

- Preoperative planning is vital for a satisfactory outcome when a peritrochanteric fracture is fixed with an ABP. Despite longer incisions and larger short tissue retraction, technically demanding ABP can result in return of anatomic alignment, no inference with hip abductors (with IMN), excellent outcomes, and minimal complications.[4,14]
- Multiple views of the intact contralateral hip and femur, as well as multiple traction views of the fractured hip, are required to properly plan the surgical sequence for this type of fixation.

- PFLP is fixed-angle devices, which may be used as an alternative to ABP or IMN. Despite early catastrophic failures with PFLP,[8,16] other studies demonstrate similar outcomes of PFLP compared to IMN.[15,30,32] The benefit of PFLP over ABP is having multiple fixed-angle screws compared to a single blade plate, which can therefore be less technically demanding.
- These plates may be used for patients who have sustained ipsilateral shaft fractures, as length-stable implants in young patients, periprosthetic fractures in combination with cerclage wires or cables when it is not possible to use intramedullary fixation or combined proximal and/or distal fracture extension with comminution.

Positioning

- When fixing a peritrochanteric fracture with an SHS device, the patient is positioned on a well-padded fracture table, with the fractured leg placed in traction using a boot. Translate the pelvis asymmetrically to the unaffected side to facilitate traction produced valgus and to avoid "peroneal post-induced varus." The two main techniques or positions are "hemilithotomy" or "scissor."
- Hemilithotomy (**FIG 6A,B**):
  - Place the contralateral leg in a well-padded lithotomy leg holder with slight ER, hip flexion, and knee flexion.
  - Benefits: lateral hip visualization
  - Disadvantages:
    - Pressure areas to leg holder
    - With prolonged cases, decreased blood inflow and increased risk of contralateral leg compartment syndrome

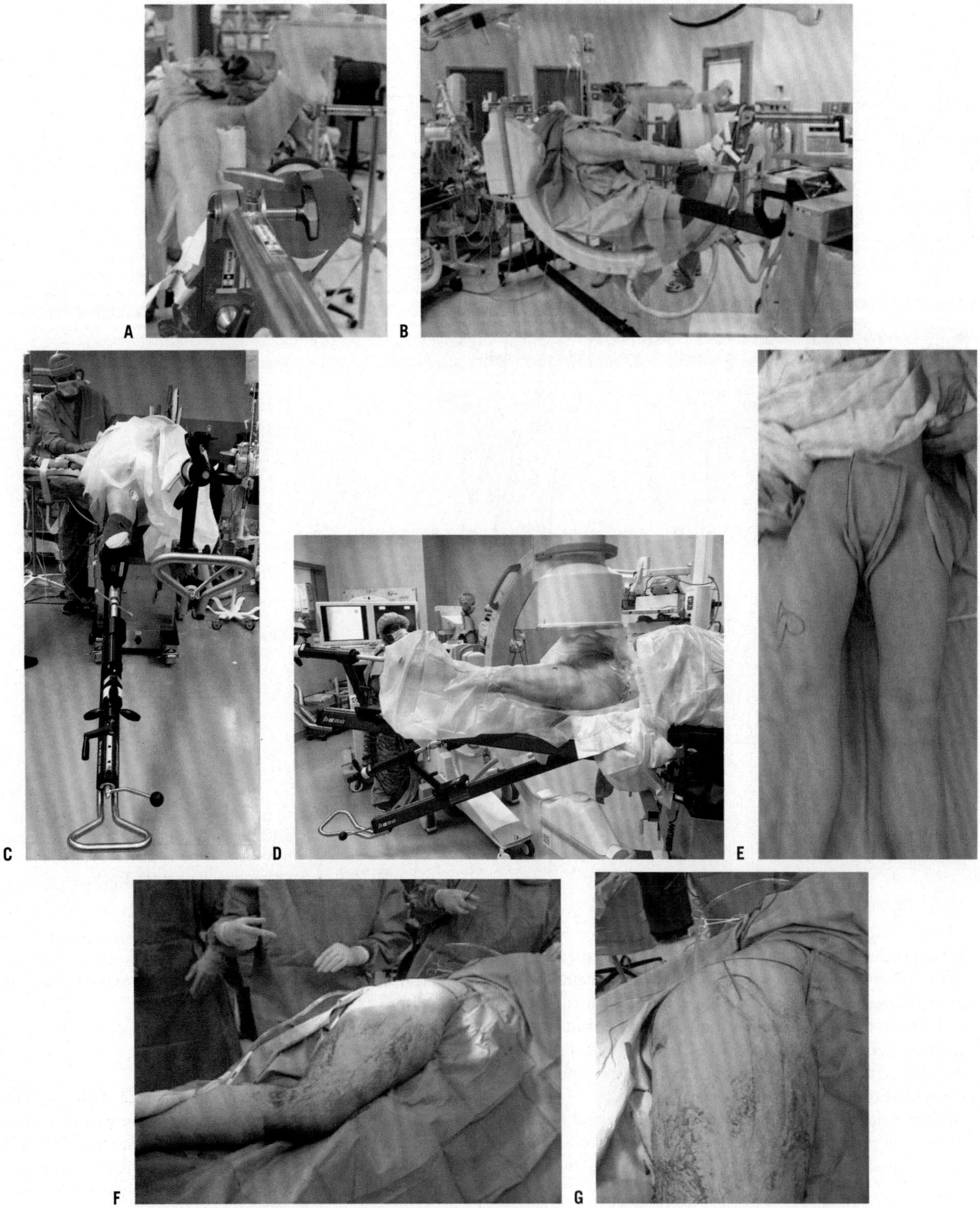

FIG 6 A. Traction table set up for right hip fracture with hemilithotomy position. Note IR of foot and patella pointing to ceiling consistent with good stable pertrochanteric closed reduction. The contralateral hip is slightly flexed and externally rotated. **B.** Extended image demonstrates lateral fluoroscopy view. **C.** Traction set up for left hip fracture with scissor technique. **D.** Note the slight extension and abduction of the contralateral right hip. **E.** Free leg setup on a radiolucent table. Small roll of towels under fractured right hip with entire right hip ready to be prepped free in preparation for right hip ABP. **F.** Free leg lateral decubitus position set up on a radiolucent table. **G.** The hip is in slight flexion, and the limb is in slight IR to offset deforming forces that facilitate fracture reduction. Also, the soft tissues fall away from the hip secondary to gravity facilitating the approach.

- Scissors (**FIG 6C,D**):
  - Place the contralateral foot in a boot holder. Slightly extend and abduct the hip. Do not place traction onto the limb.
- Benefits:
  - This position is helpful in some patients (eg, obesity, stiff contralateral hip, bilateral injuries) who may not be able to flex and externally rotate the contralateral hip to enable use of a well-leg holder and when fractures may require strong traction.
  - No pressure or inflow issues to contralateral limb.
- Disadvantages:
  - The good hip can potentially obscure fluoroscopy viewing of the fractured hip.
  - With prolonged cases, increased risk of femoral nerve stretch and injury
- Alternatively, if a fixed-angle plate is the selected implant, the patient is placed on a completely radiolucent flat-top table. The affected hip is bumped up at a 10- to 20-degree angle, and the leg is draped free (**FIG 6E**).
- In contradistinction to simple fracture patterns in elderly patients, younger patients and complex fracture patterns benefit from paralysis from anesthesia to reduce the need skeletal traction. Furthermore, lateral position with or without traction facilitates fracture reduction especially with complex fracture patterns with deformity (flexion, abduction, ER, and in obese or muscular patients (**FIG 6F,G**).[9]

FRACTURE REDUCTION

- With the patient positioned on the fracture table, the fracture is initially reduced in the coronal plane with axial traction to reestablish fracture length and attempt to fully correct the varus malalignment (**TECH FIG 1**).
  - Abduction of the leg usually corrects varus malalignment and establishes the normal neck–shaft angle.
  - Translation of the peroneal post to the contralateral ischium and lateral to the genitals will lessen the post-induced varus and improve pelvic tilt and hip valgus.
- IR of the distal extremity *usually* corrects the ER deformity at the fracture. IR also serves to align the femoral neck parallel to the floor and assist in eventual guide pin insertion.
  - In some instances, when the fracture functions as a subtrochanteric fracture, ER of the limb is necessary to achieve reduction of the rotational deformity.
  - If the fracture does not reduce with IR, additional reduction tricks will be required to reduce the fracture deformity.
- Fracture reduction is next checked in the lateral plane. Usually with unstable fracture patterns, the distal femur tends to sag or translate posteriorly while the proximal fragment is flexed and translated anteriorly by the iliopsoas. Reduction can be assisted with the following:
  - Indirectly, a crutch or mallet under the femoral shaft will translate and support the shaft.
  - Indirectly, padded attachments with some fracture tables can also support the thigh.
  - After prep and approach, direct insertion of ball spike pusher, Cobb elevator, and/or Weber clamp directly translates the shaft (**TECH FIG 2**).
- Fracture reduction is reassessed in both the AP and lateral planes and checked for neck–shaft angle, neck anteversion, rotation, and femoral shaft sag, with a goal of obtaining a near-anatomic reduction. Acceptable parameters include normal or slight valgus reduction, less than 20 degrees of angulation on the lateral radiograph, and less than 4 mm of fracture translation.[2]
- If a near-anatomic indirect, closed reduction cannot be obtained:
  - Percutaneous techniques utilizing 2.5- or 5.0-mm Schanz pins, bone hook, Weber clamp, Cobb elevator, and/or ball spike pusher can be used to manipulate fracture fragments.
  - If acceptable reduction cannot be obtained with these methods:
    - Supine, open reduction is necessary (**TECH FIG 3**).
    - Lateral, open reduction will reduce deforming forces and facilitate reduction.[9]
    - Anesthesia for complete paralysis, which is not optimal for geriatric patients

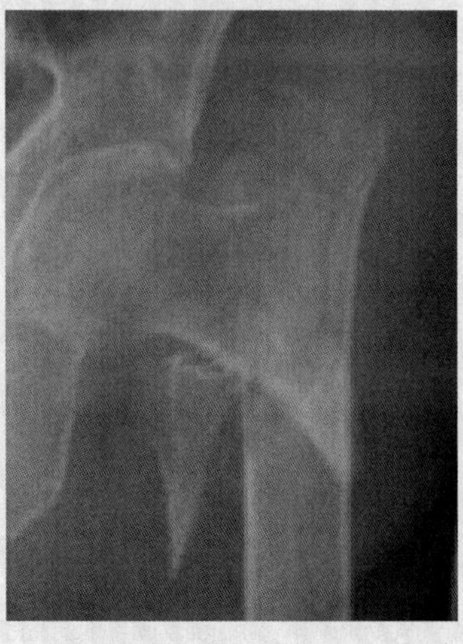

A

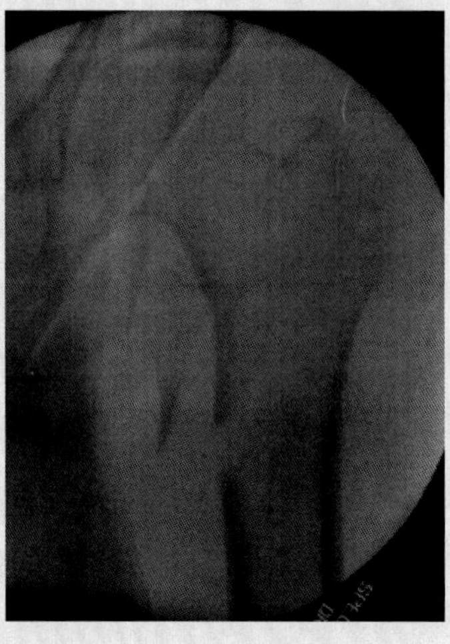

B

TECH FIG 1 A. Injury AP image demonstrates shortening and varus. **B.** Traction image demonstrates restoration of near-anatomic relationships in the AP plane.

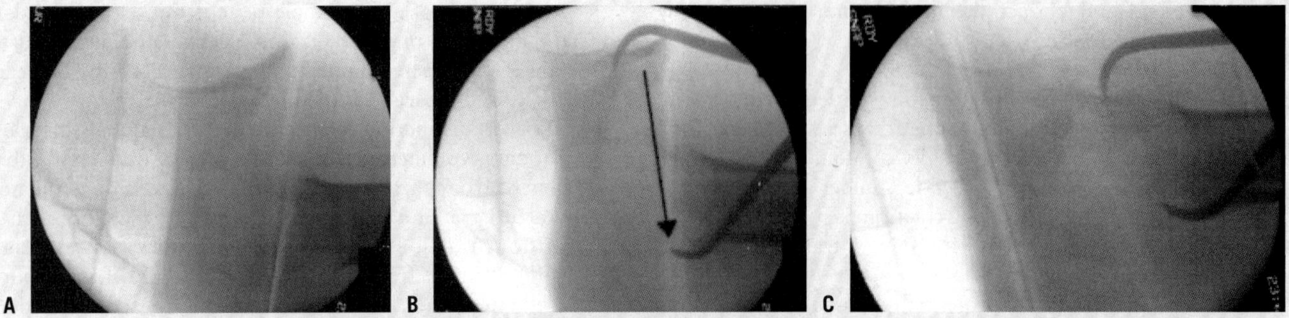

TECH FIG 2 A. Traction lateral image demonstrates the usual flexion of the proximal segment and posterior translation of the distal segment/shaft. **B.** With a small incision that will allow for perpendicular insertion of a Weber clamp, the tips of the clamp are inserted on the anteromedial neck and the posterolateral aspects of the fracture (*arrow*). **C.** With compression of the clamp, the flexion and translation deformities are corrected. The clamp is kept in position until the implant is inserted to maintain neutralization of the deforming forces.

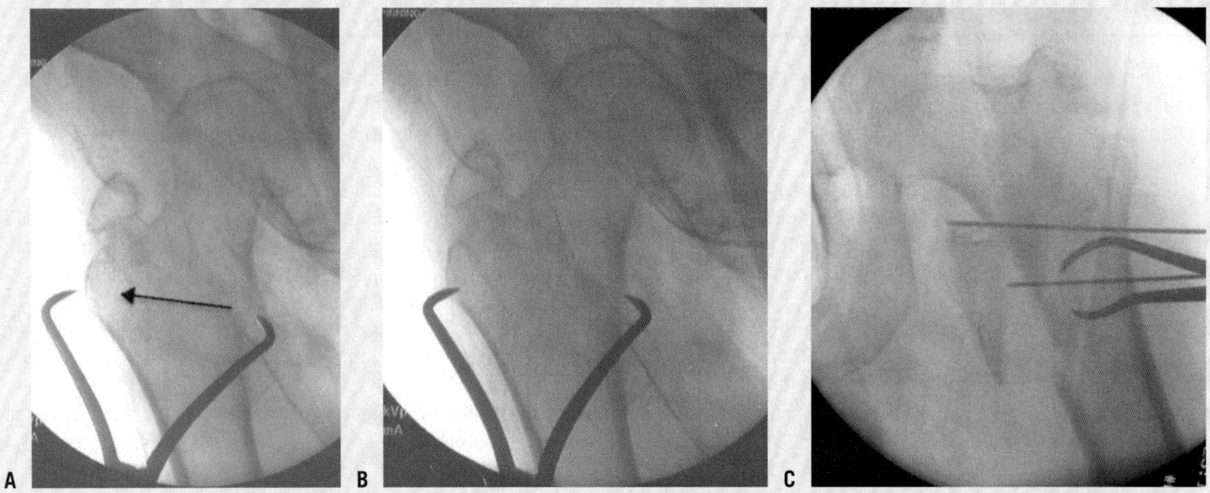

TECH FIG 3 Intraoperative AP image demonstrates translation and displacement from the calcar area. **A.** A Weber clamp is slide parallel to the anterior cortex allowing placement of the clamp tips along the inferior neck and greater trochanteric area (*arrow*). **B,C.** With compression of the clamp, the displacement and translation are corrected. The clamp is kept in position until the final implant insertion.

SIDE PLATE AND SLIDING HIP SCREW

Approach

- Because of the muscular forces exerted on the fracture fragments associated with peritrochanteric hip fractures, anatomic reduction of the fracture is close to impossible with indirect methods, especially in the coronal plane, which is often the most difficult plane to control.[1]
  - Studies have shown that absolute anatomic reduction of all fragments of these fractures is not necessary for a satisfactory functional outcome.[28]
- The primary goal of reduction of peritrochanteric hip fractures is to reestablish a normal anatomic alignment between the proximal head and neck fragment and the distal femoral shaft in the coronal, sagittal, and axial planes.
- A lateral approach to the proximal femur is the preferred approach for open reduction and internal fixation of peritrochanteric femur fractures.
- This approach may be used whether the selected implant is an SHS, ABP, or PFLP.
- The incision is centered over the lateral aspect of the femur. Its proximal extent is the palpable vastus ridge for SHS and just proximal to the tip of the greater trochanter for ABP or PFLP **(TECH FIG 4A)**.
  - The distal extent of the incision is made long enough to allow application of the plate.
  - For obese and/or muscular patients, longer incisions are preferential.
- The incision is carried through the fascia lata, posterior to the tensor muscle proximally. The vastus lateralis fascia is incised longitudinally 2 to 3 cm anterior to the linea aspera. Elevate the vastus lateralis from the posterior fascia and retract anteriorly **(TECH FIG 4B)**. Care is taken to identify and control any perforating vessels supplying the vastus lateralis muscle posteriorly.
- Proximally, the origin of the vastus lateralis is sharply released off the vastus ridge to allow atraumatic anterior retraction of the muscle to facilitate lateral femoral shaft exposure.
- Care should be taken to avoid any medial shaft dissection with stripping to maintain the vasculature to the fracture zone.

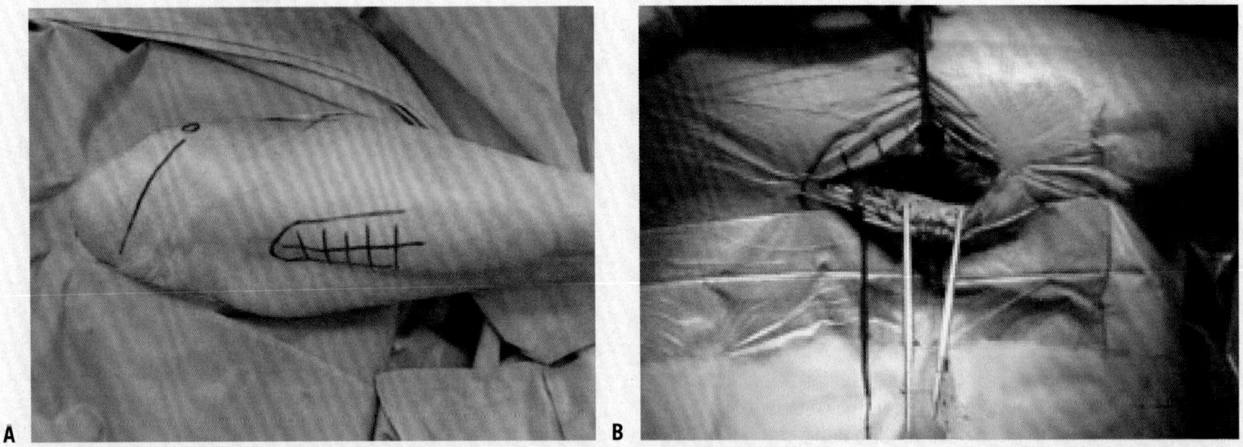

TECH FIG 4 A. For insertion of an SHS, a laterally based 8- to 10-cm incision is created just distal to the tip of the greater trochanter extending distally along the shaft. Obese or muscular patients and/or ABP and PFLP implants usually require longer incisions. **B.** Once through the fascia lata, the vastus lateralis fascia is split, and the muscle is gently dissected down to bone and then anteriorly, exposing the proximal lateral cortex of the femur.

Guide Pin Positioning for Sliding Hip Screw and Fracture Preparation

- The entrance point for the guide pin is selected once exposure of the lateral femoral cortex is completed.
  - The entrance for a 135-degree plate is typically 2 cm below the vastus ridge, opposite the midpoint of the lesser trochanter, at the level of the femoral insertion of the gluteus maximus tendon.
- Even though discouraged, the start points for the guide pin are adjusted 1 cm proximal (for lower angled devices) or distal (for higher angled devices) from the 135-degree starting point for every 5-degree adjustment in the measured neck–shaft angle.
- Insertion of a guide pin manually, through the soft tissues and capsule, external to the neck and into the femoral head can mimic femoral neck anteversion and facilitate parallel insertion of the intraosseous guide pin.
- The 135-degree angled guide is placed at the guide pin insertion site, centered in the AP plane on the femoral shaft and seated flush to the lateral cortex.
  - It is preferred to use an angled guide rather than to place the guide pin freehand to avoid levering the side plate against the lateral cortex and potentially creating a lateral wall fracture when compressing the side plate to the femur.
- The guide pin is advanced under fluoroscopic guidance, in both the AP and lateral views, to ensure central-central placement in the femoral head **(TECH FIG 5)**.
  - If the guide pin is not centered in the neck and head on both views, it must be removed and adjusted. If a terminally threaded guide pin is used, the threads create a path for pin insertion. In order to realign, the pin must be backed up, realigned, and inserted on reverse for a short section to bypass the threaded portion of the bone.
  - The fracture reduction should be reassessed, and the guide adjusted to ensure that central guide pin placement is obtained.
- Insert the guide pin within 5 mm of the articular surface in both AP and lateral projections.
- The intraosseous length of the guide pin is measured with the cannulated ruler provided in the instrument set.
  - Care must be taken when deciding on a lag screw length, especially in highly unstable fractures reduced with a substantial amount of traction. Traction can cause fracture dis-

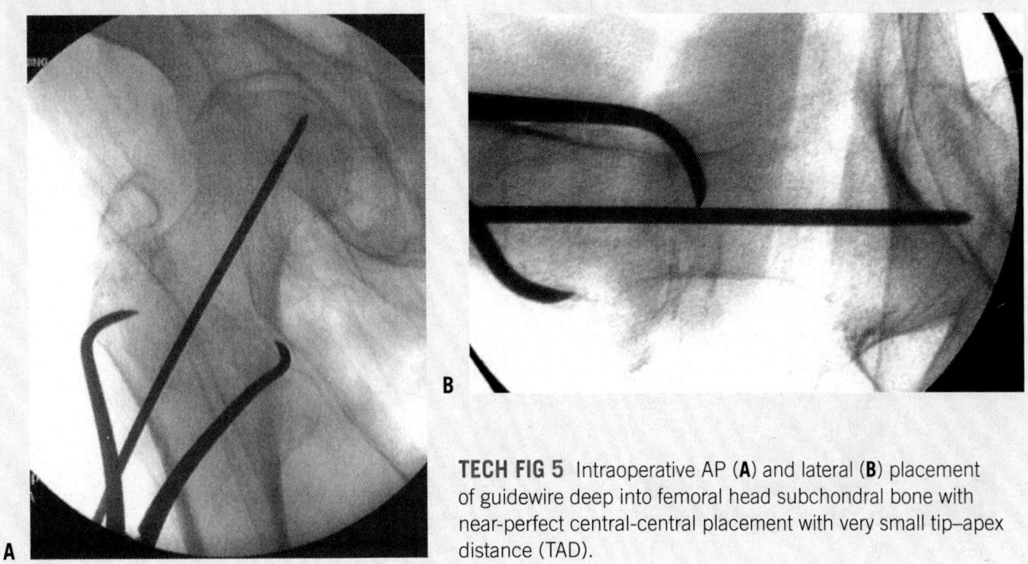

TECH FIG 5 Intraoperative AP (**A**) and lateral (**B**) placement of guidewire deep into femoral head subchondral bone with near-perfect central-central placement with very small tip–apex distance (TAD).

traction and overestimation of lag screw length, which lead to screw prominence when traction is eventually released.
  - The guide pin is then advanced into the subchondral bone to reduce the risk of inadvertent advancement into the joint or pin removal with reamer removal.
- A second guide pin can then be advanced into the femoral head proximal to the original guide pin to add stability in unstable fractures or in fractures that are reduced in anatomic alignment using excessive traction.
  - This pin acts as a derotational pin to ensure that the proximal fragment does not rotate with reaming and lag screw insertion.
- A triple reamer is used to prepare the channel in the lateral cortex, neck, and head for the lag screw and side plate barrel.
  - The reamer is set to 5 mm less than the measured lag screw length to ensure that the subchondral bone in the femoral head is not violated during reaming.
- The triple reamer is then advanced and withdrawn under fluoroscopic guidance.
  - It is important to use fluoroscopy during reaming to ensure that the guide pin is not bonded to the reamer and inadvertently advanced into the pelvis or removed upon reamer removal. Removing any potential bone remnants within the reamer, keeping the reamer running during insertion, and removal without stopping can avoid inadvertent pin advancement or removal.
- Occasionally, the intact lateral wall of the proximal femur may be fractured by the triple reamer. Occult fractures can exist. To facilitate this diagnosis, manually insert a finger within the lateral reamed hole to stress and assess an occult fracture. If this occurs, the fracture is essentially converted into a transverse or reverse oblique pattern (OTA/AO type 31-A3), and excessive fracture collapse may occur if fixed only with an SHS. In these cases, the proximal lateral wall may be buttressed with the addition of a TSP over the SHS. Alternatively, the decision may be made to convert to IMN device for fracture fixation. Therefore, because this conversion may be a possibility, prep and drape the entire leg from the iliac crest to the knee to facilitate conversion to an IMN.

Implant Insertion

- A 135-degree, two- to four-hole side plate is usually chosen for fixation **(TECH FIG 6)**.
  - Multiple clinical and cadaveric studies have shown no difference in the strength of implant fixation with side plates with more than four holes.[6,23]
- The implant is set up according to the manufacturer's specifications.
- The cannulated lag screw is then inserted over the guide pin with a centering sleeve to ensure proper positioning. Avoid toggling of the screw and centering device to reduce the risk of lateral wall fracture creation. If difficult to insert, remove the lag and try tapping before reinsertion of the lag. Careful sizing of the lag screw length is required, as noted earlier, to ensure that fracture compression and collapse does not create relative excessive screw length and lateral hardware prominence.
- Fluoroscopy and manual fracture palpation are used to ensure that the fracture is not displaced (rotated) while the lag screw is inserted.
  - If the fracture is displaced by the insertion of the lag screw:
    - Derotate the lag insertion device until the desire anatomic rotation is noted.
    - Derotate the lag and apply a clamp through the incision laterally or through a small anterior incision to compress the inferior neck, insert the lag, and then remove the clamp.
    - Remove the lag screw, a derotation screw is added cephalad, the channel is tapped, and the lag screw is reinserted. This may help, but inferior/calcar rotation/translation may still occur. If so, perform options 1 and/or 2.
- Peritrochanteric fractures of the *right hip* can displace with an *apex posterior angulation* as the lag screw is turned clockwise during insertion, whereas *left hip* fractures can displace with *apex anterior angulation* owing to the anatomic configuration and subsequent tensioning of the hip capsule with screw insertion.
- With the lag screw inserted to the desired depth of 5 to 8 mm of the femoral head articular surface, within the femoral head on the AP and lateral fluoroscopic projection, its relation to the lateral cortex is checked to ensure proper length. Laterally, the ideal position of the screw is approximately 5 to 8 mm deep to the lateral cortex.

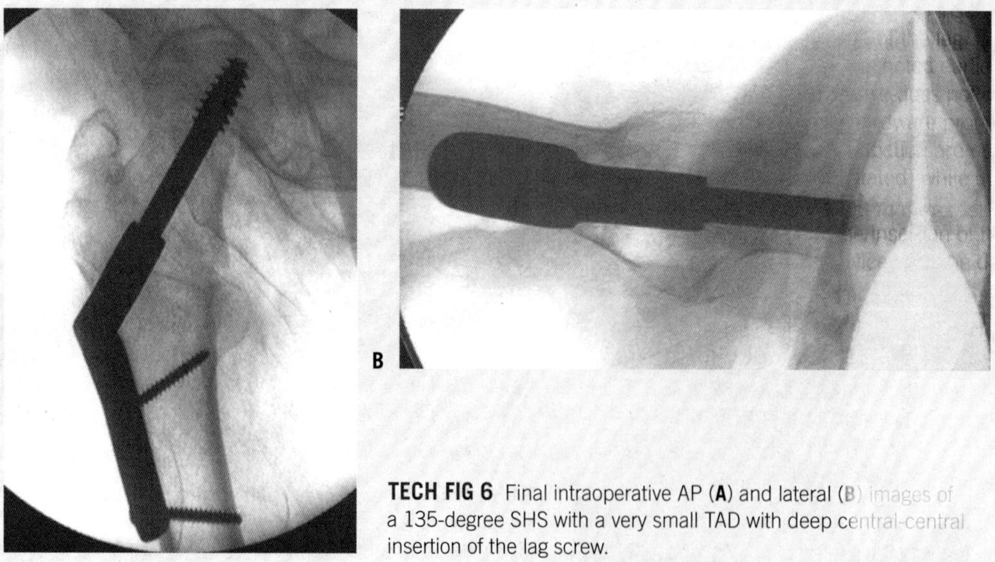

TECH FIG 6 Final intraoperative AP (**A**) and lateral (**B**) images of a 135-degree SHS with a very small TAD with deep central-central insertion of the lag screw.

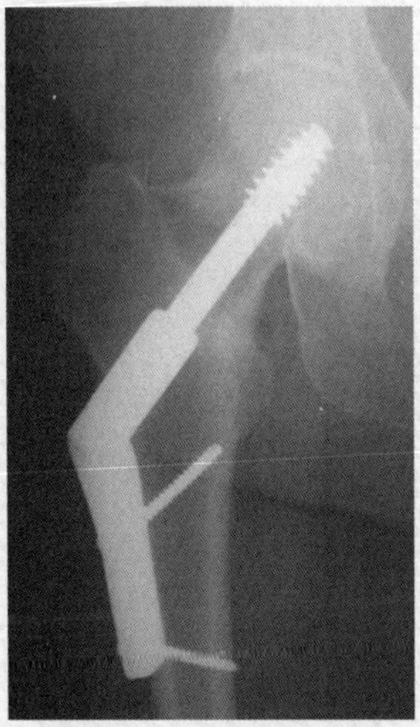

A

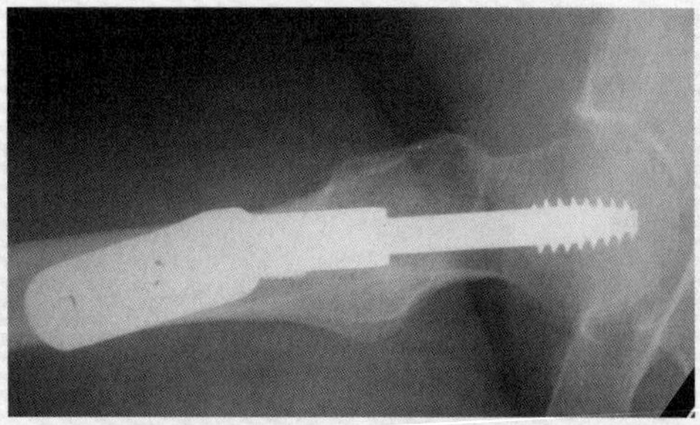

B

TECH FIG 7 Final AP (**A**) and lateral (**B**) images of a successfully treated OTA A2 fracture with a 135-degree SHS with a small amount of controlled collapse but maintenance of the neck–shaft and anteversion relationships.

- The side plate is then slid over the lag screw and inserter, so it is seated flush on the lateral cortex, and the guide pin (and derotational pin if used) is removed.
  - If lag screw length <80 mm, use a "short" instead of standard barrel length to facilitate a controlled collapse and to avoid barrel impingement before healing.
  - Assure parallel insertion of the plate barrel onto the lag screw in both planes.
  - If off plane, barrel resistance will be noted. To avoid lag screw malalignment or lateral cortex fracture, do not insert if resistance or block noted.
  - Rotating the barrel onto the screw may facilitate insertion.
  - Use the cannulated insertion device to secure plate insertion along the lateral cortex.
- Rotate the plate portion laterally to facilitate concentric placement along the shaft.
- Cortical screws are inserted to secure the plate to the femoral shaft.
- If appropriate for the fracture pattern, the lag screw compressing screw is then inserted into the barrel of the lag screw and tightened to compress the fracture in the plane of the lag screw, under fluoroscopic guidance.
  - Avoid overcompression and possible detachment of the screw from the femoral head.
  - Remove the compression screw if the fracture is oriented such that weight bearing will cause compression at the fracture site.
  - Retain the compressing screw with "short" barrel use and/or in paralytics, where there is no resting joint reaction force, and implant disengagement can occur with postoperative transfers.
- With the compression of the fracture complete, the alignment and implant position are checked once again with fluoroscopy **(TECH FIG 7)**.

ANGLED BLADE PLATE

Approach

- A lateral approach is used, as described earlier. Although the incision is more proximal, and angles toward the anterior superior iliac spine, the trochanteric block must be exposed and interval between tensor and gluteus medius must be exploited in order to visualize anterior neck. The approach is much longer distally to accommodate the full length of the plate and tensioning device.

Preparation and Implant Insertion

- With the lateral femur and trochanteric block exposed, if a direct reduction is desired, a soft tissue–sparing reduction of the trochanteric block to the proximal femur is secured with pointed bone clamps and Kirschner wires (K-wires) or small lag screws. Alternatively, an indirect reduction can be employed, relying on the proper position of the blade within the proximal segment to reduce the fracture when the plate is brought onto the shaft and compressed distally.
- Guide pins are then introduced into this reconstructed segment to facilitate proper seating of the chisel for the blade plate.
  - The first pin is placed anterior to the femoral neck and secured into the anterior femoral head to demonstrate the femoral anteversion.
  - The second pin is placed with the use of an angled guide and/or fluoroscopy near the tip of the greater trochanter and directed into the femoral head at a 90-degree angle to the femoral shaft.
  - The correct position of the chisel should be correlated and confirmed with detailed preoperative planning **(TECH FIG 8)**.
- The chisel is inserted parallel to the two guide pins, just distal to the second pin. Care must be taken to maintain the correct alignment of the chisel with the shaft of the femur because this determines the flexion–extension of the fracture, which is fixed once the chisel is inserted 1 to 2 cm.
  - Insert with a mallet and remove the chisel with the "tuning fork" every 1 to 2 cm to avoid incarceration of the chisel within the bone.
  - The chisel is directed to pass through the center of the neck and seat in the inferior portion of the femoral head.

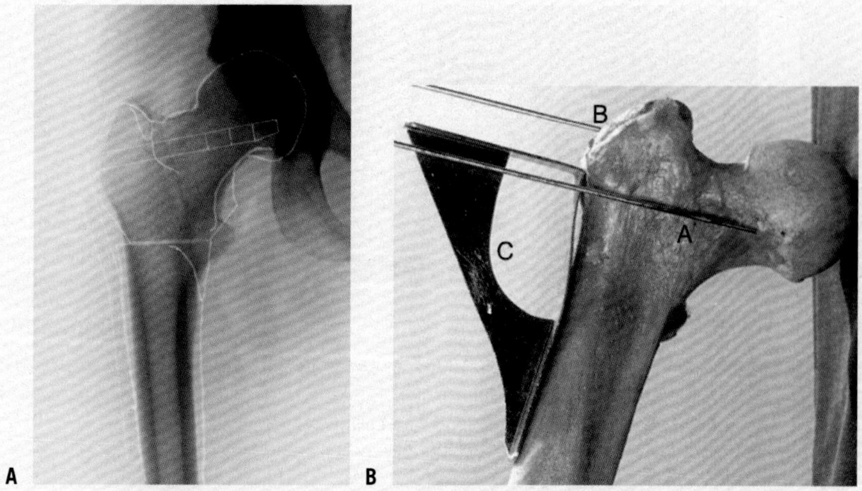

TECH FIG 8 A. With contralateral normal hip as a template, an electronic templating system is overlaid on the image demonstrating ABP start and finish locations in the head. **B.** Utilizing a cadaveric model of the proximal femur, the reference pins are used. The first pin (*A*) is slid through the soft tissues and capsule along the femoral neck into the femoral head to reference the anteversion. The second pin (*B*) is inserted into the femoral head parallel to pin (*A*) on the AP and centrally on the lateral view referencing the anteversion and centrality. The 95-degree template device (*C*) is then applied lateral to the bone parallel to both pins and at the correct position distally creating an external reference to insertion of the chisel trajectory.

Because of the anterior translation of the femoral head on the shaft, the insertion site is in the anterior half of the trochanter.
  - The position of the chisel should be frequently checked with fluoroscopy before and during its insertion.
- The chisel is carefully removed, and the appropriate-length blade plate is inserted and gently seated into the proximal fragment.
  - The insertion should be frequently checked with biplanar fluoroscopy to ensure that the blade follows the path made by the chisel.
- Once the blade is seated, the most proximal screw is placed through the implant into the medial cortex of the proximal femoral neck, rigidly securing the implant to the proximal fragment.
  - Fracture reduction is now achieved by bringing the plate to the shaft and controlling length, rotation, and compression.
- If needed, a femoral distractor may be used as a reduction tool.
  - The distractor should be fixed to the lateral aspect of the femur, with the proximal pin in the head and neck fragment and the distal pin placed distal to the end of the plate.
  - Distraction is applied across the fracture to improve fracture alignment and length through soft tissue tensioning.
  - A bone clamp is loosely applied to the distal femoral shaft fragment and plate to counteract the tendency for the fracture to be reduced into varus with the femoral distractor.
  - Pointed reduction clamps are used to reduce comminuted fragments to the plate without stripping them of soft tissue attachments.
- Fracture reduction is checked with fluoroscopy.
  - If fracture alignment is acceptable, distraction is removed while keeping clamps on allowing fragment settling and final fracture compression with the articulated tensioning device via a bicortical screw.
  - The plate is then fixed to the shaft, and fracture fragments are secured with screws in the standard manner, and lag screws are inserted where the pointed reduction clamps were previously placed **(TECH FIG 9)**.
- The final fracture alignment and length, as well as the femoral head, are examined with fluoroscopy to ensure proper fracture reduction and to make sure that there has been no head penetration by the implant.

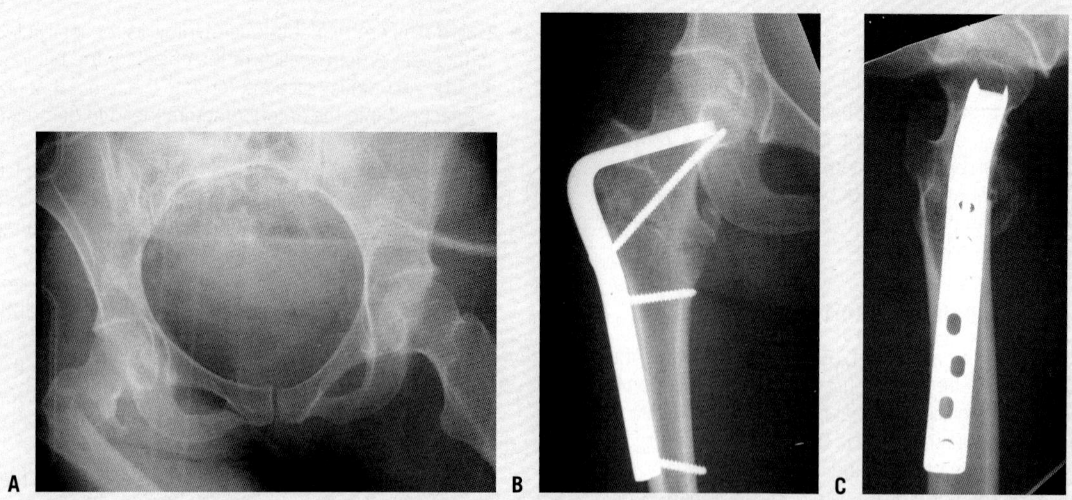

TECH FIG 9 A. Injury AP pelvis of a high-energy motor vehicle accident in a 28 year-old-female demonstrating a grossly unstable OTA A2 injury. Secondary to the marked displacement and instability in a young patient with good bone quality, a 95-degree ABP was inserted after open reduction of the fracture and preliminary clamp and pin fixation demonstrating anatomic reduction and rigid fixation on the AP (**B**) and lateral (**C**) images.

PROXIMAL FEMORAL LOCKING PLATE

Approach

- The lateral femur is exposed as noted earlier. More distal exposure may be required, depending on the length of the selected implant. In some cases, the plate may be tunneled submuscularly and fixed to the femoral shaft using small incisions.

Preparation and Implant Insertion

- If attempting direct reduction, the fracture should be reduced using a combination of traction, K-wires, reduction clamps, and Schanz pins as needed **(TECH FIG 10)**. Care should be taken to avoid interference with planned implant placement. Another option is to use Weber clamps over or through screw sites of the plate to maintain fracture reduction. Insertion interfragmentary screw before removing the clamps maintains fracture reduction.
- Once the desired reduction has been achieved, place the plate laterally centered on the shaft of the femur. The correct position of the plate proximally or distally will be determined based on desired position of the guide pins placed through threaded sleeves secured to the plate. Correct IR or ER of the plate is determined with optimal guide pin placement within the neck and head. Secondary to normal relative neck anteversion, the plate may also require slight posterior translation to improve optimal pin placement **(TECH FIG 11)**.
- Before or simultaneously securing the plate to the head with pins, temporarily secure the plate to the shaft with a drill bit through the drill sleeve, clamp, or screws to avoid shaft malreduction.
- With short stature patients, the precontoured plate may not fit well laterally, and some screws may not be able to inserted to avoid extraosseous placement.
- Many crucial elements are *required* for optimizing PFLP application and fracture healing:
  - Anatomic fracture reduction—avoidance of varus, flexion of proximal fragment
  - Fracture site compression—avoidance of distraction
    - Anatomically reduce the fracture with clamps or interfragmentary screws and then neutralize with plate.
    - Use "conical" screws instead of "locked" to compress the fracture fragments and bone–plate interval **(TECH FIG 12)**
      - Anterior superior to compress cephalad cortical contact
      - Inferior to compress calcar-shaft contact
  - Optimal plate placement to facilitate deep symmetrical placement of locking screws within the femoral head
    - Inferior or calcar pin should be central and within 5 mm of calcar bone.
    - Posterior pin should be within 5 mm of posterior neck cortex avoiding an in-out-in screw.
    - With correct plate translation in the coronal and sagittal planes, screw optimization should be obtained.
- Once fracture reduction, plate application, and pin insertion are optimized, locking screw insertion can be performed. Once the remainder of locking screws are inserted into the head, replace the conical screws for locking screws. Use 5-6 screws total within the head.
- Optimal screw depth should be within 5 mm of subchondral bone.
- Plate length and cortical shaft screw insertion should optimize balanced fixation **(TECH FIG 13)**.
- Fixation of the plate to the femoral diaphysis with adequate length restoration can be facilitated by using an articulated tensioning device, traction, or open reduction techniques **(TECH FIG 14)**.

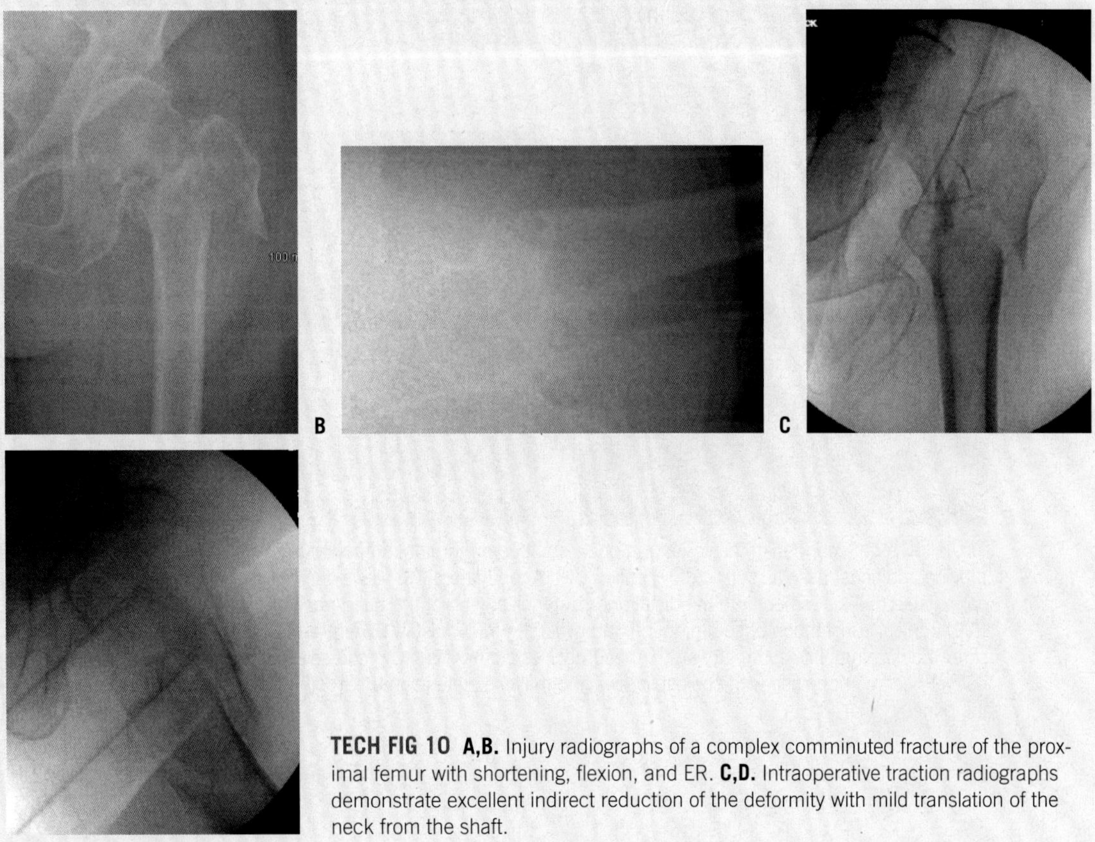

TECH FIG 10 A,B. Injury radiographs of a complex comminuted fracture of the proximal femur with shortening, flexion, and ER. **C,D.** Intraoperative traction radiographs demonstrate excellent indirect reduction of the deformity with mild translation of the neck from the shaft.

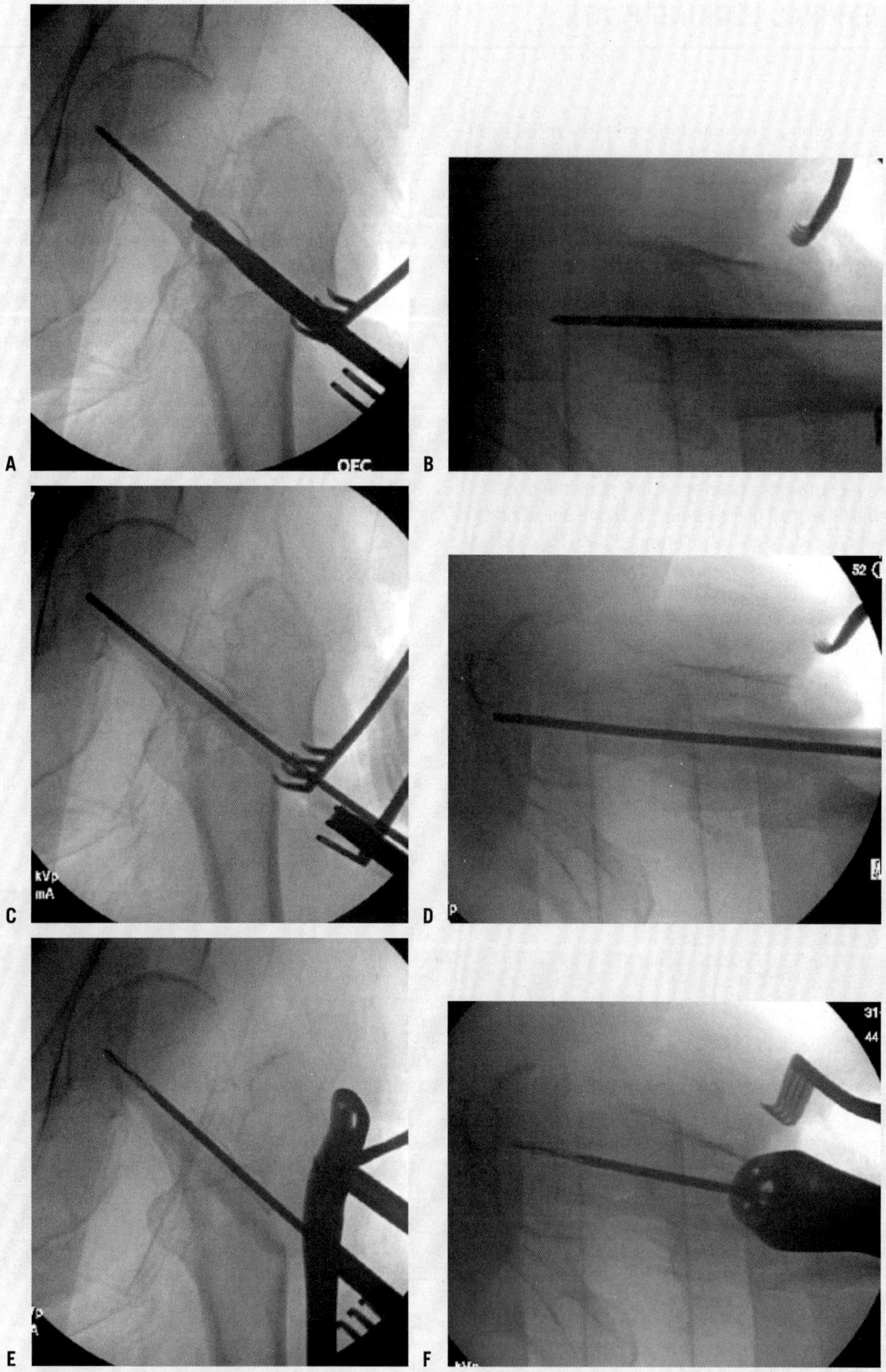

TECH FIG 11 Secondary to posterior and neck–shaft comminution, a fibular strut was inserted to provide additional biologic support for healing. AP (**A**) and lateral (**B**) views demonstrate guide pin and cannulated drill placement into the distal and posterior portion of the head/neck to perform fibular (**C,D**) cortical substitution of comminution and avoid the PFLP distal (**E**)/central (**F**) of the (alpha) locking screw confirming plate symmetry on the head/neck anatomy. Also, you can see that the fracture has not yet been compressed with conical screws and that the plate is off the trochanter/shaft portion of the bone.

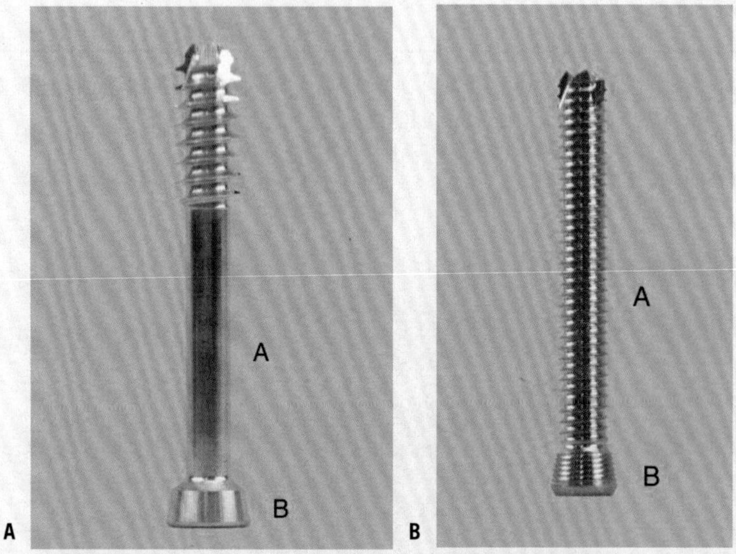

TECH FIG 12 A cannulated 6.5-mm partially threaded "conical" screw demonstrating the smooth shank (*A*) and nonthreaded screw (*B*) head (**A**) compared to a 6.5-mm fully threaded locked screw noting a threaded (*A*) locked screw (*B*) head (**B**).

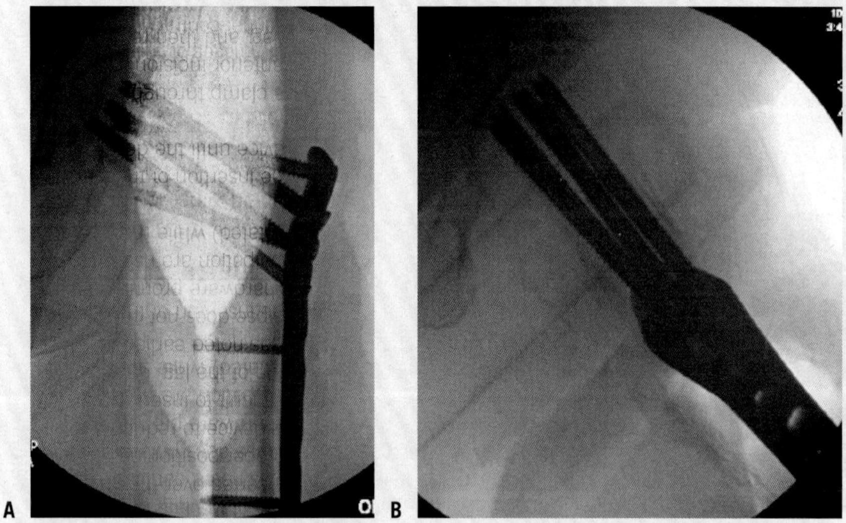

TECH FIG 13 Final AP (**A**) and lateral (**B**) intraoperative images demonstrating symmetrical screw spread within the head, screws deep to subchondral bone, and compression of the plate to the bone and of the fracture lines within neck/trochanter and transverse trochanter/shaft.

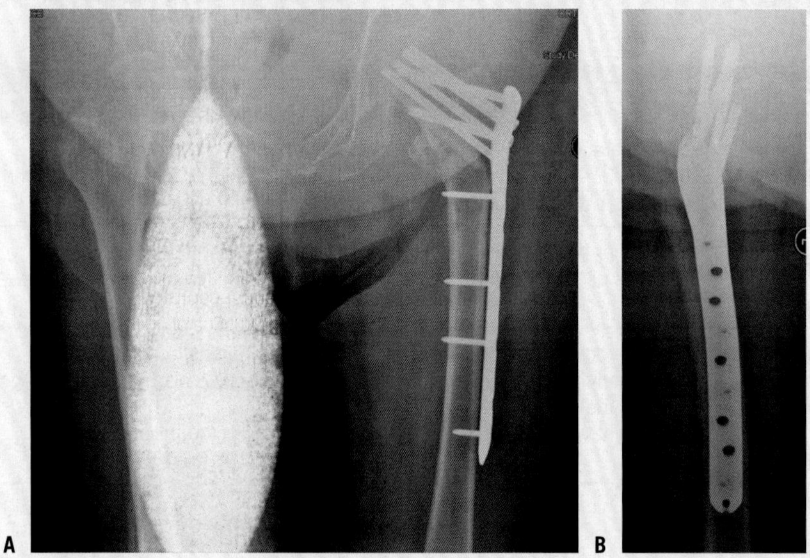

TECH FIG 14 Final standing AP (**A**) and lateral (**B**) images of complex proximal femoral fracture successfully treated with a locking proximal femoral plate. Note restoration of neck–shaft and anteversion without shortening, collapse, or displacement of the greater trochanter.

WOUND CLOSURE

- Aggressive débridement of devitalized tissue is performed before wound irrigation.
- The wound is then closed in a layered fashion; the muscle, fascia, subcutaneous tissue, and skin are repaired separately.
- Use a drain with closure or negative pressure drain (vacuum assisted closure [VAC]) for obese patients and/or prolonged surgical dissections **(TECH FIG 15)**.

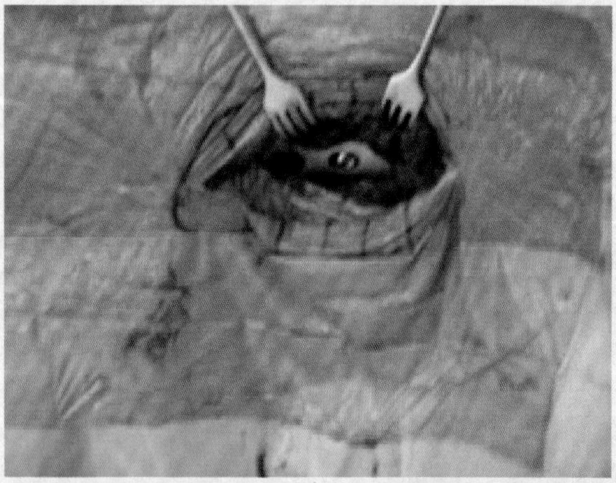
A
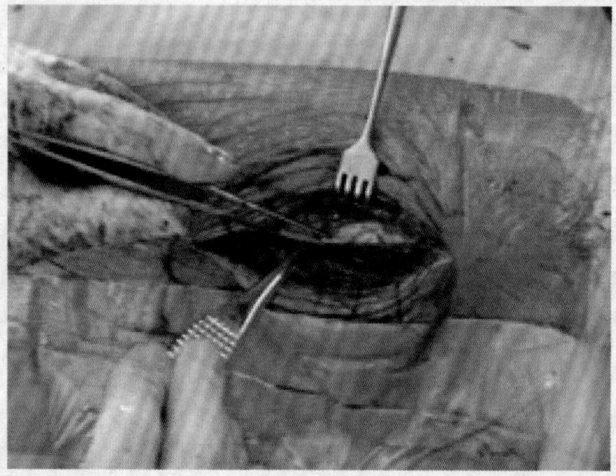
B
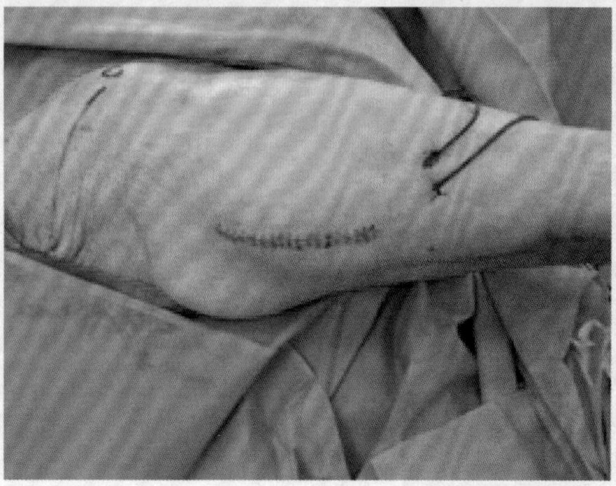
C

TECH FIG 15 After insertion of an SHS, wound closure is performed with débridement of nonviable tissue. **A.** Here, elevation of the vastus and tensor fascia exposes the plate. **B.** Restoration of muscular relationships is performed with nonbraided absorbable suture at each layer. **C.** Final closure is demonstrated with a deep and superficial drain in an elderly female who was on chronic anticoagulation therapy for cardiac issues.

TECHNIQUES

Pearls and Pitfalls

Preoperative Fracture Assessment	• The fracture pattern must be studied preoperatively so that the proper device for fixation may be chosen. Improper use of an SHS in an AO/OTA type 31-A3 fracture, for example, will lead to a higher incidence of fixation failure. Prep entire leg to prepare for potential intraoperative conversion to IMN.
Fracture Reduction	• Successful fracture reduction is mandatory for the treatment of these fractures. The rate of fixation failure increases, no matter what fixation method is used, for poorly reduced fractures. Do something to reduce fracture indirectly or directly.
Implant Selection	• Measurement of the neck–shaft angle of the normal hip must be done preoperatively to ensure that the proper-angled side plate is used. Use of an improperly angled device will prevent central and deep placement of the lag screw in the femoral head and will increase the incidence of fixation failure. • Many different device systems exist with slight variations of technique and implant design. Familiarity with the selected device is important.

<table>
<tr><td>Lag Screw Position</td><td>

- Positioning of the lag screw central-central and deep within the femoral head is one of the most important factors to protect against implant cutout.
- The tip–apex distance (TAP), as measured on AP and lateral fluoroscopy intraoperatively, should be under 25 mm to significantly decrease the incidence of fixation failure **(FIG 7)**.[2]

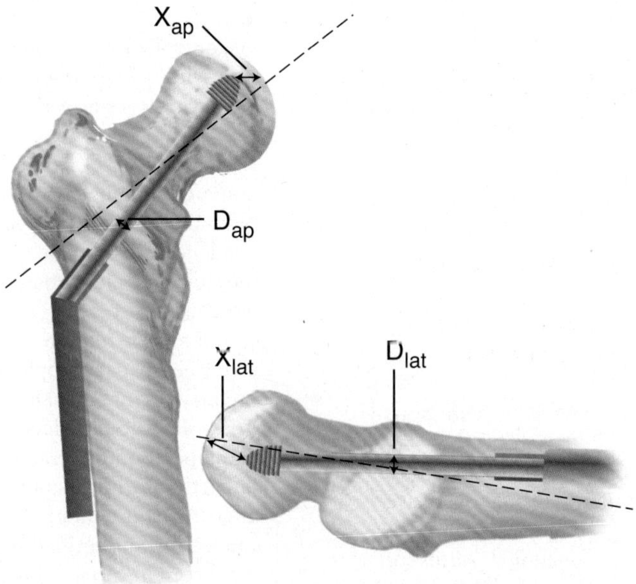

$$TAD = (X_{ap} \times \frac{D_{true}}{D_{ap}}) + (X_{lat} \times \frac{D_{true}}{D_{lat}})$$

FIG 7 Proper measurement technique for tip–apex distance (*TAD*).

</td></tr>
<tr><td>Lateral Cortical Wall Fracture</td><td>

- Missed occult or secondary intraoperative fracture with lag or plate insertion may lead to fracture overcompression or collapse resulting in inferior outcomes with SHS. When this pitfall is encountered, reestablishing the lateral cortex is crucial with the addition of trochanteric plate (TSP) to the SHS or with conversion to IMN.

</td></tr>
<tr><td>Lateral View Reduction</td><td>

- Supine reduction of peritrochanteric fractures in the lateral view is difficult. Gravity and muscular pull tend to result in an apex posterior or apex anterior position, respectively, depending on the fracture pattern. Manual adjustment of the malreduction must be performed to collinearly and anatomically reduce the fracture with pointed reduction clamps, joysticks, and/or a bone elevator. Alternatively, lateral decubitus positioning and/or paralysis will reduce these deforming forces.

</td></tr>
<tr><td>Rotational Fracture Reduction</td><td>

- Rotational reduction of peritrochanteric fractures can be challenging as well. Most simple fractures reduce with IR. Some unstable patterns and/or subtrochanteric extensions require ER especially with comminution and young patients. If in doubt, obtain a true lateral of the neck with fluoroscopy, translate the machine to the knee, and rotate the femoral condyles until approximately 10 degrees of anteversion is obtained.

</td></tr>
</table>

POSTOPERATIVE CARE

- AP and lateral radiographs of the operative hip should be obtained immediately postoperatively in the recovery room to assess implant position and fracture reduction and to ensure that no iatrogenic femur fracture was produced intraoperatively. The entire device should be included in the radiograph.
- Patients are mobilized as soon as cardiopulmonary and mental status will safely allow, usually later in the day or by postoperative day 1.
- Unrestricted immediate weight bearing facilitates mobilization and gait without an increase in fixation failure with this postoperative rehabilitation protocol.[19]
- Utilizing gait analysis, patients effectively autoregulate weight bearing based on fracture site stability; more stable constructs facilitate more weight bearing.[18]
- Don't discharge patients with draining or weeping incisions; it should be dry.
- At 2 weeks postoperative, confirm uneventful wound healing. Suture or staple removal timing should be patient specific. With a poor host, keep in longer.

- Follow-up radiographs should be obtained at 2, 6, and 12 weeks confirming controlled fracture impaction; exclude any fixation device complications; and assess fracture healing to correlate with improved mobilization and lessening pain.

OUTCOMES

- With proper fracture reduction, implant selection, and fixation device positioning, peritrochanteric hip fractures heal in up to 98% of cases.
- One-year mortality rates after fixation of peritrochanteric hip fractures range from 7% to 27%, with most studies finding a rate of 15% to 20%.[24]
- According to Medicare data, 30- and 180-day mortality rates continue to improve.
- Mortality rates depend on both preoperative and postoperative medical complications and condition as well as preoperative functional status.
- Postoperative functional status also depends on numerous variables:
  - Socioenvironmental functional status has been shown to be of great importance in determining the postoperative function status of a patient.[24]
- Longitudinal studies comparing the functional status of patients before and after hip fracture fixation have documented that roughly 40% of patients maintain their preoperative level of ambulation postoperatively.
  - Another 40% of patients have increased dependency on ambulation devices but remain ambulatory.
  - Twelve percent of patients become household-only ambulators, and 8% of patients become nonambulators postoperatively.[17]

COMPLICATIONS

- Loss of proximal fixation is defined as varus collapse and rotation of the proximal fracture fragment with migration and/or cutout of the lag screw from the femoral head **(FIG 8)**. This complication is seen in 4% to 20% of fractures, usually within 4 months of surgery.
  - Although certain fracture patterns have been shown to have a higher rate of proximal fixation loss, the fracture pattern cannot be controlled by the physician.
  - The placement of the lag screw, on the other hand, can be controlled by the physician. A central and deep position with a TAP of less than 25 mm has been shown to significantly reduce the incidence of proximal fixation loss.[3]
  - Lag screw–barrel length mismatch can create lag screw jamming, impingement, or early loss of fixation **(FIG 9)**.
  - Nonunion occurs in 1% to 2% of fractures. The low incidence is likely due to the well-vascularized nature of the cancellous peritrochanteric region of the hip through which these fractures develop. Inadequate PFLP application and/or fracture site distraction/malalignment can leap to early catastrophic failure.[8,16]
- Secondary fracture displacement (malunion)
  - With SHS, despite adequate fracture reduction and implant positioning, fractures may progress to excessive impaction, with resultant limb shortening and relative abductor shortening (abductor weakness) **(FIG 10)**. This can lead to suboptimal patient functional results. This is often seen in cases of unrecognized lateral wall fractures (either iatrogenically induced by implant placement or unrecognized from the original trauma).
  - Use of a TSP or intramedullary fixation devices and vigilant follow-up may help avoid this complication **(FIG 11)**.
- Wound dehiscence and/or infection
  - This may be lessened with removal of all nonviable tissue at time of closure.
  - Deep drains and/or VAC may lessen hematoma and/or fat necrosis drainage.
  - If drainage noted, early wound débridement, cultures, and wound management is paramount.
  - If culture positive, worse outcomes can be predicted.[10]

A

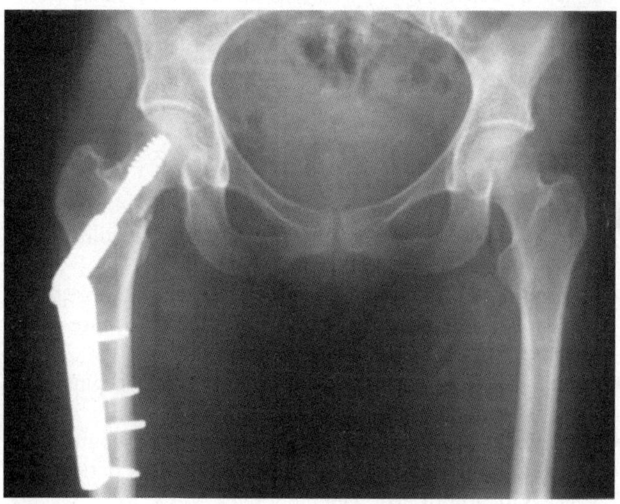

B

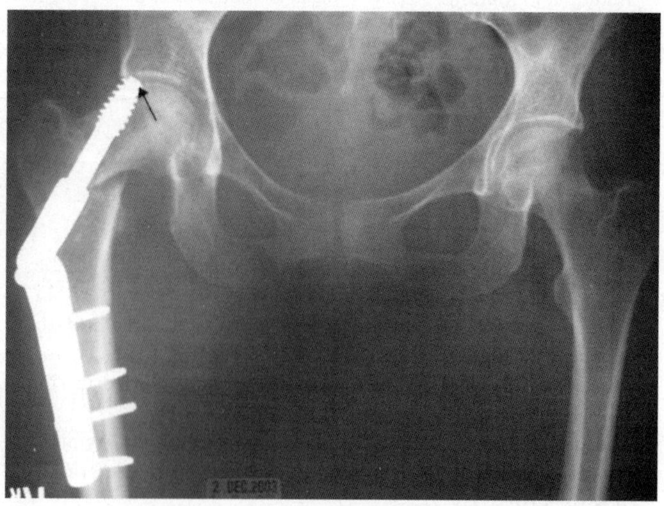

FIG 8 A simple OTA A1 pertrochanteric hip fracture is treated with an SHS with a large TAD (**A**) resulting in early failure, screw migration (*black line*), and "cut out" of the screw from the head (**B**) requiring revision surgery.

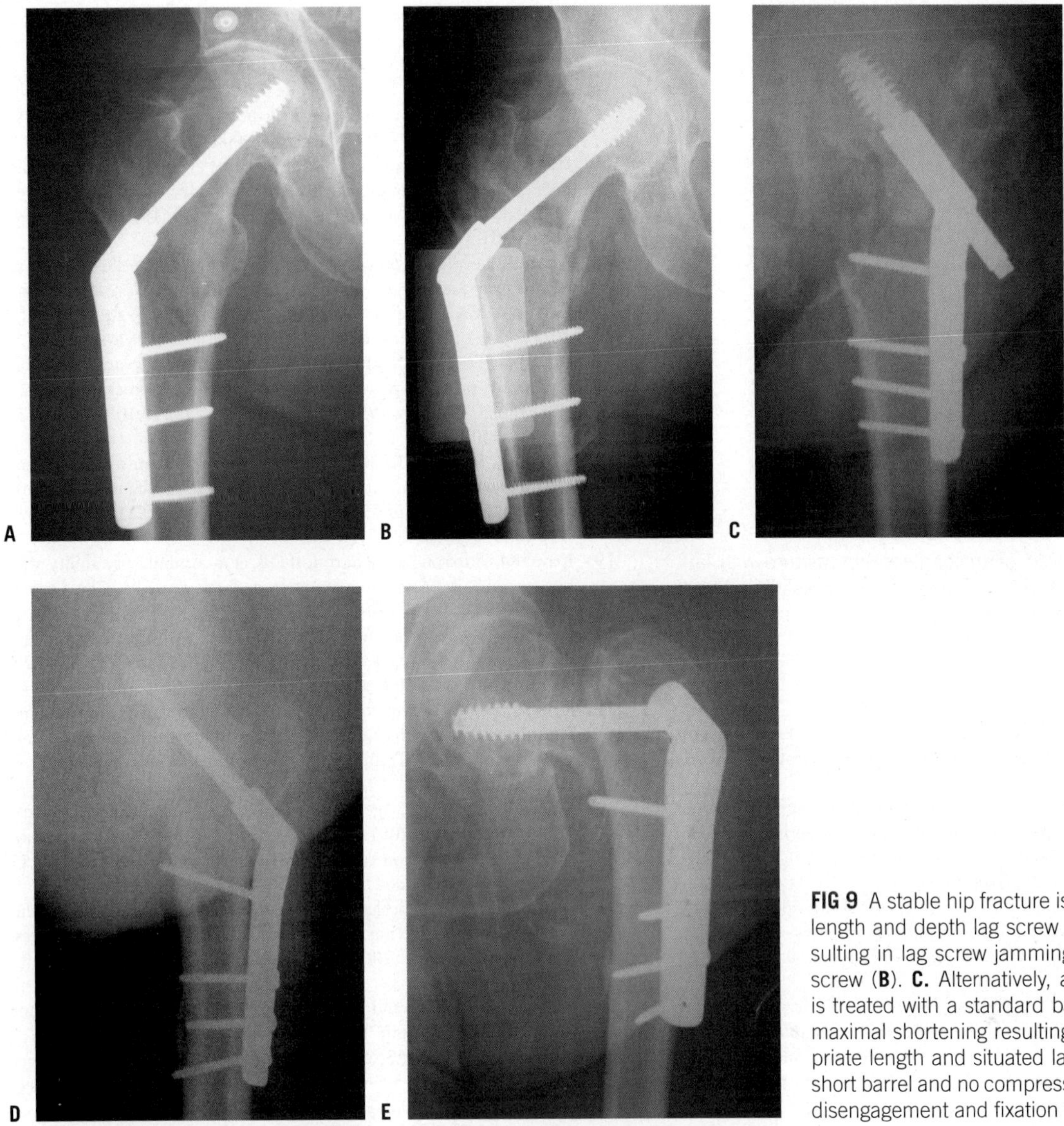

FIG 9 A stable hip fracture is treated with appropriate length and depth lag screw but a short barrel (**A**) resulting in lag screw jamming and bending of the lag screw (**B**). **C.** Alternatively, an appropriate lag screw is treated with a standard barrel, which impinges on maximal shortening resulting in nonunion. An appropriate length and situated lag screw is treated with a short barrel and no compression screw (**D**) resulting in disengagement and fixation failure (**E**).

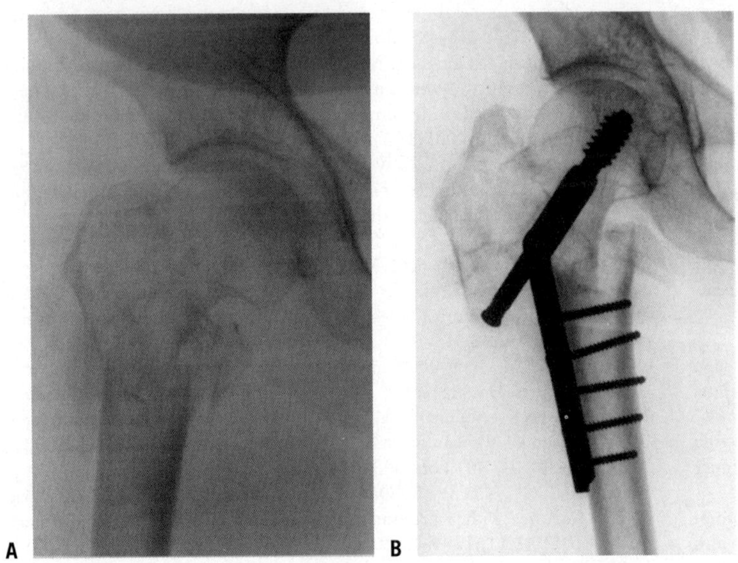

FIG 10 Injury image (**A**) demonstrating a minimally displaced pertrochanteric hip fracture with an intertrochanteric (OTA A1) and distal transverse component (OTA A2) unsuccessfully treated with an SHS (**B**) demonstrating excessive shortening and translation.

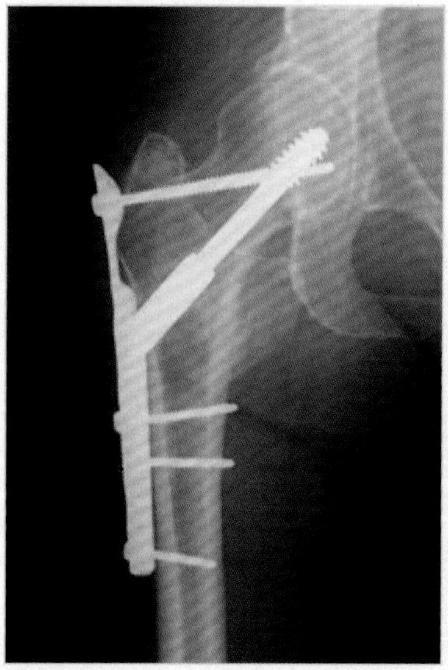

FIG 11 Postoperative healed pertrochanteric hip fracture with lateral wall extension treated with SHS and TSP successfully without excessive shortening or translation.

REFERENCES

1. Archdeacon MT, Cannada LK, Herscovici D Jr, et al. Prevention of complications after treatment of proximal femoral fractures. Instr Course Lect 2009;58:13–19.
2. Baumgaertner MR, Curtin SL, Lindskog DM, et al. The value of the tip-apex distance in predicting failure of fixation of peritrochanteric fractures of the hip. J Bone Joint Surg Am 1995;77(7):1058–1064. doi:10.2106/00004623-199507000-00012.
3. Baumgaertner MR, Solberg BD. Awareness of tip-apex distance reduces failure of fixation of trochanteric fractures of the hip. J Bone Joint Surg Br 1997;79(6):969–971. doi:10.1302/0301-620x.79b6.7949.
4. Berkes MB, Schottel PC, Weldon M, et al. Ninety-five degree angled blade plate fixation of high-energy unstable proximal femur fractures results in high rates of union and minimal complications. J Orthop Trauma 2019;33(7):335–340. doi:10.1097/BOT.0000000000001505.
5. Bhandari M, Schemitsch E, Jönsson A, et al. Gamma nails revisited: gamma nails versus compression hip screws in the management of intertrochanteric fractures of the hip: a meta-analysis. J Orthop Trauma 2009;23(6):460–464. doi:10.1097/BOT.0b013e318162f67f.
6. Bolhofner BR, Russo PR, Carmen B. Results of intertrochanteric femur fractures treated with a 135-degree sliding screw with a two-hole side plate. J Orthop Trauma 1999;13(1):5–8. doi:10.1097/00005131-199901000-00002.
7. Brauer CA, Coca-Perraillon M, Cutler DM, et al. Incidence and mortality of hip fractures in the United States. JAMA 2009;302(14):1573–1579. doi:10.1001/jama.2009.1462.
8. Collinge CA, Hymes R, Archdeacon M, et al. Unstable proximal femur fractures treated with proximal femoral locking plates: a retrospective, multicenter study of 111 cases. J Orthop Trauma 2016;30(9):489–495. doi:10.1097/BOT.0000000000000602.
9. Connelly CL, Archdeacon MT. The lateral decubitus approach for complex proximal femur fractures: anatomic reduction and locking plate neutralization: a technical trick. J Orthop Trauma 2012;26(4):252–257. doi:10.1097/BOT.0b013e31821e0b2d.
10. Duckworth AD, Phillips SA, Stone O, et al. Deep infection after hip fracture surgery: predictors of early mortality. Injury 2012;43(7):1182–1186. doi:10.1016/j.injury.2012.03.029.
11. Gómez Alonso C, Díaz Curiel M, Hawkins Carranza F, et al. Femoral bone mineral density, neck–shaft angle and mean femoral neck width as predictors of hip fracture in men and women. Osteoporos Int 2000;11(8):714–720.
12. Griffin JB. The calcar femorale redefined. Clin Orthop Relat Res 1982;(164):211–214.
13. Haidukewych GJ, Israel TA, Berry DJ. Reverse obliquity fractures of the intertrochanteric region of the femur. J Bone Joint Surg Am 2001;83(5):643–650. doi:10.2106/00004623-200105000-00001.
14. Hartline BE, Achor TS. Use of the 95-degree angled blade plate to treat a proximal femur fracture. J Orthop Trauma 2018;32(suppl 1):S26–S27. doi:10.1097/BOT.0000000000001201.
15. Hasenboehler EA, Agudelo JF, Morgan SJ, et al. Treatment of complex proximal femoral fractures with the proximal femur locking compression plate. Orthopedics 2007;30(8):618–623. doi:10.3928/01477447-20070801-18.
16. Hodel S, Beeres FJP, Babst R, et al. Complications following proximal femoral locking compression plating in unstable proximal femur fractures: medium-term follow-up. Eur J Orthop Surg Traumatol 2017;27(8):1117–1124. doi:10.1007/s00590-017-1981-1.
17. Koval KJ, Friend KD, Aharonoff GB, et al. Weight bearing after hip fracture: a prospective series of 596 geriatric hip fracture patients. J Orthop Trauma 1996;10(8):526–530. doi:10.1097/00005131-199611000-00003.
18. Koval KJ, Sala DA, Kummer FJ, et al. Postoperative weight-bearing after a fracture of the femoral neck or an intertrochanteric fracture. J Bone Joint Surg Am 1998;80(3):352–356. doi:10.2106/00004623-199803000-00007.
19. Koval KJ, Skovron ML, Aharonoff GB, et al. Ambulatory ability after hip fracture. A prospective study in geriatric patients. Clin Orthop Relat Res 1995(310):150–159.
20. Kregor PJ, Obremskey WT, Kreder HJ, et al. Unstable pertrochanteric femoral fractures. J Orthop Trauma 2014;28(suppl 8):S25–S28. doi:10.1097/BOT.0000000000000187.
21. Kyle RF, Ellis TJ, Templeman DC. Surgical treatment of intertrochanteric hip fractures with associated femoral neck fractures using a sliding hip screw. J Orthop Trauma 2005;19(1):1–4. doi:10.1097/00005131-200501000-00001.
22. Marsh JL, Slongo TF, Agel J, et al. Fracture and dislocation classification compendium—2007: Orthopaedic Trauma Association classification, database and outcomes committee. J Orthop Trauma 2007;21(10 suppl):S1–S133. doi:10.1097/00005131-200711101-00001.
23. McLoughlin SW, Wheeler DL, Rider J, et al. Biomechanical evaluation of the dynamic hip screw with two- and four-hole side plates. J Orthop Trauma 2000;14(5):318–323. doi:10.1097/00005131-200006000-00002.
24. Miller CW. Survival and ambulation following hip fracture. J Bone Joint Surg Am 1978;60(7):930–934.
25. Mitchell SM, Chung AS, Walker JB, et al. Delay in hip fracture surgery prolongs postoperative hospital length of stay but does not adversely affect outcomes at 30 days. J Orthop Trauma 2018;32(12):629–633. doi:10.1097/BOT.0000000000001306.
26. Moran CG, Wenn RT, Sikand M, et al. Early mortality after hip fracture: is delay before surgery important? J Bone Joint Surg Am 2005;87(3):483–489. doi:10.2106/JBJS.D.01796.
27. Pajarinen J, Lindahl J, Michelsson O, et al. Pertrochanteric femoral fractures treated with a dynamic hip screw or a proximal femoral nail. A randomised study comparing post-operative rehabilitation. J Bone Joint Surg Br 2005;87(1):76–81.
28. Rao JP, Banzon MT, Weiss AB, et al. Treatment of unstable intertrochanteric fractures with anatomic reduction and compression hip screw fixation. Clin Orthop Relat Res 1983(175):65–71.
29. Ruby L, Mital MA, O'Connor J, et al. Anteversion of the femoral neck. J Bone Joint Surg Am 1979;61(1):46–51.
30. Saini P, Kumar R, Shekhawat V, et al. Biological fixation of comminuted subtrochanteric fractures with proximal femur locking compression plate. Injury 2013;44(2):226–231. doi:10.1016/j.injury.2012.10.037.
31. Utrilla AL, Reig JS, Muñoz FM, et al. Trochanteric gamma nail and compression hip screw for trochanteric fractures: a randomized, prospective, comparative study in 210 elderly patients with a new design of the gamma nail. J Orthop Trauma 2005;19(4):229–233. doi:10.1097/01.bot.0000151819.95075.ad.
32. Zha GC, Chen ZL, Qi XB, et al. Treatment of pertrochanteric fractures with a proximal femur locking compression plate. Injury 2011;42(11):1294–1299. doi:10.1016/j.injury.2011.01.030.
33. Zuckerman JD, Skovron ML, Koval KJ, et al. Postoperative complications and mortality associated with operative delay in older patients who have a fracture of the hip. J Bone Joint Surg Am 1995;77(10):1551–1556. doi:10.2106/00004623-199510000-00010.

CHAPTER 38

Fixation of Periprosthetic Fractures above/below Total Hip Arthroplasty

Aaron Nauth, Amir Khoshbin, and Emil H. Schemitsch

DEFINITION

- Periprosthetic fractures about a total hip arthroplasty are fractures, which occur in the femur or acetabulum adjacent to either the femoral or acetabular component, respectively. These fractures can occur intraoperatively or postoperatively. The focus of this chapter is postoperative fractures of the femur, which occur adjacent to a well-fixed femoral component of a total hip arthroplasty.

ANATOMY

- Fractures of the femur adjacent to the femoral component of a total hip arthroplasty are most commonly described using the Vancouver classification system, which categorizes the fracture on the basis of anatomic location, stability of the femoral component, and surrounding bone stock (**TABLE 1**; **FIG 1**).[8] This classification system is simple, reliable, and serves to guide treatment.
- Vancouver type A fractures occur in the trochanteric region and involve either the greater trochanter (A_G) or the lesser trochanter (A_L).
- Vancouver type B fractures occur around or just distal to the stem of the femoral component and are subclassified based on the stability of the implant and the surrounding bone stock. Vancouver type B1 fractures occur around a stable implant. Vancouver type B2 fractures occur around a loose implant with adequate bone stock. Vancouver type B3 fractures occur around a loose implant with poor bone stock.
- Vancouver type C fractures occur well distal to a stable femoral component.

TABLE 1 Vancouver Classification of Periprosthetic Fractures of the Femur about a Total Hip Arthroplasty

Type	Fracture Description
A	Fracture around the trochanters
A_G	Greater trochanter
A_L	Lesser trochanter
B	Fracture about the stem or just distal to the stem
B1	Stable implant
B2	Loose implant with good bone stock
B3	Loose implant with poor bone stock
C	Fracture well below the implant

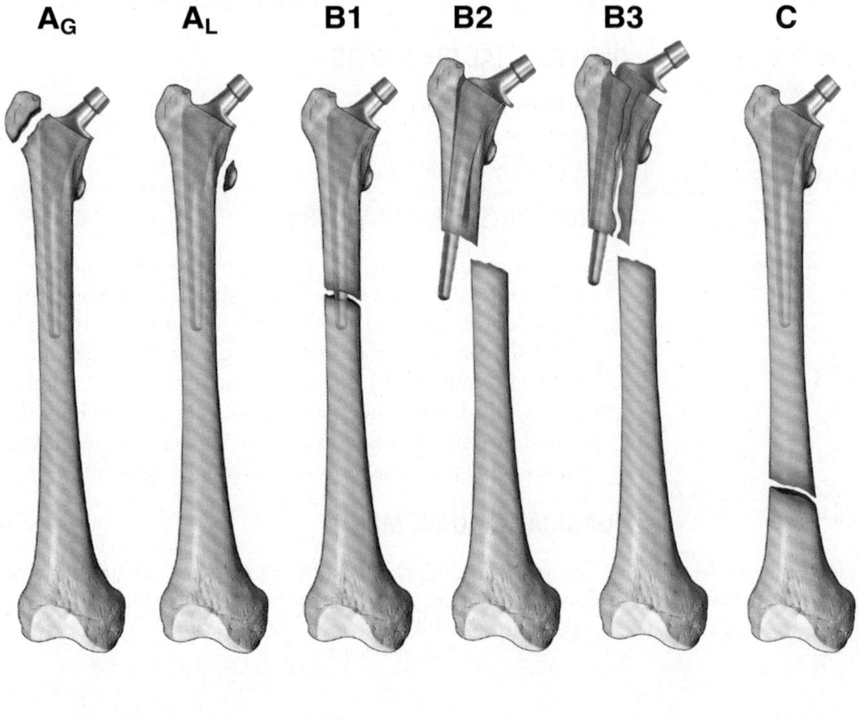

FIG 1 The Vancouver classification of periprosthetic fractures of the femur about a total hip arthroplasty.

PATHOGENESIS

- Postoperative periprosthetic fractures can occur in a variety of settings; however, major trauma accounts for a very small proportion.
- The majority of these fractures occur with a low-energy fall, and up to 25% occur without any significant trauma.
- A large proportion of these patients have pathologic and osteopenic bone due to a combination of factors including localized osteopenia of the proximal femur due to stress shielding and osteolysis (this is a particular problem with conventional polyethylene liners in long-term follow-up) as well as a high prevalence of osteoporosis in this patient population.

NATURAL HISTORY

- The vast majority of these fractures require surgical management for effective fracture healing and return of function.
- Retrospective literature has demonstrated a 1-year mortality of 11% and morbidity/mortality very similar to hip fracture patients.[1] This is an important consideration as these patients should be managed in a similar fashion to hip fracture patients by incorporating a multidisciplinary team approach (geriatrics assessment, delirium prevention, etc.), carrying out early appropriately timed surgical intervention (<48 hours from injury), and using a surgical strategy that allows early weight bearing and mobilization.

PATIENT HISTORY AND PHYSICAL FINDINGS

- It is important to obtain information regarding the mechanism of injury and level of energy imparted as well as the cause of the fall.
- A syncopal workup is often needed, although commonly, this is to be deferred until after surgery.
- Information regarding prodromal symptoms such as thigh pain with weight-bearing or start-up pain should be obtained and may indicate a preexisting loose femoral stem prior to fracture.
- A history of past infections, wound healing complications, or constitutional symptoms may indicate a periprosthetic infection.
- A social history including the patient's prior ambulatory status, use of walking aids, level of independence, and overall functionality is helpful for setting reasonable treatment goals.
- Physical examination may indicate gross deformity of the limb in a displaced fracture or the findings may be more subtle in minimally displaced fractures such as pain with range of motion or rotation of the hip, difficulty weight bearing, or weakness of the limb. Physical examination should also focus on ruling out open wounds, neurovascular injury, and associated injuries.

IMAGING AND OTHER DIAGNOSTIC STUDIES

- Investigation begins with anteroposterior (AP) and lateral radiographs of the affected femur and an AP pelvis. Radiographs should be carefully inspected for the location of fracture lines, fragment displacement, implant loosening, and quality of bone stock.
- It is *critical* to identify any evidence of implant loosening as the surgical management of a periprosthetic fracture with a loose femoral component (Vancouver type B2) typically requires revision to a long-stem component in addition to fracture fixation, whereas a fracture with a stable component (Vancouver type B1) can be readily treated with fracture fixation alone. Lindahl et al[7] reported that the most common reason for treatment failure in the fixation of Vancouver type B1 fractures was loosening of the implant, presumably due to failure to recognize that the implant was loose at the time of fracture.
- Definite signs of radiographic loosening include progressive periprosthetic or cement mantle lucency, change in position of the stem, and component or cement mantle fracture (**FIG 2**). Radiographic signs of probable loosening include greater than 2 mm of periprosthetic or cement mantle lucency, bead shedding, endosteal scalloping, and endosteal bone bridging at the tip of the stem.
- Whenever possible, preinjury radiographs should be obtained to assess for change in component position, as this is the best indication of a loose stem. Careful comparison of implant position on injury and preinjury radiographs is required, as the findings of implant subsidence can range from noticeable to relatively subtle (**FIGS 3** and **4**).
- Efforts should be made to obtain original operative reports in case revision of the implant is required.
- Infection is an important concern in the setting of a periprosthetic fracture and does require specific consideration. Careful attention should be paid to the presence of prodromal symptoms on history. Inflammatory markers such as white cell count, erythrocyte sedimentation rate (ESR), and C-reactive protein (CRP) are often elevated in the setting of trauma and, therefore, can be difficult to interpret in the setting of a fracture, unless they are significantly elevated. Despite this, these tests are routinely performed by the authors. If concern for infection exists on the basis of preinjury symptoms, a preoperative hip aspiration can be performed, or the surgeon should be prepared to proceed with a two-stage revision should obvious infection be encountered at the time of surgery (see **FIG 2**). Intraoperative cultures (multiple specimens from multiple sites) should be obtained if either the preoperative workup or intraoperative findings are suggestive of infection. The authors do not routinely use frozen sections intraoperatively.

DIFFERENTIAL DIAGNOSIS

- Periprosthetic infection
- Aseptic loosening
- Pathologic fracture

NONOPERATIVE MANAGEMENT

- Operative intervention is indicated for the vast majority of periprosthetic fractures of the femur with the exception of stable fractures of the lesser trochanter without shaft extension, minimally displaced fractures of the greater trochanter, and completely undisplaced fractures around the stem of a stable implant. In addition, minimally displaced fractures about the femoral stem in patients who are poor surgical candidates can be considered for a trial of conservative management.

SURGICAL MANAGEMENT

- The surgical management of periprosthetic femur fractures about a total hip arthroplasty is guided by the Vancouver classification.

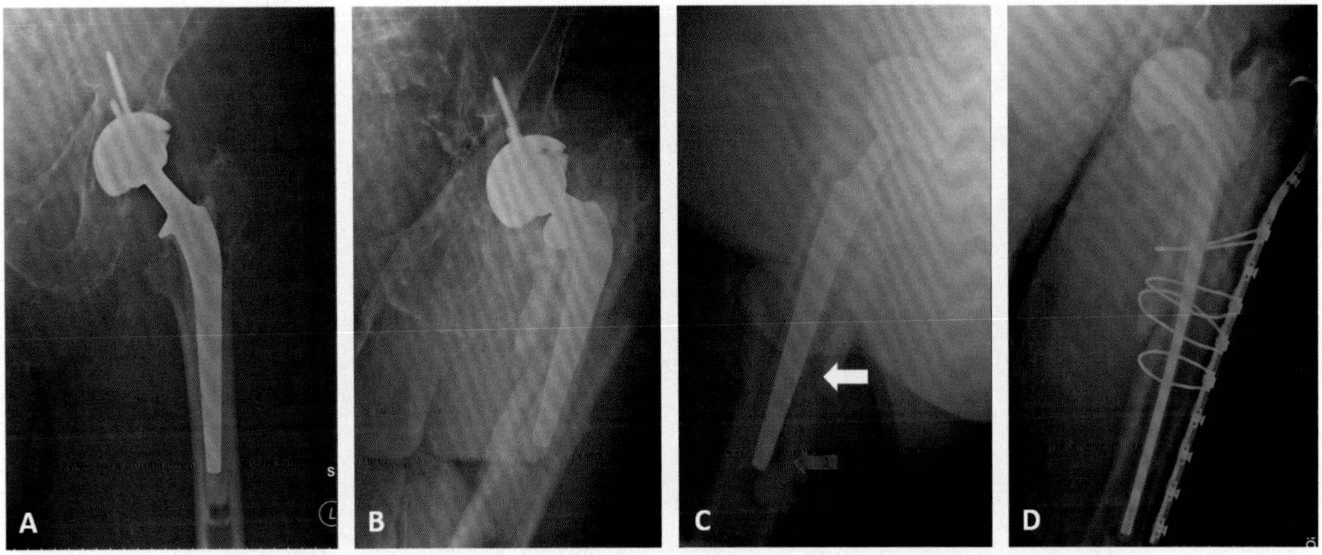

FIG 2 Radiographs of a 91-year-old male patient with a Vancouver type B2 periprosthetic femur fracture 1 year following total hip arthroplasty. Comparison with immediate postoperative radiographs (**A**) shows definite signs of loosening including progressive radiolucency of the cement–bone interface, subsidence of the implant, fracture of the cement mantle (*white arrow*), and debonding of the cement mantle around the implant (*red arrow*) (**B,C**). The patient reported a 3-month history of prodromal thigh pain and his ESR and CRP were elevated significantly. The total hip arthroplasty was presumed to be infected, and revision to an antibiotic cement spacer combined with fixation of the fracture was performed (**D**) after infection was confirmed intraoperatively. (Reproduced with permission from Nauth A, Henry P, Schemitsch EH. Periprosthetic fractures of the femur after total hip arthroplasty: cable plate and allograft strut fixation of Vancouver B1 fractures. In: Sarwark JF, ed. Knowledge Online Journal. Rosemont, IL: American Academy of Orthopaedic Surgeons, 2014;12[1].)

- Vancouver type A_L fractures of the lesser trochanter are generally managed nonsurgically as are minimally displaced Vancouver type A_G fractures of the greater trochanter. Displaced Vancouver type A_G fractures are generally managed with open reduction and internal fixation (ORIF) +/− bone grafting and polyethylene liner exchange if they are associated with osteolysis and liner wear.
- Vancouver type B1 fractures have a stable implant and are managed with fracture fixation. The focus of this techniques chapter is on the fixation of these fracture types and techniques for Vancouver type B1 fracture fixation are described in the following text in detail. There is relative controversy in the literature regarding the optimal technique for fixation of Vancouver type B1 fractures, with the main controversy centered around the use of cable plating combined with allograft strut versus isolated lateral locked plating. The biomechanical literature suggests that the use of a lateral cable plate and screws combined with the use of an anterior allograft

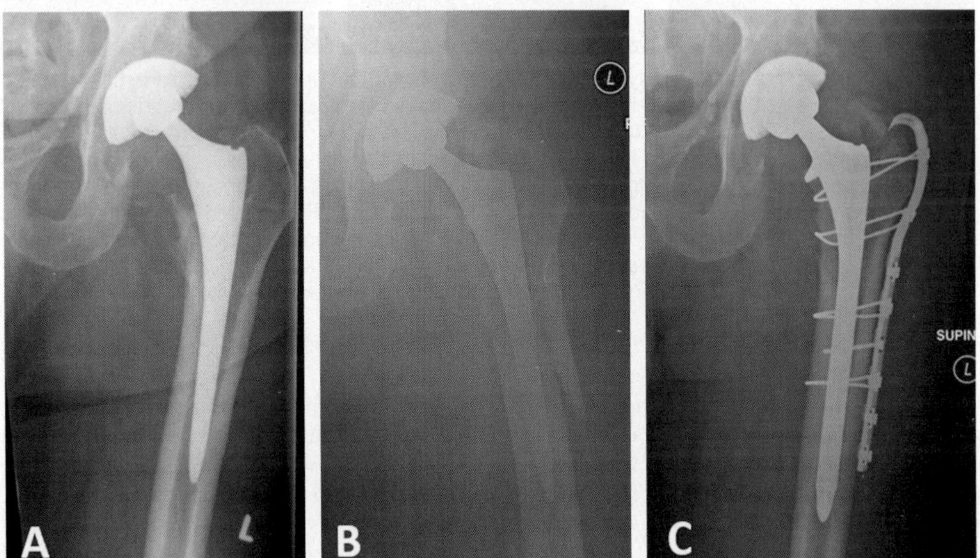

FIG 3 Vancouver type B2 periprosthetic fracture in a 75-year-old male. Comparison with preinjury radiographs (**A**) shows noticeable subsidence and change of prosthesis position confirming loosening (**B**). **C.** Revision to a long-stemmed prosthesis combined with fracture fixation was performed.

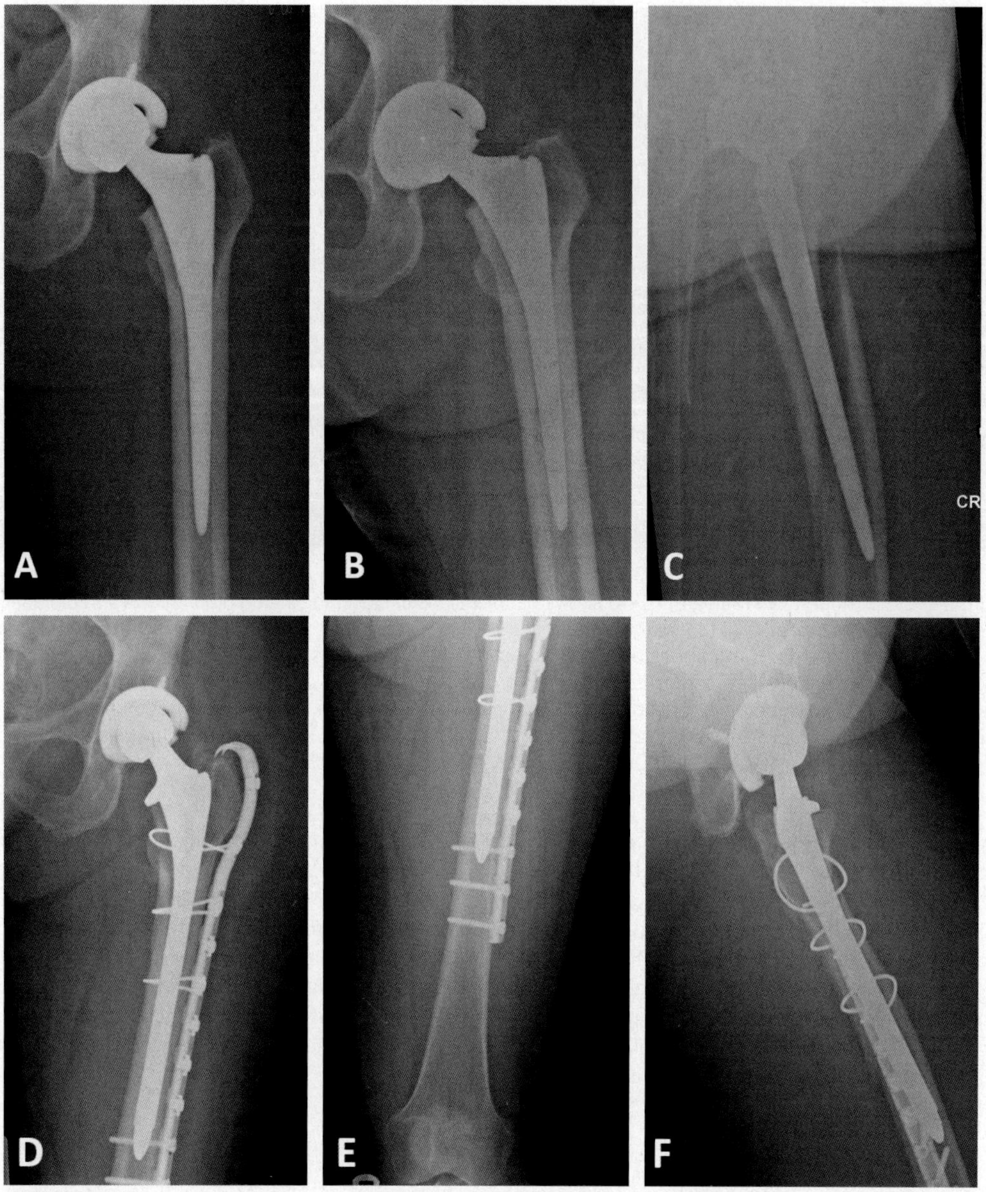

FIG 4 Radiographs of a Vancouver type B2 periprosthetic femur fracture in 52-year-old female who suffered a fall at 3 weeks postoperatively. Comparison with immediate postoperative radiographs (**A**) shows subtle subsidence of the implant (**B,C**). The patient was brought to the operating room with plans for fixation of her fracture and revision to a long-stemmed implant. Implant loosening was confirmed at the time of the operation. **D–F.** Six-month postoperative radiographs in the same patient showing revision to a long-stemmed implant with cable plate and screw fixation of the fracture. (Reproduced with permission from Nauth A, Henry P, Schemitsch EH. Periprosthetic fractures of the femur after total hip arthroplasty: cable plate and allograft strut fixation of Vancouver B1 fractures. In: Sarwark JF, ed. Orthopaedic Knowledge Online Journal. Rosemont, IL: American Academy of Orthopaedic Surgeons, 2014;12[1].)

strut (90–90 fixation) is the optimal biomechanical construct.[14] Buttaro et al[2] retrospectively reviewed a 14 patient series of Vancouver type B1 fractures treated with lateral locked plating +/− the use of a cortical strut. The authors reported a high rate of failure when isolated lateral locked plating was used (five of nine constructs) versus when lateral plating was combined with the use of a cortical strut (one of five constructs). In contrast, other authors have reported a very high rate of success when isolated lateral plating is combined with indirect reduction and biologically friendly techniques.[10] High-level prospective evidence comparing the two techniques is lacking. Irrespective of the fixation strategy used, several biomechanical and surgical principles must be adhered to when treating these fractures.

- First, it is critical that the fracture is NOT fixed with the stem in varus, as increased rates of fixation failure have been reported with varus positioning of the stem.
- Second, proximal fixation around the stem is best achieved with a combination of wires/cables and screws, and it is critical that sufficient overlap of the femoral prosthesis is obtained to avoid mechanical failure **(FIG 5)**. This generally requires fixation to the level of the greater trochanter.

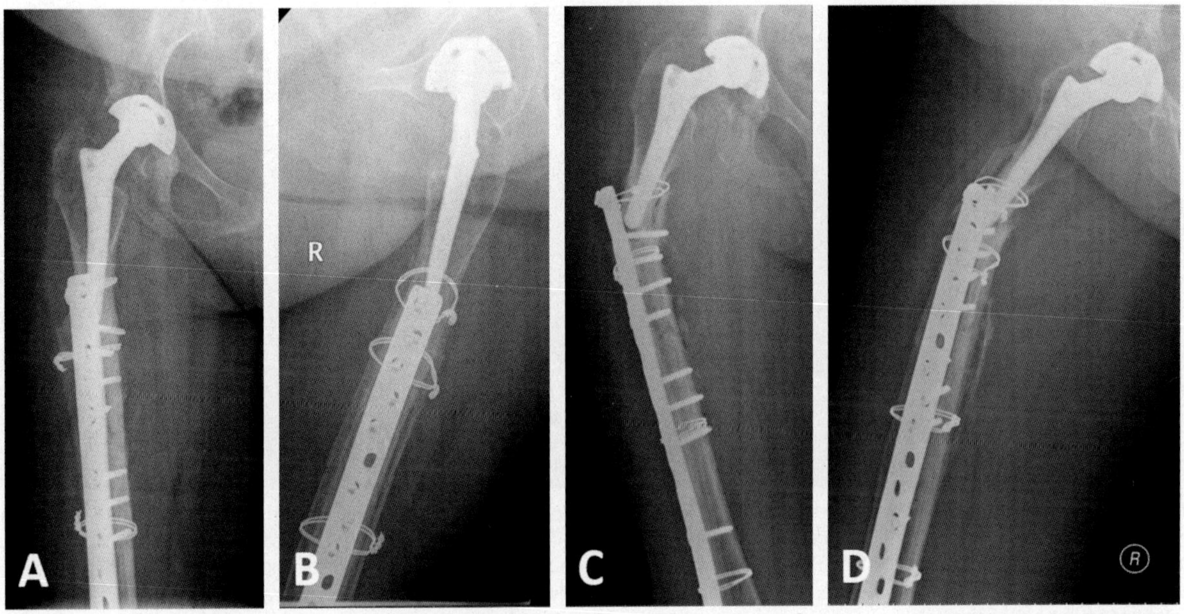

FIG 5 A,B. Radiographs of a 41-year-old female patient with a Vancouver type B1 periprosthetic fracture that was fixed with lateral locked plating and fibular strut allograft. **C,D.** Radiographs show that insufficient overlap of the femoral component was obtained with the plate and predictable failure occurred. (Reproduced with permission from Nauth A, Henry P, Schemitsch EH. Periprosthetic fractures of the femur after total hip arthroplasty: cable plate and allograft strut fixation of Vancouver B1 fractures. In: Sarwark JF, ed. Orthopaedic Knowledge Online Journal. Rosemont, IL: American Academy of Orthopaedic Surgeons, 2014;12[1].)

  - Third, it is important to remember that these fractures commonly occur in pathologic/osteopenic bone, and the use of a plate of sufficient length to stabilize the entire length of the femur is recommended to avoid future peri-implant fracture.
  - Finally, it is important to adhere to the principles of absolute versus relative stability depending on the type of fracture healing desired. In the setting of a simple transverse or spiral fracture, absolute stability and compression at the fracture site should be achieved using compression plating or lag screw fixation. This is in contrast to comminuted fractures, which require relative stability and spaced fixation to allow for fracture healing indirectly by callus formation.
- Vancouver type B2 fractures are treated with revision to a long-stemmed prosthesis and fixation of the fracture (see **FIGS 3** and **4**). The stem should bypass the fracture by at least two cortical diameters.
- Some authors have advocated for isolated ORIF without revision as an effective alternative treatment option for Vancouver type B2 fractures with the advantages of less invasive surgery, reduced surgical times, and decreased blood loss, especially in elderly patients with multiple comorbidities.[5,6,9,11–13] Joestl et al[5] compared a cohort of elderly patients that had an isolated ORIF versus revision total hip arthroplasty for the treatment of a Vancouver type B2 fracture. Fractures treated with ORIF alone all healed without complication and had equivalent follow-up mobility scores to those treated with revision arthroplasty combined with ORIF. Gitajn et al[4] reported no significant differences in revision surgery rates between patients treated with fixation alone (11%) compared with those treated with revision arthroplasty (16%). Similar results have also been replicated in cemented total hip arthroplasties.[11,12] In a recent systematic review of surgical treatment for Vancouver type B2 fractures, a total of 343 B2 fractures were reported in 14 case series.[6] Overall, 12.8% of all Vancouver B2 fractures required revision following initial treatment, with similar rates of revision surgery whether the patient was treated with a revision arthroplasty +/− internal fixation (12.4%) or internal fixation alone (13.3%).[6] ORIF of Vancouver type B2 fractures without stem revision is a viable alternative option in low-demand elderly patients with significant comorbidities **(FIG 6)**.
- Vancouver type B3 fractures require revision, ORIF, and possible structural allograft to restore bone stock.
- Vancouver type C fractures occur well below the stem and can be generally treated with isolated ORIF.

Preoperative Planning

- As indicated previously, multidisciplinary assessment is recommended to manage patient comorbidities and perioperative medical issues.
- At all times when managing periprosthetic fractures of the femur about a total hip arthroplasty, the surgeon should be prepared for the possible need for revision. This requires careful review of the initial operative report to ensure that revision implants of the appropriate type are available for possible revision of the femoral stem. Corten et al[3] reported that 20% of implants judged to be stable based on preoperative radiographs were found to be loose at the time of surgery. If any doubt exists regarding the stability of the femoral component, an arthrotomy of the hip with dislocation and stressing of the implant should be performed to rule out a loose femoral component.

Positioning

- The patient is positioned supine on a radiolucent (Jackson) table with a bump or inflated beanbag under the affected side to elevate the fractured limb **(FIG 7)**. The limb is free-draped, and intraoperative fluoroscopy is placed on the contralateral side to the fracture.

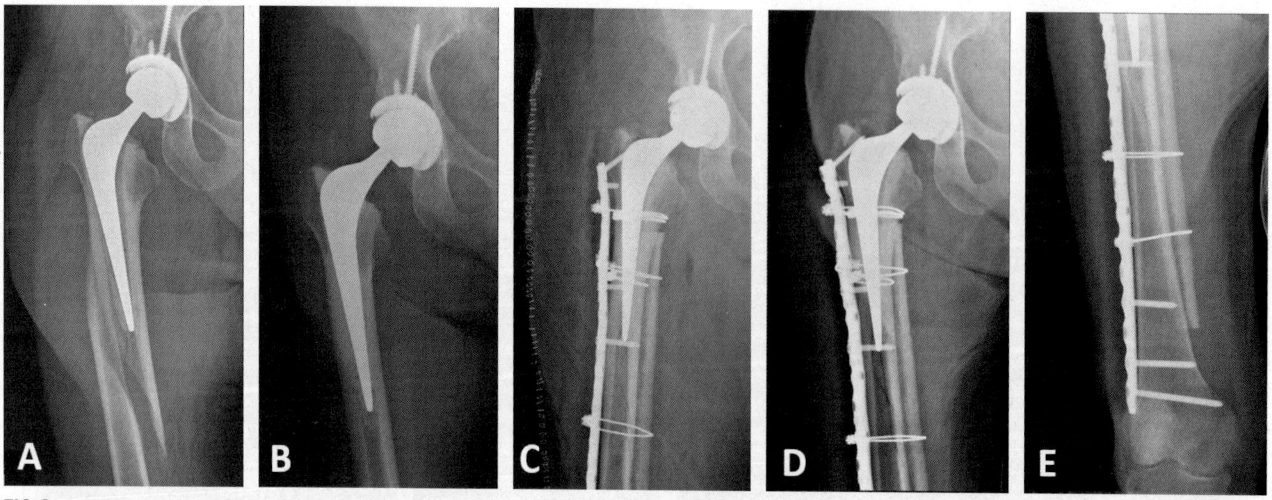

FIG 6 A. Radiograph of 90-year-old female patient with a Vancouver B2 periprosthetic fracture. Comparison with previous radiographs (**B**) shows clear evidence of loosening with fracture of the cement mantle and debonding from the polished, tapered stem. **C.** Immediate postoperative radiograph showing isolated ORIF without implant revision using a lateral locking plate and anteromedial allograft strut. The patient was made weight bearing as tolerated immediately postoperatively. **D,E.** Three-month follow-up radiographs demonstrating healing and stable component position.

- Alternatively, the patient can be positioned in the lateral decubitus position with the affected limb facing up and free-draped. This is the position of choice, if revision of the femoral component is planned or there is concern for a loose prosthesis.

Approach

- The approach involves a lateral incision using the distal aspect of the previous total hip arthroplasty incision extended distally toward the knee.
- If an arthrotomy is required for dislocation of the hip and evaluation of femoral component stability or for femoral component revision, the proximal aspect of the total hip incision can be used as well.
- If a minimally invasive approach and indirect reduction is being employed, then the distal aspect of the total hip incision is used to access the femur proximal to the fracture, and a separate distal incision is made at the lateral aspect of the distal femur for distal plate placement.

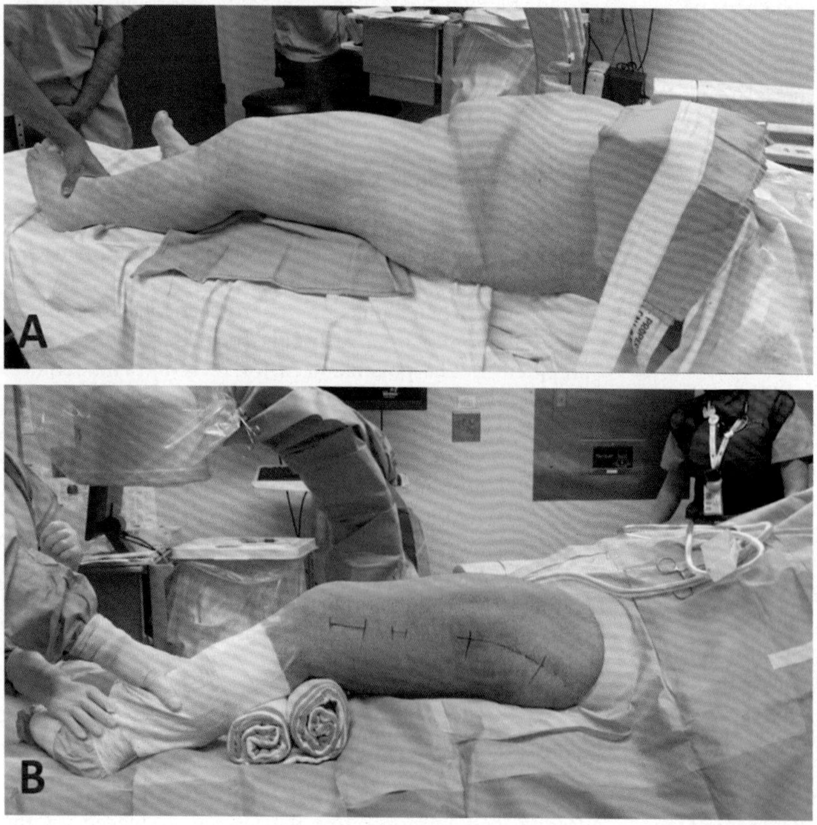

FIG 7 A,B. Intraoperative photographs showing patient positioning in the supine position with a beanbag used to elevate the operative hip and positioning of the C-arm on the patient's contralateral side.

CABLE PLATING AND ALLOGRAFT STRUT FIXATION

- Surgical exposure: A lateral exposure is carried out to expose the entire femur extending from the distal aspect of the previous total hip arthroplasty incision to the level of the distal femur. For deep dissection, the fascia lata is split in line with the skin incision, and the vastus lateralis is elevated anteriorly with dissection carried out along the posterior fibers **(TECH FIG 1C)**. Perforating vessels are identified and coagulated. The entire lateral aspect of the femur, including the fracture, is exposed from the level just below the greater trochanter to the level of the metaphyseal flair. The lateral and anterior aspects of the femur are exposed. The anterior aspect of the femur can be decorticated with a high-speed burr to promote healing between the native femur and allograft. Although the exposure is extensile, care is taken to avoid stripping the soft tissues on the posterior and medial aspects of the femur **(TECH FIG 1D)**.

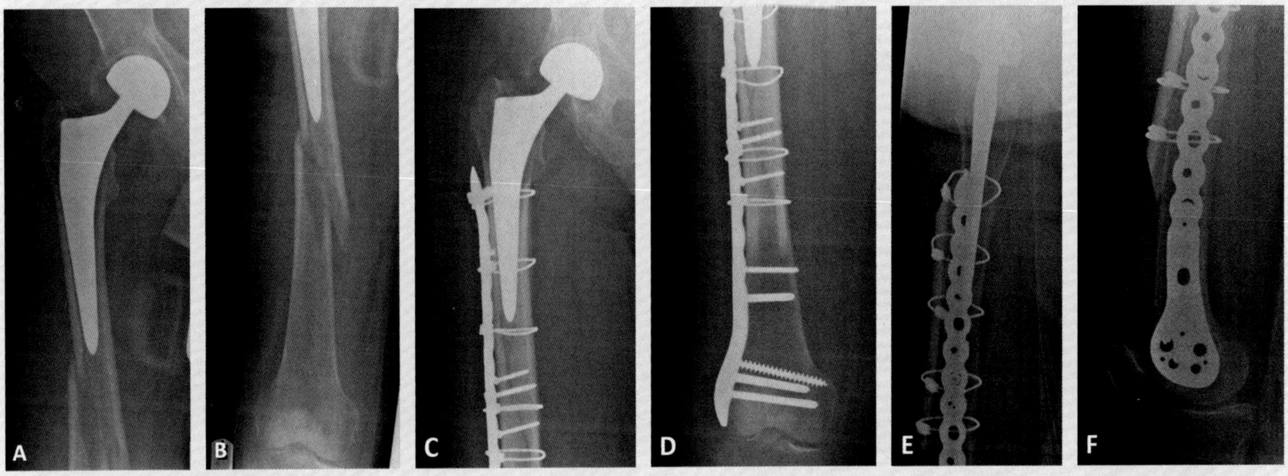

A

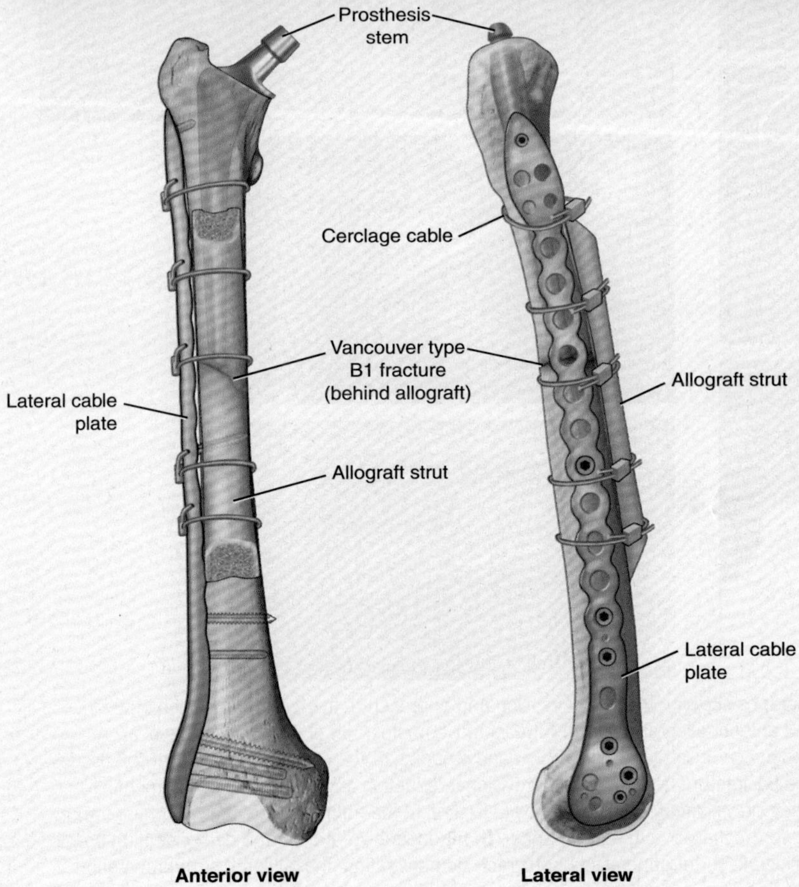

B

TECH FIG 1 **A.** Radiographs of an 82-year-old female patient with a Vancouver type B1 periprosthetic fracture at the tip of a well-fixed stem that had been functioning well prior to a fall (*A,B*). Postoperative radiographs showing fixation of the fracture with a lateral distal femoral locking plate combined with an anterior allograft strut (90–90 fixation) and cables (*C–F*). **B.** Illustration depicting the construct of a lateral cable plate and anterior allograft strut (90–90 fixation) used for fixation of a Vancouver type B1 fracture. *(continued)*

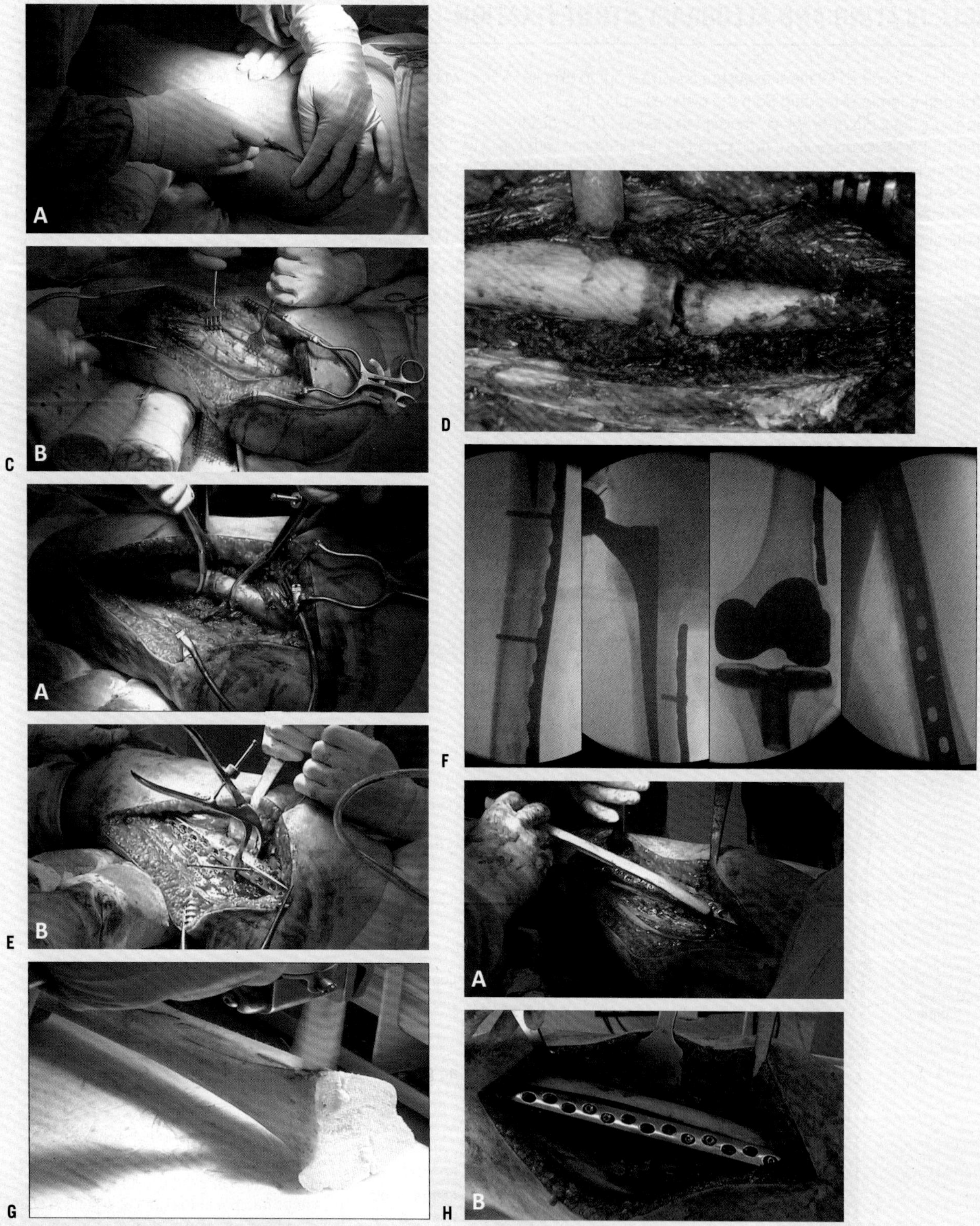

TECH FIG 1 *(continued)* **C.** Intraoperative photographs showing the lateral incision and approach to the femur for fixation of a Vancouver type B1 fracture with a cable plate and anterior allograft strut. **D.** Intraoperative photograph of the fracture site of a Vancouver type B1 fracture demonstrating the avoidance of soft tissue dissection and stripping of the posterior and medial soft tissues. **E.** Intraoperative photographs of a Vancouver type B1 fracture demonstrating provisional reduction and lateral plate placement. **F.** Intraoperative fluoroscopy pictures demonstrating provisional reduction and plate fixation of the fracture. Note that the entire femur is spanned with the plate from just below the greater trochanter to the distal femur. **G.** Intraoperative photograph demonstrating preparation of the allograft strut from a distal femoral allograft. **H.** Intraoperative photograph demonstrating final allograft strut preparation and sizing. *(continued)*

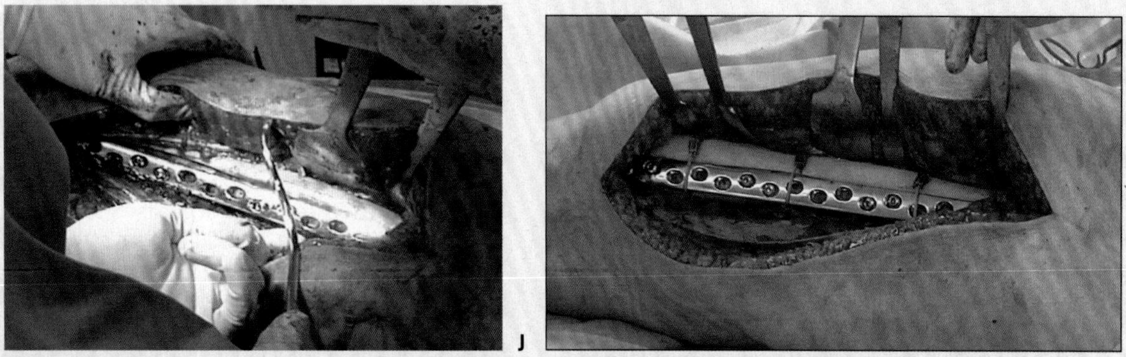

TECH FIG 1 *(continued)* **I.** Intraoperative photograph demonstrating the technique for safe cable passage around the allograft strut and lateral plate. **J.** Intraoperative photograph demonstrating the final allograft strut and cable plate construct. (**C–J:** Reproduced with permission from Nauth A, Henry P, Schemitsch EH. Periprosthetic fractures of the femur after total hip arthroplasty: cable plate and allograft strut fixation of Vancouver B1 fractures. In: Sarwark JF, ed. Orthopaedic Knowledge Online Journal. Rosemont, IL: American Academy of Orthopaedic Surgeons, 2014;12[1].)

- Fracture reduction and plate application: If doubt exists regarding the stability of the implant, the bone implant interface is carefully examined through the fracture site for any evidence of loosening. If loosening is suspected, proximal extension of the incision is carried out with an arthrotomy to evaluate implant stability at the level of the hip. Once implant stability is confirmed, fracture reduction is achieved with the use of reduction clamps **(TECH FIG 1E)**. A plate of appropriate length is chosen to span the entire femur from the distal femur to the level just below the greater trochanter or extending onto the trochanter (it is critical to ensure adequate overlap of the plate with the femoral stem to avoid mechanical failure). Plate contouring is performed as necessary depending on the plate chosen to allow application of the plate to the lateral aspect of the femur. Newer generation precontoured locking plates have a contour to accommodate the anterior bow of the native femur. Provisional screw fixation is obtained through the plate both proximal and distal to the fracture. If the fracture pattern is amenable to absolute stability, then compression at the fracture site is obtained at this stage using the compression holes in the plate, lag screws, or an articulated tensioning device. Fluoroscopy is then used to confirm anatomic reduction and alignment as well as satisfactory positioning of the plate **(TECH FIG 1F)**.
- Allograft preparation: Allograft preparation is begun as soon as the approach to the femur is complete, and both infection and implant loosening have been definitively ruled out. The authors' preference is to use the anterior cortex of a distal femoral allograft as this provides a graft, which accommodates the anterior bow of the femur and also allows for cancellous allograft to be obtained from the distal femur **(TECH FIG 1G)**. Tibial or humeral strut allografts are acceptable alternatives. A strut allograft of appropriate length to allow adequate graft overlap with the femoral prosthesis, and passage of two cables on either side of the fracture is necessary (generally, a minimum length of 25 to 30 cm is required). In addition, it is advisable to avoid ending the allograft at the same level distally as the plate and creating a stress riser. The anterior cortex of the distal femoral allograft is prepared using an oscillating saw and burr. Appropriate sizing and contouring of the graft is confirmed with provisional placement on the anterior cortex of the femur **(TECH FIG 1H)**.
- Cable passage and allograft placement: Prior to definitive allograft placement, cables are passed around the femur using a cable passer, as these are more easily passed prior to graft placement. It is critical that these cables are passed directly on the bone to avoid entrapment of neurovascular structures **(TECH FIG 1I)**. The authors typically use two cables proximal to the fracture and two cables distal to the fracture. The graft is then placed on the anterior aspect of the femur creating a 90–90 construct. The cables are then sequentially tightened, locked, and trimmed **(TECH FIG 1J)**. At this stage, supplemental screw fixation is placed proximal and distal to the fracture. Proximally, this involves placing nonlocked screws or polyaxial locking screws around the well-fixed femoral stem or the use of unicortical locking screws. Intraoperative fluoroscopy is then used to confirm anatomic reduction and alignment of the fracture and satisfactory positioning of the plate, screws, cables, and allograft strut. At this point, the wound is irrigated copiously with normal saline. Cancellous allograft harvested from the distal femoral allograft is then placed at the fracture site and at the graft–host interface. A standard closure is then performed in layers.

MINIMALLY INVASIVE ISOLATED LATERAL LOCKING PLATE FIXATION

- Surgical approach: A lateral exposure of the proximal femur is made using the distal aspect of the total hip arthroplasty incision with extension just proximal to the fracture. Deep dissection is carried out through fascia lata and posterior to vastus lateralis to expose the proximal femur from the level of the greater trochanter to just proximal to the fracture site. Care is taken to preserve the soft tissues and vascular supply at the fracture site. A distal incision of 4 to 5 cm is made at the level of the metaphyseal flare to expose the lateral aspect of the distal femur **(TECH FIG 2C)**. A Cobb elevator is then used to create a submuscular plane along the lateral aspect of the femur.

- Plate placement and indirect reduction: A lateral locking plate of appropriate length to span the entire femur is selected, contoured, and tunneled in the submuscular plane from the proximal incision to the distal incision **(TECH FIG 2D)**. An indirect reduction is performed with traction of the limb and use of the plate as a reduction aid. The plate is reduced to the femur using a nonlocking screw distally and with the use of a cable or reduction clamp proximally **(TECH FIG 2E)**. Fluoroscopy is used to confirm reduction in the coronal and sagittal planes.
- Cable placement and definitive fixation: Once reduction is confirmed fluoroscopically, definitive fixation is carried out with a combination of locking and nonlocking screws distally and the use of cables and locking screws placed around the femoral component proximally. Newer generation periprosthetic locking plates allow for the placement of polyaxial locking screws around the prosthesis, including the placement of screws into the trochanter. Both cables and screws should be used to optimize proximal fixation, with the use of two to four cables combined with two to four screws based on bone quality. Distal fixation is obtained with a combination of locking and nonlocking screws, again based on bone quality. Spaced fixation and a screw density of 50% (ie, half of the distal screw holes should be left empty) should be used to prevent a large concentration of stress over a small length of plate at the fracture site (see **TECH FIG 2A,B**). Final fluoroscopic images (see **TECH FIG 2E**) are obtained, and a standard layered closure is performed.

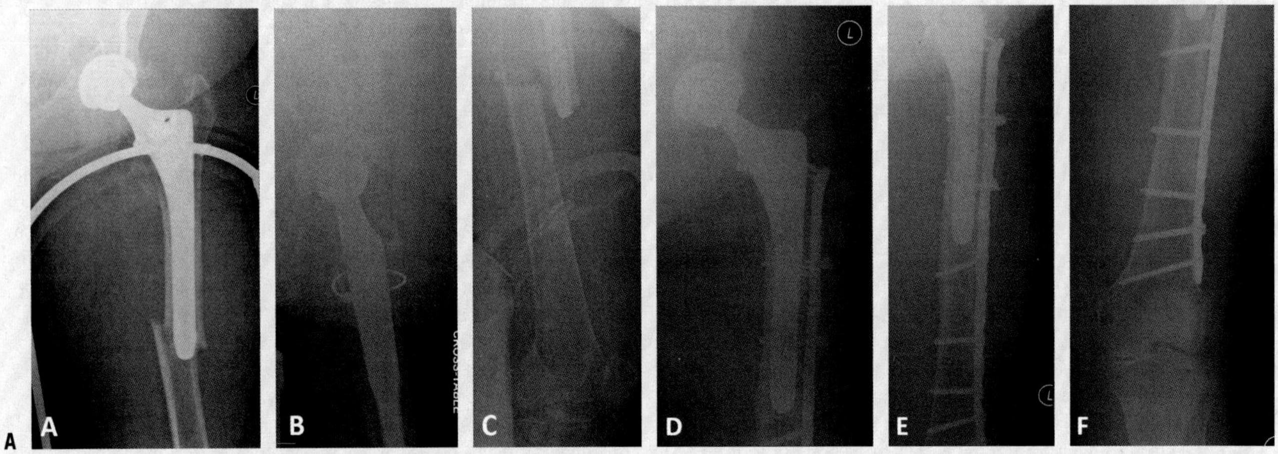

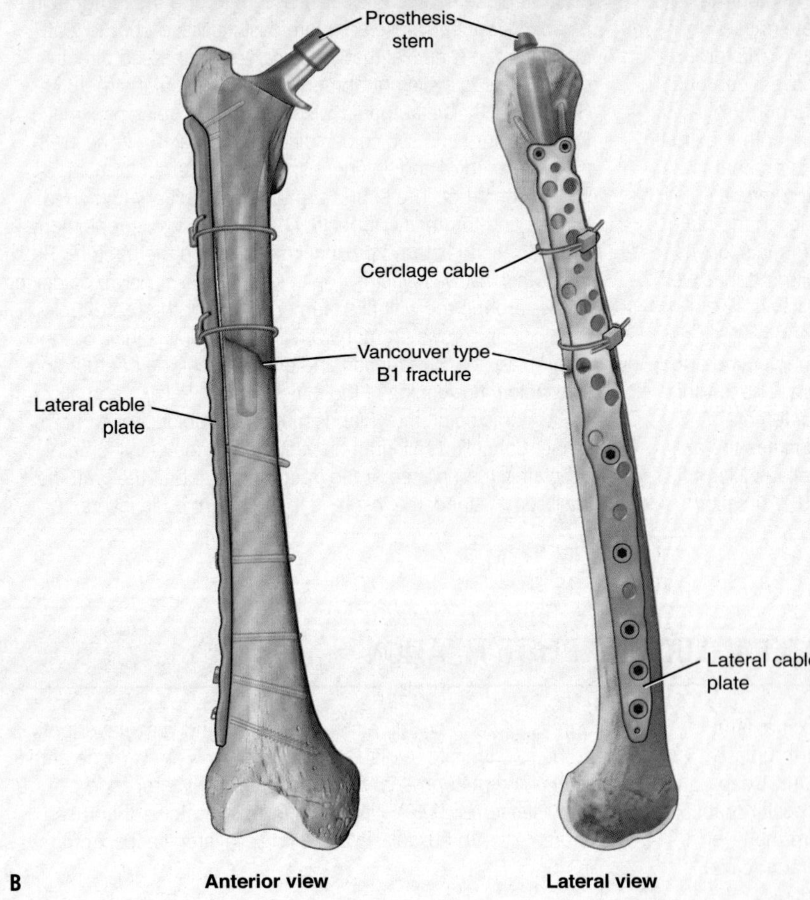

TECH FIG 2 A. Radiographs of a 78-year-old female patient with a Vancouver type B1 periprosthetic fracture at the tip of a well-fixed stem that had been functioning well prior to a fall (*A–C*). Postoperative radiographs showing fixation of the fracture with isolated lateral locked plating using a minimally invasive approach (*D–F*). **B.** Illustration depicting isolated lateral locking plate fixation of a Vancouver type B1 fracture with the use of a combination of screws and cables for proximal fixation. *(continued)*

C

D

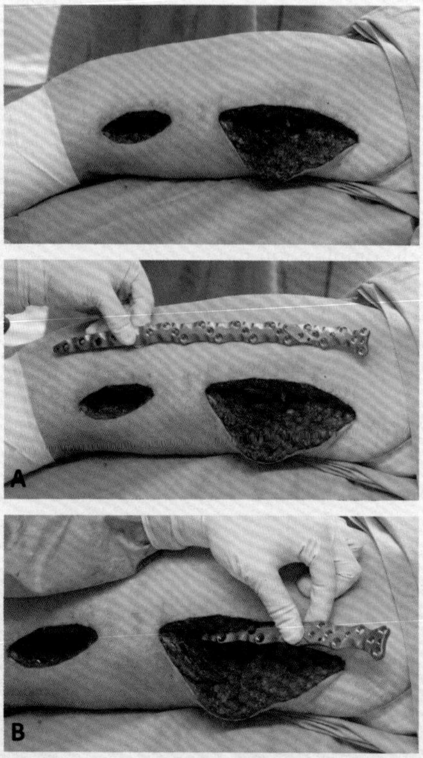

E

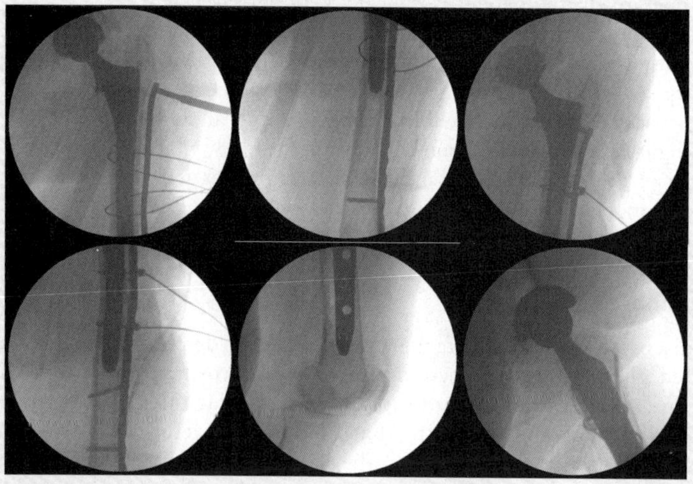

TECH FIG 2 *(continued)* **C.** Intraoperative photograph depicting the incisions for minimally invasive lateral locked plating of a Vancouver type B1 periprosthetic fracture. The skin, soft tissues, and vascular supply are left intact at the level of the fracture to preserve fracture healing biology as best as possible. **D.** Intraoperative photographs demonstrating plate selection and submuscular tunneling of the plate along the lateral aspect of the femur. **E.** Intraoperative and sequential fluoroscopic images demonstrating provisional plate placement and reduction followed by definitive fixation.

TECHNIQUES

Pearls and Pitfalls

Periprosthetic Fracture Patient Management	• These patients should be managed in a similar fashion to hip fracture patients with the following: • Multidisciplinary assessment • Expedited safe surgery (within 48 hours) • Surgical goals of early weight bearing and mobilization
Implant Loosening	• It is critical that loosening of the femoral implant is ruled out prior to proceeding with fracture fixation by careful history and radiograph review (including preinjury films if available). If doubt exists regarding implant loosening, then the stability of the implant should be assessed intraoperatively (either with visualization of the implant–bone interface at the fracture site or with a formal arthrotomy and dislocation of the hip with stressing of the femoral component) and the surgeon should be prepared to proceed with revision to a long-stemmed component if it is determined that the implant is loose.
Fracture Fixation	• There is controversy with regard to the use of isolated locked plating versus cable plating and allograft strut, and either strategy is acceptable. Irrespective of the strategy employed, it is critical that the following fixation principles are adhered to the following: • Avoid varus positioning of the femoral component. • Proximal fixation should be obtained with a combination of both cables and screws. • Sufficient overlap of the femoral component should be obtained with fracture fixation. • The entire length of the femur should be stabilized if possible. • Spaced fixation with a screw density of approximately 50% should be used distally.
Cable Plating and Allograft Strut	• If this strategy is selected, the following tips should be kept in mind: • Allograft strut can be obtained from the femur, tibia, or humerus. • Graft length should be a minimum of 25–30 cm. • Cable fixation around both the plate and allograft should be obtained with two cables, both proximal and distal to the fracture.
Isolated Lateral Locked Plating	• If this strategy is selected, the following tips should be kept in mind: • A biologically friendly surgical approach should be used to minimize disruption of soft tissues and vascular supply at the fracture site. • Proximal fixation should be obtained with a combination of cables and locking screws. • Distal fixation should be obtained with spaced fixation and a screw density of 50%.

POSTOPERATIVE CARE

- Postoperatively, the patient is typically kept partial weight bearing for a period of 6 weeks with range of motion of the knee and hip as tolerated. At 6 weeks, the patient is progressed to weight bearing as tolerated. The authors will allow patients treated with cable plating and strut allograft to weight bear as tolerated immediately after surgery, which is one of the advantages of using this construct as it facilitates more rapid mobilization and rehabilitation of the patient.

OUTCOMES

- As discussed before, Bhattacharyya et al[1] have demonstrated that patients presenting with a periprosthetic fracture about a total hip arthroplasty have similar rates of morbidity and mortality to that of the hip fracture population, with a 1-year mortality rate of approximately 11%.
- One-year mortality has been shown to be increased with delays to surgery of greater than 48 hours, and it is vital that these patients receive surgery as soon as possible.[1]

COMPLICATIONS

- Variable outcomes have been reported in the literature with regard to complication and reoperation rates. Pooled assessment of the literature on outcomes following fixation of Vancouver type B1 fractures (based on a sample size of 333 patients) suggests the following rates:
  - Overall complication rate = 15%
  - Reoperation rate = 9%
  - Nonunion or hardware failure = 9%
  - Malunion = 6%
  - Infection = 5%
- Nonunion or hardware failure is reliably treated with revision ORIF using cable plating, strut allograft, and bone grafting (or use of an osteoinductive bone graft substitute) of the nonunion site **(FIG 8)**.

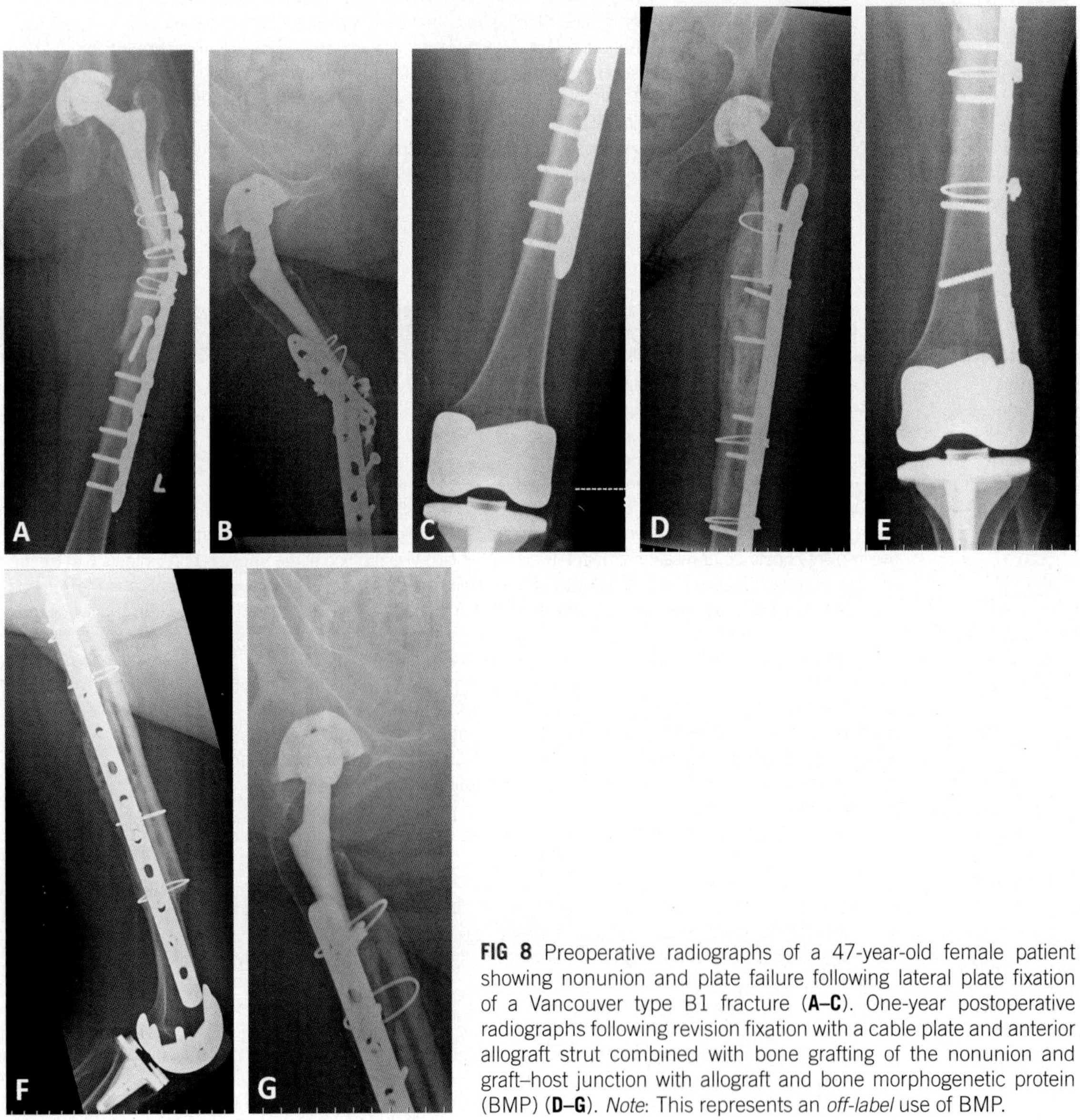

FIG 8 Preoperative radiographs of a 47-year-old female patient showing nonunion and plate failure following lateral plate fixation of a Vancouver type B1 fracture (**A–C**). One-year postoperative radiographs following revision fixation with a cable plate and anterior allograft strut combined with bone grafting of the nonunion and graft–host junction with allograft and bone morphogenetic protein (BMP) (**D–G**). *Note*: This represents an *off-label* use of BMP.

REFERENCES

1. Bhattacharyya T, Chang D, Meigs JB, et al. Mortality after periprosthetic fracture of the femur. J Bone Joint Surg 2007;89(12):2658–2662.
2. Buttaro MA, Farfalli G, Paredes Núñez M, et al. Locking compression plate fixation of Vancouver type-B1 periprosthetic femoral fractures. J Bone Joint Surg Am 2007;89(9):1964–1969.
3. Corten K, Vanrykel F, Bellemans J, et al. An algorithm for the surgical treatment of periprosthetic fractures of the femur around a well-fixed femoral component. J Bone Joint Surg Br 2009;91(11):1424–1430.
4. Gitajn IL, Heng M, Weaver MJ, et al. Mortality following surgical management of Vancouver B periprosthetic fractures. J Orthop Trauma 2017;31(1):9–14. doi:10.1097/BOT.0000000000000711.
5. Joestl J, Hofbauer M, Lang N, et al. Locking compression plate versus revision-prosthesis for Vancouver type B2 periprosthetic femoral fractures after total hip arthroplasty. Injury 2016;47(4):939–943. doi:10.1016/j.injury.2016.01.036.
6. Khan T, Grindlay D, Ollivere BJ, et al. A systematic review of Vancouver B2 and B3 periprosthetic femoral fractures. Bone Joint J 2017;99-B(4 suppl B):17–25. doi:10.1302/0301-620X.994B4.BJJ-2016-1311.R1.
7. Lindahl H, Malchau H, Odén A, et al. Risk factors for failure after treatment of a periprosthetic fracture of the femur. J Bone Joint Surg Br 2006;88(1):26–30.
8. Masri BA, Meek RM, Duncan CP. Periprosthetic fractures evaluation and treatment. Clin Orthop Relat Res 2004;(420):80–95
9. Park JS, Hong S, Nho JH, et al. Radiologic outcomes of open reduction and internal fixation for cementless stems in Vancouver B2 periprosthetic fractures. Acta Orthop Traumatol Turc 2019;53(1):24–29. doi:10.1016/j.aott.2018.10.1003.
10. Ricci WM, Bolhofner BR, Loftus T, et al. Indirect reduction and plate fixation, without grafting, for periprosthetic femoral shaft fractures about a stable intramedullary implant. J Bone Joint Surg Am 2005;87(10):2240–2245.
11. Smitham PJ, Carbone TA, Bolam SM, et al. Vancouver B2 periprosthetic fractures in cemented femoral implants can be treated with open reduction and internal fixation alone without revision. J Arthroplasty 2019;34(7):1430–1434. doi:10.1016/j.arth.2019.03.003.
12. Solomon LB, Hussenbocus SM, Carbone TA, et al. Is internal fixation alone advantageous in selected B2 periprosthetic fractures? ANZ J Surg 2015;85(3):169–173. doi:10.1111/ans.12884.
13. Spina M, Scalvi A. Vancouver B2 periprosthetic femoral fractures; a comparative study of stem revision versus internal fixation with plate. Eur J Orthop Surg Traumatol 2018;28(6):1133–1142. doi:10.1007/s00590-018-2181-3.
14. Zdero R, Walker R, Waddell JP, et al. Biomechanical evaluation of periprosthetic femoral fracture fixation. J Bone Joint Surg Am 2008;90(5):1068–1077.

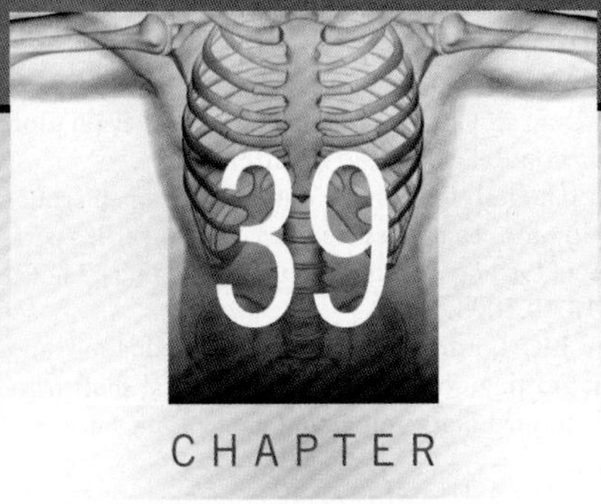

Fixation of Periprosthetic Fractures above Total Knee Arthroplasty

Richard S. Yoon, Derek J. Donegan, and Frank A. Liporace

DEFINITION

- Fractures that occur above or around the femoral component of a total knee arthroplasty (TKA).
- The rates of periprosthetic fractures for TKA vary.
- The incidence is reported to be 0.3% to 5.5% after primary TKA and up to 30% after revision TKA.[4,6,7,15]
- Supracondylar femur fractures are the most common type and the most widely reported with an incidence of 0.3% to 2.5% for primary TKA and 1.6% to 38% for revision TKA.[6,7,10,15]
- These can occur in the setting of a stable or an unstable prosthesis.
- Periprosthetic fractures are difficult to manage and have inconsistent outcomes.
- Reduction and fixation of these fractures is complicated by the preexisting implants that can obstruct reduction and placement of fixation devices.[3]
- Early mobilization is key; mortality is comparable to that of patients with hip fractures.[2]

ANATOMY

- The distal femur is a trapezoidal shape.
- The lateral distal femur is larger in the anteroposterior (AP) diameter than the medial distal femur.
- The lateral femoral condyle has a 10-degree slope in the coronal plane.
- The medial femoral condyle has a 25-degree slope in the coronal plane (**FIG 1**).
- The origin of the gastrocnemius on the distal femur acts as a deforming force leading to a recurvatum deformity.
- The insertion of the adductors on the distal femur acts as a deforming force leading to a varus deformity (**FIG 2**).

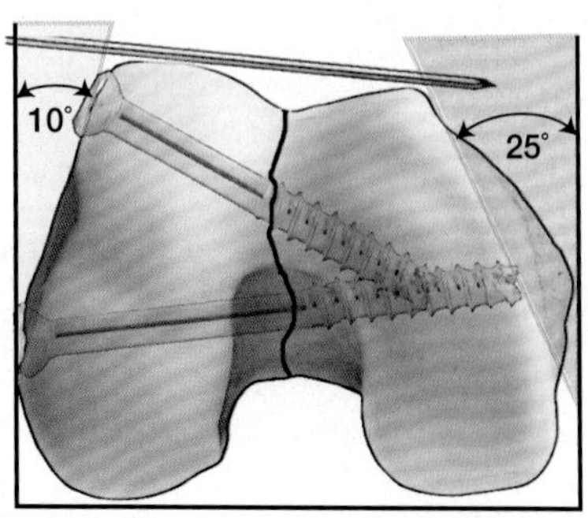

FIG 1 Schematic representation of axial of distal femoral anatomy. Note the trapezoidal shape and angular differential on lateral versus medial side.

PATHOGENESIS

- Most periprosthetic femur fractures typically result from a low-energy fall.[1]
- Multiple risk factors have been identified.
  - Metabolic issues such as osteoporosis are known risk factors for the development of periprosthetic fractures about a TKA.
  - Many studies have demonstrated a decreased bone mineral density after TKA.[13]
  - Surgical technique has also been implicated, however, not directly correlated to specifically notching of the distal femur. However, any weak spot adjacent to a stiff implant is a biomechanical risk for failure.
    - Violation of the anterior cortex of the distal femur has been thought to be an important risk factor for periprosthetic distal femur fracture after TKA.
  - There is a theoretical increased risk due to the change of the geometry of the femur and the decrease radius of curvature leading to higher stresses on the distal femur.

NATURAL HISTORY

- The goals of treatment, whether surgical or nonsurgical, are fracture healing, restoration and maintenance of knee range of motion, and pain-free function.
- In the elderly, early mobilization and achieving the ability to weight bear quickly is of paramount importance.

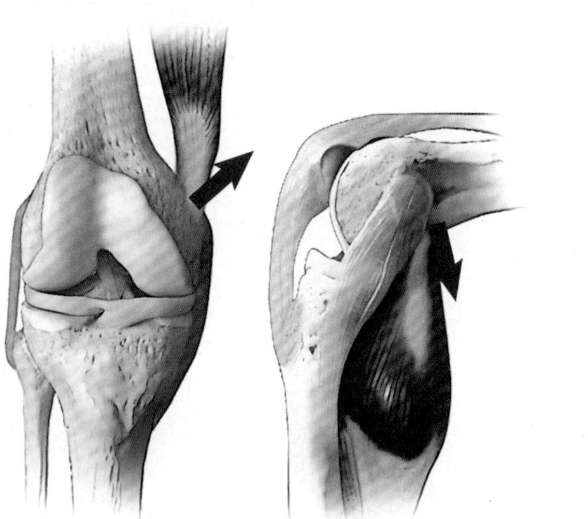

FIG 2 Schematic representation of main muscular deforming forces (*arrows*) to distal femoral fractures (adductors and gastrocnemius, respectively).

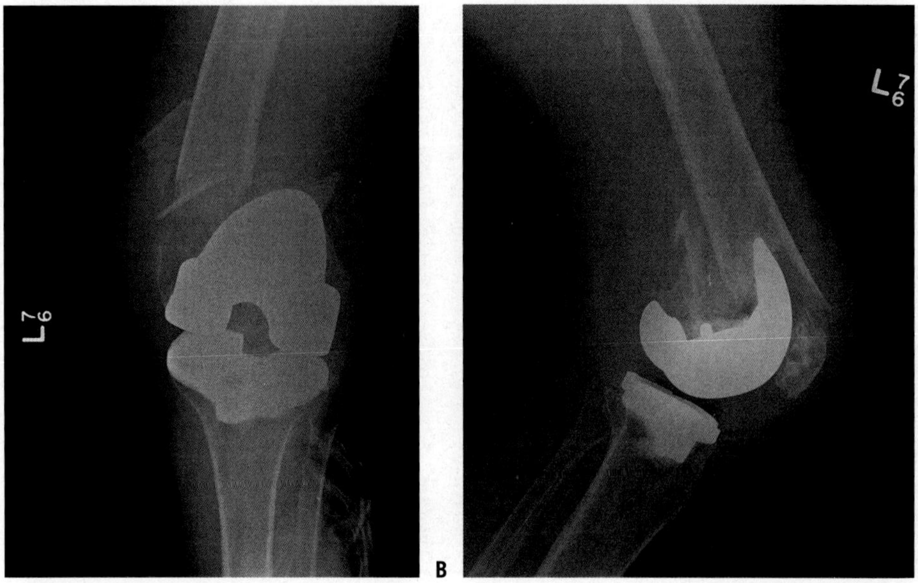

A B

FIG 3 AP (**A**) and lateral (**B**) radiographs of typical periprosthetic distal femur fracture. Note the fracture occurs at the level of the anterior flange of the total knee replacement and progress posteriorly with variable comminution.

- A good result is considered to be a minimum of 90 degrees of knee motion, fracture shortening less than or equal to 2 cm, varus–valgus malalignment less than or equal to 5 degrees, and extension malalignment less than or equal to 10 degrees with minimal to no flexion deformity.[16]
- Nonsurgical management using skeletal traction, casting, or cast bracing has been used in primary fractures; however, due to the prolonged immobility and risks associated, surgical intervention is preferred unless the patient is too sick to undergo the procedure.

PATIENT HISTORY AND PHYSICAL FINDINGS

- It is important to elicit any preexisting symptoms that may indicate whether or not an implant is loose, such as pain or instability.
- Medical records are helpful to identify surgical approach as well as type of implants.
- In the absence of a full set of records, most hospitals have an implant tracking system that can identify the implant used.
- If there is suspicion for infection based on preexisting symptoms or preinjury films demonstrating loosening, further investigation should take place to include complete blood count, erythrocyte sedimentation rate, and noncardiac C-reactive protein, and an aspiration.
- If the infection workup is suspicious, then intraoperative biopsy or staged procedures should be planned.
- Following a general medical examination, a comprehensive examination of the affected limb should be performed.
- The condition of the skin and the neurologic status of the limb should be documented.
- Vascularity should be assessed. If good pulses are not present, then an ankle–brachial index (ABI) should be performed and documented.
- An ABI less than 0.90 warrants further investigation such as a computed tomography angiography (CTA).[11]

IMAGING AND OTHER DIAGNOSTIC STUDIES

- Standard AP and lateral of the affected extremity should be obtained **(FIG 3)**.
- It is also routine practice to get images of the long bones and joints above and below the injury.
- Traction radiographs can help to demonstrate the bony anatomy and feasibility of a closed reduction.
- A CT scanogram assessing axis and leg length can also be beneficial in certain instances, such as
  - Previous history of fracture or surgery above ipsilateral implant that can aide in deformity correction in restoring mechanical axis at joint line
  - Previous history of fracture or total hip arthroplasty (THA) above ipsilateral implant with obvious leg length discrepancy can also be addressed, especially if implant is loose and revision is being considered.
- Advance imaging, specifically CT scanning, can be helpful to determine the amount of bone stock available for fixation and to evaluate the distal femoral implant for the intercondylar size if this information is not known **(FIG 4)**.

DIFFERENTIAL DIAGNOSIS

- Loose TKA
- Polyethylene failure
- Infected TKA
- Periprosthetic tibial fracture
- Periprosthetic patellar fracture
- Periprosthetic fracture around a THA/proximal intramedullary nail, otherwise known as an *interprosthetic fracture*

NONOPERATIVE MANAGEMENT

- Indication for nonoperative management includes truly nondisplaced fractures with a stable prosthesis or a patient that is too medically unstable for surgery.
- Nonsurgical management includes skeletal traction, casting, or cast bracing.
- Nonsurgical management does eliminate the surgical risks such as bleeding, infection, loss of fixation, and anesthetic complications. However, anticoagulation is needed that does introduce a different bleeding risk.
- With nonsurgical management, the extremity should be kept immobilized in extension for 4 to 6 weeks and the patient kept non–weight bearing.

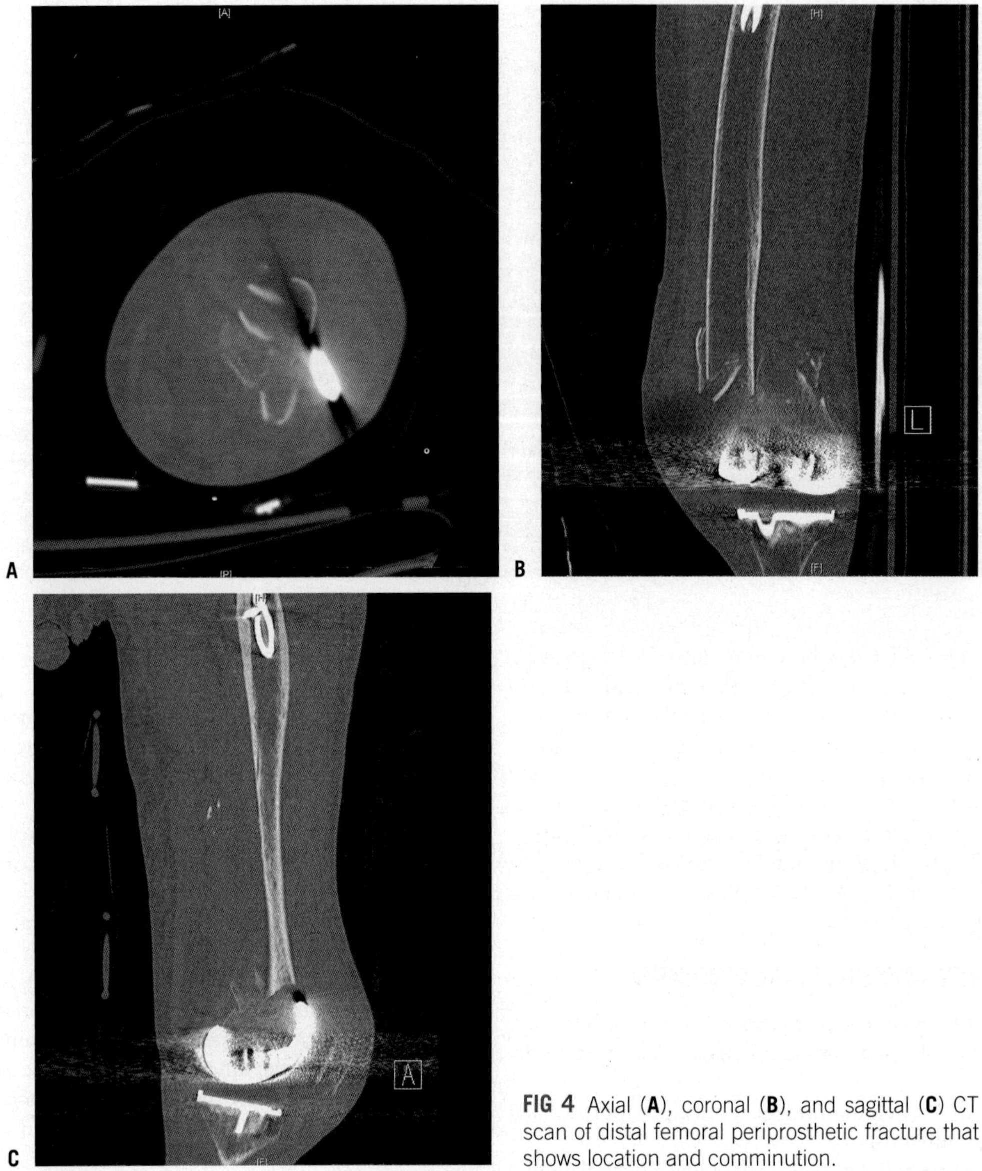

FIG 4 Axial (**A**), coronal (**B**), and sagittal (**C**) CT scan of distal femoral periprosthetic fracture that shows location and comminution.

SURGICAL MANAGEMENT

- Once surgical management has been decided, it is crucial to determine if the implant is stable or not.
- Fractures about a stable femoral component are typically treated with intramedullary nailing (IMN) or laterally based locked plating or both via nail plate combination (NPC) technique.[8,17]
- Retrograde IMN represents a good option when there is adequate bone stock and an "open box" TKA femoral component.
- Locked plates are quite helpful in the treatment of periprosthetic fractures of the distal femur.
- Advantages of locked plating include the ability for multiple fixed-angle points of fixation in osteoporotic bone, increased biomechanical strength over conventional plates, and the ability for insertion in minimally invasive techniques.[12]
- NPC can be used for those fractures with large metaphyseal involvement, especially ones with medial column comminution (NPC).
- Advantages of NPC can allow for medialization of the neutral axis to allow for reliable, immediate weight bearing; however, to date there has been no comparison of nailing versus NPC.
- When minimally invasive techniques are used, it is crucial to avoid malalignment, the most common of which are valgus and hyperextension of the distal fragment.[5]
- When periprosthetic fractures above a TKA are associated with a loose component, revision arthroplasty, which may require distal femoral replacement is the treatment of choice (this is not addressed in this chapter which is devoted to fractures around stable implants).

Preoperative Planning

- The history and physical is reviewed.
- Preinjury radiographs are reviewed if available to determine if there was any evidence of loosening or infection and to review the alignment and any potential bony deficiencies.
- Evidence of infection requires further workup as mentioned earlier.
- Prior operative reports are obtained and reviewed specifically to identify the type of implant and determine if the femoral component is an open box or not and the intercondylar size as this will influence if a nail can be placed. We have listed many of the implants in **TABLE 1**.

TABLE 1 Chart of Common Manufacturers and Implants with Representative Intercondylar Width that Limits Nail Size Usage for Retrograde Intramedullary Nailing of Distal Femoral Periprosthetic Fracture

Component	Model	Size	Intercondylar Width (mm)
Biomet	Maxim Primary		13.3
		PS Open Box	15.2
		PS Closed Box	Closed
	AGC 3000		18.0
		PS	18.0
		HPS	15.4
	Ascent Primary		18.4
		PS Open box	20.3
		PS Closed box	Closed
	Vanguard	PS	16.2
		CR	13.3
Smith & Nephew	Genesis I	CR	20.1
		PS	17.9
	Genesis II	CR 1–2	16.0
		CR 3–9	18.5
		PS	16.3
	Profix	CR	19.8
		PS	14.6
	Tricon M and C		17.0
Stryker Howmedica	Duracon		18.5
	Stabilizer		Stemmed
	Kinemax	XS	17.0
		S	18.5
		M	19.5
		L	21.0
		XL	22.5
		XXL	22.5
		Modular Condylar and Plus	Stemmed
		Modular Stabilizer and Plus	Closed
	Kinematic II		21.0
		Condylar	Stemmed
		Stabilizer	Closed
	PCA	S	16, 18
		M	15, 18
		M/L	15, 16
		L	13, 15
		XL	12, 15
	Scorpio	CR/PS 3	16.5
		CR/PS 5	16.5
		CR/PS 7	18.5
		CR/PS 9	18.5
		CR/PS 11	20.5
		CR/PS 13	20.5
		TS	Stemmed
	Series 7000 PS		20.5
		Modular	Stemmed
		Omnifit	20.5
		PS	Closed
	Triathlon CR/PS		16.0

(continued)

TABLE 1 *(continued)*

Component	Model	Size	Intercondylar Width (mm)
Zimmer, Centerpulse, Sulzer Medica	Nexgen CR	A	11.9
		B	12.1
		C	12.2
		D	12.5
		E	12.8
		F	12.9
		G	13.3
		H	13.4
	Nexgen PS/LPS	A	13.7
		B	13.7
		C	16.6
		D	16.6
		E	17.8
		F	17.8
		G	21.2
		H	21.2
	1/8 I PSCK	55	15.7
		58	15.5
		65	17.0
		66	17.1
		70	18.8
	1/8 II PSCK	54	15.3
		59	16.7
		64	18.2
		69	19.6
		74	21.0
	M/G 1	S	10.6
		S+	10.6
		Reg	12.1
		Reg+	12.3
		L	14.4
		L+	14.3
		L++	17.4
	M/G II		11.9
	Natural Knee I	0–1	12
		2	16
		3	19
		4	20
		5	22
	Natural Knee II		17
	Apollo		17
Dow Corning & Wright Medical	Axiom Primary	55	14
		60	15
		65	17
		70	18
		75	19
		80	20
		85	22
		PS 55	16
		PS 60	18
		PS 65	18
		PS 70	20
		PS 75	21
		PS 80	23
		PS 85	24
		Modular	Closed

TABLE 1 *(continued)*

Component	Model	Size	Intercondylar Width (mm)
	Advance Primary	PS 1	15
		PS 2	17
		PS 3	18
		PS 4	19
		PS 5	21
		PS 6	22
	Advantium	TC	19
		Open house	16
		PS	Closed
	Ortholoc	Standard	21
		Large	25
		Ex Large	25
	Ortholoc II		24
Synthes DePuy and J&J	PFC	CR	20
		CS 1	14.3
		CS 2	15.1
		CS 3	17.0
		CS 4–6	20.0
	PFC Sigma	CR	12.7, 17.8
		CS	17.8
	AMK	CR 1	14.2
		CR 2	16.4
		CR 2+	16.5
		CR 3	18.5
		CR 3+	17.9
		CR 4	17.6
		CR 5	20.6
	CS Congruency	1	18.7
		2	19.7
		3	21.9
		4	22
		5	24.8
	LCS Complete CR	Sm	14.4
		Sm+	15.7
		Med	16.6
		Std	17.5
		Std+	18.8
		Lrg	20.3
		Lrg+	21.9

Modified from Heckler MW, Tennant GS, Williams DP, et al. Retrograde nailing of supracondylar periprosthetic femur fractures: a surgeon's guide to femoral component sizing. Orthopedics 2007;30(5):345–348. doi:10.3928/01477447-20070501-14. Reprinted with permission from SLACK Incorporated.

- Prior operative reports should also be obtained to identify the TKA in order to have available polyethylene liners available for exchange (especially when performing retrograde intramedullary nail [rIMN] or NPC).
- Injury films are reviewed and classified **(TABLE 2)**.
- Key factors in decision-making process for operative treatment:
  - Is the bone stock adequate?
  - Does the implant have an open or closed box?
  - Is the implant loose or stable?
- If the implant is stable and there is adequate bone stock, then open reduction and internal fixation is treatment of choice:
  - If implant has open box, then both IMN and/or a laterally based locked plate can be used.
  - If implant has closed box, then a nail cannot be used easily and a laterally based locked plate is the treatment of choice.
- If the implant is loose, then revision arthroplasty is indicated. If the implant is loose, especially in octogenarian and/or severe comminution, consider distal femoral replacement.

Positioning

- When performing operative fixation of a periprosthetic femur fracture above a TKA (plate or IMN), the patient is usually positioned supine on a radiolucent flat-top Jackson table **(FIG 5)**.

TABLE 2 Chart of Classifications Commonly Used for Distal Femoral Periprosthetic Fractures

Supracondylar Periprosthetic Fractures: Classification Systems		
Study	**Type/Group**	**Description**
Neer et al	Type I	Undisplaced (<5 mm displacement and/or <5 degrees angulation)
	Type II	Displaced >1 cm
	Type IIa	With lateral femoral shaft displacement
	Type IIb	With medial femoral shaft displacement
	Type III	Displaced and comminuted
DiGioia and Rubash	Group I	Extra-articular, undisplaced (<5 mm displacement and <5 degrees angulation)
	Group II	Extra-articular, displaced (>5 mm displacement or >5 degrees angulation)
	Group III	Severely displaced (loss of cortical contact) or angulated (>10 degrees); may have intercondylar or T-shaped component
Chen et al	Type I	Nondisplaced (Neer type I)
	Type II	Displaced and/or comminuted (Neer types II and III)
Lewis and Rorabeck	Type I	Undisplaced fracture; prosthesis intact
	Type II	Displaced fracture; prosthesis intact
	Type III	Displaced or undisplaced fracture; prosthesis loose or failing

Modified with permission from Su ET, DeWal H, Di Cesare PE. Periprosthetic femoral fractures above total knee replacements. J Am Acad Orthop Surg 2004;12(1):12–20.

- Position the patient to the ipsilateral side of the table.
- One rolled blanket bump is placed under the ipsilateral hip.
- Tape the ipsilateral arm over the chest.
- Sequential compression devices on contralateral extremity
- Secure the patient with safety belt at abdomen level and 2-inch silk tape over blue towel on contralateral leg.
- Make sure all bony prominences are padded.
- C-arm will enter from contralateral side, perpendicular to the operating room (OR) table.
- A radiolucent ramp or triangle can be placed under the ipsilateral leg.
- For difficult fractures to reduce, sterile skeletal traction can be placed and weight hung off the end of the bed over a pipe bender.
- Neuromuscular blockade should be used as part of the anesthetic plan.
- Drape up proximally to include the anterior superior iliac spine to maximize exposure.

A
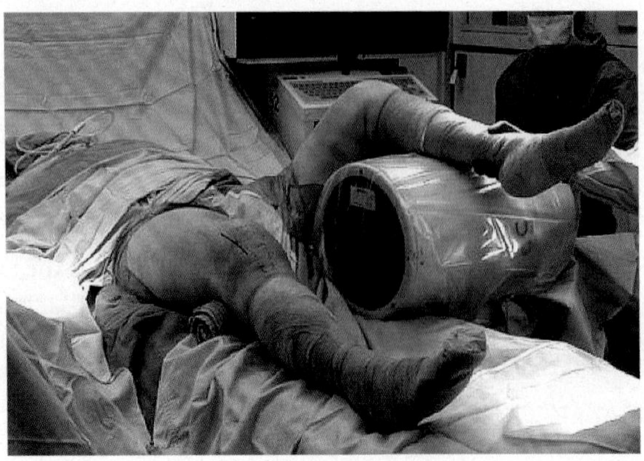
B
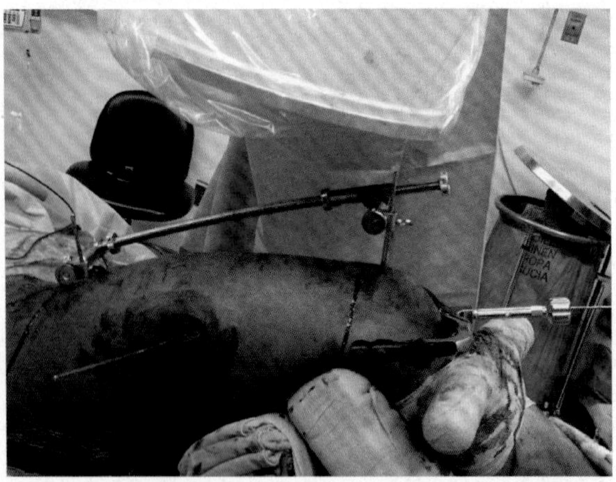

FIG 5 A. Patient positioning supine for distal femoral plate fixation. Both legs sterile prepped to allow for elevation of nonaffected extremity and prevent movement of operative extremity to allow for accurate lateral fluoroscopy without potential displacement of reduction. Note laterally drawn incision and the sterile bump under area of fracture site to aid with sagittal reduction. **B.** Positioning for retrograde nail. Note percutaneous reduction incision laterally, femoral distractor for length, proximal tibia pin for manual traction, and bump positioning for sagittal alignment. Femoral distractor placed anteriorly and medially to proposed track of ultimate IMN.

Approach

- For lateral locked plating, a standard lateral approach to the femur can be used. This can be extended into a subvastus approach if extension proximally is desired.
- For retrograde IMN, a standard midline incision can be used with a medial or lateral parapatellar arthrotomy. Full exposure is warranted to avoid damage to the polyethylene and low threshold to perform polyethylene exchange is recommended.
- For NPC, a midline approach can be used with a lateral parapatellar arthrotomy; a transtendinous approach through the patellar tendon can be used via the same window.

LATERALLY LOCKED PLATING

Exposure—Lateral Approach to Femur

- Mark out landmarks of joint line and femoral shaft/condyle **(TECH FIG 1A)**.
- Mark lateral incision in line with the femoral shaft starting at Gerdy tubercle and extending proximally to include fracture site (see **TECH FIG 1A**).
- Incise skin along marked incision down to level of iliotibial band fascia.
- Incise fascia in line with the skin.
- Expose vermillion border and/or border of femoral component.
- Be mindful to remain extra-articular and avoid violation of the joint capsule.
- If plan to bridge fracture, do not expose the fracture site.
- If plan for direct anatomic reduction, extend proximally by elevating the vastus lateralis anteriorly to directly visualize the fracture.

Reduction/Fixation

- Length, alignment, and rotation are assessed both clinically and fluoroscopically. If needed, the contralateral leg can be prepped in for comparison.
- A bump is used to control the sagittal balance. This should be placed strategically to counteract the forces of the gastrocnemius and the recurvatum deformity **(TECH FIG 1B,C)**.
- Length is achieved and maintained by longitudinal traction either manually, with the use of skeletal traction, or with a universal distractor.
- Once the length, alignment, and rotation are adequate, the appropriate length plate is determined. The goal is to have at least six holes of the plate proximal to the fracture site **(TECH FIG 1D)**.
- The plate is then slid submuscularly below the vastus lateralis along the lateral border of the femur. It is important to feel the plate contact the femur throughout the entire course.
- Using AP fluoroscopy, the appropriate plate height is determined.
- The plate is then pinned to the distal segment using a Kirschner wire (K-wire) through the center hole of the plate. Ultimately, this will be replaced with a screw that will be parallel to the distal femoral condyles, aiding in achieving appropriate coronal alignment (see **TECH FIG 1D**).
- Using fluoroscopy to get a good lateral, the sagittal plate balance is evaluated and adjusted.
- The plate is then pinned to the proximal femur in the second to last screw hole of the plate using a K-wire through perfect circle technique or an external jig and a stab incision. Unicortical screws are also useful at this stage.
- The plate height and balance is then confirmed using AP and lateral fluoroscopy.
- The plate is then secured to bone with a nonlocking screw distally to bring the plate to bone. It is important at this point to confirm that this screw did not introduce too much valgus.
- A nonlocking screw is then placed immediately proximal to the fracture site through the plate to bring the plate to bone and make fine adjustments to the coronal balance.

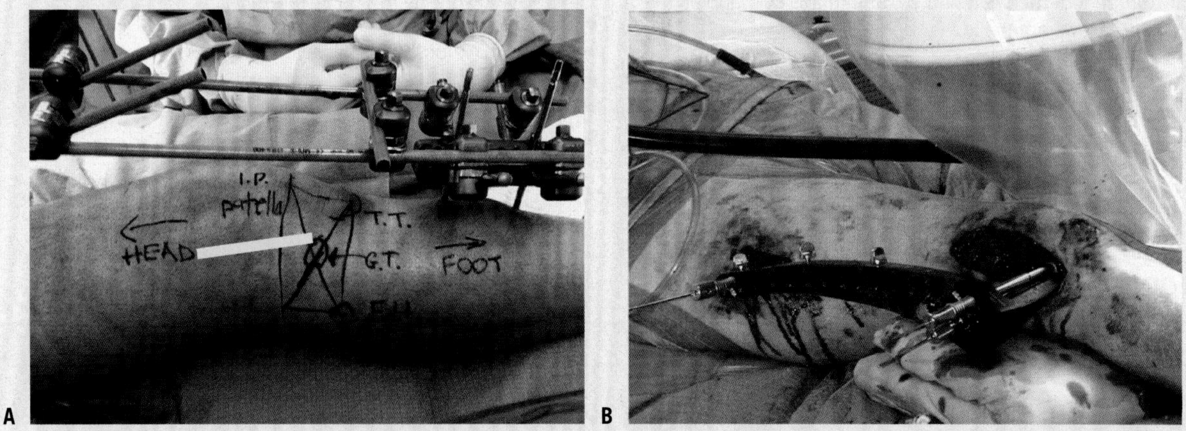

TECH FIG 1 A. Gerdy tubercle identification. Central point of "box" of distal pole of patella, fibula head, tibia tubercle, and point in line with perpendicular cross-section of first two landmarks. The yellow line indicates a utilitarian skin incision for plating distal femur fractures, beginning at Gerdy tubercle and extending proximally (about 7 cm). *FH*, fibular head; *GT*, Gerdy's tubercle; *IP*, inferior pole; *TT*, tibial tubercle. **B.** Laterally based incision distally to allow for passage of plate and proximal provisional fixation through jig to allow for box to be created. *(continued)*

TECHNIQUES

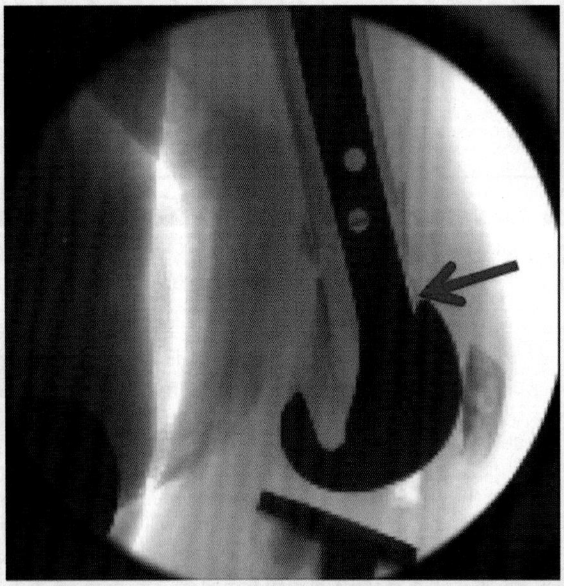
C

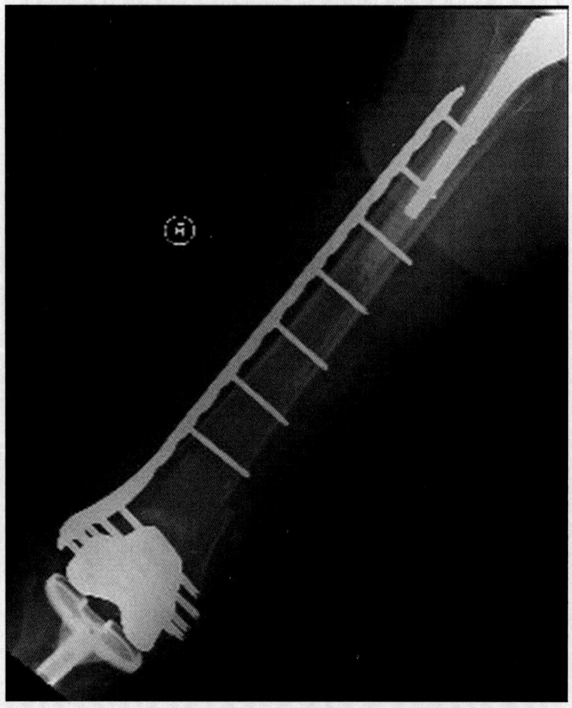
D

TECH FIG 1 *(continued)* **C.** Lateral intraoperative positioning of plate for distal femoral plating. The bump is seen at the level of the fracture to help to avoid recurvatum. Note plate is sitting as anteriorly as possible to match posterior aspect of anterior flange of implant. This is indicated with the *red arrow.* **D.** Final AP radiograph of same patient in **C**. Note distal screws in plate parallel to distal femoral condyles to allow for appropriate alignment.

- The overall length, alignment, and rotation, as well as the plate balance, are confirmed.
- The plate is then secured distally using locking screws. It is important to remember the trapezoidal shape of the distal femur as to not place screws that are too long.
- There are multiple options for proximal fixation. In good bone, unlocked screws will allow for a tight friction fit of the plate to bone. In poor bone, locked screws will result in a longer fatigue life. In general, most surgeons secured the plate proximally with hybrid fixation of nonlocked and locked screws spread evenly throughout the shaft of the plate. In this scenario all the nonlocked screws are placed first.
- An alternate technique is to use far cortical locked fixation. This can be performed by overdrilling the proximal cortex by 0.5 or 1 mm and using a locked screw or by using proprietary implants. In theory, this method may provide more lateral callus.
- The most proximal point of fixation is either a unicortical locked screw or a bicortical nonlocked screw to ease the transition of stiffness from the plated bone to the remaining host bone. If there is a concomitant hip arthroplasty, then the plate and fixation should overlap by at least two femoral cortical diameters (see **TECH FIG 1D**).
- Final fluoroscopic evaluation is performed.

Closure

- Place a Hemovac drain if necessary.
- Irrigate wounds.
- No. 1 Vicryl for the fascial layer
- A 2-0 Vicryl for superficial and subcutaneous layers
- A 3-0 nylon mattress or staples for skin
- Sterile dressing and Ace wrap from toes to thigh

RETROGRADE INTRAMEDULLARY NAILING

Exposure

- Place a sterile radiolucent triangle under the ipsilateral leg so that the knee is roughly in 30 to 40 degrees of flexion.
- Mark out landmarks: inferior pole patella, tibial tubercle, medial and lateral margins of the patellar tendon, previous TKA incision.
- Mark out new surgical incision through previous TKA incision roughly 3 cm in length (two fingerbreadths below inferior pole of patella to one fingerbreadth above the inferior pole of the patella).
- Incise skin down to paratenon of patellar tendon.
- Raise small medial flap to identify the medial border of the patellar tendon.
- Make a medial parapatellar arthrotomy to expose the intercondylar notch.

- Débride any scar tissue to clearly visualize the box of the femoral component of the TKA.
- If the area is tight, consider removing the tibial polyethylene tray.

Reduction/Fixation

- Length, alignment, and rotation are assessed using fluoroscopy.
- A bump is used to control the sagittal balance. This should be placed strategically to counteract the forces of the gastrocnemius and the recurvatum deformity (see **FIG 5B**).
- Length is achieved and maintained by longitudinal traction either manually or with the use of skeletal traction.
- Insert the guidewire through the incision to the appropriate starting point and confirm both under direct vision and fluoroscopically **(TECH FIG 2A,B)**.
  - AP view: slightly lateral to midline aiming straight up the intramedullary canal
  - Lateral view: slightly anterior aiming straight up the intramedullary canal
- Insert the guidewire until the pin is either past the fracture site and into the metaphyseal region of the femur or in deep enough to make sure that the starting point cannot move.
- Confirm location of guidewire and reduction on fluoroscopy.

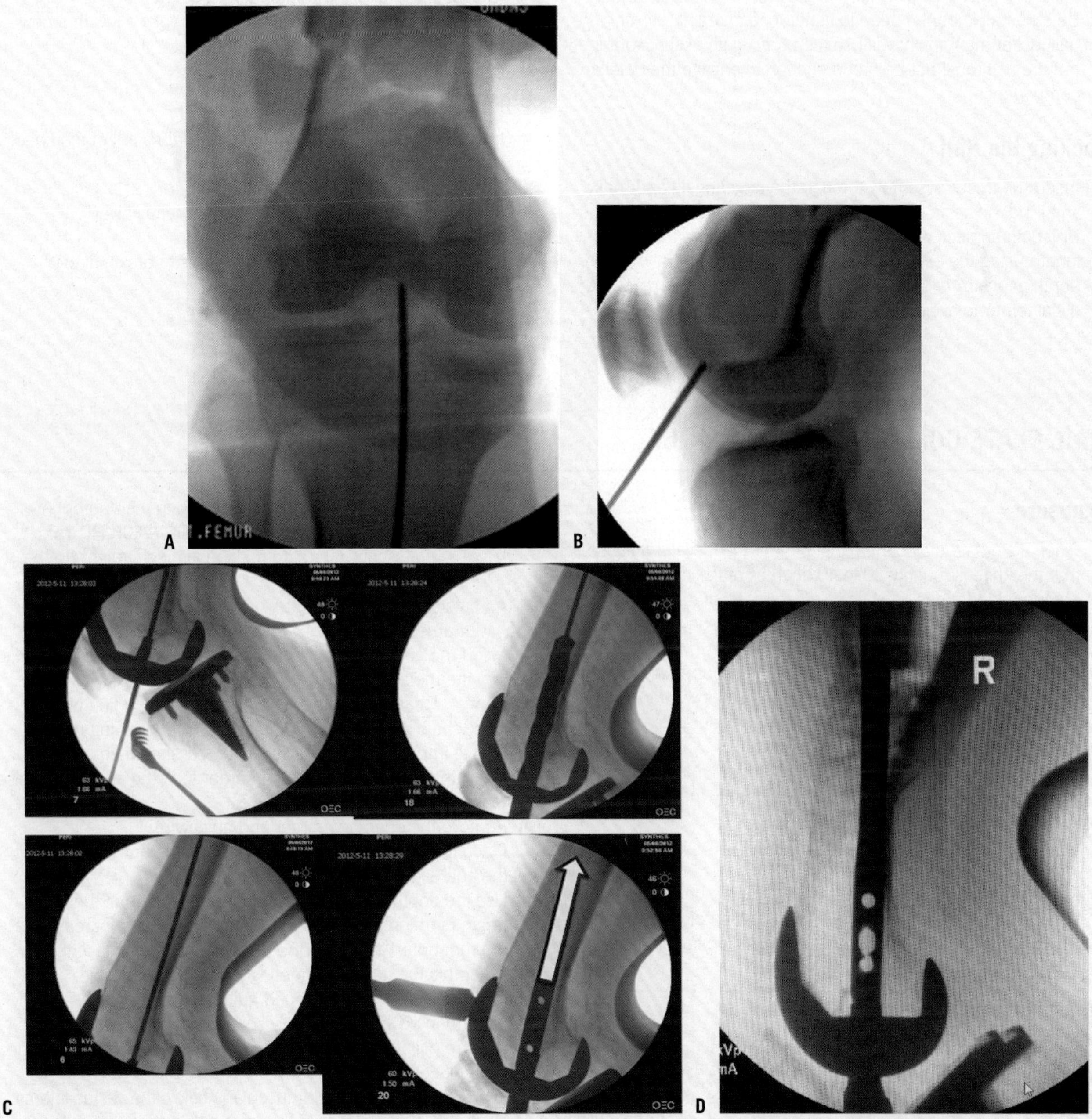

TECH FIG 2 Typical AP (**A**) and lateral (**B**) starting point for retrograde IMN without total knee replacement. There is no change in AP positioning in the face of a total knee replacement. **C.** The total knee replacement may place the starting point more posterior (*arrow*) in the lateral view. Even with a cruciate retaining implant, the trochlea part of the component may dictate a more posterior starting point. **D.** An example of an apex posterior (extension) deformity that resulted from a posteriorly based starting point.

- Open the distal femur with the appropriate opening reamer. Due to implant designs, it is sometimes necessary to enlarge the box with a metal-cutting burr in order to fit the appropriate-size reamers and nail through the box.
- Remove the opening reamer and guidewire.
- Place the ball-tipped guidewire through the entry site and up the entire length of the femur. Use intramedullary reduction tools as needed.
- Use the depth gauge and determine the length of the nail.
- Begin reaming with the end-cutting reamer and increase by 0.5 mm until 1 mm over the diameter nail being inserted.
- Assemble the nail and targeting jig on the back table.
- Insert nail over the ball-tipped guidewire as far as possible by hand then advance until fully seated with mallet assistance.
- Be sure nail is buried deep to femoral component. Leaving the nail just at the implant will use the portal to its best advantage, but the nail must not be proud enough to engage the patellar component.

Locking the Nail

- Insert the trocar assembly through the targeting jig and make small stab incision at the site of screw insertion.
- Drill both cortices with the pilot drill and measure the screw length using the calibrations on the drill and confirm with a depth gauge. Again, be aware of the trapezoidal shape of the distal femur to avoid long screws.
- Insert the appropriate length screw.
- Repeat this step for two to three interlocking screws depending on the location of the fracture.
- Confirm the length, alignment, and rotation prior to continuing with the proximal interlocking screws.
- Bring the C-arm proximally and obtain perfect circles of the proximal AP interlocking holes.
- Make small incision at the site of screw insertion. Place drill and confirm with fluoroscopy in two planes the trajectory prior to drilling.
- Drill bicortical hole.
- Use depth gauge and measure screw length and confirm on fluoroscopy.
- Insert appropriate length screws.
- Repeat steps for second interlocking screw.
- If the tibial polyethylene was removed, replace it with a new component.

Closure

- Irrigate wound and be sure to get any debris out of the knee joint to prevent third body wear.
- No. 1 Vicryl to close arthrotomy
- A 2-0 Vicryl for superficial and subcutaneous layer
- A 3-0 nylon for skin
- Sterile dressing and Ace wrap from toes to proximal thigh

NAIL PLATE COMBINATION TECHNIQUE

Exposure

- Place a sterile radiolucent triangle under the ipsilateral leg so that the knee is roughly 30 to 40 degrees of flexion.
- Mark out landmarks: inferior pole patella, tibial tubercle, medial and lateral margins of the patellar tendon, previous TKA incision.
- Mark out new surgical incision through previous TKA incision roughly 3 cm in length (two fingerbreadths below inferior pole of patella to one fingerbreadth above the inferior pole of the patella).
- Incise skin down to paratenon of patellar tendon.
- Raise small medial and lateral flaps to identify the medial and lateral border of the patellar tendon.
- Make a lateral parapatellar arthrotomy to expose the intercondylar notch.
- Débride any scar tissue to clearly visualize the box of the femoral component of the TKA as well as the polyethylene, assess for wear and if it will obstruct IMN preparation/insertion.

Reduction/Fixation

- Length, alignment, and rotation are assessed using fluoroscopy.
- A bump is used to control the sagittal balance. This should be placed strategically to counteract the forces of the gastrocnemius and the recurvatum deformity (see **FIG 5B**).
- Length is achieved and maintained by longitudinal traction either manually or with the use of skeletal traction.
- Insert the guidewire through the incision to the appropriate starting point and confirm fluoroscopically **(TECH FIG 3A)**.
  - AP view: slightly lateral to midline aiming straight up the intramedullary canal
  - Lateral view: slightly anterior aiming straight up the intramedullary canal
- Insert the guidewire until the pin is past the fracture site and into the metaphyseal region of the femur.
- Confirm location of guidewire and reduction on fluoroscopy.
- Open the distal femur with the appropriate opening reamer. Due to implant designs, it may be necessary to enlarge the box with a metal-cutting burr in order to fit the appropriate size reamers and nail through the box.
- Remove the opening reamer and guidewire.
- Place the ball-tipped guidewire through the entry site and up the entire length of the femur.
- Use the depth gauge and determine the length of the nail.
- Begin reaming with the end-cutting reamer and increase by 0.5 mm until 1 mm over the diameter nail being inserted.
- Assemble the nail and targeting jig on the back table.
- Insert nail over the ball-tipped guidewire as far as possible by hand then advance until fully seated with mallet assistance.
- Be sure nail is buried deep to femoral component; proceed to plate placement.
- The plate is then slid submuscularly below the vastus lateralis along the lateral border of the femur. It is important to feel the plate contact the femur throughout the entire course.
- Using AP fluoroscopy, the appropriate plate height is determined.

- Proximally, at the level of the vastus ridge, erring posteriorly, make an approximate 5 to 6 cm incision, split the iliotibial band longitudinally, and expose the vastus lateralis.
- In an L-typed fashion, lift the vastus lateralis anteriorly to expose the femur.
- As the plate is slide proximally, ensure that the plate is centered on the femur.
- Prior to plate sliding, depending on the patient's anatomy, custom contouring of the plate may be required in order to accommodate the vastus ridge. Preferably, contouring should include a posterior twist to avoid symptomatic hardware over the lateral greater trochanter **(TECH FIG 3B)**.
- The plate is then pinned to the distal segment using a K-wire through the center hole of the plate. Ultimately, this will be replaced with a screw that will be parallel to the distal femoral condyles, aiding in achieving appropriate coronal alignment.
- The plate height and balance is then confirmed using AP and lateral fluoroscopy.

Linking the Nail and the Plate

- Linking the two constructs can be achieved via two methods: utilizing the jig to approximate screw position and/or using perfect circle technique.
- Utilizing the jig, on a lateral, if the sleeve lines up with the plate hole, then place a lateral to medial locking screw using standard technique, however, preferably utilizing the 5.0 mm locking screw that will lock into the plate.
- If the sleeve does not line up with a screw hole, then utilizing perfect circle technique, the nearest variable angle locking hole should be aligned and targeted to create a path that can place a screw through the plate and the nail **(TECH FIG 3C).**
- One distal linked screw is recommended; if possible, two is preferable.
- No linking of the devices should be used proximally as removal of a broken screw through a nail may be dangerous if a revision is ever needed.

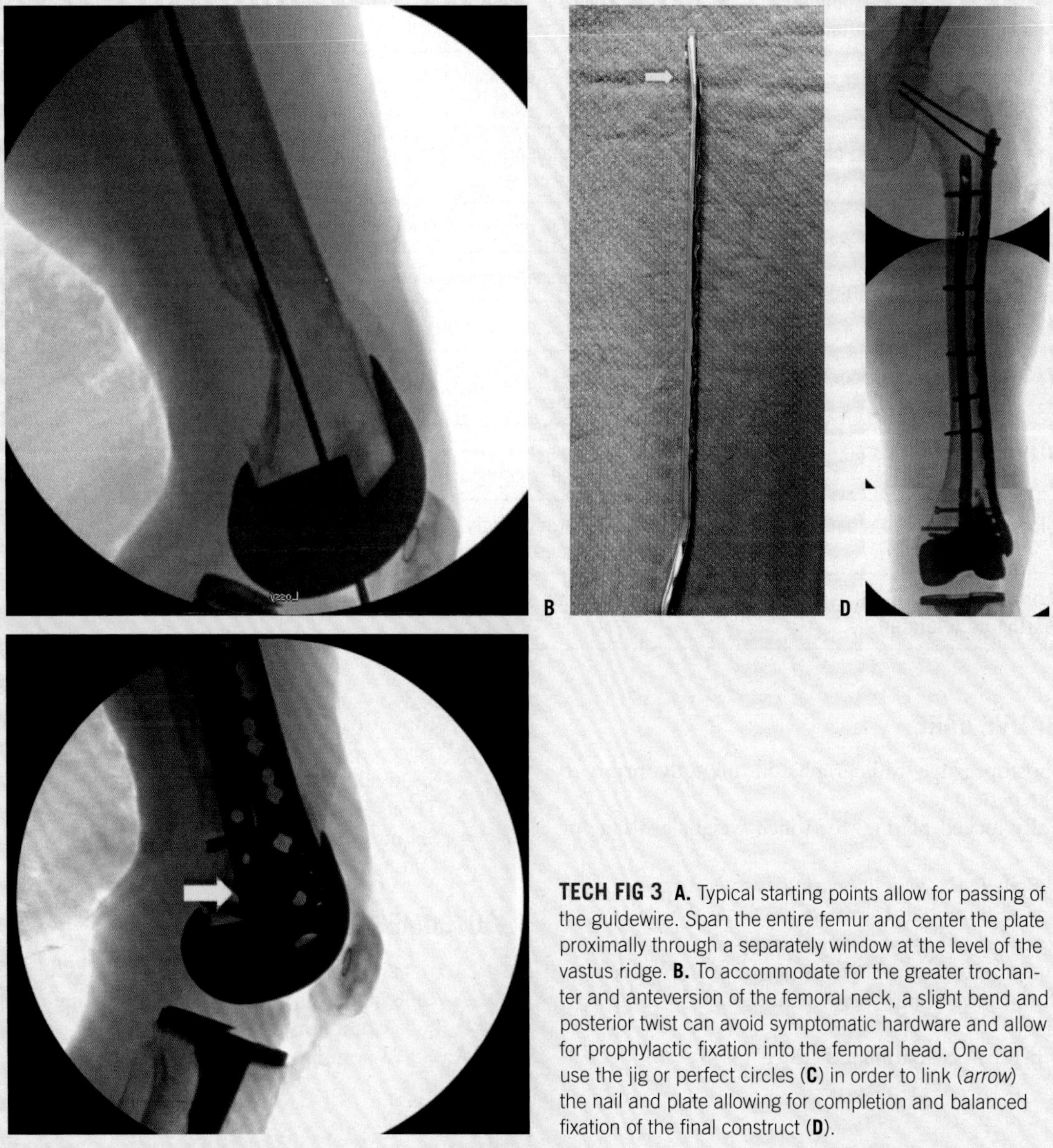

A B D C

TECH FIG 3 A. Typical starting points allow for passing of the guidewire. Span the entire femur and center the plate proximally through a separately window at the level of the vastus ridge. **B.** To accommodate for the greater trochanter and anteversion of the femoral neck, a slight bend and posterior twist can avoid symptomatic hardware and allow for prophylactic fixation into the femoral head. One can use the jig or perfect circles (**C**) in order to link (*arrow*) the nail and plate allowing for completion and balanced fixation of the final construct (**D**).

Completing the Nail Plate Combination Construct

- With the construct now linked distally, complete filling the distal locking cluster, keeping in mind the trapezoidal shape of the femur.
- Place a nonlocking screw at the apex of the fracture and/or metaphysis to get the plate down to bone.
- Move proximally to the vastus ridge window and place a nonlocking screw (preferably with the proper anteversion to prophylactically fix the neck/head, but if not able to be achieved, into the lesser trochanter)—this will also make the plate flush down to bone.
- Hybrid fixation can be achieved proximally along with percutaneous locking screws along the shaft (skipping hole) to achieve balanced fixation.
- Final fluoroscopic images are taken and saved on orthogonal views **(TECH FIG 3D)**.

Closure

- Irrigate wound and be sure to get any debris out of the knee joint to prevent third body wear.
- No. 1 Vicryl to close arthrotomy
- A 2-0 Vicryl for superficial and subcutaneous layer
- A 3-0 nylon for skin
- Sterile dressing and Ace wrap from toes to proximal thigh

TECHNIQUES

Pearls and Pitfalls

Obtain complete radiographs including mechanical axis when appropriate.	• Orthogonal films of femur, knee, and tibia. Consider computed tomography (CT) scan for preoperative planning.
If implants are stable, consider indirect reduction techniques.	• Obtain history of any pain or difficulties with the TKA prior to injury.
For retrograde IMN, be sure to check box status of implant.	• Obtain operative reports to identify implant manufacturer.
Use polyaxial locking plates.	• Allows for multiple points of fixation around the prosthesis
Do not accept axis deviation.	• Evaluate mechanical axis intraoperatively using fluoroscopy versus plain films.
Do not leave loose implants.	• If implants are loose, revise the TKA in addition to treating the fracture.
Do not use incompetent fixation.	• Assure adequate fixation and stability. Use locking constructs as determined by bone quality and fracture pattern.
Do not delay postoperative range of motion.	• Start range of motion immediately postoperatively. Assure appropriate physical therapy orders and consider use of continuous passive motion.
Do not delay surgery in the elderly.	• Medically optimize patients to allow surgery as expeditiously as possible. Communicate with medical colleagues regarding urgency of surgical intervention.
Achieve construct that will allow for weight bearing as tolerated.	• NPC spanning the entire femur can allow for immediate, reliable weight bearing.

POSTOPERATIVE CARE

- Obtain postoperative radiographs in the OR prior to waking the patient up.
- For laterally locked plating, toe-touch weight bearing for 6 weeks
- For retrograde IMN, weight bearing as tolerated
- Knee range of motion as tolerated
- Hinged knee brace for varus–valgus support
- Deep vein thrombosis prophylaxis per surgeon preference
- Twenty-four hours of intravenous antibiotics
- Pain control
- Physical therapy/occupational therapy
- Postoperative follow-up
  - Two weeks for wound check
  - Six weeks for x-rays
  - Three months for x-rays
  - Six months for x-rays
  - One year for x-rays

OUTCOMES

- A 16.4% malunion rate with rIMNs **(TECH FIG 2C,D)**[14]
- A 7.6% malunion rate with locked plating[14]
- A 3.6% nonunion rate with rIMNs[14]
- An 8.8% nonunion rate with locked plating[14]

- A 9.1% secondary surgical procedure rate with rIMNs[14]
- A 13.3% secondary surgical procedure rate with locked plating[14]
- Comparable long-term complication and survival rates compared to primary TKA[9]
- Worse midterm functional outcomes compared to primary TKA[9]

COMPLICATIONS

- Infection
- Malunion
- Nonunion
- Decrease functional outcomes
- TKA failure

REFERENCES

1. Berry DJ. Epidemiology: hip and knee. Orthop Clin North Am 1999;30:183–190.
2. Boylan MR, Riesgo Am, Paulino CB, et al. Mortality following periprosthetic proximal femoral fractures versus native hip fractures. J Bone Joint Surg Am 2018;100(7):578–585.
3. Della Rocca GJ, Leung KS, Pape HC. Periprosthetic fractures: epidemiology and future projections. J Orthop Trauma 2011;25(suppl 1):S66–S70.
4. Figgie MP, Goldberg VM, Figgie HE III, et al. The results of treatment of supracondylar fracture above total knee arthroplasty. J Arthroplasty 1990;5:267–276.
5. Haidukewych GJ. Innovations in locking plate technology. J Am Acad Orthop Surg 2004;12:205–212.
6. Healy WL, Siliski JM, Incavo SJ. Operative treatment of distal femoral fractures proximal to total knee replacements. J Bone Joint Surg Am 1993;75:27–34.
7. Inglis AE, Walker PS. Revision of failed knee replacements using fixed-axis hinges. J Bone Joint Surg Br 1991;73:757–761.
8. Liporace FA, Yoon RS. Nail plate combination technique for native and periprosthetic distal femur fractures. J Orthop Trauma 2019;33(2):e64–e68.
9. Lizaur-Utrilla A, Miralles-Muñoz FA, Sanz-Reig J. Functional outcome of total knee arthroplasty after periprosthetic distal femoral fracture. J Arthroplasty 2013;28(9):1585–1588.
10. Merkel KD, Johnson EW Jr. Supracondylar fracture of the femur after total knee arthroplasty. J Bone Joint Surg Am 1986;68:29–43.
11. Mills WJ, Barei DP, McNair P. The value of the ankle-brachial index for diagnosing arterial injury after knee dislocation: a prospective study. J Trauma 2004;56(6):1261–1265.
12. Nauth A, Ristevski B, Bégué T, et al. Periprosthetic distal femur fractures: current concepts. J Orthop Trauma 2011;25(suppl 2):S82–S85.
13. Platzer P, Schuster R, Aldrian S, et al. Management and outcome of periprosthetic fractures after total knee arthroplasty. J Trauma 2010;68:1464–1470.
14. Ristevski B, Nauth A, Williams DS, et al. Systematic review of the treatment of periprosthetic distal femur fractures. J Orthop Trauma 2014;28(5):307–312.
15. Ritter MA, Faris PM, Keating EM. Anterior femoral notching and ipsilateral supracondylar femur fracture in total knee arthroplasty. J Arthroplasty 1988;3:185–187.
16. Rorabeck CH, Taylor JW. Periprosthetic fractures of the femur complicating total knee arthroplasty. Orthop Clin North Am 1999;30:265–277.
17. Yoon RS, Patel JN, Liporace FA. Nail and plate combination fixation for periprosthetic and interprosthetic fractures. J Orthop Trauma 2019;33(suppl 6):S18–S20.

CHAPTER 40

Retrograde Intramedullary Nailing of the Femur

Ross K. Leighton

DEFINITION

- Retrograde femoral nailing can be defined as any femoral nailing technique with a distal entry from the condyles or through an intercondylar, intra-articular starting point.
- For this chapter, *retrograde femoral nailing* will refer to nails with an intercondylar starting point that extend through the shaft region to the proximal femur.

Strong Indications for a Retrograde Nail versus an Antegrade Nail

1. Intercondylar supracondylar fractures that can be nailed
2. Distal fractures with less than 5 cm between the fracture and the old epiphyseal line
3. Ipsilateral displaced femoral neck and shaft fractures
4. Periprosthetic fractures around a stable total knee prosthesis. In this case, the decision would be plate **(FIG 1A,B)** versus retrograde nail **(FIG 1C,D)**.

Relative Indications

- These have changed substantially with the move from entirely fracture table procedures to antegrade nails that can be done on a radiolucent frame. It is much easier to set up and do multiple fractures on the radiolucent table. Many of these used to be absolute indications for retrograde nails.

1. Obesity
2. Ipsilateral femur and tibia fractures (floating knee)
3. Distal third femoral shaft fractures
4. Nondisplaced ipsilateral femoral neck fractures with associated displaced shaft fractures. This is controversial, as some would carefully perform a cephalomedullary nail.
5. Bilateral femoral shaft fractures
6. Treatment of a nonunion of a supracondylar fracture following a failed plate fixation **(FIG 2A,B)**.

- See **TABLE 1** for expanded list of relative indications for a retrograde femoral nail.

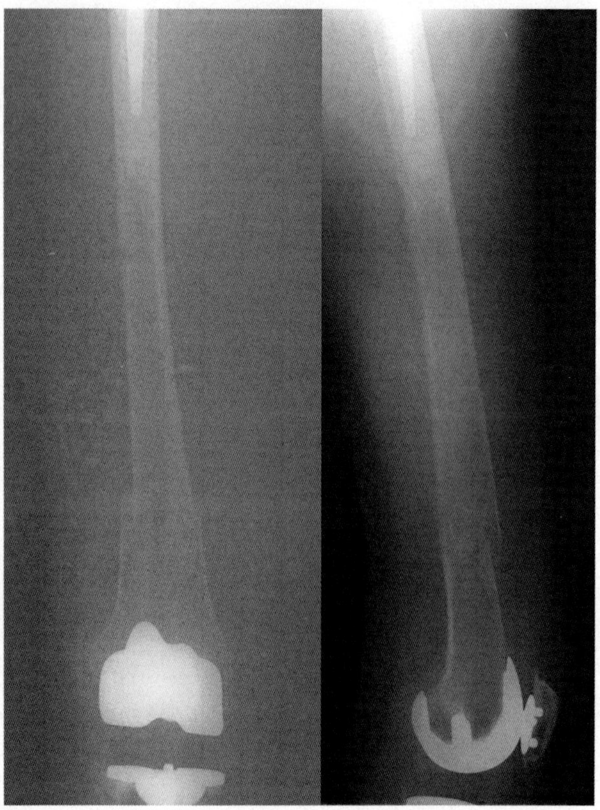

A

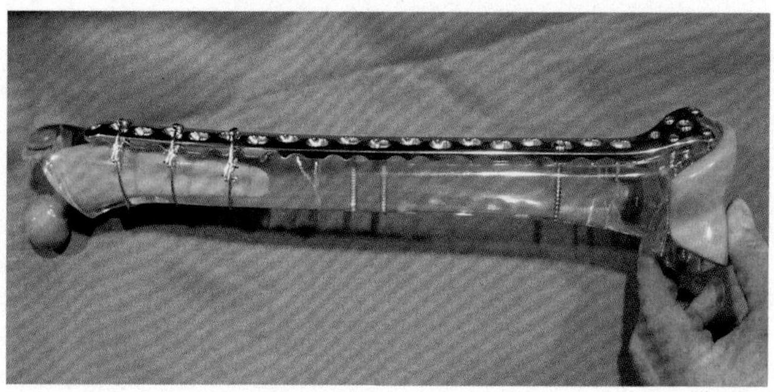

B

FIG 1 Periprosthetic fracture treated with a plate. **A,B.** Images indicating the proper plating with extended plate protecting the whole bone from a new fracture. *(continued)*

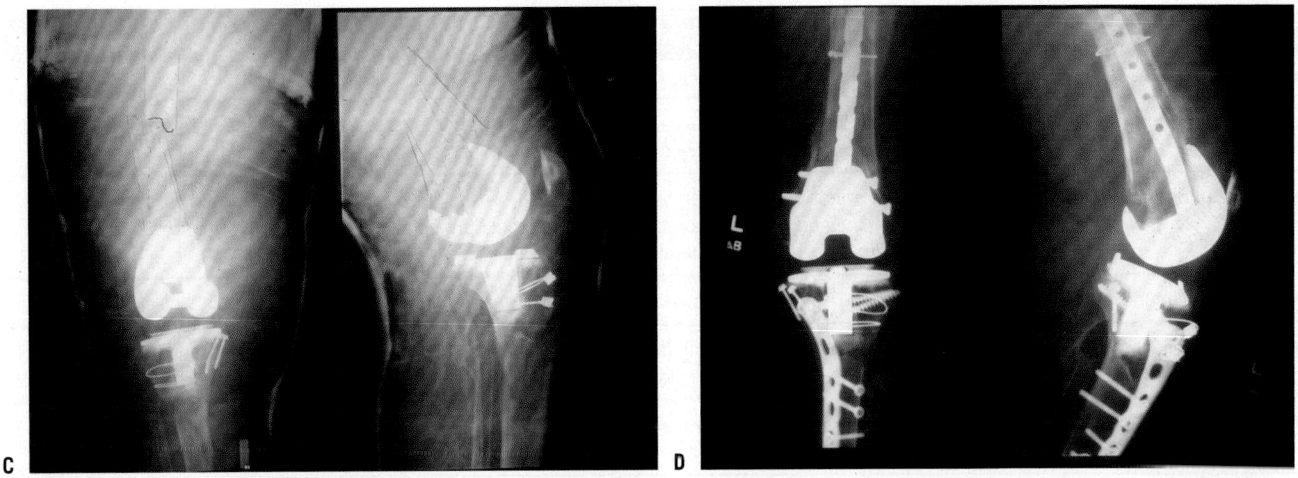

FIG 1 *(continued)* **C,D.** Illustrate periprosthetic knee fracture in a very obese patient treated with an intramedullary nail for the femur and the tibia is plated.

ANATOMY

- The femoral shaft is tubular in shape over the extent of the isthmus, gradually flaring infraisthmally into the distal femur, which is trapezoidal in cross-section.
- The entry point for the retrograde femoral nail is located at the distal end of the patellofemoral grove, just anterior to the posterior cruciate ligament insertion **(FIG 3A)**.
  - Radiographically, this is located in the midline or just medial to the midline between the condyles on the anteroposterior (AP) view and laterally just anterior to the line of Blumensaat, as it meets the trochlear grove **(FIG 3B,C)**.[5,12,14,15,19] This flat articular area has minimal to no contact with the patella until 120 degrees of flexion.[1,5]
- Pertinent proximal anatomy includes neurovascular structures anterior to the proximal femur, close to interlocking screw insertion sites.[25]
  - The femoral artery is medial to the proximal femur, with branches that cross the anterior femur more than 4 cm distal to the lesser trochanter.
  - Branches of the femoral nerve cross more proximal starting 4 cm distal to the piriformis fossa.
  - Damage to neurovascular structures caused by proximal locking screw insertion can be avoided or minimized by avoiding medial dissection and with placement at or above the lesser trochanter **(FIG 4A,B)**.

PATHOGENESIS

- Femoral shaft fractures are markers of high-energy injuries.[10,12–14,24,28]
- Studies have shown that 38% of trauma patients diagnosed with a femoral shaft fracture have additional injuries.[3,7,8,27]
  - In femur fracture patients with associated injuries, the most common findings are other musculoskeletal injuries (93%), thoracic injuries (62%), head injuries (59%), abdominal injuries (35%), and facial injuries (16%).[7]
  - Ipsilateral femoral neck fractures occur in 1% to 6% of all femoral shaft fractures and are initially missed

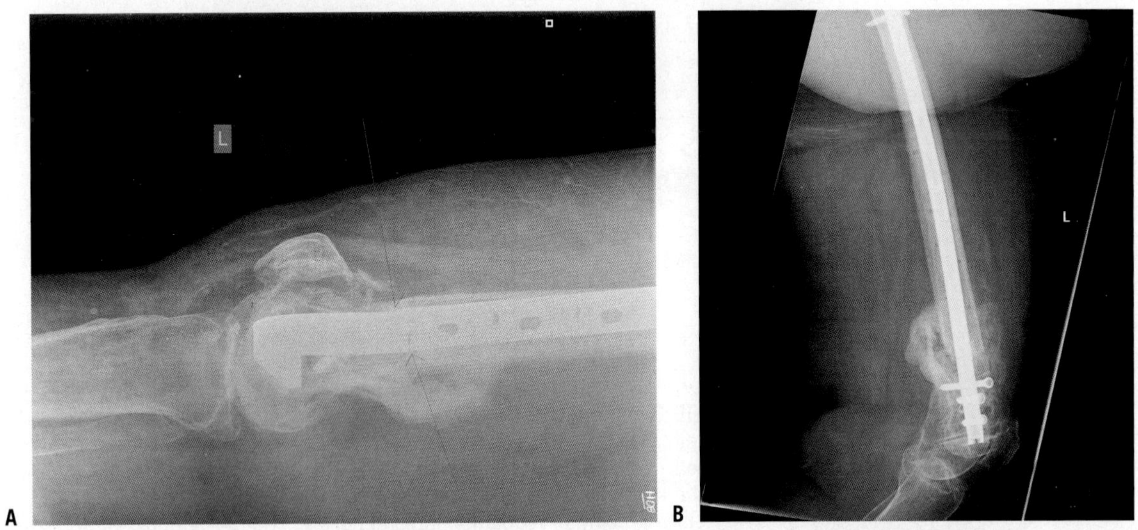

FIG 2 A. Nonunion of a distal femoral fracture with a broken plate. **B.** Intramedullary nail of the nonunion with compression of the nonunion site with stable fixation distal to the fracture.

TABLE 1 Expanded List of Relative Indications for Retrograde Intramedullary Nailing of the Femur

Indication	Rationale
All femoral shaft fractures	Shown in multiple studies to have equivalent union rates and outcomes to antegrade intramedullary nailing. Antegrade nailing is still the most common due to new less invasive techniques.
Bilateral femur fractures	Decreased overall operative time because the lower extremities can be prepared and draped together, eliminating the need to reposition for the second procedure. Limited with new techniques in 2019; more fracture dependent vs. the bilateral nature of the injury
Floating knee injuries	Single surgical approach; still a valid indication but relative not absolute
Polytrauma patient	Supine positioning without bump allows for multiple surgical team approach to patient. The radiolucent table technique has limited this indication.
Unstable spine injuries	Supine positioning without bump affords ability to maintain spine precautions throughout the procedure. The radiolucent table technique has made this more fracture dependent than spine-fracture dependent.
Acetabular or pelvic fractures	Avoids surgical incision about the hip that may limit future surgical approaches
Ipsilateral hip and femoral shaft fractures	Allows each fracture to be treated with the optimal implant
Ipsilateral femoral shaft fracture below a total hip replacement stem	Short supracondylar retrograde nails can be used to treat the fracture with a minimally invasive technique. Locked plating with a submuscular technique would be much more common in 2019.
Morbid obesity	Can be easier and more limited surgical approach but both antegrade and retrograde techniques can work well
Soft tissue wounds about the hip	Avoids surgical approach of compromised soft tissues. Burned tissue is a common example.

in up to 20% to 50% of cases.[30] Recognition of these injuries before intramedullary stabilization is important to minimize potential complications (refer to Imaging and Other Diagnostic Studies section). A preoperative computed tomography (CT) scan may be performed on each femoral neck on presentation with a femoral shaft fracture in order to rule out this associated injury. In lieu of a CT scan, some orthopaedic surgeons use cephalomedullary nails in all young patients with femoral shaft fractures to avoid missing an undisplaced femoral neck fracture **(FIG 5)**.

- All trauma patients should undergo the standard advanced trauma life support examination to rule out associated life-threatening injuries.

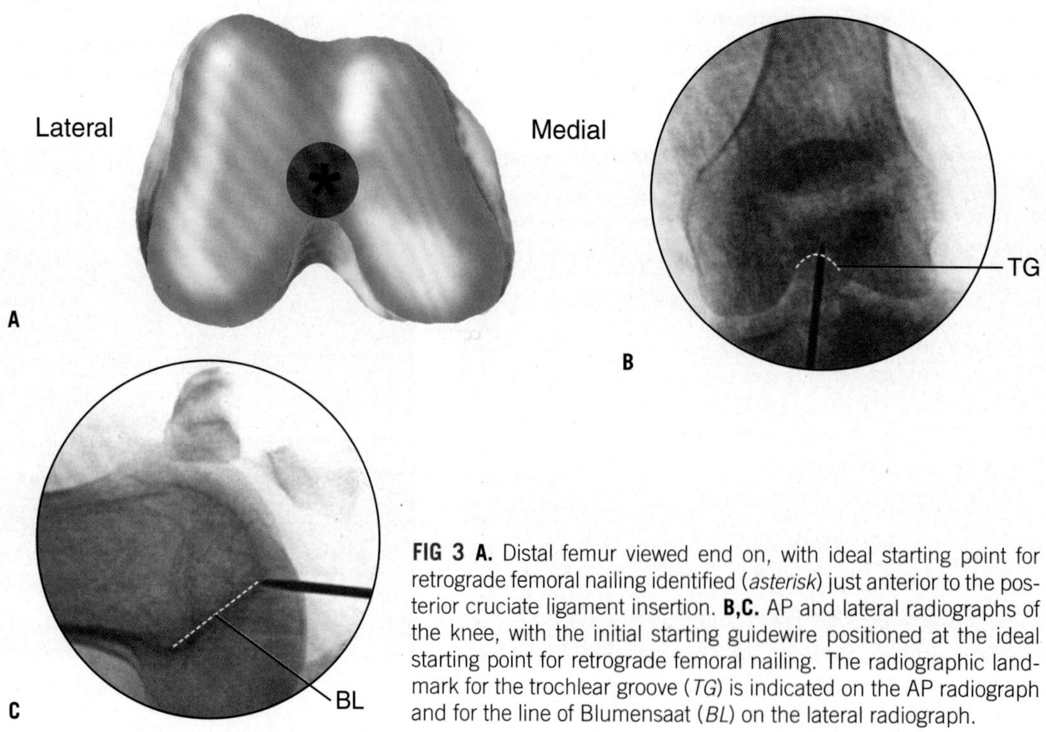

FIG 3 A. Distal femur viewed end on, with ideal starting point for retrograde femoral nailing identified (*asterisk*) just anterior to the posterior cruciate ligament insertion. **B,C.** AP and lateral radiographs of the knee, with the initial starting guidewire positioned at the ideal starting point for retrograde femoral nailing. The radiographic landmark for the trochlear groove (*TG*) is indicated on the AP radiograph and for the line of Blumensaat (*BL*) on the lateral radiograph.

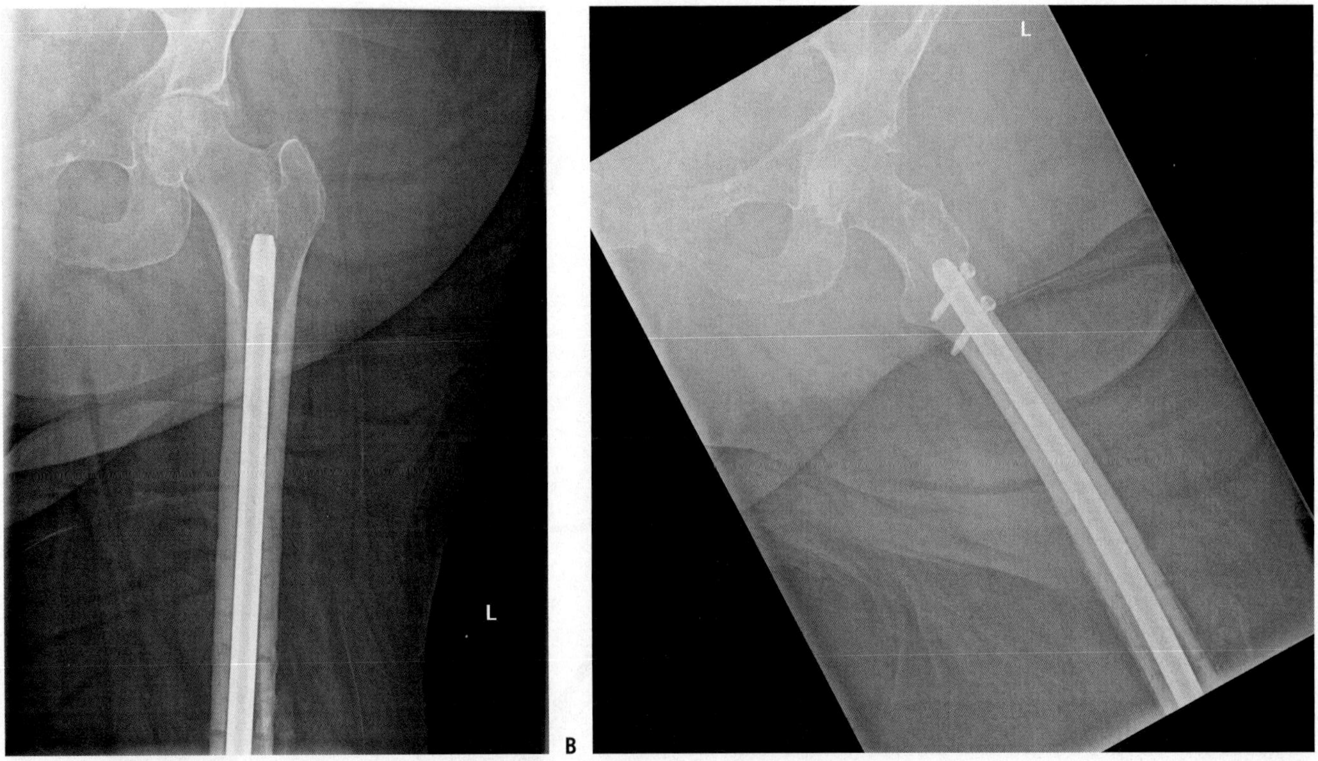

FIG 4 A. AP of proximal locking indicating the proper height at the lesser trochanter. **B.** Lateral, or slightly oblique, indicating the safe area to place the proximal screws in a retrograde nail.

- Although less common, femoral shaft fractures can occur in isolated sports injuries and in low-energy injuries associated with pathologic bone, such as with osteoporosis, metastatic bone disease, or associated bisphosphonate stress fractures.

PATIENT HISTORY AND PHYSICAL FINDINGS

- Pain and deformity of the thigh are usually obvious but may be obscured in the morbidly obese patient.
- The fractured limb should be closely examined to avoid missing any open wounds, particularly in the posterior aspect of the thigh. Skin abrasions and less obvious minor wounds should be assessed to determine if they communicate with the fracture.
- Swelling is a common finding with femoral shaft fractures. Compartment syndrome of the thigh is rare but can occur.[29]

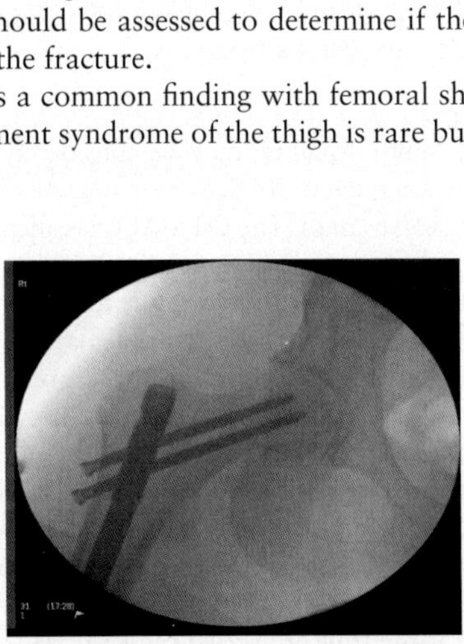

FIG 5 AP view indicates nice cephalomedullary nail as a routine for young patients with major trauma to avoid missing a subtle neck fracture.

- The entire lower extremity and pelvis needs to be evaluated because of the high rate of associated musculoskeletal injuries.
- A thorough neurologic and vascular examination must also be performed. Although femoral nerve damage is very unusual, sciatic nerve damage can occur. A complete neurologic exam must be documented preoperatively and should be repeated postoperatively.[4,6,35]
- Associated ligamentous injuries of the knee are common but may be difficult to assess until definitive stabilization of the femur has been obtained. Therefore, this examination should be repeated intraoperatively immediately after nailing the femoral shaft fracture.[32,33]

IMAGING AND OTHER DIAGNOSTIC STUDIES

- AP and lateral radiographs of the full length of the femur are essential as well as formal AP and lateral radiographs of the hip and knee. The full-length films should be one image to be certain that excessive bowing can be recognized when present.
  - Lateral knee radiographs should be closely evaluated for subtle patellar impaction fractures or nondisplaced fractures.
  - Hip radiographs should be closely examined to rule out an associated femoral neck fracture, which has been shown to occur in 1% to 6% of femoral shaft fractures.[30]
- The current recommendation is that a routine CT scan examination of the femoral neck as part of the trauma scan to rule out a femoral neck fracture. Fine cut CT are needed. Even with this specific advanced imaging, some surgeons advocate cephalomedullary nailing for these fractures.[30]
  - A reported 20% to 50% of these injuries are missed on the initial plain radiographic examination.[30]

- Because of the high association of missed coronal fractures in high-energy injuries, a CT scan of the knee should be obtained whenever formal knee radiographs reveal a supracondylar distal femur fracture, and there is consideration for retrograde nailing.[18]
  - Any coronal fractures seen on CT examination should be considered a relative contraindication for retrograde nailing owing to the possibility of compromising the distal interlocking screw fixation.

SURGICAL MANAGEMENT

Classifications and Relative Indications

- As discussed earlier, it is important to assess the extent of the fracture both proximally and distally with proper radiographs.
  - Proximally, CT scans can supplement plain radiographs to determine fracture line extension into the pertrochanteric region and to check for occult femoral neck fractures.
  - Distally, CT imaging is helpful to assess intra-articular extension and to check for coronal plane fractures.[18]
- All femoral shaft fractures, as classified by the Winquist system,[34] are technically suitable for retrograde femoral nailing **(FIG 6)**.
- Retrograde femoral nailing is considered as one option in the standard of care for treatment of midshaft femur fractures.
- It is less often used in subtrochanteric fractures, but in certain patient circumstances, a burn patient with skin issues proximally; it may be the treatment of choice **(TABLE 1)**.
  - Subtrochanteric fractures with the lesser trochanter and piriformis fossa intact, Russell-Taylor IA fracture **(FIG 7)**,[26] may be amenable to retrograde femoral nailing if other patient factors favor a retrograde approach. This would be considered a very relative indication for a retrograde nail as almost all would be treated with a cephalomedullary antegrade nail.
  - If the subtrochanteric fracture has proximal extension, including either the lesser trochanter or piriformis fossa, this would be an absolute contraindication to a retrograde nail.

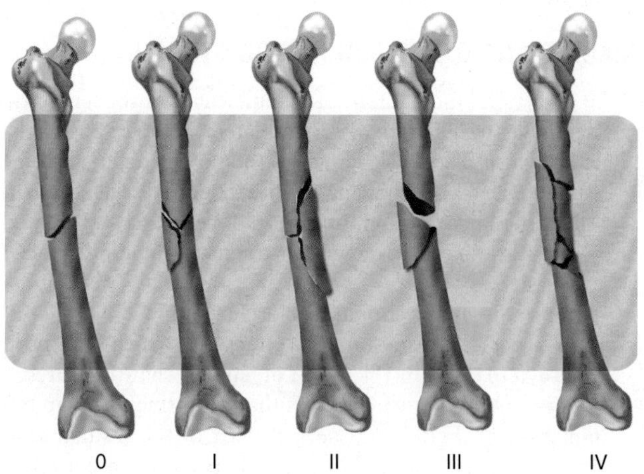

FIG 6 Winquist femoral shaft fracture classification system. All fracture patterns in this system are amenable to retrograde femoral nailing. (Reprinted with permission from Wiss DA, Brien WW, Stetson WB. Interlocked nailing for treatment of segmental fractures of the femur. J Bone Joint Surg Am 1990;72A: 724–728. Copyright © 1984 by The Journal of Bone and Joint Surgery, Incorporated.)

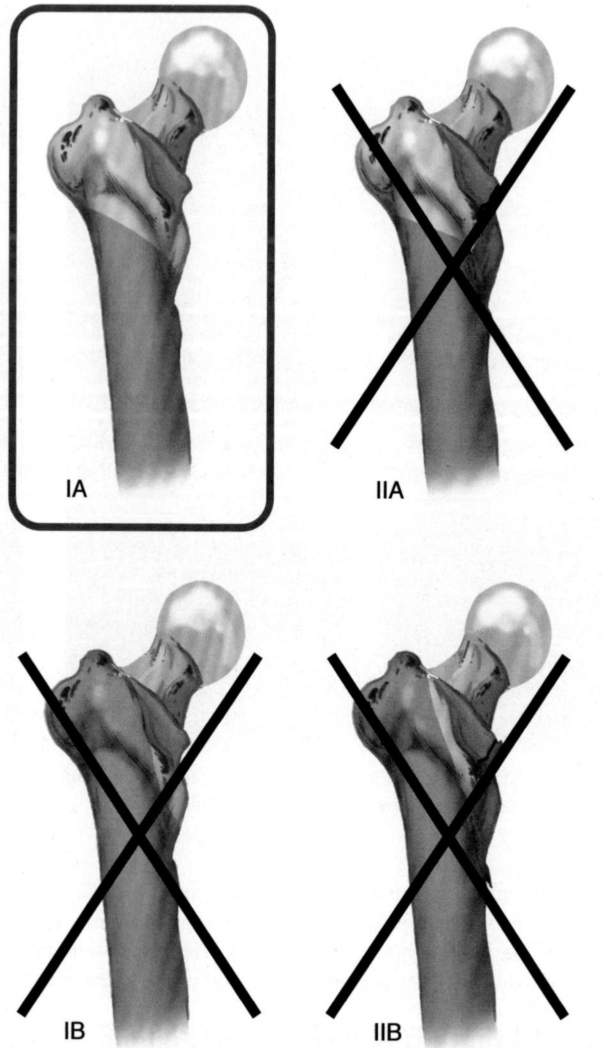

FIG 7 Russell-Taylor classification system of subtrochanteric femur fractures, with fracture patterns amenable to retrograde femoral nailing highlighted. (Reprinted from Russell TA. Subtrochanteric fractures of the femur. In: Browner B, Jupiter JB, Levine A, et al, eds. Skeletal Trauma: Basic Science, Management, and Reconstruction, ed 3. Philadelphia: Saunders, 2003:1832–1878. Copyright © 2003 Elsevier. With permission.)

- Retrograde femoral nailing may be considered in certain supracondylar distal femoral fractures (a relative indication, long locked plate versus nail). The OTA/AO classification system of distal femoral fractures[17] best elucidates which of these fractures can be addressed with retrograde femoral nailing **(FIG 8)**.
- Consideration for retrograde femoral nailing can be given for all extra-articular (A subgroup) fractures.
  - It is important to know the distance between the distal interlocking screw holes and the insertional end of the nail in the retrograde nail system that is being used.
  - The recommendation is to be able to obtain "at least" two bicortical interlocking screws below the most distal fracture line for distal fractures. Three screws are recommended if the fracture is metaphyseal, as the nail has no interference fit in this area **(FIG 9)**.
  - Nails with oblique distal interlocking options (three or four screws) can be advantageous because of increased stability and potentially less screw head prominence.

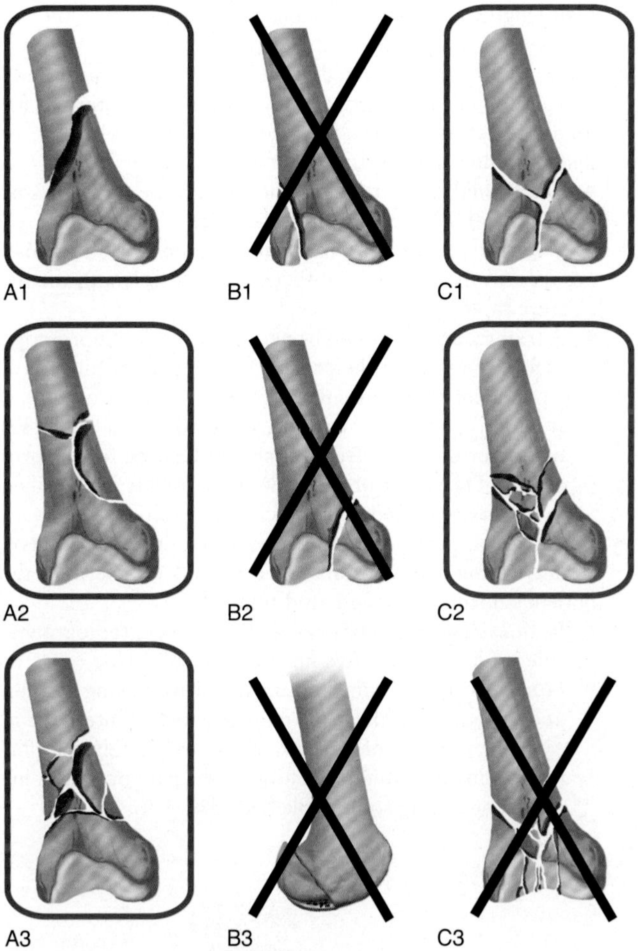

FIG 8 Müller's AO classification system of distal femoral fractures,[17] with fracture patterns amenable to retrograde femoral nailing highlighted.

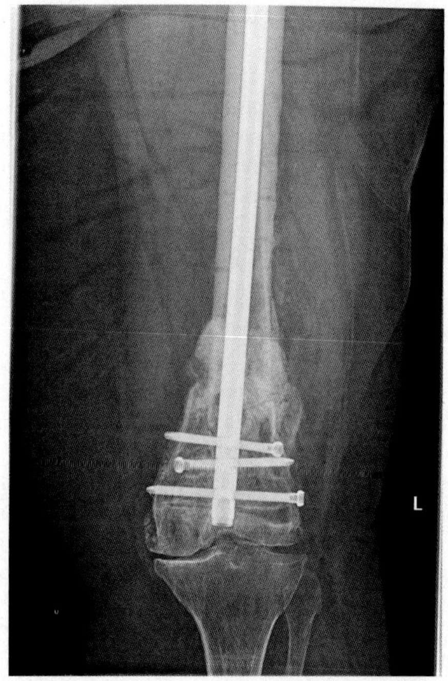

FIG 9 AP of the distal femur indicating the correct three-screw fixation in very distal fractures of the distal femur.

- Consideration for retrograde femoral nailing can be given to simple transverse articular fracture patterns (C1 and C2 subgroups).
  - This should be performed with an open medial or lateral parapatellar approach to the knee in lieu of a percutaneous approach. Articular reduction must first be obtained and then maintained with bicortical screw fixation placed outside of the planned path for the retrograde nail **(FIG 10)**.
- Partial articular fractures (all B subgroups) are a contraindication, and complex articular fractures (C3 subgroups) should not be routinely considered for retrograde femoral

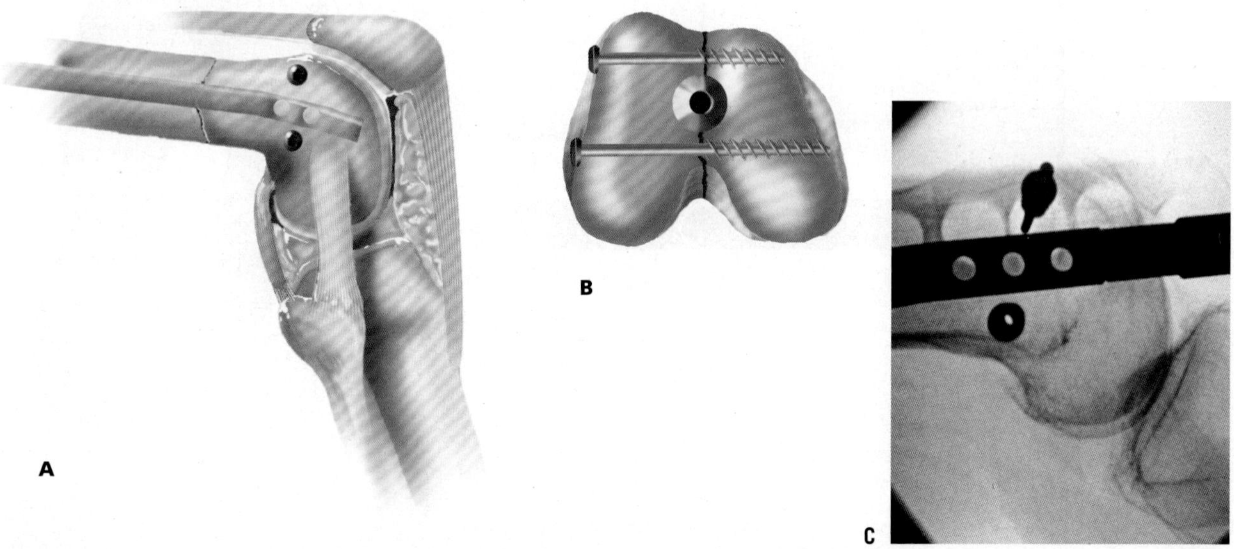

FIG 10 A. Diagram of lateral aspect of distal femur, with potential sites for intra-articular screw fixation out of the path of the retrograde femoral nail identified. **B.** Diagram of distal femur end on, with potential sites for intra-articular screw fixation out of the path of the retrograde femoral nail identified. **C.** Intraoperative lateral radiograph of a supracondylar-intracondylar (C1) distal femur fracture with intra-articular screw fixation and retrograde nail in place.

nailing but still can be considered with the right patient and surgeon combination.
- Patients with osteopenic distal fractures may be best treated with a locking screw device, whether that be a nail or a plate.
  - If a nail is chosen, those designed with multiaxial screws or the use of supplemental blocking screws may augment the distal fixation.

Contraindications to a Retrograde Nail

- Preoperative knee stiffness preventing 40 to 60 degrees of flexion
- Active knee sepsis
- Grossly contaminated soft tissue wounds about the knee remain a relative contraindication, but recent literature has shown that retrograde nailing of open fractures does not increase the incidence of postoperative knee sepsis.[23]
- Skeletally immature patients with open growth plates
- Fractures extending to the level of the lesser trochanter and more proximally unless combined with a secondary fixation device

Preoperative Planning

- AP and lateral radiographs are used to measure the diameter of the femoral canal isthmus and thus determine the approximate nail diameter. Most intramedullary nail systems come in diameters ranging from 10 to 13 mm. Typically, a 10 mm nail is large enough for most patients.
- Nail lengths are often determined intraoperatively but can be ascertained by imaging the contralateral femur.
- Radiographs are evaluated to determine the location and morphology of the fracture; they should be scrutinized for nondisplaced secondary fracture lines that could become displaced during operative treatment.
  - Occasionally, fracture fragments may be stuck in the canal and may need to be pulled out.
- In the case of fractures that show significant shortening preoperatively, it may be difficult to restore length off the fracture table.
  - A trial reduction should be performed under fluoroscopy before the start of the procedure; the patient must have a complete neuromuscular blockade for the procedure.
  - If length is difficult to restore manually, then a femoral distractor or a fracture table should be used for the procedure. Placement of the femoral distractor is described in the Fracture Reduction Techniques section.
- Before preparing and draping the injured limb, the surgeon should examine the contralateral extremity to determine the patient's normal leg length and rotation.
  - Femoral length can be evaluated by using a radiographic ruler and intraoperative fluoroscopy **(FIG 11A)**.
  - Normal rotation can be determined by flexing the hip and knee and checking the patient's normal internal and external rotation of the hip and by examining the normal resting position of the foot, as the patient lies supine on the operating room table **(FIG 11B)**.

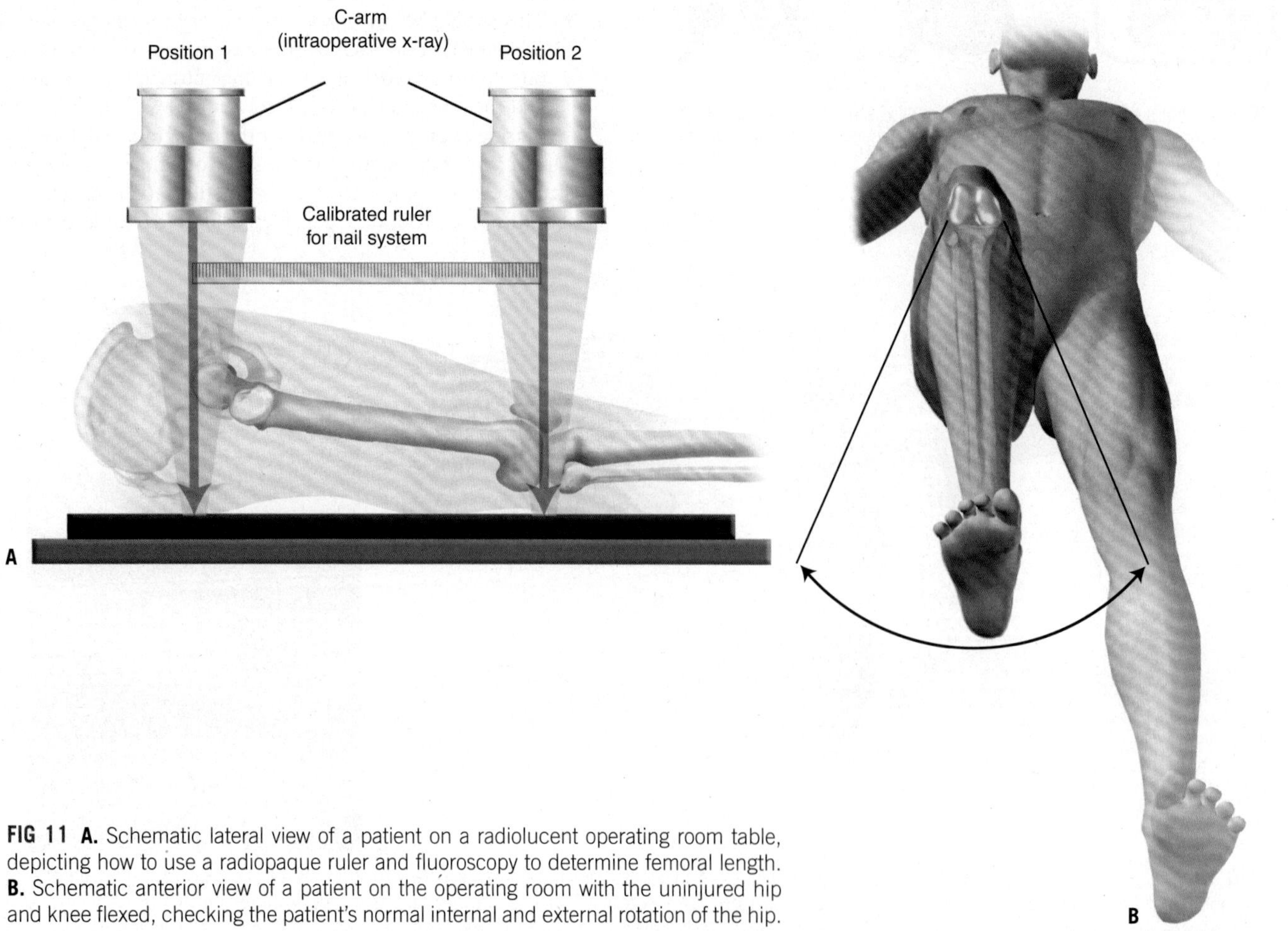

FIG 11 A. Schematic lateral view of a patient on a radiolucent operating room table, depicting how to use a radiopaque ruler and fluoroscopy to determine femoral length. **B.** Schematic anterior view of a patient on the operating room with the uninjured hip and knee flexed, checking the patient's normal internal and external rotation of the hip.

Positioning

- The patient is positioned supine on a radiolucent table (OSI fracture table or flat-top table) with no bump or a small flannel under the hip.
- A foam ramp with flannels or tenant flexible ramp, to allow maintenance of the anterior bow of the femur while reaming the femur, should be done before prepping and draping. Extension of the knee within 20 degrees of full extension must also be available to place in the proximal locking screws. Alternately, sterile triangles or bumps may be used that are removed for locking at the hip.
- The surgeon should ensure that the entire femur, from hip to knee, can be imaged on AP and lateral fluoroscopy.
- The extremity should be draped free from the anterior superior iliac spine to the ankle. The entire hip should be included in the preparation in case any femoral neck fractures are identified during or after treatment of the femoral shaft fracture.
- Radiolucent sterile towels, sheets, or a radiolucent triangle or the tenant frame are used to create a bump under the knee, allowing for about 40 to 60 degrees of knee flexion and placing the patella anterior for correct rotational alignment.[1,15]
- Intraoperative fluoroscopy should come in from the contralateral side.

Approach

- The knee should be flexed about 40 to 60 degrees to avoid injury to the proximal tibia and the patella.[15]
- Intraoperative fluoroscopy is used to obtain a perfect lateral of the knee. The line of Blumensaat should be clearly identified (see **FIG 3C**).
- A radiopaque guidewire can be used to identify the center of the long axis of the femur in order to determine the correct level of the skin incision.
- The guide pin is used to center a 1.5- to 2.5-cm incision just medial to the midline.
- A medial parapatellar incision is created using subcutaneous dissection. A medial peritendinous arthrotomy is then made to allow entrance of the initial starting guidewire into the intracondylar notch.

TECHNIQUES

PLACING THE GUIDEWIRE

- The surgeon confirms the correct placement of the initial starting guidewire on the AP and lateral fluoroscopic radiographs.
  - On the lateral image, the initial starting guidewire should be situated at the apex of the line of Blumensaat, in line with the femoral shaft (see **FIG 3C**).
  - On the AP image, the guidewire should be centered or just medial to the midline in the trochlear groove, in line with the femoral shaft (see **FIG 3B**).
  - On the AP image, the fluoroscope is moved proximally to be certain the guidewire is directed at the center of the canal.
- When starting to drill the initial guidewire, the surgeon's hand should drop slightly to prevent the wire from falling into the posterior cruciate ligament insertion; the hand is raised once the wire enters the cortex, so as to be in line with the femoral shaft.
- Once the initial starting guidewire is centered on the AP and lateral images, the wire is passed into the distal femoral shaft.
- A soft tissue retractor is placed over the initial starting guidewire to protect the patellar tendon during reaming.

CREATING AND REAMING THE STARTING HOLE

- The initial starting reamer is used to create the starting hole. (Alternatively, an awl or a step drill can be used to make the starting hole using the principles described earlier.)
- Once the starting hole has been made, a reduction tool is used to reduce and pass by the fracture site. A ball-tip guidewire is passed to the level of the femur above the lesser trochanter.

FRACTURE REDUCTION TECHNIQUES

- Traction is used to restore length. The surgeon must ensure that adequate anesthesia (full paralysis) is employed.
- There are many deforming muscle forces, depending on the level of the fracture. If the fracture cannot be reduced by manual traction, use of bumps, pulling with sheets wrapped around the proximal or distal thigh, or pushing with mallets plus an intramedullary reduction device plus the right flexion in the ramp usually allows nice reduction.
  - The iliopsoas muscle will flex and internally rotate proximal-third femoral shaft fractures by its pull on the lesser trochanter. Inserting a unicortical 5-mm Schanz pin through a percutaneous incision in the lateral cortex just above the fracture or in the greater trochanter can gain excellent control of the proximal fracture fragment.
- Distal fractures tend to angulate into recurvatum through the pull of the gastrocnemius muscle. Bumps placed under the knee to flex the knee can help relax the gastrocnemius muscle. One can also use blocking screws in distal fractures to surgically create a narrow "canal" in the metaphyseal region in line with the canal of the femoral shaft so that the

intramedullary reduction device can help with reduction of the fracture.

- The following techniques are less common but can prove useful:
  - The abductor muscles will abduct and externally rotate the proximal femur after high subtrochanteric and proximal shaft fractures. Inserting a unicortical 5-mm Schanz pin through a percutaneous incision in the lateral cortex just above the fracture or in the greater trochanter can gain excellent control of the proximal fracture fragment.
  - The adductor muscles span most shaft fractures and exert a strong axial and adduction force. Sometimes, midshaft transverse fractures can be the most difficult to reduce. Inserting a unicortical 5-mm Schanz pin through a percutaneous incision in the lateral cortex just above and just below the fracture can gain excellent control of the proximal and distal fracture fragments.
- Alternatively, a femoral distractor can assist with obtaining and maintaining fracture reduction for a fracture at any level. It can be placed laterally, inserted proximally at the greater trochanter, and distally in either the posterior aspect of the femoral condyle or in the proximal tibia. Alternatively, some surgeons recommend anterior placement to avoid potential posterior angulation of distal fracture patterns.
- Lastly, some fractures require opening of the fracture site to obtain reduction, with the finding of the muscle interposed within the fracture. We recommend laterally based incisions unless otherwise dictated by an open fracture wound.
- Restoration of length and correct rotation can be assessed clinically as well as radiographically by closely scrutinizing the diameter of the medial and lateral femoral cortex, ensuring they are of equal diameter proximal and distal to the fracture.
- If a radiolucent table or extension table is used, one can examine rotation intraoperatively once one locking screw has been inserted proximally and distally. This can allow corrections if required and is a major advantage over a fracture table in "hard to align" fractures.

PASSING THE GUIDEWIRE

- Once the fracture is reduced on the AP and lateral images, the surgeon passes the guidewire to end just below the level of the piriformis fossa.
- If translation is present at the fracture site, most systems have an intramedullary alignment guide that can be used to pass the guidewire after reaming the distal segment.
- A ball-tip guidewire is used to ensure that reaming is performed past the level of the lesser trochanter because the reamers stop at the ball-tipped portion of the guidewire.

REAMING

- Reaming should begin with an end-cutting reamer (typically size 8 or 9 mm in diameter).
- Fracture reduction must be maintained throughout the reaming process to minimize eccentric reaming.
- Reaming should be performed slowly with a low-pressure and low-temperature, acorn-shaped designed reamers in 0.5-mm increments to prevent thermal necrosis.
- Alternately, a reamer irrigator aspirator device can be used as a one pass reamer to ream and also gather bone graft. This technique is used primarily to obtain bone graft and not recommended in acute fractures unless a patient's lung function is severely compromised.
- The approximate nail diameter is selected based on the preoperative measurement of the femoral isthmus. The final nail diameter should be selected based on the size of the reamer that provides the initial cortical chatter. It should also be the nail size that allows a minimum diameter of 5.0-mm locking screws to reduce the incidence of broken screws.
- The canal is reamed to 1.5 to 2.0 mm over the selected nail diameter depending on the make of the nail.
- Nail length can be determined multiple ways:
  - A radiolucent ruler can be placed on the anterior aspect of the femur. The nail should end above the level of the lesser trochanter on the AP radiograph and should be measured so that it is deep to the apex of the line of Blumensaat on the lateral view (see **FIG 3C**).
  - Alternatively, a second guidewire of the same length can be inserted into the knee to end just deep to the apex of the line of Blumensaat on the lateral fluoroscopic image.
    - This additional guidewire is clamped at the level of the guidewire already in place.
    - The portion distal to the guidewire in place is measured to equal the amount of guidewire in the femoral canal (**TECH FIG 1**).
  - In addition, many nailing systems have "system-specific reverse measurement guides" that are outlined in their

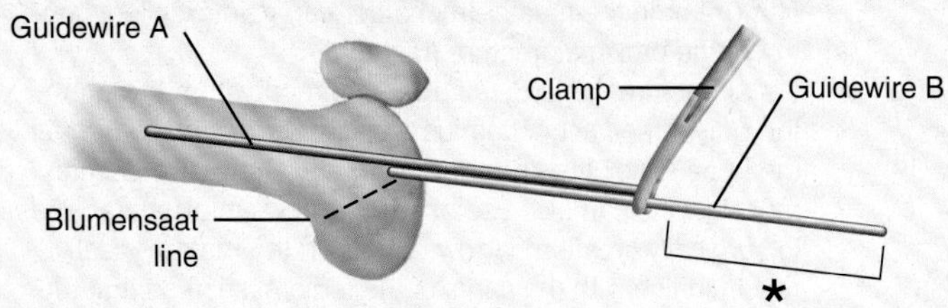

TECH FIG 1 Schematic diagram of a lateral view of the knee, obtaining femoral length measurement using the two-guidewire technique. The amount of guidewire B (*asterisk*) indicated by the bracket equals the amount of guidewire A in the femoral canal.

technique manuals. The lateral x-ray is the most important x-ray to determine leg length, as the nail must be countersunk proximal to the apex of the line of Blumensaat to ensure subchondral placement.

- If the measurement is between nail sizes, the shorter nail is selected. End caps are rarely used, as they tend to make nail removal much more difficult.

PLACING THE NAIL

- Once the nail size is selected, the nail is inserted over the guidewire.
- Most current systems allow the ball-tip guidewire to pass through the cannulated nail. If an older system is being used, then the ball-tip guidewire must be exchanged for a smooth-tip guidewire using an exchange tube.
- If guidewire exchange is required, the surgeon ensures correct placement of the smooth-tip guidewire on the AP and lateral images before nail insertion.
- The nail is inserted over the guidewire and should pass relatively easily.
  - If the nail does not advance easily, the surgeon performs a careful AP and lateral fluoroscopic assessment of the fracture reduction and nail placement.
- Nail insertion depth is assessed on the lateral knee radiograph.
  - The nail should end proximal to the apex of the line of Blumensaat to ensure subchondral placement **(TECH FIG 2A)**.
- The surgeon confirms that fracture length and alignment have been restored on the AP and lateral radiographs.
- The surgeon confirms that the nail length selected puts the proximal tip of the nail ending at or above the level of the lesser trochanter **(TECH FIG 2B)**.
  - The nail is advanced if the proximal tip does not end at or above the level of the lesser trochanter.
  - If this leaves the nail countersunk, end caps can be selected to gain nail length but are rarely used by most surgeons, as it makes removal much more difficult.
  - Care must be taken to remain below the piriformis fossa to avoid proximal nail protrusion.
- The nail is locked distally using the distal interlocking guides.
  - We typically use one lateral to medial distal interlocking screw for transverse midshaft femoral fractures, and a second anterolateral to posteromedial distal interlocking screw for comminuted or distal femoral fractures.
  - A third screw is used for distal femoral fractures running from anteromedial to distal lateral for triangular fixation (see **FIG 9**).
  - Using live fluoroscopy, the fluoroscopic machine is rotated about the knee to assess the length of the

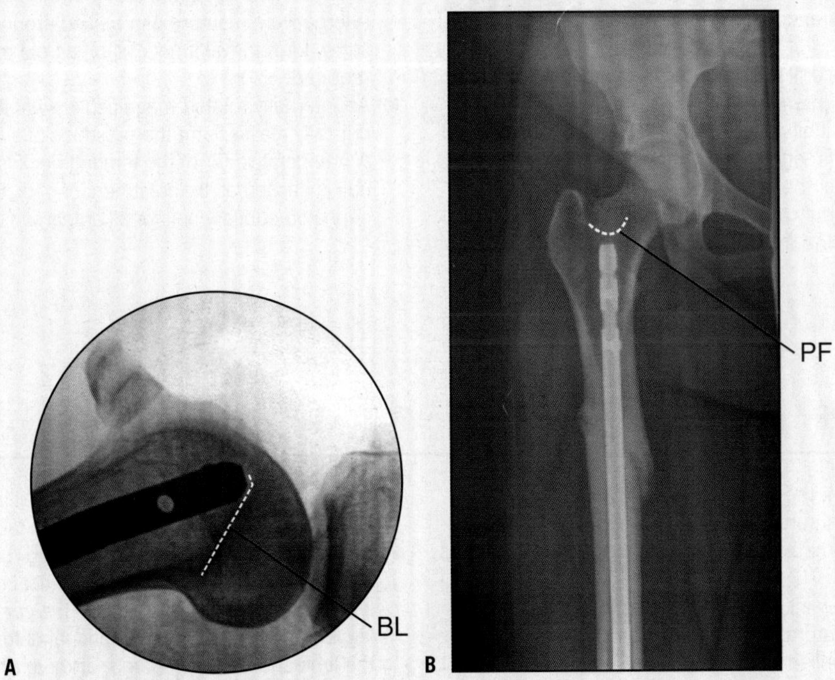

TECH FIG 2 **A.** Postoperative lateral radiograph of the knee, showing correct retrograde femoral nail insertion depth deep to the line of Blumensaat (*BL*). **B.** Postoperative AP radiograph of the hip, showing correct retrograde femoral nail insertion depth above the lesser trochanter of the femur but below the radiographic landmark for the piriformis fossa (*PF*).

interlocking screws. Because of the trapezoidal shape of the distal femur, screws are often prominent but not well recognized on the AP radiograph.
- The surgeon could consider using washers, a medial locking nut, or a locking end cap (which locks the most distal interlocking screw to the nail) as option for osteoporotic bone. These are not usually required with more modern nail design.
- Once distal interlocking screw fixation is complete, the surgeon reassesses the fracture reduction fluoroscopically.
  - If any shortening has occurred, length can be regained by manual traction or by backslapping the nail with the insertion guide nail removal attachment (the surgeon must exercise caution when using this technique in patients with osteoporotic bone).

SCREW FIXATION

- Proximal interlocking screw fixation is performed in the anterior to posterior plane using the freehand perfect circle technique.[7]
- First, a magnified AP image of the proximal femur is obtained.
- The fluoroscopy machine is rotated until the proximal interlocking hole is seen as a "perfect circle" (also discussed in Chap. 41, Antegrade Intramedullary Nailing of the Femur; Tech Fig 4, Distal interlocking screw placement).
- A 2-cm incision is made in the proximal aspect of the thigh, anteriorly centered over the two proximal interlocking holes, as visualized on the AP radiograph.
- Careful blunt dissection exposes the anterior femur.
- The drill tip should have a nonslip pointed tip to avoid slipping on the hard cortical bone of the proximal femur. The pointed soft tissue guides from large external fixation systems can be used to prevent slipping off of the anterior cortex.
- The femoral artery lies 1 cm medial to the femur at the level of the lesser trochanter, so the surgeon must avoid slipping off the femur medially.
- Once the drill passes through the first cortex, it is removed from the drill bit to confirm radiographically that it will pass though the nail by the appearance of a perfect circle within the proximal interlocking hole.
- Small changes in the drill angle can be made to ensure correct passage through the interlocking hole.
- With a mallet, the drill bit can be gently tapped through the nail hole. The drill is then reattached to complete drilling through the posterior aspect of the proximal femur.
- Because of the proximity of the sciatic nerve, care should be taken to ensure that the drill is not advanced too far past the posterior cortex.
- Before removing the drill, the surgeon must reconfirm correct rotational alignment by flexing the hip and knee and assessing the hip's internal and external rotation profile.
  - It is compared with the normal internal and external rotation of the contralateral uninjured hip that was examined preoperatively.
- Screw length measurement can be confirmed with a frog-leg lateral or a true lateral view with flexing of the hip to clear the contralateral leg.
- Two proximal interlocking screws should be used for all fractures.
  - The usual length of the proximal interlocking screw is 25 to 35 mm.
  - A second proximal interlocking screw should be used to reduce the chance of implant failure and must be used for more proximal fracture patterns. The author would suggest using a minimum of two screws proximally and distally for all locked intramedullary nails.
- A locking screwdriver, locked into the screw head, should be used to avoid losing the screw in the proximal soft tissues. Alternatively, a suture can be tied around the head of the screw for retrieval if necessary; an old method but works well if required.
- An internally rotated magnified view of the hip is obtained to critically reassess for the presence of a femoral neck fracture. A preoperative CT of the femoral neck is a must if a retrograde nail is chosen as the treatment of choice. The author uses a cephalomedullary nail for all antegrade nails.

WOUND CLOSURE

- After wound irrigation, the knee fascial layer is closed with a 0 or 1-0 absorbable suture. The subcutaneous layer is then closed with 2-0 absorbable suture. The skin can then be closed with surgical staples.
- The interlocking screw incisions can be closed with 2-0 absorbable subcutaneous sutures and skin staples.
- Soft dressings are applied.
- Before undraping the patient, the rotational alignment and length should be checked against measurements made on the unoperated limb preoperatively. If any leg length discrepancy or rotational deformity is appreciated, the limb should be corrected by changing the proximal interlocking screw or screws (if an OSI table or radiolucent table is used).
- If a fracture table and traction is used, before moving the patient off the operating table, it is critical to assess the achieved length and rotation compared to the contralateral limb. If any leg length discrepancy or rotational deformity is appreciated, the limb should be prepared, draped, and corrected by changing the proximal interlocking screws. This should be rare on a radiolucent table if the step earlier is performed.
- A repeat examination of knee stability is performed at the same time interval to determine knee stability.

Pearls and Pitfalls

Fracture Reduction	• The surgeon should request full relaxation with anesthesia to facilitate length restoration. • The surgeon should beware of the potential for shortening of the femur with retrograde insertion. Before placing the proximal interlocking screws, the surgeon should scrutinize the intraoperative radiographs of the fracture site to ensure that correct length has been obtained. Length may be regained by using the femoral distractor, or by using the guide to backslap the nail after distal interlocking screw placement, or by manual traction.
Nail Insertion: Avoiding Poor Starting Direction	• The surgeon should ensure that the initial starting guidewire is centered in line with the femoral shaft on the AP and lateral images. Due to the overhang of the posterior condyles, there is a tendency to err too far posterior because of the normal valgus of the distal end of the femur, there is a tendency to aim too medial, and a varus deformity can be created.
Nail Insertion: Avoiding Slipping Off	• When starting to drill the initial guidewire, the surgeon should drop his or her hand slightly to prevent the wire from falling into the posterior cruciate ligament insertion; the hand is raised once the surgeon enters the cortex, so as to be in line with the femoral shaft.
Nail Insertion: Avoiding Distal Nail Prominence	• Before inserting the distal interlocking screws, the surgeon should confirm the subchondral position of the nail on the lateral intraoperative radiograph just deep to the apex of the line at Blumensaat (see **TECH FIG 2A**).
Nail Insertion: Problems with Proximal Locking Screws	• The proximal femoral cortex is thick and strong. It is easy to strip proximal locking screws during their insertion. If difficulties are encountered on insertion, the surgeon should replace it with a new screw. This can help avoid significant issues if screw or nail removal is ever required.
Use of Distal End Cap	• Some systems have a locking distal end cap that can lock the most distal screw in place; this is a useful feature for osteoporotic bone. • End caps are not used (or very rarely) at this time. • Nail removal is accomplished by placing the threaded pin into the nail on AP and lateral views. • Take out the screws closest to the removal end. Ream over the pin. • Place in the guide rod and insert the nail extractor. Once seated, take out the screws on the other end of the nail. • This sequence permits seating of the extractor without rotating the nail. • As with any nail insertion, if an end cap is used, it should be specifically mentioned in the operative note for review in the event of future screw or nail removal.
Avoiding Distal Interlocking Screw Prominence	• Before removing the insertion jig, the distal femur is rotated under live fluoroscopy to evaluate the length of the distal interlocking screws. Screw length changes are made if necessary. • Accurate measurement for locking screws minimizes postoperative hardware irritation. • Off-axis screws are used when the option is available, particularly in very distal fractures of the femur.
Associated Injuries	• The surgeon should always check the preoperative images and intraoperative C-arm images for ipsilateral fractures of the femoral neck. • Cephalomedullary nails are used for most femoral fractures to prevent issues going forward, particularly with respect to the femoral neck. • The surgeon should remember to do a knee ligamentous examination after the femoral fracture is stabilized. • When using an associated simultaneous hip screw side plate implant, the surgeon should try to overlap proximal hardware for improved mechanical properties and to avoid a stress riser.[11]
Specific Fracture	• **TABLE 2** lists alternative techniques patterns.

POSTOPERATIVE CARE

- Physical therapy for active and passive knee range of motion may be started on the first postoperative day, as can ambulation.
- Weight bearing is prescribed based on the fracture pattern and associated injuries. For most femoral shaft fractures, even those with comminution, weight bearing as tolerated can be safely initiated in the immediate postoperative period.
- Routine postoperative deep vein thrombosis prophylaxis, such as low-molecular-weight heparin, may be safely initiated on postoperative day 1 and prescribed for 6 weeks, thereafter.
- Twenty-four hours of antibiotic prophylaxis is standard for closed fractures. Patients with open fractures remain on antibiotics for 48 to 72 hours after the final intraoperative débridement has been performed.

OUTCOMES

- The long-term effects of retrograde nailing on knee function are not known, but recent literature reports that knee function following retrograde and antegrade nailing to stabilize femoral shaft fractures was comparable.[2]
- Two prospective, randomized trials comparing reamed antegrade and retrograde nailing of femoral shaft fractures showed no difference in knee pain or knee function at time of fracture union.[20,31] As expected, early postoperative knee pain was higher in the retrograde femoral nailing groups,

TABLE 2 Alternative Techniques

Fracture Type	Pros	Cons	Technique
Ipsilateral femoral shaft and neck fractures	Optimal fixation for each fracture pattern	Two separate surgical procedures and implants	Stabilize hip fracture first, using cannulated screws or dynamic hip screw. Select four-hole side plate to overlap nail placement. Do not fill distal holes until after femoral nail is placed. Select femoral nail length to end at or above lesser trochanter.[22]
Subtrochanteric femoral shaft fractures	Antegrade percutaneous treatment compared to plating techniques; lower incidence of malunion than antegrade nailing technique[9,20]	Less stable proximal fixation	Use small lateral incisions at the level of the fracture to place pointed reduction clamps without muscle stripping in fracture reduction. Place two proximal cephalomedullary screws.
Periprosthetic fractures below a hip stem	Percutaneous treatment compared to plating techniques Plating is preferred by many using long plates and a submuscular approach.	Stress riser created between end of hip stem and nail	Standard technique except for shorter nail insertion If a nail is chosen, a short anterior plate may be required to reduce the stress riser effect between the nail and the femoral prosthesis.
Supracondylar femur fractures	Percutaneous treatment compared to plating techniques	Longer times to union Less stable implants than with current locking plate	Judicious use of blocking screws to ensure center placement of guidewire, reamer, and nail; important to maintain alignment during reaming
Supracondylar femur fractures with a simple sagittal fracture	Percutaneous treatment compared to plating techniques	Longer times to union has been reported. Less stable implants than with current locking plate, which may be good in some cases	As earlier, with an open parapatellar approach to knee to ensure anatomic knee reduction. (Refer to **FIG 10** for screw placement.)
Periprosthetic fractures above a total knee	Percutaneous treatment compared to plating techniques	Limited points of distal fixation, but relative stability may be a positive feature	Preoperatively, determine if femoral component has open box design; routine nail insertion technique There are charts that will note the diameter of open boxes for each type of total knee system.
Ipsilateral femoral shaft and tibial shaft fractures ("floating knee injuries")	Single approach and incision for treatment of both injuries	None	Routine insertion technique Always do the femur first and then the tibia.

but by the time of union, there was no significant difference between the two approaches.

- Fracture healing rates seem to be equivalent except in the more distal supracondylar femur fractures, which have taken longer to achieve union with antegrade nails, and even with retrograde nails, the healing is slower. The retrograde nailing technique, when used on all femoral shaft fractures appears to produce slightly higher malunion rates, with external rotation, shortening, and distal varus malalignment being the most common deformities.[21,24,31]

COMPLICATIONS

- The most common complications can often be prevented with meticulous surgical techniques.
  - Paying close attention to the proper nail insertion starting point and ensuring that the distal portion of the nail remains subchondral are two key technical points to avoiding potential knee problems.
- Distal interlocking screw prominence is common, and a relatively high percentage of patients elect to have these removed as a secondary procedure.[20,21,24]
- Malunions can be avoided when blocking screws are used judiciously for the more distal fracture patterns. Close attention is paid to ensure that the fracture reduction is first obtained and then maintained during the entire reaming process.
- Shortening and malrotation can be readily assessed at the end of the procedure and corrected immediately by revising placement of the proximal interlocking screws.
- Selecting larger diameter nails with a minimal screw diameter of 5 mm, based on feedback of cortical chatter during reaming, seems to improve union rates when the retrograde nailing technique is used.
- Subtrochanteric fractures have occurred after retrograde femoral nailing.[16] Usually, an exchange to an antegrade cephalomedullary nail is performed to provide stability for the old fracture and the new complication.

ACKNOWLEDGMENT

- We gratefully acknowledge the contributions of Laura S. Phieffer and Ronald Lakatos for portions of this chapter written for the previous edition of this book.

REFERENCES

1. Aglietti P, Insall JN, Walker PS, et al. A new patella prosthesis: design and application. Clin Orthop Relat Res 1975;107:175–187.
2. Andrzejewski K, Panasiuk M, Grzegorzewski A. Comparison of knee function in patients with a healed fracture of the femoral shaft fixed with retrograde and antegrade intramedullary nailing. Ortop Traumatol Rehabil 2013;15(5):395–405.
3. Arneson TJ, Melton LJ III, Lewallen DG, et al. Epidemiology of diaphyseal and distal femoral fractures in Rochester, Minnesota, 1965–1984. Clin Orthop Relat Res 1988;234:188–194.
4. Britton JM, Dunkerley DR. Closed nailing of a femoral fracture followed by sciatic nerve palsy. J Bone Joint Surg Br 1990;72B:318.
5. Carmack DB, Moed BR, Kingston C, et al. Identification of the optimal intercondylar starting point for retrograde femoral nailing: an anatomic study. J Trauma 2003;55:692–695.
6. Christie J, Court-Brown C, Kinninmonth AW, et al. Intramedullary locking nails in the management of femoral shaft fractures. J Bone Joint Surg Br 1988;70B:206–210.
7. Court-Brown CM. Femoral diaphyseal fractures. In: Browner B, Jupiter JB, Levine A, et al, eds. Skeletal Trauma: Basic Science, Management, and Reconstruction, ed 3. Philadelphia: Saunders, 2003:1879–1956.
8. Court-Brown CM, Rimmer S, Prakash U, et al. The epidemiology of open long bone fractures. Injury 1998;29:529–534.
9. French BG, Tornetta P III. Use of an interlocked cephalomedullary nail for subtrochanteric fracture stabilization. Clin Orthop Relat Res 1998;348:95–100.
10. Gregory P, DiCicco J, Karpik K, et al. Ipsilateral fractures of the femur and tibia: treatment with retrograde femoral nailing and unreamed tibial nailing. J Orthop Trauma 1996;10:309–316.
11. Harris T, Ruth JT, Szivek J, et al. The effect of implant overlap on the mechanical properties of the femur. J Trauma 2003;54:930–935.
12. Herscovici D Jr, Whiteman KW. Retrograde nailing of the femur using an intercondylar approach. Clin Orthop Relat Res 1996;332:98–104.
13. Moed BR, Watson JT. Retrograde intramedullary nailing, without reaming, of fractures of the femoral shaft in multiply injured patients. J Bone Joint Surg Am 1995;77A:1520–1527.
14. Moed BR, Watson JT, Cramer KE, et al. Unreamed retrograde intramedullary nailing of fractures of the femoral shaft. J Orthop Trauma 1998;12:334–342.
15. Morgan E, Ostrum RF, DiCicco J, et al. Effects of retrograde femoral intramedullary nailing on the patellofemoral articulation. J Orthop Trauma 1999;13:13–16.
16. Mounasamy V, Mallu S, Khanna V, et al. Subtrochanteric fractures after retrograde femoral nailing. World J Orthop 2015;6(9):738–743.
17. Müller ME, Nazarian S, Koch P, et al. The Comprehensive Classification of Fractures of Long Bones. Heidelberg, Germany: Springer-Verlag, 1990.
18. Nork SE, Segina DN, Aflatoon K, et al. The association between supracondylar-intercondylar distal femoral fractures and coronal plane fractures. J Bone Joint Surg Am 2005;87A:564–569.
19. Ostrum RF. Retrograde femoral nailing: indications and techniques. Op Tech Orthop 2003;13:79–84.
20. Ostrum RF, Agarwal A, Lakatos R, et al. Prospective comparison of retrograde and antegrade femoral intramedullary nailing. J Orthop Trauma 2000;14:496–501.
21. Ostrum RF, DiCicco J, Lakatos R, et al. Retrograde intramedullary nailing of femoral diaphyseal fractures. J Orthop Trauma 1998;12:464–468.
22. Ostrum RF, Tornetta P III, Watson JT, et al. Ipsilateral proximal femur and shaft fractures treated with hip screws and a reamed retrograde intramedullary nail. Clin Orthop Relat Res 2013;472(9):2751–2758.
23. O'Toole RV, Riche K, Cannada LK, et al. Analysis of postoperative knee sepsis after retrograde nail insertion of open femoral shaft fractures. Orthop Trauma 2010;24(11):677–682.
24. Ricci WM, Bellabarba C, Evanoff B, et al. Retrograde versus antegrade nailing of femoral shaft fractures. J Orthop Trauma 2001;15:161–169.
25. Riina J, Tornetta P III, Ritter C, et al. Neurologic and vascular structures at risk during anterior-posterior locking of retrograde femoral nails. J Orthop Trauma 1998;12:379–381.
26. Russell TA. Subtrochanteric fractures of the femur. In: Browner B, Jupiter JB, Levine A, et al, eds. Skeletal Trauma: Basic Science, Management, and Reconstruction, ed 3. Philadelphia: Saunders, 2003:1832–1878.
27. Salminen ST, Pihlajamaki HK, Avikainen VJ, et al. Population-based epidemiologic and morphologic study of femoral shaft fractures. Clin Orthop Relat Res 2000;372:241–249.
28. Sanders R, Koval KJ, DiPasquale T, et al. Retrograde reamed femoral nailing. J Orthop Trauma 1993;7:293–302.
29. Schwartz JT Jr, Brumback RJ, Lakatos R, et al. Acute compartment syndrome of the thigh: a spectrum of injury. J Bone Joint Surg Am 1989;71A:392–400.
30. Tornetta P III, Kain MS, Creevy WR. Diagnosis of femoral neck fractures in patients with a femoral shaft fracture: improvement with a standard protocol. J Bone Joint Surg Am 2007;89A:39–43.
31. Tornetta P III, Tiburzi D. Antegrade or retrograde reamed femoral nailing: a prospective, randomised trial. J Bone Joint Surg Br 2000;82B:652–654.
32. Vangsness CT Jr, DeCampos J, Merritt PO, et al. Meniscal injury associated with femoral shaft fractures: an arthroscopic evaluation of incidence. J Bone Joint Surg Br 1993;75B:207–209.
33. Walling AK, Seradge H, Spiegel PG. Injuries to the knee ligaments with fractures of the femur. J Bone Joint Surg Am 1982;64A:1324–1327.
34. Winquist RA, Hansen ST, Clawson DK. Closed intramedullary nailing of femoral fractures: a report of 520 cases. J Bone Joint Surg Am 1984;66A:529–539.
35. Wiss DA, Brien WW, Stetson WB. Interlocked nailing for treatment of segmental fractures of the femur. J Bone Joint Surg Am 1990;72A:724–728.

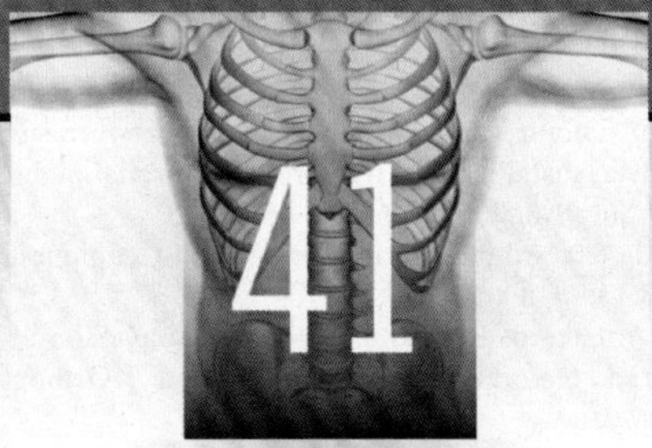

CHAPTER 41

Antegrade Intramedullary Nailing of the Femur

Patrick K. Cronin, John G. Esposito, and Mitchel B. Harris

DEFINITION

- A femoral shaft fracture is any fracture of the femoral diaphysis originating from 5 cm below the lesser trochanter to within 6 to 8 cm of the distal femoral articular surface.
  - Fractures whose essential fracture element is diaphyseal with an extension into the outer regions are different from fractures whose essential fracture element is subtrochanteric or supracondylar with extension into the diaphysis.
  - This essential "personality" of a fracture is important to keep in mind as it may inform treatment decisions and surgical approach. In some circumstances, proximal and/or distal femur involvement may warrant a different treatment (ie, lateral approach, plate fixation, etc.) as opposed to the more traditional intramedullary nailing.
- For the purposes of this chapter, we focus on fractures that are amenable to antegrade nailing.[47]
- The Abbreviated Injury Scale score for an isolated femoral shaft fracture is three, thus making the Injury Severity Score for an isolated femoral shaft fracture nine.
- Open fractures of the femur require substantially more energy than open fractures of the other extremities because of the more robust soft tissue envelope around a femur than other long bones.
- The fracture classification used most commonly is the AO Foundation/Orthopaedic Trauma Association (AO/OTA) classification.[33,59] In the AO/OTA classification, the femur is number 32 and further subdivided in simple, wedge, and complex fractures as shown **(FIG 1)**.

ANATOMY

- The femur is the longest bone in the body.
- The subtrochanteric region is subject to very high stresses because of the need to transition the forces of body weight via a lever arm (the femoral neck) into axial-directed forces distally.[26]
  - The femoral shaft is cylindrical on the anterior, medial, and lateral surfaces but coalesces posteriorly to form the linea aspera.
  - The linea aspera is a thick fascial structure in the setting of femoral shaft fractures; it frequently remains in continuity but may dissociate from the bone. It may also block reduction of the fracture if it wraps around a bone end.
  - The linea aspera protects the perforating branches of the deep femoral artery after they have passed through the adductor magnus muscle to supply a rich anastomotic network of periosteal vessels supplying the femur itself.[19]
- There are three thigh compartments: anterior, posterior, and medial separated by the medial, lateral, and posterior intermuscular septae.
  - Blunt trauma and femur fracture are the most common causes of thigh compartment syndrome accounting for approximately 49% of cases.[35] The anterior compartment is most commonly involved.[32]

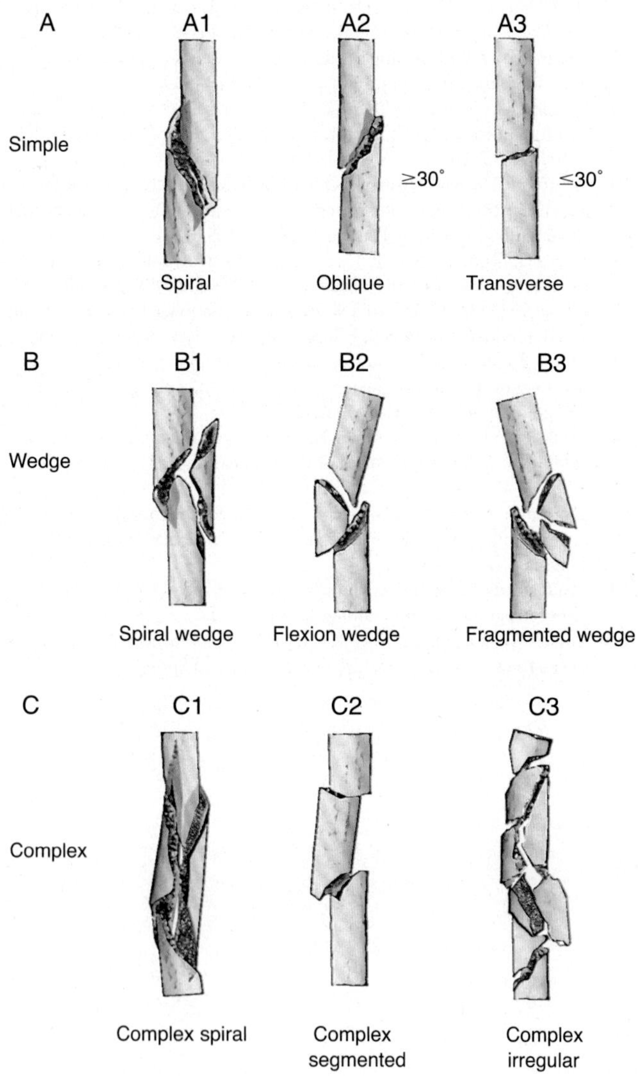

FIG 1 AO/OTA classification of femoral shaft fractures.

- Release of the anterior and posterior compartments can be performed from a single lateral incision.[52]
- The proximity of the gluteal compartment also places it at risk for compartment syndrome and should be considered, assessed, and released, if necessary.
- The femur has an anterior bow.
  - The anterior bow has an average radius of curvature of about 120 cm. African Americans tend to have a slightly larger radius of curvature (less bowed) than Caucasians.[17]
  - Part of preoperative planning for any nailing of the femur includes evaluating a full-length lateral radiograph for excessive bowing that may make accommodations necessary in the nailing procedure. This is especially true as the radii of curvature for most nails are larger than that of the femur itself.
  - In cases of aberrant femoral bowing, plate fixation may be considered; if nailing is undertaken, then bending the nail or an osteotomy to allow safe nail passage should be considered.[33]
- The endosteal diameter is important to identify, especially with young or sclerotic bone.
- Normal aging and osteoporosis result in a biomechanical adaptation of enlarged inner diameter. Thus, elderly individuals have a larger diameter femoral shaft with a thinner cortex than young patients.
- The vascular supply to the femur stems from a richly vascularized soft tissue envelope.
  - A majority (>50%) of femurs have two-nutrient foramen with nutrient arteries originating from perforating branches of the deep femoral artery. These foramina have variable locations, but on average are approximately 23 and 17 cm proximal to the femoral condyle.[29]
  - Normally, these periosteal arterial branches supply the outer one-quarter to one-third of the cortex.
  - The direction of blood flow is directed centrifugally from the high-pressure medullary arterial system to the low-pressure periosteal system.[42]
  - Once fracture occurs, a reversal of blood flow occurs with blood flowing centripetally from periosteal vessels directed radially inward (because the higher pressure intramedullary system is disrupted).[41]
- The femur is nearly entirely encased in muscle; the attachments and resting tone of which dictates deformity pattern following fracture
  - Femoral shortening is nearly always observed due to the pull of the hamstring and quadriceps muscles.
  - Proximal (subtrochanteric) fractures generally present with the proximal fragment flexed abducted and externally rotated due to the deforming unopposed muscular forces of the iliopsoas, gluteus medius, and short external rotators, respectively.
  - Mid-diaphyseal fractures tend to present with proximal fragment flexion secondary to the iliopsoas and neutral to valgus angulation due to the broad insertion of the adductor musculature.

PATHOGENESIS

- Femoral shaft fractures are high-energy injuries in the young.
- In the elderly, simple falls from ground level can be sufficient to fracture the femur, although most of these fragility fractures manifest as fractures in the peritrochanteric region.
- Fracture patterns give clues to the mechanism.
  - Transverse fracture with a butterfly fragment results from a bending force.
  - Spiral fracture patterns are usually due to torsional forces.
- Blunt injuries
  - Indirect high-energy mechanisms, such as a fall from a height or motor vehicle crashes
  - Although significant displacement occurs during the fracture process, the active and passive recoil of the soft tissue envelope decreases the initial deformity.
  - The extent of soft tissue injury can be difficult to appreciate given that the zone of injury tends to be much larger than a simple survey of the skin may indicate.
- Pathologic fractures
  - Atypical fractures, a type of stress fracture, are usually seen after the use of an antiresorptive agent. These fractures are most commonly seen in the subtrochanteric region, are transverse, and have lateral beaking.
  - Neoplasms, metastatic disease, and myelophthisic diseases can result in fractures with minimal force.
- Penetrating injuries
  - Direct mechanism of injury from ballistic injuries or other discreet weapons
  - Less initial displacement of the fracture and soft tissues than blunt force injuries
  - The extent of soft tissue injury can still be deceiving, especially in ballistic injuries where the shock and cavitation can result in extensive tissue necrosis

NATURAL HISTORY

- For the majority of human history, femoral shaft fracture management was nonoperative.
  - These methods resulted in high rates of malunion and morbidity.
- In the 1300s, Guy de Chauliac introduced isotonic skin traction as a method for femoral shaft fracture treatment.
- In the 1850s, Frank Hastings Hamilton reviewed a series of 83 fractures of the shaft of the femur and noted only 9 had a perfect result.[40] The remainder healed in malunion due to shortening, angulation, rotational deformity, and developed significant knee stiffness.
- These problems persisted even with the introduction of pin traction in 1907 by Steinmann.[40]
- Other nonoperative means for treatment such as functional bracing yielded similar issues with fracture shortening, angulation, and knee stiffness.[51]
- 1930–1940s:
  - Interest in the use of intramedullary fixation increased.
  - In 1940, Küntscher developed a V-shaped stainless steel antegrade nail.
    - The V-shaped evolved into a clôverleaf design by the late 1940s. Küntscher's original technique used open nailing (ie, exposing the fracture site to facilitate nail passage).
- 1950–1970s:
  - Intramedullary reamers and interlocking screws were developed with Modny and Bambara introducing the transfixion intramedullary nail in 1953.
  - In the 1960s, intramedullary nailing enthusiasm declined in favor of compression plating.

    - By the late 1970s, renewed interest in developing closed nailing techniques appeared in the setting of early weight bearing and minimally invasive procedures.[5,33]
- 1980s:
    - Küntscher's method was resurrected by S. Hansen and M. Chapman, who popularized Küntscher's "closed" femoral nailing technique. Locked nails were not in general use in the United States until mid-1980s.
    - In the late 1980s, Brumback and colleagues[11,12] reported the high success rate (98%) of reamed, statically locked intramedullary nails.
    - The success using closed technique resulted in low morbidity and began a change in practice to what is performed today.
    - Early studies outlined the benefits of reamed femoral nailing.
- 1990s–present:
    - Survival of traumatized patients increased, and a subset of patients who may benefit from "subacute" nailing began to be identified.
    - At-risk patients, like those with pulmonary involvement, high injury burden, or head trauma benefitted from temporizing stabilization while addressing life-threatening injuries and resuscitation before definitive fixation.
    - This paradigm shift reflects the evolution of early total care to damage control orthopaedics.[4,38,48,50]

PATIENT HISTORY AND PHYSICAL FINDINGS

- Relevant history includes age, mechanism of injury, associated injuries (ie, chest/head/bilateral injuries), loss of consciousness, weakness, paralysis, loss of sensation, history of malignancy, and antiresorptive medications as well as other medications.[30]
- Patients should be evaluated according to the Advanced Trauma Life Support guidelines.
- Hypotension should prompt early consideration for initiation of a massive transfusion protocol in multiply injured patients with femoral shaft fractures.[46]
    - Femur fractures can be associated with up to 1000 to 1500 mL of blood loss and are a notable contributor to hypotension.
- Upon evaluation by first responders, the limb should be aligned and placed in a traction device, such as a Sager or Thomas splint.
- Upon arrival to the definitive treatment location, these initial splints should be removed to facilitate complete evaluation of the injury.
    - After this initial evaluation, a care provider may determine the appropriate immobilization method depending on the specific clinical concerns.
        - Options include replacement of splint-based traction, initiation of skeletal traction, or tolerated immobilization without traction.
    - Traction improves comfort, restores physiologic length, and tightens the surrounding muscles. The taut surrounding musculature decreases potential space for accumulation of blood loss, provides a tamponade effect to hemorrhage, and serves as a soft tissue stabilizer to the fracture fragments.[13] When tolerated, immobilization without traction may be appropriate in some elderly patients; traction is generally well tolerated without many contraindications.
- It is essential to inspect the affected limb for any open wounds, swelling, and ecchymosis.
    - The extent of the open wound does not always correlate with the degree of soft tissue or fascial stripping known as the *zone of injury*.
- Vascular evaluation should include manual palpation of the popliteal, posterior tibial, and dorsalis pedis pulses.
    - The limb should be aligned before vascular examination.
    - A Doppler ultrasound device should be used in cases where a pulse cannot be readily palpated.
    - Asymmetric or absent pulses warrant a measurement of the ankle–brachial index (ABI). An ABI less than 0.9 is abnormal.
        - In cases with abnormal ABIs, arteriography should be considered to rule out vascular injury, even in the face of a perfused limb.
- Neurologic evaluation includes motor and sensory function of the femoral and sciatic nerve.
    - The femoral nerve may be difficult to examine secondary to pain associated with the fracture.
    - Sciatic nerve function can be evaluated for both peroneal and tibial branches.
        - The peroneal branch is tested with ankle and toe dorsiflexion and sensation on the top of the foot.
        - Tibial branch function is tested with ankle and toe plantarflexion as well as sensation to the sole of the foot.

IMAGING AND OTHER DIAGNOSTIC STUDIES

- Good anteroposterior (AP) and lateral views of the hip, femur, and knee are required.
    - Such films are essential in planning because the presence of a femoral neck fracture or a fracture about the knee will greatly change the operative tactic.[27]
    - Attempts should be made to get an internal rotation AP view of the femoral neck, particularly for proximal fractures.
        - These images can be evaluated alongside a pelvic computed tomography (CT) scan to fully evaluate the femoral neck. The scan should be viewed before deciding on the surgical tactic.[54]
        - Fine cut CT scans of the abdomen that include the femoral neck have been found to be sensitive enough to identify most occult femoral neck fractures.[54]

DIFFERENTIAL DIAGNOSIS

- Other injuries frequently occur concomitantly with femur fractures, including pelvic fractures, acetabular fractures, femoral neck fractures, and ligamentous injuries to the knee.
- In the absence of a reasonable mechanism, other causes for fracture such as metabolic bone disease or metastatic (or primary) fracture should be ruled out.

NONOPERATIVE MANAGEMENT

- Nonoperative management has typically been reserved for patients who are unfit for surgery, patients who are quadriplegic or paraplegic, patients in whom the benefits do not outweigh the risks, or other precluding factors (eg, active infection).
    - Nonoperative management consists of bed rest and skeletal traction (either through the distal femur or proximal tibia) starting with 15% to 20% of body weight.

- Infants and young children are treated nonoperatively because of their ability to remodel.
- Nondisplaced stress fractures in a compliant and able patient may also be considered for nonoperative treatment.
- Attention should be given to mechanical and pharmacologic venous thromboembolism prophylaxis.
  - Despite the recommendations for systemic anticoagulation for deep vein thrombosis prophylaxis in trauma patients, the appropriate type of prophylaxis, dose, and duration remain unclear.[7,31]
  - In a survey of 185 orthopaedic traumatologists, Sagi et al[44] found wide variations in venous thromboembolism prophylaxis administration.

SURGICAL MANAGEMENT

- Isolated femur fractures are not emergent and do not need to be definitively treated during off hours unless some other reason is driving the operative decision making (eg, polytrauma or vascular injury).
  - Patients with isolated femur fractures should have some method of traction, pain control, and deep vein thrombosis prophylaxis while awaiting surgical intervention.
- Appropriate evaluation and medical optimization should be performed to stabilize the patient prior to definitive fixation.
- Ideally, definitive fixation should be performed before 24 hours; otherwise, there is increased risk of pulmonary embolism and required longer hospital stay, although without a difference in mortality.[14]
- In the multiply injured patient with substantial pulmonary compromise or a blossoming head injury, definitive (intramedullary nailing) fracture fixation should be delayed until suitably cleared for surgical intervention. This represents the ideal opportunity for damage control techniques with temporary external fixation or skeletal traction.[3,6,34]
- Lactate, pH, and base excess should be monitored and included in the decision-making algorithm for early total care or damage control.[36,58]
  - Definitive fixation should be performed when the patient has achieved adequate resuscitation with improvement in acidosis as indicated by lactate less than 4.0 mmol/L, pH greater than 7.25, or base excess between −5.5 mmol/L and 5.5 mmol/L.[57]
- Currently, statically locked femoral nailing with limited reaming is the standard of care.
  - The studies by Brumback et al[8–12] determined that statically locked nails do not affect healing and avoid the problems of malrotation and shortening.
  - The reamer-irrigator-aspirator device developed to minimize the pressure-induced embolization from the marrow during reaming was shown to have a modest reduction of embolic debris during reaming and nail insertion.
    - However, these findings were not able to be correlated with any physiologic significance in a prospective randomized controlled trial, and union rates may be lower.[21]
  - Although unreamed nails are faster and theoretically avoid the pulmonary risks of emboli during reaming, the increased risk of acute respiratory distress syndrome has not been clearly born out in comparison of reamed versus unreamed nails.[53]
  - Unreamed nails have a slightly higher risk of perioperative complication.[45]
    - Iatrogenic comminution of the fracture, hardware misplacement, and rotational malalignment were the recorded perioperative complications.[45]
  - Currently, the "ream-to-fit" technique is a preferred method for the authors.[56]
- Open fractures can be safely nailed if a thorough irrigation and débridement is performed.
  - Similarly, retrograde femoral nailing following open fracture can be safely performed with a low risk for septic arthritis.[37]
  - Absorbable antibiotic beads (calcium sulfate, not calcium phosphate, mixed with vancomycin or tobramycin) can be used at the time of definitive closure to provide local antibiotic delivery.[43]
- In severely contaminated fractures, a staged approach using temporary antibiotic beads (using polymethylmethacrylate mixed with heat stable antibiotics) and external fixation, followed by nailing as soon as feasible thereafter (with or without use of absorbable beads), can be employed.
  - If there is no pin tract infection, conversion from external fixation to intramedullary nailing is best performed within 14 days of external fixator placement to minimize infection risk.[16]
  - In the case of draining pin sites where infection is suspected, staged conversion to definitive fixation is frequently used with a period of skeletal traction until the pin site drainage has declined.[34]
- Because of deforming forces in proximal femur fractures, the proximal segment tends to flex and externally rotate.
  - Care should be taken to ensure that the posterior cortex of the proximal fragment is not inadvertently reamed away. This may occur when the fracture is not aligned during reaming.
- In distal fractures, the fracture goes into recurvatum from the pull of the gastrocnemius.
  - Care should be taken to avoid varus or valgus malreduction, which can occur when the opening of the medullary canal distally does not have intimate contact with the nail and does not "self-align."
- In skeletally mature adolescents, intramedullary nailing offers the same benefits as in adults.
  - Attention should be paid to adolescents with very valgus neck angles, as some have hypothesized that this can increase the risk of avascular necrosis of the femoral head.
    - With newer implants such as trochanteric entry or lateral entry nails, many of these concerns can be alleviated. However, the studies supporting these techniques are not large series so this decision should be undertaken only after a full discussion with the family. Many surgeons use either retrograde nails or flexible fixation for adolescents.
  - Skeletally immature children may still be considered for some form of intramedullary treatment after considering remaining growth, type of fracture, and benefits over other methods of treatment.[1,18]

Preoperative Planning

- All femur fracture injury films should be reviewed, with specific attention paid to the possibility of an ipsilateral femoral neck fracture or other fracture extension.

- Strong consideration should be given to checking fine-cut CT scans to evaluate the femoral neck prior to surgical intervention.
- The overall condition of the patient and any associated injuries should be contemplated before embarking on a surgical tactic.
- If suitable, antegrade nailing in the supine position can be safely performed with proper positioning and knowledge.
  - In the presence of pelvic or acetabular fracture, pregnancy, or obesity, one should consider other tactics, such as retrograde nailing, to accommodate for the unique concerns.
- Several options have to be considered during preoperative planning. They include the following:
  - Table: fracture table or radiolucent
  - Position: supine or lateral
  - Entry point: trochanteric/lateral entry or piriformis
  - Type of nail: cephalomedullary or standard
  - Use of traction: skeletal, boot, or manual
- Reduction tools such as ball spike pushers, 5.0- or 6.0-mm Schanz screws with T-handles, a mallet, or an F tool should be available.
  - Conventional reduction clamps should be available, if not open in the room, for the scenario that the fracture must be opened to obtain the reduction.
- Before the surgeon leaves the operating room, he or she should ensure that femoral intramedullary nail fixation has resulted in satisfactory: (1) length, (2) alignment, and (3) rotation. Finally, the femoral neck should be confirmed to be intact or have been reduced and stabilized.

Positioning

- Fracture table
  - Standard fracture tables (eg, those used commonly for hip fractures) can be used for antegrade femoral nailing.
  - A large and well-padded perineal post should be used.
  - Traction should be used sparingly and only when needed.
    - Pudendal nerve palsy is associated with higher total traction forces and duration of traction.[9]
  - The legs should be scissored to facilitate imaging and allow for appropriate countertraction.
    - Placing the opposite leg in lithotomy position can allow rotation of the pelvis when traction is applied and risk compartment syndrome of the unaffected leg.
  - The ability to image all aspects of the femur should be verified before preparing and draping **(FIG 2A)**.
    - If the contralateral femur is going to be imaged for rotation comparison, this should be accounted for during patient positioning to facilitate radiographic evaluation.
- Radiolucent tables
  - Allow free image intensifier access to the lower extremity.
  - Some of the tables (Jackson table [Mizuho OSI, Orthopaedic Systems, Inc., Union City, CA]) also provide traction assemblies. These types of tables are suitable for multiple limb operations **(FIG 2B)**.
  - A radiolucent table with traction apparatus and lateral positioning can help to minimize deforming forces, control soft tissue in obese patients, and facilitate open conversion, when needed, without difficulty **(FIG 2C)**.

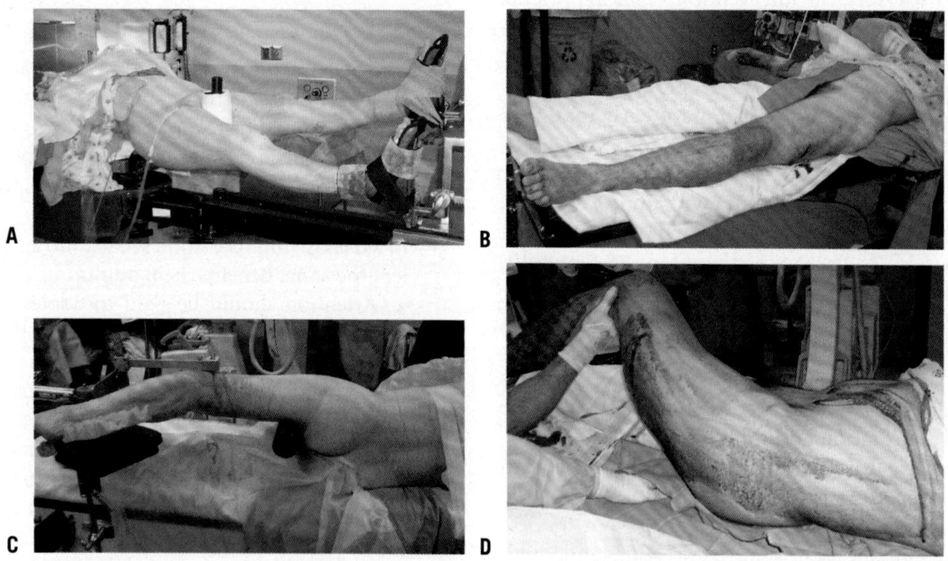

FIG 2 A. Supine positioning on a fracture table with legs scissored. Slight obliquity using a bump under the sacrum helps with hip visualization. **B.** Supine position without traction on flat-top table. The ipsilateral hip should be close to the edge, and a bump under the sacrum will help with visualization. Standard lateral views of the hip for entry points can be used but so can frog-leg laterals. **C.** Lateral position with traction. Skeletal traction in the proximal tibia or distal femur can be used. The perineal post is pictured here in the perineum, which is best for proximal fractures. In fact, little traction is usually needed and the post is frequently positioned under the apex of the fracture and used to overcome gravitational sagging. If traction will be needed, we have found that placing a blanket on the "down" leg and securing the contralateral thigh with a sling of tape coursing in a proximal and oblique fashion will resist moderate amounts of traction. **D.** Preparation and draping of the leg using a flat-top table without traction should include posterior sections of the buttocks.

- Supine position
  - The supine position may be easier for surgeons to visualize anatomic relationships.
    - However, in obese patients, it can be more difficult to properly position and gain the needed exposure.
  - Supine positioning is preferred in patients with spinal cord injuries.
  - If supine (floppy) positioning on a radiolucent table is chosen, it helps to position the patient at the edge of the bed with a small bolster under the pelvis—with the upper torso slightly adducted. Supine nailing can also be performed on a fracture table to allow traction.
  - If the patient is supine with the leg free, preparing and draping should include the posterior aspect of the gluteal area and access to the medial groin, in case access to the femoral vessels becomes necessary during the case (**FIG 2D**).
- Lateral position
  - The lateral position facilitates positioning and exposure in obese patients.
  - The ability to flex the hip reduces the deforming forces placed on the fracture fragments and can therefore facilitate reduction.
  - When using the lateral position, the pelvis is rolled forward about 15 degrees to allow lateral imaging of the proximal femur.
  - Care should be taken during positioning for proper padding and spinal precautions if occult spinal injury may be present.
- Traction
  - If traction is used, it frees an assistant and the length and rotation can be "set."
  - If manual traction is used, the length and rotation need to be checked before final interlocking.
  - Skeletal traction can be via the proximal tibia or distal femur.
    - The surgeon should be careful if there is any concern for ligamentous instability of the knee, as suggested by a knee effusion or other sign of injury.
    - If ligamentous injury is suspected, distal femoral traction can be used with preparations to drape the traction apparatus into the operative field.
    - Use of distal femoral traction can complicate distal interlocking because of the proximity of the traction apparatus with the interlocking site.
  - Boot traction is a common alternative to skeletal traction but requires the leg to be straight as opposed to the slightly flexed position when skeletal traction is used (see **FIG 2A**).
  - Care should be taken to avoid pudendal nerve traction injury (eg, avoid prolonged and excessive traction).
    - Pudendal palsy is associated with the use of small perineal post and correlates with the duration of surgery and the force of the traction applied.
    - If traction is used, it should be first applied to determine the "reducibility" of the fracture. Then, it should be reduced during prepping and applied only as needed.
    - Large and well-padded perineal posts should be used whenever possible.[9,28]
    - Pudendal nerve palsies tend to improve, but they can be very anxiety provoking and take months to resolve.
- Regardless of patient position, the surgeon should ensure that the patient has complete muscle relaxation to facilitate reduction.

SOFT TISSUE DISSECTION

- Whether using a cephalomedullary nail or piriformis fossa nail, the surgical approach is similar.
- The surgeon palpates the greater trochanter.
- For trochanteric entry, the skin incision is based about 4 to 10 cm above the trochanter in line with the femur.
  - The tensor fascia is incised, and the abductor musculature is gently separated.
  - The tendinous insertion of the gluteus medius is frequently more distal, and this tendon can be gently spread to identify a bursal area just below the medius and above the minimus.
- For piriformis entry, the incision is made about a handbreadth along the line between the trochanter and the posterior superior iliac spine.
  - Once the gluteus maximus is gently separated, the access to the piriformis fossa is posterior to the gluteus medius.
  - The piriformis fossa can be easily palpated as a "dimpled ledge" behind the trochanter. This anatomic feature is used during the percutaneous approach for proprioceptive feedback during pin placement.

TROCHANTERIC AND PIRIFORMIS FOSSA ENTRY

- After soft tissue dissection, the tip of the greater trochanter is palpated. The piriformis fossa is palpated medially.
- The ideal starting point for a piriformis fossa nail is in the fossa along the medial upslope of the greater trochanter because this is most in line with the shaft.
  - This point may vary between patients and should be confirmed with intraoperative fluoroscopy. The guidewire or awl should be directly in line with the center of the femoral shaft. This position is typically in the posterior half of the femoral neck.
  - The surgeon can have an assistant adduct the extremity to aid in exposing this spot (**TECH FIG 1A**).
- Once the starting point is identified by palpation and confirmed with fluoroscopy, the cortex is penetrated with either an awl or a threaded guidewire.
  - Every effort should be given in establishing an accurate starting point (ie, one that is in line with the femoral shaft).
  - If this is not possible, as long as the *entry* site is collinear with the shaft, the pin can be directed anteriorly. In these cases, care should be taken not to perforate the anterior cortex (**TECH FIG 1B**).
- In supine nailing, especially with obese patients, this can be very difficult. Adduction of the limb may not always be possible because of body habitus and setup and especially with proximal fractures.

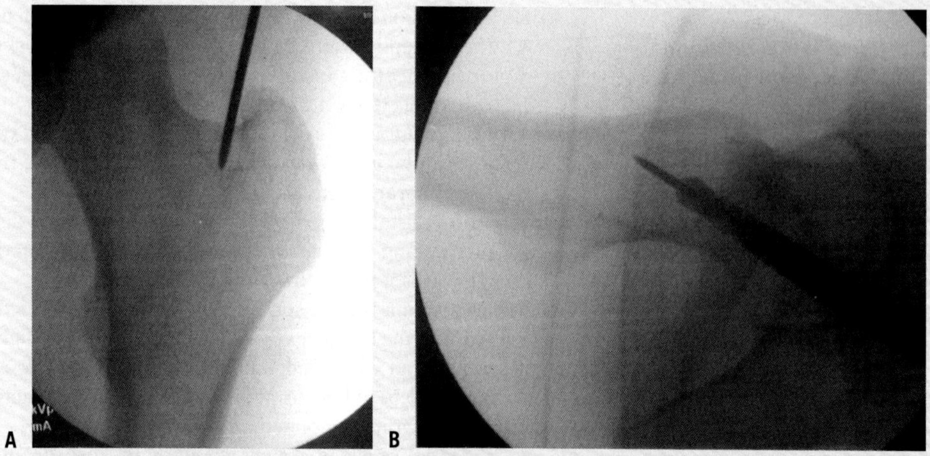

TECH FIG 1 A. AP image of the correct position of a guide pin for piriformis entry. **B.** Lateral image of piriformis starting point. The pin needs only to start in the piriformis; it will frequently course anterior, and care should be taken not to penetrate the anterior cortex. The rigid reamer needs only to open the top of the bone for access to medullary canal.

- In these cases, preparing under the buttock and accessing from a more posterior approach may allow access to the fossa.
- The lateral positioning allows the easiest access, with very few problems. In fact, nailing can be performed percutaneously (described in the following text) with little problem when using the lateral position.
- Recent literature has demonstrated no significant difference in functional outcome between patients treated with a piriformis-entry nail versus a trochanteric-entry nail.[49]
- The authors would like to emphasize that many later intraoperative complications with intramedullary nailing of the femur originate from a poor starting spot; it is worth investing the time to ensure this portion of the procedure is performed correctly.

PERCUTANEOUS METHOD OF NAILING

- The percutaneous method of nailing[61] uses cutaneous landmarks to identify the ideal entry site, which is usually about one full handbreadth (8 cm) from the posterior corner of the trochanter toward the posterior superior iliac spine **(TECH FIG 2A)**.
- A guide pin is advanced to the trochanteric bursa **(TECH FIG 2B)**.
- The pin is "rolled" off the posterior slope of the trochanter and then advanced distally and anteriorly **(TECH FIG 2C,D)**.
- A very distinct resistance is felt, as if on a pedestal or ledge of bone. The tip of the pin provides proprioceptive feedback when this occurs, and it can be felt that there are structures anteriorly and medially, which constitute the "walls" of the fossa.
- At this point, image verification is performed.
  - If the pin is not coaxial with the femur, what is most important is that the tip of the pin is centered.
- The pin is advanced to engage the cortex, and then a 9- to 12-mm rigid reamer is used to open the proximal femoral cortex **(TECH FIG 2E)**.
  - This reamer needs only to be advanced enough to open the cortex and provide access to medullary contents. Care should be taken not to ream too deeply and perforate the cortex of the proximal femur anteriorly (see **TECH FIG 1**).
- Once this step is accomplished, the remainder of the procedure can be done with standard methods, and instruments are passed via the keyhole skin incision **(TECH FIG 2F–H)**.

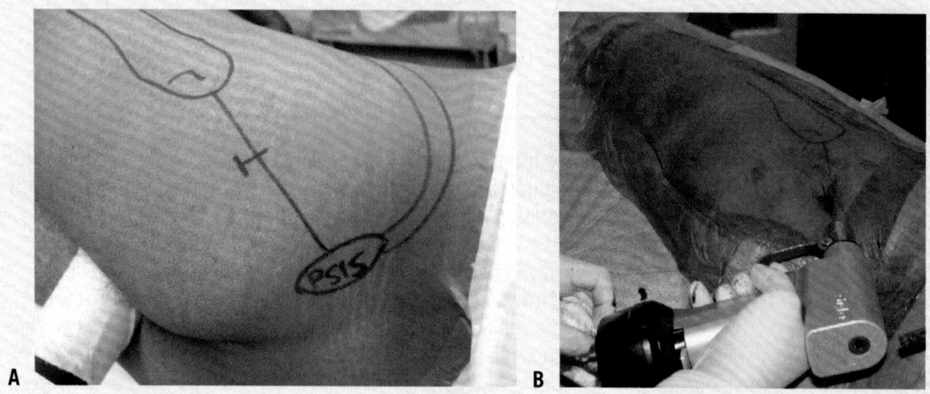

TECH FIG 2 A. The cutaneous site for percutaneous nailing, situated about midway and slightly posterior to midpoint between tip of trochanter and posterior superior iliac spine (*PSIS*). **B.** Photograph showing pin driven into piriformis via percutaneous wound. *(continued)*

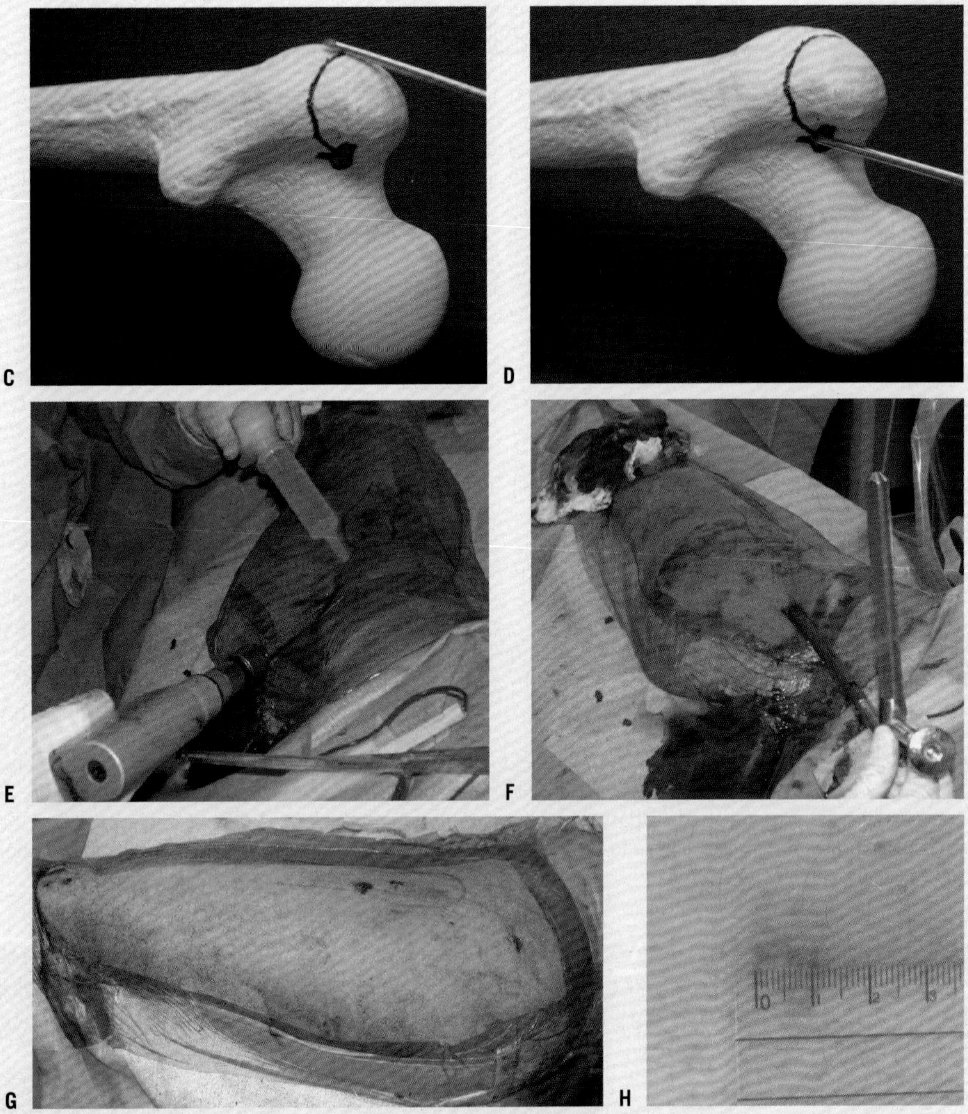

TECH FIG 2 *(continued)* **C.** The pin usually finds the trochanteric bursa. It is then rolled off the back and advanced anterior and distal until a distinct resistance is felt. It should rest on the "ledge" of bone known as the *piriformis fossa*. **D.** The pin has a resistance to anterior and distal advancement but can move medial and posterior. **E.** The rigid reamer advances over the pin to enter the proximal femur. Use of irrigation will help prevent soft tissue catching. **F.** Insertion of the nail over the guidewire. With use of a bent guidewire and ream-to-fit technique, the likelihood of an incarcerated reamer is very low, and exchange of the guidewire with a chest tube is not needed (unless a ball-tipped guidewire is used). **G.** Intraoperative photo of final wounds. **H.** Entry site wounds are usually about 1.5 cm.

TROCHANTERIC ENTRY, GUIDEWIRE PLACEMENT, AND FRACTURE REDUCTION

- After soft tissue dissection (as described previously), the surgeon palpates the tip of the greater trochanter and its AP dimensions.
- When placing the incision, ensure the anterior bow of the femur is accounted for. Failure to do so will result in an incision that is too anterior for appropriate starting position.
- Because of the inherent anatomy of the proximal femur, the ideal starting spot for a trochanteric entry nail is at the medial aspect of the tip of the greater trochanter at the junction of the anterior one-third and posterior two-thirds of the greater trochanter.
  - This spot may vary from person to person, but the correct starting point is one that is in line with the femoral shaft.
  - Once the correct starting spot is identified, the outer cortex is penetrated with either an awl or a pointed guidewire **(TECH FIG 3A)**.
- In this method, because the abductor mechanism is being split, soft tissue protection is important.
- After the starting point is identified, a guidewire is placed into the proximal femur and passed down the canal.
  - Forceful and jerking motions can be avoided by firmly twisting the guidewire through the cancellous bone.
  - A gentle J bend at the distal 1 cm of the wire allows the wire to be "bounced" off cortices and to be "steered" in metaphyseal areas **(TECH FIG 3B)**.
  - The proprioceptive feedback of a wire passing along the medullary canal is similar to the sensation of pushing a stick on a sidewalk.
- If the fracture is not reduced sufficiently to easily pass the wire across, there are several techniques available to facilitate reduction and wire passing.
  - Some nail systems provide a cannulated rod that is placed over the wire and passed into the proximal femur. This rigid wire holder functions as a wand to manipulate the proximal fragment as the wire approaches the fracture so that it can easily be passed across **(TECH FIG 3C)**.
  - An F or H bar, a crutch, or both can also be useful to manipulate the proximal and distal fragments **(TECH FIG 3D)**.
- Sometimes, the fracture cannot be perfectly reduced, but enough provisional alignment can be established to pass the guidewire.
  - If the fracture is unstable and difficult to reduce after numerous attempts, a small incision can be made along the lateral thigh over the fracture and the fracture can be digitally reduced and provisionally aligned. This maneuver should not require any significant soft tissue stripping.
  - In some cases, the incision can be lengthened to allow placement of pointed reduction clamps.
- Alternatively, 3-mm threaded guide pins can also be used **(TECH FIG 3E)**. Other methods include the use of unicortical "joystick" half-pins from an external fixator set (usually a 5-mm half-pin) **(TECH FIG 3F,G)**.
- The guidewire position in the distal segment is confirmed with intraoperative fluoroscopy.
  - The guidewire should be passed down to the distal femur physeal scar and should be center–center on both the AP and lateral views. A bend in the tip of the guidewire can facilitate achieving a satisfactory position in the distal femur.

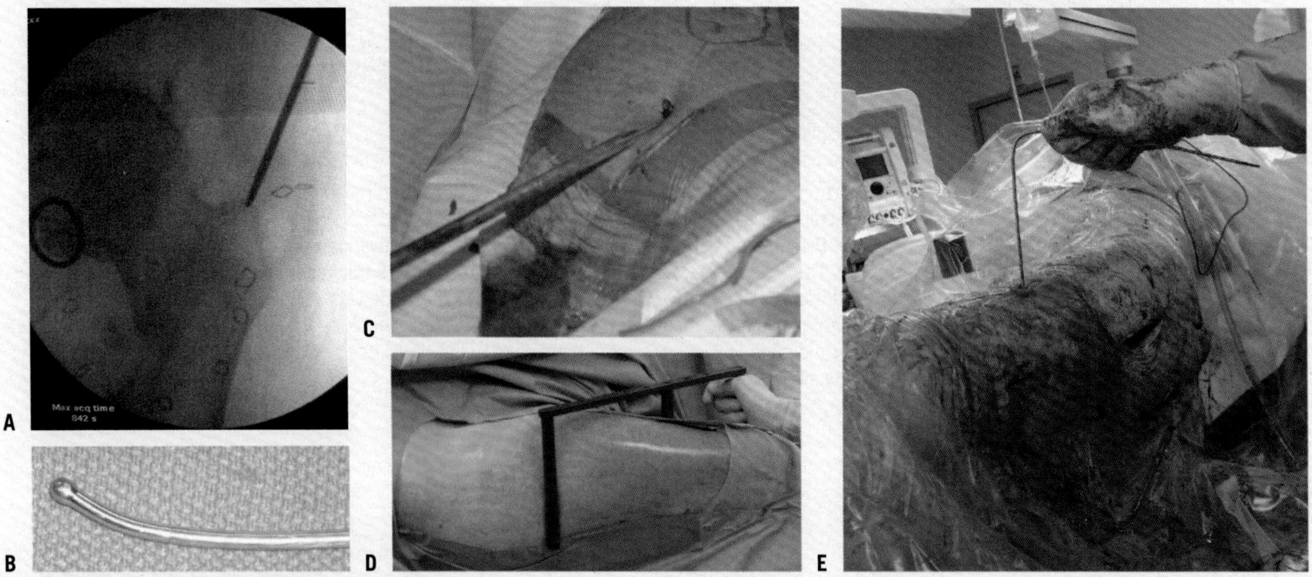

TECH FIG 3 A. The entry point for the trochanter is usually at the tip of the trochanter on the AP view and the junction of the anterior one-third and posterior two-thirds on the lateral view (not shown). **B.** Guidewire with "J bend." This helps to "steer" the wire in metaphyseal bone and will prevent reamer heads from disengaging (relevant only in modular designs). **C.** The "wand." It is available on some sets or can be performed with some extraction rods. It is placed over the guidewire into the proximal segment, down to the level of the lesser trochanter. It can manipulate the proximal fragment to aim it into the distal segment, after which the guidewire is advanced into the distal fragment. This is much more desirable than struggling with manual methods. **D.** F bar. This can be placed around the thigh to effect the desired translation. In out-of-plane deformities, the bar can find the "ideal" orientation and effect a reduction. **E.** The joystick method. Small terminally threaded wires can be drilled into the cortex of each segment and used to manipulate the fragments into reduction. Small external fixator pins can also be used and have been previously described. *(continued)*

F
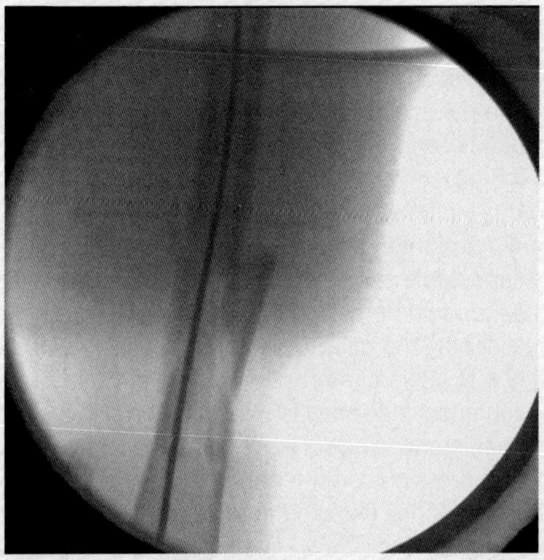

G
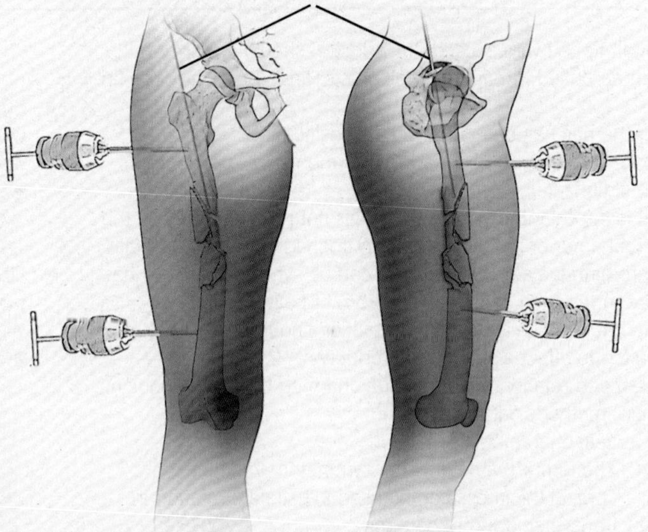

TECH FIG 3 *(continued)* **F.** Intraoperative image of guidewire passed across fracture. **G.** Illustration demonstrating unicortical placement of external fixation Schanz pins to manipulate the fracture. These pins can be placed laterally or anteriorly and should be unicortical so that the guidewire can pass.

MEASUREMENT AND REAMING

- Once the guidewire has been placed, the length of the nail is measured either with a measuring device (usually supplied by the intramedullary nail system) or by using a guidewire of the same length.
  - Placing the second wire at the entry site and measuring what is not overlapping with the inserted wire provides nail length.
  - Before measuring, the surgeon confirms the proximal position of the ruler on the greater trochanter.
  - The surgeon should make sure that there is no soft tissue between the ruler and the top of the greater trochanter, as this can artificially increase the length of the nail chosen. After the length is determined at the hip, the surgeon should determine if there is a fracture gap that he or she may backslap to achieve direct cortical contact of the fracture. If this is the case, then a slightly shorter nail should be used to account for the nail's migration proximally.
- Using the radiographs of the femur, the surgeon can estimate the beginning reamer size.
  - With "tight" canals, reaming should begin with lower sizes, and sequential reaming can begin starting with the lowest end-cutting reamer size available (usually 8.5 or 9 mm).
  - When starting to ream, the surgeon should pay particular attention to keep the reamer medial in the proximal femur to prevent reaming out the posterior or lateral cortex.
  - If the reamer does not pass easily, the surgeon should check its position with fluoroscopy because the reamer may be hitting cortical bone (usually anteriorly).
- Reaming can be increased by 1.0-mm increments until distinct "chatter" is encountered, after which it should increase in 0.5-mm increments.
- Once endosteal chatter is encountered, reaming should continue until the canal is reamed 1.5 to 2.0 mm over the proposed nail diameter.
  - With modern nail designs, most patients can be treated with 10- to 11-mm nails.
- Care should be taken when there is a tendency for a deforming force to allow for "eccentric" reaming (eg, proximal fractures).
  - In these cases, without attention, eccentric reaming can remove cortical bone and create defects that result in deformity or a nail outside the bone.
- Intramedullary reaming has a detrimental effect on the endosteal blood supply, but this effect has not translated into a less satisfactory clinical outcome. Reaming should be performed at slow driving speeds and high revolutions with sharp reamer heads to minimize intramedullary pressure and heat.[43]
- Fat embolism syndrome is always a possible concern during intramedullary reaming and is characterized by acute hypoxia (respiratory signs/symptoms), confusion (cerebral signs/symptoms), and a petechial rash. Intravascular fat continues in the circulation of the lungs, kidneys, and brain for 72 hours after reaming.

TECHNIQUES

NAIL PLACEMENT

- If a ball-tipped wire is used, the surgeon should confirm that it can be pulled through the nail or exchanged for a smooth-tip wire.
- After the nail has been inserted, its position is checked distally, at the fracture site, and proximally near its insertion site.
  - It is important to ensure the nail is not prominent above the trochanter or piriformis fossa. A trochanteric entry nail with prominence as small as 1 cm can be symptomatic and has been reported in as many as 25% of patients.[23]
- If the fracture site is distracted, traction should be reduced or adjusted to effect a satisfactory reduction.
- Length and rotation need to be reconfirmed before interlocking. Several methods can be used.[24,25,55,56]
  - Cortical characteristics
    - The femur diameter is not symmetric. Variances in cortical thickness can be used to estimate rotation in transverse fracture patterns.
    - Fracture lines can also be used to estimate correct rotation.
  - Radiographic methods
    - One method to determine rotational alignment is to check a lateral view of the contralateral hip and distal femur. These lateral views of the normal hip are then compared to the affected extremity's lateral proximal/distal femur views. The measured difference should be mirrored in the fractured side if rotation is correct.
    - In cases of comminution or bilateral fractures, another method can be used to determine or set the rotation. A true lateral of the distal femur is obtained, and the intensifier is then moved orthogonal to this position, and the proximal femur is visualized to obtain a profile of the lesser trochanter. The images are saved for reference and mirrored on the fractured side or contralateral side if bilateral.[55]
    - Baseline rotation can also be determined clinically. If the patient is positioned supine with the leg draped free, preoperatively, the surgeon should "eyeball" the baseline rotation of the contralateral leg. During or at the end of the case, the surgeon can then compare the affected extremity's rotation and length compared to the contralateral side.
- Surprisingly, rotational deformities appear to be well tolerated, with an average of 28% of patients having a deformity of more than 15 degrees.
  - In all cases, a clinical examination of rotation of both legs with the pelvis supine and the hip flexed to 90 degrees can be used to estimate symmetry.
- Unless the patient is in extremis or the surgeon is using a compression nail, all nails should be statically locked.
  - The order of interlocking should be considered.
  - In axially stable cases, the distal segment should be interlocked, and compression is applied to the fracture site by backslapping the nail; some intramedullary nails allow the surgeon to use a compression screw. In these cases, the distal interlocking screw is placed in the static position. The proximal interlocking screw is placed in the dynamic hole. The compression screw is then used and essentially "pulls" the nail, which is fixed to the distal bone fragment via the distal interlocking screw, proximally to abut against the proximal fracture fragment. Again, if this type of nail will be used with a compression screw, a slightly shorter nail should be inserted because these nails allow up to 10 mm of axial compression. Similarly, if a slot is used and the screw placed on the far side from the fracture, the fracture will compress with weight bearing.
  - The authors find that certain fracture patterns are more amenable to compression than others. Transverse femoral shaft fractures may benefit from axial compression due to their inherent rotational instability if they are gapped. Short oblique fractures, if "keyed-in" and reduced, benefit from cortical compression. If the spiral oblique fracture is out to length but not reduced, then compression is not advised as it may shorten the femur—especially if the oblique fracture pattern is prone to shear. These fracture patterns tend to heal due to the large surface area between the fracture fragments. Fracture patterns with butterfly fragments may or may not benefit from compression.
  - In unstable cases, traction and alignment should be maintained until interlocking is complete.[8,60]

PROXIMAL INTERLOCKING SCREW PLACEMENT

- There are guides with each system that allow placement of proximal screws. In general, at least one screw should be placed.
- The static screw hole should be used, and the hole closest to the fracture is preferred. In stable fracture patterns, one proximal and one distal static interlocking screw is the accepted standard of care. If the surgeon is using a compression nail and there is a fracture gap, then the surgeon can place the proximal screw in the proximal aspect of the dynamic hole; once he or she then uses the compression screw, the nail will be "pulled" up along with the distal fracture fragment and close the fracture gap.

DISTAL INTERLOCKING SCREW PLACEMENT

- Distal screw placement is usually done with a freehand technique, but other methods are now available. Each system has its own technique, and the surgeon should be aware of the methods available to diminish radiation to the patient.
  - Only one static distal interlocking screw is necessary.[20] Freehand locking can be challenging.
- In general, setup and image positioning can greatly facilitate this part of the procedure.
- Using the concentric circle concept, the image intensifier or the leg is rotated to obtain a perfect circle.
  - If the image is oval or shaped like an eye, the image intensifier is not perpendicular to the axis of the nail or, in other words, parallel or coaxial with the axis of the screw hole.
  - The goal is to align the axis of the image intensifier/beam source with that of the screw hole. Obtaining perfect circles with fluoroscopy imaging is the first critical step. The surgeon will either have to abduct or adduct the extremity or internally/externally rotate the extremity to achieve perfect circles.
    - In **TECH FIG 4A**, the image intensifier is not aligned in the coronal plane (varus or valgus to the femoral nail).
    - In **TECH FIG 4B**, the image intensifier is not aligned in the axial–transverse plane (rotationally to the nail).
    - In **TECH FIG 4C**, both screw holes in the nail line up, giving the "perfect circle" wherein the image intensifier is colinear to the axis of the screw hole in the nail.
- Next, a drill or scalpel is used to determine the cutaneous location for an incision, which should go through the fascia and to bone.
  - A drill is centered over the hole and held securely **(TECH FIG 4D)**.
  - The axis of the drill bit should be aligned with the center of the image intensifier's beam source (which is parallel to that of the hole). Thus, if the drill tip is centered over the hole and aligned with the center of the beam source, it should be coaxial with the axis of the hole.
  - Once the drill tip penetrates the first cortex and advanced slightly, fluoroscopic verification should be obtained again. At this point, subtle changes in the drill bit trajectory can be made by gently malleting the drill bit in the desired direction. For example, if the drill bit appears to be heading posterior to the nail hole, then the surgeon can gently "guide" it anteriorly by redirection with a mallet. This "fine-tuning" step can be very helpful in using a less than ideal starting hole in the bone.
  - If the drill bit "kicks" or jerks into a different direction or cannot be advanced, it is likely that it either glanced off the

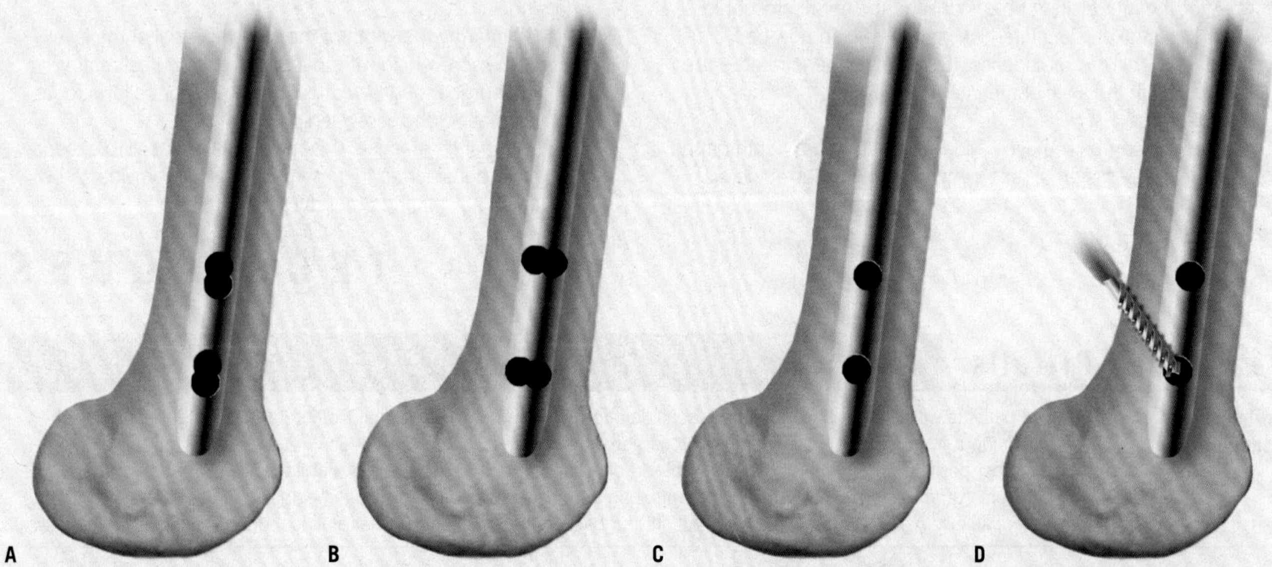

TECH FIG 4 **A.** The perfect circle method for freehand interlocking. If the image appears as two circles overlapped, the shape of an 8 will appear. The central area is elliptical and indicates that the image intensifier axis is not collinear with the axis of the screw holes. The appropriate corrective direction is parallel to the short axis of the central ellipse (or perpendicular to the long axis). In this case, the correction would be in the coronal plane (proximal to distal). **B.** In this situation, the rotation of the image does not match. It will need to be corrected along an arc parallel to the short axis of the central ellipse. **C.** The image of a perfect circle. **D.** The drill point should be in the middle of the circle. Then, the axis of the drill can be made collinear with that of the image intensifier. *(continued)*

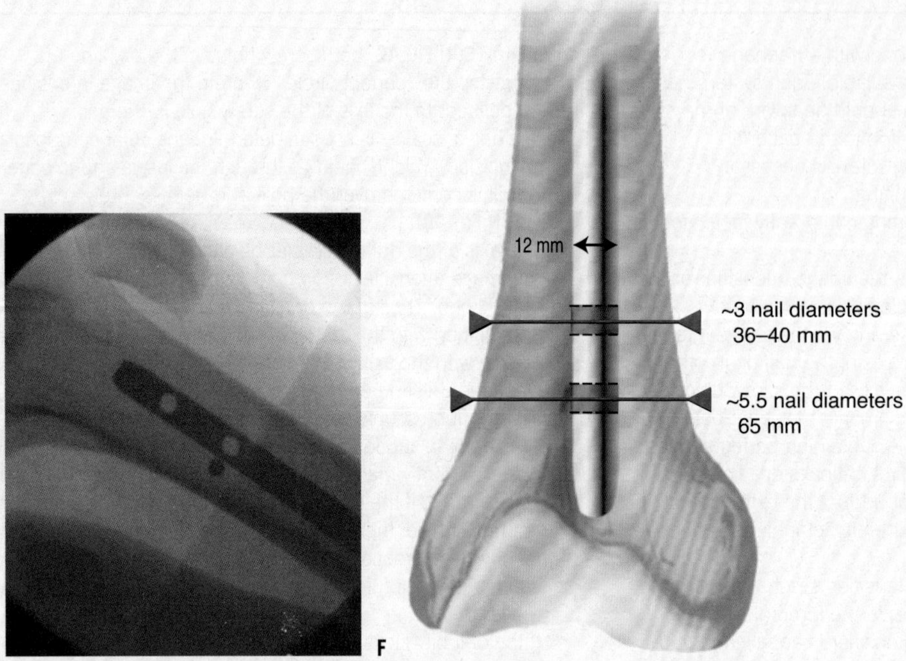

E F

TECH FIG 4 *(continued)* **E.** The drill can pass anterior or posterior to the nail and "feel" pretty good. Care should be taken to make sure the drill point does not drift during this motion. Proprioceptive feedback will frequently indicate when the drill passes through the nail and the contralateral cortex. If the drill kicks in one direction (anterior or posterior), it may have missed the nail. If it is not aligned in the coronal plane, it may hit the nail. It is important to verify all implant positions before leaving the operating room. **F.** A method of measuring using the nail as a "yardstick." If the diameter of the nail is known, then the diameter of the bone at the level of the interlocking hole can be estimated by seeing how many multiples of the nail will fit in that segment. With some practice, the accuracy of this technique is impressive: We estimate our accuracy to exceed 90% using this technique.

nail (missed the hole anteriorly or posteriorly) or is hitting the nail (proximally or distally) **(TECH FIG 4E)**.
  - After the interlocking hole is drilled, another fluoroscopic image is taken. The interlocking hole should now be "lighter," or less radiodense, if the drill bit penetrated both cortices at the level of the interlocking hole.
- Measurement
  - The drill can be removed and measured with a depth gauge or, in many systems, read directly from the drill guide or monitor.
  - An alternate method, which we have used with surprising accuracy, is to use the known diameter of the nail as a legend.
    - Comparing the width of the femoral canal at the level of the screw hole with that of the nail and estimating the number of nail widths in that segment allows for an estimate of the screw length.
    - With a little practice, this method is fairly reliable, especially considering that many companies provide screws only in 5-mm increments **(TECH FIG 4F)**.

TECHNIQUES

Pearls and Pitfalls

Preoperative Considerations	• In patients with chest or head injuries, consideration may be given to external fixation; a team-oriented approach with input from general surgery and neurosurgery is warranted. • Correct position and traction are chosen based on patient size and assistant availability. • Ensure complete muscle relaxation and antibiotic administration before the case begins. • Have an external fixation set in the room not only for backup fixation but also for facilitating reduction (ie, joystick maneuver).
Intraoperative Considerations	• Spend time on (1) obtaining the correct starting point, (2) ensuring a satisfactory reduction, and (3) satisfactory position of the guidewire center–center in the distal femur if possible; many later complications can be avoided by obtaining the correct starting point. • During nail placement, if the nail is not advancing down the intramedullary canal, stop. Check fluoroscopy to ensure it is not hitting a cortex. If there is distraction at the fracture site, consider using a shorter nail and "sink" it further down the canal—in anticipation of locking distally and backslapping the nail to decrease the fracture gap. • If backslapping is performed, two distal interlocking screws may be beneficial in case one screw breaks. • For fracture patterns that the surgeon cannot reliably key-in or reduce using fluoroscopy, that is, transverse, ensure the correct rotation by using contralateral views (ie, lesser trochanter, etc.). • After nail insertion, the surgeon should always check length, alignment, rotation, and the femoral neck (iatrogenic fracture).
Postoperative Care	• After fixation of any long bone fracture, the authors prefer to obtain full-length plane films of the femur to ensure satisfactory alignment. • Prescribe satisfactory physical therapy to ensure strengthening of the abductors, quadriceps mechanism, and gait training.

POSTOPERATIVE CARE

- Postoperative radiographs should be obtained to check fracture length, alignment, rotation, implant placement, and integrity of the femoral neck.
- A clinical examination for rotation of the hip and a thorough knee examination are needed to rule out occult knee injury.
- Most femoral fractures, irrespective of comminution, can be allowed weight bearing as tolerated.
  - Care should be taken when fracture lines are within 6 to 8 cm of the interlocking sites. In these cases, higher stresses can result in complications of the nail or delayed healing, and weight bearing can be initiated with radiographic initiation of healing (callus).
- Patients should be provided with physiotherapy for range of motion of the knee and hip and encouraged to exercise the abductors as well. Specific therapeutic protocols should be developed for these patients to strengthen hip abduction, gait training, and quadriceps control.[39]
- Deep vein thrombosis prophylaxis should be considered for all patients, unless contraindicated.

OUTCOMES

- The femur can be expected to heal in about 95% of cases, with an infection rate of about 1% (**FIGS 3** and **4**).
- Knee motion should return to normal by 12 weeks postoperatively but may be limited in head-injured or polytrauma patients owing to heterotopic bone formation or lack of early motion.[24]

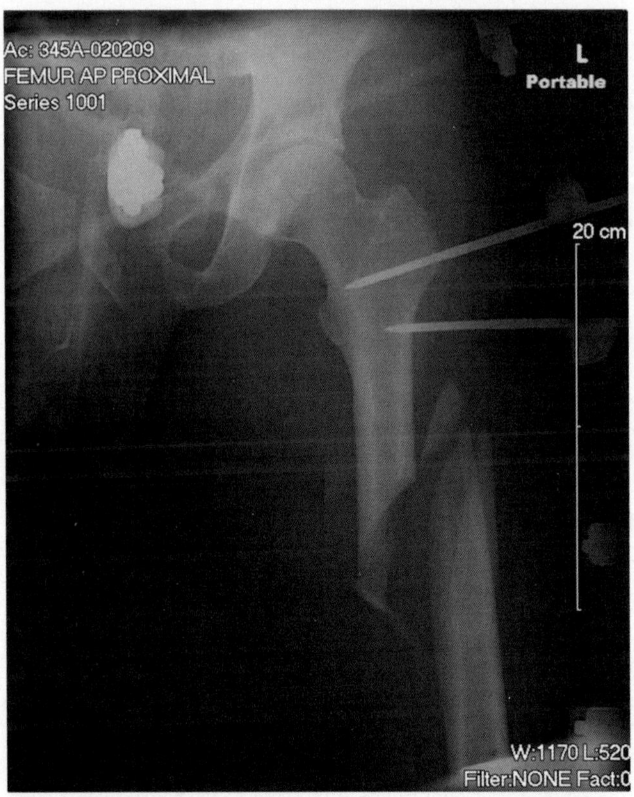

FIG 3 Radiograph demonstrating initial damage control measures using external fixation. The one proximal pin was advanced to gain bicortical purchase.

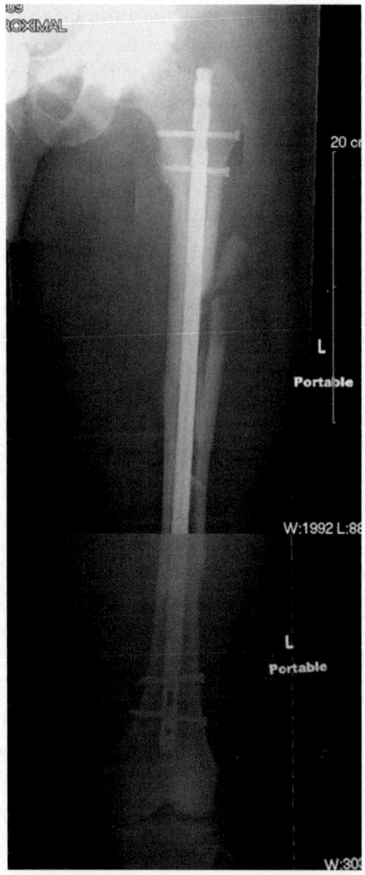

FIG 4 Final radiographs demonstrating final fixation.

- Although healing rates are good, there is almost always an objective deficit in outcomes, which may or may not be clinically relevant.
  - Objective examination can reveal deficits in endurance and strength; weather-related symptoms; or residual hip, thigh, and knee pain.
  - Much like tibial nailing, the causes of such symptoms have not been well elucidated. A recent study has investigated the use of cephalomedullary nails in select patients after femoral shaft fractures to prevent "missed" femoral neck fracture and to prophylactically protect the femoral neck.[15] This discussion is outside the scope of this chapter, but this treatment option warrants consideration in select patients.

COMPLICATIONS

- Iatrogenic femoral neck fracture
  - If the piriformis fossa is used for nail entry, the surgeon should check an AP pelvis with the femur in internal rotation at the end of the case to ensure there is no iatrogenic femoral neck fracture.
- Malunion
  - These deformities can occur in very distal rather than proximal femoral shaft fractures, where the intramedullary nail can "toggle" in the medullary space. Malalignment can also occur in highly comminuted femoral shaft fractures in which the surgeon cannot key-in or reduce

the fracture. Varus/valgus deformity (>5 degrees in coronal or sagittal planes) can be prevented by ensuring reduction *before* placement of the guidewire (ie, open reduction, Schanz pins, etc.) and reaming—especially in difficult fracture patterns. Accurate guidewire placement is also important because passage of the nail down an eccentric path can potentially cause fracture displacement in these unstable segments.

- Whereas varus/valgus malalignment can be visually/radiographically determined to some degree, rotational deformity can be more difficult to assess. As discussed earlier, rotational deformity can be prevented by paying close attention to cortical thickness because the femur is not perfectly cylindrical and cortical thickness varies. At the end of the procedure, hip rotation can be checked while the patient is still anesthetized. Differences in the rotational arc from the normal side should prompt specific fluoroscopic comparison of the rotation of both femurs. Up to 15 degrees of rotational malalignment can be well tolerated, but greater than 15 degrees should be corrected. External rotation causes more functional limitations than internal rotation, especially with demanding activities.[24,25]
    - The overall rate of malalignment is 7% to 11%, with most angular deformities occurring at the proximal and distal thirds of the femur.[33]

- Nonunion
    - The incidence of femoral shaft nonunion after intramedullary nailing varies based on the literature, but union rates range from 90% to 100%. Although outside the scope of this chapter, treatment entails dynamization, exchange nailing, plate augmentation, or external fixation.
- Limb length discrepancy
    - Up to 1.5 cm of leg length discrepancy may be well tolerated. Beyond 2 cm, many patients will eventually complain of symptoms of malalignment (eg, back, knee, or ankle pain). Although symptoms should resolve with simple shoe modifications, most patients are not able to maintain compliance.
- Infection: The risk is less than 1% in closed fractures and is an infrequent but devastating complication. It can be treated by several methods.
    - If the infection is early and fixation is stable, local and systemic antibiotic treatment with nail retention may be considered.
    - If the infection is extensive, a staged procedure should be considered with use of a temporary custom-fabricated, antibiotic-impregnated intramedullary device, possibly an external fixator, and a course of intravenous antibiotics.
    - If the infection is delayed and the fracture is partially healed, one can also consider an exchange nail with reaming and placement of a nail of greater size (usually 2 mm).
- Deep vein thrombosis
    - Most femur fractures should be considered for a combination of mechanical and pharmacologic prophylaxis against deep vein thrombosis.
- Fat emboli
    - Symptomatic fat emboli are a rare occurrence after intramedullary nailing. Care should be used especially during opening reaming and nail insertion to limit likelihood of emboli. Most importantly, patients should be normotensive during reaming and nail placement; hypotension should be avoided.
- Pain/limp
    - Decreased hip function and muscle weakness of the hip abductors and external rotators, along with trochanteric pain, thigh pain, and limp, may occur. Literature has demonstrated that antegrade nailing can affect hip kinematics—specifically with hip abduction, knee extension, and gait abnormalities.[2,22]
    - Although hip dysfunction still occurs with even retrograde nailing, the incidence seems to be greater with antegrade nails.
    - As mentioned, functional outcomes seem to be equivalent for both piriformis-entry and trochanteric-entry femoral nails.[48]
- Heterotopic ossification
    - Heterotopic ossification may occur in 9% to 60% of patients, with the most commonly associated factor being head injury.
- Implant failure
    - Failed hardware or refracture usually indicates a nonunion. In some cases, fracture of locking screws serves to "autodynamize" the fracture and healing often ensues. There is no need for hardware removal or additional surgery if the fracture heals with minimal deformity.
- Nerve injury
    - Femoral, sciatic, or pudendal nerve injuries are relatively rare. Stretch injury of the sciatic nerve due to prolonged traction during intramedullary nailing can be avoided with judicious use of traction. Pudendal nerve palsy (if intramedullary nailing is performed on a fracture table) can occur when excessive traction and a small perineal post are used. Most femur fractures can be brought to length easily, and traction should be limited to the time of reduction and nail passage and interlocking. Use of a large, well-padded perineal post, judicious traction, or a lateral distractor can avoid this problem. Treatment consists of expectant and supportive treatments.
- Compartment syndrome
    - Compartment syndrome of the thigh (especially in intubated, polytrauma victims) may occur, especially with crush injuries or prolonged hypotension. Clinical signs should be used to dictate treatment, and release of the anterior compartment is generally sufficient. If compartment pressures are to be monitored, threshold pressure is within 30 mm Hg of the patient's diastolic blood pressure if no examination is possible.

REFERENCES

1. Anglen JO, Choi L. Treatment options in pediatric femoral shaft fractures. J Orthop Trauma 2005;19(10):724–733.
2. Archdeacon M, Ford KR, Wyrick J, et al. A prospective functional outcome and motion analysis evaluation of the hip abductors after femur fracture and antegrade nailing. J Orthop Trauma 2008;22(1):3–9.
3. Bone LB, Anders MJ, Rohrbacher BJ. Treatment of femoral fractures in the multiply injured patient with thoracic injury. Clin Orthop Relat Res 1998;(347):57–61.
4. Bone LB, Johnson KD, Weigelt J, et al. Early versus delayed stabilization of femoral fractures. A prospective randomized study. J Bone Joint Surg Am 1989;71(3):336–340.
5. Bong MR, Koval KJ, Egol KA. The history of intramedullary nailing. Bull NYU Hosp Jt Dis 2006;64(3–4):94–97.

6. Bosse MJ, Mackenzie EJ, Riemer BL, et al. Adult respiratory distress syndrome, pneumonia, and mortality following thoracic injury and a femoral fracture treated either with intramedullary nailing with reaming or with a plate. A comparative study. J Bone Joint Surg Am 1997; 79(6):799–809.
7. Brox WT, Roberts KC, Taksali S, et al. The American Academy of Orthopaedic Surgeons evidence-based guideline on management of hip fractures in the elderly. J Bone Joint Surg Am 2015;97(14): 1196–1199.
8. Brumback RJ. The rationales of interlocking nailing of the femur, tibia, and humerus. Clin Orthop Relat Res 1996;(324):292–320.
9. Brumback RJ, Ellison TS, Molligan H, et al. Pudendal nerve palsy complicating intramedullary nailing of the femur. J Bone Joint Surg Am 1992;74(10):1450–1455.
10. Brumback RJ, Ellison TS, Poka A, et al. Intramedullary nailing of femoral shaft fractures. Part III: long-term effects of static interlocking fixation. J Bone Joint Surg Am 1992;74(1):106–112.
11. Brumback RJ, Reilly JP, Poka A, et al. Intramedullary nailing of femoral shaft fractures. Part I: decision-making errors with interlocking fixation. J Bone Joint Surg Am 1988;70(10):1441 1452.
12. Brumback RJ, Uwagie-Ero S, Lakatos RP, et al. Intramedullary nailing of femoral shaft fractures. Part II: fracture-healing with static interlocking fixation. J Bone Joint Surg Am 1988;70(10):1453–1462.
13. Bumpass DB, Ricci WM, McAndrew CM, et al. A prospective study of pain reduction and knee dysfunction comparing femoral skeletal traction and splinting in adult trauma patients. J Orthop Trauma 2015; 29(2):112–118.
14. Byrne JP, Nathens AB, Gomez D, et al. Timing of femoral shaft fracture fixation following major trauma: a retrospective cohort study of United States trauma centers. PLoS Med 2017;14(7):e1002336.
15. Collinge C, Liporace F, Koval K, et al. Cephalomedullary screws as the standard proximal locking screws for nailing femoral shaft fractures. J Orthop Trauma 2010;24(12):717–722.
16. Della Rocca GJ, Crist BD. External fixation versus conversion to intramedullary nailing for definitive management of closed fractures of the femoral and tibial shaft. J Am Acad Orthop Surg 2006;14:S131–S135.
17. Egol KA, Chang EY, Cvitkovic J, et al. Mismatch of current intramedullary nails with the anterior bow of the femur. J Orthop Trauma 2004;18(7):410–415.
18. Flynn JM, Schwend RM. Management of pediatric femoral shaft fractures. J Am Acad Orthop Surg 2004;12(5):347–359.
19. Grob K, Manestar M, Lang A, et al. Effects of ligation of lateral intermuscular septum perforating vessels on blood supply to the femur. Injury 2015;46(12):2461–2467.
20. Hajek PD, Bicknell HR Jr, Bronson WE, et al. The use of one compared with two distal screws in the treatment of femoral shaft fractures with interlocking intramedullary nailing. A clinical and biomechanical analysis. J Bone Joint Surg Am 1993;75(4):519–525.
21. Hall JA, Mckee MD, Vicente MR, et al. Prospective randomized clinical trial investigating the effect of the reamer-irrigator-aspirator on the volume of embolic load and respiratory function during intramedullary nailing of femoral shaft fractures. J Orthop Trauma 2017; 31(4):200–204.
22. Helmy N, Jando VT, Lu T, et al. Muscle function and functional outcome following standard antegrade reamed intramedullary nailing of isolated femoral shaft fractures. J Orthop Trauma 2008;22(1):10–15.
23. Hu S-J, Chang S-M, Ma Z, et al. PFNA-II protrusion over the greater trochanter in the Asian population used in proximal femoral fractures. Indian J Orthop 2016;50(6):641–646.
24. Jaarsma RL, Pakvis DFM, Verdonschot N, et al. Rotational malalignment after intramedullary nailing of femoral fractures. J Orthop Trauma 2004;18(7):403–409.
25. Jaarsma RL, van Kampen A. Rotational malalignment after fractures of the femur. J Bone Joint Surg Br 2004;86(8):1100–1104.
26. Johnson KD, Tencer AF, Sherman MC. Biomechanical factors affecting fracture stability and femoral bursting in closed intramedullary nailing of femoral shaft fractures, with illustrative case presentations. J Orthop Trauma 1987;1(1):1–11.
27. Jones CB, Walker JB. Diagnosis and management of ipsilateral femoral neck and shaft fractures. J Am Acad Orthop Surg 2018;26(21): e448–e454.
28. Kao JT, Burton D, Comstock C, et al. Pudendal nerve palsy after femoral intramedullary nailing. J Orthop Trauma 1993;7(1):58–63.
29. Kirschner MH, Menck J, Hennerbichler A, et al. Importance of arterial blood supply to the femur and tibia for transplantation of vascularized femoral diaphyses and knee joints. World J Surg 1998; 22(8):845–852.
30. Kobbe P, Micansky F, Lichte P, et al. Increased morbidity and mortality after bilateral femoral shaft fractures: myth or reality in the era of damage control? Injury 2013;44(2):221–225.
31. Lewis CG, Inneh IA, Schutzer SF, et al. Evaluation of the first-generation AAOS clinical guidelines on the prophylaxis of venous thromboembolic events in patients undergoing total joint arthroplasty: experience with 3289 patients from a single institution. J Bone Joint Surg Am 2014;96(16):1327–1332.
32. Mithöfer K, Lhowe DW, Vrahas MS, et al. Clinical spectrum of acute compartment syndrome of the thigh and its relation to associated injuries. Clin Orthop Relat Res 2004;(425):223–229.
33. Nork S. Femoral shaft fractures. In: Bucholz R, Heckman J, Court-Brown C, eds. Rockwood & Green's Fractures in Adults, ed 7. Philadelphia: Lippincott Williams & Wilkins, 2010;1656–1718.
34. Nowotarski PJ, Turen CH, Brumback RJ, et al. Conversion of external fixation to intramedullary nailing for fractures of the shaft of the femur in multiply injured patients. J Bone Joint Surg Am 2000; 82(6):781–788.
35. Ojike NI, Roberts CS, Giannoudis PV. Compartment syndrome of the thigh: a systematic review. Injury 2010;41(2):133–136.
36. O'Toole RV, O'Brien M, Scalea TM, et al. Resuscitation before stabilization of femoral fractures limits acute respiratory distress syndrome in patients with multiple traumatic injuries despite low use of damage control orthopedics. J Trauma 2009;67(5):1013–1021.
37. O'Toole RV, Riche K, Cannada LK, et al. Analysis of postoperative knee sepsis after retrograde nail insertion of open femoral shaft fractures. J Orthop Trauma 2010;24(11):677–682.
38. Pape HC, Hildebrand F, Pertschy S, et al. Changes in the management of femoral shaft fractures in polytrauma patients: from early total care to damage control orthopedic surgery. J Trauma 2002;53(3): 452–461.
39. Paterno MV, Archdeacon MT. Is there a standard rehabilitation protocol after femoral intramedullary nailing? J Orthop Trauma 2009; 23(suppl 5):S39–S46.
40. Peltier LF. A brief history of traction. J Bone Joint Surg Am 1968;50(8):1603–1617.
41. Reichert I, McCarthy I, Hughes S. The acute vascular response to intramedullary reaming. Microsphere estimation of blood flow in the intact ovine tibia. J Bone Joint Surg Br 1995;77(3):490–493.
42. Rhinelander FW, Peltier LF. Effects of medullary nailing on the normal blood supply of diaphyseal cortex. Clin Orthop Relat Res 1998;350:5–17.
43. Rudloff MI, Smith WR. Intramedullary nailing of the femur: current concepts concerning reaming. J Orthop Trauma 2009;23(suppl 5): S12–S17.
44. Sagi HC, Ahn J, Ciesla D, et al. Venous thromboembolism prophylaxis in orthopaedic trauma patients: a survey of OTA member practice patterns and OTA expert panel recommendations. J Orthop Trauma 2015;29(10):e355–e362.
45. Shepherd LE, Shean CJ, Gelalis ID, et al. Prospective randomized study of reamed versus unreamed femoral intramedullary nailing: an assessment of procedures. J Orthop Trauma 2001;15(1):28–33.
46. Sisak K, Manolis M, Hardy BM, et al. Epidemiology of acute transfusions in major orthopaedic trauma. J Orthop Trauma 2013;27(7): 413–418.
47. Smith R, Giannoudis P. Femoral shaft fractures. In: Browner B, Levine A, Jupiter J, eds. Skeletal Trauma, ed 4. Philadelphia: Saunders, 2009:2035–2072.
48. Sprague MA, Yang EC. Early versus delayed fixation of isolated closed femur fractures in an urban trauma center. Bull Hosp Jt Dis 2004; 62(1–2):58–61.
49. Stannard JP, Bankston L, Futch LA, et al. Functional outcome following intramedullary nailing of the femur: a prospective randomized comparison of piriformis fossa and greater trochanteric entry portals. J Bone Joint Surg Am 2011;93(15):1385–1391.

50. Steinhausen E, Lefering R, Tjardes T, et al. A risk-adapted approach is beneficial in the management of bilateral femoral shaft fractures in multiple trauma patients: an analysis based on the trauma registry of the German Trauma Society. J Trauma Acute Care Surg 2014;76(5):1288–1293.
51. Suman RK. Treatment of fractures of the femoral shaft with early cast bracing. Injury 1981;13(3):239–243.
52. Tarlow SD, Achterman CA, Hayhurst J, et al. Acute compartment syndrome in the thigh complicating fracture of the femur. A report of three cases. J Bone Joint Surg Am 1986;68(9):1439–1443.
53. The Canadian Orthopaedic Trauma Society. Reamed versus unreamed intramedullary nailing of the femur: comparison of the rate of ARDS in multiple injured patients. J Orthop Trauma 2006;20(6):384–387.
54. Tornetta P III, Kain MSH, Creevy WR. Diagnosis of femoral neck fractures in patients with a femoral shaft fracture: improvement with a standard protocol. J Bone Joint Surg Am 2007;89(1):39–43.
55. Tornetta P III, Ritz G, Kantor A. Femoral torsion after interlocked nailing of unstable femoral fractures. J Trauma 1995;38(2):213–219.
56. Tornetta P III, Tiburzi D. Anterograde interlocked nailing of distal femoral fractures after gunshot wounds. J Orthop Trauma 1994;8(3):220–227.
57. Vallier HA, Wang X, Moore TA, et al. Timing of orthopaedic surgery in multiple trauma patients: development of a protocol for early appropriate care. J Orthop Trauma 2013;27(10):543–551.
58. Weinberg DS, Narayanan AS, Moore TA, et al. Assessment of resuscitation as measured by markers of metabolic acidosis and features of injury. Bone Joint J 2017;99-B(1):122–127.
59. Winquist RA, Hansen ST Jr. Comminuted fractures of the femoral shaft treated by intramedullary nailing. Orthop Clin North Am 1980;11(3):633–648.
60. Yang E. Inserting distal screws into interlocking IM nails. Orthop Rev 1992;21:779–781.
61. Ziran BH, Smith WR, Zlotolow DA, et al. Clinical evaluation of a true percutaneous technique for antegrade femoral nailing. Orthopedics 2005;28(10):1182–1186.

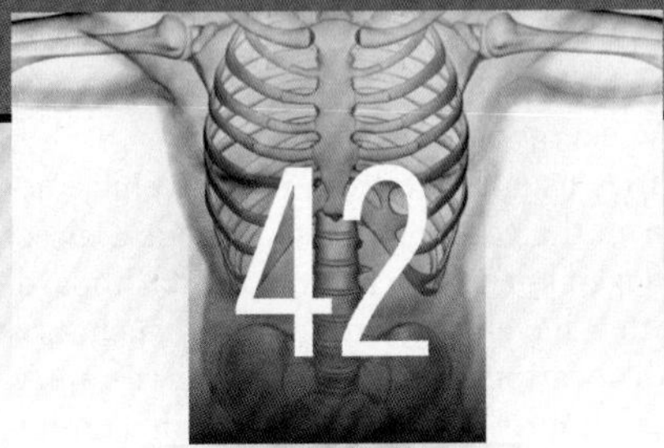

CHAPTER 42

Open Reduction and Internal Fixation of the Distal Femur

Animesh Agarwal

DEFINITION

- Distal femur fractures are complex injuries that can result in poor outcomes.
- The distal part of the femur is considered the most distal 9 to 15 cm of the femur and can involve the articular surface. The intra-articular injury can vary from a simple split to extensive comminution.
- Articular involvement can lead to posttraumatic arthritis.
- These fractures constitute 4% to 7% of all femur fractures.
  - If the hip is excluded, they represent nearly one-third of all femur fractures.
  - There is a bimodal distribution defined by the mechanism of injury (see the following discussion).

ANATOMY

- The supracondylar area of the femur is the zone between the femoral condyles and the metaphyseal–diaphyseal junction.
- The metaphyseal bone has some important structural characteristics.
  - The predominant bone is cancellous.
  - The cortices are thinner than in diaphyseal bone.
  - There is a wide intramedullary canal.
- It is also important to understand the unique bony architecture of the distal femur (**FIG 1**).
  - It is trapezoidal in shape, and hence, the posterior aspect is wider than the anterior aspect. There is a gradual decrease by 25% in the width from posterior to anterior.
  - The medial femoral condyle has a larger anterior to posterior dimension than the lateral condyle and extends farther distally.
  - The shaft is in line with the anterior half of the distal femoral condyles.
- The normal mechanical and anatomic axes of the lower limb must be understood so that the alignment of the limb can be reestablished (**FIG 2**).
  - The mechanical femoral axis, which is from the center of the femoral head to the center of the knee, is 3 degrees off the vertical. The mechanical axis of the entire limb continues to the center of the ankle.
  - The anatomic femoral axis differs from the mechanical femoral axis with an average of 9 degrees of valgus at the knee. This results in an anatomic femoral axis of the lateral distal femur of 81 degrees or an anatomic femoral axis of the medial distal femur of 99 degrees.
  - The mechanical and anatomic axes of the tibia are for practical purposes identical, going from the center of the knee to the center of the ankle.
- The treatment of distal femur fractures is affected by the various muscle attachments, which can impede or hamper proper fracture reduction.
  - The quadriceps and hamstrings result in fracture shortening; thus, muscle paralysis must be obtained for proper reduction.
  - The medial and lateral gastrocnemius results in posterior angulation and displacement of the distal segment.

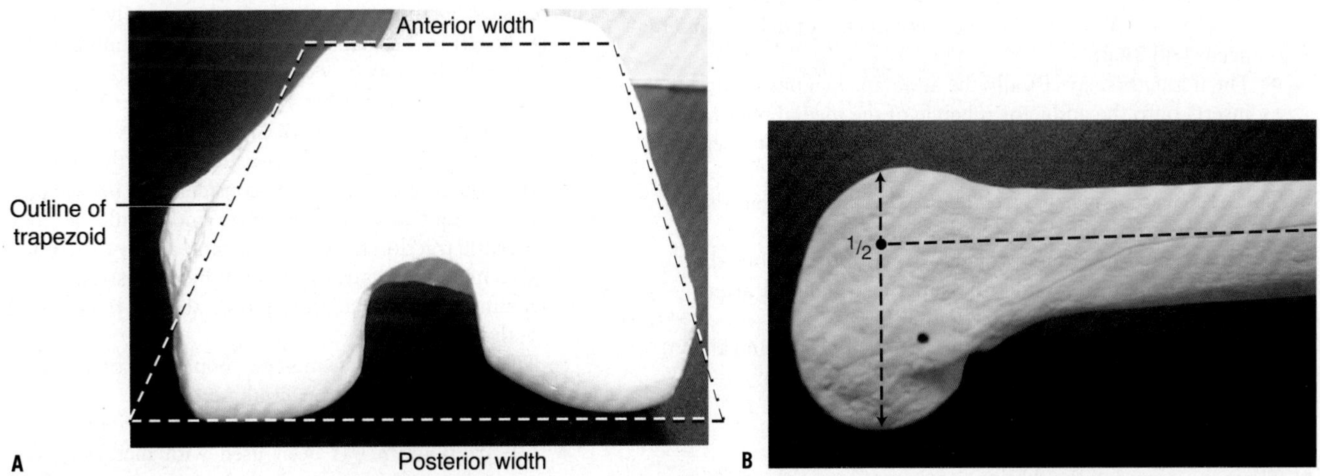

FIG 1 **A.** View of the distal femur showing the wider posterior aspect and trapezoidal shape. **B.** Lateral view of the distal femur; the shaft is in line with the anterior half of the distal femoral condyles.

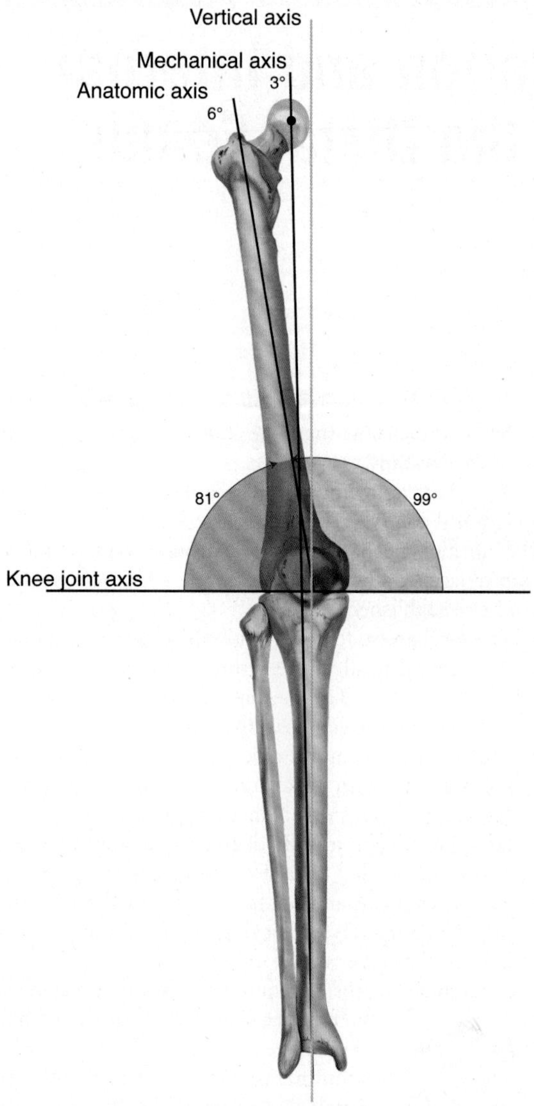

FIG 2 Mechanical and anatomic axes of the lower extremity; the 9 degrees of valgus at the knee is noted.

The distal femur "extends," resulting in an apex posterior deformity. If an intercondylar extension is present, rotational deformities of the individual condyles can occur **(FIG 3A,B)**.

- The adductors, specifically the adductor magnus, which inserts onto the adductor tubercle of the medial femoral condyle, can lead to a varus deformity of the distal segment **(FIG 3C)**.
- The neurovascular structures about the knee are at risk when an injury of the distal femur occurs.
  - At the canal of Hunter, roughly 10 cm proximal to the knee on the medial side, the superficial femoral artery enters the popliteal fossa (see **FIG 3C**).
  - Posterior to the knee, both the popliteal artery and the tibial nerve are at risk at the fracture site **(FIG 3D)**.

PATHOGENESIS

- There is a bimodal distribution in terms of age in the epidemiology of distal femur fractures. This relates to the mechanism of injury.
- High-energy and low-energy injuries occur.
  - High-energy injuries usually are from motor vehicle accidents and occur in the young patient. There is a direct impact onto the flexed knee, such as from the dashboard. These patients often have associated injuries such as a hip fracture or dislocation or vascular or nerve injury. These high-energy injuries generally result in comminuted fractures, mostly of the metaphyseal region. The comminution can be articular as well.
  - Low-energy injuries usually occur in the elderly patient who falls from a standing height. The axial loading is accompanied by either varus or valgus with or without rotation. The osteoporotic bone in these individuals leads to fracture. The fracture pattern can vary from the simplest extra-articular type to the most complex intra-articular injury. Owing to the gastrocnemius complex, an apex posterior deformity of the condyles occurs as the fragments are flexed because of the muscle attachment.

NATURAL HISTORY

- Fractures of the distal femur that have intra-articular displacement can lead to severe posttraumatic arthritis if left untreated.
- Operative treatment has led to a 32% decrease in poor outcomes.[40]

PATIENT HISTORY AND PHYSICAL FINDINGS

- Direct physical examination of the knee with a distal femur fracture is limited primarily because of pain and the obvious nature of the injury.
  - The patient presents with a swollen and tender knee after either a fall or some high-energy trauma (motor vehicle or motorcycle accident).
  - A large hemarthrosis is present.
  - Any attempts at range of motion result in severe pain, and significant crepitus is usually noted with palpation.
- If there is concern for an open knee joint, the joint can be injected after a sterile preparation to see whether the knee joint communicates with any wound. If a computed tomography (CT) scan is obtained prior to going to the operating room for temporary stabilization, air may be apparent on the imaging, which is indicative of an open knee joint.
- The physical examination is directed primarily at ascertaining the neurovascular status of the lower limb and determining whether any associated injuries exist, especially the hip (see Exam Table for Pelvis and Lower Extremity Trauma at the end of the book).
  - If there are any small wounds or tenting of the skin anteriorly, the fracture should be considered as being open.
  - It is important to check for pulses and should be done with gentle traction to realign the limb as any deformity/displacement may cause kinking of blood vessels.
    - If diminished or absent, pulses should be assessed with Doppler.
    - The ankle–brachial indices should be obtained if there is a concern for arterial injury.
    - Any value less than 0.9 warrants an arteriogram.
    - CT arteriogram has been used with increasing frequency as well in cases where there is concern **(FIG 4)**.
  - Nerve function should be checked. Sensation and both active dorsiflexion and plantarflexion must be assessed.

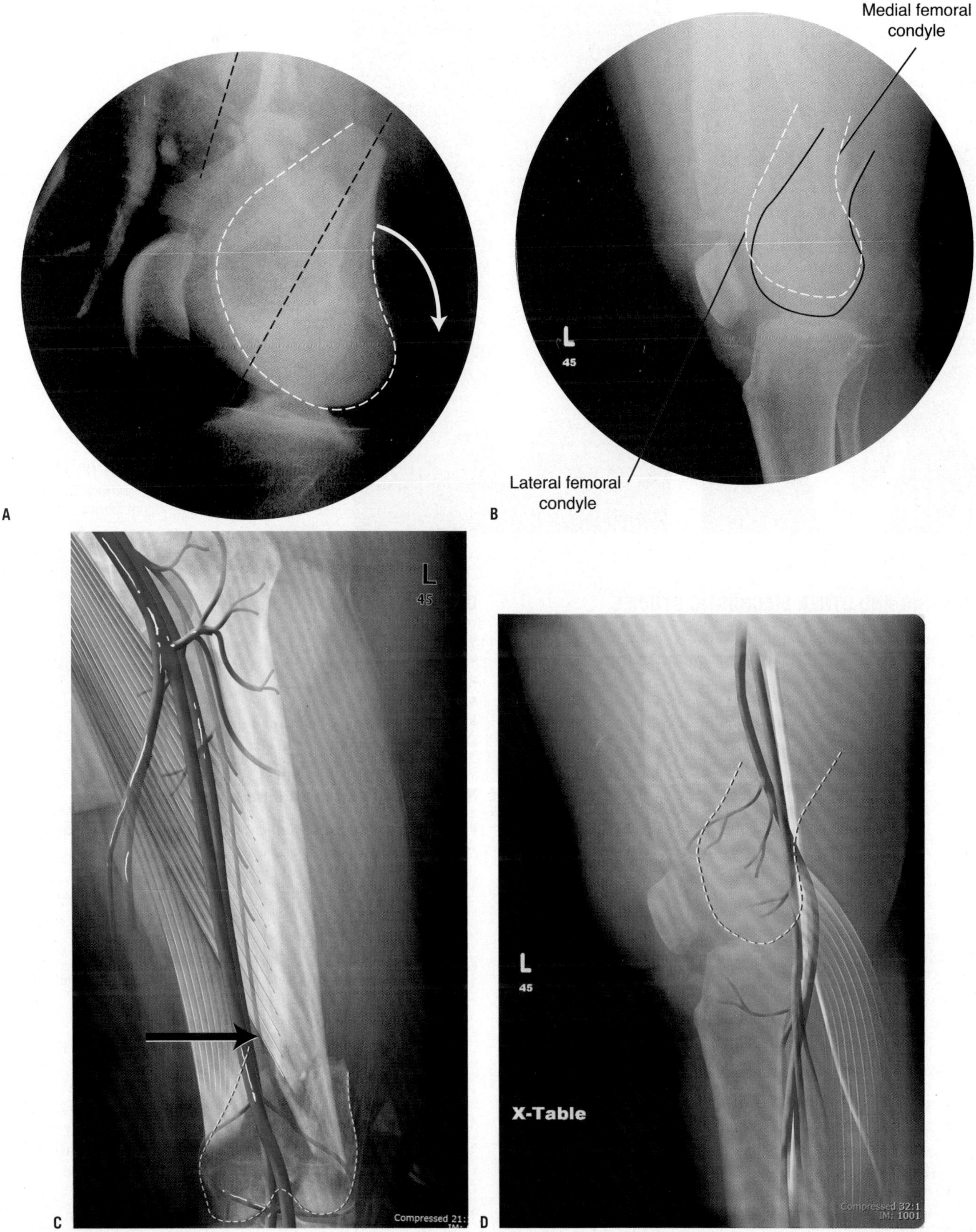

FIG 3 **A.** Patient with a grade IIIA open distal femur with extruded fragment; the "extension" of the femoral condyles is outlined. **B.** Patient with a distal femur fracture with intercondylar extension showing the subtle rotational deformities of the individual condyles. **C.** The muscle forces are shown on the distal femur, as is the femoral artery and vein entering the canal of Hunter (*arrow*). The adductor magnus inserts on the adductor tubercle, leading to a varus deformity of the distal segment. **D.** A lateral image of the same patient with the popliteal artery and tibial nerve drawn in to show the relative proximity to the fracture ends.

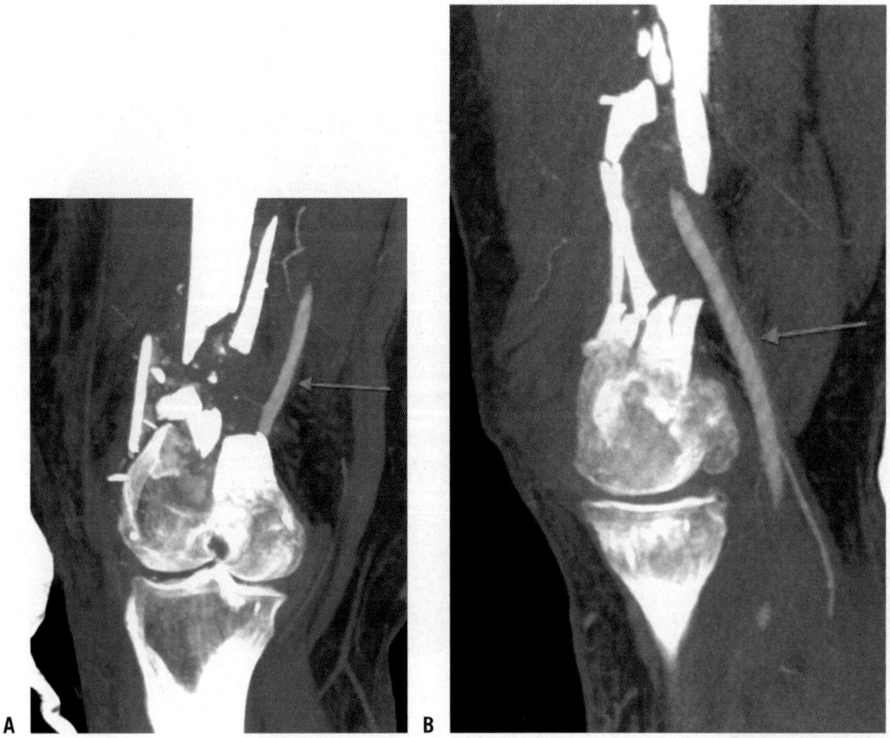

FIG 4 Coronal (**A**) and sagittal CT (**B**) angiography images showing intact femoral artery in a severely comminuted distal femur fracture (*red arrows*).

IMAGING AND OTHER DIAGNOSTIC STUDIES

- The initial imaging study is always plain radiographs. Anteroposterior (AP) and lateral radiographs of the knee should be obtained initially.
  - Traction films should be obtained if there is severe comminution of either the metaphysis or articular surface. This aids in the preoperative planning.
  - Dedicated knee films should always be obtained in the assessment of distal femur fractures. Additionally, the entire femur, to include the hip and knee, should be imaged to look for possible extension and associated injuries and to allow for preoperative planning **(FIG 5)**.
  - In cases of severe comminution, radiographs of the contralateral knee can aid in preoperative planning as well.
- A dedicated CT scan is an important adjunct to the preoperative planning when there is articular involvement **(FIG 6)**.
- Generally, extra-articular distal femur fractures do not require a CT scan. However, it has been shown that coronal fractures may be missed on plain films, and thus, there is a low threshold for obtaining a CT scan for fractures of the distal femur.[21]
  - If the fracture pattern warrants a temporary bridging external fixator, it is best to obtain the CT scan after placement of such a fixator for better definition.
  - Coronal and sagittal reconstructions should be requested.
  - Three-dimensional images can be created from most CT scans. This can also aid in the preoperative planning **(FIG 7A,B)**.
  - Subtle sagittal plane rotational malalignment between condyles can be assessed **(FIG 7C)**.
- If associated soft tissue injury is suspected, such as ligamentous tears or tendon ruptures, then magnetic resonance imaging (MRI) may be indicated. Routine use of MRI, however, is not needed.

DIFFERENTIAL DIAGNOSIS

- Proximal tibia fracture
- Femoral shaft fracture
- Septic knee
- Patella fracture
- Anterior cruciate ligament rupture
- Knee dislocation

NONOPERATIVE MANAGEMENT

- There are few relative indications for nonoperative management of distal femur fractures:
  - Poor overall medical condition
    - Patient has severe comorbidities and is too sick for surgery.
    - Patient has extremely poor bone stock.
  - Spinal cord injury (paraplegia or quadriplegia)
  - Some special situations may warrant nonoperative care on case-by-case basis.
    - Nondisplaced or minimally displaced fracture
    - Select gunshot wounds with incomplete fractures
    - Extra-articular and stable
    - Unreconstructable
    - Lack of experience by the available surgeon or lack of equipment or appropriate facility to adequately treat the injury. Transfer is indicated in these situations; otherwise, nonoperative treatment may be the only option.
- There are several methods for nonoperative treatment.
  - Skeletal traction
  - Cast bracing
  - Knee immobilizer
  - Long-leg cast

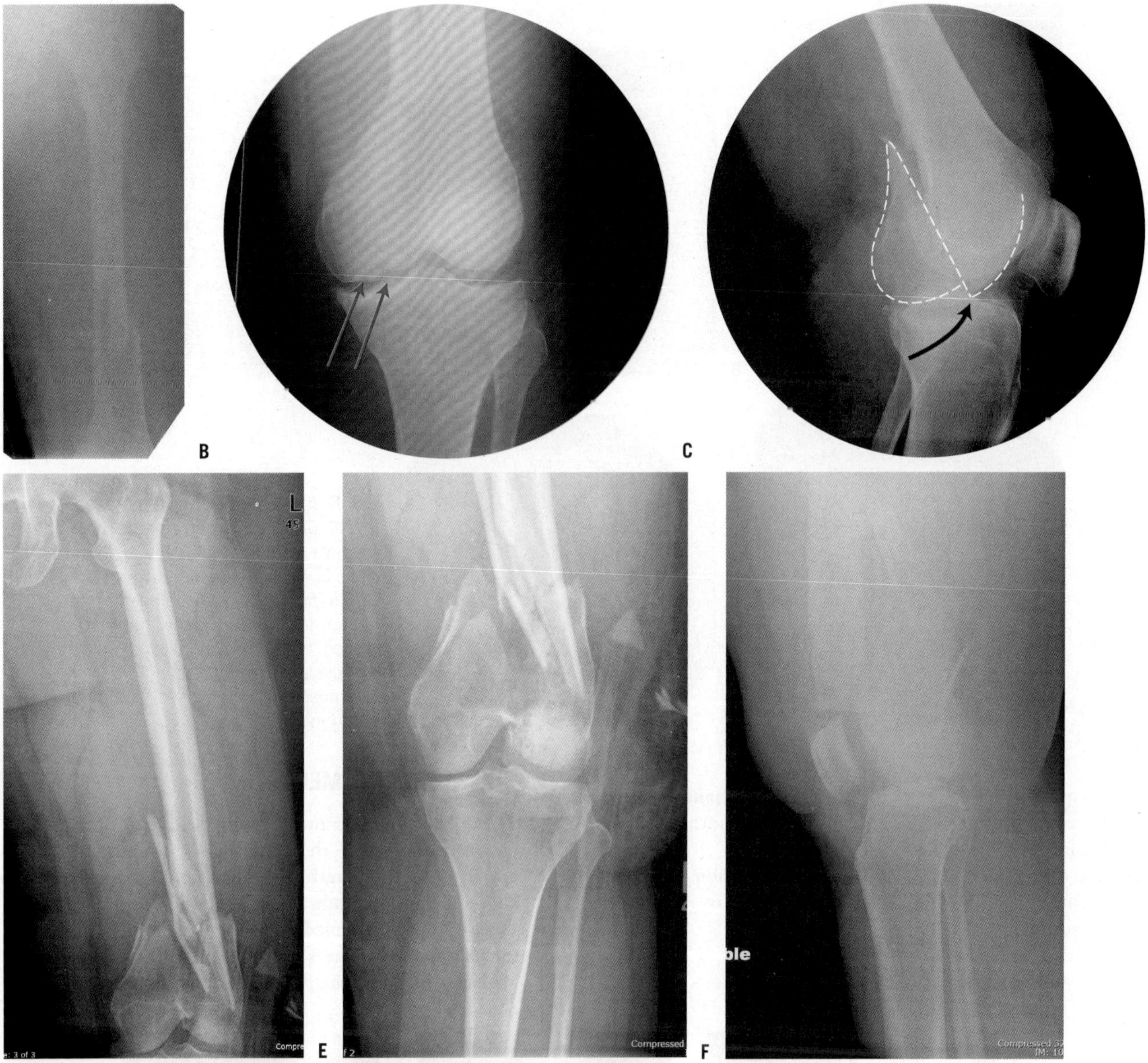

A B C D E F

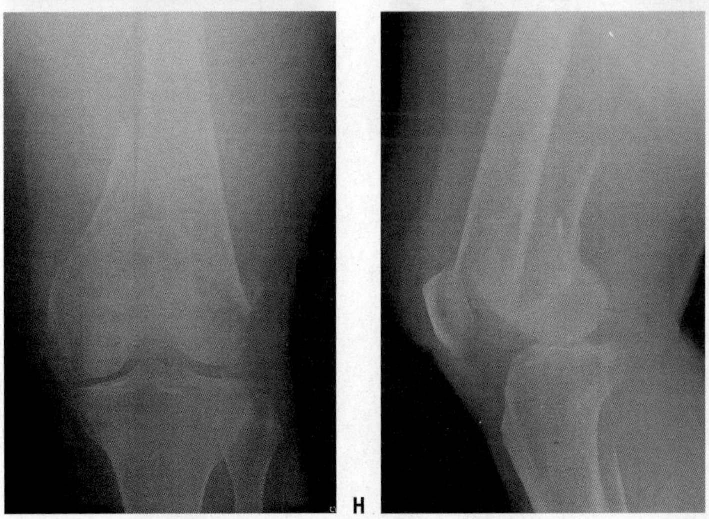

G H

FIG 5 A–C. Patient with a spiral distal-third femur fracture that appears to be extra-articular. **A.** In the AP radiograph, the knee is not fully visualized. **B.** A dedicated knee AP radiograph shows the spiral distal-third femur fracture. Note the intra-articular injury and the gap at the fracture (*arrows*). **C.** Lateral view of the knee. Again, note the coronal fracture of the medial femoral condyle (type B3). **D–F.** Plain radiographs of a patient with a grade II open distal femur fracture. **G,H.** Patient with a closed femur fracture that was initially thought to be extra-articular.

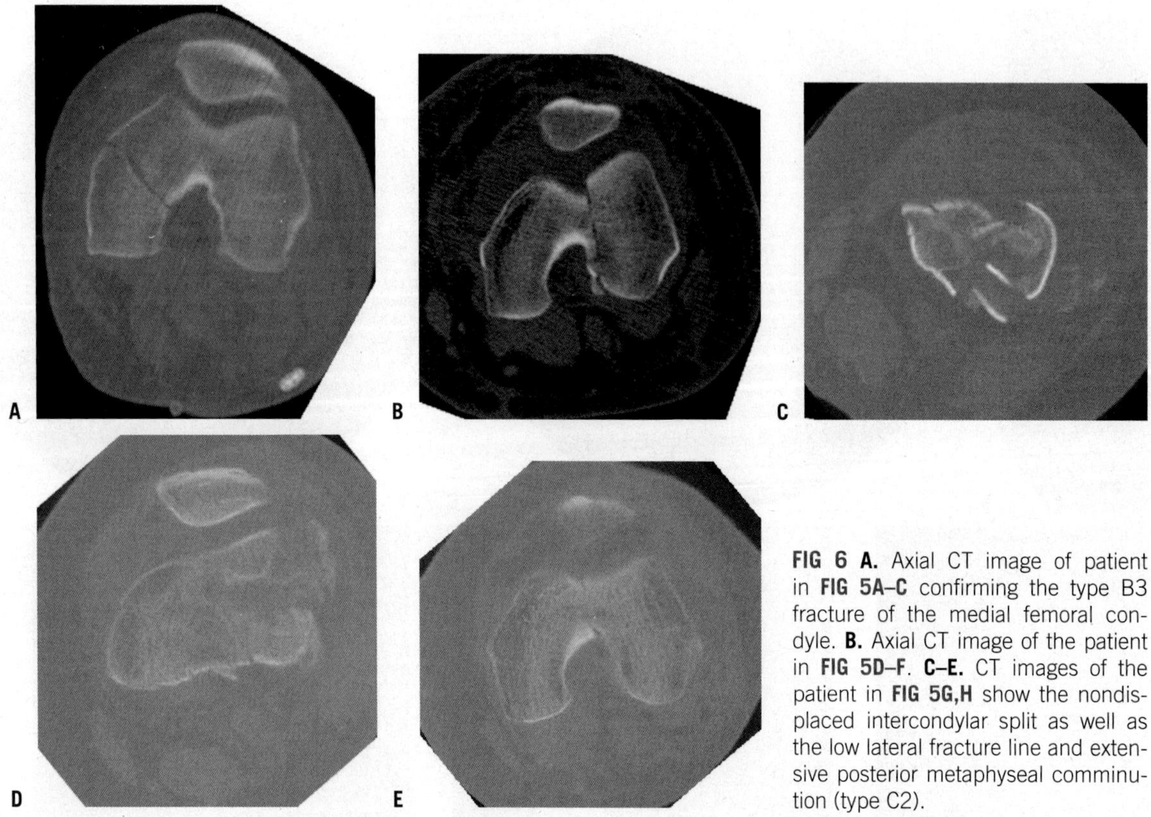

FIG 6 **A.** Axial CT image of patient in **FIG 5A–C** confirming the type B3 fracture of the medial femoral condyle. **B.** Axial CT image of the patient in **FIG 5D–F**. **C–E.** CT images of the patient in **FIG 5G,H** show the nondisplaced intercondylar split as well as the low lateral fracture line and extensive posterior metaphyseal comminution (type C2).

- There are acceptable limits for nonoperative management:
  - Seven degrees of varus or valgus from the normal valgus position
  - Ten degrees of anterior or posterior angulation. A flexion deformity is less well tolerated than an extension deformity.
  - Up to 1 to 1.5 cm of shortening
  - Two to 3 mm of step-off at the joint surface

SURGICAL MANAGEMENT

- The goal of any treatment, nonoperative or operative, is to maintain or restore the congruity of the articular surface and restore the length and alignment of the femur and, subsequently, the limb.
- Once surgery is deemed appropriate for the patient and the particular injury, the surgical technique options available are determined by the particular fracture pattern.

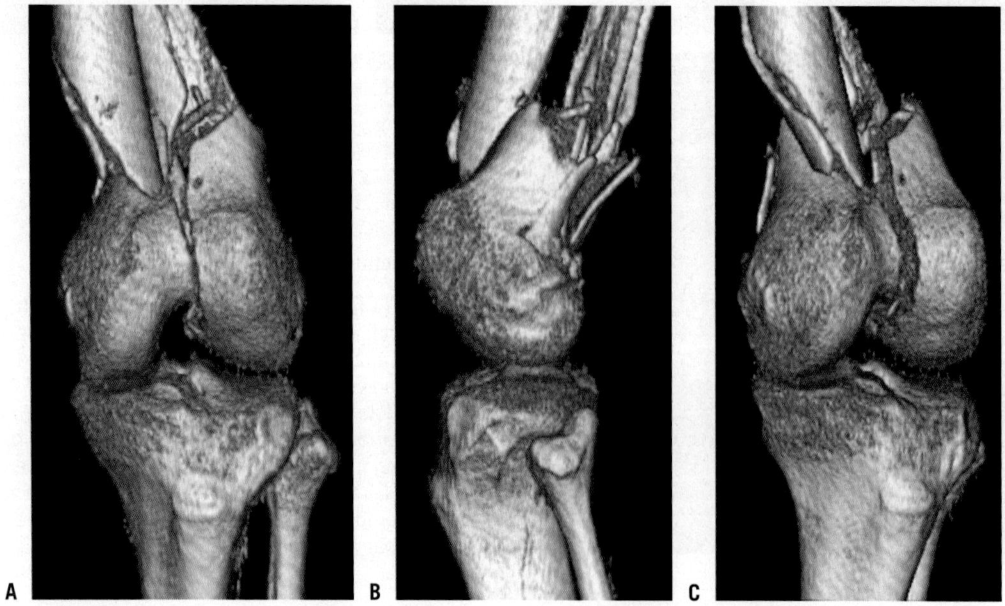

FIG 7 AP (**A**) and lateral (**B**) views of a three-dimensional (3-D) CT reconstruction of the patient in **FIG 3B** with a distal femur fracture. The fracture is well defined. **C.** An oblique 3-D CT reconstruction view showing the same patient and the rotational malalignment between condyles.

- Distal femur fractures have been classified several ways.
  - The OTA/AO classification is probably the most widely accepted classification system and allows some guidance on which techniques are best **(FIG 8; TABLE 1)**.
- Treatment also must be determined based on factors other than the classification alone.
  - The degree of comminution and injury to both the articular surface and bone
  - The amount of fracture displacement
  - The soft tissue injury
  - Associated injuries, other fractures, and injury to neurovascular structures
  - Patient's overall condition and injury to other organ systems. This may affect the timing of surgery or the positioning of the patient.
- There are several principles for the surgical management of distal femur fractures.
  - The articular surface must be reduced anatomically, which usually requires direct visualization through an open exposure (arthrotomy). Simple intra-articular splits may be treated with closed reduction and percutaneous fixation.

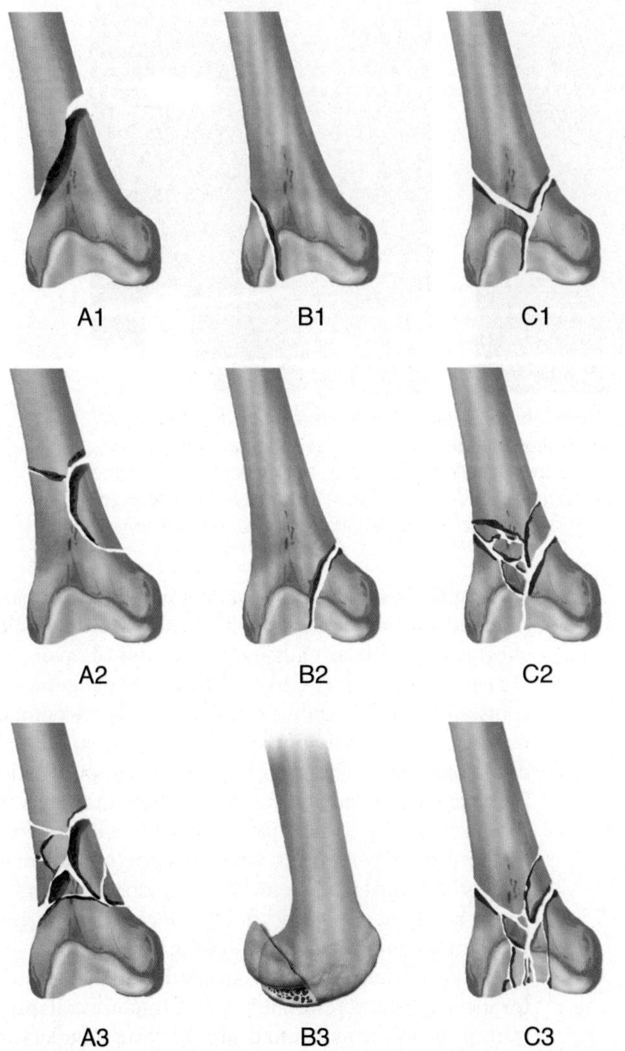

FIG 8 OTA/AO classification for distal femur fractures (types 33A, B, and C).

TABLE 1 OTA/AO Classification of Femoral Fractures

Classification	Description
Type A	Extra-articular
A1	Simple or two-part fracture
A2	Metaphyseal butterfly or wedge fracture
A3	Metaphysis is comminuted
Type B	Partial articular
B1	Sagittal plane fracture of the lateral femoral condyle
B2	Sagittal plane fracture of the medial femoral condyle
B3	Any frontal or coronal plane fracture of the condyle (Hoffa type)
Type C	Intra-articular
C1	Simple articular split and metaphyseal injury (T or Y fracture configuration)
C2	Simple articular split with comminuted metaphyseal injury
C3	Comminuted articular with varying metaphyseal injury

  - The extra-articular injury should be dealt with using indirect reduction techniques as much as possible to maintain a biologic soft tissue envelope. Avoidance of stripping of the tissues, especially on the medial side, is ideal.
  - The surgeon must reestablish the length, rotation, and alignment of the femur and the limb.
  - The soft tissue injury and bone quality may dictate treatment decisions.

Fixation Choices

- External fixation
  - A temporary bridging external fixator across the knee joint can be used if temporary stabilization is required before definitive fixation. This is usually the case where definitive open reduction and internal fixation (ORIF) is planned. This could be in cases where the soft tissues prevent immediate fixation.
  - Definitive management with bridging or nonbridging external fixation can be used for nonreconstructible joints, very severe soft tissue injuries, or severe osteopenia.
  - Bridging external fixation can be used when definitive ORIF is problematic in certain patient populations, such as Jehovah's witnesses, where additional blood loss can lead to increased morbidity or mortality. This can be done temporarily until the patient's condition improves or until healing **(FIG 9)**.
- Intramedullary nailing
  - This can be performed fairly acutely; temporary bridging external fixation is not necessary.

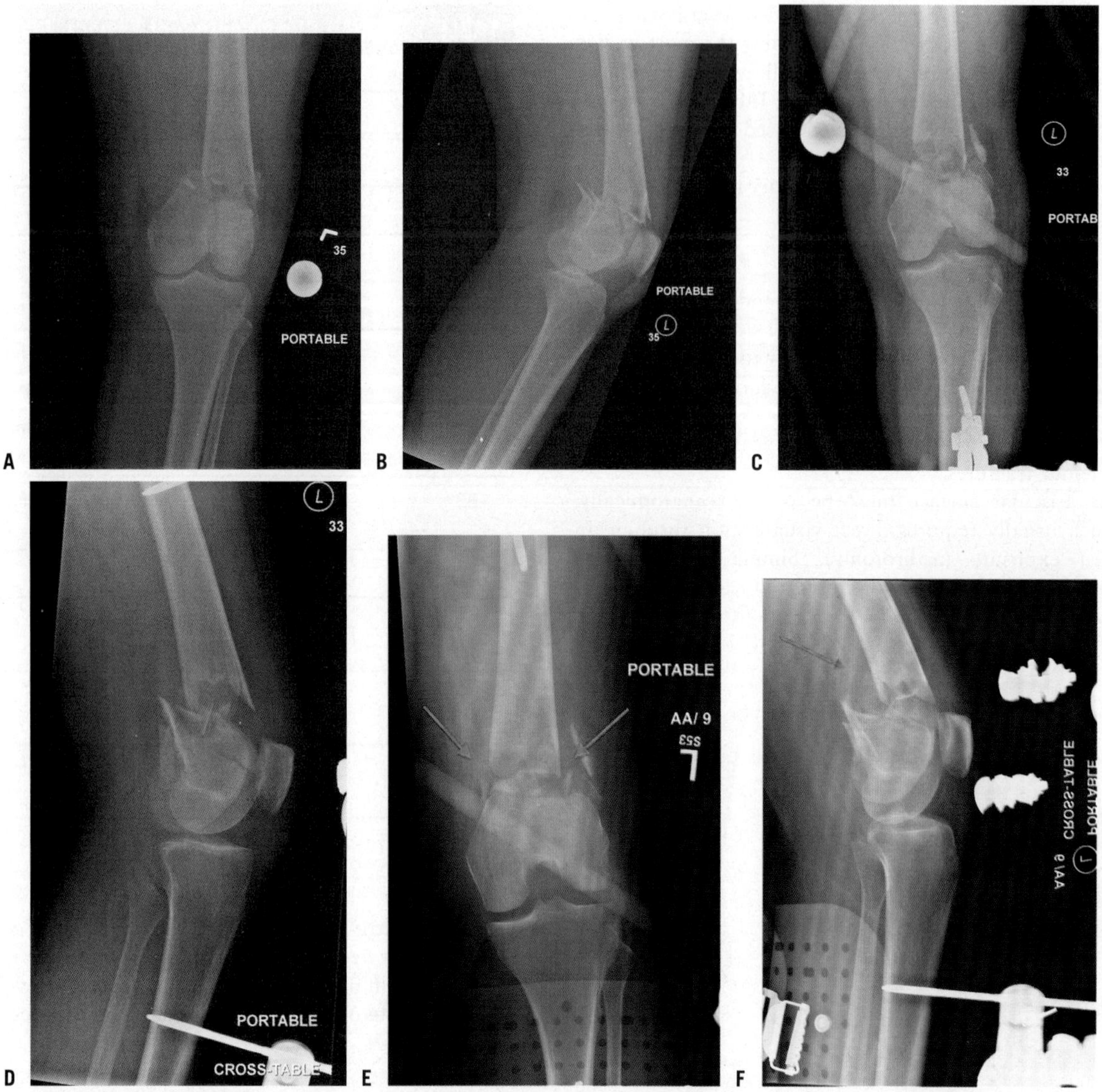

FIG 9 Critically ill elderly polytrauma Jehovah's witness patient with left C1 distal femur fracture. **A,B.** Initial injury AP and lateral views. **C,D.** Due to extremely low hematocrit, external fixation was the only surgical option allowed to minimize blood loss. Radiographs in bridging external fixation. The AP shows excellent alignment, but the lateral shows the expected extension deformity secondary to pull of gastrocsoleus complex. **E,F.** After 5 weeks in an external fixator, AP and lateral radiographs show callus formation (*red arrows*). Patient is now cleared for definitive surgical intervention.

- Antegrade intramedullary nailing has been described and can be used for distal fractures with a large enough distal segment to allow for two locking screws. Malalignment has been a problem, as has adequate fixation.[10,14]
- Retrograde intramedullary nailing can be used in the following cases **(FIG 10)**:
  - All extra-articular type A fractures greater than 4 cm from the joint. This minimal length of the distal femur allows for multiplanar interlocking in the distal fragment.
  - Type C1 or C2 fractures where the articular fracture can be anatomically reduced closed or with limited exposure. Percutaneous screws are used for the articular injury.
  - Periprosthetic fractures around a total knee arthroplasty with an "open box" femoral component
  - Most surgeons prefer to use a long nail, but short supracondylar nails are available as well. Multiple-hole short supracondylar nails have fallen out of favor.
  - Due to the wide metaphyseal region, malalignment, translation, or instability can occur with retrograde nailing due to the size of the nail in comparison to the capacious canal. The use of blocking screws can aid in the reduction and add stability in these situations.[22] Biomechanically, it was found that blocking screws in the proximal segment were superior to blocking screws in the distal segment.[1] In a retrospective cohort study, however, no significant differences in alignment were found with the use of blocking screws.[37]
  - In a biomechanical study, a retrograde nail that allows for locked distal screws showed less fracture collapse, translation of the nail, and degree of varus angulation after cyclic loading and thus may be beneficial.[34]

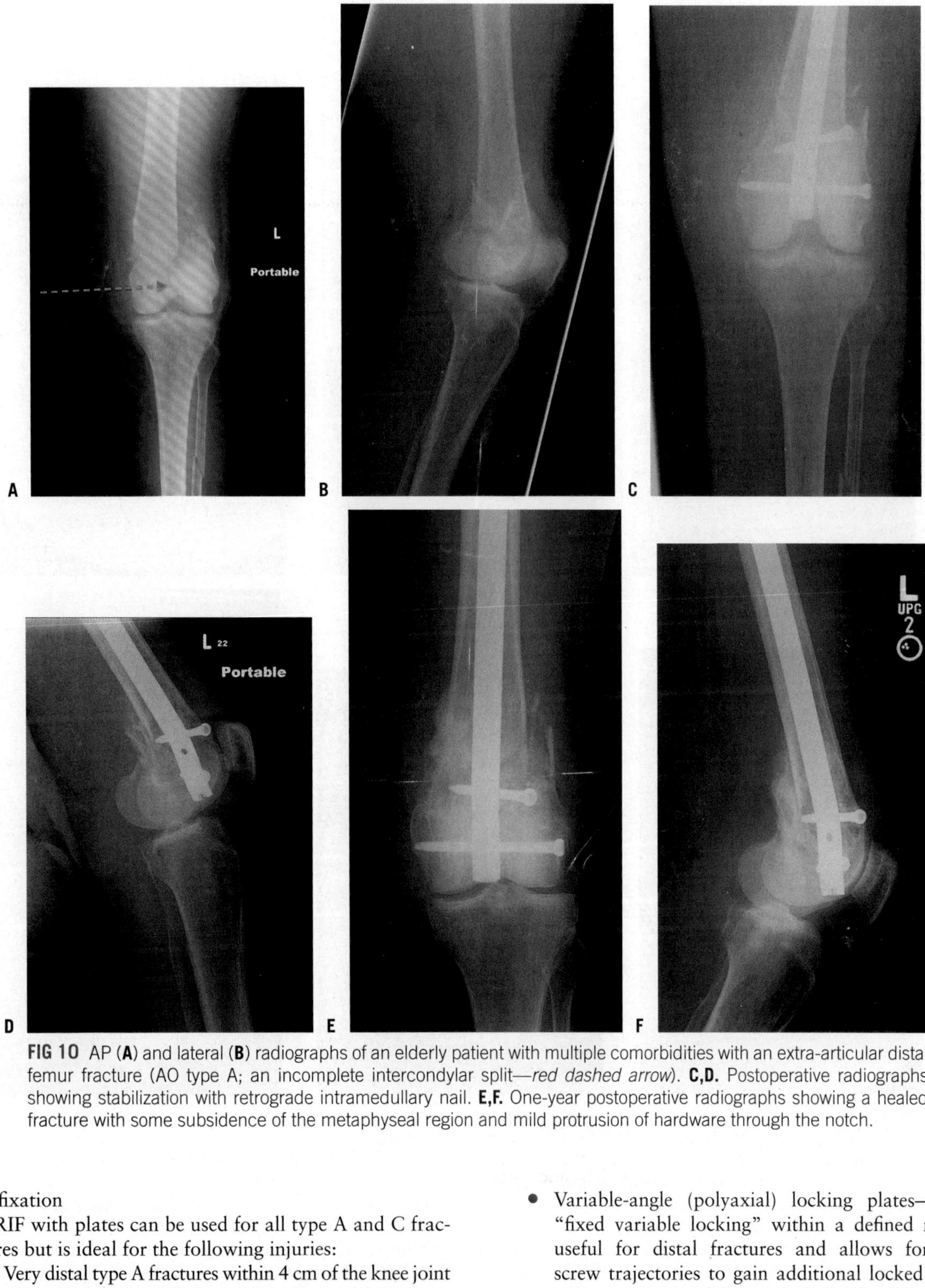

FIG 10 AP (**A**) and lateral (**B**) radiographs of an elderly patient with multiple comorbidities with an extra-articular distal femur fracture (AO type A; an incomplete intercondylar split—*red dashed arrow*). **C,D.** Postoperative radiographs showing stabilization with retrograde intramedullary nail. **E,F.** One-year postoperative radiographs showing a healed fracture with some subsidence of the metaphyseal region and mild protrusion of hardware through the notch.

- Plate fixation
  - ORIF with plates can be used for all type A and C fractures but is ideal for the following injuries:
    - Very distal type A fractures within 4 cm of the knee joint
    - All articular type C fractures, but almost all C3 types
    - Periprosthetic fractures about a "closed box" femoral component of a total knee arthroplasty
    - The partial articular type B1 or B2 if an antiglide plate is needed
- Plate options (preferred to least preferred; fixed-angle devices preferred)
  - Fixed-angle locking plates (percutaneous jigs are advantageous and allow for minimally invasive techniques)
- Variable-angle (polyaxial) locking plates—allow for "fixed variable locking" within a defined range. It is useful for distal fractures and allows for increased screw trajectories to gain additional locked fixation in short segments, which may not be feasible with fixed-angle trajectory plates, although this is uncommon (**FIG 11**).
  - Recently, significantly higher failure rates with the use of variable technology in the management of OTA/AO type C3 fractures has been reported.[33] In other studies, these plates have been shown to have similar results as fixed angle locking plates and felt to be safe and effective.[9,19]

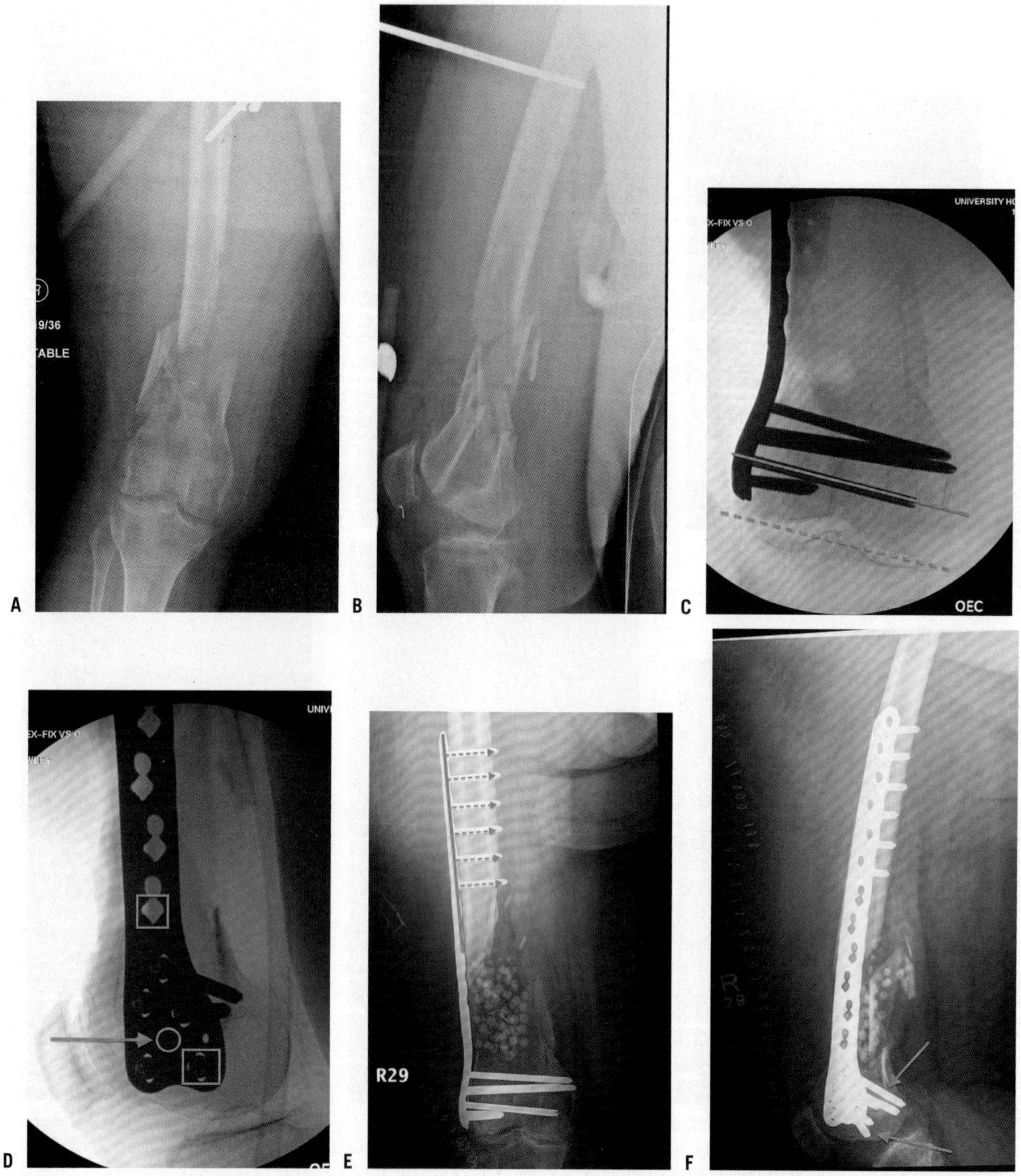

FIG 11 Morbidly obese female with a severely comminuted and open right distal C3 femur fracture. AP (**A**) and lateral (**B**) radiographs showing the amount of comminution, bone loss, and distal nature of the injury after the initial irrigation, débridement, and bridging external fixation. **C,D.** Intraoperative fluoroscopic images during application of a variable-angle locking plate. The AP shows the "central screw" to aid in reestablishment of the anatomic axis of the femur (*parallel lines solid*, screw; *dashed*, joint line). The lateral view shows the central screw, which is a fixed-angle hole (*arrow* and *circle*), as opposed to the variable-angle holes (*red box*; both for the combination holes and isolated variable-angle screws). **E,F.** Two-week postoperative radiographs. The AP view shows the proximal screws placed perpendicular (*dashed arrows*) to the plate even through the variable-angle portion of the combination holes, which was facilitated by the targeting device. Both views demonstrate the advantage of the variable-angle locking holes distally to allow for additional fixation in this short distal segment with a more posterior and distal trajectory (*solid arrows* on lateral view). The bone substitute placed for the bone defect (*white pellets*) are also clearly visualized. *(continued)*

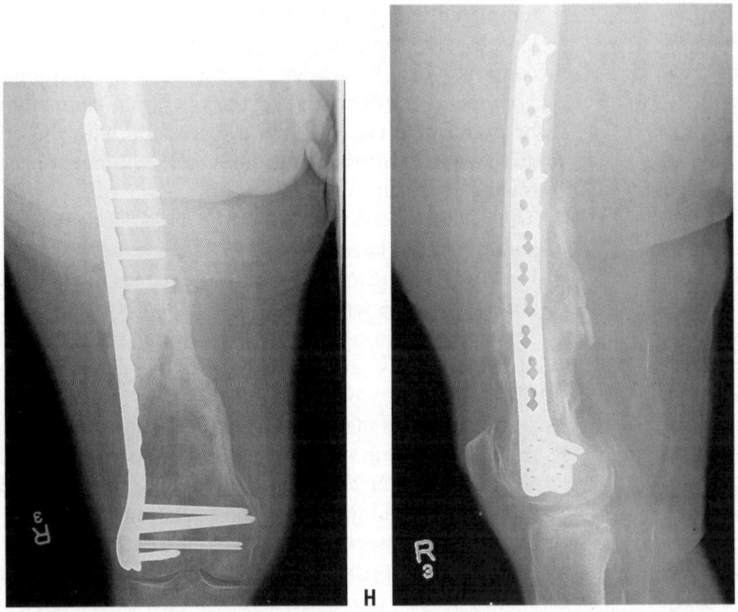

G H

FIG 11 *(continued)* **G,H.** Five-month follow-up films showing replacement of the calcium sulfate beads with successful consolidation of the metaphyseal comminution.

- Ninety-five–degree condylar screw
  - Recently, use of the 95-degree condylar screw was revisited and found to have significantly less complications and reoperations than the Less Invasive Stabilization System (LISS [™Synthes]) plate and better union rate.[7]
- Ninety-five–degree blade plate
  - Use of the angled blade plate compared to a locking plate construct was found to have less complications and nonunions.[36] This method is less applicable in fractures with intra-articular involvement, particularly in the face of coronal splits.
- Nonlocking plates with or without medial support (medial plate or external fixation)

- Limited internal fixation
  - Limited fixation with screws only can be used for partial articular type B, especially type B3.
  - The amount of open reduction required depends on the adequacy of closed reduction techniques and obtaining an anatomic reduction of the joint surface.
  - Headless screws are useful for type B3 fractures in which the screws have to penetrate the joint surface **(FIG 12)**.
  - Countersinking the screw heads can also be performed.
- Biomechanics of fixation: implant considerations
  - There has been concern that the newer locking plate constructs are too stiff, resulting in inconsistent and asymmetric callus formation.[17]
  - Constructs that are too rigid or comprised entirely of locking screws were found to contribute to nonunion.[38]
  - Some clinical evidence shows less callus formation with stainless steel plates versus titanium plates.[17] Recently, use of stainless-steel plates was found to be an independent predictor of nonunion.[27,38] However, the geometry of the plate and the construct that is built is far more important than the material of the plate.
  - Conversely, a biomechanical study has not shown a significant difference mechanically between constructs of stainless steel LISS plates with bicortical screws or titanium LISS plate with unicortical screws.[2]

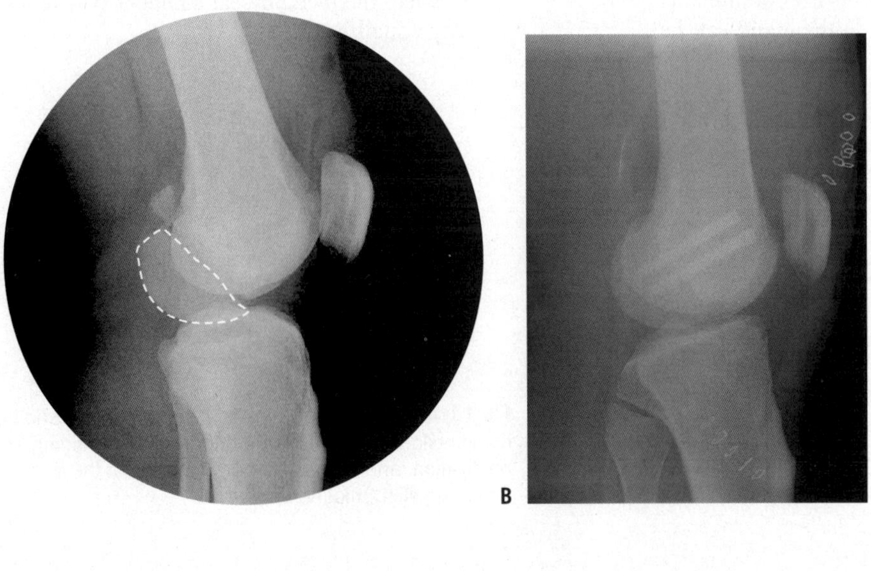

A B

FIG 12 A. Lateral radiograph of patient with a grade II open distal medial femoral condyle fracture (type B3) (*outlined*). The Hoffa fragment is outlined. **B.** Postoperative radiograph after fixation with headless screws, buried underneath the subchondral bone.

- The flexibility of fixation constructs can be increased by the use of a technique referred to as *far cortical locking* (FCL). Specialized screws are used, in which the screw locks into the plate and only engages the far cortex. Alternatively, regular locking screws can be used and the near cortex is overdrilled allowing for purchase only in the far cortex and locking into the plate. This has been thought to improve fracture healing.[11]
- Clinical observational studies have shown increased callus formation in FCL constructs when compared to standard locking.[5,15,24]
- The "polyaxial" locking plates have been shown to be biomechanically sound in the management of supracondylar femur fractures.[23,39] with similar clinical results to fixed angle locking plates[9,19] although some concerns with high failure rates have been suggested in OTA/AO type C3 fractures.[33] All "polyaxial" plates have at least one major "fixed" screw that is the primary support.

- Distal femoral replacement
  - Recently, the use of a distal femoral replacing prosthesis in the management of distal femur fractures in the elderly has been suggested but has not been widely adopted.[4]
  - Distal femoral replacement historically has been reserved for revision surgery with a periprosthetic femur fracture above a total knee arthroplasty most often with a loose prosthesis.

Preoperative Planning

- Surgical timing can be affected by the following:
  - Soft tissue issues
  - Medical condition of the patient
  - Adequacy of available operative team
  - Availability of implants
- The approach must take the following issues into consideration:
  - The ability to incorporate lacerations in open fractures into the incision (**FIG 13**) can be useful and should be considered. However, this is not always necessary or possible.
  - Soft tissue dissection should be limited.
  - Adequate exposure is important to anatomically restore the articular surface.
- Restoration of limb "anatomy" must be accomplished and allow early range of motion.
  - Stable internal fixation and length and sizes of implants should be templated. Radiographs of the injury can be templated with implant templates to ensure that proper lengths are available. A tentative plan of the fixation construct can be drawn on the image. Additionally, "preoperative planning" of the operating room should be performed; this includes a discussion with the operative team about the positioning and equipment needed for the procedure.
  - The need for bone grafting or the use of bone graft substitutes should be assessed.
  - Fracture fragments and the anticipated fixation construct should be templated.
  - The surgeon should check for coronal plane fractures of the condyles (also known as *Hoffa fragments*) (see **FIGS 5C** and **6**).
- Associated injuries may affect the treatment options.
  - An ipsilateral hip or more proximal shaft fracture may alter the implant choice. A longer plate may be needed to address both injuries, or consideration to overlap implants may be warranted to avoid a stress riser.
  - An associated proximal tibia fracture may alter the approach used. A more lateral incision incorporating a lazy S incision for the proximal tibia injury may be required.
  - Critically ill patients may require delayed fixation after temporary stabilization via bridging external fixation methods (**FIG 14**).

Positioning

- A radiolucent table should be used to allow adequate visualization with a C-arm.
- The patient is placed supine with a hip bump.
  - The rotation of the proximal segment of the fracture (hip) should be aligned before patient preparation.
    - Using the C-arm, the profile of the lesser trochanter with the corresponding knee (patella) straight up is determined on the uninjured side (**FIG 15A,B**).
    - The injured hip is imaged and internally rotated by the hip bump so that duplication of the profile of the normal side is achieved. The size of the bump may be adjusted as needed for the amount of rotation required.
    - The injured knee is placed in the patella-up position to confirm rotation.
    - This technique is helpful in comminuted metaphyseal fractures where the rotation is difficult to assess or in cases where the metaphyseal component will not be directly visualized.

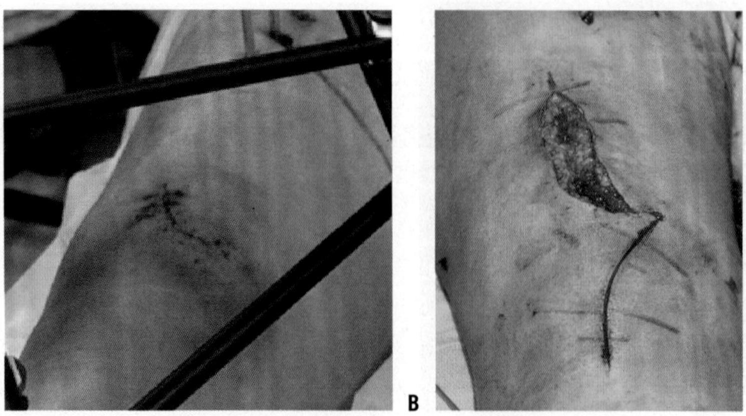

A B

FIG 13 **A.** Patient with open distal femur fracture and traumatic oblique laceration after débridement, bridging external fixation, and closure. **B.** Incorporation of the laceration into a modified midline approach.

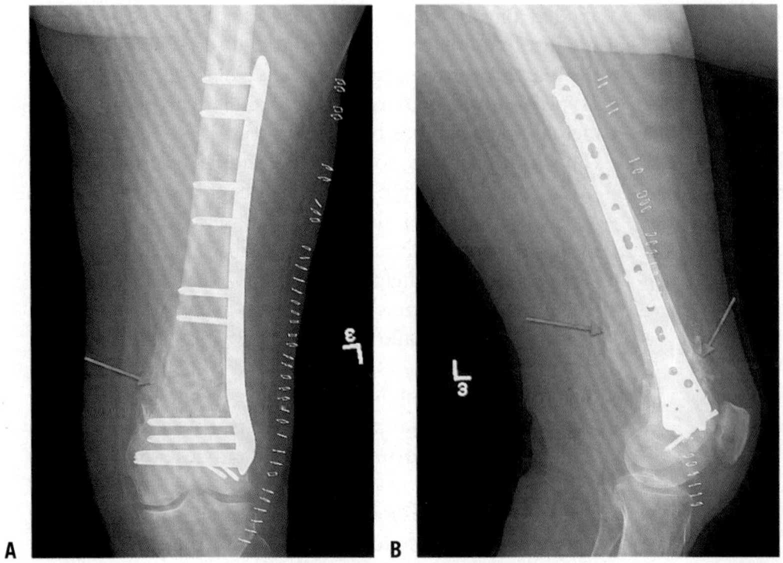

FIG 14 A,B. Two-week postoperative radiographs of patient from **FIG 9** who underwent delayed ORIF at 5 weeks post-injury. These radiographs exhibit the abundant amount of callus present (*red arrows*) after successful ORIF with reestablishment of length, alignment, and rotation was accomplished with takedown of the callus.

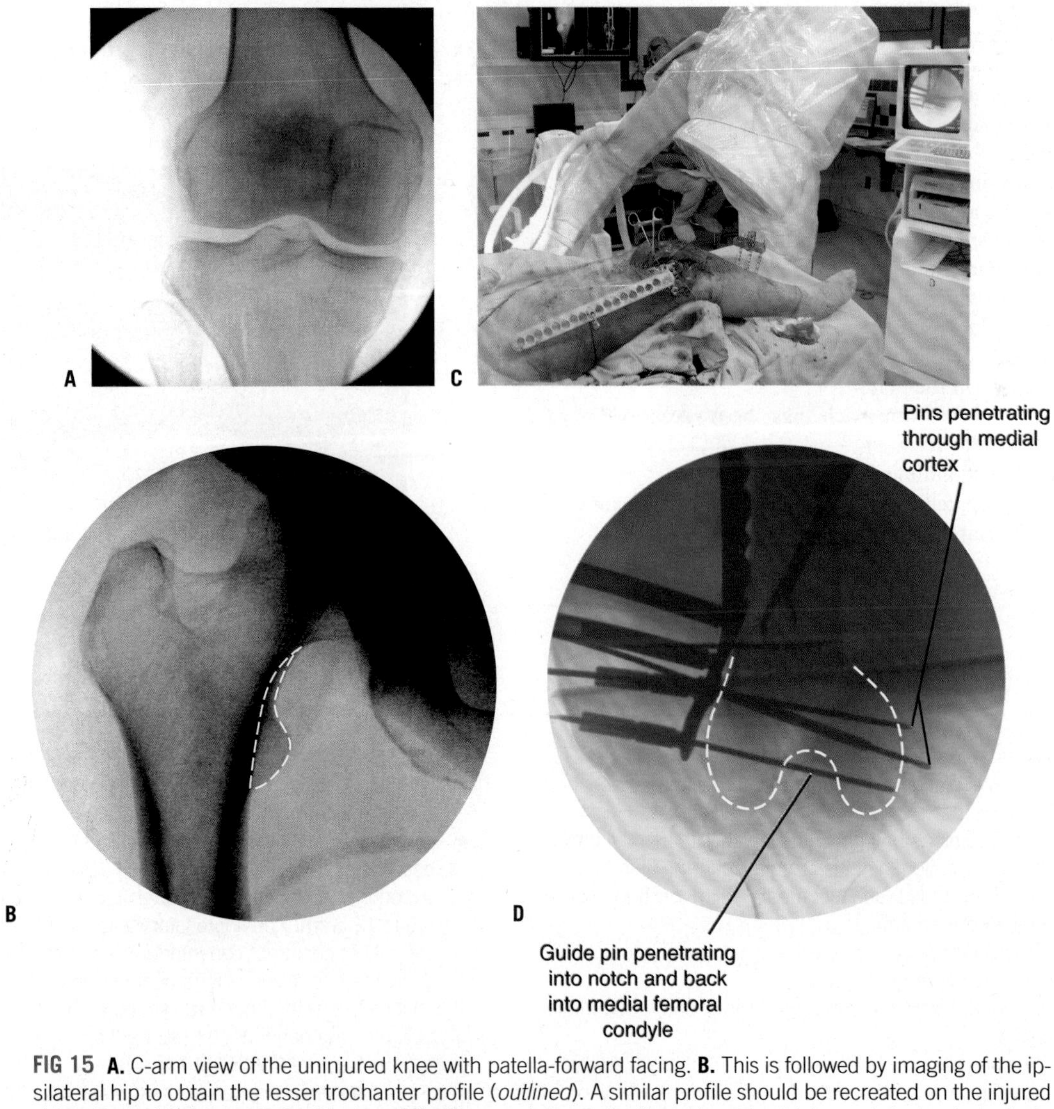

FIG 15 A. C-arm view of the uninjured knee with patella-forward facing. **B.** This is followed by imaging of the ipsilateral hip to obtain the lesser trochanter profile (*outlined*). A similar profile should be recreated on the injured side with the hip bump. **C.** Positioning of the C-arm relative to the flexed knee to obtain a notch view to evaluate for guide pin penetration in the posterior aspect. **D.** The resulting C-arm image.

- Even though the distal segment is not in "fixed" rotation, this technique is useful to minimize the chance of a malrotation during definitive fixation.
- A sterile tourniquet may be used unless a temporary fixator prevents its placement.
- A large bump or a sterile triangle is used under the knee.
  - This allows for knee flexion, relaxing the gastrocsoleus complex and facilitating the reduction.
  - A sterile and removable one is most useful.
- The C-arm is brought in from the opposite side.
  - It should be angled so that it is parallel with the femoral shaft.
  - A notch view is useful for screw trajectories in the distal femur. This is achieved by the C-arm angled roughly around 30 to 45 degrees directed cephalad, and visualization will depend on the concurrent amount of knee flexion **(FIG 15C,D)**.

Approach

- The best-known approach for the treatment of distal femur fractures has been the straight lateral approach **(FIG 16)**.
  - This is suitable for types A and C1 fractures.
  - The incision may curve distally toward the tibial tubercle, and osteotomy may be performed.
  - Newer approaches include a lateral inverted U to allow better access to the joint and to allow for plate placement.
- The minimally invasive lateral approach can be used for certain fractures and implants.
  - The joint must be visualized, reduced, and stabilized.
  - The placement of the plate on the shaft is done submuscularly, and reduction and fixation are done percutaneously under fluoroscopic guidance.
  - This is ideal for plating systems with targeting devices for the screws in the plate.
- A modified anterior approach has been described by Starr et al.[31]
  - This involves a midline incision.
  - A lateral parapatellar arthrotomy is done with elevation of the vastus lateralis as in the lateral approach.
- A medial parapatellar arthrotomy can be used for retrograde intramedullary nailing or limited screw fixation.
  - Miniarthrotomy is used for the retrograde nail.
  - Type B injuries may require a formal arthrotomy.
- A medial approach has been described.
  - This is appropriate for types B2 and B3 fractures.
  - It can be used in type C3 fractures if a second plate is being used (in conjunction with a lateral approach).
- A total knee approach has been described by Schatzker.[28]
  - This is extremely helpful for type C2 or C3 fractures.
  - It is used for plates but can be used for retrograde intramedullary nailing once the articular surface is reconstructed.
  - A midline approach is used.
  - An extended medial parapatellar arthrotomy is done.
  - This allows exposure of the condyles for articular reduction.
- A midline incision with a lateral parapatellar arthrotomy is my preferred exposure for type C2 or C3 fractures.
  - A midline approach is used.
  - A lateral parapatellar arthrotomy is done.
  - Proximal extension is made into the quadriceps tendon, enough to repair to itself.
  - Medial dislocation of patella is done.
  - This allows exposure of the condyles for articular reduction and easier lateral plate insertion.

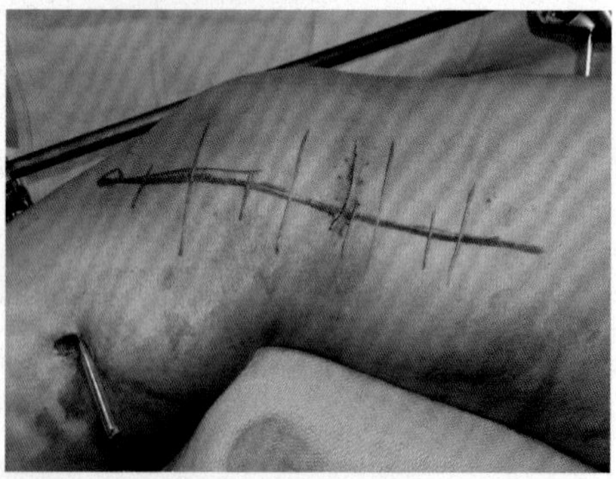

FIG 16 Skin incision for a lateral approach.

TEMPORARY BRIDGING EXTERNAL FIXATION

- A large external fixation system is used.
- A small bump is placed under the knee to place the knee in slight flexion.
- The injured extremity is brought out to length with manual traction.
- Two or three 5-mm Schanz pins are placed in the tibia in an anterior to posterior direction just medial to the crest to ensure intramedullary placement.
- Two or three 5-mm Schanz pins are placed in the femoral shaft in an anterior to posterior direction.
  - These should be placed out of the zone of soft tissue injury if possible.
  - The pins are placed while the limb is out to length so that the quadriceps is not "skewered" in a shortened position.
  - The pins can be placed outside of the anticipated plate location. This, however, has not been empirically found to be a problem. In my experience, plates have often overlapped with pin sites, and there has not been an associated problem with infections.
- The safe zone for anterior pin placement in the femur has been described as a region starting 7.5 cm proximal to the superior pole of the patella and extending proximal for another 4.5 to 12.5 cm. The entire lateral aspect of the femur is safe. Lateral pin construct can interfere with plate placement if using the frame as an "intra-operative distractor."[3]
- Pin placement in the tibia may be altered if additional uses of such pins are needed, such as traction for an associated acetabular fracture **(TECH FIG 1A)**.
- The bars can be configured in many ways, all of which provide temporary stabilization across the knee joint. I prefer a diamond configuration **(TECH FIG 1B)**.

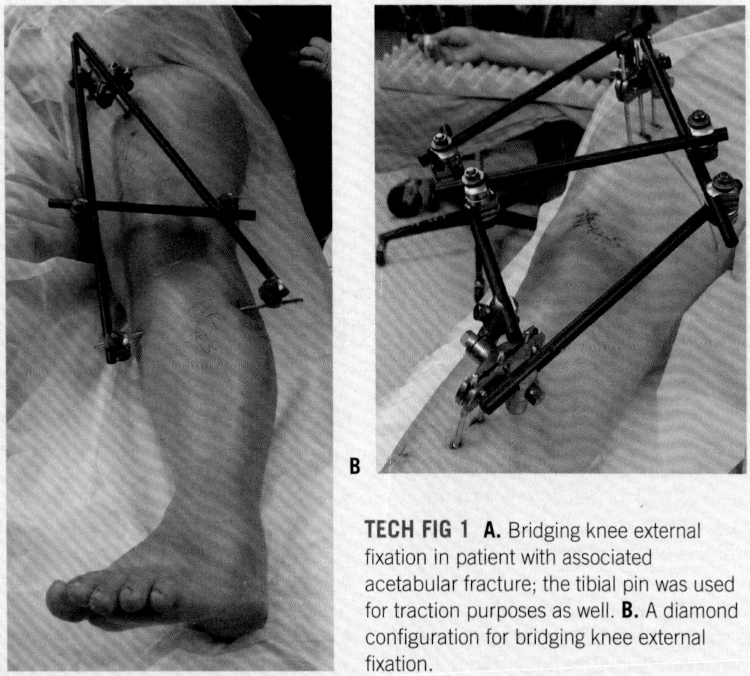

A B

TECH FIG 1 A. Bridging knee external fixation in patient with associated acetabular fracture; the tibial pin was used for traction purposes as well. **B.** A diamond configuration for bridging knee external fixation.

Reduction of the Metaphyseal Component

- Gross reduction of the metaphyseal component of the fracture should be performed with traction and manipulation of the pins.
- The fracture should be brought out to length.
  - Intraoperatively, the opposite leg can be used to help determine length.
- Postoperatively, a scanogram can be used to determine whether the length has been regained before definitive fixation if there is extensive comminution, but this is not always needed **(TECH FIG 2)**. Although the knee may be somewhat flexed, the scanogram can still be obtained and the femoral length determined as opposed to the entire leg length.

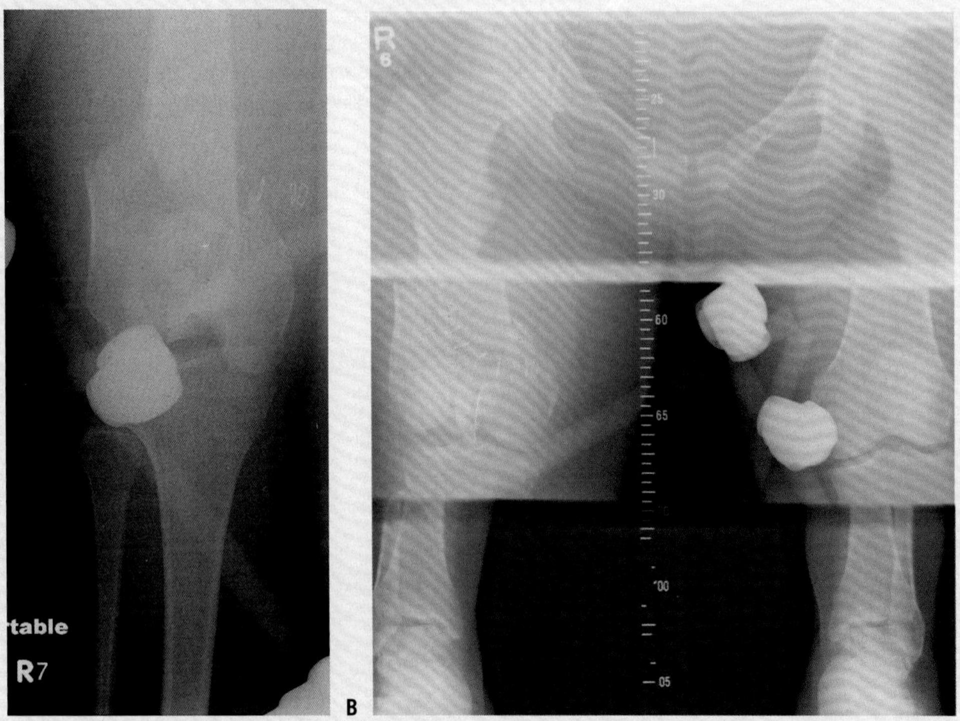

A B

TECH FIG 2 AP radiograph (**A**) and scanogram (**B**) showing that length was reestablished with the external fixator.

- The rotation should be checked once again before locking the external fixator construct, as described earlier under Positioning section. The same technique should be performed under sterile conditions.
- Varus–valgus alignment should be assessed before final tightening as well.
- This can be done by using the Bovie cord intraoperatively and assessing the mechanical axis of the limb by fluoroscopically evaluating from the hip to the ankle with the cord centered at the femoral head all the way to the ankle.
- The point at which the cord crosses the knee allows one to judge the varus–valgus alignment.

OPEN REDUCTION AND INTERNAL FIXATION OF THE DISTAL FEMUR WITH LOCKING PLATES (TYPE C FRACTURES)

- This technique can be used regardless of the locking plate system used. Each system's technique guide should be reviewed before use as each system has its own idiosyncrasies. Variations in plate application as well as reduction tools and techniques are unique to each system.
- The temporary external fixator is prepared using a "double-double" technique.
  - The fixator is first prepared with a Betadine "scrub" (7.5% povidone-iodine) solution followed by a Betadine "paint" (10% povidone-iodine) solution (Beta–Beta preparation), followed by the extremity with a second Beta–Beta preparation.
  - The surgeon then does an alcohol preparation, followed by iodine for the fixator, followed by alcohol and iodine on the skin.
  - This has been successful in our practice and allows for maintenance of traction during the preparation and aids in the actual surgery, functioning as a femoral distractor. (Chlorhexidine is used in iodine-allergic patients.)
  - An alternative is to completely remove the fixator components, except the pins, and wash, sterilize, and then reassemble the fixator on the patient after the leg has been prepared.
- If there is no temporary bridging external fixator, the metaphyseal component of the fracture can be reduced and brought out to length with a femoral distractor, a temporary simple external fixator, or manual traction if adequate help is available.
  - Rotation of the proximal segment can be manipulated with the device used.

Midline Approach with an Extended Lateral Parapatellar Arthrotomy

- A straight incision is made directly anterior about 5 cm proximal to the superior pole of the patella and distally to the level of the tibia tubercle **(TECH FIG 3A)**.
- The lateral skin flap is developed to allow for a lateral parapatellar arthrotomy **(TECH FIG 3B)**.
- The arthrotomy is performed, ensuring a cuff of tissue on the lateral aspect of the patella for repair as well as medially on the quadriceps **(TECH FIG 3C)**.
- The patella can be subluxated medially or inverted with knee flexion to allow exposure of the condyles **(TECH FIG 3D)**.
  - Additionally, a blunt Hohmann retractor can be placed on the medial side at the level of the condyle to retract the patella.
- The capsule is subperiosteally elevated off the lateral femoral condyle to allow for placement of the plate.
  - The lateral collateral ligament is preserved because the dissection is limited to the anterior two-thirds of the lateral femoral condyle and plate placement is usually proximal to the lateral epicondyle.
  - The medial side in the metaphyseal region is left undisturbed as much as possible.

A 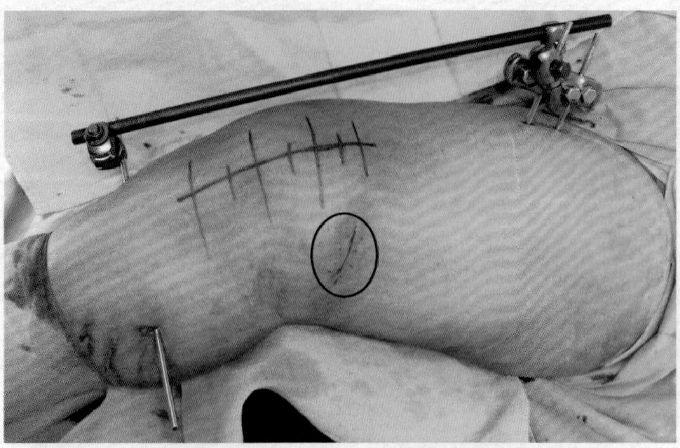

B 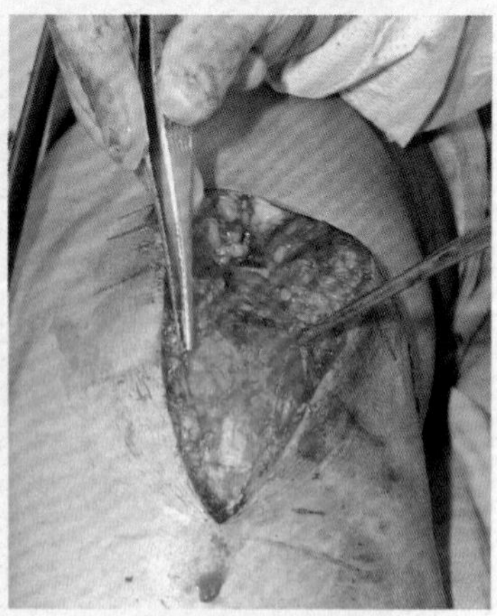

TECH FIG 3 Patient with grade II open distal femur fracture (also shown in **FIGS 5D–F**, **6B**, and **7**). **A.** Straight midline incision used—open laceration from original injury is seen on lateral aspect (*circled in black*). **B.** Lateral skin flap is developed. *(continued)*

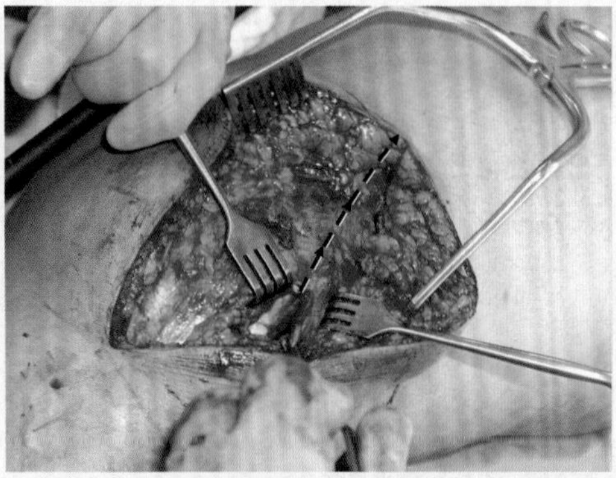

C

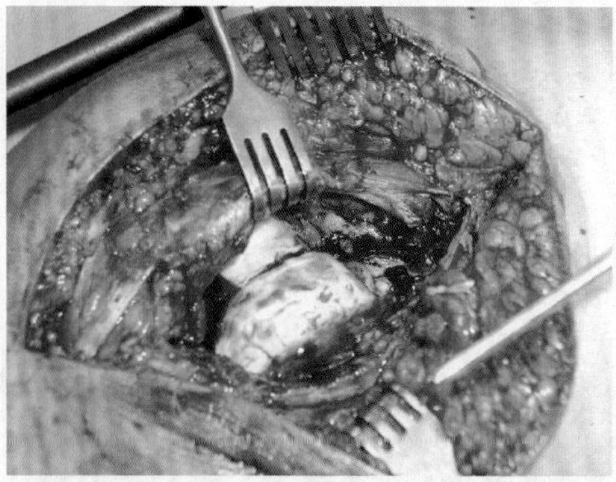

D

TECH FIG 3 *(continued)* **C.** Arthrotomy is started and then extended proximally into the quad tendon (*dashed line*). **D.** The arthrotomy is completed, and the condyles are visualized with medial subluxation of the patella.

Reduction of the Articular Surface

- The joint is evaluated to determine comminution.
- Joint reconstruction is then performed with direct reduction. Each condyle is fully assessed first for smaller fracture fragments, with the goal of restoring each condyle anatomically. Small-diameter screws (<3.0 mm) may be used and can be countersunk underneath the articular surface.
- Large coronal fracture fragments are best treated with countersunk 3.5- to 4.5-mm lag-type screws. We use headless screws.
- Once each condyle is thought to be restored, or if a simple fracture pattern is present, the condyles should be reduced to each other using a large, pointed reduction forceps **(TECH FIG 4A–C)**.
- Each fragment can be rotated relative to another; this must be addressed as discussed before.
  - The best way to assess this is under direct visualization and evaluating the reduction at the trochlear region of the patellofemoral joint.
  - Additionally, preoperative evaluation assessing the lateral radiograph can guide the surgeon. Intraoperative fluoroscopy to reassess the lateral view is also useful.
- Temporary Kirschner wires or the guide pins for the locking screws for the plate can be used for additional stabilization of the two condyles **(TECH FIG 4D)**.

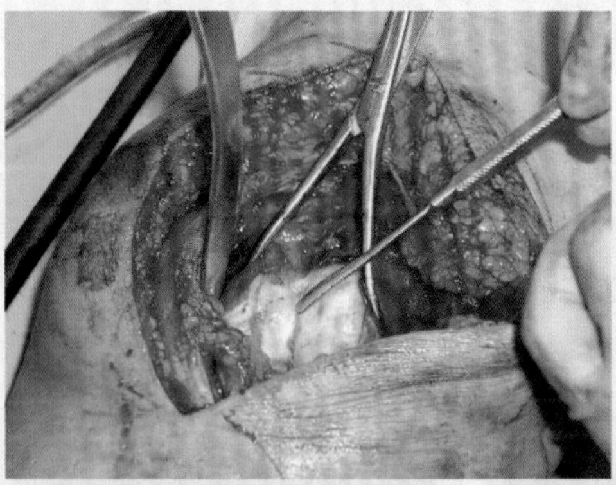

A

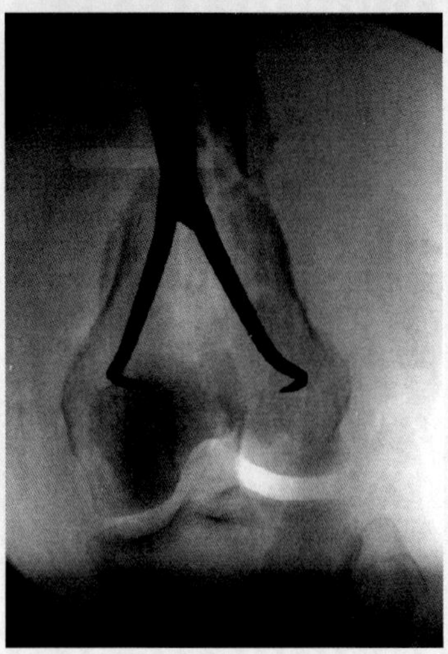

B

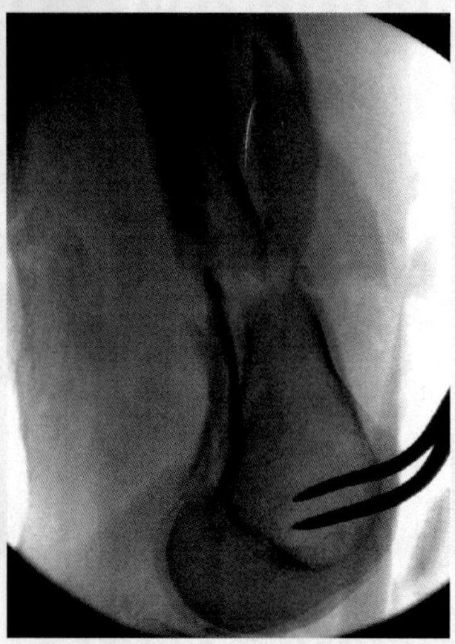

C

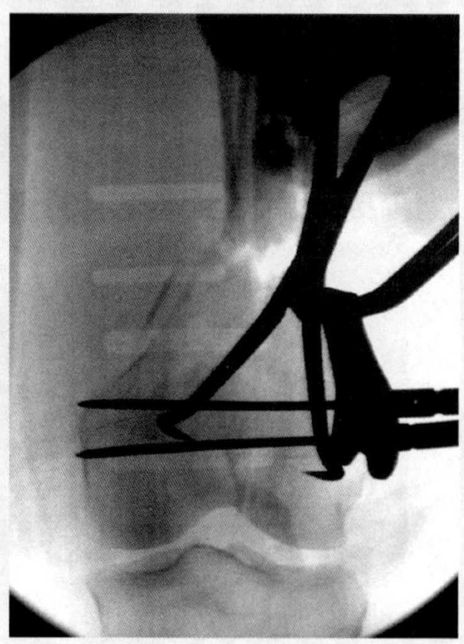

D

TECH FIG 4 The condyles are reduced under direct visualization (**A**) and confirmed with AP (**B**) and lateral (**C**) intraoperative fluoroscopic images. **D.** Guide pins through the plate template or screw trajectory guide are used to temporarily stabilize the intercondylar split.

Definitive Fixation of the Condyles

- This can be accomplished outside the plate first and supplemented with screws through the plate. The area around the proposed plate, the "periphery," can be used for the screw placement to avoid interference with the plate placement itself.
  - If this is done, then the metaphyseal fracture does not necessarily have to be properly reduced before initial screw placement.
- Screws can also be placed from medial to lateral to avoid interference with the plate.
- Definitive fixation can be accomplished through the plate also (see next section on Screw Placement).
  - If this is done, the metaphyseal component should be reduced to ensure the proper flexion–extension alignment of the shaft with the condyles.
  - This will ensure that the plate is collinear with the shaft once fixed to the distal segment. Otherwise, a malreduction in the sagittal plane will occur.
  - The temporary Kirschner wires can be left in place to stabilize the joint.

Reduction of the Shaft to the Distal Segment

- Once the articular surface is temporarily stabilized or reduced, the reduction of the shaft to the distal segment should be performed before plate application.
- This can be temporarily stabilized with Kirschner wires or Steinmann pins.
- Alternatively, precisely placed bumps underneath the distal segment can be used to correct the extension of the distal segment and align it with the shaft.
- Adjustment or loosening of the temporary external fixator can aid in reduction if needed.
- The plate can then be placed submuscularly.

Placement of the Plate

- Each fixed-angle plating system is designed to help reestablish the valgus alignment of the distal femur.
  - The screws in the distal portion of the plate are designed to be parallel to the joint surface.
  - Thus, the initial guidewires for these screws should be placed parallel and confirmed by fluoroscopy.
    - A distal "joint wire" can be placed to better evaluate this **(TECH FIG 5A)**.
  - Placing the distal screws parallel to the joint will help ensure that when the shaft is brought to the plate, the anatomic axis of the femur is restored.
  - With the variable-angle locking plates, the same technique should be employed to ensure that the plate is applied in a way to restore the anatomic axis of the femur. A fixed-angle central screw hole still exists in these plates to aid in plate application **(**see **FIG 11C**, parallel lines; see **FIG 11D**, red arrow/red circle**)**.
- A distal screw trajectory guide is provided for some systems **(TECH FIG 5B)**. This can be used to help ensure accurate placement of the plate distally, and initial guidewires can be placed through this.
  - Once the wires are placed, the guide can be removed and replaced with the plate using the wires as a guide.
  - However, the shaft portion of the plate requires submuscular insertion, and thus the plate cannot be brought to an appropriate position to allow this to occur.

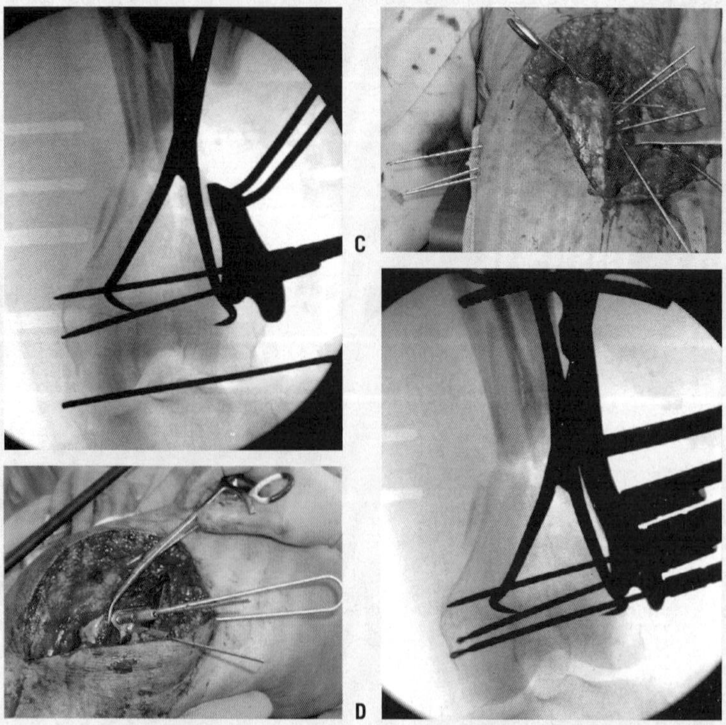
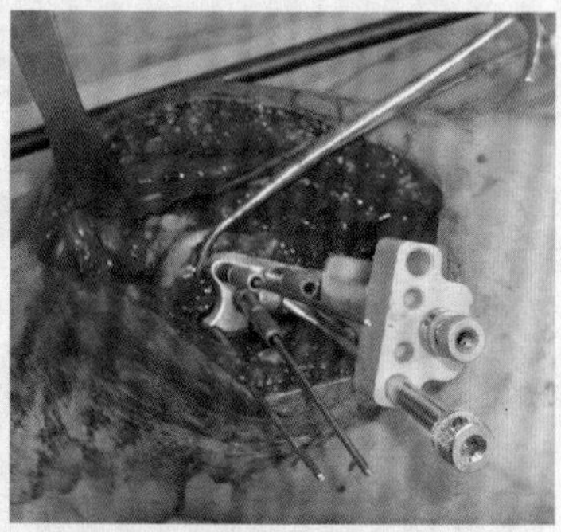

TECH FIG 5 A. Distal reference pin is placed to ensure that the proximal pin is parallel to the joint. **B.** Clinical picture depicting the guide. **C.** Different patient showing the penetration of the medial side with the guidewires to allow plate placement. **D,E.** The plate is placed with additional guide pins in place. *(continued)*

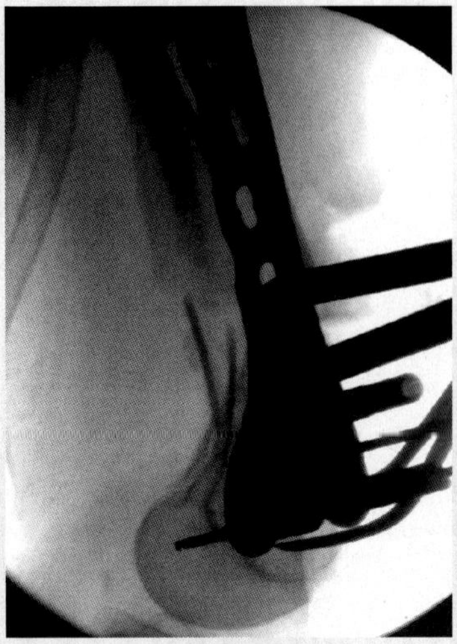
F

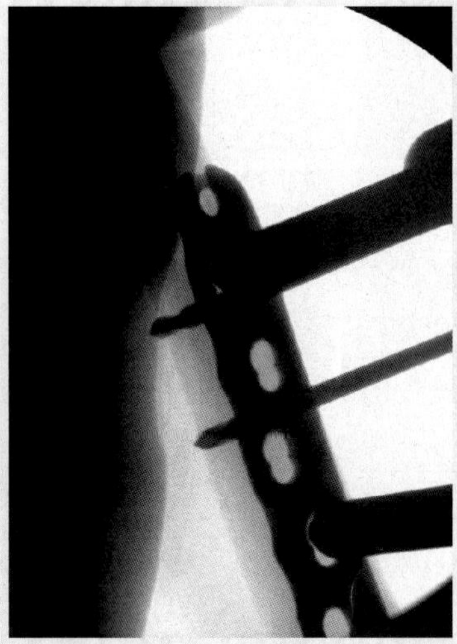
G

TECH FIG 5 *(continued)* **F,G.** Lateral intraoperative fluoroscopic images ensure proper plate placement on the femur before screw insertion.

- To solve this, the guidewires can be driven through the medial side of the knee, which is distal enough to be safe **(TECH FIG 5C)**.
- The plate can then be inserted submuscularly, and the guidewires driven back through the plate laterally, thus aligning the plate to the distal segment and ensuring proper screw trajectory and plate placement **(TECH FIG 5D,E)**.
- A single guidewire in a central hole will still allow flexion–extension placement of the plate if this needs to be adjusted.
- After placing the initial guidewire parallel to the joint distally, and ensuring the fracture is reduced, the surgeon should obtain fluoroscopic visualization of the plate proximally on the shaft to ensure that the plate is on the bone **(TECH FIG 5F,G)**.
  - To ensure placement of the plate on the bone both proximally and distally, it is best to stabilize the plate distally (where exposure is) using a guidewire in the center hole. This allows for a pivot point around which the AP positioning of the plate can be manipulated for the shaft. Fluoroscopy to image the lateral is then used to ensure placement.
  - Once the AP position is obtained, the plate is stabilized proximally.
- The plate should be temporarily stabilized to the bone proximally.
  - Before the temporary stabilization, the length and rotation must be checked. Ideally, if the temporary fixator is in place, these two parameters have been maintained during the course of the operation.
  - If no screw targeting guide is present, a percutaneous provisional fixation pin can be used to stabilize the plate.
  - If a targeting guide is used, then a soft tissue guide for the most proximal hole is placed percutaneously and a drill bit or guidewire is used to stabilize the plate.
  - The variable-angle locking plates also have proximal shaft targeting devices; however, variable locking trajectories can only be accomplished outside the targeting device and can be cumbersome. Generally, variable-angle locking is not necessary in the shaft and locking screws collinear with the hole can be placed through the targeting device. (see **FIG 11E**, red arrows showing perpendicular nature of locking screws; see **FIG 11F**, variable-angle locking screws in the shaft are useful in cases where there is a preexisting hip replacement with a femoral component.)
  - Again, the flexion–extension reduction should be checked.
  - This procedure creates our "box" construct, which aids in the placement of screws through the targeting device (if used) and in temporary stabilization of the fracture construct.

Screw Placement

- If the intercondylar split is going to be stabilized by screws through the plate, partially threaded screws or overdrilled fully threaded screws should be used first to provide interfragmentary compression.
  - Specially designed conical screws for certain systems exist, or large partially threaded screws can be used (>4.5 mm). This also compresses the plate to the bone.
- Once the articular injury is addressed, at least two additional locking screws should be placed into the distal segment to secure the plate and the alignment.
  - The trajectory of distal locking screws can be assessed on the notch view to ensure that penetration through the intercondylar notch does not occur (**TECH FIG 6**; see **FIG 15C** for C-arm setup and position for this image).
  - Before placing the locking screws, the length, rotation, and alignment must be checked again if no fixator or distractor is in place holding the fracture alignment.
  - The plate can be locked to the distal segment and then used to manipulate the distal segment relative to the shaft for the flexion–extension reduction.
    - This, however, is predicated on proper distal alignment of the plate. Otherwise, once the plate is fixed to the distal segment in a malposition and the fracture reduced, the plate may be anterior or posterior on the shaft.
    - The distal screws in a variable-angle locking plate are noncircular to allow for the variable-angle locking mechanism. Screws can be placed directly collinear or with a "variability" of 15 degrees in any direction depending on the system used (see **FIG 11D**, square outline).

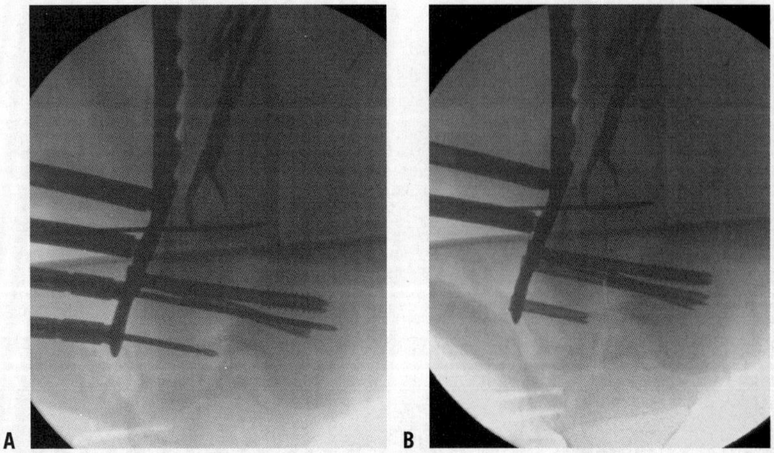

TECH FIG 6 A,B. Patient seen in **FIG 15C,D**, with the guidewire now pulled back and an appropriately sized screw placed.

Attaching the Distal Segment to the Shaft

- The distal segment is now fixed and can be attached to the shaft.
- If there is malalignment in the coronal plane but the sagittal plane alignment is reduced, the shaft can be "pulled" to the plate by means of various threaded devices or a nonlocking screw that can be placed freehand under fluoroscopic guidance or through a targeting jig **(TECH FIG 7)**.

Placement of Additional Screws

- Once proper reduction of the fracture is temporarily achieved and the plate is in proper position, additional screws can be placed.
- If the targeting screw guide is used, percutaneous locking screws can be placed through the soft tissue drill or screw guides **(TECH FIG 8A–C)**.
- If no targeting guide is available, fluoroscopic guidance and a percutaneous method can be used freehand.
- Depending on the system, locking drill guides can be placed freehand to ensure proper trajectory of the drill so that locking screws can be used.
- If that is not the case, nonlocking screws should be placed.
  - Experience is required for the freehand percutaneous method; otherwise, an open approach to the shaft should be performed.
  - The final construct should be checked with fluoroscopy on the lateral aspect as well **(TECH FIG 8D,E)**.
  - The restoration of the mechanical axis can be checked intraoperatively after temporary stabilization (preferred) or definitive stabilization using the Bovie cord.
  - **TECH FIG 8F–H** show the repair after definitive stabilization.
- The exact number of screws in each fragment has yet to be determined in the literature, but our preference has been to have at least five screws in each fragment if possible at the end of fixation.
  - A longer working length in the shaft should be used, and not all holes need to be filled.
  - Plate longer than nine holes with eight holes being proximal to the fracture has been recommended to avoid complications with hardware failure or healing.[26]
  - There is evidence that in young patients with good bone, no locking screws are needed in the diaphysis.
  - Multiple locking screws are used in the epiphysis because of the short length of these distal fragments.
  - The largest screws available for the epiphysis should be used.

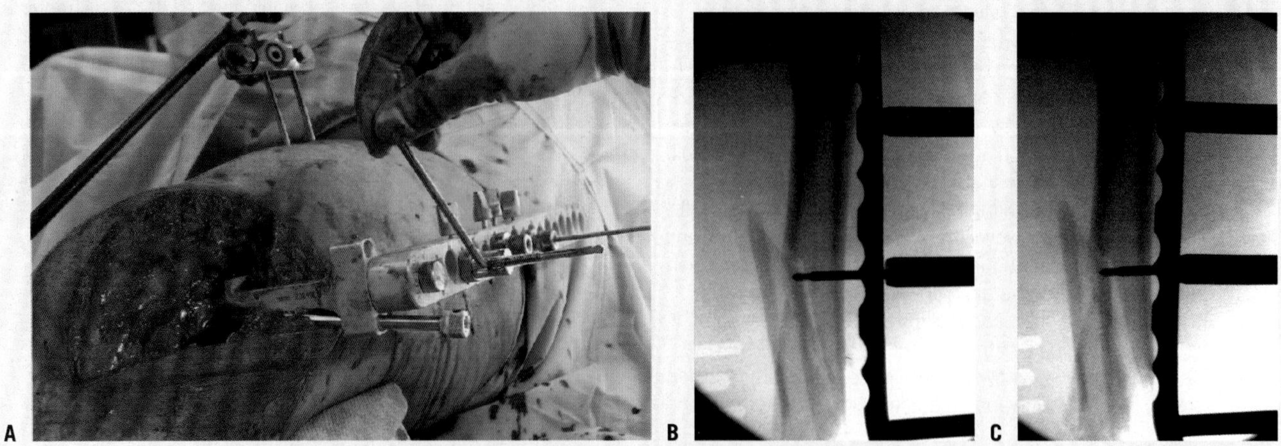

TECH FIG 7 A–C. The "whirlybird" device is tightened and the bone pulled to the plate.

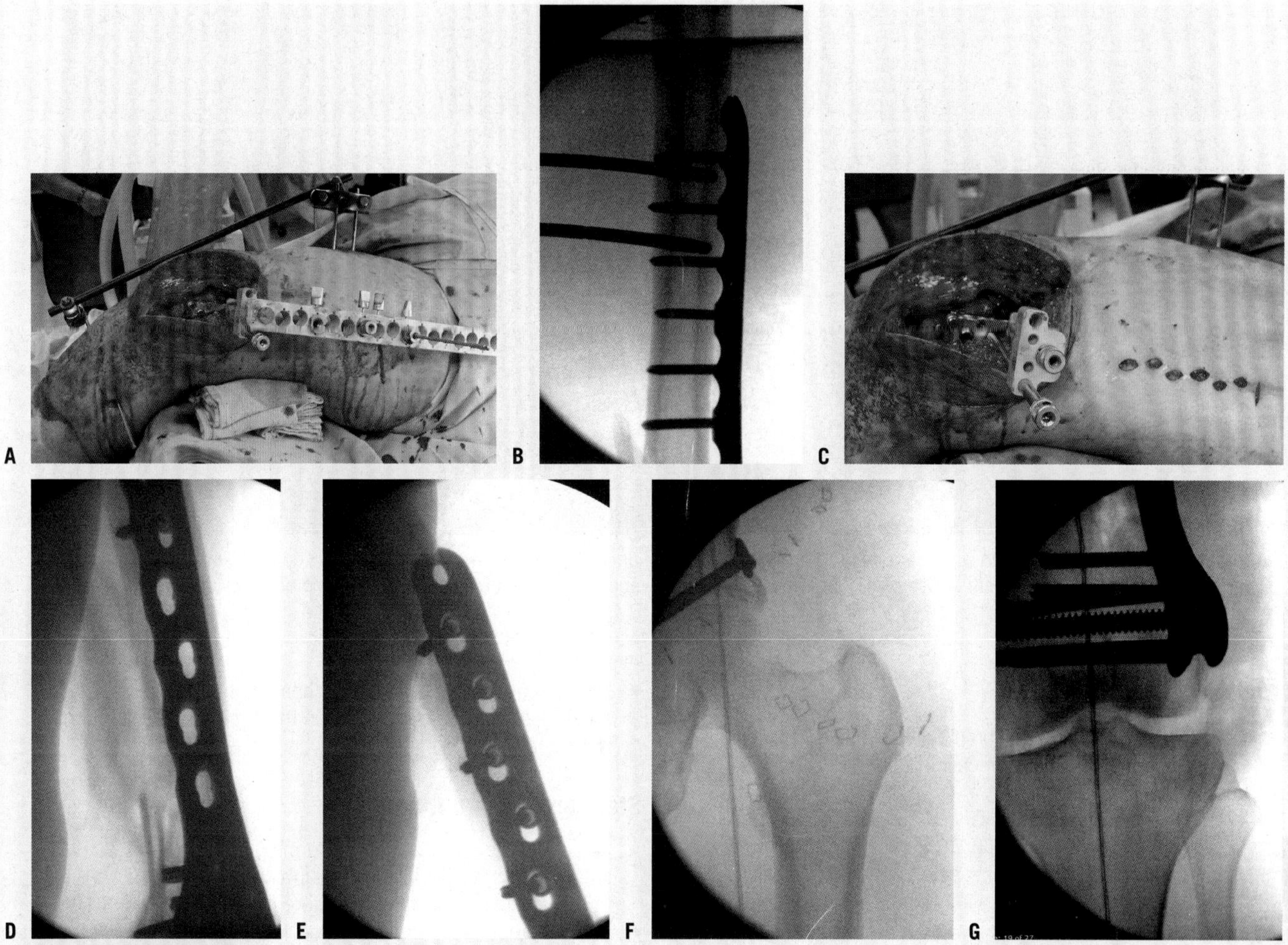

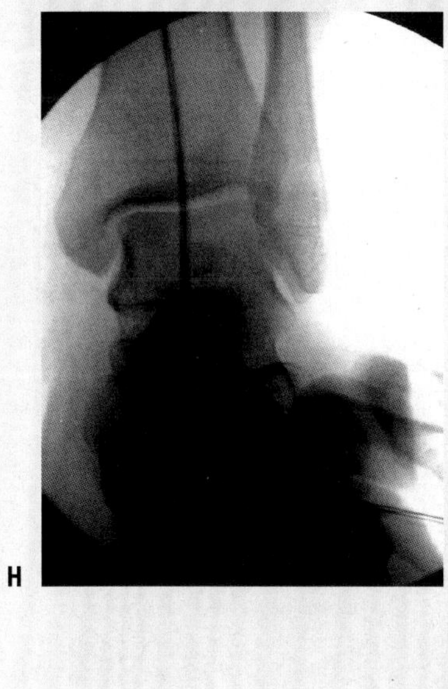

TECH FIG 8 **A.** Targeting guide for proximal screws. **B.** C-arm image of screws placed. **C.** Stab incisions used for percutaneous method. **D,E.** Plate placement on the lateral aspect is confirmed. **F–H.** Alignment is checked intraoperatively with the Bovie cord. The mechanical axis from the center of the femoral head through the middle of the knee to the middle of the ankle is confirmed.

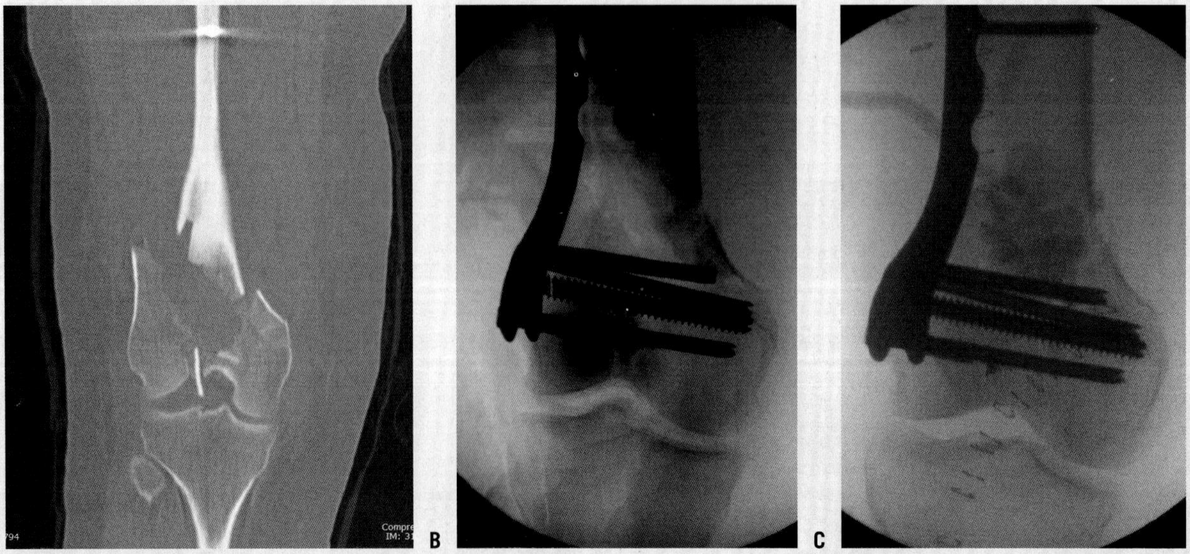

TECH FIG 9 **A.** Patient with significant metaphyseal bone loss from an open injury shown on CT scan. **B.** The postfixation radiograph shows the void. **C.** Placement of OsteoSet beads impregnated with vancomycin (off-label use) to fill the void and provide osteoconductive material for healing.

Bone Grafting

- The metaphyseal comminution may require bone grafting or the use of bone substitutes in cases of open fractures with bone loss.
  - The exact type and need vary and should be based on the surgeon's experience **(TECH FIG 9)**.
  - In closed fractures, avoiding stripping of the medial soft tissues often allows for healing without bone grafting.
  - In open fractures with significant bone loss, we have had good success with the use of bone substitutes such as calcium sulfate (+/– antibiotics mixed in; off-label use), avoiding the need for later grafting (see **FIG 11A–H**).
- Hemostasis is achieved throughout the procedure or after the tourniquet is released. A tourniquet can be used to help minimize bleeding and improve visualization, especially for articular reconstruction. Often, a sterile tourniquet is used because of the temporary bridging external fixator that is in place.
- After adequate irrigation (before bone graft or substitute placement if used), a drain is placed in the knee joint and brought out laterally.

Standard Wound Closure

- Closure of the arthrotomy is performed with figure-8 0 Vicryl sutures. This is reinforced by a running 2-0 FiberWire (Arthrex, Inc., Naples, FL) or Ethibond suture (Ethicon) **(TECH FIG 10A)**.
- The subcutaneous tissue is closed with 2-0 Vicryl.
- The skin is closed with staples, as are the percutaneous stab incisions.
- The knee is flexed and extended fully to ensure restoration of motion as well as to break any adhesions in the quadriceps that may have formed while the temporary bridging external fixator had been in place **(TECH FIG 10B,C)**.
- The final radiographs are taken in the operating room **(TECH FIG 10D–F)**.

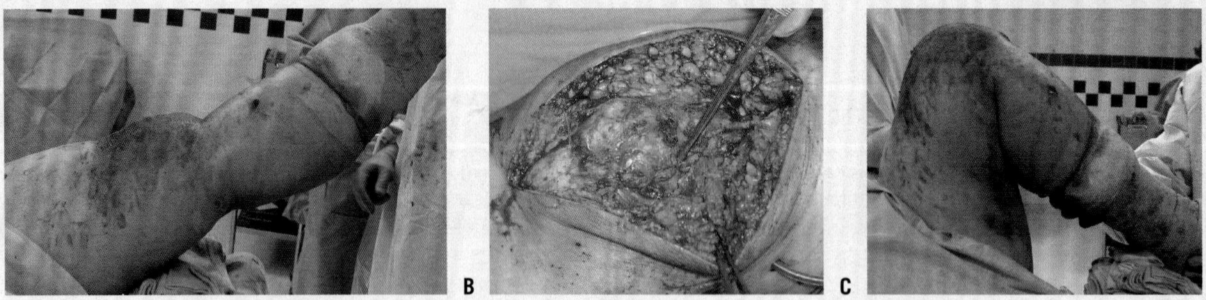

TECH FIG 10 **A.** Closure of the arthrotomy. **B,C.** Full flexion and extension of the knee after definitive fixation and closure. *(continued)*

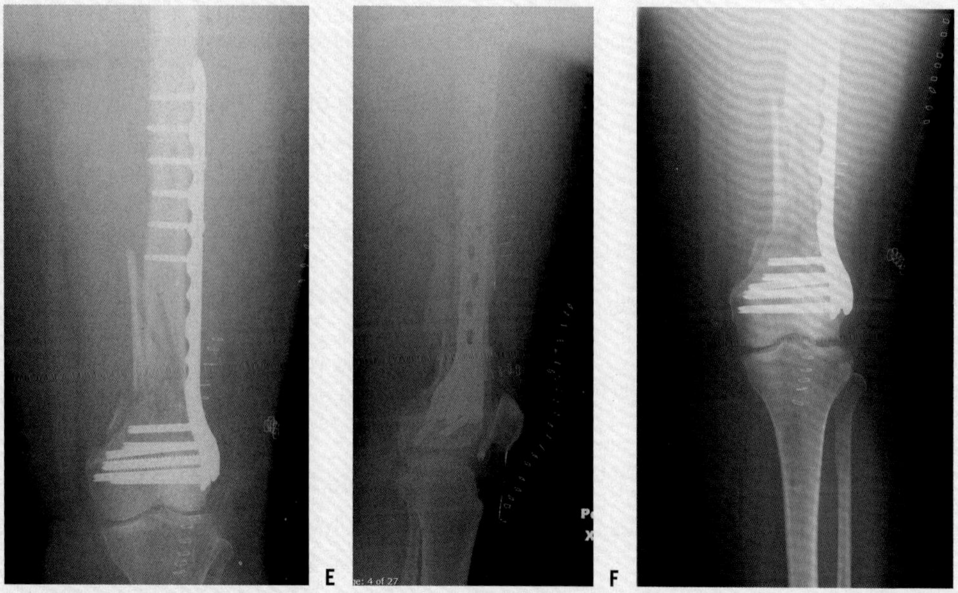

TECH FIG 10 *(continued)* As seen in final AP (**D**) and lateral (**E**) radiographs, the metaphyseal comminution is bridged and left undisturbed. **F.** AP of the knee showing proper alignment of the distal femur.

OPEN REDUCTION AND INTERNAL FIXATION OF THE DISTAL FEMUR WITH LOCKING PLATES (TYPE A OR NONDISPLACED TYPE C1 OR C2)

- This technique can be used regardless of the locking plate system used. Each system's technique guide should be reviewed before use as each system has its own idiosyncrasies. Variations in plate application as well as reduction tools and techniques are unique to each system.
- See comments earlier regarding temporary use of an external fixator or distractor.

Limited Lateral Approach

- A lateral incision measuring about 5 to 6 cm is made starting at the level of the joint and extending proximally in line with the shaft. The distal extent is curved slightly toward the tibial tubercle, as in the lateral approach **(TECH FIG 11A,B)**.
- The iliotibial band is incised in line with the skin incision **(TECH FIG 11C)**.

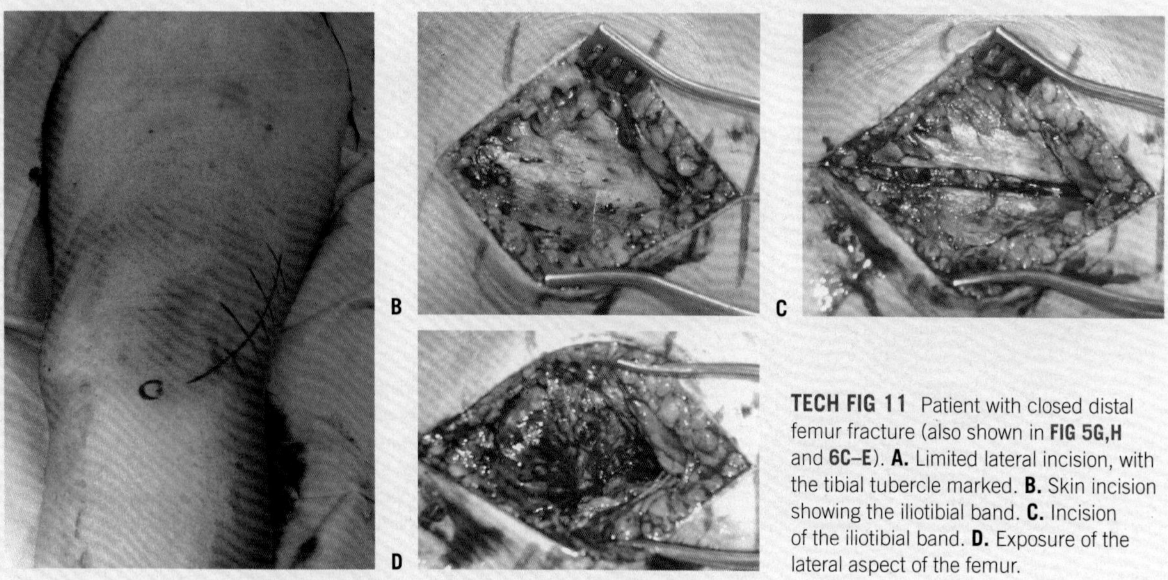

TECH FIG 11 Patient with closed distal femur fracture (also shown in **FIG 5G,H** and **6C–E**). **A.** Limited lateral incision, with the tibial tubercle marked. **B.** Skin incision showing the iliotibial band. **C.** Incision of the iliotibial band. **D.** Exposure of the lateral aspect of the femur.

- The dissection is carried down to the lateral femoral condyle. The lateral aspect is exposed enough for plate placement **(TECH FIG 11D)**.
- A Cobb elevator is used to create a plane submuscularly up the lateral shaft of the femur for placement of the plate.

Stabilizing the Articular Surface

- For nondisplaced type C1 or C2 fractures, the first priority is to stabilize the articular surface.
- Visualization of the joint may be accomplished with placement of a blunt Hohmann retractor (or similar Z retractor) **(TECH FIG 12A)**.
- A reduction forceps is placed anteriorly to hold the reduction **(TECH FIG 12B)**.
- Temporary Kirschner wires or guidewires from a cannulated system can be placed for additional stability **(TECH FIG 12C,D)**.
- All clamps, Kirschner wires, or guidewires should be placed outside the zone of plate application **(TECH FIG 12E,F)**.
- Definitive fixation of the condyles should be performed (see technique description earlier) **(TECH FIG 12G)**.

Reduction of the Distal Segment and Plate Placement

- Reduction of the distal segment to the shaft can be performed using temporary Steinmann pins **(TECH FIG 13)**.
- The plate can now be applied in a submuscular fashion (see Placement of the Plate section earlier).

Wound Closure

- Final radiographs are taken in the operating room **(TECH FIG 14)**.
- Standard wound closure is undertaken, as described in the previous section.

Retrograde Nailing (see FIG 10)

- Refer to Chapter 40 on retrograde nailing of the femur.

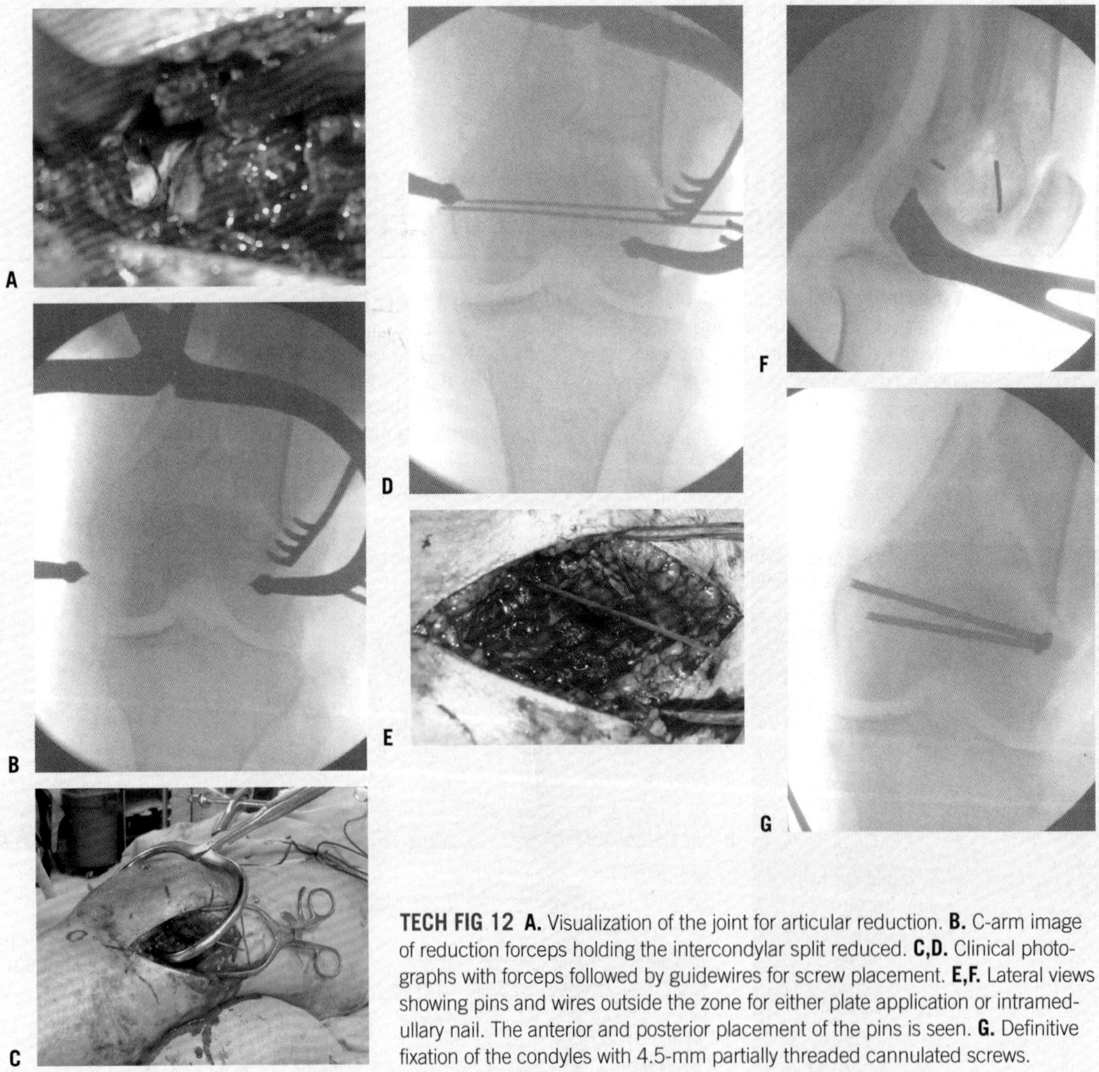

TECH FIG 12 A. Visualization of the joint for articular reduction. **B.** C-arm image of reduction forceps holding the intercondylar split reduced. **C,D.** Clinical photographs with forceps followed by guidewires for screw placement. **E,F.** Lateral views showing pins and wires outside the zone for either plate application or intramedullary nail. The anterior and posterior placement of the pins is seen. **G.** Definitive fixation of the condyles with 4.5-mm partially threaded cannulated screws.

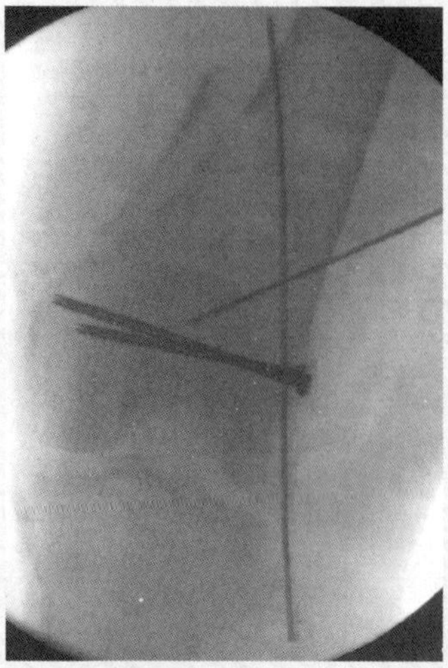

TECH FIG 13 Adjunctive temporary fixation with Steinmann pins to reduce the shaft to the distal construct; pins again are placed outside of the area for plate application.

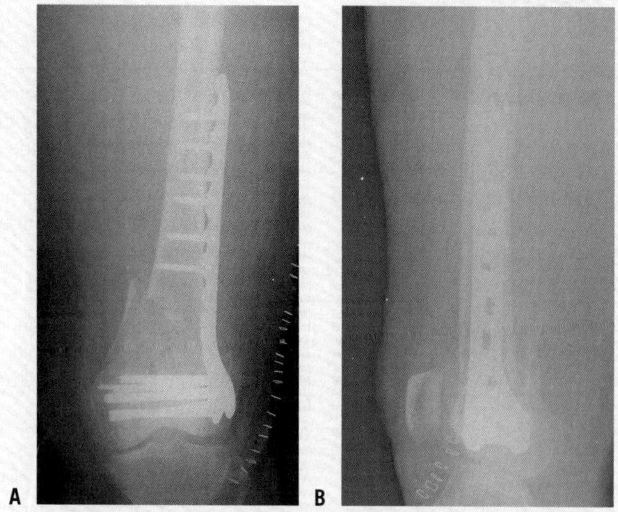

TECH FIG 14 Final AP (**A**) and lateral (**B**) radiographs reveal that the posterior and medial metaphyseal comminution is left undisturbed.

TECHNIQUES

Pearls and Pitfalls

Articular Reduction	• Direct open reduction should be used. • Fixation can be outside the plate or through the plate. • If outside the plate, screws should be out of the way of the plate to maximize fixation points through the plate. • If a nail is being used with an articular split, the screws should be placed anterior and/or posterior to the proposed nail trajectory.
Plate Application	• The initial guidewire through the central hole in the plate should be parallel to the joint. Ninety-five degrees is built into the plate. If locking screws are placed parallel to the joint, then once the plate is reduced to the shaft, the proper alignment is restored. • Rotation must be continually assessed. • The fracture should be reduced in the sagittal plane before temporary fixation or creation of a "box construct" with the plate. • In comminuted cases, a scanogram or opposite-side femur film with a ruler can be obtained to help determine the length. • Use of a long plate greater than nine holes in overall length with at least eight holes proximal to the fracture has been recommended.[14] • Anterior plate application on the shaft is linked to compromised fixation and early failure.[3] • Anterior plate application distally leads to hardware prominence and pain.[3]
Soft Tissue Handling	• The surgeon should avoid stripping the soft tissues medially. This will obviate the need for bone grafting especially in closed fractures. • The plate should be placed submuscularly.
Temporary Bridging External Fixator	• Any construct can be used. • The pins and bars should be placed in a manner such that the fixator could be used intraoperatively as a femoral distractor to hold the reduction, allowing the plating to occur. • The fixator pins in the femur should be placed while traction is applied to the limb so as to maximize the length of the quadriceps. This will ensure that difficulty regaining length is not associated with "skewering" of the quadriceps. • Anterior pins in the femur should be placed above at least 7.5 cm from the superior pole of the patella.
Periprosthetic Fractures	• The surgeon should ensure that the femoral component will allow an intramedullary nail to be placed (eg, the femoral box is open). • If the component is stemmed, then the surgeon should make sure that cables are available to help supplement plate fixation; unicortical locked screws may not be sufficient for fixation. • The new variable-angle (polyaxial) locking plates may allow for screw fixation around the stemmed components and bicortical locked fixation.

Deformity Prevention Valgus Deformity	• Placing the initial guidewire through the "central" hole for plate fixation parallel to the joint ensures proper alignment of the plate relative to the shaft. The plates are designed to recreate the normal anatomic relationship of the distal femur to the shaft. Additionally, a clamp can be placed on the distal fragment and held in the proper position as the plate is applied while adhering to the same principle as outlined earlier.
Varus Deformity	• In a similar fashion, a varus deformity can be prevented by the same technique; however, once the plate is fixed to the distal segment in its proper alignment to the distal segment, a nonlocking screw can be used in the shaft to "suck" the plate to the bone, resulting in correction of the varus.
Extension Deformity	• Because of the pull of the gastrocnemius complex, the distal fragment tends to flex downward, resulting in a relative "extension" deformity at the metaphysis. To prevent this, the knee is flexed as much as feasible to allow for operative fixation, and a bump directly underneath the apex of the deformity can help prevent the deforming forces.
"Golf Club" Deformity[3]	• Placement of the plate too posteriorly on the distal aspect will medialize the distal segment. • Placement of the plate too distal on the femur can also medialize the distal segment. • Perfect lateral fluoroscopic visualization to ensure proper placement of the plate on the lateral aspect of the femur is paramount.

POSTOPERATIVE CARE

- The goal of stable fixation is to allow early range of motion. My preference is a hinged knee brace locked in extension for 2 weeks, at which time the wound is healed and full motion is then started.
- A continuous passive motion machine can be used.
- Cold therapy products can be used.
- A drain can be used for 48 hours postoperatively as needed.
- Deep vein thrombosis prophylaxis may be indicated for certain patients:
  - Obese
  - Multiply injured
  - History of previous deep vein thrombosis
  - Patient who may not be mobile enough despite an isolated injury
  - Length of prophylaxis
    - In cases of an isolated injury to the femur, we prescribe 2 weeks of deep vein thrombosis prophylaxis for these patients and then reassess in terms of mobility.
    - In patients who have additional significant risk factors for deep vein thrombosis and in the polytrauma patient, 6 to 12 weeks is prescribed.
  - Low-molecular-weight heparin is our preferred chemoprophylaxis.
  - Inferior vena cava filter may need to be considered in those multiply injured patients who cannot be anticoagulated.
- Early protected weight bearing
  - Toe-touch weight bearing for at least 6 to 8 weeks for plate fixation
  - Followed by partial weight bearing for 4 to 6 weeks for plate fixation
  - Followed by full weight bearing
  - Immediate weight bearing can be indicated for fixation of type A fractures, with intramedullary nailing if the fracture pattern is stable and not comminuted.
  - For type C fractures treated with intramedullary nailing and screw fixation for the articular component, toe-touch weight bearing or non–weight bearing for 6 to 8 weeks is adequate, followed by full weight bearing.
  - The aforementioned time frames are purely guidelines. The time to weight bearing is based on the fracture pattern, comminution, bone quality, patient body mass index (BMI), and radiographic evidence of healing.
  - Patients having any radiographic cortical bridging by 4 months has been shown to be predictive of final union.[32]
- Patients are prescribed physical therapy for range of motion and strengthening at 2 weeks.

OUTCOMES

- Results are good to excellent in 50% to 96% of cases.[18,25,40]
  - Average range of motion is about 110 to 120 degrees.
  - About 70% to 80% of patients can walk without aids.
  - Elderly patients continue to have a higher perioperative risk of dying in the hospital from such injuries, along with poor functional long-term outcomes.[13]
  - Overall mortality has been reported as 13.4% in geriatric distal femur fractures at 1 year. There was also a significant increase in 30-day, 6-month, and 1-year mortality if operated on greater than 2 days from admission compared to less than 2 days.[20]
- It is difficult to compare the results of studies in the literature.[40]
  - There is no universally accepted classification.
  - There are varying indications.
  - Different grading systems are used.
  - Not all authors adhere to the same principles.

COMPLICATIONS

- Locking plates have become useful, but despite this newer plate technology, care must be taken to avoid common pitfalls; complications are still problematic, with overall healing problem reported as high as 32%.[8,12]
- It has been suggested that the use of a longer plate (longer than nine holes in length with eight holes proximal to the fracture) can minimize failures of fixation.[26]
- Neurovascular injuries
  - Can occur from initial trauma
  - Rare after surgery

- Infection
  - 0% to 10% rate after ORIF
  - Predisposing factors
    - High-energy injuries
    - Open fractures
    - Extensive dissection
    - Prolonged operative time
    - Inadequate fixation
- Nonunion
  - 0% to 19% rate after ORIF
  - Predisposing factors
    - Open fractures[29]
    - Bone loss or defect **(FIG 17A)**
    - High-energy injuries
    - Soft tissue stripping
    - Loss of osseous vascularity
    - Inadequate stabilization
    - No bone grafts
    - Infection[29]
    - The use of a stainless steel plate was found to be an independent predictor of nonunion.[27,38]
    - High rigidity and all locking constructs[38]
- Malunion
  - More common with nonsurgical treatment, which results in varus and recurvatum
  - Operative treatment with newer locking plates can result in valgus.
  - Malrotation has been reported as high as 38.5%.[6]
  - Treatment required to restore mechanical axis
    - Supracondylar osteotomy
    - Stable fixation
    - Early range of motion
- The incidence of hardware failure has been reported as anywhere from 0% to 22% of cases (**FIG 17B,C**, plate; **FIG 17D,E**, screws).[26,35]
  - Predisposing factors
    - Comminution of metaphyseal area
    - Older age

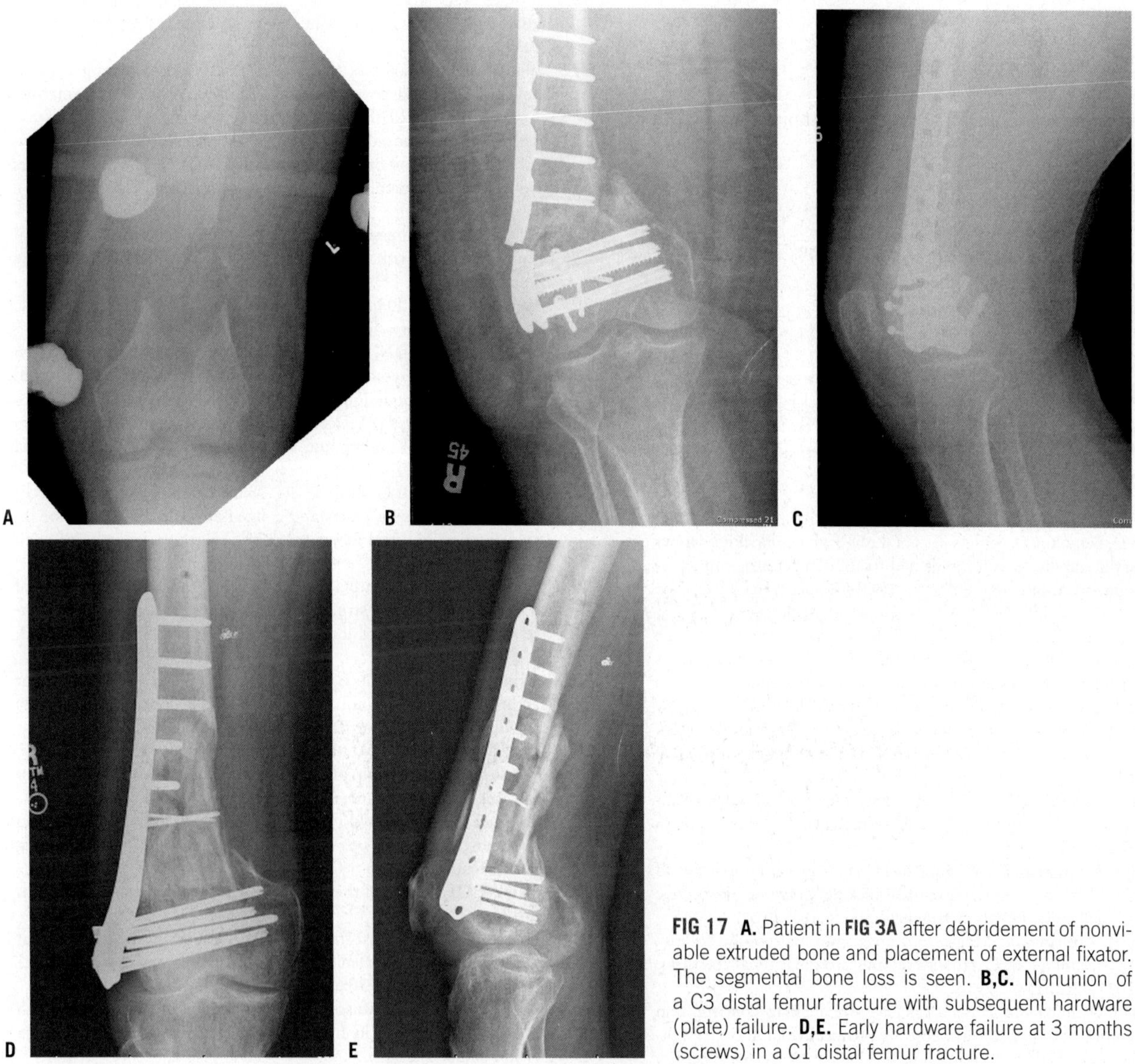

FIG 17 A. Patient in **FIG 3A** after débridement of nonviable extruded bone and placement of external fixator. The segmental bone loss is seen. **B,C.** Nonunion of a C3 distal femur fracture with subsequent hardware (plate) failure. **D,E.** Early hardware failure at 3 months (screws) in a C1 distal femur fracture.

- Very distal fracture
- Premature loading or weight bearing
- Open fractures
- Segmental bone loss
- Smoking
- Increased BMI
- Shorter plates (less than nine holes of overall length)
- Variable-angle locking technology has been suggested as a factor but controversial.[9,19,33]
- Diabetes
- Nonunion
- Infection
- A new technique using both an intramedullary nail (for endosteal substitution) and a lateral locked plate in the management of distal femur fractures in patients with morbid obesity or segmental bone loss has been described as a way to prevent hardware failure.[16,30]

- Knee stiffness: Almost all patients exhibit some loss of motion.
  - Protruding hardware (see **FIG 10E,F**)
  - Articular malreduction
  - Adhesions
    - Intra-articular
    - Ligamentous–capsular contractures
    - Muscle scarring
  - Treatment may consist of any or combination of the following:
    - Manipulation
    - Arthroscopic lysis
    - Formal quadricepsplasty
- Posttraumatic arthritis occurs in 0% to 30% of cases.
  - Predisposing factors
    - Severe articular comminution
    - Cartilage loss
    - Cartilage impaction or damage
  - Surgical factors
    - Failure of anatomic reduction
    - Malalignment of fracture

REFERENCES

1. Auston D, Donohue D, Stoops K, et al. Long segment blocking screws increase the stability of retrograde nail fixation in geriatric supracondylar femur fractures: eliminating the "Bell-Clapper effect." J Orthop Trauma 2018;32:559–564.
2. Beingessner D, Moon E, Barei D, et al. Biomechanical analysis of the less invasive stabilization system for mechanically unstable fractures of the distal femur: comparison of titanium versus stainless steel and bicortical versus unicortical fixation. J Trauma 2011;71(3):620–624.
3. Beltran MJ, Collinge CA, Patzkowski JC, et al. The safe zone for external fixator pins in the femur. J Orthop Trauma 2012;26: 643–647.
4. Bettin CC, Weinlein JC, Toy PC, et al. Distal femoral replacement for acute distal femoral fractures in elderly patients. J Orthop Trauma 2016;30:503–509.
5. Bottlang M, Fitzpatrick DC, Sheerin D, et al. Dynamic fixation of distal femur fractures using far cortical locking screws: a prospective observational study. J Orthop Trauma 2014;28:181–188.
6. Buckley R, Mohanty K, Malish D. Lower limb malrotation following MIPO technique of distal femoral and proximal tibial fractures. Injury 2011;42(2):194–199.
7. Canadian Orthopaedic Trauma Society. Are locking constructs in distal femoral fractures always best? A prospective multicenter randomized controlled trial comparing the Less Invasive Stabilization System with the minimally invasive dynamic condylar screw system. J Orthop Trauma 2016;30:e1–e6.
8. Collinge CA, Gardner MJ, Crist BD. Pitfalls in the application of distal femur plates for fractures. J Orthop Trauma 2011;25(11):695–706.
9. Dang KH, Armstrong CA, Karia RA, et al. Outcomes of distal femur fractures treated with the Synthes 4.5 mm VA-LCP curved condylar plate. Int Orthop 2019;43:1709–1714.
10. Domínguez I, Rodriguez EM, De Pedro Moro JA, et al. Antegrade nailing for fractures of the distal femur. Clin Orthop Relat Res 1998;(350):74–79.
11. Doornink J, Fitzpatrick DC, Madey SM, et al. Far cortical locking enables flexible fixation with periarticular locking plates. J Orthop Trauma 2011;25(suppl 1):S29–S34.
12. Henderson CE, Kuhl LL, Fitzpatrick DC, et al. Locking plates for distal femur fractures: is there a problem with fracture healing? J Orthop Trauma 2011;25(suppl 1):S8–S14.
13. Kammerlander C, Riedmüller P, Gosch M, et al. Functional outcome and mortality in geriatric distal femoral fractures. Injury 2012;43(7):1096–1101.
14. Leung KS, Shen WY, Mui LT, et al. Interlocking intramedullary nailing for supracondylar and intercondylar fractures of the distal part of the femur. J Bone Joint Surg Am 1991;73A:332–340.
15. Linn MS, McAndrew CM, Prusaczyk B, et al. Dynamic locked plating of distal femur fractures. J Orthop Trauma 2015;29:447–450.
16. Liporace FA, Yoon RS. Nail plate combination technique for native and periprosthetic distal femur fractures. J Orthop Trauma 2019;33:e64–e68.
17. Lujan TJ, Henderson CE, Madey SM, et al. Locked plating of distal femur fractures leads to inconsistent and asymmetric callus formation. J Orthop Trauma 2010;24(3):156–162.
18. Markmiller M, Konrad G, Südkamp N. Femur-LISS and distal femoral nail for fixation of distal femoral fractures: are there differences in outcome and complications? Clin Orthop Relat Res 2004;(426): 252–257.
19. McDonald TC, Lambert JJ, Hulick RM, et al. Treatment of distal femur fractures with the Depuy-Synthes variable angle locking compression plate. J Orthop Trauma 2019;33:432–437.
20. Myers PM, Laboe P, Johnson KJ, et al. Patient mortality in geriatric distal femur fractures. J Orthop Trauma 2018;32:111–115.
21. Nork SE, Segina DN, Aflatoon K, et al. The association between supracondylar-intercondylar distal femoral fractures and coronal plane fractures. J Bone Joint Surg Am 2005;87A:564–569.
22. Ostrum RF, Maurer JP. Distal third femur fractures treated with retrograde femoral nailing and blocking screws. J Orthop Trauma 2009;23:681–684.
23. Otto RJ, Moed BR, Bledsoe JG. Biomechanical comparison of polyaxial-type locking plates and a fixed-angle locking plate for internal fixation of distal femur fractures. J Orthop Trauma 2009;23: 645–652.
24. Plumarom Y, Wilkinson BG, Marsh L, et al. Radiographic healing of far cortical locking constructs in distal femur fractures: a comparative study with standard locking plates. J Orthop Trauma 2019;33: 277–283.
25. Rademakers MV, Kerkhoffs GMMJ, Sierevelt IN, et al. Intra-articular fractures of the distal femur: a long-term follow-up study of surgically treated patients. J Orthop Trauma 2004;18:213–219.
26. Ricci WM, Streuble PN, Morshed S, et al. Risk factors for failure of locked plate fixation of distal femur fractures: an analysis of 335 cases. J Orthop Trauma 2014;28(2):83–89.
27. Rodriguez EK, Zurakowski D, Herder L, et al. Mechanical construct characteristics predisposing to non-union after locked lateral plating of distal femur fractures. J Orthop Trauma 2016;30:403–408.
28. Schatzker J. Fractures of the distal femur revisited. Clin Orthop Relat Res 1998;(347):43–56.
29. Southeast Fracture Consortium. LCP versus LISS in the treatment of open and closed distal femur fractures: does it make a difference? J Orthop Trauma 2016;30:e212–e216.
30. Spitler CA, Bergin PF, Russell GV, et al. Endosteal substitution with an intramedullary rod in fractures of the femur. J Orthop Trauma 2018;32(suppl 1):S25–S29.

31. Starr AJ, Jones AL, Reinert CM. The "Swashbuckler": a modified anterior approach for fractures of the distal femur. J Orthop Trauma 1999;13:138–140.
32. Strotman PK, Karunakar MA, Seymour R, et al. Any cortical bridging predicts healing of supracondylar femur fractures after treatment with locked plating. J Orthop Trauma 2017;31:538–544.
33. Tank JC, Schneider PS, Davis E, et al. Early mechanical failures of the Synthes variable angle locking distal femur plate. J Orthop Trauma 2016;30:e7–e11.
34. Tejwani NC, Park S, Iesaka K, et al. The effect of locked distal screws in retrograde nailing of osteoporotic distal femur fractures: a laboratory study using cadaver femurs. J Orthop Trauma 2005;19:380–383.
35. Vallier HA, Hennessey TA, Sontich JK, et al. Failure of LCP condylar plate fixation in the distal part of the femur. A report of six cases. J Bone Joint Surg Am 2006;88:846–853.
36. Vallier HA, Immler W. Comparison of the 95-degree angled blade plate and the locking condylar plate for the treatment of distal femoral fractures. J Orthop Trauma 2012;26:327–332.
37. Van Dyke B, Colley R, Ottomeyer C, et al. Effect of blocking screws on union of infraisthmal femur fractures stabilized with a retrograde intramedullary nail. J Orthop Trauma 2018;32:251–255.
38. Wang MT, An VVG, Sivakumar BS. Non-union in lateral locked plating for distal femoral fractures: a systematic review. Injury 2019;50:1790–1794.
39. Wilkens KJ, Curtiss S, Lee MA. Polyaxial locking plate fixation in distal femur fractures: A biomechanical comparison. J Orthop Trauma 2008;22:624–628.
40. Zlowodzki M, Bhandari M, Marek DJ, et al. Operative treatment of acute distal femur fractures: systematic review of 2 comparative studies and 45 case series (1989 to 2005). J Orthop Trauma 2006;20:366–371.

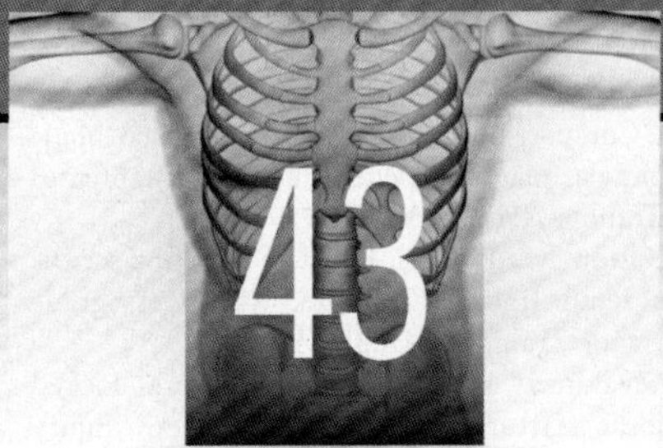

CHAPTER

Open Reduction and Internal Fixation of the Patella

Samir Mehta

DEFINITION

- The patella, the largest sesamoid bone, is an essential component for knee extension (in conjunction with the patellar and quadriceps tendons) and provides leverage to the quadriceps mechanism. Fractures of the patella have the potential to disrupt the extensor mechanism.
- Fractures of the patella can impact knee mechanics, as these are often articular injuries.
- Management of patellar fractures must restore the extensor mechanism while ensuring anatomic reconstruction of the articular surface.
- Descriptive terms (stellate or comminuted, transverse, vertical, apical or inferior pole, and sleeve) are used to classify patellar fractures.
- Fixation strategies typically focus on techniques allowing for early weight bearing and graduated range of motion.

ANATOMY

- The articular surface is composed of medial and lateral facets, with the medial facet having the most variability in size and shape. Horizontal ridges further subdivide the medial and lateral facets. An odd facet lies at the most medial aspect of the articular surface. The undulating nature of the articular surface can make interpretation of the lateral radiograph difficult, which can result in the appearance of hardware used for fracture fixation being "safe" while it is actually intra-articular. The distal pole of the undersurface is extra-articular, which is an important consideration when addressing injuries in this region as some techniques suggest advancement of the patellar tendon with concomitant excision of the inferior pole fractures **(FIG 1)**.
- The superior pole of the patella serves as an attachment for the quadriceps tendon. The most superficial portion of the quadriceps tendon courses over the anterior patellar surface and is contiguous with the patellar tendon. The patellar tendon courses from the apex of the patella to the tibial tubercle.
- The patellar retinaculum is composed of thickenings of the fascia lata of the thigh in addition to the aponeurosis of the vastus medialis and lateralis.[16] In addition to stabilizing the patella, the retinaculum acts as a secondary extensor. An intact retinaculum in the setting of a patellar fracture may allow for extension of the knee. This is particularly true in comminuted but minimally displaced fractures. The retinaculum is often torn in conjunction with an extensor mechanism injury. As a result, it is an absolute requirement that the retinaculum be repaired in conjunction with any patellar reconstruction.
- Multiple arteries about the knee supply a peripatellar plexus, although the main intraosseous blood supply is from a distal to proximal direction.[17]
- The patella acts to increase the moment arm of the extensor mechanism by displacing the quadriceps tendon anteriorly. This increased moment arm is most critical during terminal extension, when the quadriceps is otherwise at a mechanical disadvantage.[9] Terminal extension is critical to the gait cycle.
- Due to the small contact area of the articular surface and the high level of compressive forces generated by the extensor mechanism, the contact stress on the patellofemoral joint has been estimated to be higher than any other major weight-bearing joint.[5] For example, stair climbing generates sevenfold body weight forces across the patellofemoral joint.

PATHOGENESIS

- Fractures of the patella may result from direct force to the anterior knee, indirect forces transmitted through the extensor mechanism, or a combination of both.
- The patella is particularly susceptible to injury from direct blows given its superficial location and minimal soft tissue envelope.
- The portion of the patella articulating with the femur moves from distal to proximal with increasing degrees of flexion.

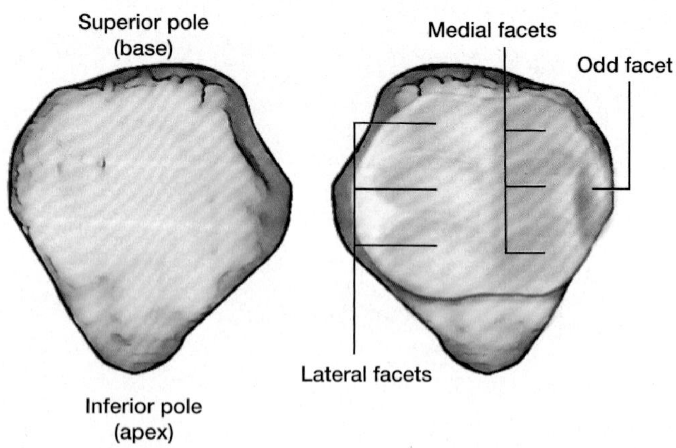

FIG 1 Patellar anatomy. The major facets include the medial, lateral, and odd facets. The medial and lateral facets are further subdivided by subtle horizontal ridges.

The fracture pattern for direct blows to the patella has been shown to correspond to the articulating portion of the patella at the time of injury, thus corresponding to the amount of knee flexion at time of injury.[1]

- Indirect forces causing fracture can be caused by unanticipated and rapid flexion of the knee while the quadriceps is also firing. Fractures from an indirect mechanism tend to be less comminuted than those from direct trauma.[5]
- Stress fractures, while possible, are a rare cause of fractures of the patella but can be seen as a result of overtraining.

NATURAL HISTORY

- Depending on the type of fracture and involvement of the retinaculum, various amounts of long-term extensor lag and weakness can be expected. The long-term effect on range of motion likewise depends on fracture pattern and displacement.
- There is an increased incidence of osteoarthritis of the knee after patellar fracture. The increased rate of arthritis may be both from initial cartilage injury and posttraumatic arthritis due to articular cartilage incongruity. Despite advances in techniques and technology, outcomes after operative fixation still show functional impairment.
- Outcomes after patellar fracture are highly dependent on the ability to restore full extension, obtaining a functional range of flexion, and a congruent, stable reduction.
- In patients with active extension and minimal meaningful articular step-off, nonoperative management is typically preferred, particularly in the older age group.

PATIENT HISTORY AND PHYSICAL FINDINGS

- Physical examination findings are as follows:
  - Often, a defect can be palpated in the patella.
  - New onset of joint effusion after injury localizes within the capsule of the knee. A knee effusion may not be present if there is disruption of the retinaculum, allowing hematoma to escape from the joint capsule. A significant effusion can increase tension on the limited soft tissue envelope resulting in necrosis of the skin.
  - The position of the patella (baja vs. alta) and palpation of defects with the patella, quadriceps tendon, or patellar tendon can help differentiate between patellar fracture and ligamentous extensor disruption.
  - Pain can limit the ability to test for active extension of the knee or for extensor lag. Introduction of local anesthesia after aspiration of hematoma can aid in assessment of extensor function. The surgeon should note any extravasation of local anesthetic to evaluate intra-articular extension of skin defects.
  - Aspiration: The surgeon notes the amount of fluid aspirated. The presence of fat lobules in the syringe signifies a fracture extending into the knee capsule.
  - Patients with patellar fractures are able to actively extend the knee (or hold the knee in extension against gravity) in marginal or longitudinal fracture types or in fractures with intact secondary extensors (ie, retinaculum). Knee extension is usually not possible with displaced transverse fractures or comminuted fractures in which the retinaculum is torn.
- History is critical in determining a direct versus indirect cause of fracture. Patellar fractures caused by a high-energy direct cause (ie, head-on motor vehicle accident with dashboard injury) are often associated with other injuries to the knee.
- Peripheral pulses and neurologic function must be examined.
- Knee stability should be evaluated. Patellar fractures may be accompanied by cruciate ligament injury or associated knee dislocation.
- Open fractures will require urgent operative management and are associated with an increased rate of nonunion and infection.[21] Open fractures also connote higher energy and an increased likelihood of associated injury.
- Physical examination must include a thorough secondary survey for other associated injuries. Distal femur fractures and acetabular injuries are commonly associated in high-energy motor vehicle accidents owing to transfer of force through the flexed knee (eg, dashboard injury).

IMAGING AND OTHER DIAGNOSTIC STUDIES

- Anteroposterior (AP) and lateral views of the knee and an axial view of the patella provide sufficient information for nearly all fracture types.
- In the trauma setting, the Merchant view[13] may be obtained **(FIG 2A)**. Alternatively, a computed tomography (CT) scan may provide additional information in the setting of significant comminution.
- CT scanning to look at the articular surface may be helpful if a patella eversion technique is being considered.
- A bipartite patella, arising from failed fusion of patellar ossification centers, can be mistaken for a fracture. Bipartite patellae are most commonly located superolaterally and occur more frequently in males. In 40% of individuals with a bipartite patella, the contralateral patella will also be bipartite **(FIG 2B,C)**.[7]
- The normal Insall-Salvati ratio (height of the patella over the distance from the inferior pole to the tibial tubercle) is about 1.0.[8]
  - Values less than 0.8 represent patella alta and possible patellar tendon rupture. Patella alta may also be seen in patellar sleeve fractures in the pediatric population.
  - Values greater than 1.2 represent patella baja and possible quadriceps tendon rupture.

DIFFERENTIAL DIAGNOSIS

- Quadriceps rupture
- Patellar tendon rupture
- Bipartite patella
- Ligamentous or meniscal injury
- Distal femur or tibial plateau fracture
- Inflammatory arthritis or septic arthritis
- Osteochondral injury
- Patellar dislocation or retinacular injury
- Severe hemarthrosis

NONOPERATIVE MANAGEMENT

- Fractures can be managed nonoperatively if they meet the following criteria:
  - No associated extensor mechanism disruption (ability to perform an active straight-leg raise or hold the leg in full extension without significant lag)
  - Less than 2 mm of displacement of the meaningful articular surface or less than 3 mm separation of the

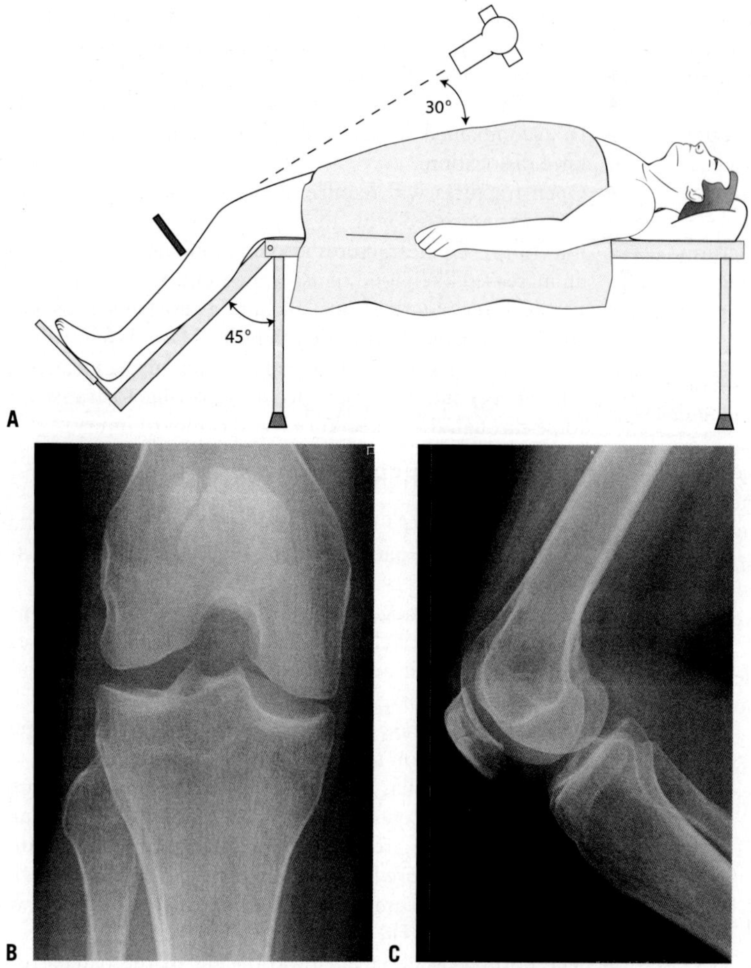

FIG 2 A. In the Merchant view, the knee is allowed to bend to 45 degrees, and the x-ray beam is angled at 30 degrees to the horizon. The x-ray cassette is placed perpendicular to the leg on the proximal tibial diaphysis. **B,C.** Bipartite patella. Note the classic superolateral position of this multipartite patella and the sclerotic margins.

fracture fragments.[3,6] Less displacement is tolerated by some authors in the presence of transverse fractures.[4]

- The described period of immobilization varies. Historically, patients were kept in a long-leg or cylinder cast for 4 to 6 weeks. Current nonoperative management involves early functional treatment with graduated increase in range of motion.
- Our preference for nonoperative treatment includes full weight bearing with crutches and a hinged knee brace.
  - The leg is maintained in extension for 3 weeks, 0 to 30 degrees of active flexion for 3 weeks, followed by full motion with physiotherapy as needed.
  - High-impact activity including contact sports is allowed at 12 weeks.
- Nonoperative management of appropriate fractures results in good overall results, with loss of flexion the most common complication.[4,5]

SURGICAL MANAGEMENT

- Operative treatment is the preferred treatment for the majority of fractures not meeting the nonoperative criteria outlined earlier. Treatment is aimed reconstruction of the extensor mechanism with anatomic reconstruction of the articular surface.
- Open reduction and internal fixation is the treatment of choice.
- Cases with severe comminution of the inferior or superior pole may be considered for partial patellectomy with reapproximation of the patellar tendon.
- Functional deficits without a patella are significant, therefore a total patellectomy should only be reserved for the most severe cases where reconstruction is not possible.
- Methods involving arthroscopy or external fixation have not gained widespread use.
- Soft tissue management is essential due to the limited soft tissue envelope covering the patella. This care for soft tissue begins in the emergency department. Splints or knee immobilizers must be accompanied by copious padding to minimize complications from pressure. Similarly, early aspiration of the hemarthrosis can prevent pressure necrosis.

Preoperative Planning

- Operative timing is dictated by patient condition, presence of open fractures, and condition of the soft tissues.
- Fracture imaging is reviewed.
- Necessary equipment for surgical stabilization should be available.
- Examination under anesthesia is critical, as evaluation of coexisting ligamentous injuries is often limited by patient pain prior to surgery. Lachman, pivot shift, posterior

drawer, and varus–valgus testing should be undertaken before preparing the surgical site.
- Concomitant injuries may be addressed in the same surgery.

Positioning

- Patients are placed in the supine position on a radiolucent table.
- A small bump (eg, rolled blanket or 1 L intravenous fluid bag wrapped in a towel) under the ipsilateral hip will internally rotate the limb placing the patella in a more advantageous surgical position.
- If a tourniquet is used, it must be placed as proximally as possible on the thigh. The quadriceps must not be trapped under the tourniquet, as this may retract the patella superiorly, hindering fracture reduction. The knee is flexed to 90 degrees before elevating the tourniquet. If the retinaculum is disrupted and the superior patella is high riding, the quadriceps should be pulled distally before inflating the tourniquet.[23]

Exposure

- Longitudinal incisions should be used. Although a transverse incision can be made, this does not allow for an extensile exposure if needed.
- We use a longitudinal incision to facilitate exposure and allow extension to the tibial tubercle for wire augmentation when needed. A longitudinal exposure is better tolerated for future reconstructive surgeries and may therefore be beneficial in elderly patients or patients with preexisting osteoarthritis (**FIG 3**).
- A transverse approach follows the skin lines and may be preferable cosmetically but has limited utility. A transverse approach does minimize risk of injury to the infrapatellar branch of the saphenous nerve. In the setting of an open wound, a transverse incision may be necessary to facilitate exposure.
- Dissection is carried through the patellar bursa to expose the fracture site. Hematoma is often encountered upon opening bursa. Hematoma is cleared from the fracture site with copious irrigation and small curettes. The fracture line is followed to the retinacular tissue; the surgeon identifies the superior and inferior leaves of retinaculum and tags them for later repair.
- The fracture edges should be defined clearly. Reapproximation of the dorsal, cortical fracture edges will allow for an indirect reduction of the articular surface, particularly in transverse fracture patterns.
- Reduction of the pieces can be obtained by hyperextending the knee (via a small bump placed under the ankle) and pointed reduction clamps on the inferior and superior pole of the patella. Direct reduction of the dorsal surface of the patella in elementary fracture patterns will facilitate indirect reduction of the articular surface. Use of a Kirschner wire as a joystick or a dental pick can also facilitate reduction (**FIG 4**).
- In severely comminuted fractures or fractures with a coronal split such that direct reduction of the dorsal surface will not affect articular reduction, direct visualization of the articular surface can be performed by everting the patella. Often, a CT is helpful in determining the severity of comminution. The patellar is everted via a lateral parapatellar arthrotomy.[14] The joint surface is visualized and then provisionally reduced with clamps, Kirschner wires, and miniscrews. Definitive fixation is often performed with miniplate stabilization of the dorsal surface.

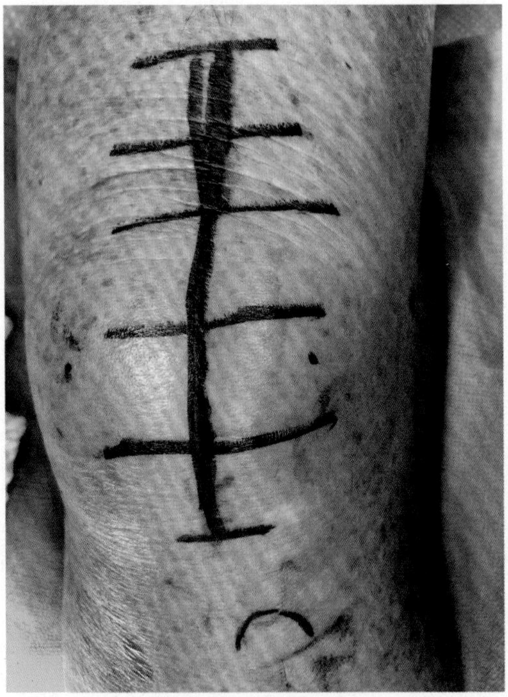

FIG 3 Longitudinal incision extending from proximal to the superior pole of the patella to distal to tibial tubercle.

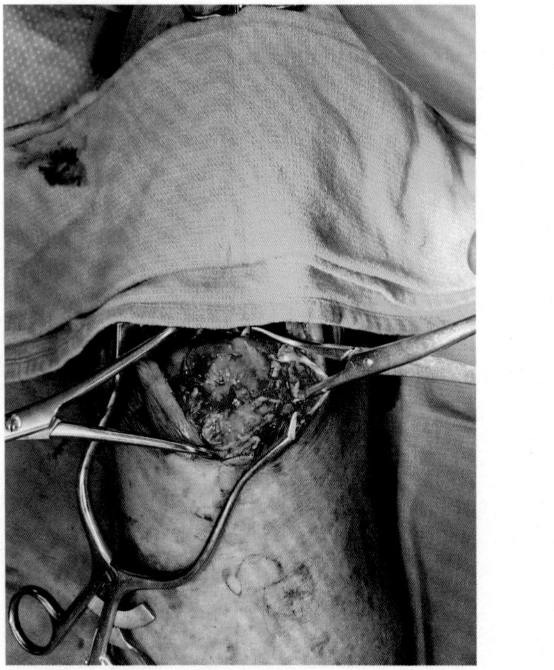

FIG 4 Multiple pointed reduction clamps to maintain reduction of the patellar fracture with fracture visualization dorsally with indirect reduction of the articular surface.

TENSION BAND WIRING

- Tension band wiring can be used to stabilize transverse fracture patterns. More complex fracture patterns can use a tension band construct if the fracture can be converted to a transverse pattern by fixation of smaller comminuted pieces with screws or Kirschner wires. Tension band constructs may also be used for more distal pole fractures, with Kirschner wires placed more closely together to capture the fragment.
- Two 1.6- to 2.0-mm Kirschner wires will span the fracture in parallel **(TECH FIG 1A)**. They can be introduced through the fracture site into the proximal fragment in a retrograde fashion or into the distal fragment in an antegrade fashion.
  - The Kirschner wire is delivered until flush with the fracture line, and the fracture reduction is obtained and held with patellar reduction clamps or Weber clamps.
  - Fracture reduction is checked by palpating the articular surface with a Freer elevator (or by finger palpation if the rent in the retinaculum allows). When encountered, small articular fragments without attached subchondral bone may be discarded. Depressed articular fragments are gently reduced by a Freer elevator.
- Once the fracture is sufficiently reduced, the Kirschner wire is delivered through the opposite fracture fragment.
  - A lateral fluoroscopic view may help to ensure appropriate fracture reduction and Kirschner wire placement.
- Ideally, the Kirschner wires will be about 5 mm below the anterior surface of the patella.[15] The Kirschner wire should be clipped to leave roughly 1 cm of prominence below the inferior pole of the patella.
- A 1.0-mm thick (18 g) cerclage wire is passed just deep to the Kirschner wires, abutting the superior pole of the patella. Care must be taken to leave little to no intervening soft tissue between the superior patella and the tension band. If the wire does not abut the bone, the patient will ultimately have an extensor lag.
  - A 16-gauge angiocatheter may be passed through the quadriceps mechanism, and the wire advanced through the catheter to aid in placement of the wire **(TECH FIG 1B)**.[23]
- The cerclage wire is passed distally in a similar fashion, ensuring the wire abuts the distal pole of the patella.
  - The wire is looped around the anterior aspect of the patella.
  - Alternatively, the wire may be crisscrossed in a figure-8 pattern.
- Prior to tensioning, the surgeon verifies that the Kirschner wires capture the cerclage wire.
- To ensure even tensioning, a two-loop tensioning technique is used. A twist is made in the cerclage wire on the opposite side of the two free ends of the wire. The free ends are gently twisted. These two loops are sequentially tightened with a large needle driver **(TECH FIG 1C)**. The loop is lifted to tension the wire and then twisted.[23]
  - Wires are sequentially tensioned until appropriate compression is visualized and palpated at the fracture site.
- The ends of the twists are clipped, bent over, and tamped into bone to minimize prominence.
- The superior portion of the Kirschner wire is bent and then cut, leaving a hook to capture the cerclage wire. The Kirschner wire is rotated and tamped into the superior pole of the patella.

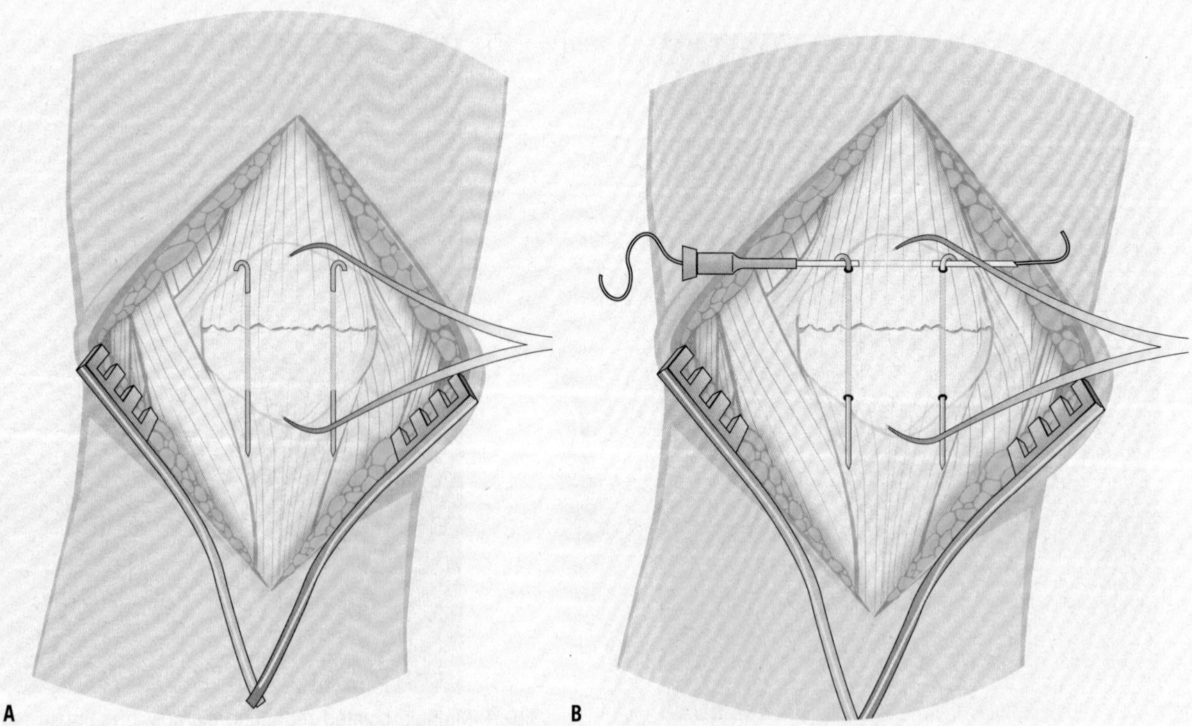

TECH FIG 1 Tension band fixation. **A.** Fracture reduction is maintained with a Weber clamp while Kirschner wires are passed. **B.** A large angiocatheter is used for ease of wire placement deep to Kirschner wires and beneath the quadriceps tendon. *(continued)*

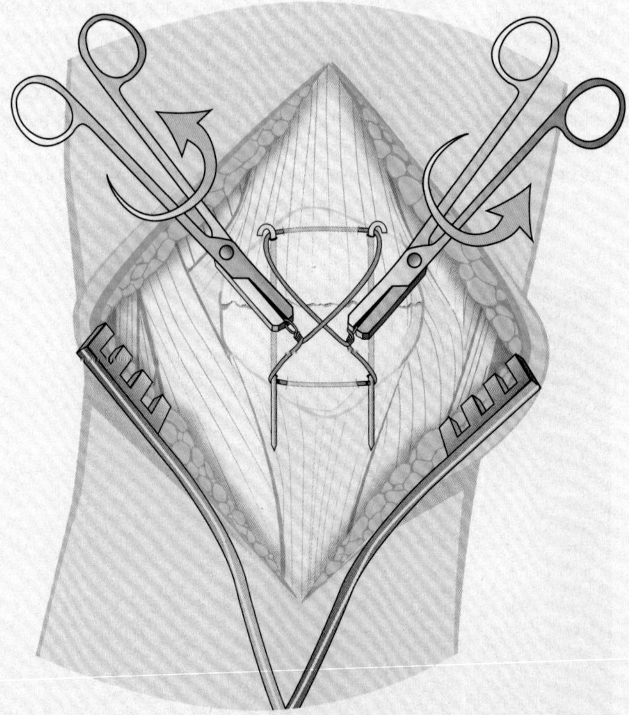

C

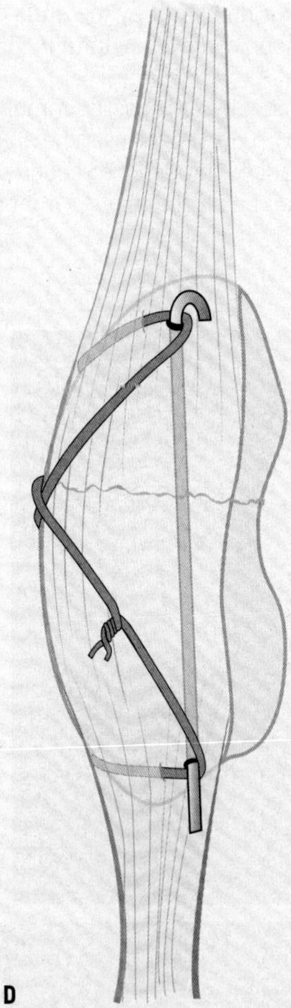

D

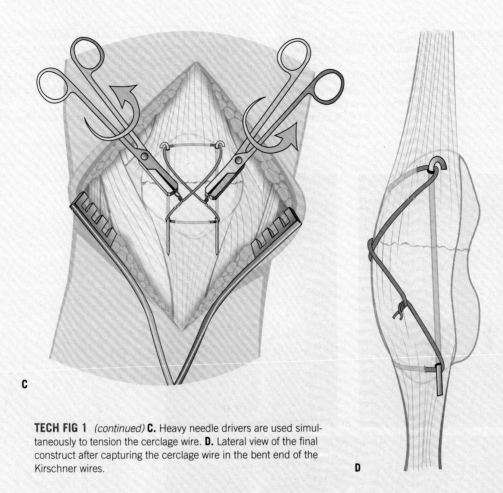

TECH FIG 1 *(continued)* **C.** Heavy needle drivers are used simultaneously to tension the cerclage wire. **D.** Lateral view of the final construct after capturing the cerclage wire in the bent end of the Kirschner wires.

The inferior tip of the wire is cut to avoid excessive length within the patella tendon while leaving enough wire to maintain position of the cerclage wire **(TECH FIG 1D)**.

- Retinacular defects are repaired with absorbable braided suture, a critical step in restoring the extensor mechanism. An intact or repaired retinaculum augments fixation of the patella and is an essential component of an extensor mechanism repair given the significant contribution of the retinaculum to the stability and strength of the extensor mechanism. After patellar fixation, both the medial and lateral sides should be examined for retinacular tears. Primary closure with heavy suture is critical. This also aids in preserving the integrity of the knee joint. Inspection of the repair should be performed prior to wound closure and any defects in the fascia should be addressed.
- After fixation and meticulous retinacular repair, the knee should be brought through a range of motion to approximately 90 degrees. If this cannot be done based on concerns of fixation, then early motion must be avoided for 6 weeks. Typically, the fixation and soft tissue repair allows for this test to be performed confirming the stability of the construct.
- The tourniquet is deflated (if used), and hemostasis is obtained. The wound is thoroughly irrigated. A suction drain is placed as needed, and the wound is closed with buried absorbable sutures followed by simple nylon sutures.
- A well-padded sterile dressing is applied with padding over the leg from the malleoli to the proximal thigh. A knee immobilizer is placed.

MODIFIED TENSION BAND WITH CANNULATED CREWS

- As advocated by Carpenter et al,[5] cannulated screws may be used in place of Kirschner wires in a tension band construct for transverse fracture patterns **(TECH FIG 2A–C)**. This construct has shown to be superior biomechanically to the Kirschner wire tension band construct, resisting larger forces and resulting in less fracture gaping with loads.[5]
- Reduction is obtained as described earlier, with the guidewires for the 4.0- or 4.5-mm partially threaded cannulated screws used in place of Kirschner wires.
- Screws are placed over the guidewires using a lag technique and are left short of the distal cortex. If the screws are long (past the cortex), the wires will not abut the bone

and are at risk for being cut by the ends of the screw. A lateral fluoroscopic view is helpful in verifying screw placement.

- A 0.8-mm (18-gauge) wire is passed through a single cannulated screw, looped back over the anterior surface of the patella, and advanced through the second screw. Alternatively, 1.6-mm cable can be placed through 4.5-mm cannulated screws.
- After bringing the two ends of the wire together, a two-loop tightening technique is used as described earlier, and the twists are buried **(TECH FIG 2D)**.
- This technique is difficult to use with more inferior fractures as the nose of the patella is narrow and two screws may not fit in the fragment.
- As previously described, the retinaculum should be inspected and repaired.

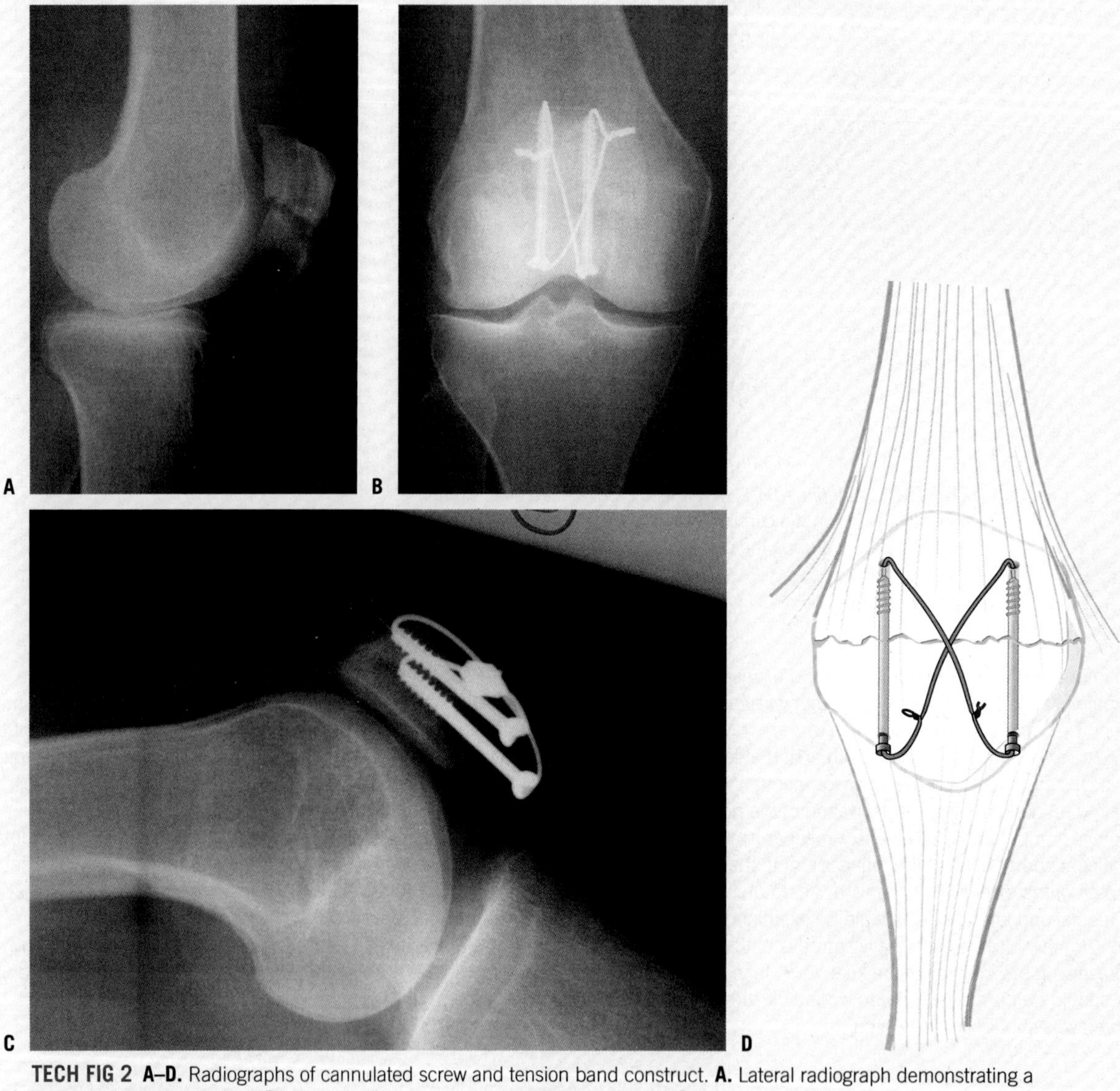

TECH FIG 2 A–D. Radiographs of cannulated screw and tension band construct. **A.** Lateral radiograph demonstrating a transverse patellar fracture. **B.** AP view of final screw and cerclage construct. **C.** Lateral view showing that the screw threads are slightly prominent and not entirely within bone. **D.** Final construct of cannulated screw with cerclage wire. The threads remain entirely within bone.

INTERFRAGMENTARY SCREWS WITHOUT TENSION BANDING

- Although occasionally used with tension band constructs to convert complex fracture patterns into transverse patterns, screw fixation can also be used alone (**TECH FIG 3**). This construct is particularly suited for simple fracture patterns with articular displacement and an intact retinaculum.
- Lag screw fixation is often the method of choice for longitudinal fractures requiring operative management. Lag screw fixation for transverse fractures is also a suitable option, especially in patients with good bone stock. Multiple biomechanical studies have shown two cortical lag screws to be nearly as strong as[2] or stronger than[5] tension band alone in good quality bone.
- After obtaining reduction with pointed forceps, 3.5- or 4.5-mm cortical screws are used in lagging fashion across fracture sites.
- Closure and retinacular repair are undertaken as described earlier with meticulous attention paid to gaining stable retinacular reapproximation.

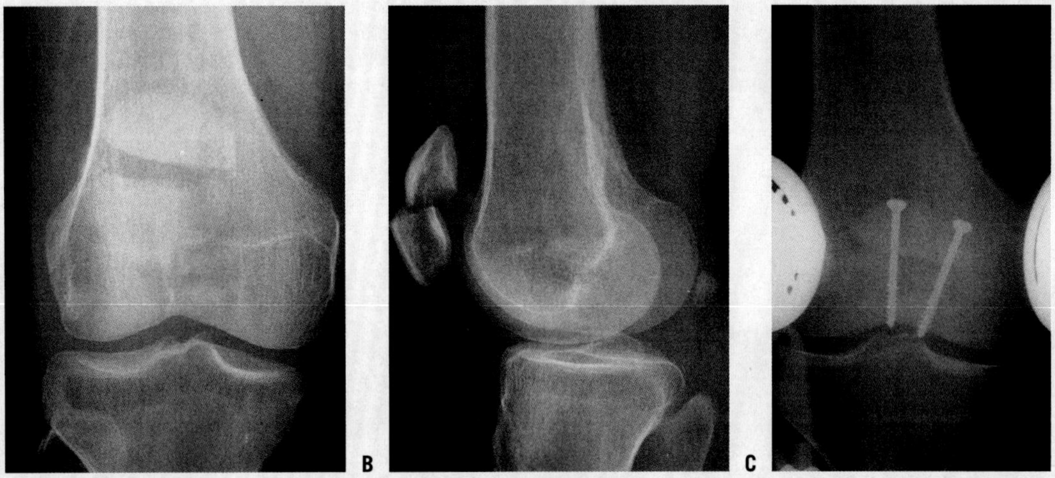

TECH FIG 3 Radiographs of lag screw construct. **A,B.** AP and lateral injury films. **C.** Postoperative radiograph. Note bicortical screw purchase.

PLATE FIXATION

- Small plate fixation of the patella with minifragment implants and fracture-specific constructs has become more prevalent.[19,22]
- Minifragment plate fixation of the patella may allow for less soft tissue irritation and fixation of complex fracture patterns.
- Severely comminuted fractures or those with bone loss may be treated with open reduction and internal fixation with minifragment plates and screws. This will allow for restoration for the extensor mechanism and prevent the need for a patellectomy.
- Provisional reduction of the fracture is obtained with Kirschner wires, reduction clamps, and minifragment screws as necessary.
- Minifragment plates are then undercontoured to fit the dorsal cortex of the patella. Usually, two to three plates are applied with necessary instrumentation to facilitate plate application (**TECH FIG 4**).
- The plate is then applied to the patella, with screw fixation through the proximal hole of the plate from the superior pole of the patella to the inferior pole. The plate is then compressed to bone distally, and a second screw is placed through the most distal hole from the inferior pole to the superior pole (**TECH FIG 5**).
- It is essential to have a well-contoured plate to limit soft tissue irritation. Locking plates can be used in poor quality bone, but the screws will not compress the plate to bone, therefore, the plates must be anatomically contoured.
- Typically, we use 2.0- or 2.4-mm plates as these provide adequate stabilization and limited soft tissue irritation (**TECH FIGS 6** and **7**).
  - As previously described, the retinaculum should be inspected and repaired.

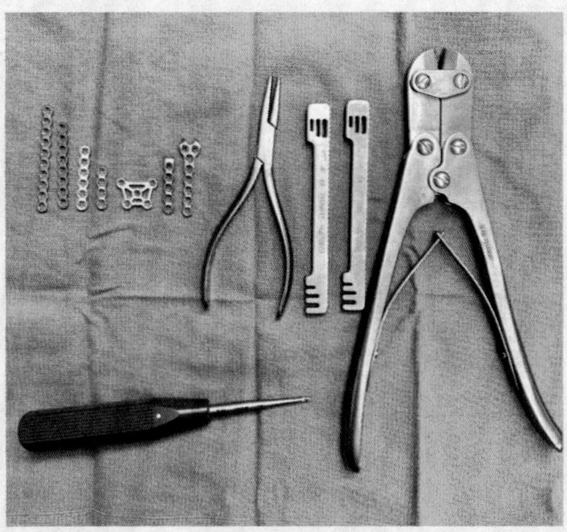

TECH FIG 4 During application of minifragment plates, several different instruments are necessary to contour and optimize plate fixation. In addition, different plate formations may be helpful in fixation strategies.

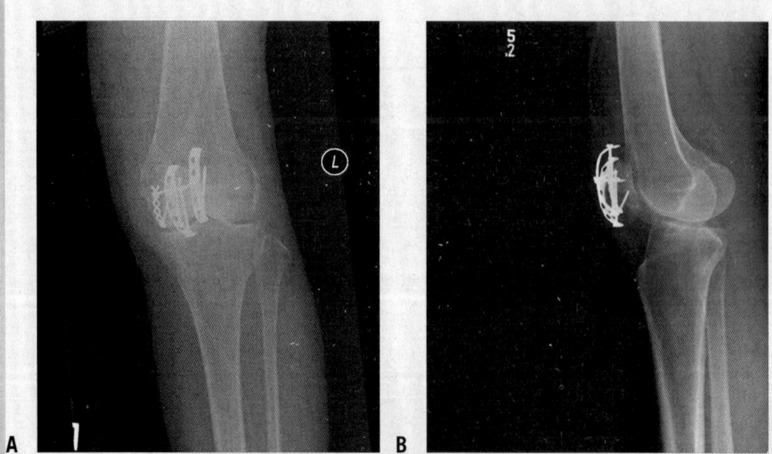

TECH FIG 5 Plate fixation. **A,B.** AP and lateral postoperative radiographs showing plate fixation using minifragment plates for fixation of a severely comminuted fracture of the patella. The plates used in this case should have been contoured to fit the superior pole better. In addition, two of the plates used in this case were 2.7-mm plates, which we no longer use in our plate constructs (opting for 2.0- or 2.4-mm plates).

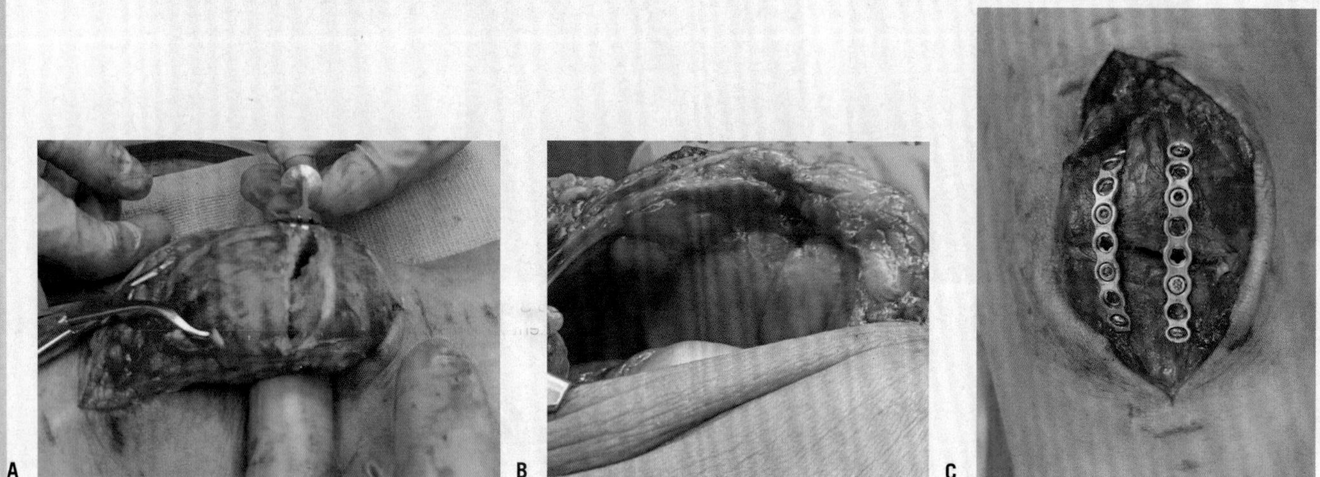

TECH FIG 6 **A.** Transverse patella fracture with nonunion treated with débridement of nonunion site. **B.** Clamp fixation of the transverse patella fracture with direct visualization of the joint surface to assess reduction. **C.** Dorsal minifragment plate application to compress articular surface and reduce fracture.

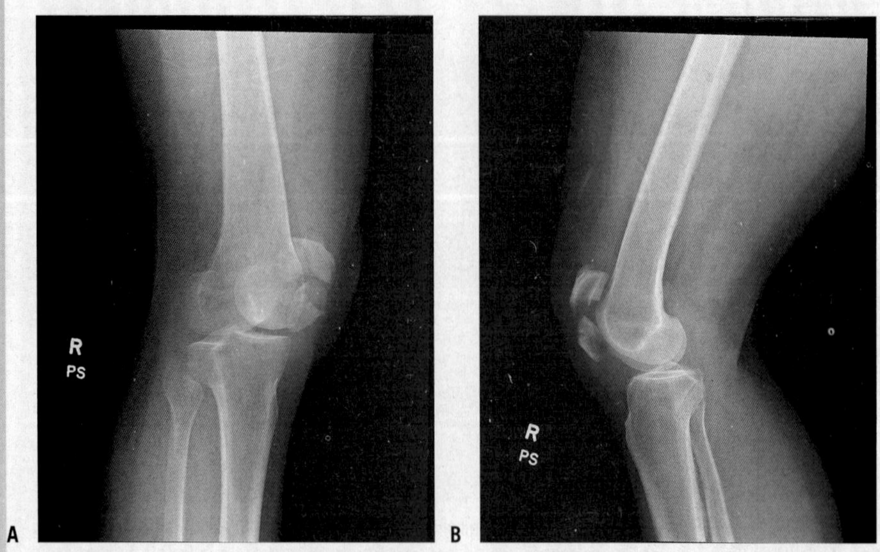

TECH FIG 7 Oblique (**A**) and lateral (**B**) radiographs of a comminuted patellar fracture. *(continued)*

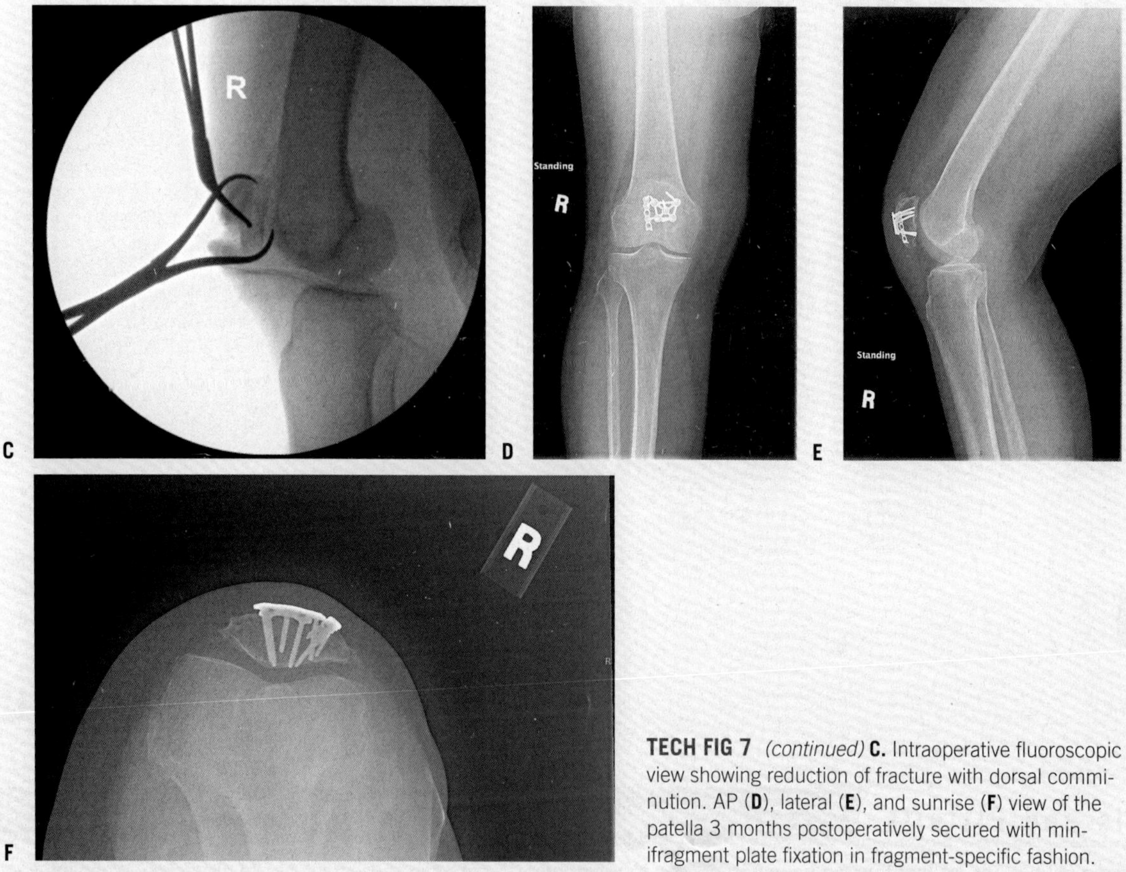

TECH FIG 7 *(continued)* **C.** Intraoperative fluoroscopic view showing reduction of fracture with dorsal comminution. AP (**D**), lateral (**E**), and sunrise (**F**) view of the patella 3 months postoperatively secured with minifragment plate fixation in fragment-specific fashion.

PARTIAL PATELLECTOMY

- Partial patellectomy is often advocated for comminuted fractures of the patella when a portion of the patella is significantly comminuted. Often, this comminution occurs at the patellar pole, with inferior pole fractures being more common.
- After a standard approach as discussed previously, the comminuted fracture fragments are identified. If restoration of the comminuted site is not possible, the comminuted fragments are removed. In some cases, the fragments may be left to facilitate healing of the soft tissue to the bone. Preservation of as large a portion of the articular surface as possible is critical.
- Multiple (usually three) longitudinal drill holes are made through the remaining portion of the patella such that the entrance point of the tendinous attachment will be as near to the articular surface as possible. The amount of holes is equal to the number of sutures plus one.
- A suture passer or anterior cruciate ligament Beath pin can be used to help facilitate passage of the suture through the bone tunnels.
- Nonabsorbable suture with a tendon-grasping stitch (eg, Krackow) is used to attach the adjacent tendon (usually patellar tendon) through the drill holes. Suture is tied with the knee in neutral or hyperextension **(TECH FIG 8)**. The suture, similar to the cerclage wires previously, must be tied directly on the bone (usually superior pole of the patella).
- Repair may be augmented by a tension band construct through the patella and tibial tubercle or by Mersilene tape, although we do not commonly perform such augmentation.
- Retinaculum is repaired with absorbable suture.
- Closure is as described earlier including the retinaculum, which will augment stability of the soft tissue repair.

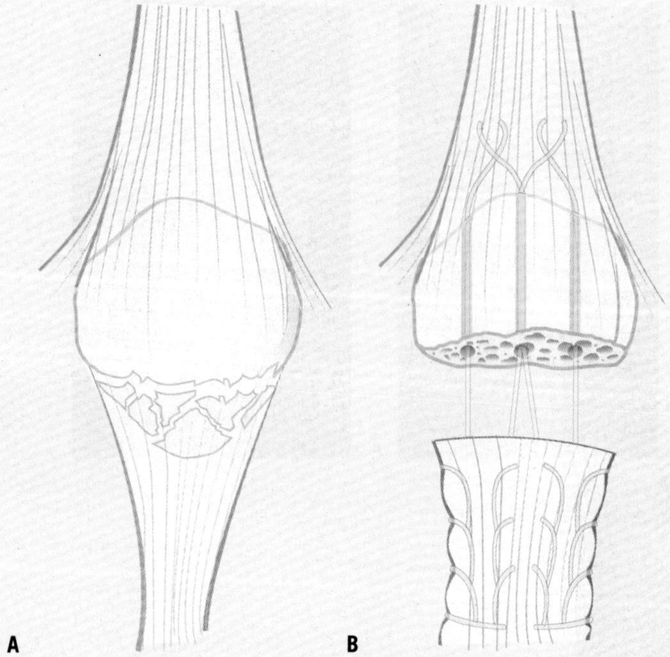

TECH FIG 8 Partial patellectomy. **A.** Comminuted distal pole of patella fracture, an ideal fracture pattern for the construct. **B.** Suture placement prior to tensioning and tying. Two sutures and three drill holes are used.

TECHNIQUES

Pearls and Pitfalls

The surgeon should ensure that tension band wires have little to no intervening tissue between the wire and the patella when passing under the Kirschner wires at the proximal and distal poles.	• This common error can cause fracture site distraction. When the fracture is loaded, the fragments can displace on the Kirschner wire until the tension band becomes taut.[5] This will leave the patient with a lag.
Cannulated screws must be left short of the far cortex if used with a tension band construct. In contrast, when using screw in a lagging fashion, bicortical purchase affords a better construct.	• Protrusion of the screw past the distal cortex creates a stress riser in the tension band.[5] Additionally, the tension band does contact the screw tip rather than the bone, lessening compression forces on the bone through the tension construct. The tension band wire can also break along the edge of the screw if the screw is protruding too far.
There is a delicate balance between early range of motion to promote better long-term range of motion and protection of fixation to avoid loss of reduction.	• Passive range-of-motion exercises ought to begin as soon as surgeon comfort allows and the wound is healed. Intraoperative knee range of motion resulting in gaping at the fracture site and poor intraoperative bone stock may lead to the decision for delayed passive range of motion.
When possible, complex fracture patterns are converted into simpler or transverse patterns.	• Fixation of longitudinal comminuted fragments with interfragmentary screws often allows the fracture pattern to be treated as a simpler transverse pattern.
Minifragment fixation or fragment-specific fixation of patella fractures can yield superior results through stable restoration of the articular surface without causing irritation of the patellar tendon or quadriceps tendon.	• Plates need to be well countered to fit the patella. Fragments need to be stabilized with either screw fixation or the use of the body of the plate to buttress and control fragments.

POSTOPERATIVE CARE

- Passive knee extension with gentle active flexion begins once soft tissue healing is ensured. We use an abundance of padding postoperatively underneath any bracing until postoperative soft tissue swelling resolves.
- The knee should be maintained in full extension (no bumps or pillows under the knee) to prevent an extensor lag.
- Patients are allowed to bear full weight with crutches and the knee fully extended in a knee immobilizer or hinged knee brace immediately postoperatively.
  - We prefer 3 weeks with the knee in extension, 3 weeks of knee flexion from 0 to 30 degrees through a hinged knee brace, and then full knee flexion out of a hinged knee brace.

- Full weight bearing out of a brace is allowed once signs of fracture healing are evident on postoperative imaging, usually around 6 weeks.
- Although straight-leg raising and quadriceps sets with the knee extended may begin immediately postoperatively, quadriceps strengthening with resistance is held until signs of fracture healing appear.
- For fracture fixation deemed unstable during intraoperative range of motion, initiation of knee motion may be held until fracture healing is evident.
- Rehabilitation must keep in mind the compressive forces on the patella during knee flexion. Compressive forces are greater than seven times body weight on each leg during stair climbing and reach nearly eight times body weight while squatting.[12]

OUTCOMES

- Outcomes depend on maintenance of fracture reduction.
- In a review of 320 patients with patellar fractures (212 treated nonoperatively) with a mean follow-up of 8.9 years, Boström[3] reported that 24% of patients did not consider themselves fully recovered; moderate or severe pain persisted in 31% of patients. The range of mobility was normal in 90% of patients, with the majority of restriction of motion in elderly patients. Ninety-one percent of patients had fracture union.
- In a series of 30 patients with isolated, unilateral patellar fractures, anterior knee pain during activities of daily living was experienced by 24 (80%) of the patients. Clinical improvement occurred over the first 6 months. However, functional impairment persisted at 12 months, with objective testing demonstrating deficits in strength, power, and endurance in the knee extensor mechanism on the injured side.[10]
- Long-term (6.5 years) functional follow-up of 40 isolated, ipsilateral patellar fractures was obtained by LeBrun et al.[11] The mean normalized 36-Item Short Form Survey physical composite score and the mean normalized Knee Injury and Osteoarthritis Outcome Scores were statistically different from reference population norms. Removal of symptomatic fixation was required in 52% of the patients, whereas 38% of those with retained fixation self-reported implant-related pain at least some of the time. Biodex dynamometric testing revealed a mean isometric extension deficit of 26% between the uninvolved and involved sides for peak torque. Extension power deficits over 30% were noted when compared with the contralateral side.[11]
- Functional outcomes after long-term follow-up of tension band wiring have been reported to be the same as age-matched standards.[18]

COMPLICATIONS

- The historical complication rate of operative intervention for patellar fractures varies in the literature. Although a recent study on perioperative complications reported a rate of 25%,[20] historical rates are much lower.[3]
- Infection rates are low and can be minimized by the use of perioperative antibiotics and careful soft tissue handling. Few postoperative infections are deep infections involving the joint.[3,20]
- Patients often note palpable hardware, given the thin overlying tissue. Although we do not routinely remove hardware, patients in whom the hardware becomes symptomatic may have hardware removal after fracture consolidation. Hardware removal rates have varied in the literature from 10% to 60% with tension band constructs.[18,20]
- Smith et al[20] reported fracture displacement of more than 2 mm in 22% of patients treated with tension band wiring. All patients with significant displacement requiring reoperation were weight bearing without bracing between 3 and 5 weeks. In the remainder of cases with loss of fixation, the most common cause was technical error.
- Nonunion with tension band techniques done technically correct is a rare complication, occurring in less than 1% of fractures fixed in this manner.[5]
- Decreased knee range of motion is another possible complication. Flexion is more commonly lost than extension. At times, this loss of motion can be due to intra-articular adhesions and can benefit from arthroscopic release.
- As with many intra-articular fractures, posttraumatic osteoarthritis develops in the injured extremity at a rate greater than that of the uninjured extremity. Reported rates of osteoarthritis vary greatly.

REFERENCES

1. Atkison PJ, Haut RC. Injuries produced by blunt trauma to the human patellofemoral joint vary with flexion angle of the knee. J Orthop Res 2001;19:827–833.
2. Benjamin J, Bried J, Dohm M, et al. Biomechanical evaluation of various forms of fixation of transverse patellar fractures. J Orthop Trauma 1987;1:219–222.
3. Boström A. Fracture of the patella. A study of 422 patellar fractures. Acta Orthop Scand Suppl 1972;143:1–80.
4. Braun W, Wiedemann M, Rüter A, et al. Indications and results of nonoperative treatment of patellar fractures. Clin Orthop Relat Res 1993;(289):197–201.
5. Carpenter JE, Kasman R, Matthews LS. Fractures of the patella. J Bone Joint Surg Am 1993;75:1550–1561.
6. Edwards B, Johnell O, Redlund-Johnell L. Patellar fractures. A 30-year follow-up. Acta Orthop Scand 1989;60:712–714.
7. Green WT Jr. Painful bipartite patellae. A report of three cases. Clin Orthop Relat Res 1975;(110):197–200.
8. Insall J, Goldberg V, Salvati E. Recurrent dislocation of the high-riding patella. Clin Orthop Relat Res 1972;88:67–69.
9. Kaufer H. Mechanical function of the patella. J Bone Joint Surg Am 1971;53(8):1551–1560.
10. Lazaro LE, Wellman DS, Sauro G, et al. Outcomes after operative fixation of complete articular patellar fractures: assessment of functional impairment. J Bone Joint Surg Am 2013;95(14):e96.8.
11. LeBrun CT, Langford JR, Sagi HC. Functional outcomes after operatively treated patella fractures. J Orthop Trauma 2012;26:422–426.
12. Matthews LS, Sonstegard DA, Henke JA. Load bearing characteristics of the patello-femoral joint. Acta Orthop Scand 1977;48:511–516.
13. Merchant AC, Mercer RL, Jacobsen RH, et al. Roentgenographic analysis of patellofemoral congruence. J Bone Joint Surg Am 1974;56(7):1391–1396.
14. Müller EC, Frosch KH. Plate osteosynthesis of patellar fractures [in German]. Oper Orthop Traumatol 2017;29(6):509–519.
15. Nerlich M, Weigel B. Patella. In: Ruedi TP, Murphy WM, eds. AO Principles of Fracture Management. New York: Thieme, 2000: 487–501.
16. Reider B, Marshall JL, Koslin B, et al. The anterior aspect of the knee joint. J Bone Joint Surg Am 1981;63(3):351–356.
17. Scapinelli R. Blood supply of the human patella. Its relation to ischaemic necrosis after fracture. J Bone Joint Surg Br 1967;49(3): 563–570.

18. Schemitsch EH, Weinberg J, McKee MD, et al. Functional outcome of patella fractures following open reduction and internal fixation. J Orthop Trauma 1999;13:279.
19. Siljander MP, Vara AD, Koueiter DM, et al. Novel anterior plating technique for patella fracture fixation. Orthopedics 2017;40(4):e739–e743.
20. Smith ST, Cramer KE, Karges DE, et al. Early complications in the operative treatment of patella fractures. J Orthop Trauma 1997;11:183–187.
21. Torchia ME, Lewallen DG. Open fractures of the patella. J Orthop Trauma 1996;10:403–409.
22. Verbeek DO, Hickerson LE, Warner SJ, et al. Low profile mesh plating for patella fractures: video of a novel surgical technique. J Orthop Trauma 2016;30(suppl 2):S32–S33.
23. Wilber JH. Patellar fractures: open reduction internal fixation. In: Wiss DA, ed. Master Techniques in Orthopaedic Surgery: Fractures. Philadelphia: Lippincott Williams & Wilkins, 1998:335–346.

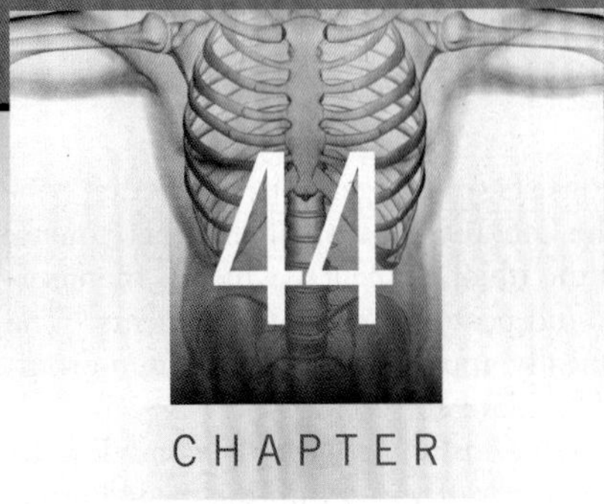

Spanning External Fixation of the Knee (Distal Femur and Proximal Tibia)

Milton Thomas Michael Little and Brandon J. Gaston

DEFINITION

- The use of knee-spanning external fixation for proximal tibia and distal femur fractures has increased with the understanding of appropriate soft tissue management and damage control orthopaedics in the care of severely injured patients.[1,2,8,10,24,27,29]
- Patients presenting with tibial plateau fractures and distal femur fractures may present with additional injuries, which preclude early definitive management leading to application of a temporizing external fixator to allow for stabilization of the patient and management of the soft tissues.[3,29]
- Understanding the indications, technique, benefits, and complications associated with application of a temporizing knee-spanning external fixator is critical to definitive management of tibial plateau fractures, distal femur fractures, and acute management of knee dislocations.

ANATOMY

Distal Femur

- The distal femur is considered the zone 7.6 to 15 cm proximal to the articular surface of the distal femur (**FIG 1**).[14]

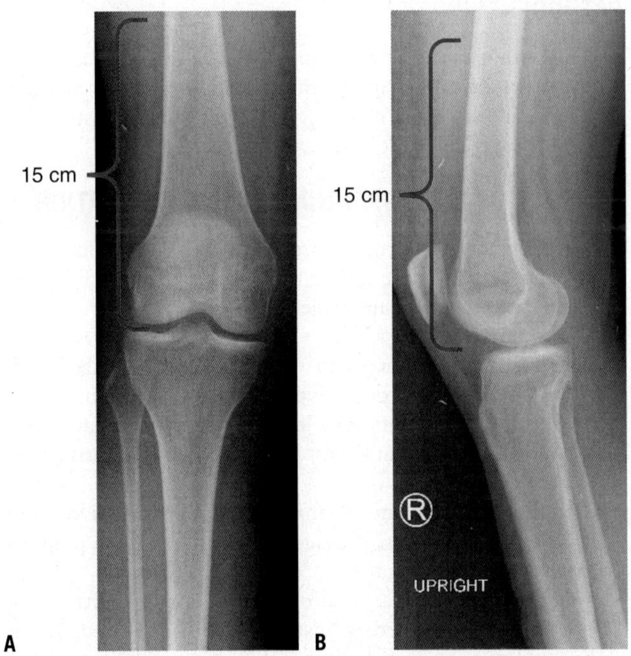

FIG 1 AP (**A**) and lateral (**B**) views of a normal knee. The distal femur marked in *red* is 7.6 to 15 cm proximal to the articular surface. The lateral tibial plateau is 2 to 3 mm higher than the medial tibial plateau.

- The coronal mechanical axis of the femur is in ~3 degrees of valgus, whereas the anatomic axis is in 9 degrees of valgus (**FIG 2**).[22]
- The distal femur is composed of a medial and lateral condyle with their associated epicondyles. The condyles are wider posteriorly than anteriorly forming the trapezoidal shape of the distal femur on axial cross-sections (**FIG 3**).[14]

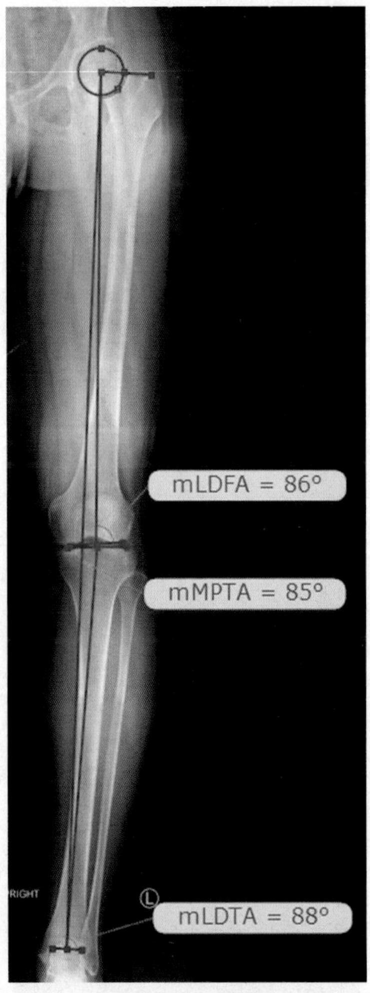

FIG 2 Long-leg lower extremity view. Mechanical axis lateral distal femoral angle (*mLDFA*) is 86 degrees. The patient's distal femur is in 4 degrees of valgus. Mechanical axis medial proximal tibial angle (*mMPTA*) is 85 degrees. The patient's tibia is in 5 degrees of varus at baseline. The mechanical angle lateral distal tibial angle (*mLDTA*) is 88 degrees.

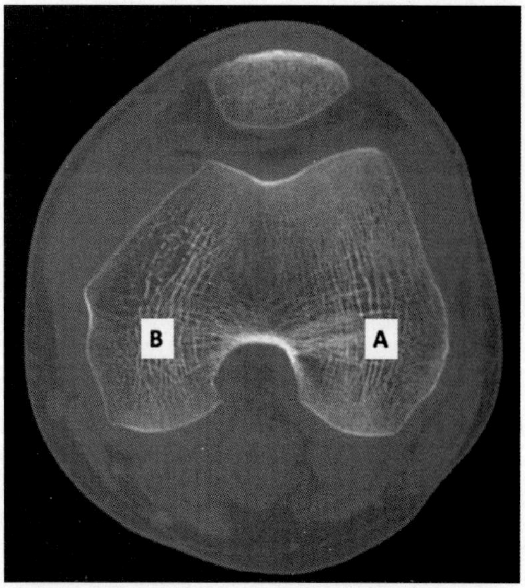

FIG 3 Axial cut of distal femur. Lateral femoral condyle (*A*) and medial femoral condyle (*B*).

- The medial femoral condyle is larger than the lateral femoral condyle, which contributes to the mechanical and anatomic axis of the femur.
- The distal femur/femoral shaft is surrounded by anterior, posterior, and medial compartments. The anterior compartment consists of the rectus femoris and vastus musculature (medial, lateralis, and intermedius) the posterior compartment consists of the biceps femoris, semimembranosus, semitendinosus. The medial compartment consists of the obturator externus, adductor brevis, adductor longus, and adductor magnus.
- The gastrocnemius originates from the medial and lateral condyles of the distal femur, and the pull of the gastrocnemius causes extension of the articular segment in distal femur fractures (**FIG 4**).

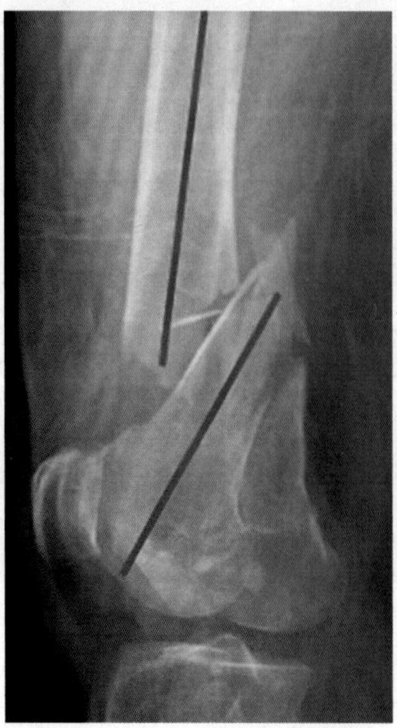

FIG 4 Gastrocnemius-induced extension deformity of the distal femur. Axis of femoral shaft marked by *red lines*.

Proximal Tibia

- The tibial plateau consists of a larger concave medial condyle as viewed on the lateral view, a smaller higher convex lateral condyle, and the tibial eminence, which is the insertion for the anterior and posterior cruciate ligaments.[4] The lateral plateau is typically approximately 2 to 3 mm proximal to the medial tibial plateau (see **FIG 1**).
- Due to the anatomic relationship between the condyles, the tibial plateau is in 3 degrees of varus with the medial proximal tibia angle ~87 degrees (see **FIGS 1** and **2**). Additionally, the tibial plateau has a variable posterior slope that averages near 9 degrees.
- The medial tibial plateau is covered with a smaller, less mobile meniscus, whereas the lateral tibial plateau is covered with a larger meniscus. The lateral meniscus covers nearly 50% of the tibial plateau and is critical in stabilizing the lateral femoral condyle. The medial tibial plateau is smaller and more dependent on the posterior horn of the meniscus to maintain stability of the medial femoral condyle.[4]

Knee Joint

- There is minimal inherent stability to the osseous components of the knee joint. The knee joint is dependent on the anterior and posterior cruciate ligaments, the medial and lateral collateral ligaments, and the posterior corner to provide stability to the joint.
- These ligaments are the critical factor in the use of external fixation for temporary stabilization of distal femur and proximal tibia fractures.
- External fixation uses traction/distraction to realign fracture fragments by taking advantage of the surrounding soft tissues and ligamentous structures. The understanding of this concept of ligamentotaxis is critical to the use of a knee-spanning external fixator.

PATHOGENESIS

- The pathogenesis of proximal tibia and distal femur fractures are discussed in depth in their respective chapters. Please refer to those chapters regarding natural history, patient history, and physical exam findings.

PURPOSE OF KNEE-SPANNING EXTERNAL FIXATION

- Knee-spanning external fixators are used to stabilize distal femur fractures, knee dislocations, and proximal tibia fractures that are length unstable (**FIG 5**).
- Without external fixation
  - Fracture shortening can occur causing increased difficulty with future definitive surgical intervention.
  - Fracture fragments may lead to skin pressure at subcutaneous surfaces and cause skin necrosis and further soft tissue injury
- The application of knee-spanning external fixators for these injuries is critical to soft tissue and cartilage rest in preparation for definitive treatment.[8,24,27]
- Additionally, external fixation improves the ability of the patients to be turned, transferred, and mobilized by the hospital nursing staff.[10] External fixation stabilizes the extremity, and patients may even be discharged with a plan to return to the hospital when soft tissues are amenable to definitive fixation.

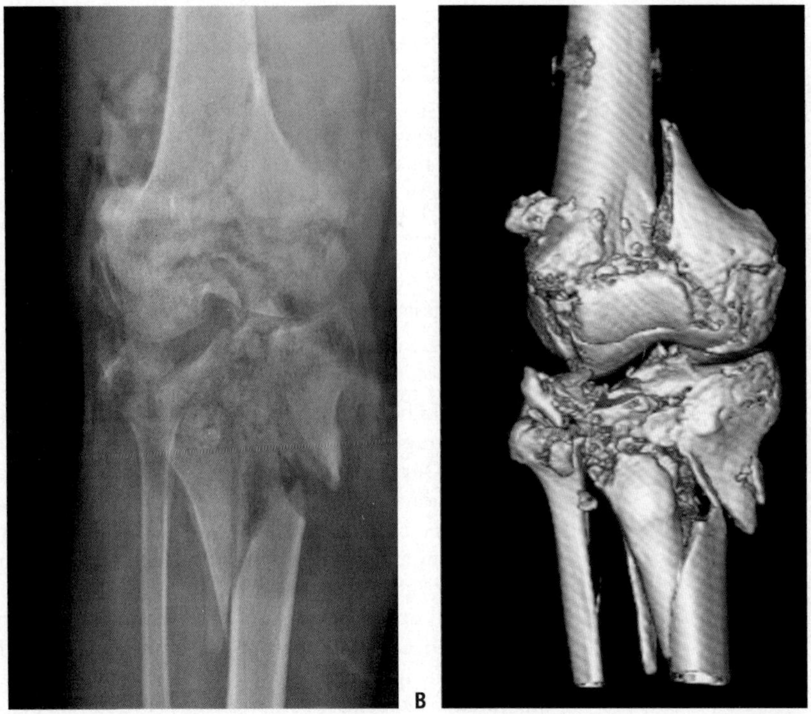

A B

FIG 5 A. AP view of high-energy distal femur and proximal tibia fracture. **B.** Three-dimensional reconstruction of high-energy distal femur and proximal tibia fracture.

IMAGING AND OTHER DIAGNOSTIC STUDIES

- Anteroposterior (AP) and lateral radiographs are the primary screening imaging for these injuries **(FIG 6)**.
- Full length AP and lateral views of the femur and the tibia should be performed to assess for associated injuries and dictate external fixator pin placement.
- Computed tomography (CT) should be delayed until after application of a knee-spanning external fixator to allow for improved visualization and interpretation. CT scan prior to external fixator application should be reserved for open fractures or fractures that may benefit from early provisional fixation to decrease soft tissue injury or tension.

INDICATIONS FOR KNEE-SPANNING EXTERNAL FIXATION

- Length unstable tibial plateau, distal femur fractures, or knee dislocations **(FIG 7)**
  - Extremity shortening
  - Increased contact pressure at cartilage
- Fracture-dislocations of the knee
- Fractures with soft tissue abnormalities
  - Open fractures requiring soft tissue coverage
  - Fracture blisters
  - Significant soft tissue swelling
  - Tented skin or skin at risk of conversion to open fracture

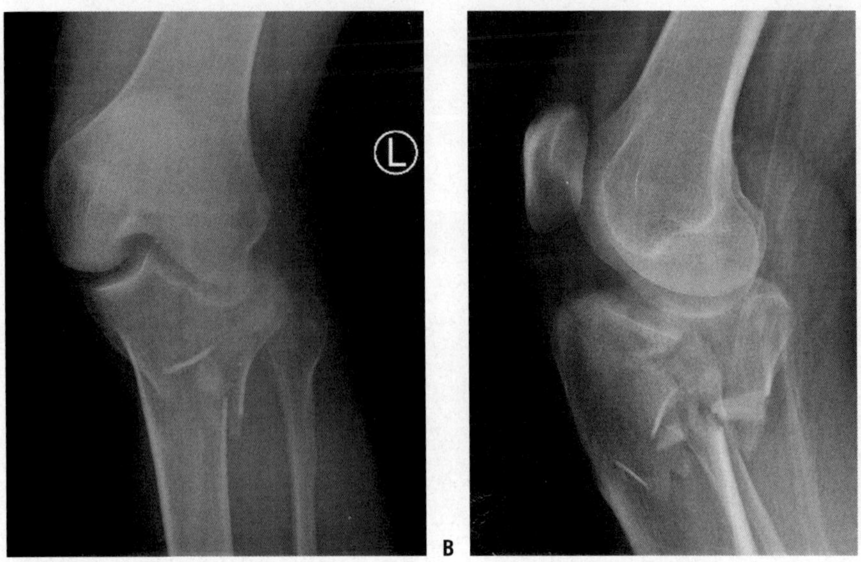

A B

FIG 6 AP (**A**) and lateral (**B**) views of a displaced shortened bicondylar tibial plateau fracture.

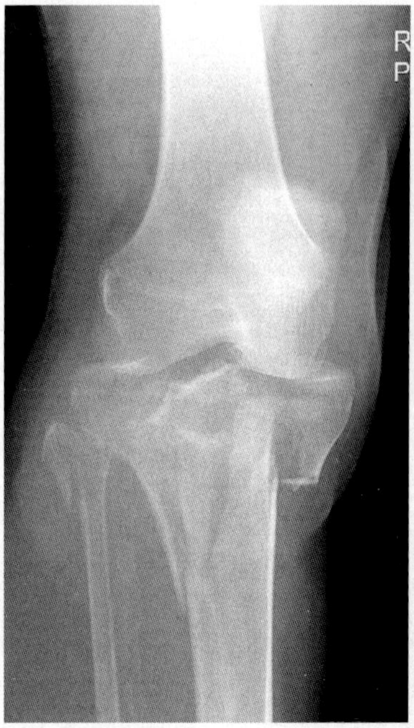

FIG 7 AP view of tibial plateau fracture with severe shortening and displacement.

- Compartment syndrome
- Fractures with vascular injury/insufficiency
- Knee dislocations that are unstable after reduction or in obese patients or those who cannot be braced

Preoperative Planning

- All imaging should be reviewed for the fracture characteristics and associated injuries, which may alter external fixator placement or construction.
- The incisions for the definitive surgical intervention should be drawn to avoid placement of external fixator pins in the surgical field **(FIG 8)**.
- Definitive surgical treatment plate length and position should be assessed to avoid overlap of definitive implants with external fixation pin sites (fluoroscopy can be used intraoperatively to confirm).
- Soft tissues should be assessed for injuries that may require soft tissue transfer or split-thickness skin grafts to determine possible donor sites following definitive fixation. Schanz pin insertion in these regions should be avoided if possible.

Positioning

- Patients should be positioned on a radiolucent table, which allows radiographic visualization from the proximal femur to the ankle. Our institution uses the Mizuho OSI Flat Jackson table (Union City, CA).
- A bump can be placed under the ipsilateral hip to keep the extremity from externally rotating and improve AP radiographic visualization.
- The ipsilateral upper extremity can be crossed over the patient's chest to avoid traction at the brachial plexus with elevation of the ipsilateral hip.
- If uninjured, a sequential compression sleeve can be placed on the contralateral extremity.
- All bony prominences should be padded to avoid skin pressure/necrosis.
- A ramp of towels or Bone Foam (Corcoran, MN) can be placed under the ipsilateral extremity to place the knee at 10 to 15 degrees of flexion **(FIG 9)**.

Approach

- Percutaneous insertion of the 5.0-mm Schanz pins should be performed based on the location in the femur and the tibia.
- A 0.5-cm incision is performed to expose the bone.

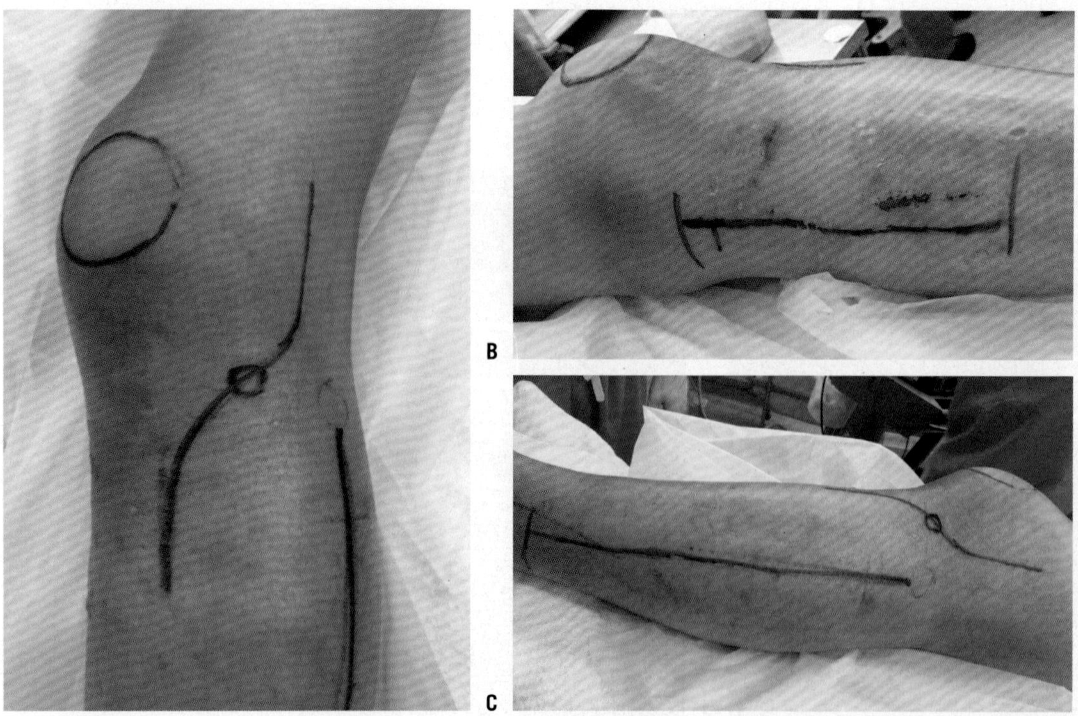
A B C

FIG 8 Preoperative planning with anterolateral (**A**), medial (**B**), and lateral fasciotomy (**C**) incisions in place.

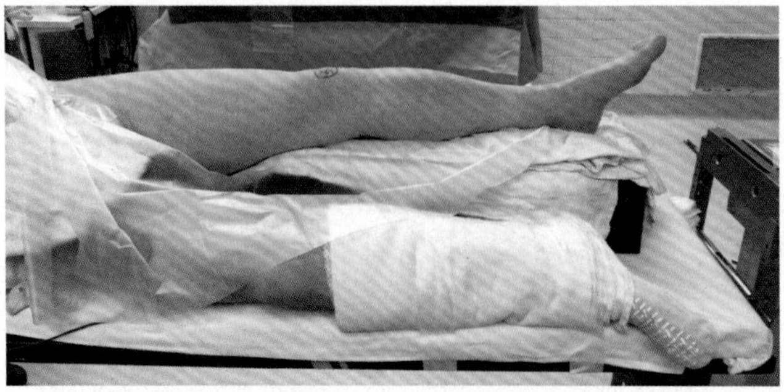

FIG 9 Patient positioning for external fixation application.

- A triple sleeve should be used to protect the skin during insertion of the pins and avoid thermal injury.
- Predrilling with a 3.5- or 3.2-mm drill (osteoporotic patients) with irrigation will decrease heat generation and decrease risk of osteomyelitis and skin necrosis with pin insertion.[20,25,30]
- The use of self-drilling and self-tapping pins without predrilling will either strip the near cortex or crack the far cortex and should be avoided.
- Standard Schanz pins can be used for hand insertion following drilling. Self-drilling/self-tapping pins can also be used but we recommend drilling for them as well to decrease heat generation (**FIG 10**).[20,25,30]

Direct Anterior Femoral Pin

- Direct anterior femoral pins are placed in line with the femoral shaft and require placement directly through the rectus femoris and vastus intermedius.
- One should spread through the quadriceps muscle and use a soft tissue sleeve during drilling and pin insertion to avoid further soft tissue injury.

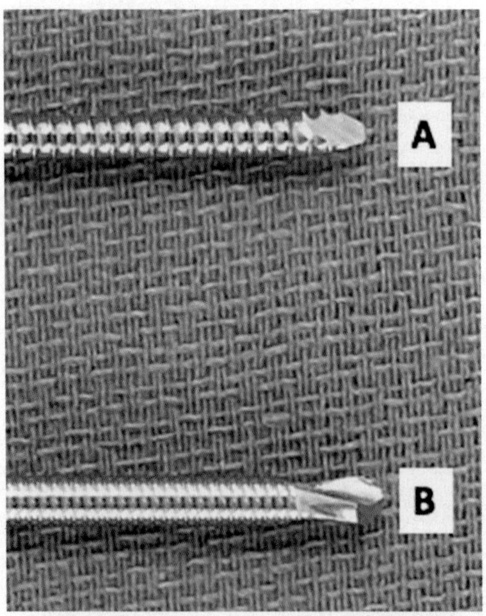

FIG 10 Non–self-drilling Schanz pin (*A*) and self-drilling/self-tapping Schanz pin (*B*). Note the drill tip present on the self-drilling Schanz pin. The lack of threads in that region of the pin require deeper insertion of the pin to achieve adequate pin purchase in the far cortex.

- Anterior pins allow for in-line reduction of tibial plateau and distal femur fractures utilizing the frame as a reduction device.[18]
- Egol et al[8] reported a 1.5% rate of quadriceps heterotopic ossification with the use of direct anterior pins in their series of staged treatment of tibial plateau fractures.
- Schanz pins should be placed in the proximal aspect of the femur approximately 5 cm distal to the lesser trochanter. Given the nature of the injury and the desire for long plating constructs, it may be difficult to avoid overlap of the definitive implant with the external fixation pin sites. Data has been mixed regarding the risks associated with pin site overlap and risk of deep infection.[16,21,26]
- Pins should never be placed close to the planned endpoint of a plate or nail to be used for fixation as it can act as a stress riser and cause a peri-implant fracture.

Anterolateral Femoral Pin

- Pins are inserted using the same soft tissue protection and drilling/irrigation techniques described earlier.
- Pins are inserted along the anterolateral aspect of the femur through the vastus lateralis to avoid rectus femoris and vastus intermedius scarring, which could inhibit knee range of motion (**FIG 11**).

Tibial Pins

- Tibial pins should be inserted along the anteromedial aspect of the tibia just medial to the tibial crest.
- The triple sleeve can allow the pins to be inserted perpendicular to the axis of the tibia despite the medial start point.
- Care should be taken to avoid unicortical pin placement to avoid excessive heat generation and osteomyelitis.[3,10]
- The surgeon should be aware of the planned length of the definitive tibial plates when placing external fixator Schanz pins. Avoid overlap of the definitive hardware with the pin sites, if possible, to minimize the risk of contamination and deep infection.[16,21,26]

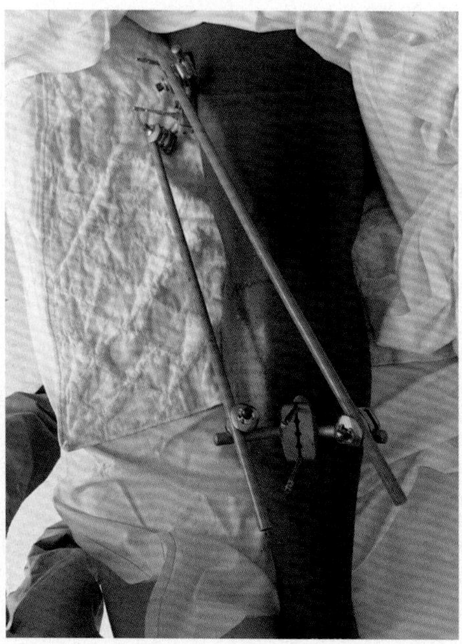

FIG 11 Anterolateral femoral pins for a knee-spanning external fixator.

KNEE-SPANNING EXTERNAL FIXATOR APPLICATION FOR A TIBIAL PLATEAU FRACTURE

Definitive Surgical Planning

- Planned surgical incisions should be drawn to avoid placement of external fixator pins in the future surgical field. Radiographs should be evaluated to determine the displacement and extent of the fracture **(TECH FIG 1)**.

Femoral Schanz Pin Insertion

- Fluoroscopy can be used to localize the lesser trochanter in preparation for proximal pin insertion.
- A 1-cm incision is made through the skin and fascia at the planned pin position.
- A tonsil is used to spread through the rectus femoris and vastus medialis down to bone.

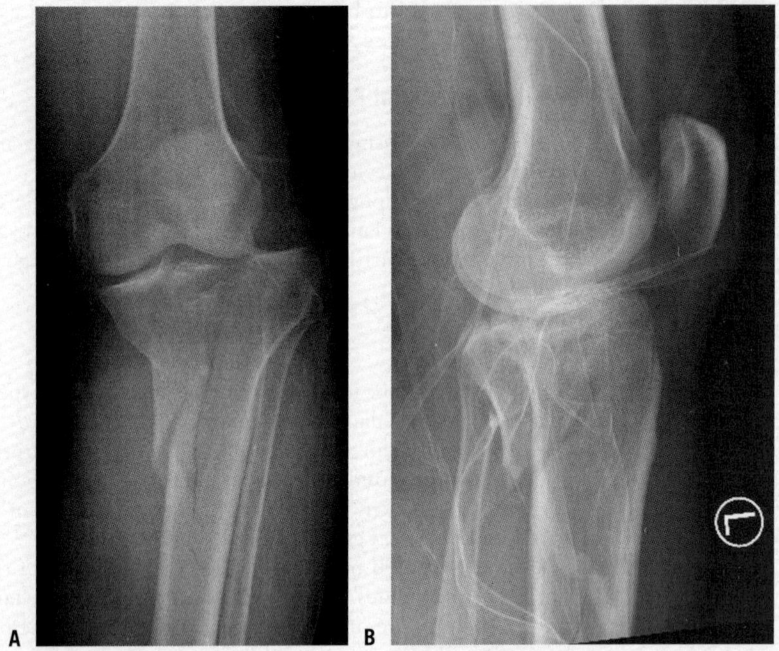

TECH FIG 1 A. AP view of proximal tibial shaft/tibial plateau fracture dislocation. **B.** Lateral view of tibial fracture.

- The triple sleeve is used to palpate the medial and lateral aspect of the femoral shaft so that the triple sleeve can be centered on the bone.
- The 3.5-mm drill is then used to drill bicortically through the bone while irrigating the drill continuously **(TECH FIG 2)**.
- The 5.0- × 200-mm standard Schanz pin is then inserted by hand with the pin inserted past the nonthreaded tip **(TECH FIG 3)**.
- The second femoral Schanz pin is inserted in the same fashion approximately 5 to 7 cm distal to the initial pin **(TECH FIG 4)**.

Proximal Bar Application

- Pin to bar clamps are applied to the two pins followed by application of a 300- to 350-mm carbon fiber rod.
- The bar should end proximal to the knee joint to avoid obscuring radiographic visualization of the joint **(TECH FIG 5)**.

Tibial Pin Insertion

- The most distal pin of the external fixation construct is then inserted after careful assessment of the planned definitive plate construct.

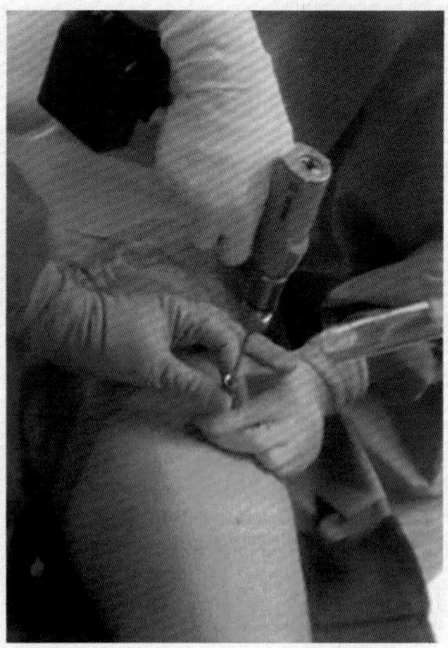

TECH FIG 2 Predrilling and irrigation to minimize heat generation during pin insertion.

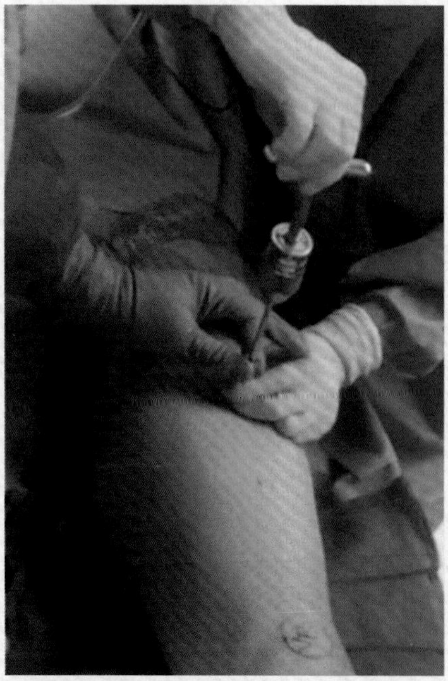

TECH FIG 3 Hand insertion of Schanz pin.

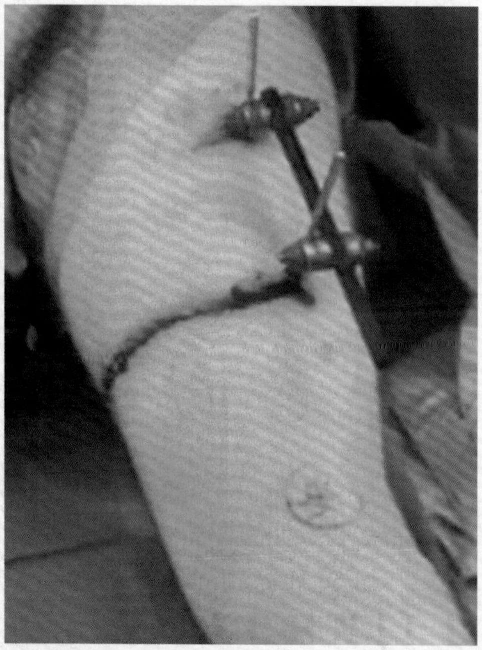

TECH FIG 5 Application of proximal carbon fiber bar.

- Following a 1-cm incision, the tonsil is used to spread down to bone followed by use of the triple sleeve tissue protector for drilling with the 3.5-mm drill.
- Continuous irrigation should be performed during drilling of the tibia. The drill should enter the bone perpendicular to the tibial shaft with care taken to drill bicortically.
- The 5.0- × 200-mm standard Schanz pin is then inserted by hand to minimize thermal injury **(TECH FIG 6)**.

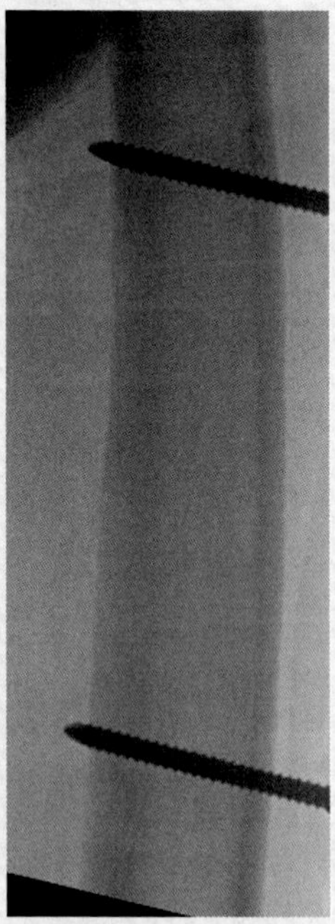

TECH FIG 4 Lateral view of femoral Schanz pins.

Establishment of Length

- A pin to bar clamp is then applied to the tibial Schanz pin, and an ~450-mm carbon fiber rod is applied to the clamp.
- Once this bar is locked into place, a loose bar to bar clamp is applied to connect the tibial pin to the femoral construct. The bar to bar clamp should not overlap the knee joint or articular surface to allow for appropriate fluoroscopy/radiographs.
- At this point, your length reduction is performed by pulling traction proximally and distally. One assistant should pull from the femur side, and a second assistant should pull from the tibial side while the surgical tech or a third assistant can tighten

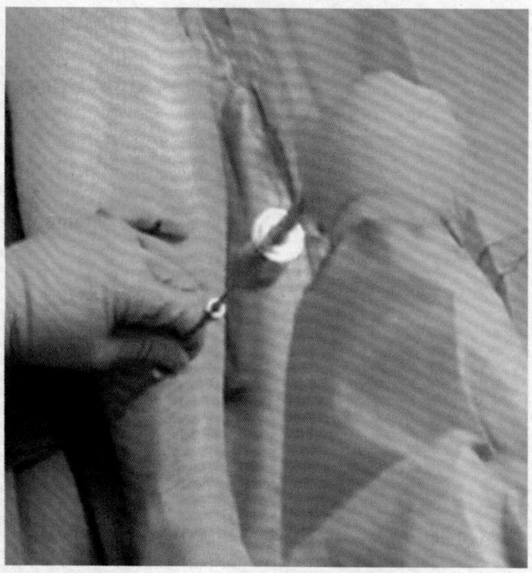

TECH FIG 6 Insertion of distal Schanz pin.

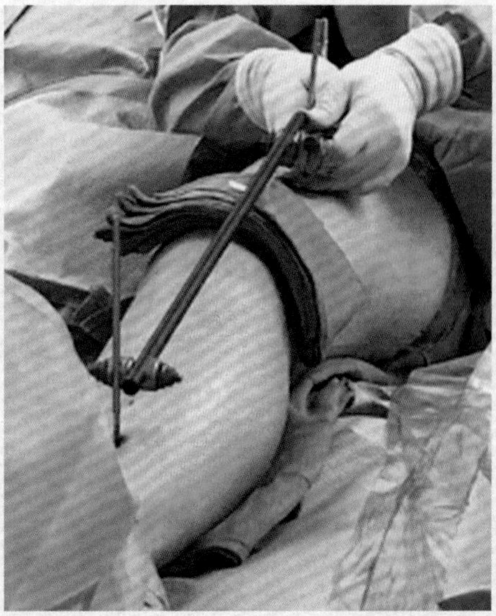

TECH FIG 7 Application of longitudinal traction to reestablish appropriate fracture length.

the bar to bar clamp once fluoroscopy confirms appropriate reestablishment of length **(TECH FIG 7)**.

- AP and lateral fluoroscopic imaging should be performed to confirm appropriate length and 10 to 15 degrees of knee flexion **(TECH FIG 8)**.

Coronal Reduction[18]

- Evaluation of the fracture on AP imaging will allow assessment of the coronal reduction and determine the force necessary to better align the fracture.
- Care should be taken to determine the final location of the definitive hardware and once that is determined, the location of the final Schanz can be chosen.
- If the fracture is in varus alignment, a pin to bar clamp can be applied to the carbon fiber bar on the lateral aspect of the bar. Placing the triple sleeve through the pin to bar clamp ensures appropriate contact and bicortical pin placement in the tibia. Placing the pin obliquely out of plane of the tibia allows the surgeon to direct a posteromedial force to the tibia to reduce the fracture **(TECH FIG 9)**.
- If the fracture is in valgus alignment, the pin can be placed on the medial aspect of the bar in the same fashion, and application of a posterolateral-directed force can better reduce the fracture.
- Final fluoroscopic imaging should be performed to confirm appropriate alignment **(TECH FIG 10)**.

Sagittal Alignment[18]

- Lateral fluoroscopy will allow the surgeon to evaluate the sagittal alignment of the fracture.
- If the fracture is in procurvatum or recurvatum, the surgeon can unlock the pin component of the pin to bar clamp allowing you to reduce the distal fragment without losing coronal alignment.
- If placing a fixator for a distal femur fracture, this process should start with placement of two tibial pins followed by placement of the most proximal femoral pin to establish length. The final steerage pin can then be applied to assist with coronal and sagittal reduction.

External Fixator Stabilization[3]

- In order to improve stability of the external fixator, the surgeon should then add an additional carbon fiber bar between the two

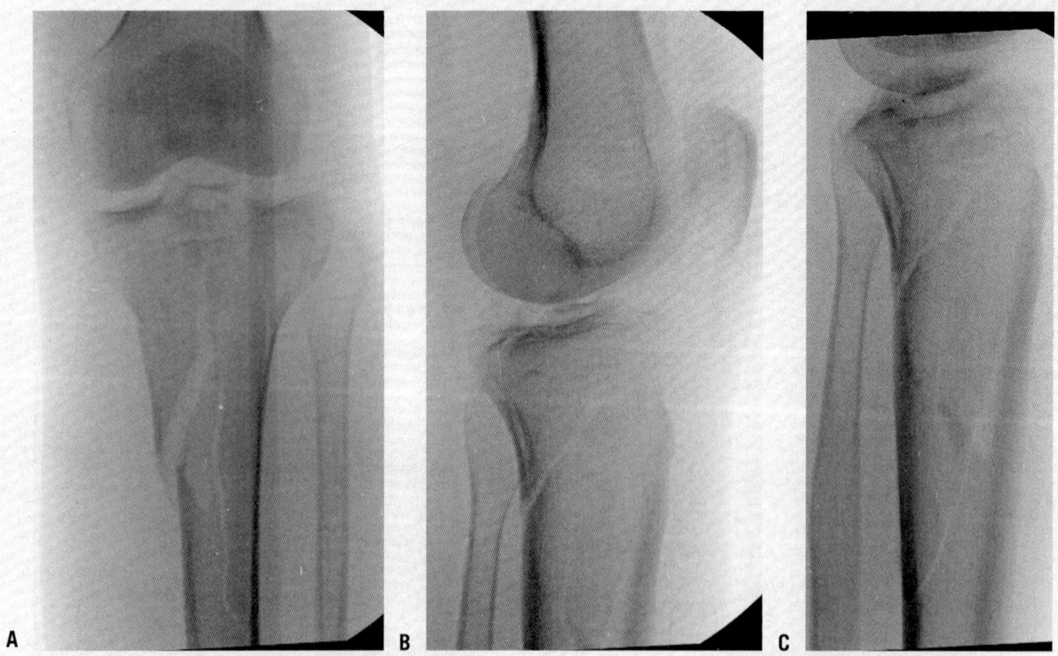

TECH FIG 8 AP (**A**) and lateral (**B,C**) views of fracture after establishment of fracture length. Note lateral translation of the tibial shaft despite appropriate fracture length.

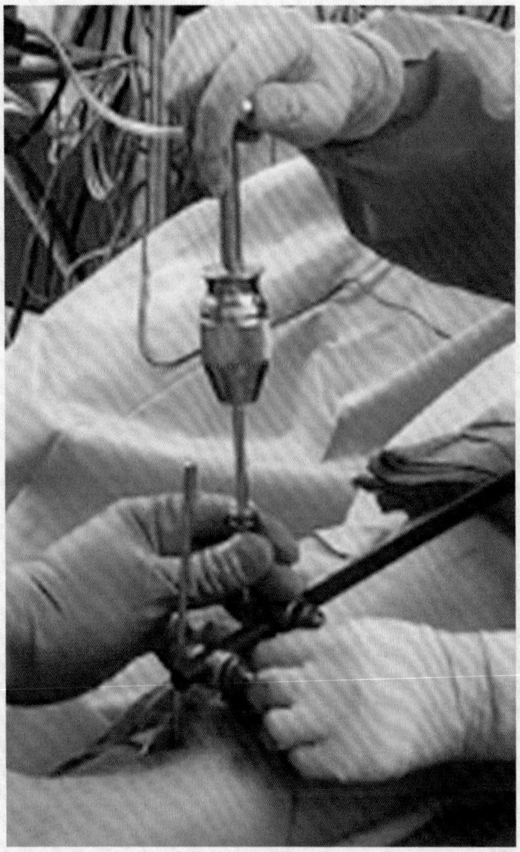

TECH FIG 9 Insertion of second tibial pin. Hand insertion of the final pin through the pin to bar clamp.

near Schanz pins with pin to bar clamps. The additional bar provides additional stability to the construct **(TECH FIG 11)**.

Examine for Compartment Syndrome

- After proximal tibia fractures are pulled out to length, some will have an increase in compartment pressure, particularly fracture dislocation patterns. Once the reduction is obtained, a careful assessment for compartment syndrome is needed. The surgeon should have a low threshold to measure the intercompartmental pressure.

Dressing Application

- The initial dressing for the pin sites includes Xeroform (Covidien: Dublin Ireland) to keep the pin sites moist and a Kerlix (Kendall: Miami, Florida) bolster to provide compression at the pin insertion sites.
- The bolster prevents motion and hematoma at pin sites and when combined with close monitoring of heat generation during drilling, has been shown to decrease the risk of pin site infection with external fixator application.[5]

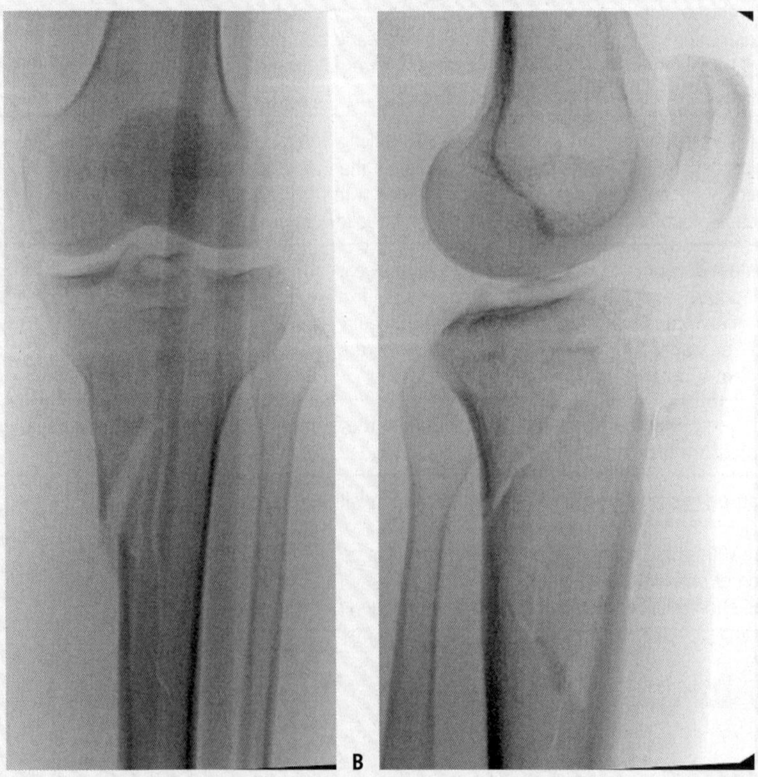

A B

TECH FIG 10 Final fluoroscopy AP (**A**) and lateral (**B**) knee images.

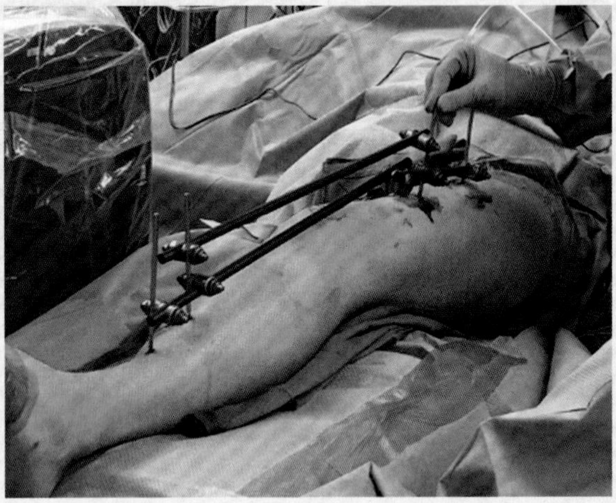

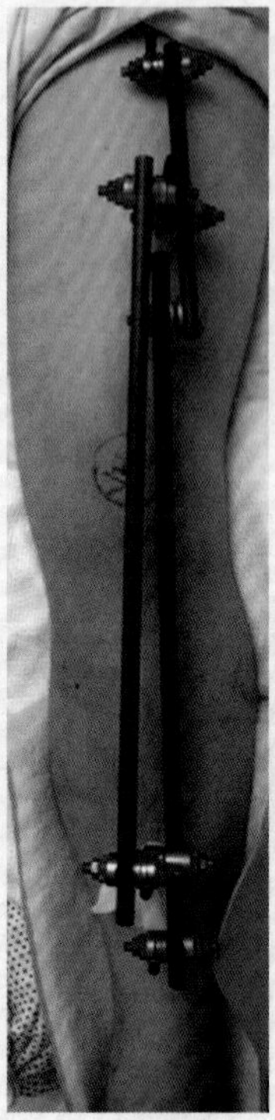

TECH FIG 11 Final external fixator construct with the addition of a second bar for increased stability. Lateral view of the external fixator (**A**) and direct anterior view of the external fixator (**B**).

TECHNIQUES

Pearls and Pitfalls

Indications	• If there are concerns with the soft tissue envelope or the hemodynamic stability of the patient, proceed with damage control/temporary spanning external fixator rather than early total care. • One should have a low threshold for application of a spanning external fixator in the setting of grossly unstable or shortened fractures.
Schanz Pin Insertion	• The triple sleeve/soft tissue guide prevents skin necrosis with drilling and pin insertion. • Predrilling with irrigation decreases heat generation and protects the soft tissues. • Bicortical pin placement is critical to decreasing heat generation with drilling and pin insertion. • All these factors decrease risk of osteomyelitis and late infection following external fixation.
Reduction	• Achieving an appropriate reduction with distraction of the joint may ease eventual conversion to definitive fixation. • Delayed treatment of fractures that have been placed in external fixators in shortened or malaligned positioned may increase the risk of skin tension, soft tissue injury, and difficulty achieving anatomic reduction. • External fixators should be applied for each patient as if it will be the definitive form of care. • Evaluate for compartment syndrome after restoration of length.
Mobilization	• Patients should be allowed to transfer and use wheelchairs with the extremity elevated to decrease risk of deep vein thrombosis and pressure ulcers.
Conversion to Definitive Fixation[11,13,21,28]	• The external fixator can be kept in place during definitive fixation without a significantly higher risk of deep infection. • Standard surgical prep with chlorhexidine or povidone-iodine has been shown to significantly decrease bacterial contamination of external fixator sites. • External fixator clamps should be reprepped following manipulation of the clamp sites.

POSTOPERATIVE CARE

- AP and lateral radiographs should be performed following completion of external fixation.
- CT following external fixation fixator will provide improved interpretation of the injury and assist with preoperative planning for the definitive surgery (**FIG 12**).
- Currently, there is no consensus on pin care for temporary spanning external fixators, but care should be taken to keep pin sites clean and dry until conversion to definitive internal fixation.[5,7,19,23]
- Pin sites can be cleaned daily with saline, soap/water, or a solution of one-half hydrogen peroxide/one-half normal saline. No pin site protocol has been determined to be superior.
- Although there is drainage from the pin sites, a Kerlix bolster may be helpful in limiting motion, drainage, and loosening of the Schanz pins.
- Care should be taken to provide a pin holiday of 5 to 7 days if a pin site becomes irritated, loose, or infected prior to intramedullary nailing or overlapping of the definitive implant with the infected pin site.
- During conversion to definitive treatment, the external fixator may be kept in place as a device to provide stability and maintain fractures reduction.
- External fixators pin sites are commonly contaminated and should be included as part of the preoperative surgical prep.[11,13,28]
- There has been no significant difference in the rate of external fixator or surgical site contamination between povidone-iodine and chlorhexidine for surgical prep.
- Manipulation of the external fixator clamps increases the number of bacteria present on an external fixator, so these regions should be decontaminated intraoperatively following manipulation of external fixator bars and clamps.[11,28]

OUTCOMES

- The use of temporary spanning external fixators as part of the two-staged treatment of tibial plateau fractures has been shown to be effective at limiting infection, wound complications, and need for additional surgical procedures (**FIG 13**).[1,2,8]

COMPLICATIONS

- Pin tract infection is the most common complication, and pin sites should be monitored closely.[17,19,23]
- Egol et al[6] showed a 1.2% risk of rectus heterotopic ossification following direct anterior external fixator application.
- Controversy exists regarding the impact of temporary spanning external fixation on knee stiffness following definitive treatment of tibial plateau fractures.[1,12,15]
- Continuous passive motion machines have been shown to decrease the risk of stiffness in patients treated with spanning external fixation.[12]
- The risk of deep infection following spanning external fixation has been shown to be as low as 1.7% in the setting of intramedullary nail placement.[21]
- Studies investigating the risk of osteomyelitis for temporary spanning external fixators are limited.
- Gillig et al[9] reported a rate of 3.5% patient sensitivity or sensation of warmth during magnetic resonance imaging (MRI) with external fixators in place. No patients had short- or long-term complications of MRI use while in spanning external fixators.[9]

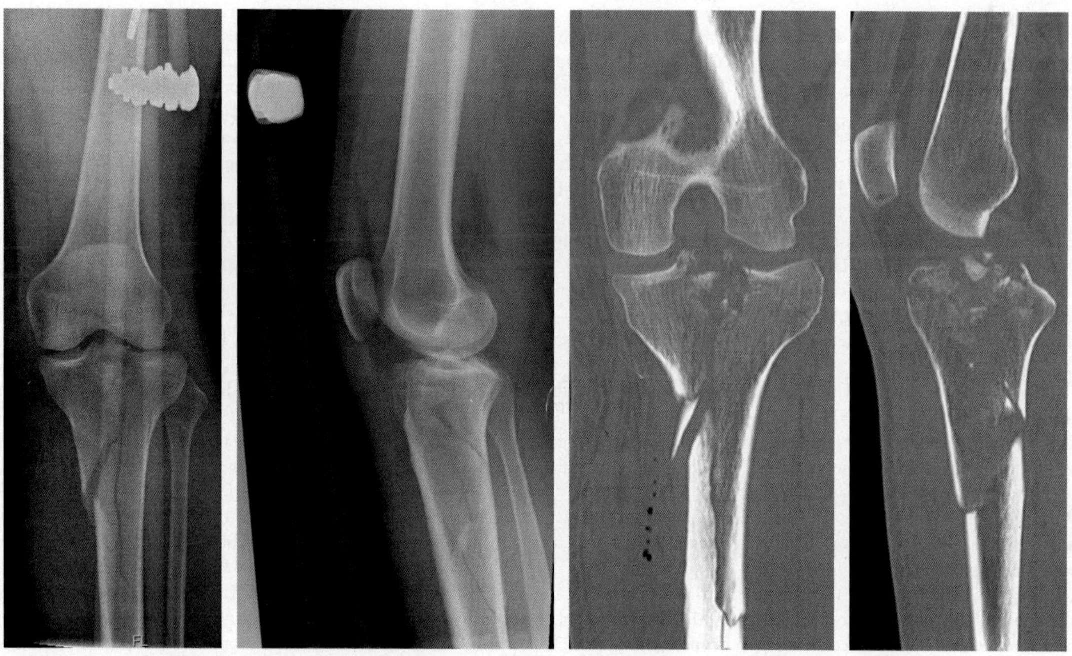

FIG 12 Radiographs and CT evaluation of fracture postexternal fixator application.

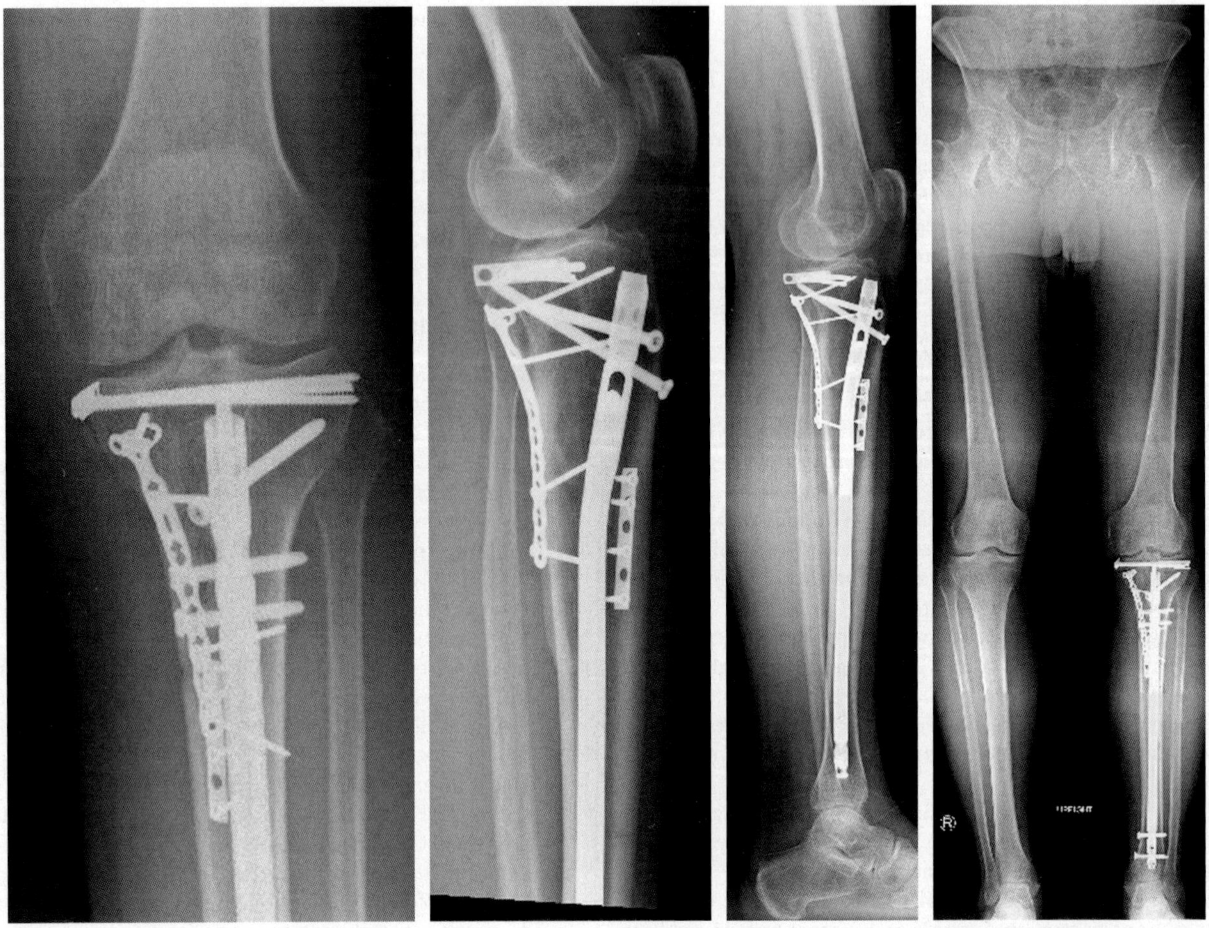

FIG 13 Final radiographs and 1-year follow-up radiographs following conversion to definitive treatment.

REFERENCES

1. Barei DP, Nork SE, Mills WJ, et al. Complications associated with internal fixation of high-energy bicondylar tibial plateau fractures utilizing a two-incision technique. J Orthop Trauma 2004;18(10):649–657.
2. Barei DP, Nork SE, Mills WJ, et al. Functional outcomes of severe bicondylar tibial plateau fractures treated with dual incisions and medial and lateral plates. J Bone Joint Surg Am 2006;88(8):1713–1721.
3. Bible JE, Mir HR. External fixation: principles and applications. J Am Acad Orthop Surg 2015;23(11):683–690.
4. Cole P, Levy B, Schatzker J, et al. Tibial plateau fractures. In: Browner BD, Jupiter JB, Levine AM, et al, eds. Skeletal Trauma: Basic Science, Management, and Reconstruction, ed 4. Philadelphia: Saunders, 2009:2201–2287.
5. Davies R, Holt N, Nayagam S. The care of pin sites with external fixation. J Bone Joint Surg Br 2005;87(5):716–719.
6. Egol KA, Bazzi J, McLaurin TM, et al. The effect of knee-spanning external fixation on compartment pressures in the leg. J Orthop Trauma 2008;22(10):680–685.
7. Egol KA, Paksima N, Puopolo S, et al. Treatment of external fixation pins about the wrist: a prospective, randomized trial. J Bone Joint Surg Am 2006;88(2):349–354.
8. Egol KA, Tejwani NC, Capla EL, et al. Staged management of high-energy proximal tibia fractures (OTA types 41): the results of a prospective, standardized protocol. J Orthop Trauma 2005;19(7):448–456.
9. Gillig JD, Goode RD, Campfield B, et al. Safety and complications associated with MRI-conditional external fixators in patients with tibial plateau fractures: a case series. J Orthop Trauma 2018;32(10):521–525.
10. Haidukewych GJ. Temporary external fixation for the management of complex intra- and periarticular fractures of the lower extremity. J Orthop Trauma 2002;16(9):678–685.
11. Hak DJ, Wiater PJ, Williams RM, et al. The effectiveness of standard povidone iodine surgical preparation in decontaminating external fixator components. Injury 2005;36(12):1449–1452.
12. Haller JM, Holt DC, McFadden ML, et al. Arthrofibrosis of the knee following a fracture of the tibial plateau. Bone Joint J 2015;97-B(1):109–114.
13. Hardeski D, Gaski G, Joshi M, et al. Can applied external fixators be sterilized for surgery? A prospective cohort study of orthopaedic trauma patients. Injury 2016;47(12):2679–2682.
14. Krettek C. Fractures of the distal femur. In: Browner BD, Jupiter JB, Levine AM, et al, eds. Skeletal Trauma: Basic Science, Management, and Reconstruction, ed 4. Philadelphia: Saunders, 2009:2073–2130.
15. Kugelman DN, Qatu AM, Strauss EJ, et al. Knee stiffness after tibial plateau fractures: predictors and outcomes (OTA-41). J Orthop Trauma 2018;32(11):e421–e427.
16. Laible C, Earl-Royal E, Davidovitch R, et al. Infection after spanning external fixation for high-energy tibial plateau fractures: is pin site-plate overlap a problem? J Orthop Trauma 2012;26(2):92–97.
17. Lethaby A, Temple J, Santy J. Pin site care for preventing infections associated with external bone fixators and pins. Cochrane Database Syst Rev 2008;(4):CD004551.
18. Liskutin T, Bernstein M, Lack W, et al. Surgical technique: achieving reduction with temporizing, knee-spanning external fixation. J Orthop Trauma 2018;32 suppl 1:S32–S33.
19. Mahan J, Seligson D, Henry SL, et al. Factors in pin tract infections. Orthopedics 1991;14(3):305–308.
20. Matthews LS, Green CA, Goldstein SA. The thermal effects of skeletal fixation-pin insertion in bone. J Bone Joint Surg Am 1984;66(7):1077–1083.

21. Nowotarski PJ, Turen CH, Brumback RJ, et al. Conversion of external fixation to intramedullary nailing for fractures of the shaft of the femur in multiply injured patients. J Bone Joint Surg Am 2000;82(6):781–788.
22. Paley D. Normal lower limb alignment and joint orientation. In: Paley D, ed. Principles of Deformity Correction. Berlin: Springer-Verlag, 2002:1–18.
23. Parameswaran AD, Roberts CS, Seligson D, et al. Pin tract infection with contemporary external fixation: how much of a problem? J Orthop Trauma 2003;17(7):503–507.
24. Patterson MJ, Cole JD. Two-staged delayed open reduction and internal fixation of severe pilon fractures. J Orthop Trauma 1999;13(2):85–91.
25. Seitz WH Jr, Froimson AI, Brooks DB, et al. External fixator pin insertion techniques: biomechanical analysis and clinical relevance. J Hand Surg Am 1991;16(3):560–563.
26. Shah CM, Babb PE, McAndrew CM, et al. Definitive plates overlapping provisional external fixator pin sites: is the infection risk increased? J Orthop Trauma 2014;28(9):518–522.
27. Sirkin M, Sanders R, DiPasquale T, et al. A staged protocol for soft tissue management in the treatment of complex pilon fractures. J Orthop Trauma 1999;13(2):78–84.
28. Stinner DJ, Beltran MJ, Masini BD, et al. Bacteria on external fixators: which prep is best? J Trauma Acute Care Surg 2012;72(3):760–764.
29. Taeger G, Ruchholtz S, Waydhas C, et al. Damage control orthopedics in patients with multiple injuries is effective, time saving, and safe. J Trauma 2005;59(2):409–417.
30. Wikenheiser MA, Markel MD, Lewallen DG, et al. Thermal response and torque resistance of five cortical half-pins under simulated insertion technique. J Orthop Res 1995;13(4):615–619.

CHAPTER 45

Open Reduction and Internal Fixation of Bicondylar Plateau Fractures

William M. Ricci

DEFINITION

- Bicondylar tibial plateau fractures involve both medial and lateral tibial condyles.
- Schatzker types V and VI fractures are each considered bicondylar fractures.
- Schatzker type V fractures (**FIG 1A,B**) involve both condyles without complete dissociation from the shaft and are usually amenable to medial and lateral buttress plate fixation.
- Schatzker type VI fractures (**FIG 1C,D**) involve both condyles with complete dissociation of the articular segment from the shaft. These fractures are typically treated with lateral locked plates or dual (lateral and medial) plating.
- Lateral fractures with associated posteromedial fragments do not fit the Schatzker classification and should be recognized as bicondylar fractures. These often require posteromedial fixation independent from lateral fixation and may be representative of fracture-dislocation (see **FIG 3**).

ANATOMY OF THE PROXIMAL TIBIA

- In the loaded knee, the medial plateau bears about 60% to 75% of the load.[7,9]
- Stronger, denser subchondral bone is found on the medial side due to increased load.
- Bony anatomy
  - The medial plateau is larger in cross-sectional area than the lateral plateau.
  - The medial plateau is concave, the lateral plateau convex. The lateral plateau is usually higher than the medial plateau.
  - In the sagittal plane, there is posterior slope of the proximal tibia articular segment that ranges from 5 to 15 degrees relative to the anatomic axis of the tibia.[3]
  - In the coronal plane, there is varus of the proximal articular segment that ranges from 0 to 5 degrees relative to the anatomic axis of the tibia.[5,6]
- Soft tissue anatomy (**FIG 2**)
  - The iliotibial band inserts on the tubercle of Gerdy.
  - The anterior cruciate ligament attaches adjacent and medial to the tibial eminence. It acts to resist anterior translation of the tibia relative to the femur. Recognizing a fracture fragment that contains this attachment can be important to reestablish stability to the knee.
  - The posterior cruciate ligament attaches about 1 cm below the joint line on the posterior ridge of the tibial plateau and a few millimeters lateral to the tibial tubercle.
  - The function of the posterior cruciate is to resist posterior tibial translation of the tibia relative to the femur. This acts as the central pivot of the knee.
- The medial collateral ligament (MCL) originates on the medial femoral epicondyle and inserts on the medial tibial condyle.
  - The MCL resists valgus force.
- The lateral collateral ligament originates on the lateral epicondyle of the femur and attaches to the fibular head.
  - The lateral collateral ligament resists varus force and external rotation of the femur.
- The menisci, medial and lateral, are crescent-shaped fibrocartilaginous structures that act to dissipate the load on the tibial plateau, deepen the articular surfaces of the plateau, and help lubricate and provide nutrition to the knee.
  - The medial meniscus is more C-shaped, and the lateral meniscus is more circular in shape.
  - The lateral meniscus is more mobile than the medial meniscus.

PATHOGENESIS OF BICONDYLAR TIBIAL PLATEAU FRACTURES

- Bicondylar tibial plateau fractures are typically caused by a high-energy mechanism with associated injury to the surrounding soft tissue.
- The mechanism responsible for injury is primarily an axial force, which may be associated with a varus or valgus moment.
- With a valgus force, the lateral femoral condyle is driven, wedge-like, into the underlying lateral tibial plateau.[6]
- The size of the fracture fragments depends on multiple factors, including localization of the impact, the magnitude of the axial force producing the fracture, the density of the bone, and the position of the knee joint at the moment of trauma.
- Ligament and meniscal injuries are very commonly associated with tibial plateau fractures.[4]
  - Repair of ligament injuries at the time of fracture fixation is controversial. Some advocate ligamentous repair at the time of fracture fixation, whereas others feel that if the fracture can be reduced, there is no need for early ligamentous repair.

NATURAL HISTORY

- Acute compartment syndrome is not infrequently associated.[11]
- Joint incongruity can predispose to arthrosis.
- Secondary varus or valgus displacement can occur, especially with osteoporotic depressed fractures.
- Range of motion loss is common.
- Joint instability can result from associated ligament injury and/or malreduction in the coronal plane.

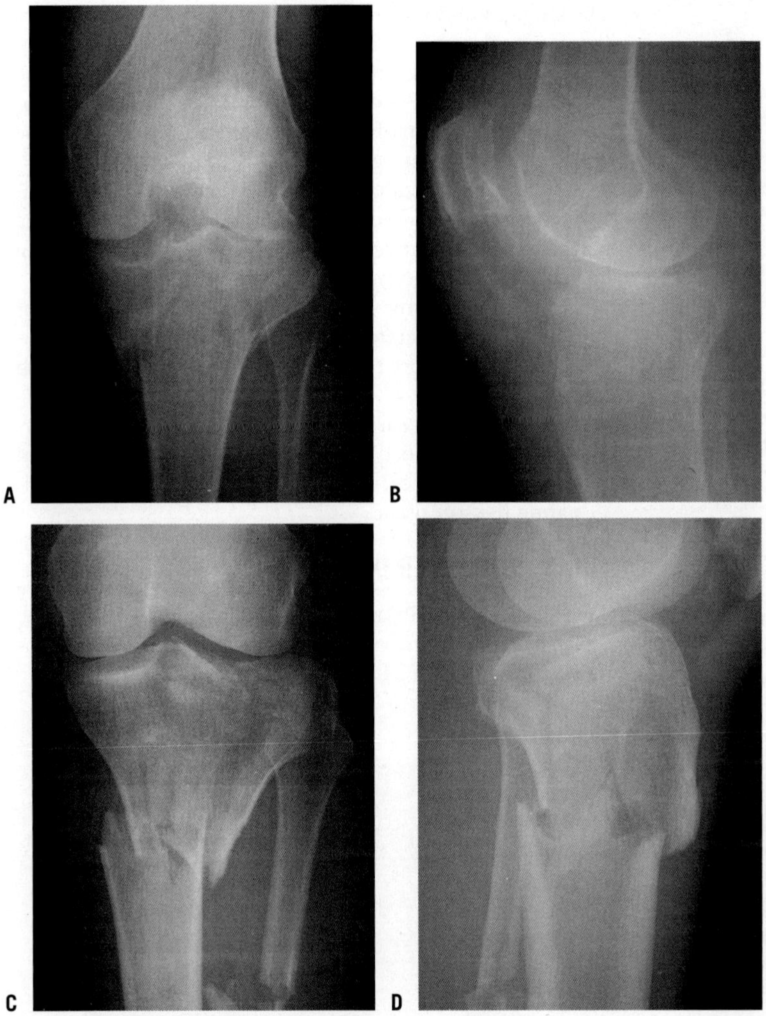

FIG 1 AP (**A**) and lateral (**B**) views of a Schatzker type V bicondylar tibial plateau fracture. AP (**C**) and lateral (**D**) views of a Schatzker type VI bicondylar tibial plateau fracture.

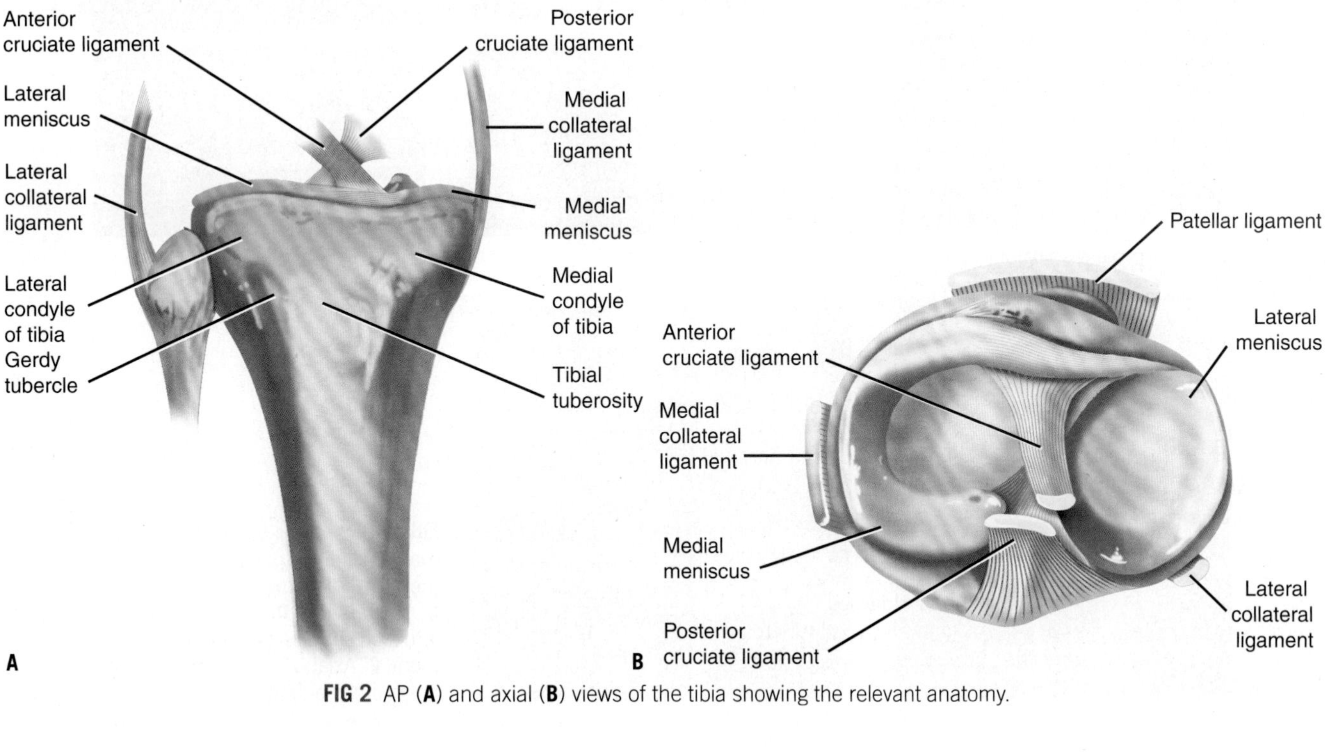

FIG 2 AP (**A**) and axial (**B**) views of the tibia showing the relevant anatomy.

PATIENT HISTORY AND PHYSICAL FINDINGS

- Generally, a bicondylar injury pattern is caused by a high-energy mechanism. It may also be seen with a low-energy mechanism, such as a fall from standing height in an older patient with osteoporosis.
- The patient will complain of a painful swollen knee and will have difficulty bearing weight on the extremity. Hemarthrosis will be present if the capsule has not been disrupted.
- The patient history should include details of the injury mechanism, preinjury ambulatory status, and any previous injury and disability.
- A complete examination should rule out other injuries. The vascular status of the limb proximal and distal to the injury should be evaluated.
- If there is an abnormality on palpation of pulses, further vascular examination is warranted.
- The ankle–brachial index of the extremity, along with ultrasound examination of the leg, can be helpful in fully evaluating the possibility of vascular injury, which occurs in about 2% of these fractures.[1,8]
- The patient is evaluated for compartment syndrome upon presentation, and in most cases for 24 hours, especially for high-energy mechanisms and highly displaced fractures.[11]
- The strength of dorsiflexion and eversion will help evaluate the peroneal nerve. It is important to examine and document peroneal nerve function before surgery because of the possibility of injury from stretch or direct impact. Motor and sensory function of the nerve proximal and distal to the injury should be assessed.
- A thorough examination of the knee ligaments and extensor mechanism is needed, but this cannot accurately be performed preoperatively owing to difficulty differentiating ligamentous from bony instability.
  - Examination of the knee ligaments and extensor mechanism should therefore take place after operative stabilization and before the patient is awake in the operating room.
  - Soft tissues need careful inspection before definitive surgical intervention can take place. The surgeon should note where surgical incisions will be located when evaluating the soft tissue.

IMAGING AND OTHER DIAGNOSTIC STUDIES

- Anteroposterior (AP) and lateral radiographs of the knee. The need for oblique views is being supplanted by computed tomography (CT) **(FIG 3A–C)**.

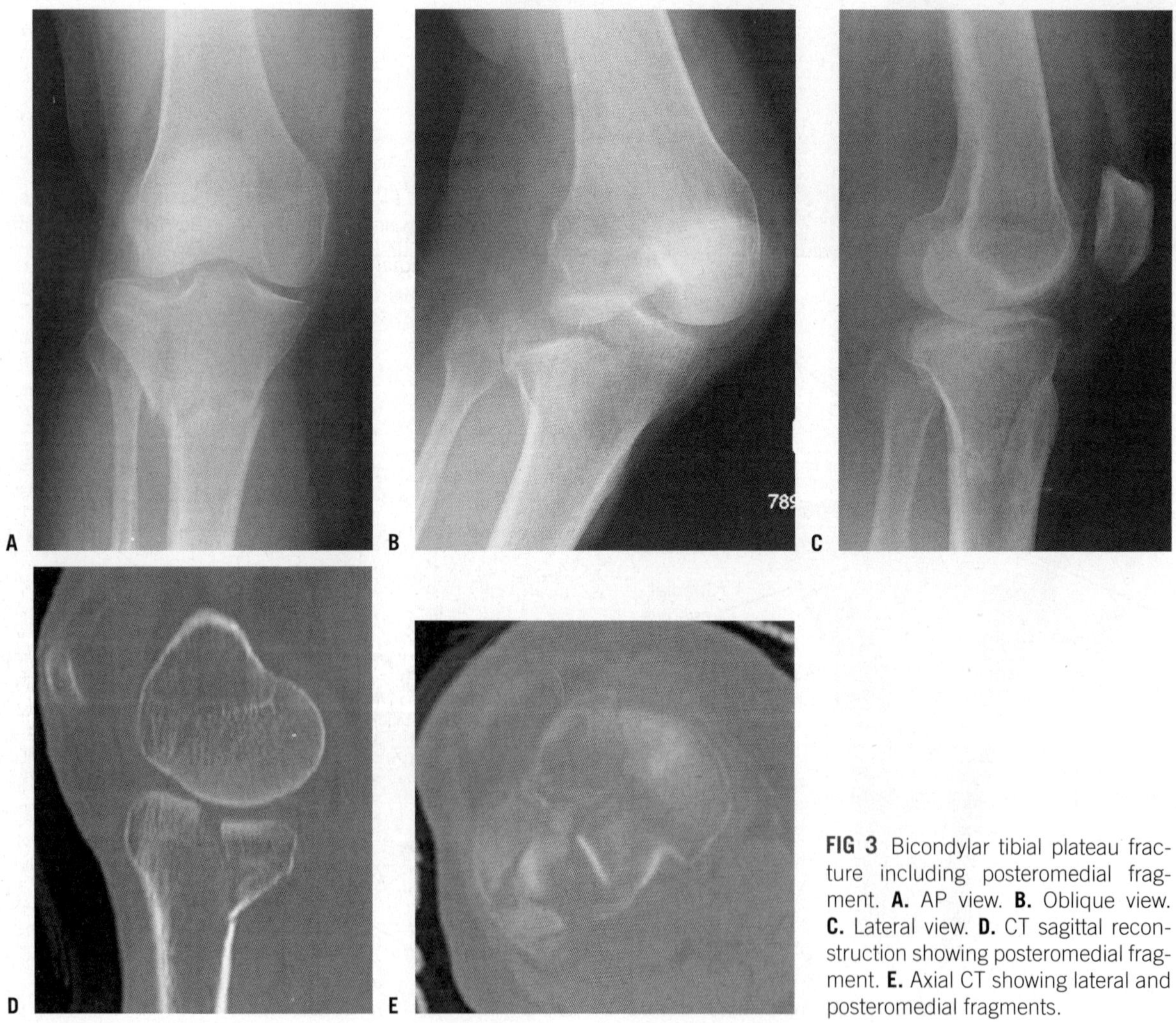

FIG 3 Bicondylar tibial plateau fracture including posteromedial fragment. **A.** AP view. **B.** Oblique view. **C.** Lateral view. **D.** CT sagittal reconstruction showing posteromedial fragment. **E.** Axial CT showing lateral and posteromedial fragments.

- CT scan with sagittal and coronal reconstruction is helpful to define complex fracture patterns and to plan surgical tactics **(FIG 3D,E)**.
- Three-dimensional CT reconstructions can be helpful, but only provides information regarding surface topography. Impacted fragments are generally better appreciated with two-dimensional CT.
- Although not routine, magnetic resonance imaging can be useful in individual circumstances when ligament and meniscal injury around the knee is suspected and may not be directly visualized during surgery.[4]

DIFFERENTIAL DIAGNOSIS

- Multiligament injury at the knee
- Proximal tibial shaft fracture
- Unicondylar tibial plateau fracture
- Patella fracture
- Extensor mechanism disruption

NONOPERATIVE MANAGEMENT

- A fracture brace, a long-leg cast, or both may be used to treat low-energy nondisplaced fractures. Nonoperative management may also be desired if patient factors (eg, comorbidities, functional status) would make operative intervention inappropriate.
  - These fractures require close observation to ensure progressive malalignment (particularly varus) does not occur.

OPEN REDUCTION AND INTERNAL FIXATION

Preoperative Planning

- The patient is examined, and imaging studies are reviewed.
- A staged protocol is considered with first-stage provisional spanning external fixation for high-energy bicondylar injuries prone to soft tissue swelling. Open reduction and internal fixation can be performed when the soft tissue envelope is amenable to the planned approach.
  - External fixation pins should be placed out of the zone of injury and, to the extent possible, out of the zone of future hardware placement.[10]
- A definitive surgical technique (eg, plating, nailing, or external fixation) is chosen.
  - A backup plan should always be in place.
- A surgical approach is planned that affords adequate exposure for reduction and stabilization of the fracture while minimizing soft tissue stripping.
- Patient positioning should be planned to ease surgical exposure. It is usually supine but can be prone when a posterior or posteromedial approach is used. This is particularly helpful if the posterior fragment is large and extends far laterally.
- The surgeon should consider whether a nonsterile or sterile tourniquet is required and the prep and draping procedure planned accordingly.
- The C-arm location should be identified. It should be placed on the contralateral side of the patient's injured limb for a lateral exposure and on the ipsilateral side for a medial exposure. The monitor is positioned for comfortable viewing.
- Consideration should be given whether a femoral distractor will be useful.
  - In bicondylar fracture patterns, joint distraction is marginal with use of a femoral distractor as distraction occurs through the fracture rather than across the joint.
- A tactic for articular and metaphyseal fracture reductions are planned based on preoperative imaging and chosen method of fixation.
  - The surgeon should decide which part of the bicondylar pattern to stabilize first: medial or lateral. The side that affords easiest anatomic reduction to the shaft fragment, typically the least comminuted side, is reduced and provisionally stabilized first. If the pattern is a variant of a fracture-dislocation, the medial side (the intact side) should be fixed first.
  - The initial fixation should not interfere with fixation of the opposite condyle.
- The opposite condyle is then reduced to the shaft and the provisionally fixed condyle.
  - Minor adjustments to both condyles are often required to obtain final reduction.
  - Care is taken to adjust coronal and sagittal plane alignment of both condyles.
- Definitive fixation is applied.
  - Required implants are inventoried and their availability confirmed.
- Additional equipment is identified, listed, and their availability confirmed.
- Postoperative immobilization is considered, and any supplies required are inventoried and their availability confirmed.

Choosing Approaches for Open Reduction and Internal Fixation

- Single lateral, dual (lateral and posteromedial), and single posteromedial approaches are most common.
- Single anterior midline incisions with medial and lateral stripping should be avoided.
  - A midline approach with medial and lateral exposure has been associated with high complication rates and should be avoided.
  - When medial and lateral exposure is required, an anterolateral exposure with the addition of a posteromedial approach is preferred.
- Metaphyseal fracture components are best treated indirectly to maximally preserve biologic potential for healing, especially when they are comminuted.

Lateral Approach Indications

- A lateral approach is standard to address the lateral component of bicondylar fractures.
- It allows for direct exposure of lateral intra-articular fractures, the lateral meniscus, and for placement of lateral plates.
- The medial component of a bicondylar fracture can be stabilized from the lateral exposure with multiple locking screws engaging the medial fragment provided there is: no medial articular incongruity necessitating a separate direct exposure, no medial metaphyseal comminution necessitating separate medial fixation, and that the medial condyle is large enough to accept the locking screws.

Medial and Posteromedial Approach Indications

- The medial component of a bicondylar fracture may be directly approached via a medial or posteromedial approach.
  - Coronal medial fractures with a typical posteromedial fragment, with or without associated lateral fractures, are common and are best managed with a posteromedial approach and posteromedial buttress plate.
  - When the entire medial condyle is involved, a posteromedial or direct medial approach can be used.

Posterior Approach Indications

- A minority of fractures, those with a posterior lateral shearing injury pattern, may benefit from a direct posterior exposure.

TECHNIQUES

OPEN REDUCTION AND INTERNAL FIXATION OF BICONDYLAR TIBIAL PLATEAU FRACTURES

Open Reduction and Internal Fixation via Dual Approaches: Lateral and Posteromedial Approaches

- The choice of order, lateral or posteromedial approach first, is determined by the fracture pattern. Generally, the side with least comminution, so an anatomic reduction to the shaft can be accomplished, is approached first.
- The patient is positioned supine on a radiolucent or fracture table, with a bump under the contralateral hip considered.
- Nonsterile high thigh tourniquet is applied.
  - Optionally, the lower extremity is exsanguinated and the tourniquet inflated to about 250 to 300 mm Hg.

Posteromedial Surgical Approach

- The incision is marked and started 1 cm posterior to the posteromedial edge of the tibial metaphysis **(TECH FIG 1A)**.
  - The saphenous vein and nerve should be carefully avoided during the dissection superficial to the fascia.
  - Deeper dissection continues to expose the pes anserine tendons **(TECH FIG 1B)**.
  - Dissection and mobilization of the tendons allow access to the fracture above, below, or between the tendons.
- The medial gastrocnemius is dissected from the posteromedial tibia.
- Subperiosteal dissection should be limited to the fracture margins to aid in confirmation of the reduction.
- The fracture margins are exposed posterior and/or anterior to the MCL. The MCL is left intact.

Medial Reduction

- Medial-sided fracture reduction is accomplished with a combination of traction, manual manipulation, and appropriately positioned reduction clamps **(TECH FIG 2A,B)**.
  - Valgus stress, due to an associated lateral condyle fracture, may not be helpful for reduction.
- The weight of the leg often contributes to varus deformity and should be neutralized with longitudinal traction either manually or via a medial femoral distractor.
- Articular fracture reduction is typically judged indirectly via cortical reduction and fluoroscopy. A submeniscal arthrotomy performed anterior to the MCL can provide a view of the anterior portion of the medial plateau.

Medial Fixation

- Medial fixation depends on the fracture pattern.
- For the common coronal posteromedial fragment, a posteromedial plate that is slightly under contoured to help buttress the fragment is used.
- The plate location for medial fractures that are complete may be either posteromedial **(TECH FIG 2C,D)** or anteromedial. Some surgeons advocate direct medial plating over the MCL.
  - Medial plating is generally posteromedial when adjunctive to lateral plating in the case of comminuted bicondylar fractures.
- Initial medial fixation should take care to avoid interfering with reduction of the lateral-sided fracture **(TECH FIG 2E,F)**.
  - Once the entirety of the fracture is reduced, fixation from the medial side should capture the lateral fracture to provide added stability.

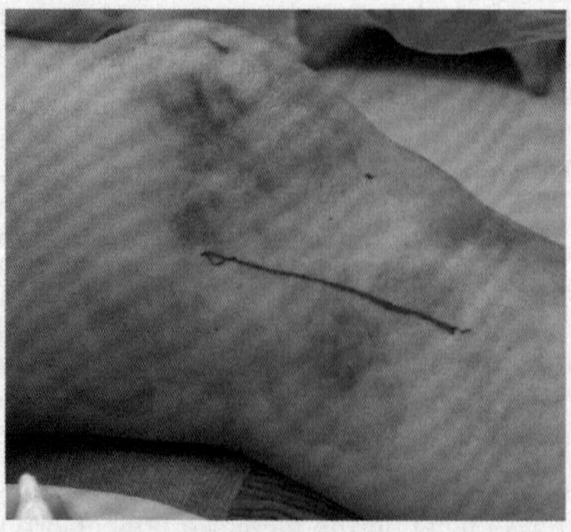

A

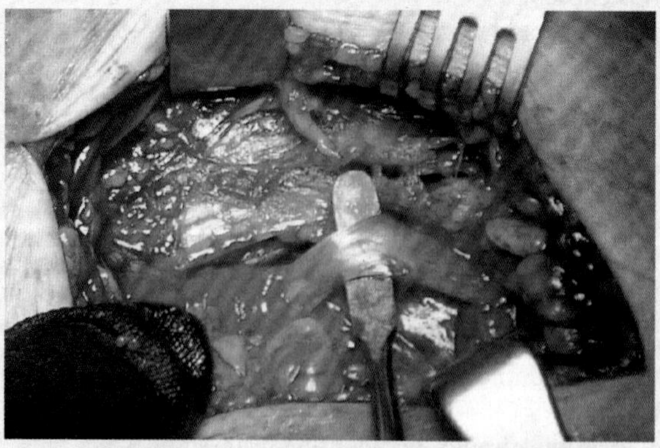

B

TECH FIG 1 A. Skin incision for posteromedial approach to tibial plateau. **B.** Deep dissection for the posteromedial approach includes exposure of the pes anserine tendons, which are preserved.

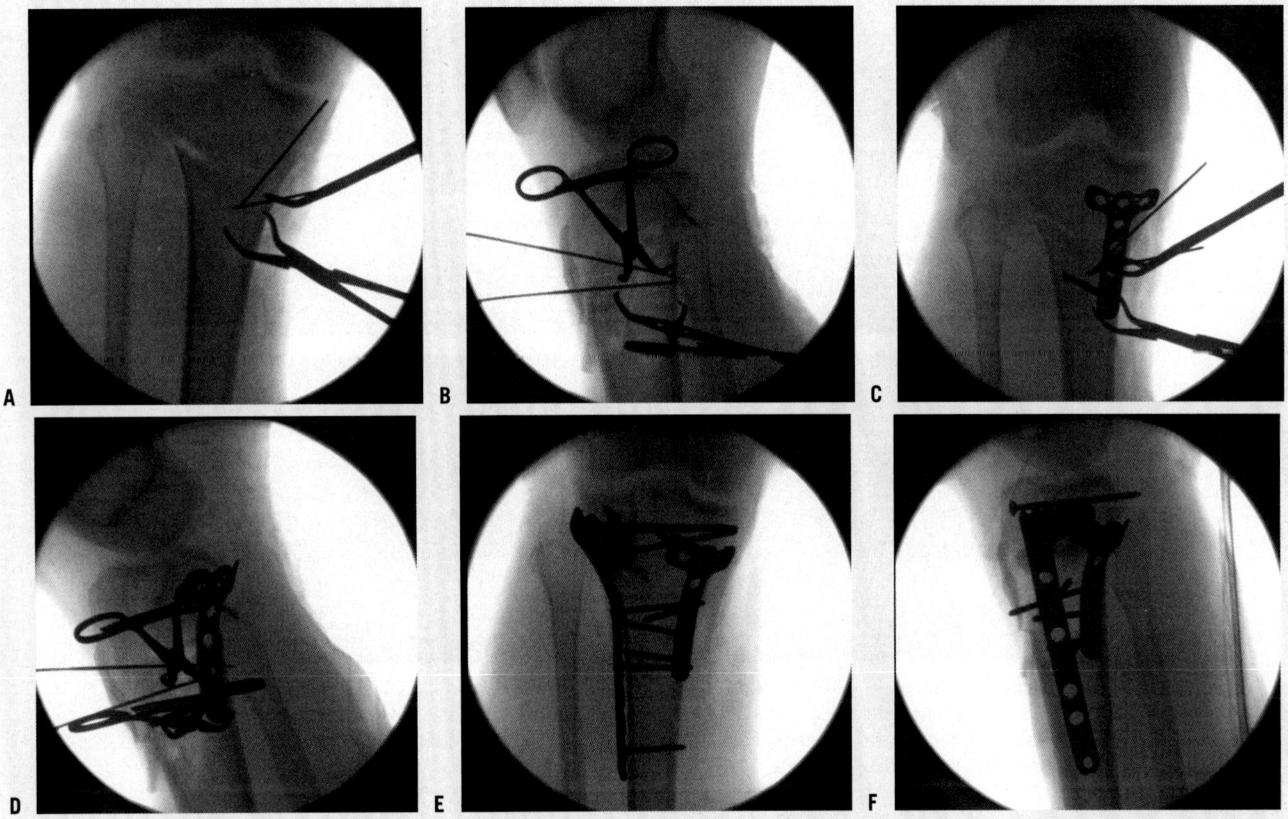

TECH FIG 2 AP (**A**) and lateral (**B**) fluoro shots showing reduction of medial condyle of bicondylar fracture. The medial side is secured first with a posteromedial plate (**C,D**). Lateral fixation supports the depressed lateral articular surface, the lateral condyle, and, by virtue of long locked screws, adds support to the medial fragment (**E,F**).

Lateral Surgical Approach

- The surgeon identifies and marks landmarks (Gerdy tubercle, tibial crest, patella, fibular head).
- The skin incision is marked beginning distally about 1 to 2 cm lateral to the tibial crest, curving posteriorly over Gerdy tubercle and then proceeding superiorly across the joint line toward the lateral femoral epicondyle **(TECH FIG 3A)**.
- The skin is incised along the marked incision, and dissection is carried to the fascia without detaching subcutaneous fat from the fascia **(TECH FIG 3B)**.
- The facia is divided parallel with the skin incision.
  - Distally, the anterior compartment fascia is feathered off the anterior fascial flap to expose the proximal lateral shaft and metaphysis.
  - Proximally, the fibers of the iliotibial band are split longitudinally without disrupting the capsule **(TECH FIG 3C)**.
  - Centrally, the iliotibial band is elevated from the tubercle of Gerdy anteriorly and posteriorly.
- If required for lateral articular reduction, a lateral submeniscal arthrotomy is made by incising the capsule horizontally **(TECH FIG 3D)**.
  - The meniscus is elevated, inspected for tears, and repaired as needed.
  - Most of the meniscal injuries are peripheral rim tears and may be repaired in a horizontal mattress fashion to the capsule.

Lateral Reduction

- Note that simultaneous exposure of the medial side may be required if medial reduction is not already obtained.
- Intra-articular lateral fracture fragments are visualized directly (via the submeniscal arthrotomy) and indirectly (with the aid of fluoroscopy) while reduction is obtained.
- Articular reduction is obtained with aid of reduction clamps, tamps, and joysticks and are provisionally held with Kirschner wire fixation and/or a large periarticular reduction forceps.
- Condylar width is restored with aid of a large periarticular reduction clamp.
- Metaphyseal fracture components should be indirectly reduced with fluoroscopic guidance such that the articular block is aligned relative to the shaft.

Lateral Fixation

- A laterally applied plate is useful to support lateral condylar fragments and to support depressed articular fragments (via the raft effect of multiple proximal screws placed subchondrally) (see **TECH FIG 2E**).
- Support of the medial side can be provided via a lateral plate when the medial fragment is of sufficient size and location that multiple screws from the lateral plate engage the medial fragment **(TECH FIG 4A,B)**.
  - Locking screws provide superior resistance to medial subsidence and are preferred to nonlocking screws for this application.

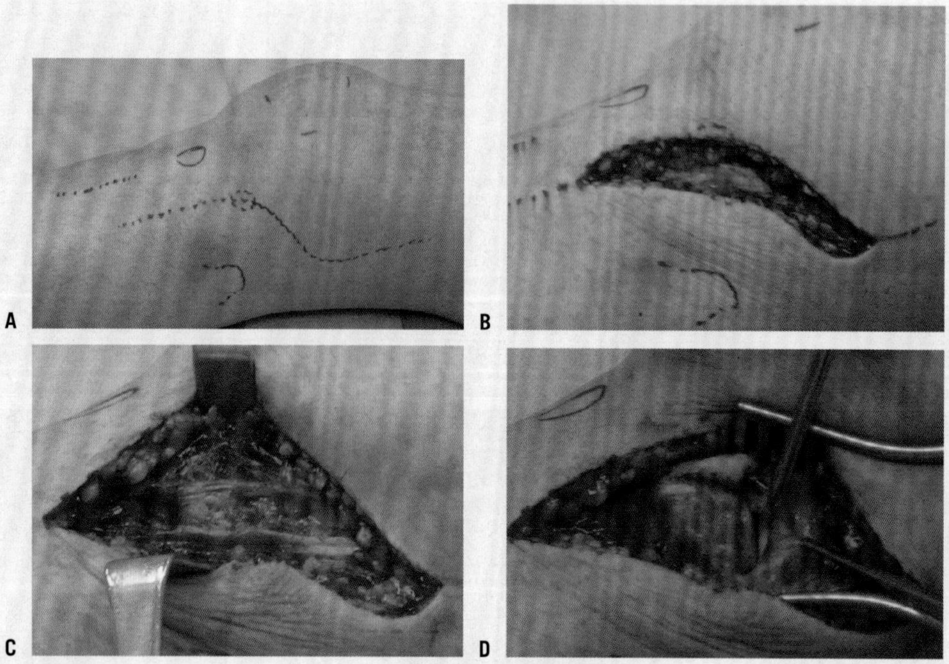

TECH FIG 3 **A.** Landmarks (patella, tibial tubercle, tubercle of Gerdy, and fibula) for the anterior lateral approach. **B.** Anterior lateral approach superficial dissection. **C.** Deep lateral exposure with iliotibial band incised parallel to its fibers centered over tubercle of Gerdy. **D.** Submeniscal arthrotomy provides direct access to the lateral articular surface.

- When compression is required between the medial and lateral fragment, nonlocked lag screws should be used before placing locked screws across the fracture line.
- When the medial fragment is of such size and location that multiple locked screws from a lateral plate cannot engage this fragment, separate medial fixation is required.
  - This is most commonly the case with posteromedial fragments that are amenable to separate posteromedial buttress plate fixation.

Management of Lateral Subchondral Defects

- Subchondral defects should be grafted with allograft, autograft, or bone substitute.

Closure

- Layered closure of the wounds are performed in standard fashion. A deep drain that can decompress the knee joint is considered.
  - If postoperative compartment syndrome is a risk, leaving the deep fascia open or extending the facial incision to create a prophylactic fasciotomy should be considered.

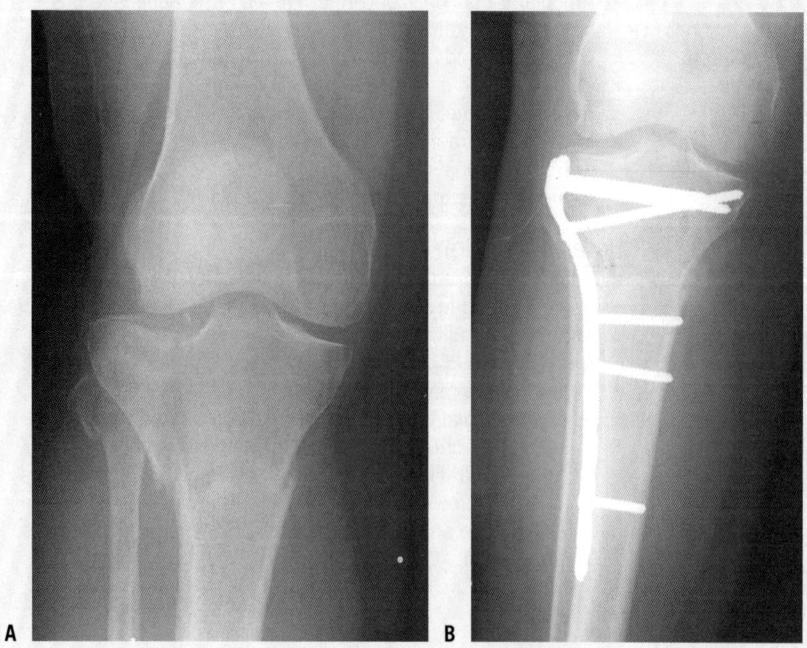

TECH FIG 4 Bicondylar tibial plateau fracture with a large medial fragment (**A**) supported with a single lateral locking plate (**B**).

Open Reduction and Internal Fixation via the Posterior Approach (Posterior Shearing Fracture)

Posterior Surgical Approach

- The patient is positioned prone with a high thigh tourniquet.
- An S-shaped incision starts midline superiorly and extends medial distally. The incision is centered on the popliteal fossa, with the transverse component made at the joint line **(TECH FIG 5A–C)**.
- The surgeon identifies and protects the common peroneal nerve, popliteal artery and vein, tibial nerve, and medial sural cutaneous nerve (see **TECH FIG 5C**).
- The lateral head of the gastrocnemius is dissected bluntly and its blood supply protected distally. The tendon is divided proximally, leaving a stump for repair.
- The lateral gastrocnemius is retracted medially **(TECH FIG 5D)**.
- The popliteus and soleus origin are elevated off the posteromedial aspect of the proximal tibia.

Reduction

- The articular surface is elevated through the fracture site and the reduction assessed indirectly with fluoroscopy and by the cortical reduction. Direct visualization of the articular surface is difficult.

Fixation

- A relatively thin plate is contoured to buttress the fragments. Lag screw technique is used to compress the fragments **(TECH FIG 5E,F)**.

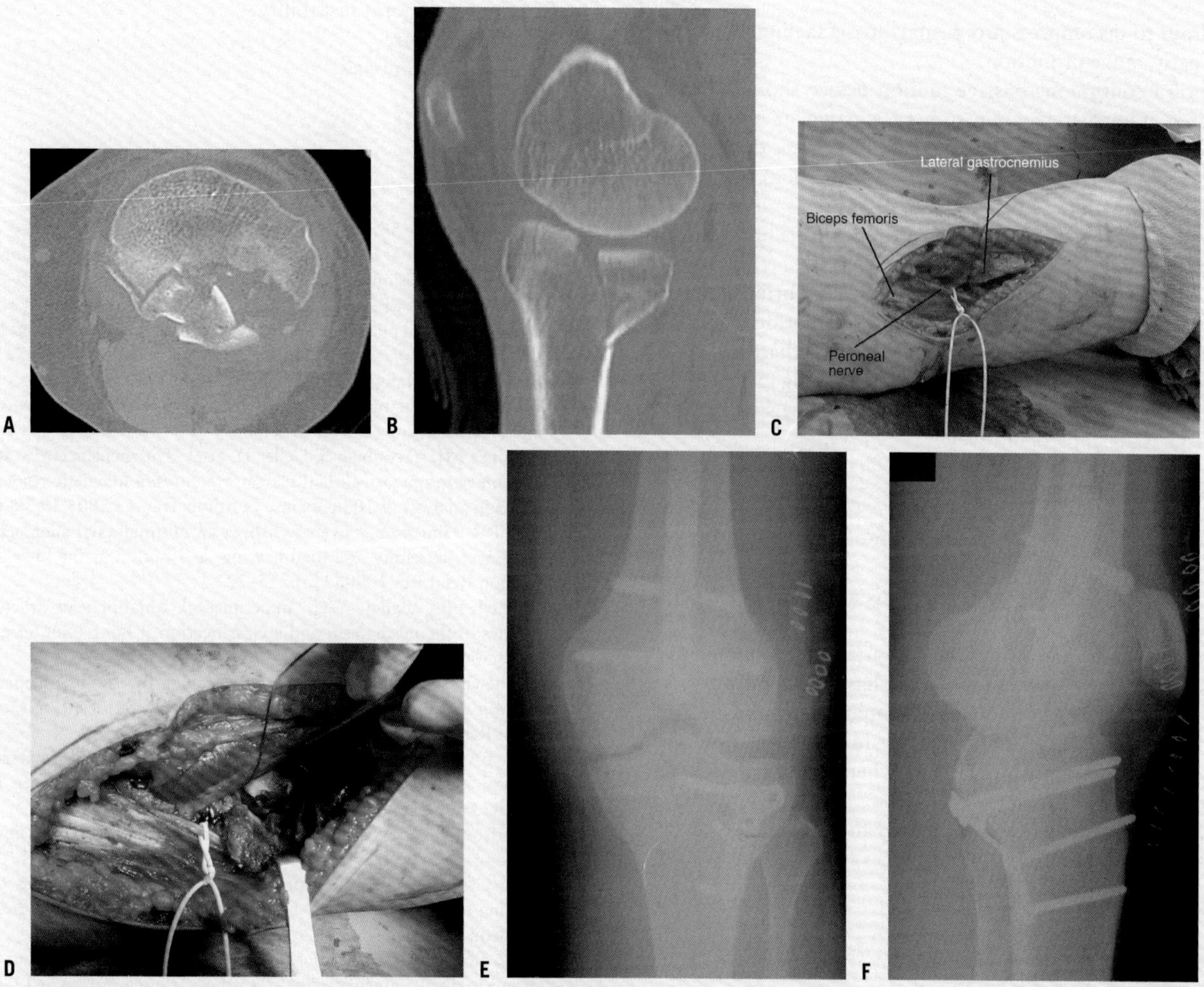

TECH FIG 5 Axial (**A**) and sagittal (**B**) CT scans demonstrating posterior shearing injury. **C.** Posterior S-shaped incision starting midline superiorly, transverse at the joint line, and extending to the medial side in the distal aspect of the incision. **D.** The lateral gastrocnemius is released after identification of neurovascular structures and elevated medially. Postoperative AP (**E**) and lateral (**F**) radiographs demonstrating posterior plating.

Pearls and Pitfalls

With medial metaphyseal comminution, do not rely on a lateral locked plate to support the medial side.	• A laterally applied plate is useful to support lateral condylar fragments and to support depressed articular fragments (via a raft effect of multiple proximal screws placed subchondrally). Separate medial fixation is indicated in the described situation.
Posteromedial vertical intra-articular shear fractures benefit from buttress plates.	• Support of the medial side can be provided via a lateral plate when the medial fragment is of such a size and location that multiple screws from the lateral plate engage the medial fragment. Posterior medial fragments as described are not well supported from the lateral side.
Schatzker type V fractures are usually amenable to relatively thin medial and lateral buttress plates.	• Schatzker type VI fractures have more metaphyseal/diaphyseal involvement and typically require stronger plates than type V fractures.
Sagittal plane alignment of the medial and lateral condyles should have relatively equal posterior slope.	• An AP radiograph tilted to accommodate the posterior slope (about 8–10 degrees) should equally profile the subchondral bone of both the medial and lateral condyles.

POSTOPERATIVE CARE

- A drain to decompress any hemarthrosis facilitates obtaining early range of motion.
- Use of a continuous passive motion device should be considered immediately after surgery starting at about 0 to 40 degrees. Flexion is advanced 5 to 10 degrees during each of three 2-hour sessions per day, with the goal being 0 to 90 degrees within 24 to 36 hours.
- Chemical deep vein thrombosis prophylaxis is provided for approximately 4 weeks.
- Initial physical therapy concentrates on restoring range of motion with closed-chain active range-of-motion exercises.
- Toe-touch weight bearing is permitted immediately.
- Weight bearing is advanced and strengthening exercises are initiated upon evidence of fracture healing, usually about 8 to 12 weeks postoperatively.

OUTCOMES

- Satisfactory articular reduction (step-off or gap of 2 mm or less) is obtained in 62.1% of cases.[2]
  - There were 91.2% who had satisfactory coronal plane alignment.
  - Also, 72.1% had satisfactory sagittal plane alignment.
- Bicondylar tibial plateau fractures have a significant negative effect on leisure activities, employment, and general mobilization. Significant residual dysfunction was observed out to 51 months postoperatively when compared with the general population.[2]
- Decreased arc of motion compared to the uninvolved extremity is common.

COMPLICATIONS

- Compartment syndrome
- Infection (7% to 8.4%)[1]
- Superficial and deep wound complications
- Residual knee joint instability
- Painful hardware
- Deep vein thrombosis
- Arthrosis
- Loss of motion

REFERENCES

1. Barei DP, Nork SE, Mills WJ, et al. Complications associated with internal fixation of high-energy bicondylar tibial plateau fractures utilizing a two-incision technique. J Orthop Trauma 2004;18:649–657.
2. Barei DP, Nork SE, Mills WJ, et al. Functional outcomes of severe bicondylar tibial plateau fractures treated with dual incisions and medial and lateral plates. J Bone Joint Surg Am 2006;88:1713–1721.
3. Brandon ML, Haynes PT, Bonamo JR, et al. The association between posterior-inferior tibial slope and anterior cruciate ligament insufficiency. Arthroscopy 2006;22:894–899.
4. Gardner MJ, Yacoubian S, Geller D, et al. The incidence of soft tissue injury in operative tibial plateau fractures: a magnetic resonance imaging analysis of 103 patients. J Orthop Trauma 2005;19:79–84.
5. Hsu RW, Himeno S, Coventry MB, et al. Normal axial alignment of the lower extremity and load-bearing distribution at the knee. Clin Orthop Relat Res 1990;(255):215–227.
6. Kennedy JC, Bailey WH. Experimental tibial-plateau fractures. Studies of the mechanism and a classification. J Bone Joint Surg Am 1968;50:1522–1534.
7. Lachiewicz PF, Funcik T. Factors influencing the results of open reduction and internal fixation of tibial plateau fractures. Clin Orthop Relat Res 1990;(259):210–215.
8. Levy BA, Zlowodzki MP, Graves M, et al. Screening for extermity arterial injury with the arterial pressure index. Am J Emerg Med 2005;23:689–695.
9. Morrison JB. The mechanics of the knee joint in relation to normal walking. J Biomech 1970;3:51–61.
10. Shah CM, Babb PE, McAndrew CM, et al. Definitive plates overlapping provisional external fixator pin sites: is the infection risk increased? J Orthop Trauma 2014;28:518–522.
11. Ziran BH, Becher SJ. Radiographic predictors of compartment syndrome in tibial plateau fractures. J Orthop Trauma 2013;27:612–615.

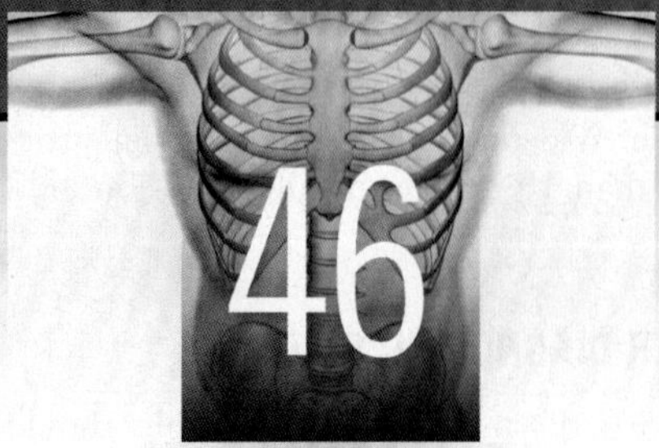

CHAPTER 46

Lateral Tibial Plateau Fractures

Daniel Bravin and Philip R. Wolinsky

DEFINITION

- Tibial plateau fractures are intra-articular fractures that can result in malalignment of the articular surface and/or limb, with the risk of subsequent arthritis.

ANATOMY

- The tibial plateau consists of three osseous structures: the lateral plateau, the medial plateau, and the intercondylar eminence.
  - The lateral plateau is smaller and convex, the medial plateau is larger and slightly concave. Both plateaus are covered by a meniscus, which serves as a shock absorber and improves the congruency of the femorotibial joint.
  - The lateral plateau sits slightly higher than the medial joint surface and forms an angle of 3 degrees of varus with respect of the tibial shaft. This is helpful to identify the lateral plateau on the lateral radiograph.
  - The lateral tibial plateau has variable width, and contralateral radiographs are helpful to evaluate patients' individual morphology.
  - The anatomy of the tibial plateau leads to an eccentric load distribution. The lateral plateau bears 40% of the knee's load.[1] This asymmetric weight bearing results in increased medial subchondral bone formation and a stronger, denser medial plateau.
  - The central, nonarticular intercondylar eminence serves as the tibial attachment of the anterior and posterior cruciate ligaments.
  - The knee joint stability is provided by the cruciate and collateral ligaments as well as the capsule.
- The tibial tuberosity and Gerdy tubercle are bony prominences located adjacent to the lateral tibial plateau that the patellar tendon and the iliotibial tract attach to. These are important landmarks for planning surgical incisions.

PATHOGENESIS

- Several factors are thought to contribute to the higher incidence of lateral as opposed to medial plateau fractures.
  - The relative softness of the subchondral bone of the lateral plateau, the valgus axis of the lower extremity, and the susceptibility of the leg to a medially directed force (people tend to get hit on the outside of their knees) lead to the higher prevalence of lateral plateau fractures.[1]
- Tibial plateau fractures are due to either direct trauma to the proximal tibia/knee joint or to indirect axial forces.
  - The most frequent mechanism of a lateral plateau fracture is a direct laterally based force applied to the proximal tibia region. This causes a valgus force and drives the lateral femoral condyle into the softer lateral tibial plateau.
  - Indirect axial forces may occur in high-energy injuries and are associated with complex tibial plateau fractures.
  - Twisting injuries account for only 5% to 10% of tibial plateau fractures and are most commonly sporting injuries (eg, skiing).
  - Geriatric tibial plateau fractures are becoming more common. These typically are a result of lower energy mechanisms (eg, a ground-level fall).
- Split or wedge fractures are more rare and occur in younger patients with harder bone, whereas joint depression fractures occur more frequently in older patients with more osteoporotic or osteopenic bone, which is less able to withstand compression.

NATURAL HISTORY

- The natural history of lateral tibial plateau fractures depends on the degree of articular depression and knee stability. Knee instability may result not only from the fracture but also from any accompanying soft tissue injuries such as meniscal injuries or rupture of a cruciate or collateral ligaments.
- The prognosis of nondisplaced or minimally displaced fractures is favorable, but displaced fractures, especially in combination with knee instability, may result in early posttraumatic arthritis.
- Meniscal injuries have been reported in up to 50% of tibial plateau fractures. Meniscal injuries are a major determinant of prognosis because meniscal integrity is important for joint stability and may compensate for articular incongruity.
- Patients evaluated with magnetic resonance imaging (MRI) have been found to have high rates of soft tissue injuries around the knee including meniscal and ligamentous injuries ranging between rates of 47% and 99%.[12]

PATIENT HISTORY AND PHYSICAL FINDINGS

- The physical examination should always include a thorough assessment of the soft tissue envelope.
- The thin soft tissue envelope of the proximal tibia predisposes to open fractures and development of tissue ischemia or necrosis. It is important to assess the soft tissue injury because it may not allow for early definitive fixation of the fracture and require temporary external fixation.
- A compartment syndrome may be present. Clinical findings of compartment syndrome include increasing pain, paresthesias, pain with passive stretch, paresis, in the setting of

intact pulses, and pink skin coloring. Pain out of proportion to the injury, increasing narcotic requirements, and agitation are frequently the first indicators.
  - A compartment syndrome requires a fasciotomy.
- Measuring compartment pressures may be helpful when the clinical symptoms of a compartment syndrome are unclear or unobtainable.
  - A pressure difference between the preoperative diastolic blood pressure and the compartment pressure of less than 30 mm Hg are diagnostic of a compartment syndrome and require a fasciotomy.
  - Typically, as soon as a compartment syndrome is diagnosed, operative intervention is required.
- The neurovascular status of the extremity must be carefully evaluated, although concomitant injuries of neurovascular structures are uncommon for lateral plateau fracture, they do occur.
  - Palpation of peripheral pulses (should be present and symmetrical)
  - Doppler ultrasound
  - An ankle–brachial index less than 0.9 indicates that vascular injury is likely.
- Examination of knee stability prior to surgical stabilization, is difficult, so it should be tested under anesthesia after fracture fixation.
  - Assessment of knee stability is difficult on initial examination because of the instability due to the fracture(s), the intracapsular hematoma, and pain.
  - Varus and valgus stress radiographs of the knee in near-full extension can be performed with sedation or under general anesthesia. Widening of the femoral–tibial articulation of more than 10 degrees in full extension indicates instability.

IMAGING AND OTHER DIAGNOSTIC STUDIES

- Plain anteroposterior (AP) and lateral radiographs should be centered on the knee, with the AP view angled 10 degrees in a craniocaudal direction to approximate the posterior slope of the plateau (plateau view).
- The standard tool for analyzing tibial plateau fractures is a thin-cut computed tomography (CT) scan with two- and three-dimensional reconstructions because the extent of this is underestimated on plain radiographs **(FIG 1A–D)**.[6]
- Although MRI evaluates both osseous and soft tissue injuries, it has not yet become a standard tool in analyzing tibial plateau fractures. It may be helpful for identifying meniscal and ligamentous injuries.
- Contralateral films can be obtained preoperatively or intraoperatively and provide important information such as the patients slope, condylar width, and unique morphology **(FIG 1E,F)**.

DIFFERENTIAL DIAGNOSIS

- Ligamentous injuries of the knee
- Knee dislocation
- Meniscal injury
- Bone bruise
- Compartment syndrome

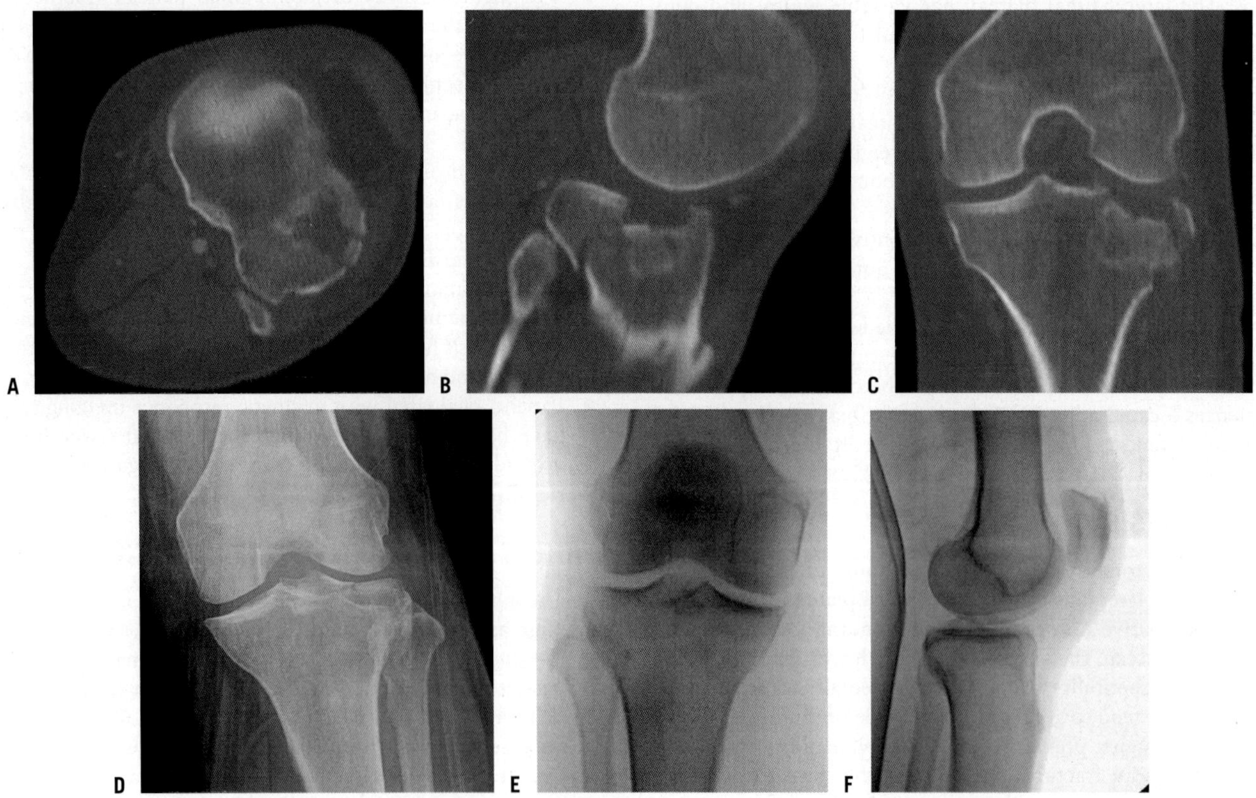

FIG 1 A–D. Preoperative CT scans and x-rays and a showing a lateral tibial plateau split depression fracture pattern. **E,F.** Intraoperative fluoroscopy of the contralateral knee, including an AP slope view of the proximal tibia and a lateral image demonstrating the tibial slope (the leg is adducted a small amount past a perfect lateral to see the different medial and lateral tibial plateau slopes).

NONOPERATIVE MANAGEMENT

- For nondisplaced or minimally displaced fractures, the indications for surgical treatment are controversial and vary widely in the literature. The range of acceptable articular depression varies from 2 mm to 1 cm.
- Nondisplaced or minimally displaced tibial plateau fractures with a stabile knee joint can be managed nonoperatively.
- Different protocols exist, but generally toe-touch weight bearing is recommended for 6 to 8 weeks with progressive weight bearing at that time point.
- In the absence of ligamentous injury or instability, bracing is not required.
- Isometric quadriceps exercises and progressive passive, active-assisted, and active range-of-knee motion exercises are recommended to avoid substantial muscle atrophy.
- Failure to maintain reduction with nonoperative management is an indication for surgical fracture stabilization. Therefore, frequent surveillance radiographs are required for the management of these patients.

SURGICAL MANAGEMENT

- The primary management of tibial plateau fractures is usually dictated by the soft tissue injury and by the fracture type.
- Absolute indications for surgery are open fractures, fractures with vascular or neurologic lesions, and/or fractures with compartment syndrome. Surgery is also recommended for displaced articular injuries and fractures with valgus instability.
- The goals in the surgical treatment of tibial plateau fractures are restoration of the articular surface, mechanical axis, meniscal integrity, and axial stability to avoid or postpone the development of posttraumatic arthritis. Fracture stability allows early rehabilitation and supports long-term full recovery.[8]
- The degree of soft tissue injury and the general condition of the patient are important factors in surgical decision making.
  - If there is severe soft tissue damage or a polytraumatized patient, a temporary external fixator can be applied to regain and maintain gross length, rotation, and alignment until definitive fixation can be performed.
  - Definitive fracture stabilization with open reduction and internal fixation is delayed until soft tissue damage or the patient's systemic issues have been resolved.

Preoperative Planning

- Review radiographs, CT, and MRI.
- Surgical approach and placement of implants
  - Plate fixation is recommended for almost all fractures. In young patients with pure split patterns and excellent bone, screw osteosynthesis alone can be considered.
  - Whether a cortical window is required depends on the degree and location of impaction and the presence or absence and location of a cortical split. Condylar widening is a good radiologic sign for the requirement of articular elevation with a tamp via a cortical window.
  - Options to assess and reduce the articular surface include performing a submeniscal arthrotomy for visualization of the articular surface and either opening and working through a fracture line, or creating a cortical window or performing an osteotomy, or using fluoroscopic imaging. Arthroscopy is also an option, although rarely required.
  - Lateral meniscus tears are associated with lateral tibial plateau fractures and are most commonly bucket-handle tears originating at the meniscocapsular junction. These should be repaired at the time of fracture fixation.
  - Meniscal and ligamentous injuries require either open or arthroscopic surgery for repair or reconstruction. These can be performed on a delayed basis.
- The surgeon should be aware of the need for bone grafting (autograft, allograft, bone graft substitute) when there is depression of articular fragments that require elevation to fill the void.
- Separate classifications of open fracture and the degree of closed soft tissue injuries exist.
  - Open fractures are classified according to Gustilo et al.[4]
  - The soft tissue injury can be classified according to Tscherne and Oestern.[11]
- The *Arbeitsgemeinschaft für Osteosynthesefragen* (AO) Orthopaedic Trauma Association classification for proximal tibial fractures distinguishes between extra-articular, partial articular, and complete articular fractures and further subdivides them based on the level of comminution **(TABLE 1)**.
- The Schatzker classification distinguishes between lateral and medial plateau fractures **(TABLE 2)**.
  - In general, types I through III are low-energy injuries affecting the lateral plateau.
  - Types IV through VI are higher energy injuries that involve the medial plateau and/or both plateaus, with or without ligamentous injuries.

Positioning

- Supine position
- A bump (ie, rolled blanket) can be put under the ipsilateral hip, so the patella is facing straight up to "fight" the tendency of the limb to externally rotate. A ramp should be used to elevate the operative leg and assist with fluoroscopy (contralateral limb is out of the way when getting lateral images).

TABLE 1 AO Classification for Proximal Tibial Fractures

Classification	Description
AO 41-A	Extra-articular fractures
AO 41-B	Partial intra-articular fractures
B1	Split fracture of the lateral plateau
B2	Depression fracture of the lateral plateau
B3	Split depression fracture of the lateral plateau
AO 41-C	Complete articular fractures
C1	Simple bicondylar fracture with simple metaphyseal fracture
C2	Simple bicondylar fracture with comminuted metaphyseal fracture
C3	Comminuted articular and metaphyseal fracture

AO, *Arbeitsgemeinschaft für Osteosynthesefragen.*

TABLE 2 Schatzker Classification of Tibial Plateau Fractures

Type	Description
I	Split fracture of the lateral tibial plateau
II	Split depression fracture of the lateral tibial plateau
III	Pure central depression fracture of the lateral tibial plateau
IV	Split (type A) or depression (type B) fracture of the medial plateau
V	Bicondylar tibial plateau fracture
VI	Comminuted tibial plateau fracture with dissociation between the metaphysis and the diaphysis

- The knee should be slightly bent (about 30 degrees) to reduce tension of collateral ligaments **(FIG 2)**.
- A tourniquet may be used to minimize blood loss and to improve fracture visualization.
- Use a radiolucent operating table to allow intraoperative imaging.
- Ipsilateral iliac crest is prepared and draped if autologous bone graft is needed; however, autograft is increasingly rarely used.

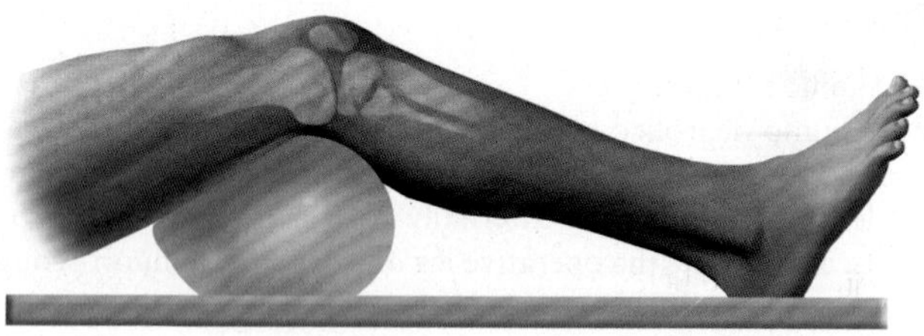

FIG 2 Leg position to reduce collateral ligament tension.

Approach

- The surgical approach and fixation plan for lateral tibial plateau fractures require
  - Good visualization of the lateral plateau
  - Preservation of anatomic structures
  - Minimal soft tissue and osseous devitalization
- It can be summarized as follows:
  - Elevation of the meniscus
  - Reduction of the fracture
  - Temporary fixation with Kirschner wire or small fragment screw fixation
  - Final stabilization with lag screws, conventional plate, or angular stable plate
- The incision must be planned to avoid implant location directly underneath the skin incision. Important landmarks are the joint line, Gerdy tubercle, the tibial tubercle, the fibular head, and the lateral femoral epicondyle **(FIG 3)**.
- The standard approach for lateral tibial plateau fractures is the anterolateral approach, which provides excellent exposure of the lateral plateau and allows good soft tissue coverage of the implant.
- The posterolateral approach is an option for posterior fractures of the lateral plateau.

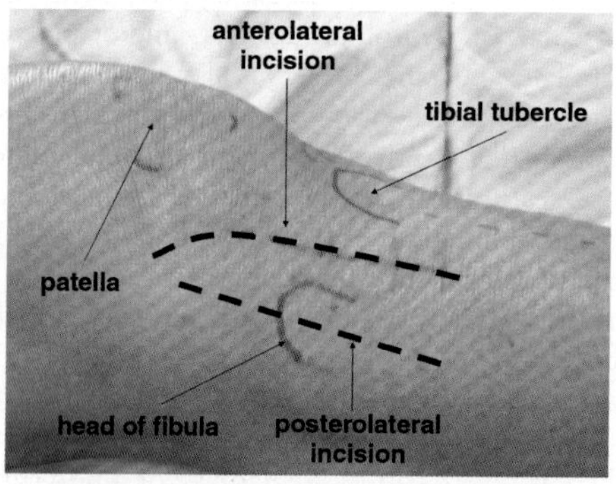

FIG 3 Landmarks for skin incision.

TECHNIQUES

ANTEROLATERAL APPROACH

- A straight, hockey stick, or lazy S incision (about 10 cm long) with the knee in 30 degrees of flexion is made.
- The incision is extended down through the iliotibial band proximally and the fascia of the anterior compartment distally.
- The tibialis anterior muscle is elevated off the proximal tibia to the level of the capsule and the coronary ligament is incised **(TECH FIG 1)**.
- To expose the lateral tibial plateau, a submeniscal arthrotomy is created, and the lateral meniscus is raised with holding sutures after incision of the coronary ligament.
- Assessment of the articular reduction is critical. Restoring condylar width is vital. A temporary universal distractor or external fixator placed into the distal femur and tibia allow for distraction and direct visualization of the articular surface through the submeniscal arthrotomy.

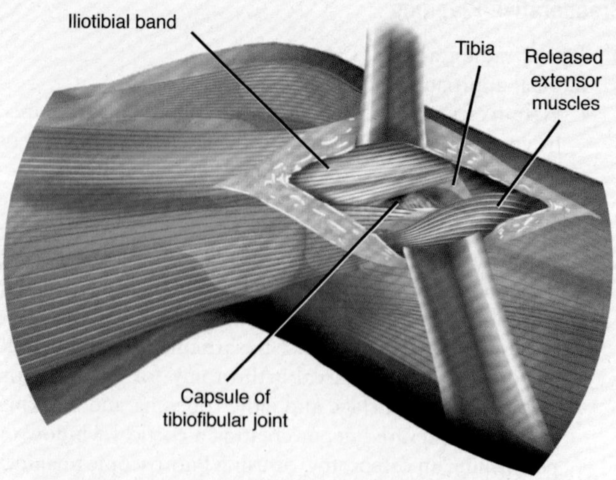

TECH FIG 1 Anterolateral approach to the lateral tibial plateau.

POSTEROLATERAL APPROACH

- The patient is placed in a lateral decubitus position.
- A longitudinal incision is made, about 3 cm proximal to the joint line, and carried down along the fibula **(TECH FIG 2)**.[3]
- Dissection is carried anterior in the incision similar to a standard anterolateral approach with a submeniscal arthrotomy.
- The peroneal nerve is dissected posteriorly and mobilized.
- Blunt dissection is carried out between the lateral head of the gastrocnemius and the soleus.
- The popliteus muscle is exposed and retracted medially. The popliteal artery and vein are protected deep to the lateral head of the gastrocnemius.
- The inferior geniculate artery may need to be ligated.
- A subperiosteal dissection is performed posteriorly, elevating off the soleus (can be carried out about 4 to 5 cm distally).
- The posterolateral approach has limited excursion distally because of the trifurcation of the vessels.
- Newer techniques, such as epicondylar osteotomy or other osteotomies, allow greater exposure to the posterior lateral plateau.

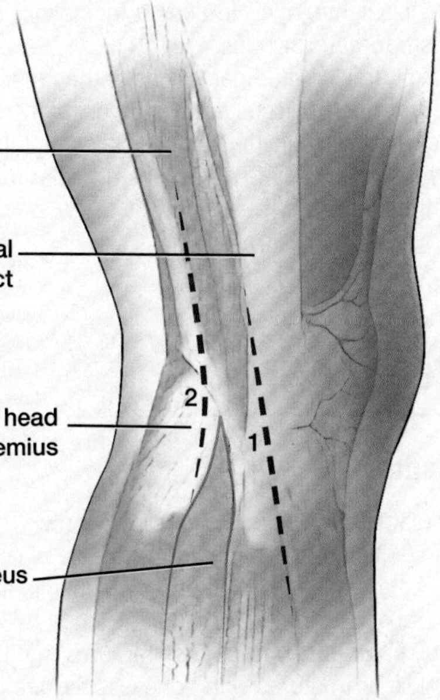

TECH FIG 2 Posterolateral approach to the lateral tibial plateau.

REDUCTION

- Careful treatment of the soft tissue and periosteum is mandatory.
- Reduction is aided by ligamentotaxis. An external fixator or a distractor may be a helpful tool.
- Displaced fragments are reduced.
  - One technique is to use a tamp, which can be inserted through a distal tibial bone window **(TECH FIG 3A)**.
  - Reduction is temporarily maintained with Kirschner wires or lag screws **(TECH FIG 3B)**.
- Depressed fragments need to be elevated.
  - Elevation is achieved by carefully hitting the tamp (eg, with a mallet) under fluoroscopy until the contour of the subchondral bone is reestablished.
  - Direct visualization of the articular surface is still recommended.
- Defects created by depression should be filled with bone graft (most commonly allograft) or bone graft substitute **(TECH FIG 3C)**.

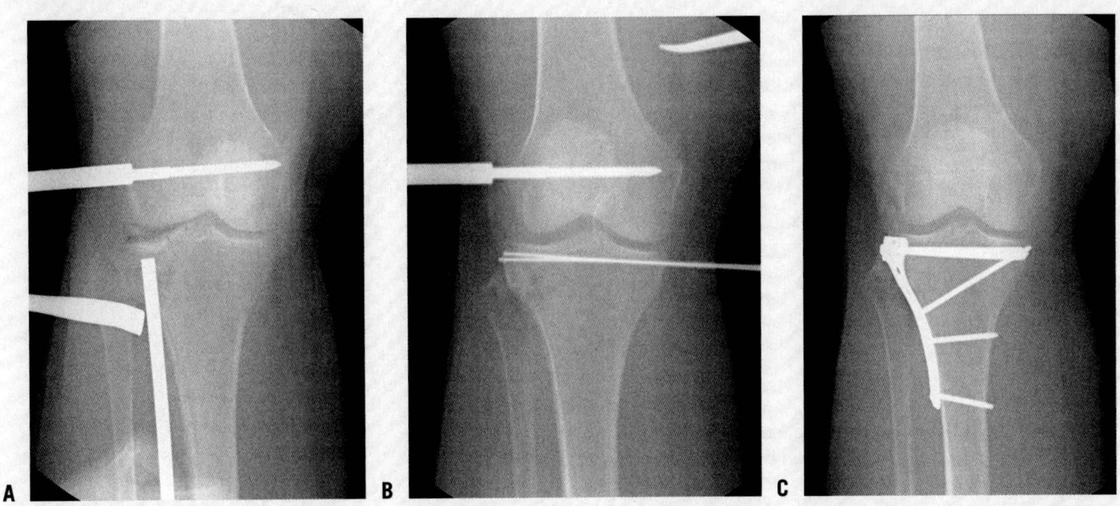

TECH FIG 3 A. Tamp-assisted fracture reduction. **B.** Temporary reduction held in place with Kirschner wires. **C.** Final reduction and fixation construct.

MENISCAL REPAIR

- Meniscal integrity is important for stability and to avoid posttraumatic arthritis.
- Peripheral longitudinal lesions of the anterior and intermediate part of the meniscus are fixated using the "outside-in suture" technique. The joint is open at this point through the submeniscal arthrotomy to assess the articular reduction and integrity of the meniscus.
- Lateral meniscus tears tend to be at the meniscocapsular junction. There is also bare area at the popliteal hiatus where the meniscus is not attached to the capsule.
- Peripheral longitudinal lesions of the posterior meniscus are fixated using the "all-inside" technique to avoid injury to the neurovascular structures in the popliteal area.
- Complex meniscal lesions in the avascular area require resection.

OSTEOSYNTHESIS

Implants

- Implants may include cancellous screws, cortical screws, conventional plates, or angular stable plates.
  - Lateral plating, locking or nonlocking, should be used in most cases.
- Multifragmentary fractures, fractures that breach the lateral cortex, or fractures with bone loss require plate osteosynthesis.
- For multifragmentary fractures or fractures with bone loss, no evidence-based advantage of locking plates versus nonlocking plates has been shown. However, locking plates in these types of plateau fractures are advisable:
  - Elderly patients with poor bone quantity and quality
  - The stability of angular stable plates does not depend on friction between the plate and the bone. There is also a theoretical advantage of less compression of the periosteum, with consequent better blood supply to the fracture area.
- Precontoured locking or nonlocking plates are available and make plate application easier.
- A minimally invasive technique can sometimes be used by sliding the plate beneath an intact soft tissue envelope and placing the distal screws percutaneously.

Pure Split Fractures of the Lateral Plateau (AO 41-B1 or Schatzker I)

- For fixation, two large, partially threaded cancellous screws or lag screws with/without washers can be used in younger patients, with great bone and minimally displaced fractures **(TECH FIG 4)**.
- Plate fixation in a buttress position is commonly used and is biomechanically stronger than screws alone.
- In general, a B type, partial articular fracture is treated with buttress plating (B is for buttress).
- In elderly or osteopenic patients, plate fixation is strongly recommended.

Pure Depression Fractures of the Lateral Plateau (AO 41-B2 or Schatzker III)

- The depression is elevated through a cortical window or osteotomy. The fracture may be fixed with subchondral cancellous screws, but in general, plate fixation with rafting screws is recommended. In cases of bone loss and/or voids left after fragment elevation/reduction, bone graft or bone graft substitute is recommended.
- In osteopenic patients, plate fixation with filling of any voids (bone graft or substitute) is recommended.

Split Depression Fracture of the Lateral Plateau (AO 41-B3 or Schatzker II)

- The depression is elevated by working through the split component and insertion of bone graft/bone void filler.
- The articular surface should be reduced, and the joint surface compressed.
- Screws are placed in the subchondral bone to support the elevated joint surface (rafting), and a locking plate or buttress plate is applied **(TECH FIG 5)**.

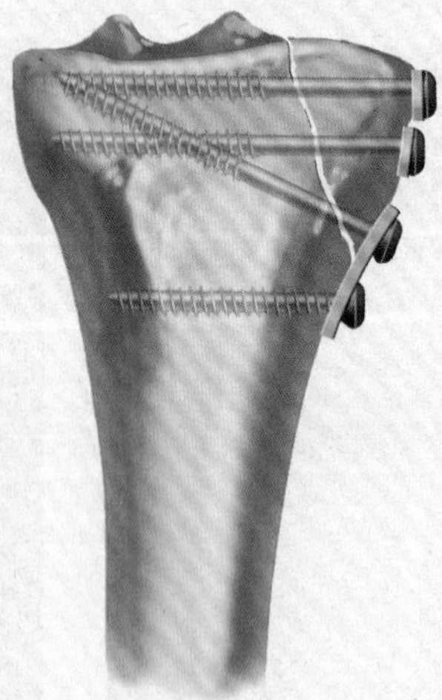

TECH FIG 4 Stabilization of B1 or Schatzker I fracture with two lag screws and two-hole plate in antiglide position.

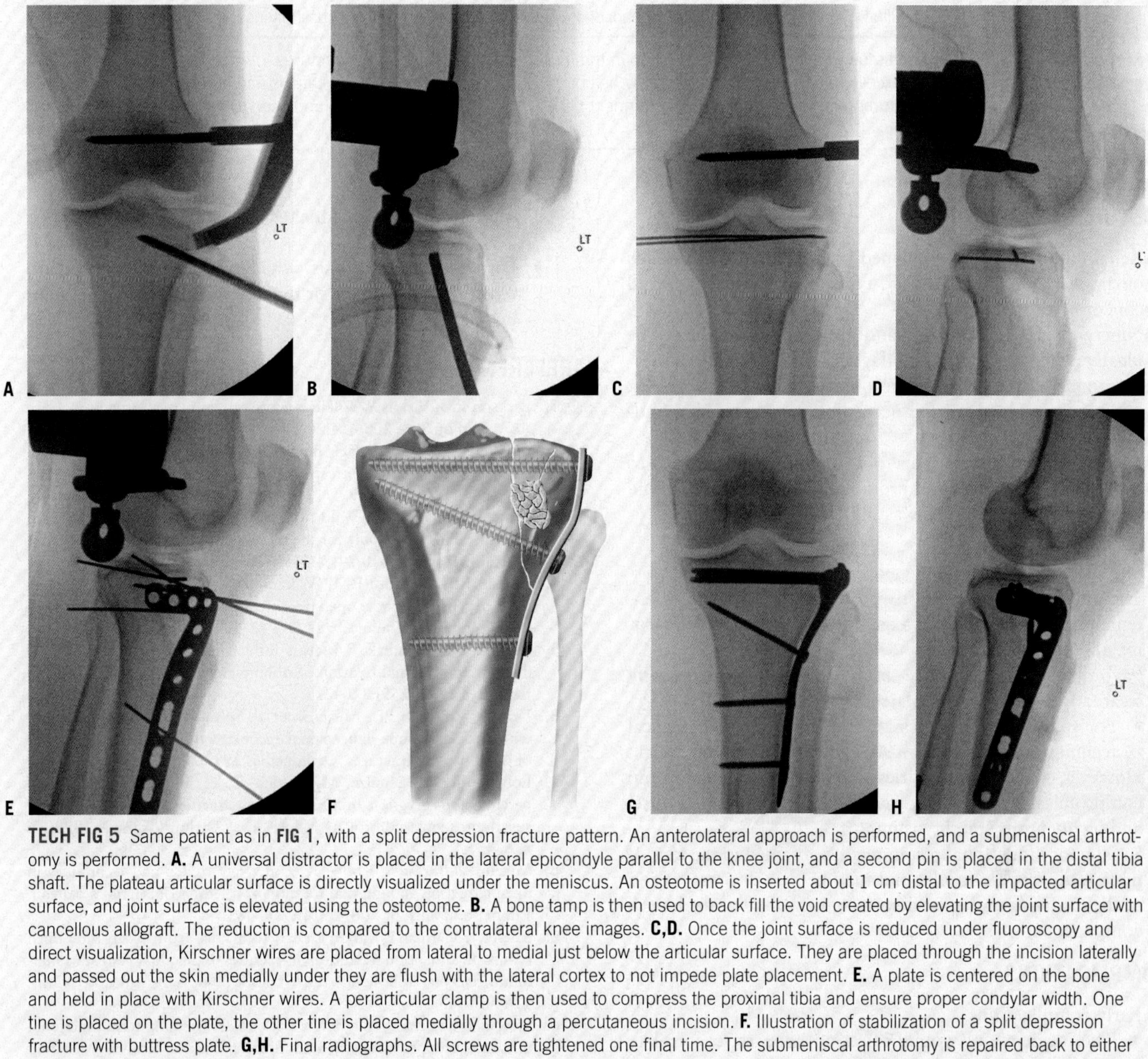

TECH FIG 5 Same patient as in **FIG 1**, with a split depression fracture pattern. An anterolateral approach is performed, and a submeniscal arthrotomy is performed. **A.** A universal distractor is placed in the lateral epicondyle parallel to the knee joint, and a second pin is placed in the distal tibia shaft. The plateau articular surface is directly visualized under the meniscus. An osteotome is inserted about 1 cm distal to the impacted articular surface, and joint surface is elevated using the osteotome. **B.** A bone tamp is then used to back fill the void created by elevating the joint surface with cancellous allograft. The reduction is compared to the contralateral knee images. **C,D.** Once the joint surface is reduced under fluoroscopy and direct visualization, Kirschner wires are placed from lateral to medial just below the articular surface. They are placed through the incision laterally and passed out the skin medially under they are flush with the lateral cortex to not impede plate placement. **E.** A plate is centered on the bone and held in place with Kirschner wires. A periarticular clamp is then used to compress the proximal tibia and ensure proper condylar width. One tine is placed on the plate, the other tine is placed medially through a percutaneous incision. **F.** Illustration of stabilization of a split depression fracture with buttress plate. **G,H.** Final radiographs. All screws are tightened one final time. The submeniscal arthrotomy is repaired back to either soft tissue from the proximal tibia or the plate.

TECHNIQUES

Pearls and Pitfalls

Meniscal Repair	• Meniscal repair is crucial to reduce the incidence of degenerative changes after tibial plateau fractures. Even a failed meniscal repair that requires subsequent meniscotomy can be protective of the underlying cartilage.
Articular Depression	• Articular depression is a major determinant of posttraumatic arthritis. After surgical management, no articular depression should be present. However, secondary articular depression may occur due to loss of fixation. To prevent secondary articular depression, sufficient bone graft or bone graft substitute should be used together with internal fixation to stabilize tibial plateau depression fractures. However, tibial plateau depression fractures with a poorer articular reconstruction may still have a good functional outcome if meniscal integrity is preserved. • Excessive soft tissue stripping may increase the risk for infection and nonunion. Therefore, soft tissue preserving techniques with the least possible soft tissue stripping should be used.

Bone Grafting	• Iliac crest bone grafting is always an option but is used less often now than in the past. Allograft bone graft is recommended due to decreased donor site morbidity and has equivalent outcomes. Bone substitutes such as coralline hydroxyapatite and calcium phosphate cements have also been successfully used.
Soft Tissue Assessment	• Soft tissue assessment is a pivotal step in the management of tibial plateau fractures. • An excellent reduction and fixation may be compromised by soft tissue complications and/or infection. • Fractures with severe soft tissue impairment benefit from external stabilization and secondary open reduction and internal fixation.

POSTOPERATIVE CARE

- Rehabilitation must be planned individually and depends on patient age, bone quality, type of osteosynthesis, and concomitant injury.
- Ninety degrees of flexion and full extension should be ideally achieved by 10 to 14 days.
- Toe-touch weight bearing is recommended for 6 to 8 weeks, with progression thereafter according to radiographic findings and symptoms.
- Early mobilization and range-of-motion exercises are key to the successful treatment of proximal tibia fractures to avoid knee stiffness and muscle wasting.

OUTCOMES

- The outcome depends mostly on the restoration and maintenance of the mechanical axis, knee stability, joint congruity, and meniscal integrity.
- Favorable outcomes have been reported for surgically treated low-energy tibial plateau fractures.[10]
  - For split and split depression fractures, adequate surgical techniques yield more than 90% good and excellent results.[7]
- However, concomitant injuries of ligaments and menisci can compromise the outcome. Therefore, maintaining menisci and ligamentous stability is important.
- Satisfactory functional results can be obtained in the face of poor radiographic results and may be due to preservation of the meniscus and its ability to bear the load of the lateral compartment.

COMPLICATIONS

- Early complications
  - The incidence of wound infection appears to correlate with the injury severity, soft tissue damage, surgical techniques, and the amount of hardware implanted and ranges from 0% to 32%.[13]
  - Deep vein thrombosis rates are reported to be 5% to 10%, and pulmonary embolus occurs in 1% to 2% of patients.[2,5]
- Late complications
  - Loss of fixation with axial malalignment and valgus deformity
  - Malunion as a consequence of inadequate reduction or loss of reduction
  - Posttraumatic arthrosis, which may result from the initial chondral damage or may be related to residual joint incongruity[9]

REFERENCES

1. Berkson EM, Virkus WW. High-energy tibial plateau fractures. J Am Acad Orthop Surg 2006;14:20–31.
2. Blokker CP, Rorabeck CH, Bourne RB. Tibial plateau fractures. An analysis of the results of treatment in 60 patients. Clin Orthop Relat Res 1984;(182):193–199.
3. Frosch KH, Balcarek P, Walde T, et al. A new posterolateral approach without fibula osteotomy for the treatment of tibial plateau fractures. J Orthop Trauma 2010;24(8):515–520.
4. Gustilo RB, Mendoza RM, Williams DN. Problems in the management of type III (severe) open fractures: a new classification of type III open fractures. J Trauma 1984;24:742–746.
5. Lachiewicz PF, Funcik T. Factors influencing the results of open reduction and internal fixation of tibial plateau fractures. Clin Orthop Relat Res 1990;(259):210–215.
6. Liow RY, Birdsall PD, Mucci B, et al. Spiral computed tomography with two- and three-dimensional reconstruction in the management of tibial plateau fractures. Orthopedics 1999;22:929–932.
7. Lobenhoffer P, Schulze M, Gerich T, et al. Closed reduction/percutaneous fixation of tibial plateau fractures: arthroscopic versus fluoroscopic control of reduction. J Orthop Trauma 1999;13:426–431.
8. Musahl V, Tarkin I, Kobbe P, et al. New trends and techniques in open reduction and internal fixation of fractures of the tibial plateau. J Bone Joint Surg Br 2009;91(4):426–433.
9. Saleh KJ, Sherman P, Katkin P, et al. Total knee arthroplasty after open reduction and internal fixation of fractures of the tibial plateau: a minimum five-year follow-up study. J Bone Joint Surg Am 2001;83(8):1144–1148.
10. Stevens DG, Beharry R, McKee MD, et al. The long-term functional outcome of operatively treated tibial plateau fractures. J Orthop Trauma 2001;15:312–320.
11. Tscherne H, Oestern HJ. A new classification of soft-tissue damage in open and closed fractures (author's transl) [in German]. Unfallheilkunde 1982;85:111–115.
12. Warner SJ, Garner MR, Schottel PC, et al. The effect of soft tissue injuries on clinical outcomes after tibial plateau fracture fixation. J Orthop Trauma 2018;32(3):141–147.
13. Young MJ, Barrack RL. Complications of internal fixation of tibial plateau fractures. Orthop Rev 1994;23:149–154.

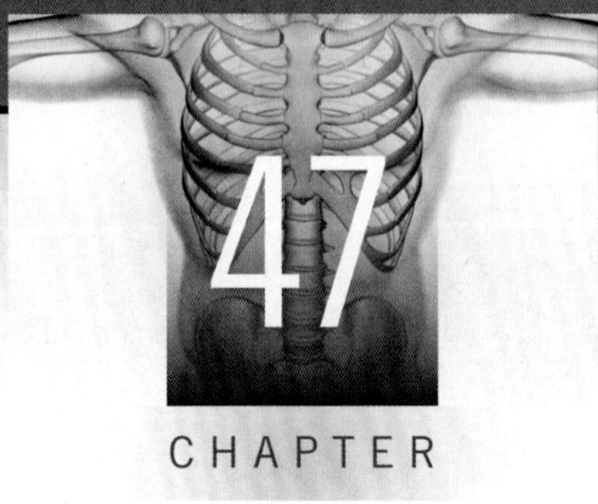

CHAPTER 47

Fixation of Posterior Tibial Plateau Fractures via Posterior Approaches

Stephen A. Kottmeier, Amanda C. Pawlak, and Erik Noble Kubiak

DEFINITION

- When managing articular fractures of the proximal tibia, the goals toward achieving a favorable long-term outcome include the preservation of motion, strength, stability, and painless function.[26,36]
- Required objectives include the operative restoration of both articular congruity and the limb mechanical axis.[32]
- Surgical requisites when executing osseous fixation include the preservation of regional blood supply to both osseous and soft tissue structures. The avoidance of complications demands a stable fixation construct that respects the vulnerability of the surrounding soft tissue envelope.[1,9,11,29,39]
- Until recently, posterior surgical approach strategies to the proximal tibial plateau have been met with understandable trepidation. Indications, once vague, are presently more clearly defined and approaches respecting the vulnerable regional anatomy increasingly familiar.
- Posteromedial approaches have been advocated for the treatment of posteromedial tibial plateau fractures and fracture-dislocations.[13–15] This can be combined with an anterolateral approach for bicondylar tibial plateau fractures during staged management, but it is difficult to perform concurrently with an anterolateral tibial plateau approach owing to patient positioning.
- Carlson[6] offered the posterolateral approach in combination with the posteromedial approach for the successful treatment of posterior dominant bicondylar shear fractures.

ANATOMY

- Anatomically, the posterior aspect of the proximal tibia affords three tissue planes: medial, middle, and lateral, all of which are part of the extensile posterior approach.
- The medial tissue plane is bounded superiorly by the semimembranosus muscle, the medial head of the gastrocnemius laterally, and the soleus and popliteus inferiorly. The inferior medial geniculate neurovascular bundle is at risk during this dissection if not disrupted by fracture displacement **(FIG 1A)**.

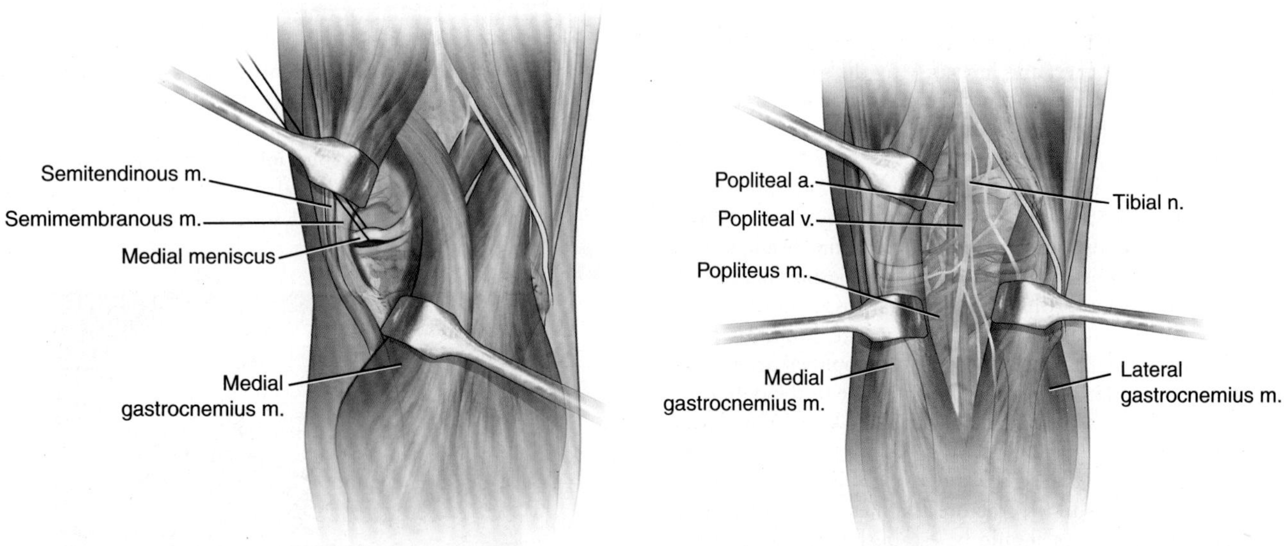

A **B**

FIG 1 A. Posteromedial tibial plateau approach described by Lobenhoffer.[25] The posteromedial approach offers easy access to the posterior aspect of the medial tibial plateau. Reduction and application of buttress fixation of medial coronal plane fractures within the medial plateau are facilitated by this exposure, which is posterior to the hamstring tendons and the medial collateral ligament. Visualization of the concave surface of the medial plateau is difficult. Reduction is provisionally performed via cortical reads, and the reduction of the articular surface is confirmed radiographically. **B.** Extensile posterior approach to the proximal tibia as described by Trickey[34] and more recently by Tscherne and Johnson.[22] Access to the posterior tibial plateau via the extensile posterior approach. Surgical access to the PCL insertion and origin is gained. *(continued)*

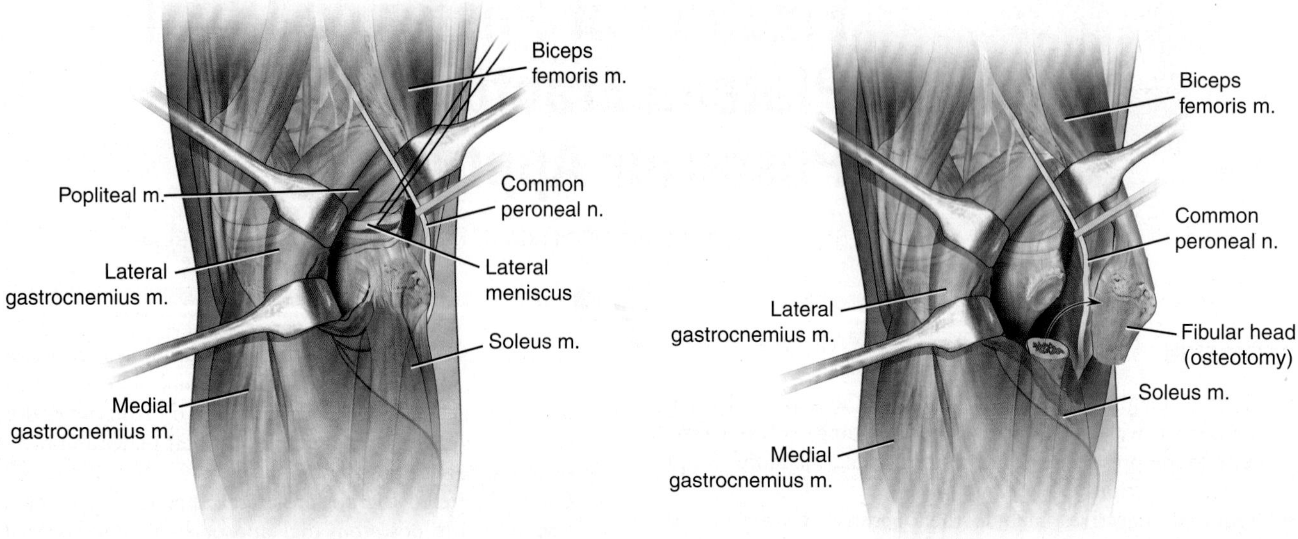

C D

FIG 1 *(continued)* **C.** Posterolateral approach to the proximal tibia. Note the position of the fibular head tends to obscure much of the view. This approach offers limited access to the posterolateral tibial plateau. Improved access can be obtained by a fibular osteotomy. **D.** Fibular osteotomy improves the view of the posterolateral plateau.

- The middle tissue dissection is bounded medially by the medial head of the gastrocnemius, laterally by the lateral head of the gastrocnemius, and inferiorly by the popliteus muscle. The posterior tibial nerve, artery, and venous drainage are at greatest risk during this approach. The rich venous return coming from the gastrocnemius heads is tedious to dissect during this approach plane **(FIG 1B)**.[40]
- The lateral dissection is bounded superiorly by the popliteus muscle, medially by the lateral head of gastrocnemius, laterally by the posterior aspect of the fibula and the common peroneal nerve, and inferiorly by the soleus. The common peroneal nerve and popliteal artery and nerve are at risk **(FIG 1C)**. Proximal fibular osteotomy can be used to improve exposure **(FIG 1D)**.[42]
- The popliteal artery passes through the popliteal fossa terminating at the lower border of the popliteus muscle, whereupon it divides into its two terminal branches: the anterior and posterior tibial arteries. The popliteal artery passes obliquely through the popliteal fossa and then travels between the gastrocnemius and popliteal muscles of the posterior compartment of the leg. The popliteal artery gives off five genicular branches that contribute to the periarticular genicular anastomosis that supply the knee joint capsule and ligaments.
- Ligaments/tendons/menisci: Owing to the proximity of regional soft tissues to fracture fragments, the integrity of regional soft tissues should be established (physical examination, imaging, operative inspection). Required surgical access to fracture components should not render these soft tissues at risk.
- Osseous anatomy: Because of an increased recognition of the limitations of surgical approaches and implant design, the concept of anatomic osseous columns or quadrants has emerged. This has endorsed classification schemes based on an axial perspective.
- Pathoanatomy
  - Conventional two-dimensional (coronally based) classifications suffer with regard to the characterization of posterior shearing or coronal plane fractures that involve the retrotibial proximal articular surface. Such classifications endorse primarily medial and/or lateral fixation.
  - Contemporary classifications of tibial plateau fractures have increasingly adopted an axially based "three-column" scheme or one consisting of "quadrants." This perspective has provided surgeons with a better understanding of plausible and often necessary circumferential access to the proximal tibia.[7,20,23,27,41]
  - Luo et al[27] described a three-column, CT-based classification for complex multiplanar tibial plateau fractures **(FIG 2)**. Using axial CT analysis, the tibial plateau is divided into three regions: lateral, medial, and posterior columns.

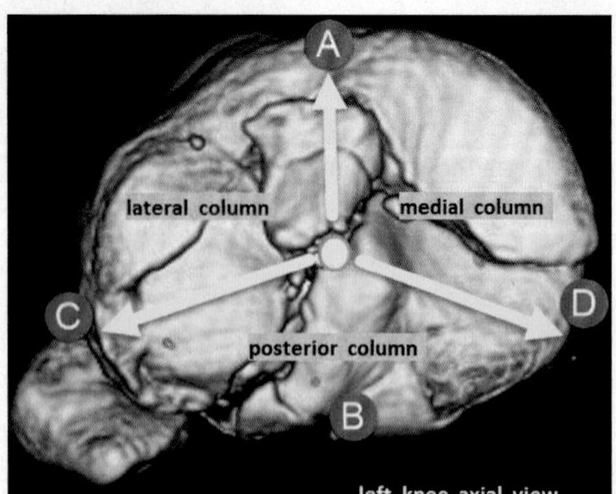

FIG 2 Three-column classification.[27] Recently evolving classification schemes emphasize an axial rather than sagittal or coronal perspective.

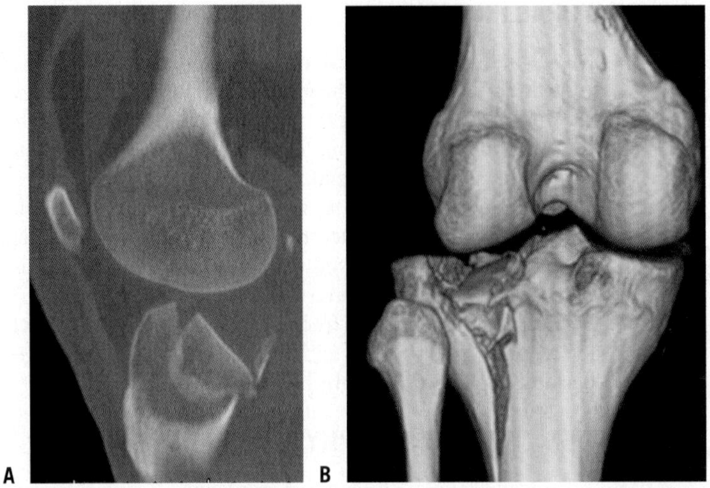

FIG 3 Posterolateral tibial plateau fracture. **A.** CT scan sagittal view shows large vertically oriented fragment within lateral compartment. **B.** 3-D CT posterior perspective shows large vertically oriented fragment within lateral compartment.

To conform to the three-column fracture assignment, at least one independent articular fragment must remain within each of the three columns. Alternatively, Chang et al[7] offered a four-quadrant scheme with similar requisites.

PATHOGENESIS

- Posterolateral unicondylar fractures
  - Usually, the result of low-energy mechanisms of axial compression with the knee in a flexed position.
  - Typically comminuted with a large, vertically oriented articular portion, which is often not appreciated on conventional radiographs compared to posteromedial "shear" patterns **(FIG 3A)**.
  - The vertical orientation of the articular portion favors posterolateral access; however, this exposure offers only a small aperture for safe reduction and fixation **(FIG 3B)**.
- Medial fracture-dislocations (Moore type 1)
  - Moore type 1 fractures can be mistakenly interpreted as a lateral or bicondylar fracture pattern and subsequently accessed and fixated inadequately **(FIG 4A)**.
  - These fractures may present with articular extension within the lateral compartment; yet, the lateral cortical column remains intact. This may be confirmed with review of a preoperative computed tomography (CT) scan **(FIG 4B)**.
  - Unicondylar, sagittally oriented fractures are receptive to conventional, anterior midline approaches.[12] Conversely, those with oblique or primarily coronally oriented fracture planes require posterior retrocondylar access and fixation **(FIG 4C)**.
- Bicondylar fractures with coronally oriented posteromedial fractures
  - Posteromedial fragments of significance may be present in 60% to 70% of Orthopaedic Trauma Association

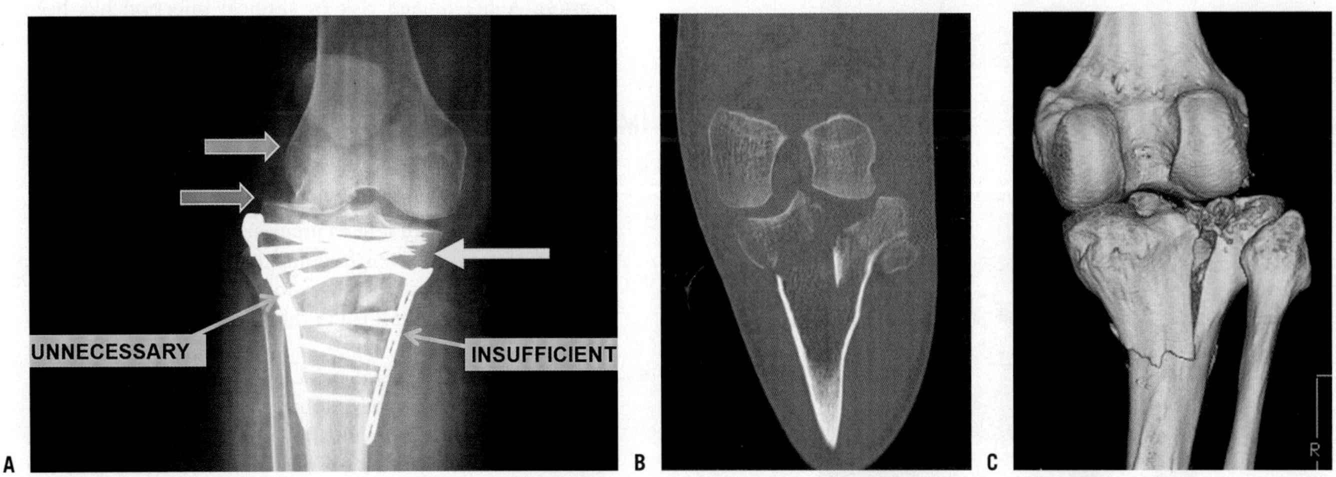

FIG 4 A. Right knee AP postoperative radiograph of Moore type 1 medial fracture-dislocation after improper assessment and fixation. This fracture was misinterpreted as a bicondylar variant. The lateral plate serves no purpose, and the medial condyle (*yellow arrow*) is inadequately reduced and fixated. The overlying asymmetry of the lateral articular surfaces (*blue arrows*) is secondary to medial condylar malreduction. There is no fracture involving the lateral condyle other than some articular impaction. **B.** In a different patient, a coronal view CT scan shows a Moore type 1 medial fracture of the right knee with no breach of the lateral cortical column. **C.** A posterior perspective 3-D CT scan reveals a medial condylar fragment in typical varus and an entrapped fragment within the osseous surfaces, which may inhibit reduction.

(OTA) C-type bicondylar fractures and may encompass as much as 25% of the entire joint surface.[2,19]
  - Unrecognized or inadequate fixation of a posteromedial fragment may result in articular incongruity and limb malalignment.[37]
  - Contemporary laterally applied locking plates may not offer sufficient fixation or engage the posteromedial fragment.[41] Plate design and placement may influence the capture of the posteromedial fragment. Plates introduced in a buttress mode to the retrocondylar surface may obviate these concerns.
- Combined "dual" posterior (medial and lateral) shear fractures
  - Secondary to axial loading of the knee in flexion resulting in both posteromedial and posterolateral fracture patterns, often without any compromise of the anterior cortical osseous elements of the proximal tibia.
  - With more force applied, anterior subluxation of the tibia on the femur may result in compromise to the lateral meniscus and anterior cruciate ligament (ACL). The potential for popliteal vessel injury exists and should be observed for.
  - The medial component is typically not comminuted and is often coronally oriented. The posterolateral fragment is typically comminuted with a vertically oriented articular component **(FIG 5)**.
  - Reduction and fixation is performed with dual simultaneous posteromedial and posterolateral exposures performed with the patient in the prone position.

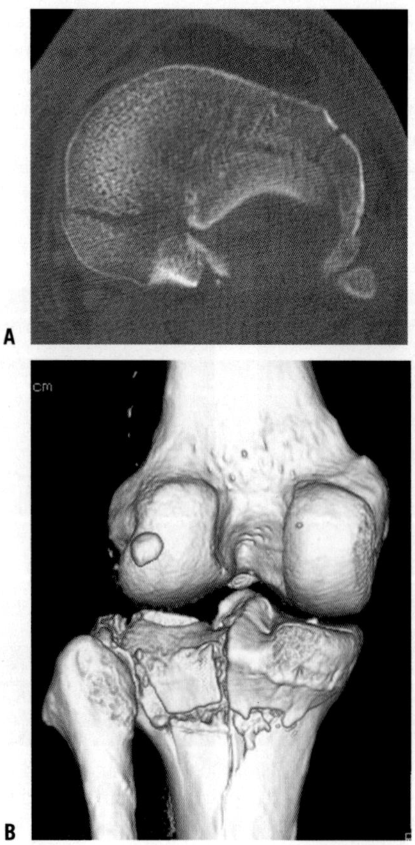

FIG 5 Combined ("dual") posterior bicondylar shear fractures of the left knee. **A.** Axial view CT scan shows a coronal split medial fracture/vertically oriented lateral fracture. **B.** Posterior perspective 3-D CT scan.

NATURAL HISTORY

- Most high-energy periarticular injuries are treated in a staged manner wherein the knee is initially stabilized in an external fixator, allowing the soft tissue envelope to evolve to the point that swelling is resolving and any fracture blisters have reepithelialized.
- The decision to proceed with open reduction and internal fixation can be made once the soft tissue envelope is less vulnerable and has moved past the acute inflammatory phase (typically more than 5 days).
- Healing of metaphyseal fractures generally occurs slowly by creeping substitution and therefore requires prolonged periods of protected weight bearing (10 to 12 weeks).

PATIENT HISTORY AND PHYSICAL EXAMINATION

- Advanced trauma life support guidelines. Comprehensive physical examination to determine all associated injuries.
- Patient history detailing the mechanism of injury. High- versus low-energy mechanisms must be considered.
- Assessment of any additional extremity, spine, pelvic, and closed cavity lesions. Prone positioning may be contraindicated in polytraumatized individuals.
- Adequate history detailing social history, medical comorbidities, and an assessment of anticipated patient compliance with postsurgical protocols.
- Thorough examination of the affected lower leg including documenting the neurovascular status of the limb. Fracture patterns (Moore type 1 and bilateral posterior shear) properly indicated for posterior access are at heightened risk for associated traumatic vascular compromise. Ankle–brachial indices should be obtained; values less than 0.9 should trigger a vascular consult.
- Soft tissue injuries should be documented as well as previous scars noted and their origins documented. A high index of suspicion should be maintained for compartment syndrome before and after placement of external fixation, if employed. Fasciotomy wounds should be strategized to accommodate subsequent staged surgical access and fixation. A heightened risk of surgical infection has been demonstrated in the presence of open fractures and closed degloving injuries.

IMAGING AND OTHER DIAGNOSTIC STUDIES

- Conventional radiographs
  - Orthogonal radiographs of the knee to include anteroposterior (AP) and lateral images.
  - Contralateral knee orthogonal images: AP and lateral. Contralateral radiographs allow the surgeon to reconstruct the fractured knee in the mirror image of its uninjured partner.
- CT scan analysis: general principles—posteromedial, posterolateral, and combined fracture variants
  - CT of the knee is invaluable in determining the exact pathoanatomic characteristics of the articular fracture pattern.
  - More contemporary classification systems describe high-energy tibial plateau fractures in terms of quadrants or columns, which may enhance circumferential conceptualization of the fracture pattern.[27]
  - If a staged approach is selected, the CT scan should be obtained after application of the spanning external fixator.

A distraction CT scan taken after transarticular external fixation determines
- The size and location of columnar components
- Regions and degree of articular impaction
- Osteoarticular fragment plane
- Integrity and location of inferior cortical apical spikes that may dictate preferential access and orientation of implants
- Incarcerated fragments that may preclude reduction

- MRI has been found to improve the detection of associated meniscal and ligamentous injuries occurring with tibial plateau fractures.[31] The role if any of preoperative MRIs to assess osseous and articular soft tissue lesions remains controversial.
- Venous Doppler studies: Fracture patterns of considerable complexity are often referrals and transferred from other facilities and consequently may be of several days or more chronicity. The treating surgeon must maintain a high index of suspicion for possible venous thromboembolism.

DIFFERENTIAL DIAGNOSIS

- Moore 1 versus Schatzker 4
  - Moore type 1 fractures represent a fracture-dislocation with the fracture fragment commonly obliquely oriented and in the semicoronal plane.
  - Schatzker type 4 fractures are sagittally oriented medial condyle fractures.
- "Bicondylar"—incorrect fracture type designation
  - Moore type 1 lesions incorrectly designated as bicondylar fractures
  - Moore type 1 present with an intact lateral cortical column
  - The perceived incongruence of the lateral condyle is due to impaction of the lateral femoral condyle within the central portion of the tibial eminence.
- Associated diagnoses
  - ACL injuries
  - Posterior cruciate ligament (PCL) injuries
  - Lateral and medial meniscus injuries
  - Popliteal artery intimal tear
  - Peroneal or posterior tibial nerve injuries
  - Deep vein thrombosis
  - Compartment syndrome

NONOPERATIVE MANAGEMENT

- Less than 2 mm of joint depression
- Less than 10 degrees of valgus or varus instability
- No evidence of tibial subluxation relative to the femur on AP and lateral images
- Knee immobilizer for 2 weeks, followed by initiation of active-assisted knee range of motion in a hinged knee brace. Non–weight bearing for 6 weeks, followed by progressive weight bearing to full weight bearing over a 4-week period.

SURGICAL MANAGEMENT

- Fracture-pattern specific reduction and fixation techniques and maneuvers
  - Moore type 1 medial fracture-dislocations
  - Bicondylar tibial fractures with staged fixation strategies
  - Isolated posterolateral fractures
  - Dual posterior shear fractures

Preoperative Planning

- Careful review of the radiographs and axial CT scan images to determine the injury pattern and location of joint impaction is key to determining a preferential surgical tactic.
- Injuries to the posterior lateral and/or medial plateau fractures are accessible via direct posterior approaches.

Positioning

- Posterior surgical approaches to the proximal tibia require proper patient preparation, positioning, and imaging. Posteromedial and posterolateral approaches are both receptive to prone positioning (described). Alternatively, the posteromedial approach can be performed in the supine position and the posterolateral in the lateral position. Similarly, a "floating" knee position, in which simultaneous approaches can be performed concurrently, has been described but offers considerable obstacles as well.[7,27]
- With the patient in the supine position (before prone positioning), a urinary catheter is inserted and a proximal thigh tourniquet applied. The patient is then placed prone with the affected limb on a well-padded support to allow unencumbered lateral imaging (FIG 6).

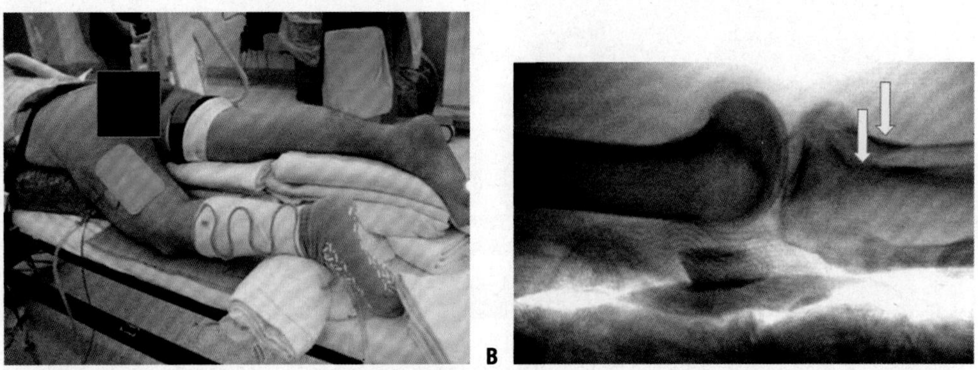
A B

FIG 6 Patient positioning. **A.** The surgeon is positioned opposite the affected limb, which is elevated to permit unobscured lateral fluoroscopic imaging. **B.** Lateral fluoroscopic imaging. Proper elevation and limb rotation permit satisfactory lateral imaging. The readily appreciated corresponding osseous surfaces (*arrows*) aid in reduction assessment.

- Bolsters are placed under the chest to allow the abdomen to remain free and the patient's face to remain free of compression. Attention needs to be paid to not inadvertently extend and retract the shoulders during positioning to avoid unnecessary traction on the brachial plexus.
- Hip hyperextension is avoided to prevent femoral neurapraxia. The image intensifier is situated on the affected side, and adequate AP and lateral images are confirmed.
- While prone, the affected extremity tends to assume a posture of external rotation. To obtain a true lateral image, a combination of hip hemipelvic bolsters and proper table rotation is required.
- When performing the Lobenhoffer (posteromedial) approach, the surgeon is positioned on the opposite side of the affected extremity.

Approach

- Posterolateral approach
- Posteromedial (Lobenhoffer) approach

POSTEROLATERAL APPROACH

- An 8- to 10-cm linear skin incision is performed along the medial border of the fibular head, beginning 2 cm above the popliteal crease **(TECH FIG 1A)**. Alternatively, an inverted L-shaped incision can be employed traversing the popliteal crease just superior to it. The subcutaneous tissue and popliteal fascia are next incised by sharp dissection.
- The peroneal nerve is identified along the posterior aspect of the biceps femoris muscle and tendon within the investing fascia and adipose tissue posterior to it **(TECH FIG 1B)**. It is exposed proximally and distally and mobilized distally to the level of the peroneal tunnel adjacent to the fibular neck. It is carefully protected to the lateral side. The lateral sural cutaneous nerve, a division of the peroneal nerve, sends a medial branch at the popliteal level, which is identified and protected medially **(TECH FIG 1C)**.
- The interval between the lateral head of the gastrocnemius and the peroneus longus is bluntly dissected to reveal the popliteus tendon overlying the origin of the soleus **(TECH FIG 1D)**. The lateral gastrocnemius muscle is retracted medially, and the soleus muscle is divided from its posterior attachment to the proximal fibula and tibia, from lateral to medial as needed to gain access to the fracture.
  - Vigorous retraction of the soleus should be avoided to prevent injury to the posterior neurovascular structures that lie on the dorsal surface of the soleus and are tethered to the tibia as the popliteal artery trifurcates.
  - The distal dissection distally should be limited to no more than 2.5 to 5 cm below the articular level. Inferior to this is the anterior tibial vessel, a main branch of the

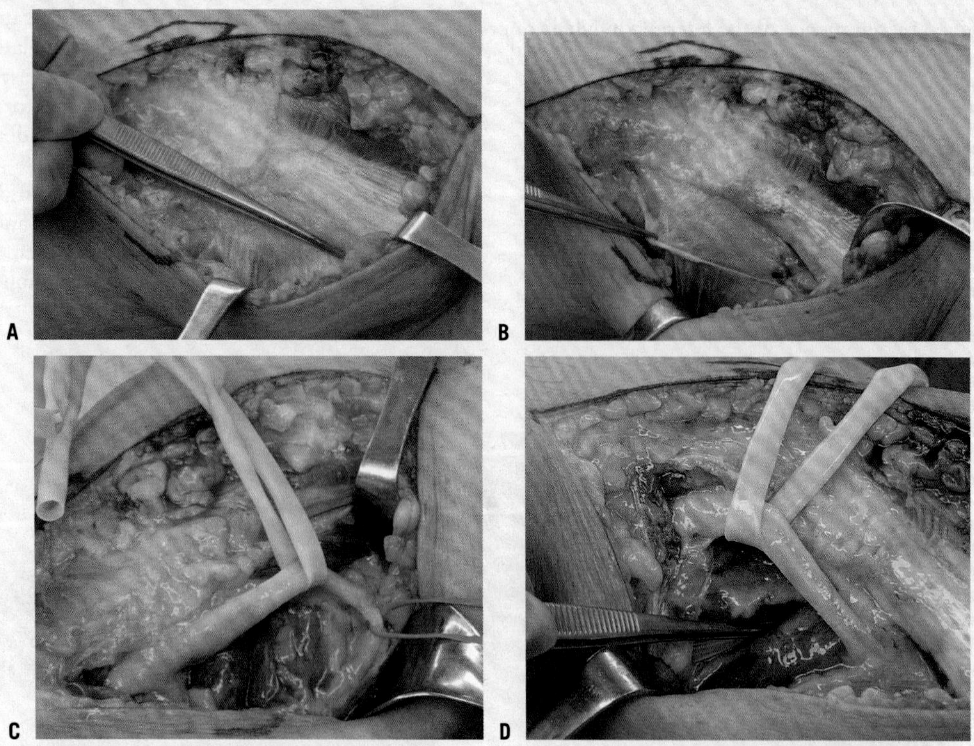

TECH FIG 1 Posterolateral approach to the left knee. **A.** The skin incision is along medial border of fibular head. **B.** Incision of the investing fascia posterior to the biceps reveals the underlying peroneal nerve. **C.** The peroneal nerve is mobilized and is within the penrose drain. Depicted within the blue vessel loop is the lateral sural cutaneous nerve. **D.** Intermuscular interval is developed. *(continued)*

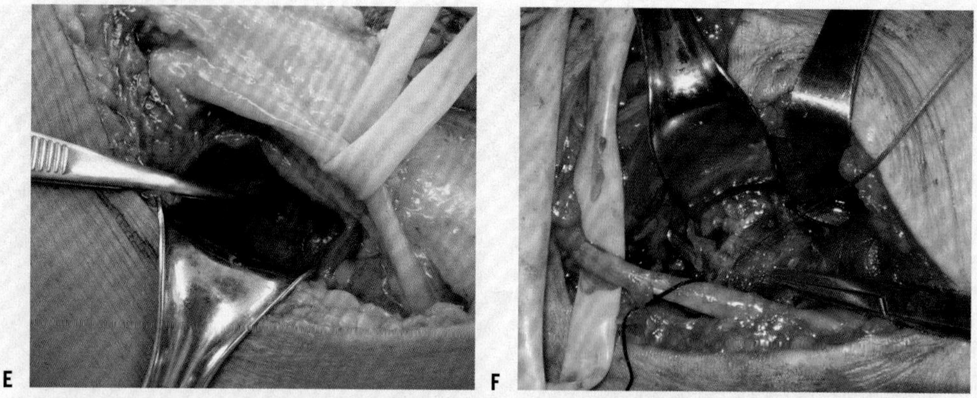

TECH FIG 1 *(continued)* **E.** Inferolateral genicular vascular bundle is identified and ligated. **F.** Popliteus tendon overlying clamp is tenotomized and secured with ligature for subsequent repair.

popliteal vessel, traversing between the tibia and fibular head within the upper margin of the interosseous membrane to reach the anterior compartment. Both surgical dissection and placement of retractors render it at risk.[18]

- The inferolateral genicular vascular bundle is identified and ligated **(TECH FIG 1E)**. The inferior margin of the popliteus muscle is dissected and mobilized superiorly. Alternatively, a tenotomy of the popliteus can be performed with subsequent repair upon completion of the procedure **(TECH FIG 1F)**. If further distal exposure is required for placement of a plate, the soleus origin may be partially elevated. The posterior ligamentocapsular complex is incised transversely and the lateral meniscus elevated superiorly to allow inspection of the posterior articular surface. Fracture fragment soft tissue attachments should be maintained to preserve osseous blood supply.
- Interposition of soft tissues, hematoma and osseous debris are evacuated with the knee in a position of flexion. Osteoarticular fracture fragment reduction can be performed and confirmed indirectly by assessing reduction of apical cortical spikes.

POSTEROMEDIAL (LOBENHOFFER) APPROACH

- Operative landmarks include the readily palpable and identifiable medial head of the gastrocnemius and hamstring tendons.
- Vertical, S-, and L-shaped incisions have all been described to initiate the operative exposure to the posterior aspect of the proximal tibia.[4,5,13,17] Commonly, a 6- to 8-cm linear incision is established medially just posterior to the palpable posteromedial tibial border **(TECH FIG 2A)**. It should be adjacent and colinear to the medial border of the medial head of the gastrocnemius. The incision ascends to, or just cranial to, the medial joint line.
- The short saphenous vein is identified within the sulcus between the two gastrocnemius heads. Full-thickness fasciocutaneous flaps are established to protect both the sural nerve and vein. With deeper dissection, the medial head of the gastrocnemius is next visualized, mobilized, and retracted laterally. The pes tendons and their attachments may be maintained or divided as necessary **(TECH FIG 2B)**.

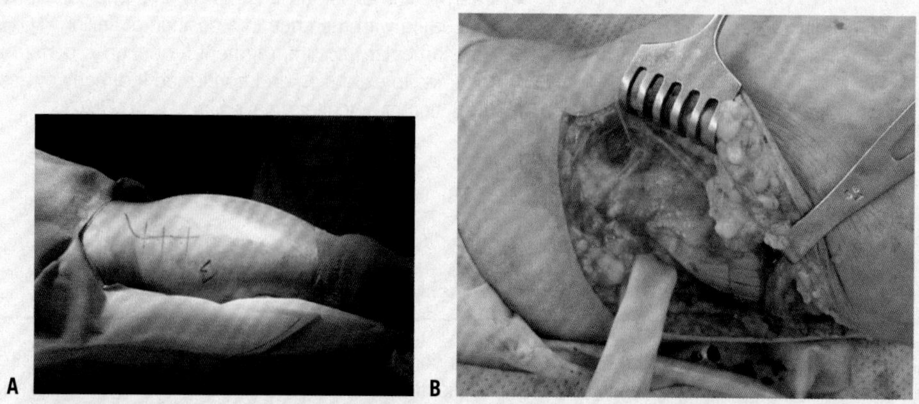

TECH FIG 2 Posteromedial (Lobenhoffer) approach to the right knee. **A.** A straight or curvilinear skin incision is made posterior to the palpable posterior tibial border. **B.** The medial gastrocnemius is bluntly developed and mobilized laterally. Pes tendons are pictured in penrose drain. *(continued)*

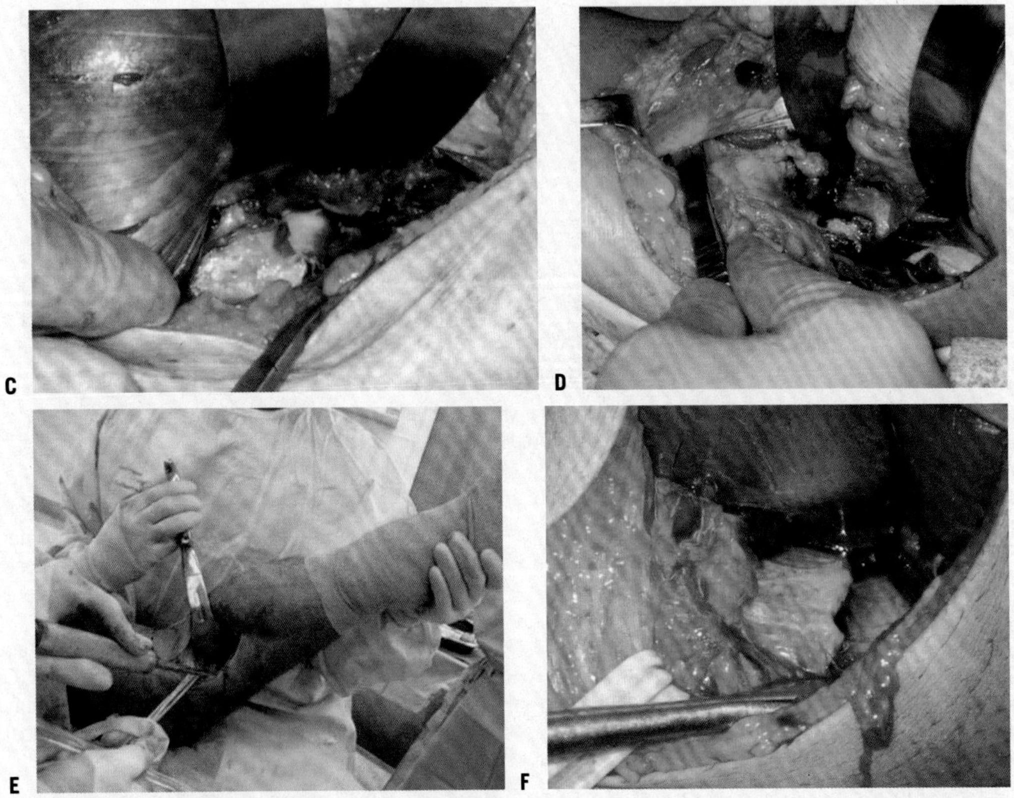

TECH FIG 2 *(continued)* **C.** Retractors are applied gently to lateral tibial border. **D.** The medial gastrocnemius tendon overlying instrument may be developed and divided as necessary to enhance lateral access. **E.** Knee flexion permits evacuation of interposed soft tissues and fracture hematoma. **F.** Knee extension facilitates reduction.

- The popliteal neurovascular bundle remains undissected. Medial to lateral dissection beneath the popliteus serves to protect it.
  - The popliteal vessels are neither formally encountered nor mobilized.
- The popliteus and soleus are elevated as required to gain access to the posterior column. The popliteus is mobilized laterally beginning at its medial margin. Retractors are positioned on the lateral tibial osseous margin, and gentle retraction is used to limit the risk of venous thrombosis and neurovascular injury **(TECH FIG 2C)**.
  - Surgical dissection within proximity of the proximal tibiofibular joint is discouraged to avoid injury to the posterior tibial recurrent artery.
- If exposure proves insufficient to gain adequate fracture site access, or implant insertion proves difficult, an alternative option includes conversion to a more extensile exposure. The skin incision is extended laterally in a curvilinear fashion across the popliteal crease. The tendon of the medial gastrocnemius is divided, with a retained stump, to aid in its subsequent reattachment **(TECH FIG 2D)**. Division of the tendon must remain inferior to its vascular contribution from the arterial trifurcation.
  - This more extensile modification affords increased lateral access, facilitating both reduction and fixation of those fracture variants extending within the lateral compartment.
- Interposition of soft tissues, hematoma and osseous debris are evacuated with the knee in a position of flexion **(TECH FIG 2E)**. Osteoarticular fracture fragment reduction is performed with the knee in extension and confirmed indirectly by assessing reduction of apical cortical spikes **(TECH FIG 2F)**.

REDUCTION AND FIXATION OF POSTEROLATERAL FRACTURES

- A standard lateral approach is not suitable to address the required exposure, reduction, and fixation of posterolateral shearing fractures. Reduction with conventional exposures may prove difficult in the absence of an intact posterior cortex. Fixation techniques employing lag screws introduced from anterior to posterior are insufficient. Biomechanical principles require the application of a direct posterolateral antiglide buttress plate.[8]
- Posterolateral exposure affords direct fracture visualization, permitting elevation and anatomic reduction of the vertically oriented posterolateral articular fragment. Grafting of the resultant

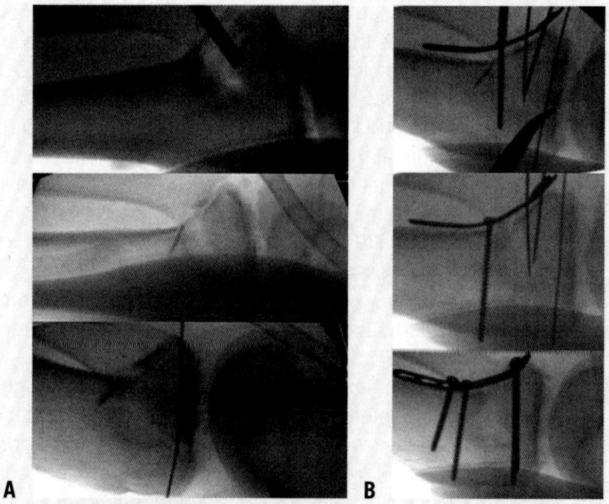

TECH FIG 3 Reduction and fixation of posterolateral fractures. **A.** Elevation and temporary transfixation with smooth Kirschner wires. **B.** Undercontoured plate secured with pull screws.

void is followed by buttress plating, permitting maintenance of reduction, and resistance to axial load.

- Medial retractors are carefully introduced to avoid shearing injuries to the geniculate vascular bundles. The popliteus muscle is identified, and the inferior lateral genicular artery traversing the muscular surface is ligated.
- The lateral head of the gastrocnemius is retracted laterally, and the popliteal muscle is bluntly elevated to enhance exposure of the posterior aspect of the proximal tibia. The popliteus muscle and the lateral head of gastrocnemius are retracted medially to expose the lateral aspect of proximal tibia and tibiofibular joint.
- The inferior border of the popliteus muscle is dissected and retracted superiorly, and the posterolateral wedge of the fracture is fully exposed. The posterior ligamentocapsular complex is opened transversely, and the meniscus is elevated and the fracture pattern examined. Division of the popliteus tendon may prove necessary if visualization of fracture site is compromised.
- The gastrocnemius, popliteus, and soleus should be mobilized bluntly to avoid compromising the oblique popliteal ligament. The soleus takes its origin from the posterior aspect of the fibula and tibia more distally than is generally required for an adequate exposure. Its origin may be partially elevated if further distal exposure is required for plate placement. Trifurcation vessels traversing the interosseus membrane limit safe dissection to within 5 to 10 cm distal to the lateral joint line.
- Anatomic reduction is achieved under direct visualization by hyperextension with axial traction and elevation of the fragment with the aid of a periosteal elevator or right angle clamp. For split-depression fractures, the articular surface is elevated by working through the cortical fracture site under direct vision to assess the quality of reduction. Cortical fracture fragment soft tissue attachments are preserved to preserve blood supply. The horn of lateral meniscus can be elevated and retracted to permit posterior articular surface visualization.
- The reduced fracture is fixed preliminarily with two or three Kirschner wires of 2.0-mm thickness, and the reduction is assessed fluoroscopically with posteroanterior (PA) and lateral projections **(TECH FIG 3A)**. The articular surface is anatomically restored by using a posterolateral buttress plate and void filler (autograft, allograft osteoplastic agents). Precontoured or modified conventional plates are introduced in buttress mode. With the inclusion of "pull" screws, intentionally undercontoured plates conform well to the retrocondylar osseous surface **(TECH FIG 3B)**. Subchondral screws are placed to support the elevated joint surface. Screws should not exit the anterior cortex, unless required for stability, as they may prove symptomatic.

REDUCTION AND FIXATION OF MOORE TYPE 1 MEDIAL FRACTURE-DISLOCATIONS

- Definition: obliquely or coronally oriented isolated fragment that involves a substantial portion of the posteromedial condyle.
- Frequently present as a fracture-dislocation with potential for associated concerning osseous and soft tissue injury.[10,28]
- May be mistakenly interpreted as a lateral tibial plateau fracture and incorrectly characterized as a "bicondylar" tibial plateau fracture. Careful scrutiny of imaging studies, particularly CT scans, will identify an intact cortical column laterally. The use of a laterally based approach with primarily lateral fixation likely will result in inadequate reduction and insufficient fixation. Isolated posteromedial split fractures of the tibial plateau are preferentially managed with a posteromedial (Lobenhoffer) approach with the patient placed in the prone position.[13,14,25]
- The posteromedial fracture is mobilized to allow for extraction of interposed hematoma, soft tissue, and osteochondral debris. Mobilization of the posteromedial fracture is facilitated by placing the patient's knee in a position of flexion. Placing the patient's knee in extension facilitates reduction. The inferior apex of the retrocondylar medial fracture serves as an indirect reduction aid and a means for effective fixation with the use of antiglide techniques.
- Occasionally, fracture patterns may extend laterally within the subchondral region of the lateral tibial condyle. This lateral

extension occurs in the absence of any lateral cortical compromise. Accurate reduction may necessitate extraction or reduction of these lateral osteochondral components, which require a more extensile version of the posteromedial (Lobenhoffer) approach.

- In such circumstances, the medial gastrocnemius tendon is sectioned proximally to enhance exposure, reduction, and subsequent fixation.[4] Sectioning of the gastrocnemius tendon should be performed inferior to its origin to limit compromise to its arterial supply.
- Fixation constructs may be extended laterally with the posteromedial (Lobenhoffer) approach to allow for reduction and fixation of the lateral articular components of these primarily medially oriented fractures.

Moore Type 1 Medial Fracture-Dislocation

- Isolated posteromedial split fractures and medial fracture-dislocations of the tibial plateau may be preferentially managed with a posteromedial (Lobenhoffer) approach with the patient placed in the prone position.
- A distraction CT scan obtained after transarticular external fixation determines the size and location of the medial condyle fracture and serves to direct ideal fixation strategy. Three-dimensional (3-D) CT reconstructions demonstrate the site of apical discontinuity. This facilitates the strategic placement of antiglide devices at the apex inferiorly. The inferior apex of the retrocondylar medial fracture serves as an indirect reduction aid and as means for effective fixation with the use of antiglide techniques **(TECH FIG 4A,B)**.
  - The reduction assessment is indirect and judged based on the adequacy of reduction of the apex of the fracture in addition to articular reduction demonstrated with intraoperative fluoroscopy.
- With the knee in a flexed position, the posteromedial fragment is mobilized and interposed soft tissue, osteochondral debris, and hematoma evacuated **(TECH FIG 4C)**. The articular surface is elevated by working through the fracture site under fluoroscopic guidance to assess the quality of reduction. Additionally, a linear incision within the medial collateral ligament may further confirm articular reconstitution.

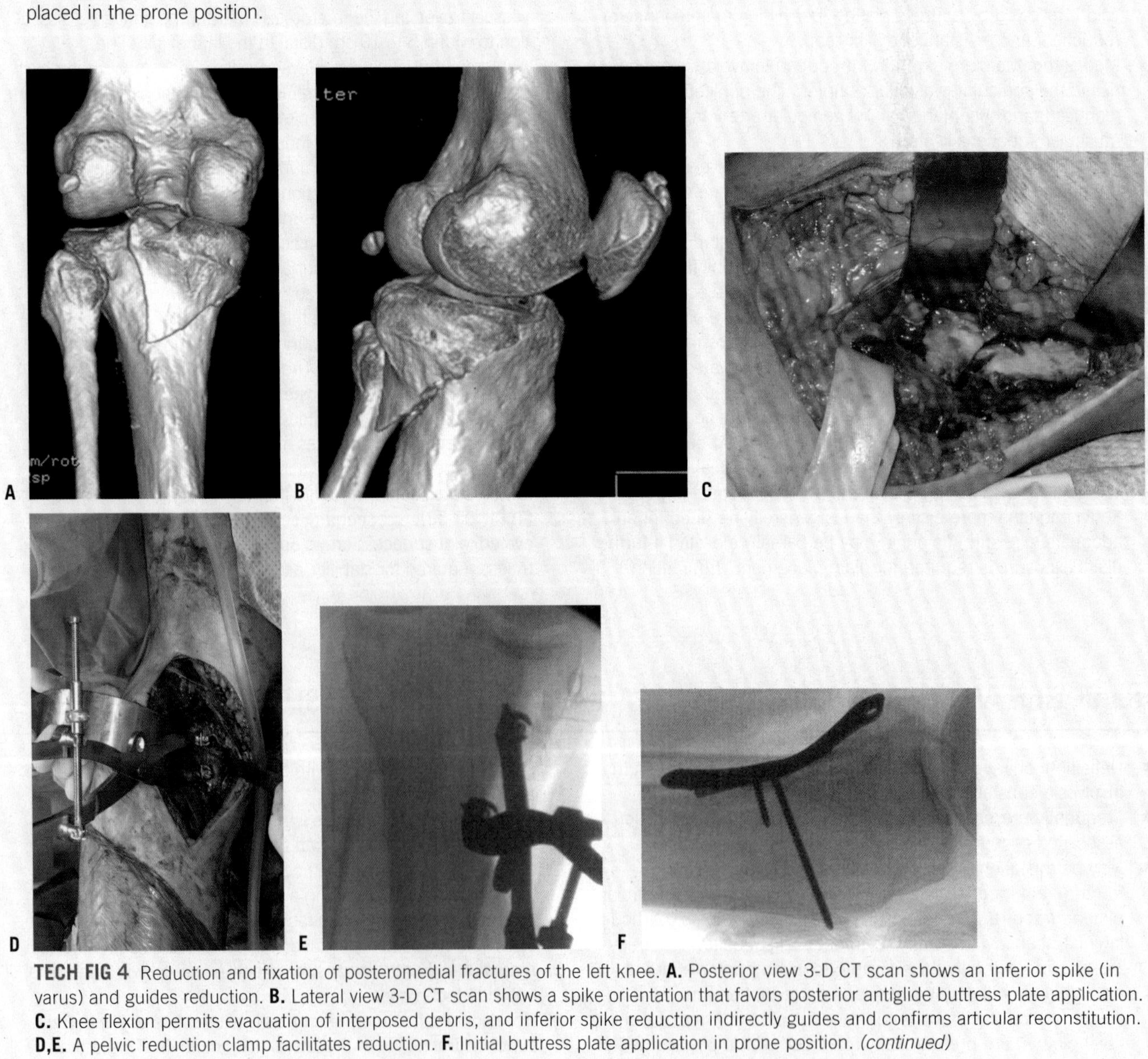

TECH FIG 4 Reduction and fixation of posteromedial fractures of the left knee. **A.** Posterior view 3-D CT scan shows an inferior spike (in varus) and guides reduction. **B.** Lateral view 3-D CT scan shows a spike orientation that favors posterior antiglide buttress plate application. **C.** Knee flexion permits evacuation of interposed debris, and inferior spike reduction indirectly guides and confirms articular reconstitution. **D,E.** A pelvic reduction clamp facilitates reduction. **F.** Initial buttress plate application in prone position. *(continued)*

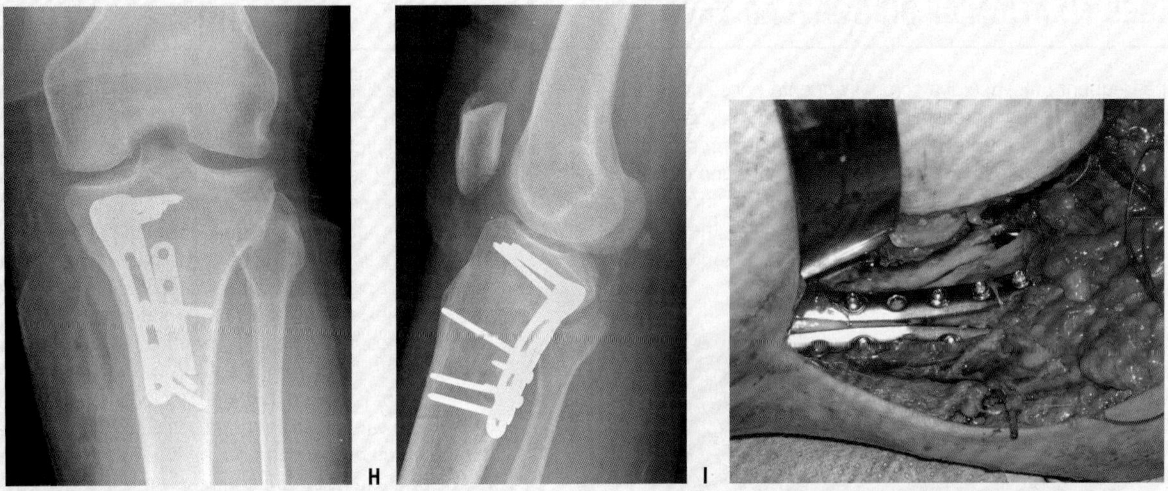

G H I

TECH FIG 4 *(continued)* **G,H.** AP and lateral views showing final reduction employing lag screw and buttress plate fixation. **I.** Medial column orthogonal plate construct.

- Reduction of the fracture is performed with imparted extension and valgus force to the knee, axial traction, and an anteriorly directed force to the fracture fragment (ball spike pusher or periosteal elevator). The introduction of a small pelvic reduction clamp (Jungbluth clamp) secured to temporary screws within each fracture component offers a powerful means toward overcoming varus force and regaining length **(TECH FIG 4D,E)**.
- The prone position (in contrast to supine) readily accommodates the extended knee position and valgus applied force facilitating reduction as well as the trajectory of implant insertion devices (drills, depth gauges, and screws) **(TECH FIG 4F)**.
- The reduced fracture is fixed preliminarily with two or three Kirschner wires, and the reduction is assessed by fluoroscopy in PA and lateral views.
- Stable fixation is attained using standard principles of lag screw technique and buttress plating where indicated **(TECH FIG 4G,H)**. Modified conventional plates, site-specific plates or, alternatively, angular stable dorsal antiglide plates may be employed.
  - On occasion, the fracture pathoanatomic characteristics (bone quality, comminution, fracture obliquity) may be requiring of orthogonal plate constructs **(TECH FIG 4I)**.

Moore Type 1 Medial Fracture-Dislocation with Lateral Intra-articular Extension

- Occasionally, fracture patterns may extend laterally within the subchondral region of the lateral femoral condyle **(TECH FIG 5A)**. This lateral extension occurs in the absence of any lateral cortical compromise. Accurate reduction may necessitate extraction or reduction of these lateral osteochondral components, which require a more extensile version of the posteromedial (Lobenhoffer) approach.
- In such circumstances, the medial gastrocnemius tendon is sectioned proximally to enhance exposure, reduction, and subsequent fixation. Division of the medial gastrocnemius tendon is performed inferior to its origin to limit compromise to its arterial supply. The medial head of the gastrocnemius muscle is then mobilized and retracted laterally.
- Access to articular components within the posterolateral tibial plateau is addressed by first mobilizing the medial condylar fragment, affording access to them. Fixation constructs may be extended laterally with the posteromedial approach to allow for reduction and fixation of the lateral extensions of these primarily medially oriented fractures **(TECH FIG 5B,C)**.

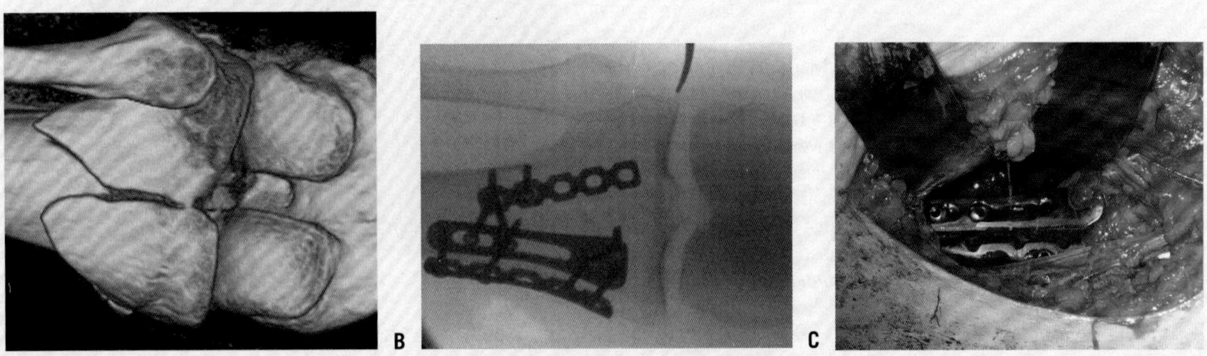

A B C

TECH FIG 5 Medial column fractures with lateral intra-articular extension. **A.** Unique fracture patterns with lateral columnar involvement may be receptive to extensile modification of the medial Lobenhoffer approach with or without medial gastrocnemius tendon tenotomy. **B,C.** PA fluoroscopic and intraoperative views show laterally applied plate introduced via posteromedial approach.

STAGED FIXATION OF BICONDYLAR VARIANTS

- The frequent presence of a coronally oriented posteromedial fragment has been increasingly appreciated in bicondylar fracture patterns. If unrecognized or inadequately reduced and fixated, articular incongruity and limb malalignment with compromised clinical outcomes may result.[37]
- To provide an adequate and preserved reduction, the surgeon may perform dual plate fixation, which uses both anterolateral and posteromedial approaches performed simultaneously in the supine position.[1,3,16]
- Typically, medial condyle reduction is performed first because the medial condyle is often less comminuted than its lateral counterpart and serves as a foundation on which to build the lateral articular and lateral column components.
- Adequate reduction and fixation of the posteromedial fragment with the patient placed in the supine position may be complicated by knee extension that is required for reduction as well as the limited exposure and conflicts with screw and drill trajectory **(TECH FIG 6)**.[38]
  - If the patient is placed in the supine position, the knee tends to drift into varus, which complicates both reduction and the maintenance of reduction during fixation. In this situation, valgus and extension are commonly required to provide effective reduction. Although overcome with some effort, these deforming forces are increasingly problematic as fracture complexity increases.
- Initial posteromedial column fixation performed in the prone position may overcome these obstacles if anticipated **(TECH FIG 7A)**. Implants initially introduced to afford posteromedial fixation should not conflict with subsequent constructs introduced laterally ("implant gridlock").
- Reduction and stabilization of the medial column **(TECH FIG 7B)** is followed by repositioning the patient supine and repreparation of the limb (same setting) for lateral column and lateral articular surface fixation **(TECH FIG 7C–E)**.[24]

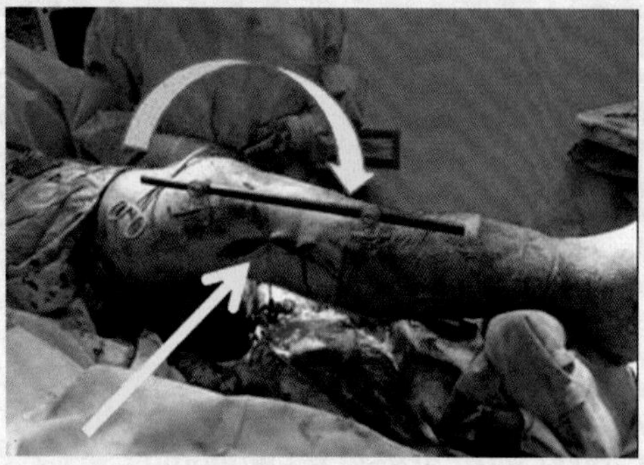

TECH FIG 6 Fixation of medial columnar fractures in the supine position may be hindered by required valgus and extension forces (*curved arrow*) as well as implant trajectory (*straight arrow*). In addition, the supine knee tends to fall into varus and flexion, which conflicts with required valgus and extension to contribute to reduction. The trajectory of implant insertion devices is often off axis, contributing to insertion difficulties.

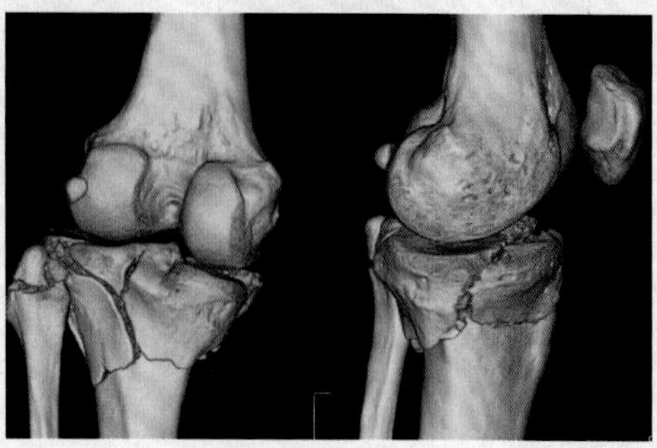

A

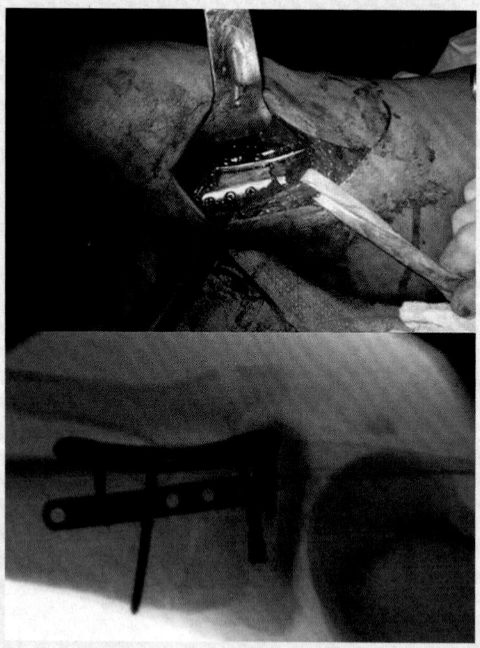

B

TECH FIG 7 Staged bicondylar reduction and fixation ("flip" prone then supine) of the left knee. **A.** 3-D CT reconstruction of a bicondylar variant in which stage fixation may prove desirable (posterior and medial sagittal perspectives). **B.** Left knee prone; the first stage is medial columnar reconstruction. Introduced implants should not conflict with subsequent implant insertion performed laterally while supine. *(continued)*

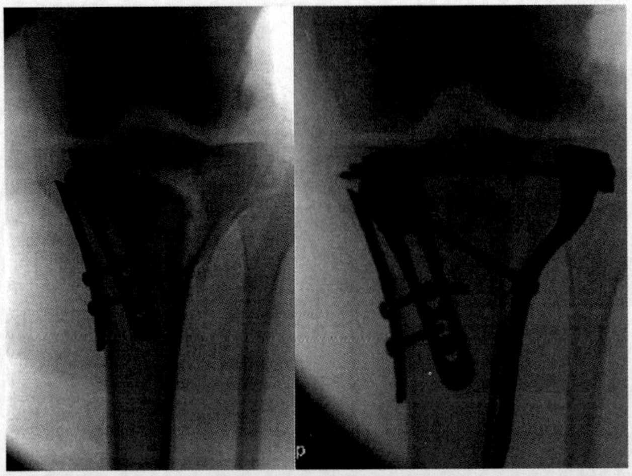
C

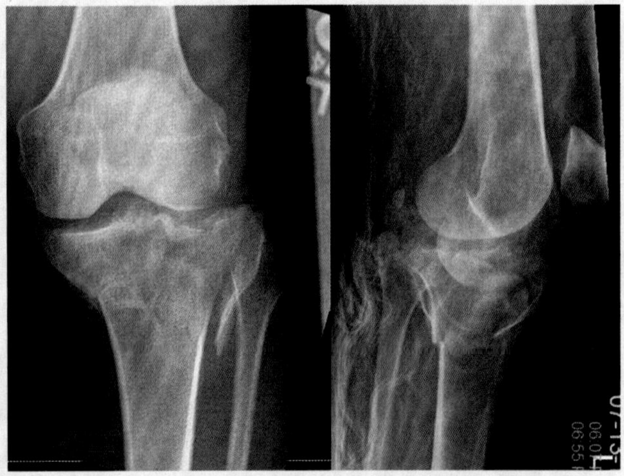
D

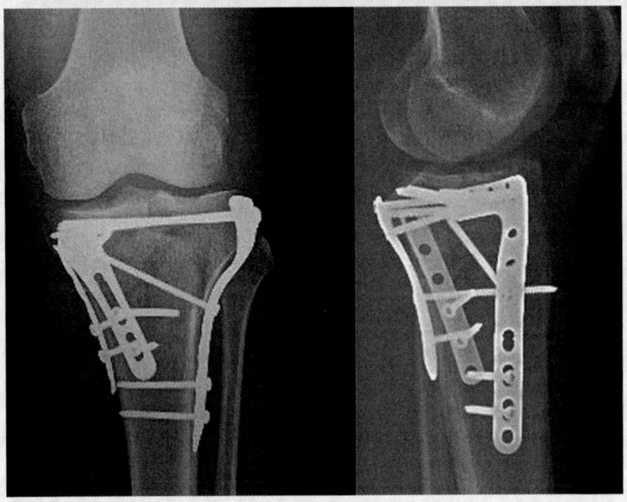
E

TECH FIG 7 *(continued)* **C.** Left knee medial columnar restoration (fluoroscopic view). The patient is repositioned supine followed by lateral reconstruction. **D.** AP and lateral preoperative radiographs. **E.** AP and lateral postoperative radiographs.

REPAIR OF POSTERIOR BICONDYLAR TIBIAL PLATEAU FRACTURES

- Description
  - Medial compartment; coronal shear, little or no comminution
  - Lateral compartment; comminuted and a significant vertically oriented articular fragment
- Surgical exposure
  - Combined posteromedial (linear incision) and posterolateral (curvilinear). Dual surgical skin incisions can be configured as required.
  - Dual exposure performed simultaneously in prone position **(TECH FIG 8A,B)**
    - It is beneficial to leave both exposures (posteromedial and posterolateral) open during the reduction and osteosynthesis. This permits resolution of implant conflicts ("gridlock") and offers the opportunity for minor reduction and fixation adjustments **(TECH FIG 8C,D)**.

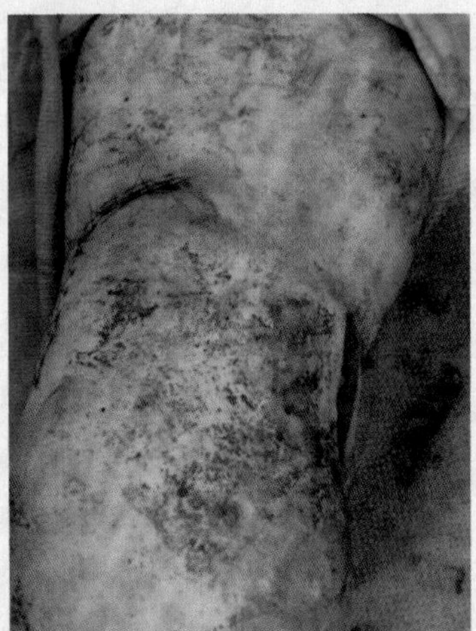
A

TECH FIG 8 Posterior bicondylar ("shear") fracture of the left knee). **A.** A lateral curvilinear incision or medial linear incision is made. *(continued)*

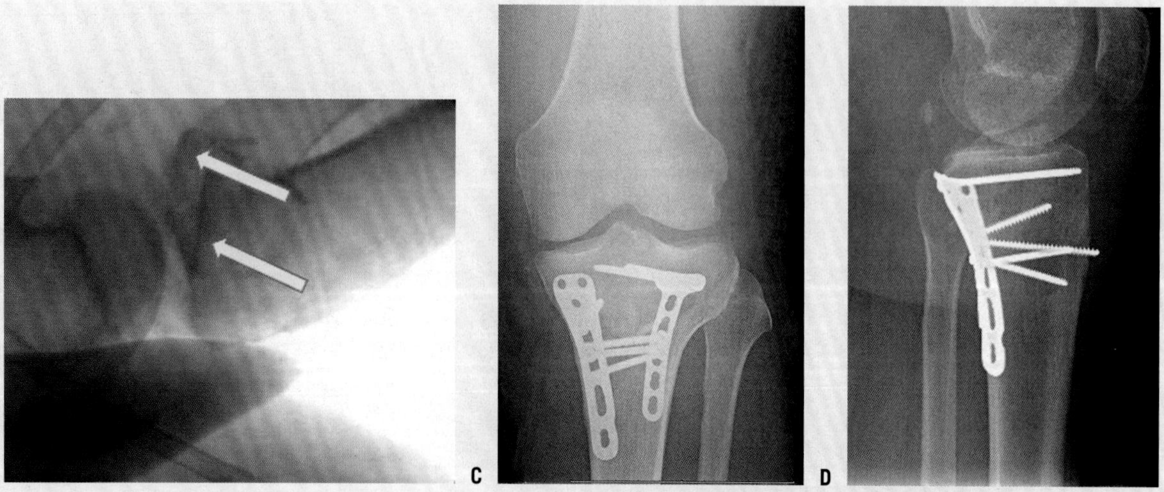

TECH FIG 8 *(continued)* **B.** Lateral fluoroscopic projection shows medial and lateral components both semivertically oriented (*arrows*). **C,D.** Postoperative AP and lateral radiographs. (Note symptomatic excessively long screw on lateral projection.)

COMPLETION

- The meniscal insertions are repaired as indicated with braided suture.
- Any performed tenotomies (medial gastrocnemius/popliteus) are repaired.
- The skin and subcutaneous tissues are closed in layers with either absorbable or nonabsorbable suture.
- A well-padded dressing is applied, and the patient is then placed in a knee immobilizer after they are returned to a supine position.
- Immobilization in flexion ("to limit tension on the posterior wound") is discouraged as this may compromise short- and long-term restoration of knee extension.

Pearls and Pitfalls

Foley Catheter	• Patient may be in the prone position for an extended period of time.
Flexion Contractures of the Knee	• Avoid immobilization in position of flexion to limit extension loss. • Employ transverse incision extension with discretion as this may have a role in extension loss.
Confirmation of Adequate Limb Position	• Proper limb position as described unencumbered by the opposite limb • Proper rotation of limb and C-arm as well as table tilt
Deep Vein Thrombosis	• Consider surveillance Doppler pre- and postoperatively as vessels are mobilized and retracted for an extended period of time.
Moore Type 1 Medial Fracture/Fracture-Dislocations	• Can be misinterpreted as a bicondylar fracture

Staged Bicondylar Fixation Strategy

- Posteromedial column must be anatomically restored to provide an accurate foundation for subsequent lateral fixation efforts.
- Possible obstacles:
  - Significant varus of the posteromedial fragment (**FIG 7A**)
  - Comminuted or primarily posteriorly oriented posteromedial apical spike (**FIG 7B**)
  - Incarcerated posterior fragments (**FIG 7C**)
- In addition to the inconveniences of patient and limb repreparation, the staged strategy does not allow for simultaneous reduction of the medial and lateral condylar components. Furthermore, the staged strategy mandates accurate and anatomic reduction of the medial condyle before subsequent fixation of the lateral condyle. Initial prone positioning required for staged management may be inapplicable in the polytraumatized individual.

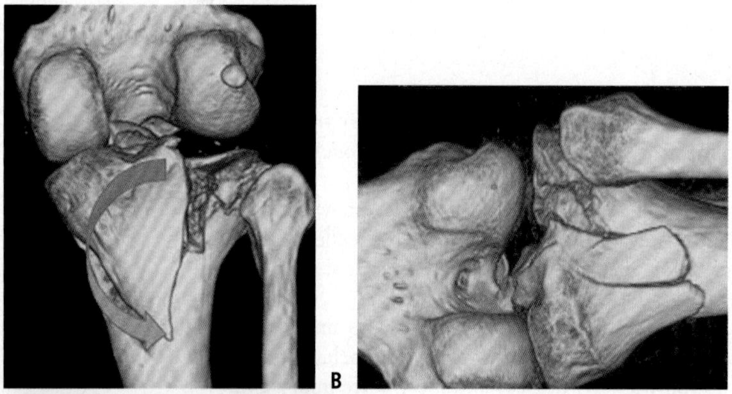

A B

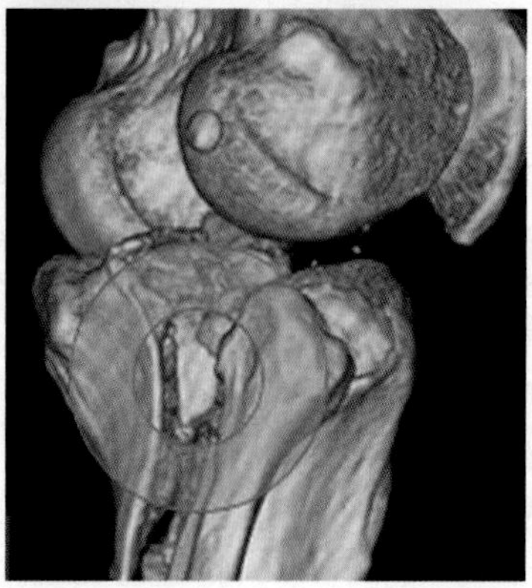

C

FIG 7 Obstacles to reduction. **A.** Significant varus of the posteromedial fragment. **B.** Comminuted or primarily posteriorly oriented posteromedial apical spike. **C.** Incarcerated posterior fragments.

Implant Gridlock

- Staged procedures initiated with medial fixation should not conflict with subsequent lateral fixation construct.

Removal of Hardware (Lateral)

- Efforts toward extracting previously introduced posterolateral implants may be complicated by considerable operative blood loss.[21]

Posteromedial (Lobenhoffer) Approach

- Surgeon is positioned on the unaffected side.
- Extensile approach with medial gastrocnemius tenotomy affords access to the lateral retrocondylar surface.

Implant-related Discomfort Secondary to Screw Length (see TECH FIG 8D)

- Screws introduced posterior to anterior, particularly with intentionally undercontoured plates, may prove of excessive length and a source of discomfort anteriorly, particularly with kneeling activities.

Posterolateral Approach

- Avoid excessive distal dissection in proximity to interosseous vessels.
- Identify and ligate inferior lateral geniculate artery.

POSTOPERATIVE CARE

- Non–weight bearing on the injured lower extremity for at least 6 to 8 weeks followed by a 4-week period of progressive weight bearing
- Early passive and active-assisted range of motion to start in the hospital. Constant passive motion machine are used during the inpatient stay.
- Knee immobilizer for use at night. Special attention is paid to maintaining full knee extension after direct posterior approaches that tend to develop flexion contractures.
- Deep venous thrombosis prophylaxis; most commonly Lovenox for 4 weeks unless contraindicated by preexisting patient medical conditions

OUTCOMES

- The overall clinical success rates for the open treatment of tibial plateau fractures via a posterior approach are reported as excellent.
- Yu et al[43] report in a limited series of 15 patients who were treated via a posterolateral prone approach excellent modified Hospital for Special Surgery (HSS) knee scores (mean HSS knee score 93.4, range 86 to 100).
- Row et al[30] report a series of 28 patients who underwent fixation utilizing a staged prone–supine approach. Average range of motion was 123 degrees and mean knee injury and osteoarthritis outcome score (KOOS) was 78 out of 100.
- Fakler et al[13] report two cases of Moore type 1 fracture-dislocations using a direct posterior approach. Both patients recovered full range of motion without complication at 1 year of follow-up.
- Tao et al[33] report use of a modified posterolateral approach in 11 patients with posterolateral shearing fractures. Mean HSS knee score at 1 year postoperatively was 93 (range 84 to 97) with average range of motion of 123 degrees.
- Carlson[6] report five patients with posterior bicondylar tibial plateau fractures who underwent fixation using dual posteromedial and posterolateral incisions with average range of motion of 121 degrees. All patients returned to near full activities.
- Chang et al[7] report 12 patients treated with dual posteromedial and anterolateral incisions with triple plate fixation. Mean HSS knee score at 1 year postoperatively was 87.3 (range 78 to 95).
- Higher rates of conversion to total knee arthroplasty are observed in bicondylar injuries and patients older than 48 years, although the total conversion rate was only 7.3%.[35]

COMPLICATIONS

- Common peroneal nerve palsy
- Deep venous thrombosis
- Knee flexion contracture
- Arthrofibrosis
- Retinal injury secondary to prolonged prone positioning
- Insufficient fixation and malreduction resultant from an exposure, which is unfamiliar and not readily extensile
- Symptomatic hardware requiring subsequent removal of hardware

REFERENCES

1. Barei DP, Nork SE, Mills WJ, et al. Complications associated with internal fixation of high-energy bicondylar tibial plateau fractures utilizing a two-incision technique. J Orthop Trauma 2004;18(10):649–657.
2. Barei DP, O'Mara TJ, Taitsman LA, et al. Frequency and fracture morphology of the posteromedial fragment in bicondylar tibial plateau fracture patterns. J Orthop Trauma 2008;22(3):176–182.
3. Bendayan J, Noblin JD, Freeland AE. Posteromedial second incision to reduce and stabilize a displaced posterior fragment that can occur in Schatzker type V bicondylar tibial plateau fractures. Orthopedics 1996;19(10):903–904.
4. Bhattacharyya T, McCarty LP III, Harris MB, et al. The posterior shearing tibial plateau fracture: treatment and results via a posterior approach. J Orthop Trauma 2005;19(5):305–310.
5. Brunner A, Honigmann P, Horisberger M, et al. Open reduction and fixation of medial Moore type II fractures of the tibial plateau by a direct dorsal approach. Arch Orthop Trauma Surg 2009;129(9):1233–1238.
6. Carlson DA. Posterior bicondylar tibial plateau fractures. J Orthop Trauma 2005;19(2):73–78.
7. Chang SM, Wang X, Zhou JQ, et al. Posterior coronal plating of bicondylar tibial plateau fractures through posteromedial and anterolateral approaches in a healthy floating supine position. Orthopedics 2012;35(7):583–588.
8. Chang SM, Zheng HP, Li HF, et al. Treatment of isolated posterior coronal fracture of the lateral tibial plateau through posterolateral approach for direct exposure and buttress plate fixation. Arch Orthop Trauma Surg 2009;129(7):955–962.
9. Colman M, Wright A, Gruen G, et al. Prolonged operative time increases infection rate in tibial plateau fractures. Injury 2013;44(2):249–252.
10. De Boeck H, Opdecam P. Posteromedial tibial plateau fractures. Operative treatment by posterior approach. Clin Orthop Relat Res 1995;(320):125–128.
11. Egol KA, Tejwani NC, Capla EL, et al. Staged management of high-energy proximal tibia fractures (OTA types 41): the results of a prospective, standardized protocol. J Orthop Trauma 2005;19(7):448–456.
12. Espinoza-Ervin CZ, Starr AJ, Reinert CM, et al. Use of a midline anterior incision for isolated medial tibial plateau fractures. J Orthop Trauma 2009;23(2):148–153.
13. Fakler JK, Ryzewicz M, Hartshorn C, et al. Optimizing the management of Moore type 1 postero-medial split fracture dislocations of the tibial head: description of the Lobenhoffer approach. J Orthop Trauma 2007;21(5):330–336.
14. Galla M, Lobenhoffer P. The direct, dorsal approach to the treatment of unstable tibial posteromedial fracture-dislocations [in German]. Unfallchirurg 2003;106(3):241–247.
15. Galla M, Riemer C, Lobenhoffer P. Direct posterior approach for the treatment of posteromedial tibial head fractures [in German]. Oper Orthop Traumatol 2009;21(1):51–64.
16. Georgiadis GM. Combined anterior and posterior approaches for complex tibial plateau fractures. J Bone Joint Surg Br 1994;76(2):285–289.
17. He X, Ye P, Hu Y, et al. A posterior inverted L-shaped approach for the treatment of posterior bicondylar tibial plateau fractures. Arch Orthop Trauma Surg 2013;133(1):23–28.
18. Heidari N, Lidder S, Grechenig W, et al. The risk of injury to the anterior tibial artery in the posterolateral approach to the tibia plateau: a cadaver study. J Orthop Trauma 2013;27(4):221–225.
19. Higgins TF, Kemper D, Klatt J. Incidence and morphology of the posteromedial fragment in bicondylar tibial plateau fractures. J Orthop Trauma 2009;23(1):45–51.
20. Higgins TF, Klatt J, Bachus KN. Biomechanical analysis of bicondylar tibial plateau fixation: how does lateral locking plate fixation compare to dual plate fixation? J Orthop Trauma 2007;21(5):301–306.
21. Huang YG, Chang SM. The posterolateral approach for plating tibial plateau fractures: problems in secondary hardware removal. Arch Orthop Trauma Surg 2012;132(5):733–734.

22. Johnson EE, Timon S, Osuji C. Surgical technique: Tscherne-Johnson extensile approach for tibial plateau fractures. Clin Orthop Relat Res 2013;471(9):2760–2767.
23. Kottmeier SA, Jones CB, Tornetta P III, et al. Locked and minimally invasive plating: a paradigm shift? Metadiaphyseal site-specific concerns and controversies. Instr Course Lect 2013;62:41–59.
24. Kottmeier SA, Watson JT, Row E, et al. Staged fixation of tibial plateau fractures: strategies for the posterior approach. J Knee Surg 2016;29(1):2–11.
25. Lobenhoffer P, Gerich T, Bertram T, et al. Particular posteromedial and posterolateral approaches for the treatment of tibial head fractures [in German]. Unfallchirurg 1997;100(12):957–967.
26. Lowe JA, Tejwani N, Yoo BJ, et al. Surgical techniques for complex proximal tibial fractures. Instr Course Lect 2012;61:39–51.
27. Luo CF, Sun H, Zhang B, et al. Three-column fixation for complex tibial plateau fractures. J Orthop Trauma 2010;24(11):683–692.
28. Moore TM. Fracture–dislocation of the knee. Clin Orthop Relat Res 1981;156:128–140.
29. Morris BJ, Unger RZ, Archer KR, et al. Risk factors of infection after ORIF of bicondylar tibial plateau fractures. J Orthop Trauma 2013;27(9):e196–e200.
30. Row ER, Komatsu DE, Watson JT, et al. Staged prone/supine fixation of high-energy multicolumnar tibial plateau fractures: a multicenter analysis. J Orthop Trauma 2018;32(4):e117–e122.
31. Stannard JP, Lopez R, Volgas D. Soft tissue injury of the knee after tibial plateau fractures. J Knee Surg 2010;23(4):187–192.
32. Streubel PN, Glasgow D, Wong A, et al. Sagittal plane deformity in bicondylar tibial plateau fractures. J Orthop Trauma 2011;25(9):560–565.
33. Tao J, Hang DH, Wang QG, et al. The posterolateral shearing tibial plateau fracture: treatment and results via a modified posterolateral approach. Knee 2008;15(6):473–479.
34. Trickey EL. Rupture of the posterior cruciate ligament of the knee. J Bone Joint Surg Br 1968;50(2):334–341.
35. Wasserstein D, Henry P, Paterson JM, et al. Risk of total knee arthroplasty after operatively treated tibial plateau fracture: a matched-population-based cohort study. J Bone Joint Surg Am 2014;96(2):144–150.
36. Watson JT. High-energy fractures of the tibial plateau. Orthop Clin North Am 1994;25(4):723–752.
37. Weaver MJ, Harris MB, Strom AC, et al. Fracture pattern and fixation type related to loss of reduction in bicondylar tibial plateau fractures. Injury 2012;43(6):864–869.
38. Weil YA, Gardner MJ, Boraiah S, et al. Posteromedial supine approach for reduction and fixation of medial and bicondylar tibial plateau fractures. J Orthop Trauma 2008;22(5):357–362.
39. Xu YQ, Li Q, Shen TG, et al. An efficacy analysis of surgical timing and procedures for high-energy complex tibial plateau fractures. Orthop Surg 2013;5(3):188–195.
40. Yin Z, Yang W, Gu Y, et al. A modified direct posterior midline approach for the treatment of posterior column tibial plateau fractures. J Knee Surg 2020;33:646–654.
41. Yoo BJ, Beingessner DM, Barei DP. Stabilization of the posteromedial fragment in bicondylar tibial plateau fractures: a mechanical comparison of locking and nonlocking single and dual plating methods. J Trauma 2010;69(1):148–155.
42. Yu B, Han K, Zhan C, et al. Fibular head osteotomy: a new approach for the treatment of lateral or posterolateral tibial plateau fractures. Knee 2010;17(5):313–318.
43. Yu GR, Xia J, Zhou JQ, et al. Low-energy fracture of posterolateral tibial plateau: treatment by a posterolateral prone approach. J Trauma Acute Care Surg 2012;72(5):1416–1423.

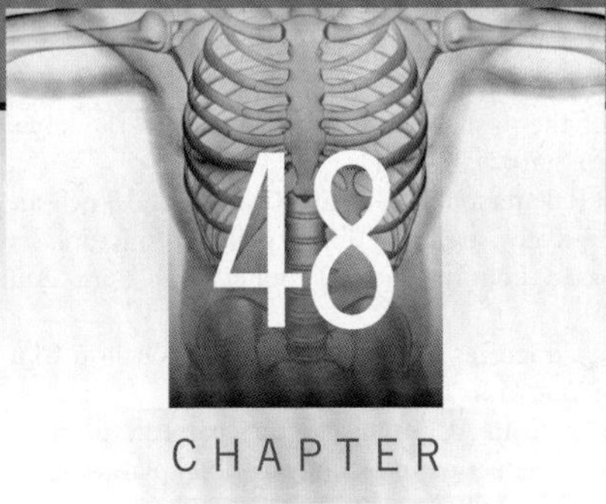

Leg

External Fixation of the Tibia

Midhat Patel and J. Tracy Watson

DEFINITION

- Indications for external fixation of the tibial shaft in trauma applications include the treatment of open fractures with extensive soft tissue devitalization and contamination. Other indications include the stabilization of closed fractures with high-grade soft tissue injury or compartment syndrome. External fixation is favored when the fracture configuration extends into the metaphyseal/diaphyseal junction or the joint itself, making other treatment options problematic.
  - For patients with multiple long bone fractures, external fixation has been used as a method for temporary, if not definitive, stabilization.[7]
  - With the introduction of circular and hybrid techniques, indications have been expanded to include the definitive treatment of complex periarticular injuries, which include high-energy tibial plateau and distal tibial pilon fractures.[9]
  - Hexapod fixators can be used to perform gradual reductions of the tibial shaft or periarticular injuries in cases of severe soft tissue injury, where soft tissue coverage procedures are contraindicated and in cases of delayed presentation, where acute distraction and reduction would compromise neurovascular elements.[24]
- Contemporary external fixation systems in current clinical use can be categorized according to the type of bone anchorage used.
  - Fixation is achieved either using large threaded pins, which are screwed into the bone, or by drilling small-diameter transfixion wires through the bone. The pins or wires are then connected to one another through the use of longitudinal bars or circular rings.
  - The distinction is thus between monolateral external fixation (longitudinal connecting pins to bars) and circular external fixation (wires and/or pins connecting to rings).
- Acute trauma applications primarily use monolateral frame configurations and are the focus of techniques described here.
  - The first type of monolateral frame is modular with individual components: separate bars, attachable pin–bar clamps, bar-to-bar clamps, and Schanz pins **(FIG 1A,B)**. These "simple monolateral" frames allow for a wide range of flexibility with "build-up" or "build-down" capabilities.

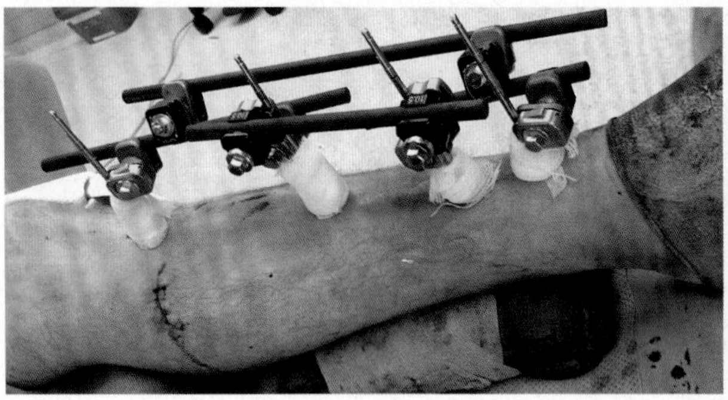
A

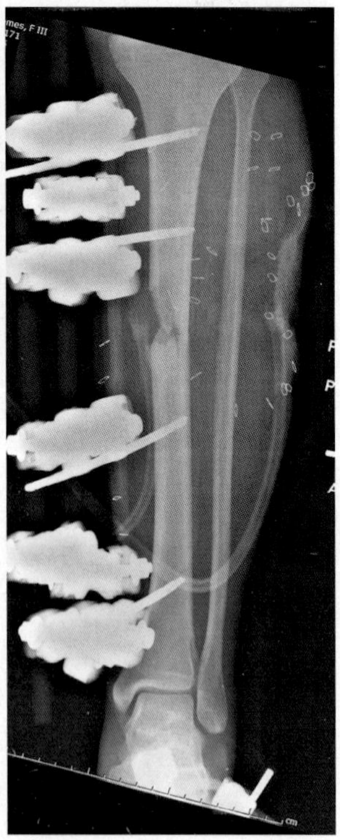
B

FIG 1 **A.** Simple monolateral four-pin frame with a double-stack connecting bar to increase frame stability. **B.** X-ray demonstrating ability to connect the fixation pins to each limb segment in a variety of ways to achieve a congruent reduction. *(continued)*

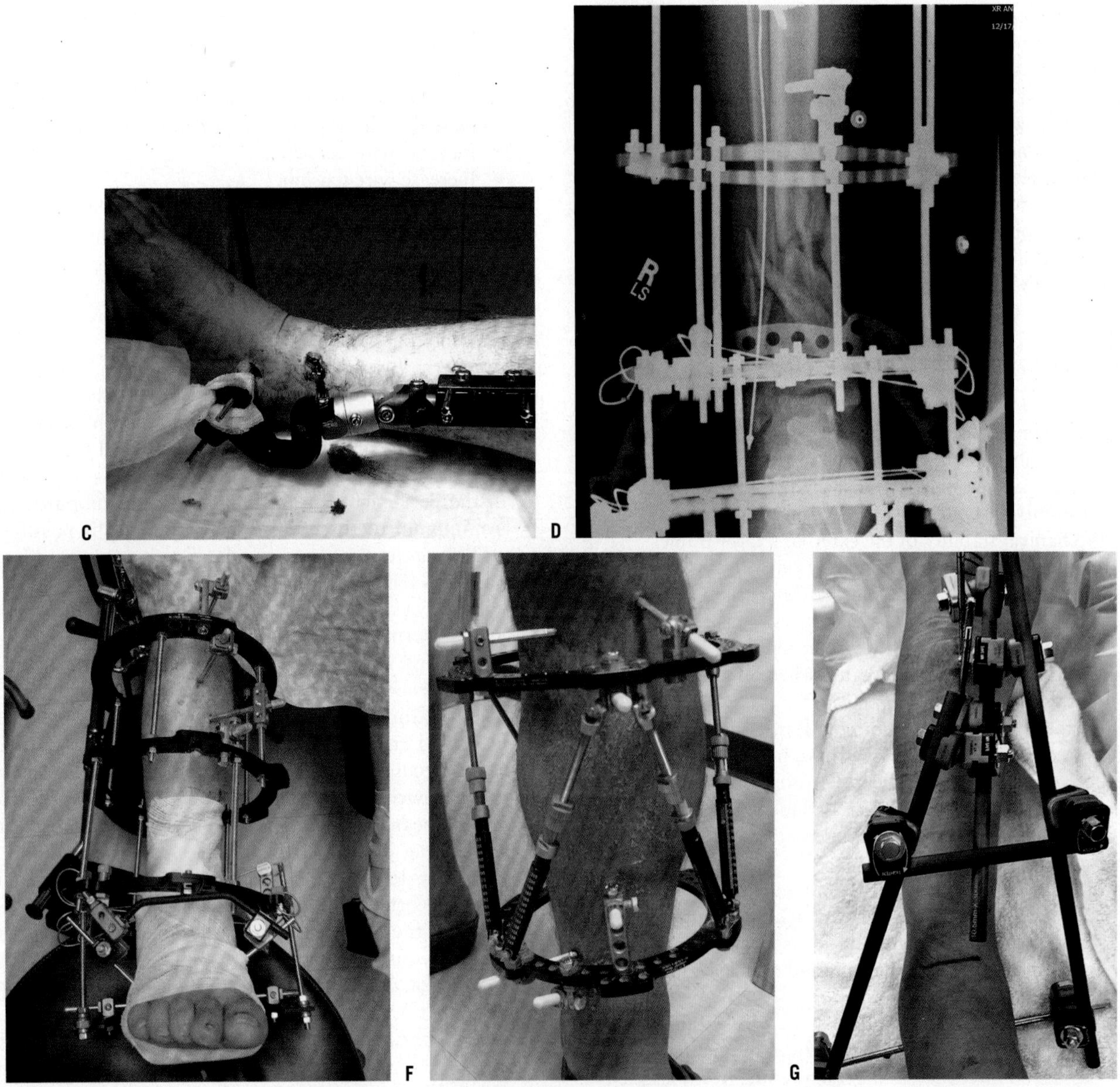

FIG 1 *(continued)* **C.** Large monotube fixator spanning the ankle for a severe pilon fracture. This was applied to temporize the soft tissues before definitive open stabilization of the injury. **D,E.** Small tensioned wire circular fixator used for definitive management of a distal tibial periarticular fracture with proximal shaft extension. The versatility of these frames allows for spanning into the foot to maintain a plantigrade position. **F.** A hexapod frame attached to the bone with large Schanz pins. This frame allows for gradual correction of fracture displacement over time by adjusting the six distractors. **G.** Ankle-spanning "delta" frame with medial, lateral triangular support bars connecting to the calcaneal pin to maintain distraction across the joint.

  - The second type of monolateral frame is a more constrained type of fixator that comes preassembled with a multipin clamp at each end of a long rigid tubular body. The telescoping tube allows for axial compression or distraction of this so-called monotube-type fixator **(FIG 1C)**.
- For diaphyseal injuries, the most common type of fixator application is the monolateral frame using large pins for skeletal stabilization.
  - Simple monolateral fixators have the distinct advantage of allowing individual pins to be placed at different angles and varying obliquities while still connecting to the bar. This is helpful when altering the pin position to avoid areas of soft tissue compromise (ie, open wounds or severe contusion).[21]
  - The advantage of the monotube-type fixator is its simplicity. Pin placement is predetermined by the multipin clamps. Loosening the universal articulations between the body and the clamps allows these frames to be easily manipulated to reduce a fracture.
- Many high-energy fractures involve the metaphyseal regions, and transfixion techniques using small tensioned wires are ideally suited to this region. They have better mechanical stability and longevity than traditional half-pin techniques.
  - Small tensioned wire circular frames or hybrid frames (frames using a combination of large half-pins and transfixion wires) can be useful in patients with severe tibial metaphyseal injuries that occur in concert with other

conditions such as soft tissue compromise or compartment syndrome or in patients with multiple injuries **(FIG 1D,E)**.
  - Hexapod fixators are ring fixators consisting of six distractors and 12 ball joints, which allow for 6 degrees of freedom of bone fragment displacement. By adjusting the simple distractors, gradual three-dimensional corrections or acute reductions are possible without the need for complicated frame mechanisms **(FIG 1F)**.
- Fracture-dislocations of the ankle such as pilon fractures can initially be managed with a delta-frame construct **(FIG 1G)**.

Monolateral External Fixators

- The stability of all monolateral fixators is based on the concept of a simple "four-pin frame."
  - Pin number, pin separation, and pin proximity to the fracture site, as well as bone bar distance and the diameter of the pins and connecting bars, all influence the final mechanical stability of the external fixator frame.[5]
- Large pin monolateral fixators rely on stiff pins for frame stability. On loading, these pins act as cantilevers and produce eccentric loading characteristics. Shear forces are regarded as inhibitory to fracture healing and bone formation, and this may be accentuated when all pins are placed in the same orientation.
- After stable frame application, the soft tissue injury can be addressed. Once the soft tissues have healed, conversion to definitive internal fixation can be safely accomplished. In some cases, the external device is the definitive treatment. Dynamic weight bearing is initiated at an early stage once the fracture is deemed stable.
  - In fractures that are highly comminuted, weight bearing is delayed until visible callus is achieved and sufficient stability has been maintained. As healing progresses, active dynamization of the frame may be required to achieve solid union.
- Dynamization converts a static fixator, which seeks to neutralize all forces including axial motion, to one that allows the passage of forces across the fracture site. As the elasticity of the callus decreases, bone stiffness and strength increase and larger loads can be supported.[17] Thus, axial dynamization helps to restore cortical contact and to produce a stable fracture pattern with inherent mechanical support.[6] This is accomplished by making adjustments in the pin–bar clamps with simple monolateral fixators or in releasing the body on a monotube-type fixator.
- Bony healing is not complete until remodeling of the fracture has been achieved. At this stage, the visible fracture lines in the callus decrease and subsequently disappear. The fixator can be removed at this point.

Circular External Fixation

- Circular or semicircular fixators allow for multiple planes of fixation, which minimizes the harmful effects of cantilever loading and shear forces, while accentuating axial micromotion and dynamization.[25]
- Ring fixators are built with longitudinal connecting rods between rings to which the small-diameter tensioned wires are attached. Alternatively, the bone fragments may be attached to the rings by half-pins. The connecting rods may incorporate universal joints, which give these frames their ability to produce gradual multiplanar angular and axial adjustments **(FIG 2A)**.
- Several component-related factors can be manipulated to increase the stability of the ring fixation construct:
  - Increase wire diameter.
  - Increase wire tension.
  - Increase pin-crossing angle to approach 90 degrees.
  - Decrease ring size (distance of ring to bone).
  - Increase number of wires per segment.
  - Use of olive or drop wires.
  - Close ring position to either side of the fracture site.
  - Centering bone in the middle of the ring
- The term *hybrid* when applied to external fixation denotes the use of half-pins and wires in the same frame mounting as well as using a combination of rings and monolateral connecting bars. Stable hybrid frames should include a ring incorporating multiple levels of fixation in the periarticular fragment. This is accomplished with a minimum of three tensioned wires and if possible, an additional level of periarticular fixation using adjunctive half-pins **(FIG 2B)**.[1,2]
- The use of a single bar connecting the shaft to the periarticular ring places significant stresses on the single connecting clamp and accentuates the harmful off-axis forces generated with weight bearing. This type of hybrid fixator construct has been shown to have much less axial and bending stiffness compared to a standard axial circular fixator. This is the reason that most of these devices tend to lose reduction with progressive weight bearing.[19] A hybrid circular frame with *multiple* connecting bars is superior to a single monolateral bar. However, full circular frames with a minimum of four half-pins attached to the shaft component and two complete rings connected by four threaded rods are superior to both constructs.[1,2]
- Distraction osteogenesis is the mechanical induction of new bone that occurs between bony surfaces that are gradually pulled apart. Ilizarov described this as "the tension-stress effect."[13–15] Osteogenesis in the gap of a distracted bone takes place by the formation of a physis-like structure. New bone forms in parallel columns extending in both directions from a central growth region known as the *interzone*. Recruitment of the tissue-forming cells for the interzone originates in the periosteum.[15]
- Distraction, accomplished through the use of a ring fixator or a stable monotube device, initiates the histogenesis of bone, muscle, nerves, and skin.[14,15] This facilitates the treatment of complex orthopedic diseases, including osteomyelitis, fibrous dysplasia, and significant segmental bone loss (see **FIG 2A**). Other conditions that have been historically refractory to standard treatments such as congenital pseudoarthrosis, severe hemimelias, and significant leg length discrepancies can also be addressed.[15,16,26,28]
- Bone transport methodologies can replace large skeletal defects with normal healthy bone structure, which is well vascularized and is relatively impervious to stress fractures. The ability to correct significant angular, translational, and axial deformities simultaneously through relative percutaneous techniques, as well as perform these corrections in an ambulatory outpatient setting, adds to the attractiveness of this methodology.[3]

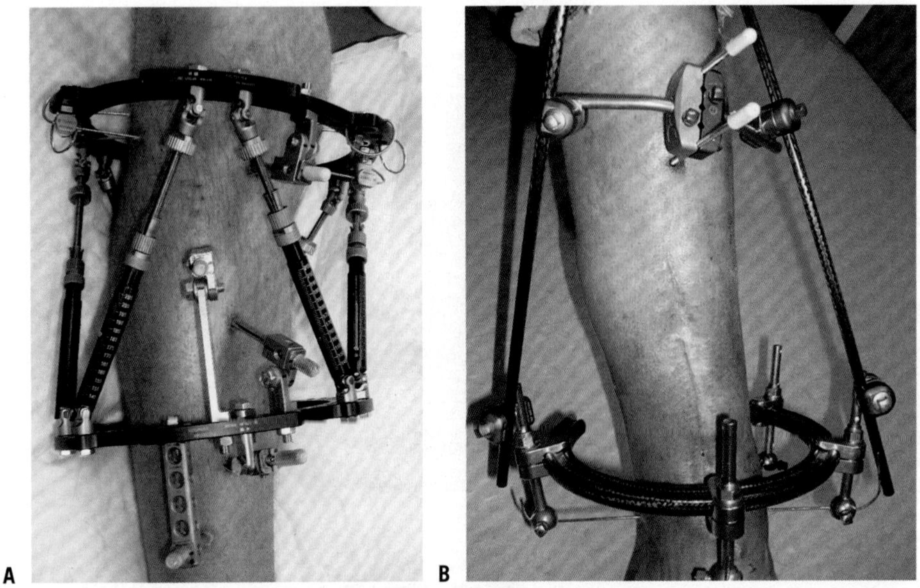

FIG 2 **A.** A contemporary ring fixator with a combination of half-pin fixation in the diaphysis and tensioned wires in the metaphyseal regions. Rings are connected to each other with six hexapod struts, which can be individually adjusted to affect a six-axis correction. This configuration can be used for a host of conditions including the gradual reduction and realignment of acute fractures, correction of malunion nonunion with deformity, and to perform limb lengthening and bone transport. **B.** Hybrid fixator applied to a tibial plateau fracture and pilon fracture (half ring fixator at the metaphyseal regions and half monolateral fixator in the diaphyseal component). These frames combine diaphyseal half-pins with multiple metaphyseal tensioned wires. These frames may be mechanically insufficient to neutralize harmful cantilever bending and thus should be applied with great care.

ANATOMY

- The bulk of the tibia is easily accessible in that most of the diaphyseal portions are subcutaneous.
  - The hard cortical bone found in this location is ideally suited to the placement of large pins that achieve excellent mechanical fixation.
  - The cross-sectional anatomy of the diaphysis and the lateral location of the muscular compartments allow placement of half-pins in a wide range of subcutaneous locations. This facilitates pin placement "out of plane" or divergent to each other, which helps achieve excellent frame stability **(FIG 3)**.
- The proximal and distal periarticular metaphyseal regions of the tibia are also subcutaneous except for their lateral surfaces. The bone in these locations is primarily cancellous, with thin cortical walls.
  - The mechanical stability achieved with half-pins depends on cortical purchase and therefore may not be adequate for fixation in this cortex-deficient region.
  - If half-pins are used, they are typically angled and larger, with a cancellous pitch.
  - Excellent stability is afforded in these areas by using small-diameter tensioned transfixion wires in conjunction with circular external fixators. Metaphyseal transfixion wires can be combined with diaphyseal half-pins can be combined to produce frames for periarticular fracture fixation for complex pilon and plateau fractures.

PATHOGENESIS

- Open tibial diaphyseal fractures are primarily candidates for closed intramedullary nailing, but there are occasions when external fixation is indicated.
  - External fixation is favored when there is substantial contamination and severe soft tissue injury or when the fracture configuration extends into the metaphyseal–diaphyseal junction or the joint itself, making intramedullary nailing problematic.
- The choice of external fixator type depends on the location and complexity of the fracture as well as the type of wound present when dealing with open injuries.
  - The less stable the fracture pattern (ie, the more comminution), the more complex a frame needs to be applied to control motion at the bone ends.
  - If possible, weight bearing should be a consideration.
  - If periarticular extension or involvement is present, the ability to bridge the joint with the frame provides satisfactory stability for both hard and soft tissues.
  - It is important that the frame be constructed and applied to allow for multiple débridements and subsequent soft tissue reconstruction. This demands that the pins are placed away from the zone of injury to avoid potential pin site contamination with the operative field.
- Fractures treated with external fixation heal with external bridging callus. External bridging callus is largely under the control of mechanical and other humoral factors and is highly dependent on the integrity of the surrounding soft

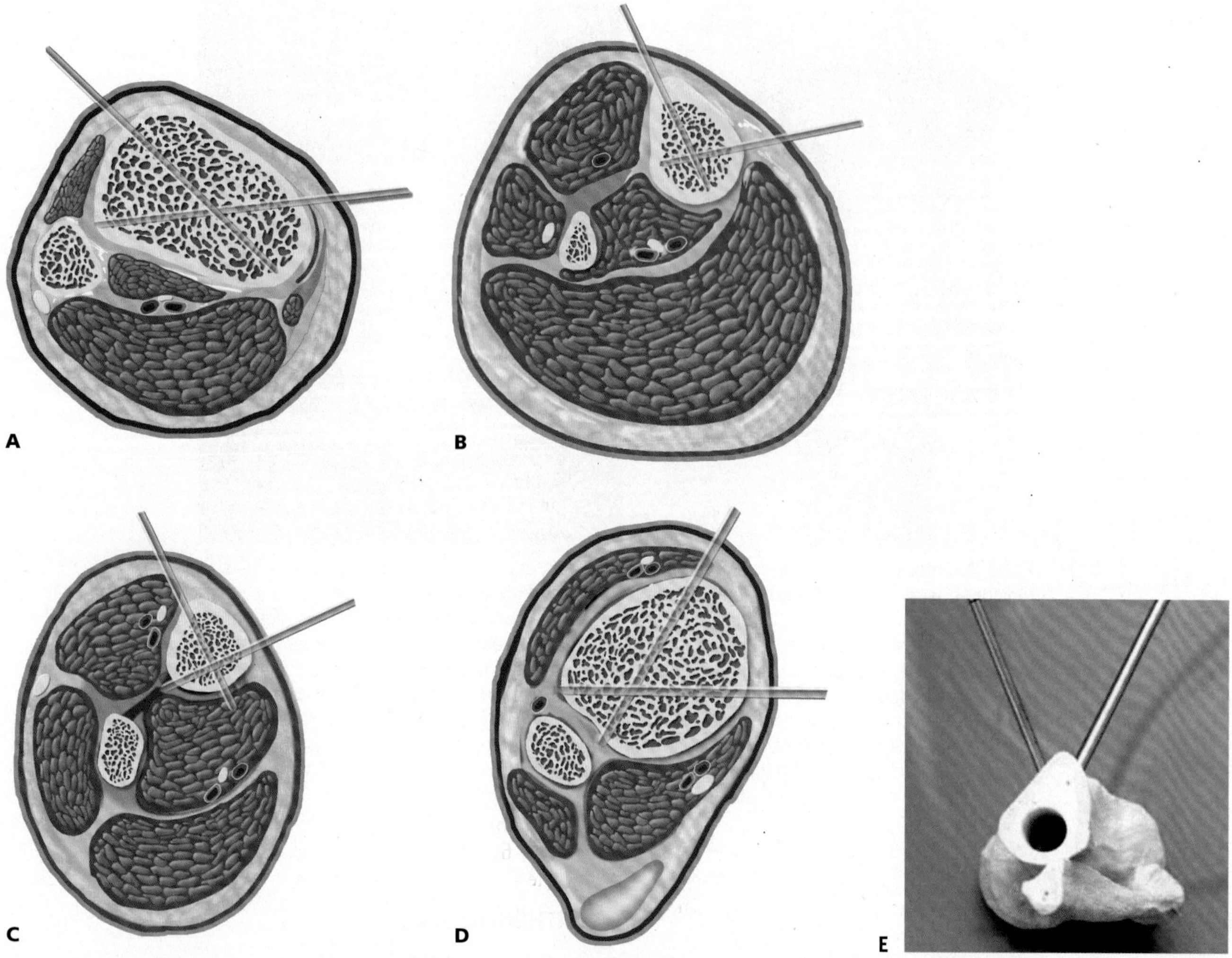

FIG 3 A–D. Cross-sectional anatomy of the tibia at all levels. The proximal cross-section demonstrates the ability to achieve at least 120 degrees of pin divergence in this region with progressively smaller diversion angles as the pins are placed distally. It is important to avoid tethering of any musculotendinous structures. To accomplish this, pins are placed primarily along the subcutaneous border of the tibia. **E.** Model showing similar pin placement avoiding the anterolateral and posterior muscular compartments. Posterior cortex pin protrusion is minimal to avoid damaging any posterior neurovascular structures.

tissue envelope. This type of fracture healing has the ability to bridge large gaps and is very tolerant of movement.

- Micromotion with the external fixator construct has been found to accentuate fracture union. It results in the development of a large callus with formation of cartilage due to the greater inflammatory response caused by increased micromovement of the fragments.
- There appears to be a threshold at which the degree of micromotion becomes inhibitory to this overall remodeling process, however, so hypertrophic nonunion can result from an unstable external frame.

- Temporary spanning fixation for complex articular injuries is used routinely. The ability to achieve an initial ligamentotaxis reduction substantially decreases the amount of injury-related swelling and edema by reducing large fracture gaps.
  - It is important to achieve an early ligamentotaxis reduction: A delay of more than a few days will result in an inability to disimpact and adequately reduce displaced metaphyseal fragments with distraction alone.
  - Once the soft tissues have recovered, definitive open reconstruction can be accomplished with relative ease as the operative tactic can be directed to the area of articular involvement.[27]
- Application of these techniques in a polytrauma patient is valuable when rapid stabilization is necessary for a patient in extremis. Simple monolateral or monotube fixators can be placed rapidly across long bone injuries, providing adequate stabilization to facilitate the management and resuscitation of the polytrauma patient (**FIG 4**).

PATIENT HISTORY AND PHYSICAL FINDINGS

- History should focus on the mechanism of injury.
  - Determining whether the injury was high energy versus low energy gives the surgeon an idea of the extent of the soft tissue zone of injury and will help determine the possible location of fixation pins.

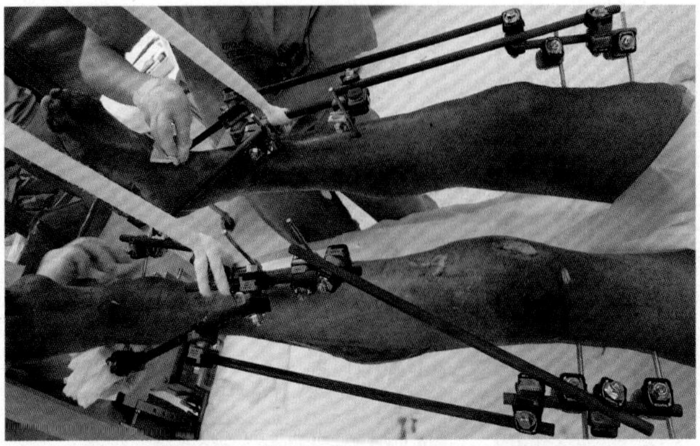

FIG 4 Polytrauma patient with bilateral temporary spanning fixators. External fixation on the *right side* spans bicondylar tibial plateau fracture with an ipsilateral pilon fracture. The left knee is bridged to stabilize a tibial plateau fracture and a severe bimalleolar ankle fracture. The left leg injury is complicated by a compartment syndrome with open fasciotomy wounds.

- Determining the location of the accident is helpful in cases of open fracture (ie, open field with soil contamination vs. slip and fall on ice and snow).
  - These parameters give the surgeon an idea as to the extent of intraoperative débridement that might be required to cleanse the wound and the necessary antibiotic coverage for the injury.
- The neurovascular status should be documented, specifically the presence or absence of the anterior and posterior tibial pulses at the ankle.
  - A weak or absent pulse may be an indication of vascular injury and may dictate further evaluation with ankle–brachial indices, compartment pressure evaluation, or a formal arteriogram.
  - Evaluation of compartment pressures is often indicated in open fractures and closed high-energy fractures with severe soft tissue contusion.
- Evaluation of soft tissues and grading of the open fracture with regard to the size, orientation, and location of the open wounds aid in decision making about pin placement and the configuration of the fixator to allow access to open wounds (**FIG 5**).

IMAGING AND OTHER DIAGNOSTIC STUDIES

- Imaging of the tibia should include at least two orthogonal views, anteroposterior and lateral.
  - Radiographs of the knee and ankle are necessary to evaluate any articular fracture involvement or associated knee or ankle subluxation or dislocation.
  - Identifying any occult fracture lines aids in the preoperative planning of potential pin placement.
  - Many patients with high-energy tibial fractures have associated foot injuries, and views of the foot and ankle are necessary to identify this injury pattern.
- Traction radiographs of articular injuries of the tibia are useful to identify the nature and orientation of metaphyseal fragments as well as degree of articular impaction. This aids in determining whether a joint-spanning fixator is necessary.
- Distraction computed tomography (CT) scans should be obtained *after* the knee- or ankle-spanning fixator has been applied. These studies indicate the effectiveness of the ligamentotaxis reduction. This allows the surgeon to determine the preoperative plan for definitive fixation once the soft tissues have recovered (**FIG 6**).[29]

SURGICAL MANAGEMENT

- The surgical decisions relate to the configuration of the external device to be applied. These generally fall into two categories of treatment options.
- The first category is a temporary device intended to allow the soft tissues to recover or the patient's overall condition to improve until definitive fixation of the injury can be safely carried out.
  - Temporary frames include knee- or ankle-spanning fixators used in cases of periarticular injuries requiring ligamentotaxis reduction and relative stabilization and simple frames spanning a tibial shaft fracture in the case of a polytrauma patient who needs emergent stabilization of injuries. These frames in diaphyseal injuries are

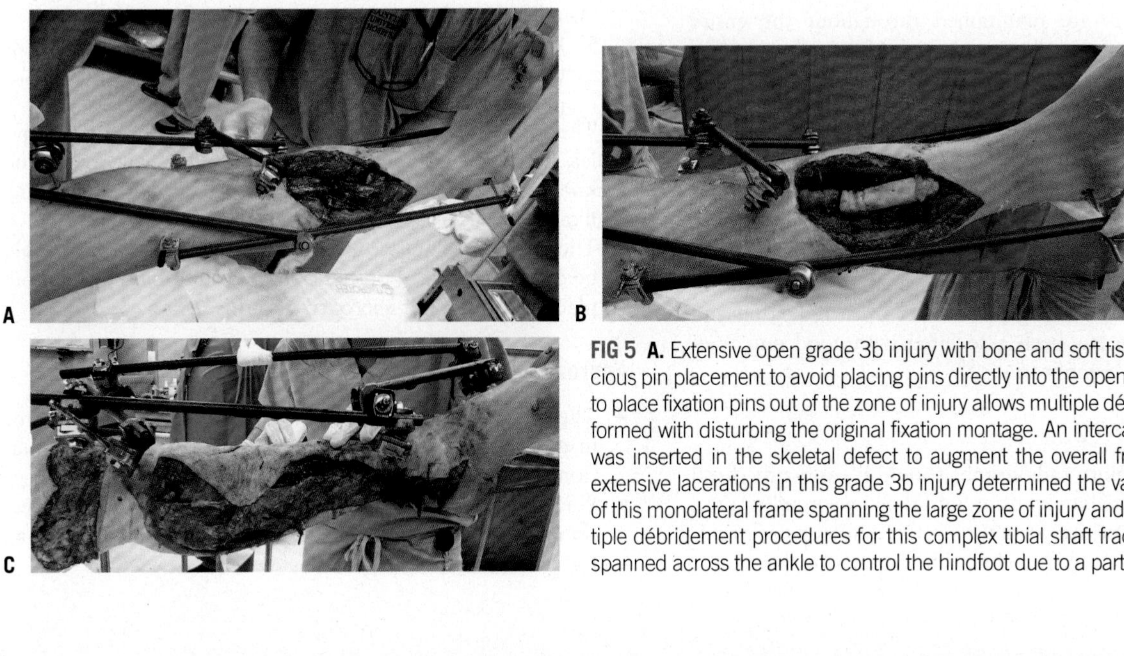

FIG 5 A. Extensive open grade 3b injury with bone and soft tissue loss dictates judicious pin placement to avoid placing pins directly into the open wound. **B.** The ability to place fixation pins out of the zone of injury allows multiple débridements to be performed with disturbing the original fixation montage. An intercalary antibiotic spacer was inserted in the skeletal defect to augment the overall frame stability. **C.** The extensive lacerations in this grade 3b injury determined the variable pin placement of this monolateral frame spanning the large zone of injury and helped facilitate multiple débridement procedures for this complex tibial shaft fracture. The frame was spanned across the ankle to control the hindfoot due to a partial heel pad avulsion.

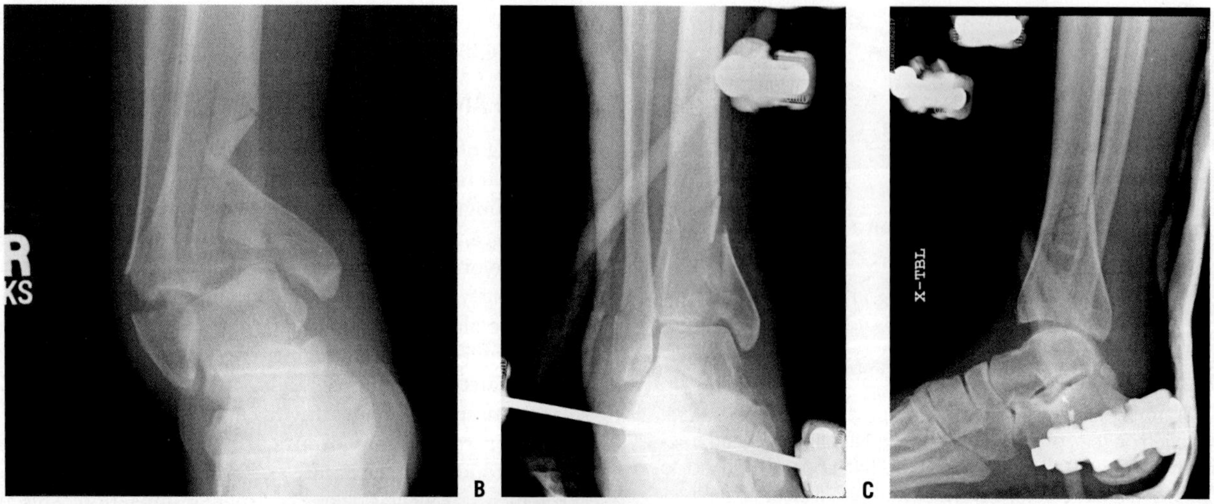

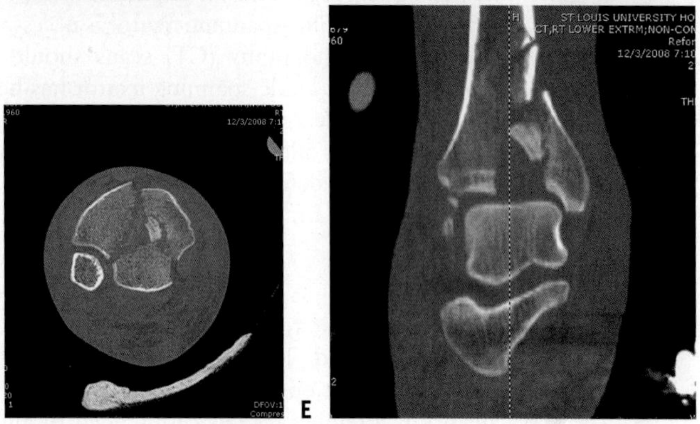

FIG 6 A–C. Injury and post–external fixation films demonstrating an ankle-spanning frame stabilizing a complex pilon fracture. **D,E.** CT scans obtained after distraction in the frame provide valuable information to help determine the preoperative plan for delayed definitive reconstruction once the soft tissues have recovered.

later converted to intramedullary nails once the patient can undergo additional surgery.[12] Intra-articular fractures are converted to open reduction and internal fixation with plates and screws or the frame is modified with internal fixation as definitive treatment.
  - They are simplistic and not intended for long-term treatment times.
- Definitive treatment fixators are primarily applied to diaphyseal injuries with severe soft tissue compromise (open and closed).
  - These devices are maintained throughout the entire treatment period to allow access to soft tissues and facilitate secondary procedures such as rotational or free flap coverage as well as delayed bone grafting.
  - These frames are more involved and are intended to remain in place for the entire treatment period (ie, hexapod fixators).
  - These devices allow for adjustments in all planes throughout the healing process to help prevent malunion.
- In distal tibia fractures, maintenance of external fixation in the initial bone healing phase after open reduction and internal fixation has been associated with good outcomes and low rate of complications.[20]

Preoperative Planning

- Evaluation of injury radiographs should identify any distal or proximal articular extension into the knee or ankle joint.
- Location of the primary fracture is noted in terms of proximal or distal locations to help decide on a particular fixator construct and to help determine if a joint-spanning fixator is required.

Positioning

- The patient's entire lower extremity is elevated using bumps or a beanbag patient positioner under the ipsilateral hip. This elevates the tibia off the operating table (**FIG 7**).
- The foot can be supported with a sterile bump, thus suspending the limb and allowing full 360-degree access and visualization of the limb.
  - Elevating the limb positions, the nonoperative leg below the operative limb, which aids in placing out-of-plane pins as well as circular frame components
- The image intensifier is positioned opposite the operative leg. This aids in fluoroscopic visualization of the femur and knee, which is important when applying a knee-spanning fixator for a severe tibial plateau fracture.
- The location of any proposed periarticular incisions should be carefully marked on the skin to ensure that eventual pin placement does not encroach into this region.[18]

Approach

- The integrity of the pin–bone interface is a critical factor in determining the longevity of an applied external fixation pin.
- Pin insertion technique is important in achieving an infection-free, stable pin–bone interface and thus maintaining frame stability.

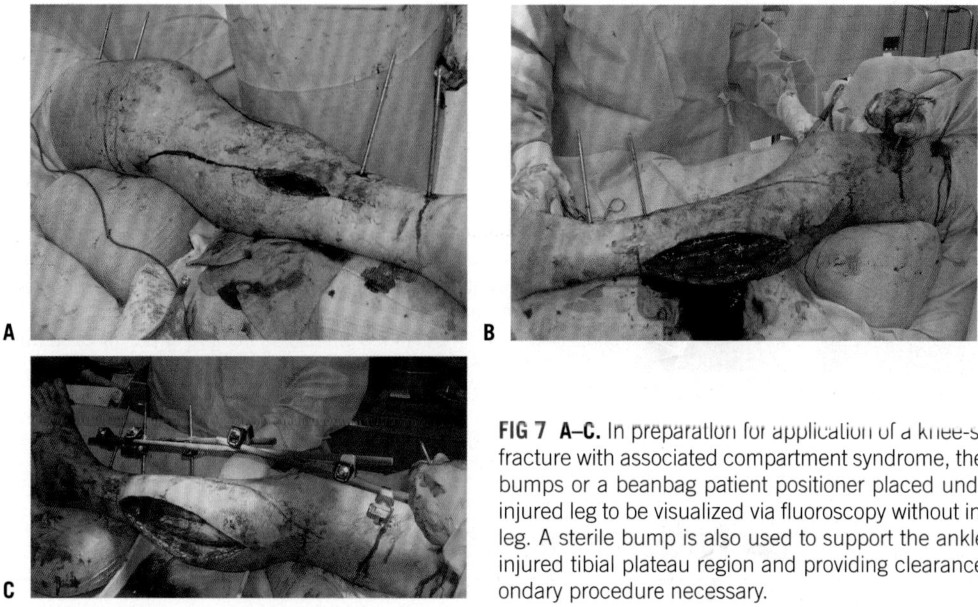

FIG 7 A–C. In preparation for application of a knee-spanning frame for a complex plateau fracture with associated compartment syndrome, the injured limb is elevated using sterile bumps or a beanbag patient positioner placed under the ipsilateral hip. This allows the injured leg to be visualized via fluoroscopy without interference from the opposite "down" leg. A sterile bump is also used to support the ankle, allowing 360-degree access to the injured tibial plateau region and providing clearance for any fixator configuration or secondary procedure necessary.

PIN INSERTION TECHNIQUE

- The correct insertion technique involves incising the skin directly at the side of pin insertion.
- After a generous incision is made, dissection is carried directly down to bone, and the periosteum is incised where anatomically feasible **(TECH FIG 1A)**.
- A small Penfield-type elevator is used to gently reflect the periosteum off the bone at the site of insertion **(TECH FIG 1B)**. Extraneous soft tissue tethering and necrosis is avoided by minimizing soft tissue at the site of insertion.
- A trocar and drill sleeve are advanced directly to bone, minimizing the amount of soft tissue entrapment that might be encountered during predrilling **(TECH FIG 1C,D)**. A sleeve should also be used if a self-drilling pin is selected.
- After predrilling, an appropriate-size depth of pin is advanced by hand to achieve bicortical purchase. Any offending soft tissue tethering should be released with a small scalpel **(TECH FIG 1E,F)**.
- Fluoroscopy is used to ensure that transcortical pin placement is avoided **(TECH FIG 1G)**.

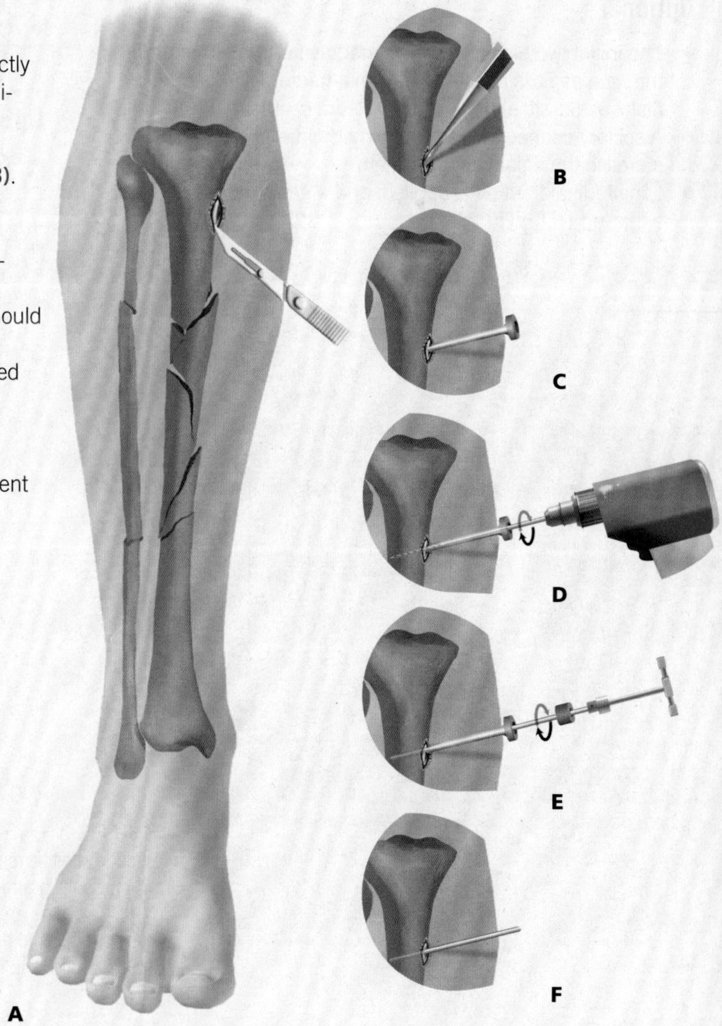

TECH FIG 1 Proper pin insertion technique. **A.** A generous incision is made over the location of the pin site. **B.** A small elevator is used to elevate all soft tissues, including the periosteum, off the bone to help avoid the tethering of excessive soft tissues during predrilling and pin insertion. **C.** A trocar is advanced to bone to protect the soft tissues. **D.** The pin site is predrilled through the trocar to avoid incarcerating and tethering soft tissues. **E,F.** A T-handle insertion chuck is used to hand torque the pin into position, achieving purchase in both the near and far cortices. *(continued)*

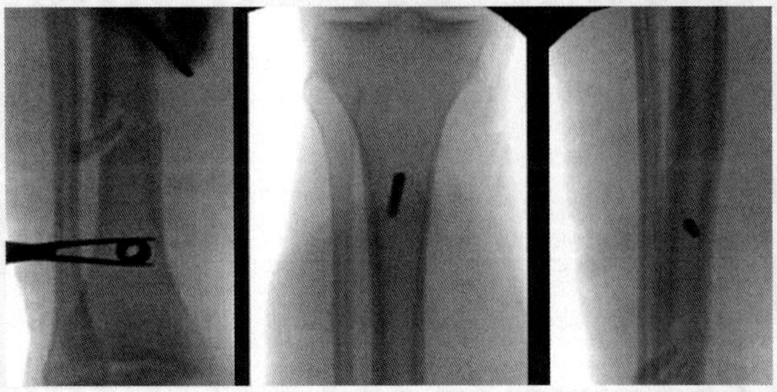

G

TECH FIG 1 *(continued)* **G.** It is important to place the trocar over the center of the medullary canal and confirm its location to ensure that the pin captures the near cortex, medullary canal, and far cortex. This confirms that a transcortical pin is avoided, as these pins can be stress risers and may lead to pin-related fracture or pin infection due to the drilling and placement in only hard, dense cortical bone.

MONOLATERAL FOUR-PIN FRAME APPLICATION FOR TIBIAL SHAFT FRACTURE

- Contemporary simple monolateral fixators have clamps that allow independent adjustments at each pin–bar interface, allowing wide variability in pin placement, which helps to avoid areas of soft tissue compromise.
  - Because of this feature, simple four-pin placement may be random on either side of the fracture.

Option 1

- The initial two pins are first inserted as far away from the fracture line as possible in the proximal fracture segment and as distal as possible in the distal fracture segment **(TECH FIG 2A)**.
- A solitary connecting rod is attached close to the bone to increase the rigidity of the system.
- Longitudinal traction is applied, and a gross reduction is achieved **(TECH FIG 2B–F)**.
- The intermediate pins can then be inserted using the pin fixation clamps attached to the rod to act as templates with drill sleeves as guides.
- These pins should not encroach on the open wound or severely contused skin in the immediate zone of injury.
- After placement of these two additional pins, the reduction can be achieved with minimal difficulty by additional manipulation of the fracture.
- Once satisfactory reduction has been accomplished, the clamps are tightened, and reduction is confirmed via fluoroscopy.

Option 2

- Alternatively, all the fixation pins can be inserted independent of each other, with two pins proximally and two pins distally **(TECH FIG 3)**.
- The two proximal pins are connected to a solitary bar, and the distal two pins are connected to a solitary bar.
- Both proximal and distal bars are then used as reduction tools to manipulate the fracture into alignment.
- Once reduction has been achieved, an additional bar-to-bar construct between the two fixed-pin couples is connected.
- Reduction is confirmed under fluoroscopy.

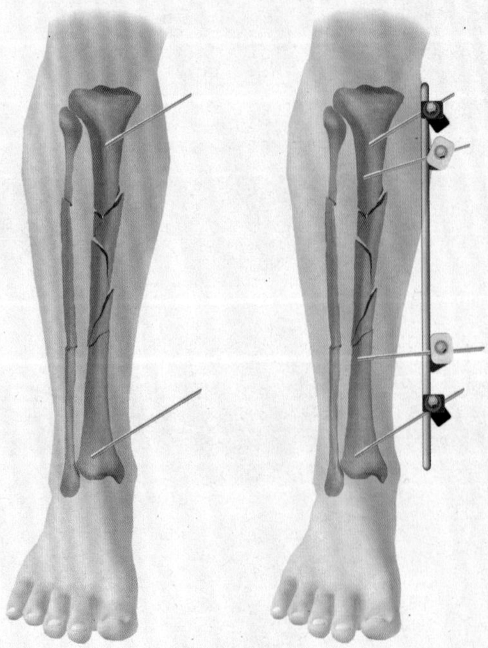

A B

TECH FIG 2 Placement of a simple four-pin monolateral fixator. **A.** Two pins are placed on either side of the fracture as far from the fracture as possible. A connecting bar is then attached to the two pins (**B**), and a gradual reduction is performed (**C–F**). Two pins are then placed as close to the fracture as possible on either side, after longitudinal traction has accomplished a reduction. The inner pins are then attached, and the reduction is fine-tuned. *(continued)*

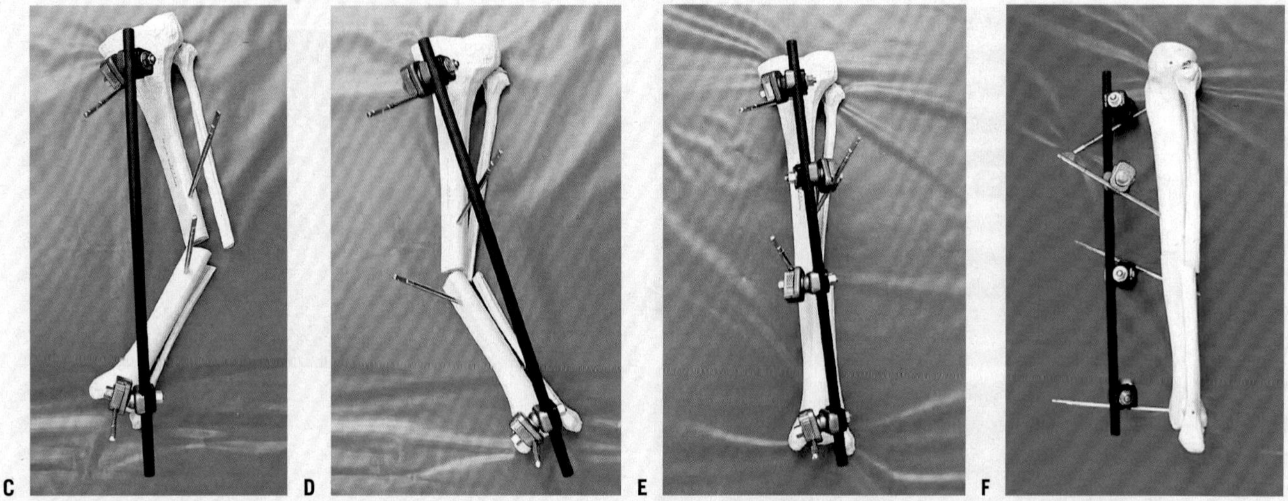

TECH FIG 2 *(continued)*

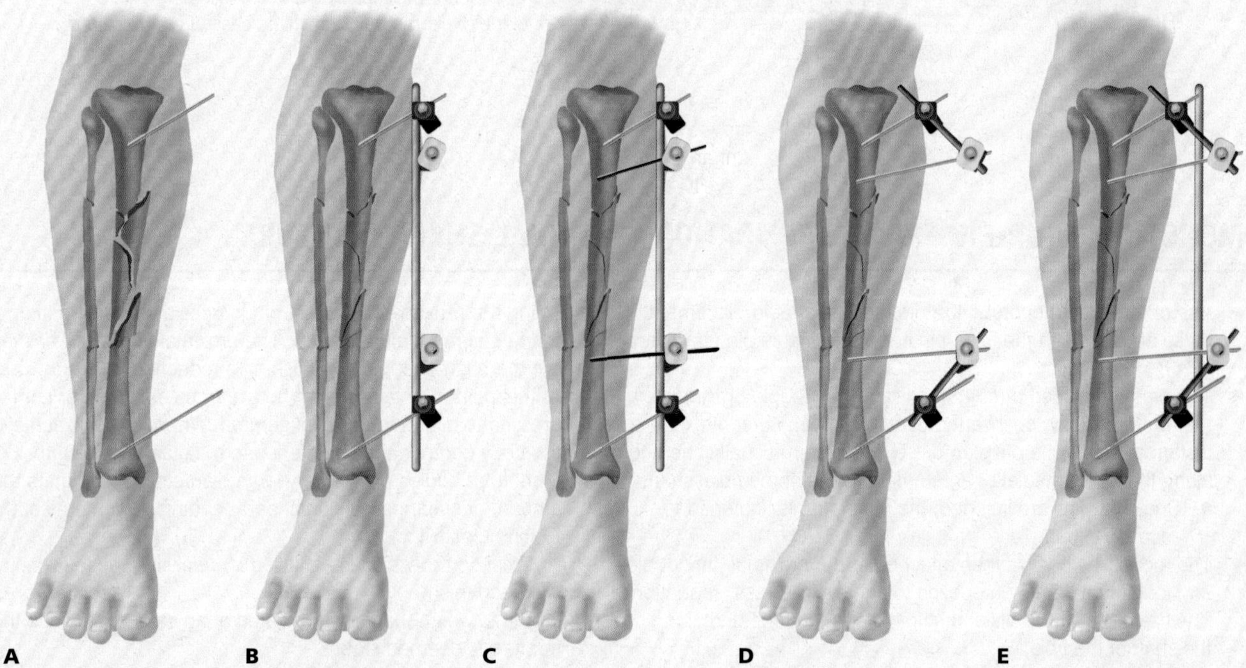

TECH FIG 3 Alternative method for simple four-pin monolateral fixator. **A,B.** Once the bar is attached, two intercalary clamps can be positioned as templates for the placement of the interior pins. **C.** Final construct after interior pin placement. **D.** The proximal and distal two pins can be attached to each other by a solitary bar. These bars can then be used as tools to reduce the fracture. **E.** The two bars are then connected by a solitary bar, and the fracture reduction is maintained. *(continued)*

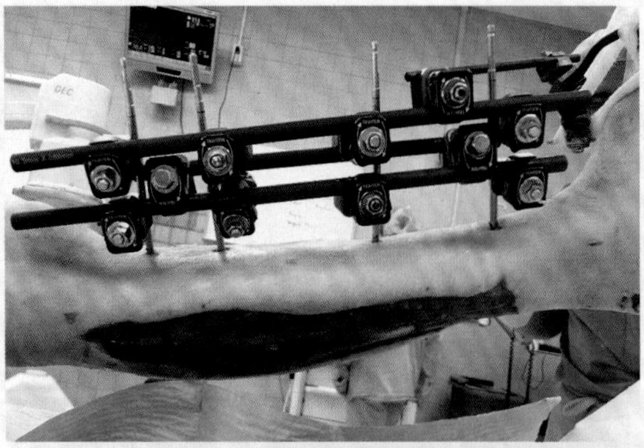

F

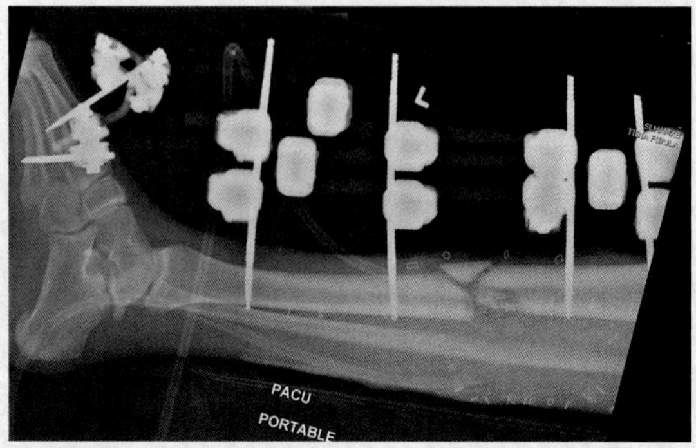

G

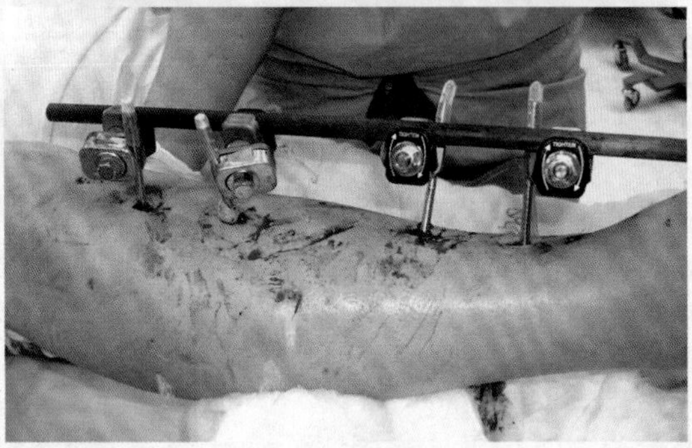

H

TECH FIG 3 *(continued)* **F,G.** Closed fracture with associated compartment syndrome is reduced and stabilized using a four-pin fixator with a double stack bar for stability, and the foot is spanned to maintain a plantigrade foot. **H.** Similar tibial fracture reduced with four pins and a single bar. Note pins out of plane to each other to facilitate ease of pin insertion.

MONOTUBE FOUR-PIN FRAME APPLICATION FOR TIBIAL SHAFT FRACTURE

- Use of the large monotube fixators facilitates rapid placement of these devices, with the fixed-pin couple acting as pin templates **(TECH FIG 4)**.
- Two pins are placed through the fixator pin couple proximal to the fracture. They are inserted parallel to each other at fixed distances set by the pin clamp itself. These are usually oriented along the direct medial or anteromedial face of the tibial shaft.
  - Once the pins are inserted, the pin clamp is tightened to secure them in place.
- The monotube body is then attached to the proximal pin couple and longitudinal traction applied to achieve a "gross" reduction. The fixator body and distal multipin clamp are oriented along the shaft of the tibia.
  - The proximal and distal ball joints should be freely movable with the telescoping body extended.
- Two pins are placed through the pin couple distal to the fracture and tightened.
  - Care must be taken to allow adequate length of the monotube frame before final reduction and tightening of the body.[23]
- Using the proximal and distal pin clamps as reduction aids, the fracture is manually reduced. The proximal and distal ball joints are then tightened, accomplishing a reduction.
- At this point, the telescoping body can be extended or compressed to dial in the axial alignment. When length is achieved, the body component is tightened to maintain axial length.
- Monotube bodies have a very large diameter, which limits the amount of shearing, torsional, and bending movements of the fixation construct.
  - Axial compression is achieved by releasing the telescoping mechanism.
- Dynamic weight bearing is initiated at an early stage once the fracture is deemed stable.
  - In fractures that are highly comminuted, weight bearing is delayed until visible callus is achieved, and sufficient stability has been maintained.
- The telescopic body allows dynamic movement in an axial direction, which is a stimulus for early periosteal healing.

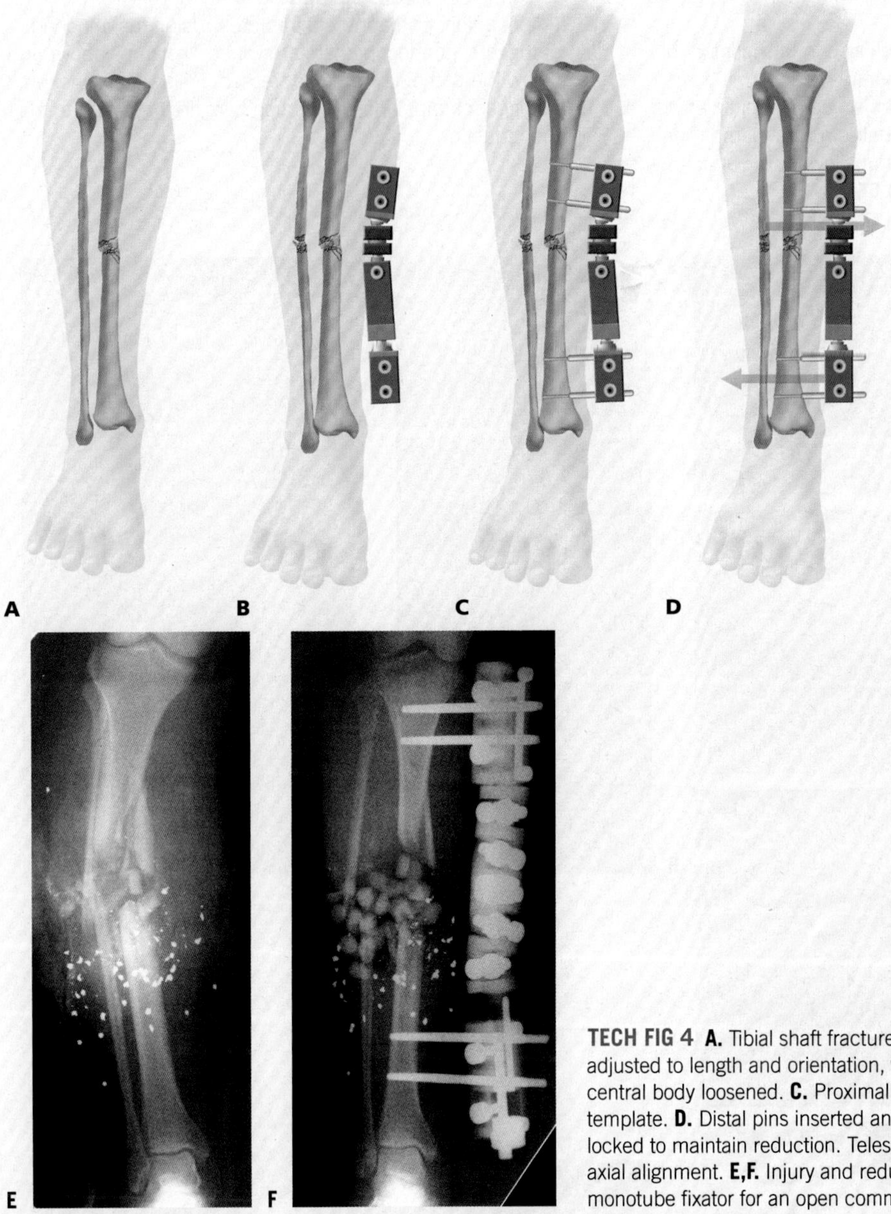

TECH FIG 4 **A.** Tibial shaft fracture with displacement. **B.** Monotube fixator adjusted to length and orientation, with all ball joints and the telescoping central body loosened. **C.** Proximal two pins applied using pin couple as template. **D.** Distal pins inserted and fracture reduced with all ball joints locked to maintain reduction. Telescoping body is also locked to maintain axial alignment. **E,F.** Injury and reduction radiographs using a large-body monotube fixator for an open comminuted tibial shaft fracture.

KNEE-SPANNING FIXATOR OF TIBIAL PLATEAU FRACTURE

- Two half-pins are placed along the anterolateral thigh. These pins are placed in the midshaft region of the femur **(TECH FIG 5A–C)**.
- Two half-pins are then inserted into the midshaft and distal tibia.
- Apply the tibial pins far enough away from the distal extension of the proximal tibia such that any future incisions required to perform definitive open reduction and internal fixation of the plateau fracture would not impinge on the pins.
- A solitary bar can then be used to span all pins **(TECH FIG 5D,E)**.
  - Longitudinal traction is applied and reduction confirmed under fluoroscopy.
  - Slight flexion of the knee is maintained, and all connections are tightened to maintain the ligamentotaxis reduction.
- Alternatively, the proximal two femur pins can be connected using a single bar and the two tibial pins with a second bar. These two bars can then be manipulated to achieve a reduction of the plateau, and a third bar connecting the proximal femoral

and distal tibial bars is then attached and tightened to maintain the reduction.

- A large monotube fixator can also be used in this fashion to span the knee and maintain a temporary reduction.
- Newer frame designs allow the use of single multipin clamps. These are applied with at least two half-pins per clamp. The clamps have integrated outriggers that allow for the attachment of longer connecting bars **(TECH FIG 5F–H)**.
- The multipin clamps are applied above and below the joint (knee, ankle, or diaphyseal fractures. Using the attached outriggers, connecting bars are joined to clamps above and below the pathology to be addressed. Following reduction, the outrigger clamps and connecting bars are tightened to maintain the reduction.

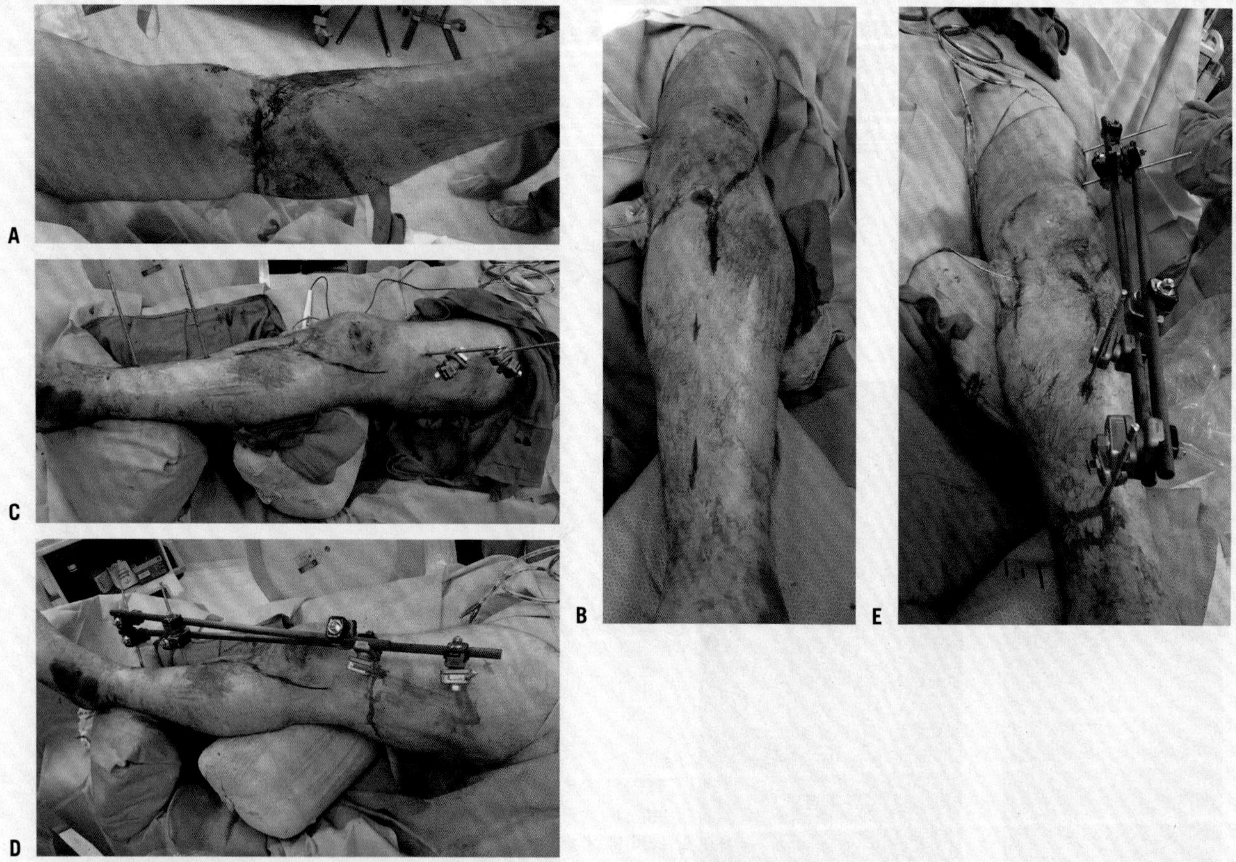

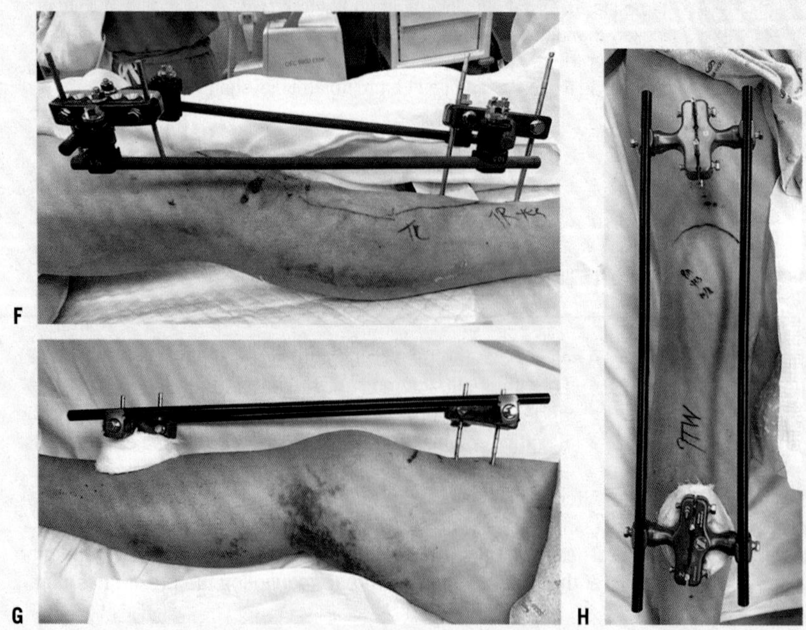

TECH FIG 5 **A.** Open tibial plateau fracture to be stabilized with knee-spanning fixator. **B.** Following a gentle manual reduction, the proposed locations for eventual fixation incisions, as well as proposed pin sites, are marked on the skin. **C.** Two pins each above (distal femur) and below (midtibia) the plateau fracture zone of injury are applied. **D,E.** One single bar connects the proximal two pins to the distal two pins. The fracture is then reduced and the clamps tightened. A second bar was added for stability, bridging the fracture. **F–H.** In a different patient, a knee-spanning frame was applied using multipin clamps with integrated outriggers. Pin couples were placed above and below the knee with medical and lateral connecting bars spanning the knee. Following traction and reduction, the clamps are tightened, maintaining the spanning fixator.

ANKLE-SPANNING FIXATOR FOR TIBIAL PILON FRACTURE

- Two Schanz pins are placed into the midshaft tibial region **(TECH FIG 6A,B)**.
  - Avoid any compromised soft tissues and possible fracture extension if spanning the ankle for a severe pilon fracture with shaft extension.
- A centrally threaded transfixion pin is then placed through the calcaneal tuberosity from medial to lateral, avoiding the posterior tibial artery.
  - The appropriate location for this pin is 1.5 cm anterior to the posterior aspect of the heel and 1.5 cm proximal to the plantar aspect of the heel.
  - This location is confirmed via fluoroscopy.
- A solitary bar is connected to the tibial pins.
- Medial and lateral bars are then connected to each side of the heel pin, making a triangular configuration **(TECH FIG 6C,D)**.
  - Longitudinal traction is carried out to obtain length, and care is taken to achieve appropriate anteroposterior reduction.
- To maintain a plantigrade foot and to maintain alignment, a pin is placed into the base of the first or second metatarsal and, in some cases, the fifth metatarsal as well.[30]
  - This forefoot pin is then connected to the main frame with a connecting bar, and the foot is held in neutral dorsiflexion.
  - As with knee-spanning fixators, new designs have integrated outriggers that allow for the attachment of longer connecting bars **(TECH FIG 6E)**.

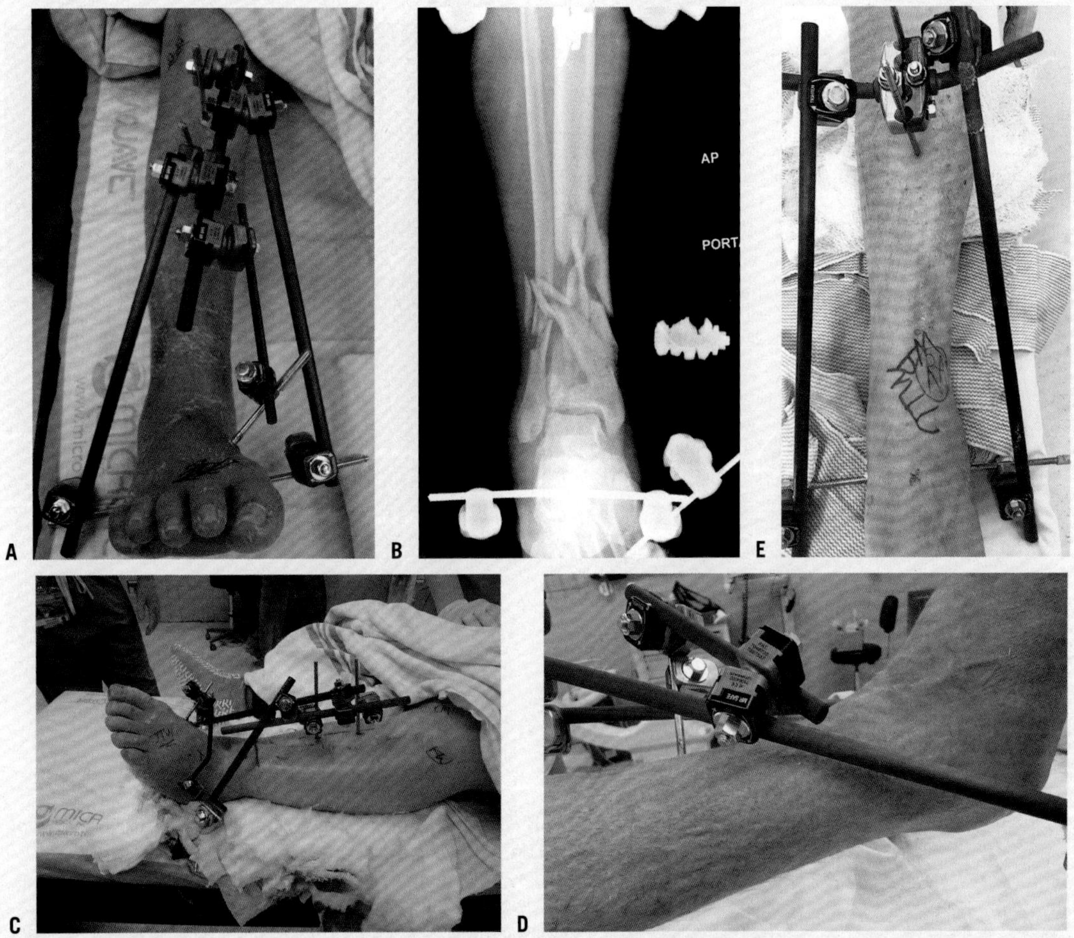

TECH FIG 6 Ankle-spanning fixators bridging a severe pilon fracture. **A,B.** Two pins are placed into the proximal tibia, out of the distal fracture zone of injury. A calcaneal transfixion pin is placed through the calcaneal tuberosity, and subsequent medial-lateral triangulation connecting bars are attached. Longitudinal traction is applied, and all bars are tightened to maintain reduction. A forefoot pin is placed into the first metatarsal to maintain the foot in a neutral position and avoid equinus contracture. **C.** Similar pin configuration with a triangular frame. First and fifth metatarsal pins with a forefoot bar were applied to maintain a neutral foot position. **D.** Skin demonstrates wrinkles and at this time is amenable to formal open reconstructive procedures. **E.** An ankle-spanning frame using a multipin clamp with integrated outriggers and connecting bars spanning the ankle in a different patient. Multipin clamps are attached using a minimum of two half-pins to prevent frame rotation and instability around the pin.

TWO-PIN FIXATOR: TEMPORARY STABILIZATION FOR TIBIAL SHAFT, PILON, OR PLATEAU FRACTURES

- This is a temporary frame designed for rapid distraction and gross reduction used for all types of tibial pathology.
- A proximal centrally threaded transfixion pin is applied one fingerbreadth proximal to the tip of the proximal fibula. It is inserted from lateral to medial **(TECH FIG 7A,B)**.
  - Alternatively, this pin can be placed into the distal femur at the level of the midpatella along the midlateral condyle of the femur.
- A second transfixion pin is placed through the calcaneal tuberosity, similar to the ankle-spanning frame described earlier.
- Two long connecting bars are then attached to the pins on each side of the leg.
  - Longitudinal traction is applied, and a gross reduction is achieved.
- In some circumstances, a third pin is placed into the tibial shaft and attached to one of the longitudinal bars by a third connecting bar **(TECH FIG 7C,D)**. This is done to add stability to this very simple frame **(TECH FIG 7E–G)**.

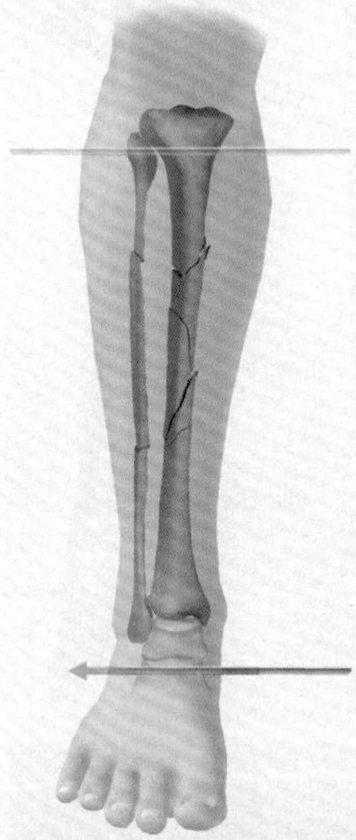
A
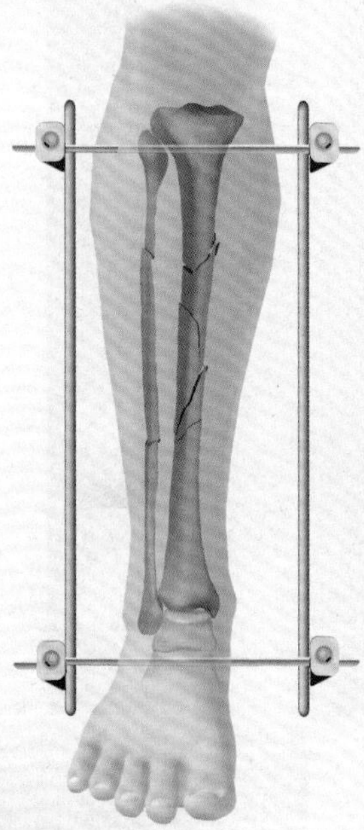
B
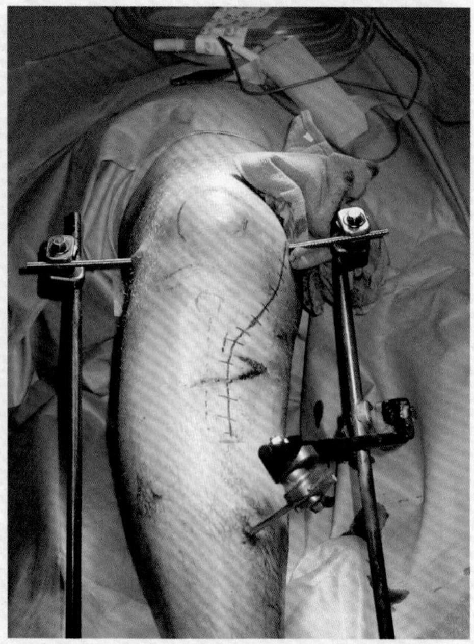
C
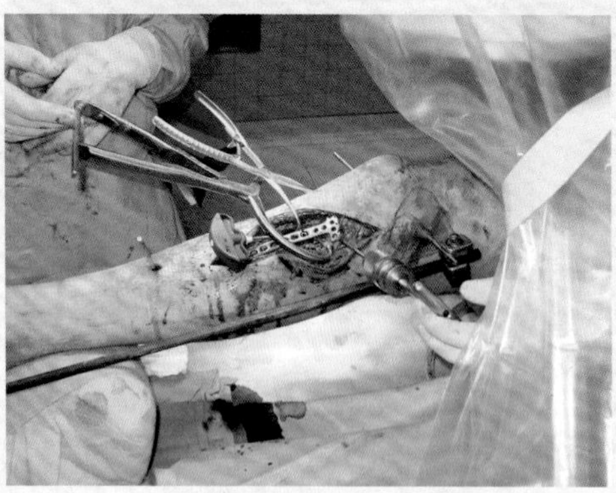
D

TECH FIG 7 A,B. Application of spanning two-pin fixator "traveling traction" with attachment of medial and lateral bars. This is used as a very temporary frame to stabilize a variety of conditions. **C,D.** Two-pin fixator used to stabilize a severe plateau fracture. A third pin was inserted into the distal third of the tibia to provide additional stability. The frame is prepped directly into the operative field at the time of secondary surgery to definitively stabilize the fracture using a medial buttress plate. *(continued)*

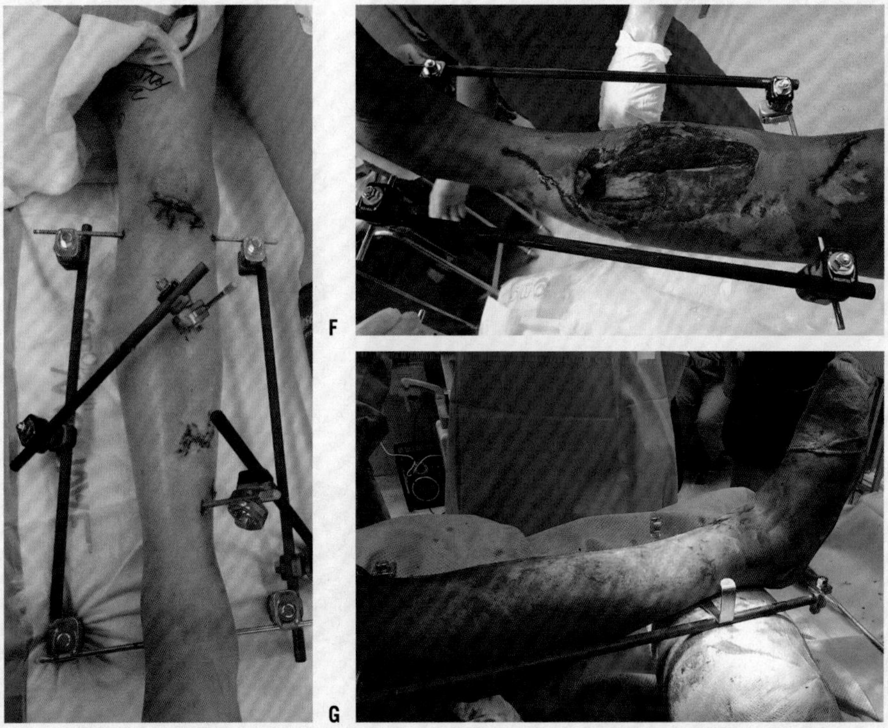

E F G

TECH FIG 7 *(continued)* **E.** Modified two-pin fixator with an additional half-pin placed above and below the fracture for added stability prior to intramedullary nailing of the shaft injury. **F.** Spanning two-pin frame providing initial stabilization to a severe open tibia with soft tissue and bone loss. This temporizes the injury and allows for additional staging procedures. **G.** Simple two-pin frame previously applied and now used as a reduction aid at the time of definitive intramedullary nailing.

TECHNIQUES

Pearls and Pitfalls

Pin Placement Location	• Areas of soft tissue compromise, open wounds, and occult fracture lines as identified on CT scans should be avoided. This prevents any associated pin tract infection from involving the fracture site. The frame must be constructed and applied to allow for multiple débridements, subsequent soft tissue reconstruction, and definitive secondary internal fixation conversions. Thus, the pins must be placed away from the zone of injury to avoid potential pin site contamination with the operative field. (Mark proposed incisions on skin prior to pin placement.)
Pin Insertion Technique	• Adequate skin release is provided to avoid tethering or bunching of soft tissues around pins. Pins are overwrapped with small gauze wrap to provide a stable pin–skin interface and to avoid excessive pin–skin motion and development of tissue necrosis and infection.
Temporary frames require adjunctive splinting of knee, leg, ankle, and foot.	• Temporary spanning frames are *not* excessively rigid and require additional splinting to maintain the foot in neutral and to avoid the development of equinus contractures. Alternatively, span frame into foot using metatarsal pins to maintain a plantigrade foot.
Delta Frame Temporary Ankle-Spanning Fixator	• The weakest part of a monolateral system is the junction between the fixator clamp and the Schanz pins. Insufficient holding strength on a pin by a clamp can result in a decrease in the overall fixation rigidity as well as increased motion and cortical bone reaction at the pin–bone interface. Cyclic loading will loosen the tightened screws in the pin clamps. One needs to be aware of the mechanical yield characteristics of the clamps, bars, and pins throughout the course of treatment.[8] • A simple monolateral frame can be configured in a triangular-type construct about the distal tibial and ankle region in an effort to achieve relative stability to temporize unstable pilon, ankle, and very distal tibial fractures. These are usually constructed with two or three pins in the mid- to distal tibia and a single transversely placed centrally threaded calcaneal tuberosity pin. These tibial pins are then connected in a triangular fashion with distraction across the calcaneal pin, effecting a ligamentotaxis reduction at the distal tibia (see **FIG 1G**). • The triangular external fixator construct can obscure the site of injury on radiographs, and unbeknownst to the surgeon as the clamps "creep," the reduction can be lost as the foot construct subluxes posteriorly (**FIG 8A**). Because most ankle spanning frames have a solitary calcaneal pin, the bars attached to the foot "pinwheel" around this axis pin and rotate posteriorly with ambulation and the shaft translates anteriorly, putting more pressure on the soft tissues as the reduction is lost (**FIG 8B,C**). • A blocking bar placed across the triangular configuration may inhibit this "pinwheel" effect (**FIG 8D**). Application of forefoot pins and stabilization of the foot in neutral position not only prevents rotation with calcaneal pin loosening but also maintains the foot in neutral and prevents the common complication of forefoot equinus (**FIG 8E**).[4]

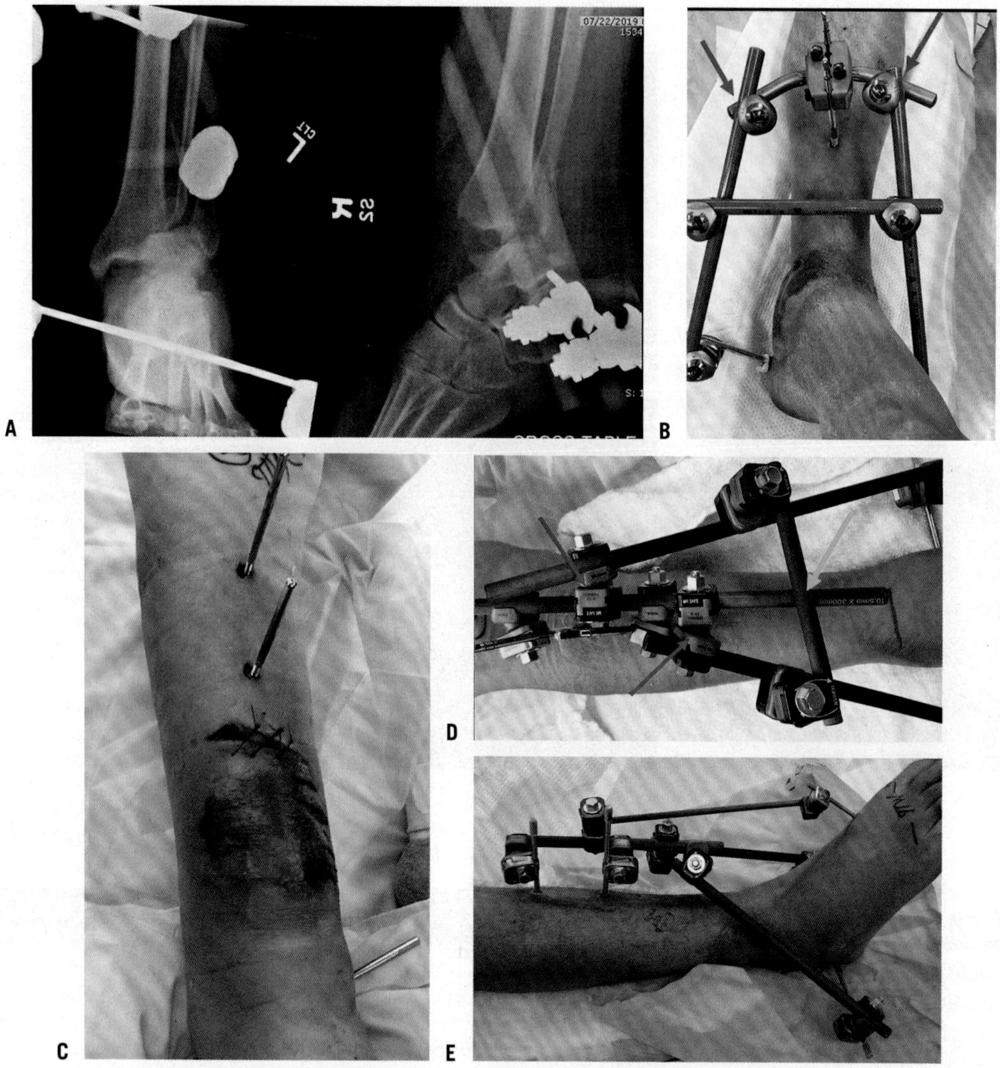

FIG 8 **A.** Ankle fracture 6 days postoperatively in a spanning ankle external fixator. **B.** The bar-to-bar connections (*red arrows*) gradually loosened, allowing the medial and lateral distraction bars connected to the calcaneus pin to rotate around the proximal bars. This resulted in posterior redislocation of the ankle with soft tissue compromise and blisters on the anterior skin due to the posteriorly subluxed ankle. **C.** Anterior skin necrosis resulting from unrecognized gradual posterior subluxation of the foot and ankle in a triangular external fixator construct in a different patient. **D.** Bar-to-bar clamps (*red arrows*) are attaching the medial and lateral triangular connecting bars to the calcaneal pin. These are subject to gradual creep and loosening, which can lead to gradual posterior subluxation of the foot and ankle. A blocking bar (*green arrow*) has been added to the construct that is resting on the main longitudinal bar. This blocking bar will prevent the foot and ankle from pinwheeling around the proximal connections and dislocating the ankle, should these bar-to-bar clamps undergo gradual creep. **E.** Spanning frame with medial lateral bars and a forefoot pin to maintain ankle in neutral and prevent posterior subluxation.

POSTOPERATIVE CARE

- A compressive dressing should be applied to the pin sites immediately after surgery to stabilize the pin–skin interface and thus minimize pin–skin motion, which can lead to the development of necrotic debris.
- Compressive dressings can be removed within 10 days to 2 weeks once the pin sites are healed.
- If appropriate pin insertion technique is used, the pin sites will completely heal around each individual pin. Once healed, only showering, without any other pin cleaning procedures, is necessary.[22]
  - Removal of a serous crust around the pins using dilute hydrogen peroxide and saline may occasionally be necessary.
- Ointments should not be used for pin care. They tend to inhibit the normal skin flora and alter the normal skin bacteria and may lead to superinfection or pin site colonization.

- If pin drainage does develop, pin care should be provided three times a day.
  - This may also involve rewrapping and compressing the offending pin site in an effort to minimize the abnormal pin–skin motion.
- Following a standardized protocol that involves precleaning the external fixator frame, followed by alcohol wash, sequential povidone-iodine preparation, paint, and spray with air drying followed by draping the extremity and fixator directly into the operative field, additional surgery can be safely performed without an increased rate of postoperative wound infection.
- Definitive treatment with an external fixator demands close scrutiny of the radiographs to ensure that the fracture has completely healed before frame removal. Various techniques have been described, including CT scans, ultrasound, and bone densitometry, to determine the adequacy of fracture healing.
- There is no consensus among trauma surgeons to define fracture healing. The most common criteria considered are cortical apposition of at least three cortices, obliteration of fracture line, ability to bear weight without pain, and no palpation with tenderness.
  - In general, the patient should be fully weight bearing with minimal pain at the fracture site. The frame should be fully dynamized such that the load is being borne by the patient's limb rather than by the external fixator.

OUTCOMES

- Staged management of high-energy tibial plateau and tibial pilon fractures using spanning external fixation to allow the recovery of soft tissues has reduced the overall rates of soft tissue complications. With secondary plating procedures after soft tissue recovery, infection rates have been reported to be less than 5% for complex plateau fractures and less than 7% for complex pilon fractures.
- No severe complications related to the temporary external fixator alone have been reported.
- Immediate external fixation followed by early, closed, interlocking nailing has been demonstrated to be a safe and effective treatment for open tibial fractures if early (<21 days after injury) conversion to intramedullary nailing is performed.
- Early soft tissue coverage and closure is the primary determinant of delayed infection, highlighting the need for effective soft tissue management and early closure of open injuries.
- Definitive treatment of open tibial fractures with external fixation has a higher rate of malunion compared with intramedullary nailing. No difference in union rates is noted. Slightly higher rates of infection are noted in the external fixation group.
  - The severity of the soft tissue injury rather than the choice of implant appears to be the predominant factor influencing outcome. External fixation is preferentially used in patients with the most severe soft tissue injuries or wound contamination.
- Definitive treatment of extra-articular distal tibia fractures with Ilizarov external fixation versus plate osteosynthesis has the benefits of immediate postoperative weight bearing with lower rates of malunion, nonunion, and delayed union.[10]

COMPLICATIONS

- Wire and pin site complications include pin site inflammation, chronic infection, loosening, or metal fatigue failure.
  - Minor pin tract inflammation requires more frequent pin care consisting of daily cleansing with mild soap or half-strength peroxide and saline solution.
  - Occasionally, an inflamed pin site with purulent discharge will require antibiotics and continued daily pin care.
- Severe pin tract infection consists of serous or seropurulent drainage in concert with redness, inflammation, and radiographs showing osteolysis of both the near and far cortices.
  - Once osteolysis occurs with bicortical involvement, the offending pin should be removed immediately, with débridement of the pin tract.[11]
- Late deformity after removal of the apparatus usually presents as a gradual deviation of the limb. This often occurs if the patient and surgeon become "frame weary," which results in frame removal before healing is complete.
  - One should always err on the conservative side and leave the frame on for an extended time to ensure that the fracture has healed.
- When late deformity occurs, it usually has an unsatisfactory outcome unless collapse is detected early and the frame is reapplied.
  - If untreated, the resulting malunion requires secondary osteotomy procedures.
  - Early detection of delayed union often requires adjunctive bone grafting for previously open shaft fractures.

REFERENCES

1. Akilapa O, Gaffey A. Hydroxyapatite pins for external fixation: is there sufficient evidence to prove that coated pins are less likely to be replaced prematurely? Acta Orthop Traumatol Turc 2015;49(4):410–415.
2. Ali AM, Yang L, Hashmi M, et al. Bicondylar tibial plateau fractures managed with the Sheffield hybrid fixator. Biomechanical study and operative technique. Injury 2001;32(suppl 4):SD86–SD91.
3. Aronson J, Johnson E, Harp JH. Local bone transportation for treatment of intercalary defects by the Ilizarov technique. Biomechanical and clinical considerations. Clin Orthop Relat Res 1989;(243):71–79.
4. Barrett MO, Wade AM, Della Rocca GJ, et al. The safety of forefoot metatarsal pins in external fixation of the lower extremity. J Bone Joint Surg Am 2008;90(3):560–564.
5. Behrens F, Johnson W. Unilateral external fixation. Methods to increase and reduce frame stiffness. Clin Orthop Relat Res 1989;(241):48–56.
6. Chao EY, Aro HT, Lewallen DG, et al. The effect of rigidity on fracture healing in external fixation. Clin Orthop Relat Res 1989;(241):24–35.
7. Della Rocca GJ, Crist BD. External fixation versus conversion to intramedullary nailing for definitive management of closed fractures of the femoral and tibial shaft. J Am Acad Orthop Surg 2006;14(10):S131–S135.
8. Drijber FL, Finlay JB. Universal joint slippage as a cause of Hoffmann half-frame external fixator failure [corrected]. J Biomed Eng 1992;14(6):509–515.
9. Egol KA, Tejwani NC, Capla EL, et al. Staged management of high-energy proximal tibia fractures (OTA types 41): the results of a prospective, standardized protocol. J Orthop Trauma 2005;19:448–456.
10. Fadel M, Ahmed MA, Al-Dars AM, et al. Ilizarov external fixation versus plate osteosynthesis in the management of extra-articular fractures of the distal tibia. Int Orthop 2015;39(3):513–519.
11. Green SA. Complications of External Skeletal Fixation: Causes, Prevention, and Treatment. Springfield, IL: Charles C Thomas, 1981.

12. Haidukewych GJ. Temporary external fixation for the management of complex intra- and periarticular fractures of the lower extremity. J Orthop Trauma 2002;16:678–685.
13. Ilizarov GA. The tension-stress effect on the genesis and growth of tissues. Part I. The influence of stability of fixation and soft-tissue preservation. Clin Orthop Relat Res 1989;(238):249–281.
14. Ilizarov GA. The tension-stress effect on the genesis and growth of tissues: part II. The influence of the rate and frequency of distraction. Clin Orthop Relat Res 1989;(239):263–285.
15. Ilizarov GA. Transosseous Osteosynthesis. Theoretical and Clinical Aspects of the Regeneration and Growth of Tissue. Berlin, Germany: Springer-Verlag, 1992.
16. Kashiwagi N, Suzuki S, Seto Y, et al. Bilateral humeral lengthening in achondroplasia. Clin Orthop Relat Res 2001;(391):251–257.
17. Kenwright J, Richardson JB, Cunningham JL, et al. Axial movement and tibial fractures. A controlled randomised trial of treatment. J Bone Joint Surg Br 1991;73:654–659.
18. Laible C, Earl-Royal E, Davidovitch R, et al. Infection after spanning external fixation for high-energy tibial plateau fractures: is pin site-plate overlap a problem? J Orthop Trauma 2012;26(2):92–97.
19. La Russa V, Skallerud B, Klaksvik J, et al. Reduction in wire tension caused by dynamic loading. An experimental Ilizarov frame study. J Biomech 2011;44(8):1454–1458.
20. Lavini F, Dall'oca C, Mezzari S, et al. Temporary bridging external fixation in distal tibial fracture. Injury 2014;45(suppl 6):S58–S63.
21. Lenarz C, Bledsoe G, Watson JT. Circular external fixation frames with divergent half pins: a pilot biomechanical study. Clin Orthop Relat Res 2008;466(12):2933–2939.
22. Lethaby A, Temple J, Santy J. Pin site care for preventing infections associated with external bone fixators and pins. Cochrane Database Syst Rev 2008;(4):CD004551.
23. Marsh JL, Bonar S, Nepola JV, et al. Use of an articulated external fixator for fractures of the tibial plafond. J Bone Joint Surg Am 1995;77(10):1498–1509.
24. Nho SJ, Helfet DL, Rozbruch SR. Temporary intentional leg shortening and deformation to facilitate wound closure using the Ilizarov/Taylor spatial frame. J Orthop Trauma 2006;20(6):419–424.
25. Podolsky A, Chao EY. Mechanical performance of Ilizarov circular external fixators in comparison with other external fixators. Clin Orthop Relat Res 1993;(293):61–70.
26. Rozbruch SR, Pugsley JS, Fragomen AT, et al. Repair of tibial nonunions and bone defects with the Taylor spatial frame. J Orthop Trauma 2008;22(2):88–95.
27. Sirkin M, Sanders R, DiPasquale T, et al. A staged protocol for soft tissue management in the treatment of complex pilon fractures. J Orthop Trauma 1999;13:78–84.
28. Tetsworth KD, Paley D. Accuracy of correction of complex lower-extremity deformities by the Ilizarov method. Clin Orthop Relat Res 1994;(301):102–110.
29. Watson JT, Moed BR, Karges DE, et al. Pilon fractures. Treatment protocol based on severity of soft tissue injury. Clin Orthop Relat Res 2000;(375):78–90.
30. Ziran BH, Morrison T, Little J, et al. A new ankle spanning fixator construct for distal tibia fractures: optimizing visualization, minimizing pin problems, and protecting the heel. J Orthop Trauma 2013;27(2):e45–e49.

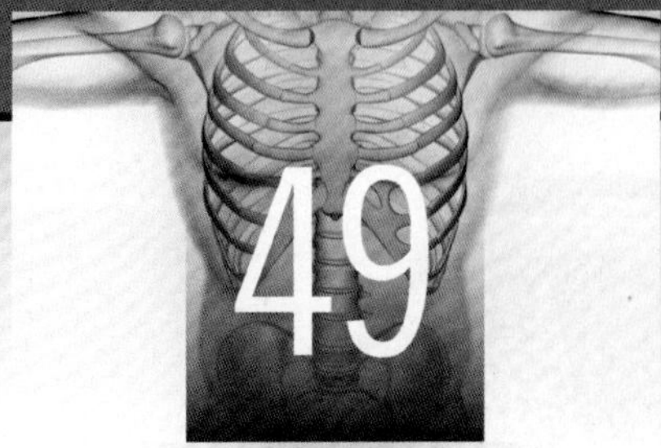

CHAPTER 49

Intramedullary Nailing of the Tibia

Daniel S. Horwitz and Erik Noble Kubiak

DEFINITION

- Intramedullary nailing techniques are typically used for closed and open displaced diaphyseal tibial fractures.
- The indications for intramedullary nailing can be extended to proximal and distal metaphyseal tibia fractures, including those associated with simple articular involvement.
- Both traditional peripatellar tendinous and semiextended approaches are used to attain the entry site for nailing all levels of tibial fractures.

ANATOMY

- The triangular-shaped proximal tibia is narrowest medially, and the proximal medial tibial cortex is obliquely oriented to the frontal plane. The medullary canal of the tibia exits at the margin of the lateral articular facet. As a result of this complex proximal anatomy, there is less sagittal plane space for an intramedullary nail within the tibia metaphysis with a medial or central insertion path. With a medial start site, the nail can deflect the anteromedial metaphyseal cortex or fail to contact the lateral proximal cortex and create a valgus deformity. Due to these factors, a start site corresponding to the medial aspect of the lateral tibial spine on the anteroposterior (AP) view is recommended.
- The patellar tendon inserts on the tibial tubercle and extends the proximal fracture segment in proximal fracture patterns. This displacement is accentuated with further flexion of the knee, which typically is required to attain the proper starting point for intramedullary nailing utilizing a standard flexed technique (**FIG 1A**).
- Gerdy tubercle—the origin of the anterior compartment muscles and insertion site of the iliotibial band—is palpable along the proximal lateral tibia. In addition to the deforming forces of the patellar tendon, the anterior compartment muscles and the iliotibial band contribute to the shortening and valgus deformity typically seen with more proximal fractures.
- The anterior tibial crest corresponds to the vertical lateral surface of the tibia. When it is palpable, it is an excellent reference for the anatomic axis and nail path (**FIG 1B**).
- The anteromedial tibial surface is subcutaneous and often is the site of traumatic open wounds.
- The anterior neurovascular bundle and tibialis anterior tendon are at risk with anterior to posterior distal interlocking screw paths; limited internal rotation of the nail may decrease the risk of iatrogenic nerve injury, but excessive rotation may put the posterior neurovascular bundle at risk from medial to lateral interlocks (**FIG 1C**).[5]
- The Hoffa fat pad and intermeniscal ligament are commonly injured during all tibial intramedullary nail insertion techniques, especially during lateral parapatellar tendinous and patellar tendon-splitting approaches.[33,40]

PATHOGENESIS

- Tibial shaft fractures may occur from high-energy mechanisms of injury, as when a pedestrian is struck by a motor vehicle. Many fractures, however, result from low-energy mechanisms such as simple falls in elderly patients or those with poor bone quality or sports-related injuries (common in soccer players) in younger patients.[8]
- In this low-energy fracture group, elderly patients are more likely to have comminuted and open fractures due to simple falls.

NATURAL HISTORY

- The long-term outcome of tibial malunion is not clearly defined in the trauma literature.
  - A weak association is seen between a tibial shaft fracture malunion and ipsilateral knee and ankle arthritis.[15,23,38]
- Knee pain is reported in up to 58% of cases after intramedullary nailing. This pain typically is anterior, associated with activity, and exacerbated by kneeling activities.[8,14]
  - Knee pain improves in about 50% of patients after hardware removal.[8]
  - Attempts to detect a correlation between start sites and knee pain have been inconclusive, and comparative evaluations between traditional start sites and semiextended start sites (ie, suprapatellar) are underway. Recent publications suggest a lower incidence of knee pain with semiextended approaches, potentially due to the avoidance of an incision and scar directly in the kneeling contact pathway.[1,2,4,5]

PATIENT HISTORY AND PHYSICAL FINDINGS

- Understanding the mechanism of injury and the environment in which the injury occurred is important for evaluating a patient's risk for associated injuries and compartment syndrome. In open fractures, it can help determine the choice of prophylactic antibiotic therapy.
- All patients who sustain tibial shaft fractures from high-energy mechanisms should undergo standard advanced trauma and life support protocol to have a thorough examination for life- and other limb-threatening injuries. Seventy-five percent of patients with open tibia fractures have associated injuries.[2]

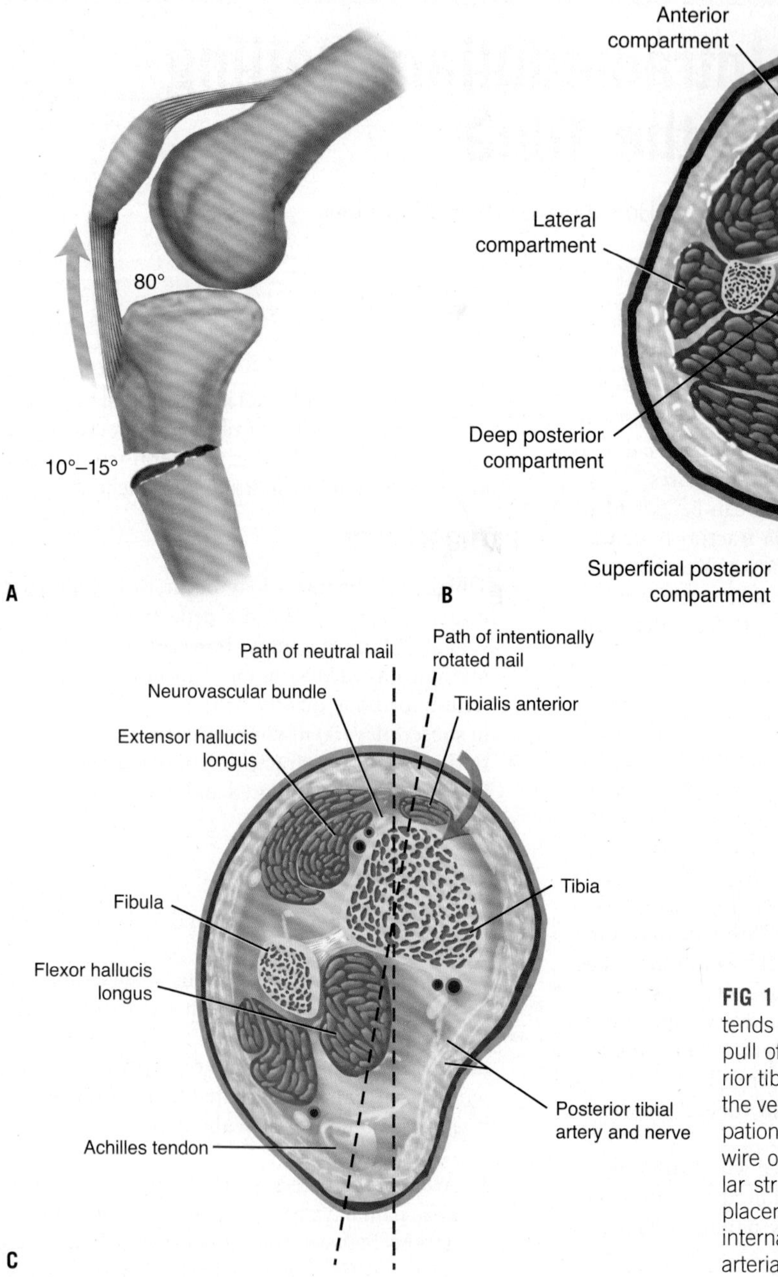

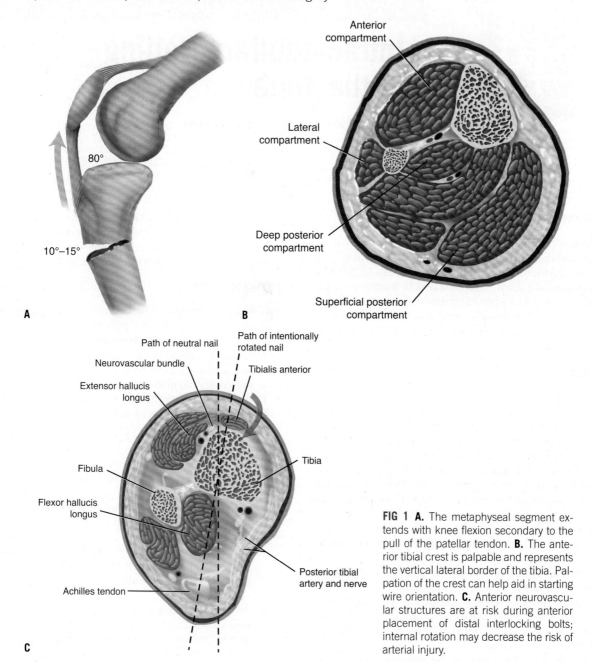

FIG 1 **A.** The metaphyseal segment extends with knee flexion secondary to the pull of the patellar tendon. **B.** The anterior tibial crest is palpable and represents the vertical lateral border of the tibia. Palpation of the crest can help aid in starting wire orientation. **C.** Anterior neurovascular structures are at risk during anterior placement of distal interlocking bolts; internal rotation may decrease the risk of arterial injury.

- To evaluate a patient's risk for potential complications, other medical conditions should be investigated, including a history of diabetes mellitus, renal disease, inflammatory arthropathies, tobacco use (which increases healing time by up to 40%), and peripheral vascular disease.[6]
- It also is important to determine the patient's normal activities and employment requirements to give them a reasonable expectation for when they will be able to resume those activities.
- Pain at the fracture site, swelling, and deformity are common findings in patients with tibial shaft fractures.
- A thorough examination of the skin is important to avoid missing open fracture wounds.
- Evaluation of the soft tissue envelope for abrasions, contusions, and fracture blisters can help determine whether definitive treatment can be done primarily or if a staged or delayed approach is required.
- A detailed neurovascular examination is critical to avoid the devastating complications associated with compartment syndrome, which can occur in both closed and open fractures (see Chap. 51).

IMAGING AND OTHER DIAGNOSTIC STUDIES

- Full-length AP and lateral plain radiographs are necessary to adequately evaluate the tibia and fibula. Complete orthogonal views of the tibia and fibula help evaluate for concurrent fractures or dislocation and any preexisting deformity or implants.
    - Orthogonal radiographic views of the knee and ankle are required to rule out articular involvement.
- Axial computed tomography (CT) scan can be used for proximal and distal fractures to rule out intra-articular

fracture extension. The association between distal one-third oblique tibial shaft fractures and tibial plafond involvement has led some authors to recommend standard CT scanning of all oblique distal third fractures.[6,19]
  - Nondisplaced fracture lines are common.
  - Gunshot wounds may merit CT evaluation to rule out intra-articular bullet fragments and intra-articular fracture extension.
- Magnetic resonance imaging is not useful for most diaphyseal or metadiaphyseal fractures.
- Ankle–brachial index (systolic pressure in injured leg below injury divided by systolic pressure of the brachium) after fracture reduction should be used to rule out vascular injuries in severely displaced fractures or fractures with severe soft tissue injury. Values of less than 0.9 may be indicative of vascular injury, requiring further investigation.[22]
- Compartment pressure evaluation with a commercially available handheld single-stick monitor or with a side-ported catheter connected to a pressure monitor (using the arterial line setup) is indicated in patients who have severe or increasing swelling and are not able to comply with physical examination and questioning. In patients who are alert and responsive the diagnosis should be based on clinical examination, not on measured compartment pressures.
  - Observe for early signs of compartment syndrome in all patients with tibial diaphyseal fractures.
  - Open fracture does not preclude development of compartment syndrome.
  - Measure the pressure difference between the diastolic pressure and the intracompartmental pressure—a differential value of less than 30 mm Hg is considered an indication for a four-compartment fasciotomy.[21]

NONOPERATIVE MANAGEMENT

- Nonoperative management may be indicated in ambulatory patients for closed and open fractures that do not require flap coverage and that do not present with excessive initial shortening or unacceptable angulation when a cast is applied **(FIG 2)**.
- An intact fibula with an axially unstable fracture pattern (ie, short oblique, butterfly fragment, or comminuted) is at risk for shortening and varus deformities and is a relative contraindication to nonoperative management.
- A higher rate of malunion and nonunion with nonoperative management is seen in higher energy fractures.[4,12]
- Joint stiffness, especially hindfoot, is common with all forms of prolonged immobilization.[9,26]
- Multiple studies have demonstrated earlier return to work and higher function with operative treatment of these fractures.
- Initial treatment includes ~2 weeks of a long-leg splint and then a long-leg cast for 2 to 4 weeks.
  - When the initial swelling has subsided, the patient is graduated to a patellar tendon or functional brace. Weight bearing is allowed and encouraged.
  - Radiographs are evaluated at 1- to 2-week intervals over the first month of treatment to confirm maintenance of acceptable alignment.
  - The treating surgeon must be adept at the use of wedging casts in order to attain acceptable alignment and must be committed to frequent reevaluation as noted earlier.

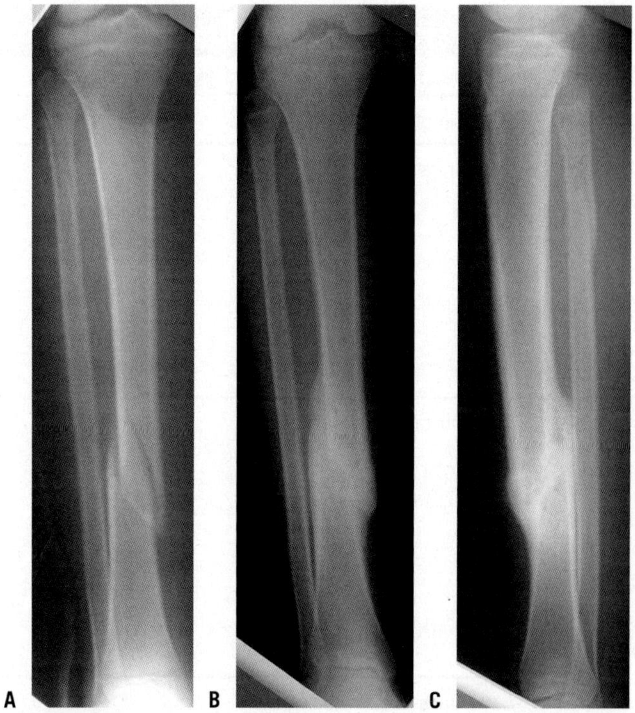

FIG 2 A–C. An oblique diaphyseal tibial shaft fracture treated nonoperatively to union. (Courtesy of Paul Tornetta III, MD.)

SURGICAL MANAGEMENT

Classification and Relative Indications

- Tibia fractures usually are classified according to the AO Foundation and Orthopaedic Trauma Association classification **(TABLE 1)**.
- Several relatively well-accepted indications and contraindications have been established for the intramedullary nailing of tibia fractures **(TABLE 2)**.
- A thorough evaluation of the patient's soft tissue envelope will determine when the patient can proceed with definitive fixation.
- Complete orthogonal radiographs of the entire tibia and fibula are important to determine whether the patient's intramedullary canal is large enough to accommodate an intramedullary nail (approximately 8 mm) and identify any preexisting deformity that may preclude nail placement. Most modern cannulated nail designs start near 8 mm in diameter. Complete radiographs also identify any proximal or distal articular involvement.
  - Preoperative measurement of the intramedullary canal and the length of the tibia will help determine which size nail can be used.
    - The lateral radiograph is the most accurate to use for measuring the appropriate nail length.
    - Measuring the narrowest diameter of the diaphysis on the AP and lateral views will determine the appropriate nail diameter and what degree of intramedullary reaming will be necessary.
- Orthogonal radiographs of the uninjured tibia can be used as templates for determining the appropriate length, alignment, and rotation in comminuted fractures or open fractures with bone loss.

TABLE 1 The AO Foundation and Orthopaedic Trauma Association Classification of Diaphyseal Tibial Fractures

Classification	Description	Illustration	Classification	Description	Illustration
42-A	Simple		42-B3	Fragmented wedge	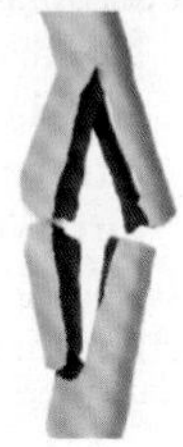
42-A1	Spiral	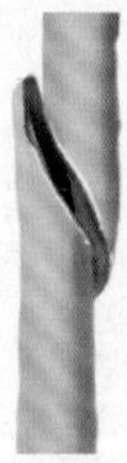	42-C	Complex	
42-A2	Oblique (≥30 degrees)	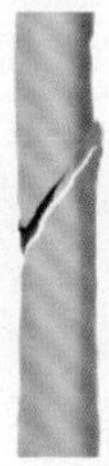	42-C1	Spiral	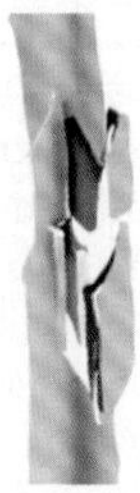
42-A3	Transverse (<30 degrees)	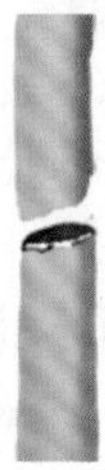	42-C2	Segmented	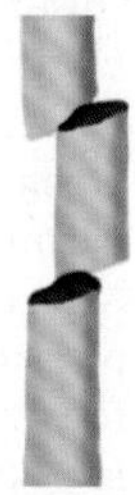
42-B	Wedge		42-C3	Irregular	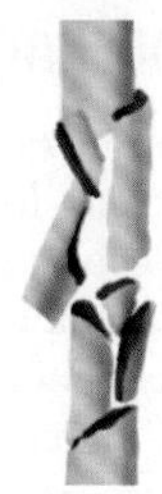
42-B1	Spiral wedge	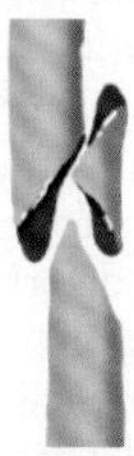			
42-B2	Bending wedge	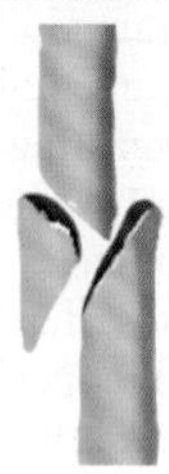			

Positioning

- Supine positioning is standard.
- A fracture table can be used with boot traction, calcaneal traction, or an arthroscopy leg holder that supports the leg and provides mechanical traction when no assistants are available. However, knee hyperflexion is difficult, and the guidewire insertion angle is suboptimal for proximal fractures **(FIG 3A)**.[20] This technique has largely been replaced by the use of a femoral distractor with medial to lateral pins placed in the posterior aspect of the proximal and distal metaphysis close to the articular surface. This technique allows "inline traction" while leaving entry and interlock sites clear **(FIG 3C)**.

TABLE 2 Relative Indications and Contraindications for Intramedullary Nailing of Tibial Fractures

Relative Indications

- High-energy mechanism
- Moderate to severe soft tissue injury precluding cast or brace
- Angular deformity ≥5–10 degrees
- Rotational deformity ≥5–10 degrees
- Shortening >1 cm
- Displacement >50%
- An ipsilateral fibula fracture at the same level
- An intact fibula
- Compartment syndrome
- Ipsilateral femoral fracture
- Inability to maintain reduction
- Older age, inability to manage with cast or brace

Contraindications

- Intramedullary canal diameter <6 mm
- Gross contamination of intramedullary canal
- Severe soft tissue injury where limb salvage is uncertain
- Preexisting deformity precluding nail insertion
- Ipsilateral total knee arthroplasty or knee arthrodesis
- Significant articular involvement
- Previous cruciate ligament reconstruction

- The patient is placed on the radiolucent table in one of the following positions:
  - Supine with the leg free **(FIG 3B)**
    - Mechanical traction is helpful to achieve reduction when the leg is draped free **(FIG 3C,D)**.
    - The proximal posterior Schanz pin **(FIG 3E)** is inserted medial to lateral and parallel to the tibial plateau.
    - The distal Schanz pin **(FIG 3F)** is inserted parallel to the plafond and inferior to the projected end of the nail.
  - Supine with the leg flexed over a bolster or radiolucent triangle **(FIG 3G)**
    - Maximizing knee flexion makes it easier to attain a start site and to obtain an optimal insertion vector, which approaches a parallel path with the anterior tibial border, but suboptimal for more proximal fractures.
  - Semiextended position
    - For proximal fractures, extending the knee to 20 to 30 degrees of flexion counters the pull of the patellar tendon and helps reduce the flexion deformity that is typical for these fractures.[32] Either a radiolucent triangle or bolster can be used **(FIG 3H)**. A distinction must be made between the suprapatellar approach and parapatellar (either medial and lateral).

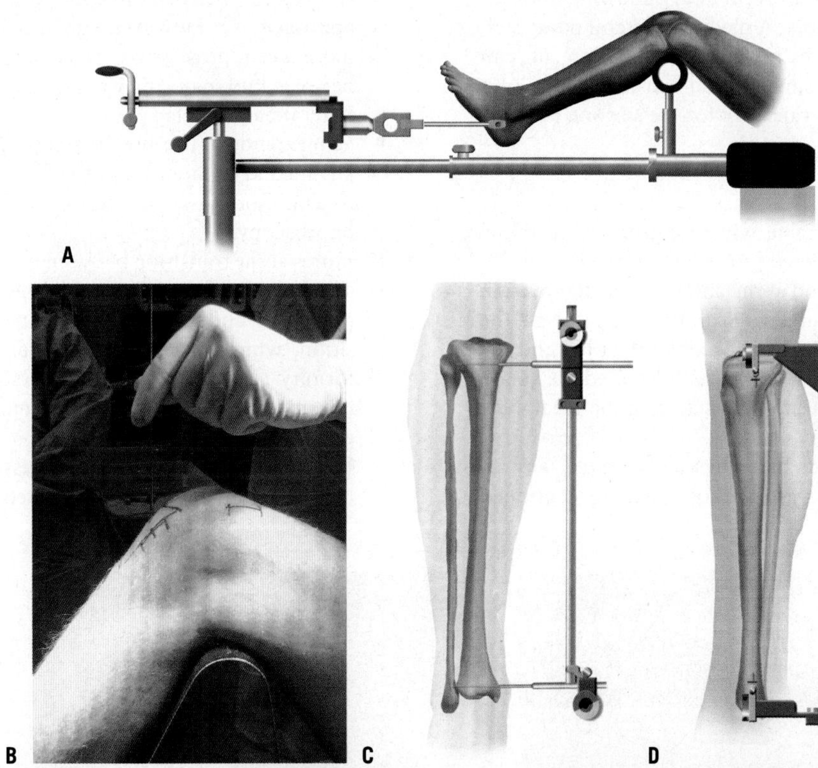

FIG 3 **A.** The fractured leg is positioned in calcaneal skeletal traction on the fracture table. This provides excellent mechanical traction but limits limb mobility, especially knee flexion. **B.** The knee is flexed over a positioning triangle in preparation for the surgical approach. **C,D.** The tibial fracture is distracted and reduced using a mechanical distraction device with proximal and distal half-pins. *(continued)*

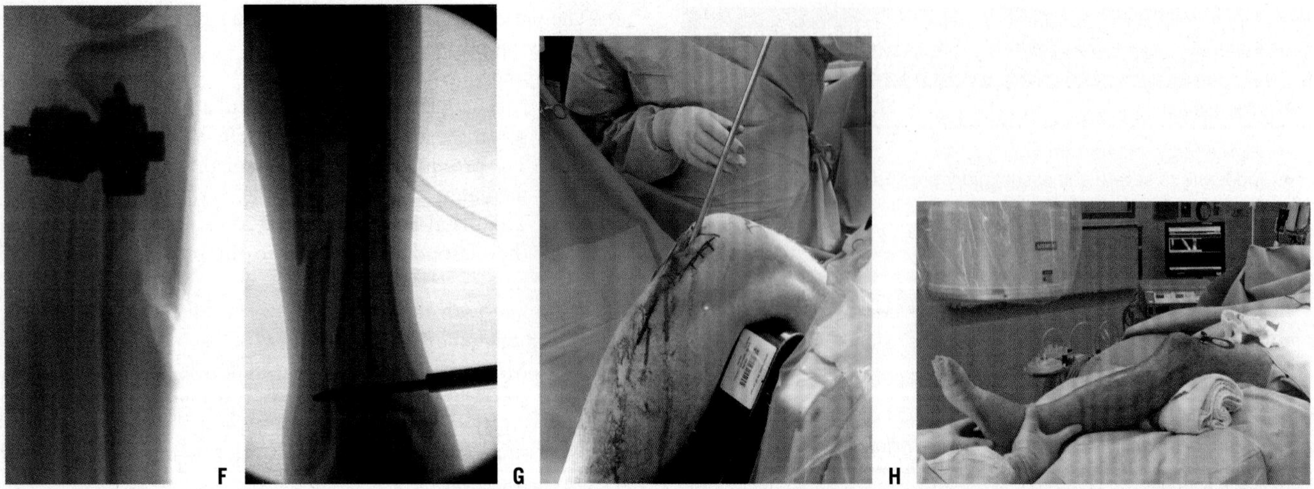

E F G H

FIG 3 *(continued)* **E.** A posteriorly positioned half-pin can be placed behind the projected nail path. **F.** A distal half-pin placed just over and parallel to the plafond can be helpful for aligning the distal fragment and lies inferior to the projected end of the nail. **G.** The knee is maximally flexed over the triangle to allow for the proper starting wire insertion angle. **H.** Typical setup for semiextended nailing with a small bolster for limited knee flexion and easy access to the limb for reduction and imaging.

The suprapatellar approach by definition requires specialized equipment and often requires near-complete knee extension in order to obtain access below the patella. As a result, it is not possible to obtain the correct starting point and the correct trajectory that is required for successful nailing of proximal fractures unless there is an ACL injury allowing anterior translation of the tibia. A medial or lateral parapatellar approach requires no specialized equipment, can be done through a similar sized incision, and allows reliable access and trajectory for the starting point.

Approach

- Use fluoroscopy to determine which approach will allow the starting point to be placed just medial to the lateral tibial spine on the AP view and at the anterior articular margin on the lateral view.[33] A guidewire can be used to assess the relationship between the anatomic axis of the tibia and the appropriate start site (**FIG 4**). Externally rotated views are common and can be misleading in selecting the ideal start point.[39]
- For diaphyseal and distal metaphyseal fractures, any of the following approaches are appropriate. As mentioned earlier, the patient's anatomy and fracture deformity can be used to determine which approach allows for appropriate starting point placement.
  - Medial parapatellar/paratendinous
  - Transpatellar tendon (This approach may be avoided by some surgeons due to previous retrospective series that showed an increased likelihood of knee pain with this approach.[14,25] However, other retrospective series and more recent prospective trials have found no association between knee pain and the surgical approach used.[7,35–37])
  - Lateral parapatellar
  - Semiextended. The use of a suprapatellar or parapatellar (medial or lateral) approach may be of benefit when nailing more distal fractures as it facilitates the ease of fluoroscopy.
- Fractures at the transition between metaphysis and diaphysis
  - The lateral parapatellar tendinous approach allows for guidewire and nail placement in the more lateral position, which is beneficial in countering the valgus deformity associated with these fractures. It also allows intramedullary nailing in the familiar hyperflexed knee position.
    - The semiextended position assists for reduction of the flexion deformity associated with these fractures.

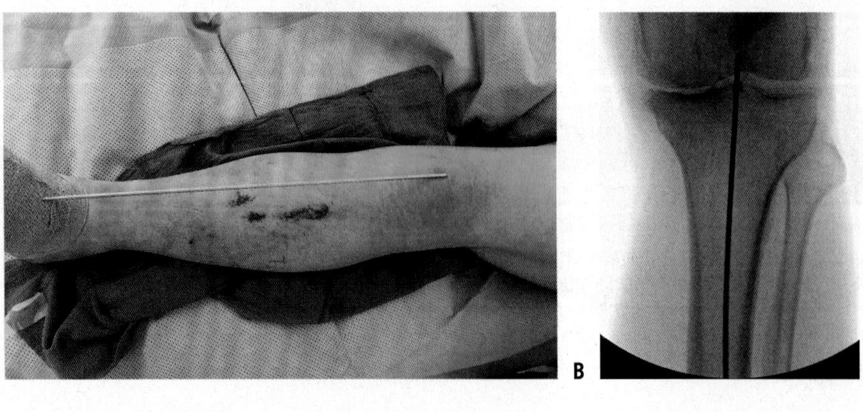

A B

FIG 4 Clinical and fluoroscopic examples demonstrating usage of a guidewire to determine tibial anatomic axis and appropriate start site. **A.** Guidewire placed along tibial crest. **B.** Correlating fluoroscopic AP view showing guidewire at the medial aspect of the lateral tibial spine.

- The limited or formal medial parapatellar/paratendinous approach may be used if the surgeon is unfamiliar with the suprapatellar approach and special instrumentation is not available. Alternatively, a parapatellar approach with or without arthrotomy can be used, and this is the authors' preferred method for proximal fractures.
- If the suprapatellar approach is being performed, a superomedial or superior midline incision is used, and special instrumentation is required. In cases where the suprapatellar approach is chosen and the surgeon is unable to obtain an acceptable starting point or wire trajectory, the incision can be extended slightly inferiorly and medial, and a "medial snip" of the superior medial retinaculum can be performed. This maneuver routinely mobilizes the patella enough to allow proper wire placement and orientation.
- All of the surgical approaches are performed with the knee in the semiextended position.

SURGICAL APPROACH

Medial Parapatellar Tendon Approach

- Palpate and mark the medial border of the patellar tendon (**TECH FIG 1**).
- Incise the skin at the medial border of the patellar tendon.
- Full-thickness skin flaps are developed.
- Dissection is carried down to the retinaculum.
- The retinaculum is then split, and the patellar tendon is retracted laterally.
- Do not incise the capsule.

Transpatellar Tendon Approach

- Palpate and mark the medial and lateral borders of the patellar tendon, the inferior border of the patella, and the tibial tubercle (see **TECH FIG 1**).
- Incise the skin starting at the inferior margin of the patella and continue distally in the middle of the patellar tendon.
- Full-thickness skin flaps are developed.
- Incise the paratenon in the midline and elevate medial and lateral flaps to identify the margins of the patellar tendon.
- Make a single full-thickness incision in the midline of the patellar tendon. Do not incise the capsule and avoid injuring the menisci at the inferior margin of the incision.

Lateral Parapatellar Tendon Approach

- Palpate and mark the lateral border of the patellar tendon (see **TECH FIG 1**).
- Incise the skin at the lateral border of the patellar tendon.
- Full-thickness skin flaps are developed.
- Dissection is carried down to the retinaculum.
- The retinaculum is then split, and the patellar tendon is retracted medially.
- Do not incise the capsule.

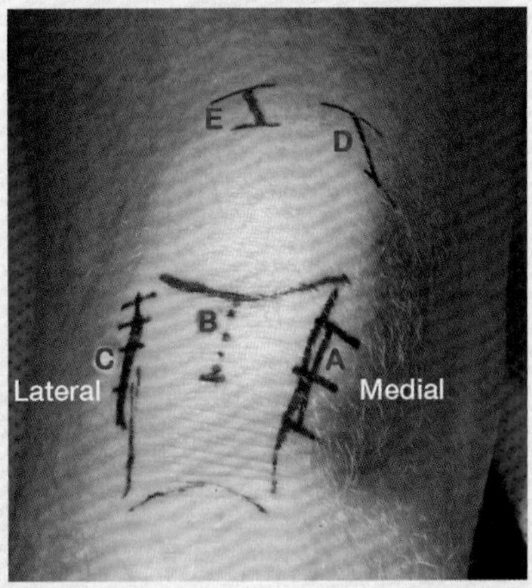

TECH FIG 1 Options for surgical incisions in relation to the patella and patellar tendon. Medial parapatellar tendon incision (*A*). Transpatellar tendon incision (*B*). Lateral parapatellar tendon (*C*). Superomedial Patellar Incision (*D*). Suprapatellar incision (*E*).

Semiextended Position[32]

Medial Parapatellar Approach

- Either a standard midline or limited medial skin incision can be used (**TECH FIG 2**).
- Full-thickness skin flaps are developed.
- The distal portion of the quadriceps tendon is incised, leaving a 2-mm cuff of tendon medially for later repair.
- A formal medial arthrotomy is done extending around the patella, leaving a 2-mm cuff of capsule and retinaculum for later repair, and continuing along the medial border of the patellar tendon.

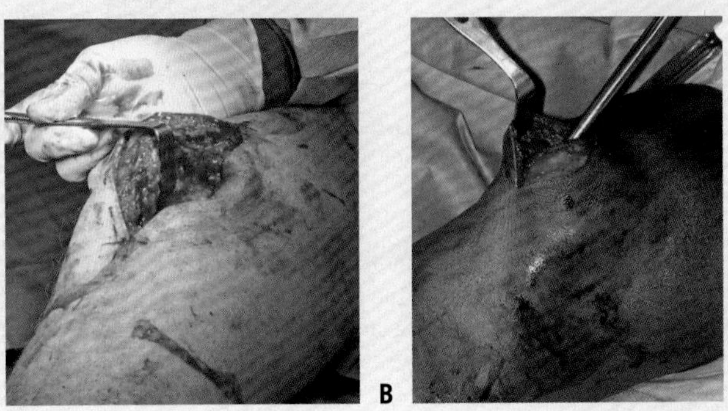

A B

TECH FIG 2 **A.** A formal full medial parapatellar approach allows for easy patellar subluxation and start site localization but requires significant dissection. **B.** The alternative is a limited medial approach. (**B:** Courtesy of Paul Tornetta III, MD.)

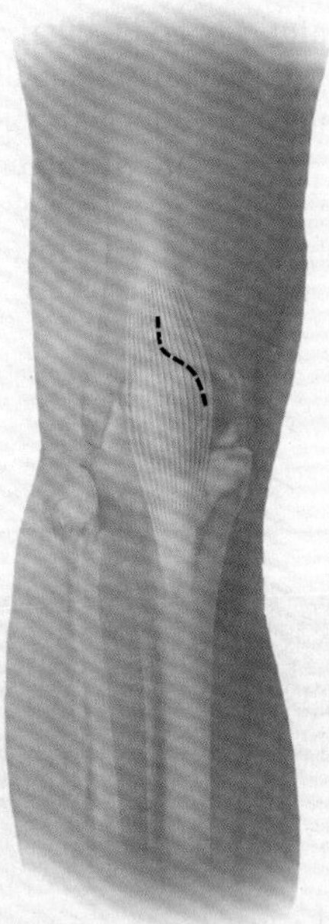

TECH FIG 3 A partial medial parapatellar arthrotomy that is carried into the intermedius allows enough subluxation of the patella to perform semiextended nailing. (Courtesy of Paul Tornetta III, MD.)

Suprapatellar Approach[34]

- The suprapatellar approach requires special nail insertion instrumentation as well as cannulas for guide pin placement and reaming.
- The skin incision is made at the superomedial edge of the patella **(TECH FIG 3)**.
  - Full-thickness skin flaps are developed.
  - Make a superomedial arthrotomy large enough to place the special instrumentation.
  - At times when there is no sufficient patella mobility to allow for cannula passage under the patella, the superior portion of a medial parapatellar approach is developed to allow for mobilization of the patella to protect the patella femoral joint. This maneuver, known as a *medial snip*, can help avoid an anterior starting point or an excessively posteriorly angulated trajectory.
- An alternative skin incision can be made extending from the midline of the superior pole of the patella proximally (see **TECH FIG 1**).
  - Full-thickness skin flaps are developed.
  - Incise the quadriceps tendon in the midline, extending proximally from the superior pole of the patella, and make an arthrotomy.
  - Mobilize the patella and free up any adhesions in the patellofemoral joint.

Extra-articular Extended[17]

- Semiextended nailing is performed with the goal of remaining outside knee synovium/joint.
  - Medial or lateral parapatellar approach is selected based on patellar laxity. Most commonly, this will be a lateral approach. A complete lateral release is performed preserving the synovium if possible. The intact synovium limits the iatrogenic injury to the cartilage overlaying the femoral condyle. The incision should be biased toward the superior pole of the patella to prevent skin damage.
  - A curvilinear incision begins at the inferior third of the patella and extends proximally to the level of the proximal pole.
  - Dissect synovium from retinaculum; divide retinaculum sharply.

Standard Intramedullary Nailing

Initial Guidewire Placement

- Drape the leg free, including the proximal thigh. Draping the leg more distally can limit knee flexion due to bunching of the drapes.
- Flex the knee over a bolster or radiolucent triangle.
  - A padded thigh tourniquet can be applied and inflated during the surgical approach, but it must not be inflated during reaming because of the risk of thermal injury to the intramedullary canal. For this reason, a thigh tourniquet is usually omitted.
- The starting guidewire is placed on the skin and radiographically aligned with the anatomic axis and in line with the lateral tibial spine on a true AP fluoroscopic image. The skin can be marked along the guidewire path to allow visualization of the anatomic axis without fluoroscopy **(TECH FIG 4A)**.
- The appropriate surgical approach is performed.

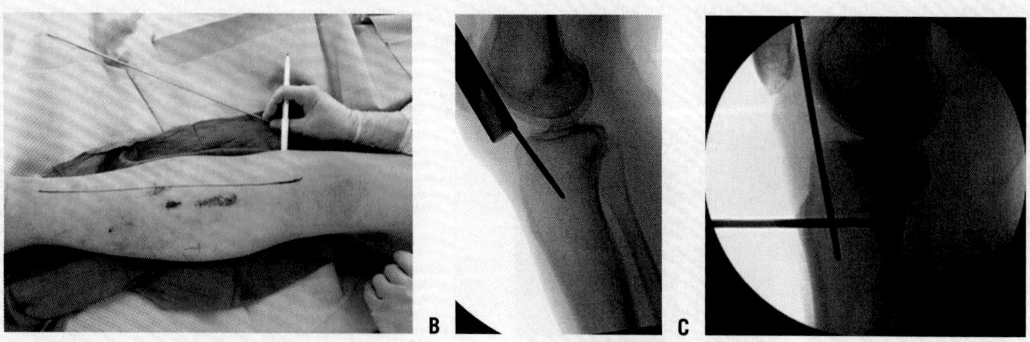

A B C

TECH FIG 4 A. Marking the skin along the crest can assist in aligning the guidewire with the path of the intramedullary canal and lessen the need for fluoroscopic guidance. **B.** Ideal proximal extra-articular start site as seen on lateral fluoroscopic image; this is near the articular margin. **C.** An ideal insertion vector approaches a parallel path with anterior cortex and minimizes the likelihood of fragment extension with seating of the nail.

- The knee is maximally flexed, and the guidewire is aligned with the anatomic axis of the tibia.
  - Typically, achieving an appropriate insertion vector will require the wire to be pushed against the patella or the peripatellar tissues.
- The anterior tibial crest is palpated for frontal plane wire alignment.
- Lateral plane fluoroscopy is necessary to place the wire at the proximal and superior aspect of the "flat spot" and near-parallel with the anterior tibial cortical line **(TECH FIG 4B)**.
- The guidewire is directed 8 to 10 cm into the metaphysis.
  - Guidewire position is verified in the AP and lateral planes.
  - The frontal plane wire position should be in line with the anatomic axis and proximally should be just medial to the lateral tibial spine. Lateral alignment should be nearly parallel with the anterior tibial cortex, and all efforts should be made to avoid a posteriorly directed vector **(TECH FIG 4C)**.

Creating and Reaming the Starting Hole

- The opening reamer (matching the proximal nail diameter) is introduced via a tissue sleeve and inserted while carefully maintaining knee hyperflexion and biplanar alignment. Some authors favor the use of an awl over a powered reamer as it is less likely to damage surrounding tissues. This is only an option when performing traditional flexed nailing.
- If the knee is allowed to extend or posterior pressure is not maintained on the tissue sleeve, the starting hole will become enlarged anteriorly, and the proximal anterior cortex will be violated.
- All semiextended nailing should be performed with a 6-inch bolster under the knee to prevent knee extension and anterior migration of the entry portal.
  - Imprecise reaming technique leads to anteriorization of the nail and violation of the proximal anterior cortex **(TECH FIG 5)**.

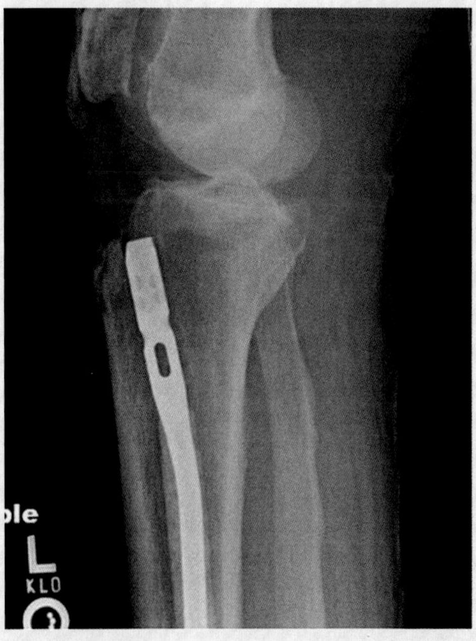

TECH FIG 5 If flexion is not maintained during reaming, or reaming is started before entrance into the starting hole, the anterior tibial cortex will be violated by the reamer, and an anterior nail path will be produced.

- Place a 15-degree bend 2 cm from the distal extent of the ball-tipped guidewire to allow for directional control during wire advancement.
  - Alternatively, a straight ball-tipped guidewire can be used with an intramedullary reduction instrument (ie, a cannulated finger device), which can precisely direct the wire and simplify passage across the fracture.
- A ball-tipped guidewire is introduced into the proximal segment, and the knee is slightly extended for fracture reduction and instrumentation.

Fracture Reduction

Simple Middle Diaphyseal Fractures (Transverse or Short Oblique)

- Manual traction with gross manipulation will reduce simple transverse middiaphyseal fractures.
- Medially based external fixation or distraction with a large universal distractor is helpful for reduction when no assistants are available, in large patients, or when used for provisional fixation.
- Muscular paralysis is necessary to simplify fracture reduction.
- Placement of percutaneous pointed reduction forceps can be helpful in oblique and short oblique patterns to achieve anatomic or near-anatomic reduction.
  - Use fluoroscopy to mark the level and orientation of the fracture on the skin to facilitate the reduction clamp orientation and ideal placement of skin incisions.
  - Introduce a small or large pointed clamp under and through skin stab wounds; care must be taken to maintain clamp points against bone **(TECH FIG 6A–C)**.
  - Typically, the spike on the distal fragment is posterolateral.
  - A surgical dissection down to the fracture to facilitate a timely and accurate reduction of the fracture is preferred to accepting a malreduction and injuring the soft tissue envelope with multiple errant percutaneous clamp attempts **(TECH FIG 6D,E)**.[3,7,8]

Highly Comminuted Middle Diaphyseal Fractures

- Have comparison radiographic images of the uninjured extremity available to be used as a template for length and rotational reduction landmarks.
- Mechanical traction with medially based half-pin fixation is very helpful **(TECH FIG 7 A,E,F-H)**.
  - A large external fixator or large universal distractor is equally effective.
  - The proximal Schanz is placed posteriorly and parallel to the tibial plateau **(TECH FIG 7B,C)**.
  - The distal Schanz pin is placed just above and parallel to the plafond **(TECH FIG 7D)**.
- The intramedullary reduction tool available in most nail or reamer sets can be used to manipulate the proximal fragment in order to advance the tool across the fracture, which achieves fracture reduction and guidewire placement.

Open Middle Diaphyseal Fractures

- Large segmental and butterfly fragments that are completely devitalized and void of soft tissue attachments should be removed and cleaned of contamination.
- These pieces can be reintroduced into the fracture site and used to perform anatomic open reduction following passage of the intramedullary rod and interlocking. These pieces should be removed after fixation is completed because they represent a large amount of nonviable material in a high-risk wound.

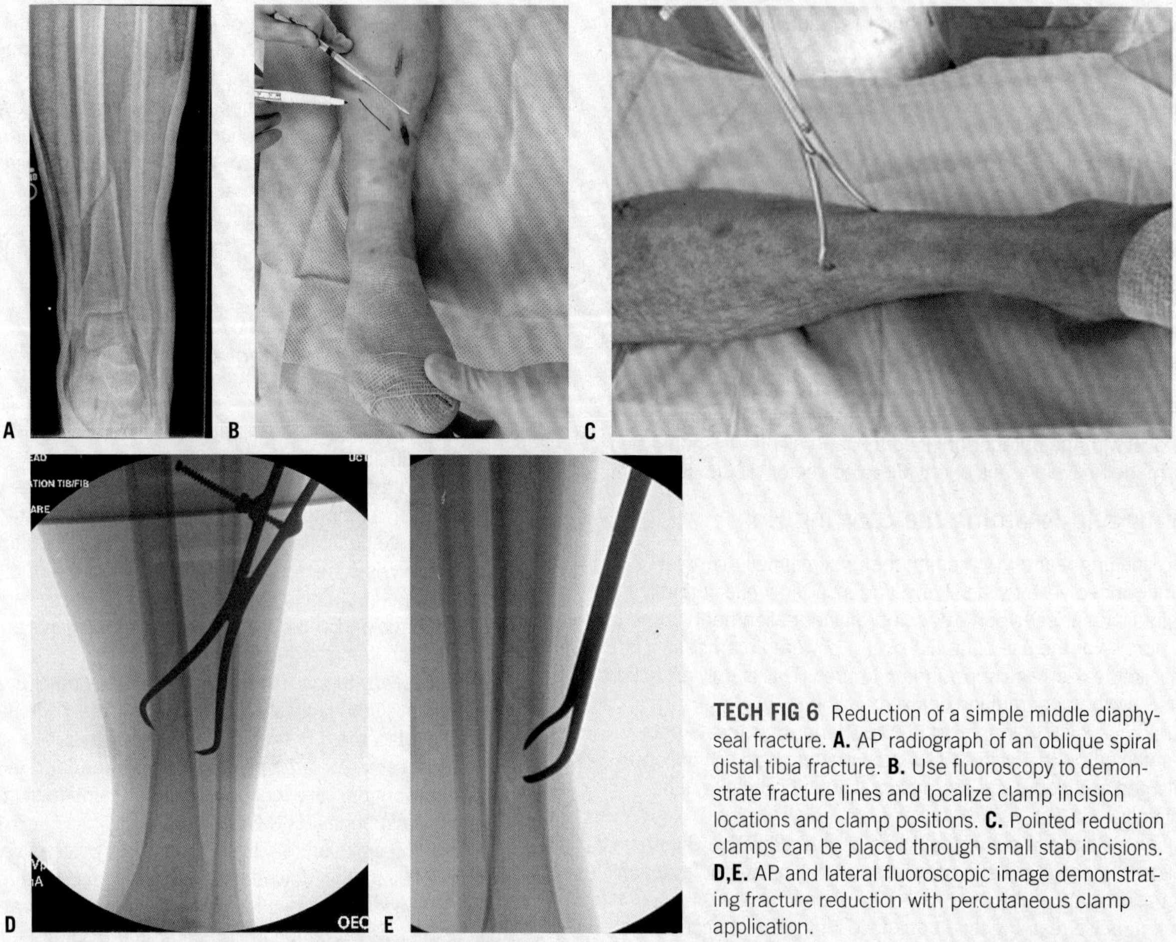

TECH FIG 6 Reduction of a simple middle diaphyseal fracture. **A.** AP radiograph of an oblique spiral distal tibia fracture. **B.** Use fluoroscopy to demonstrate fracture lines and localize clamp incision locations and clamp positions. **C.** Pointed reduction clamps can be placed through small stab incisions. **D,E.** AP and lateral fluoroscopic image demonstrating fracture reduction with percutaneous clamp application.

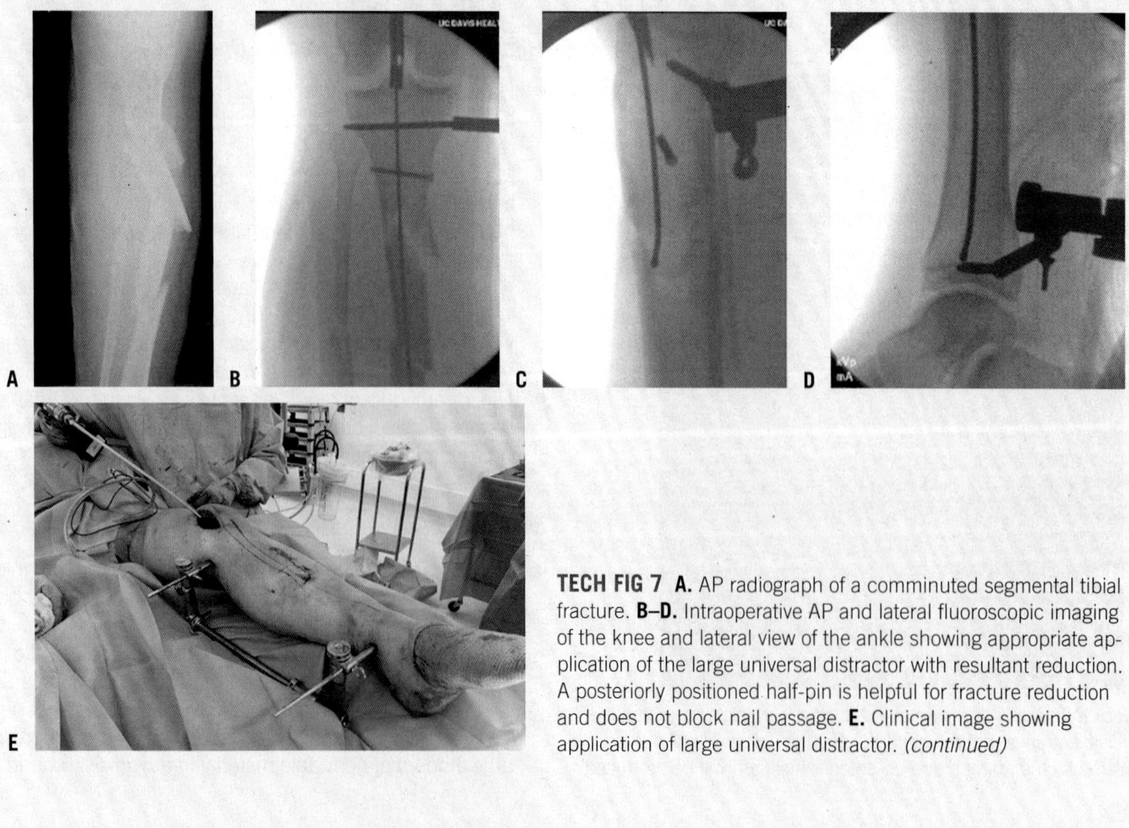

TECH FIG 7 **A.** AP radiograph of a comminuted segmental tibial fracture. **B–D.** Intraoperative AP and lateral fluoroscopic imaging of the knee and lateral view of the ankle showing appropriate application of the large universal distractor with resultant reduction. A posteriorly positioned half-pin is helpful for fracture reduction and does not block nail passage. **E.** Clinical image showing application of large universal distractor. *(continued)*

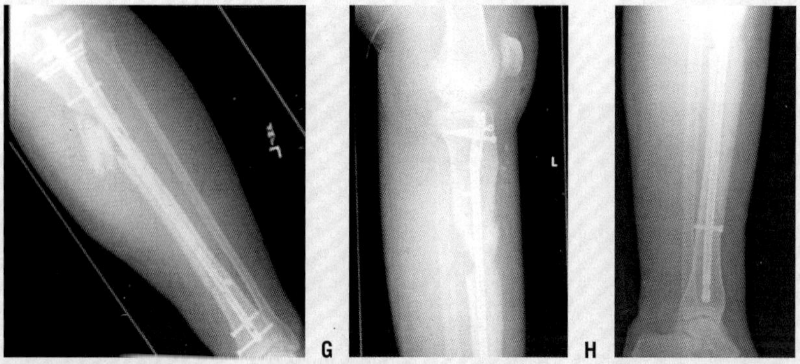

F G H

TECH FIG 7 *(continued)* **F–H.** Postoperative AP and lateral radiographs of the knee and tibia showing successful fixation.

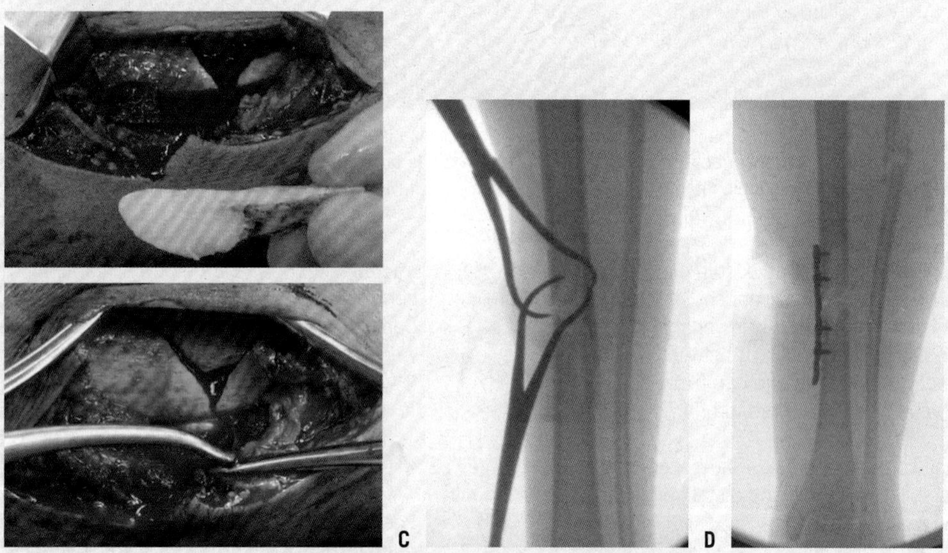

A B C D

TECH FIG 8 Reduction of an open middle diaphyseal fracture. **A.** A large segment of stripped cortical bone has been removed and cleaned on the back table. **B.** The cortical fragment has been placed into the fracture site and clamped in reduced position to reduce the fracture anatomically. **C.** Intraoperative fluoroscopic image of the fracture with the fracture fragment clamped in reduced position; note that this fragment will be removed after reaming and nail passage. **D.** Unicortical plates are useful for maintaining reduction during nail passage.

- Occasionally, an osteotome is required to free near-circumferential fragments **(TECH FIG 8A–C)**.
- If reduction is difficult, a small fragment unicortical plate can be used to maintain the reduction during reaming and nail placement. Once interlocking is completed, the plate should be removed **(TECH FIG 8D)**.
- Consider leaving the unicortical plate when the reduction is lost after its removal, and antibiotic spacer is being employed to manage a large bone defect. The plate will help maintain the reduction and contain the antibiotic spacer. It will be removed when future staged bone grafting is performed.[10]

Passing the Guidewire

- Once optimal AP and lateral plane reduction is achieved, the wire is advanced past the level of the fracture. Verify that the wire is within the canal on both the AP and lateral views to avoid advancing too far and damaging extramedullary structures.
- In metadiaphyseal fractures, the wire must be centered in the metaphyseal segment.
  - In proximal and distal fractures, blocking screws or pins may be required to ensure centralized positioning of the guidewire **(TECH FIG 9A)**.
- Once centralized, the ball-tipped wire must be impacted into the subchondral bone of the tibial plafond at the level of the physeal scar. This decreases the risk of inadvertently removing the guidewire during reaming.
- To assure an accurate reduction, the wire should be centered at the entrance and exit of all fracture segments.
- Nail length measurement is performed using supplied length gauges and should be verified with lateral fluoroscopic measurement **(TECH FIG 9B,C)**. The lateral view is used because it is more accurate in determining the level of the articular surface and avoiding nail prominence.
  - Alternatively, inserting a guidewire of the same length to the nail entry site and then measuring the length differential

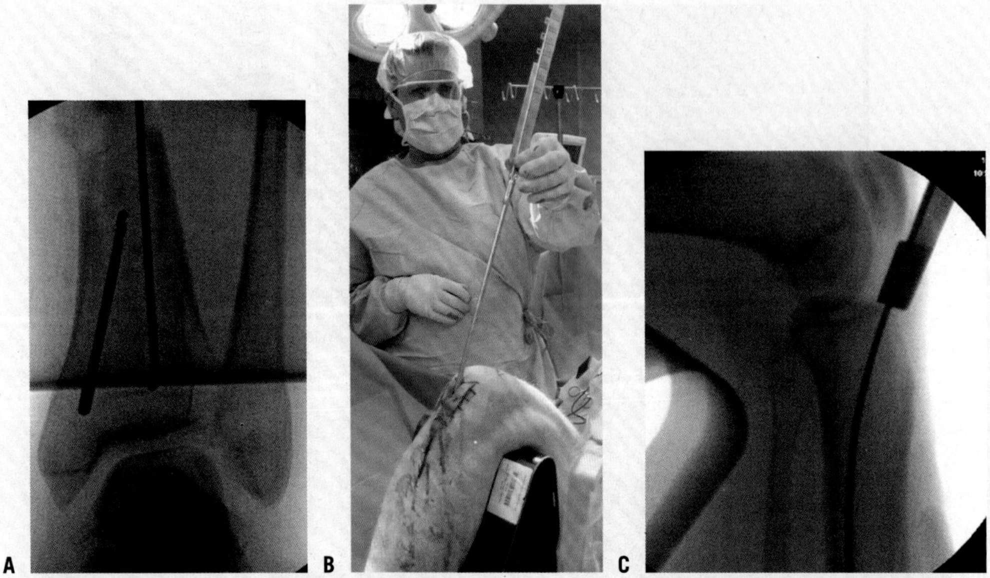

TECH FIG 9 **A.** A drill bit is used to ensure the guidewire is placed centrally in the distal segment of this distal metadiaphyseal fracture. **B,C.** The nail length guide is pushed to the opening of the tibia and verified with lateral fluoroscopic imaging.

between wires also provides an accurate measurement. However, this introduces the significant cost of a second guidewire.
- Device manufacturers supply nails in variable increments. When a length measurement falls in between lengths, choose the shorter length. A threaded end cap (usually 5, 10, and 15 mm) can be used if it is desired to bring the nail to top of the canal opening.
- Leaving the nail countersunk below the bone surface does not compromise stability in middle and distal fractures but may complicate future nail extraction.

Reaming the Canal

- Before reaming, estimate the narrowest canal diameter using both AP and lateral plain radiographs. Alternatively, intramedullary reamer sets typically have a radiolucent ruler that allows for intraoperative fluoroscopic verification, which should be done on both the AP and lateral views. The canal typically is reamed at least 1 mm over the isthmic diameter to minimize the risk of nail incarceration. When nailing metaphyseal fracture, overream 2 mm at least to facilitate an easy nail insertion.
- Reaming should begin with an end-cutting reamer—the 8.5- or 9-mm size in most systems.
- Reamer heads should be evaluated before insertion and should be sharp and free of defects.
- Insert the reamer head into the proximal metaphysis with the knee in maximal flexion before applying power to avoid distorting the entrance hole **(TECH FIG 10A)**.
- Reamers are advanced at a slow pace under full power.
  - If the reamer shafts are not solid, but are wound, be sure to avoid using reverse when drilling as this may cause the reamers to unwind if resistance is encountered within the intramedullary canal.
- Reduction should be maintained during power reaming. Reamed malreductions will persist after nail insertion. When the nail is being used to reduce a diaphyseal fracture, do not power ream the fracture site but, instead, push the reamer across the fracture site then resume power reaming. This is facilitated by gently tapping the drill or reamer shaft.
- Care must be taken not to inadvertently extract the guidewire when the reamers are removed.
  - Multiple techniques are used. First, manual downward pressure can be applied to the wire with specialized instruments, medicine cups, or cleaning cannulas **(TECH FIG 10B)**.
  - Once the reamer has cleared the opening, it can be clamped and held in position **(TECH FIG 10C)**.
- For the minimally reamed technique, a single end-cutting reamer (usually 9 mm) is passed down the canal to ensure the smallest diameter nail can pass through the narrowest segment of the intramedullary canal.
- In an effort to minimize thermal damage to the endosteal cortex, reaming should be discontinued within 0.5 to 1 mm of hearing the reamer head catching ("chatter") on the endosteal cortex.
  - Care also should be used when there is butterfly or oblique fracture fragments. Continued reaming after encountering chatter may result in iatrogenic comminution and loss of reduction.

Unreamed Technique

- There are limited indications for this technique. Nail incarceration is a significant risk.
- Limited reaming with passage of a single 9-mm end-cutting reamer should always be considered in lieu of undreamed nailing.
- Standard preparation technique is used for the starting hole, and the fracture is reduced.
- Precise evaluation of the lateral isthmic diameter is repeated, and a small-diameter nail is selected, typically in the 7- to 9-mm range.
- A good guideline is to use a nail 1 to 1.5 mm smaller than the narrowest measure of the isthmus on the lateral radiograph.
- If lateral plane imaging is suggestive of canal diameter very close to nail size, a single pass with an end-cutting reamer usually is performed to decrease the possibility of nail incarceration.

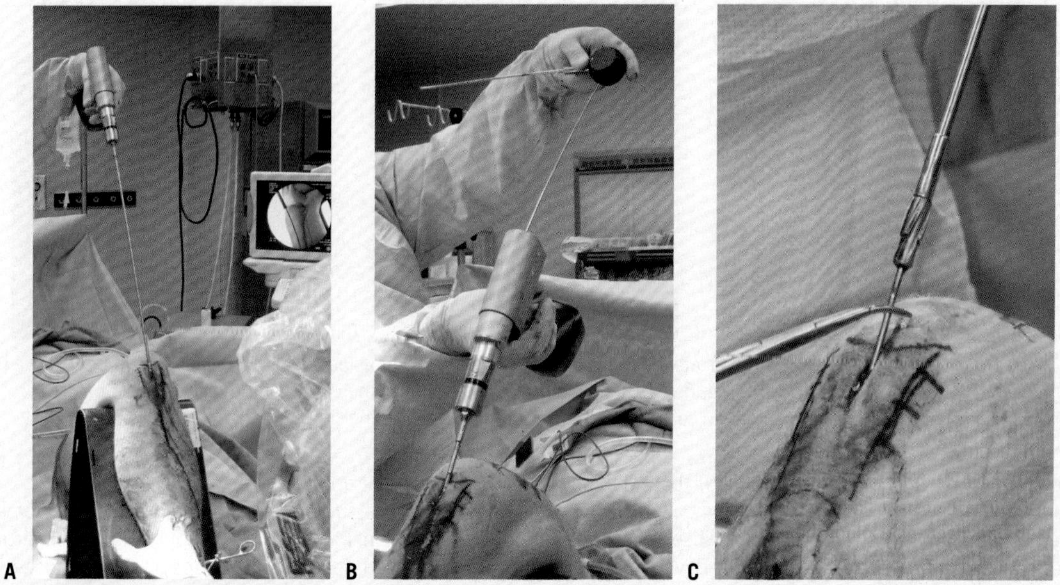

TECH FIG 10 **A.** Maintenance of maximal knee flexion protects the entrance hole from being inadvertently enlarged by the reamer. **B.** If the guidewire is rotating during reaming, it must be held down as the reamer is pulled back to avoid inadvertent removal of the guidewire. **C.** A clamp can be used to grasp the guidewire when the reamer head clears the soft tissues.

- The nail is inserted and impacted in standard fashion. If significant resistance is encountered when the nail reaches the isthmus, the nail is removed to avoid incarceration or iatrogenic fracture propagation. A reamer 0.5 to 1.0 mm larger than the nail is passed down the canal, and nail passage is attempted again.

Nail Insertion

- Once the nail insertion handle is attached, pass a drill through the proximal screw insertion attachment and screw insertion cannulas before inserting the nail to ensure accurate alignment of the attachment jig.
- Nails with chisel tips or distal additional bends ease insertion when started 180 degrees from final position during initial metaphyseal entry then rotated into final position once in the tibia.
- Maintain nail rotation during insertion by aligning the center of the insertion handle with the tibial crest. Consider internal rotation of the nail if distal AP interlocking bolts are deemed necessary to minimize damage to distal neurovascular structures.
  - Maintain knee hyperflexion during nail insertion to minimize the risk of posterior cortical abutment and iatrogenic fracture.
  - When semiextended nailing is chosen, maintain a bolster under the knee and gentle elevation of the nail jig during insertion to minimize iatrogenic cartilage injury.
- Impact the nail to the final depth using lateral plane fluoroscopy.

Interlocking Bolt Insertion

- In simple transverse fractures, place distal interlocks first to allow for backslapping for interfragmentary compression and gap minimization. Alternatively, proximal interlocks can be placed first, and the nail can be gently forward slapped to avoid gapping at the fracture site.
- Usually, distal interlock bolts are placed medial to lateral.
- Position the leg in slight extension and stable neutral rotation.
- Rotate the C-arm to lateral imaging position and pull the tube back away from the medial side of the leg to allow for drill placement.
- Rotate the leg and C-arm individually and sequentially to create a perfect circle image; optimize this view before drilling attempts **(TECH FIG 11A)**.
- After localizing the interlocking hole using a clamp and fluoroscopy, make an incision large enough to place the locking bolt. Use blunt clamp dissection until the cortex is reached.
- Use a sharp drill point and place the center of the point in the center of the circle.
  - Hold the drill obliquely to the nail axis to simplify repositioning **(TECH FIG 11B)**.
  - Gently tapping the end of the drill is helpful in "seating" the tip in the correct position before initiating power, especially when using a brad tip design.
- Once the central location is achieved; align hand and drill with imaging axis.
  - Fluoroscopes with laser alignment guides can be helpful to assist with alignment by centering the laser on the skin incision and then placing the laser in the center of the back of the drill when preparing to drill the hole **(TECH FIG 11C)**.
  - Drill to the midsagittal point in the tibia. Then, disengage the drill from the drill bit and check the fluoroscopic image.
    - If the drill is accurately positioned in the center of the hole, advance the drill bit with power through the far cortex; avoid broaching the far cortex by impacting with a mallet to avoid iatrogenic fracture.
    - Drill the second interlock hole using the same technique but maintaining a parallel axis with the first successful drill passage.
- Replace the drill with the appropriate depth gauge and check an AP image before screw length selection.

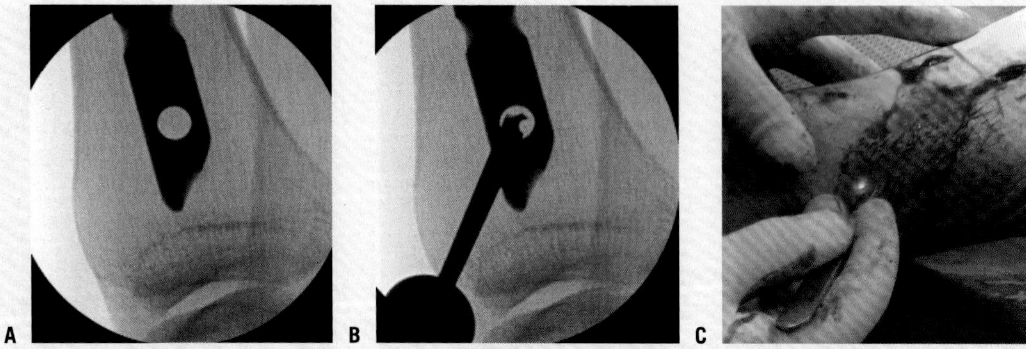

TECH FIG 11 **A.** A perfectly rotated lateral fluoroscopic image will appear as a perfect circle and should be achieved before drilling is attempted. **B.** The drill point must be aligned in the center of the perfect circle before drilling. **C.** The laser alignment guide can be helpful for localizing the skin incision.

- Once interlock lengths and position are verified, "backslapping" can occur to optimize compression.
  - Using the slotted mallet attachment on the insertion handle, superiorly directed mallet blows can be used while pressure is applied to the foot in order to compress the fracture site. Fluoroscopy should be used to monitor the amount of compression and the nail position proximally. If backslapping is planned, the nail should be slightly over inserted to avoid nail prominence after compression is performed.
- Place proximal interlocks through drill guides.
  - Because the tibia is a triangle, oblique views may be used to more accurately judge screw length for transverse locking bolt measurement.
  - If oblique locking bolts are chosen proximally, oblique fluoroscopic views should be used prior to insertion handle removal to avoid placing long screws that are particularly symptomatic on the medial side of the knee and to avoid injury to the peroneal nerve posterolaterally.

Lateral Parapatellar Tendon Approach

- After completing the lateral parapatellar approach described, the standard patient positioning is used.
- The lateral parapatellar approach allows the guide pin to be more easily placed just medial to the lateral tibial spine on the AP view and along the lateral cortex to correct the valgus angulation.
  - If a true AP view is not obtained and the leg is externally rotated, the starting point will be more medial than desired.[6]
- It is important to get enough knee flexion over the radiolucent triangle or bolster to allow for the guide pin to be placed as proximal as possible and parallel along the anterior tibial cortex to help correct the typical flexion deformity.[24]

Semiextended Technique

- The benefit of the semiextended technique is that the leg position helps neutralize the associated flexion deformity.[32]
- The patient is placed in the semiextended position as described earlier.
- The open medial parapatellar approach can be used (see **TECH FIG 2**).
  - Using the previously described surgical approach, the patella is subluxated to allow for guide pin placement, reaming, and nail placement, with the knee remaining in the semiextended position.
  - No special instruments are required.
- Suprapatellar approach[34]
  - Either the superomedial or direct superior approach is used.
  - Special instrumentation is required; which instrumentation is needed depends on the specific system used.
  - The patella is subluxated using an elongated cannula **(TECH FIG 12A)**.
  - The cannula is advanced to the standard starting point using fluoroscopy.
  - The guide pin is placed in the standard position **(TECH FIG 12B)**.
  - The typical steps—using the opening drill, placing the guidewire, and reaming—are all completed through the elongated cannula.
  - Standard intramedullary reamers can be used, but reamer extensions are helpful, especially in taller patients.
  - Fracture reduction and passing of the guidewire are performed before reaming.
  - A special elongated nail insertion handle is required for nail insertion **(TECH FIG 12C)**.
  - Proximal locking bolt insertion is done using the aiming arm.
  - Distal locking bolts are placed using the standard freehand technique, as previously described.
  - It is critical that the reamer is in the metaphysis before power reaming with all semiextended techniques to prevent anterior entry portal migration.
  - Flex the knee to remove the insertion jig with all semiextended techniques. The anterior pressure of the femoral condyles on the jig causes binding between the inflexible jig and the relatively flexible nail, which can make remove of the jig extremely difficult unless the knee is flexed. This should not be a "white knuckle situation." The jig bolt can break or strip if the knee is not flexed.

Adjunct Reduction and Fixation Techniques

Blocking/Pöller Screws

- Screws can be placed across the intramedullary canal to create a "false" cortex outside of the isthmus that narrows the potential space for the nail. This aids in both fracture reduction as the nail is being placed and maintenance of the reduction once the nail is seated.[16,28]
- Locking bolts found in the nailing set or small fragment screws should be used. If possible, use the smallest diameter locking bolts available for the nail system.

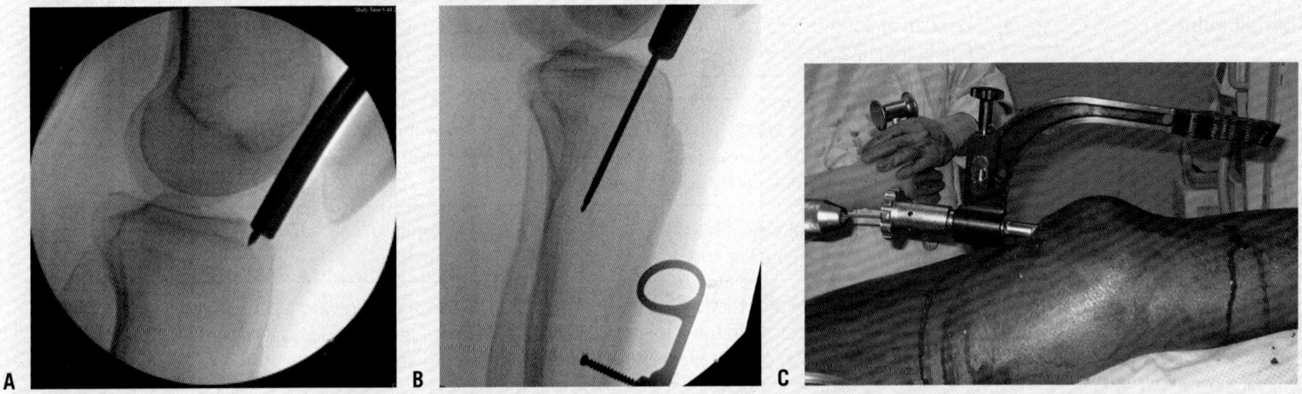

TECH FIG 12 A. Suprapatellar approach: A specially designed cannula is used to subluxate the patella and pass through the patellofemoral joint and is positioned at the appropriate starting point. **B.** The guide pin is advanced appropriately, and the cannula is used for the opening reamer, guidewire placement, and intramedullary reaming—but not nail insertion. Long reamer extensions are helpful for intramedullary reaming. **C.** A specialized, long insertion handle is required for suprapatellar techniques to reach the tibial start site.

- Blocking screws can either be placed prior to initial nail insertion or, if the nail is inserted and residual deformity exists, the nail can be removed and blocking screws can be inserted.
  - Coronal and sagittal plane correction can be performed by placing a screw at the concavity of the deformity.
    - To correct valgus, the screw is placed laterally **(TECH FIG 13A)**. To correct lateral plane extension, the screw is placed posteriorly **(TECH FIG 13B)**.
  - The appropriately sized drill bit is placed with fluoroscopic assistance.
  - The appropriately sized screw replaces the drill bit.
  - The guidewire is then inserted and seated distally.
  - Intramedullary reaming is necessary to ensure the nail follows the newly created path.
    - When a screw that blocks the way is encountered, simply push the reamer head past the screw without reaming. This avoids dulling the reamer head and potentially displacing the blocking screw. Be conservative with the constriction of the nail path when using blocking screws; err on the side of leaving room to prevent iatrogenic comminution of the fracture when passing the reamers or the nails.
    - Once passed the screw, resume reaming.
    - After reaming is complete, insert the intramedullary nail.
    - If the displacement has not been corrected, it will be necessary to remove the nail, and additional screws may be added. Reaming and reinsertion of the guidewire are required before reinserting the nail.
- Interlocking bolts through the nail are placed in the standard fashion **(TECH FIG 13B,C)**.

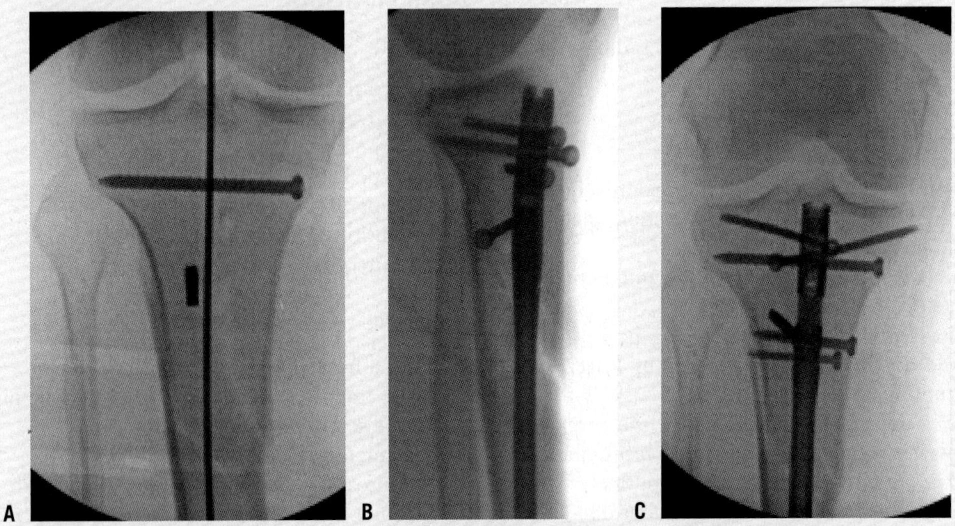

TECH FIG 13 A. A blocking screw positioned just lateral to the ideal nail path to prevent valgus deformation. **B.** A posterior blocking screw limits proximal fragment extension by limiting the effective anterior to posterior canal diameter. **B,C.** Lateral and AP fluoroscopic imaging showing oblique and medial to lateral interlocking bolts placed through the nail.

Pearls and Pitfalls

Starting Point	• The starting point should be at the anterior articular margin and just medial to the lateral tibial spine. Starting too medial and distal for proximal metaphyseal fractures results in a valgus and flexed malunion.
Centering the Guidewire	• Center the guidewire distally on the AP and lateral views. If not centered, the nail will follow the path of the reamer and guidewire, which will malreduce the fracture. Many modern nail have a distal additional bend, and they will sit slightly anterior in the distal tibia. Also, remember that the center of the tibial diaphysis projects to slightly lateral in the tibial metaphysis.
Measuring Nail Length	• Measure on the lateral view. Measuring on the AP view will potentially lead to a nail that is too long, with articular prominence causing knee pain or articular surface damage.
Femoral Distractor or External Fixator for Reduction	• Half-pins can be placed outside of the path of the nail. The best positions are posterior in the proximal tibia and distally very close to the subchondral bone of the tibial plafond. Placement of the proximal pin too anteriorly and the distal pin too proximally may impede reaming and nail insertion.
Unicortical Plates for Reduction	• Metadiaphyseal plates contribute to stability and maintenance of reduction and removal can lead to loss of reduction after nail passage. Diaphyseal reduction plates, however, should be removed to prevent rigid fixation of the fracture gap.
Blocking Screws/Pöller Screws	• Use interlocking bolts from nail instrumentation or small fragment screws and use great care during nail passage to avoid iatrogenic comminution. • Do not remove screws because they provide stability and help maintain reduction. • Use caution when using a drill bit because it is prone to breakage during nail insertion and removal after nail passage may destabilize the construct.
Posterior Malleolus	• Critically evaluate the posterior malleolus in distal diaphyseal and metaphyseal fractures pre-, intra-, and postoperatively. • If a posterior malleolar fracture or articular involvement is missed, ankle subluxation or displacement of the articular surface can occur with weight bearing.

POSTOPERATIVE CARE

- Weight bearing as tolerated, unless there is articular involvement
- Posterior splint or cam walker
- Early range of motion
- Suture removal at 2 to 3 weeks postoperatively.
- Strengthening after at 6-week clinic visit
  - Consider a quadriceps-specific program.
- After the 6-week visit, return clinic visits are made at 6- to 8-week intervals until the bone is clinically and radiographically healed.

OUTCOMES

- Long-term follow-up of patients treated nonoperatively reveals persistent functional deficits and dysfunction, including stiffness, pain, and loss of muscle power.[9,18,26,27]
- Anterior knee pain is common (50% to 60%), and patients should be informed of this preoperatively.[7,14]
  - This knee pain is more common in young patients. It typically is mild and may be exacerbated by kneeling, squatting, or running.
  - Its occurrence is not clearly dependent on the surgical approach; however, using a semiextended technique is recommended in patients who must kneel routinely.[29,30]
  - Nail removal leads to pain resolution in about one-half of patients and decreased pain in another one-fourth.[8]
- At late follow-up after tibial nailing, patients' function is comparable to population norms, but objective and subjective evaluation shows persistent sequelae, including knee pain, persistent swelling, muscle weakness, and arthritis—many of which are not insignificant.
- Malunion has an unclear association with development of arthritis.
  - Some authors have associated even mild deformity with increased risk of osteoarthritis.[15,38]

COMPLICATIONS[6,31]

Infection

- Closed fractures: about 1%
- Open fractures
  - Type I: 5%
  - Type II: 10%
  - Type III: over 15%
- Condition of the soft tissues is key for risk of infection and for outcome.

Nonunion

- Closed fractures: 3%
- Open fractures: about 15% and may be higher, depending on the soft tissue injury
- Risk factors[10]
  - Unreamed smaller diameter nails with smaller locking bolts are associated with delayed or nonunion and an increased risk of locking bolt breakage.
  - Closed fractures carry a risk of severe soft tissue injury, that is, internal degloving.

- Open fractures may be accompanied by severe soft tissue injury.
  - Delayed bone grafting may be warranted for treatment of bone loss.
  - The use of recombinant human bone morphogenetic protein 2 is U.S. Food and Drug Administration approved in open tibia fractures.[11] It decreases the nonunion rate by 29% and decreases secondary interventions. Bone morphogenetic protein 2 combined with allograft for delayed bone grafting procedures in tibia fractures with cortical defects have shown a similar rate of healing to autograft with the benefit of decreased donor site morbidity.[13]
- Compartment syndrome
- Fracture pattern—transverse
- Host factors
  - Tobacco use
  - Medications: bisphosphonates, nonsteroidal anti-inflammatory drugs
  - Diabetes mellitus
  - Vascular disease
  - Malnutrition—albumin level lower than 34 g per L and a lymphocyte count below 1500 per mm^3
- Infection

Malunion

- Occurs in up to 37% of all tibial nailing procedures
  - Malunion is seen in as many as 84% of patients with proximal metaphyseal tibia fractures.
  - These can be avoided with proper surgical techniques.

REFERENCES

1. Bakhsh WR, Cherney SM, McAndrew CM, et al. Surgical approaches to intramedullary nailing of the tibia: comparative analysis of knee pain and functional outcomes. Injury 2016;47(4):958–961.
2. Baumgartner M, Tornetta P, eds. Orthopaedic Knowledge Update: Trauma 3. Rosemont, IL: American Academy of Orthopaedic Surgeons, 2005.
3. Bishop JA, Dikos GD, Mickelson D, et al. Open reduction and intramedullary nail fixation of closed tibial fractures. Orthopedics 2012;35(11):e1631–e1634.
4. Bone LB, Sucato D, Stegemann PM, et al. Displaced isolated fractures of the tibial shaft treated with either a cast or intramedullary nailing. An outcome analysis of matched pairs of patients. J Bone Joint Surg Am 1997;79(9):1336–1341.
5. Bono CM, Sirkin M, Sabatino CT, et al. Neurovascular and tendinous damage with placement of anteroposterior distal locking bolts in the tibia. J Orthop Trauma 2003;17:677–682.
6. Cannada LK, Anglen JO, Archdeacon MT, et al. Avoiding complications in the care of fractures of the tibia. J Bone Joint Surg Am 2008;90(8):1760–1768.
7. Court-Brown CM, Gustilo T, Shaw AD. Knee pain after intramedullary tibial nailing: its incidence, etiology, and outcome. J Orthop Trauma 1997;11:103–105.
8. Court-Brown CM, McBirnie J. The epidemiology of tibial fractures. J Bone Joint Surg Br 1995;77(3):417–421.
9. Digby JM, Holloway GM, Webb JK. A study of function after tibial cast bracing. Injury 1983;14:432–439.
10. Drosos GI, Bishay M, Karnezis IA, et al. Factors affecting fracture healing after intramedullary nailing of the tibial diaphysis for closed and grade I open fractures. J Bone Joint Surg Br 2006;88(2):227–231.
11. Govender S, Csimma C, Genant HK, et al. Recombinant human bone morphogenetic protein-2 for treatment of open tibial fractures: a prospective, controlled, randomized study of four hundred and fifty patients. J Bone Joint Surg Am 2002;84:2123–2134.
12. Hooper GJ, Keddell RG, Penny ID. Conservative management or closed nailing for tibial shaft fractures. A randomised prospective trial. J Bone Joint Surg Br 1991;73(1):83–85.
13. Jones AL, Bucholz RW, Bosse MJ, et al. Recombinant human BMP-2 and allograft compared with autogenous bone graft for reconstruction of diaphyseal tibial fractures with cortical defects. A randomized, controlled trial. J Bone Joint Surg Am 2006;88(7):1431–1441.
14. Keating JF, Orfaly R, O'Brien PJ. Knee pain after tibial nailing. J Orthop Trauma 1997;11:10–13.
15. Kettelkamp DB, Hillberry BM, Murrish DE, et al. Degenerative arthritis of the knee secondary to fracture malunion. Clin Orthop Relat Res 1988;(234):159–169.
16. Krettek C, Miclau T, Schandelmaier P, et al. The mechanical effect of blocking screws ("Poller screws") in stabilizing tibia fractures with short proximal or distal fragments after insertion of small-diameter intramedullary nails. J Orthop Trauma 1999;13:550–553.
17. Kubiak EN, Widmer BJ, Horwitz DS. Extra-articular technique for semiextended tibial nailing. J Orthop Trauma 2010;24(11):704–708.
18. Kyrö A, Lamppu M, Böstman O. Intramedullary nailing of tibial shaft fractures. Ann Chir Gynaecol 1995;84:51–61.
19. Marchand LS, Rane AA, Working ZM, et al. Radiographic investigation of the distal extension of fractures into the articular surface of the tibia (The RIDEFAST study). J Orthop Trauma 2017;31(12):668–674.
20. McKee MD, Schemitsch EH, Waddell JP, et al. A prospective, randomized clinical trial comparing tibial nailing using fracture table traction versus manual traction. J Orthop Trauma 1999;13:463–469.
21. McQueen MM, Christie J, Court-Brown CM. Acute compartment syndrome in tibial diaphyseal fractures. J Bone Joint Surg Br 1996;78(1):95–98.
22. Mills WJ, Barei DP, McNair P. The value of the ankle-brachial index for diagnosing arterial injury after knee dislocation: a prospective study. J Trauma 2004;56:1261–1265.
23. Milner S, Greenwood D. Degenerative changes at the knee and ankle related to malunion of tibial fractures. J Bone Joint Surg Br 1997;79(4):698.
24. Nork SE, Barei DP, Schildhauer TA, et al. Intramedullary nailing of proximal quarter tibial fractures. J Orthop Trauma 2006;20:523–528.
25. Orfaly R, Keating JE, O'Brien PJ. Knee pain after tibial nailing: does the entry point matter? J Bone Joint Surg Br 1995;77(6):976–977.
26. Pun WK, Chow SP, Fang D, et al. A study of function and residual joint stiffness after functional bracing of tibial shaft fractures. Clin Orthop Relat Res 1991;(267):157–163.
27. Puno RM, Teynor JT, Nagano J, et al. Critical analysis of results of treatment of 201 tibial shaft fractures. Clin Orthop Relat Res 1986;(212):113–121.
28. Ricci WM, O'Boyle M, Borrelli J, et al. Fractures of the proximal third of the tibial shaft treated with intramedullary nails and blocking screws. J Orthop Trauma 2001;15:264–270.
29. Rothberg DL, Daubs GM, Horwitz DS, et al. One-year postoperative knee pain in patients with semi-extended tibial nailing versus control group. Orthopedics 2013;36(5):e548–e553.
30. Ryan SP, Steen B, Tornetta P III. Semi-extended nailing of metaphyseal tibia fractures: alignment and incidence of postoperative knee pain. J Orthop Trauma 2014;28(5):263–269.
31. Schmidt A, Finkemeier CG, Tornetta P. Treatment of closed tibia fractures. In: Tornetta P, ed. Instructional Course Lectures: Trauma. Rosemont, IL: American Academy of Orthopaedic Surgeons, 2006:215–229.
32. Tornetta P III, Collins E. Semiextended position of intramedullary nailing of the proximal tibia. Clin Orthop Relat Res 1996;(328):185–189.
33. Tornetta P III, Riina J, Geller J, et al. Intraarticular anatomic risks of tibial nailing. J Orthop Trauma 1999;13:247–251.

34. Tornetta P III, Steen B, Ryan S. Tibial metaphyseal fractures: nailing in extension. Presented at Orthopaedic Trauma Association Annual Meeting, Denver, October 16–18, 2008.

35. Väistö O, Toivanen J, Kannus P, et al. Anterior knee pain after intramedullary nailing of fractures of the tibial shaft: an eight-year follow-up of a prospective, randomized study comparing two different nail-insertion techniques. J Trauma 2008;64:1511–1516.

36. Väistö O, Toivanen J, Kannus P, et al. Anterior knee pain and thigh muscle strength after intramedullary nailing of a tibial shaft fracture: an 8-year follow-up of 28 consecutive cases. J Orthop Trauma 2007;21:165–171.

37. Väistö O, Toivanen J, Paakkala T, et al. Anterior knee pain after intramedullary nailing of a tibial shaft fracture: an ultrasound study of the patellar tendons of 36 patients. J Orthop Trauma 2005;19:311–316.

38. van der Schoot DK, Den Outer AJ, Bode PJ, et al. Degenerative changes at the knee and ankle related to malunion of tibial fractures. 15-year follow-up of 88 patients. J Bone Joint Surg Br 1996;78:722–725.

39. Walker RM, Zdero R, McKee MD, et al. Ideal tibial intramedullary nail insertion point varies with tibial rotation. J Orthop Trauma 2011;25:726–730.

40. Weninger P, Schultz A, Traxler H, et al. Anatomical assessment of the Hoffa fat pad during insertion of a tibial intramedullary nail—comparison of three surgical approaches. J Trauma 2009;66:1140–1145.

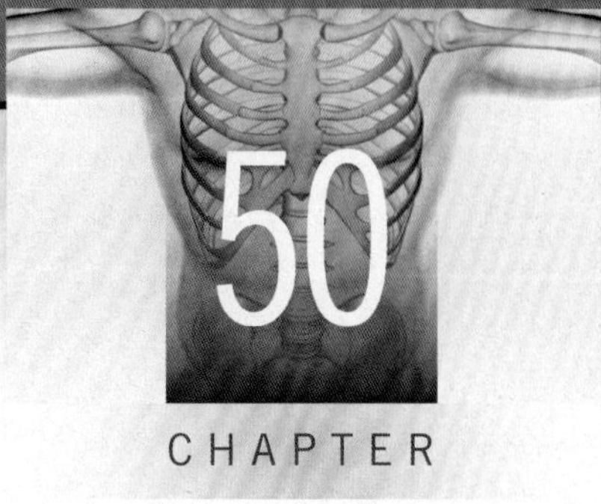

Intramedullary Nailing of Metaphyseal Proximal and Distal Fractures

Robert Ostrum and Michael Quackenbush

DEFINITION

- A fracture of the proximal or distal tibial metaphysis can occur from a variety of high- and low-energy trauma.
- Fractures may be confined to the metaphysis or extend into the articular surface.
- Simple fractures suggest lower energy injuries, whereas comminution signifies a greater amount of energy and a higher velocity mechanism.

ANATOMY

- Proximal metaphyseal fractures of the tibia are those that occur proximal to the isthmus of the tibia (**FIG 1A**).
- Distal metaphyseal fractures of the tibia are those that occur distal to the isthmus of the tibia (**FIG 1B**).

PATHOGENESIS

- Common causes of tibial fractures include high-energy collisions (pedestrian vs. car bumper) such as an automobile or motorcycle crash.
- Lower energy injuries, such as certain sports injuries or falls, can also cause fractures of both the proximal or distal tibial metaphysis.

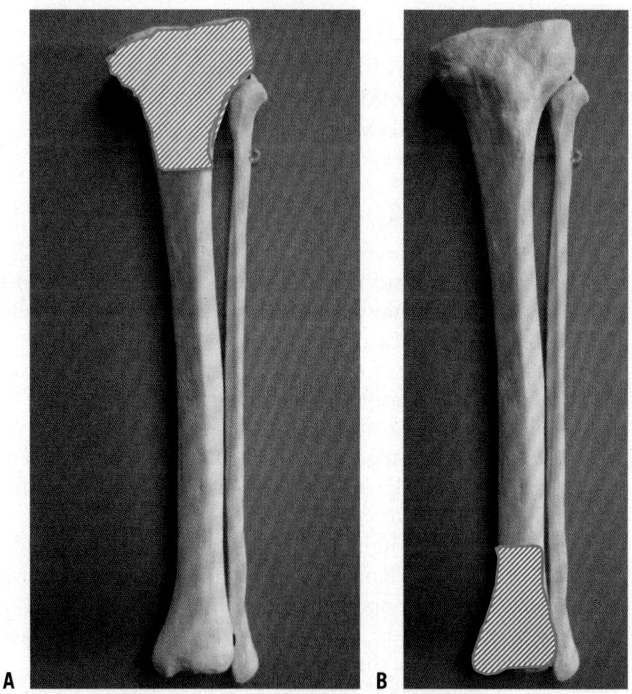

FIG 1 A. AP view of synthetic tibia model. *Shading* of the proximal tibial metaphysis is shown. **B.** AP view of synthetic tibia model. *Shading* of the distal tibial metaphysis is shown.

NATURAL HISTORY

- Fractures of the tibia can occur in all age groups and from a variety of mechanisms.
- Goals of treatment should include restoration of length, rotation, and alignment of the tibia with a return to previous level of activity and function.
- Recognition and treatment of associated injuries including those to nerves, blood vessels, or compartment syndrome should be an integral part of the assessment and treatment to prevent complications.

PATIENT HISTORY AND PHYSICAL FINDINGS

- Patients will often present with a recent history of trauma.
- Tibial fractures may present with a variety of findings:
  - Pain in the affected extremity with an inability to bear weight
  - Leg length inequality
  - Visual deformity including tenting of the skin
  - Contusions/abrasions
  - Nerve injury
  - Open fractures
  - Compartment syndrome
  - Sensory deficits in the foot (less common)

IMAGING AND OTHER DIAGNOSTIC STUDIES

- Diagnosis of a proximal or distal tibia (**FIG 2**) fracture can usually be made with standard orthogonal anteroposterior (AP) and lateral x-rays.
  - Dedicated knee and ankle x-rays are necessary to decrease the chance of missing a fracture at the articular surface.
- Fractures that extend proximally or distally into the articular surface may require a computed tomography (CT) scan to evaluate joint involvement and/or displacement to aid in preoperative planning (**FIG 3**).

DIFFERENTIAL DIAGNOSIS

- Trauma
  - Fractures of the knee
  - Fractures of the ankle
- Soft tissue injury
  - Ankle injury
  - Knee injury
- Compartment syndrome

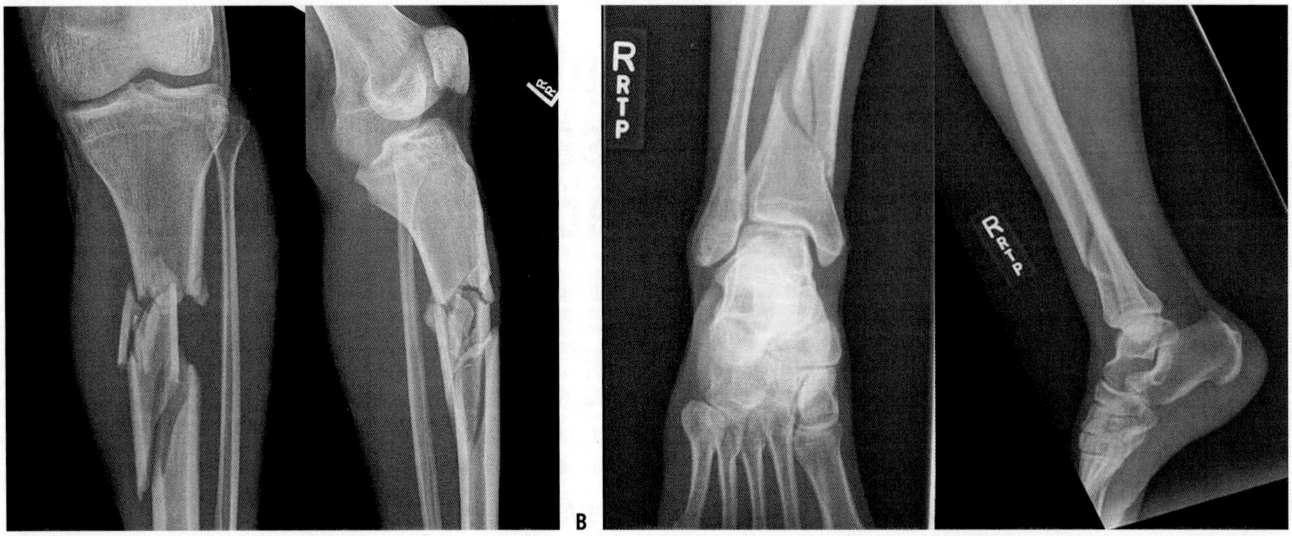

A B

FIG 2 **A.** AP and lateral x-rays of a proximal tibia fracture. **B.** AP and lateral x-rays of a distal tibia fracture.

- Peripheral vascular injury
- Pathologic process (tumor/malignancy)
- Infection

NONOPERATIVE MANAGEMENT

- Nonoperative management is normally reserved for lower energy injuries with minimal or no displacement.
- Patients with low functional demands (ie, paraplegic) or significant medical comorbidities can be successfully treated without surgical intervention.
- Nonoperative management of the proximal or distal tibia often involves a long-leg splint with conversion to a long-leg cast once swelling has resolved.
  - Distal fractures may be converted to a short-leg cast or brace once there is radiographic evidence of healing.
- Non–weight bearing for the first 6 weeks with progression to full weight bearing, with or without a brace, once there is physical evidence of healing (decrease in pain) and/or radiographic evidence of healing (callus formation)

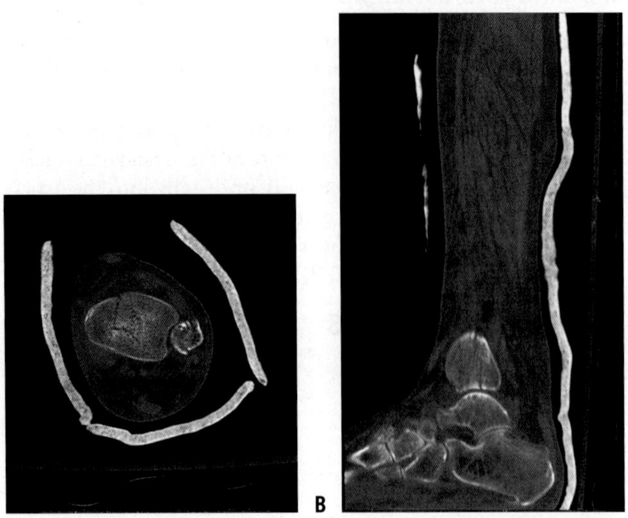

A B

FIG 3 **A.** CT of distal tibia with axial cut demonstrating intra-articular extension of distal tibia fracture. **B.** CT of distal tibia with sagittal cut demonstrating intra-articular extension of distal tibia fracture.

SURGICAL MANAGEMENT

Proximal Tibia Fractures

- The proximal tibia presents a challenge for intramedullary (IM) nailing due to deforming forces from the patella and the eccentric starting point for the IM nail.
- Flexion of the knee past 60 degrees to allow access to the tibial nail starting point causes the quadriceps, patella, and patellar tendon to extend the proximal fracture fragment leading to an extreme procurvatum deformity.
  - In addition, starting the IM nail in the center of the tibial spines, in the coronal plane will produce a valgus deformity. Techniques to prevent these deformities include the following:
    - Starting portal close to the lateral spine
    - Judicious use of blocking screws
    - Suprapatellar IM nailing
    - Semiextended IM nailing
    - Clamps, plates for reduction prior to IM nailing

Preoperative Planning

- A review of all images will help to plan the surgical approach.
- Fractures that extend into the proximal plateau or across the distal plafond may require closed or open reduction and fixation prior to IM nailing.
  - Large lag screws, from 4.5 to 6.5 mm placed in the coronal plane posteriorly in the tibial plateau will be out of the way of the tibial nail and its entry site.
  - Depending on the fixation required, small fragment screws and/or plates should be readily available for distal fractures.
- Obtaining and maintaining the reduction may require additional equipment. Planning ahead of time will avoid unnecessary delays in the operating room.
  - Some examples of other items you may wish to have available include the following (**FIG 4**):
    - Clamps, "spike" pushers, Kirschner wires
    - Small fragment set (for provisional plate fixation)
    - Large fragment (4.5- to 6.5-mm) screws
    - External fixator/universal distractor
    - Skeletal traction tray (calcaneal traction)

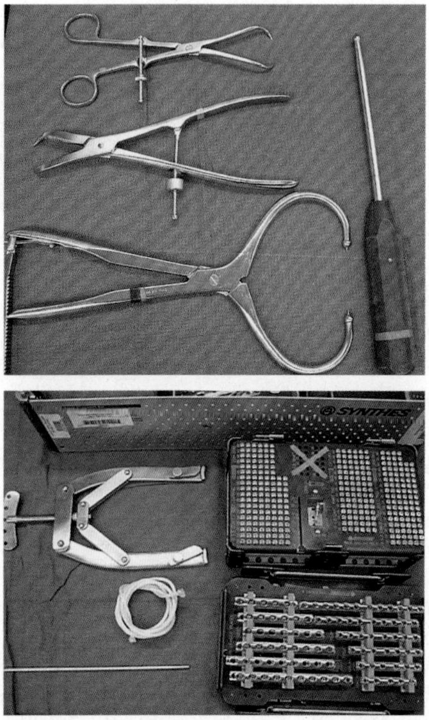

FIG 4 A,B. Preoperative planning may include additional equipment. This may include small fragment plates and screws (DePuy Synthes, Paoli, PA), specific clamps, or traction sets.

Positioning

- Patients are positioned in the supine position on a radiolucent table. A bolster may be placed under the ipsilateral hip.
- Radiolucent triangles may be used to assist with flexion of the knee for standard nailing **(FIG 5)**, whereas smaller bumps may be placed under the knee for semiextended approaches **(FIG 6)**.

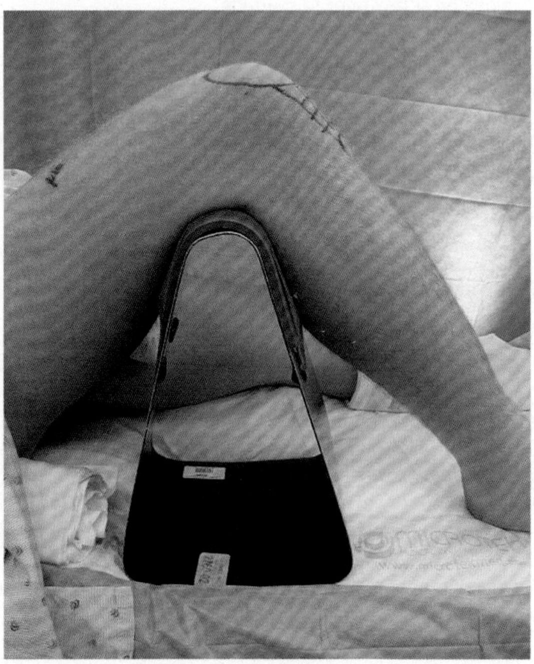

FIG 5 Standard tibial nailing requires flexion of the knee. Radiolucent triangles may help with positioning.

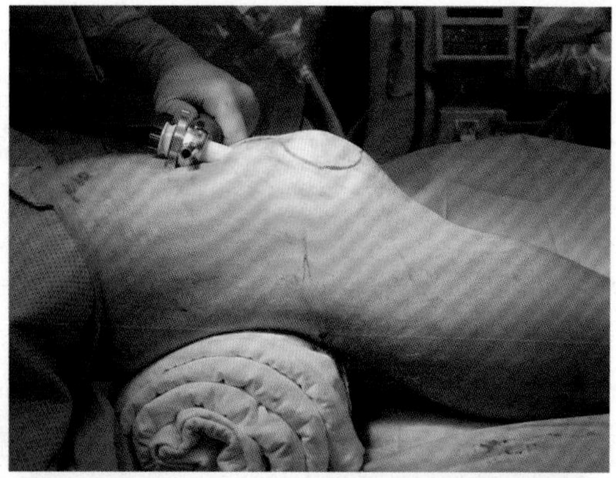

FIG 6 Patient positioning for semiextended or suprapatellar nailing. Notice a small bump under the knee to provide 30 to 40 degrees of knee flexion. Suprapatellar nailing requires specific instruments seen here.

Approach

- Standard nailing uses an incision between the inferior pole of the patella and the tibial tubercle **(FIG 7)**.
- Incision is carried down through skin and subcutaneous tissue and should be carried distally to the proximal tibia.
- The patellar tendon is identified, and an incision can be made medial to the patellar tendon or through the tendon.
  - Guidewire placement and correct starting point are extremely important, especially with proximal fractures.
  - Avoid an incision too medial, which could make it difficult to achieve the correct starting point.
  - Semiextended nailing may use various surgical approaches.
  - If a suprapatellar portal is chosen, the incision is made from the superior pole of the patella proximally in line with the quadriceps tendon **(FIG 8)**. A deeper incision is then made through the quadriceps tendon.
  - If the knee joint is too tight to enter through this portal, the skin incision can be carried distally, and a medial parapatellar arthrotomy can be made to help elevate the patella out of way and provide access to the correct starting point. This approach is described as being performed in full extension, which does not allow for both the proper portal and trajectory. At least 25 degrees of flexion is needed to obtain both.

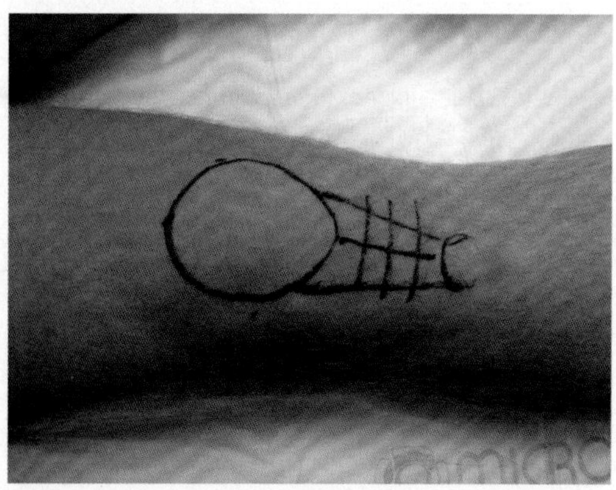

FIG 7 Skin incision for standard tibial nailing from inferior pole of the patella to the tibial tubercle.

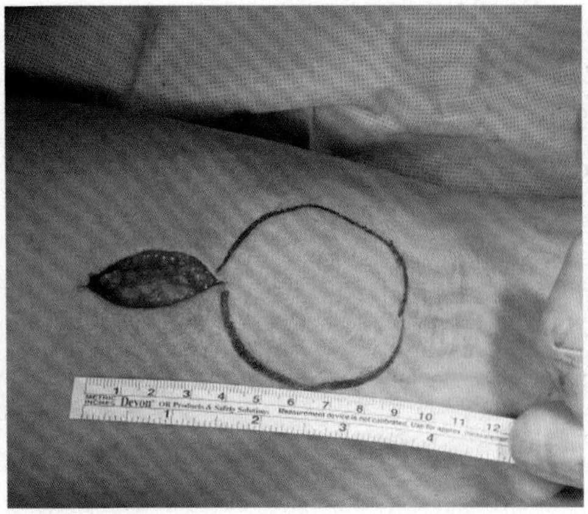

FIG 8 Skin incision used for a suprapatellar tibial nail is from the superior pole of the patella proximal approximately 3 cm centered over the quadriceps tendon.

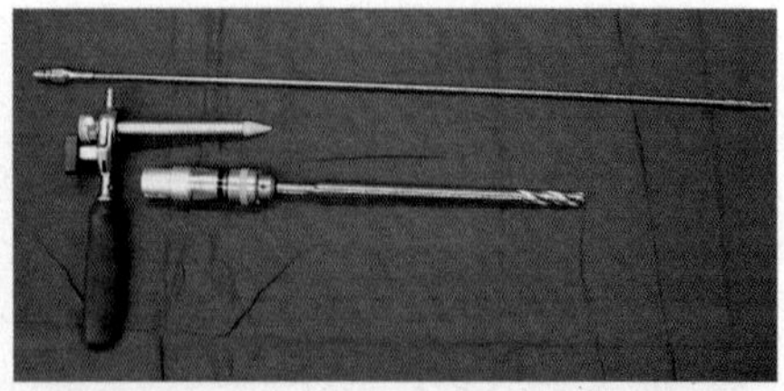

FIG 9 Suprapatellar nailing requires specific instrumentation. Specifically, it requires longer cannulas to protect the cartilage of the patellofemoral joint, a longer opening reamer, and longer reamer rods.

- The other option is to make a 4-cm incision over the patella and do a release of the retinaculum on the medial side of the patella to allow it to be mobilized. This approach allows for both the proper portal placement and trajectory for the nail.
- The semiextended approaches require specific instrumentation **(FIG 9)** and soft tissue guides to help protect the cartilage in the patellofemoral joint and to avoid unnecessary damage to the joint surface.
- Guide pin placement and starting point are dependent on whether the tibia fracture is proximal or distal.
  - For distal fractures, a starting point just medial to the lateral tibial eminence on the frontal plane and along the proximal anterior portion of the tibia anterior to the cruciate insertion is appropriate.
  - The wire should be aiming down the center of the canal in the AP plane and traversing parallel to the anterior cortex on the lateral view.
- For proximal fractures, the starting guide pin should be slightly more lateral, in line with the lateral tibial eminence, and parallel to the lateral cortex of the proximal tibia.
- On the lateral view, a starting point that appears on the articular surface allows for proper anterior trajectory, avoids the meniscus attachments, and avoids anterior angulatory deformity.

PROXIMAL TIBIA FRACTURES

- The starting point for IM nailing of fractures of the proximal tibia must be modified from the "classic" entry portal.
- The IM nail for proximal fractures is inserted at the superior part of the tibial plateau and more lateral, at the lateral tibial spine, in line with the lateral cortex of the proximal tibia.
- On the sagittal view, the IM nail should be traversing parallel to the anterior cortex to avoid deformity **(TECH FIG 1A)**.
- If, despite proper proximal tibial insertion site technique, deformity still occurs, then the next best intraoperative solution is the application of blocking screws.
  - These are usually the locking screws from the IM tibial nail set and are placed to prevent the IM nail from going posteriorly and causing the procurvatum deformity.
  - In the sagittal plane, the blocking screws are placed posterior to the IM nail to force it off of the posterior cortex and parallel to the anterior cortex **(TECH FIG 1B)**.
  - If the deformity is present with the IM guidewire in place after fracture reduction, then the blocking screw can be placed to "block" the guidewire to a more anterior position prior to reaming.
  - Sometimes, the guidewire is so far posterior that the blocking screw has to be placed anterior to the wire that lies on the posterior proximal tibial cortex. In this case, the blocking screw is inserted in its proper position and then the guidewire is pulled back and reinserted anterior to the blocking screw prior to reaming.
  - The reamer must either hit the blocking screw or be forcibly pushed past it for the screw to work.
- Similarly, a lateral blocking screw can be added to redirect the nail centered in the proximal fragment on the coronal view **(TECH FIG 1C,D)**. This strategy is most commonly employed when the proximal tibia is nailed with the knee flexed greater than 60 degrees over a triangle and a too medial starting point has been employed.

Additional Strategies

- Two other strategies for proper insertion site and trajectory are to perform the IM nailing with the knee in less flexion to prevent the extremes of proximal deformity.
- The semiextended position allows for a small paramedian arthrotomy, with the knee in only slight flexion, and subluxation of the patella allows for a straight trajectory in the proximal fragment and a more anterior line of insertion. This insertion technique has been shown to have an equivalent incidence of knee pain to hyperflexion nailing of the tibia.[5]
- The second option is suprapatellar IM nailing. This has gained popularity lately but requires special extra-long insertion

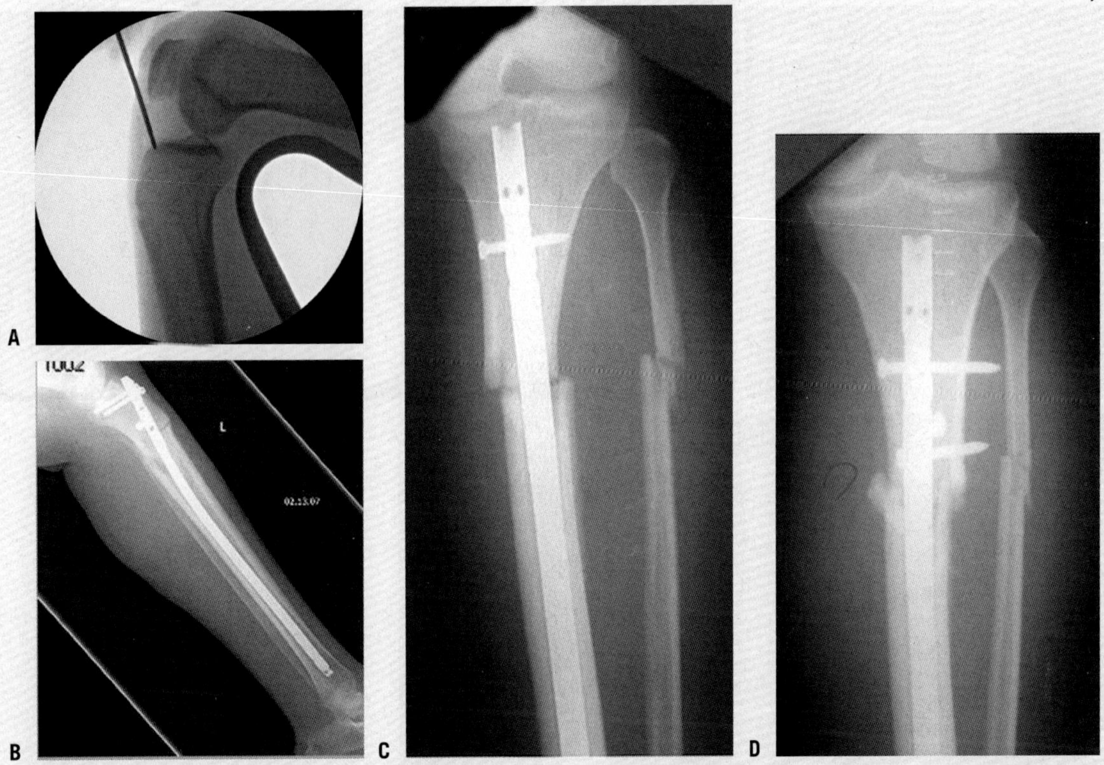

TECH FIG 1 **A.** Guidewire positioning for proximal tibia fractures at the flat anterior part of the tibial plateau and more lateral, at the lateral tibial spine, in line with the lateral cortex of the proximal tibia. On the sagittal view, the IM nail should be traversing parallel to the anterior cortex to avoid deformity. **B.** A blocking screw in the proximal tibia will help guide the nail into the right position and aid in reduction of this common deformity. **C.** An AP radiograph demonstrating common valgus deformity with a medial starting point. **D.** Correction of the deformity can be seen with a laterally placed blocking screw in the proximal fragment. The nail will "bounce" off of the nail and center itself in the proximal deformity.

instruments and caution so as not to cause damage to the patellofemoral cartilage.

- The best insertion angle is between 20 and 50 degrees of knee flexion, but up to 22% articular damage has been reported. A small insertion site is created just above the superior pole of the patella, and a cannula is inserted in the patellofemoral groove.
- A guide pin is then placed just proximal on the "flat portion" of the proximal tibia just superior to the anterior slope.
- This pin is directed in a direction that centers the pin in both planes using the more proximal and lateral starting points previously described.
- All reaming is done through the cannula to prevent articular damage.
- Bolsters are used under the knee and, with the knee in only slight flexion, the fracture stays reduced during the IM nailing procedure **(TECH FIG 2A–D)**.

- Finally, direct reduction of the fracture through small incisions can be performed prior to IM nailing. If a suprapatellar approach is chosen augmentation of the reduction is often needed as the trajectory will be too posterior (see **TECH FIG 2C**).
  - A ball spike "pusher" can be used with a small anterior incision to push the proximal fragment down and inhibit the flexion deformity **(TECH FIG 2E)**.
  - Percutaneous clamps **(TECH FIG 2F)** through very small incisions, without stripping of soft tissues, that are placed to reduce the fracture allow for the surgeon to ream and place the IM nail with the fracture reduced.
  - A small fragment plate, usually a one-third tubular plate, can be placed safely through a small incision **(TECH FIG 2G)** to reduce the fracture precisely prior to IM nailing.
    - An anterolateral incision centered over the proximal fracture and under the muscle mass allows for the placement of a five-hole plate with two screws on either side of the fracture line. The screws can be directed into the anterior cortex or placed unicortical to allow the subsequent passage of the IM nail. These plates can be left in place after IM nailing if adequate soft tissue coverage is present.

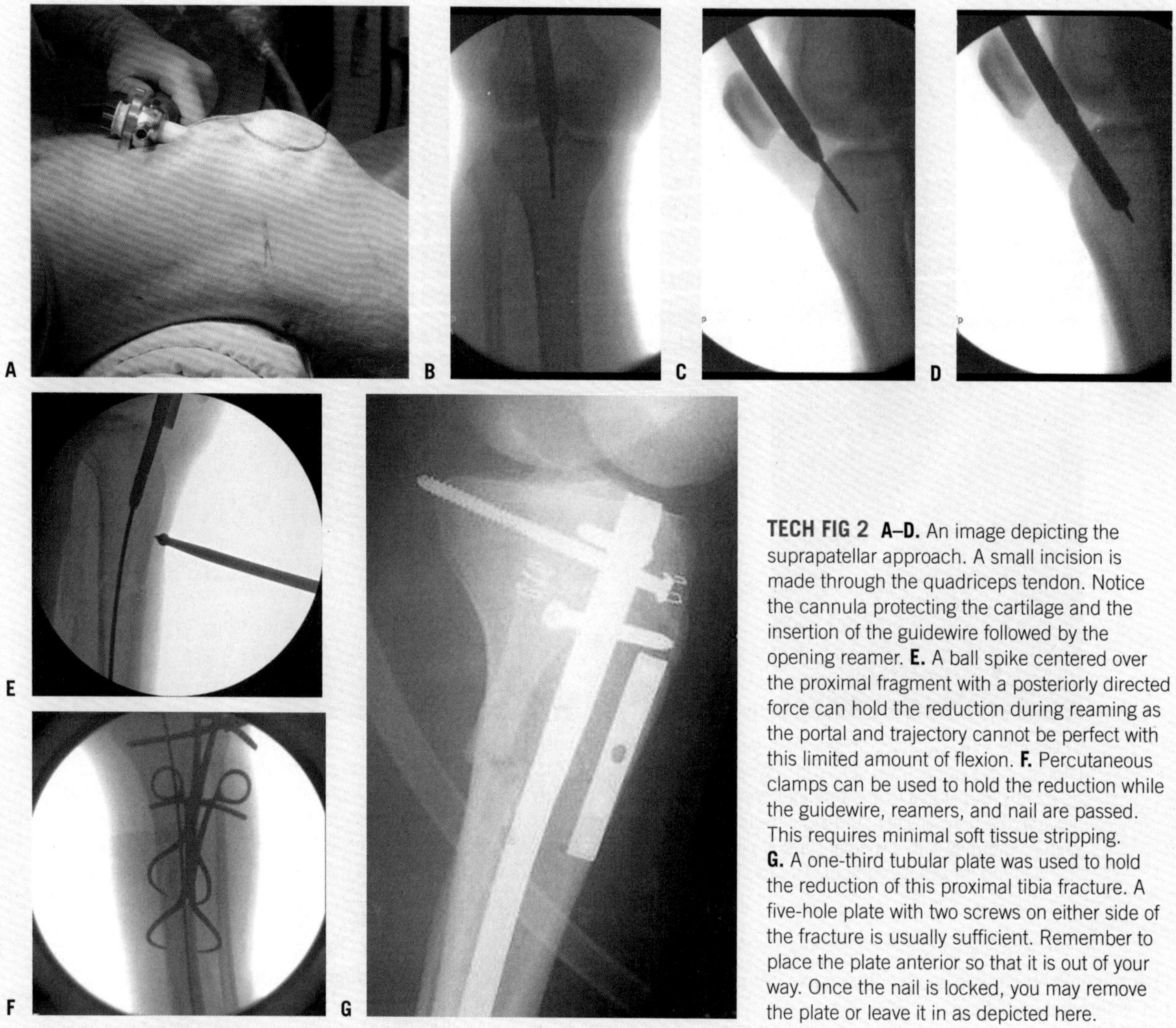

TECH FIG 2 A–D. An image depicting the suprapatellar approach. A small incision is made through the quadriceps tendon. Notice the cannula protecting the cartilage and the insertion of the guidewire followed by the opening reamer. **E.** A ball spike centered over the proximal fragment with a posteriorly directed force can hold the reduction during reaming as the portal and trajectory cannot be perfect with this limited amount of flexion. **F.** Percutaneous clamps can be used to hold the reduction while the guidewire, reamers, and nail are passed. This requires minimal soft tissue stripping. **G.** A one-third tubular plate was used to hold the reduction of this proximal tibia fracture. A five-hole plate with two screws on either side of the fracture is usually sufficient. Remember to place the plate anterior so that it is out of your way. Once the nail is locked, you may remove the plate or leave it in as depicted here.

DISTAL FRACTURES

- Similarly to proximal fractures, reduction is the key to IM nailing of distal tibia fractures.
- The placement of the tip of the IM nail in the distal tibia is crucial. The nail should be centered or just lateral to the midportion of the talus.[8]
- A closed reduction can be performed but is often difficult with spiral fractures that have an intact fibula or those with a proximal fibula fracture.
- One should always be aware that distal rotational tibial fractures have a high incidence of posterior malleolar fracture. If present, these should be fixed prior to the nailing. Additionally, a clamp from anteromedial to posterior supporting the fragment is advised during reaming and nailing even if fixation is present.
- For oblique fractures a pointed reduction clamp is routinely used, with minimal soft tissue stripping, to maintain the reduction during the entire procedure.
- The guidewire should not be bent as the tip of common nails area straight, and a curve in the distal segment of the guidewire will eccentrically ream.
- To correct varus or lateral translation, a blocking screw can be inserted just medial to the guidewire in the distal fragment **(TECH FIG 3A)**.
  - This is done using the same drill bit and screws from the IM nailing set and should be close enough to the guide rod that the reamers and IM nail will bounce off of it.

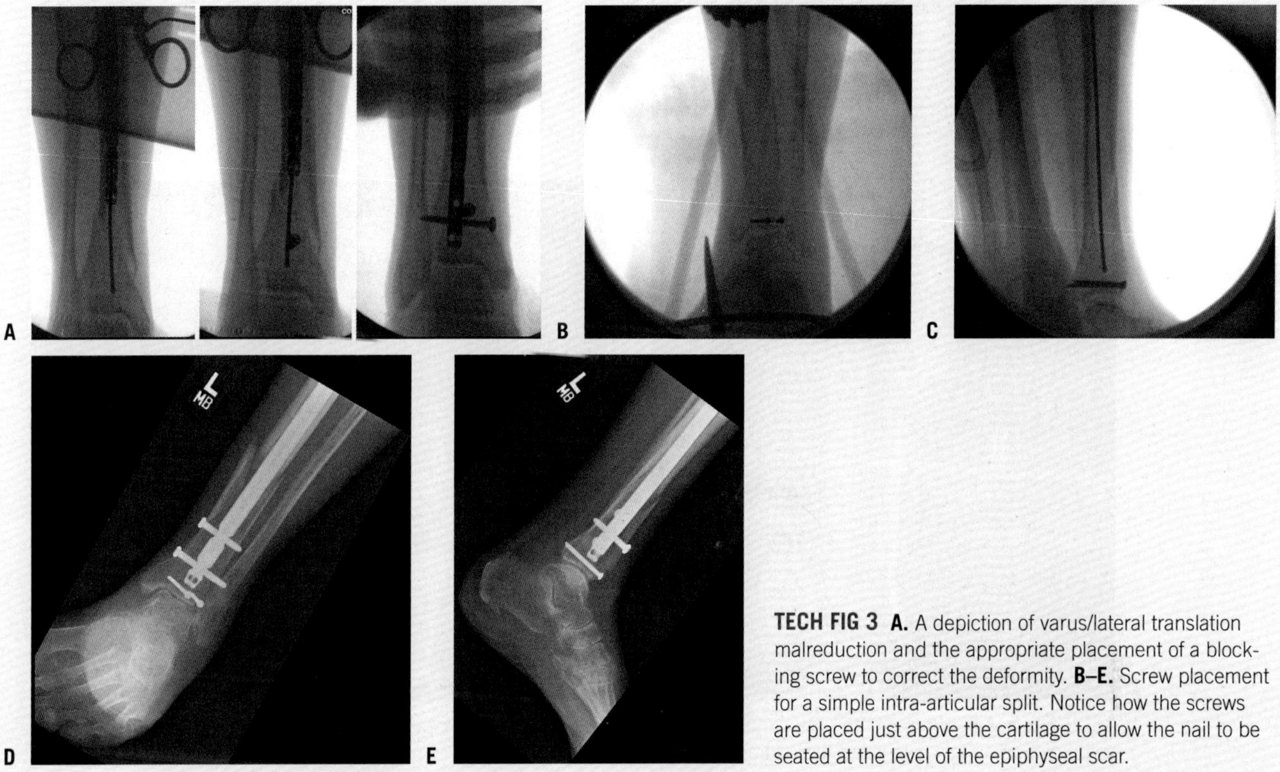

TECH FIG 3 **A.** A depiction of varus/lateral translation malreduction and the appropriate placement of a blocking screw to correct the deformity. **B–E.** Screw placement for a simple intra-articular split. Notice how the screws are placed just above the cartilage to allow the nail to be seated at the level of the epiphyseal scar.

- The other option is fixation of the fibula fracture, especially in distal one-third tibia and associated fibula fractures. Although attention to proper alignment in the operating room may preclude the need for fibular fixation.[3] There are pros and cons to this approach.
  - For the pros, the surgeon can get rotation and length correct and make the IM nail procedure much easier.
  - The cons relate to the fact that a malreduction of a comminuted fibula can lead to deformity and malunion of the tibia (**TECH FIGS 4** and **5**).
- Further, if tibial metaphyseal comminution is present, fixation of the fibula may not allow this area to compress and consolidate and later exchange procedures require an osteotomy of the fibula to allow for tibial compression and subsequent union.
- Adjunctive plating of the distal tibia with subsequent IM nailing is to be avoided as the skin of the distal leg has a limited blood supply as does the tibia; incisions with plate and subsequent IM nail insertion could lead to disastrous skin and bone healing issues.
- Regardless of the method of reduction, reaming is typically only 0.5 mm over the size of the nail in the distal segment and 1.5 to 2.0 mm over the size of the nail in the isthmus.
- For distal fractures, two interlocking screws should be inserted through the IM nail into the distal fragment, preferably with screws at 90 degrees or oblique to each other as these out-of-plane screws allow for early motion and lessen the chance of screw loosening and loss of distal fixation. Recently, authors have suggested a mini-open technique for anterior screw placement to avoid tendon or nerve injury.[4]

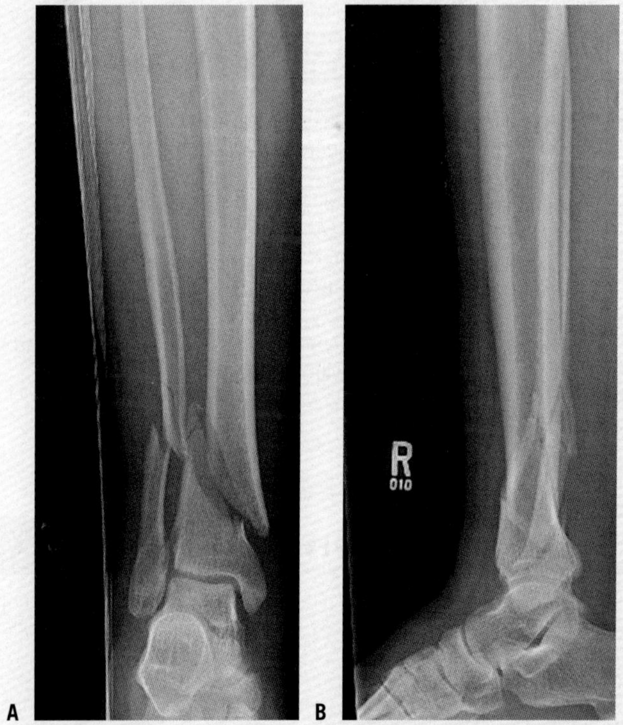

TECH FIG 4 **A,B.** A 30-year-old male who twisted right leg while running down a dock. AP and lateral radiographs showing a displaced fracture of the very distal right tibia and associated comminuted fibula fracture.

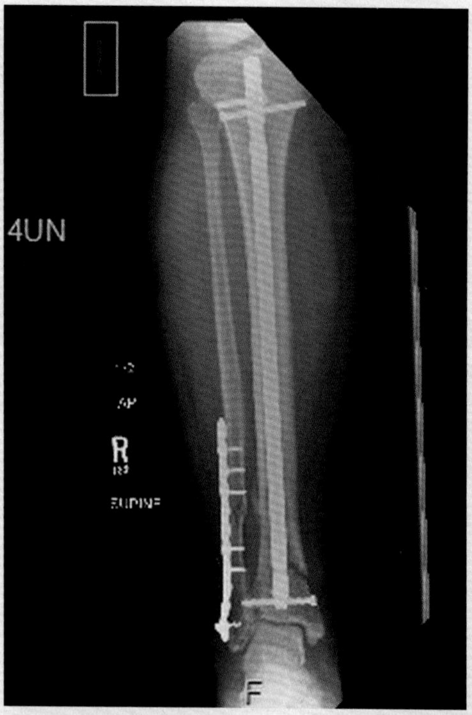

A

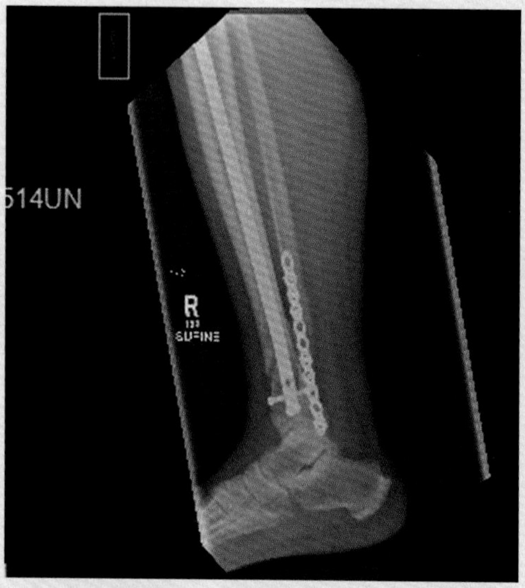

B

TECH FIG 5 A,B. Three-month postinjury x-rays show the use of a dynamic compression plate on the fibula with union and slight valgus but healed fracture of the very distal right tibia.

INTRA-ARTICULAR SPLITS

- Proximal and distal intra-articular splits associated with a metaphyseal fracture can be treated by percutaneous clamp and screw fixation.
- For proximal fractures, these are most commonly sagittal splits, and 4.5- to 6.5-mm screws with washers can be placed across the split from lateral to medial as long as the screw is at the midportion of the plateau or posterior to this line.
  - Because the IM nail enters anteriorly, the posteriorly placed screw will not interfere with IM nail passage.
- For distal fractures, the plane of the fracture needs to be identified. If the fracture is not completely visible or understood on plain x-rays, then a CT scan is performed to elucidate the fracture configuration and morphology.
  - Once the fracture is identified, a percutaneous clamp and a partially threaded cancellous screw or fully threaded screw can be inserted perpendicular to the fracture line at the level of the epiphyseal scar.
  - This distal screw insertion site allows for the IM nail placement as far distal as possible up to this screw **(TECH FIG 3B–E)**.

TECHNIQUES

Pearls and Pitfalls

Proximal tibia fractures behave differently than diaphyseal fractures.	• Correct starting point is essential to eliminating valgus and flexion deformity; slightly more lateral and proximal than the conventional starting point
The starting point makes all the difference.	• "High on the tibia, at the edge of the articular surface of the knee, just medial to the lateral tibial spine"[7]
Reduce and hold the reduction prior to reaming and inserting the nail.	• The nail will not reduce the fracture if it is in the proximal or distal metaphysis due to a canal–nail size mismatch. Reduce and hold the reduction and then ream and insert the IM nail. Percutaneous clamps with minimal soft tissue stripping can hold proximal and distal fractures reduced during reaming and nailing.

Nailing of proximal fractures with the knee in extension may be technically easier.	• With semiextended position, there is less pull on the proximal fragment through the patellar tendon and less deformity. Suprapatellar nailing requires specialized equipment, and there is the possibility of cartilage damage.
Proximal plate fixation can be extremely helpful.	• You can use any variety of plates, just be sure that it is out of the way of your nail; can be left in, but be cautious of making an incision through the zone of injury.
Beware of the intra-articular extension.	• Any questions about the extent of the fracture should be further investigated with a CT scan. If there is intra-articular involvement, address that first and then continue with the IM nail.
Blocking screws can help direct the nail and alleviate malreductions that come with bone/implant mismatch.	• They are minimally invasive, and you can use the same screws as your interlocking screws. Placed in the right position, they can help redirect your nail and guide it in the right direction.

POSTOPERATIVE CARE

- After surgery, immobilization of the limb can be achieved by placement of a splint or boot for soft tissue protection along with elastic bandage compression, ice, and elevation.
  - The splint is typically removed prior to discharge once the patient's pain allows range of motion (ROM). This may help avoid an acquired equinus contracture.
- Antibiotics are generally discontinued after 24 hours but may continue until all wounds are closed in the presence of an open fracture or with fasciotomies performed secondary to compartment syndrome.
- Although full weight bearing is generally protected until there is radiographic evidence of healing (10 to 12 weeks), aggressive ROM including heel cord stretching and mobilization are essential to provide optimal outcomes.
  - Partial weight bearing can be started at 6 weeks, depending on the progression of healing and the inherent stability of the fracture–nail construct.
- A course of deep venous thrombosis (DVT) prophylaxis is recommended for at least 2 weeks, with longer duration for patients who may have multiple injuries or who are otherwise slow to mobilize.
  - Low-molecular-weight heparin is often used in multiply injured patients or those who are high risk, whereas low-dose aspirin may be sufficient for the ambulatory patient.
- Follow-up is generally at 2 weeks for suture removal, 6 weeks for radiographic follow-up and to assess ROM, and 3 months for advancement to weight bearing as tolerated.
- Follow-up beyond that may be every 6 to 12 weeks thereafter, depending on healing and return to function.

OUTCOMES

- Closed tibial fractures should be expected to heal by 24 weeks.
- There is little information about the long-term, patient-reported outcomes of tibial shaft fractures.
- Factors such as smoking, comminution, quality of reduction, and whether or not the fracture is open can influence the patient's ability to heal a tibia fracture.
- Those fractures associated with intra-articular extension may have decreased joint motion despite aggressive postoperative therapy.
- Tibial IM nailing, whether using a medial patellar tendon incision or a midline tendon split, has been shown to cause knee pain in as high as 50% of patients with hardware removal alleviating pain in half of the patients.
- For distal fractures, to prevent valgus and procurvatum the IM nail should be centered in the plafond or slightly posterolateral.[2]
- A slightly larger incision with retraction of the tendons and neurovascular bundle is recommended for placement of the distal AP interlocking screw in the IM nail.
- Semiextended, suprapatellar, and infrapatellar approaches have similar rates of knee pain and alignment.[6]

COMPLICATIONS

- Similar to other orthopaedic surgery
  - Infection
  - DVT
  - Malunion
  - Nonunion
  - Hardware irritation/pain (knee pain)
- Malunion can be avoided with proper starting point and ensuring that you have appropriate reduction prior to IM nailing.
  - In some instances, leaving intraoperative adjunctive fixation (ie, plate, blocking screws) indefinitely may provide additional stability and aid in healing and prevention of late deformity.
- Nonunions are not uncommon in tibia fractures and increase if the fracture is comminuted or is an open fracture with extensive soft tissue stripping.
  - Recent studies have suggested avoiding reoperations until at least 6 months after surgery in absence of infection or catastrophic failure[1] as these fractures may simply require longer to achieve union.
- Hypertrophic nonunions are usually a result of a canal–nail mismatch and instability.
  - These are most readily treated with a dynamic exchange nailing often with a fibular osteotomy to allow for compression at the nonunion site. The nonunion in these cases does not need to be débrided.
  - IM cultures should be done in all nonunions, open or closed, to rule out infection as a cause of the nonunion.

- Atrophic or oligotrophic nonunions may need an increase in stability as well, but most require the addition of bone graft.
    - Options include autograft, allograft, or a combination of these adjuvants to obtain union.

REFERENCES

1. Bhandari M, Guyatt G, Tornetta P III, et al. Randomized trial of reamed and unreamed intramedullary nailing of tibial shaft fractures. J Bone Joint Surg Am 2008;90:2567–2578.
2. Brinkmann E, DiSilvio F, Tripp M, et al. Distal nail target and alignment of distal tibia fractures. J Orthop Trauma 2019;33(3):137–142.
3. De Giacomo AF, Tornetta P III. Alignment after intramedullary nailing of distal tibia fractures without fibula fixation. J Orthop Trauma 2016;30(10):561–567.
4. Mitchell PM, Collinge CA, Barcak E, et al. Proximity and risks of the anterior neurovascular and tendinous anatomy of the distal leg relative to anteriorly applied distal locking screws for tibia nailing: a plea for open insertion. J Orthop Trauma 2017;31(7):375–379.
5. Ryan SP, Steen B, Tornetta P III. Semi-extended nailing of metaphyseal tibia fractures: alignment and incidence of postoperative knee pain. J Orthop Trauma 2014;28(5):263–269.
6. Sanders RW, DiPasquale TG, Jordan CJ, et al. Semiextended intramedullary nailing of the tibia using a suprapatellar approach: radiographic results and clinical outcomes at a minimum of 12 months follow-up. J Orthop Trauma 2014;28(suppl 8):S29–S39.
7. Schmidt AH, Templeman DC, Tornetta P, et al. Anatomic assessment of the proper insertion site for a tibial intramedullary nail. J Orthop Trauma 2003;17:75–76.
8. Triantafillou K, Barcak E, Villarreal A, et al. Proper distal placement of tibial nail improves rate of malalignment for distal tibia fractures. J Orthop Trauma 2017;31(12):e407–e411.

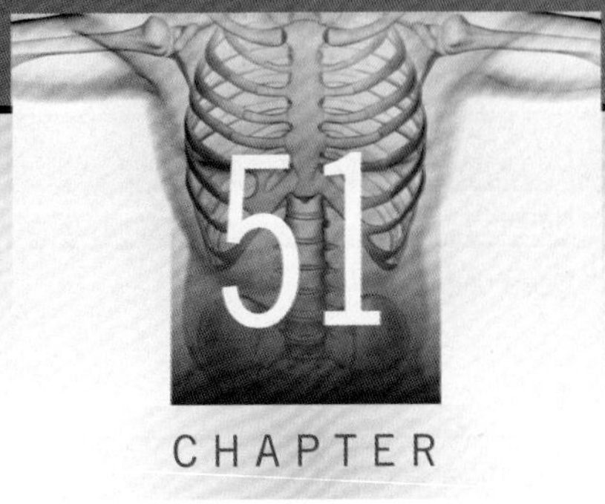

Fasciotomy of the Leg for Acute Compartment Syndrome

George Partal, Andrew Furey, and Robert V. O'Toole

DEFINITION

- Compartment syndrome remains one of the most devastating orthopaedic conditions if not treated appropriately. The potential clinical sequelae and medicolegal implications of possible missed compartment syndrome make it one of the most important entities in all of orthopaedic surgery.[5]
- Compartment syndrome is a condition, with numerous causes, in which the pressure within the osteofascial compartment rises to a level that exceeds intramuscular arteriolar pressure, resulting in decreased blood flow to the capillaries, decreased oxygen diffusion to the tissue, and, ultimately, cell death. This is the rare orthopaedic emergency for which evidence indicates that delay in treatment results in worse outcomes.[10,13,29–31,34]
- The clinical sequelae of missed compartment syndrome can be life- and limb-threatening. Myonecrosis can lead to acute renal failure and multiorgan failure if not appropriately managed.[24]
- Any situation that leads to increased pressure within the compartment can result in compartment syndrome.
  - The impermeable fascia prevents fluid from leaking out of the compartment and also prevents an increase in volume that could reduce pressure within the compartment.
- The incidence of compartment syndrome is 7.3 per 100,000 male patients and 0.7 per 100,000 female patients.
- This chapter describes acute compartment syndrome (ACS), in contrast to exertional compartment syndrome.
  - Exertional compartment syndrome is a transient chronic condition brought on by exercise. Unlike ACS, exertional compartment syndrome is not an emergency, and its treatment is beyond the scope of this chapter.

ANATOMY

- The lower leg has four compartments: anterior, lateral, superficial posterior, and deep posterior (**FIG 1**; **TABLE 1**).
- The anterior compartment is bound anteriorly by fascia, laterally by the anterior intermuscular septum, and posteriorly by the interosseous membrane between the fibula and tibia.
  - The four muscles in this compartment are the tibialis anterior, extensor digitorum longus, extensor hallucis longus, and peroneus tertius.
  - The neurovascular bundle includes the deep peroneal nerve and the anterior tibial artery.
  - The deep peroneal nerve provides sensation to the first dorsal web space of the foot and motor function to all the muscles in the anterior compartment.
  - The anterior tibial artery travels in this compartment just anterior to the tibiofibular interosseous membrane and continues in the foot as the dorsalis pedis artery.

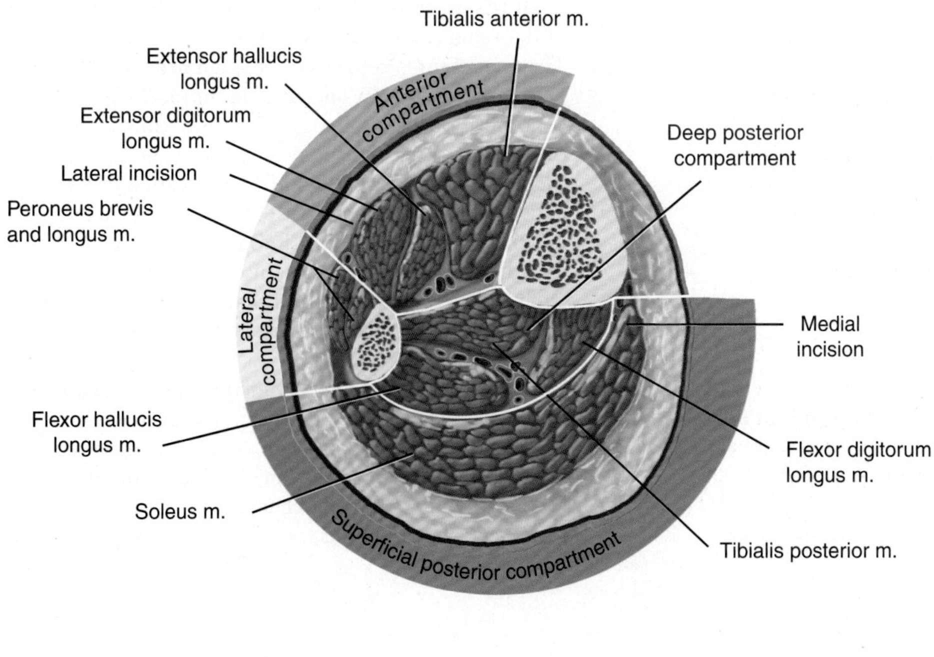

FIG 1 Cross-section of the lower leg at midtibial level.

TABLE 1 Compartments of the Lower Leg

Compartment	Muscles	Major Arteries	Nerves
Anterior	Tibialis anterior Extensor hallucis longus Extensor digitorum longus Peroneus tertius	Anterior tibial	Deep peroneal
Lateral	Peroneus brevis Peroneus longus	None	Superficial peroneal Deep peroneal (proximal in leg)
Deep Posterior	Posterior tibialis Flexor hallucis longus Flexor digitorum longus	Posterior tibial Peroneal	Tibial
Superficial Posterior	Gastrocnemius Soleus	None	None

- The lateral compartment is bordered anteriorly by the fascia, posteriorly by the posterior intermuscular septum, and medially by the fibula.
  - The lateral compartment has only two muscles: the peroneus longus and the peroneus brevis.
  - The major nerve supply to the lateral compartment is the superficial peroneal nerve, which supplies the two muscles of the compartment. The nerve supplies sensation to the dorsum of the foot, except the first dorsal web space.
  - Because the deep peroneal nerve courses proximally around the fibular head, both the deep and superficial peroneal nerves travel proximally within this compartment.
  - No main vessels are present in this compartment, and the muscles receive their blood supply from the peroneal and anterior tibial arteries.
- The deep posterior compartment contains the flexor digitorum longus, tibialis posterior, and flexor hallucis longus muscles. Popliteus is thought to lie within this compartment proximally.
  - Although it is not considered a separate compartment, the tibialis posterior muscle can have its own fascial covering.
  - The deep posterior compartment contains the main neurovascular bundle of the posterior compartment, which consists of the tibial nerve, posterior tibial artery and vein, and peroneal artery and vein.
- The superficial posterior compartment contains the gastrocnemius, soleus, and plantaris muscles, which are supplied by branches of the tibial nerve, posterior tibial artery, and peroneal arteries.
  - No major artery travels in this compartment.

PATHOGENESIS

- Although the exact pathophysiology is not completely understood, the syndrome is thought to be the result of either a decrease in the space available for the tissues within the fixed compartment or an increase in the size of the tissues within the compartment.
  - Either case can result in an increase in pressure above a critical value.
- Increased fluid content and swelling of damaged muscles can be caused by the following:
  - Bleeding into the compartment (from fractures, large vessel injury, or bleeding disorders)
    - Fractures are the most common cause of compartment syndrome. It is estimated that 9.1% of tibial plateau fractures develop compartment syndrome.[7]
    - Blunt trauma is the second most common cause, accounting for 23% of cases.[19]
  - Increased capillary permeability (eg, burns, ischemia, exercise, snake bite, drug injection, intravenous fluids)
- Decreased compartment size can be caused by the following:
  - Burns
  - Tight circumferential wrapping, dressings, casts
  - Localized external pressure, such as lying on the limb for an extended period of time or from pressure on the "well leg" in the lithotomy position on the fracture table
- Elevated pressure prevents perfusion of the tissue from the capillaries and results in anoxia and necrosis.
  - The impermeable fascia prevents fluid from escaping, causing a rise in compartment pressure, such that it exceeds the pressure within the veins, resulting in collapse of the veins or an increase in venous pressure.[22]
  - The final event is cellular anoxia and necrosis.[24]
  - During necrosis, an increase in intracellular calcium concentration occurs, coupled with a subsequent shift of water into the tissue, causing the tissue to swell further, adding to the pressure.[12] This "capillary leakage" adds to the increased pressure in the compartment, thus creating a vicious cycle. Lindsay et al[17] reported that prolonged ischemia of the muscle results in adenosine triphosphate breakdown and that the amount of energy depletion during ischemia determines the extent of the ischemic damage.
- The effects on muscle and nerve function are time dependent.
  - Prolonged delay results in greater loss of function.
  - Red muscle fibers (eg, anterior compartment of the leg), which rely predominantly on aerobic metabolism, are far more vulnerable to ischemia than "white" muscle fibers (eg, gastrocnemius muscle), which rely on anaerobic metabolism.[14]

- After sustained elevation of compartment pressures for more than 6 to 8 hours, nerve conduction is blocked.[10] In animal studies,[13,30] irreversible muscle damage occurred after 8 to 12 hours.
- The exact pressure at which change within the compartment occurs has been the subject of debate and has evolved over time.
  - Initially, the pressure of 30 mm Hg was reported to be the maximum pressure above which irreversible muscle damage occurred.[40]
  - Currently, clinicians have recognized the importance of the patient's blood pressure when considering the compartment pressure and use an absolute difference between diastolic blood pressure and compartment pressure of less than 30 mm Hg as an indicator of ACS.[18]
- Animal studies have highlighted the importance of the systemic pressures relative to the compartment pressure.
  - Whitesides and Heckman[40] found that irreversible ischemic changes occurred when the compartment pressure was elevated within 30 mm Hg of the mean arterial pressure and within 20 mm Hg of the diastolic pressure.
  - Research[4] on limb ischemia at the University of Pennsylvania led to similar conclusions. Bernot et al[4] coined the term *delta P*, referring to the difference between the mean arterial pressure minus the compartment pressure, with a lower number reflecting less blood flow. The authors[4] found that cellular anoxia and death occur with pressure within 20 mm Hg of the mean arterial pressure; however, at pressures within 40 mm Hg, oxygen tension was reduced, but anoxia was not indicated and aerobic metabolism persisted.
  - McQueen et al[18] used the cutoff of compartment pressure within 30 mm Hg of the diastolic blood pressure as a fasciotomy threshold. No adverse clinical outcomes occurred as a result of not releasing compartments with pressures that were more than 30 mm Hg from the diastolic blood pressure, and this has come to be the value currently used most often as a threshold for compartment syndrome.

NATURAL HISTORY

- The outcome of compartment syndrome depends on location, trauma to the tissue, and time to intervention.
  - Six hours of ischemia currently is the accepted upper limit of viability. Rorabeck and Macnab[31] reported almost complete recovery of the limb function when fasciotomies were performed within 6 hours of the onset of symptoms.
  - Muscle undergoes irreversible change after 8 hours of ischemia, whereas nerves can incur irreversible damage in 6 hours.[10]
- Compartment syndrome can have broad effects on multiple systems.
  - As muscle necrosis occurs, myoglobin, potassium, and other metabolites are released into circulation.
  - As a result, several metabolic conditions can arise, including myoglobinuria, hypothermia, metabolic acidosis, and hyperkalemia. In turn, these biochemical phenomena can cause renal failure, cardiac arrhythmias, and, potentially, death.

PATIENT HISTORY AND PHYSICAL FINDINGS

- Diagnosis of compartment syndrome is a clinical challenge, and significant variation among clinicians likely exists.[25] Studies of diagnosis in patients are limited by lack of a reliable gold standard other than "fasciotomy was performed," which is what typically is used in the literature.
- Compartment syndrome is, for the most part, still a clinical diagnosis. However, the use of physical examination findings to diagnose compartment syndrome has not been well validated.[38]
- The key to successful handling of compartment syndrome is early diagnosis and treatment. Therefore, the orthopaedic surgeon must be familiar with the risk factors and signs and symptoms of the diagnosis, obtain a detailed documented history, and perform a thorough physical examination.

Risk Factors for Compartment Syndrome

- The patient's history is critical. Certain aspects of the patient's history render the syndrome more likely.
- Risk factors for compartment syndrome include age younger than 35 years, male gender, and mechanism of sport injury.[19,26,43]
- The most common cause of ACS is fracture, and the second most common cause is soft tissue injury.
- Tibial fractures are associated with a high rate of compartment syndrome, with rates for shaft fractures ranging from 1% to 11%.[25,38] Proximal tibial fractures are at particular risk, especially high-energy tibial plateau fractures, with rates of approximately 15% to 28%[3,9,33] and fracture-dislocations reported to be as high as 53%.[20,36] Ballistic proximal fibular fractures[20] also have been shown to be at particular risk for developing compartment syndrome.
  - It should be noted that open fractures can still develop ACS, and some authors have found no difference in incidence of ACS with open compared with closed fractures.[18,19]
  - The existence of any of the following characteristics should heighten the surgeon's suspicion: high-energy injury mechanism, a patient receiving anticoagulation medication, or a patient with a tight circumferential dressing.

Physical Examination of Acute Compartment Syndrome

- Little rigorous data exist regarding the validation of clinical examination findings. The most widely cited review of the literature on this topic includes only four patients with compartment syndrome.[38]
- The classic "Ps" taught in medical schools (pain out of proportion, pain with passive range of motion, paresthesias, pulselessness, pallor, paralysis, and pressure on palpation) for diagnosing compartment syndrome are not equally useful, and little validation work has been conducted.[38]
- Pain out of proportion to the injury is a classic symptom of the diagnosis. Patient injury severity and perception and expression of pain vary substantially, rendering this judgment difficult in clinical practice. The amount of pain medicine needed by the patient is a useful predictor of compartment syndrome in a pediatric setting.[2]

- Patients in whom pain might be difficult to ascertain include those with head injuries; those using ethanol or drugs; those who are intubated or sedated; those who have major distracting injuries, such as long bone fracture; those receiving large amounts of pain medicine; and those with any other factor that might alter the patient's ability to accurately sense and communicate pain levels.
  - Pain perception can also be altered by anesthesia, and some work suggests that patients receiving epidural anesthesia are four times more likely to develop compartment syndrome than those receiving other forms of pain control.[23]
  - This type of anesthesia results in a sympathetic nerve blockade, thereby increasing the blood flow, compounding the local tissue pressures and extremity swelling.
- Similarly, local anesthesia combined with narcotics has been shown to increase the risk of compartment syndrome.[8,23]
  - Pulselessness typically is not helpful because the presence of a pulse does not rule out compartment syndrome. Most patients with ACS have normal pulses.
  - Pallor typically is not helpful either. Pallor also reflects loss of arterial flow and rarely is present during physical examination.
- Pain with passive range of motion of the muscles of the compartment is another classic sign of compartment syndrome.[12] For tibial fractures, for example, motion of the toes does not typically cause substantial pain.
- Zones of paresthesia can be a useful, but confusing, symptom of compartment syndrome.
  - It has been shown, however, that nerve function is altered after only 2 hours of ischemia; therefore, paresthesia represents a potential early symptom.[11]
- Light touch is a better indicator because it indicates change in the ability of the nerves to detect a threshold force, as opposed to two-point discrimination. Two-point discrimination is a test of nerve density, which might not change until later in the process.
  - With increased pressure in a compartment, the sensory nerves are affected first and then the motor nerves (eg, in the anterior compartment, the deep peroneal nerve is affected quickly and patients report loss of sensation between the first two toes).
  - Considering that small fiber nerves are affected first, light touch will be affected before pressure and proprioception.
- Decreased motor function of muscles in the compartment is another classic sign. However, it can be caused by ischemia, guarding, pain, or a combination of these factors, particularly in patients with distracting extremity injuries, such as tibial shaft fracture.
  - Muscle force should be documented in all compartments when ruling out compartment syndrome. Documenting that the patient "wiggles toes" is not adequate because that indicates only that either the flexors or extensors are firing. "NVI" is not useful either because it does not state the exact muscle groups that were tested.
- Palpation of tight compartments has been thought to be an important indicator of compartment syndrome. The deep posterior compartment cannot be directly palpated because of its location deep to the superficial posterior compartment. Recent data have questioned clinicians' ability to evaluate pressure based on palpation alone.[35]
- Serial examinations are critical. All complaints should be thoroughly investigated, and all findings should be carefully documented in the chart such that subsequent examiners can refer to the record as a tool for diagnosis.

IMAGING AND OTHER DIAGNOSTIC STUDIES

- The diagnosis of compartment syndrome typically is made clinically. Intracompartmental pressure measurements are the most common data used to aid in diagnosis, particularly in patients with limited physical examinations.
- Once a patient is diagnosed with compartment syndrome, fasciotomies should be performed emergently. Any workup that could substantially delay this process should be undertaken with great caution.

Intracompartmental Pressure Measurements

- If the patient cannot provide clinical clues because he or she is sedated or for other reasons, or if the diagnosis is in question, compartment pressures can be measured.
- The exact pressure that defines compartment syndrome is still debated, although a pressure measurement should be obtained with reference to the diastolic blood pressure.[18]
  - Some authors have argued that using single-pressure measurements alone might result in high rates of false-positive diagnoses using the standard delta P of 30 mm Hg threshold.[27,41] Therefore, in our opinion, compartment pressure checks should not be performed on patients in whom there is no clinical concern for ACS.
  - The technique of measuring compartment pressures must be mastered by the surgeon.
  - Inexperience with the technique can lead to inaccurate data and potentially missed compartment syndrome.
  - When measuring the pressure, the surgeon must be familiar with the local anatomy and able to accurately measure all the compartments.
  - Location of the measurement is important.
  - Whitesides and Heckman[40] reported that the highest pressures were within 5 cm of the fracture site; pressures decreased as the measurements were obtained distally and proximally to the fracture.

Measurement of the Compartment Pressure

- Several techniques to measure compartment pressure have been described, including the Whiteside infusion technique, the STIC technique, the Wick catheter technique, and the slit catheter technique. The two most commonly used instruments are the Whiteside side port needle and the slit catheter device.
- Numerous digital pressure monitors are commercially available and frequently used. The Stryker pressure monitor is in common clinical use (**FIG 2**).
- Inserting an arterial line (16- to 18-gauge needle) is easy to do in the operating room, but the pressure measured with a simple needle is thought to be 5 to 19 mm Hg higher than the pressure measured with a side port or wick catheter.[21]
- Pressure values should be recorded for all four compartments. Typically, each compartment is checked twice. If a fracture is present, the value will be highest within 5 cm of the fracture.[40] The contralateral limb can be checked as a control. Normal resting internal compartment pressure is approximately 8 mm Hg in adults and 13 to 16 mm Hg in children.

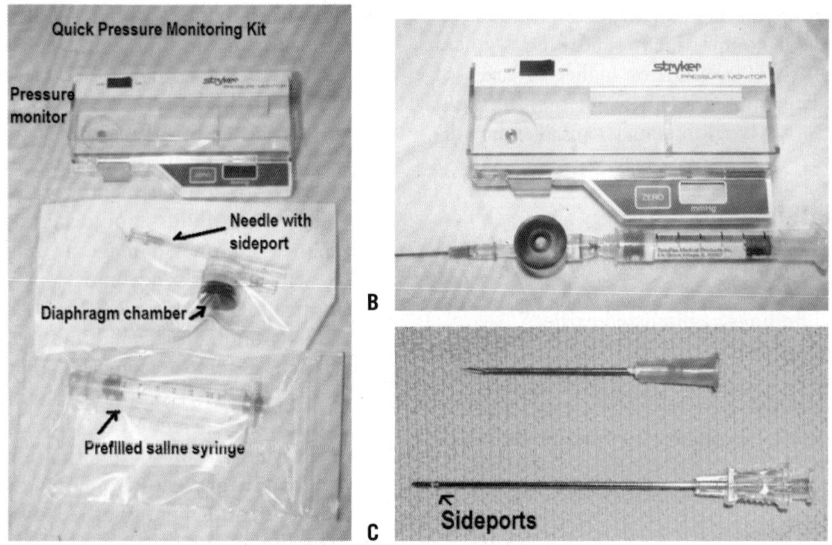

FIG 2 Stryker intracompartmental pressure monitor. **A.** Quick pressure monitoring kit containing the intracompartmental pressure monitor, a prefilled saline syringe, a diaphragm chamber (transducer), and a needle. **B.** The assembled pressure monitor. To assemble the monitor kit, the needle is attached to the tapered end of the tapered chamber stem (transducer). The blue cap from the prefilled syringe is removed, and the syringe is screwed into the remaining end of the transducer, which is a Luer-lock connection. The cover of the monitor is opened. The transducer is placed inside the well (black surface down). The snap cover is closed. Next, the clear end cap is pulled off the syringe end, and the monitor is ready to use. To prime the monitor, the needle is held 45 degrees up from the horizontal and the syringe plunger is pushed slowly to purge air from the syringe. The monitor is then turned on. The assembled monitor is tilted at the approximate intended angle of insertion of the needle into the skin. The zero button is pressed to set the display at zero. The needle is then inserted into the appropriate location in the compartment. **C.** The intracompartmental pressure monitor needle has side ports to prevent soft tissue from collapsing around the needle opening. This is different from a regular needle that has only one opening at the end.

- Delta P (diastolic blood pressure minus intracompartmental pressure) is measured.
  - A delta P of less than 30 mm Hg generally is accepted as an indication for fasciotomy based on the work conducted by McQueen et al[19] that showed that all patients with a delta P greater than 10 mm Hg in whom fasciotomy was not performed had normal function at follow-up. Clinicians should interpret this study with caution considering it used continuous pressure measurement values averaged over 12 hours (not one-time pressure measurements, as are obtained in common clinical practice) and considering only three patients in that study had compartment syndrome.
  - Although some animal data indicate that lower thresholds might be safe and although some concern might exist that this threshold leads to a high false-positive rate,[27,41] clinicians should be reassured that delta P of 30 mm Hg seems to be highly sensitive to avoid missing any compartment syndromes.
  - Unless the patient will be in the operating room for a prolonged time period, preoperative values of diastolic pressure should typically be used because diastolic blood pressure decreases 20 points, on average, with anesthesia.[15]
- McQueen et al[19] have advocated routine continuous pressure monitoring in the anterior compartment of tibial fractures. It is their center's technique for continuous monitoring that has been extrapolated to determine our current threshold of 30 mm Hg delta P even though the measurement technique used does not currently include continuous measurement. Continuous monitoring of routine tibial shaft fractures has not gained clinical popularity in North America as of yet, likely because of logistical difficulties in setting up the monitoring and some clinicians' concerns regarding the false positives associated with monitoring.[27,41]
- Near-infrared spectroscopy is a noninvasive and continuous method that determines tissue oxygenation by comparing the light emitted when comparing the concentration of venous blood oxyhemoglobin and deoxyhemoglobin. It might ultimately be a tool to monitor patients with evolving compartment syndrome, making it useful in the setting of critically ill patients.[1,28] This technology has not been validated and is not currently in routine clinical use.
  - Laboratory studies should include a complete metabolic profile, a complete blood count with differential, creatine phosphokinase (CPK), urine myoglobin, serum myoglobin, urinalysis (which might be positive for blood but negative for red blood cells, indicating myoglobin in the urine caused by rhabdomyolysis), and a coagulation profile (prothrombin time, partial thromboplastin time, international normalized ratio).
- Obtaining a complete laboratory panel should not delay operative treatment in a diagnosed case of compartment syndrome.

- Elevated CPK or creatine kinase in an intubated trauma patient might be a sign of compartment syndrome. Typical CPK values are 1000 to 5000 μg/L or higher in cases of ACS. One recent study proposed a CPK value of 4000 μg/L as indicative of ACS.[39] Myoglobinemia can also be observed in some cases.

DIFFERENTIAL DIAGNOSIS

- Compartment syndrome is diagnosed in a patient with either of the following:
  - Suspicious clinical findings as discussed earlier
  - Pressure in a compartment within 30 mm Hg of the diastolic blood pressure
- Other diagnoses to consider
  - Normal pain response secondary to fracture or other trauma
  - Low pain tolerance secondary to preoperative substance abuse
  - Muscle rupture
  - Deep venous thrombosis and thrombophlebitis
  - Cellulitis
  - Coelenterate and jellyfish envenomations
  - Necrotizing fasciitis
  - Peripheral vascular injury
  - Peripheral nerve injury
  - Rhabdomyolysis
- Of special note, recent studies have shown that in the case of envenomations, compartment syndrome is multifactorial and fasciotomy might not prevent myonecrosis, which can be caused by the direct toxic effect of the venom and the inflammatory response.
  - In these cases, antivenom should be administered; this has been shown to decrease limb hypoperfusion.

NONOPERATIVE MANAGEMENT

- All patients suspected of having ACS should undergo emergent fasciotomies performed in the operating room or at the bedside.
- Nonoperative treatment of ACS is almost never appropriate unless operative treatment would risk the patient's life. ACS is a life- and limb-threatening injury; the successful treatment of which is based on limiting the time until fasciotomy is performed.
- Considering that ischemic injury is the basis for compartment syndrome, additional oxygen should be administered to the patient diagnosed with compartment syndrome because it will slightly increase the blood partial pressure of oxygen.
  - The surgeon must ensure that the patient is normotensive because hypotension reduces perfusion pressure and leads to further tissue injury.
- Any circumferential bandages or casts should be removed from patients at risk for development of compartment syndrome.
  - Compartment pressure falls by 30% when a cast is split on one side and by 65% when a cast is spread after splitting. Splitting the padding reduces the pressure by an additional 10% and complete removal of the cast by another 15%. A total of 85% to 90% reduction in pressure can be achieved by removing the cast.[42]
- Elevating the limb above the heart decreases mean arterial pressure in the limb without changing the intracompartmental pressure. Thus, the affected extremity should not be elevated.
  - As shown by Wiger et al,[42] after an elevation of 35 cm, the mean perfusion pressure decreased by 23 mm Hg but the intracompartmental pressure stayed the same.
- Intravenous fluids should be administered to decrease the chance of kidney damage from myoglobin.
  - The "crush syndrome" is a sequela of muscle necrosis (ie, high CPK level, above 20,000 IU) that manifests as nonoliguric renal failure, myoglobinuria, oliguria, shock, acidosis, hyperkalemia, and cardiac arrhythmia.
  - Treatment is supportive, with ventilatory support, hydration, correction of acidosis, and dialysis.
  - It is important in this situation to decrease the metabolic load by preventing ongoing tissue necrosis and performing débridement of all dead tissue.
- The use of narcotics should be closely recorded and monitored for any patient suspected of having compartment syndrome.
  - The use of local, spinal, or epidural anesthesia for postoperative pain control generally is discouraged in patients at high risk for compartment syndrome because it limits the ability of the clinician to perform serial examinations.

Late Presentation of Acute Compartment Syndrome

- Nonoperative treatment of missed compartment syndrome is reserved for patients presenting very late after missed compartment syndrome who already have irreversible muscle necrosis.
  - One school of thought is that these patients should not be treated operatively because doing so would increase the chance of infection and lead to amputation.
  - It often is difficult to know when compartment syndrome has occurred, however, so in situations in which it is unclear, it is probably wise to release the compartments.
  - One school of thought is that if compartment syndrome has run its course, fasciotomies should not be performed unless the pressure in the compartment is within 30 mm Hg of diastolic pressure, but this recommendation is controversial and without support in the literature.

SURGICAL MANAGEMENT

- All patients with ACS should be treated with emergent fasciotomies of the affected compartments because compartment syndrome is limb-threatening and potentially life-threatening if allowed to progress to myonecrosis and renal failure.
- Time to diagnosis and surgical treatment of compartment syndrome is critical; nerve damage after 6 hours of ischemia might be irreversible.
- Patients with compartment syndrome should be given the highest priority, and the condition should be treated as an operative emergency.
- Fasciotomy of the involved compartment is the standard of care for ACS.
  - In a trauma setting, typically all four compartments of the leg are released, regardless of evidence of involvement of the other compartments.

- Fasciotomies ideally should be performed in the operating room.
  - If the patient is too ill to be transported to the operating room or if no operating room is available, fasciotomies can be performed at the bedside in as sterile an environment as possible.
- The only common contraindication to fasciotomy in the face of compartment syndrome is delayed presentation, in which a patient with missed compartment syndrome presents late, after irreversible injury has set in (see Nonoperative Management section).
- Fasciotomies are also often performed in a prophylactic manner for any patient with an ischemic limb for more than 6 hours to prevent reperfusion injury.

Preoperative Planning

- Once compartment syndrome is diagnosed, every effort should be directed at getting the patient to the operating room as quickly as possible for fasciotomies.
  - All further workup should be deferred until fasciotomies are complete, except workup that is needed for a potential life-threatening injury.
  - Little preoperative planning is required for this component of the patient's treatment.
- Radiographs should be reviewed to rule out fractures and dislocations; however, additional radiographs can be obtained in the operating room after fasciotomies have been completed.
- Only essential preoperative workup should be conducted before the patient is taken to the operating room. The case should not be delayed for additional, nonessential radiographic workup.

Positioning

- The patient usually is positioned supine on the operating room table to facilitate fasciotomies. A small bump can be placed under the hip on the affected side.
- The leg is prepared in a sterile fashion, and a thigh tourniquet is applied but not inflated.

Approach

- Two separate techniques have been used for decompression of the lower leg compartments.
  - The two-incision technique is the most commonly used method, but a one-incision technique involving a lateral (perifibular) approach also exists.
  - The two-incision technique is more straightforward and requires less experience to ensure a complete compartment release and is therefore typically advocated. Draw both planned incisions on the skin before making them to avoid a narrow skin bridge.
  - Some have argued that the one-incision technique can be useful in cases of defined anterior tibial artery injuries to help prevent loss of anterior skin.

DOUBLE-INCISION TECHNIQUE

TECHNIQUES

Anterolateral Incision

- The anterolateral incision decompresses the anterior and lateral compartments.
  - The anterolateral incision is made halfway between the fibula and the crest of the tibia and lies just above the intermuscular septum dividing the anterior and lateral compartments **(TECH FIG 1A)**.
- Fasciotomies have also been accomplished through small incisions. However, we prefer using generous incisions to allow for full decompression of the compartments.
  - We recommend incisions that typically are at least 15 to 20 cm both medially and laterally.
- A small transverse incision is made to identify the intermuscular septum, after which scissors are used to split the fascia of the anterior and lateral compartments.
  - Care must be taken to avoid injuring the superficial peroneal nerve by making separate incisions in each compartment and not cutting the intermuscular septum **(TECH FIG 1B–F)**.

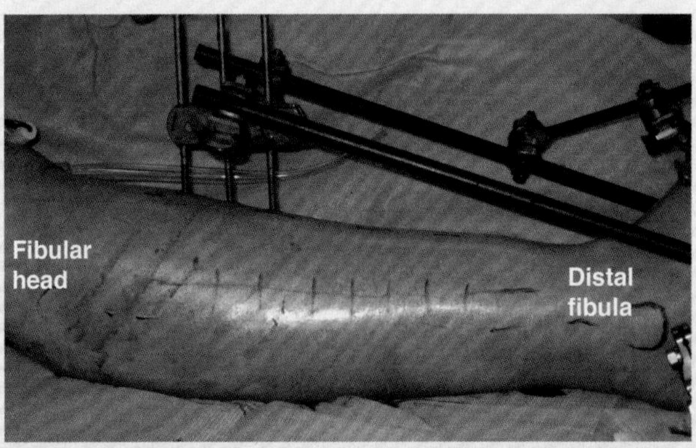

A

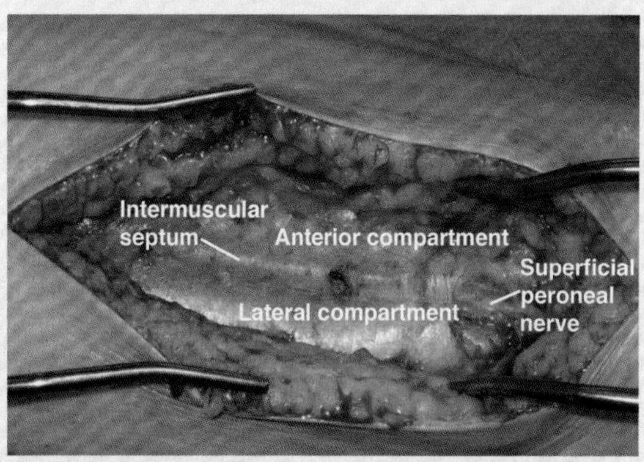

B

TECH FIG 1 Lateral incision of the two-incision technique. **A.** The anterolateral incision is made halfway between the fibula and the tibial crest overlying the intermuscular septum dividing the anterior and lateral compartments. **B.** Close-up picture of the fasciotomy site after skin incision before the fascia is open, showing the intermuscular septum between the lateral and anterior compartments and the course of the superficial peroneal nerve. *(continued)*

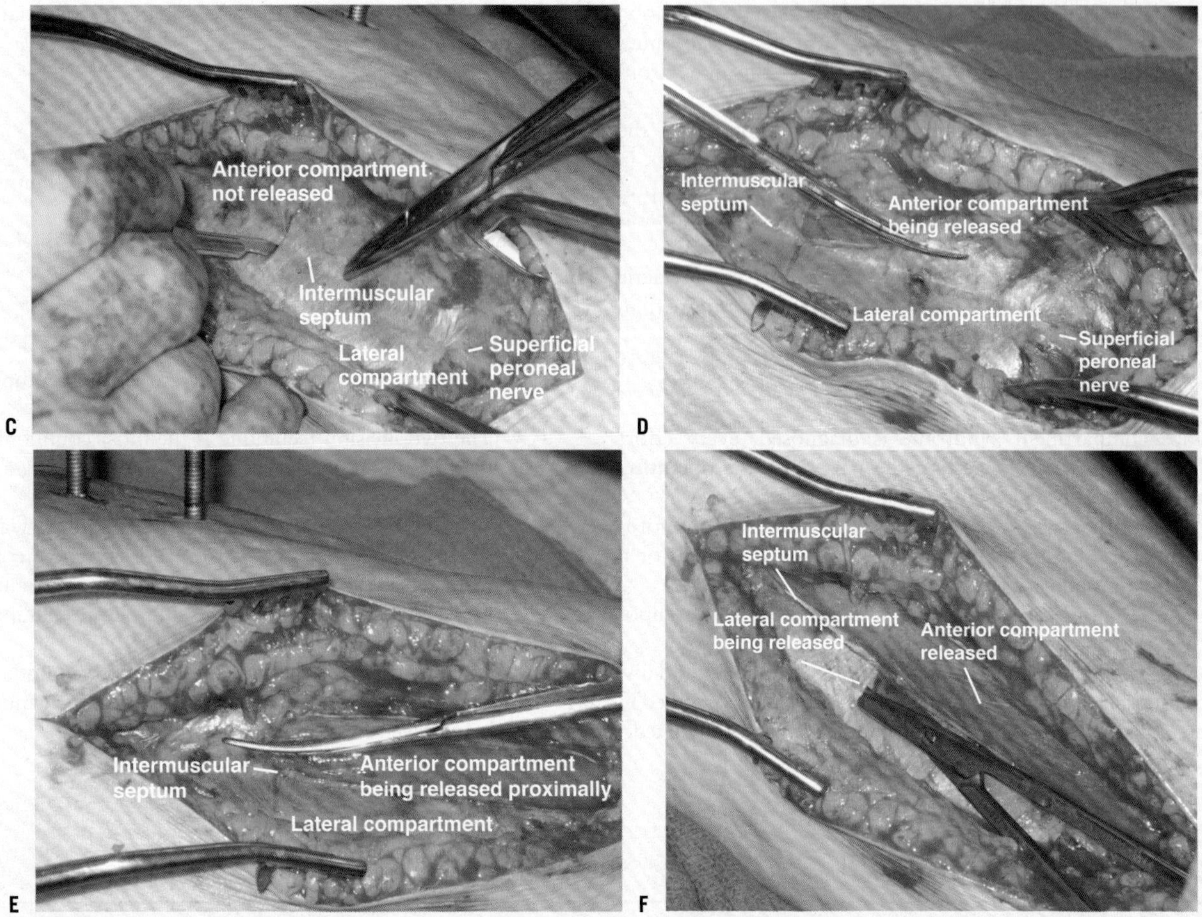

TECH FIG 1 *(continued)* **C.** With a knife, a small transverse incision is made over the intermuscular septum. Care is taken to avoid injury to the superficial peroneal nerve. **D.** The surgeon inserts the tips of the scissors into the small rent in the fascia, and, keeping the tips of the scissors up and away from the superficial peroneal nerve, the surgeon incises the fascia over the anterior compartment distally. **E.** The scissors are turned with the tips proximally, and the fascia of the anterior compartment is released proximally. **F.** The tips of the scissors are then inserted into the rent created in the fascia of the lateral compartment. Keeping the tips of the scissors up and away from the superficial peroneal nerve, the surgeon releases the fascia over the lateral compartment proximally and distally.

Posteromedial Incision

- The posteromedial approach decompresses the superficial and deep posterior compartments.
  - The incision lies approximately 2 cm posterior to the posterior tibial margin **(TECH FIG 2A)**.
  - Care is taken to avoid injury to the saphenous vein and nerve, which are retracted anteriorly.
- Each fascia of the deep and superficial posterior compartments is incised longitudinally in line with the incision **(TECH FIG 2B–E)**.
- The deep posterior compartment is initially released distally, and then the scissors are oriented proximally through and under the soleus bridge. If the posterior tibia is visualized, the deep posterior compartment has been released.
- Some surgeons release the soleus attachment to the tibia more than halfway. Also, the fascia over the posterior tibial muscle should be released.
- One useful tip is to keep the tips of the scissors away from major neurovascular structures.

One-Incision Technique

- The one-incision technique often requires more careful dissection around major neurovascular structures and can prove to be more challenging. For this reason, it is less often used. Bible et al[6] showed no difference in infection or nonunion rates between a one- and two-incision fasciotomy technique.
- A straight lateral incision is created that originates just posterior and parallel to the fibula at the level of the fibular head (protecting the peroneal nerve) to a point above the tip of the lateral malleolus **(TECH FIG 3A)**.
- Posterior to the fibula, access is gained to the deep and superficial posterior compartments **(TECH FIG 3B)**.
  - The fascia between the soleus and flexor hallucis longus is identified distally and released proximally to the level of the soleus origin **(TECH FIG 3C)**.[16]
- Anterior to the fibula, the anterior and lateral compartments are decompressed, taking care to avoid injury to the superficial peroneal nerve.

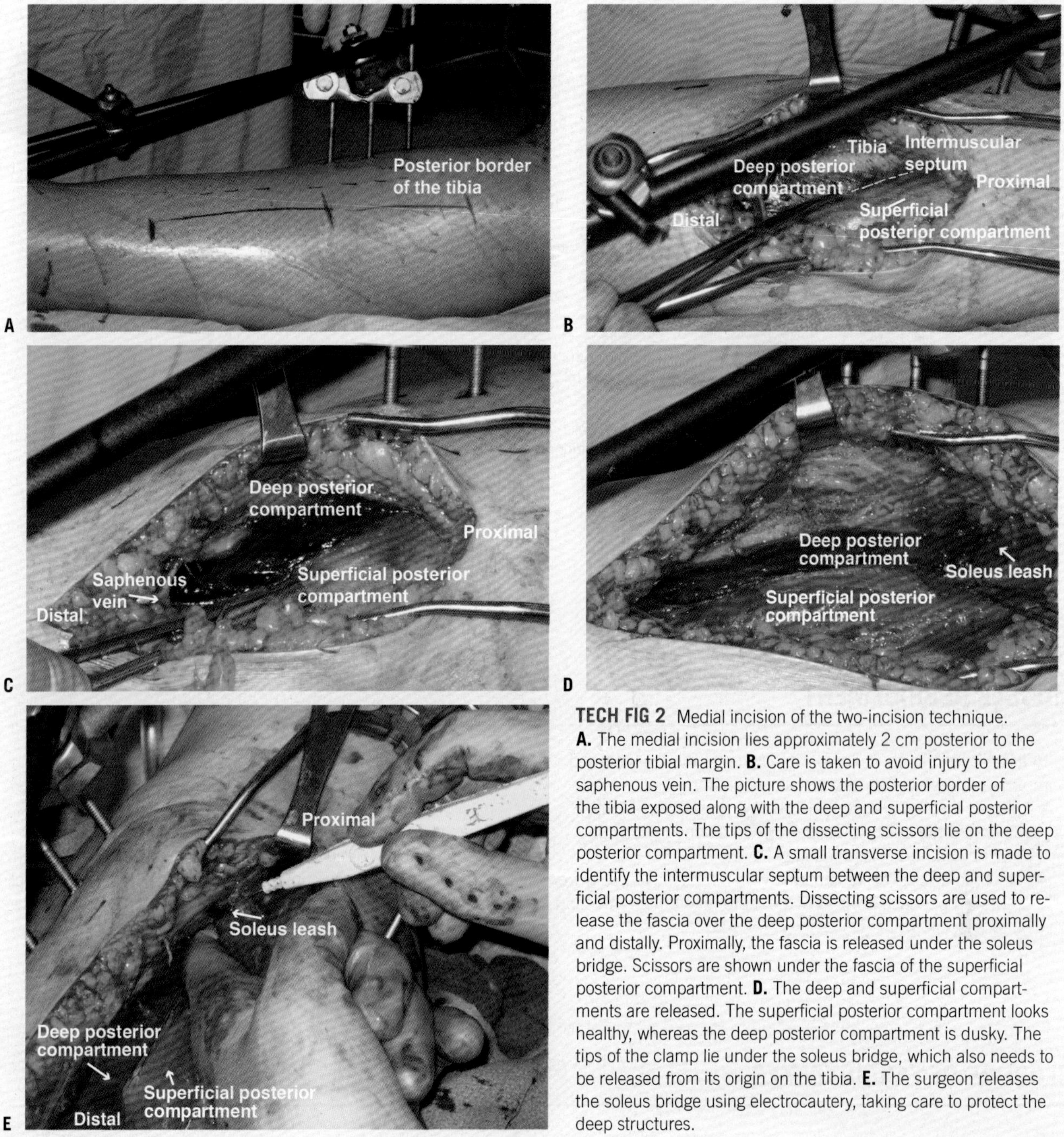

TECH FIG 2 Medial incision of the two-incision technique. **A.** The medial incision lies approximately 2 cm posterior to the posterior tibial margin. **B.** Care is taken to avoid injury to the saphenous vein. The picture shows the posterior border of the tibia exposed along with the deep and superficial posterior compartments. The tips of the dissecting scissors lie on the deep posterior compartment. **C.** A small transverse incision is made to identify the intermuscular septum between the deep and superficial posterior compartments. Dissecting scissors are used to release the fascia over the deep posterior compartment proximally and distally. Proximally, the fascia is released under the soleus bridge. Scissors are shown under the fascia of the superficial posterior compartment. **D.** The deep and superficial compartments are released. The superficial posterior compartment looks healthy, whereas the deep posterior compartment is dusky. The tips of the clamp lie under the soleus bridge, which also needs to be released from its origin on the tibia. **E.** The surgeon releases the soleus bridge using electrocautery, taking care to protect the deep structures.

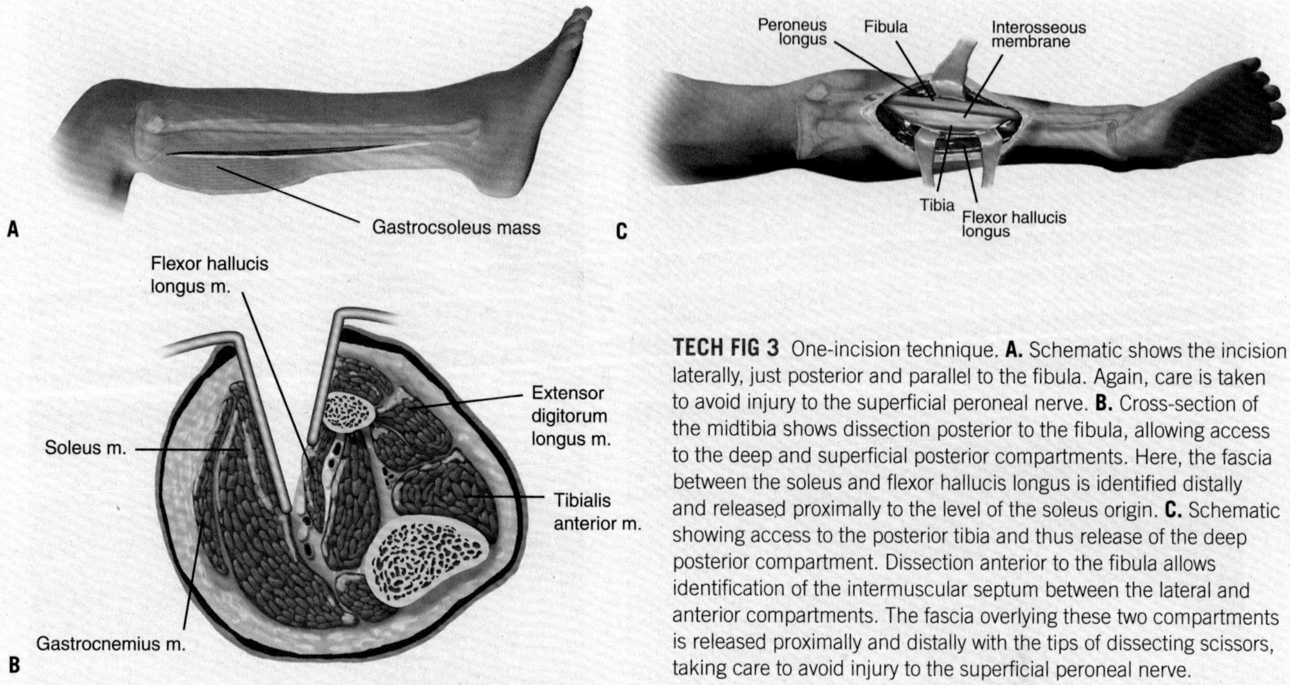

TECH FIG 3 One-incision technique. **A.** Schematic shows the incision laterally, just posterior and parallel to the fibula. Again, care is taken to avoid injury to the superficial peroneal nerve. **B.** Cross-section of the midtibia shows dissection posterior to the fibula, allowing access to the deep and superficial posterior compartments. Here, the fascia between the soleus and flexor hallucis longus is identified distally and released proximally to the level of the soleus origin. **C.** Schematic showing access to the posterior tibia and thus release of the deep posterior compartment. Dissection anterior to the fibula allows identification of the intermuscular septum between the lateral and anterior compartments. The fascia overlying these two compartments is released proximally and distally with the tips of dissecting scissors, taking care to avoid injury to the superficial peroneal nerve.

MUSCLE DÉBRIDEMENT

- Regardless of the choice of fasciotomy performed, devitalized muscle undergoes débridement as necessary.
  - Muscle viability is ascertained by the presence of healthy color and the ability to contract when pinched gently or touched with the electrocautery.
  - Necrotic muscle serves no function and must eventually be removed because it will form a culture medium for infection after fasciotomy.
- Extensive débridement typically is not undertaken until the second look at 36 to 72 hours, when muscle viability is more readily determined.
- When fasciotomies are performed in the setting of fractures, the fractures are stabilized with either internal or external fixation, which eliminates the need for constrictive casts and allows access for clinical examination, repeat pressure measurements, and wound care.
  - Fixation of fractures can trigger compartment syndrome through traction and reaming.

CLOSURE OF FASCIOTOMIES

- Fasciotomies typically are not closed acutely because the skin itself can constrict muscle.
- Most often, fasciotomy wounds are either packed with moist dressings **(TECH FIG 4A)** or covered with a sterile vacuum sponge and kept under suction until the next débridement procedure **(TECH FIG 4B)**.
- After a lower leg fasciotomy, a useful technique has been the shoelace closure, which involves using a vessel loop and skin staples to gradually close large areas of gaping skin.
  - This allows gradual approximation of the skin edges over the course of several days, thus potentially obviating the need for a skin graft **(TECH FIG 4C)**.
- It is our opinion that if two surgical wounds are present, the surgeon should attempt to close the medial wound secondarily before the lateral wound.
  - The lateral side of the leg has better soft tissue coverage and consequently is easier to skin graft over if one of the wounds cannot be closed.
- Sometimes, small relaxing incisions around the fasciotomy wound can decrease the tension, enhancing the chance of healing **(TECH FIG 4D)**.

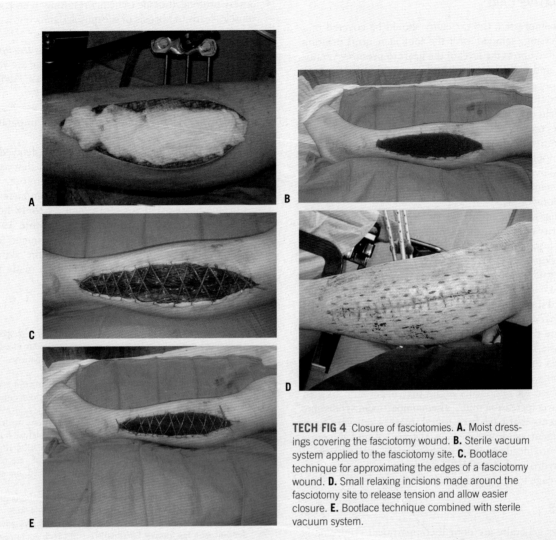

TECH FIG 4 Closure of fasciotomies. **A.** Moist dressings covering the fasciotomy wound. **B.** Sterile vacuum system applied to the fasciotomy site. **C.** Bootlace technique for approximating the edges of a fasciotomy wound. **D.** Small relaxing incisions made around the fasciotomy site to release tension and allow easier closure. **E.** Bootlace technique combined with sterile vacuum system.

TECHNIQUES

Pearls and Pitfalls

Medicolegal Pitfalls	• When in doubt, the surgeon should measure and document pressure in all compartments of the involved extremity. The surgeon should clearly document in the patient's chart that the patient does not have compartment syndrome at this time if the clinical examination findings and pressures are negative.
	  • In 1993, the average litigation award was $280,000 for eight cases of missed compartment syndrome (in all eight cases, no compartment pressures had been measured).[37]
	• The surgeon should consider the possibility of equipment error.
	  • Needles can be misplaced in tendons, fascia, or the wrong compartment. All pressure readings must be interpreted within the context of the clinical presentation.
	• The surgeon should fully release all four compartments along with the soleal leash and posterior tibial fascia.
	• No tight postoperative dressings should be used.
	• Skin can cause increased pressure, so the surgeon should not close acutely.

POSTOPERATIVE CARE

- Once decompressed, the extremity should be covered in a bulky dressing, splinted with the foot in neutral position and elevated above the level of the heart to promote venous drainage and reduce interstitial fluid.
  - The foot should be splinted in neutral position to prevent equinus contracture.
- The patient must be closely monitored for the systemic effects of compartment syndrome. See the discussion in the Nonoperative Management section regarding administration of supplemental oxygen, intravenous hydration, mannitol, and hyperbaric oxygen.
  - Intravenous hydration is important to help prevent rhabdomyolysis.
- The timing of skin closure varies depending on the cause and severity of compartment syndrome.
  - Most fasciotomies can be closed in 5 to 7 days.
  - If the skin is not easily closed secondarily, a split-thickness skin graft is needed to prevent excessive granulation and to lessen exposure of muscle and tendon. A flap might be needed if nerves, vessels, or bone is exposed.
  - If delayed primary closure is planned, a small relaxing incision can be made.
- Hyperbaric oxygen has been used because it reduces tissue edema through oxygen-induced vasoconstriction while maintaining and increasing oxygen perfusion.
  - However, its opponents argue that hyperbaric oxygen leads to reperfusion injury after compartment syndrome.
- Other agents that have been found to affect recovery from compartment syndrome include allopurinol and oxypurinol, superoxide dismutase, deferoxamine, and pentafraction of hydroxyethyl starch. These agents are antioxidants that scavenge for damaging free radicals.

OUTCOMES

- Outcomes generally are poor if compartment syndrome is diagnosed and treated in a delayed fashion. Results are better with earlier treatment.
- In a study by Sheridan and Matsen,[34] 50% of patients underwent decompression within 12 hours and 50% underwent decompression after 12 hours. Sixty-eight percent of the patients who underwent decompression within 12 hours had normal leg function, whereas only 8% of the delayed group had normal function.
- If untreated, Volkmann ischemic contractures develop, leading to claw toes, weak dorsiflexors, sensory loss, chronic pain, and, eventually, amputation.
- ACS results in hospital stays that are increased threefold and hospital charges that are more than doubled. It is important in this day and age to avoid unnecessary fasciotomies.[32]

COMPLICATIONS

- Most patients (77%) complain of altered sensation within the margins of the wound.[18]
- Forty percent report dry, scaly skin; 33%, pruritus; 30%, discolored skin; 25%, swollen extremity; 26%, tethered scars; 13%, recurrent ulcerations; 13%, muscle herniation; 10%, pain related to the wound; and 7%, tethered tendons.
- Severe prolonged tissue ischemia resulting in necrosis of the muscles leads to fibrosis of the muscles and contracture that can continue over a period of several weeks.
  - This is known as *Volkmann ischemic contracture*.
- The late sequelae of compartment syndrome are weak dorsiflexors, claw toes, sensory loss, chronic pain, and, eventually, amputation.
- Delayed fasciotomy beyond 12 hours is associated with a reported infection rate of 46% and an amputation rate of 21%.[34]
  - The complication rate associated with delayed fasciotomies is also much higher (54%) than that associated with early fasciotomies (4.5%). Therefore, the current recommendation is that if the compartment syndrome has existed for more than 24 to 48 hours and the compartment pressures are not within 30 mm Hg of diastolic pressure, supportive treatment for acute renal failure should be considered, the skin should not be violated, and plans should be made for later reconstruction.

REFERENCES

1. Arbabi S, Brundage SI, Gentilello LM. Near-infrared spectroscopy: a potential method for continuous, transcutaneous monitoring for compartmental syndrome in critically injured patients. J Trauma 1999;47:829–833.
2. Bae DS, Kadiyala RK, Waters PM. Acute compartment syndrome in children: contemporary diagnosis, treatment, and outcome. J Pediatr Orthop 2001;21:680–688.
3. Barei DP, Nork SE, Mills WJ, et al. Complications associated with internal fixation of high-energy bicondylar tibial plateau fractures utilizing a two-incision technique. J Orthop Trauma 2004;18:649–657.
4. Bernot M, Gupta R, Dobrasz J, et al. The effect of antecedent ischemia on the tolerance of skeletal muscle to increased interstitial pressure. J Orthop Trauma 1996;10:555–559.
5. Bhattacharyya T, Vrahas MS. The medical-legal aspects of compartment syndrome. J Bone Joint Surg Am 2004;86:864–868.
6. Bible JE, McClure DJ, Mir HR. Analysis of single-incision versus dual-incision fasciotomy for tibial fractures with acute compartment syndrome. J Orthop Trauma 2013;27:607–611.
7. Blick SS, Brumback RJ, Poka A, et al. Compartment syndrome in open tibial fractures. J Bone Joint Surg Am 1986;68:1348–1353.
8. Dunwoody JM, Reichert CC, Brown KL. Compartment syndrome associated with bupivacaine and fentanyl epidural analgesia in pediatric orthopaedics. J Pediatr Orthop 1997;17:285–288.
9. Egol KA, Tejwani NC, Capla EL, et al. Staged management of high-energy proximal tibia fractures (OTA types 41): the results of a prospective, standardized protocol. J Orthop Trauma 2005;19:448–455.
10. Hargens AR, Romine JS, Sipe JC, et al. Peripheral nerve-conduction block by high muscle-compartment pressure. J Bone Joint Surg Am 1979;61:192–200.
11. Hargens AR, Schmidt DA, Evans KL, et al. Quantitation of skeletal-muscle necrosis in a model compartment syndrome. J Bone Joint Surg Am 1981;63:631–636.
12. Heppenstall RB, McCombs PR, DeLaurentis DA. Vascular injuries and compartment syndromes. In: Bucholz RW, Heckman JD, eds. Rockwood and Green's Fractures in Adults, vol 1, ed 5. Philadelphia: Lippincott Williams & Wilkins, 2001:331–352.
13. Heppenstall RB, Scott R, Sapega A, et al. A comparative study of the tolerance of skeletal muscle to ischemia. Tourniquet application compared with acute compartment syndrome. J Bone Joint Surg Am 1986;68:820–828.
14. Jennische E. Ischaemia-induced injury in glycogen-depleted skeletal muscle. Selective vulnerability of FG-fibres. Acta Physiol Scand 1985;125:727–734.

15. Kakar S, Firoozabadi R, McKean J, et al. Diastolic blood pressure in patients with tibia fractures under anaesthesia: implications for the diagnosis of compartment syndrome. J Orthop Trauma 2007;21:99–103.
16. Kelly RP, Whitesides TE Jr. Transfibular route for fasciotomy of the leg. J Bone Joint Surg Am 1967;49:1022–1023.
17. Lindsay TF, Liauw S, Romaschin AD, et al. The effect of ischemia/reperfusion on adenine nucleotide metabolism and xanthine oxidase production in skeletal muscle. J Vasc Surg 1990;12:8–15.
18. McQueen MM, Christie J, Court-Brown CM. Acute compartment syndrome in tibial diaphyseal fractures. J Bone Joint Surg Br 1996;78:95–98.
19. McQueen MM, Gaston P, Court-Brown CM. Acute compartment syndrome. Who is at risk? J Bone Joint Surg Br 2000;82:200–203.
20. Meskey T, Hardcastle J, O'Toole RV. Are certain fractures at increased risk for compartment syndrome after civilian ballistic injury? J Trauma 2011;71:1385–1389.
21. Moed BR, Thorderson PK. Measurement of intracompartmental pressure: a comparison of the slit catheter, side-ported needle, and simple needle. J Bone Joint Surg Am 1993;75:231–235.
22. Morrow BC, Mawhinney IN, Elliott JR. Tibial compartment syndrome complicating closed femoral nailing: diagnosis delayed by an epidural analgesic technique—case report. J Trauma 1994;37:867–868.
23. Mubarak SJ, Wilton NC. Compartment syndromes and epidural analgesia. J Pediatr Orthop 1997;17:282–284.
24. Olson SA, Glasgow RR. Acute compartment syndrome in lower extremity musculoskeletal trauma. J Am Acad Orthop Surg 2005;13:436–444.
25. O'Toole RV, Whitney A, Merchant N, et al. Variation in diagnosis of compartment syndrome by surgeons treating tibial shaft fractures. J Trauma 2009;67:735–741.
26. Park S, Ahn J, Gee AO, et al. Compartment syndrome in tibial fractures. J Orthop Trauma 2009;23:514–518.
27. Prayson MJ, Chen JL, Hampers D, et al. Baseline compartment pressure measurements in isolated lower extremity fractures without clinical compartment syndrome. J Trauma 2006;60:1037–1040.
28. Reisman WM, Shuler MS, Kinsey TL, et al. Relationship between near infrared spectroscopy and intra-compartmental pressures. J Emerg Med 2013;44:292–298.
29. Rorabeck CH. The treatment of compartment syndromes of the leg. J Bone Joint Surg Br 1984;66:93–97.
30. Rorabeck CH, Clarke KM. The pathophysiology of the anterior tibial compartment syndrome: an experimental investigation. J Trauma 1978;18:299–304.
31. Rorabeck CH, Macnab L. Anterior tibial-compartment syndrome complicating fractures of the shaft of the tibia. J Bone Joint Surg Am 1976;58:549–550.
32. Schmidt AH. The impact of compartment syndrome on hospital length of stay and charges among adult patients admitted with a fracture of the tibia. J Orthop Trauma 2011;25:355–357.
33. Shah SN, Karunakar MA. Early wound complications after operative treatment of high energy tibial plateau fractures through two incisions. Bull NYU Hosp Jt Dis 2007;65:115–119.
34. Sheridan GW, Matsen FA III. Fasciotomy in the treatment of the acute compartment syndrome. J Bone Joint Surg Am 1976;58:112–115.
35. Shuler FD, Dietz MJ. Physicians' ability to manually detect isolated elevations in leg intracompartmental pressure. J Bone Joint Surg Am 2010;92:361–367.
36. Stark E, Stucken C, Trainer G, et al. Compartment syndrome in Schatzker type VI plateau fractures and medial condylar fracture-dislocations treated with temporary external fixation. J Orthop Trauma 2009;23:502–506.
37. Templeman D, Varecka T, Schmidt R. Economic costs of missed compartment syndromes. Paper presented at: Annual Meeting of the American Academy of Orthopaedic Surgeons; February 1993; San Francisco, CA.
38. Ulmer T. The clinical diagnosis of compartment syndrome of the lower leg: are clinical findings predictive of the disorder? J Orthop Trauma 2002;16:572–577.
39. Valdez C, Schroeder E, Amdur R, et al. Serum creatine kinase levels are associated with extremity compartment syndrome. J Trauma Acute Care Surg 2013;74:441–445.
40. Whitesides TE, Heckman MM. Acute compartment syndrome: update on diagnosis and treatment. J Am Acad Orthop Surg 1996;4:209–218.
41. Whitney A, O'Toole RV, Hui E, et al. Do one-time intracompartmental pressure measurements have a high false-positive rate in diagnosing compartment syndrome? J Trauma Acute Care Surg 2014;76(2):479–483.
42. Wiger P, Blomqvist G, Styf J. Wound closure by dermatotraction after fasciotomy for acute compartment syndrome. Scand J Plast Reconstr Surg Hand Surg 2000;34:315–320.
43. Wind TC, Saunders SM, Barfield WR, et al. Compartment syndrome after low-energy tibia fractures sustained during athletic competition. J Orthop Trauma 2012;26:33–36.

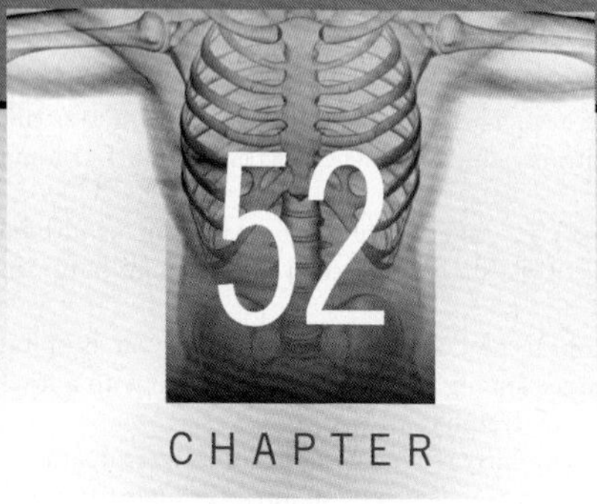

CHAPTER 52

Above-Knee (Transfemoral) Amputation

Israel Dudkiewicz and Jacob Bickels

BACKGROUND

- Limb sparing is feasible in most bone and soft tissue sarcomas of the femur and thigh. Some tumors may, however, be associated with extensive bone destruction, extensive soft tissue contamination, and neurovascular involvement, at which point they will require an above-knee amputation (AKA) **(FIG 1)**.
- An AKA is a transfemoral amputation of the lower extremity that is classified by the height of the femoral osteotomy: high (just below the lesser trochanter), standard or midfemur (diaphyseal), or low distal femur (supracondylar) **(FIG 2)**.
- The margins of resection of the underlying tumor dictate the amputation height, but optimal function will be achieved if at least 50% of the femoral length can be spared.

ANATOMY

- The major anatomic structures that require identification and manipulation are the femoral vessels and sciatic and femoral nerves.
  - The key muscle groups are transected and reconstructed to cover the femoral stump and to allow function.
- High AKA
  - Proximally, the femoral artery lies beneath the sartorius muscle, anterior to the adductor longus muscle and anterior to the femur.
  - The profunda femoris artery lies posterior to the adductor longus muscle, and the femoral artery is lateral to the femoral vein at this level.
  - The sciatic nerve lies posterior to the adductor magnus and anterior to the long head of the biceps.

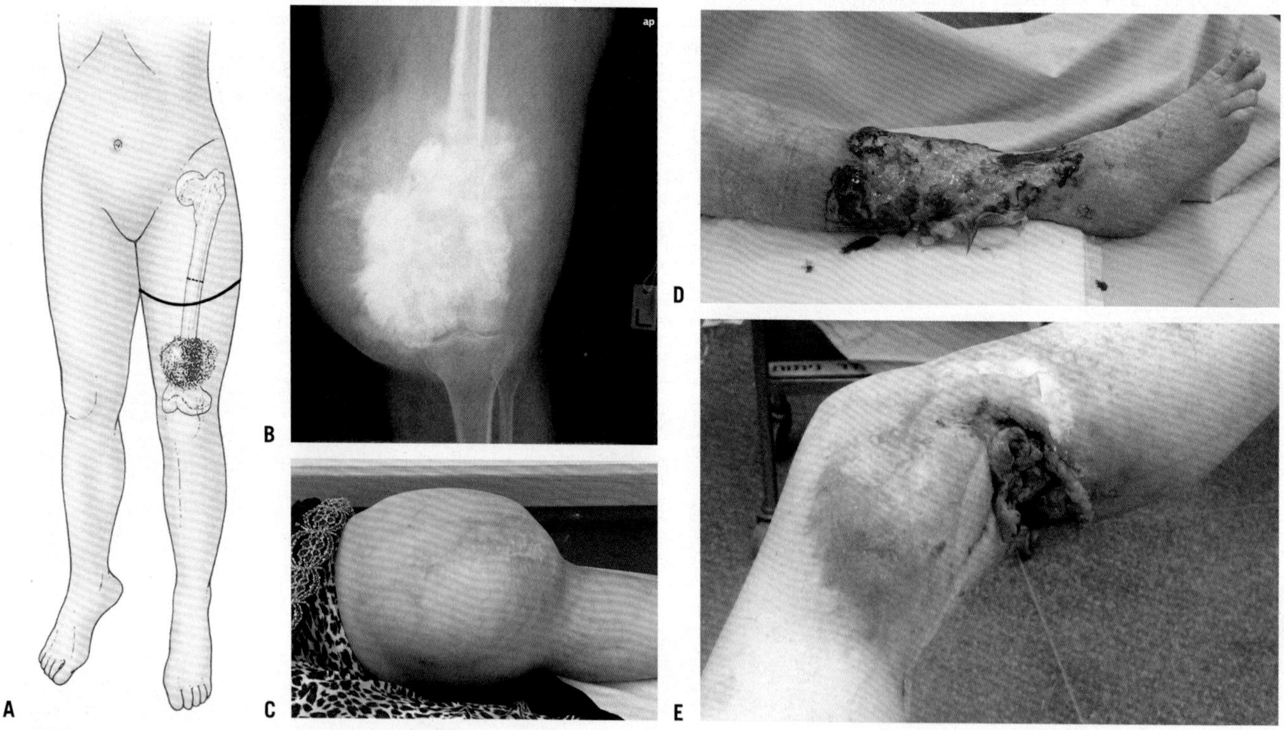

FIG 1 **A.** Primary bone sarcoma of the distal femur. Plain radiograph (**B**) and clinical photograph (**C**) showing an extensive osteosarcoma of the distal femur with massive bone destruction and soft tissue extension. **D.** Locally disseminated, fungating high-grade soft tissue sarcoma of the leg. **E.** Fungating squamous cell carcinoma of the popliteal fossa.

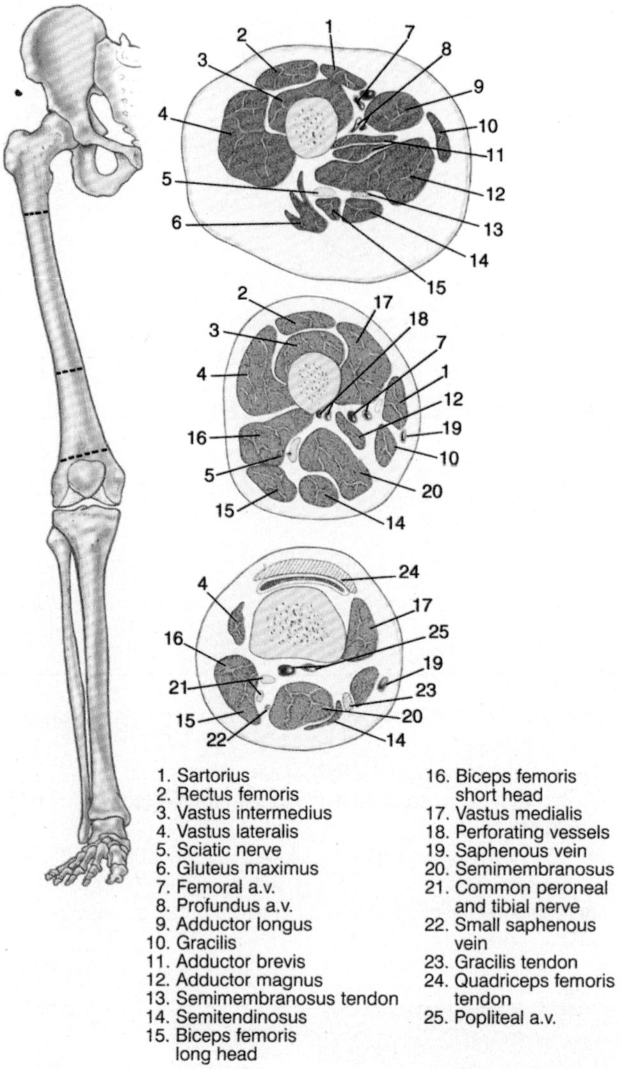

FIG 2 Level of osteotomy and cross-sectional anatomy of supracondylar, mid femur, and high AKA.

- Midfemur AKA
  - The femoral artery lies between the vastus medialis and the adductor magnus and is medial to the femur in the mid thigh area.
  - The femoral vein is lateral to the artery in this region.
  - The sciatic nerve lies between the short head of the biceps and the semimembranosus muscle.
- Supracondylar AKA
  - The femoral artery is directly posterior to the femur. After passing the canal of Hunter, the femoral artery joins the sciatic nerve in the popliteal fossa. The artery is deep and medial to the sciatic nerve.

INDICATIONS

- An AKA is carried out for a primary or locally recurrent tumor where limb salvage would not effectively remove the disease or yield a functional limb because of:
  - Extensive soft tissue involvement that precludes adequate prosthetic coverage **(FIG 3A)**
  - Vascular involvement with invasion of the major blood vessels **(FIG 3B)**
  - Tumors of the distal lower extremity with major nerve involvement, such as tumors of the popliteal space
  - Infection, particularly in the case of tumor ulceration, which prevents limb-sparing resection, or persistent periprosthetic infections.
  - Skeletal immaturity, which often leads to significant limb-length discrepancies when limb-sparing procedures are done on skeletally immature patients.

IMAGING AND OTHER STAGING STUDIES

- Plain radiographs often provide the initial estimation of the extent of tumoral mass and establish the necessity to perform an amputation and its level.
- Computed tomography and magnetic resonance imaging (MRI) studies provide an accurate determination of osseous, intramedullary, and soft tissue involvement.
  - MRIs of the entire femur and thigh are mandatory to rule out the presence of skip metastases and neurovascular involvement and thereby determine the level of amputation.
  - MRI angiography demonstrates the vascular anatomy of the affected limb and defines the extent of vascular involvement.

SURGICAL MANAGEMENT

Preoperative Planning

- When AKAs are done for oncologic indications, the extent of tumor involvement ultimately determines the level of amputation. Beyond that consideration, retaining as much length as possible will facilitate prosthetic fitting.
- When planning the types of flaps that will be used for the amputation, the surgeon should consider the extent of the soft

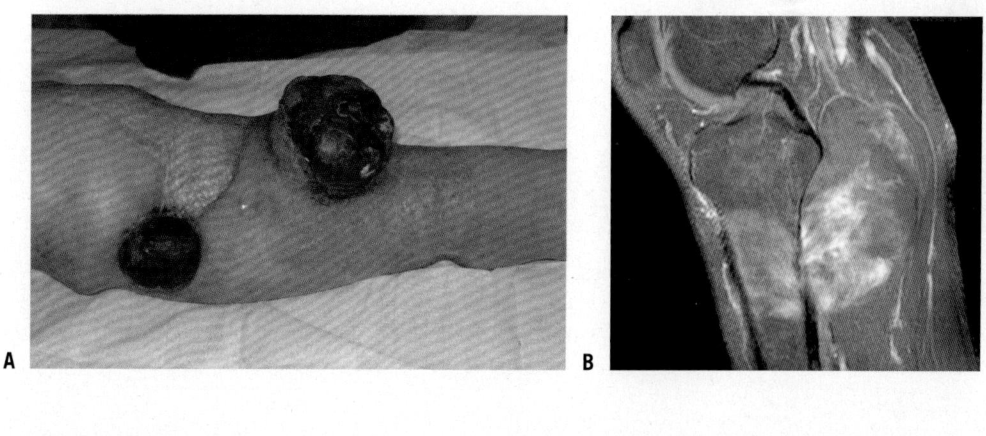

FIG 3 A. Multicentric recurrent soft tissue sarcoma of the leg. **B.** Sagittal MRI view showing synovial sarcoma of the popliteal fossa occupying the neurovascular bundle and extending into the proximal tibia.

tissue component of the tumor, the external skin quality, any prior radiation fields, and the presence of previous incisions.
- The most common type of flap is the anterior and posterior fish-mouth flap. However, the types of flaps may vary depending on the extent of the distal femoral tumor, which may preclude the classical fish-mouth incision.
- Preoperatively, patients should be evaluated by a physical medicine and rehabilitation team together with the assigned prosthetist in order to manage expectations, answer specific questions regarding daily activities and function, and lower the level of anxiety.

Positioning

- Patients are placed supine on the operating table with the operative extremity in flexion and abduction.
- The ipsilateral gluteus should be slightly elevated to allow better access to the posterior thigh **(FIG 4)**.

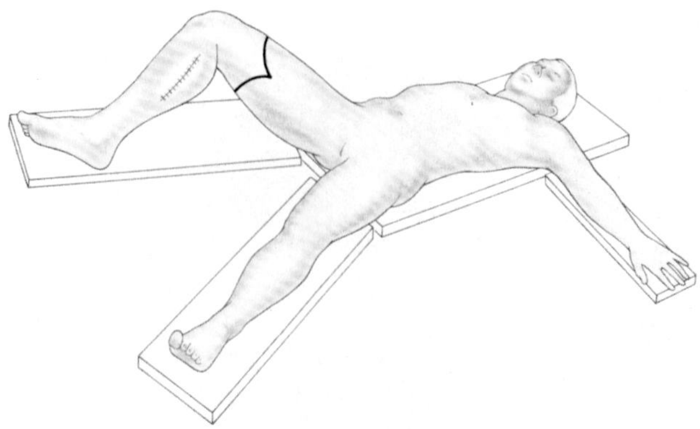

FIG 4 The patient is supine. The operated extremity is in flexion and abduction.

TECHNIQUES

DISSECTION

- The incision is marked on the skin **(TECH FIG 1A,B)**, and the cut is done vertically through the skin edges, subcutaneous tissue, and superficial fascia.
- The major muscles should be carefully transected by means of electrocautery in order to reduce bleeding and marked for later use in soft tissue reconstruction **(TECH FIG 1C,D)**.
  - The level of the amputation will determine which muscles will be transected, but portions of the quadriceps, hamstrings, and adductors are cut at almost all levels.
- The deep femoral artery and vein are dissected, suture ligated, and transected.
- Nerves should be pulled gently to a length of about 2 cm, ligated with nonabsorbable sutures, and transected with a knife **(TECH FIG 1E)**.
  - The nerves should then be allowed to retract back to the muscle mass.
- An epineural injection of bupivacaine 0.5% can be considered.

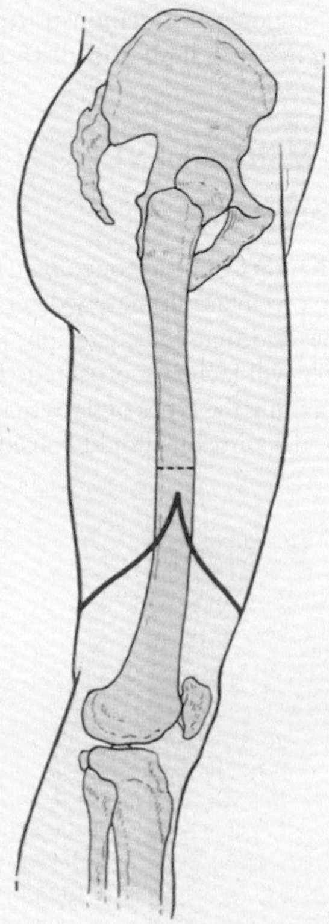

A

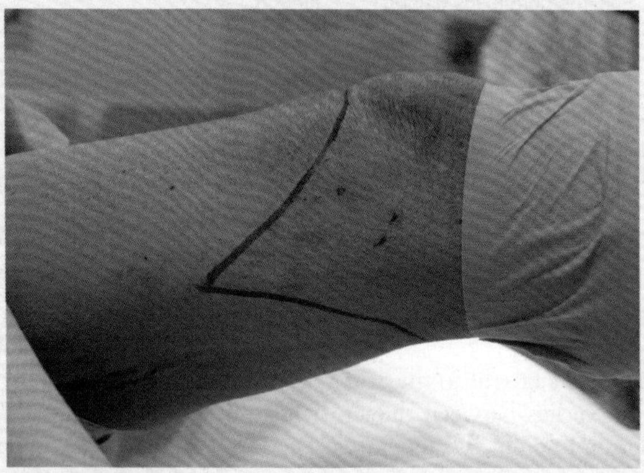

B

TECH FIG 1 **A,B.** The planned fish-mouth incision line. *(continued)*

C

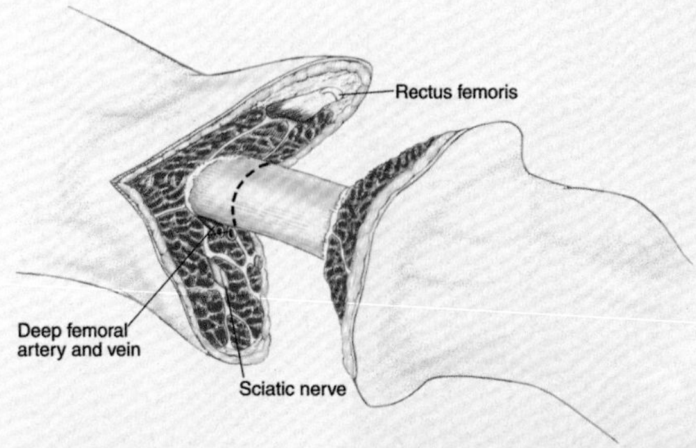

D

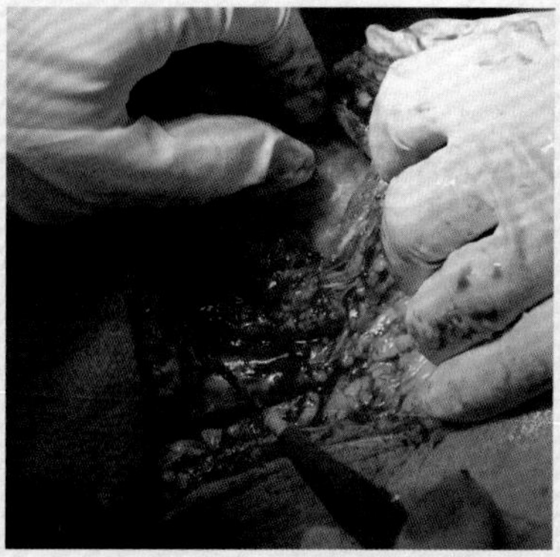

E

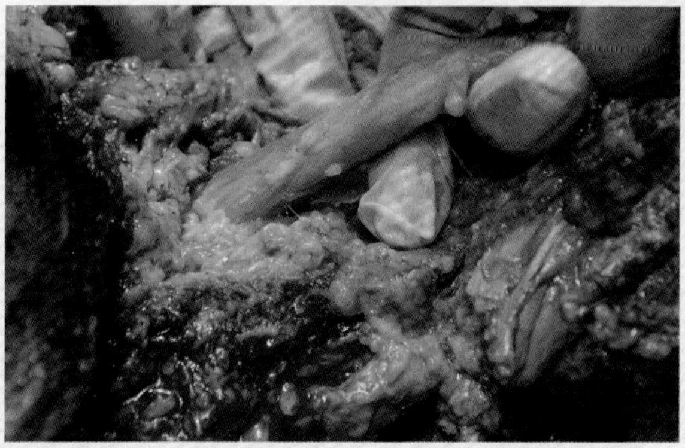

TECH FIG 1 *(continued)* **C,D.** The incision through the skin, superficial fascia, and subcutaneous tissue vertical to the skin edges. Muscles are beveled in their transection down to bone by means of electrocautery. **E.** The sciatic nerve prior to its ligation and dissection.

AMPUTATION AND STUMP MANAGEMENT

- The bone is cut with an oscillating or Gigli saw. A retractor placed around the femur can prevent damage to the soft tissue and flaps **(TECH FIG 2A)**.
- A frozen section from the remaining intramedullary canal should be done if the margins of resection are questionable with regard to being tumor free.
- The femoral edge is beveled with a saw or rasp in order to smooth the remaining edge and to leave a less prominent point of contact for the prosthesis **(TECH FIG 2B,C)**.
- Gelfoam or bone wax is placed in the distal femoral stump canal to prevent large hematomas from occurring as a result of continuous intraosseous bleeding after surgery (this is more common in children and young adults).
- Excess muscle and fat tissue should be removed to allow the desired conical shape of the stump.
- To balance the orientation of the femoral stump and preserve muscle function and strength, drill holes can be made in the femur to tenodese the overlying muscles.
    - Alternatively, a purse-string suture of the overlying muscle may be used.

A

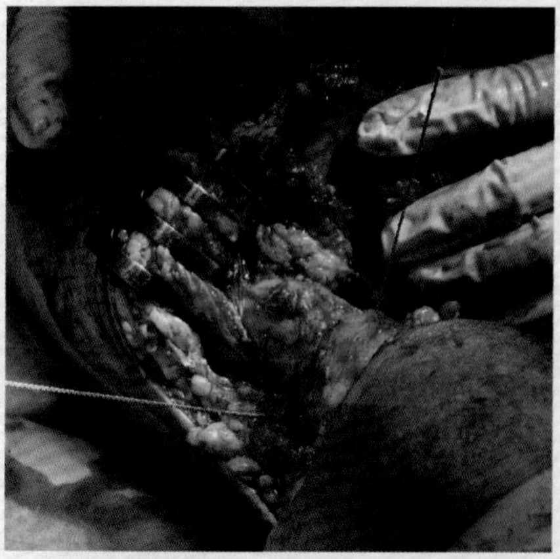

TECH FIG 2 **A.** The femur is cut with a Gigli saw. A retractor is placed anteriorly to prevent damage to the adjacent soft tissues. *(continued)*

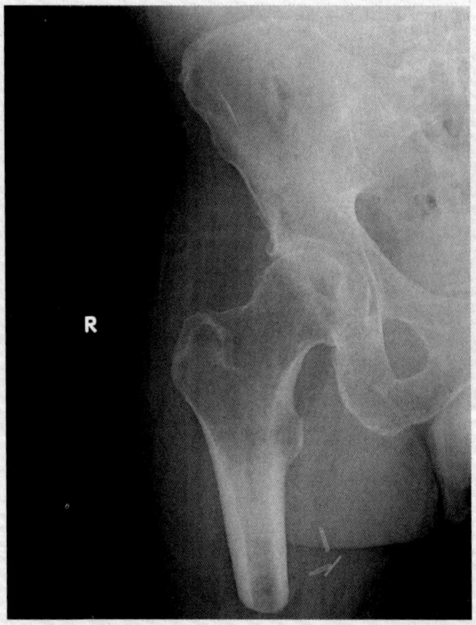

B

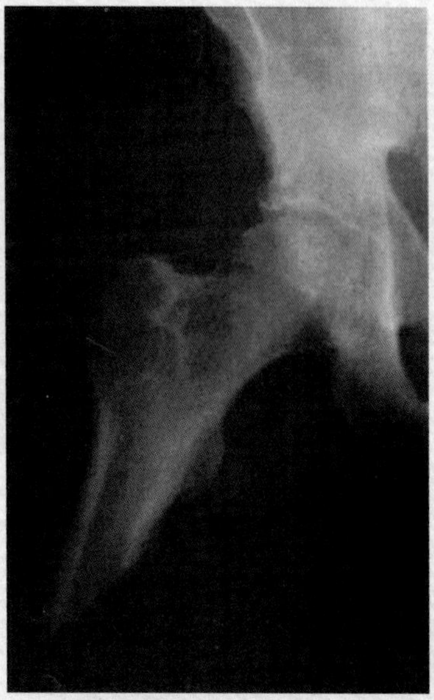

C

TECH FIG 2 *(continued)* Postoperative radiographs showing appropriate smooth edges of the femoral stump (**B**), and an inappropriate sharp edge (**C**), which can become extremely painful, especially when pressure from a prosthetic socket is applied.

COMPLETION

- Meticulous hemostasis may prevent the need for drain placement.
- The superficial fascia should be tightly closed **(TECH FIG 3A)**.
- While closing the skin edges, the surgeon should take care to avoid leaving residual excess tissue and large skin folds, both of which can later interfere with optimal prosthetic fitting.
- When required, a single drain is positioned as distally as possible and preferably on the lateral aspect of the stump **(TECH FIG 3B)**.
  - The drain should be removed as soon as possible to decrease the risk of infection.
- A rigid dressing should be applied at the completion of the amputation to reduce swelling and prevent the development of a flexion contracture **(TECH FIG 3C)**.

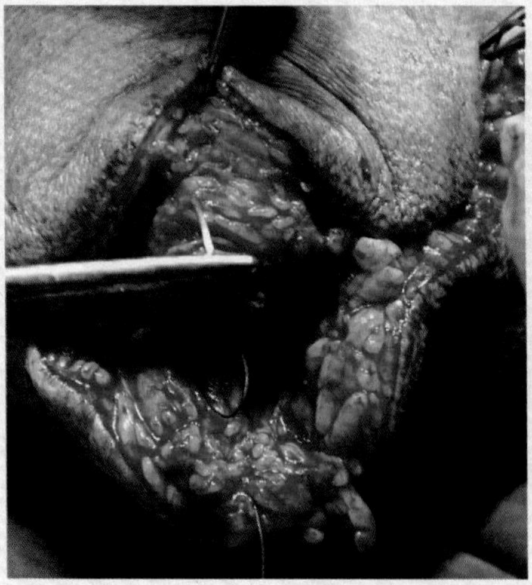

A

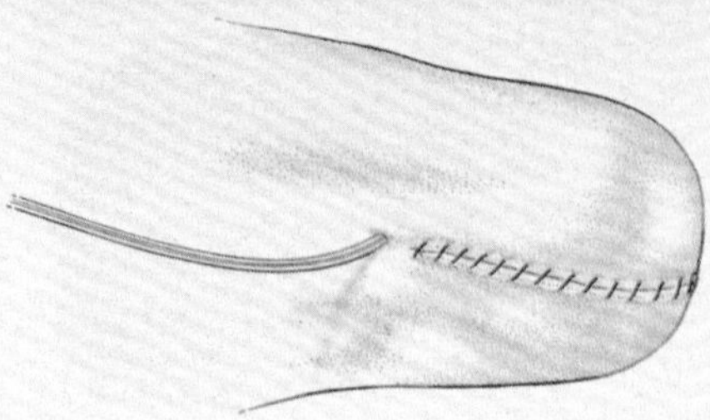

B

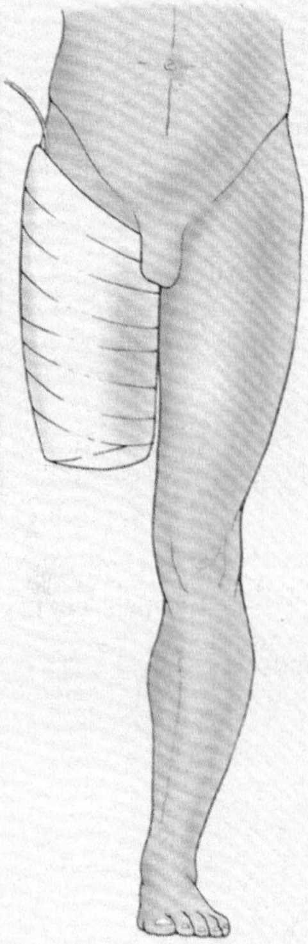

C

TECH FIG 3 A. The superficial fascia is tightly sutured. Skin folds should be avoided. **B.** A closed suction drain is positioned at the lateral aspect of the incision. **C.** Application of a rigid dressing.

Pearls and Pitfalls

Postoperative Flexion	• Flexion contractures can be prevented with the use of proximal casting or immobilization at the groin level, with the stump suspended in place with a belt, if necessary.
Adductor Myodesis	• After AKA, the iliopsoas and hip abductors can cause the stump to go into flexion and abduction. Tenodesing the adductor magnus prevents this deformity and helps prevent the loss of hip adduction power, which has been estimated to be up to 70% less without myodesis. Myodesis acts as an insertion site and facilitates muscle contraction and function.
Muscle Balance	• Managing muscle group imbalances through myoplasty also improves the function of the amputee. Because the hip flexors are stronger than the extensors, the hamstrings should be cut longer than the quadriceps and be attached to one another.
Neuroma	• Nerves should be cut with a blade as proximally as possible and buried within muscular tissue, and bupivacaine 0.5% should be injected to control postoperative pain.
Phantom Pain	• It is important to identify and diagnose pain type and origin early and manage it aggressively.
Skin Pressure from Bone Edges	• The distal anterior cortical edge of the femur should be beveled to prevent pressure arising from bone edges, particularly with prosthetic use.

POSTOPERATIVE CARE

- A compressive dressing applied to the stump site reduces postoperative swelling at the stump site.
- Proximal extension of the postoperative immobilizer or splint, prone positioning, and physical therapy help to prevent flexion contracture.
- Fitting for an initial or temporary prosthesis soon after wound healing and swelling resolution is most often associated with increased compliance with prosthetic use.
- Because the energy requirements of AKAs are about 60% to 100% greater than that required for nonamputees, many amputees require the use of assistive devices for ambulation.
- Phantom limb pain and sensations can diminish over time.
  - However, when phantom pain persists, physical and occupational therapies, narcotics, and drugs with effects on nerves, such as gabapentin (Neurontin), may be helpful.

OUTCOMES

- Through effective multidisciplinary care, most patients are able to ambulate and return to normal daily activities, including driving. Some are also able to participate in sporting activities.
- Outcome studies that compare patients treated with amputations versus those treated with limb salvage procedures found that AKA amputees were more limited in their mobility and community activities compared to those with limb salvage, but they reported less muscle weakness.
- Assessments by numerous psychological measures have demonstrated that AKA amputees generally have approximately the same overall quality of life compared to patients who undergo limb-sparing surgery.

COMPLICATIONS

- Wound-healing problems can arise but are not as common as in amputations performed for vascular or ischemic problems.
  - Wound problems after amputations performed for tumors are most likely due to preoperative host factors, such as comorbidities and nutritional status.
  - Special care should be given in cases when the amputation is carried out in a previously irradiated field.
- Phantom pain or causalgia syndromes may occur and are difficult to predict, and it should be borne in mind that patients with significant preoperative pain complain of postoperative pain more often.
  - It is important to identify and diagnose these painful syndromes early and manage them aggressively.

SUGGESTED READINGS

Duzcu S, Ilaslan H, Joyce MJ, et al. Stump neuroma. Orthopedics 2015;38(12):720, 769–770.

Furtado S, Grimer RJ, Cool P, et al. Physical functioning, pain and quality of life after amputation for musculoskeletal tumors: a national survey. Bone Joint J 2015;97-B(9):1284–1290.

Renard AJ, Veth RP, Schreuder HW, et al. Function and complications after ablative and limb-salvage therapy in lower extremity sarcoma of bone. J Surg Oncol 2000;73(4):198–205.

CHAPTER 53

Below-Knee Amputation

Israel Dudkiewicz and Jacob Bickels

BACKGROUND

- Bone and soft tissue tumors of the distal leg, ankle, and foot may require a below-knee amputation (BKA) to achieve wide margins of resection.
- A limb-salvage attempt in these cases may not be possible or may result in a dysfunctional extremity due to a massive loss of muscles and neurovascular elements.
- Advances in prosthetic design and engineering have enabled BKA amputees to be very active in a variety of activities, often more active than patients who have had limb-sparing procedures for similar tumors.

INDICATIONS

- Primary, locally recurrent, or metastatic and infiltrative bone and soft tissue tumors of the leg, calf, ankle, and foot, which are not suitable for limb salvage resection and have not responded to preoperative chemotherapeutic and radiation treatment protocols **(FIG 1)**
- Palliation of intractable pain associated with infiltrative tumors of the leg, calf, ankle, and foot that are not suitable for limb salvage resection

IMAGING AND OTHER STAGING STUDIES

- Magnetic resonance imaging is the imaging modality of choice for evaluating the extents of bone and soft tissue tumor involvement and the relation of the tumor to the neurovascular structures of the lower extremity.
  - These data had traditionally been gained by the combined use of plain radiographs, computed tomography, and angiography.

SURGICAL MANAGEMENT

Preoperative Planning

- The major anatomic structures that require identification and manipulation include the tibial and peroneal neurovascular bundles. Key muscle groups will need to be transected and reconstructed to cover the tibial and fibular stumps and to allow optimal function and future prosthetic fitting.
- The ideal level of surgical resection for a BKA is at the musculocutaneous junction of the gastrocnemius muscle. This provides better soft tissue padding and usually a more reliable blood supply for the posterior flap.
- The recommended length for a BKA stump for optimal prosthetic fitting is between 12.5 and 17.5 cm. However, tumor extent and margin widths will ultimately determine the length of the stump for a given patient.
- Careful flap selection is important in achieving a functional BKA stump. Because of the subcutaneous location of the tibia and sparse musculature of the anterior leg compartment, use of a long posterior flap is preferable to a fish-mouth flap.
- Preoperative referrals to a psychologist and prosthetist are often useful in helping patients prepare for their upcoming life adjustments.

Positioning

- The patient is placed supine on the operating table with the operated extremity slightly elevated.
- The initial approach is made anteriorly in most cases.
- The knee can be flexed and abducted or adducted to gain exposure of its posterior elements.

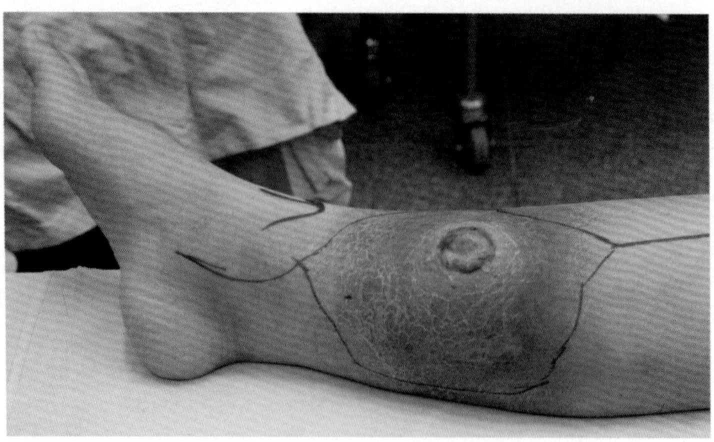

FIG 1 Fungating soft tissue sarcoma of the leg. BKA is required to achieve wide margins of resection.

INCISION AND FLAP SELECTION

- Because of the subcutaneous location of the tibia and the minimal musculature of the anterior leg compartment, a long posterior flap is preferable to the classic fish-mouth flap.
  - The anterior flap is angled backward by approximately 1 cm to prevent skin protuberance (dog-ear flap) upon flap closure **(TECH FIG 1A)**.
  - The junction between the anterior and posterior flaps is at the level of the fibula. Proper adjustment of the surgical flaps is critical for both wound healing and prosthetic fitting.
- The planned surgical incision is marked, and a midline vertical line is drawn along the anterior and posterior flaps to allow their optimal opposition upon wound closure **(TECH FIG 1B)**.
- In the initial incision, flaps of the skin, superficial fascia, and subcutaneous tissue up to the level of the tibia are cut perpendicular to the skin surface.
- The osteotomy line on the tibia is marked with electrocautery **(TECH FIG 1C)**.

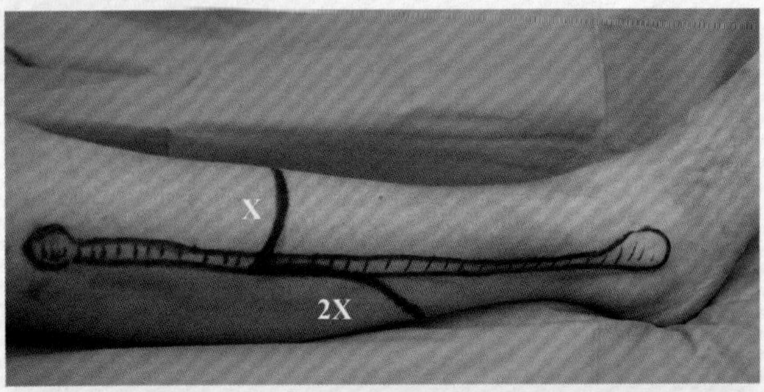

A

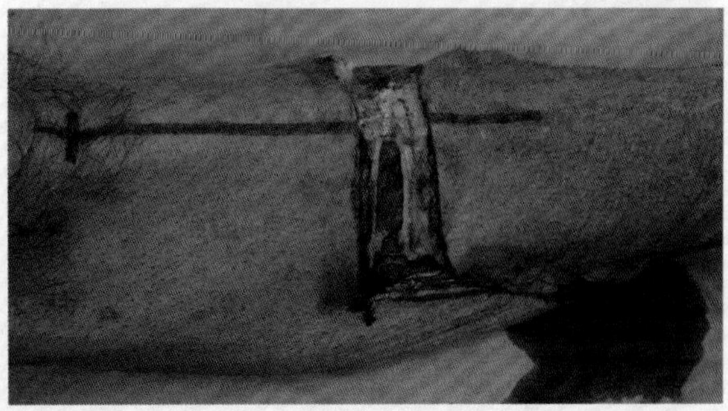

B

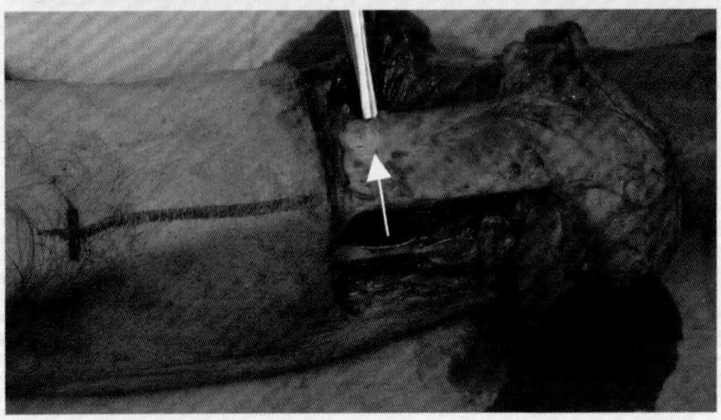

C

TECH FIG 1 **A.** Flap design for BKA includes short anterior and long posterior flaps, joined at the level of the fibular diaphysis. The length of the posterior flap is approximately twice the length the anterior flap, which is angled backward to avoid skin protuberance upon flap closure. **B.** A midline vertical line is made along the anterior and posterior flaps to allow accurate adjustment upon flap closure. Skin, superficial fascia, and subcutaneous tissue cut is perpendicularly done up to the level of the tibia. **C.** The osteotomy line on the tibia is marked with electrocautery (*arrow*).

SOFT TISSUE DISSECTION

- The muscles of the anterior, lateral, and deep compartments of the leg are transected by electrocautery to minimize bleeding **(TECH FIG 2A)**.
  - Vascular structures are ligated and divided. Major blood vessels are suture ligated **(TECH FIG 2B,C)**.
  - The large muscle groups are tapered so that they can be secured over the cut ends of the bone.
- Nerves are meticulously dissected and gently pulled at least 2 cm out of their surrounding muscle mass.
  - They are doubly ligated with monofilament nonabsorbable suture.
- Prior to cutting the nerves, anesthetics are injected locally proximal to the ligation site in order to reduce the risk of neuropathic pain.
- The nerves are cut by a blade and not by scissors or electrocautery because a sharp incision line is traumatic to the nerve tissue and associated with lower risk of neuroma formation.
- The nerve endings are then deeply embedded within muscle tissue as proximally as possible in order to decrease the likelihood of neuroma formation and neuropathic pain. In the event a neuroma is formed, it will be protected from pressure related to the prosthetic socket by the surrounding muscles.

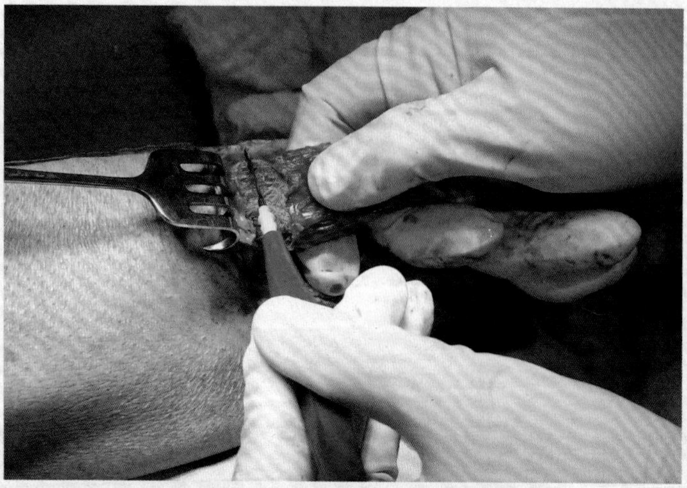

A

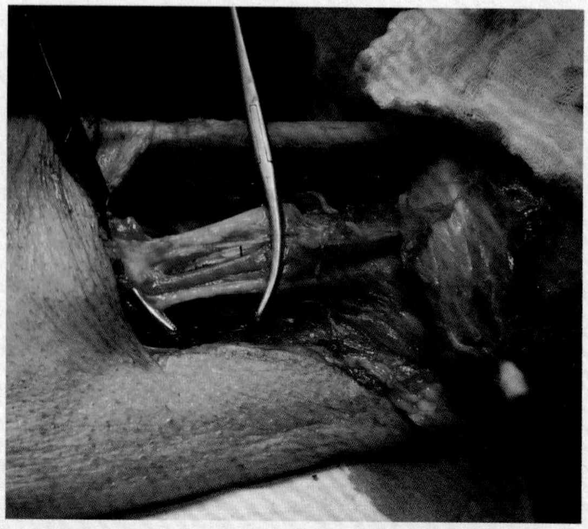

C

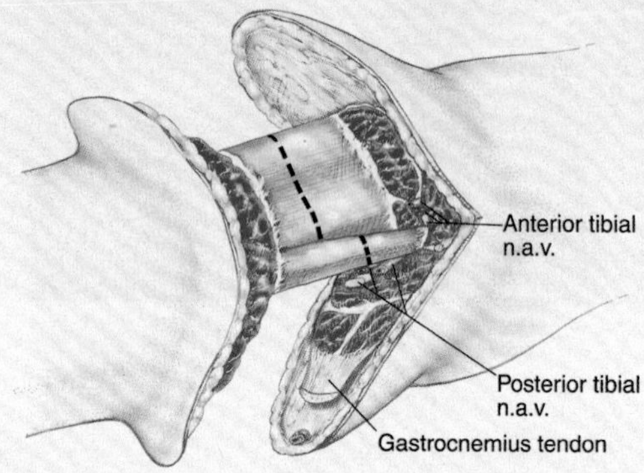

B

TECH FIG 2 **A.** Muscle compartments are transected using electrocautery. **B,C.** Vascular structures are ligated in continuity and divided. Dashed lines represent the levels of osteotomies.

BONE TRANSECTION AND STUMP MANAGEMENT

- The tibia is osteotomized by an oscillating or Gigli saw **(TECH FIG 3A)**.
- The fibula is resected 1 to 2 cm proximal to the tibial osteotomy to create a more tapered stump **(TECH FIG 3B)**.
- The cut edge of the tibia is beveled by means of a saw or a rasp in order to smooth the edges and contour the bone for a better prosthetic fit **(TECH FIG 3C)**.
- Intramedullary content taken from the edge of the stump should be sent for histopathologic evaluation to verify that it is free of tumor.
  - If the amputation is performed for a soft tissue sarcoma, soft tissues from the surgical margins should be assessed in a similar manner.
- The major muscle groups of the posterior flap are attached anteriorly to the stump by means of heavy sutures to cover the bone through drill holes in the distal tibia.
  - The remaining muscle layers are used to make a circumferential covering layer **(TECH FIG 3D)**.

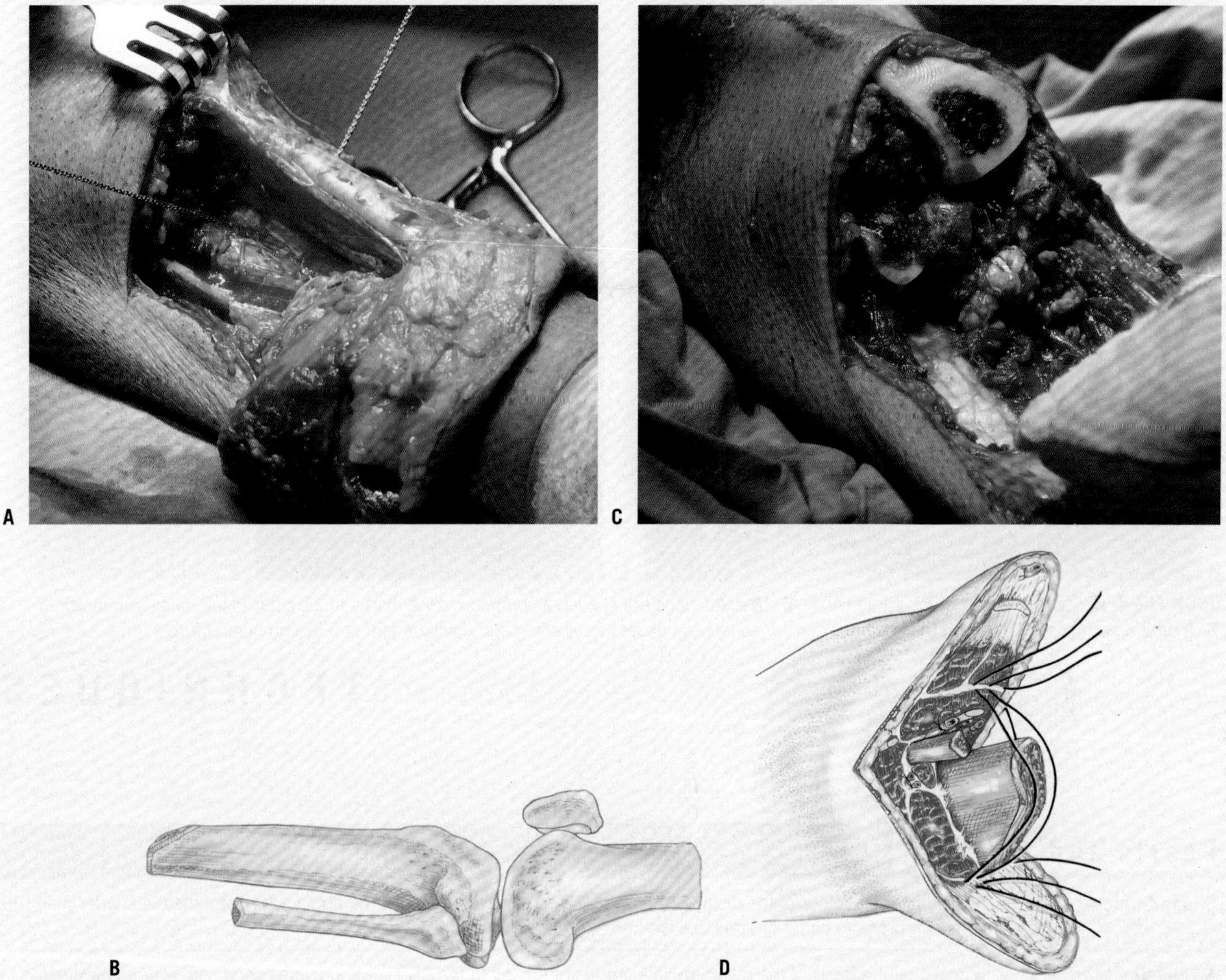

TECH FIG 3 **A.** Tibial osteotomy is done using a Gigli saw. Alternatively, an oscillating saw can be used for this purpose. **B.** The fibula is resected 1 to 2 cm proximal to the tibial osteotomy. **C.** The cut edge of the tibia is beveled using a saw or rasp. **D.** The major muscle groups of the posterior flap are attached anteriorly to the tibia to cover the bony stump using heavy sutures.

COMPLETION

- Prevention of hematoma and seroma development is critical. Although the use of drains is still common practice, meticulous hemostasis and the use of a properly fitted compression dressing may obviate the need for their use.
  - These complications can delay wound healing and, in some cases, delay adjunctive treatments, such as chemotherapy and radiation therapy.
- In most cases, wounds can be closed without suction drains following meticulous hemostasis.
  - If needed, closed suction drains can be placed beneath the fascial layer and brought out of the medial and lateral aspects of the incision.
- The superficial fascia is tightly closed **(TECH FIG 4A)**.
- Skin and subcutaneous tissue should be precisely closed to avoid tension or, alternatively, excess tissue and large skin folds, which may cause wound complications and interfere with optimal prosthetic fitting **(TECH FIG 4B)**.
  - Skin may be closed with either sutures or clips, which have shown equivalent long-term results in terms of wound healing and functional outcome.
- A rigid dressing is applied at the completion of the procedure with the knee in extension to prevent excessive swelling and development of a flexion contracture **(TECH FIG 4C)**.
- After the initial rigid dressing is removed (usually 10 to 14 days after surgery), a stump-shrinker sock can be worn to decrease any remaining swelling.

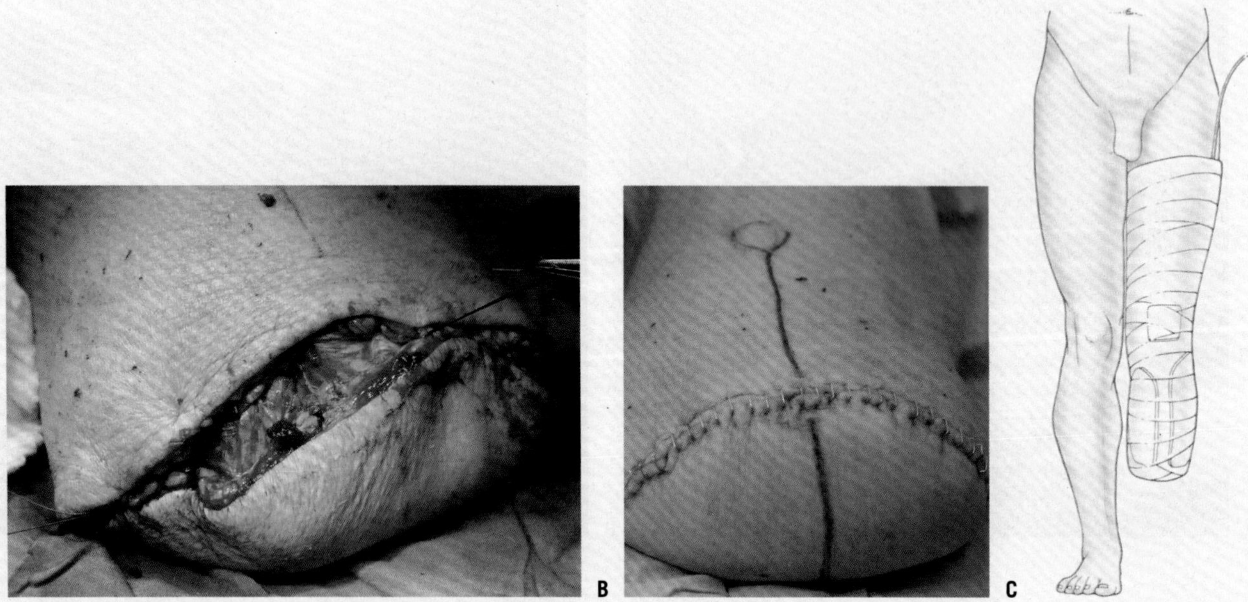

TECH FIG 4 **A.** Superficial fascia is sutured tightly. **B.** Muscles flaps are aligned along the midline marks made prior to the initial skin incision. **C.** A rigid dressing is applied with the knee in extension to prevent excessive swelling and development of a flexion contracture.

Pearls and Pitfalls

Stump Contour	• Rounding the contour of the distal end of the tibial stump and resecting the fibula a few centimeters shorter than the tibia can promote better fit and ease with prosthesis use.
Myodesis	• Functional myodesis of the major muscle groups of the leg to the distal tibia provides good soft tissue coverage for the stump while allowing functional range of motion.
Wound Healing Problems	• Healing can be compromised by preoperative chemotherapy. Attention to detail with wound closures can help avoid these problems as well as hematoma and seroma development, which can delay other adjuvant treatments.
Postoperative Flexion Contracture	• The use of a knee immobilizer or custom splint can prevent the development of a flexion contracture.
Phantom Pain and Causalgia	• Nerves should be cut as proximally as possible and buried within muscular tissue. Bupivacaine 0.5% should be injected to control postoperative pain. It is important to identify and diagnose pain type and origin early and manage it aggressively.

POSTOPERATIVE CARE

- Once the initial postoperative dressing is removed, a stump-shrinker sock can be worn to minimize swelling.
- Patients should be counseled that the transition to prosthesis fitting and use will be slow and gradual and will occur over a period of about 3 to 6 months. Once an initial prosthesis can be fitted, wear time is gradually increased to build tolerance.

OUTCOMES

- Similar to other lower extremity amputations, BKAs have been shown to be effective in palliation and improving the quality of life in cancer patients.
- As might be expected, patients after BKAs report fewer limitations than their above-knee amputation counterparts and are less likely to ambulate with walking aids or a limp.

- The vast improvements in prosthetic design for BKA amputees allow them to be highly functional in terms of mobility. They can participate in almost any recreational activity of their choice without limitations associated with the amputation.

COMPLICATIONS

- Hematoma and seroma development can cause serious wound healing problems that sometimes require additional surgeries. This is a major problem when the amputation has been done for a primary bone or soft tissue sarcoma and adjuvant chemotherapy is needed. Such wound problems can delay the initiation of these important treatments and, ultimately, delay prosthetic fitting as well.

SUGGESTED READINGS

Davis AM, Devlin M, Griffin AM, et al. Functional outcome in amputation versus limb sparing of patients with lower extremity sarcoma: a matched case-control study. Arch Phys Med Rehabil 1999;80:615–618.

Paradasaney PK, Sullivan PE, Portney LG, et al. Advantage of limb salvage over amputation for proximal lower extremity tumors. Clin Orthop Relat Res 2006;444:201–208.

Sugarbaker P, Malawer M. Hip disarticulation. In: Malawer MM, Sugarbaker PH, eds. Musculoskeletal Cancer Surgery: Treatment of Sarcomas and Allied Diseases. Boston: Kluwer, 2001:363–369.

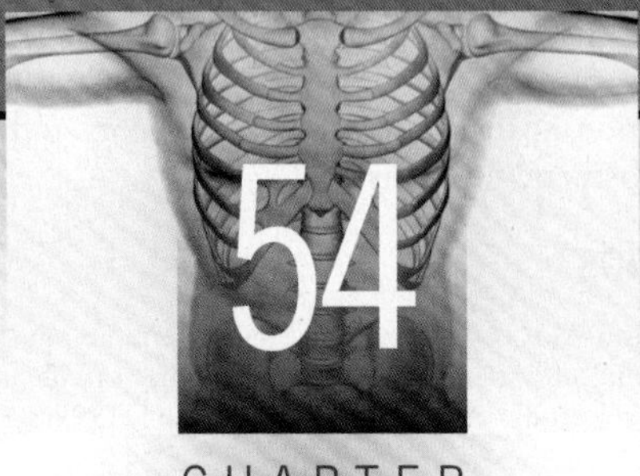

CHAPTER

Foot and Ankle

Open Reduction and Internal Fixation of the Pilon

Hans P. Van Lancker

DEFINITION

- In orthopaedic surgery, the terms *pilon* and *plafond* have been loosely translated and interchangeably used to describe the weight-bearing portion of the distal tibial articular surface.
- These injuries account for approximately 1% of all lower extremity fractures and 5% to 10% of tibial fractures.
- Most orthopaedic surgeons will encounter these injuries during the course of their practice, thus a basic understanding of their characteristics and their management possibilities is important for any practicing orthopaedist exposed to trauma.
- Open reduction with internal fixation (ORIF) remains the basis by which most pilon fractures are definitively stabilized.
- The temporary use of closed reduction and external fixation is an important tool in managing soft tissue tension and decreasing complications in this area prone to difficult coverage options.
- The definitive use of a ring frame fixator remains a useful tool in cases involving considerable soft tissue or bone loss and/or contamination.
- As established by Ruedi and Allgower,[16] the goals of any surgery for pilon fractures should include precise articular reconstruction, restoration of extremity length and alignment, stable fracture fixation, and early joint motion.
- ORIF presents difficulties during the management of pilon fractures as it may further compromise the thin soft tissue envelope surrounding the distal tibia, that is, wound complications and infection.
- Minimally invasive techniques such as percutaneous plating, combination intramedullary nailing and plating and the use of interfragmentary cannulated screws may help to avoid soft tissue injury and reduce infectious complications (see **FIGS 3C,D** and **4E,F**).

ANATOMY

- Pilon fractures involve the weight-bearing articular surface of the distal tibia. In the majority of cases, there is an associated distal fibular fracture and/or syndesmotic injury.
- The talus is predominantly cartilage covered and sits in the ankle mortise beneath the tibial pilon and is restrained medially and laterally by the malleoli.

PATHOGENESIS

- The mechanism of injury for articular fractures of the distal tibia usually involves some degree of axial compression as the dense talus impacts into the tibia's distal articular surface, this can be independent or often combined with a torsional force.
- The distinction between fracture patterns is thus attributed to a number of other associated variables, such as the amount of rotational forced involved, foot (talus) position during loading, bone quality, and energy of impact.
- Highly comminuted articular injuries usually occur due to high-energy axial loading forces, whereas spiral fractures with minimal articular injury are presumed to result from lower energy rotational forces. True bending injuries are seen less commonly and may be caused by low- or high-energy mechanisms.
- Despite the absence of a clear spectrum of injury severity, an estimation of the energy involved in a pilon fracture can be assumed from aspects other than the tibial fracture pattern itself (eg, history, soft tissue injury, associated injuries).
- Open injuries occur in approximately 15% to 40% of pilon fractures, reflecting the severity of the injury and the necessity for aggressive soft tissue management.
- Associated injuries should be carefully investigated as 5% to 10% of pilon fractures are bilateral, 30% have ipsilateral lower extremity injuries, and 15% have injuries to the spine, pelvis, or upper extremities.
- Although a number of injury combinations is possible in the distal tibia, characteristic patterns can often be identified. Understanding the pattern of injury is critical to formulating an optimal treatment plan.
- Lower energy metaphyseal or diaphyseal involvement of the tibia is typically spiral in nature with a cortical spike that can guide the reduction.
- Metaphyseal comminution just above the articular pilon is resultant of high-energy axial loading, as the talus impacts into the corresponding weight-bearing surface of the tibia. In such injuries, the anterior plafond is often comminuted and impacted into the adjacent metaphysis.
- The Orthopaedic Trauma Association's (OTA) Committee for Coding and Classification has developed its alphanumeric system[7] from the Arbeitsgemeinschaft für Osteosynthesefragen–Association for the Study of Internal Fixation (AO/AOF). This alphanumeric system is popular among fracture surgeons and is used in most current reports of fracture treatment.
- Distal tibial fractures are designated as types 43-A, 43-B, and 43-C, with further subgrouping based on specific fracture characteristics (**FIG 1**).
  - The three major types—A (extra-articular), B (partial articular), and C (intra-articular extension with complete separation between the articular fracture fragments and the tibial shaft)—are further divided into subgroups based on the amount of fracture comminution, articular depression, and overall displacement.

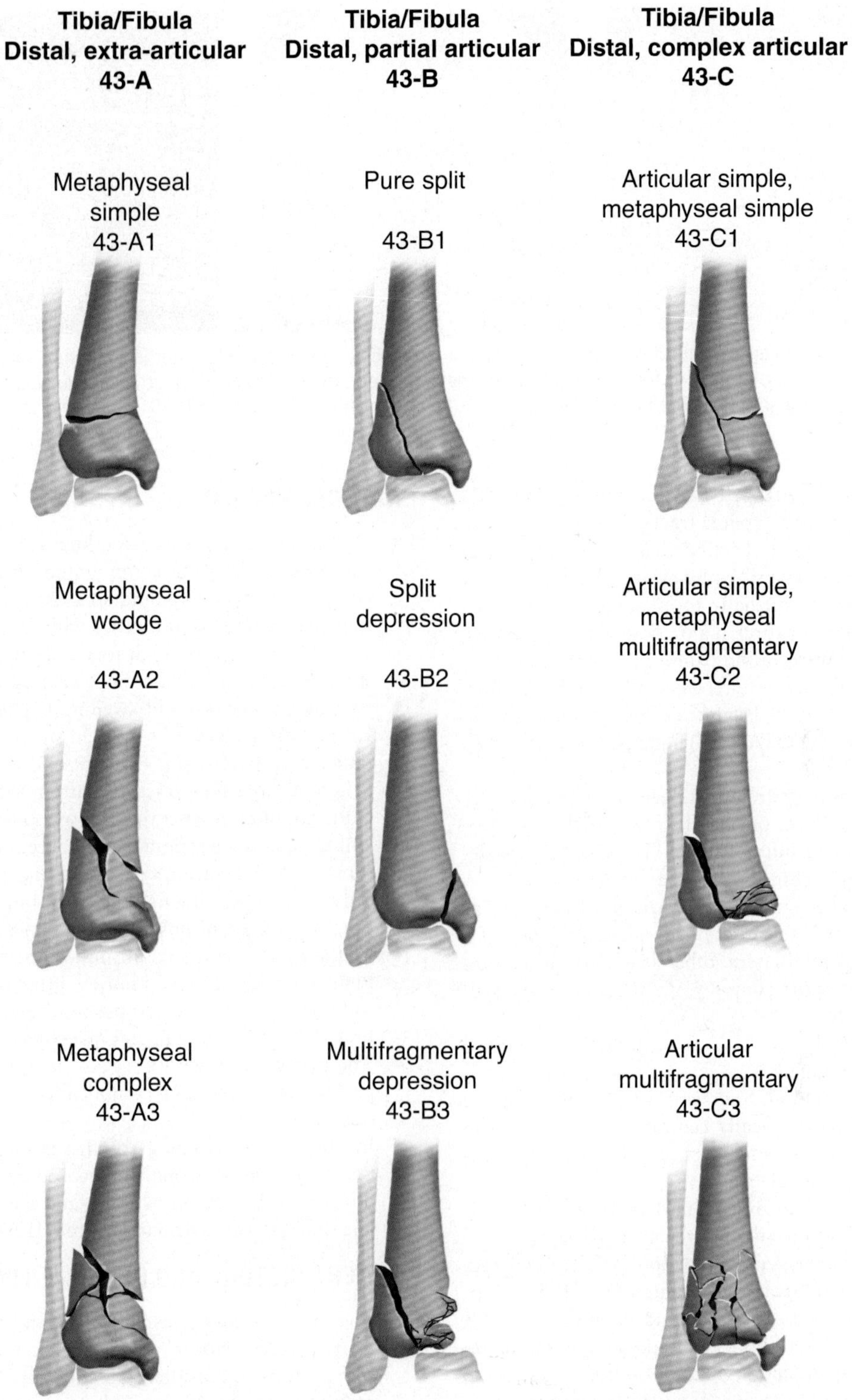

FIG 1 The OTA's alphanumeric classification of distal tibia fractures (OTA 43) are grouped into types 43-A (extra-articular), 43-B (partial articular), and 43-C (complete articular). Each type is subgrouped based on specific fracture characteristics.

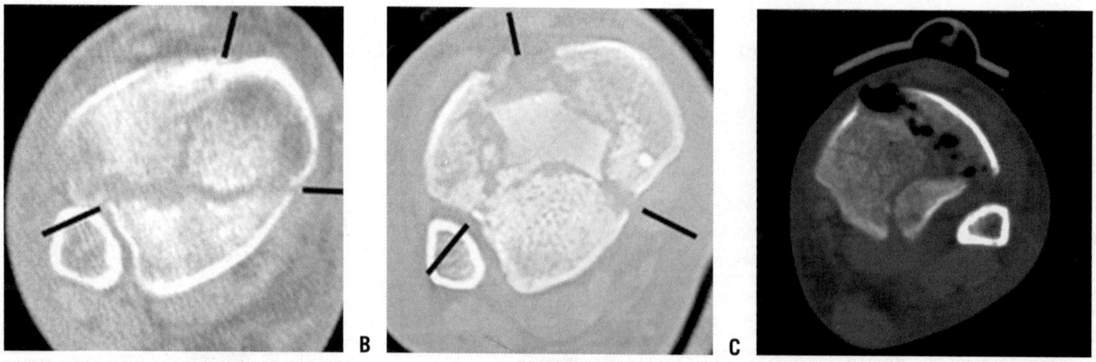

FIG 2 A–C. CT images from 43-C3 plafond injuries demonstrating typical fracture patterns with anterolateral, medial malleolus, and posteromedial fragments. Variable amounts of central or anterocentral articular impaction and comminution are commonly seen. Take notice of the air apparent in the CT image of **FIG 2C**, suggesting this is an open fracture injury.

- Cole and associates[5] mapped 38 consecutive AO/OTA 43-C3 (complex articular) pilon fractures with computed tomography (CT) scans and found that all pilon fractures in this category exited the tibiofibular joint laterally and at two separate locations medially to create a coronally oriented "Y" pattern with three major fragments **(FIG 2A–C)**. Additionally, there were varying amounts of articular comminution anterolaterally or anteromedially (see **FIG 2B,C**).
- The three "major" pilon fragments seen in comminuted complete articular (AO/OTA 43-C) injuries can be described as follows:
  - First, a posterior pilon fragment develops with a fracture line exiting 1 to 4 cm proximal to the articular surface (in partial articular injuries [AO/OTA 43-B], the posterior pilon often remains intact).
  - An anterolateral pilon fracture fragment of varying size separates with its anteroinferior tibiofibular ligament attachment. This anterolateral tubercle of Chaput requires fixation to restore the anatomy and function of the syndesmosis complex.
  - A medial malleolar fracture is identified as the third characteristic fragment.
  - Isolated osteochondral fragments of variable size are often encountered (typically central to anterolateral in location; see **FIG 2B,C**) and constitute the remaining portion of the articular surface.
- High-energy injuries can extend into the tibial diaphysis with fibular fractures proximal to the articular level.
- Finally, the syndesmosis will be functionally disrupted, secondary to the fibular fracture and anterolateral pilon separation. The syndesmosis anatomy and function can often be restored by fixation of both the fibula and anterolateral pilon. As such, syndesmotic fixation is rarely required. However, a radiographic external rotation stress test or a Cotton test can be used to confirm syndesmotic stability. If the syndesmosis remains disrupted and widened after fracture fixation, it should be reduced and reinforced with screw or suture button fixation (see **FIG 3C,D**).
- In contrast to high-energy patterns, rotational injuries **(FIG 3)** cause spiral fractures of the distal tibia and fibula. The fibular fracture commonly originates at the articular level. Intra-articular injury, if present, is typically simple and without comminution or impaction. This can coincide with a syndesmotic injury.

NATURAL HISTORY

- On one end of the spectrum, high-energy vertical compression injuries result in comminuted articular fractures with compromised surrounding soft tissues. On the other end, low-energy rotational injuries with minimal axial compression produce more straightforward spiral fractures with less soft tissue damage and a more favorable prognosis.
- Soft tissue reaction and swelling is patient dependent and varies considerably. The mechanism does not always potentiate a comparable soft tissue reaction.
- Where a particular fracture pattern falls within this spectrum can often predict the eventual outcome of the injury.
- Unfortunately, determining the outcomes from these fractures is not straightforward as existing classification systems fail to clearly distinguish the spectrum of injury, making a fair comparison of published outcomes difficult to achieve.
- The surgeon maintains an important role in affecting the final outcome of these injuries, principally by designing a treatment plan that accomplishes the surgical goals detailed previously while minimizing the risks of complications.
- The timing of surgery in regard to the soft tissue injury is paramount in avoiding complications that can lead to poor outcomes.
- In addition to avoiding soft tissue complications, the patient's outcome is strongly influenced by the quality of the reduction of the articular surface and the axial and rotational alignment of the articular surface relative to the tibial shaft.

PATIENT HISTORY AND PHYSICAL FINDINGS

- The injury history is usually clear and often involves a fall from heights, motor vehicle crash, motorcycle crash, or sports injury. Occasionally, a patient will simply misstep on stairs or a curb. A simple, low-energy mechanism should prompt consideration for osteoporosis evaluation.
  - These patients are usually injured by high-energy means and should be evaluated as trauma patients and according to advanced trauma life support protocols.
- All associated injuries must be identified and formulated into the global treatment plan.
- Comorbidities such as diabetes mellitus, vascular disease, tobacco usage, and chronic immune or inflammatory disease may affect treatment and risk stratification. The medication profile should be assessed for blood thinners,

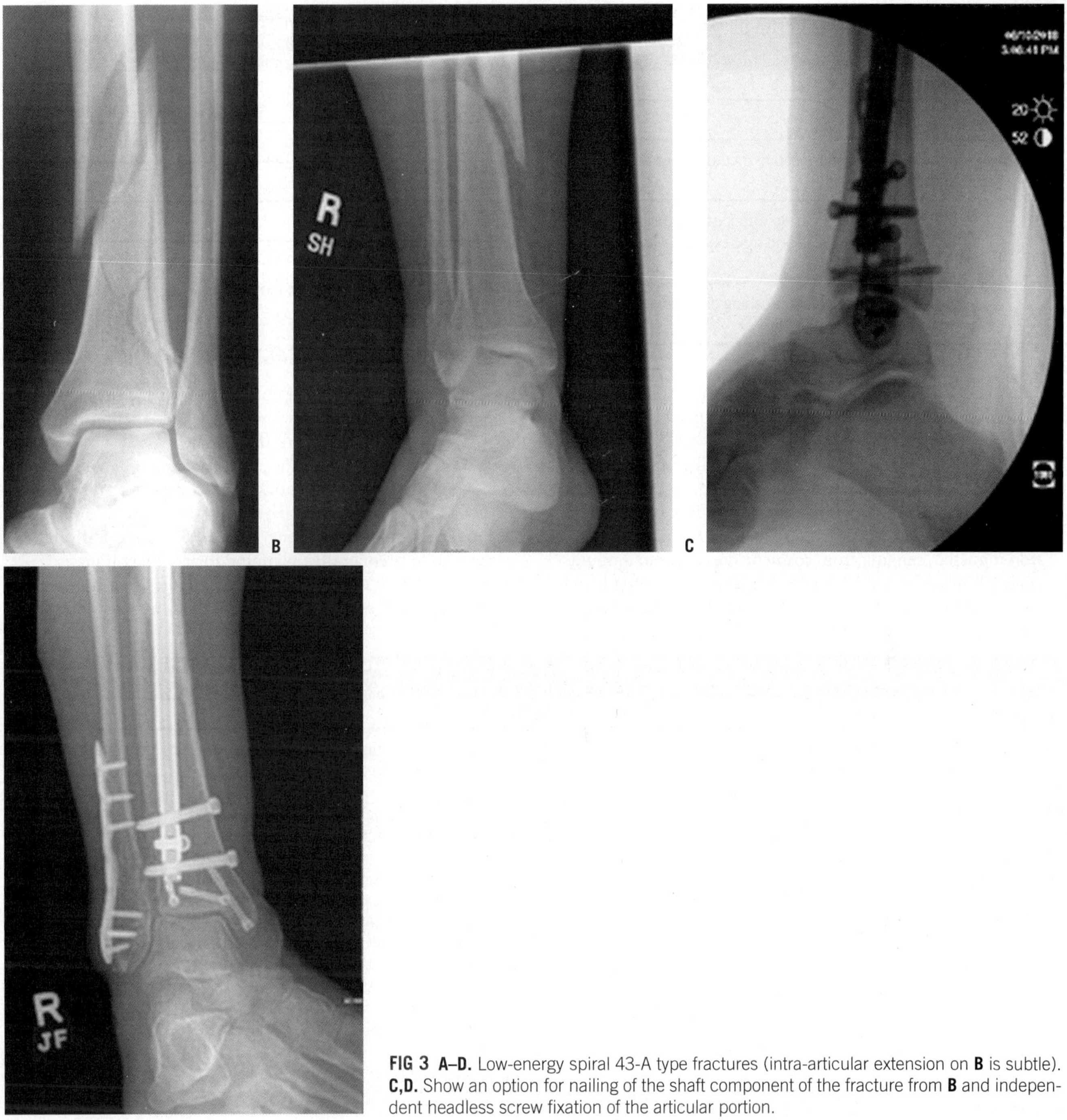

FIG 3 A–D. Low-energy spiral 43-A type fractures (intra-articular extension on **B** is subtle). **C,D.** Show an option for nailing of the shaft component of the fracture from **B** and independent headless screw fixation of the articular portion.

anti-inflammatories, and others that may affect surgical risk or bone metabolism.

- A meticulous examination with special attention to soft tissue and neurovascular status is important in the evaluation and classification of these fractures **(TABLES 1–3)**.
  - With wound complication rates having a historic potential of 50%,[13,21] recognition and appropriate management of the soft tissue injury cannot be overemphasized.
  - Inspect and document wounds, swelling, ecchymosis, blisters, ischemic skin, and chronic skin/vascular changes.
  - Identify open fractures.
  - Establish the personality of both the bony and soft tissue injuries.
- A careful vascular examination is important in evaluating patients with high-energy pilon injuries, as arterial compromise appears to be more common than previously appreciated (which may help explain the relatively high complication rates seen with early ORIF).
  - Findings of vascular compromise may be subtle (such as a one vessel injury, eg, anterior tibial artery) due to

TABLE 1 Tscherne and Gotzen Grading System for Closed Fractures

Grade	Description
0	Little/no soft tissue injury
1	Superficial abrasion and mild to moderately severe fracture configuration
2	Deep, contaminated abrasion with local contusional damage to skin or muscle and moderately severe fracture configuration
3	Extensive skin contusion or crushing or muscle destruction and severe fracture

collateral/retrograde flow patterns. Arterial compression testing (Allen test) about the ankle, ankle–brachial indices, or the addition of angiography to CT may be a useful tools to further evaluate the local vasculature.

- While rare, compartment syndrome may occur creating the need for urgent operative intervention. Compartment syndrome has devastating consequences for patient function if missed, ranging from cosmetic deformity to amputation. All pilon fractures should be assessed and monitored for compartment syndrome. Compartment syndrome can occur pre- or postoperatively and is more common in high-energy injuries.

TABLE 2 Gustilo and Anderson System for Grading Open Fractures

Grade	Type of Trauma	Wound Size	Soft Tissue Injury
I	Low energy	<1 cm	Minimal
II	Intermediate energy	>1 cm	Moderate
III	High energy	>10 cm	Severe, with crushing

IMAGING AND OTHER DIAGNOSTIC STUDIES

- The diagnosis of tibial pilon fracture is initially evaluated with three radiographic views of the ankle (anteroposterior [AP], mortise, and lateral) **(FIG 4A,B)**.
  - These views should be repeated after all "reductions" including application of temporizing external fixation.
- CT scans have been clearly shown to improve a surgeon's understanding of the injury (see **FIGS 2** and **4G–J**) and are critical to preoperative planning for complex injuries.[22]
- For displaced, comminuted pilon fractures, the best time to obtain a CT scan is after temporizing external fixation is

TABLE 3 Methods for Examining the Distal Leg

Examination	Technique	Grading	Significance
General appearance	Observation for swelling, blisters, wounds, ecchymosis	Closed injury (Tscherne and Gotzen): 0: Injury from indirect forces with negligible soft tissue injury 1: Superficial contusion/abrasion, simple fractures 2: Deep abrasions, muscle/skin contusion, direct trauma 3: Excessive skin contusion, crushed skin/muscle, subQ degloving, compartment syndrome Open injury (Gustilo and Anderson): 1: Low energy, <1 cm wound 2: Intermediate energy, 1–10 cm wound 3: High-energy, blast/crush, contaminated, >10 cm 3a: Adequate soft tissues for coverage 3b: Inadequate soft tissues; requires soft tissue reconstruction 3c: Associated vascular injury requiring repair	Increased surgical risks until soft tissues have improved.
Vascular	Palpating pulses and Doppler tones. Compare to contralateral side. "Allen test of the leg" to assess for a single vessel injury (eg, anterior tibial artery), compress posterior tibia artery while palpating dorsalis pedis (DP) artery. If the DP pulse disappears, there is likely injury to the anterior tibial artery and DP flow is occurring retrograde through the forefoot collateral arch.	Pulse grading: 0: Absent 1+: Barely palpable 2+: Normal 3+: Enlarged 4+: Aneurysmal	Increased surgical risks for wound problems, infection, failed treatment; alternative approaches
Neurologic	Light touch and motor examination	Quantify light touch	Charcot problems
Associated injury (foot, talus, knee, hip, lumbar spine)	Observation, palpation, and ROM	N/A	Avoid missed injury.

SubQ, subcutaneous; ROM, range of motion; N/A, not applicable.

performed **(FIG 4C–E)**, when the fracture length is restored. This tends to grossly reduce many parts of the fracture, making the pathoanatomy of the injury more understandable **(FIG 4G–J)**.

- The addition of angiography to CT is considered for assessing the arterial tree of the distal leg before pilon reconstruction if vascular injury is suspected. Occult vascular injuries, especially of the anterior tibial artery, do occur with some frequency in high-energy pilon fractures and may contribute to wound complications postoperatively if not recognized.
- Three-dimensional (3-D) CT reconstructions can be useful in preoperative planning and teaching. Advanced imaging such as this can help to guide the surgical approach and choice of fixation to allow for less invasive surgery without compromising the reduction or fixation.

DIFFERENTIAL DIAGNOSIS

- Tibial shaft fracture
- Ankle fracture or dislocation
- Talus fracture

NONOPERATIVE MANAGEMENT

- Nonoperative treatment should be reserved for nondisplaced or minimally displaced fractures that are determined to be stable and have little comminution and soft tissue injury.
  - This scenario is uncommon, however, as the amount of energy necessary to fracture the tibial pilon usually results in significant fracture displacement and resultant instability.

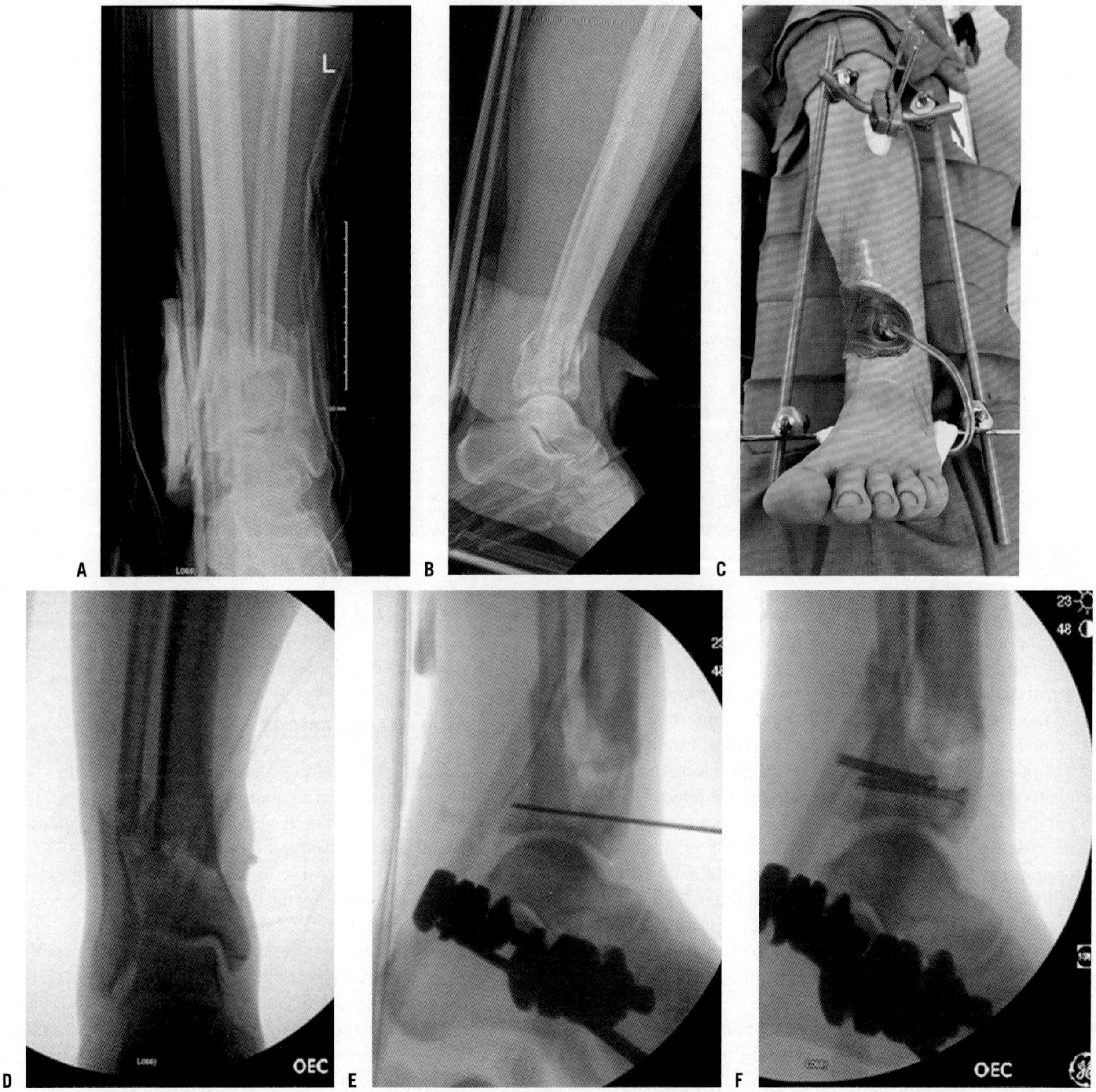

FIG 4 Case example of an open 43-C3 tibial plafond injury. **A,B.** Injury radiographs. **C.** Clinical picture of travelling traction ankle-spanning external fixation with an incisional vacuum assisted closure (VAC) for an open fracture wound. **D–F.** Radiographs of ankle after closed reduction and application of external fixator and simultaneous percutaneous articular ORIF. *(continued)*

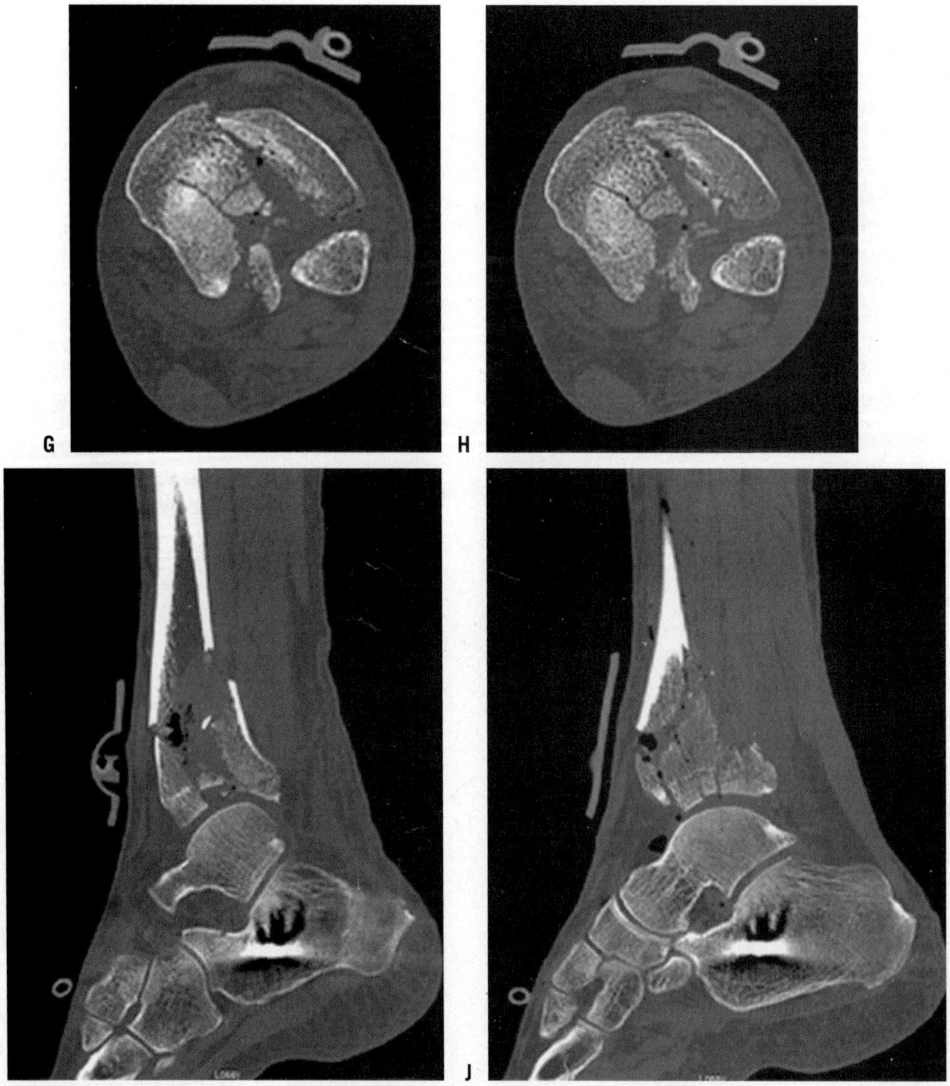

G H I J

FIG 4 *(continued)* **G–J.** Axial and sagittal CT images showing articular injury pattern.

  - Some consideration may be given to nonoperative treatment in the infirmed or neuropathic patient, although the risks of splinting or casting are often greater than for operative treatment. Shared and informed decision making with the patient and/or their family is especially important in these patients that may be less than ideal surgical candidates.
- Attempts at casting or splinting unstable pilon fractures in patients considered to be poor candidates for operative treatment (ie, elderly, diabetics, vasculopaths, etc.) are fraught with risks for progressive deformity, skin breakdown, and amputation. Despite the surgical risks minimally invasive methods to restore metaphyseal alignment may be warranted.
- The presence of other musculoskeletal injuries becomes a strong relative indication for surgical treatment of the pilon fracture as surgical stabilization may allow for easier mobilization and rehabilitation.
- Reasonable conservative treatment options include non–weight bearing with casting or bracing until radiographic signs of healing are visualized.
- Regular follow-up and radiographic vigilance is needed to ensure that articular congruity and axial alignment of the lower leg remain satisfactory.
- Protected weight bearing (PWB) must be individualized in each case, but usually, greater than 10 to 12 weeks of PWB is necessary to safely maintain alignment.

SURGICAL MANAGEMENT

- Displaced tibial pilon fractures generally require surgery. ORIF is the preferred method of treatment for such displaced fractures to achieve the goals of a congruent, stable, and well aligned joint.
- ORIF of pilon fractures should be delayed until the soft tissues will allow for primary closure, but within a reasonable time frame (ie, 5 to 21 days from the injury).
- Low-energy fractures with little comminution or soft tissue compromise may be candidates for immediate ORIF. In many cases, however, the degree of soft tissue injury is not fully appreciated at the time of presentation and waiting for soft tissues to manifest the extent of their injury may be prudent.
- Early application of ankle-spanning external fixation or "travelling traction" and staged ORIF of the pilon has been successful at reducing major complication rates from 50% to 0% to 10%.[14,19]

- External fixation can accelerate the recovery of soft tissues by providing better axial support and alignment than can be achieved with splinting or casting. External fixation also ensures distraction of the joint to a more anatomic position preventing continued pressure on the cartilage.
- A simple external fixation construct linking the tibial diaphysis (proximal to area of proposed plate placement) to the calcaneus suffices for the temporary fixator in most cases (see **FIG 4C**). Pins in the first and fifth metatarsals to prevent cavovarus deformity of the foot is helpful if the frame will be on more than a week or if the foot sits in a plantarflexed position.
  - This method brings the limb out to length and allows the tissues to recover under more physiologic conditions.
  - When being use for temporary stabilization, the external fixator pins should be positioned away from the zone of definitive fixation to avoid potential contamination of the surgical site and definitive hardware.
- An associated fibular fracture may be stabilized (surgeon's discretion) in the initial setting along with temporizing external fixation until definitive ORIF is appropriate.
  - If the fibula is to be repaired in this manner, its reduction must be anatomic or there may be difficulty with reducing the tibia at the time of staged pilon reconstruction.
  - ORIF of an associated fibular fracture at the time of temporizing external fixation has shown to have an increased risk of fibular wound breakdown.
  - Fixation of the fibular fracture done after anatomic fixation of tibial plafond can be done percutaneously with plate, screw, or intramedullary (IM) nail fixation (**FIG 6E** and **7G** are examples of percutaneous IM screw fixation of the fibula).
- Early ORIF through a posterior lateral approach of displaced posterior distal fragment(s) at the time of external fixation with delayed anterior ORIF can also be considered to improve articular reduction.
- The patient should return at regular intervals after temporary external fixation to schedule and undergo definitive fixation.
- The return of skin wrinkles, blister epithelialization, and ecchymosis resolution are several parameters to observe when staging the open tibial procedure.
- In many cases, the external fixator may be used as a distractor during the definitive fixation and then removed.
- In instances of considerable soft tissue loss, damage or wound contamination, external fixation can be used for definitive fixation. In these instances pins close to the fracture should be used for greater stability. If pins will be in a long time, there may be an advantage to hydroxyapatite-coated pins in the metaphysis and/or fine wires with a ring or hybrid frame.

Preoperative Planning

- Understanding the personality of the injury including soft tissue problems, patient/host issues, as well as the fracture configuration is critical to formulating an optimal treatment plan.
- Preoperative planning allows the surgeon to work through the case "on paper" while minimizing risk and often preventing unnecessary delays during the surgery.
- A preoperative tracing (**FIG 5**) or a computer-based template can help to determine instrumentation needs, surgical approaches, anticipated reduction methods, and implant strategies (selection and placement).
- CT and 3-D reconstructions often allow the surgeon to choose the optimal approach to address the articular pathology and apply implants (eg, anteromedial vs. anterolateral approaches for most AO/OTA 43-C fractures). As mentioned earlier, this can help provide for more focused less invasive soft tissue dissection.
  - **FIGS 6** and **7** demonstrate this decision process.

Positioning

- Pilon fractures are often approached through one of the three primary anterior approaches; thus, the patient is positioned supine on a radiolucent table.

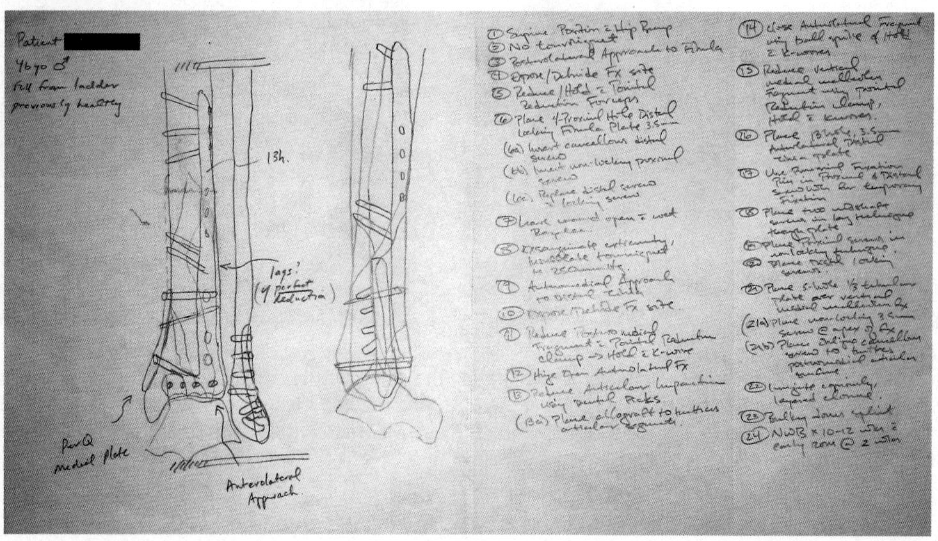

FIG 5 Preoperative plan and templating for tibial plafond fracture reconstruction.

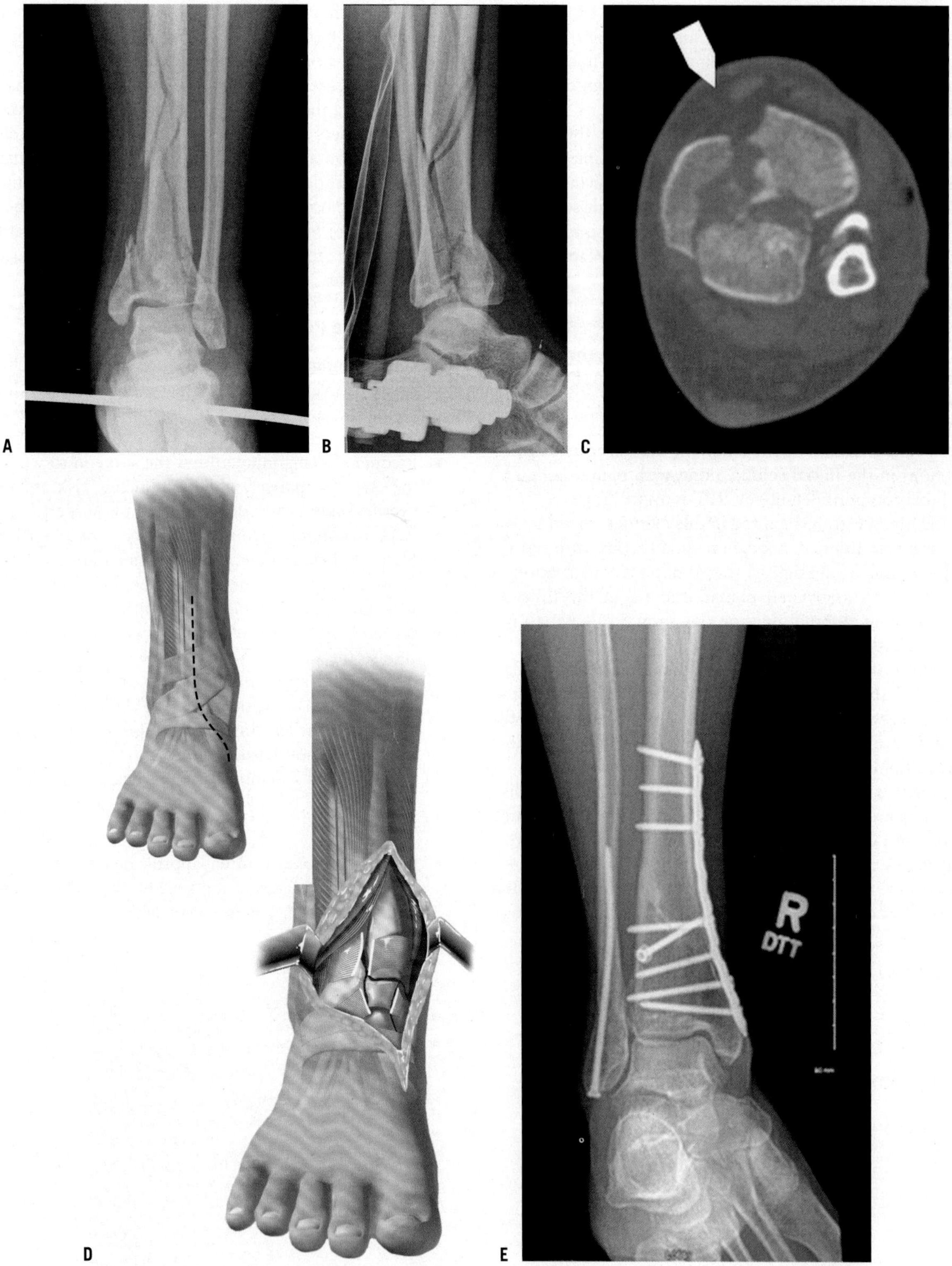

FIG 6 A,B. Injury x-rays of a 43-C fracture with medial-sided articular comminution and anterior cortical split. **C.** Corresponding axial CT slice. **D.** Schematic demonstrating the anteromedial approach. The incision is located over the anterior compartment, lateral of the palpable crest of the tibia, and curving gently medially at the ankle joint. **E.** Postoperative radiographs of a healed 43-C2 fracture approached through an anterior medial approach with percutaneous fixation of the fibula fracture.

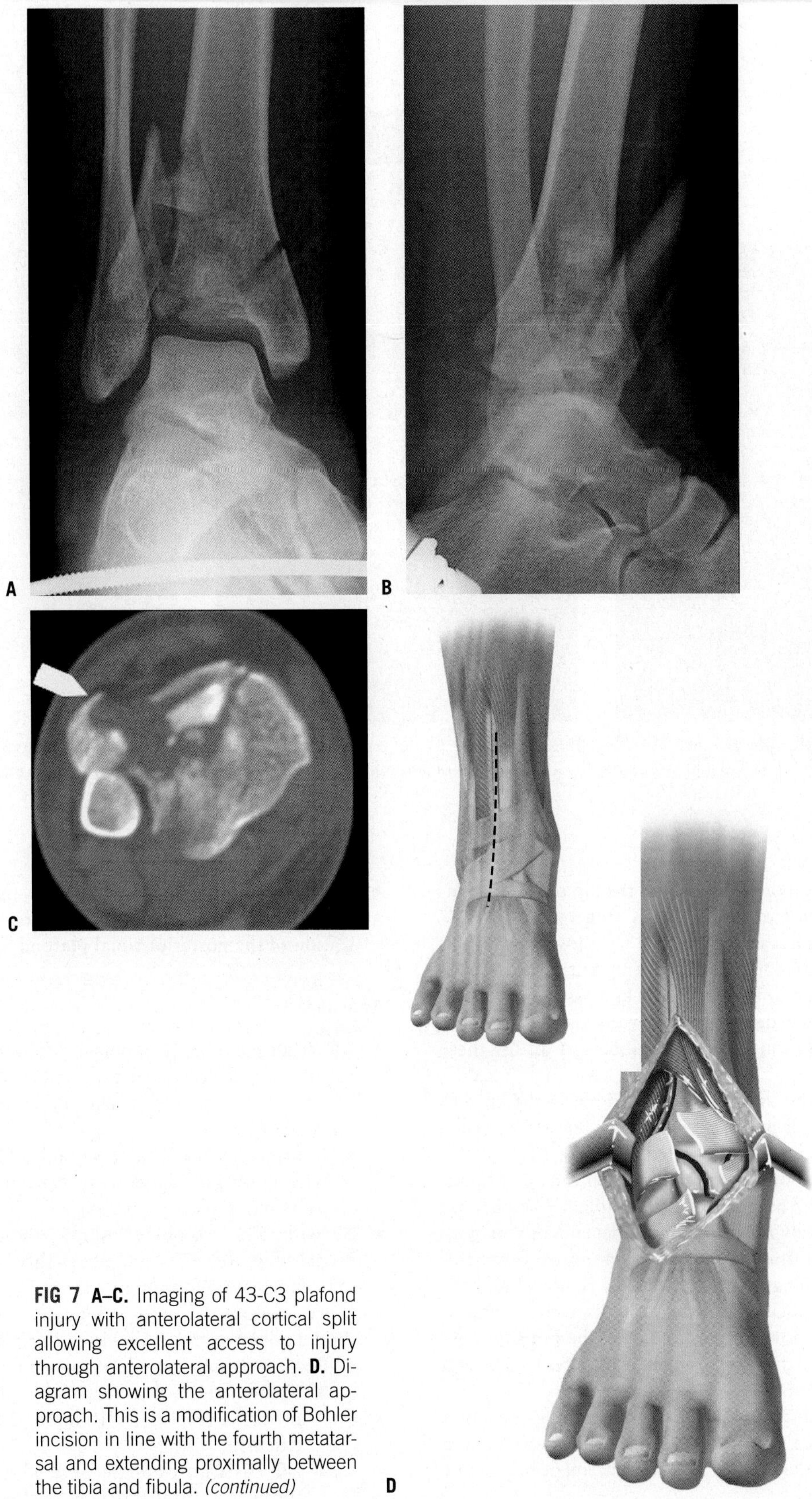

FIG 7 A–C. Imaging of 43-C3 plafond injury with anterolateral cortical split allowing excellent access to injury through anterolateral approach. **D.** Diagram showing the anterolateral approach. This is a modification of Bohler incision in line with the fourth metatarsal and extending proximally between the tibia and fibula. *(continued)*

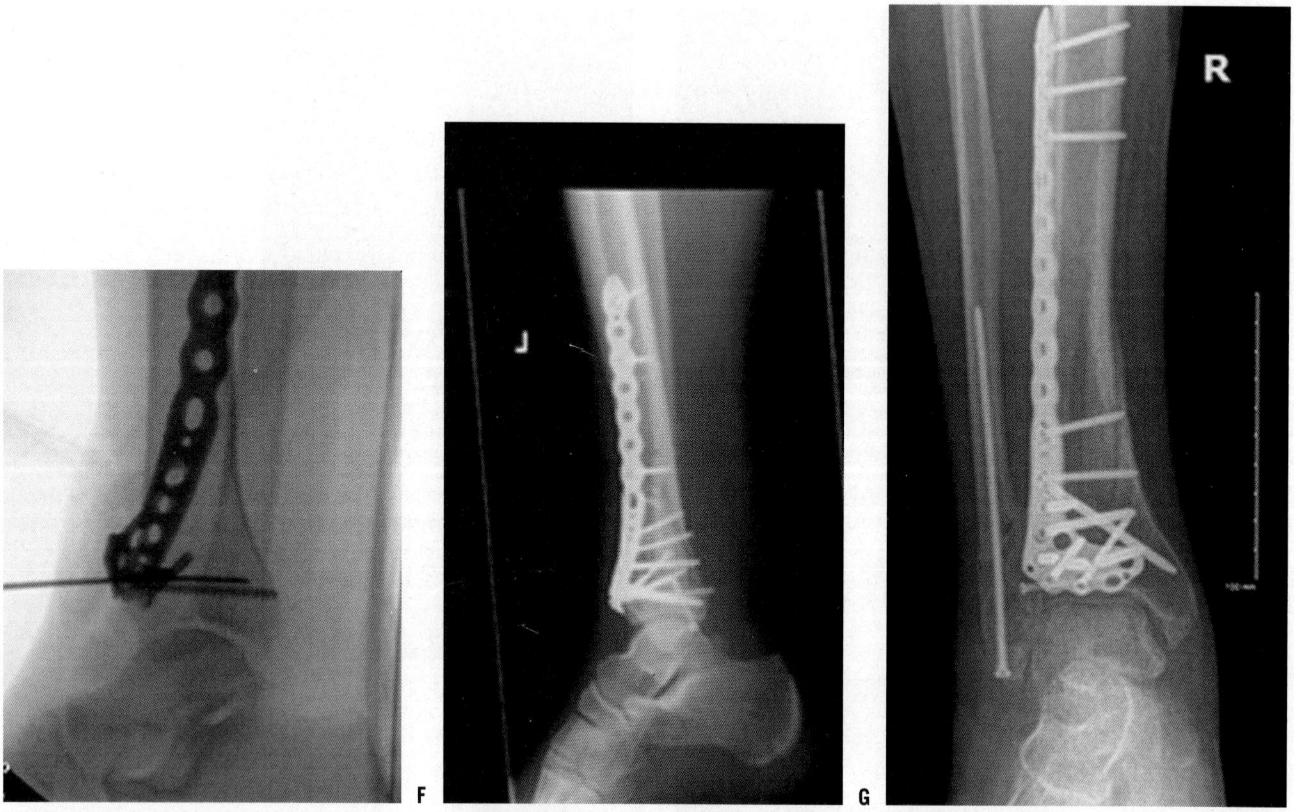

E F G

FIG 7 *(continued)* **E,F.** Intraoperative and postoperative radiographs of a 43-C2 injury fixated through an anterolateral approach **G.** Postoperative radiographs of a 43-C3 injury repaired through an anterolateral approach with cannulated articular screws and percutaneous screw fixation of the fibula.

- A gel or blanket roll or bump behind the hip may help control external rotation of the leg during surgery.
- Tourniquet control can be helpful to allow for visualization, particularly of the ankle joint but is not necessary and should be limited as much as possible to ensure adequate antibiotic delivery and avoid tissue ischemia. Many surgeons no longer use tourniquets at all for these procedures.
- The preparation and draping are carried above the knee to make Gerdy tubercle and the distal femur region accessible if any autogenous bone graft is needed.
- If needed, the temporary external fixation pins can be incorporated into the preparation and draping. The pins are used intraoperatively for distraction independently or with a universal (femoral) distractor. Pins that appear erythematous or with drainage should always be removed and the sites isolated from the surgical area. Alternatively, some surgeons prefer to remove all pins and keep the pin sites covered in an occlusive dressing, using new pin sites for skeletal distraction if needed.
- Pin or manual distraction is helpful in obtaining reduction and provisional stabilization of the articular surface and can also be used during initial plate placement and screw fixation.
- If a posteromedial approach is planned, the patient may still be positioned supine, but the surgeon may need to externally rotate the leg or place a bump under the contralateral hip for access.
- If a posterolateral approach is used, the patient is best positioned prone (or lateral) to allow the surgeon ideal visualization of the posterior tibial plafond and/or fibula.

Approaches

- Although historically, a single "utilitarian" approach was popular in the reconstruction of the tibial pilon, a variety of surgical approaches are currently used to treat these fractures **(FIG 8)**.
  - In principle, less dissection and soft tissue retraction as well as optimal implant placement should be possible using more direct approaches.
- As with other complex injuries, the selection of an approach that addresses the personality of each injury is recommended for pilon fractures.
- More customized and minimally invasive approaches should adhere to the following principle:
  - Respect of soft tissue intervals and vascularity
    - Maintenance of a reasonable skin bridge between incisions (especially if these incisions are long or extensile).
    - **FIG 7G** is an example of a 43-C3 fracture repaired through a distal articular level anterolateral incision and a separate, more proximal incision to fixate the superior plate.
- Making skin incisions directly over bone should be avoided when possible. Thus, if skin problems occur, resultant

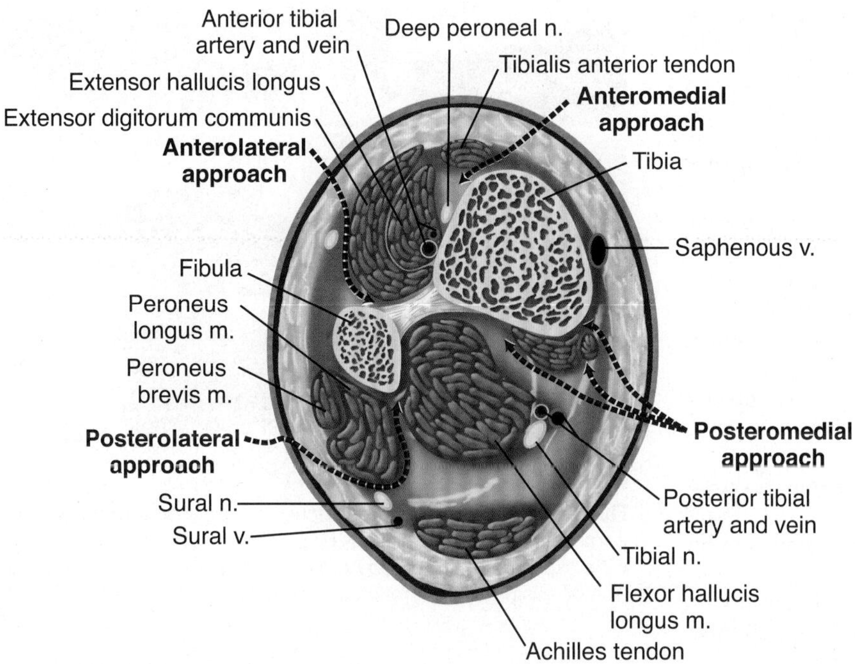

FIG 8 Approaches to the tibial plafond are probably best tailored to match the injury pattern. Over 90% of plafond fractures are well approached anteriorly (anteromedially or anterolaterally), but other approaches are sometimes useful.

defects can be reconstructed with a simple skin graft or fasciocutaneous flap as opposed to a free soft tissue transfer.

- Thoughtfully chosen incisions to access and reduce the important fracture fragments is requisite. Skin bridges should be made as wide as possible, overlapping longitudinally only as much as necessary. Using a 1:1 ratio is safe with respect to the random pattern flap that is created between any two incisions. Undermining the skin should be minimized, and respectful soft tissue handling maintained throughout the procedure.[11]

Anterolateral Approach

- The anterolateral approach has become common for pilon injuries in which the primary displaced fragments of the injury are more laterally located (see **FIGS 7** and **8**).
  - This approach to the ankle has been nicely described by Herscovici and associates.[10]
- The dissection proceeds just lateral to the extensor digitorum longus and peroneus tertius. The anterior tibial neurovascular bundle remains medial.
- Superficial peroneal nerve branches will be encountered and should be protected. Potential iatrogenic injury or neuropraxia should be discussed with the patient preoperatively.
- If a narrow skin bridge occurs between this approach and the fibular incision, this approach should be kept short (eg, 4 to 5 cm) and used for the articular reduction alone. However, this is another reason not to perform initial ORIF of the fibula until the definitive plan is made.
- The fibula fracture can be approached with percutaneous intramedullary fixation (with a long screw or nail) or a percutaneous plate and screw fixation if feasible given the fracture type (see **FIGS 4E,F**; **6E**; and **7G**).
- In some cases, the articular injury can be addressed through a small anterolateral approach and attachment of the reconstructed articular segment to the intact diaphysis accomplished by insertion of an anterolateral submuscular or anteromedial subcutaneous plate (see **FIG 7G**).
  - Proximal fixation can then be applied in a more "open" manner outside the zone of injury using a standard anterolateral approach to the tibia.
  - It can be beneficial for the soft tissue closure to have a separate incisions for the articular reduction distally and the plate fixation proximally.
- Alternatively, if the fibula and pilon are being repaired at the same operative visit, a single gently curved skin incision placed over the syndesmosis can be used to access both bones.
  - With this modification the superficial peroneal nerve will be encountered and should be protected.
- A similar deep approach that could be considered a superficial modification of the anterolateral approach is the lateral approach as described by Grose et al.[8] It is reserved for situations with compromised anteromedial soft tissue envelope or more laterally based fractures.
  - The skin incision is made at the anterior fibular border from the most proximal fracture line (either fibular or tibial) to approximately 4 cm distal to the joint.
  - Blunt dissection to the posterior fibular border allows for ORIF of fibular shaft fracture. Addressing the tibial fracture first, however, allows use of the fibular fracture interval for visualization of the tibia.
  - Blunt dissection over the anterior edge of the fibula leads to the interosseous membrane.
  - Blunt dissection between the interosseous membrane and the overlying contents of the anterior compartment allows for visualization of the tibial articular surface.

Anteromedial Approach

- The traditional anteromedial approach to the distal tibia uses an anteromedial incision directed longitudinally a centimeter

or so lateral to the anterior tibial crest and follows medially to the tibialis anterior tendon to the navicular to allow for careful medial column exposure (see **FIGS 6A–E** and **8**).
  - An anteromedial approach such as this can be used for injuries where the primary articular fracture is medial and/or it propagates from anterior to medial up the distal tibia.
- Accessing the far lateral joint surface using this approach requires a fairly vigorous retraction of the anterior ankle soft tissues. Alternatively, a small anterolateral incision can be used concomitantly with the anteromedial approach or vice versa to reduce and/or stabilize the smaller fragment.
- Dissection is full thickness and carried medial to the tibialis anterior tendon so as not to create multiple tissue dissection planes.
- Careful handling of the skin and subcutaneous tissue is essential.
- The paratenon of the tibialis anterior tendon should not be disrupted.
- Extensive periosteal stripping of fracture fragments is avoided, and fragments should be carefully hinged on their soft tissue attachments to preserve their vascularity.
- Hinging open the anterior fragments like a book using a small lamina spreader can help reveal the involvement and displacement of the central and posterior articular pilon and metaphysis.
  - Once the extent of the fracture is appreciated, reduction and fixation can be performed piece by piece with fragment specific screws or simultaneously with contoured plate and screw fixation.

Posterolateral and Posteromedial Approaches

- Additional described approaches include the posteromedial and posterolateral approaches (see **FIGS 8–10**).
  - The need for these approaches is specific to certain fracture patterns, and they can be useful in combination with other approaches.
  - These approaches allow for specific and minimized access to only portions of the articular surface. Complex intra-articular injuries are not typically well addressed through these approaches alone, and they are best viewed as accessory incisions.[12]
  - They are best suited for aiding in reduction of hard-to-reduce posterior fragments and applying antiglide or push plates that aid in reduction and provide fixation stability for individual posterior articular segments (**FIG 10** gives an example of the usefulness of these approaches for a specific injury).
  - The posterolateral approach is commonly used in the fixation of isolated type-B partial articular posterior injuries.
- To use the posterolateral approach to the distal tibia, the patient is best positioned prone with a bump under the opposite pelvis to keep the ankle in neutral to enhance lateral imaging.
  - The skin incision is placed 1 to 2 cm posterior to a standard fibular incision and can also be used for posterior or posterolateral fibular reduction and repair.

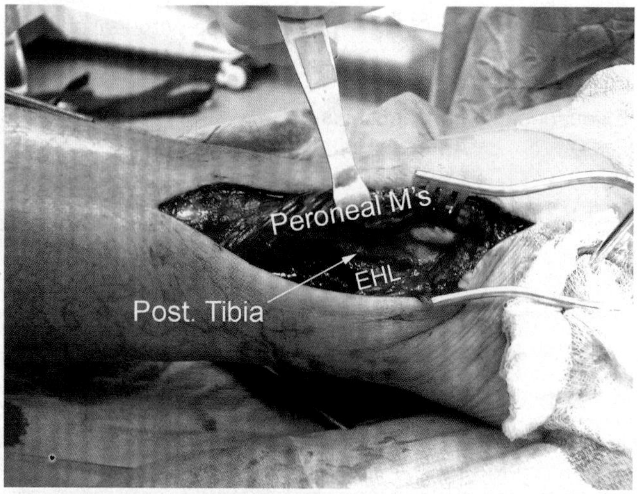

FIG 9 The posterolateral approach uses the interval between the peroneal and extensor hallucis longus (*EHL*) muscles and allows for wide exposure of the posterior distal tibia. Access to the fibula can also be easily gained through this incision.

  - The sural nerve is typically directly under the incision and must be identified and protected throughout the procedure.
  - This approach uses the interval between the peroneal tendons and flexor hallucis longus to approach the posterior tibia. During the deep dissection, the peroneal artery should be identified and protected.
  - If fibular reduction and fixation is planned, it is best done after the tibia is fixed as the fibular fixation may impede imaging or reduction of the joint surface. The fibula may be approached on either the medial or the lateral side of the peroneal tendons (**FIGS 9** and **10**; see also **FIG 8**).
  - The posterior cortex fracture apex is rarely comminuted and can be used to gauge reduction. Small or minifragment buttress plates are often useful here (see **FIG 10**). Precontoured plates designed for posterior distal tibial application are also available. The reduction of the joint is indirect and should be confirmed fluoroscopically.
- The posteromedial approach uses a skin incision posterior to the medial aspect of the tibia and requires mobilization of (and risk to) the posterior tibial tendon and posterior tibial neurovascular bundle (see **FIGS 8** and **10**).
  - There are three intervals that can be used to access the posteromedial tibia via this approach depending on the fracture configuration and how far posterior on the tibia the exposure needs to be
    - Anterior to the posterior tibial tendon
    - Between the posterior tibial and the flexor digitorum communis tendons
    - Between the flexor digitorum communis tendon and the posterior tibial neurovascular bundle
  - This approach can be useful in reduction and minifragment plate or isolated screw fixation of articular fragments.
  - The posterior retinaculum is incised and then repaired at the time of wound closure.

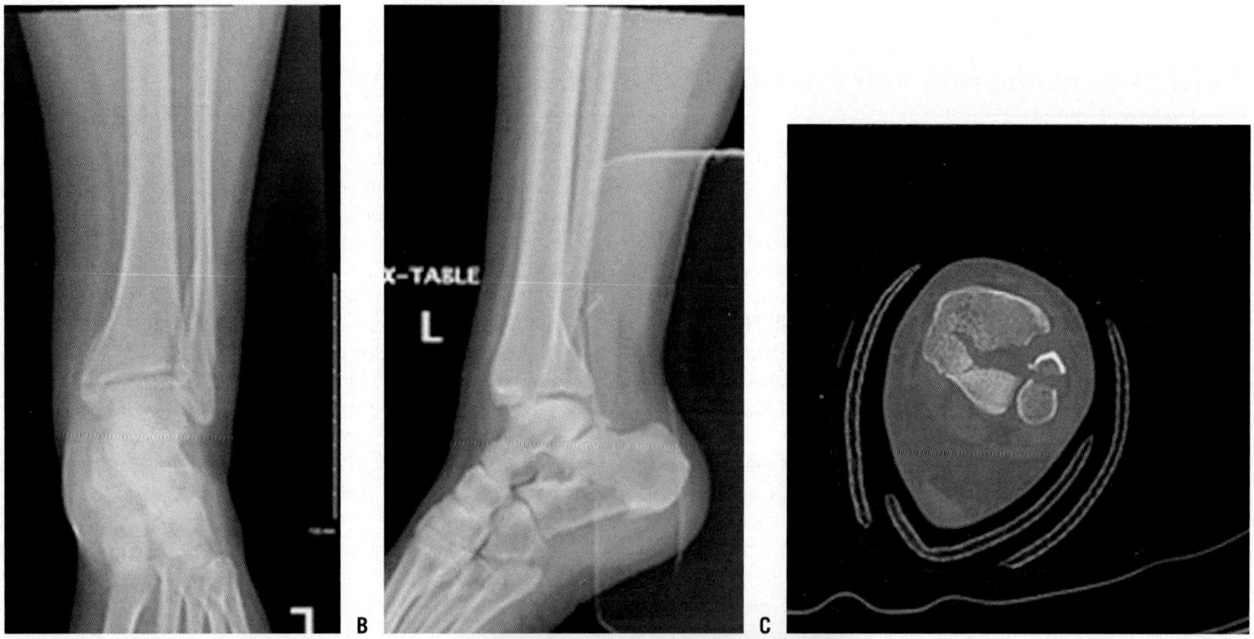

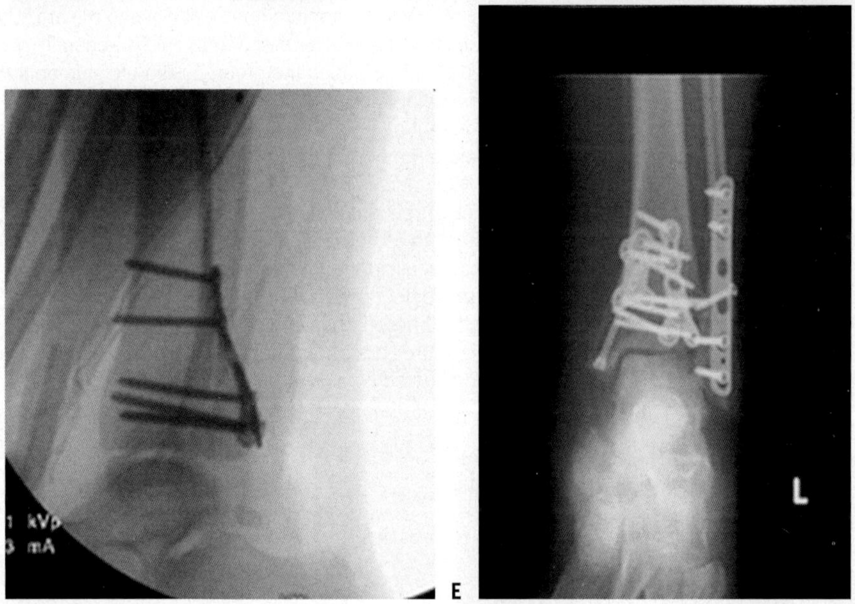

FIG 10 Case example of a 43-B3 injury benefiting from a posterior medial and posterior lateral approach. **A,B.** Emergency department radiographs. **C.** Post reduction CT scan. **D.** Intraoperative radiographs demonstrating reduction of the posterior fragment. **E.** Postoperative radiographs of the injury demonstrating multiple small fragment plate and cannulated screw fixation.

REDUCTION AND FIXATION OF THE FIBULA

- Consideration for the timing and incision placement during the fibular repair must be thoughtful to prevent soft tissue issues or competing approaches.
- The fibula can be reduced and fixed first to indirectly reduce the tibia fracture. This is most helpful in cases with substantial lateral or valgus displacement.
- In this context, the fibula *must* be anatomically reduced or it will impede the plafond reduction.
- If staged treatment is employed with external fixation applied at a referring hospital, most tertiary centers prefer the fibula to remain unfixed, allowing for maximal flexibility for the surgeon providing definitive treatment.
- If separate approaches are to be used for tibial and fibular repair, the fibular incision is often made posterolateral to maintain an optimal distance from anticipated anteromedial or anterolateral incisions.
- The posterolateral approach to the distal fibula is also desirable as it falls between the major distributions of the sural and superficial peroneal nerves.
- Percutaneous approaches can be used for simple fibula injuries with intramedullary screw or nail fixation to further help avoid soft tissue issues (see **FIGS 6E** and **7G**).

ARTICULAR REDUCTION AND FIXATION OF THE PILON

- The first priority in ORIF of complex articular injuries is accurate realignment of the joint surface with rigid internal fixation of the articular surface.
- As previously described, approach is based on the injury pattern to optimize access to the important pathoanatomy, such as using anteromedial approach for fractures with a medial split and medially concentrated articular injury **(TECH FIG 1A–C)**.
- Once stabilized, the articular segment is then attached to the tibial diaphysis through open or minimally invasive plating (see **FIG 7G**), intramedullary nailing (or external fixation) (see **FIGS 3C,D** and **4C–F**).
- Often, reduction of the articular segment and meta-diaphysis can be performed simultaneously (see **FIGS 4D,E** and **7E**), and in some cases, it is necessary to perform these together.
- Nonreconstructible small articular fragments and discarded as they have no vascularity.
- Larger articular fragments should be preserved even if they have no soft tissue attachments.
- Regardless of the approach chosen as the most appropriate by the surgeon, careful and precise articular reconstruction must be achieved.
  - An anatomic reconstruction is always the goal; however, this may not be possible if there are many small articular fragments. All attempts should be made to restore the joint and its alignment.
- With joint distraction (using an assistant, femoral distractor or external fixator), the anterior two-thirds of the joint should be readily accessible through an anterior approach.
- A small lamina spreader is helpful for booking open vertical cortical fractures to access impacted articular fragments **(TECH FIG 1D,E)**.
- One articular fragment can be definitively or temporarily reconstructed to another with screws, Kirschner wires (K-wires), or resorbable pins until all important fragments are addressed. Any intact articular surface can serve as the basis of the reduction.
- When necessary, the talar dome can be used as a template for the articular reduction.
  - The reconstruction can be provisionally stabilized with multiple K-wires and clamps **(TECH FIG 1F,G)**.
- Direct visualization of the joint and/or fluoroscopic guidance should be critically evaluated with each step in fixation.
- The posterior plafond can be difficult to reduce from an anterior-based exposure. Ankle positioning can affect the position of this fragment.
  - Wire joystick manipulation, the use of a sharp pick, or careful pointed clamp application is at times necessary to obtain an adequate reduction of the posterior fragments.
  - Posterior approaches may also be necessary, especially if displaced posterior fracture lines exit close to the articular surface, creating smaller fragments. This is generally performed as a first step in the prone position to gain an intact posterior joint to work to from the front.
- Small and minifragment screws are useful and should be placed before removal of the provisional wires **(TECH FIG 1H,I**; see **FIGS 4D,E**; and **10E)**.
- Once articular reconstruction is complete, the disimpacted metaphyseal area is evaluated for bone grafting needs.
- In most cases, allograft or bone graft substitute is used as metaphyseal defects heal well.
- If autograft is chosen, the Gerdy tubercle region is an easily accessible source and is less painful than the iliac crest. This can be augmented by allograft or graft substitutes.

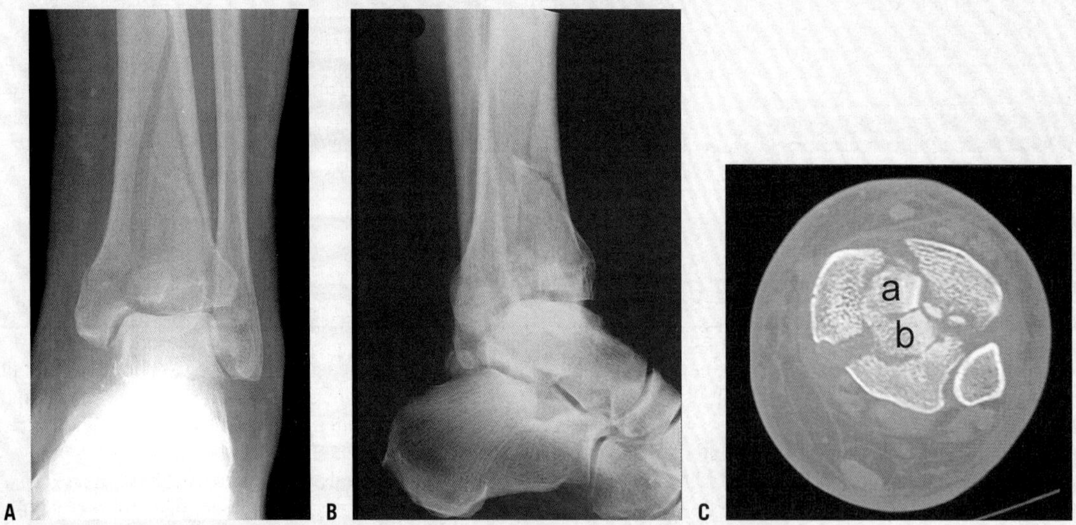

TECH FIG 1 A–C. Typical case example of a 43-A3 plafond injury. Please take notice of specific fragments *a* and *b*. The articular surface of these fragments is rotated 90 deg from the normal anatomic position towards the lateral side of the leg. Recognizing this is essential to appropriate reduction and fixation. *(continued)*

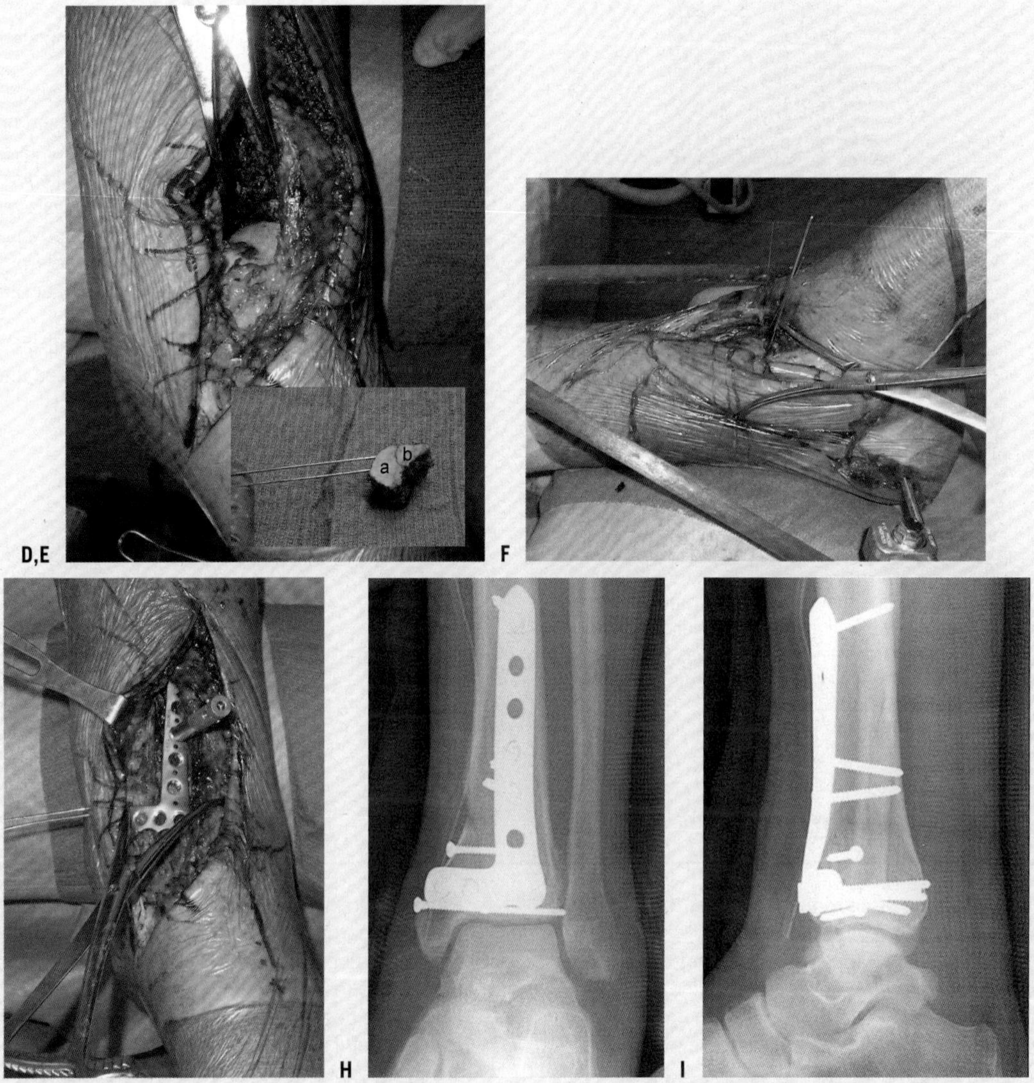

TECH FIG 1 *(continued)* **D,E.** The anterior cortical split is opened like a book and held with a lamina spreader. Dissection is limited to that necessary for reduction and plating. Direct visualization of the anterior two-thirds of the joint is typically available and may be enhanced with use of a distractor (or the external fixator). In some extreme cases such as this (*inset*), major articular fragments are reconstructed with K-wires, minifragment screws, and/or absorbable pins on the back table. **F.** Clamps and provisional fixation with K-wires can be placed through the wounds or percutaneously (carefully) (see **FIG 4E,F** as well). **G.** Intraoperative photos show lag screws, and anterior plating is performed to optimize fixation of the articular segment with a raft of AP screws. Autograft from Gerdy tubercle was used above the disimpacted articular surface. **H,I.** Corresponding postoperative radiographs.

EXTRA-ARTICULAR (METAPHYSEAL) REDUCTION AND FIXATION OF THE PILON

- Once the articular reduction is completed, reattaching the distal articular segment to the diaphysis is accomplished (often, this is done simultaneously).
- Plate fixation is most common, although external fixation, ring frame, or an intramedullary nail can be combined with a limited ORIF of the articular surface.
- Currently, anatomically contoured low-profile, small fragment plates (with locking capability) designed for the distal tibia are available from most implant vendors.
- The anatomic design of these implants affords a satisfactory match to the anterior, anteromedial, or anterolateral (**TECH FIG 2**; see also **TECH FIG 1F**) surface of the distal tibia.

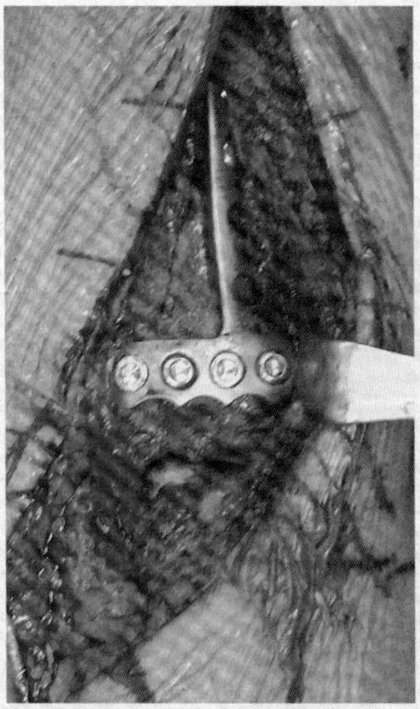

TECH FIG 2 Intraoperative photos show lag screws, and anterior plating is performed to optimize fixation of the articular segment with a raft of AP screws. Autograft from Gerdy tubercle was used above the disimpacted articular surface, but allograft or substitutes may be used.

- Nonlocking screws are used first to bring the plate in close apposition to bone in order to minimize the plate's prominence against the soft tissues.
- Subsequent insertion of locking screws, creating a hybrid internal fixation construct, is determined based on factors such as bone quality, comminution, and patient factors that may influence the expected time to healing. Locked screws, when used, are typically used only in the metaphysis with lag fixation at the joint and unlocked fixation in the diaphysis.
- An anterior plate location (direct anterior, anteromedial, or anterolateral) is often best for neutralization or buttressing of complex intra-articular fractures.
- Once intraoperative radiographs reveal a satisfactory reduction and position of implants, the incision is closed after copious irrigation.

WOUND CLOSURE AND CARE

- Retinacular layers are reapproximated to cover the underlying bone and implants.
- A drain or incisional negative pressure dressing can be considered to minimize pressure on the incision line from fluid accumulation under the wound.
- Vancomycin powder or paste can be left in the wound for improved infection prophylaxis.
- The subcutaneous layer is closed with an absorbable suture before skin closure.
- 4-0 or 3-0 nylon or Prolene interrupted sutures, a carefully tensioned running suture, or a subcuticular 3-0 Monocryl and skin glue can typically be used along with atraumatic soft tissue handling during wound closure. The Allgöwer-Donati technique is a good option for high-tension wounds or areas of soft tissue injury **(TECH FIG 3)**.[17]
- Closing an anteromedial incision, if chosen, without tension is critically important. Any substantial tension on the anterior skin edges after closure will likely result in some degree of soft tissue necrosis. Rarely, accomplishing this step may require relaxation of the lateral incision, pie crusting, or a return trip to the operating room for delayed closure.
- Minimally invasive or separate articular and shaft incisions can make closure easier.
- The skin can be reprepped at the end of the procedure with an iodine-based preparation before application of the dressing and splint.
- A lightly compressive bulky dressing and three-sided plaster splint or boot should be applied with the ankle in neutral position.
- Prophylactic incisional negative pressure wound therapy (low pressure) can help prevent infection and wound dehiscence in cases with considerable soft tissue injury or in open fractures.[20]
- Elevation is resumed on pillows, a bump, or blankets before leaving the operating room (OR) to minimize swelling.
- Ice is a useful adjunct to improve swelling pre- and postoperatively thought should be used on a specific schedule to avoid burns.
- The dressing can be left on until postoperative follow-up unless saturated.

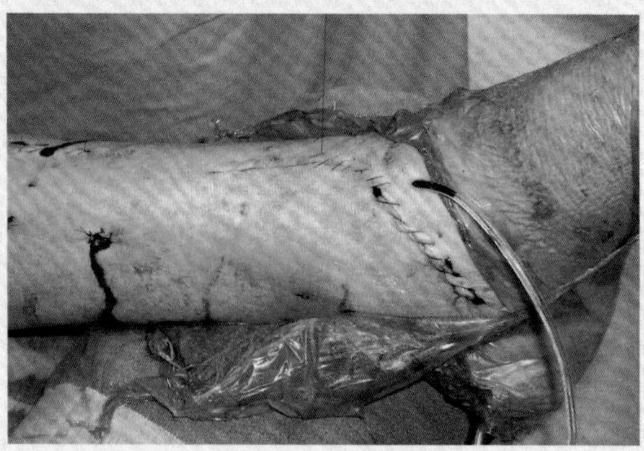

TECH FIG 3 Wound closure is performed with a traumatic technique with the superficial layers closed using fine nylon or Prolene suture.

Pearls and Pitfalls

Minimizing Risk for Major Complications	• Prior to modern methods of soft tissue handling, open treatment of high-energy tibial pilon fractures was associated with high complication rates (~50%). Many of these complications are potentially preventable, thus tibial pilon fractures present the orthopaedic surgeon with a concrete opportunity to influence a patient's ultimate outcome. • Contemporary fracture treatment principles (eg, staged treatment protocols, tailored surgical approaches, careful soft tissue handling, indirect reduction, and biologic fixation) have reduced the rate of complications to an acceptable level (approximately 0%–10%) for these fractures.
Surgical Goals	• The goals of surgery for pilon fractures include precise articular reconstruction, restoration of extremity length, alignment and rotation, stable fracture fixation, and early joint motion. The avoidance of complications is critical to consistently achieving optimal clinical results.
Soft Tissue Management	• The soft tissues must be notably improved at the time of pilon ORIF. • Staged treatment protocols, tailored surgical approaches, careful soft tissue handling, and indirect reduction should be used routinely for these injuries.
Articular Reduction Tricks	• The articular reduction is of paramount importance and is usually performed first, followed by the metaphyseal–diaphyseal reduction. • Longitudinal traction with an external fixator or femoral distractor allows for indirect fracture reduction and joint visualization. Articular fragments may be disimpacted with small osteotomes or elevators. These fragments should be kept as large as possible, and any voids created by disimpaction are considered for grafting. Small devascularized irreparable free fragments should be removed. A well-positioned talar dome may be useful as a template for articular reduction. Multiple K-wires and carefully placed pointed clamp may be helpful in gaining and maintaining reduction. Provisional cannulated screw or minifragment fixation can be a useful tool for maintaining the articular reduction to then be reinforced with larger plates or an intramedullary nail. Fracture reduction should be carefully scrutinized using direct visualization and/or fluoroscopy before and after fixation so that changes can be made prior to leaving the OR.
Metaphyseal Reduction Tricks	• Often, reducing the joint fragments will simultaneously realign the metaphysis. • Pointed clamps, small push plates, and lag screws are very useful for the metaphyseal reduction. Axial alignment must be carefully scrutinized clinically and radiographically. A well-repaired fibula is an excellent guide for restoring tibial length.
Fixation Problems	• The 2.4-, 2.7-, and 3.5-mm screws, lag screws, and occasionally absorbable pins are used for fixation of the articular fragments. These are often placed in subchondral bone to gain optimal stability of osteochondral fragments. Anatomically, contoured pilon plates with locking capability are nice tools for use in complete articular injuries or osteoporotic bone but are not necessary (or desirable) for all injuries.

POSTOPERATIVE CARE

- Elevation of the extremity should continue for the next few weeks to protect the closure of the incisions. Patient education is important to maximize the patient's understanding of wound risks along with compliance with elevation and other postoperative treatments.
- Aggressive respiratory care and supplemental oxygen are continued until the patient is fully awake and off intravenous narcotics (respiratory depressants).
- Immobilization is maintained for approximately 10 to 14 days or until adequate healing of the incisions has occurred. A well-padded postoperative splint should be kept in place until outpatient follow-up and will aid in wound recovery. The use of an incisional VAC dressing can be useful on tenuous wounds/incisions.
- At the time of suture removal, ankle range-of-motion exercises are initiated, and the limb is placed in a removable fracture brace or boot.
- Non–weight bearing or toe-touch weight bearing is continued with advancement in weight bearing made when radiographic evidence of fracture consolidation is adequate, typically at 10 to 12 weeks after surgery. With combined intramedullary nail and articular fixation weight bearing can begin once healing of the articular fractures has been achieved (at times, this may occur before the metaphyseal or diaphyseal fracture segment).

OUTCOMES

- The philosophy for ORIF of pilon fractures is a direct extension of Ruedi and Allgower's[16] original recommendations.
- Historically, early poor results with ORIF were primarily related to the disruption of the soft tissue envelope and not the fixation of the bony fracture itself.[13,21]
  - These failures were the result of the fragility of the thin soft tissue envelope in this area; misunderstandings of the soft tissue injury severity; overly aggressive soft tissue stripping during surgery; and the use of prominent, large fragment implants for stabilization.
- More modern techniques of pilon fracture management have led to more satisfactory complication rates for pilon fractures.
  - Sirkin et al[19] and Patterson and Cole[14] both retrospectively analyzed a staged protocol for management of C-type pilon fractures with early stabilization of the fibular fracture and temporary spanning external fixation of the tibia across the ankle joint. Formal open reconstruction of the tibial fracture with plating was performed when soft tissues normalized (average of 13 days and 24 days, respectively). Results of this two-staged technique for the treatment of these high-energy pilon fractures resulted in deep infections of in 6% and 0% of patients, respectively.

- Short- to medium-term results of open pilon fractures treated with staged ORIF showed functional outcomes were below age-matched norms, despite low complication rates (3%).[3]
- A recent report on AO/OTA type C pilon fractures showed that treatment with early, definitive ORIF (88% within initial 48 hours) was generally safe: Deep infection or wound complications developed in 6%, requiring additional operative intervention.[23]
- The authors concluded that this protocol is safe and effective if used by experienced orthopaedic trauma surgeons.
- There are a few limited studies that have compared staged ORIF to other methods for treating tibial pilon fractures.
- Three different management protocols for severe pilon fractures (92% 43-C fractures) were retrospectively compared[2]:
  - Primary ORIF (n = 15, reserved for patients with closed fractures without severe soft tissue trauma)
  - Primary minimally invasive osteosynthesis of the articular surface with long-term (minimum of 4 weeks) transarticular external fixation of the ankle (n = 28). Two-stage procedure with primary minimally invasive osteosynthesis of the articular surface combined with ankle-spanning external fixation, followed by staged subcutaneous plating (n = 8).
  - Although the incidence of wound infection did not differ significantly among the three groups, this study found that patients who had undergone two-stage surgery did better in terms of pain, ankle motion, activities of daily living, and the need for secondary arthrodesis compared to the other groups.
- Results of 50 patients with tibial pilon fractures treated by ORIF were compared to 17 patients treated with minimally invasive osteosynthesis or external fixation.[1] Three parameters significantly influenced results: the severity of fracture, the quality of surgical reduction, and the procedure by which the fracture was managed (ORIF did better).
- Functional outcomes of 63 patients after operative treatment of 43-B or C pilon fractures treated with ORIF were compared versus 16 treated with limited open articular reduction and wire ring external fixation.[9] The greatest impairment in outcome was noted after type C3 fractures regardless of the method of treatment employed. ORIF was associated with fewer complications and less posttraumatic arthritis when compared to external fixation, but this finding possibly reflected a selection bias as open injuries and the more severely comminuted fractures were all managed with external fixation.
- Three studies that have reported intermediate- or long-term patient outcomes after ORIF of tibial pilon fractures.
- Thirty patients who completed the 36-Item Short Form Survey (SF-36) greater than 18 months after ORIF of a tibial pilon fracture showed deficits in every SF-36 subcategory, with the largest differences in outcomes seen in the areas of physical function and physical role function.[18]
- Eighty patients evaluated with the SF-36 greater than 2 years after ORIF of a pilon injury diminished also showed diminished scores in all eight functional domains of the SF-36, including markedly abnormal scores for physical function, physical role function, and bodily pain.[15] They also noted that 35% of patients reported substantial ankle stiffness, 29% had persistent swelling, and 33% described ongoing pain. Of the participants who had been employed before the injury, 43% were not working at final follow-up.
- Ninety-nine patients with pilon fractures were evaluated over 11 years. Seventy-two percent of these patients were satisfied with their outcome.[6]

COMPLICATIONS

- Tibial pilon fractures are often complex injuries that have a high potential for complications if not managed thoughtfully.
- As many of these complications are somewhat preventable, tibial pilon fractures present the orthopaedic surgeon with an opportunity to positively influence a patient's ultimate outcome.
- Although we cannot alter the severity of a particular injury, appropriate surgical timing and soft tissue handling, along with exact articular reduction and stable fixation to allow for early motion, offer the best chance of obtaining good results with few complications for patients with these fractures.
- Long surgery or tourniquet use may increase the likelihood of infection or wound healing issues. If a tourniquet is used, timing of the tourniquet inflation needs to not prevent systemic antibiotic delivery to the surgical area. Most of these fractures can be reduced and fixated completely without the use of a tourniquet.
- Wound problems resulting from these procedures should be treated aggressively to prevent deep infection. A low threshold to comanage these issues with a wound care physician or nurse can aid in the successful resolution of the wound issue.
- For superficial marginal wound necrosis, successful management can be achieved with local wound care with or without oral antibiotics. At times, a negative pressure wound VAC can be useful in achieving healing of these wounds (see **FIG 4C**).
- Full-thickness necrosis (eschar) formation can be followed as well in reliable patients. They are educated to return immediately for any worsening of wound problems. Once the eschar begins to detach or drain (becomes an "unstable" eschar), it will require removal along with antibiotic therapy and potential VAC treatment. If healing beneath the eschar is inadequate at the time of its unroofing, the patient may require formal débridement and soft tissue coverage with a simple skin graft, fasciocutaneous flap, or free soft tissue transfer, depending on the area and size of the wound and how much "biology" will be necessary to aid healing and prevent infection.
- Anteromedial wounds of this sort are more problematic than anterolateral wounds or others because the underlying tibia and plate will be exposed in the anteromedial case. This has led to the anterolateral approach being preferred whenever possible.
- A preoperative chlorhexidine scrub and reprepping of the skin with iodine after closure but before dressing application may help avoid superficial wound complications.
- Silver-impregnated dressings and wound stabilization with splinting or skin glue have been shown to be anecdotally effective in helping to decrease superficial wound complications.
- Established deep infection is a limb-threatening problem and usually requires intravenous antibiotics, staged surgeries

including external fixation, soft tissue coverage (often through free-tissue transfer), and possibly late bone grafting.

- Importantly, not all patients are good candidates for such complex reconstructive procedures, and, in these cases, early below-the-knee amputation is a useful means for restoring predictable function in an expeditious manner. This is especially true in cases of documented or anticipated noncompliance.
- Malunion typically occurs in varus. It occurs if malalignment is accepted or unrecognized, union is not achieved, and/or the fixation fails.
- Prevention is important and should focus on providing adequate initial and ongoing medial column support against an intact, plated, or healed fibula.
- Some surgeons avoid fixation of the fibula entirely. This method is typically coupled with external fixation for the tibia fracture after limited open articular reconstruction.
- Avoiding fibular stabilization, however, does not convincingly decrease and perhaps even increases the chance of angular deformity. Additionally, maintaining appropriate length is more difficult with the use of external fixation alone.
- Intramedullary fixation of the fibula with a guidewire, long small-fragment screw or fibula specific nail is emerging as an option in these injuries to percutaneously maintain fibular length and reduction.
- Malalignment of the tibia or fibula may adversely affect ankle function and result in painful ankle arthrosis.
- Most authors use less than 5 degrees of varus/valgus and less than 5 or 10 degrees of recurvatum/procurvatum as a limit for acceptable alignment.
- Malunion surgery is typically associated with adjustment of the fixation and requires careful preoperative planning and perhaps referral to a surgeon with experience in posttraumatic reconstruction.
- Percutaneous reduction and fixation of the fibula to prevent malalignment or collapse can aid in preventing these complications (see **FIGS 6E** and **7G**).
- Nonunion or delayed union occurs in about 5% or more of patients and may occur in combination with malalignment.
- Injury and host factors are generally implicated in problems with union of the tibial pilon.
- Deep infection of a previously operated on tibial pilon nonunion should always be considered as a cause, and the appropriate lab work and cultures at the time of revision should be performed.
- Significant metaphyseal comminution, open fractures, and bone loss are factors prone to causing healing problems. Adjunctive measures should be considered in these cases.
- Smoking cessation and avoidance of nonsteroidal anti-inflammatory medications should be routinely discussed with patients to decrease the likelihood of these complications.
- Immediate or early-staged (4 to 8 weeks) bone grafting may advance tibial metaphyseal healing in high-risk fractures. External bone stimulation can also be considered early (for acceleration of fresh fracture healing) or late (as an adjunct to nonunion surgery) in the treatment course.
- Treatment of an established distal tibial nonunion requires a comprehensive plan including consideration of the soft tissues, local biology and mechanics, presence of infection, condition of the ankle joint, and others.
- Repair frequently requires realignment of the limb axis, followed by rigid fixation with or without bone grafting.
- Posttraumatic arthritis should be addressed by an initial course of conservative care with anti-inflammatories, injections, physical therapy, and bracing. Ankle arthrodesis (method by surgeon preference) is often chosen once nonoperative treatment measures have been exhausted. Trial of a lace up ankle brace is a good technique to determine how a patient will tolerate a fusion.
- Recent advances in total ankle arthroplasty may hold promise in carefully selected patients but is not currently a standard recommendation.
- Rarely, a primary arthrodesis is considered for limb salvage in severe fractures in which the articular surface cannot be salvaged.[4]
- The combination of metaphyseal nonunion and ankle arthritis is particularly difficult because the intercalary segment of tibia (between the nonunion site and the ankle joint) is often small and of poor bone quality.
- Treatment options for this condition include amputation (especially if infection is present), resection with distraction osteogenesis, or internal fixation spanning both the nonunion and arthritic ankle along with bone grafting.

REFERENCES

1. Babis GC, Vayanos ED, Papaioannou N, et al. Results of surgical treatment of tibial plafond fractures. Clin Orthop Relat Res 1997;(341):99–105.
2. Blauth M, Bastian L, Krettek C, et al. Surgical options for the treatment of severe tibial pilon fractures: a study of three techniques. J Orthop Trauma 2001;15:153–160.
3. Boraiah S, Kemp TJ, Erwteman A, et al. Outcome following open reduction and internal fixation of open pilon fractures. J Bone Joint Surg Am 2010;92:346–352.
4. Bozic V, Thordarson DB, Hertz J. Ankle fusion for definitive management of non-reconstructable pilon fractures. Foot Ankle Int 2008;29:914–918.
5. Cole PA, Mehrle RK, Bhandari M. The pilon map: assessment of fracture lines and comminution zones in AO C3 type pilon fractures. Presented at: Orthopedic Trauma Association Annual Meeting; October 8–10, 2004; Hollywood, FL.
6. Duckworth AD, Jefferies JG, Clement ND, et al. Type C tibial pilon fractures: short- and long-term outcome following operative intervention. Bone Joint J 2016;98-B(8):1106–1111.
7. Fracture and dislocation compendium. Orthopaedic Trauma Association Committee for Coding and Classifications. J Orthop Trauma 1996;10(suppl 1):v–ix, 1–154.
8. Grose A, Gardner MJ, Hettrich C, et al. J Orthop Trauma 2007;21(8):530–537.
9. Harris AM, Patterson BM, Sontich JK, et al. Results and outcomes after operative treatment of high-tibial plafond fractures. Foot Ankle Int 2006;27:256–265.
10. Herscovici D Jr, Sanders RW, Infante A, et al. Bohler incision: an extensile anterolateral approach to the foot and ankle. J Orthop Trauma 2000;14:429–432.
11. Howard JL, Agel J, Barei D, et al. Challenging the dogma of the 7-cm rule: a prospective study evaluating incision placement and wound healing for tibial plafond fractures. Presented at: Orthopaedic Trauma Association Annual Meeting; October 5–7, 2006; Phoenix, AZ.
12. Ketz K, Sanders R. Staged posterior tibial plating for the treatment of Orthopaedic Trauma Association 43C2 and 43C3 tibial pilon fractures. J Orthop Trauma 2012;26(6):341–347.
13. McFerran MA, Smith SW, Boulas HG, et al. Complications encountered in the treatment of pilon fractures. J Orthop Trauma 1992;6:195–200.

14. Patterson MJ, Cole JD. Two-staged delayed open reduction and internal fixation of severe pilon fractures. J Orthop Trauma 1999;13:85–91.
15. Pollak AN, McCarthy ML, Bess RS, et al. Outcomes after treatment of high-energy tibial plafond fractures. J Bone Joint Surg Am 2003;85(10):1893–1900.
16. Ruedi T, Allgower M. Fractures of the lower end of the distal tibia into the ankle joint. Injury 1969;1:92–99.
17. Sagi HC, Papp S, Dipasquale T. The effect of suture pattern and tension on cutaneous blood flow as assessed by laser Doppler flowmetry in a pig model. J Orthop Trauma 2008;22(3):171–175.
18. Sands A, Grujic L, Byck DC, et al. Clinical and functional outcomes of internal fixation of displaced pilon fractures. Clin Orthop Relat Res 1998;(347):131–137.
19. Sirkin M, Sanders R, DiPasquale T, et al. A staged protocol for soft tissue management in the treatment of complex pilon fractures. J Orthop Trauma 1999;13:78–84.
20. Stannard JP, Volgas DA, McGwin G III, et al. Incisional negative pressure wound therapy after high-risk lower extremity fractures. J Orthop Trauma 2012;26(1):37–42.
21. Teeny SM, Wiss DA. Open reduction and internal fixation of tibial plafond fractures. Variables contributing to poor results and complications. Clin Orthop Relat Res 1993;292:108–117.
22. Tornetta P III, Gorup J. Axial computed tomography of pilon fractures. Clin Orthop Relat Res 1996;(323):273–276.
23. White TO, Guy P, Cooke CJ, et al. The results of early primary open reduction and internal fixation for treatment of OTA 43.C-type tibial pilon fractures: a cohort study. J Orthop Trauma 2010;24:757–763.

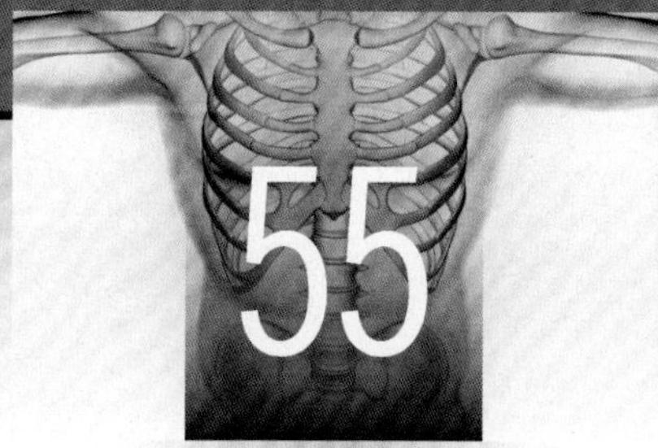

CHAPTER 55

Open Reduction and Internal Fixation of the Medial and Lateral Malleoli

Christopher Del Balso and David W. Sanders

DEFINITION

- The ankle is a modified hinge joint, which relies on a congruently reduced mortise to provide optimal function.
- Maintenance of normal tibiotalar contact is essential if one is to maintain function.
- Surgical treatment of displaced, unstable ankle fractures centers on anatomic restoration of the bony and ligamentous relationships that make up the ankle mortise.[12]
- This chapter focuses on the treatment of a specific pattern of injury to the ankle, specifically, the bimalleolar fracture pattern.

ANATOMY

- The anatomy of the distal tibia and ankle joint must be taken into account when considering ankle fractures. As the tibial shaft flares in the supramalleolar region, the dense cortical bone changes to metaphyseal cancellous bone **(FIG 1A)**.
- The shape of the tibial articular surface is concave, with distal extension of the anterior and posterior lips.
  - This surface has been called the *tibial plafond*, which is French for ceiling.
- The talar dome is wedge-shaped and sits within the mortise. It is wider anteriorly than posteriorly.
- The medial end of the tibia is the medial malleolus.
  - The medial malleolus is composed of the anterior and posterior colliculi, separated by the intercollicular groove **(FIG 1B)**.
  - The anterior colliculus is the narrower and most distal portion of the medial malleolus and serves as the origin of the superficial deltoid ligaments.
  - The intercollicular groove and the posterior colliculus, which is broader than the anterior colliculus, provide the origin of the deep deltoid ligaments.
  - The insertions of the deltoid ligaments (medial tubercle of the talus, navicular tuberosity, and sustentaculum tali) can also be considered as part of the medial malleolar osteoligamentous complex.
- The lateral malleolus is the distal end of the fibula. It extends approximately 1 cm distally and posteriorly compared to the medial malleolus.
- The syndesmotic ligament complex unites the distal fibula with the distal tibia. The following ligaments make up the syndesmotic complex: the anteroinferior tibiofibular ligament, the posteroinferior tibiofibular ligament, the inferior transverse ligament, and the interosseous ligament **(FIG 1C)**.

PATHOGENESIS

- The majority of bimalleolar ankle fractures are secondary to rotation of the body about a supinated or pronated foot. They are best defined by the classification of Lauge-Hansen **(FIG 2)**.[5]
- The supination–external rotation pattern of ankle fracture is divided into four stages.
  - The stage I injury is tearing of the anteroinferior tibiofibular ligaments.
  - As the external rotation force continues laterally, a spiral fracture of the fibula occurs. On lateral radiograph, the fracture line will pass from the anteroinferior cortex to the posterosuperior cortex.
  - The third stage occurs when the posteroinferior tibiofibular ligaments avulse or fracture off the posterior malleolus.
  - The final stage results in a medial malleolar osteoligamentous complex injury with either a deep deltoid ligament tear or a fracture of the medial malleolus.
- The pronation–external rotation variant also has four stages. Because of the pronated position of the foot at injury, however, the medial structures are injured in the early stages.
  - The fibula fracture pattern seen with this mechanism is usually suprasyndesmotic, and the fracture pattern is an anterosuperior to posteroinferior fracture line as seen on the lateral radiograph.
- The supination–adduction pattern is heralded by a low transverse fibular fracture and a vertical shearing pattern medially. This pattern is also associated with tibial plafond impaction.
- Finally, the pronation–abduction pattern is identified by the avulsion of the medial malleolus and a transverse or laterally comminuted fibular fracture above the syndesmosis secondary to a direct bending moment.

PATIENT HISTORY AND PHYSICAL FINDINGS

- Most patients who present with ankle pain following trauma will describe a twisting type of injury. Less frequently, they will report a direct blow to the ankle.
- Proper medical history should include the patient's current comorbid medical conditions, such as peripheral vascular disease, diabetes, or peripheral neuropathy.
- Physical examination should center on inspection, palpation, and neurovascular examination.
  - It is important to note any gross deformity, which may signify dislocation. If dislocation is present, the ankle should be reduced and splinted as soon as possible to prevent skin tenting (and subsequent skin necrosis) and neurovascular compromise.

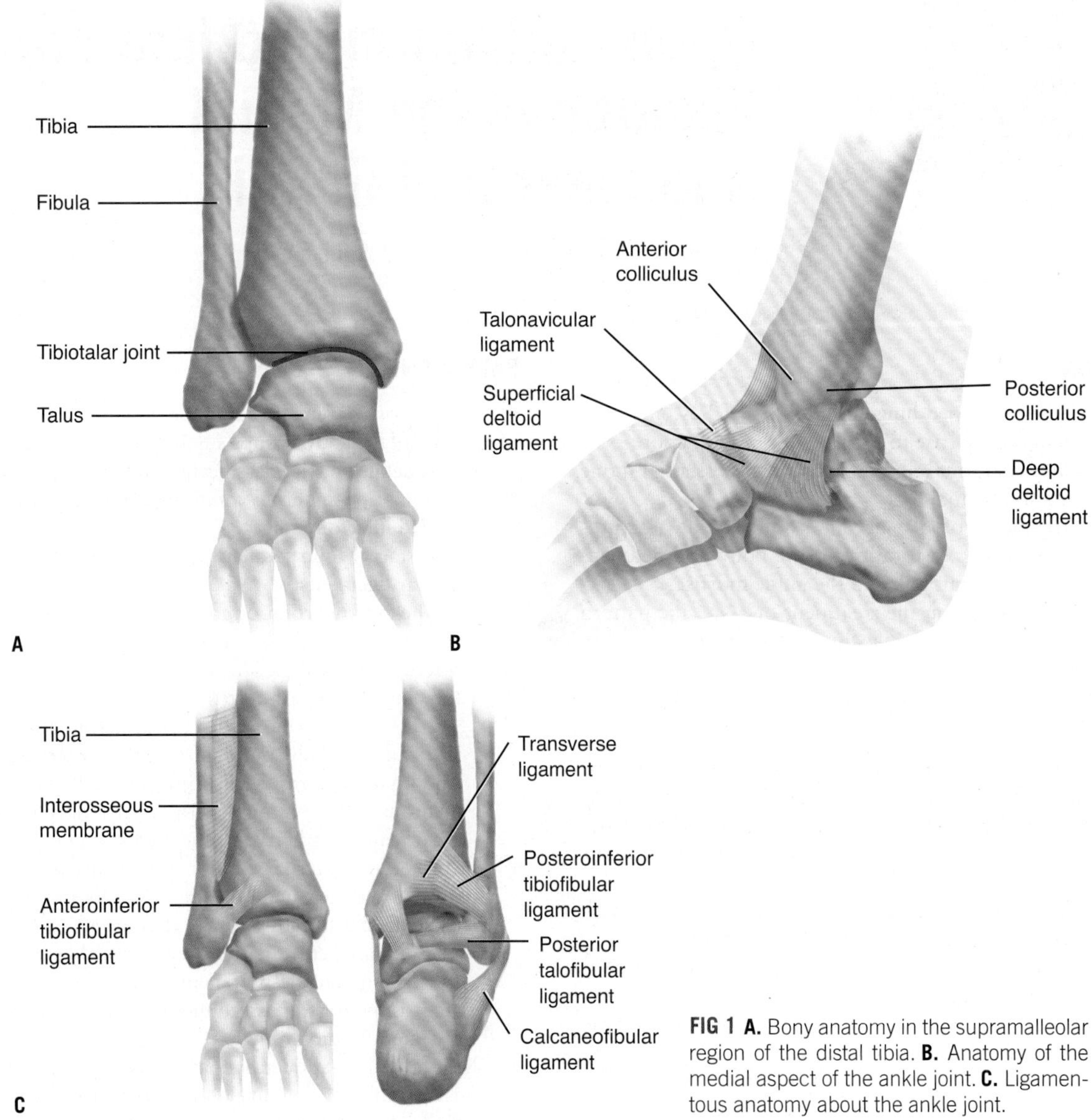

FIG 1 A. Bony anatomy in the supramalleolar region of the distal tibia. **B.** Anatomy of the medial aspect of the ankle joint. **C.** Ligamentous anatomy about the ankle joint.

- Inspection for any open wound about the ankle is critical as well. Open fractures imply a surgical urgency. Swelling, ecchymosis, and tenderness about the malleoli should be recorded.
- For patients with a supination–external rotation pattern isolated fibula fracture who present with an intact mortise, the stress examination can be revealing. Stress views are performed through external rotation of the foot with the ankle in dorsiflexion and the leg stabilized or by supporting the patient's leg with a pillow or cushion and allowing the ankle to rotate with the force of gravity. Greater than 4 mm of medial clear space widening in association with a lateral malleolus fracture signifies an unstable pattern.[7,9,17]
- Weight-bearing radiographs may alternatively be obtained in supination–external rotation patterns with isolated fibula fracture. Radiographs should be obtained 7 to 10 days following injury. Increased medial clear space relative to superior joint space indicates an unstable fracture.[1]
- Pain at the ankle along the syndesmosis during a squeeze test implies injury to the syndesmosis.
- The proximal fibula, knee, and tibia should also be examined. Palpation of pulses, detection of capillary refill, and a careful neurosensory examination must be documented prior to manipulation.

IMAGING AND OTHER DIAGNOSTIC STUDIES

- Radiographic examination includes the ankle trauma series: anteroposterior (AP), lateral, and mortise view **(FIG 3A–C)**.
- In patients with isolated lateral malleolar fractures with clinical signs of medial injury, or if there is any question of ankle stability in a supination–external rotation fracture pattern, a manual external rotation stress test, gravity stress radiograph, or weight-bearing radiographs should be obtained to assess for instability.[1,2,7]
  - The tibia is held internally rotated 15 degrees with the ankle in dorsiflexion to produce a gentle external rotation moment at the ankle under fluoroscopy **(FIG 3D)**.[11] Greater than 4 mm of medial clear space widening that is more than 1 mm greater than the superior joint space

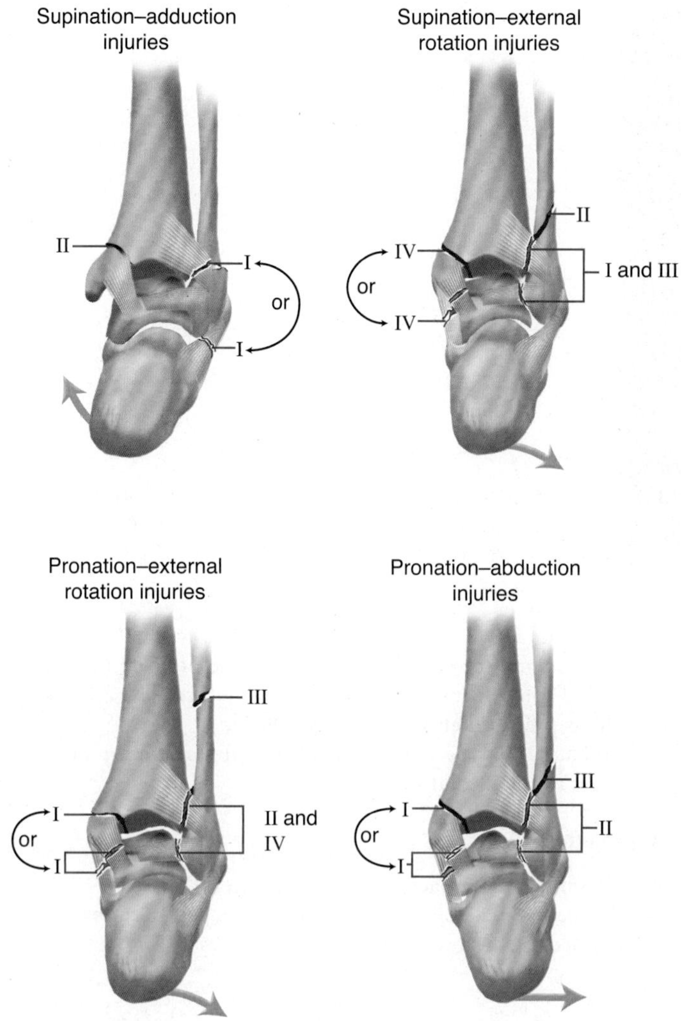

FIG 2 Lauge-Hansen classification of ankle fractures. *Arrows* (pink) indicate direction of applied stress/force.

in association with a lateral malleolus fracture signifies an unstable pattern **(FIG 3E)**.

- At 7 to 10 days postinjury, weight-bearing radiographs may be obtained. Increased medial clear space relative to superior joint space on the mortise view indicates an unstable fracture pattern.[1]
- If clinically warranted, full-length tibia–fibula radiographs should be obtained.
- Restoration of medial ankle stability depends on the size and location of the medial malleolar fragment.
  - The size of the medial fragment is key to stability.
  - Anterior collicular fractures only have the superficial deltoid attached. In about 25% of supination–external rotation type 4 injuries, there will be an associated deep deltoid rupture.[10] Thus, fixation of this fragment will not enhance stability.
  - The lateral radiograph is the key. If the fragment is greater than 2.8 cm wide (supracollicular fracture), the deep deltoid will be attached, and stability is restored after fixation. If the fragment is less than 1.7 cm wide (anterior collicular or intercollicular fracture), then stability is not restored with fixation. For fractures in between, an intraoperative external rotation stress examination should be performed following malleolar fixation.
- Computed tomography (CT) scanning may be helpful in assessing posterior malleolar fragment size in rotational ankle fractures (see Chap. 56).
- Magnetic resonance imaging may have some use if there is an isolated lateral malleolus fracture with signs of medial injury and an equivocal stress examination.

DIFFERENTIAL DIAGNOSIS

- Ankle sprain
- Lateral malleolus fracture
- Medial malleolus fracture
- Maisonneuve fracture
- Bimalleolar ankle fracture
- Trimalleolar ankle fracture
- Lateral process talus fracture
- Anterior process calcaneus fracture
- Subtalar dislocation

NONOPERATIVE MANAGEMENT

- Ankle fractures in which the ankle mortise remains stable can be treated nonoperatively.
  - Isolated lateral malleolus fractures without evidence of medial-sided injury are considered supination–external rotation type 2 injuries and can be treated with functional bracing and weight bearing as tolerated.

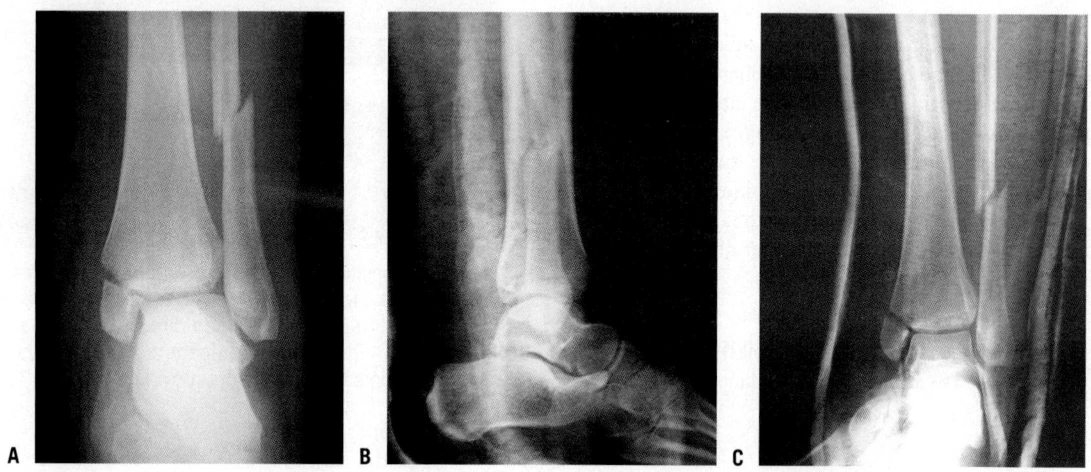

FIG 3 Radiographic evaluation with an ankle trauma series: AP (**A**), lateral (**B**), and mortise (**C**) views. *(continued)*

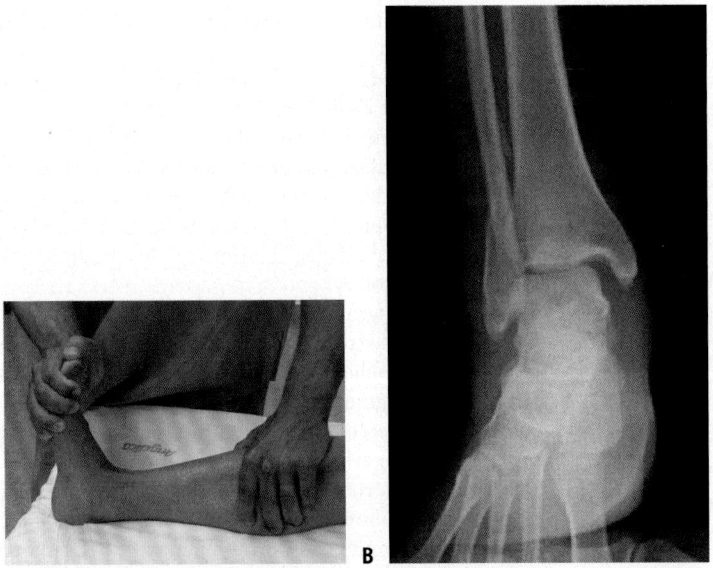

A B

FIG 3 *(continued)* Clinical (**D**) and radiographic (**E**) demonstration of a physician-assisted external rotation stress examination of the ankle.

- Unstable patterns, such as supination–external rotation type 4, either ligamentous or a true bimalleolar or trimalleolar ankle fracture, can also be treated nonoperatively in patients who are poor surgical candidates (eg, insulin-dependent diabetics), who have severe soft tissue problems, or who do not wish to undergo surgical stabilization.
- If nonoperative treatment is chosen, it is crucial to ensure anatomic mortise reduction throughout treatment until healing.
- Unstable injuries should be treated in a well-molded short-leg cast and checked on a weekly basis to ensure continued mortise reduction.

SURGICAL MANAGEMENT

- Any fracture of the ankle in which there is residual talar tilt or talar subluxation such that the ankle mortise is not anatomically reduced is an indication for surgical stabilization.

Preoperative Planning

- Surgical anatomy should be reviewed prior to entering the operating room, including the bony and ligamentous structures.
  - The neurovascular anatomy about the ankle should be reviewed, including the course of the saphenous vein medially and the superficial peroneal nerve laterally.
- Equipment to be used includes a small fragment plate and screw set, large pelvic reduction clamps, small-diameter Kirschner wires, and 3.5- to 4.0-mm cannulated screw sets. If the nature of the fracture is still in question, radiographic stress examination may be performed under anesthesia.

Positioning

- The patient is positioned supine with a small bump under the ipsilateral hip to ease access to the fibula.
- A pneumatic tourniquet is applied to the affected thigh if desired for use during the surgical procedure. The affected limb is prepared and draped free **(FIG 4)**.
- The bump may be removed after lateral fixation for easier access to the medial side.

Approach

- The fibula is approached via a direct lateral incision.
- The medial malleolus is approached via a gently curved anteromedial incision.

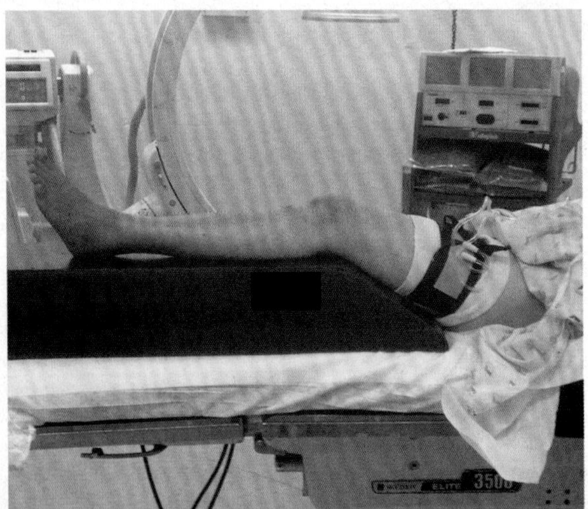

FIG 4 Supine positioning of the injured ankle. A thigh tourniquet is applied, a rolled sheet bump is placed under the hip to internally rotate the leg, so the patella is pointed directly anterior, and the ankle is elevated on an inclined bump (foam bump or sheets) to allow for lateral fluoroscopic images without moving the ankle.

DIRECT LATERAL APPROACH TO THE FIBULA

Exposure

- The incision is kept just off the posterior border of the fibula but may be adjusted slightly based on soft tissue considerations **(TECH FIG 1A)**.
  - Deeper tissues are incised in line with the skin incision **(TECH FIG 1B)**.
  - Care must be taken proximally in the wound to avoid injury to the superficial peroneal nerve, which crosses the field about 7 cm proximal to the distal tip of the fibula **(TECH FIG 1C)**.
- Next, the peroneal fascia is divided, and the peroneal tendons and musculature are retracted posteriorly.
  - With gentle elevation of the periosteum about the fracture site, the fibula should be exposed.
  - Care should be taken to avoid excessive stripping of fracture fragments as well as iatrogenic disruption of the syndesmotic ligaments as they insert anteriorly on the fibula.

Lateral Plating

- Following exposure of the fracture, the first step involves cleaning the fracture site **(TECH FIG 2A)** followed by fracture reduction.
- Usually, reduction is afforded by a small "lion jaw" clamp or pointed reduction forceps.
  - If reduction is difficult, manual traction with pronation and internal rotation will allow for fracture alignment in supination–external rotation patterns.
  - Care should be taken to avoid placing clamps over fracture spikes to prevent inadvertent comminution **(TECH FIG 2B)**.
- If the clamps make it difficult to place a lag screw, provisional Kirschner wires may be placed across the fracture and the clamps removed **(TECH FIG 2C)**.
- At this point, if a lateral plate is chosen, the lag screw is placed in the anterior to posterior direction, perpendicular to the fracture.
  - If a posterior plate (antiglide) is chosen, the lag screw is placed through the plate in a posterior to anterior direction.
  - In either case, the near cortex is overdrilled with a 3.5-mm drill bit followed by drilling of the far cortex with a 2.5-mm drill bit **(TECH FIG 2D)**.
- The length of the screw is measured, and a self-tapping 3.5-mm screw is placed across the fracture in the screw track.
- Next, a one-third tubular plate is placed directly lateral on the fibula (neutralization) **(TECH FIG 2E)**.
- The proximal screw holes are filled with bicortical 3.5-mm screws after drilling with the 2.5-mm drill bit.
- Distally, unicortical cancellous screws are placed, with care not to penetrate the distal tibia–fibula joint. In osteoporotic bone, locking screws can be used distally (one-third tubular locking plate used in this example) **(TECH FIG 2F,G)**.
- The wound is closed **(TECH FIG 2H)**.

Posterior Antiglide Plating

- The procedure proceeds as for lateral plating until the time of lag screw placement.
- A one-third tubular plate is positioned posteriorly (antiglide), and reduction is afforded by a small "lion jaw" clamp or pointed reduction forceps.
- The lag screw is placed through the plate in a posterior to anterior direction.
  - The near cortex is overdrilled with a 3.5-mm drill bit followed by drilling of the far cortex with a 2.5-mm drill bit.
  - The length of the screw is measured, and a self-tapping 3.5-mm screw is placed across the fracture in the screw track.
- The proximal screw holes are filled with bicortical 3.5-mm screws after drilling with the 2.5-mm drill bit.
- Distally, bicortical 3.5-mm screws can be placed as the posterior to anterior trajectory reduces the risk of intra-articular penetration.
- The wound is closed.

Obtaining Fibular Length

- In cases in which the fibula is significantly shortened (high-energy, late presentation of fracture in which callus is present), adjunctive techniques may be necessary to achieve anatomic fibular length.
  - A small bone distractor can be placed proximally to the plate in the proximal segment and through the plate in the distal segment with appropriate distraction applied to achieve fibular length **(TECH FIG 3A)**.
  - Alternatively, a laterally placed fibular plate can be secured to the distal segment with a screw and a push–pull screw (3.5-mm cortical screw) can be placed proximal to the plate in the proximal segment. A laminar spreader can then be used to push the proximal end of the plate distally, which will then distract the fracture site to the appropriate fibular length **(TECH FIG 3B)**.
  - Fibular length assessment may be performed intraoperatively using fluoroscopy. Three measurements are used to ascertain whether the correct fibular length has been restored. They are the talocrural angle,[16] the tibiofibular (or Shenton) line,[8] and the dime sign.[18]

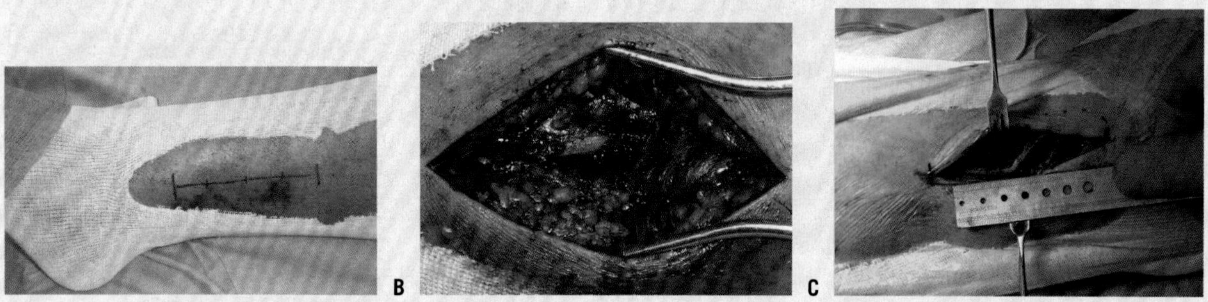

A B C

TECH FIG 1 Surgical approach to the fibula, directly lateral. **A.** Skin incision marked out just along the posterior border of the fibula, centered about the level of the fracture. **B.** Incision through the peroneal (lateral compartment) fascia, exposing the fracture site. **C.** Identification of the superficial peroneal nerve as it crosses proximally in the wound.

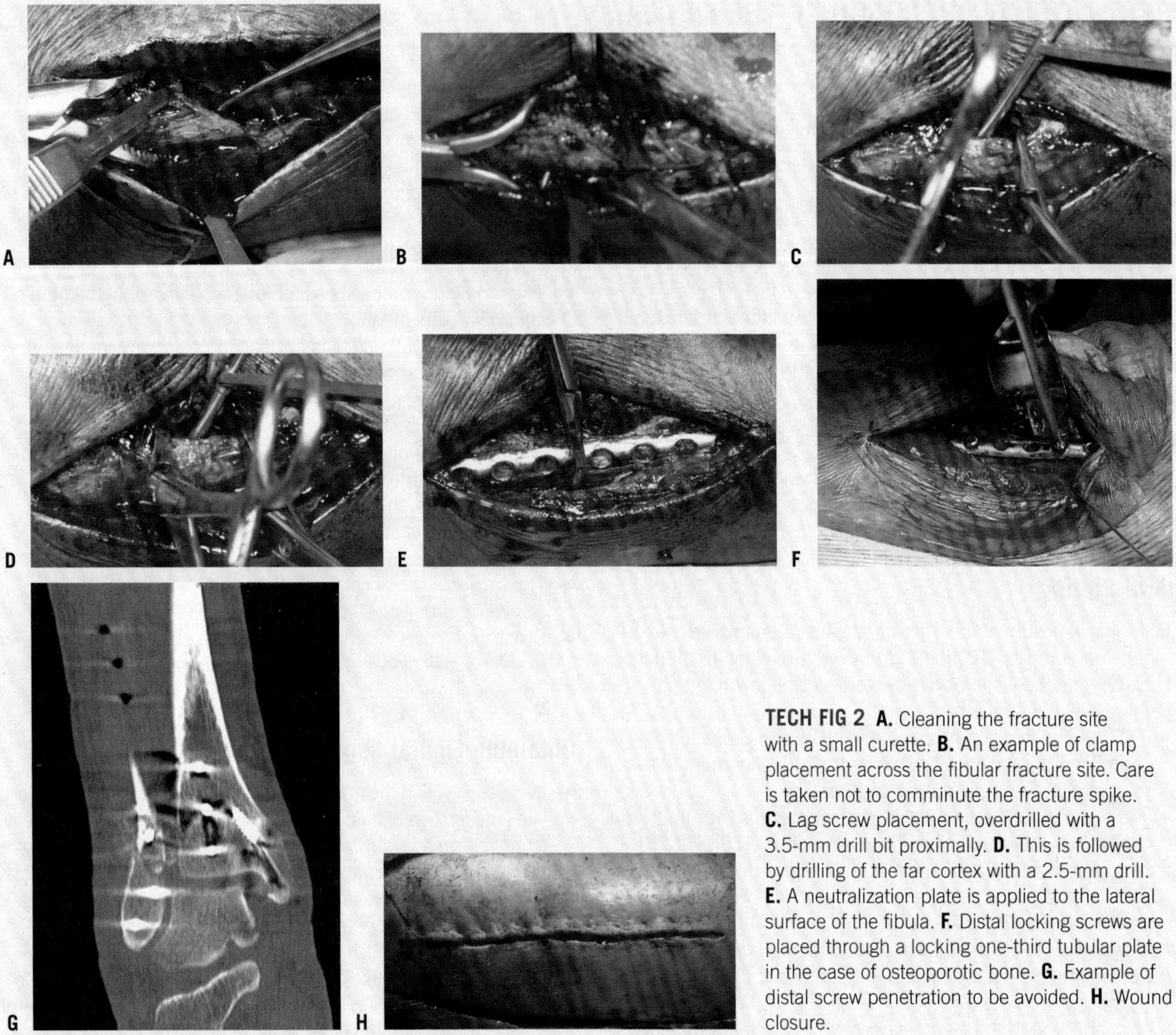

TECH FIG 2 A. Cleaning the fracture site with a small curette. **B.** An example of clamp placement across the fibular fracture site. Care is taken not to comminute the fracture spike. **C.** Lag screw placement, overdrilled with a 3.5-mm drill bit proximally. **D.** This is followed by drilling of the far cortex with a 2.5-mm drill. **E.** A neutralization plate is applied to the lateral surface of the fibula. **F.** Distal locking screws are placed through a locking one-third tubular plate in the case of osteoporotic bone. **G.** Example of distal screw penetration to be avoided. **H.** Wound closure.

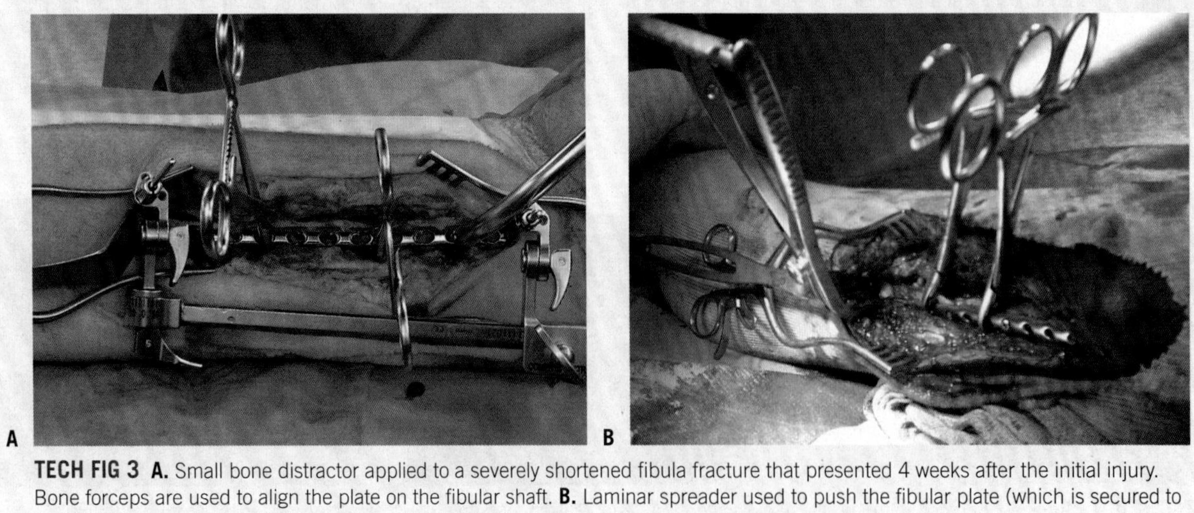

TECH FIG 3 A. Small bone distractor applied to a severely shortened fibula fracture that presented 4 weeks after the initial injury. Bone forceps are used to align the plate on the fibular shaft. **B.** Laminar spreader used to push the fibular plate (which is secured to the distal fragment only) distally causing distraction at the fracture site.

ANTEROMEDIAL APPROACH TO THE MEDIAL MALLEOLUS

Exposure

- The medial malleolus is approached via a gently curved anteromedial incision **(TECH FIG 4A)**.
  - An incision is made parallel to the saphenous vein that is either concave anteriorly or concave posteriorly to allow visualization of the anteromedial joint.
- After dissection of the skin, the subcutaneous tissues should be carefully dissected to prevent injury to the saphenous vein and nerve **(TECH FIG 4B)**.
- With the dissection carried down sharply to the bone, the periosteum is elevated for 1 mm proximally and distally.
- The fracture should be booked open to allow visual inspection of the talar dome for chondral injury.
- The joint and medial gutter should be irrigated through the fracture for any loose hematoma or debris that may impede reduction **(TECH FIG 4C)**.

Operative Stabilization

- Following exposure, the medial malleolar fragment (usually one large piece) can be reduced with the aid of a dental tool or small, pointed reduction clamp **(TECH FIG 5A)**.
- The fragment can be provisionally stabilized with small-diameter (1.25-mm) Kirschner wires placed in parallel. Alternatively, two 2.5-mm drill bits can be used to drill paths for two parallel screws, leaving the drill bits in place to gain rotational control of the malleolar fragment **(TECH FIG 5B)**.
- After radiographic documentation of the reduction and wire placement, cannulated screws of appropriate length may be placed over the wires after drilling of the out cortices with a cannulated drill. Alternatively, noncannulated screws may be used independent of the provisional stabilization.
- Usually, 4.0-mm partially threaded cancellous screws can be placed. Alternatively, two bicortical 3.5-mm screws placed in lag mode.[14]
- Two screws are recommended for rotational control. If the fragment is too small, however, one screw may suffice owing to the inherent stability of the undulating fracture line.
- Countersinking the screw heads medially may help to alleviate painful prominent hardware.
- Comminuted fractures that are not amenable to screw fixation may benefit from a small buttress plate or a "suture tension band" technique using the deltoid ligament for fixation.
  - The suture or wire tension band is anchored about a more proximal screw placed parallel to the articular surface.

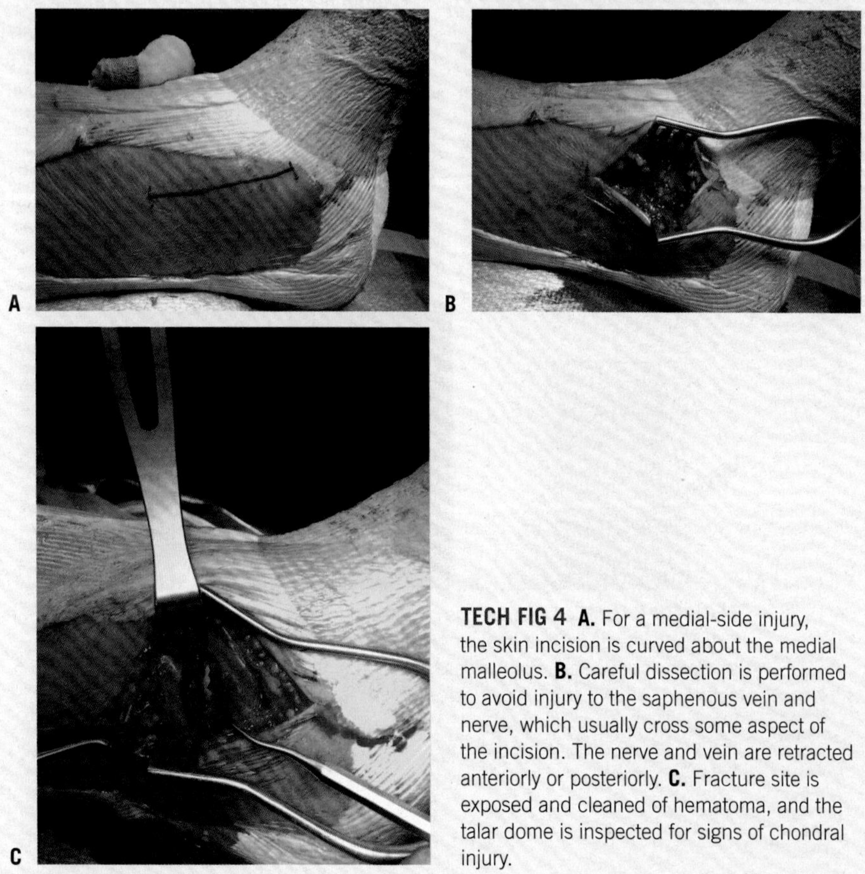

TECH FIG 4 **A.** For a medial-side injury, the skin incision is curved about the medial malleolus. **B.** Careful dissection is performed to avoid injury to the saphenous vein and nerve, which usually cross some aspect of the incision. The nerve and vein are retracted anteriorly or posteriorly. **C.** Fracture site is exposed and cleaned of hematoma, and the talar dome is inspected for signs of chondral injury.

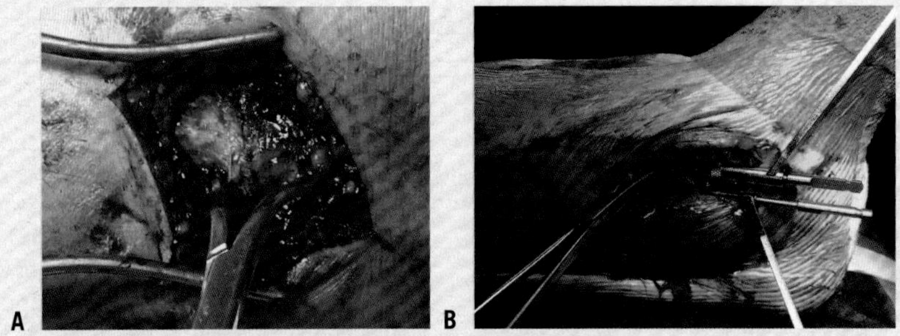

TECH FIG 5 **A.** Reduction is achieved with a pointed reduction clamp. **B.** Two 2.5-mm drills are placed across the fracture site in parallel fashion and left in place to maintain rotational control. One drill is left in place as the first partially threaded screw is placed.

Syndesmosis Fixation

- After stabilization of the medial and lateral sides of the ankle, syndesmotic integrity should be assessed.
  - The Cotton test involves providing a lateral force on the fibula with a bone hook or bone clamp **(TECH FIG 6A)**.
  - The stress external rotation test can also be used to assess for syndesmotic integrity.
  - Lateral displacement that allows more than a few millimeters of tibiofibular widening is considered pathologic and an indication for syndesmotic fixation.
  - The lateral radiograph should be scrutinized to assess the relationship of the fibula to the articular surface of the ankle joint. In general, on a true lateral view of the ankle, the tip of the fibula should be anterior to the posterior border of the diaphyseal tibia and comparisons to the contralateral ankle can be assessed.
- With a bolster behind the ankle, a large tenaculum clamp is placed across the tibiofibular joint, with one tine on the distal tibia and the other on the fibula **(TECH FIG 6B)**.
- Reduction is confirmed on the AP, mortise, and lateral radiographic views.
- Although dorsiflexion of the talus has been recommended in the past to prevent overtightening of the syndesmosis, more recent studies have shown that it is virtually impossible to over-tighten an anatomically reduced mortise.
- Direct reduction of the syndesmosis with visualization of the anterior distal fibula seated within the tibial incisura should be performed if there is concern for malreduction.
  - The incidence of syndesmosis malreduction is as high as 40% and is associated with worse functional outcomes.[14,15]
- Fixation choices range from one or two screws, with three or four cortices drilled and 3.5- or 4.5-mm screw diameters used. Although the size and number of screws remain controversial, some parameters are agreed on.
  - Screws can be placed adjacent to the joint and, as they are positional, do not need to be parallel to the joint.
  - The screw should not be placed in lag mode.
  - If a lateral plate is used, the screw is placed through one of the distal holes.
  - If a posterior plate is used, the syndesmosis screw(s) are placed outside the plate on the lateral cortex.

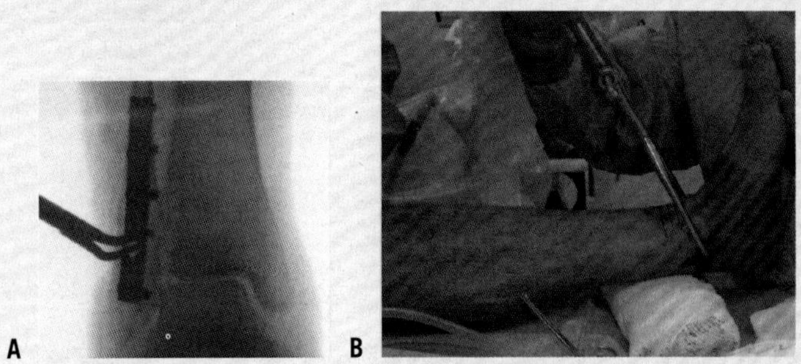

TECH FIG 6 **A.** The Cotton test is performed following fibular fixation by pulling laterally with a hook or clamp to assess the integrity of the syndesmosis. **B.** Reduction and stabilization of the syndesmosis is achieved with a clamp placed across the distal tibiofibular joint and a bump placed under the leg.

Pearls and Pitfalls

Damage or Entrapment of Superficial Peroneal Nerve	• Care must be taken to expose and mobilize the nerve proximally if in the surgical field **(FIG 5A)**. This will help minimize the chance of damage during surgery and closure.
Failure to Obtain Fibular Length	• This will lead to persistent medial widening. • A plate is used to push the distal fragment with a laminar spreader. The distal tibiofibular anatomic relationship is assessed, and the contralateral ankle is used for comparison.
Presence of Osteoporotic Bone	• Supplementary Kirschner wires • Multiple syndesmosis screws • Posteriorly placed fibula plate with bicortical screws proximal and distal to fracture • Locked plate
Intra-articular Hardware Penetration	• Careful intraoperative radiographic assessment is important. • Distal screws in the lateral fibular plate must be unicortical. • AP radiograph is best to evaluate medial malleolus fixation.
Malreduction of the Syndesmosis	• Bolster is placed under ankle, not the foot, as this will cause anterior displacement **(FIG 5B)**. • A good lateral radiograph is obtained to assess reduction. • It is impossible to overtighten an anatomically reduced syndesmosis.
Fibular Fracture Comminution (Inability to Place a Lag Screw)	• Preoperative recognition of pronation–abduction injuries that can result in regional comminution • Bridge plating with bone grafting • Extraperiosteal bridge plating allows indirect fracture reduction, secondary bone healing, and reduces periosteal striping of comminuted fracture fragments, obviating the need for bone grafting.
Peroneal Tendinitis and Painful Hardware	• Laterally placed fibular hardware is associated with a higher incidence of painful hardware. • Posteriorly placed fibular fixation is associated with a higher incidence of peroneal tendinitis.

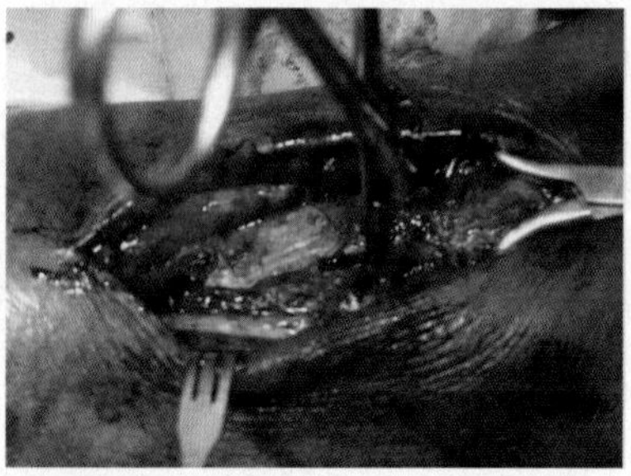

A

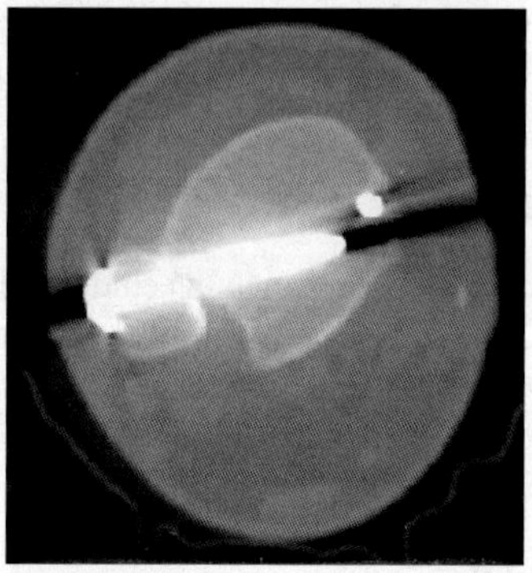

B

FIG 5 A. Identification and protection of the superficial peroneal nerve within the anterior flap. **B.** CT scan showing malreduction of the syndesmosis.

POSTOPERATIVE CARE

- All ankles should be splinted in the neutral position and elevated for at least 24 hours postoperatively.
- The postoperative splint is removed at 10 or 14 days, and sutures are removed.
- Patients are then placed into a removable functional brace or cast boot that allows them to begin early active-assisted and passive range of ankle motion.
- All patients are kept non–weight bearing for at least 6 weeks.
- At 6 weeks, patients are progressed to weight bearing as tolerated based on radiographic criteria.
  - Weight bearing can be delayed for slow healing and presence of a syndesmotic screw. In general, weight-bearing status is not delayed because of syndesmotic injury, and syndesmosis screw removal is not routine prior to progression to weight bearing as tolerated, but patients should be advised of the possibility of screw breakage following weight bearing.[6]
- Patients are restricted from operating an automobile for 9 weeks following right-sided ankle fracture.[3]

OUTCOMES

- One year after ankle fracture surgery, patients generally do well, with most experiencing little or mild pain and few restrictions in functional activities. They have significant improvement in function compared with 6 months after surgery.
  - Younger age, male sex, absence of diabetes, and a lower American Society of Anesthesia class are predictive of functional recovery at 1 year following ankle fracture surgery.[4]

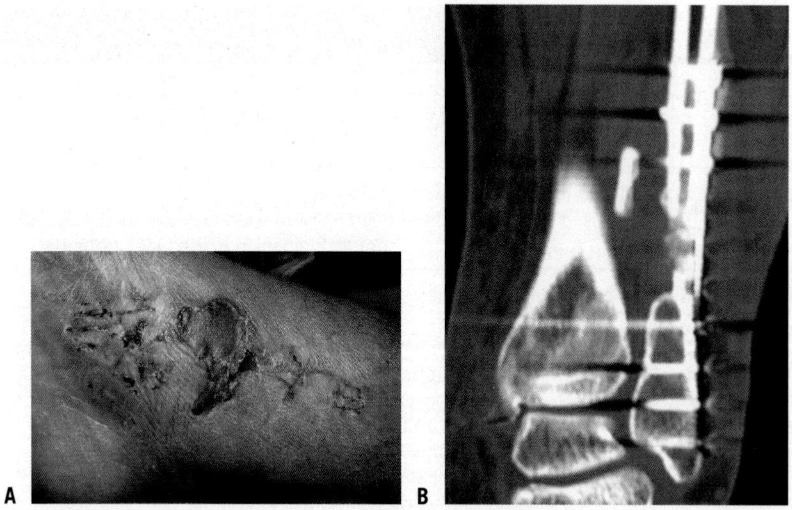

FIG 6 **A.** Skin necrosis and slough following surgical intervention. **B.** CT scan demonstrating fibular nonunion at 6 months following open reduction and internal fixation of a pronation–abduction injury.

  - It is important to counsel patients and their families on the expected outcome after injury with regard to functional recovery.
- Looking specifically at elderly patients (older than 60 years), functional outcomes steadily improved over 1 year of follow-up, albeit at a slower rate than in the younger patients.[4]
  - Operative fixation of unstable ankle fractures in the elderly can provide a reasonable functional result at the 1-year follow-up.

COMPLICATIONS

- Minor complications include epidermolysis **(FIG 6A)**, superficial infection, and peroneal tendinitis with painful hardware.[13]
- Major problems include nonunion **(FIG 6B)**, hardware failure, deep infection, and compartment syndrome.[13]

REFERENCES

1. Dawe EJ, Shafafy R, Quayle J, et al. The effect of different methods of stability assessment on fixation rate and complications in supination external rotation (SER) 2/4 ankle fractures. Foot Ankle Surg 2015;21(2):86–90.
2. Egol KA, Amirtharajah M, Tejwani NC, et al. Ankle stress test for predicting the need for surgical fixation of isolated fibular fractures. J Bone Joint Surg Am 2004;86(11):2393–2398.
3. Egol KA, Sheikhazadeh A, Mogatederi S, et al. Lower-extremity function for driving an automobile after operative treatment of ankle fracture. J Bone Joint Surg Am 2003;85(7):1185–1189.
4. Egol KA, Tejwani NC, Walsh MG, et al. Predictors of short-term functional outcome following ankle fracture surgery. J Bone Joint Surg Am 2006;88(5):974–979.
5. Lauge-Hansen N. Fractures of the ankle. II. Combined experimental-surgical and experimental-roentgenologic investigations. Arch Surg 1950;60(5):957–985.
6. Manjoo A, Sanders DW, Tieszer C, et al. Functional and radiographic results of patients with syndesmotic screw fixation: implications for screw removal. J Orthop Trauma 2010;24(1):2–6.
7. McConnell T, Creevy W, Tornetta P III. Stress examination of supination external rotation-type fibular fractures. J Bone Joint Surg Am 2004;86(10):2171–2178.
8. Morris M, Chandler R. Fractures of the ankle. Tech Orthop 1987;2(3):10–19.
9. Pakarinen H, Flinkkilä T, Ohtonen P, et al. Intraoperative assessment of the stability of the distal tibiofibular joint in supination-external rotation injuries of the ankle: sensitivity, specificity, and reliability of two clinical tests. J Bone Joint Surg Am 2011;93(22):2057–2061.
10. Pankovich AM, Shivaram MS. Anatomical basis of variability in injuries of the medial malleolus and the deltoid ligament. I. Anatomical studies. Acta Orthop Scand 1979;50(2):217–223.
11. Park SS, Kubiak EN, Egol KA, et al. Stress radiographs after ankle fracture: the effect of ankle position and deltoid ligament status on medial clear space measurements. J Orthop Trauma 2006;20(1):11–18.
12. Pettrone FA, Gail M, Pee D, et al. Quantitative criteria for prediction of the results after displaced fracture of the ankle. J Bone Joint Surg Am 1983;65(5):667–677.
13. Phillips WA, Schwartz HS, Keller CS, et al. A prospective, randomized study of the management of severe ankle fractures. J Bone Joint Surg Am 1985;67(1):67–78.
14. Ricci WM, Tornetta P, Borrelli J Jr. Lag screw fixation of medial malleolar fractures: a biomechanical, radiographic, and clinical comparison of unicortical partially threaded lag screws and bicortical fully threaded lag screws. J Orthop Trauma 2012;26(10):602–606.
15. Sagi HC, Shah AR, Sanders RW. The functional consequence of syndesmotic joint malreduction at a minimum 2-year follow-up. J Orthop Trauma 2012;26(7):439–443.
16. Sarkisian JS, Cody GW. Closed treatment of ankle fractures: a new criterion for evaluation—a review of 250 cases. J Trauma 1976;16(4):323–326.
17. Seidel A, Krause F, Weber M. Weightbearing vs gravity stress radiographs for stability evaluation of supination-external rotation fractures of the ankle. Foot Ankle Int 2017;38(7):736–744.
18. Weber BG, Simpson LA. Corrective lengthening osteotomy of the fibula. Clin Orthop Relat Res 1985;(199):61–67.

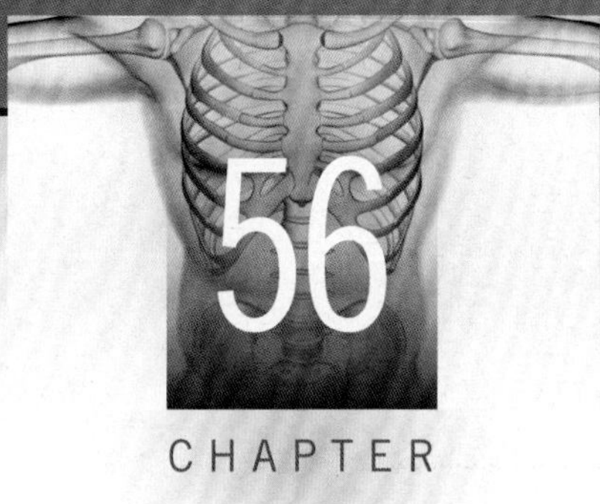

CHAPTER 56

Surgical Management of Posterior Malleolus Fractures

Malcolm R. DeBaun, L. Henry Goodnough, Sean T. Campbell, Thomas Githens, and Michael J. Gardner

DEFINITION

- The ankle is a modified hinge joint and relies on a congruent tibiotalar joint to provide optimal function.
- The posterior lip of the tibial plafond extends distally in the sagittal plane and forms the posterior malleolus or Volkmann tubercle.
- The posterior malleolus is important for tibiotalar articular congruence and syndesmotic stability.

ANATOMY

- The anatomy of the distal tibia and ankle joint must be taken into account when considering ankle fractures (**FIG 1**). As the tibial shaft flares in the supramalleolar region, the dense cortical bone changes to metaphyseal cancellous bone.
- The shape of the tibial articular surface is concave, with distal extension of the anterior and posterior lips.
- The posterior malleolus is the posterior aspect of the tibial plafond and contains an attachment point of the postero-inferior tibiotalar ligament (PITFL), a component of the syndesmosis.
- The PITFL is composed of a deep and superficial ligament and originates from the posterior malleolus and runs laterally to insert onto the posterior aspect of the distal fibula.

PATHOGENESIS

- Most posterior malleolar fractures are associated with a rotational ankle injury in a supinated or pronated foot.
- Often, the fibula and possibly the medial malleolus are fractured as the rotational deforming forces propagate around the ankle mortise.
- Lauge-Hansen classification can helpful to extrapolate mechanism of injury and predict intraoperative findings based on foot position at time of injury and vector of rotational force.[11]
    - This classification system fails to describe all fracture patterns about the ankle involving the posterior malleolus and should be interpreted with discernment.[9]
    - Posterior malleolar fractures are implicated in external rotational injury patterns.

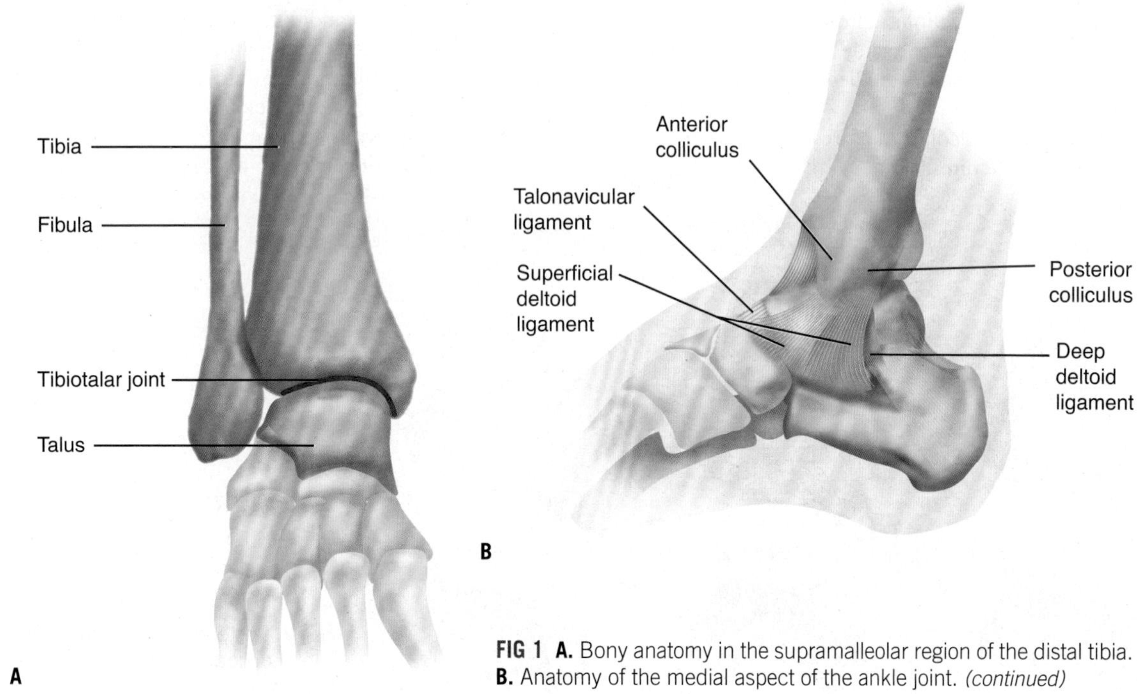

FIG 1 **A.** Bony anatomy in the supramalleolar region of the distal tibia. **B.** Anatomy of the medial aspect of the ankle joint. *(continued)*

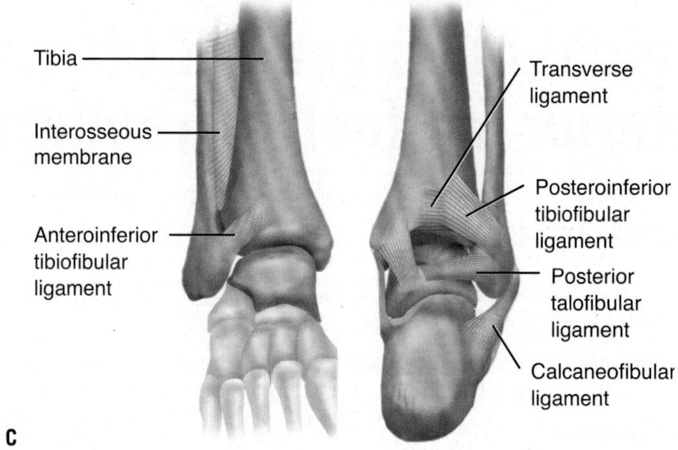

FIG 1 *(continued)* **C.** Ligamentous anatomy about the ankle joint.

- The supination–external rotation variant is divided into four stages:
  - Stage 1: rupture of the anteroinferior tibiofibular ligaments
  - Stage 2: spiral fracture of the fibula at level of syndesmosis
  - Stage 3: posterior malleolus fracture with an intact PITFL attachment or PITFL rupture
  - Stage 4: medial malleolus fracture or deep deltoid injury
- The pronation–external rotation variant also has four stages. Because of the pronated position of the foot at injury, however, the medial structures are injured initially.
  - Stage 1: medial malleolus fracture or deep deltoid injury
  - Stage 2: anteroinferior tibiofibular ligament rupture
  - Stage 3: spiral fracture of fibula above level of syndesmosis
  - Stage 4: Posterior malleolus is fractured with an intact PITFL attachment or the PITFL ruptures without posterior malleolus fracture.
- Some posterior malleolar fractures are also associated with a supination plantarflexion injury. This typically occurs in combination with an oblique anterior distal to posterior superior fibula fracture at the same level and a more transverse fracture of the posterior malleolus that takes with it a large portion of the joint.
- Isolated posterior malleolar fractures are associated with distal tibia spiral fractures.[4]
- The posterior malleolus can be a significant component of pilon fractures.
- The morphology of the posterior malleolus fracture can be variable **(FIG 2)**.[10]
  - Posterolateral oblique
  - Medial extension
  - Small shell

PATIENT HISTORY AND PHYSICAL FINDINGS

- Most patients who present with a malleolar fracture following a traumatic incident will describe a twisting type of injury. Less frequently, they will report a hyperplantarflexion injury or a direct blow to the ankle.
  - High-energy mechanisms with axial load to the ankle can lead to pilon injuries, which may have posterior malleolar involvement.
- Proper medical history should include the patient's current comorbid medical conditions, such as peripheral vascular disease, diabetes, peripheral neuropathy, and the use of anticoagulation.
- Physical examination should center on inspection, palpation, and neurovascular examination.
  - It is important to note any gross deformity, which may signify dislocation. If dislocation is present, the ankle

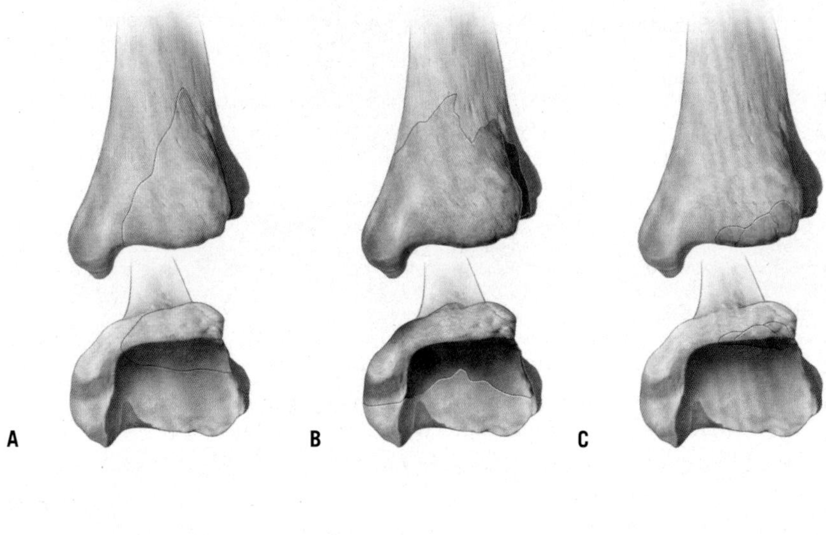

FIG 2 Posterior malleolus variants: posterolateral oblique (**A**), medial extension (**B**), and small shell (**C**).[10]

should be reduced and splinted as soon as possible to prevent skin tenting (and subsequent skin necrosis) and neurovascular compromise.

- Swelling, ecchymosis, and tenderness about the malleoli should be recorded.
  - Soft tissue assessment is critical to inform management with respect to timing of definitive surgery and need for staged fixation for soft tissue rest.
- Inspection for any open wound about the ankle is critical as well. Open fractures imply a surgical urgency. If there is an open fracture, intravenous antibiotics should be administered with verification of updated tetanus vaccination. The wound should be cleared of gross contamination, the fracture is then reduced, sterile dressing is applied, and the limb is splinted.
- The proximal fibula, knee, tibia, and foot should also be examined for external signs of injury and tenderness. Palpation of pulses, detection of capillary refill, and a careful neurosensory examination should be documented prior to manipulation.

IMAGING AND OTHER DIAGNOSTIC STUDIES

- Radiographic examination includes the ankle trauma series: anteroposterior, lateral, and mortise views.
- In the setting of pain and deformity of the leg, full-length orthogonal tibiofibular radiographs should be obtained, which may reveal a distal tibia spiral fracture with concomitant posterior malleolus fracture or a more proximal segmental injury.
- If a posterior malleolus fracture is diagnosed on radiographs or suspected secondary to mechanism (rotational injury resulting in distal third spiral tibia fracture), postreduction and splinting computed tomography (CT) of the injured ankle is recommended.
  - CT scans, especially axial and sagittal cuts, can be helpful to understand the morphology of the posterior malleolus fracture, and thus, inform the approach and reduction strategy.[2,10]
  - Presence of intercalated fragments, displacement, degree of comminution, articular impaction, and fracture obliquity can be assessed preoperatively for planning.

DIFFERENTIAL DIAGNOSIS

- Ankle sprain
- Lateral malleolus fracture
- Medial malleolus fracture
- Pilon fracture
- Maisonneuve fracture
- Bimalleolar ankle fracture
- Trimalleolar ankle fracture
- Lateral process talus fracture
- Anterior process calcaneus fracture
- Subtalar dislocation

NONOPERATIVE MANAGEMENT

- Our preference is to treat small posterior malleolar fragments not amenable to buttress plating or lag screw fixation nonoperatively.
  - In this scenario, stable fixation of the fibula with or without syndesmotic fixation (depending on intraoperative stress testing) suffices to stabilize the tibiotalar joint.
  - We do not use a specific percentage of tibial plafond involvement to quantitatively dictate surgical decision making.
- After closed reduction, a short-leg splint is applied and molded to hold the reduction.
  - The ankle is preferably splinted in neutral position.
  - However, there are certain fracture patterns (eg, those with a large posterior malleolus fragment and posterior tibiotalar instability) that may benefit from slight plantarflexion temporarily to relax the pull of the gastrocnemius–soleus complex, thus preventing posterior subluxation of the tibiotalar joint. This should be confirmed with postreduction radiographs.
- A repeat postreduction neurovascular examination should be documented.

SURGICAL MANAGEMENT

- Definitive indications for operative management of posterior malleolar fractures are controversial.
- Timing of surgery is dependent on status of the soft tissues and energy of the injury.
  - Either before significant swelling that precludes skin closure and/or fracture blister formation
  - After edema has subsided and/or fracture blisters have epithelized and skin about the ankle wrinkles when pinched
  - Lower energy rotational injuries without a dislocation often have less dramatic soft tissue injury and may be amendable to early definitive fixation.
- General principles to guide surgical decision making
  - Restore articular congruity.
  - Remove intraarticular debris
  - Reduction of the syndesmosis by restoring position of the posterior complex
  - Stabilization of syndesmosis (attachment of PITFL and restoration of incisura anatomy)
  - Prevent posterior tibiotalar instability.
  - Preserve biology while achieving stable fixation to allow for early functional rehabilitation.

Preoperative Planning

- Preoperative CT scanning is helpful to guide management.
  - Determine degree of articular injury.
  - Intercalated fracture fragments that would interfere with indirect reduction techniques may guide surgeon towards an open reduction.
  - Axial images can inform surgical approach.
    - If there is medial extension or obliquity, a posteromedial approach may be chosen.
  - Minimally or nondisplaced posterior malleolar fractures identified on CT may benefit from either nonoperative treatment or indirect reduction techniques and percutaneous lag screw fixation to avoid unnecessary biologic cost associated with formal open reduction methods.
  - Size and morphology of the fragment can inform fixation strategy.
- Surgical anatomy should be reviewed prior to entering the operating room, including the bony and ligamentous structures that will be encountered, fracture pattern, and obliquity.

- The neurovascular anatomy about the ankle should be reviewed, including the course of the saphenous vein and nerve medially and the superficial peroneal nerve laterally as well as the posteromedial neurovascular bundle and sural nerve depending on the approach.
- If other malleoli are fractured, the order of reduction and fixation should be planned preoperatively.
- Methods for reduction and provisional fixation should be planned, with backup plans available.
- Perfect mortise and lateral of the well leg can be taken prior to prep and drape for later comparison, especially if a syndesmotic injury is suspected.
- Preoperative CT scan should be scrutinized to determine approach, reduction, and fixation strategy.
- Equipment typically used includes small pointed reduction clamps, ball-spike pushers, sharp hooks/dental picks, and elevators for reduction; Kirschner wires (K-wires) for provisional fixation; small and minifragment plates and screws for definitive (or provisional) fixation.

Positioning

- Radiolucent cantilever table
- Thigh tourniquet per surgeon preference
- Supine ("floppy lateral")
  - Posterolateral approach
    - Ipsilateral hip bump
    - Operative leg placed on foam wedge or blanket ramp to facilitate lateral intraoperative imaging and leg rotation
    - Table can be airplaned toward contralateral leg to facilitate access.
  - Posteromedial approach
    - No hip bump or contralateral bump
    - Operative leg placed on foam wedge or blanket ramp to facilitate lateral intraoperative imaging
    - Table can be tilted down toward ipsilateral leg, hip can be externally rotated, or, occasionally, knee can be flexed to facilitate additional access.
- Prone (posterolateral or posteromedial approach) is the preferred position, particularly if the fracture has comminution that benefits from an open reduction.
  - Bump contralateral pelvis while prone to internally rotate operative leg and facilitate prone lateral and mortise view and exposure of medial malleolus
  - Ankle positioned on the end of the table with foot hanging free for intraoperative dorsiflexion and anterior translation
    - A sterile pillow or towel bump can be placed anterior to the ankle to facilitate more dorsiflexion. Before prepping, a perfect lateral fluoroscopic view should be obtained with an anterior translator force on the foot to make sure that the contralateral ankle does not block the view.
  - Care must be taken to ensure adequate padding of all bony prominences including knees and elbows.
  - Shoulder flexed/abducted and elbows flexed less than 90 degrees

Approach

- Posterolateral approach[17]
  - Most common approach for posterolateral malleolar fractures
  - Posterolateral aspect of fibula and posterior malleolus can be exposed for reduction and fixation through same skin incision.
  - Can be performed prone (recommended) or supine depending on surgeon preference
- Posteromedial approach[1]
  - Indicated for posterior malleolar fractures with medial extension
    - Some posterior malleolar fractures with primarily lateral obliquity can be accessed via a posteromedial approach for reduction, but drilling angles for posterior to anterior screws can be challenging, necessitating alternative fixation techniques (see **TECH FIG 5**).
  - Can be performed supine or prone depending on surgeon preference

TECHNIQUES

EXPOSURE

Posterolateral Approach

- Incision is centered between posterior border of fibula and lateral border of Achilles tendon.
- Blunt dissection is undertaken to the fascia.
  - Care must be taken to avoid injury to the sural nerve, which is superficial and typically lies medially in the distal wound.
- Crural fascia incised sharply to expose interval between peroneal and flexor hallucis longus (FHL) fascia.
  - Avoid incising investing fascia of either muscle group.
  - When done properly, no muscle fibers should be seen.
  - The peroneal tendons can later be retracted laterally for access to the fibula.
- FHL is elevated and retracted medially, exposing the posterior malleolus fracture (**TECH FIG 1**).
  - Peroneal artery bifurcates into anterior perforating peroneal and lateral calcaneal branches on average 8 mm proximal to plafond.
  - The posterior branch lies on the interosseous membrane and is often tethered to the FHL with elevation.
    - Care taken to avoid injury with proximal dissection or implant placement[12]
  - The posterior syndesmotic ligaments are protected by carefully elevating the FHL off the ligaments.

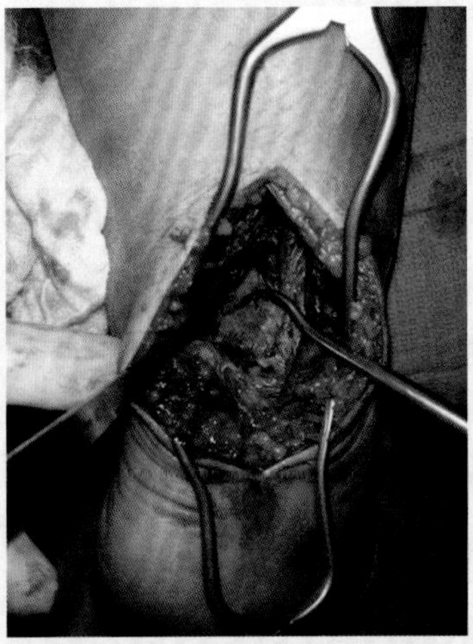

TECH FIG 1 Clinical photograph demonstrating exposure of the posterior malleolus via a posterolateral approach. The muscle belly of the FHL is elevated and retracted medially with a small Hohmann retractor. A shoulder hook is mobilizing the posterior malleolus fragment in preparation for anatomic reduction.

Posteromedial Approach

- Incision made halfway between the posterior margin of the medial malleolus and medial border of the Achilles tendon **(TECH FIG 2)**.
- Blunt dissection to undertaken to the fascia
- Multiple deep intervals can be exploited.
  - Access to posterior fracture fragment
    - Fascia is carefully incised over the posteromedial neurovascular bundle.
    - Bundle is controlled with a vessel loop allowing for access to the fracture from either side.
    - FHL is mobilized to access the posterior fracture.
    - Arthrotomy can be performed to access the articular surface.
  - Access to posteromedial fragment
    - Retinaculum overlying the tibialis posterior (TP) and the flexor digitorum longus (FDL) can be incised sharply.
    - Posteromedial fragment can be visualized between the TP and FDL or anterior to the TP, depending on morphology of the fracture.

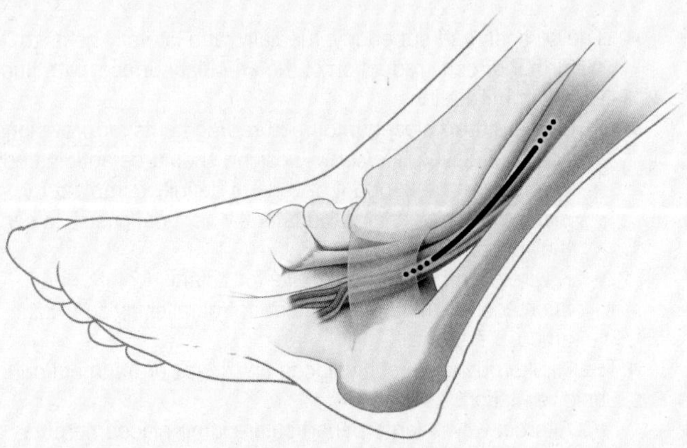

A

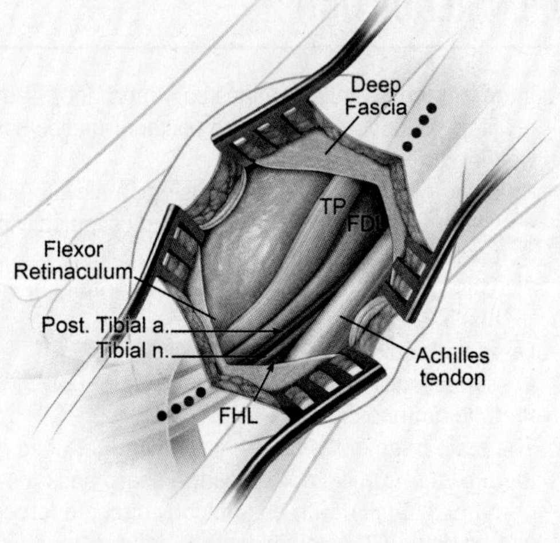

B

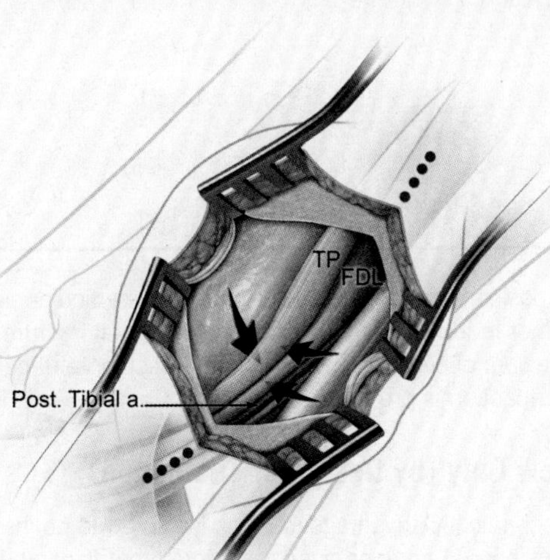

C

TECH FIG 2 Posteromedial approach. **A.** The incision is made halfway between the posteromedial border of the tibia and the Achilles tendon. **B.** Deep dissection. *TP*, tibialis posterior; *FDL*, flexor digitorum longus; *FHL*, flexor hallucis longus. **C.** Intervals to access posteromedial fractures. *(continued)*

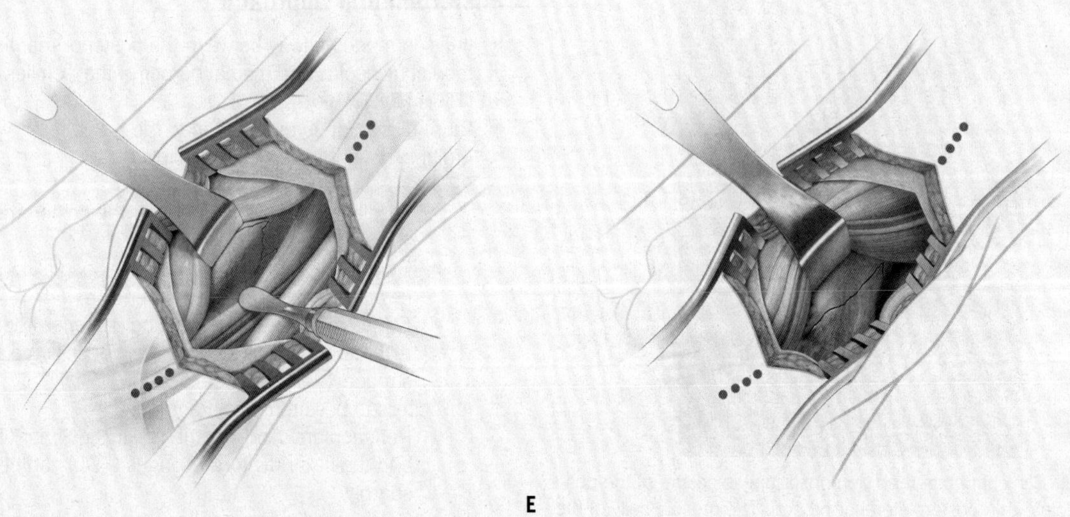

TECH FIG 2 *(continued)* **D.** Window between the posterior tibial tendon and the FDL, revealing a posterior malleolus fracture with medial extension. **E.** Posterior window exposing a posterolateral-oblique variant.

OPEN REDUCTION

- Interfragmentary callus, periosteum, and debris are cleared to facilitate reduction by elevating posterior malleolus distally and working through the fracture.
- Articular impaction is reduced, using an elevator, tamp.
  - Often, this must be monitored fluoroscopically if using the posterolateral approach.
  - This step is often best visualized prior to plate fixation of the fibula.
- Large metaphyseal defects are grafted.
  - Cancellous allograft
  - Calcium phosphate
- The main fragment is hinged closed and reduced often using the proximal cortical apical read. A sharp hook for manipulation or manual traction with an anteriorly directed force on the ankle can be helpful. If gaining length is difficult, then fixation of the fibula may help obtain the reduction, but plates on the fibula may block fluoroscopic visualization of the joint.
- The cortical read superiorly, medially, and laterally helps to confirm indirectly reduction of the articular surface, with fluoroscopic confirmation.
- K-wires are then placed into fracture fragments for provisional fixation. Definitive plate/screw position should be anticipated.
  - K-wires can be kept out of zone of definitive implant by placing them medially and laterally as "goal posts" to center the vertical buttress plate.
  - K-wires can be placed parallel to the ankle joint under fluoroscopic guidance as guide for parallel lag screws at articular surface.
- Ball spike pusher directly placed on the major fragment can hold reduction.
  - Alternatively, a large periarticular clamp placed percutaneously anteriorly on the tibia can be used to maintain reduction.

FIXATION

Buttress Plate

- Flexible tubular or minifragment plate
- Undercontoured but flexible to allow autocontouring and fracture compression
- Axillary screw is inserted first, buttressing the distal fragment and generating compression.
- At least two points of fixation proximal to the fracture **(TECH FIG 3)**
- Lag or position screws can be inserted above articular surface through or independent to the plate in the distal fracture.
  - Be aware of overcompression of the articular surface if voids or impaction is present.

Lag Screw Only (by Design or Technique)

- It is mechanically advantageous for a lag screw to be inserted from posterior to anterior given that more threads can be engaged into the intact segment.

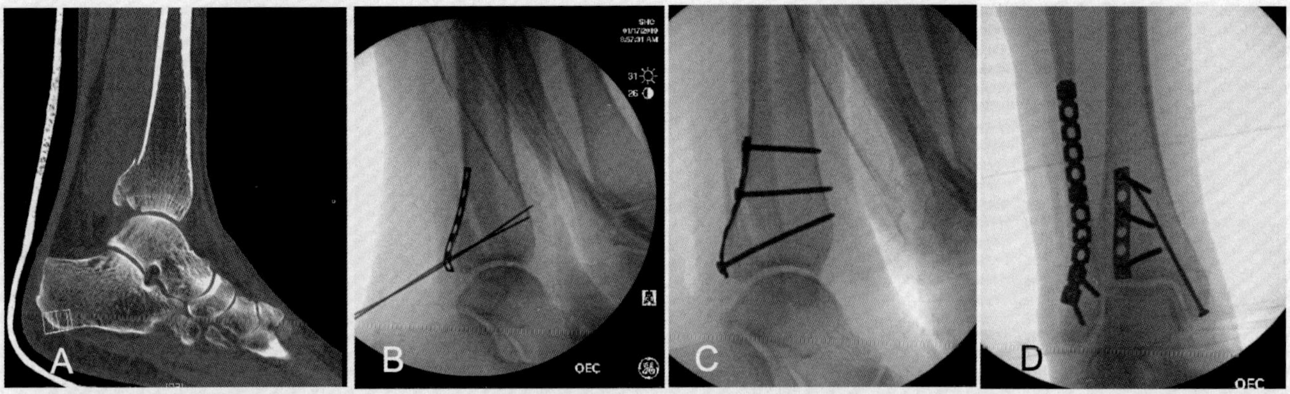

TECH FIG 3 Posterior buttress plate. **A.** Sagittal CT scan of a displaced posterior malleolus fragment with intra-articular impaction. **B.** Intraoperative fluoroscopy demonstrating reduction of the posterior malleolus and provisional fixation with K-wires to allow for placement of the buttress plate. **C,D.** Definitive fixation of posterior malleolus with a buttress plate. Note that the posterior malleolus was fixed prior to lateral and medial malleolus fixation to facilitate assessment of articular reduction on lateral imaging without obstruction from fibular implants.

- Useful for nondisplaced or minimally displaced fractures that can be reduced indirectly with manual traction
  - Occasionally useful for fractures reduced through a posteromedial approach but with insufficient medial obliquity to allow drilling angles and application of a buttress plate
    - In presence of a medial malleolar fractures
    - If surgeon desires to avoid prone positioning
  - If anterior to posterior lag screw placement, safe percutaneous technique is crucial to avoid neurovascular injury **(TECH FIG 4)**.
    - Incise skin only, blunt dissection to the bone with clamp, and spreading clamp upon extraction to create safe pathway
    - Drill sleeves are mandatory.
    - Oscillate function on drill avoids entangling critical structures.
- Care taken not to make screw length too long
- If using partially threaded screws, the threads should not cross the fracture when inserted into final position.
- Alternatively, for cannulated screws, a guidewire can be inserted anterior to posterior by oscillating to protect soft tissue structures.
  - The guidewire can be pulled through the posterior side until it sits flush with the anterior cortex.
  - A small incision is made to accommodate a partially threaded cannulated screw. The path of the screw is bluntly dissected.
  - The screw length can be determined using a measuring device that slides on top of the guidewire **(TECH FIG 5)**.

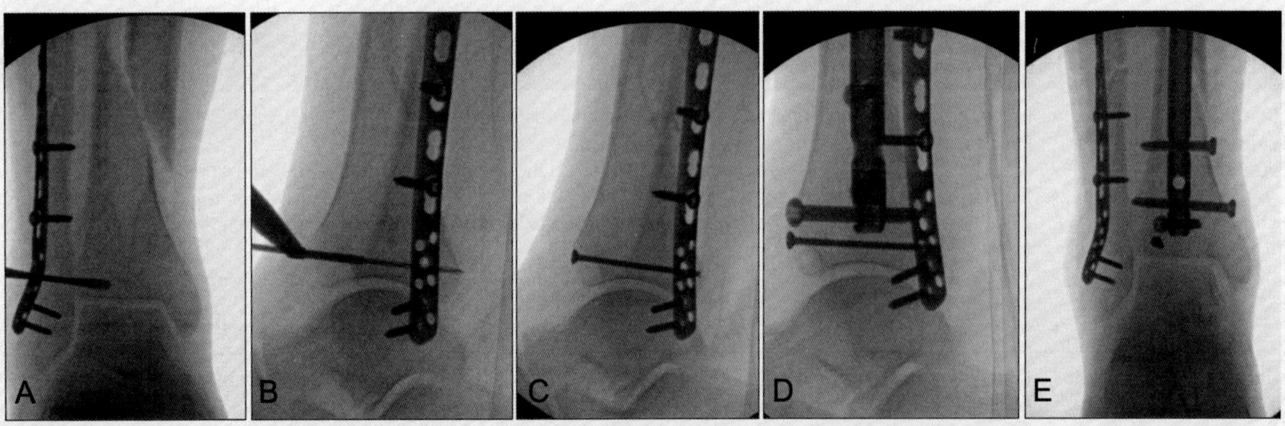

TECH FIG 4 Anterior to posterior percutaneous lag screw. **A.** Posterior malleolar fracture below a distal tibia fracture, fluoroscopy used to plan lag screw placement while avoiding the path of intramedullary implant. **B.** Percutaneous lag by technique under fluoroscopic guidance. **C.** Solid core lag screw by technique. **D,E.** Tibial nail with three distal interlocks unencumbered by previous lag screw placement.

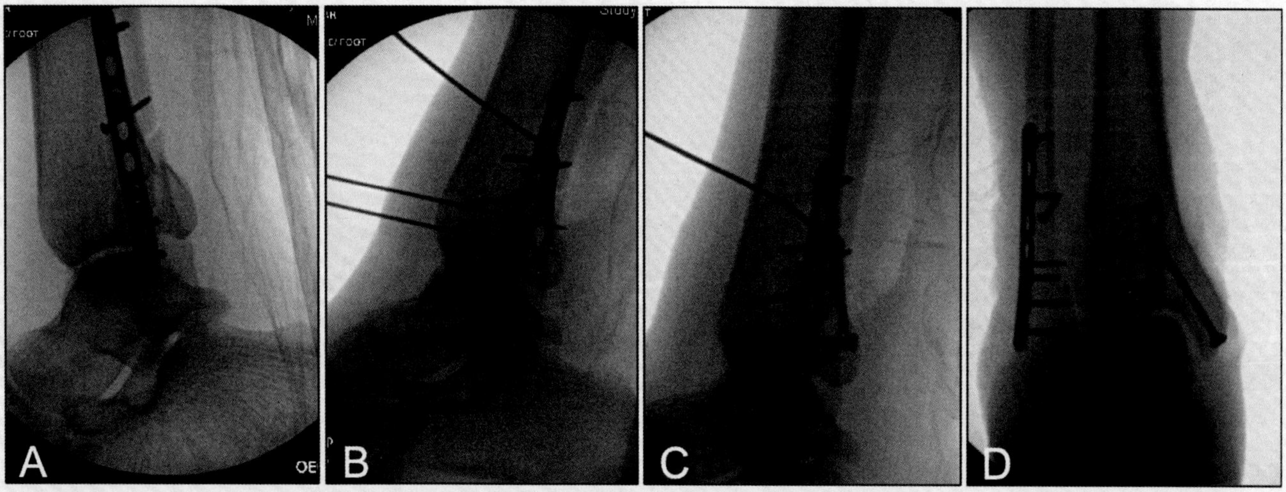

TECH FIG 5 Posterior to anterior percutaneous lag screw. **A.** Lateral view of displaced posterior malleolus fracture. **B.** Directly reduced and provisionally fixed posterior malleolus fracture with minifragment antiglide plating via a posteromedial approach (patient was supine) and K-wires inserted from anterior to posterior. **C,D.** Independent lag screw (by design) inserted over guidewire to supplement posterior malleolus fixation without additional dissection.

WOUND CLOSURE

- The peroneal or posterior tibial tendon sheaths are repaired using absorbable suture.
- Nylon suture in vertical mattress or Allgower-Donati configuration is used for the skin.
  - Excessive absorbable suture in the subcutaneous layer is avoided.
- When possible, knots are placed on the posterior aspect of the incision due to more robust blood flow.
- Aggressive manipulation of the skin with instruments is avoided.

TECHNIQUES

Pearls and Pitfalls

Concurrent Lateral Malleolus Fractures	• In the presence of a concomitant operative lateral malleolus fracture, we recommend addressing the posterior malleolus first. • Articular surface of the tibia is adequately visualized on the lateral image, which can be obscured by a fibular plate. • Stability of the syndesmosis can be restored by fixing the posterior malleolus fracture often obviating the need to place independent syndesmotic fixation; however, the ankle should be stressed after fixation is complete to confirm stability using fluoroscopy.[8,13] • The fibula can be reduced and fixed by retracting the peroneal tendons laterally or medially depending on desired plate positioning through the same posterolateral approach skin incision. • If posteromedial approach was employed, a separate lateral incision is used to approach the fibula.
Concurrent Distal Tibial Spiral Fracture	• If there is a distal tibial spiral fracture with associated posterior malleolus fragment, the posterior malleolus should be surgically addressed prior to fixing the extra-articular tibia fracture. • Take care to not place posterior malleolus fixation in the pathway of the intramedullary nail or future screw/interlock fixation.

POSTOPERATIVE CARE

- All ankles should be immobilized in neutral position and elevated for at least 24 hours postoperatively.
- We remove the sutures at 10 to 14 days.
- Patients are then placed into a removable boot (if not already in one) that allows them to begin early active-assisted and passive range of ankle motion.[5]
- Patients are also allowed to begin isometric strengthening exercises.
- Patients are typically kept non–weight bearing for the first 6 weeks.
- At 6 weeks, patients are progressed to weight bearing as tolerated without the functional brace.
- Patients are restricted from operating an automobile for 9 weeks following right-sided ankle fracture.[6]

OUTCOMES

- Ankle fractures with posterior malleolus involvement are associated with poorer outcomes compared to ankle fractures with an intact posterior malleolus.[15–16]
- Surgical management of posterior malleolar fractures restores syndesmosis anatomy, avoids a painful malunion of the incisura, and improves distribution of tibiotalar joint contact pressures.[7,8]
- Compared to screw only fixation for the posterior malleolus, buttress plating is more biomechanically stable and demonstrates superior clinical outcomes. No differences have been shown with respect to ankle range of motion or development of posttraumatic arthritis between both fixation strategies,[3,14] but high-level evidence does not exist.
- In the absence of articular impaction, intercalated fragments, and persistent posterior subluxation of the talus despite reduction of medial/lateral malleolus fractures, definitive operative indications to improve clinical outcomes in patients after posterior malleolus fractures is controversial.

REFERENCES

1. Bali N, Aktselis I, Ramasamy A, et al. An evolution in the management of fractures of the ankle: safety and efficacy of posteromedial approach for Haraguchi type 2 posterior malleolar fractures. Bone Joint J 2017;99-B:1496–1501.
2. Bartoníček J, Rammelt S, Tucek M. Posterior malleolar fractures: changing concepts and recent developments. Foot Ankle Clin 2017;22:125–145.
3. Bennett C, Behn A, Daoud A, et al. Buttress plating versus anterior-to-posterior lag screws for fixation of the posterior malleolus: a biomechanical study. J Orthop Trauma 2016;30:664–669.
4. Boraiah S, Gardner MJ, Helfet DL, et al. High association of posterior malleolus fractures with spiral distal tibial fractures. Clin Orthop Relat Res 2008;466:1692–1698.
5. Egol KA, Dolan R, Koval KJ. Functional outcome of surgery for fractures of the ankle. A prospective, randomised comparison of management in a cast or a functional brace. J Bone Joint Surg Br 2000;82:246–249.
6. Egol KA, Sheikhazadeh A, Mogatederi S, et al. Lower-extremity function for driving an automobile after operative treatment of ankle fracture. J Bone Joint Surg Am 2003;85:1185–1189.
7. Evers J, Fischer M, Zderic I, et al. The role of a small posterior malleolar fragment in trimalleolar fractures: a biomechanical study. Bone Joint J 2018;100-B:95–100.
8. Gardner MJ, Brodsky A, Briggs SM, et al. Fixation of posterior malleolar fractures provides greater syndesmotic stability. Clin Orthop Relat Res 2006;447:165–171.
9. Gardner MJ, Demetrakopoulos D, Briggs SM, et al. The ability of the Lauge-Hansen classification to predict ligament injury and mechanism in ankle fractures: an MRI study. J Orthop Trauma 2006;20:267–272.
10. Haraguchi N, Haruyama H, Toga H, et al. Pathoanatomy of posterior malleolar fractures of the ankle. J Bone Joint Surg Am 2006;88:1085–1092.
11. Lauge-Hansen N. Fractures of the ankle. II. Combined experimental-surgical and experimental-roentgenologic investigations. Arch Surg 1950;60:957–985.
12. Lidder S, Masterson S, Dreu M, et al. The risk of injury to the peroneal artery in the posterolateral approach to the distal tibia: a cadaver study. J Orthop Trauma 2014;28:534–537.
13. Miller AN, Carroll EA, Parker RJ, et al. Posterior malleolar stabilization of syndesmotic injuries is equivalent to screw fixation. Clin Orthop Relat Res 2010;468:1129–1135.
14. O'Connor TJ, Mueller B, Ly TV, et al. "A to P" screw versus posterolateral plate for posterior malleolus fixation in trimalleolar ankle fractures. J Orthop Trauma 2015;29:e151–e156.
15. Swiontkowski MF, Engelberg R, Martin DP, et al. Short musculoskeletal function assessment questionnaire: validity, reliability, and responsiveness. J Bone Joint Surg Am 1999;81:1245–1260.
16. Tejwani NC, Pahk B, Egol KA. Effect of posterior malleolus fracture on outcome after unstable ankle fracture. J Trauma 2010;69:666–669.
17. Tornetta P III, Ricci W, Nork S, et al. The posterolateral approach to the tibia for displaced posterior malleolar injuries. J Orthop Trauma 2011;25:123–126.

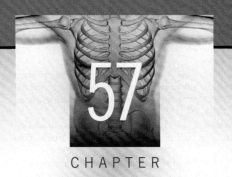

57

CHAPTER

Open and Fluoroscopic Reduction of the Syndesmosis

Elizabeth A. Martin and Paul Tornetta III

DEFINITION

- The syndesmosis is a ligamentous complex that stabilizes the distal articulation of the tibia and fibula.
- Injury to the syndesmosis can confer instability to the ankle joint.
- Reduction of the syndesmosis can be difficult to assess, and iatrogenic malreduction can occur in several directions including rotation, translation, compression, and length.

ANATOMY

- The syndesmosis consists of the shallow bony articulation between the distal fibula and tibia and its associated ligamentous support.[14]
- The distal fibula sits in a groove on the distal lateral tibia known as the *incisura fibularis*.
- The depth and shape of the incisura vary between individuals, and this anatomic variability may contribute to malreduction of the syndesmosis.[2,4]
  - Shallow incisura and those with anteversion are prone to anterior translation.
  - Deep incisura may be more constrained or lead to posterior translation if the posterior lip is not as deep as the anterior lip.
- Four main ligaments constitute the tibiofibular syndesmosis (**FIG 1**).
  - Anterior inferior tibiofibular ligament
  - Posterior inferior tibiofibular ligament
  - Inferior transverse ligament
  - Intraosseous ligament

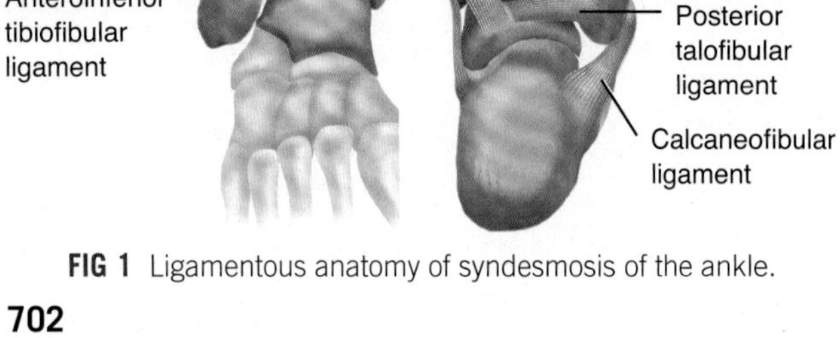

FIG 1 Ligamentous anatomy of syndesmosis of the ankle.

- These ligaments allow for a small amount of motion between the tibia and fibula, mainly functioning to stabilize the fibula within the incisura with tibiotalar joint motion. The fibula externally rotates and migrates proximally with dorsiflexion of the ankle.

PATHOGENESIS

- Syndesmotic injuries typically result from an external rotation or pronation force applied to the ankle through an indirect mechanism.
- Can be purely ligamentous or associated with fractures
  - Pronation abduction (PA) and pronation external rotation (PER) injuries typically injure the syndesmosis. Supination–external rotation (SER) injuries injure the syndesmosis in between 20% and 40% of cases.[13]

NATURAL HISTORY

- As there are multiple ligaments stabilizing the syndesmosis, the injury encompasses a spectrum of stability and severity.[5]
- The untreated unstable syndesmotic injury can lead to tibiotalar joint instability, incongruity, and early degenerative change.[15]
  - Tibiotalar incongruity during weight bearing of as little as 1 to 2 mm can cause a change in joint contact forces.
- Outcomes following treated syndesmotic injury can vary based on quality of reduction as well as type and severity of initial injury and associated articular injury.

PATIENT HISTORY AND PHYSICAL FINDINGS

- Patient history may include the following:
  - An indirect injury to the ankle, typically in rotation
  - Swelling and ecchymosis diffusely about the ankle
  - Inability to bear weight, particularly in the setting of associated fracture
- Physical examination methods include the following:
  - Palpation of the ankle including the deltoid ligament medially and anterior syndesmotic ligaments
  - Examination of the ipsilateral knee and leg for tenderness at the proximal fibula and shaft
  - Physical exam maneuvers performed at the ankle are more useful in the absence of ankle fracture, as fracture-related pain can elicit a positive test without syndesmotic injury.
- Clinical tests for syndesmotic injury include the following[28]:
  - Pain with palpation of the syndesmosis
  - Syndesmotic squeeze test: pain reproduced at the ankle with application of transverse compression of the tibia and fibula at midcalf level

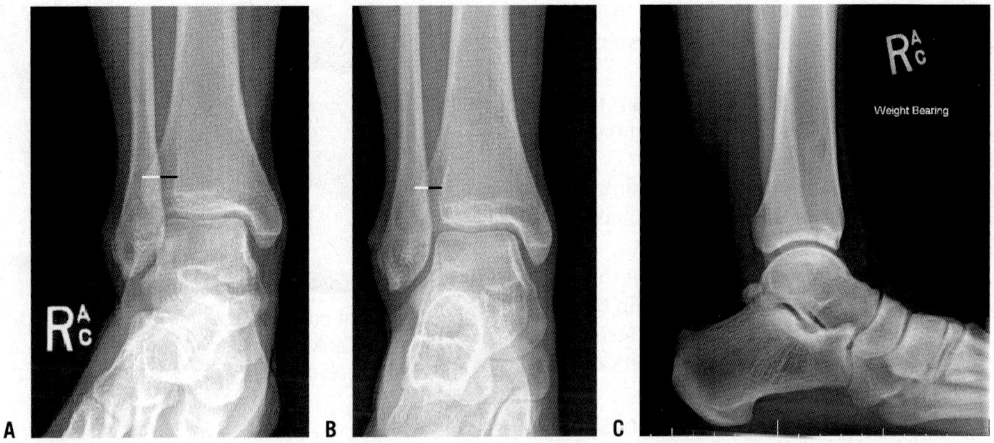

FIG 2 A. AP view of the ankle demonstrating tibiofibular overlap greater than 6 mm (*white line*) tibiofibular clear space less than 6 mm (*black line*) and symmetric medial and superior clear space. Tibiofibular overlap and clear space are measured 1 cm above the plafond. **B.** Mortise view of the ankle demonstrating tibiofibular overlap greater than 1 mm (*white line*) tibiofibular clear space less than 6 mm (*black line*) and symmetric medial and superior clear space. **C.** True lateral view of the ankle demonstrating fibula in the posterior half of the tibia and superimposed medial and lateral aspects of the talar dome. The amount of posterior malleolus visualized behind the fibula and shape and location of the fibula are compared to the contralateral ankle intraoperatively to gauge reduction.

- Pain with passive dorsiflexion and external rotation of the ankle
- Hop test: pain elicited at the syndesmosis with attempted single-leg hop

IMAGING AND OTHER DIAGNOSTIC STUDIES

- Plain radiographs including anteroposterior (AP), mortise and lateral views of the ankle, and AP and lateral views of the tibia and fibula should be obtained.
- Radiographic parameters for evaluating syndesmotic instability:
  - On an AP and mortise radiograph, the medial clear space, tibiofibular clear space, and tibiofibular overlap can be measured **(FIG 2A,B)**.
    - Tibiofibular overlap varies based on the rotation of the ankle but is measured 1 cm above the plafond and should be at least 6 mm on the AP and 1 mm on the mortise view.
    - The tibiofibular clear space, measured 1 cm above the tibiotalar joint, is more consistent with rotation and should be less than 6 mm on both AP and mortise views.
    - The medial clear space should be equal to or less than the superior clear space, typically 5 mm or less.
  - On a lateral radiograph, the position of the fibula relative to the talus and posterior malleolus on a true lateral should be assessed **(FIG 2C)**. This should be symmetric to the normal uninjured ankle.
- Stress radiographs are critical to evaluate for unstable syndesmotic injury in the setting of a stable-appearing mortise on injury films.
- Manual external rotation, gravity, and weight-bearing stress radiographs have been described. The gravity stress view may overestimate the medial clear space as the ankle is typically in a plantarflexed position and is therefore not recommended.
- Radiographs of the contralateral ankle are often performed to compare and assess accuracy of ankle fracture and syndesmotic reduction, including AP, mortise, and lateral views. In operative cases, the perfect lateral view is easier obtained in the operating room.
- Computed tomography (CT) scan can be used to further evaluate the alignment of the fibula within the incisura as well as the associated fracture if indicated.
- Bilateral axial CT can allow for side-to-side comparison in both injury characterization and planning the reduction.
- Weight-bearing CT scan is an emerging modality that can allow for evaluation of syndesmotic alignment in injuries able to undergo weight-bearing stress.[12]
- Magnetic resonance imaging can be used to evaluate for ligamentous and articular injury.

DIFFERENTIAL DIAGNOSIS

- Lateral ankle ligamentous injury
- Isolated bony injury
- Deltoid ligament injury
- Peroneal tendon subluxation/rupture

NONOPERATIVE MANAGEMENT

- Stable syndesmotic injuries can be treated with closed management.

SURGICAL MANAGEMENT

- Surgical fixation of a syndesmotic injury is indicated in the setting of instability.
- Numerous syndesmotic reduction techniques have been described, including open reduction with palpation, open

reduction by direct visualization, reduction using arthroscopic visualization, and closed reduction using radiographic parameters.
- Although the syndesmosis is malreduced in up to 52% of cases,[9] little attention has been paid to open reduction techniques.
- Techniques involving visualization of the incisura and of the anterolateral joint have been described, as have open palpation techniques.[12,22,23,29]
- Direct inspection of the anterolateral corner of the ankle joint allows for visualization of the relationship between the talus, tibia, and fibula. The articular surface of the anterolateral tibial plafond and the anteromedial fibula can then be directly aligned.
- The anterior and posterior inferior tibiofibular ligaments have a reproducible distance from the superior margin of the distal articular cartilage, so it has been suggested that these cartilage surfaces could serve as a landmark for syndesmotic reduction.[18]

- Various fixation techniques can be employed including screw fixation, suture button fixation, hybrid fixation, and direct repair.
- Goals of treatment
  - Restore fibular length and rotation, stabilizing fracture if indicated.
  - Restore ankle mortise and syndesmotic alignment.
  - Minimize soft tissue trauma.
  - Protect at-risk structures.
    - Superficial peroneal nerve
    - Peroneal tendons
    - Peroneus tertius tendon
    - Saphenous structures
  - Prevent iatrogenic complications.
    - Malreduction of fracture or syndesmosis
    - Shortening of the fibula
    - Inadequate fixation
    - Disruption of lateral ankle ligaments

Preoperative Planning

- All imaging studies are reviewed.
- Surgical anatomy should be reviewed, including the path of the saphenous structures, superficial peroneal nerve, and ligamentous anatomy.
- Fixation of associated fractures should be planned and performed concurrently as indicated, prior to syndesmotic fixation.
- It is critical that length and rotation of the fibula be restored either by direct fixation of the fibula or indirectly by anatomically fixing the syndesmosis.
- If the injury pattern requires a lateral or posterolateral fibular incision, reduction by palpation and radiographic guidance may be more appropriate than open reduction and direct visualization to avoid additional anterolateral incision and additional dissection.
- Alternately, the lateral incision can curve anteriorly distally to expose the anterior portion of the joint.
- In the most common pattern, the Weber B SER 4 fracture, the syndesmosis generally lines up quite well after anatomic reduction of the fibula as long as the heel is not resting on a bump.

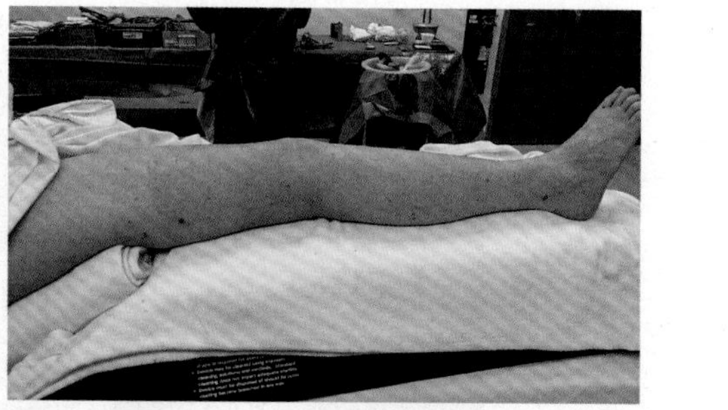

FIG 3 Patient positioned supine with bump under the ipsilateral hip to rotate the ankle into neutral position. Bump can be placed under the heel to prevent posterior translation of the talus.

- Imaging of the contralateral ankle is routinely used to plan and assess reduction of the ankle and syndesmosis. The authors prefer a perfect lateral of the unaffected side in the operating room to make sure that the view is tangent to the plafond and that the joint is not rotated at all.

Positioning

- Position the patient supine on a radiolucent table with bump under the operative hip to keep the ankle in a position of neutral rotation **(FIG 3)**.
  - Patient can alternatively be laterally positioned if needed, externally rotating the hip to place the ankle in neutral rotation and visualize the syndesmosis anteriorly.
- A C-arm image intensifier is used to assist in the operative procedure. Standard C-arm is most often used and should be positioned contralateral to the injured extremity.
- If formal radiographs of the contralateral ankle have not been performed preoperatively, or if they are malrotated or of poor quality, comparison mortise and perfect lateral images are obtained prior to positioning and draping.
- A calf or thigh tourniquet is not required but may be used based on surgeon preference.
- External rotation stress radiograph is performed intraoperatively prior to making an incision in the absence of gross instability.

Approach

- The articular approach to reduction of the syndesmosis with direct visualization removes the anatomic variation of the incisura. Also, there is a smaller difference in width of the tibia compared to the fibula at the plafond versus the incisura. Thus, because visualization is performed only anteriorly, measuring at the joint level may provide better translational alignment of the syndesmosis versus using the incisura.[29] Additionally, shortening can be identified at this level.
- The open anterolateral approach is most appropriate in the setting of a Weber C or Maisonneuve injury, when a lateral approach to the distal fibula is not performed.
- If a lateral incision is made, then it can be extended to visualize the anterolateral joint if needed. If a posterolateral incision is made, then a separate small anterolateral incision can be added if needed.

REDUCTION OF THE SYNDESMOSIS

Reduction with Direct Visualization

- The incision should be placed anterolaterally at the level of the joint, lateral to the peroneus tertius in line with the lateral gutter **(TECH FIG 1A)**.
- Longitudinal incision is performed over the distal aspect of the incisura and lateral gutter.
- The intermediate dorsal cutaneous branch of the superficial peroneal nerve must be protected anteriorly.
- Dissection proceeds down to the level of the joint capsule. The capsule is incised in line with the lateral gutter and protected for later repair **(TECH FIG 1B)**.
- The anterolateral corner of the ankle joint including tibiotalar, distal tibiofibular, and proximal talofibular articulations are then directly visualized anteriorly.
- The syndesmotic relationship is restored **(TECH FIG 1C)** by aligning the articular surfaces of the anterolateral distal tibia and anteromedial distal fibula.
- The reduction is stabilized with a Kirschner wire from fibula into the tibia **(TECH FIG 1D)**, avoiding the path of planned syndesmotic fixation.
- The incisura can be viewed from this approach as well **(TECH FIG 1E)**; however, the authors perform this tibiotalar articular method to mitigate anatomic differences in the incisura and better judge length and translation at the joint level.[29]
- Although a clamp can be used to stabilize if placed carefully, it may be associated with iatrogenic malreduction, even if preoperative CT is used to guide clamp trajectory.[6,19] Thus, the authors only rarely use clamps in acute cases.
- The reduction is visualized again after provisional fixation to ensure the position did not change.
- The incisura and anterolateral joint can also be visualized if a lateral fibular incision is used to fix the fibula **(TECH FIG 1F,G)**.

Reduction Using Palpation

- Palpation of the syndesmosis is an alternative reduction method accessed during a lateral or posterolateral approach to the fibula. This can be used when intraoperative stress testing demonstrates syndesmotic injury, and separate anterolateral approach is not or cannot be performed.
- After the fibula is reduced and fixed with anatomic length and rotation, the incisura and anterolateral joint can be palpated anteriorly through the lateral incision to guide syndesmotic reduction.
- On palpation, the anterior tibiofibular relationship should be congruent at the incisura without translation or diastasis.
- If this technique is used, the radiographic reduction method in the following text should also be used.

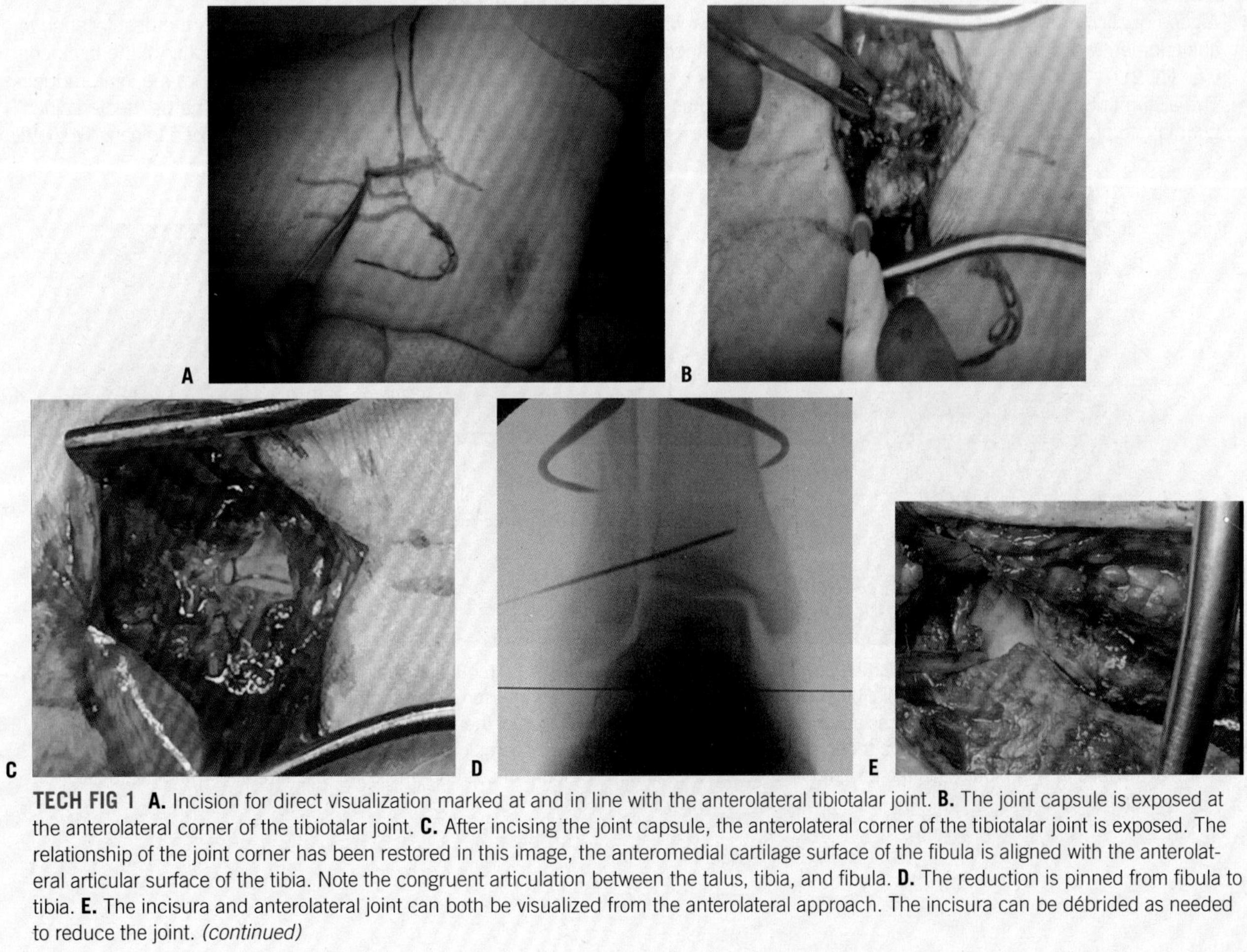

TECH FIG 1 **A.** Incision for direct visualization marked at and in line with the anterolateral tibiotalar joint. **B.** The joint capsule is exposed at the anterolateral corner of the tibiotalar joint. **C.** After incising the joint capsule, the anterolateral corner of the tibiotalar joint is exposed. The relationship of the joint corner has been restored in this image, the anteromedial cartilage surface of the fibula is aligned with the anterolateral articular surface of the tibia. Note the congruent articulation between the talus, tibia, and fibula. **D.** The reduction is pinned from fibula to tibia. **E.** The incisura and anterolateral joint can both be visualized from the anterolateral approach. The incisura can be débrided as needed to reduce the joint. *(continued)*

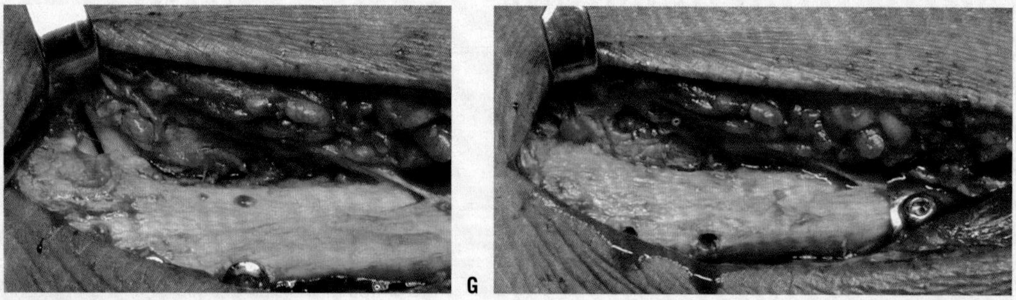

F G

TECH FIG 1 *(continued)* **F.** The incisura and anterolateral joint can also be visualized through a lateral approach and débrided if needed, such as in this revision case. Malreduction is pictured—with screw fixation in place, gapping is noted between the tibia, talus, and fibula. **G.** Following screw removal and reduction of the syndesmosis.

RADIOGRAPHIC ASSESSMENT OF REDUCTION

- Once the syndesmosis is reduced, intraoperative imaging is used to assess reduction.
- The same radiographic parameters are used regardless of reduction maneuver.
- If an open reduction with direct visualization or palpation cannot be performed, such as in cases of marked soft tissue trauma, the radiographic assessment is used to guide reduction.
- A good quality, properly rotated intraoperative mortise view with ankle in neutral dorsiflexion and true lateral view are obtained (see **FIG 2**).
- The alignment of the contralateral unaffected side is used as a template to provide a direct comparison.
- On the mortise view, the tibiofibular clear space should be less than 6 mm, medial clear space should be equal or less than the superior clear space, and talofibular articulation should be congruent **(TECH FIG 2A)**.
- On the lateral view, the fibula should be in the posterior half of the tibia, using the contralateral side as a guide for position of the fibula relative to the talus and posterior malleolus **(TECH FIG 2B)**.
- If the posterior malleolus is not damaged, the best location to assess the reduction is using the relationship of the back cortical edge of the fibula to the back corner of the joint, reducing the affected side to appear the same as the unaffected side.
- If intraoperative CT is available, it can be used to gauge reduction.

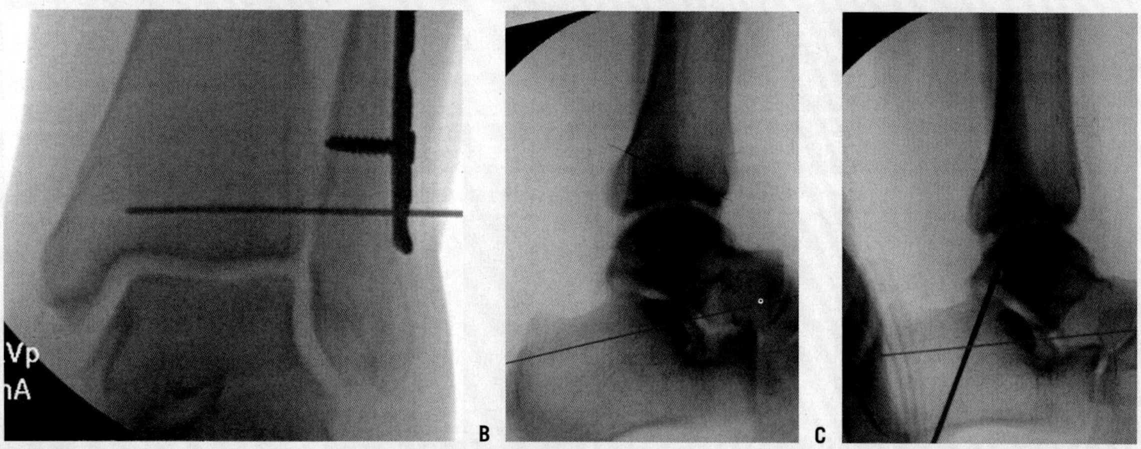

A B C

TECH FIG 2 **A.** Intraoperative mortise view assessing the pinned syndesmotic reduction. Note the restoration of symmetric medial and superior joint spaces and tibiofibular clear space less than 6 mm. Comparison to the contralateral side should have symmetric appearance of these spaces as well as symmetric length and rotation of the fibula. **B,C.** Intraoperative lateral views of both ankles assessing the syndesmotic reduction. Note the true lateral view with complete overlap of the medial and lateral aspects of the talar dome. Fibula is in the posterior half of the tibia, and the amount of posterior malleolus visualized is symmetric to the contralateral ankle.

INTERNAL FIXATION

- Once the reduction has been evaluated visually and radiographically, the syndesmosis is stabilized with screw or suture button fixation.
- It has been demonstrated that if the reduction is accurate, there is no advantage of one method over the other. Suture button methods are much more expensive, and this factor should be considered. In cases where the surgeon is unable to accurately reduce the syndesmosis, the flexible technique may provide an advantage but should never be used if the fibula is not out to length.
- For the open reduction technique, fixation can then be placed percutaneously or with a small posterolateral incision.

Screw Placement

- The authors prefer a two-screw construct when fibular fracture is not fixed, using 3.5- or 4.0-mm cortical screws, with distal screw approximately 1 to 2 cm proximal to the tibiotalar joint **(TECH FIG 3A)**.
- In poor bone, a short, thin plate can be used as a large washer.
- The correct starting position is identified using fluoroscopy, and small incision is made, dissecting bluntly to the fibula **(TECH FIG 3B)**.
- Using fluoroscopic guidance, the start point is confirmed, and drill is advanced.
- It is dogma that the drill must be parallel to the tibiotalar joint line in approximately 30 degrees posterior to anterior trajectory. In reality, these screws are placed as positional screws across a reduced syndesmosis, so their direction is not relevant. However, if the screws are being used to provide a compression reduction, then the direction of the screw must be perpendicular to the displacement of the tibiofibular articulation **(TECH FIG 3C)**.
- Screws can be placed in tricortical or quadricortical fashion depending on surgeon preference.[32]

Suture Button Fixation

- Suture button fixation is flexible, and if the surgeon cannot accurately reduce the joint, then the flexibility will allow for some translation and autocorrection.[27]
- The syndesmosis is approached, reduced, and held manually or provisionally pinned as earlier.
- Guidewire for the suture button device is placed at the lateral fibula, approximately 1.5 cm proximal to the plafond. Suture button can also be placed through a compatible plate.
- Care is taken to ensure the appropriate angle and trajectory, parallel with the plafond and approximately 30 degrees posterior to anterior, along the transmalleolar axis **(TECH FIG 4A)**.
- Drill, or guidewire and cannulated drill, for the suture button device is then driven from the lateral fibula through the anteromedial tibia using image intensifier.
- Suture button device is then passed through the drilled tunnel from the fibula to the tibia.
- The device is passed from lateral to medial, until the medial button is pulled from the tibia. The path of the saphenous structures must be avoided when exiting into the medial soft tissues.
- Gentle backward tension is placed on the device laterally to flip and seat the medial button on the tibia. The device should be held proximal to the lateral button to avoid inadvertently tightening during this step.
- Care must be taken to ensure that the button is lying completely flush on the tibia with no interposed soft tissues **(TECH FIG 4B,C)**.
- A small incision can be made at the exit point of the tibial tunnel, and blunt dissection can be used to expose the exit point if needed. This can both protect the saphenous structures and clear interposed soft tissue to ensure the medial button is lying directly on the tibial cortex.
- Once the button is flush medially, the device is tightened by applying alternating tension to the lateral sutures to remove all

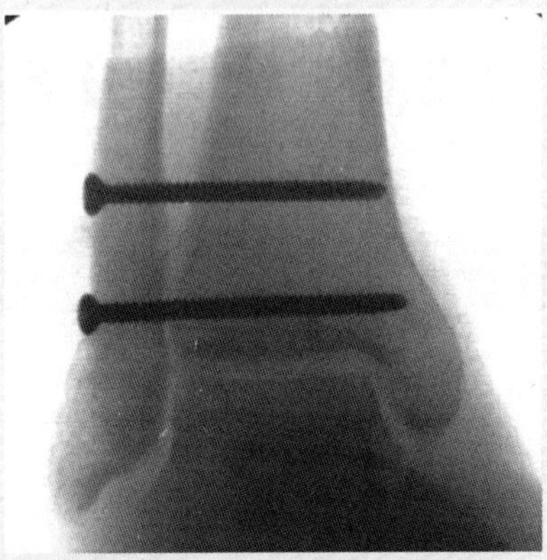
A

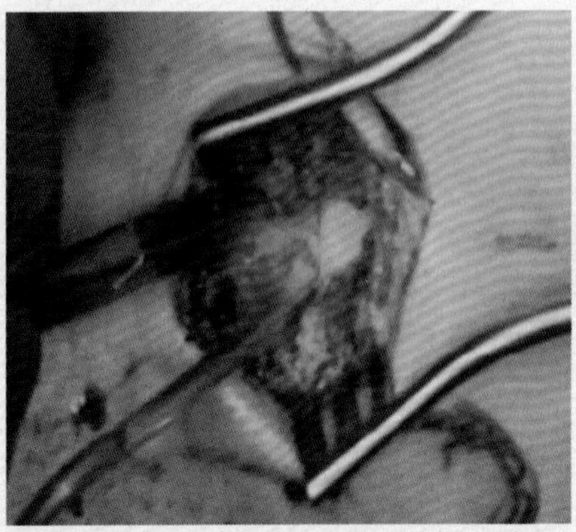
B

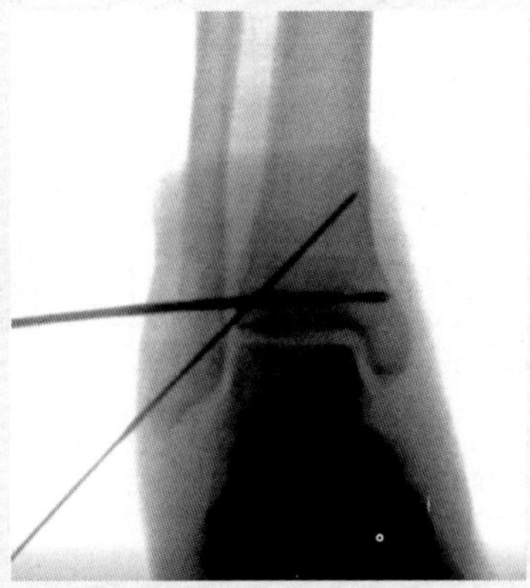
C

TECH FIG 3 A. Two-screw configuration with distal screw approximately 1 cm from the tibiotalar joint. **B.** Image demonstrating reduced joint with congruent articular surfaces of the anterolateral distal tibia and anteromedial distal fibula and two percutaneous incisions for syndesmotic screws over the lateral fibula. **C.** Appropriate trajectory for syndesmotic screw with drill parallel to the tibiotalar joint.

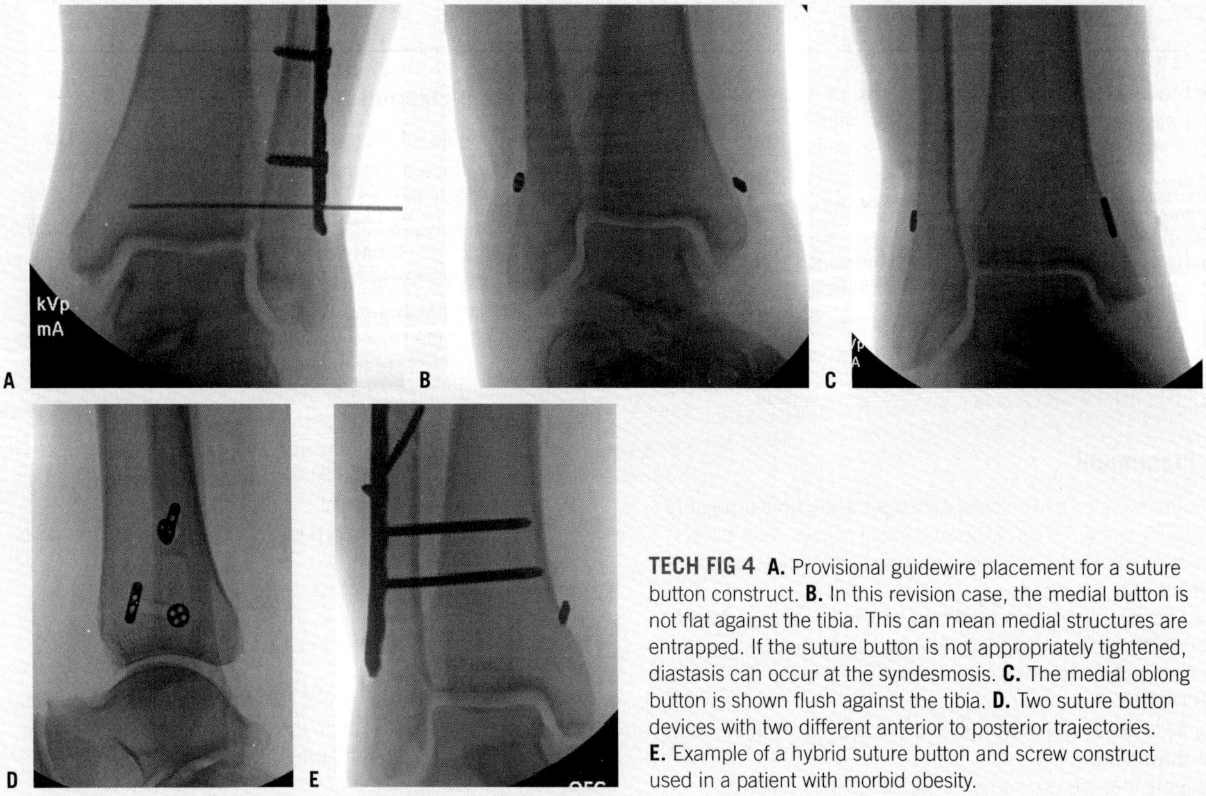

TECH FIG 4 **A.** Provisional guidewire placement for a suture button construct. **B.** In this revision case, the medial button is not flat against the tibia. This can mean medial structures are entrapped. If the suture button is not appropriately tightened, diastasis can occur at the syndesmosis. **C.** The medial oblong button is shown flush against the tibia. **D.** Two suture button devices with two different anterior to posterior trajectories. **E.** Example of a hybrid suture button and screw construct used in a patient with morbid obesity.

slack from the device. The medial and lateral buttons must lie flush. A curved clamp can be placed under the lateral button to maintain even tension and removed when the button reaches the fibula. Sutures are tied if needed or are cut if knotless device is used.

- Single or multiple devices can be used depending on surgeon preference. If more than one device is used, the second device should be placed on a different posterior to anterior trajectory **(TECH FIG 4D)**.
- Suture button fixation in isolation is not recommended with a length-unstable fibula fracture. The fracture should first be repaired if suture button is used.
- Alternatively, flexible fixation can be combined with screw fixation for a fibula fracture with axial instability.[25]
  - In this case, the suture button is placed first, approximately 1.5 cm proximal to the joint, followed by a screw in the more proximal position. Reduction is held until the proximal screw is placed **(TECH FIG 4E)**.

Pearls and Pitfalls

Indications	• The unstable syndesmosis must be identified and stabilized. • Suture button fixation should not be used in isolation in an axially unstable injury.
Reduction	• Malreduction of the fibula fracture will likely result in malreduction of the syndesmosis. • Restoration of fibular length and rotation of the fibula is critical. • The syndesmosis must be reduced prior to placing fixation device. • Good intraoperative films must be obtained to judge reduction, including a properly rotated mortise and a true lateral.
Fixation	• The fibular length must be maintained with the chosen fixation method; length is best maintained with static fixation of the fibula or syndesmosis. • Suture button must be flush against the tibial cortex, and flush to the fibula or lateral plate with no slack, to prevent diastasis. • A small medial incision can be used in suture button fixation to clear interposed soft tissues if the medial button does not lie flush.

POSTOPERATIVE CARE

- Immobilization in a well-padded splint and strict elevation are recommended in the immediate postoperative period. Immobilization continues until sutures or staples are removed at 2 weeks or longer in those with impaired wound healing potential such as diabetics and smokers.
- Transition into a tall walker boot with active range of motion at 2 weeks. Cast immobilization is maintained in patients with diabetes and neuropathy and considered in osteoporosis, smoking, and if concern for compliance with restrictions.
- Non–weight bearing is maintained for at least 6 weeks, longer if needed for associated fractures or comorbidities.
  - Earlier weight bearing at 2 to 4 weeks has been described without major complications; however, most surgeons prefer at least 8 weeks of non–weight bearing. This may be modified based on bone quality, expected compliance, and the weight of the patient.[24]
- Weight bearing is initiated progressively as tolerated with assistive device with weaning from assistive device at 3 months.
- Return to full activity, especially competitive athletics, is allowed when complete healing is observed on radiographs and when symptoms allow.
- Syndesmotic screw removal is debated, although the literature does not support improved outcomes with routine removal.[7]

OUTCOMES

- There is no universal method to reduce, fix, or measure malreduction of the syndesmosis.
- Comparing outcomes following syndesmotic injury is complicated by inconsistency between studies. Areas of variability include injury definition and severity, reduction methods, fixation constructs, and parameters to measure reduction accuracy and functional outcomes.
- Syndesmotic injuries have been shown to be associated with worse functional outcomes compared to ankle fractures without syndesmotic disruption.[8,31]
  - Outcomes in Weber B SER patterns are similar in those with and without syndesmotic injury.[16]
- The association between inaccurate reduction of the syndesmosis and functional outcome is not clearly defined.
  - Several studies have shown an association between syndesmotic malreduction and worse clinical outcomes.[1,21,26]
  - Others have not been able to demonstrate a significant relationship between poorer outcomes and syndesmotic malreduction in the short term[4,30] or have shown a trend toward poorer outcomes without statistical significance.[17,32]
  - Although the degree of syndesmotic malreduction in each direction that leads to poorer outcomes is unclear, small changes in ankle joint alignment can lead to changes in contact forces.
- Open reduction, palpation, and closed reduction have been evaluated clinically and biomechanically.
  - Direct visualization via the incisura was shown to have lower rates of malreduction than indirect reduction.[20]
  - Open reduction with direct visualization at the distal articular cartilage was shown to provide more accurate reduction than visualizing the incisura.[29]
  - In an intact fibula model, no significant difference in reduction quality using direct visualization or palpation was noted.[23]
  - Trends toward external rotation and anteromedial translation with direct visualization and fibular external rotation and posterolateral translation with palpation
- Using a clamp to reduce can lead to syndesmotic overcompression and/or malreduction when compared to palpation or direct visualization, even if preoperative CT scan is used to plan the clamp trajectory.[6,19]
- Fixation methods have also been compared, including screw fixation, suture button fixation, and ligament reconstruction.
  - No difference in outcomes has been shown between one or two screws, fixation through three or four cortices, or size of screw used for fixation.
  - No clear difference has been shown in outcomes if syndesmotic screws are left in place, are allowed to break, or are removed.[10]
  - The literature does not support improved outcomes with routine screw removal,[7] and retained screws may not contribute to stiffness or impaired ankle dorsiflexion.[3]
  - Suture button devices have been shown to have lower rates of malreduction than screw fixation.[11,27]
  - Functional outcomes following suture button versus screw fixation have been similar or favoring suture button.
    - A recent randomized trial was unable to ascertain a difference but was underpowered for functional outcome.[27]

COMPLICATIONS

- Malunion
- Recurrence
- Deep infection
- Hardware failure
- Painful hardware
- Ankle instability
- Tibiotalar arthrosis
- Tibiofibular synostosis

REFERENCES

1. Andersen MR, Diep LM, Frihagen F, et al. Importance of syndesmotic reduction on clinical outcome after syndesmosis injuries. J Orthop Trauma 2019;33(8):397–403.
2. Boszczyk A, Kwapisz S, Krümmel M, et al. Correlation of incisura anatomy with syndesmotic malreduction. Foot Ankle Int 2018;39(3):369–375.
3. Briceno J, Wusu T, Kaiser P, et al. Effect of syndesmotic implant removal on dorsiflexion. Foot Ankle Int 2019;40(5):499–505.
4. Cherney SM, Cosgrove CT, Spraggs-Hughes AG, et al. Functional outcomes of syndesmotic injuries based on objective reduction accuracy at a minimum 1-year follow-up. J Orthop Trauma 2018;32(1):43–51.
5. Clanton TO, Williams BT, Backus JD, et al. Biomechanical analysis of the individual ligament contributions to syndesmotic stability. Foot Ankle Int 2017;38(1):66–75.
6. Cosgrove CT, Spraggs-Hughes AG, Putnam SM, et al. A novel indirect reduction technique in ankle syndesmotic injuries: a cadaveric study. J Orthop Trauma 2018;32(7):361–367
7. Dingemans SA, Rammelt S, White TO, et al. Should syndesmotic screws be removed after surgical fixation of unstable ankle fractures? A systematic review. Bone Joint J 2016;98(11):1497–1504.
8. Egol KA, Pahk B, Walsh M, et al. Outcome after unstable ankle fracture: effect of syndesmotic stabilization. J Orthop Trauma 2010;4(1):7–11.
9. Gardner MJ, Demetrakopoulos D, Briggs SM, et al. Malreduction of the tibiofibular syndesmosis in ankle fractures. Foot Ankle Int 2006;27(10):788–792.

10. Gennis E, Koenig S, Rodericks D, et al. The fate of the fixed syndesmosis over time. Foot Ankle Int 2015;36(10):1202–1208.
11. Grassi A, Samuelsson K, D'Hooghe P, et al. Dynamic stabilization of syndesmosis injuries reduces complications and reoperations as compared with screw fixation: a meta-analysis of randomized controlled trials. Am J Sports Med 2020;48(4):1000–1013.
12. Hagemeijer NC, Chang SH, Abdelaziz ME, et al. Range of normal and abnormal syndesmotic measurements using weightbearing CT. Foot Ankle Int 2019;40(12):1430–1437.
13. Haller JM, Githens M, Rothberg D, et al. Syndesmosis and syndesmotic equivalent injuries in tibial plafond fractures. J Orthop Trauma 2019;33(3):e74–e78.
14. Hermans JJ, Beumer A, de Jong TA, et al. Anatomy of the distal tibiofibular syndesmosis in adults: a pictorial essay with a multimodality approach. J Anat 2010;217(6):633–645.
15. Hunt KJ, Goeb Y, Behn AW, et al. Ankle joint contact loads and displacement with progressive syndesmotic injury. Foot Ankle Int 2015;36(9):1095–1103.
16. Kortekangas T, Flinkkilä T, Niinimäki J, et al. Effect of syndesmosis injury in SER IV (Weber B)-type ankle fractures on function and incidence of osteoarthritis. Foot Ankle Int 2015;36(2):180–187.
17. Laflamme M, Belzile EL, Bédard L, et al. A prospective randomized multicenter trial comparing clinical outcomes of patients treated surgically with a static or dynamic implant for acute ankle syndesmosis rupture. J Orthop Trauma 2015;29(5):216–223.
18. Lilyquist M, Shaw A, Latz K, et al. Cadaveric analysis of the distal tibiofibular syndesmosis. Foot Ankle Int 2016;37(8):882–890.
19. Miller AN, Barei DP, Iaquinto JM, et al. Iatrogenic syndesmosis malreduction via clamp and screw placement. J Orthop Trauma 2013;27(2):100–106.
20. Miller AN, Carroll EA, Parker RJ, et al. Direct visualization for syndesmotic stabilization of ankle fractures. Foot Ankle Int 2009;30:419–426.
21. Naqvi GA, Cunningham P, Lynch B, et al. Fixation of ankle syndesmotic injuries: comparison of tightrope fixation and syndesmotic screw fixation for accuracy of syndesmotic reduction. Am J Sports Med 2012;40:2828–2835.
22. Pang EQ, Bedigrew K, Palanca A, et al. Ankle joint contact loads and displacement in syndesmosis injuries repaired with tightropes compared to screw fixation in a static model. Injury 2019;50(11):1901–1907.
23. Pang EQ, Coughlan M, Bonaretti S, et al. Assessment of open syndesmosis reduction techniques in an unbroken fibula model: visualization versus palpation. J Orthop Trauma 2019;33(1):e14–e18.
24. Pyle C, Kim-Orden M, Hughes T, et al. Effect of early weightbearing following open reduction and internal fixation of unstable ankle fractures on wound complications or failures of fixation. Foot Ankle Int 2019;40(12):1397–1402.
25. Riedel MD, Miller CP, Kwon JY. Augmenting suture-button fixation for Maisonneuve injuries with fibular shortening: technique tip. Foot Ankle Int 2017;38(10):1146–1151.
26. Sagi HC, Shah AR, Sanders RW. The functional consequence of syndesmotic joint malreduction at a minimum 2-year follow-up. J Orthop Trauma 2012;26(7):439–443.
27. Sanders D, Schneider P, Taylor M, et al. Improved reduction of the tibiofibular syndesmosis with tightrope compared with screw fixation: results of a randomized controlled study. J Orthop Trauma 2019;33(11):531–537.
28. Sman AD, Hiller CE, Rae K, et al. Diagnostic accuracy of clinical tests for ankle syndesmosis injury. Br J Sports Med 2015;49(5):323–329.
29. Tornetta P III, Yakavonis M, Veltre D, et al. Reducing the syndesmosis under direct vision: where should I look? J Orthop Trauma 2019;33(9):450–454.
30. Warner SJ, Fabricant PD, Garner MR, et al. The measurement and clinical importance of syndesmotic reduction after operative fixation of rotational ankle fractures. J Bone Joint Surg Am 2015;97(23):1935–1944.
31. Weening B, Bhandari M. Predictors of functional outcome following transsyndesmotic screw fixation of ankle fractures. J Orthop Trauma 2005;19(2):102–108.
32. Wikerøy AK, Høiness PR, Andreassen GS, et al. No difference in functional and radiographic results 8.4 years after quadricortical compared with tricortical syndesmosis fixation in ankle fractures. J Orthop Trauma 2010; 24(1):17–23.

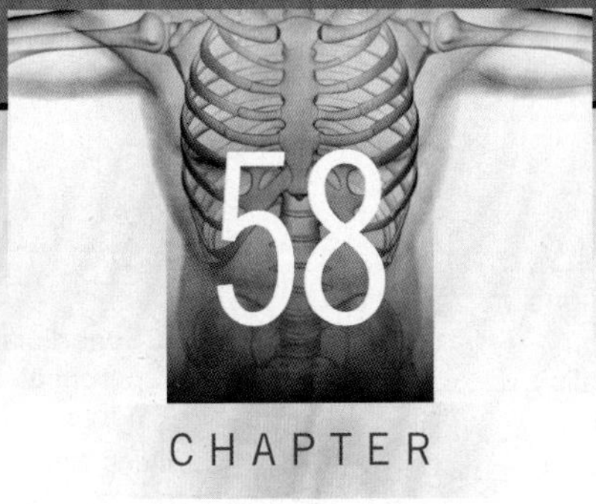

Hindfoot Fusion Nail for Geriatric Indications

Paul Andrzejowski and Peter V. Giannoudis

DEFINITION

- A hindfoot nail, otherwise known as a *retrograde tibial nail*, or tibiotalocalcaneal (TTC) nail is a load-sharing device inserted through the hindfoot (os calcis, otherwise known as the *calcaneum*, and talus) into the tibia, in order to achieve relative stability across the tibiotalar and talocalcaneal joint surfaces, rendering them immobile.
- Fusion is the process of different bones joining to become one; this occurs as a part of normal development, but can also be surgically induced (arthrodesis), which we discuss in this chapter. For fusion to occur, the bones concerned must be kept in close contact and firmly fixed in a stable position using a strong construct such as a TTC nail.

ANATOMY

- The hindfoot is formed from the calcaneus and talus, and through communication with the midfoot anteriorly, contributes to two bony arches, which allow for normal ambulation: medial arch (calcaneus, talus, navicular, three cuneiforms, three medial metatarsals) and lateral arch (calcaneus, cuboid, two lateral metatarsals).
  - In normal physiology, strong ligaments are integral to joining bony structures throughout the foot, including the hindfoot. Insertion of a nail bypasses these, assuming their function of stabilizing the ankle mortise **(FIG 1A)**.
- The calcaneal tuberosity, on its plantar aspect, is the primary weight-bearing point of the hindfoot, posteroinferior in relation to the talus, which lies above.
  - It can be palpated clearly under the skin and used as a landmark when planning incision to the plantar aspect for nail insertion.
- The talus sits on top of the calcaneus and through three articulations forms the ankle joint: superiorly at the trochlear ridge with the inferior tibia, medially with the medial malleolus of the tibia, and laterally with the lateral malleolus of the fibula. Anteriorly, it communicates with the midfoot at the talonavicular joint.
  - The talar body is somewhat wider anteriorly, which means that in full dorsiflexion it locks between the medial and lateral malleoli, but in plantarflexion slight laxity allows for sideways tilt: an important consideration for positioning throughout the operation **(FIG 1B)**.
- The tibia is the main weight-bearing structure of the lower leg, communicating with the talus at tibiotalar joint, which has two facets; in normal circumstances, the superior facet permits dorsiflexion and plantarflexion at the ankle. At the junction between the middle and distal third of the tibia, there is a narrowing (isthmus), and the tibia has an anterior bow, which can be marked in some individuals.
  - These factors must be taken into account during preoperative planning and assessed using anteroposterior (AP) and lateral x-rays.

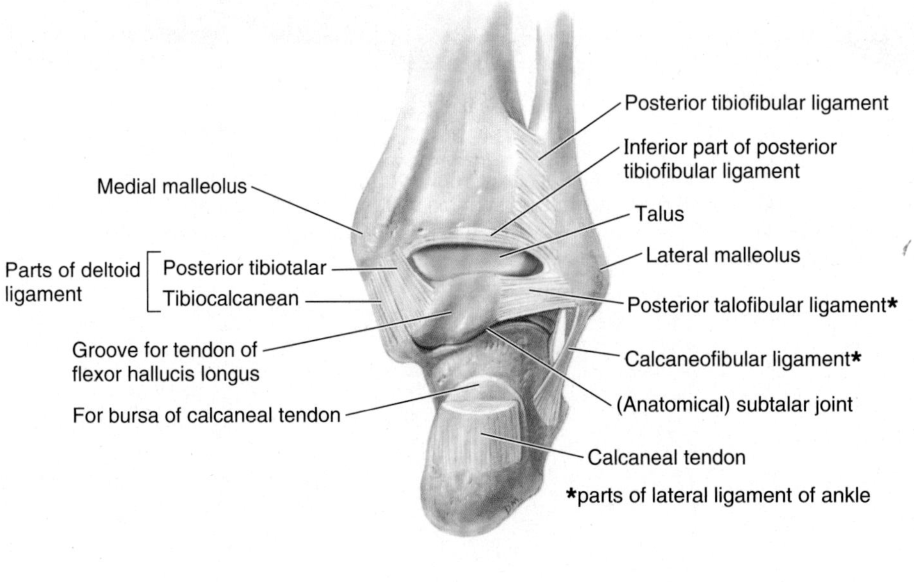

A

FIG 1 Foot and ankle anatomy. **A.** Posterior view of the ligaments and bony alignment. *(continued)*

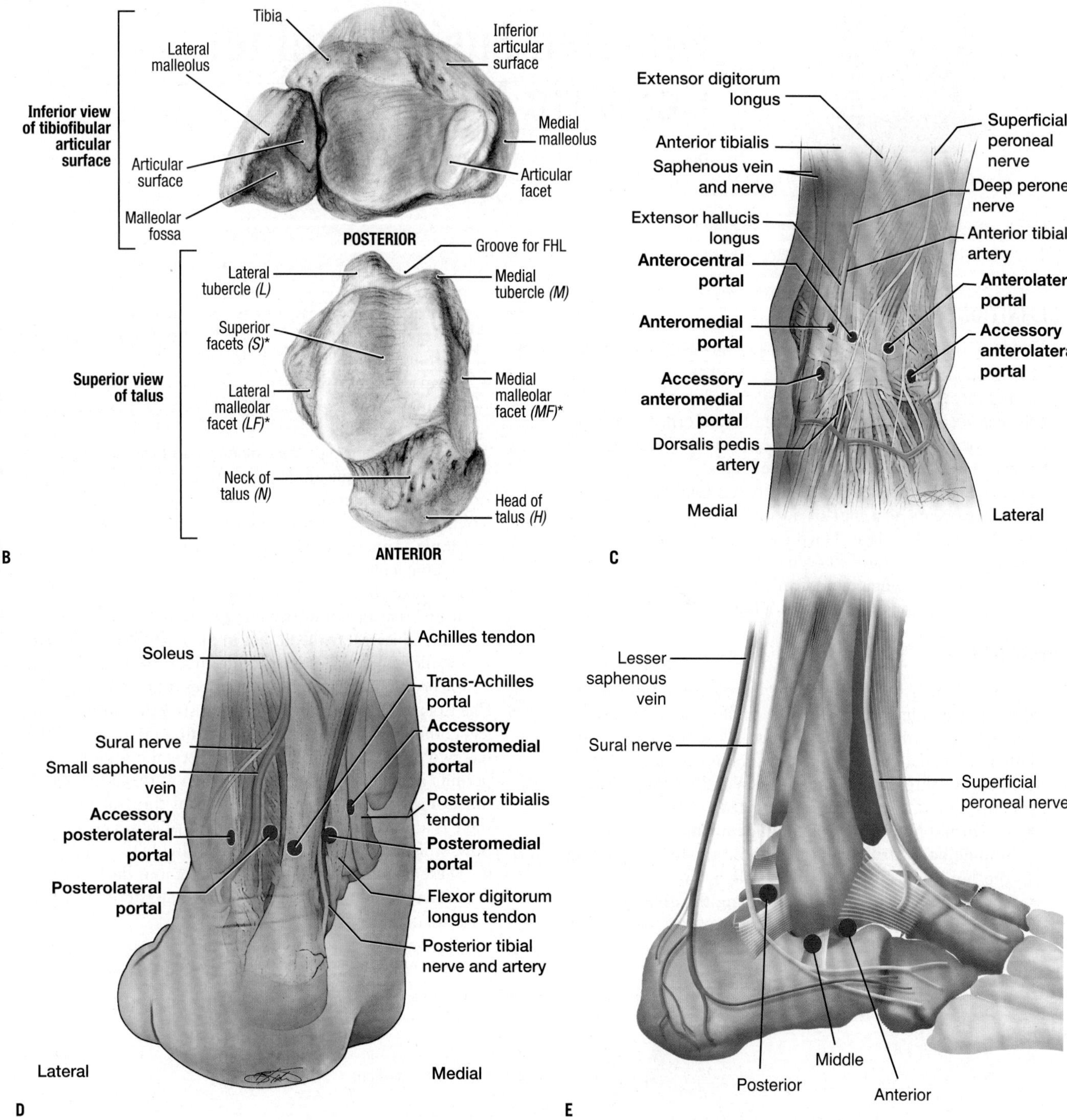

FIG 1 *(continued)* **B.** Superior and inferior talus articulations. *FHL*, flexor hallucis longus. Anterior (**C**), posterior (**D**), and Lateral aspect (**E**) ankle neurovascular anatomy and portal positions. (**A:** Reprinted with permission from Moore KL, Dalley AF, Agur AMR. Clinically Oriented Anatomy, ed 7. Baltimore: Lippincott Williams & Wilkins, 2014. Figure 6-28A. **B:** Reprinted with permission from Agur AMR, Dalley AF. Grant's Atlas of Anatomy, ed 14. Baltimore: Wolters Kluwer, 2017. Figure 6-83.)

- The distal fibula forms the lateral malleolus of the ankle joint and is important for its stability. When fusing the ankle, this can be used as graft material.
- There is a natural 12 degrees of hindfoot valgus and 5 to 10 degrees of external rotation with respect to the tibial crest, which one should seek to replicate as closely as possible with a TTC nail.[24]
- Anterior to the medial malleolus lies the long saphenous vein and nerve, posteriorly lie the tibial nerve and posterior tibial artery and vein **(FIG 1C–E)**. On the lateral aspect, the superficial peroneal nerve crosses the fibula 5 to 15 cm above the lateral malleolus, and the sural nerve passes posteriorly in between the peroneus longus and Achilles tendon.
  - Severing nerves can lead to painful neuroma formation and numbness, and injury to vascular structures can lead to impaired blood supply and potential ischemia.
- Blood supply to the hindfoot comes from the rich reticular network, which receive their origins from the anterior and posterior tibial arteries, with sensory nerve supply derived from all nerves crossing the region, including the sural, saphenous, tibial, superficial, and deep peroneal nerves.

PATHOGENESIS

- Trauma: The nature of fractures to the foot and ankle are directly correlated to the amount of force transmitted through bone and soft tissue structures during an injury. Higher energy injuries lead to more widespread damage, with injury pattern being related to the route of energy transmission through the ankle mortise, as defined in the Lauge-Hansen classification.[31]
  - In geriatric patients, a significant number of ankle fractures come from low-energy injuries in osteoporotic bone—which breaks either just above or just below the level of the syndesmosis, which is usually stronger than the bone which surrounds it—and often involve the tibia and fibula at the same level, making them unstable.[2,17]
- Osteoarthritis (OA) refers to a degenerative joint process that can be multifactorial in origin.
  - It is characterized by loss of joint space, osteophyte formation, subchondral cysts, and sclerosis. In the ankle, unlike the hip and knee, almost 70% of ankle OA is posttraumatic.[13,15,29]
- Loss of joint space is secondary to cartilage wear and destruction; as a consequence of aging there is a loss of water and proteoglycans from the collagen fibrils that make up the cartilage, which leads to a stiffening, which predisposes it to subsequent damage and subsequent inflammatory cascade, which leads to further chondrolysis.[29]
- Osteophytes are fibrocartilage capped bony outgrowths seen at diarthrodial subchondral joint margins. It is debated whether they are caused by a physiologic reaction (adaption) to abnormal weight-bearing pattern through the joint (ie, have a cause) or are produced secondary to the hyperinflammatory state of the joint with overactivation of the osteochondral repair and growth mechanisms via mesenchymal stem cells in the synovial or periosteal lining (dysregulation of normal repair mechanisms).[13,28,29]
- Subchondral cyst formation is also not fully understood, but two main theories predominate.[6,16,29]
  - In some cases, synovium is seen to extend into the bone, and abnormal cartilage is seen over and within the cysts, which suggests their origin may be due to "synovial intrusion."
  - In other cases, however, there is no communication between the cyst and joint. The "bone contusion theory" postulates that microfractures are caused by impact and friction between opposing bone ends in a joint with degenerate protective cartilage; the subsequent osteoclastic resorption of necrotic bone allows synovial fluid to enter the subchondral space from the joint capsule. This is exacerbated by abnormal remodeling and repair mechanisms seen in OA.
- Subchondral sclerosis can be seen on x-rays in later stages of OA. It represents an increase in bone volume density seen at subchondral bone interfaces, but actual mineralization and therefore strength and stiffness are reduced.
  - It is theorized that the increase in amount of bone is generated to compensate for lack of strength in the bone itself and other deformities such as cysts, which weaken bone further in themselves and can therefore be considered to represent a mechanoregulatory response.[18]
- Avascular necrosis (AVN) in the hindfoot is most commonly seen following high-energy injury, which strips the blood supply from bony structures, in particular, the talus, with dislocation resulting in a high rate of AVN.[20,21,27]

NATURAL HISTORY

- Trauma: If a patient has normal biology surrounding a fracture site, with bone ends of the fracture fragments in close association, and held in a cast in relative stability, they will generally proceed to unite. Depending on the nature of the fracture, however, especially in unstable fractures, this can result in malunion, which could lead to subsequent arthritis, or even nonunion, which has been reported as high as 48% to 73% in patients older than 60 years.[17]
  - It is these cases for which surgery is an absolute indication in most circumstances. Surgery will also allow for earlier return to active range of motion and function. Generally, after 6 weeks, if relatively stable and left untouched, fractures will heal by indirect healing, and hematoma surrounding the fracture will have consolidated into hard callus, at which point a patient will be able to ambulate freely with few restrictions. In cases of operative fixation, total time to fracture healing may be longer depending on the nature of fixation applied due to interruption of the fracture hematoma, but as the fixation device will be load sharing, in a position of either absolute or relative stability, patients are usually able to get back to normal function earlier, which is one of the main indications to operate.[4]
- AVN, if left unmanaged, leads to collapse of bony structures and significant pain, with potential instability, especially in the ankle joint.[27]
- OA is generally a slowly progressive, chronic condition; however, in cases of major trauma to the joint, this process can be accelerated. There is classically activity-related swelling,

sprains, and pain; stiffness; altered foot alignment with time; and altered anatomic axis of foot structures.

- On examination, this manifests itself with ankle effusion; weak ligament and tendon complexes; generalized tenderness; reduced range of motion; any direction of abnormal alignment of hindfoot, midfoot, or forefoot structures; and alterations of the coronal or sagittal axes of the foot or swelling of any of the small joint complexes. If symptoms progress to a stage resulting in disability, operative intervention may be the only means of restoring a normal baseline level of function.[15]

PATIENT HISTORY AND PHYSICAL FINDINGS

Acute Trauma

- A formal advanced trauma life support approach, with primary and secondary surveys should be taken initially to rule out any life- or limb-threatening injuries. Mechanism of injury must be established, in particular any fall from height, which may have led to injury anywhere up the patient's vertical column, including lower limbs, hips, pelvis, and spine.
- Concerning the ankle and hindfoot, it is essential to assess for skin integrity and viability, looking for evidence of fracture blisters, whether the fracture is open or closed, and assess distal neurovascular status. Compartment syndrome must also be ruled out. Severity of injury will broadly be determined by the mechanism and energy of injury sustained (higher energy = worse injury pattern and higher risk of compartment syndrome).
- In particular, fracture-dislocations in the hindfoot pose a significant risk for soft tissue degloving and neurovascular compromise. Very careful attention must be paid to this; it should be regularly monitored and not forgotten about.
- If there is good skin integrity, and no concern of soft tissue compromise or compartment syndrome, more time can be taken to plan subsequent management accordingly.

Elective

- History of management of chronic illnesses, whether this can be diabetes, rheumatoid disease, end-organ disease or other, will need to be elicited. It is important to make sure the patient is stable before proceeding, which may require discussion with their specialist physicians.
- Examination of the ankle and hindfoot is critical if the patient has underlying disorders.
- Assessment of skin integrity and viability, including neuropathic and vascular ulceration
- Neurologic examination of lower limbs, including assessing for peripheral neuropathy, "glove and stocking" distribution of numbness, and level of fine-touch pressure sensation using a 5.07 per 10 g monofilament device, pinprick sensation using a Neurotip (Owen Mumford Ltd, Brook Hill, Woodstock, Oxfordshire, OX20 1TU, United Kingdom), vibration perception using a 128-Hz tuning fork, and ankle reflexes, proprioception, and thermal (hot/cold) discrimination[10,23]
- Posterior tibial and dorsalis pedis pulse, distal capillary refill time assessment, as well as characterization of waveforms using a Doppler probe as necessary
- Ankle–brachial pressure index assessment
- Rule out obviously infected joint (rubor/dolor/calor/tumor),[11] investigating further as appropriate, as this would be a contraindication to fusion nailing.

IMAGING AND OTHER DIAGNOSTIC STUDIES

- Baseline blood tests
  - Complete blood count, including white cell differential, platelets, hemoglobin level, and concentration, to assess fitness and infection risk
  - Urea, creatinine, and electrolytes to assess fitness
  - Liver function, bone profile (calcium, phosphate, alkaline phosphatase) to assess fitness and bone healing potential
  - Vitamin D and trace elements to assess fitness, soft tissue, and bone healing potential
  - Coagulation screen to rule out coagulopathy
  - C-reactive protein and erythrocyte sedimentation rate to assess for infection
  - Diabetes blood tests: fasting glucose and hemoglobin A1c
- Imaging **(FIG 2)**
  - At a minimum, plain film radiographs should be obtained, with AP, mortise, and lateral views.
  - Depending on the nature of the ankle/hindfoot, computed tomography (CT) scanning may also be required for preoperative planning purposes.
  - Magnetic resonance imaging of ankle/hindfoot to assess for AVN, also magnetic resonance angiogram, may be required in cases of concerning vasculopathy. In rare cases where the indication for surgery is part of a tumor resection operation, need for vessel embolization can be assessed and planned.
  - If malignancy involved, consider staging CT scanning and bone scans in liaison with the oncology multidisciplinary team.
  - Imaging can also be used to estimate length and width of nail required, using templating software.

DIFFERENTIAL DIAGNOSIS

- Any erosive or inflammatory arthritis, commonly rheumatoid
- Degenerative end-stage osteoarthritis
- Posttraumatic arthritis
- Chronic infection or septic arthritis, with chondrolysis and loss of joint space
- Charcot neuroarthropathy
- Diabetic neuroarthropathy of other cause
- Talus collapse with avascular necrosis
- Bone tumor
- Acquired or congenital rigid equinovarus deformity
- Failed ankle or hindfoot arthrodesis
- Failed total ankle arthroplasty
- Trauma

NONOPERATIVE MANAGEMENT

- Traumatic ankle fractures may be suitable for nonoperative management in either a walker boot or cast depending on their severity and stability, and physical state of the patient, with the risks of surgery weighed up against the benefits of surgery, which include a quicker resolution of pain and return to function, and healing in an improved position than if managed conservatively. It should be noted that nonoperative management of unstable ankle fractures can have seriously deleterious consequences, with malunion of up to 73% and secondary displacement seen in up to 23% of cases, which can have severely disabling long-term consequences.[22]
- Most cases of osteoarthritis are managed nonsurgically, with oral analgesia, anti-inflammatory agents, and local

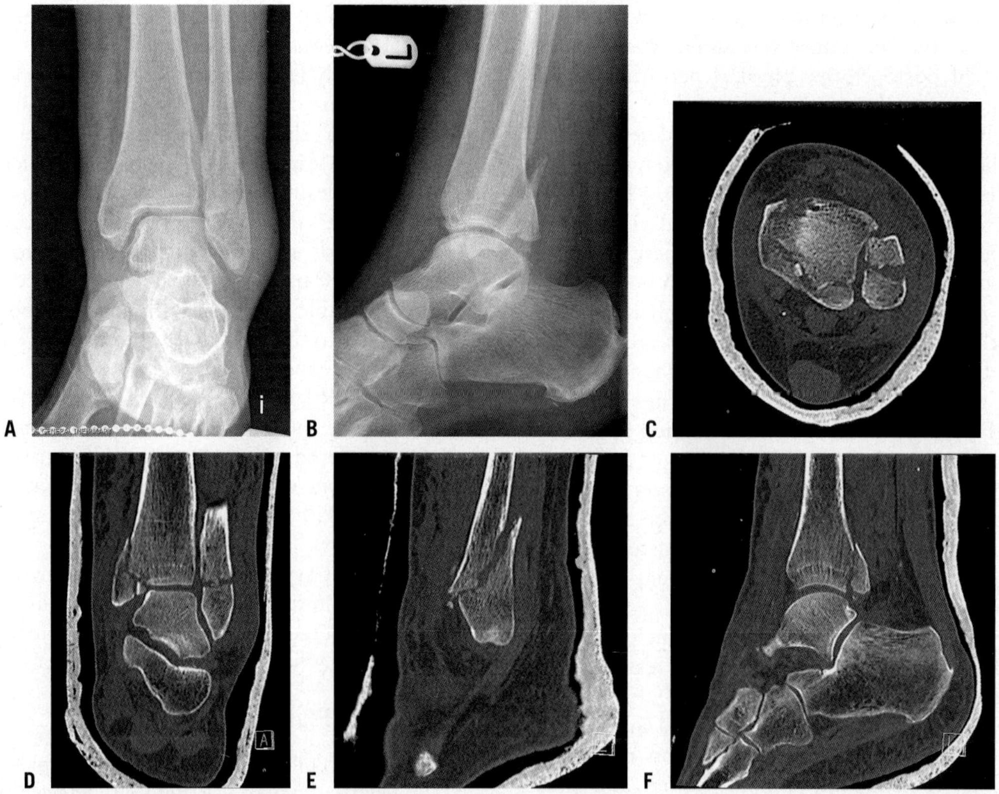

FIG 2 AP (**A**) and lateral (**B**) radiographs and axial (**C**), coronal (**D**), and sagittal (fibula in **E**, tibia in **F**) CTs of an ankle fracture repaired using TTC nailing.

steroid injections alongside physiotherapy and orthotic support. Depending on the functional demand of the patient concerned, for some patients, this may not satisfy their functional requirements, however.

- AVN, depending on the severity and pain, can be managed conservatively in the first instance, unless surgery can improve the final outcome and potentially restore blood supply, in which case, pursuing a conservative course would be inadvisable.

SURGICAL MANAGEMENT

Indications (TABLE 1)

- The decision to manage a fracture with a hindfoot nail in the acute setting rests on two main factors: the nature of both the injury and the patient. Hindfoot nailing is a viable treatment option for any patient regardless of age, especially where there is extensive soft tissue injury or more complicated fracture configuration, such as Arbeitsgemeinschaft für Osteosynthesefragen/Orthopedic Trauma Association (AO/OTA) type 43-C pilon fractures, talus fracture-dislocations, or calcaneal fractures.[25]
- In geriatric populations, one must consider the injury in the context of the host (patient); the geriatric population is one that naturally poses various challenges, and the relevant risks and benefits of any procedure must be weighed against these. Wherever possible, the various treatment options should be discussed with the patient directly, or where unable, their relatives, to come to a sensible management decision. Every procedure comes with different potential positive and negative outcomes attached, and depending on

TABLE 1 Indications for Retrograde Tibial Nailing

Acute Pathology: Trauma
Injury-related
• Complex fracture pattern to ankle joint, tibial plafond (pilon), or hindfoot fracture-dislocation
• Irreversible cartilage injury
• Extensive soft tissue injury
Patient-related
• Wound- or fracture-healing risk factors: immunocompromise, vascular disease, neuropathy (eg, diabetes)
• Smoking status
• Low level of patient compliance with postoperative rehabilitation (eg, dementia)
• Low level of functional outcome required (poor baseline mobility)
Elective Pathology
• Erosive or inflammatory degeneration, with chondrolysis and arthralgia (eg, rheumatoid arthritis, septic arthritis)
• Cartilage/bone destruction or abnormality to hindfoot or ankle of any other cause (eg, Charcot/diabetic neuropathy, posttraumatic arthritis, end-stage osteoarthritis, talar AVN with collapse, acquired or congenital rigid equinovarus deformity, bone tumor)
• Iatrogenic (eg, failed ankle or hindfoot arthrodesis, failed total ankle arthroplasty)

AVN, avascular necrosis.

the patient's baseline function and their expectations following treatment, they may have very different ambitions for their level of postoperative physical performance, to balance against potential risks of surgery.

- The nature of the fracture itself must be considered.
  - In cases where the injury has caused, or is likely to lead to irreversible cartilage injury, ankle fusion may be preferable to the long-term arthralgia from chondral damage.
  - Hindfoot nails can also be used in cases where complete reconstruction would be inadvisable due to host factors or used as part of a staged reconstruction plan.[25,32]
  - Many ankle fractures in geriatric patients are fragility fractures due to osteoporotic bone, which pose challenges for traditional open reduction and internal fixation (ORIF), a problem that is circumvented by use of a TTC nail.[26]
  - In cases in which there has been extensive soft tissue injury in a closed fracture, which would pose a risk for infection and wound breakdown if incised to operate, or in open fractures where metalwork may interfere with wound management or a stable zone of injury is required for soft tissue cover, a hindfoot nailing procedure to allow fracture union (with or without fusion) is an acceptable treatment option.[2,3,5,12,14,17,22,26]
- In most cases in which the procedure is used in geriatric populations, however, it is often patient factors that drive decision making. Concomitant pathophysiology alongside the injury can have profound consequences for success of both wound and fracture healing. Patients with any form of immunocompromise, vasculopathy, or neuropathy are at higher risk for delayed wound healing, infection, and nonunion. Diabetic patients and those who smoke are particularly at risk for postoperative complications. Insertion of a hindfoot nail requires significantly less soft tissue dissection than for traditional ORIF, with a much lower risk for problems with wound healing and infection postoperatively.[1,26,30]
- Finally, and importantly, the social context must be considered. Patients who have a low baseline of physical function and therefore who put low cyclical loads through their ankle joint are less likely to require full range of active motion following repair of their fracture. It is important in patients with poor mobility to maintain this level as best as possible and return to fully weight bearing as swiftly as possible following surgery to maintain muscle tone and keep mobile.[12,22] Depending on the nature of the fracture, traditional foot/ankle ORIF operations can require up to 6 weeks of immobilization afterward to achieve safe, reliable results. In patients with poor muscle tone and baseline mobility, this consigns the patient to inevitable disuse sarcopenia and higher risk of thromboembolic events as well as impairing return to preinjury functional status. It also puts patients who are unable to comply with this postoperative rehabilitation plan, whether through dementia or domestic/other circumstances, at risk for failure of fixation and thereby further surgery.[12]
- End-stage destructive osteoarthritis can be very disabling, and in such cases, operative intervention may be required. The operation offered will depend on the patient's baseline functional level.[7,20]
  - For younger, more middle-aged and generally active older patients, a total ankle arthroplasty must be considered as an alternative treatment option and form part of the informed consent discussion.
  - In elderly frail patients, however, a hindfoot fusion nail procedure can offer good pain relief and a good level of function relative to their baseline mobility.
- In cases of severe avascular necrosis, which lead to almost complete destruction of bony architecture, commonly of the talus, a salvage operation is often required. There are a number of management options, including ankle fusion using a TTC nail, with the talus itself used as bone graft. It offers a stable construct with generally positive outcomes, preferable to the difficult symptoms that patients with these conditions experience daily.
- A total ankle replacement (TAR) is one of the treatment options for end-stage joint erosion, which would generally be offered to more functionally active patients. When this fails, one of the treatment options is to fuse the ankle with a TTC nail, to reduce pain and symptoms of ankle instability.
  - A recent systematic review has shown that TAR has a revision rate of up to 23%,[19] and ankle fusion often represents a more reliable method of managing severe ankle arthritis, with fewer overall complications.

Preoperative Planning

- The initial concern with preoperative planning is the type and length of nail to use. Before the development of specialist hindfoot fusion nails, it was common to use short nails that had been designed for distal femoral supracondylar fractures, curved humeral nails, or longer tibial intramedullary nails inverted and used in a retrograde fashion. Studies show broadly good results with all of these methods, but newer nail designs account for physiologic valgus at the ankle joint and provide multiple hindfoot-specific locking options.
- Some studies have suggested that longer nails have favorable biomechanics, as they passed through the isthmus so were more stable and reduced the risk of periprosthetic fracture; however, modern fusion nail designs that have stable cross-locking options take this into account, and there is no longer the need to cross the isthmus in all cases, although this is still a valid consideration, and studies have shown good results using longer hindfoot nails.[2]
- Hindfoot-specific nailing systems range from 150 to 300 mm in length, to provide a nail that bypasses the isthmus, should this be advantageous or preferred. In cases of severe osteoporosis and poor bone stock, it may be necessary to cross the isthmus to achieve adequate stability that comes with the longer working length of the nail.
- Specific operative techniques vary depending on which nail is chosen, and one must be familiar with the particular system chosen, consulting the respective manual beforehand. Photos shown demonstrate the Phoenix Ankle Arthrodesis Nail System (Zimmer Biomet, Warsaw, IN) used to manage an ankle fracture.
- Other popular systems include the T2 Arthrodesis Nailing System (Stryker, Kalamazoo, MI), the TRIGEN Fusion Nail (Smith & Nephew, Memphis, TN), and the VALOR Hindfoot Fusion Nail System (Wright Medical Group N.V., Arlington, TN) among several others.

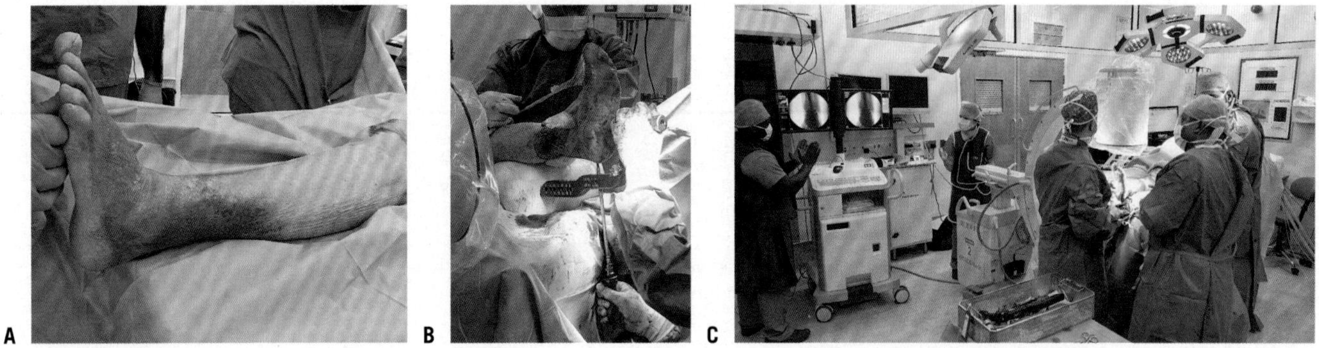

FIG 3 A. Preoperative positioning of patient, with foot 5 to 8 cm off end of operating table, to allow adequate access to hindfoot. **B.** Technique of holding foot in plantigrade using sterile iodine plastic incision drapes and jig insertion facilitating PA nail insertion. **C.** General operating room and fluoroscopic x-ray setup.

Positioning

- Patients can either be positioned lateral or supine.
- Lateral position offers the advantage of making posteroanterior (PA) screw insertion easier and facilitating lateral insertion of other screws without having to move the patient.
- Our preferred method is supine on a radiolucent table, with a sandbag or bolster underneath the ipsilateral buttock, with a high tourniquet placed on the thigh.
- It is vital that the heel of the foot is able to hang off the end of the table, in order to achieve good access to the hindfoot, and facilitate PA screw insertion **(FIG 3A)**.
- A bolster can be used as required underneath the calf to help with access.
- The surgeon should be positioned at the end of the table and assistant as needed. Our preferred method for retracting the foot is shown in **FIG 3B**. Once prepped, the toes are blocked off with an Ioban antimicrobial incision drape, and this used as a sling to hold the foot in position.
- This positioning provides good access to all aspects of the ankle joint for bone resection or joint preparation as needed as well as the plantar aspect of the foot for nail and PA screw insertion and allows easy insertion and manipulation of targeting jigs. It is also simpler when dealing with patients of a larger body habitus and checking ankle rotation with respect to the contralateral side.
- The C-arm x-ray machine is set up to come in from the contralateral side, with fluoroscopy screens placed here also **(FIG 3C)**.

Approach

- The approach varies slightly depending on which nail is used, and the relevant operative technique booklet must be consulted when using unfamiliar kit. It also depends on whether preparation of the joint surface is to be performed or not.
- Furthermore, consideration must be made whether an open or closed approach is to be used for the joint surface preparation.
- Portals for ankle joint preparation, if this technique is to be used, can be made through any of the standard approaches. We find anteromedial and anterolateral portal sites the most useful **(FIG 4A)**.
- In general, for open approaches, incisions must be made centered over lateral and/or medial malleoli for joint preparation and autograft harvest as well as on the plantar aspect of the heel for TTC nail insertion, posteriorly for PA screw insertion, and in various positions on the lower leg for locking screw insertion **(FIG 4B,C)**.

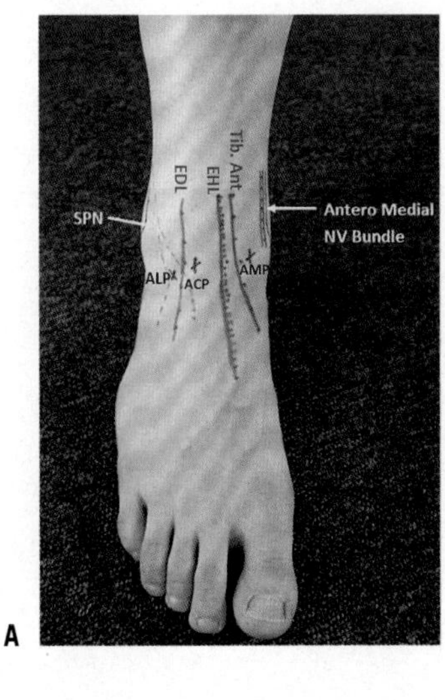

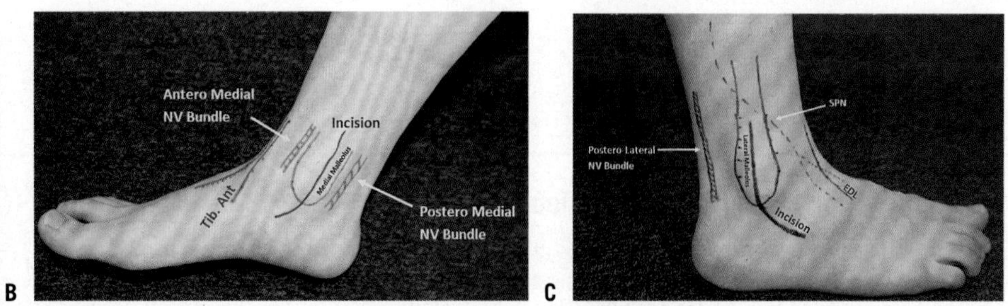

FIG 4 Surface anatomy of anterior (**A**), medial (**B**), and lateral (**C**) aspects of ankle, with arthroscopic portal approaches marked as a black cross. Tendons are in *red*, nerves in *yellow*, and portals and incisions in *blue*. *EDL*, extensor digitorum longus; *EHL*, extensor hallucis longus; *Tib Ant*, tibialis anterior; *SPN*, superficial peroneal nerve; *NV*, neurovascular; *ALP*, anterolateral portal; *ACP*, anterocentral portal; *AMP*, anteromedial portal.

LATERAL INCISION

- The first incision should be made laterally, curving over the lateral malleolus, distally along the peroneus tendon, from 2 to 3 cm above to the sinus tarsi distally to allow subtalar joint exposure (see **FIG 4C**).
- Care should be taken to protect the superficial peroneal nerve anteriorly from 5 to 15 cm above the lateral malleolus, and the sural nerve posteriorly, as well as the peroneal muscle tendons and the lateral peroneal artery, which is sometimes present near the syndesmosis.
- Care should also be taken to preserve the peroneal tendons, which run posteriorly.

DISTAL FIBULA OSTEOTOMY

- Harvest the distal 5-cm of fibula using either a bone saw or drill followed by osteotome, with a cut 2 cm above the tibiotalar joint, at an angle superolateral to inferomedial to improve healing and postoperative irritation from prominent bone ends (**TECH FIG 1**).
- After harvest, the resected fibula should be morselized to use as autologous bone graft, using either a bone saw or reamer.
- Once the lateral approach and distal fibula resection are completed, access to the joint can be obtained for preparation.

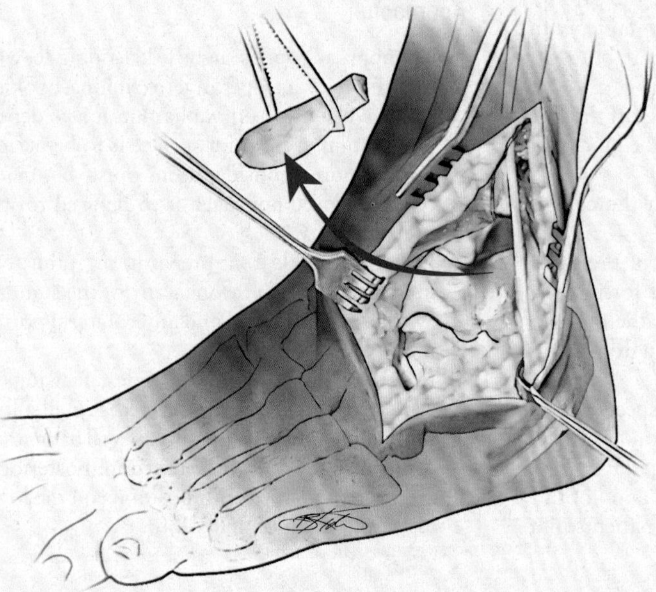
A

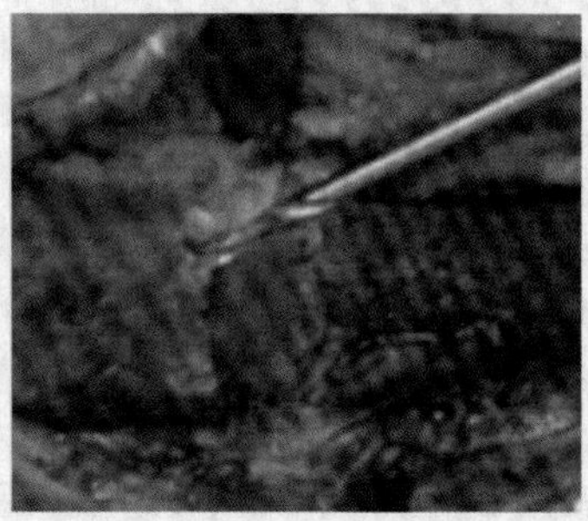
B

TECH FIG 1 Illustration *(red arrow)* (**A**) and intraoperative image (**B**) demonstrating distal fibular resection.

JOINT PREPARATION

Method 1: Joint Congruent Resection

- The aim is to preserve the natural shape of the ankle joint as much as possible and minimize shortening of the limb while removing all remaining joint cartilage.
- This can be done open or arthroscopically.
- Open
  - Articular cartilage is then removed from the distal tibia and proximal talus, moving from lateral to medial, down to fresh bleeding bone, using osteotomes, curettes and bone nibblers.
  - Deformities such as osteophytes are removed accordingly, and using arthrotomies from anteromedial/lateral aspects, any ankle deformity can also be corrected as required.
- Arthroscopic
  - Usually, ankle joint débridement with synovectomy is performed through anterolateral and anteromedial port sites at the tibiotalar joint and should also be extended to include the subtalar joint using appropriate portals (**TECH FIG 2A**).
  - If an arthroscopic approach is to be taken, this will have to be completed prior to fibular resection or the decision made to perform arthroscopic fibula resection (**TECH FIG 2B–E**), which has also been shown to have good results.[7]

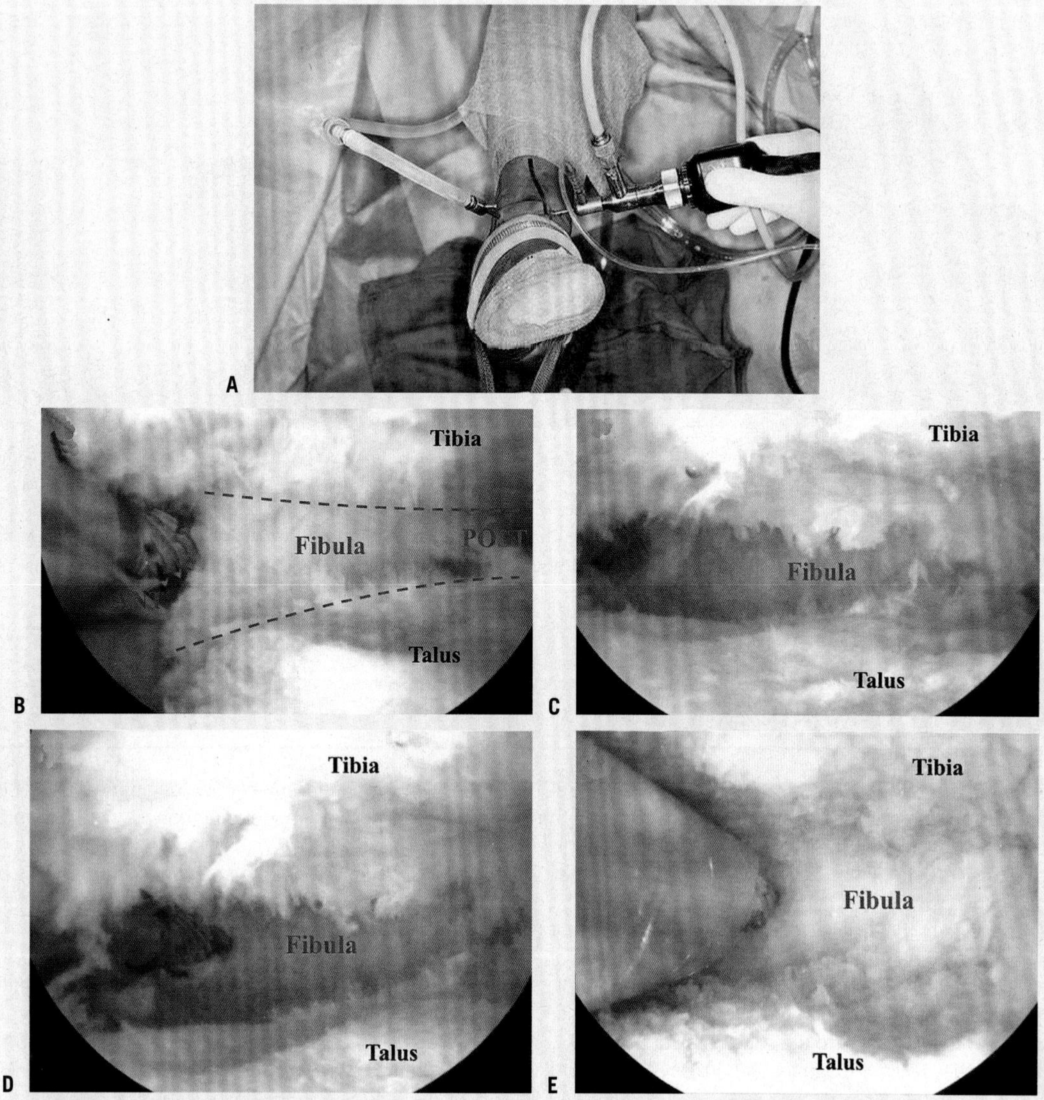

TECH FIG 2 **A.** Anterior ankle arthroscopic portals in situ. **B–E.** Arthroscopic arthrodesis with tibiotalar osteotomy in a right ankle. **B.** Initially burr placed anterior (*ANT*) to fibula. **C.** The area to be débrided is marked. **D,E.** Fibula osteotomized anterior to posterior (*POST*). (Reprinted from Bernasconi A, Mehdi N, Lintz F. Fibular intra-articular resection during arthroscopic ankle arthrodesis: the surgical technique. Arthrosc Tech 2017;6[5]:e1865–e1870. Copyright © 2017 by the Arthroscopy Association of North America. With permission.)

Method 2: Flat Cut Resection

- Using the lateral or medial incision for access, a cut is made transversely across the distal tibia using a bone saw. An incision can also be made over the medial aspect to remove the medial malleolus if required, which can also be incorporated into the bone graft material **(TECH FIG 3A)**.
- The ankle must then be held in strict plantigrade position.
- A matching cut should be made transversely in the proximal talar dome.
- Posterior and lateral surfaces of the talus are then decorticated using osteotomes.
- Excise articular surface from subtalar joint.
  - This method aims to increase the fusion surface and also allows for more precise positioning: The distal tibia can be moved medially to align the hindfoot more directly in relation to the tibia **(TECH FIG 3B,C)**.
- The subchondral bone surfaces should then be drilled with a 2.5-mm drill bit, to encourage a fresh-bleeding surface.

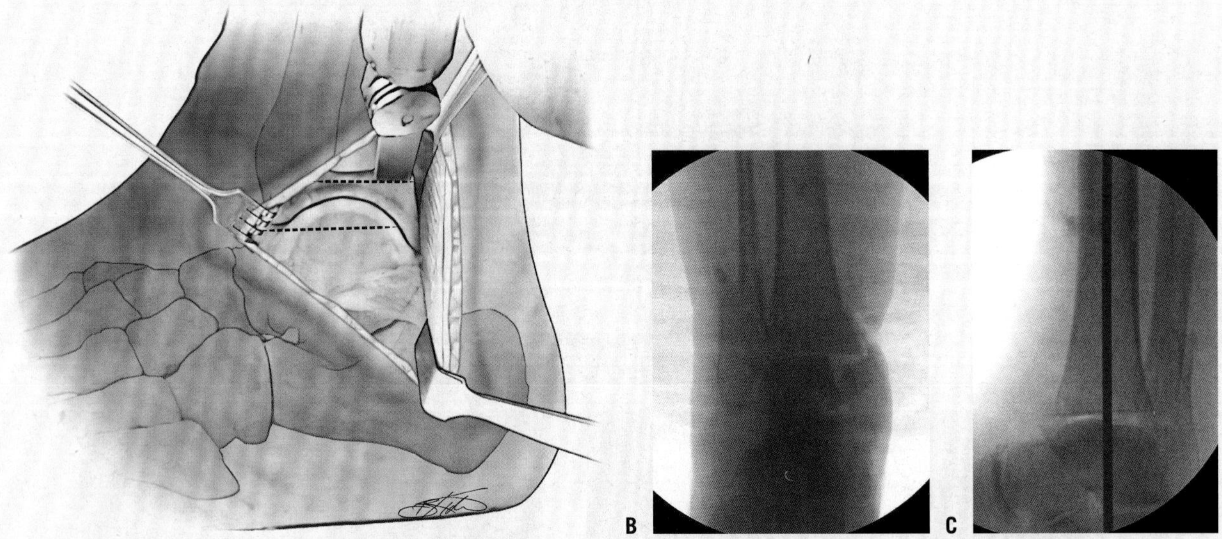

TECH FIG 3 A. Illustration of flat-cut tibiotalar resection. Intraoperative AP (**B**) and lateral (**C**) radiographs of flat-cut tibial plafond.

INCISION AND ENTRY POINT FOR NAIL

- When positioning the joint, the overall aim is to achieve neutral dorsiflexion, 3 to 5 degrees of hindfoot, and external rotation the same as the other foot or 5 to 10 degrees in relation to the tibial crest. The second ray should be parallel with the anteromedial crest of the tibia **(TECH FIG 4A,B)**.
- Put a Kirschner wire or metal instrument on the plantar aspect of the foot, at the boundary of the lateral third, and take an axial heel view with x-ray—aim to align this with the central longitudinal axis of the calcaneus. Use a skin marker to note this position.
- Next, move the wire/instrument to the lateral aspect of the ankle and swing the C-arm through for lateral x-rays to confirm position, aiming for the central longitudinal axis of the tibia, and mark this position—extending down onto the plantar aspect **(TECH FIG 4C,D)**.
- These two lines should intersect and form a cross on the bottom of the foot, just anterior to the subcalcaneal fat pad, well in front of the calcaneal tuberosity.
- Make a skin incision and use blunt dissection down to plantar fascia and then use the knife to cut in line with its fibers **(TECH FIG 4E)**.
- Sweep the intrinsic foot muscles aside and aim to visualize and protect the neurovascular bundle present nearby **(TECH FIG 4F)**.

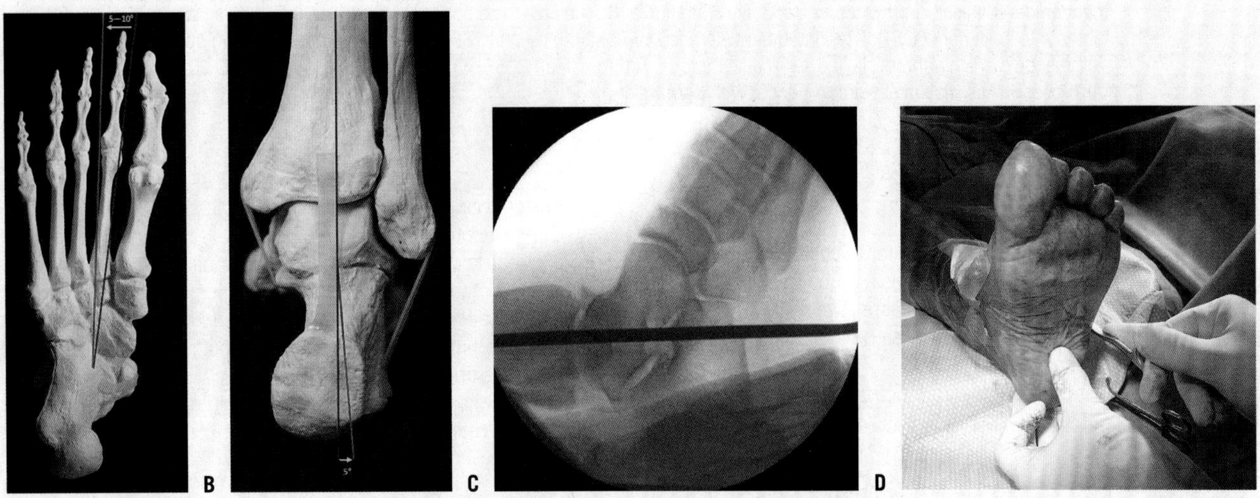

TECH FIG 4 Position of external rotation (**A**) and hindfoot valgus (**B**) required for ankle fusion. Intraoperative lateral radiograph (**C**) and photo (**D**) demonstrating method of locating incision and entry point using metal instrument. *(continued)*

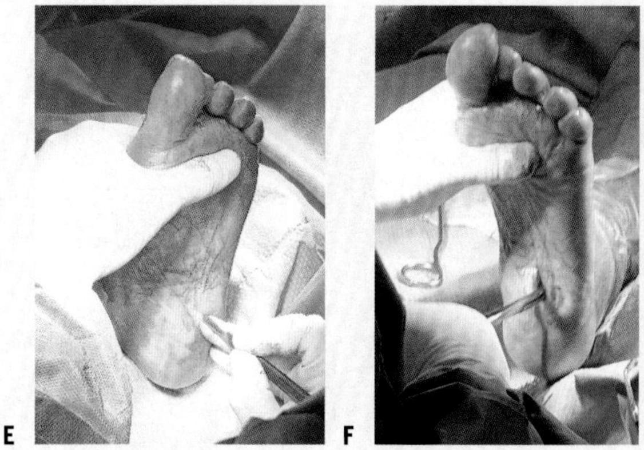

TECH FIG 4 *(continued)* **E.** Careful entry incision following check with fluoroscopic guidance. **F.** Dissection down to bone of calcaneus under direct vision, with careful attention to neurovascular structures.

WIRE INSERTION AND REAMING

- An entry guidewire is then used to obtain the correct position for subsequent reaming and nail insertion, these vary by kit but are generally 3 mm in diameter and 240 to 340 mm in length.
- Careful, repeated x-rays should guide the wire insertion, starting roughly 2 cm behind the articulation of calcaneum with transverse tarsal joints, and aim to be through the center of the talar dome and center–center up the medullary canal of the tibial shaft on AP and lateral x-rays. If position is not satisfactory, the "pepperpot" or wire offset guide can be used to improve placement of the guidewire **(TECH FIG 5A–E)**.
- It is critical that this is done with the foot angled in the correct position as discussed earlier from here onward, or else nail position and subsequent foot orientation will be wrong: if along the anterior tibial wall, there will be increased dorsiflexion and anterior translation of the foot with the opposite if along the posterior wall. If put along the lateral or medial walls, there will be abnormal valgus or varus position of the foot, respectively.
- A cannulated drill should then be used to ream over the entry guidewire, through a soft tissue protector **(TECH FIG 5F)**.
  - This will vary according to manufacturer, from 7 to 12.5 mm in diameter, up to 200 mm in length.
- Remove the entry guidewire and swap to the ball-tip guidewire in its place (reamer cannot pass beyond this point).
- Following this, using the modular reamer heads with a flexible modular reamer system. The starting diameter will depend on the initial entry reamer width and aim to ream 0.5 to 1.5 mm wider than the chosen nail, through a soft tissue protector **(TECH FIG 5G)**.
- Continue to screen as this is performed to ensure correct size and reduce risk of fracture **(TECH FIG 5H)**.

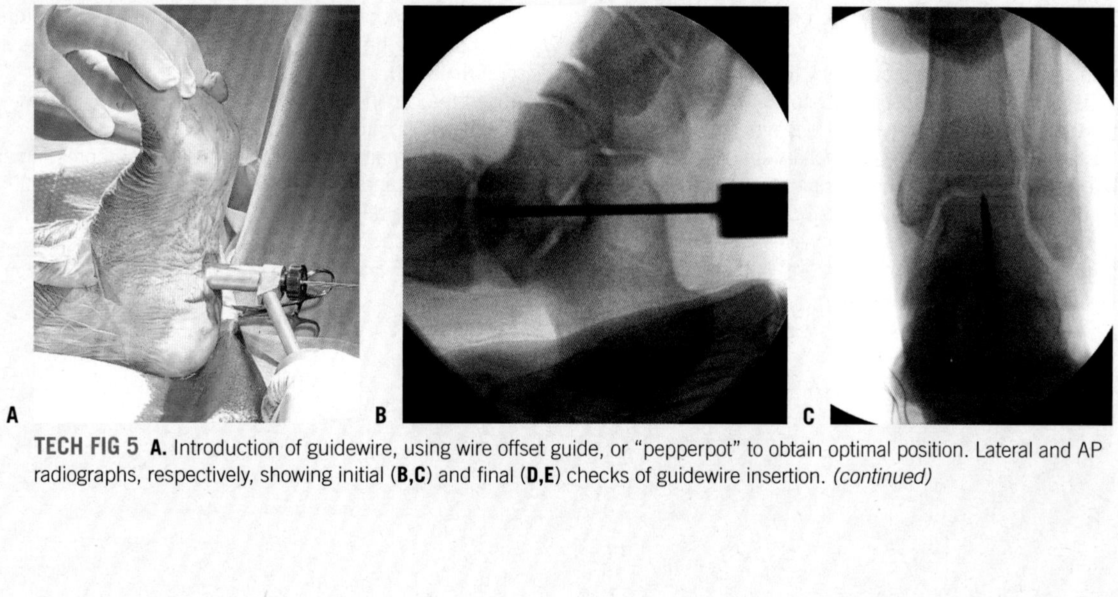

TECH FIG 5 **A.** Introduction of guidewire, using wire offset guide, or "pepperpot" to obtain optimal position. Lateral and AP radiographs, respectively, showing initial (**B,C**) and final (**D,E**) checks of guidewire insertion. *(continued)*

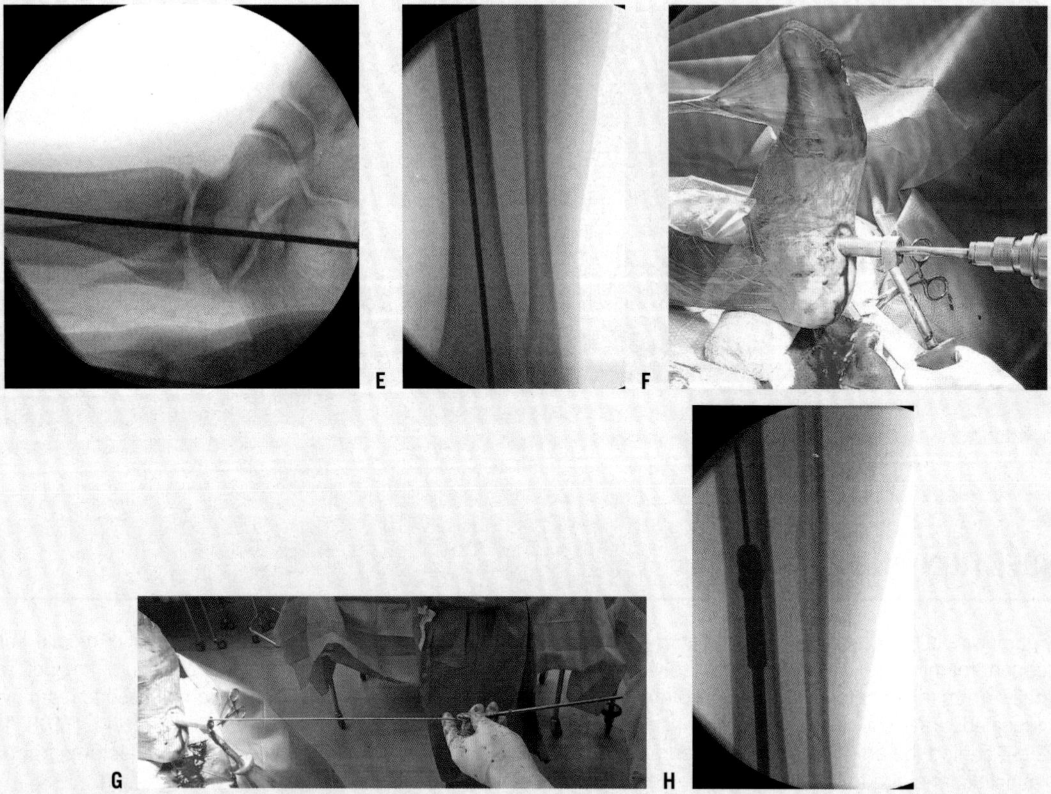

TECH FIG 5 *(continued)* **F.** Entry reaming. **G.** Sequential reaming of tibial canal. Note brass-colored cutting reamer, on flexible drill driver, which follows the path of the ball-tipped guidewire. **H.** AP radiograph of reamer over guidewire in tibial canal.

NAIL SELECTION AND INSERTION

- In cases of poor bone, we recommend using a longer nail in order to achieve a longer working length if there is poor-quality bone stock available more distally and proceed to pass the isthmus as required.
- Using the measuring device provided by the manufacturer—typically a telescopic depth gauge or a measuring ruler calibrated for length of the guidewire—to determine length of nail required.
- When determining length, the proximal aspect of the nail should extend 5 cm beyond any possible stress risers in the cortex, such as holes from previous removal of metal, tibial fractures, nonunion sites, or osteotomy sites. The distal aspect should usually be countersunk up to 1 cm into the calcaneus; this is to facilitate compression later.
- The chosen nail must now be connected to the outrigger jig **(TECH FIG 6A)**.
- The alignment of all drill sleeves from the jig into their respective holes on the nail must be checked before proceeding **(TECH FIG 6B)**.
- Insert the nail in the desired position over the guidewire, using the jig to help guide the position **(TECH FIG 6C–F)**.
- Countersink nail 5 to 10 mm to facilitate compression at the joint surface and avoid potentially painfully prominent metalwork postoperatively.
- Remove guidewire.

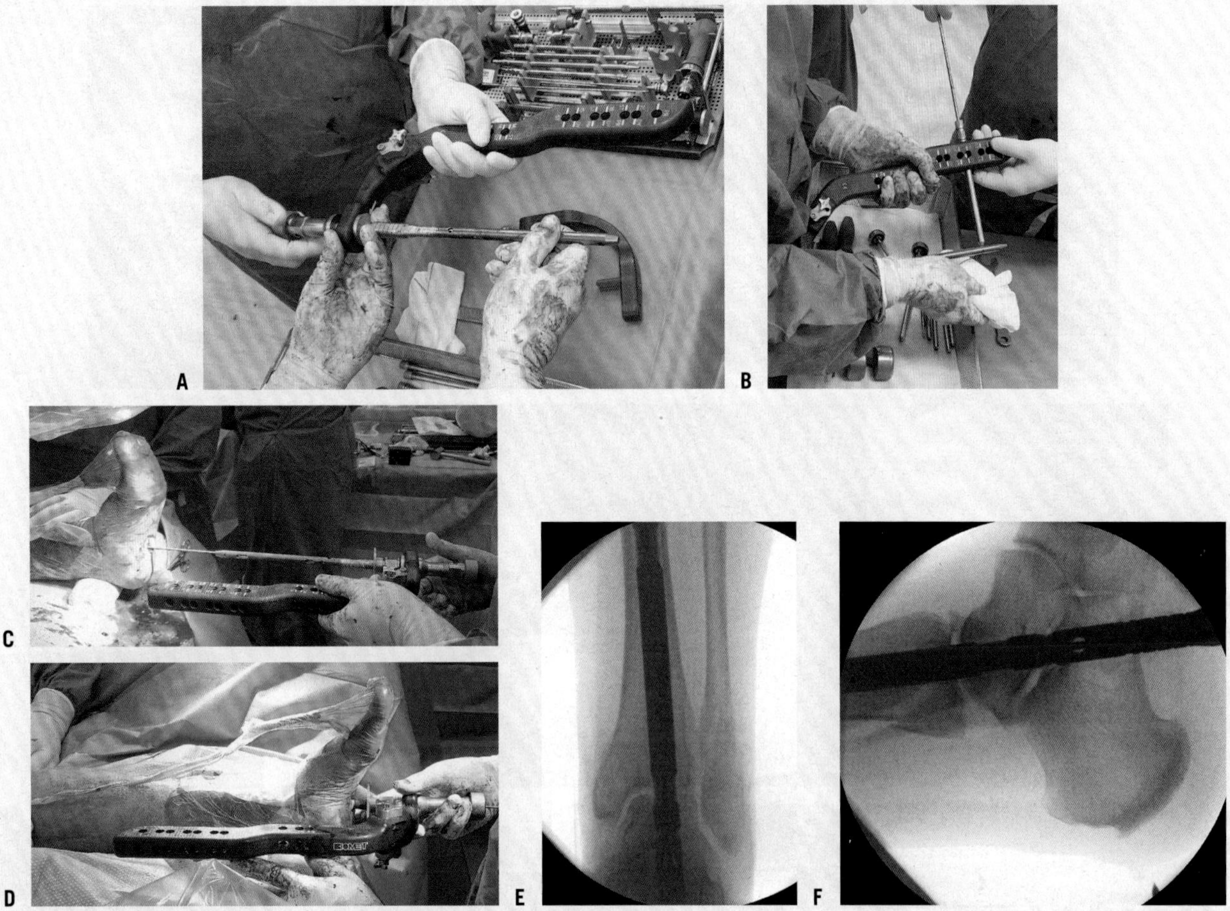

TECH FIG 6 A. Outrigger jig assembly. **B.** Ensuring outrigger jig holes align with nail. First (**C**) and second (**D**) stages of nail insertion over guidewire. AP (**E**) and lateral (**F**) radiographs checking insertion nail over guidewire.

SCREW PLACEMENT AND COMPRESSION

- Screw placement and order of recommended insertion vary according to manufacturer; however, either a fixed locking screw is placed in the talus and a dynamic locking screw placed in the proximal aspect of the nail, or vice versa. It may be easier to place the talar screw first if for any reason there is very limited bone, as when the joint is compressed the surgeon has to be sure that they will be able to lock the talus in position. These should be bicortical, confirmed using radiography **(TECH FIG 7A,B)**.
- Before placement of the second screw position, manually impact the joint surfaces together **(TECH FIG 7C–E)**.
- All systems come with an outrigger jig to aid screw placement, but with most systems, if a longer nail is used, the jig may not be long enough to guide drilling for the most proximal screw sites, and these will have to be done freehand.
- After this has been achieved, tighten the *internal* compression mechanism present inside the nail from the distal aspect. Depending on system, this can compress the tibiotalar joint up to 7 mm.
- Following this, apply *external* compression to the plantar aspect of the calcaneum, using whichever device is provided by the manufacturer, usually this involves a ratcheting mechanism to turn, connected through the nail to locking screws in the talus and tibia. Make sure that if this step is to be used that the correct arrangement of screws in their respective dynamic/locking holes have been placed or else this could generate problems.
- When satisfactory compression is achieved at the talocalcaneal joint, a bicortical distal locking screw must be inserted, usually into the calcaneum.
- The PA screw must then be inserted as guided by the jig, with some systems also offering an additional oblique locking screw from the calcaneum, through the talus and into tibia **(TECH FIG 7F,G)**.
- Finally, the end cap should be attached, and usually, several different lengths are available for this depending on the level of countersink **(TECH FIG 7H)**.

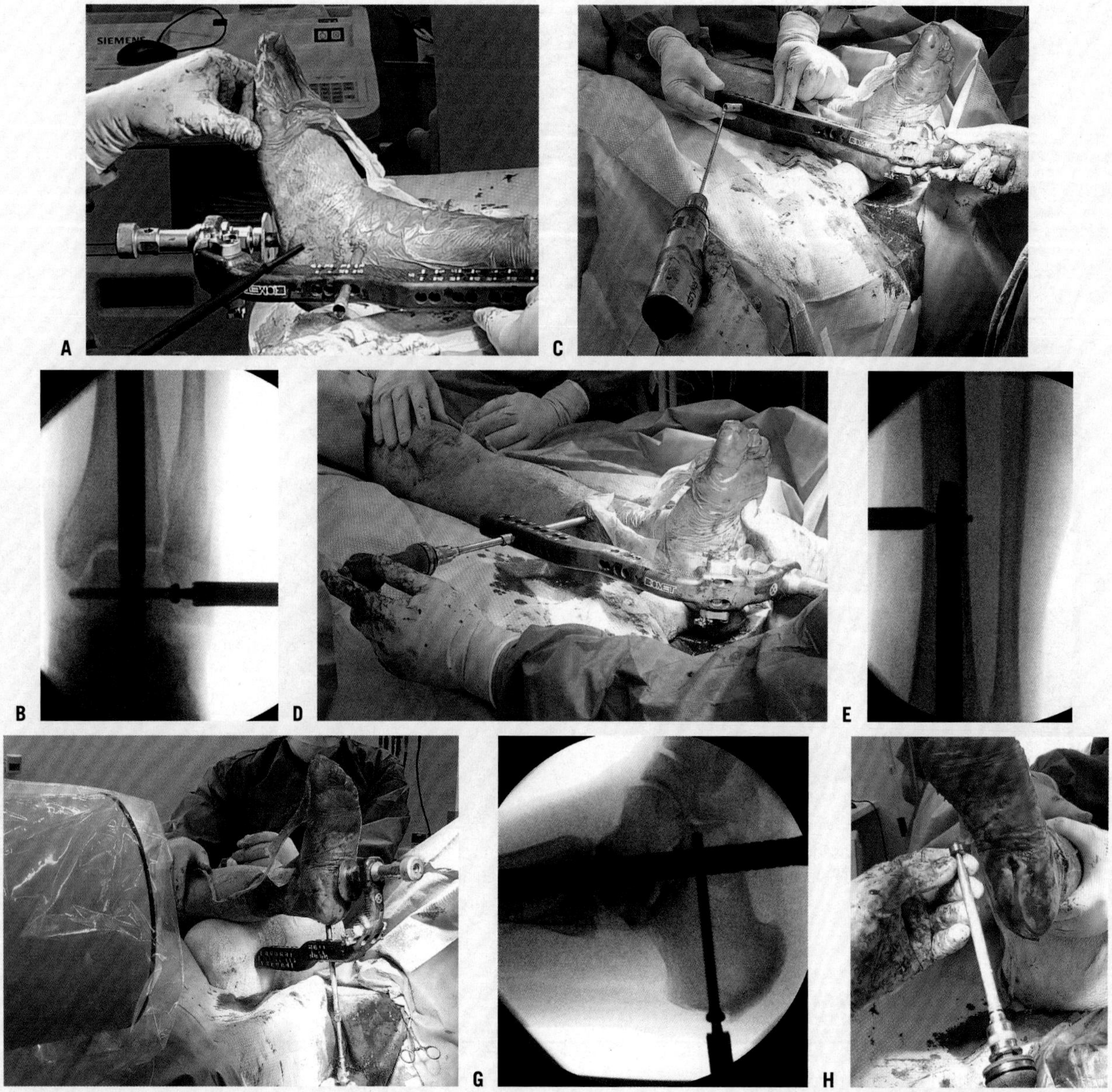

TECH FIG 7 **A.** Talar locking screw, ready for insertion via outrigger jig. **B.** AP radiograph checking to ensure bicortical purchase of talar locking screw. **C.** Drilling proximal locking screw hole using outrigger jig to guide placement. **D.** Inserting proximal locking screw using outrigger jig. **E.** AP radiograph of proximal screw insertion. **F.** Insertion of PA locking screw into calcaneum. Note position of fluoroscopic x-ray for screening. **G.** Lateral radiograph of PA screw insertion. **H.** End cap on end of screwdriver, ready for application.

FIBULA BONE GRAFT APPLICATION AND COMPLETION

- The morselized fibula graft taken earlier should now be applied around all aspects of the prepared joint surface, especially at the posterior aspect where the tibia and calcaneus should be further decorticated to provide a larger surface area for bone grafting. The more graft available, the better the outcomes.[9]
- Graft material can be augmented using commercially available allograft or calcium phosphate–based bridging substitute **(TECH FIG 8A)**.
- This should be contained as best as possible with closure in layers.
- Prior to final closure, check x-rays must be taken using the image intensifier **(TECH FIG 8B–D)**.

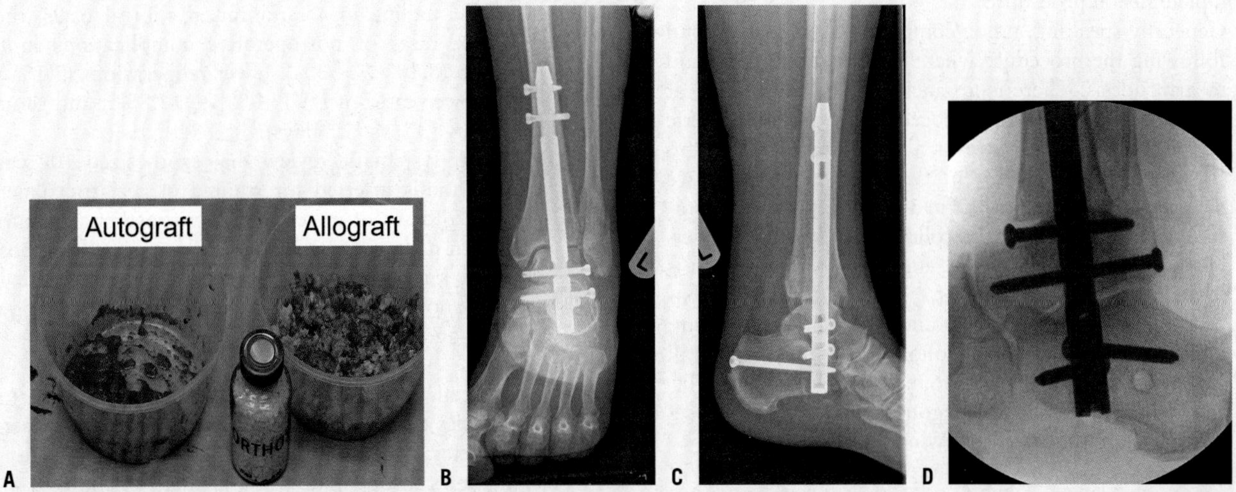

TECH FIG 8 **A.** Autograft and allograft material, ready for implantation. Final AP (**B**) and lateral (**C**) x-rays of ankle repair using TTC nail to manage a fracture. **D.** Final intraoperative radiograph in a different patient in whom flat-cut resection with an intent to fuse was performed.

Pearls and Pitfalls

Retraction of Foot/ Positioning	• The technique shown in **FIG 3B**, using the incision drape attached to surgical tape, is a simple way of maintaining good retraction and plantigrade position. Keeping the foot off the end of the table also helps with PA screw insertion and fitting the jig.
Intraoperative X-Rays (Image Intensifier)	• Ensure there is careful note made throughout of repeated AP and lateral x-rays, to ensure good positioning of metalwork, especially the guidewire before reaming.
Positioning	• Once reaming has begun, position cannot be changed. Therefore, one must make sure that the foot is in complete plantigrade position. This is dictated by the wire position. Be aware that the nail position can then change as it goes up the tibial canal. Unless it is inserted straight through the middle on the lateral x-ray view, there is a risk that the nail might hit the posterior cortex and therefore apply a slight plantarflexed position to the hindfoot. Also, depending on the nail design, there may be a built-in angulation, which must be taken into account.
Use of Dynamic/ Locking Screws into Nail	• If intending to compress at the ankle joint, using the mechanisms available with the various types of nail/kit, one must plan carefully where screws will be placed. If the incorrect combination of locking/dynamic screws are inserted prior to the compression stage(s), it will introduce potential complications, so avoid this with good preparation.

POSTOPERATIVE CARE

- Our preferred method for patients undergoing a full fusion procedure is for the patient to be non–weight bearing in a backslab, which should remain in place for 2 weeks until review of wounds in clinic and changed into a below-knee full cast, and remain non–weight bearing for a further 4 weeks at which point x-rays are taken to assess for union.
- If no sign of union, patients will be kept non–weight bearing for a further 6 weeks, at which point they will be put into a walker boot and allowed progressive weight bearing with the help of physiotherapy, and followed up until full union, and thereafter as appropriate.
- It can often take up to 12 weeks for satisfactory evidence of union before weight bearing is allowed.
- Metalwork is not usually removed in these patients unless it is causing irritation or follow-up x-rays show sign of infection.
- Although the patient is non–weight bearing, it is essential to have performed a venous thromboembolism risk assessment and prescribed appropriate thromboprophylaxis.
- For patients in whom the joint surface is *not prepared for fusion*, for example, geriatric patients with ankle fractures, they are allowed to weight bear as tolerated postoperatively. In our center, we routinely aim to remove nails at around 6 months, after radiographic signs of union, to avoid metalwork failure, although elsewhere good outcomes have been achieved even when metalwork is left in situ. This depends largely on the functional status of the patient.

OUTCOMES

- Complete fusion procedure
  - Generally speaking, union/complete fusion is successful following the procedure where careful attention is paid to arthrodesis. There is a paucity of studies looking at outcomes following this procedure in purely geriatric patient populations, however, although these concord to the general trend where reported. From the evidence we have available, summarized in a recent report and literature review by Wukich and colleagues,[30] looking at overall success of the procedure, successful overall fusion is reported to be an average of 79% in patients with diabetic or Charcot neuropathy and 86% in those without, and up to 100% in some cohorts. The average overall success of limb salvage was found to be 97%. Recent literature published suggests a good overall return to baseline work and function following the procedure.[8,24,30]
- Partial fusion procedure (no joint preparation)
  - Most of the data available in geriatric patients for this procedure comes from trauma series, where fusion nails were used as a means of stabilizing the ankle mortise to allow fracture healing. In younger and more active populations, it is recommended either to always remove the nail after fracture union, or formally fuse the joint surface, to reduce the risk of metal fatigue, failure, and pain. In older patients, practice varies, with excellent subjective results reported regardless of whether formal fusion has been performed or not, with radiologic union reported in 74% to 96% of cases, and 78% to 94% of these patients achieving a return to baseline function.[2,3,5,12,14,22,25,26]
  - In older, frailer populations, there seems to be little difference in outcomes whether the nails are left in or planned to be removed, and in fact, in one study half of the patients requested for the nails to be left in as they felt their ankles were more stable than before their fracture,[17] although it must be borne in mind that a small risk does exist for periprosthetic fracture if the nails are left in, especially if they are not specifically designed for the hindfoot.[2]
  - Generally speaking, after insertion of a hindfoot nail without the intent to fuse, patients are able to fully bear weight soon afterward, and so return to relative level of normality, which for many is a significant advantage.[25] In fact, the only randomized controlled trial to compare traditional ORIF versus TTC nailing showed no difference in pre- and postoperative functional outcome scores between the procedures performed in elderly patients and the TTC group being able to mobilize sooner after surgery.[12]

COMPLICATIONS

- Overall, complication rates vary between 11% and 100%, depending on patient cohort, with an average of 40% overall complication risk, including 13% overall risk of infection, depending on the study and patient characteristics.[30] In a multicenter study reporting complications in 38 patients in TTC nails inserted for primary fusion (mean age 55 years, range 27 to 81 years), there were 2 cases of metalwork failure, 6 cases of nonunion requiring revision, 2 cases of wound infection, no deep wound infection, 1 systemic infection, and 1 case requiring implant removal.[24]
- When looking at complication rates following nails inserted for trauma in geriatric patients and comparing ORIF versus TTC nailing in a randomized clinical trials, there were lower rates of postoperative complications in the TTC group (8.1% vs. 33%), fewer reoperations (2.1% vs. 13.8%), fewer cases of DVT (0% vs. 13.8%), and shorter hospital stay (3.1 vs. 5.2 days).[12]
  - A recent systematic review that synthesized 102 cases of TTC nails inserted for trauma in geriatric patients showed 6 cases of infection, 3 periprosthetic fractures, 2 broken nails, 5 loose screws, 1 deep vein thrombosis, 1 below-knee amputation (in a vasculopathic patient), 2 valgus nonunions, 1 case of displacement requiring renailing, and 1 case of delayed union.[5]
- Infection
  - Superficial (infection of wound, manageable with oral antibiotics): This is significantly related to the presence of diabetes, which was seen to increase the risk by up to eight times in one study (non–diabetes mellitus: 1.8%, diabetes mellitus: 13.1%).[30]
  - Deep (infection affecting metalwork or bone, requiring admission for intravenous antibiotics and possibly débridement): This varies by whether there was trauma or not, with higher rates of infection seen in open fractures and higher energy injuries, and one must ensure thorough management with washout and débridement, with consideration given to application of local antibiotic-releasing cement.[26]
- Nonunion in cases of fracture are generally quite low, in the region of 1% to 10%, with overall good healing seen with a stable ankle mortise.[5,12,14,25,26]
- Perioperative talar split is a rare but serious potential complication, which can be avoided by good preoperative planning and careful sequential reaming of the talus.
- Tibial stress-riser (periprosthetic) fracture is generally rare but can be seen in older short nail designs in particular.[25]
- Hardware failure overall is rare, but this can include broken locking screws or nails, which are often asymptomatic in themselves and can be removed if required after fracture union.
- Valgus alignment of the ankle can occur due to the nail design of slight malalignment on nail insertion and can be readily corrected subsequently.[3]
- Skin ulcer complications can be a problem especially in diabetic or vasculopathic patients, with an increased risk of infection.
- Prominent metalwork and nail protrusion can occur, in which cases if troublesome can be removed following fracture union in cases of fracture, or arthrodesis/union in elective cases.
- Deep vein thrombosis and venous thromboembolic complications postoperatively are always a risk, and suitable thromboprophylaxis must be put in place.

REFERENCES

1. Aigner R, Salomia C, Lechler P, et al. Relationship of prolonged operative time and comorbidities with complications after geriatric ankle fractures. Foot Ankle Int 2017;38(1):41–48.
2. Al-Nammari SS, Dawson-Bowling S, Amin A, et al. Fragility fractures of the ankle in the frail elderly patient: treatment with a long calcaneotalotibial nail. Bone Joint J 2014;96-B(6):817–822.
3. Amirfeyz R, Bacon A, Ling J, et al. Fixation of ankle fragility fractures by tibiotalocalcaneal nail. Arch Orthop Trauma Surg 2008;128(4): 423–428.

4. Andrzejowski P, Giannoudis PV. The "diamond concept" for long bone non-union management. J Orthop Traumatol 2019; 20(1):21.
5. Ap N. A systematic review of the evidence for intramedullary hindfoot nailing in elderly patients with unstable ankle fractures. Orthop Rheumatol 2018;12(5):1–7.
6. Audrey HX, Abd Razak HRB, Andrew THC. The truth behind subchondral cysts in osteoarthritis of the knee. Open Orthop J 2014; 8:7–10.
7. Bernasconi A, Mehdi N, Lintz F. Fibular intra-articular resection during arthroscopic ankle arthrodesis: the surgical technique. Arthrosc Tech 2017;6(5):e1865–e1870.
8. Buchner M, Sabo D. Ankle fusion attributable to posttraumatic arthrosis: a long-term followup of 48 patients. Clin Orthop Relat Res 2003;(406):155–164
9. DiGiovanni CW, Lin SS, Daniels TR, et al. The importance of sufficient graft material in achieving foot or ankle fusion. J Bone Joint Surg Am 2016;98(15):1260–1267.
10. Dros J, Wewerinke A, Bindels PJ, et al. Accuracy of monofilament testing to diagnose peripheral neuropathy: a systematic review. Ann Family Med 2009;7(6):555–558.
11. Freire MO, Van Dyke TE. Natural resolution of inflammation. Periodontol 2000 2013;63(1):149–164.
12. Georgiannos D, Lampridis V, Bisbinas I. Fragility fractures of the ankle in the elderly: open reduction and internal fixation versus tibio-talo-calcaneal nailing: short-term results of a prospective randomized-controlled study. Injury 2017;48(2):519–524.
13. Hintermann B, Knupp M, Zwicky L, et al. Total ankle replacement for treatment of end-stage osteoarthritis in elderly patients. J Aging Res 2012;2012:345237.
14. Jonas SC, Young AF, Curwen CH, et al. Functional outcome following tibio-talar-calcaneal nailing for unstable osteoporotic ankle fractures. Injury 2013;44(7):994–997.
15. Le V, Veljkovic A, Salat P, et al. Ankle arthritis. Foot Ankle Orthop 2019;4(3):247301141985293.
16. Lee JH, Dyke JP, Ballon D, et al. Subchondral fluid dynamics in a model of osteoarthritis: use of dynamic contrast-enhanced magnetic resonance imaging. Osteoarthritis Cartilage 2009;17(10): 1350–1355.
17. Lemon M, Somayaji HS, Khaleel A, et al. Fragility fractures of the ankle: stabilisation with an expandable calcaneotalotibial nail. J Bone Joint Surg Br 2005;87(6):809–813.
18. Li G, Yin J, Gao J, et al. Subchondral bone in osteoarthritis: insight into risk factors and microstructural changes. Arthritis Res Ther 2013;15(6):223.
19. Maffulli N, Longo UG, Locher J, et al. Outcome of ankle arthrodesis and ankle prosthesis: a review of the current status. Br Med Bull 2017;124(1):91–112.
20. McBride DJ, Ramamurthy C, Laing P. The hindfoot: calcaneal and talar fractures and dislocations. Part II: fracture and dislocations of the talus. Curr Orthop 2005;19(2):101–107.
21. Mohammad HR, A'Court J, Pillai A. Extruded talus treated with reimplantation and primary tibiotalocalcaneal arthrodesis. Ann R Coll Surg Engl 2017;99(4):e115–e117.
22. Persigant M, Colin F, Noailles T, et al. Functional assessment of transplantar nailing for ankle fracture in the elderly: 48 weeks' prospective follow-up of 14 patients. Orthop Traumatol Surg Res 2018;104(4):507–510.
23. Pop-Busui R, Boulton AJM, Feldman EL, et al. Diabetic neuropathy: a position statement by the American Diabetes Association. Diabetes Care 2017;40(1):136–154.
24. Rammelt S, Pyrc J, Agren P-H, et al. Tibiotalocalcaneal fusion using the hindfoot arthrodesis nail: a multicenter study. Foot Ankle Int 2013;34(9):1245–1255.
25. Tarkin IS, Fourman MS. Retrograde hindfoot nailing for acute trauma. Curr Rev Musculoskelet Med 2018;11(3):439–444.
26. Taylor BC, Hansen DC, Harrison R, et al. Primary retrograde tibiotalocalcaneal nailing for fragility ankle fractures. Iowa Orthop J 2016;36:75–78.
27. Tenenbaum S, Stockton KG, Bariteau JT, et al. Salvage of avascular necrosis of the talus by combined ankle and hindfoot arthrodesis without structural bone graft. Foot Ankle Int 2015;36(3):282–287.
28. van der Kraan PM, van den Berg WB. Osteophytes: relevance and biology. Osteoarthritis Cartilage 2007;15(3):237–244.
29. Wen C, Lu WW, Chiu KY. Importance of subchondral bone in the pathogenesis and management of osteoarthritis from bench to bed. J Orthop Translat 2014;2(1):16–25.
30. Wukich DK, Mallory BR, Suder NC, et al. Tibiotalocalcaneal arthrodesis using retrograde intramedullary nail fixation: comparison of patients with and without diabetes mellitus. J Foot Ankle Surg 2015;54(5):876–882.
31. Yde J. The Lauge Hansen classification of malleolar fractures. Acta Orthop Scand 1980;51(1):181–192.
32. Zak L, Wozasek GE. Tibio-talo-calcaneal fusion after limb salvage procedures—a retrospective study. Injury 2017;48(7):1684–1688.

CHAPTER 59

Open Reduction and Internal Fixation of the Talus

Heather A. Vallier

DEFINITION

- Fractures of the talus are severe injuries affecting ankle and hindfoot joint function.
- Displaced fractures of the talus are a surgical challenge to orthopaedic surgeons. The injuries are infrequent, and the fracture anatomy may be concealed by adjacent osseous structures.
  - Open reduction and internal fixation of displaced fractures is recommended to restore articular and axial alignment.
- Clinical and functional outcomes of talus fractures are related to severity of articular and soft tissue injury and may be optimized with accurate reduction and meticulous soft tissue handling. Despite this, ankle and subtalar joint stiffness, posttraumatic arthrosis, and osteonecrosis occur commonly.

ANATOMY

- Two anatomic factors play important roles in the outcome of talus fractures.
  - Seventy percent of the bone is covered by articular cartilage, precluding extraosseous perfusion through those areas.
  - Disruption of blood supply to the talus is based on initial fracture displacement, and with open or comminuted fractures, which are associated with higher risk of osteonecrosis. The blood supply to the talar body enters through the inferior talar neck via the artery of the tarsal canal. This key vessel originates from the posterior tibial artery. Secondary blood supply to the body is derived from the anterior tibial artery, as the artery of the tarsal sinus, which enters inferior to the lateral neck and anastomoses with the artery of the tarsal canal. Circulation to the dorsal neck and head is supplied via small branches from the anterior tibial artery. Posterior talar blood supply originates from perforating branches of the peroneal artery **(FIG 1)**.[5]
- Recent latex injection cadaveric study evaluated talar vascularity using gadolinium-enhanced magnetic resonance imaging (MRI) followed by gross dissection.[8] Results showed the following:
  - Peroneal artery contributed 17% of talar perfusion.
  - Anterior tibial artery contributed 36% of talar perfusion.
  - Posterior tibial artery contributed 47% of talar perfusion.
- Substantial vascular contribution to the posterior talus support reasons why talar neck fractures may not result in avascular necrosis. Furthermore, in the presence of an associated medial malleolus fracture, the deltoid ligament and deltoid artery may remain intact, fostering perfusion to the medial body.
- The talus has seven articulations.
  - Three superior surfaces articulate with the tibia plafond and the medial and lateral malleoli.
  - Three surfaces articulate with the calcaneus via the anterior, middle, and posterior facets of the subtalar joint.
  - The final articulation of the talar head with the navicular represents an important articulation for midfoot motion.
- Predictable stiffness and posttraumatic arthritic changes are experienced with severe fractures of the talus.

PATHOGENESIS

- Fractures of the talus present in varying patterns depending on the mechanism of injury.

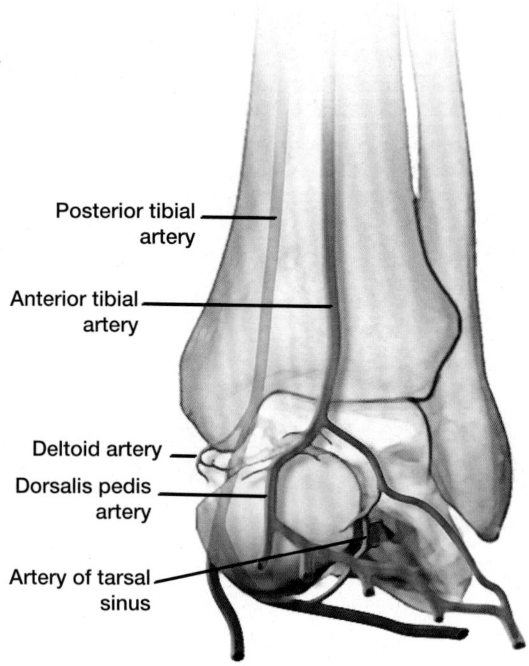

A

FIG 1 Blood supply to the talus originates from all three major arteries in the leg. **A.** Anteroposterior view. *(continued)*

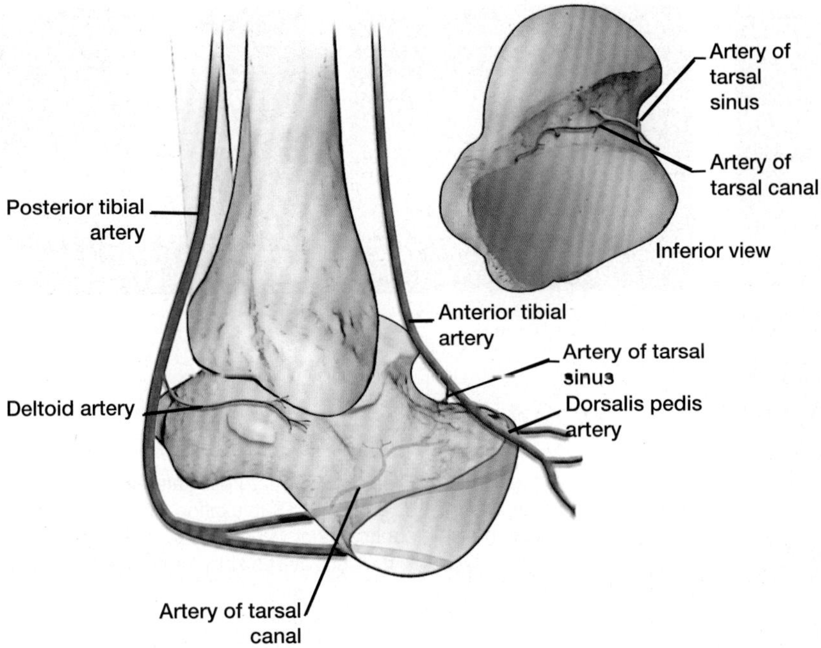

FIG 1 *(continued)* **B.** Lateral view.

- Fractures of the talar head are intra-articular and the result of axial load to the talonavicular joint with the foot positioned in plantarflexion.
  - These fractures constitute up to 10% of all fractures of the talus.
  - They are uncommon but may be associated with talonavicular or subtalar dislocation.
- Talar neck fractures occur in the frontal plane and result from dorsiflexion of the foot against the anterior lip of the distal tibia. The fracture begins transversely along the medial talar neck due to an associated supination force to the hindfoot. The fracture line extends laterally. The fracture may be extra-articular, intra-articular, or both. With increased energy, the hindfoot supination force generates a fracture of the medial malleolus of the ankle.
  - After completion of the neck fracture, continued dorsiflexion and axial load to the body of the talus may force dislocation of the talar body posteriorly, disrupting extraosseous circulation.
- Fractures of the body of the talus occur with approximately 20% of talus fractures. The mechanism of injury is the same for body fractures as for fractures of the talar neck.
  - Fracture patterns of the body of the talus include coronal, sagittal, horizontal shear, and crush fractures of the weight-bearing surface. Coronal fractures extending into the anterior portion of the talar body are classified as talar body fractures when the primary fracture line extends posterior to the lateral process.
- Process fractures of the talar body are described by anatomic location.
  - Lateral and posterior process fractures are sustained by inversion and eversion mechanisms of the ankle, respectively. These fractures are often missed on plain radiographs of the ankle and may be diagnosed as ankle sprains.
    - Hawkins[6] classified lateral process fractures into avulsion, isolated, and comminuted types.
  - Posteromedial and posterolateral process fractures may occur on either side of the flexor hallucis longus (FHL) tendon. These are commonly intra-articular fractures of the inferior surface of the posterior talus.

NATURAL HISTORY

- Fractures of the head of the talus are commonly nondisplaced because of powerful capsular attachments.
- Displaced fractures of the talar head have a 10% incidence of osteonecrosis and can lead to posttraumatic arthrosis.[6]
- Fractures of the neck of the talus are defined as fractures anterior to the lateral process. Hawkins[6] described injury of vascular perfusion to the bone by delineating three groups of fractures of the talar neck.
  - Group I is nondisplaced. Disruption of blood flow is limited to the anterolateral region of the bone.
    - Although Hawkins reported a 13% incidence of osteonecrosis after these injuries, more recent work suggests osteonecrosis very rarely occurs with this pattern.
  - Group II fractures involve displacement of the talar dome fragment with associated subluxation or dislocation of the talar body.
    - Hawkins classification was recently modified to denote IIA and IIB groups, with subluxation and dislocation, respectively.[13]
    - The original report of this subclassification noted osteonecrosis to occur only after IIB fractures. However, a composite of literature suggests a 20% to 50% risk of osteonecrosis when displacement at the subtalar joint is present **(FIG 2A,B)**.[4,11,13]
  - In group III, the talar neck fracture is associated with dislocation of the tibiotalar and subtalar joints. The incidence of osteonecrosis of the talar body is 50% to 100% **(FIG 2C)**.
  - Hawkins classification was modified by Canale and Kelly[3] to include a fourth type of injury. In addition to the type III fracture-dislocation, there is associated

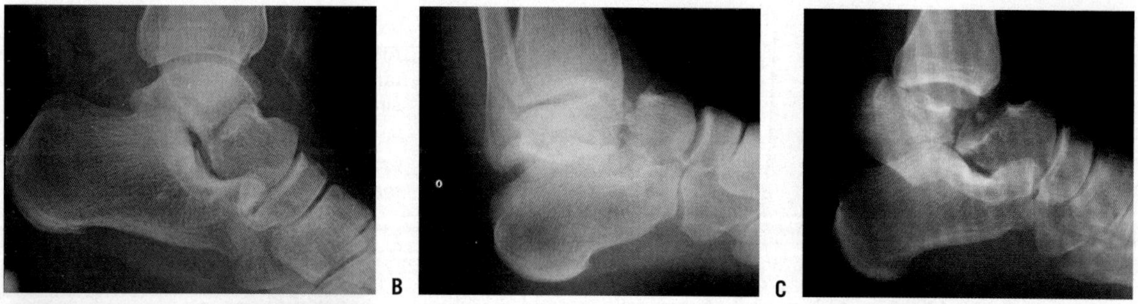

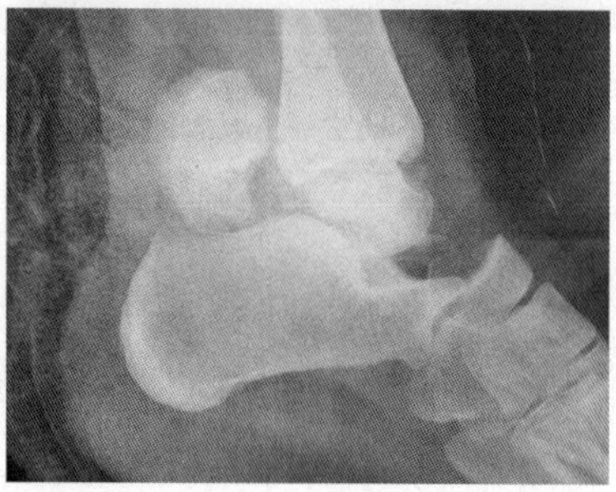

A B C D

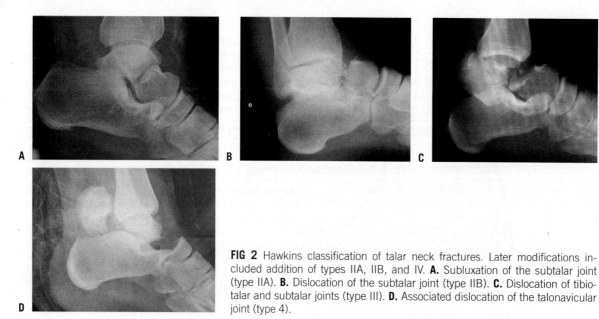

FIG 2 Hawkins classification of talar neck fractures. Later modifications included addition of types IIA, IIB, and IV. **A.** Subluxation of the subtalar joint (type IIA). **B.** Dislocation of the subtalar joint (type IIB). **C.** Dislocation of tibiotalar and subtalar joints (type III). **D.** Associated dislocation of the talonavicular joint (type 4).

talonavicular dislocation. All extraosseous blood flow to the talus is considered disrupted.
  - The prognostic value of Hawkins classification is the increasing incidence of osteonecrosis based on initial fracture displacement **(FIG 2D)**.[3,6]
- Talar body fractures are defined as fractures extending into or posterior to the lateral process.

PATIENT HISTORY AND PHYSICAL FINDINGS

- Fractures of the talus are commonly associated with vehicular trauma and falls.
  - The relationship of severe lower extremity trauma and airbags is well known. After airbag deployment, the torso and lower extremities are directed toward the floor panel of the car.
  - High-energy hindfoot trauma has increased over time. Globally, transport-related injuries remain the leading cause of disability from injury. By 2020, traffic injuries will increase from a current ninth position to third regarding disability-adjusted life-years lost.[2]

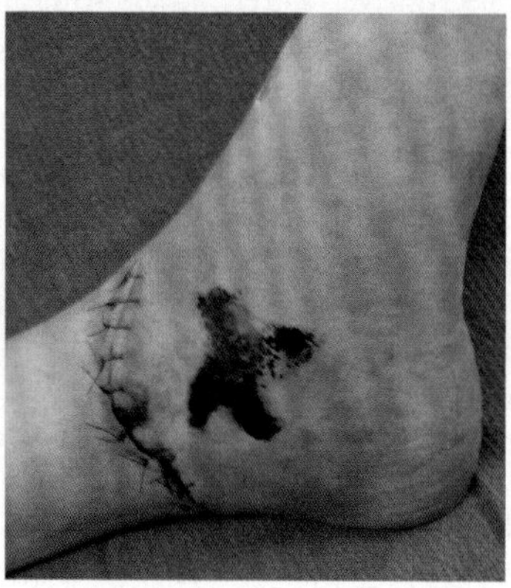

FIG 3 A young woman presented several hours after open talar neck fracture with associated tibiotalar and subtalar dislocations. Despite urgent reduction of the talar body, she developed full-thickness skin necrosis over the lateral ankle.

- Optimizing initial care of the bony and soft tissue injuries will mitigate infectious complications and generate anatomic talar articular and axial alignment to provide best long-term patient outcome.
  - On the initial examination, the physician should note pain, deformity, soft tissue swelling, open fractures, and associated fractures of adjacent bones to the foot and ankle and should perform complete neurologic and vascular evaluations of the extremity.
- Detailed documentation of the talus fracture pattern and local soft tissue injury is paramount.
  - Soft tissue local pressure phenomenon, commonly found anterolaterally in closed type III fractures of the talar neck, may precipitate full-thickness skin necrosis if not decompressed early **(FIG 3)**.
  - Severe swelling of the ankle is common in the acute fracture of the talus and may progress to serous and hemorrhagic fracture blister formation, delaying safe execution of extensile operative incisions.
  - Open fractures will be apparent by laceration of the ankle or hindfoot. Expeditious intravenous antibiotics are indicated. Dislocations should be reduced, and saline dressings and splints should be applied, with attention to urgent surgical débridement.

IMAGING AND OTHER DIAGNOSTIC STUDIES

- Three plain radiographic views are necessary to evaluate talus fractures: anteroposterior (AP), mortise (15-degree internal rotation view), and lateral images of the ankle.
  - The AP and mortise views of the ankle demonstrate alignment of the talar body in the ankle mortise. The lateral view depicts the sagittal outline of the talus.
- The Canale view is used to assess varus or valgus malalignment of the talar neck, primarily used in the operating room to assess reduction.[3] The knee must be flexed and the foot in equinus and pronation, with the x-ray tube directed 15 degrees caudally **(FIG 4A,B)**.
- Because of the high-energy nature of fractures of the talus, AP and oblique views of the foot should be a standard

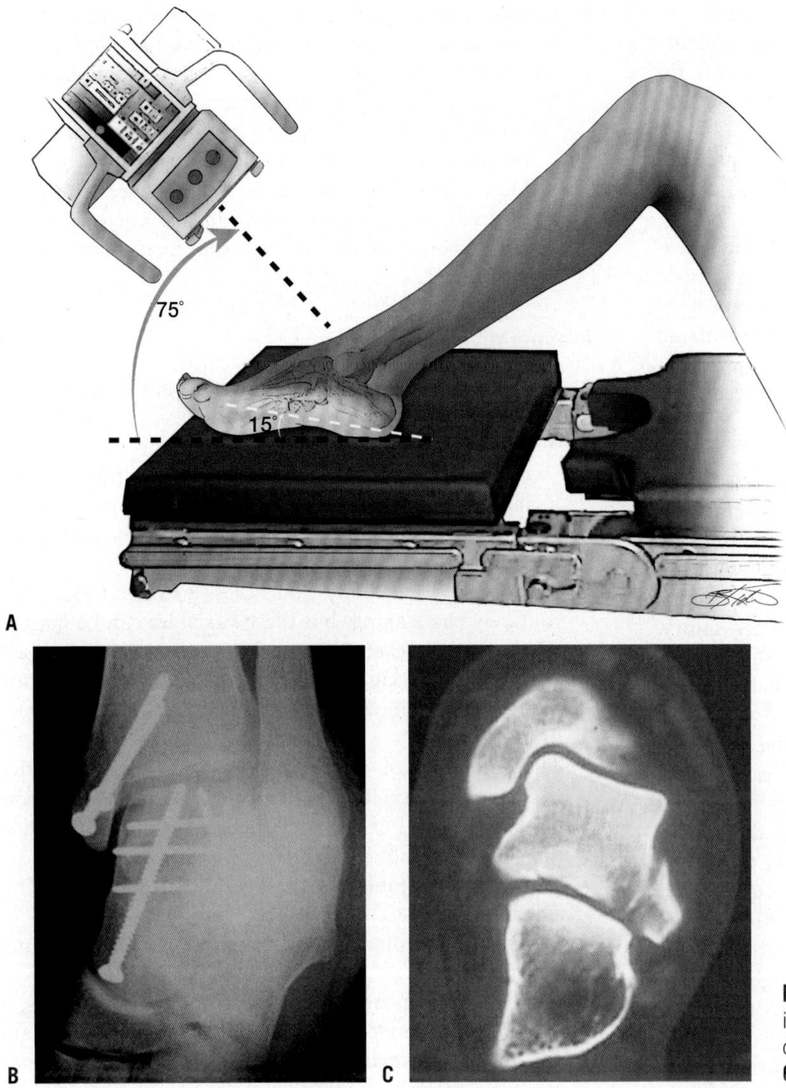

FIG 4 A. The Canale view is obtained with the foot in equinus and pronation. **B.** Canale radiography demonstrates the axial alignment of the talus. **C.** Lateral process fracture as shown on CT scan.

addition to the three-view plain film ankle protocol so as not to miss associated midfoot and forefoot injuries.

- Computed tomography (CT) provides important additional information to the three-view plain film series of the ankle. Thirty-degree coronal and paraxial CT imaging is important to confirm Hawkins type I fracture of the talar neck and to plan treatment of talar body fractures with extension posterior to the lateral process.
- Reconstructions of both sagittal and coronal CT studies provide valuable information about incremental pathoanatomy of the entire talus, medial to lateral and anterior to posterior, respectively.
- In addition, confirmation of a process fracture that is not clearly viewed by plain film is easily diagnosed by CT **(FIG 4C)**.

DIFFERENTIAL DIAGNOSIS

- Process fracture of the talus
  - Lateral process fracture
  - Posterior process fracture
- Head of talus fracture
- Neck of talus fracture
- Body of talus fracture
- Neck and body of talus fracture
- Fracture-dislocation of talus
  - Involving body
  - Involving neck and body
- Extruded talus
- Any of these injuries to the talus may be open fractures, affecting management.

NONOPERATIVE MANAGEMENT

- Fractures of the talus include a spectrum of injury, ranging from isolated regions of the talus (eg, lateral process) to severely comminuted talus fractures involving all parts of bone, making nonoperative management inappropriate.
  - High-energy mechanisms that cause talus fractures precipitate fracture displacement and joint surface incongruity.
- Posterior and lateral process fractures, minimally displaced (<2 mm) and involving less than 1 cm of bone, are commonly managed nonoperatively.
  - These injuries are treated acutely in well-padded, compressive dressings with posterior splints and non–weight

bearing. Swelling and immediate pain in the ankle improve within 7 to 10 days. The patient is subsequently converted to a short-leg, non–weight-bearing cast for 6 weeks followed by progressive range of ankle and subtalar motion and return to weight bearing.
  - If the process fracture is severely comminuted, precluding surgical reconstruction, the same initial and definitive nonoperative management is employed.
- Isolated fractures of the head of the talus without dislocation and without displacement are largely stable fractures. These injuries require plain radiographic evaluation of both the ipsilateral foot and ankle to confirm the isolated nature of the injury. Consider CT scan (axial and transverse views of foot and ankle) to rule out associated midfoot pathology.
  - Acutely, a nondisplaced talar head fracture is splinted for 7 to 10 days with subsequent short-leg casting in neutral plantarflexion with non–weight bearing for 4 weeks. Intermittent daily ankle and subtalar motion with Achilles tendon stretching should follow with application of a removable splint. The patient remains non–weight bearing until 6 to 8 weeks after injury. Next, progressive weight bearing, range of motion, stretching, and strengthening of the entire lower extremity are recommended.
- The Hawkins type I fracture of the neck of the talus is a nondisplaced talar neck fracture. The talus remains anatomically positioned in the ankle and subtalar joint with minimal potential for disruption of perfusion to the bone.
  - If there is displacement of the neck fracture, the injury will be considered Hawkins type II, which requires surgical treatment to obtain and maintain the reduction.
- Truly nondisplaced fractures of neck of the talus can be treated nonoperatively in a short-leg, non–weight-bearing cast for 6 to 8 weeks. Close follow-up is recommended to identify any displacement of the neck fracture. At 6 to 8 weeks after the injury, progressive weight bearing, range of motion, stretching, and strengthening are initiated.
- Fractures to the dome of the talus are usually severe, causing articular displacement, and are an indication for surgery. Open fractures of the talus, even with no displacement, are best managed with rigid surgical stabilization to allow for wound care and early motion.

SURGICAL MANAGEMENT

- The timing of operative management of talus fractures was previously an area of controversy.
  - Recent studies confirm that definitive fixation of the talus is not an emergency and specifically that delay is not associated with osteonecrosis.[4,7,9,11,13]
  - However, fracture-dislocations generate threat of pressure phenomenon to the skin, and possible plantar nerve dysfunction. Dislocations of the talus should be urgently reduced.
- Regarding general guidelines for fractures of the body, neck, and head of talus fractures, surgical management is indicated with fracture displacement, malalignment, subluxation, dislocation, or instability.
- Regarding surgical indications for process fractures of the talus include displaced fractures with large fragments showing extension into the subtalar joint.
- For patients with severe open fractures of the talus or closed injuries in which soft tissue compromise precludes immediate, definitive fixation, definitive surgery should be delayed.
  - Initial splinting will often maintain the peritalar joints in suitable position. This may avoid contamination of the surgical field with wires or Schanz pins.
  - Occasionally, provisional Kirschner wires or spanning external fixation may maintain alignment more effectively than a splint, until internal fixation can be safely performed.

Preoperative Planning

- Operative planning for talus fractures requires understanding of all major fracture fragments.
  - A preoperative CT scan of the fracture is helpful for a comminuted talar body fracture or for fractures of the lateral or posterior processes. The surgeon must become familiar with the morphology of the bone and its many contours to facilitate reconstruction.
- Intraoperative visibility and access to talar fragments are routinely challenging, but these variables can be largely facilitated by correct patient positioning, surgical approaches, adequate operating room lighting (headlamp), attention to reduction techniques, and strategic selection and placement of implants.
- The principles of open treatment are restoring articular congruity and axial alignment, maximizing the revascularization potential of the bone, and allowing early motion of the ankle and subtalar joints.
- The operating table should be radiolucent, absent metal side bars.
- A headlamp promotes optimal visualization for complex fractures.
- A tray of fine-tipped, sharp and strong bone elevators; dental probes; Freer elevators; small bone clamps; small lamina spreaders; and small distractors or external fixation equipment is essential.
- Small fragment (3.5-mm) and minifragment (2.0-, 2.4-, or 2.7-mm) screw/plate instrumentation are used for fixation.
  - An extra-long minifragment screw (2.0 to 2.7 mm) inventory is recommended, with screws up to 50 mm long. These implants are particularly helpful when reconstructing comminuted fractures.
  - Contemporary minifragment systems are predominantly stainless steel.
  - Some authors have suggested using titanium implants to allow use of MRI to assess osteonecrosis; however, the role of MRI in postoperative evaluation is unclear because presence of osteonecrosis would not impact weight bearing or other standard care.
  - Consider tapping long screws (>30 mm) directed through dense talar body bone to avoid difficulty with insertion or shearing of mini-screw head.
  - Small osteochondral fragments can be fixed with, cruciform screws inset into the articular cartilage or with bioabsorbable pegs or headless articular screws.

Positioning

- Displaced fractures of the head, neck, body, and lateral process of the talus are best reconstructed with the patient in

the supine position with a bump under the ipsilateral buttock to point the foot straight upward.
  - Supine positioning allows medial, anterolateral, and direct lateral incisions to be performed with ease.
  - Intraoperative fluoroscopy is conveniently performed with the patient in this universal position.
- Fractures of the posterior body of the talus are performed through a posteromedial approach.
  - Placing a bump beneath the contralateral hip in a supine patient will cause the injured leg to externally rotate, placing the medial ankle and hindfoot in ideal position (**FIG 5**).
  - A bump beneath the injured lower leg and foot will elevate the talus sufficiently to avoid the other leg when imaging.

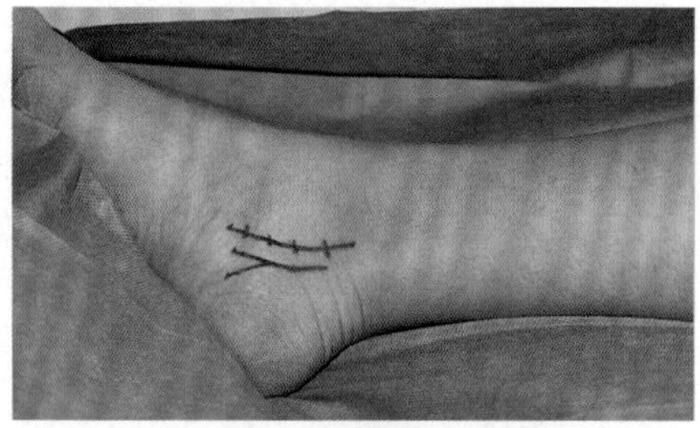

FIG 5 The patient is positioned supine with a contralateral hip bump for the posteromedial approach to the talar body.

Approach

- Anatomic reduction of displaced head, neck, and body fractures requires visualization of both medial and lateral surfaces of the talus. Anteromedial and anterolateral (dual-incision) approaches effectively prevent malreduction of the talar neck.
  - The two incisions also facilitate strategic placement of implants.
- A surgeon's initial impression of the dual-incision approach to talus fractures may be perceived to disregard the biology of the bone and its limited extraosseous blood supply. With attention to detail, however, neither the plantar nor the direct dorsal blood supply to the talus is violated. Care must be taken not to violate the deltoid ligament or the inferior surface of the talar neck.
- Anatomic reduction of complex talus fractures is achieved by working from side to side through both incisions.
- An important modification of the medial approach to the talus is the medial malleolar osteotomy. In displaced body or complex talar neck fractures, the osteotomy will improve exposure and will facilitate reduction and fixation.
- An isolated posteromedial body fracture or posterior process fracture of the talus may require a posteromedial approach.

EXPOSURE

TECHNIQUES

Anteromedial and Anterolateral Approaches

- The anteromedial incision extends from the tip of the medial malleolus along the axis of the talar neck over the tarsal navicular to the edge of the medial cuneiform (**TECH FIG 1A,B**).
  - This incision is between the tibialis anterior and tibialis posterior tendons.
  - The distal extension promotes exposure of the medial surface of the talar head, neck, and distal body. A small rongeur can remove bone from the dorsomedial aspect of the navicular. This will allow for insertion of wires and screws along the long axis of the talus, placing them directly through the medial aspect of the talar head articular surface.
- Bone removed from the navicular may be used as autogenous graft to dorsal and medial neck deficits, later in the procedure.
- The approach may be lengthened proximally to improve visibility of the medial body.

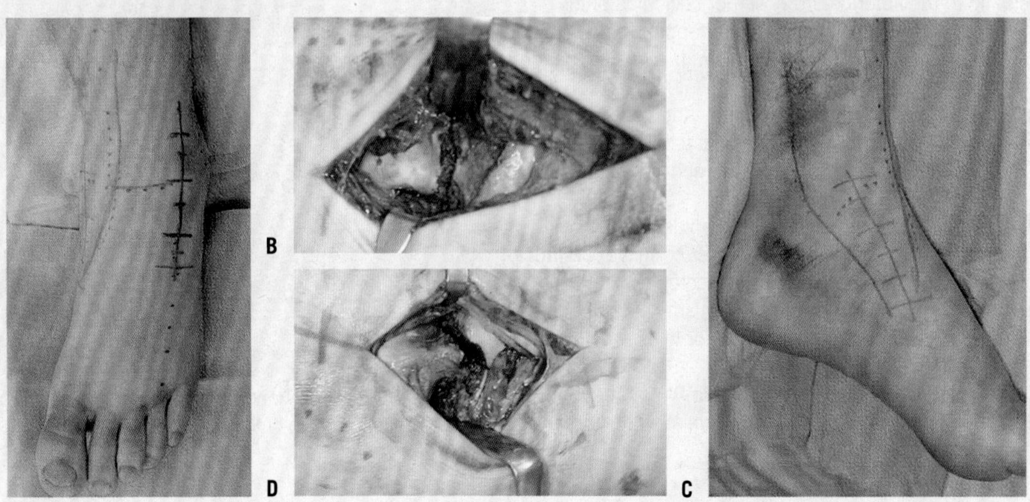

TECH FIG 1 A. Anteromedial approach to the talus. **B.** Anteromedial dissection to the talar neck. **C.** Anterolateral approach to the talus. **D.** Anterolateral dissection to the talar neck. (**A,C:** From Vallier HA, Nork SE, Benirschke SK, et al. Surgical treatment of talar body fractures. J Bone Joint Surg Am 2004;86-A[suppl 1][pt 2]:180–192.)

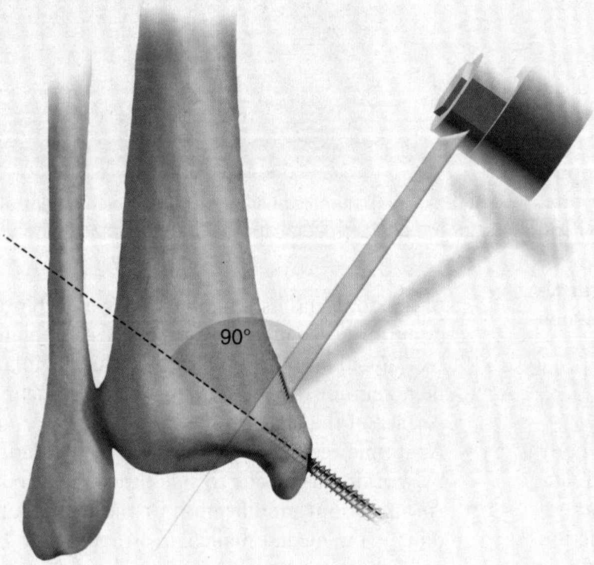

A

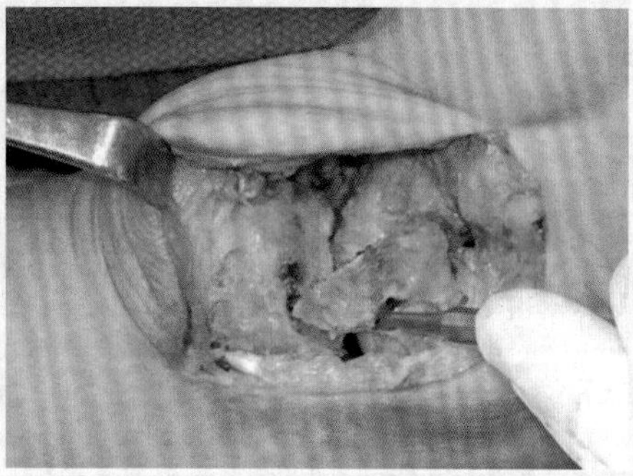

B

TECH FIG 2 A. Orientation and location of medial malleolar osteotomy. **B.** Improved visualization of the medial talar body after osteotomy.

- The anterolateral incision extends from the tip of the distal fibula toward the base of the fourth metatarsal. This exposes the lateral process and lateral neck **(TECH FIG 1C,D)**.
  - If a lateral talar body fracture is present, the incision should originate 1.5 cm more proximally.
  - The lateral retinaculum is sharply incised, and the extensor digitorum brevis muscle is reflected distally off its proximal origin, allowing access to the lateral capsule of the talus.
  - The lateral capsulotomy is made in line with the axis of the neck of the talus.
  - The lateral process is easily accessed through this exposure.
  - Anatomic reduction of complex talus fractures is achieved by working from side to side through both incisions.

Transmalleolar Approach

- The medial incision is extended longitudinally, over the anterior aspect of the medial malleolus.
- After exposing the malleolus, without violating the periosteum, the distal tip of the anterior and posterior colliculus of the medial malleolus must be predrilled and tapped for two parallel, 3.5-mm interfragmentary cortical or 4.0-mm partially threaded cancellous screws.
- An oblique osteotomy directed toward the shoulder of the medial ankle mortise is performed using a very thin oscillating saw blade, advancing only to the level of the medial subchondral bone.
  - The osteotomy is completed into the ankle joint by gentle insertion of a thin osteotome on the inner cortex **(TECH FIG 2)**.
  - Completing the osteotomy with an osteotome minimizes chondral damage and improves irregularity of the deep bone to ease reduction of the osteotomy prior to its repair at the end of the procedure.
- The anterior ankle capsule is released from the anterior border of the medial malleolus to allow inferior mobilization of the malleolus. The deltoid vessels perfusing the medial body of the talus are protected with gentle retraction.

Posterior Approach

- The incision is curved and extends along the course of the posterior tibialis tendon and just posterior to it. Depending on the size and location of the fracture, the interval posterior to the flexor digitorum longus and adjacent to the neurovascular bundle may be used.
  - Alternatively, a small process fracture may be more accessible by using the interval between the neurovascular bundle and the FHL **(TECH FIG 3)**.
- When making the incision through the deep posterior compartment fascia, the surgeon must take care to identify and gently retract the medial neurovascular structures.
- After safely retracting the nerve and artery, the FHL tendon represents a landmark directly posterior to the body of the talus.

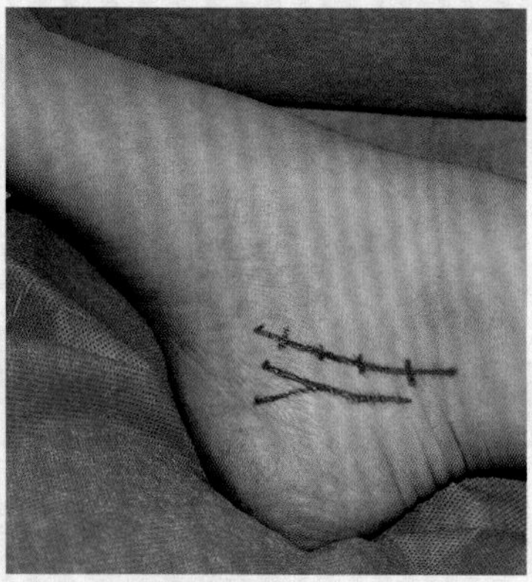

TECH FIG 3 Marked incision for posteromedial exposure to the talus and the relationship of the neurovascular bundle.

OPEN REDUCTION AND INTERNAL FIXATION OF THE NECK OF THE TALUS

Reduction

- After completion of the medial approach, limited sharp dissection is performed only along the medial neck and head to remove extraosseous soft tissue attachments and expose the talar body, neck, and head and the talonavicular joint.
- The medial fracture line is commonly found to have comminution that affects understanding of the true length and alignment of the medial column of the bone.
  - Inserting a mini-lamina spreader to gently disimpact the medial talar neck fracture allows restoration of length and alignment of the medial and dorsal surface of the neck.
  - Anatomic alignment is achieved using the dental probe and small elevators as reduction tools.
- If the talar neck fracture is intra-articular with extension into the subtalar joint, the body fragment routinely assumes a flexed, malrotated position.
  - A Weber clamp to secure the talar head fragment may be inserted with the tines located one in each of the two incisions. This provides excellent control of the talar head fragment to restore length, angulation, and rotation.
  - Often, the best reduction read is along the cortical bone of the lateral neck, just anterior to the lateral process. Usually, anatomic alignment can be established in this area, often revealing bony defects in the dorsal and medial neck, depending on the energy of injury and baseline bone quality.

Trial Fixation

- Once the talar neck is reduced, the next step is to advance Kirschner wires retrograde through the talar head, across the fracture into the posterior body, to hold the position of the talar neck fracture.
  - If no bony reduction keys are visible along the medial talar neck due to comminution, the mini-lamina spreader is inserted in the fracture medially while the surgeon patiently reduces the medial talar neck alignment. The lateral cortical read described earlier is particularly helpful, when available.
- After reduction, retrograde Kirschner wires are advanced through the lateral talar head and across the fracture, provisionally fixing the medial and lateral sides of the talus fracture.
- Talar neck fluoroscopy is necessary to evaluate translation and alignment of the fracture. This important step establishes the true length and alignment of the medial talar neck.
- A Canale view should be obtained. If the provisional fixation is tenuous, the Canale view can be modified by keeping the leg on the table and adjusting the gantry of the C-arm appropriately (see **FIG 4**).

Screw Fixation

- Definitive fixation of the medial talar neck fracture is achieved by gently subluxing the medial talonavicular joint to expose the articular surface of the talar head **(TECH FIG 4A–C)**.

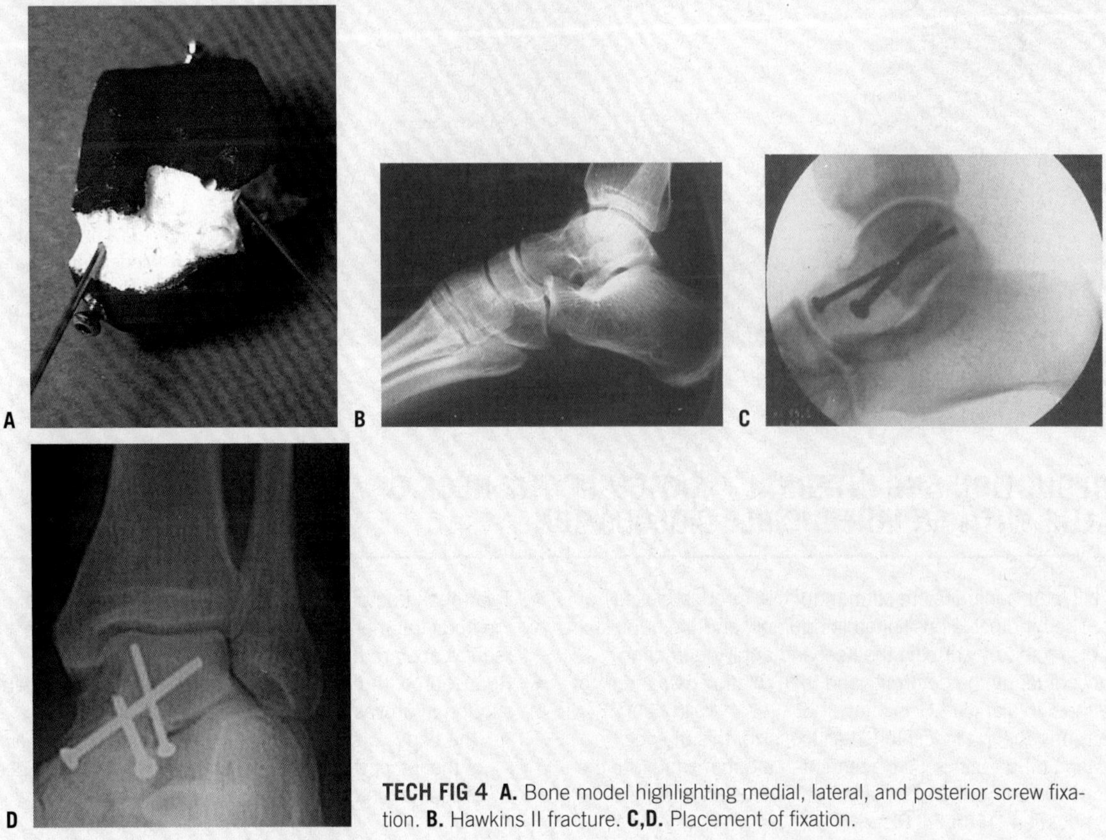

TECH FIG 4 A. Bone model highlighting medial, lateral, and posterior screw fixation. **B.** Hawkins II fracture. **C,D.** Placement of fixation.

- A countersunk 3.5- or 2.7-mm screw is advanced to the posterior body of the talus.
- Laterally, very dense cortical bone along the proximal neck presents an excellent extra-articular location for advancing a second longitudinal screw.
- Comminution within the neck of the talus may preclude compression with interfragmentary screws; rather, the longitudinal screws should be placed as positional screws.
  - The medial screw is more easily directed posterolaterally, and lateral screws are more easily directed posteromedially **(TECH FIG 4D)**.

Plate Fixation

- Talar neck fractures that are comminuted may be effectively treated with minifragment plate fixation.
  - These plates are easily contoured and may be applied along medial and/or lateral neck surfaces **(TECH FIG 5)**.
  - The medial side offers a very narrow corridor for implant placement, avoiding encroachment onto the medial body articular surface.
  - Lateral plates may be curved to capture the lateral process, which is effective when a concurrent lateral process fracture is present.

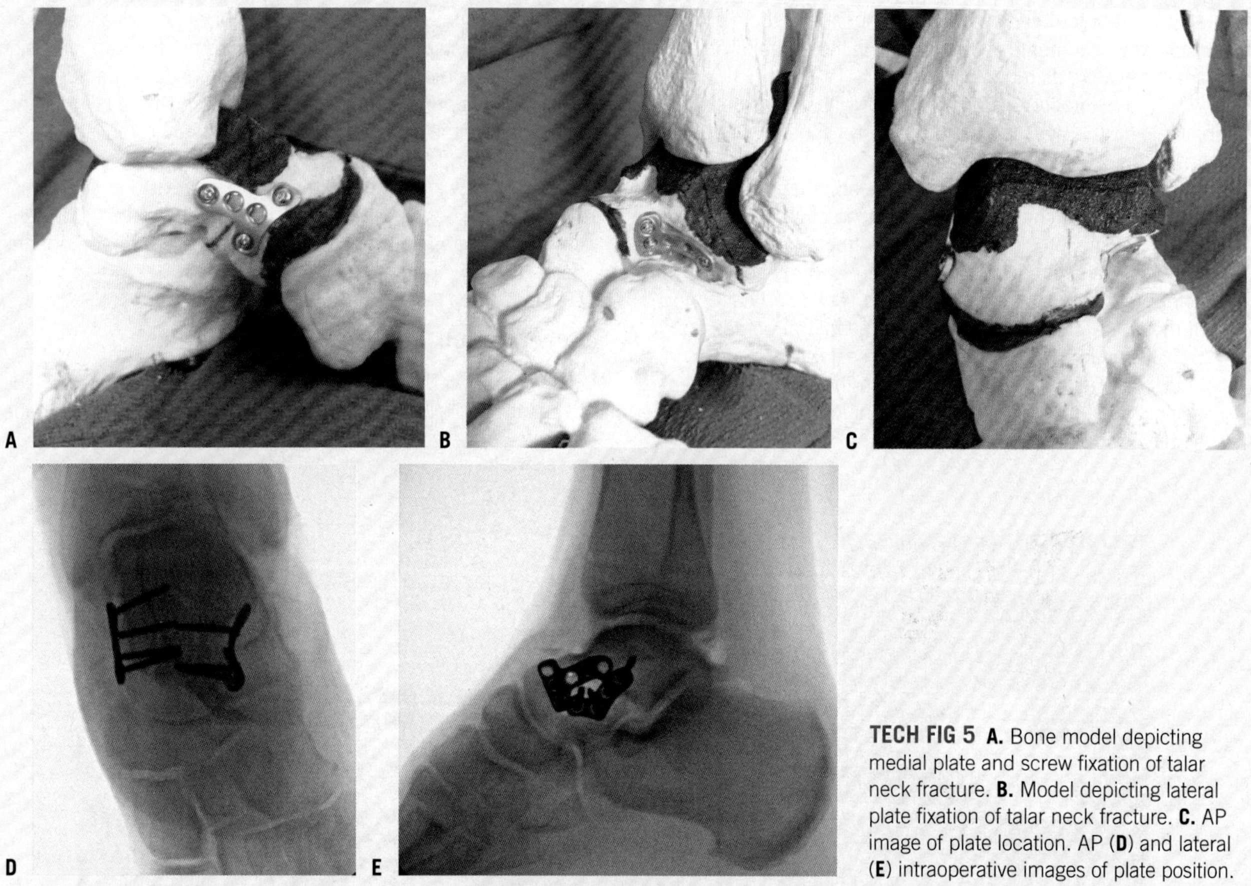

TECH FIG 5 A. Bone model depicting medial plate and screw fixation of talar neck fracture. **B.** Model depicting lateral plate fixation of talar neck fracture. **C.** AP image of plate location. AP (**D**) and lateral (**E**) intraoperative images of plate position.

OPEN REDUCTION AND INTERNAL FIXATION OF THE NECK OF THE TALUS WITH AN IRREDUCIBLE DISLOCATION

- Hawkins type IIB injuries are often reducible through closed means. The hindfoot is positioned in equinus, and the subtalar joint is distracted by gripping the heel and applying traction while accentuating the deformity and then rotating calcaneus to reduce the subtalar joint.
- On occasion, due to swelling or small foot size, this may be more difficult. Percutaneous placement of a Schanz pin into the calcaneus will improve control of the calcaneus and may aid closed reduction **(TECH FIG 6)**.
- Talar neck fractures with associated posterior dislocation of the body fragment may be difficult to reduce and most always require open reduction.
- Reduction of the body is an immediate goal to eliminate pressure on neurovascular structures and skin.
  - The body commonly dislocates posteromedially because of the intact deep deltoid ligament. However, the body may dislocate directly posteriorly or posterolaterally.

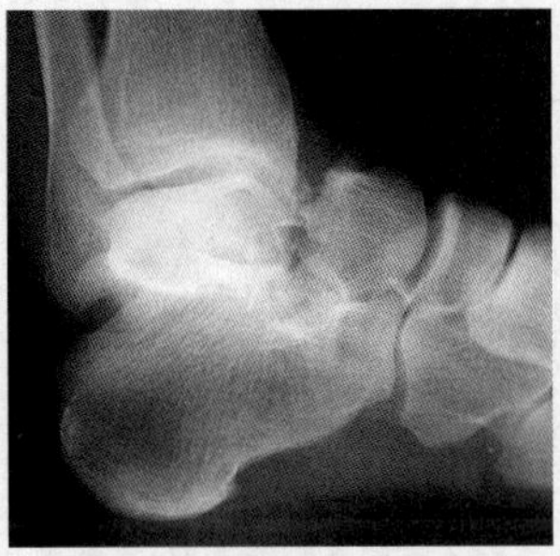

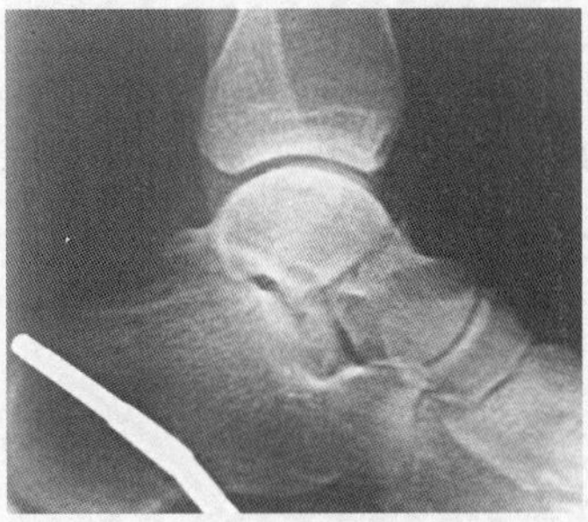

A B

TECH FIG 6 A 38-year-old man who sustained a talar neck fracture with dislocation of the subtalar joint in a motorcycle accident presented to the hospital more than 12 hours after the injury with severe soft tissue swelling and fracture blisters. **A.** Lateral radiograph made at the time of presentation. **B.** Lateral radiograph made after closed reduction, which was facilitated with percutaneous insertion of a calcaneal pin. Seventeen days later, after some improvement in the soft tissue injury, the patient underwent open reduction and internal fixation. (From Vallier HA, Nork SE, Barei D, et al. Talar neck fractures: results and outcomes. J Bone Joint Surg Am 2004;86[8]:1616–1624.)

- An open fracture-dislocation allows the surgeon access to the body fragment through the common transverse medial traumatic wound.
- Associated medial or lateral malleolus fracture of the ankle aids reduction of the talar body dislocation, particularly with disruption of the syndesmotic ligament. These situations effectively increase the space available through which to reduce the talar body.
- Reduction of the dislocated body fragment may be attempted in the emergency room using radiographic information and conscious sedation.
  - A well-controlled, single attempt at closed reduction is reasonable.
  - The hindfoot is positioned in equinus, and the subtalar joint is distracted by gripping the heel and applying traction. Next, the dislocated talar body fragment is pushed anteriorly.
- If the closed reduction is unsuccessful, closed or open reduction under general anesthesia is recommended immediately in the operating room.

Open Reduction of the Talar Dome Fragment

- Reduction of the talar dome fragment, recalcitrant to a closed or percutaneous reduction is undertaken, using the anteromedial approach. General anesthesia with complete muscular paralysis must be maintained.
  - After completion of the anteromedial approach, a lamina spreader or universal distractor is applied medially, distracting the ankle and subtalar joints **(TECH FIG 7)**.
  - Manual pressure over the talar body may reduce it. Release of the posterior ankle capsule with a no. 15 blade, followed by percutaneous tendo Achilles lengthening will increase the space of that interval and will decrease the difficulty of reduction.
  - If these measures fail, a 3.5-mm Schanz pin can be inserted directly into the talar body through the surgical wound, and the talus can be pulled back into the ankle joint **(TECH FIG 8)**.
- Once the head, neck, and body fragments are reducible, reduction is performed, followed by lag screw or plate fixation.
- If the patients' soft tissues are severely damaged, it may be prudent to close the wounds after the dislocations are reduced. Definitive fixation can be undertaken in 1 to 2 weeks once swelling has subsided. Additionally, some multiply injured patients may be underresuscitated and/or have severe intracranial pressure or medical reason precluding lengthy surgery. Such patients are better managed definitively on a delayed basis, once dislocations are reduced.

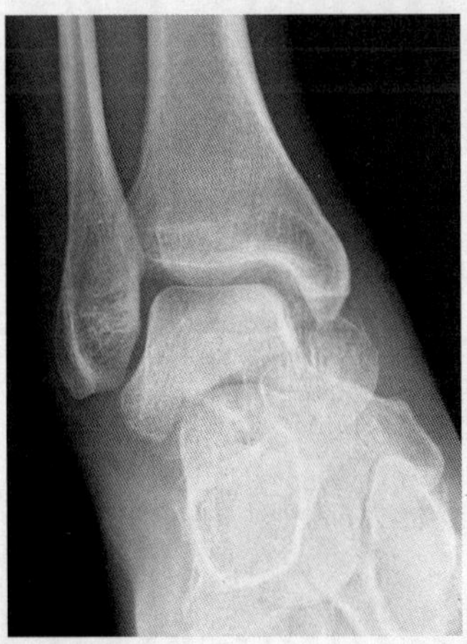

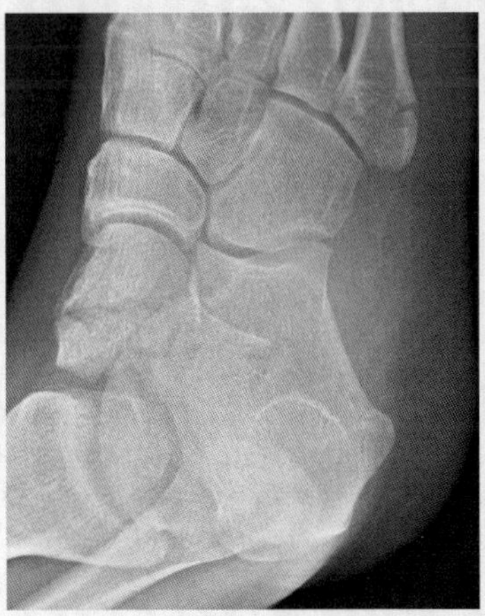

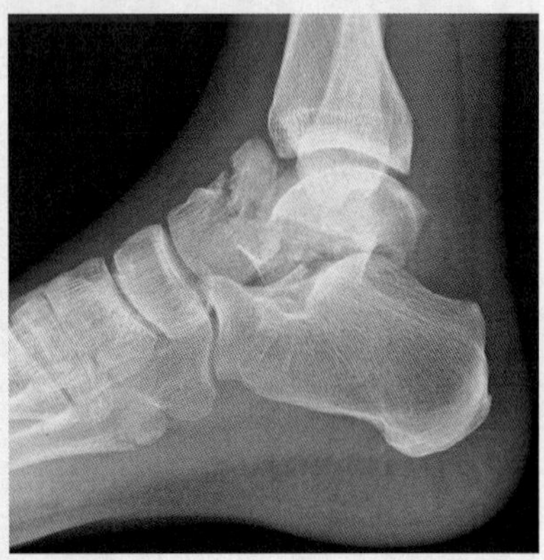

A B C

TECH FIG 7 A–C. Injury radiographs show talar neck fracture with subtalar dislocation in a patient who presented 3 weeks after injury. Closed reduction was not possible. Open reduction was undertaken using dual anteromedial and anterolateral exposures. *(continued)*

TECHNIQUES

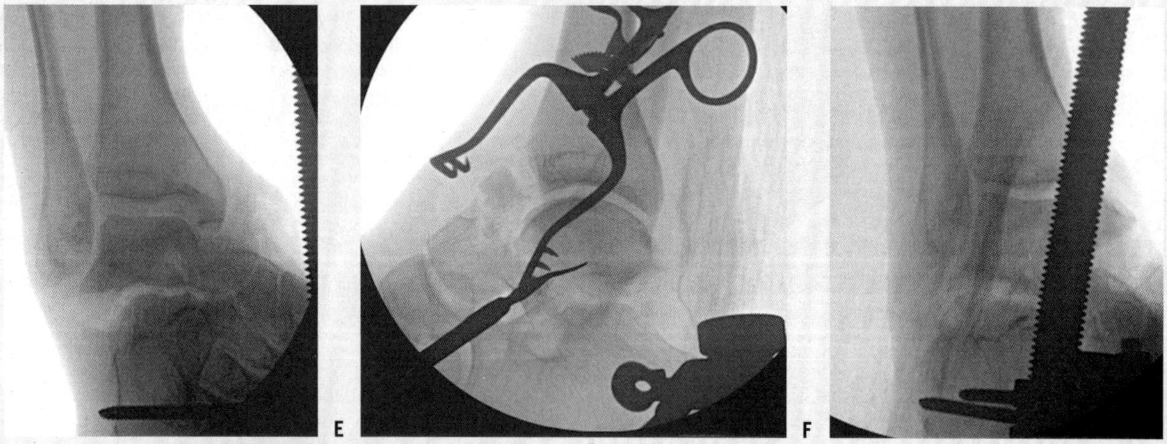

D E F

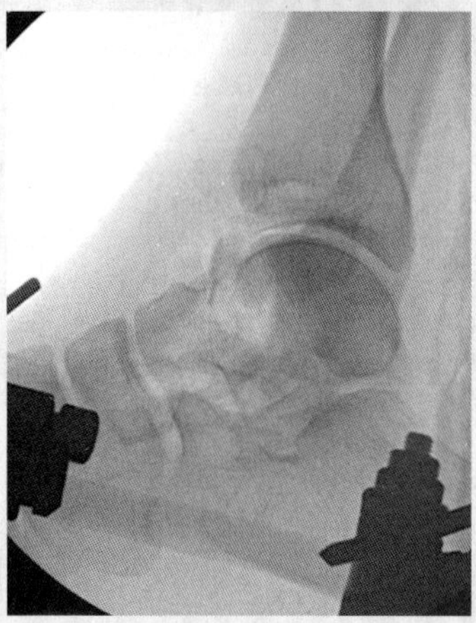

G

TECH FIG 7 *(continued)* **D–G.** A Universal distractor was placed with Schanz pins in the medial distal tibia and calcaneus facilitating distraction of the ankle and subtalar joints. The ankle capsule was released, and the Achilles tendon was percutaneously lengthened.

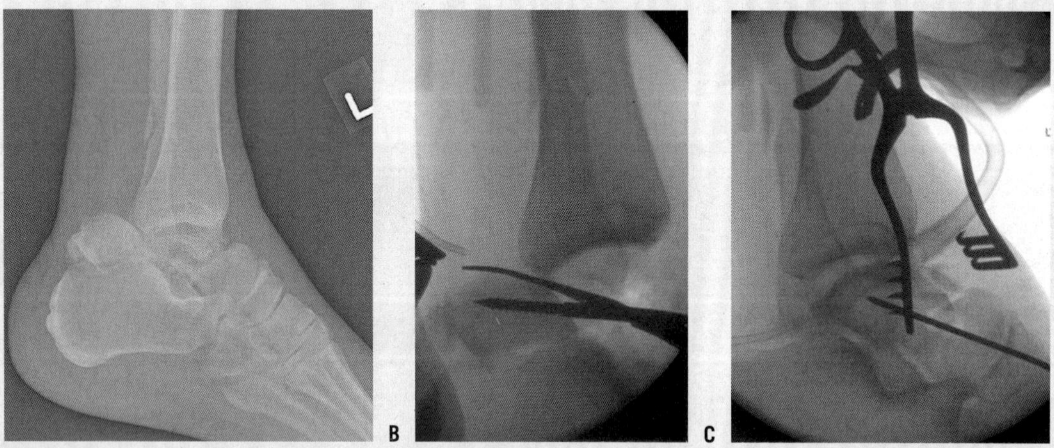

A B C

TECH FIG 8 **A.** Posteromedial dislocation of the talar body was initially irreducible even with attempted open reduction using an anteromedial exposure. A Schanz pin was inserted into the talar body (**B**), permitting direct reduction of the talar body (**C**).

OPEN REDUCTION AND INTERNAL FIXATION OF THE BODY OF THE TALUS

- Reconstruction of talar body fractures is best performed using dual anteromedial and anterolateral approaches with the addition of the medial malleolar osteotomy.
  - Unless the fracture line is transverse and very anterior, allowing reasonable access by a standard dual approach, a transmalleolar approach is planned.
- Fracture patterns to the body of the talus occur in both sagittal and coronal planes. Regardless of the fracture plane, the principle is to work through the fenestration provided by the medial malleolar osteotomy, using fine-tipped dental probes, sequentially reducing the posterior portion of the body to the anterior body fragments.
- Small, smooth Kirschner wires are inserted, provisionally fixing the body.
- Associated fractures of the neck of the talus are provisionally fixed after reduction of the body fracture.
  - Interfragmentary, countersunk, minifragment screws (2.0, 2.4, or 2.7 mm) are sequentially inserted, fixing the body fragment.
    - Headless screws can also be used for this fracture.
  - Finally, countersunk, interfragmentary small fragment and/or minifragment plate and screw constructs are used to fix the talar neck fracture.
  - Talar body fracture-dislocations with associated ankle malleolar fractures present a more complex case requiring much attention to appropriate soft tissue dissection; yet, the ankle injury often allows the surgeon better exposure to medial and lateral components of the fractured talar body **(TECH FIG 9)**.
  - Fixation of the malleolar fractures commonly begins with the plate fixation of the lateral malleolus through a separate longitudinal direct lateral or posterolateral approach. The medial malleolus is routinely fixed last **(TECH FIG 10)**.

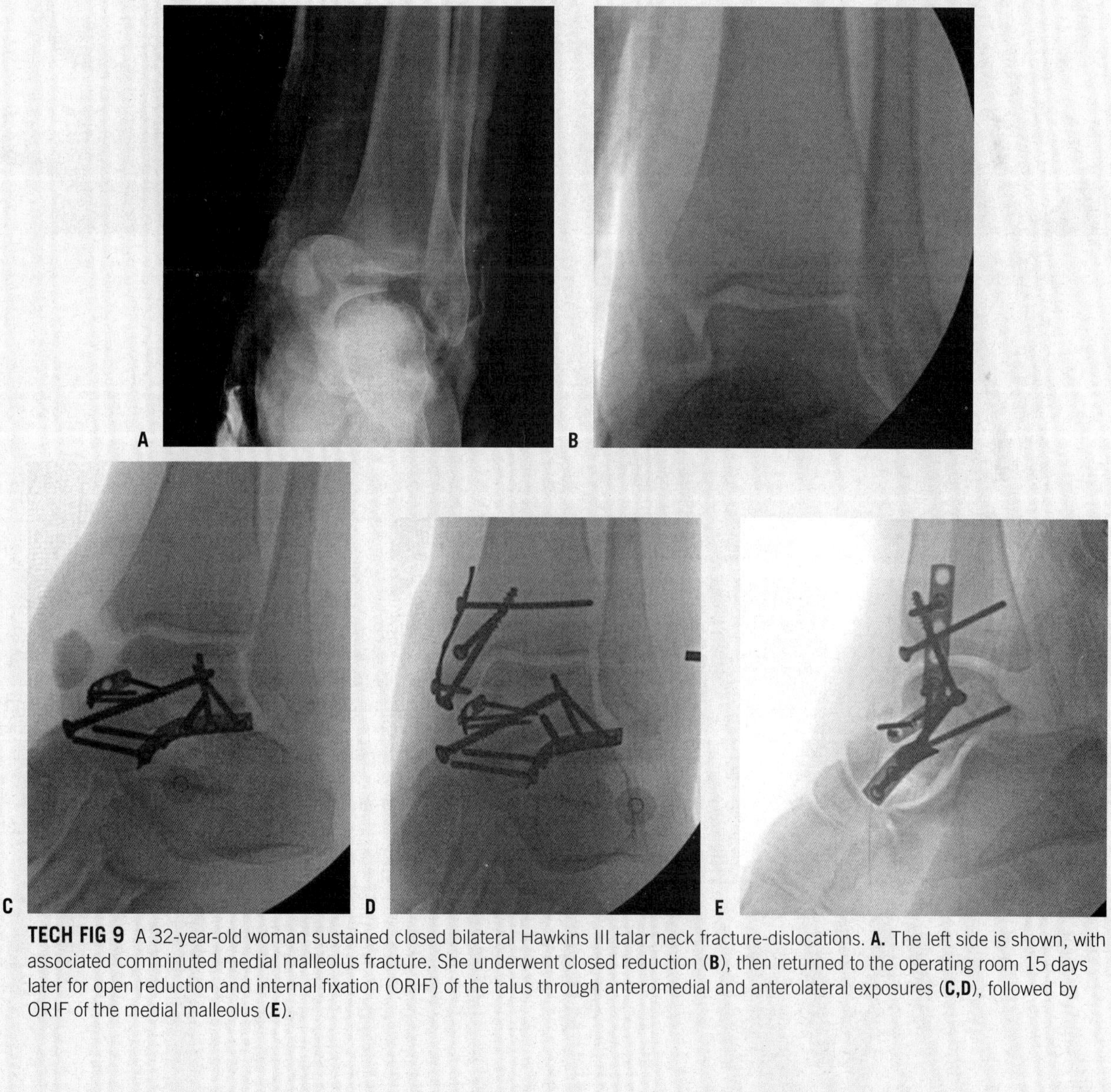

TECH FIG 9 A 32-year-old woman sustained closed bilateral Hawkins III talar neck fracture-dislocations. **A.** The left side is shown, with associated comminuted medial malleolus fracture. She underwent closed reduction (**B**), then returned to the operating room 15 days later for open reduction and internal fixation (ORIF) of the talus through anteromedial and anterolateral exposures (**C,D**), followed by ORIF of the medial malleolus (**E**).

TECHNIQUES

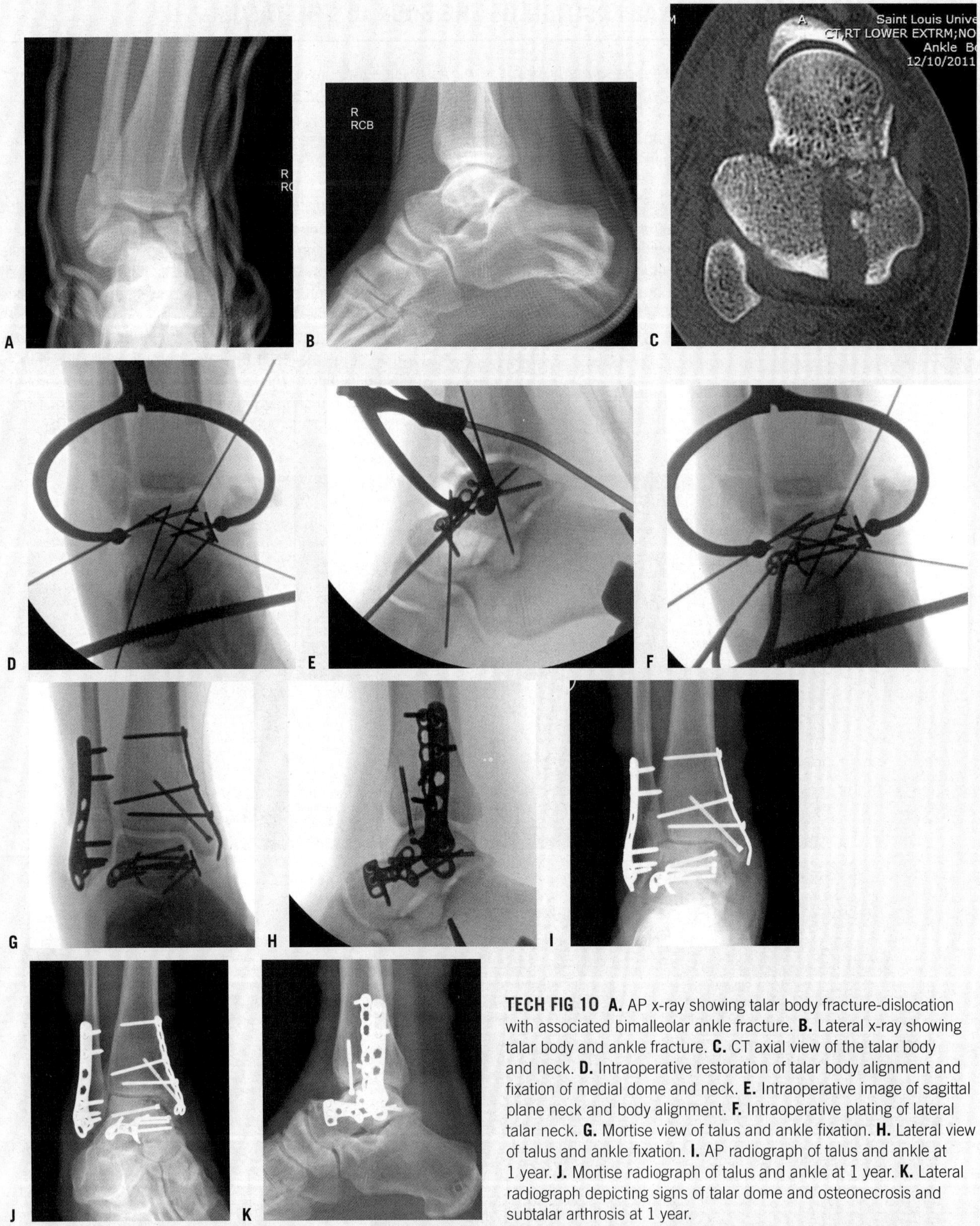

TECH FIG 10 A. AP x-ray showing talar body fracture-dislocation with associated bimalleolar ankle fracture. **B.** Lateral x-ray showing talar body and ankle fracture. **C.** CT axial view of the talar body and neck. **D.** Intraoperative restoration of talar body alignment and fixation of medial dome and neck. **E.** Intraoperative image of sagittal plane neck and body alignment. **F.** Intraoperative plating of lateral talar neck. **G.** Mortise view of talus and ankle fixation. **H.** Lateral view of talus and ankle fixation. **I.** AP radiograph of talus and ankle at 1 year. **J.** Mortise radiograph of talus and ankle at 1 year. **K.** Lateral radiograph depicting signs of talar dome and osteonecrosis and subtalar arthrosis at 1 year.

OPEN REDUCTION AND INTERNAL FIXATION OF THE POSTERIOR BODY TALUS

- Displaced, intra-articular posterior talar body fractures present largely in the coronal plane **(TECH FIG 11)**.
  - Supine positioning with a contralateral bump facilitates external rotation of the injured leg. This effectively places the ankle in excellent position for a lateral view once the fluoroscopy machine is pushed into place (see **FIG 5**).
- The fracture is fixed either by interfragmentary, parallel screw fixation, or a well-contoured plate and positional screws.

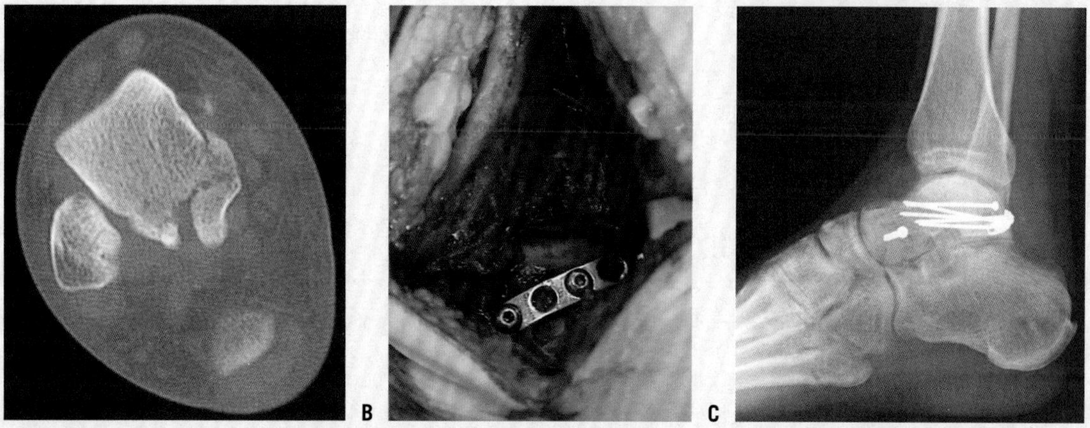

A B C

TECH FIG 11 **A.** Injury CT of posterior talus fracture. **B.** Intraoperative plate fixation. **C.** Postoperative lateral view.

OPEN REDUCTION AND INTERNAL FIXATION OF THE LATERAL PROCESS OF THE TALUS

- Open reduction and internal fixation of fractures of the lateral process of the talus may be performed with the patient positioned supine.
- After completing the anterolateral approach, the surgeon carefully evaluates the lateral process fracture **(TECH FIG 12)**.
  - The subtalar joint is assessed and chondral flaps and nonreconstructable fragments from the talus and calcaneus are removed.
  - Only very small fragments should be removed.
  - Larger fragments, even those without soft tissue attachments, are needed to restore the structure of the lateral process in any closed fracture of the lateral process of the talus.
- Occasionally, intercalary fragments are too small to be reduced and stabilized. If these fragments are impacted, and disimpaction and elevation of them will result in losing ability to retain them, they may be left in place. The surrounding lateral process architecture can then be restored to foster congruity of the lateral portions of the talus with the corresponding area of the calcaneus.
- Alternatively, these tiny fragments may be excised and the remaining lateral portion of the lateral process may be medialized so that it is continuous with the talar body, while ensuring that the articular alignment of the two fragments is positioned anatomically.

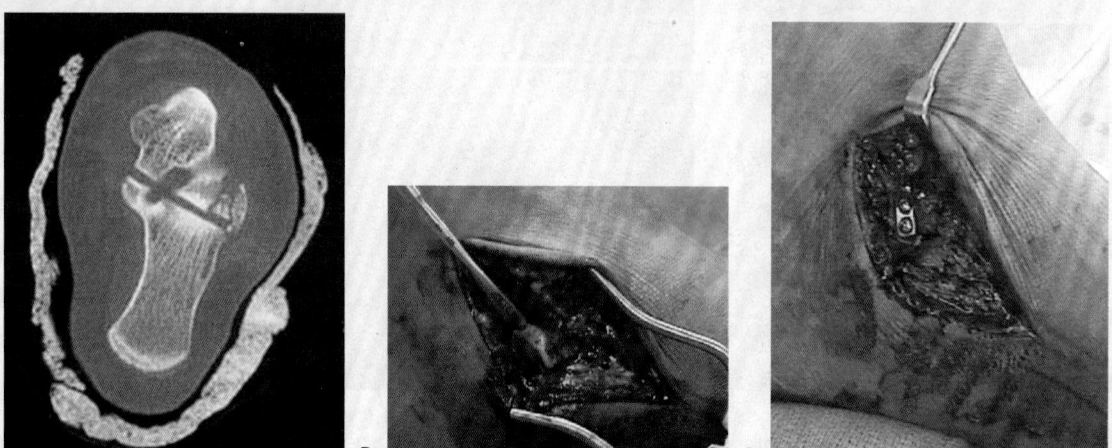

A B C

TECH FIG 12 Lateral process fracture of talus. **A.** Preoperative CT image. **B.** Intraoperative view of fracture. **C.** Intraoperative view of fixation. *(continued)*

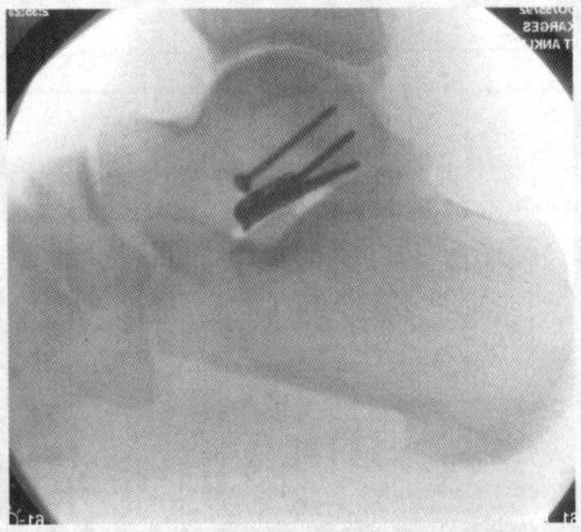

D

TECH FIG 12 *(continued)* **D.** Postoperative image.

- Any anterior or posterior osteochondral fragments are reduced and provisionally fixed with small, smooth Kirschner wires.
  - A Freer elevator is helpful to determine the anatomic subtalar joint line.
  - Final reduction of the direct lateral fragments of the lateral process is provisionally fixed by Kirschner wires.
- Isolated lateral process fractures without comminution are best fixed by interfragmentary screw fixation.
- Comminuted fractures should be buttressed by minifragment plate fixation to resist displacement against axial loads to the process.

MANAGEMENT OF PANTALAR DISLOCATION

- A complete dislocation of the talus at the tibiotalar, subtalar, and talonavicular joints is very rare.[1,10] Most of these injuries are open, with lateral wounds occurring most often.
- Closed pantalar dislocations are unlikely to be reduced via closed means. These injuries place a severe amount of stress on the adjacent neurovascular structures and surrounding soft tissues and should be reduced urgently.
- After general anesthesia, closed reduction may be attempted. More effective would be percutaneous assistance with a steerage Schanz pin in the calcaneus.
- Distraction of the ankle, subtalar, and talonavicular joints using external fixation and/or universal distractors is another method that may foster reduction.
- More often open reduction will be necessary, and the anteromedial exposure is an effective starting point, followed by percutaneous aids, possibly including strategic placement of external fixation distractors.
- Once the talus is reduced and all adjacent joints are congruous, external fixation, possibly using the pins already placed, is an excellent definitive means of maintaining alignment.
  - Injuries to capsule and retinacular tissues are repaired.
- In the case of open pantalar dislocation, talus devoid of soft tissue attachments should be immediately placed in a Bacitracin or chlorhexidine solution and transported to the operating room.
- After preparation and draping, the talus is gently scrubbed with chlorhexidine and débrided of contaminated soft tissue before reimplantation.
- A foot and ankle external fixator is constructed **(TECH FIG 13)**.
  - A medial triangular frame works nicely. This may consist of Schanz pins placed into the medial distal tibia, medial calcaneus, and the cuneiforms.
  - Definitive external fixation is retained for approximately 12 weeks to promote healing of the surrounding capsular and other soft tissues.
  - External fixation is preferable to Kirschner wires traversing the injured joints. Wires may directly contaminate the joints, and they are less stiff and more easily displaced than an external fixator.

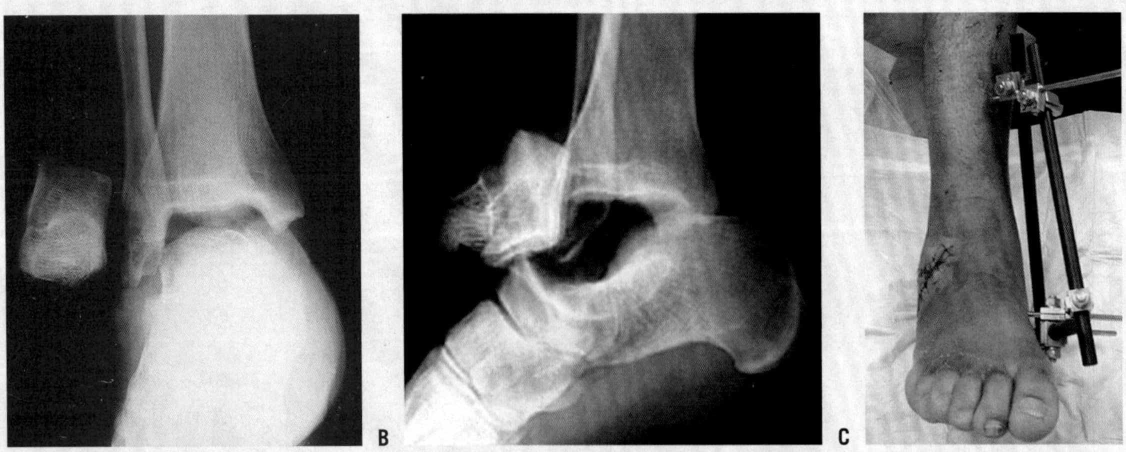

A B C

TECH FIG 13 A,B. A 30-year-old man sustained open pantalar dislocation in motorcycle crash. He underwent urgent débridement and open reduction. **C.** A triangular external fixator was placed with Schanz pins in the distal tibia, calcaneus, and cuneiforms.

Pearls and Pitfalls

Avoid medial dissection of the neck plantar to the insertion of the posterior tibial tendon.	• The tuberosity of the tarsal navicular is an important landmark identifying the plantar limit to the medial approach. Immediate swelling obscures palpation of this landmark.
The neck of the talus is aligned eccentrically medial in the hindfoot.	• The proximal portion of the anterolateral surgical approach should be directed more anteriorly if managing concurrent talar dome or tibia plafond fractures.
A medial malleolar osteotomy performed distal to the shoulder of the medial ankle mortise gives poor visualization of the talar dome.	• The osteotomy should be made at the level of the joint using a thin saw blade and completed with an osteotome. The surgeon should protect the soft tissues posterior to the malleolus during the osteotomy.
Beware of fixing the neck of the talus in varus malalignment and/or talar neck extension.	• The surgeon should view the Canale image intraoperatively with C-arm fluoroscopy (flexed knee, everted foot in equinus, and C-arm tube directed 15 degrees caudad). A true lateral image of the talus will avoid fixing the neck in extension.
Medial screw fixation of talar neck fractures, not countersunk in the talar head, commonly achieves poor fixation in the metaphyseal bone. Such screws are also not well-aligned with the longitudinal axis of the talus.	• The surgeon should avoid placement of isolated screws within the medial talar neck.
Do not use posterior to anterior screw fixation, with the patient in the prone position, for a displaced talar neck fracture.	• Posterior to anterior fixation does not facilitate anteromedial and anterolateral exposures to accurately reduce a displaced fracture.

POSTOPERATIVE CARE

- The goal of operative and nonoperative treatment of talus fractures is to achieve union and to restore hindfoot function.
- Immediate postoperative treatment consists of sterile ankle dressings and a well-padded, short-leg dressing with a posterior plaster splint.
  - The ankle is positioned in neutral plantarflexion.
  - In 2 to 3 weeks, once the swelling has subsided and the wounds are healed, ankle and subtalar motion exercises are recommended.
  - Upper and contralateral lower extremity strengthening may be valuable during the initial, subacute postinjury period.
- Partial osteonecrosis of the lateral dome of the talus is common. This may be seen because only the medial deep deltoid blood supply to the talar body remains intact after the injury.
  - The Hawkins sign is an early subchondral radiolucent line indicating blood supply to the body of the talus. Its presence, seen on an AP radiograph within 6 to 8 weeks, indicates bone resorption from disuse osteopenia, which is an active process requiring vascularity **(FIG 6)**.[6]
  - Fortunately, patients with isolated regional osteonecrosis of the talar dome rarely experience late collapse.
  - There are no data to support extended periods of non–weight bearing in patients with osteonecrosis. Currently, the impact of weight bearing on the progression of osteonecrosis is unknown. Procedures designed to revascularize the talus, such as core decompression, are not recommended.
- By 3 months, the fractures should be healed enough to permit gradual advancement of weight bearing as tolerated.
- Nonoperative management of talus fractures requires cast immobilization for 6 weeks.
  - After cast immobilization, the injury should be treated with stretching exercises and advancement of weight bearing.
- Follow-up postoperative management requires a three-view plain radiographic ankle series.

OUTCOMES

- Risk factors that lead to worse functional outcomes include comminution, a higher Hawkins classification, open fracture, and associated ipsilateral lower extremity injuries.
  - Osteonecrosis of the talus, posttraumatic arthrosis, joint stiffness, and varus malalignment also have a negative impact on the outcome.[9,12,13]
- The incidence of osteonecrosis of the talar body has been shown to increase with the severity of injury. Recent studies evaluating talar neck fractures identify an overall 50%

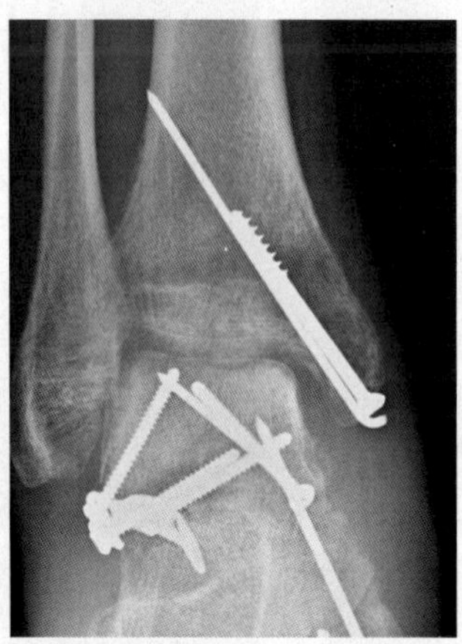

FIG 6 Two months after reduction and fixation of comminuted talus fractures, Hawkins sign is seen on mortise radiography, noted as lucency in the subchondral bone of the talar dome, consistent with disuse osteopenia with intact perfusion.

incidence of osteonecrosis, with evidence of collapse of the talar dome approximately half of cases.[11,13]

- Posttraumatic arthrosis secondary to these injuries is more common than osteonecrosis and most often presents in the subtalar joint.
  - Ankle arthrosis does not occur as an isolated outcome; it is seen in association with subtalar arthritis and is more frequent after talar body fracture.[11]
- No consensus exists regarding the most appropriate treatment of the extruded talus. This is a rare injury with an intuitively poor prognosis.
- Two recent studies evaluated reimplantation of the talus if possible.[1,10] Infection rates were low in both reports, supporting that reimplantation is usually effective.

COMPLICATIONS

- Soft tissue complications associated with talus fractures are predominantly superficial.
  - If full-thickness slough occurs, however, a formal wound débridement is mandatory followed by rotational or free flap coverage.
- The incidence of delayed union or nonunion of fractures of the talar neck varies in the literature between 0% and 10%.[4,9,13] The presence of osteonecrosis is a primary cause of nonunion. Nonunion of the talar neck fracture may also result from poor fixation.
  - If the cause of nonunion is unclear, the nonunion should be studied by MRI or CT scan. Every effort should be made to revise fixation with autogenous bone graft when possible.
  - Osteonecrosis of the body of the talus poses a challenging reconstruction because the bone is necrotic and not suitable for arthrodesis or as a stable bed for arthroplasty. Osteonecrosis with collapse requires removal of the body fragment and tibiocalcaneal fusion with or without structural autograft or allograft to address leg length discrepancy (**FIG 7**).
- Nonoperative management of comminuted lateral or posteromedial process fractures is unpredictable.
  - If pain persists long after the patient has returned to full weight bearing and radiographic or CT imaging suggests nonunion, resection of these fragments is routinely helpful. Pain may be secondary to fibrous nonunion.
- Malunion of the talus is predominantly due to varus malalignment. Malalignment of the talar neck is best prevented using dual anteromedial and anterolateral approaches in combination with the Canale image intraoperatively.

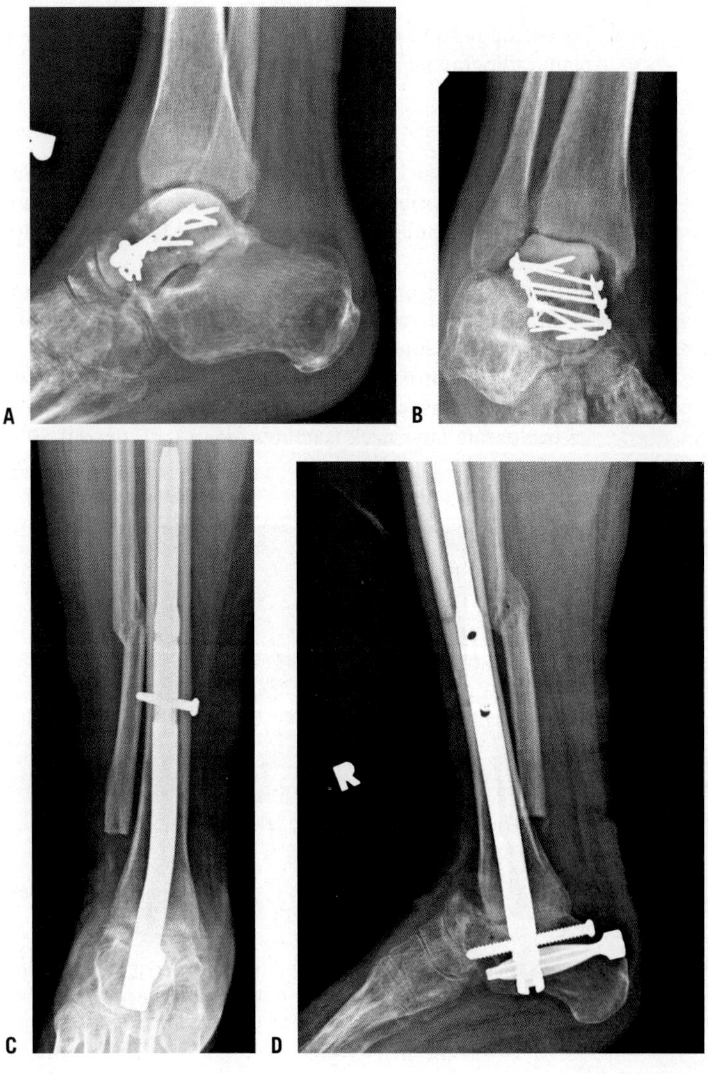

FIG 7 Patient with medial open talar neck fracture-dislocation was treated with immediate irrigation and débridement, reduction of body of talus, primary closure of wound, and temporary foot and ankle external fixator until soft tissue swelling resolved, allowing safe open reduction internal fixation. **A,B.** Healed talar neck injury with painful osteonecrosis of body of talus. **C,D.** Transfibular resection of talar body, tibiocalcaneal arthrodesis with intramedullary implant.

- Subtalar and ankle arthrosis is the most common complication associated with fractures of the talus, especially fractures that involve the body.[4,9,12,13] The incidence of subtalar arthrosis is greatest and can be routinely managed by conservative measures and occasionally with subtalar arthrodesis.
  - Arthritic symptoms can be managed effectively with nonsteroidal anti-inflammatories. The arthritic hindfoot is also benefited by custom ankle bracing or orthotics.
  - If symptoms of arthrosis are not improved nonoperatively, the patient may be evaluated by selective hindfoot and ankle lidocaine injection. Relief of joint pain, whether unifocal or bifocal, will allow the surgeon to counsel the patient on reconstructive treatment.

ACKNOWLEDGMENT

- The author would like to thank David E. Karges for his outstanding work on the previous edition chapter.

REFERENCES

1. Boden KA, Weinberg DS, Vallier HA. Complications and functional outcomes after pantalar dislocation. J Bone Joint Surg Am 2017;99:666–675.
2. Burgess AR, Dischinger PC, O'Quinn TD, et al. Lower extremity injuries in drivers of airbag-equipped automobiles: clinical and crash reconstruction correlations. J Trauma 1995;38:509–516.
3. Canale ST, Kelly FB Jr. Fractures of the neck of the talus. Long-term evaluation of seventy-one cases. J Bone Joint Surg Am 1978;60(2):143–156.
4. Dodd A, Lefaivre KA. Outcomes of talar neck fractures: a systematic review and meta-analysis. J Orthop Trauma 2015;29:210–215.
5. Haliburton RA, Sullivan CR, Kelly PJ, et al. The extra-osseous and intra-osseous blood supply of the talus. J Bone Joint Surg Am 1958;40-A(5):1115–1120.
6. Hawkins LG. Fractures of the neck of the talus. J Bone Joint Surg Am 1970;52(5):991–1002.
7. Lindvall E, Haidukewych G, DiPasquale T, et al. Open reduction and internal fixation of isolated, displaced talar neck and body fractures. J Bone Joint Surg Am 2004;86:2229–2234.
8. Miller AN, Prasarn ML, Dyke JP, et al. Quantitative assessment of the vascularity of the talus with gadolinium-enhanced magnetic resonance imaging. J Bone Joint Surg Am 2011;93(12):1116–1121.
9. Sanders DW, Busam M, Hattwick E, et al. Functional outcomes following displaced talar neck fractures. J Orthop Trauma 2004;18:265–270.
10. Smith C, Nork S, Sangeorzan B. The extruded talus: results of reimplantation. J Bone Joint Surg Am 2006;88(11):2418–2424.
11. Vallier HA, Nork SE, Barei DP, et al. Talar neck fractures: results and outcomes. J Bone Joint Surg Am 2004;86:1616–1624.
12. Vallier HA, Nork SE, Benirschke SK, et al. Surgical treatment of talar body fractures. J Bone Joint Surg Am 2003;85(9):1716–1724.
13. Vallier HA, Reichard SG, Boyd AJ, et al. A new look at the Hawkins classification for talar neck fractures: which features of injury and treatment are predictive of osteonecrosis? J Bone Joint Surg Am 2014;96:192–197.

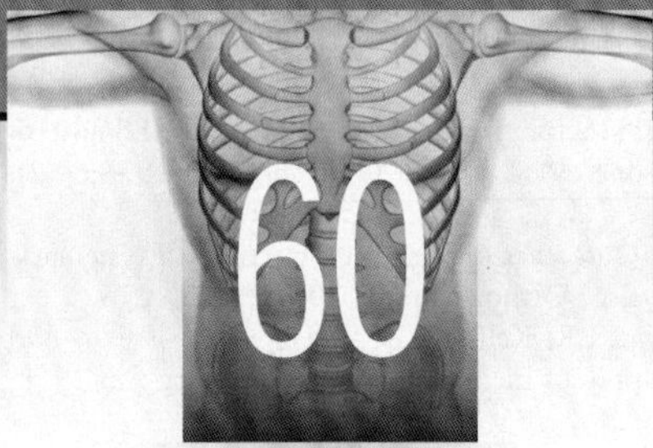

CHAPTER 60

Surgical Treatment of Calcaneal Fractures

Richard S. Yoon and Joshua R. Langford

DEFINITION

- An intra-articular calcaneus fracture is an injury that involves the joint surfaces of the calcaneus, usually with displacement.
- A fracture-dislocation of the calcaneus occurs when the superior lateral fragment of the posterior facet dislocates from beneath the talus to a position beneath the fibula or interposed between the fibula and the lateral talus. It carries a poor prognosis if treated nonoperatively. Therefore, all patients with this injury should be treated operatively, unless their medical condition precludes surgery.
- Anterior process fractures are injuries involving only the anterior portion of the calcaneus. When nondisplaced, they can be treated nonoperatively. Displaced fragments usually require surgery.
- A fibular rim fracture represents an avulsion of the superior peroneal retinaculum and is indicative of peroneal tendon instability.

ANATOMY

- The calcaneus is the largest bone in the foot. It has a complex shape that must be understood to make surgical reconstruction predictable.
- The calcaneus functions to transmit weight-bearing forces of the leg into the foot.
- The articular facets of the calcaneus combined with the corresponding facets on the talus form the subtalar joint. This joint along with the calcaneocuboid joint has a shock absorber function, thus allowing the foot to accommodate to variations in terrain.
- The four articular facets of the calcaneus include posterior, anterior, middle, and cuboid. Exact articular alignment is required for full function of this four-joint complex.
- The internal structure of the calcaneus reflects its weight-bearing role.
  - There is particularly dense trabecular bone in the juxta-articular regions, especially below the posterior facet (the thalamic trabecular system).
  - The tendo-Achilles insertion also has dense trabecular bone.
  - There exists a normal area of relatively little trabecular bone directly below the angle of Gissane called the *neutral triangle*. For this reason, filling this area with bone graft after fixation of a calcaneus fracture is rarely necessary.
- Cortical bone of 3 to 4 mm in thickness occurs in the superomedial region (sustentaculum area) and in the superolateral strut of bone that runs between the cuboid and posterior facets (anterolateral fragment). These regions of cortical bone will come into play when discussing the internal fixation of the calcaneus (**FIG 1**).
- The soft tissues of the calcaneus are easily damaged by trauma. This is especially true in the case of displaced tongue and tuberosity fractures, which can lead to pressure necrosis of the posterior soft tissue. Management of this injury component is essential to avoid iatrogenic surgical complications. The peroneal tendons traverse the retrofibular groove and are located on the lateral aspect of the calcaneus. The sural nerve courses along the lateral calcaneus and can be injured during any lateral exposure of the calcaneus.
- The blood supply to the lateral soft tissues of the calcaneus includes the lateral calcaneal artery, the lateral malleolar artery, and the lateral tarsal artery.
  - In both the extensile lateral exposure and the sinus tarsi approach, the lateral calcaneal artery is at risk for injury.
  - The lateral calcaneal artery must be preserved to prevent wound healing problems at the apex of the extensile lateral approach.

PATHOGENESIS

- Despite the seemingly infinite varieties of fractures that occur, stereotypic fracture lines, fragments, and displacements can be recognized.
- The calcaneus is fractured by a combination of shear and compression forces generated by the talus descending on the calcaneus.

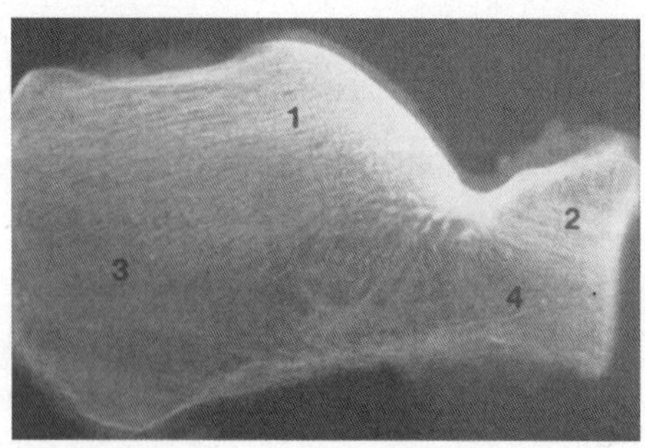

FIG 1 A lateral radiograph of a calcaneus specimen sectioned in the sagittal plane. The trabecular systems are visualized and numbered *1* to *4*. The densest bone is in the juxta-articular regions. Thick cortical bone also is present in the anterolateral fragment and medial wall in the sustentacular region. *1*, thalamic trabecular system; *2*, anterior apophyseal trabecular system; *3*, posterior plantar trabecular system; *4*, anterior plantar trabecular system. These regions provide optimal bone for internal fixation.

- Two primary fracture lines occur.
  - The first occurs in the angle of Gissane and divides the calcaneus into anterior and posterior fragments. It can split either the middle or anterior facet, and the fracture continues on the lateral wall in an inverted Y shape **(FIG 2)**.
  - The second fracture divides the calcaneus into medial and lateral halves and shears the posterior facet into two or more fragments.
    - As the talus continues to compress the calcaneus, the lateral half of the posterior facet is impacted into the body of the calcaneus, with the recoil producing a step-off in the posterior facet.

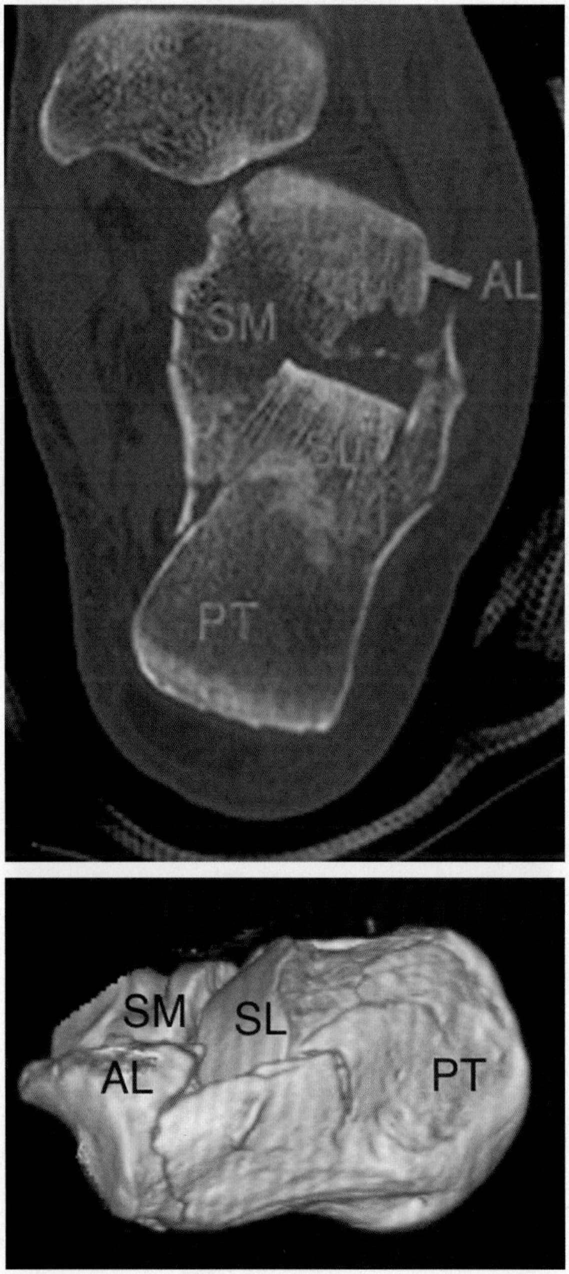

A
B

FIG 2 A,B. CT scans showing pattern of joint depression calcaneal fractures and main fragments. *AL*, anterolateral fragment; *SM*, superomedial fragment; *SL*, superolateral fragment; *PT*, posterior tuberosity.

    - This same fracture line commonly continues into the cuboid facet and, in combination with the first primary fracture line, produces the anterolateral fragment and superomedial fragment.
    - In this way, these two fracture lines produce fracture components that include the superomedial fragment, anterolateral fragment, posterior facet, and tuberosity.
  - The posterior facet is fractured into a superolateral fragment, occasional central fragments, and a portion connected to the sustentaculum tali (the superomedial fragment).
  - The portion connected to the sustentaculum tali is often referred to as the *constant fragment* because of the fact that it is rarely displaced to a significant extent. However, a recent study has demonstrated that the "constant fragment" frequently has some displacement and fracture lines.
- Characteristic displacements of these components occur.
  - The tuberosity is driven up between the pieces of the posterior facet, can tilt into valgus or varus, and is usually translated laterally. The tuberosity acts as a wedge that prevents reduction of the posterior facet **(FIG 3A)**.
  - The lateral posterior facet fragments are impacted and rotated plantarly into the body of the calcaneus **(FIG 3B)**.
  - The posterior facet breaks into one of three patterns, which form the basis of the Sanders classification:
    - Sanders II: two main pieces **(FIG 3C)**
    - Sanders III: three main pieces **(FIG 3D)**
    - Sanders IV: multifragmentary
  - The superomedial fragment retains alignment to the talus by means of its ligamentous attachments but can be subtly displaced by overlap with the anterior portion of the calcaneus. This overlap occurs along the primary fracture line that occurs in the sinus tarsi.
  - The anterolateral fragment displaces superiorly a variable amount. It typically extends into the cuboid facet, with varying degrees of displacement **(FIG 3E)**.
- The lateral calcaneal wall is displaced outward in the area of the trochlear tubercle. This, in combination with tuberosity translation, accounts for the heel widening and peroneal impingement that occur.
- In certain cases with significant lateral wall blowout, especially high-energy open fractures, the peroneal tendons will dislocate and may require stabilization **(FIG 3F)**.
- The first fracture types recognized were the joint depression and tongue-type patterns, which are readily identified on a lateral heel radiograph.
  - The tongue fracture maintains a connection between the tuberosity and the posterior facet, whereas the joint depression separates the fractured joint surface from the tuberosity **(FIG 4A,B)**.
  - Because of this anatomy, certain tongue fractures have a large portion, or even the entire posterior facet, in continuity with the tuberosity (AO Orthopaedic Trauma Association 73 C1). Thus, reduction of the tuberosity will reduce indirectly the posterior facet and restore the angle of Böhler. This particular pattern is well suited for small incision or percutaneous techniques **(FIG 4C,D)**.
- Tuberosity fractures involve the insertion of the Achilles tendon. They do not involve the posterior facet.

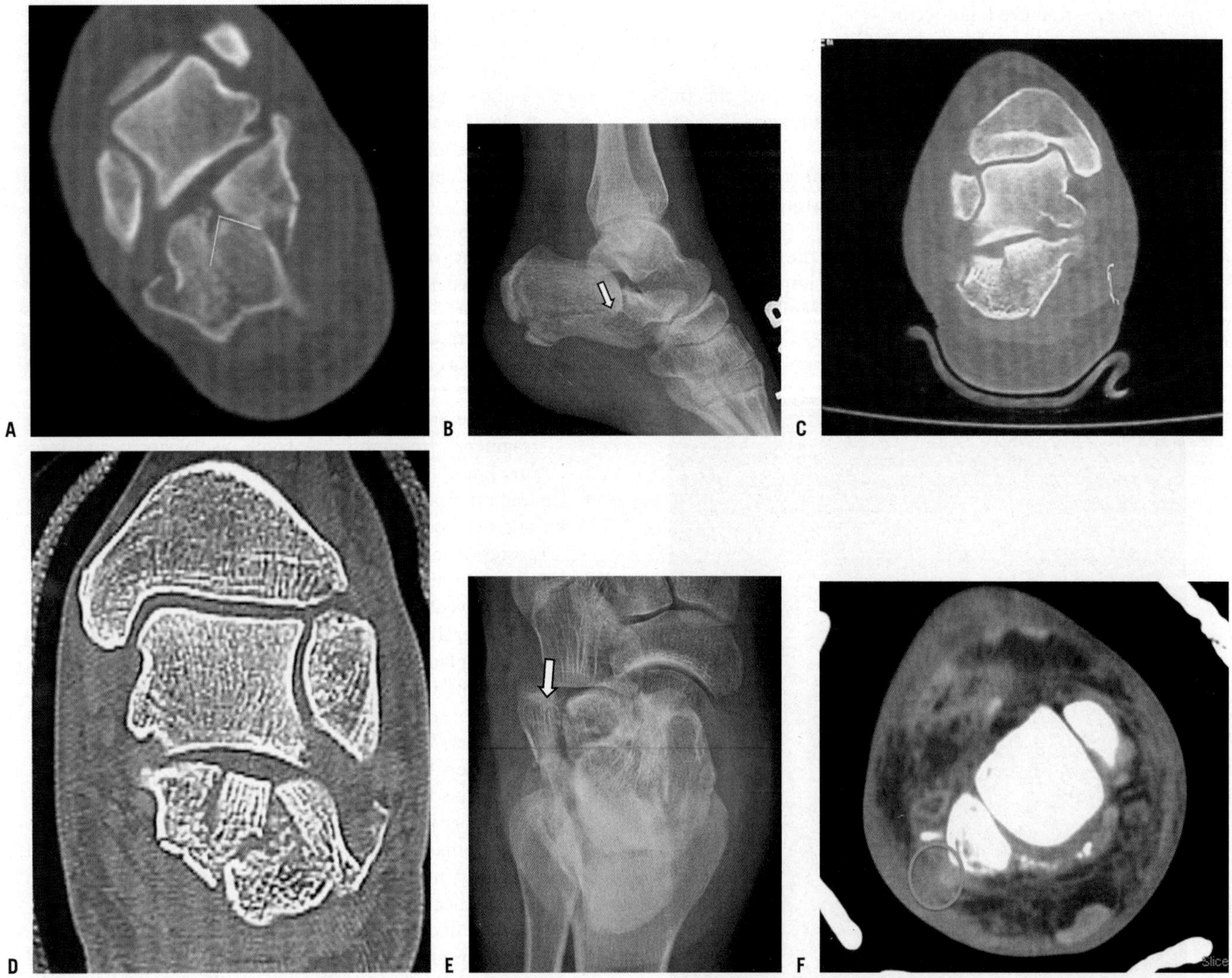

FIG 3 A. Coronal CT scan demonstrating how the posterior tuberosity acts as a wedge to separate the superomedial and superolateral fragments. **B.** The posterior facet displaces and rotates in a plantar direction (*arrow*). **C,D.** Coronal CT scans showing a Sanders II fracture with a large superomedial fragment (**C**) and a Sanders III fracture (**D**). **E.** The primary fracture line extends into the calcaneal cuboid facet. The anterolateral fragment is represented by the most lateral piece (*arrow*). **F.** Axial CT showing dislocated peroneal tendons. (**E:** Courtesy of Paul Tornetta, III, MD.)

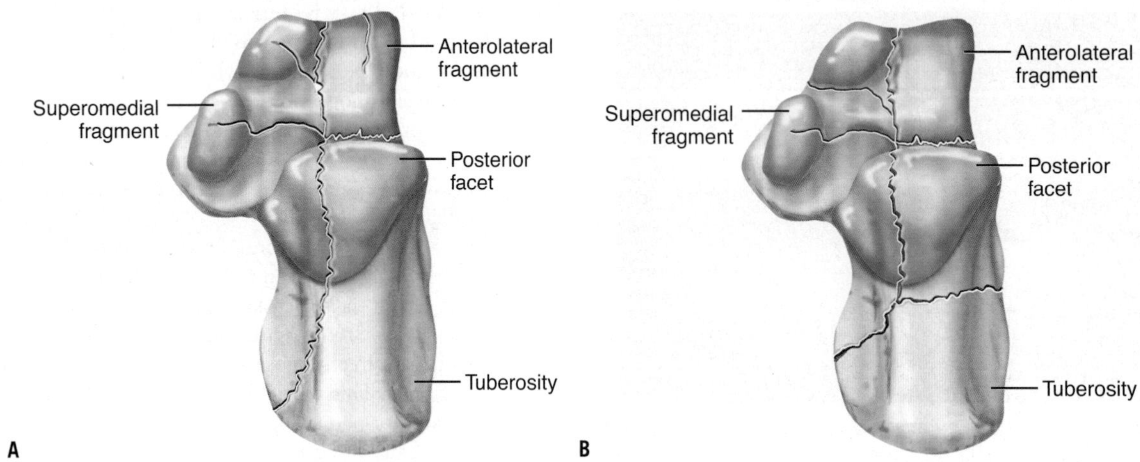

FIG 4 Calcaneus fracture patterns: tongue (**A**) and joint depression (**B**). *(continued)*

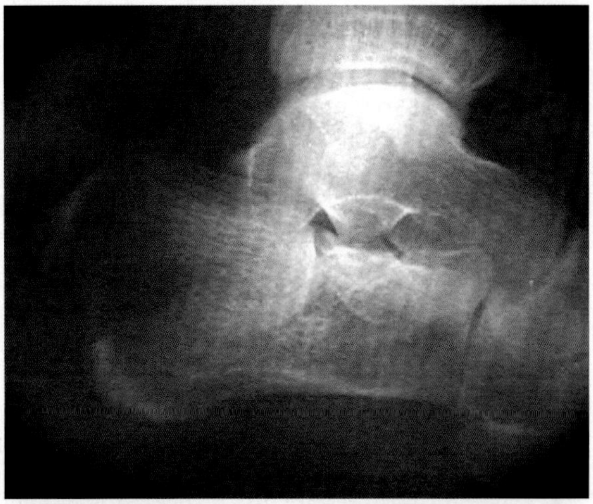

C

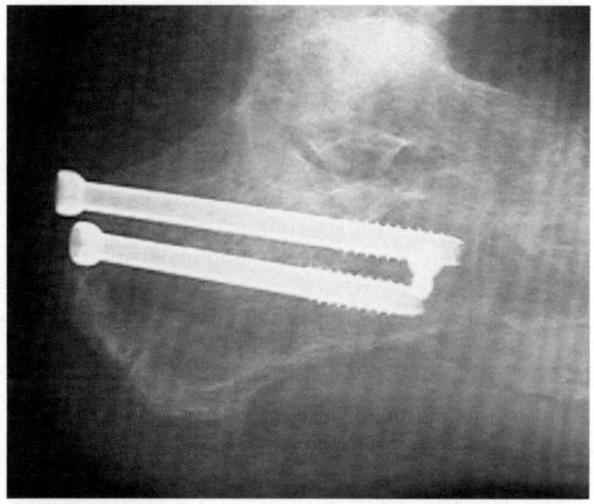

D

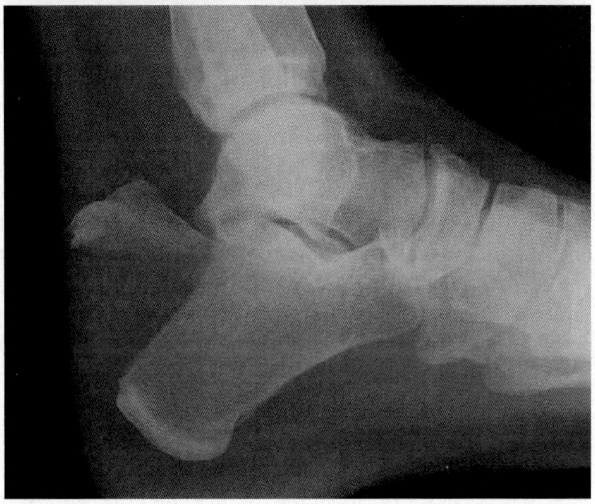

E

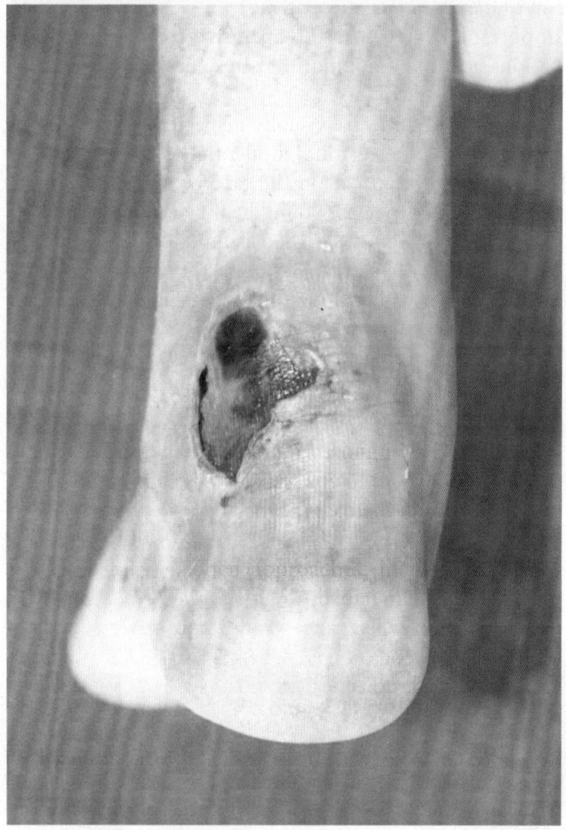

F

FIG 4 *(continued)* Lateral x-rays of tongue fracture: preoperative (**C**) and postoperative (**D**). Lateral x-ray of tuberosity fracture (**E**) and clinical picture of same patient demonstrating skin necrosis (**F**).

- Secondary to pressure on the skin, tuberosity and tongue fractures will frequently lead to skin breakdown. Therefore, they must be treated in an emergent manner **(FIG 4E,F)**.
- Reduction of a joint depression pattern is best performed with an open reduction.

NATURAL HISTORY

- An intra-articular fracture of the calcaneus is a serious injury that will diminish foot function.
- Nonoperative treatment is with early motion and delayed weight bearing 6 to 8 weeks after injury. This method has the least chance of iatrogenic injury.
- In a classic review by Lindsay and Dewar, only 17% of patients had no foot symptoms with long-term follow-up.
- The loss of ability to perform manual labor is common, with an average time off work of 4 to 6 months for laborers.
- Loss of subtalar motion to varying extents will occur.
- Tibiotalar impingement and anterior ankle pain can be produced if the crush deformity is severe enough, leading to settling of the talus into the body of the calcaneus.
- It can take 18 to 24 months for the foot symptoms to maximally improve after this injury. Most improvement occurs in the first 12 months.
- The key concept here is that patients who continue to improve symptomatically can be observed until maximum improvement occurs.

- A recent randomized study found that the need for late subtalar arthrodesis is five to six times greater if nonoperative treatment is used on all injuries. However, the rate of fusion for nonoperatively treated fractures was only 17%.
  - If a subtalar fusion is used to treat posttraumatic arthrosis after a calcaneus fracture that was treated without surgery and allowed to go on to a malunion, it is more difficult to reconstruct the entire external anatomy. The fusion will require a calcaneal osteotomy in addition to a fusion to restore the central point of the weight-bearing surface and the height of the bone.

PATIENT HISTORY AND PHYSICAL FINDINGS

- The history is typically one of a fall or vehicle crash. However, calcaneal fractures can occur and are frequently misdiagnosed after minor trauma in older osteoporotic patients and in diabetics with neuropathy.
  - Important risk factors for operative treatment complications include smoking, diabetes, peripheral vascular disease, and steroid use.
  - The foot and ankle are visually inspected.
  - Swelling is graded as mild, moderate, or severe.
    - Operative treatment in the face of severe soft tissue swelling is prone to wound healing complications.
    - Fracture blisters are graded as fluid- or blood-filled. If unhealed, fracture blisters are a source of skin bacterial colonization. Blood-filled blisters denote a deeper dermal injury.
    - Skin contusion is noted.
    - If present, the wrinkle sign is noted. This is defined as wrinkles appearing with dorsiflexion of the foot. This sign indicates that the swelling is resolving and surgical incisions are less likely to experience complications.
    - Open wounds are noted and, if present, represent a surgical emergency.
- The physician palpates the foot and ankle, looks for spine injuries or ipsilateral fractures, and performs a secondary survey for other injuries.
  - Spine injuries are said to accompany up to 10% of all calcaneal fractures.
- The physician assesses for compartment syndrome. Look for pain with passive flexion and extension of the toes, significant foot swelling, and elevated compartment pressure measurements (pressures within 30 mm Hg of diastolic pressure).
  - Compartment syndrome can occur in 5% to 10% of all calcaneal fractures.
- The physician performs a neurologic examination to check the sensory function of the foot and toes, including light touch and pinprick.
  - Calcaneal fractures, especially fractures with open wounds medially, can damage the posterior tibial nerve and vessels.
- Calcaneal fractures are also associated with lumbar spine injuries, and a full examination of the spine is necessary.

IMAGING AND OTHER DIAGNOSTIC STUDIES

- Anteroposterior (AP) and lateral **(FIG 5A,B)** foot radiographs are the initial screening study.
  - The axial (Harris) view should also be obtained **(FIG 5C)**. This view will demonstrate the medial wall and show the relation of the superomedial fragment to the tuberosity.
  - Broden views are radiographs that focus on the subtalar joint. They are taken with the foot internally rotated and the x-ray beam angled to varying degrees cephalad **(FIG 5D,E)**. By using different degrees of cephalad angulation, different parts of the posterior facet may be imaged. They are best used intraoperatively to judge the reduction of the posterior facet and the medial wall of the calcaneus.
- Three views of the ankle are also helpful. The AP and mortise views can demonstrate fibular rim fractures (indicative of peroneal instability) and fracture-dislocations (superolateral fragment may be displaced into the lateral gutter) **(FIG 5F,G)**.

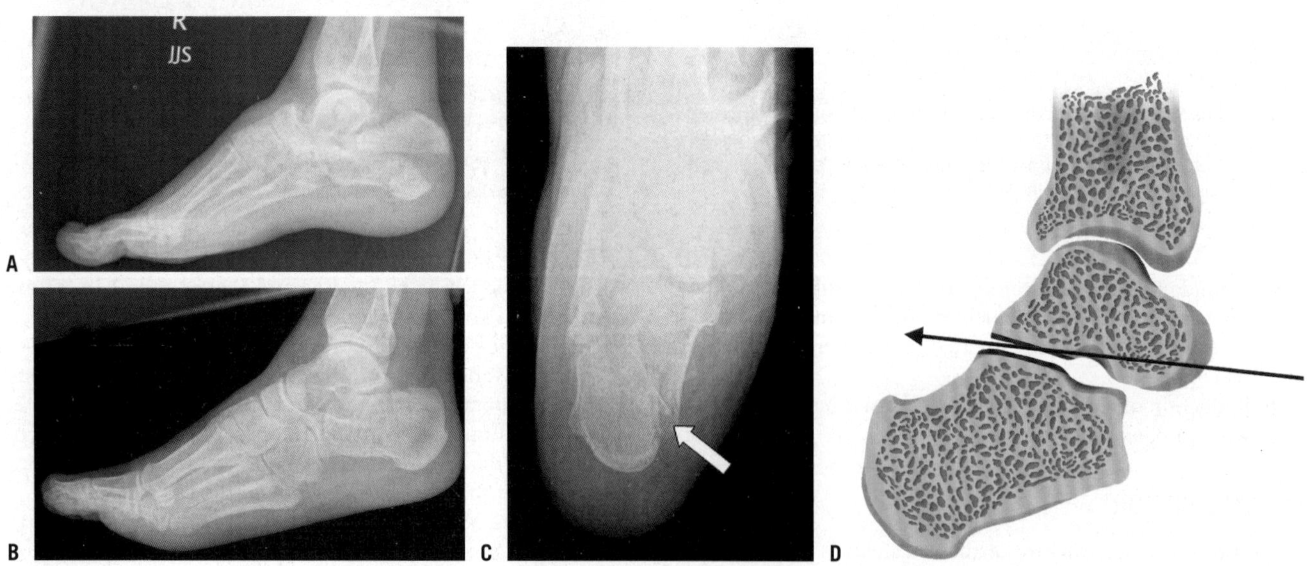

FIG 5 A,B. Lateral radiographs showing a severely displaced tongue-type Sanders II fracture of the calcaneus with midfoot dislocation (**A**) and a Sanders III fracture (**B**). **C.** The axial Harris view demonstrates displacement of the medial wall (*arrow*). Reduction of this pathoanatomy is the basis for the medial approach. **D.** Broden views are obtained by centering the x-ray beam on the posterior facet, internally rotating the foot, and directing the beam cephalad (*red arrow*). *(continued)*

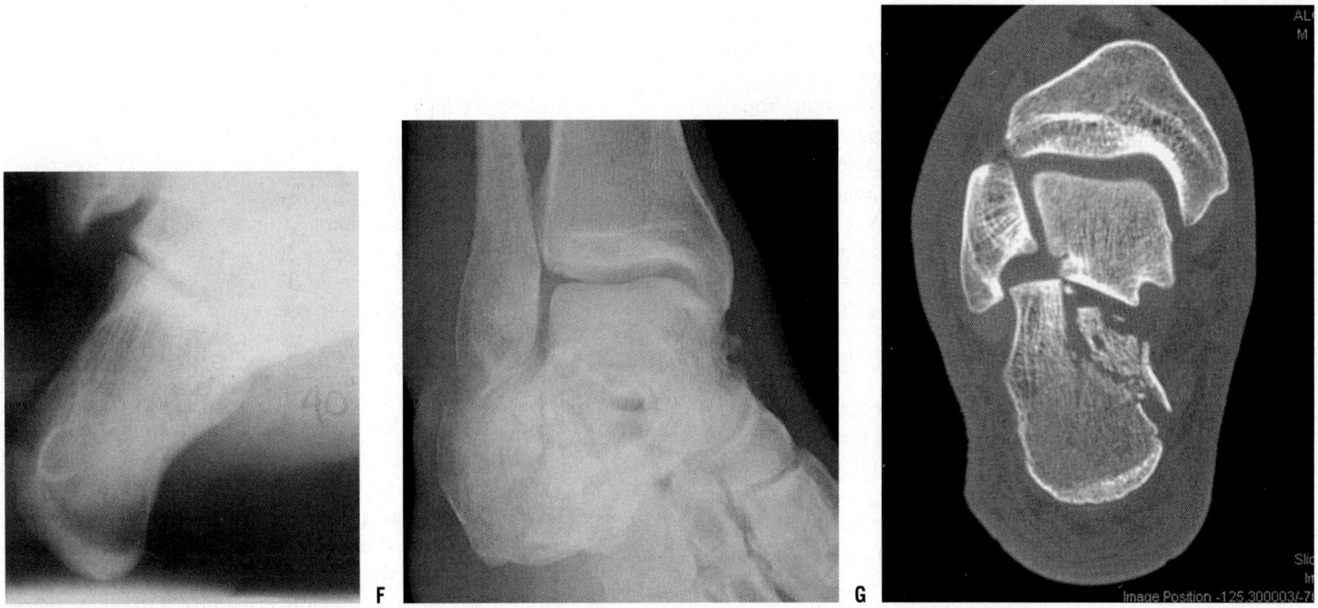

E F G

FIG 5 *(continued)* **E.** As the beam is aimed cephalad, more anterior portions of the posterior facet are visualized. Also note the medial wall on profile. As the x-ray is tilted more, the view becomes a true Harris axial view (if the internal rotation is removed). **F.** Ankle mortise showing a fracture-dislocation. **G.** Coronal CT scan of the same patient with a fracture-dislocation.

- If a fracture appears to be nondisplaced or minimally displaced but uncertainty exists about the alignment at the joint surface, a computed tomography (CT) scan is ordered.
- If the fracture is displaced, a CT scan is needed to define the anatomy and plan surgery (see **FIG 3A,C,D,F**).
  - A CT scan with biplanar cuts and reconstructions is needed. This will best delineate the fragments and displacements. The most important view is the plane perpendicular to the posterior facet of the talus (30-degree semicoronal view).

DIFFERENTIAL DIAGNOSIS

- Lateral process of talus fracture
- Severe ankle sprain
- Subtalar dislocation
- Stress fractures of the calcaneus can masquerade as a soft tissue disorder of the hindfoot (eg, plantar fasciitis).

NONOPERATIVE MANAGEMENT

- The indications for nonoperative treatment include posterior facet displacement less than 2 mm and medical conditions such as peripheral vascular disease or poorly controlled diabetes.
- Some surgeons consider smoking a relative contraindication as it predisposes to a higher wound complication rate.
- Minimal-incision techniques may be used in this setting with lower risk of wound complications.
- Severe fracture blisters or severe soft tissue injury can preclude operative treatment, although open reduction and internal fixation can be performed as late as 4 weeks after injury.
- The recommended nonoperative treatment is compression wrapping, early motion, and delayed weight bearing at 6 to 8 weeks after injury. This offers the least iatrogenic risk to the patient while optimizing chances for subtalar motion.
- During the first 2 to 3 weeks, the patient should be placed into a cam boot or splint at all times to prevent the development of an equinus contracture.
- Once weight bearing is started, the patient continues with range-of-motion exercises.
  - Strengthening of the foot and ankle muscles is added as fracture consolidation progresses.
- A well-cushioned shoe usually offers the best pain relief. Two different shoe sizes may be needed in extreme cases.
  - A rocker-bottom sole can be added to assist with the toe-off stance phase of gait.
- If posttraumatic arthrosis develops, various orthotics can be used in an attempt to relieve symptoms.
- Nonoperative treatment is not recommended for calcaneal fracture-dislocations, as a painful deformed foot is practically guaranteed if it is left unreduced.

SURGICAL MANAGEMENT

- The displaced intra-articular calcaneal fracture presents a difficult challenge.
- Foot pain and stiffness are common even with the best of treatment, and iatrogenic problems such as infection can result in loss of limb in extreme circumstances, and at the least, predispose to a poor result.
- Thus, a careful, individualized approach is recommended, with a priority on avoiding iatrogenic problems while attaining an anatomic alignment of the calcaneus.
- Indications include displacement of the posterior facet of more than 2 mm and calcaneus fracture-dislocation.
  - Research shows that certain patient groups, such as those receiving worker's compensation, are predisposed to a poor result with operative treatment but that does not obviate the benefits of obtaining anatomic foot alignment and lessening the chances of late subtalar fusion.

  - In addition, not all patients receiving worker's compensation do poorly, and some do return to gainful employment, although with restrictions in some settings.
- The choice of any surgical approach or technique should always have the goal of total anatomic restoration, although extreme comminution can compromise attainment of this goal.
- Furthermore, choosing between percutaneous technique, temporary fixation staged to definitive fixation, sinus tarsi, or extensile lateral approach is dependent on fracture severity and associated soft tissue status. This chapter focuses on the limited incision and sinus tarsi approaches.

Preoperative Planning

- Once operative treatment has been elected, the surgical approach is chosen based on a number of factors, including the surgeon's training and experience and the pathoanatomy present.
- The timing of surgery differs between minimal-incision techniques and the extensile lateral approach. The timing is in general when the wrinkle sign develops and the soft tissue envelope is optimal.
- When using a sinus tarsi or similar minimal-incision approach, surgery should be performed before 2 weeks. If the soft tissue envelope is not ready in that time frame, then an extensile lateral approach should be used once the soft tissues are optimal.
- The injury pathoanatomy is analyzed first by looking at the posterior facet pattern (Sanders II, III, or IV), displacement, and location of the primary fracture line in the posterior facet.
  - Fractures that are more medial are more difficult to visualize, and more fragments involving the posterior facet are more difficult to fixate anatomically.
  - Fractures that separate the entire posterior facet and have a tongue pattern are amenable to percutaneous Essex-Lopresti techniques.
  - Conversely, joint depression fractures require open reduction of the posterior facet.
  - A highly comminuted Sanders IV fracture should be treated with open reduction and primary fusion through a sinus tarsi or extensile lateral exposure.
- The other fracture components to be analyzed for displacement are the superomedial fragment, anterolateral fragment, and tuberosity. The surgical plan should address each of these pathologies for reduction strategy and fixation.
- The typical reduction order is first to correct any superomedial fragment subluxation.
  - Next, the superomedial fragment is reduced and held to the tuberosity.
  - The posterior facet is then reduced and fixed.
  - Finally, the anterolateral fragment is reduced and fixed.
- The size and integrity of the superomedial fragment is critical, as fixation techniques largely center on screw placement into its substance. A small or comminuted superomedial fragment makes rigid fixation harder to achieve and may call for alternative techniques.
  - A significantly displaced superomedial fragment may require a separate medial incision to assist with reduction and fixation.
  - Restoration of the superomedial fragment to the tuberosity will restore the calcaneal shape and make room for reduction of the displaced posterior facet fragments.
  - The superomedial fragment may be incarcerated in the sinus tarsi and subtly subluxated. This is recognized by the preoperative CT scan on the sagittal reconstructions and by the lack of congruence of the superomedial fragment with the undersurface of the talus.
    - Failure to correct this subluxation makes posterior facet reduction very difficult.
- The anterolateral fragment should key into location just in front of the reduced posterior facet and restores lateral column length. This is assessed by assuring reconstruction of the hard cortical bone that represents the crucial angle of Gissane.
  - It can be fixed with either lag screws into the superomedial fragment or a minifragment plate. Some of the perimeter plates have a small extension to pull this fragment into place.
  - The fixation chosen depends on the approach taken. Fractures splitting the posterior facet will require lag screws inserted from lateral to medial; they range in size from 2 to 4 mm, depending on the fractures present.
  - Sanders III fractures are converted into two major pieces with the use of countersunk minifragment screws or bioabsorbable pins that fix the intermediate piece to the more medial piece.
- The plate chosen depends on the approach.
  - Strategic placement of small and minifragment plates, technique-specific plates, and occasionally lag screws alone is used in minimal-incision techniques.
- Plans must be made for imaging, most typically, fluoroscopy. This will allow control of the AP, lateral, axial, and Broden views intraoperatively.
  - Arthroscopy can also help visualize the posterior facet. It allows for more accurate reduction in fractures managed with either the extensile lateral or minimal-incision approaches.
    - Correlation between fluoroscopy and arthroscopy is critical to ensure accurate reduction.

Positioning

- Open reduction and internal fixation procedures are performed in the lateral decubitus position with the injured foot placed behind the uninjured foot and supported on a stable base of sheets or foam. A thigh tourniquet is applied.
- The fluoroscope is brought in from the side opposite the surgeon regardless of the surgical approach.
- The same position can be used for percutaneous manipulations of tongue fractures. This allows conversion to the extensile lateral approach if needed, as recommended by Tornetta.
- Minimal-incision approaches may performed supine with a bump under the ipsilateral hip. A thigh tourniquet is placed.
  - The injured leg is elevated on a stable base of sheets or foam. This allows for easier lateral imaging with fluoroscopy and easier medial external fixator placement, which may be used to assist with reduction.
- For bilateral injuries treated with a sinus tarsi approach, the patient is placed supine.
- The arthroscope is placed with the monitor on the same side as the C-arm, toward the head of the bed.

Approach

- Minimal-incision techniques will address most but not all calcaneal pathologies but require a firm understanding of the fragments, displacements, and deforming forces present.
  - All small-incision techniques are not the same.
  - The Essex-Lopresti maneuver is applicable only to fractures with a tongue pattern.
  - Techniques involving multiple small incisions for joint reduction and screw placement are best suited for simple joint depression patterns without significant displacement.
- Sinus tarsi approaches allow adequate visualization of the posterior facet and can be used for Sanders II and IV fractures as we recommend fusion for type IV injuries.
  - Certain but not all Sanders III fractures can also be treated with this approach but should only be treated by surgeons with extensive knowledge of calcaneal fracture management.
  - Ideally, a surgeon should perform many cases with an extensile lateral approach prior to attempting minimal-incision techniques such as the sinus tarsi approach. This allows for a much better understanding of the complex calcaneal anatomy.

MINIMAL-INCISION REDUCTION AND FIXATION OF TONGUE FRACTURES

- If performed acutely, minimal-incision reductions can be technically easier and do not increase the risk of infection in our experience.
  - If there is any question, the surgeon should use the presence of the wrinkle sign and healing of fracture blisters.
- This technique is ideally indicated for tongue patterns that have a large percentage of the posterior facet connected to the tuberosity (Sanders IIC) **(TECH FIG 1A)**.
  - The technique can be used for Sanders IIA and IIB patterns, but the facet reduction is more difficult if done percutaneously.
  - The surgery is often performed on an urgent basis secondary to pressure necrosis of the posterior skin that can occur secondary to the displaced posterior tuberosity **(TECH FIG 1B)**.
- This surgery can be performed in either a supine or lateral position, with the addition of a sinus tarsi incision to visualize the posterior facet if exact reduction cannot be confirmed on fluoroscopy.
  - If possible conversion to the extensile lateral approach is suspected, lateral positioning will facilitate this approach if percutaneous methods fail.
- The patient is placed supine with a generous bump under the ipsilateral hip to assist access to the heel.
- A popliteal block is placed by the anesthesia team. This will allow for outpatient surgery management of this injury.
- Two small incisions are used, one just medial and one just lateral to the Achilles insertion.
  - A stout Steinmann pin or guidewire for a 6.5-mm or larger cannulated screw is introduced into the calcaneus from the posterior tuberosity.
  - The guide pin is drilled directly toward the distal end of the displaced posterior facet fragment **(TECH FIG 1C)**.
  - The pin is then used as a levering tool to restore the Böhler angle of the fractured calcaneus **(TECH FIG 1D)**.
- Taking a lateral view of the normal heel and saving it on the fluoroscope provides a comparison to judge reduction.
- Once the fracture is reduced, a second guide pin is drilled from the second incision into the anterior calcaneus and the reduction guide pin, which is bent in the reduction process, is exchanged for a new pin, which is also drilled into the anterior calcaneus.
  - Cannulated screws are introduced from the tuberosity into the anterior portion of the calcaneus **(TECH FIG 1E–G)**.

A
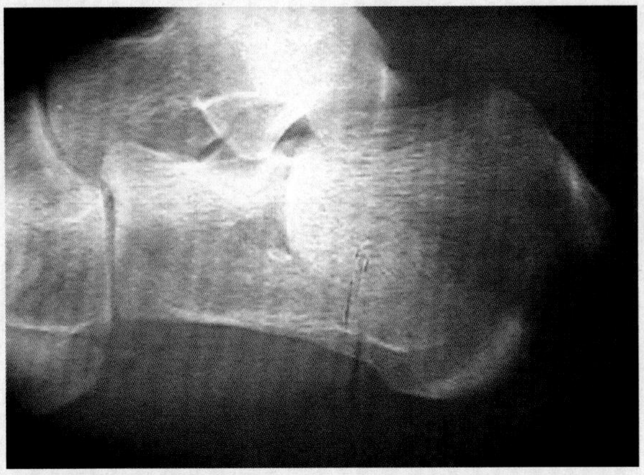
B
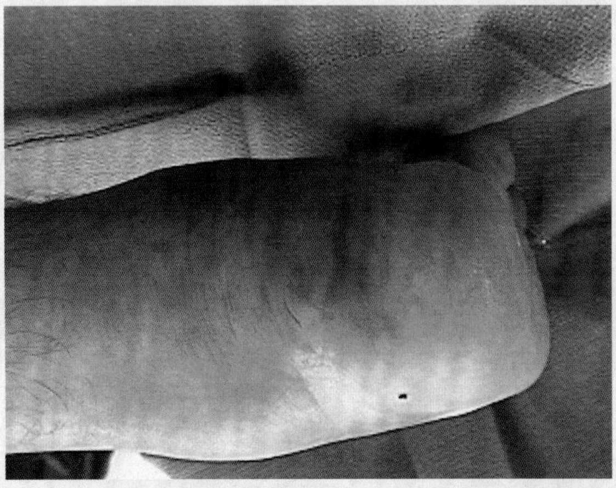

TECH FIG 1 A. A displaced tongue fracture demonstrates the typical displacement and location of an injury amenable to percutaneous reduction. The anterior process is not comminuted but does have a sagittal fracture line requiring lag screw fixation. **B.** Clinical picture demonstrating skin blistering and early pressure changes. *(continued)*

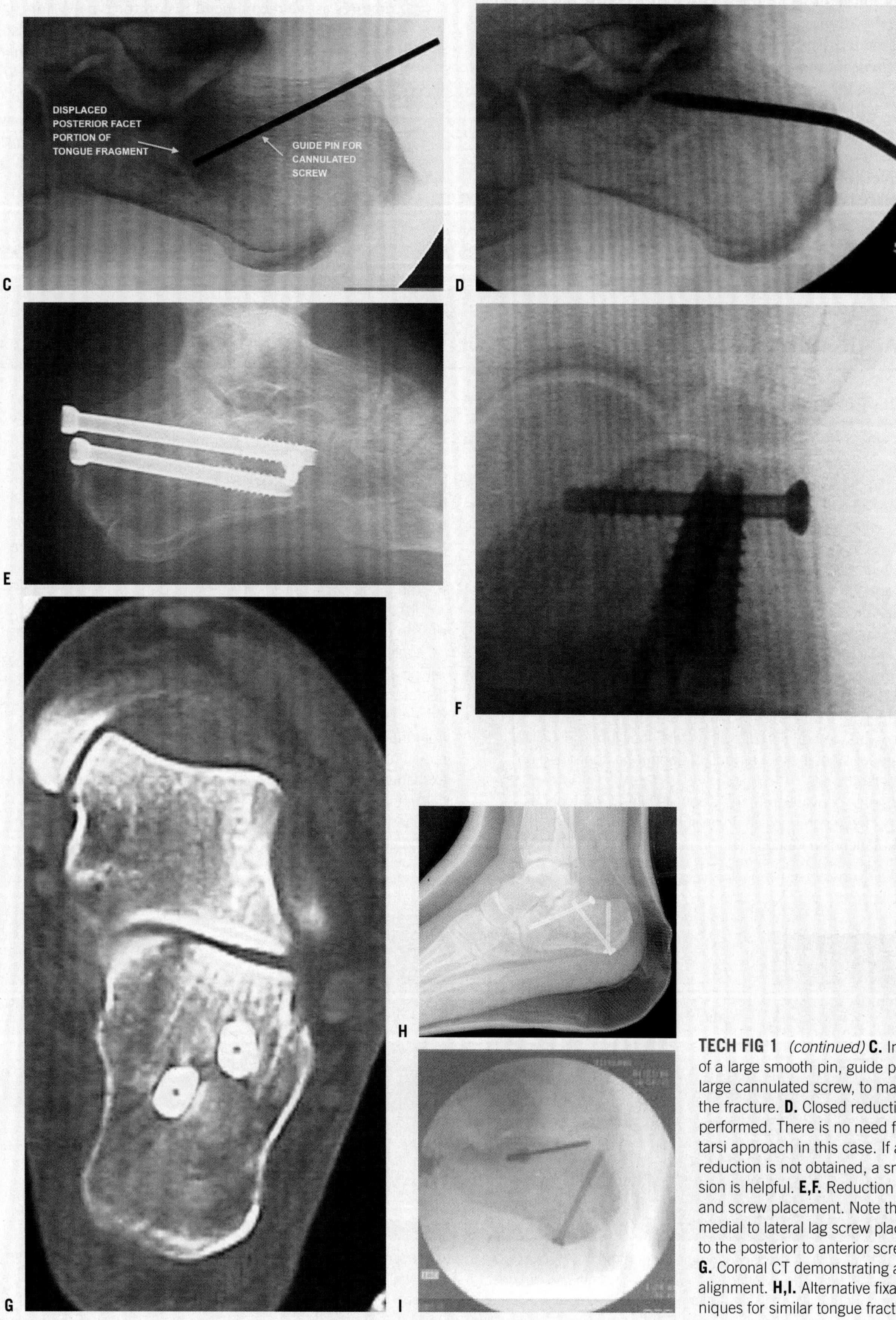

TECH FIG 1 *(continued)* **C.** Introduction of a large smooth pin, guide pin for a large cannulated screw, to manipulate the fracture. **D.** Closed reduction is performed. There is no need for a sinus tarsi approach in this case. If adequate reduction is not obtained, a small incision is helpful. **E,F.** Reduction obtained and screw placement. Note the anterior, medial to lateral lag screw placed prior to the posterior to anterior screws. **G.** Coronal CT demonstrating adequate alignment. **H,I.** Alternative fixation techniques for similar tongue fractures.

- Alternative or adjunctive fixation strategies include placing a 4.0-mm screw from the plantar tuberosity into the dorsal calcaneus surface. This resists plantar displacement of the tongue fragment.
- Lag screws can also be used to stabilize the posterior facet from the lateral calcaneus into the superomedial fragment and to stabilize sagittal fracture lines in the anterior calcaneus **(TECH FIG 1H,I)**.

PROVISIONAL PERCUTANEOUS PIN FIXATION

- Reserved for severe Sanders III/IV fractures with significant posterior facet depression and/or lateral wall blow out
- Purpose of temporary wire fixation is to restore height and valgus (if possible) while waiting for soft tissue swelling to resolve.
- Temporarily, maintaining height allows the soft tissue to mature in an elongated position, allowing for easier closure of a staged open approach, decreasing soft tissue tension, and theoretically, decreasing soft tissue complications.
- Utilizing the equatorial talar line (ETL) **(TECH FIG 2A)**, if the posterior tuberosity falls above the ETL, this is predictive of Sanders III/IV fracture and may benefit from temporary fixation **(TECH FIG 2B,C)**.
- Skin becomes amenable in the desired "elongated" position, allowing for less tension and easier closure for uncomplicated healing.

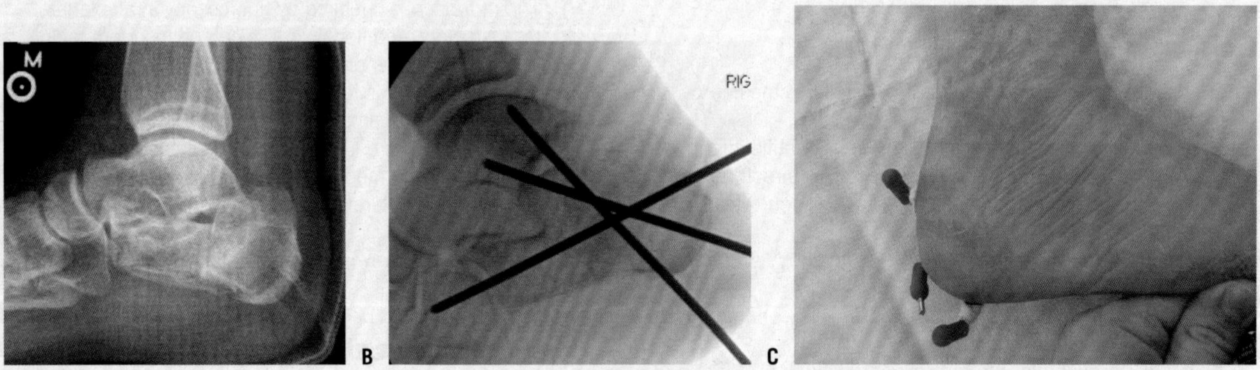

A B C

TECH FIG 2 A–C. The ETL draw from the anterior talar process to the posterior process (**A**) can help to determine if fracture pattern is amenable to provisional pin fixation prior to definitive extensile lateral approach. If the posterior calcaneal process is above the ETL, then this is predictive of Sanders III/IV fracture and would be amenable. Provisional pin fixation is done to restore as much height and valgus as possible (**B,C**) to allow for the skin to mature in an "elongated" positions to allow for less soft tissue tension when definitive fixation is performed.

OPEN REDUCTION

- If the Böhler angle is not reducible, or if a step-off remains in the posterior facet, an open reduction is performed.
  - We prefer a small sinus tarsi incision approach to aid in the reduction.
- A 4- to 6-cm sinus tarsus incision is made to expose the posterior facet, the anterolateral fragment, and a portion of the lateral calcaneal wall **(TECH FIG 3)**.
- The posterior facet is reduced under direct vision, and the reduction is confirmed with fluoroscopy. An arthroscope is helpful as well.
- A traction pin in the tuberosity can help restore calcaneal height.
- Laterally to medially directed lag screws are placed across the posterior facet. A minifragment plate is used to bridge the posterior facet to the anterolateral fragment.
- The lateral wall should be manually compressed at this point.
- Layered closure is performed.

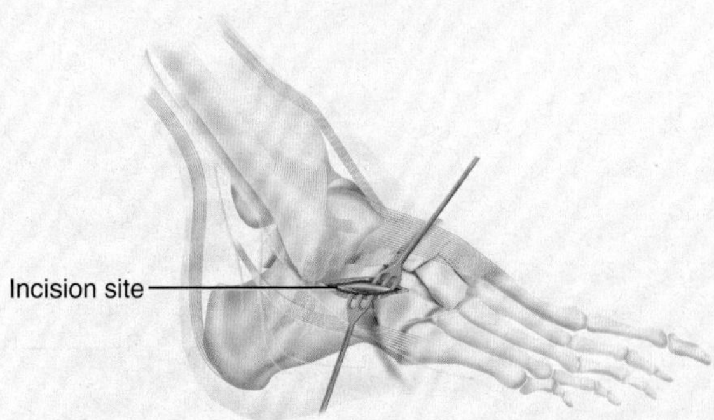

TECH FIG 3 Lateral approach for the small-incision technique.

SIMULTANEOUS MEDIAL AND LATERAL APPROACHES

- Combined medial and lateral approaches are rarely required.
  - One exception would be in a fracture involving significant displacement of the sustentaculum tali that cannot be reduced from the lateral approach.
  - Otherwise, modern implants and techniques obviate the need for a separate medial incision in most cases.
- If a surgeon wishes to proceed with a combined approach, the following points are taken into consideration.
- In general, except for open fractures, timing should be guided by the presence of the wrinkle sign and healing of fracture blisters.
- This technique is ideally indicated for Sanders II fractures with greater than 2 mm of displacement of the posterior facet and a large superomedial fragment. It can be applied to nearly any fracture pattern, but the limited exposure makes posterior facet reduction more difficult for Sanders III and IV patterns.
- A generous bump is placed under the ipsilateral hip. The heel is left slightly off the end of the bed to facilitate the placement of axially directed fixation.
- A popliteal block is placed by the anesthesia team.

Incisions and Dissection

- The medial approach is posterior and parallel to the neurovascular bundle (**TECH FIG 4A**).
  - The medial calcaneal sensory branch is identified deep to the flexor retinaculum and preserved. This directly exposes the superomedial fragment and keeps the neurovascular bundle in the anterior flap.
- The lateral sinus tarsi approach extends anteriorly 4 to 6 cm from the tip of the fibula (see **TECH FIG 2**).
  - This will provide exposure of the posterior facet and anterolateral fragment.
  - It is performed after the medial approach.
- At this point, all fracture fragments are identified and cleaned of debris.
- The posterior facet is partly reduced to avoid obstruction of the superomedial fragment and tuberosity reduction.
- The posterior tuberosity requires distraction. This can be accomplished with different techniques, including application of a 1.6-mm Steinmann pin. The pin is introduced into the tuberosity of the calcaneus in a medial to lateral direction. The pin is tensioned with a Kirschner bow, and an assistant distracts the tuberosity allowing for correction of shortening (**TECH FIG 4B**).
- The medial fracture fragments are cleaned of debris, and landmarks for reduction are identified.

Medial Reduction and Fixation

- Reduction and fixation can be done with one of two strategies.
- The first is with an antiglide 2.7-mm plate.
  - One can predrill a hole on the tuberosity fragment next to the fracture site and to the length measured.
  - With use of distraction and manipulation, an approximate reduction of the superomedial fragment and tuberosity is obtained, particularly with respect to length.
  - A 2.7-mm five-hole T plate or similar plate is then placed on the bone, and the premeasured screw is inserted. As the plate tightens to the bone, it will help reduce any tuberosity translation (**TECH FIG 5**).
  - The reduction is checked by fluoroscopy in all planes.
  - If satisfactory, additional screws can be inserted, taking care to avoid the posterior facet.
- The second method is to obtain a reduction by traction and translation of the tuberosity.
  - One can then introduce axial cannulated screws—one up the inside of the medial wall and the other as a lag screw from the inferolateral tuberosity into the superomedial fragment.
  - This latter lag screw is a useful adjunct to a medial antiglide plate.

Lateral Reduction and Fixation

- Once the medial side is reduced, the lateral side is addressed.
- The posterior facet is manipulated and reduced. The reduction is checked with Broden views and the arthroscope (**TECH FIG 6**).
- It is common to approximate one portion of the facet, only to have another portion malreduced.
- Once an anatomic reduction is obtained, provisional fixation with Kirschner wires is performed. Two lateral to medial directed

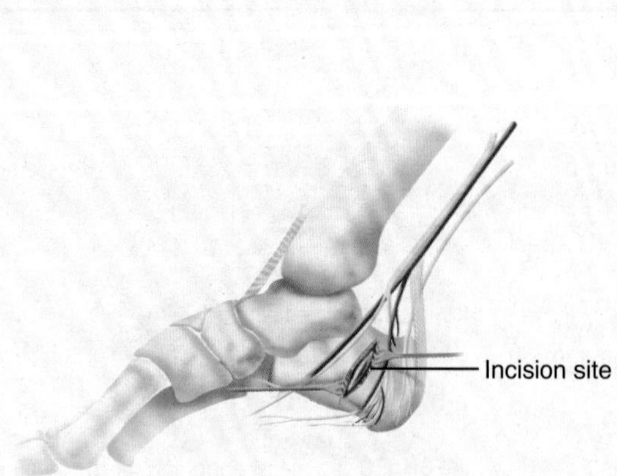

A

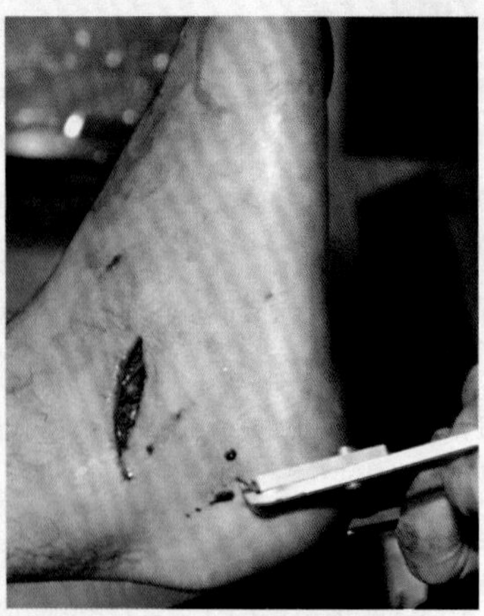

B

TECH FIG 4 **A.** Medial approach for the small-incision technique. **B.** A tensioned 1.6-mm smooth Kirschner wire is placed in the inferior tuberosity and is used to apply traction to the calcaneus. The heel is slightly off the end of the bed to facilitate placement of axial fixation.

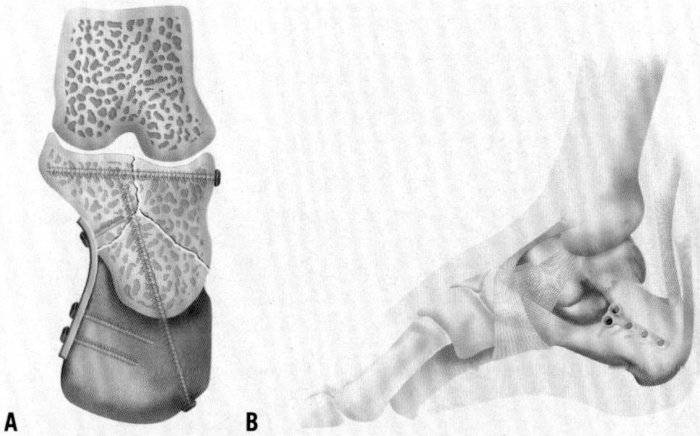

TECH FIG 5 Axial (**A**) and medial (**B**) views of fixation with a medial plate and lateral screws.

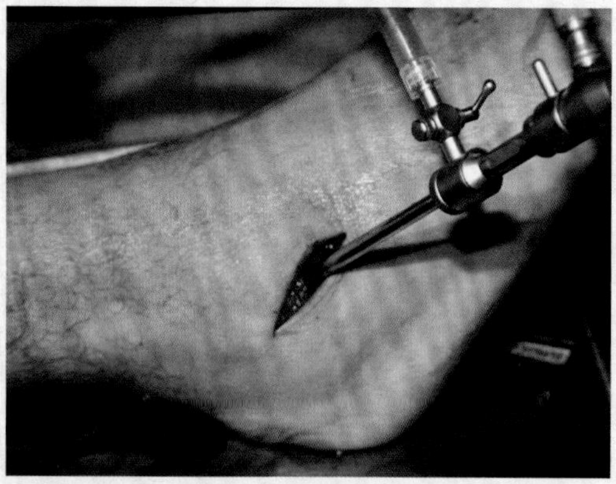

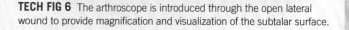

TECH FIG 6 The arthroscope is introduced through the open lateral wound to provide magnification and visualization of the subtalar surface.

lag screws are then inserted just beneath the articular surface of the posterior facet.

- The anterolateral fragment will now reduce anatomically to the posterior facet. It can be fixated with either a minifragment plate that bridges from the posterior facet to the anterolateral fragment, in essence crossing the crucial angle of Gissane or lag screws can be used. These screws can be placed from the anterolateral fragment to the superomedial fragment or from the posterior tuberosity into the anterior calcaneus.
- The lateral wall should be manually compressed at this point.
- Layered closure is performed.

SINUS TARSI APPROACH

- In an effort to decrease the risk of wound healing problems and subsequent infections, various surgeons have pursued open treatment and internal fixation of joint depression fractures through a minimal-incision technique using an incision centered over the sinus tarsi.
- This approach is ideally suited for Sanders II and IV fractures **(TECH FIG 7)**.
  - Some Sanders III fractures with an anteriorly located central fragment can also be treated.
  - Caution should be exercised when treating Sanders III fractures with a posteriorly located central fragment.

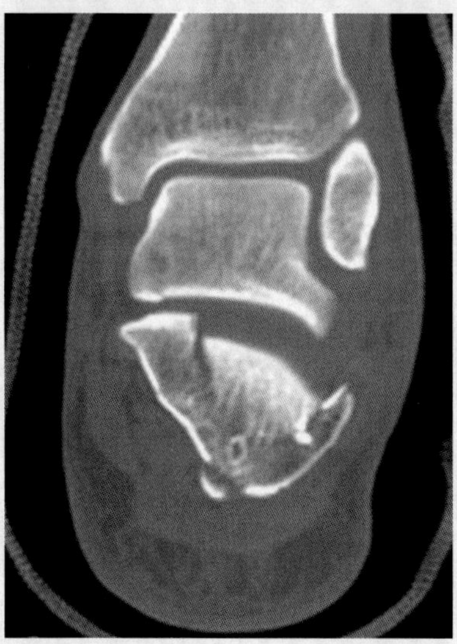

TECH FIG 7 Sanders II part joint depression fracture.

These fractures are extremely difficult to reduce from a sinus tarsi incision even with the assistance of an arthroscope and special instruments and implants.
    - In the end, a small incision with poor reduction does not lead to optimal results.
  - Open fractures are ideally treated with this more biologically friendly approach.
- Surgical timing is extremely important. Fractures should be treated prior to approximately 14 days, if the soft tissues will allow.
  - If swelling and blisters prevent surgery in this time frame, consideration should be given to proceeding with an extensile lateral exposure when the soft tissues are optimal.
- The patient is placed supine with the operative extremity elevated on a support. A thigh tourniquet is used.
- Regional blocks are useful for postoperative pain relief.

Preliminary Reduction

- In an effort to facilitate open treatment and internal fixation through a sinus tarsi approach, the posterior tuberosity must be reduced to the sustentacular fragment prior to attempting reduction of the posterior facet.
  - Multiple techniques can be used. These include manual distraction, reduction, and then internal fixation with temporary wires or a fully threaded noncompression screw from the posterior tuberosity into the sustentacular fragment.
  - The easiest and most reproducible maneuver to date has been application of a temporary, medially placed external fixator **(TECH FIG 8)**.
  - This is accomplished with a small pin to bar frame system and a universal clamp.

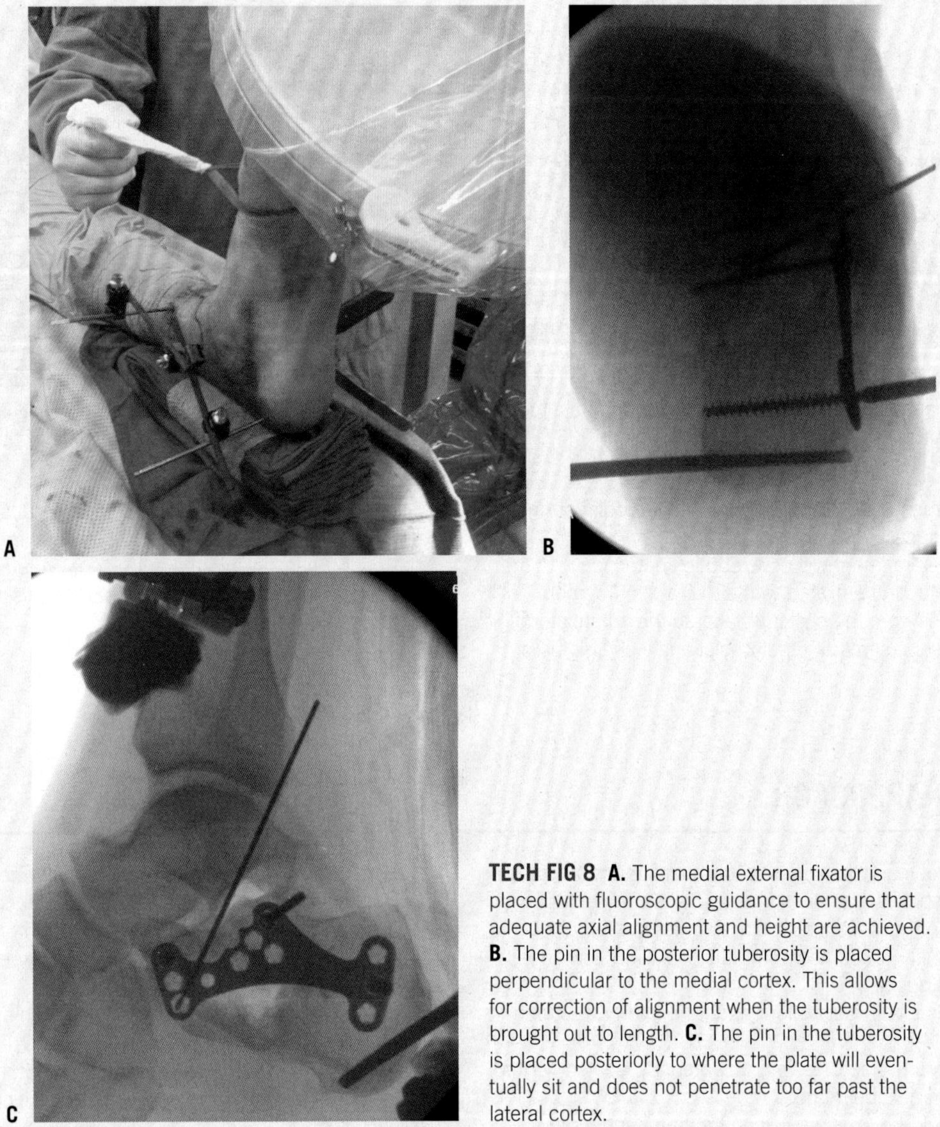

TECH FIG 8 **A.** The medial external fixator is placed with fluoroscopic guidance to ensure that adequate axial alignment and height are achieved. **B.** The pin in the posterior tuberosity is placed perpendicular to the medial cortex. This allows for correction of alignment when the tuberosity is brought out to length. **C.** The pin in the tuberosity is placed posteriorly to where the plate will eventually sit and does not penetrate too far past the lateral cortex.

- A 4-mm half-pin is placed in the tibial metadiaphyseal region (bicortical), taking care not to injure the saphenous vein and nerve. The pin is placed from medial to lateral.
- A second 4-mm half-pin is placed from medial to lateral in the posterior tuberosity under fluoroscopic guidance.
  - The pin must be placed posterior to all fracture lines.
  - The pin should be placed posterior to where the plate will sit.
- Each pin is connected to a bar, and then the bars are connected with a universal clamp.
- A closed reduction is performed, bringing the posterior tuberosity out of varus or valgus and back to the appropriate height. Translation is also corrected. With fluoroscopic imaging, adequate alignment is achieved.
  - The external fixator may need adjustment throughout the case to facilitate reduction.

Incision and Dissection

- Different sinus tarsi incisions have been described in the literature. We prefer a slightly longer incision. This allows for easier reduction and hardware placement with less tension on the skin. This ultimately leads to improved wound healing.
  - The incision starts 1 cm above the tip of the lateral malleolus and extends to 1 cm distal to the anterior process of the calcaneus. It is located just anterior to the peroneal tendon sheath **(TECH FIG 9A)**.
- After sharp dissection through the skin, bluntly dissect down, taking precautions not to injure any branches of the sural nerve. The extensor digitorum brevis is elevated anteriorly, and the joint capsule to the posterior facet is incised, exposing the displaced articular fragments and hematoma.
  - The lateral wall is exposed by elevating the peroneal tendons while attempting to keep them within their sheath **(TECH FIG 9B)**.
  - The calcaneofibular ligament is also elevated but left attached to the fibula.
  - Multiple small fragments of the wall will need to be gently teased away from the overlying soft tissues and either placed into a sterile container with saline or simply impacted back into the body.
    - The entire lateral wall does not need to be removed as in the extensile lateral approach, secondary to adequate visualization of the displaced posterior facet from the sinus tarsi.

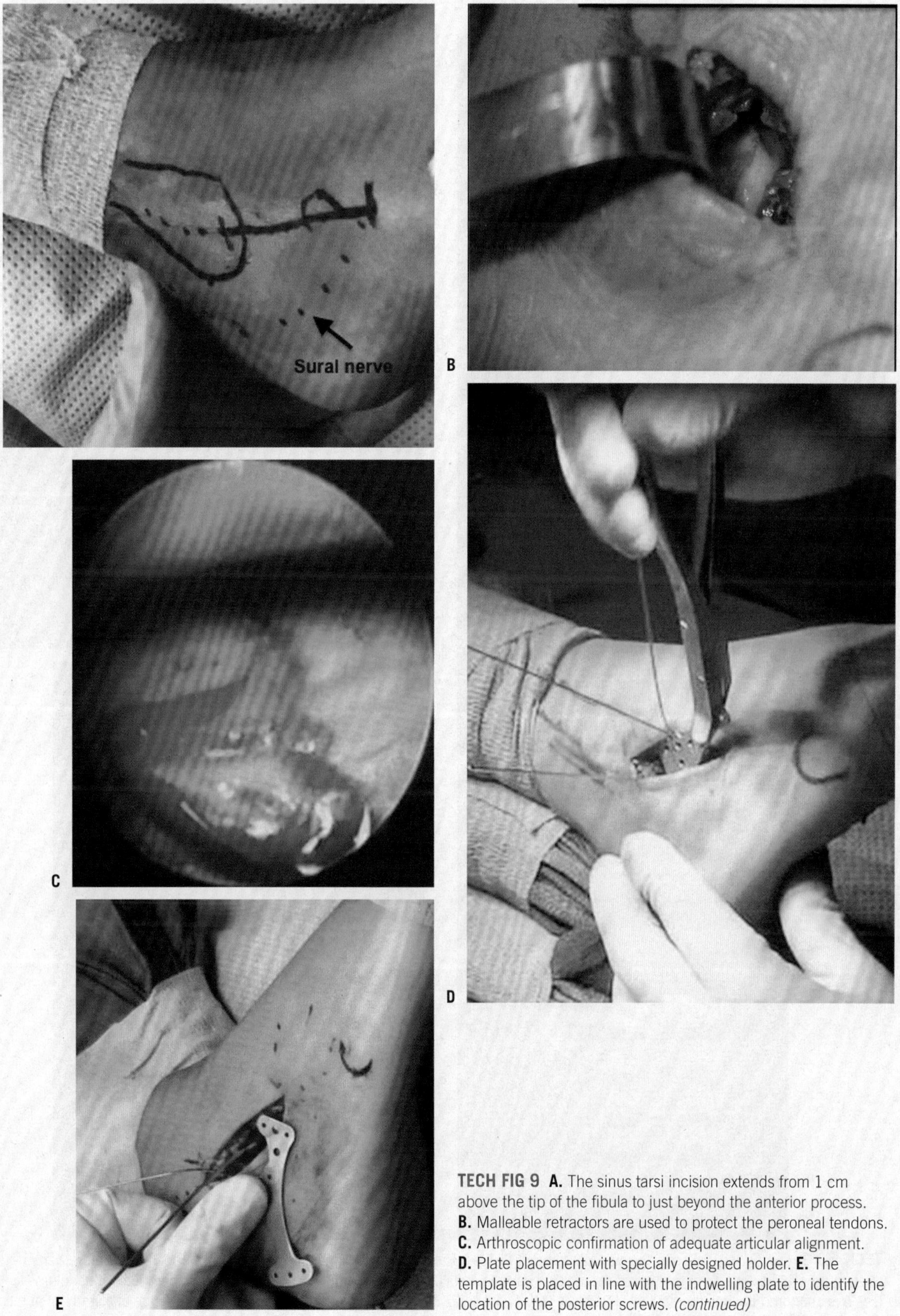

A B C D E

TECH FIG 9 **A.** The sinus tarsi incision extends from 1 cm above the tip of the fibula to just beyond the anterior process. **B.** Malleable retractors are used to protect the peroneal tendons. **C.** Arthroscopic confirmation of adequate articular alignment. **D.** Plate placement with specially designed holder. **E.** The template is placed in line with the indwelling plate to identify the location of the posterior screws. *(continued)*

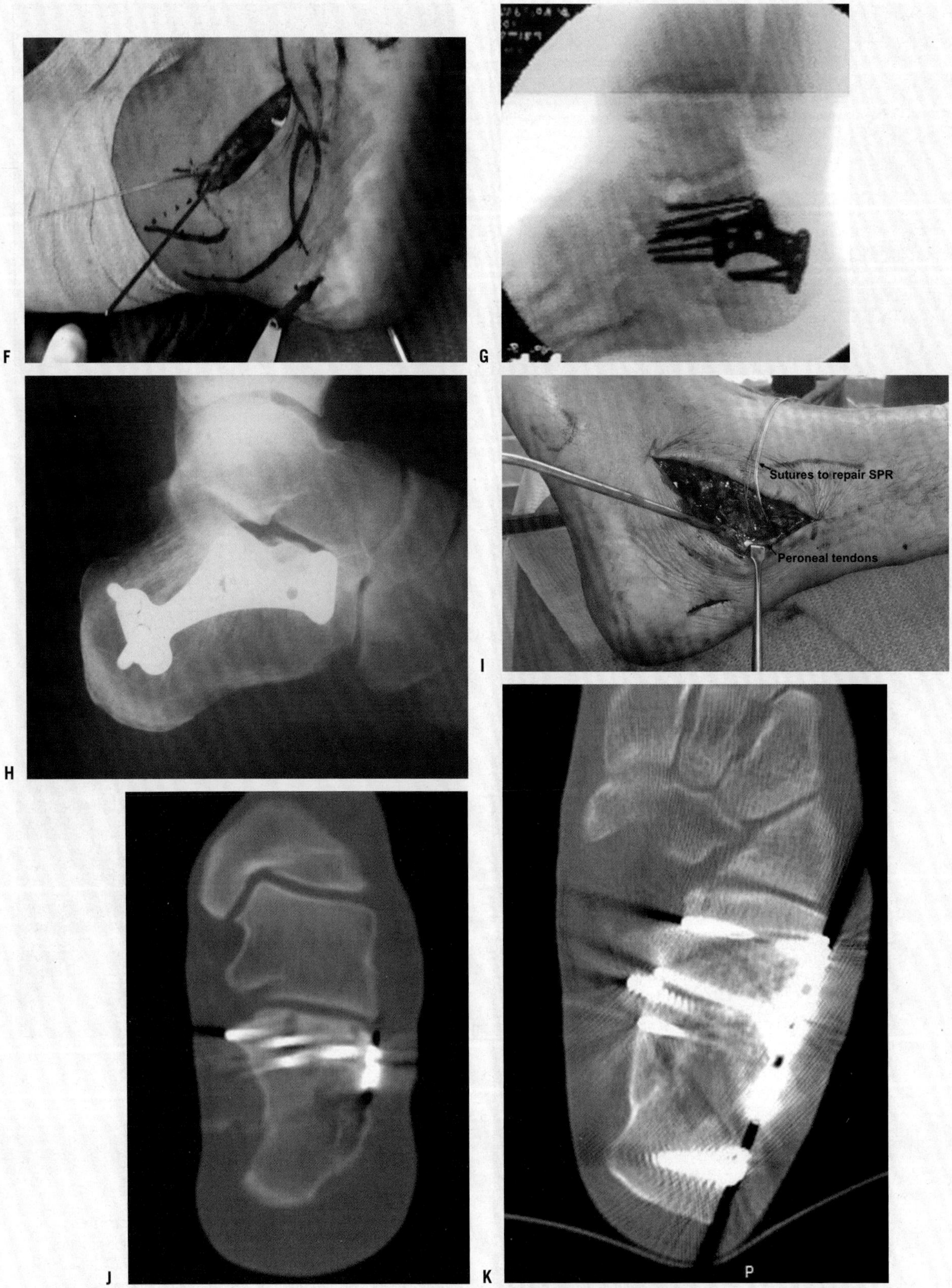

TECH FIG 9 *(continued)* **F.** Posterior screw placement. **G.** Final Broden view. **H.** Final lateral view. **I.** Intraoperative picture demonstrating proximal extension of the sinus tarsi incision used to stabilize the peroneal tendons. The superior peroneal retinaculum (*SPR*) is anchored back to the fibula with sutures. **J,K.** CT scan 2 years after surgery demonstrates maintenance of alignment at the articular surface and correction of varus.

- If a plate is going to be used, which will fixate all portions of the calcaneus, then a path must be created along the lateral aspect of the posterior tuberosity. This is performed with a broad blunt elevator.
- The anterior portion of the calcaneus is similarly exposed with either sharp dissection or blunt elevator dissection below the peroneal tendons.

Reduction and Fixation

- The posterior facet is reduced first. Any central fragments are reduced to the sustentacular (superomedial) fragment and stabilized with temporary wires.
- If reduction is adequate based on both fluoroscopy and arthroscopy, small absorbable pins are placed. The superolateral fragment is elevated out of the body, taking care not to damage the articular cartilage. It is reduced to the sustentacular fragment and stabilized with temporary wires.
- If adequate reduction is confirmed with both fluoroscopy and arthroscopy, small lag screws are placed perpendicular to the fracture line just below the articular surface **(TECH FIG 9C)**.
  - These can be 2- to 3-mm screws in most cases.
  - Care should be taken to position them so that they do not interfere with later plate placement.
- The goal is to place the screws into the good-quality bone of the sustentaculum. If good fixation is not available because of the small size of the sustentacular fragment, the screw angle must be changed. The further distal to the articular surface the starting point for the screw, the easier is the placement into the widest portion of the sustentaculum. The ideal starting point is approximately 10 to 15 mm distal to the articular surface. Be careful not to penetrate the medial articular surface. Once the posterior facet is reconstructed, the anterior calcaneus must be reduced and fixated to the posterior facet reestablishing the crucial angle of Gissane.
- The posterior tuberosity must then be definitively reduced and fixated to the remainder of the reconstructed calcaneus.
  - This can be accomplished with either multiple screws or a plate and screws. In simple terms, the three main portions of the calcaneus need to be brought together, and any manner of stable internal fixation is acceptable.
- A plate that connects all three segments is preferred. This eliminates multiple screw heads in the posterior tuberosity, which may be painful.
  - After determining plate size based on template placement under fluoroscopy, the final plate is placed through the incision while protecting and elevating the peroneal tendons. It is aligned into appropriate position, and the screws are placed **(TECH FIG 9D)**.
  - The first screw is placed into the anterior calcaneus just proximal to the calcaneocuboid joint. The anterior calcaneus is then reduced to the posterior facet, and screws are then placed to fixate the posterior facet. A second and, if necessary, third screw are then placed into the anterior portion of the calcaneal plate.
  - The same sized template or a second plate of similar size is then laid over the skin in line with the implanted plate **(TECH FIG 9E)**. This allows for determination of the location of the holes in the plate overlying the posterior tuberosity.
  - A small incision is made over the posterior plate. Even though these holes should be posterior to the sural nerve, care is taken during dissection and screw placement to avoid injury to any aberrant branches of the sural nerve **(TECH FIG 9F)**.
  - A final axial fluoroscopic image is obtained prior to screw placement, and if adequate alignment is noted, two or three screws are placed. If adequate alignment is not noted, the external fixator is adjusted prior to screw placement.
  - Nonlocking screws are usually sufficient, but in cases of comminution or poor bone quality, locking screws can be used.
  - Final imaging is performed to confirm adequate hardware placement and reduction **(TECH FIG 9G,H)**.
- If the peroneal tendons are unstable, the incision is extended in line with the distal fibula. The tendons are then reduced and stabilized by reconstructing the superior peroneal retinaculum. Groove deepening is rarely needed **(TECH FIG 9I)**.
- Bone grafting is usually not necessary.
- A layered closure is performed. A drain is not needed.
- A well-padded splint is placed holding the ankle in neutral.
- CT scan can be obtained postoperatively. This will help surgeons determine how well they executed their operative plan and help them fine-tune their skills **(TECH FIG 9J,K)**.

HIGHLY COMMINUTED SANDERS IV FRACTURES

- Special consideration must be given to these high-energy fractures. Open reduction and internal fixation alone lead to very poor results. For this reason, open reduction and internal fixation is combined with primary subtalar fusion **(TECH FIG 10A–D)**.
- Whether the reduction and fixation are performed through a sinus tarsi approach or an extensile lateral approach, the reduction of the body and the articular surfaces must be accomplished, as this is not an in situ fusion.
- The fusion is performed by removing cartilage from the opposing surfaces of the posterior and medial facets of the calcaneus and talus. The subchondral bone is then drilled, and cancellous bone graft is used to fill any voids. The fusion is then performed with two screws placed from the posterior tuberosity in to the talus.
- The screws can be cannulated or solid, fully threaded or partially threaded, and are placed to miss the hardware already in position.
  - Advocates of fully threaded screws site the benefit of avoiding compression and subsequent displacement.
  - Partially threaded screws can be used without the risk of leading to displacement by placing one locking screw in each of the three segments of the reconstructed calcaneus (anterior, posterior facet, and posterior tuberosity). This technique provides a stable calcaneus against, which the talus can be compressed **(TECH FIG 10E,F)**.

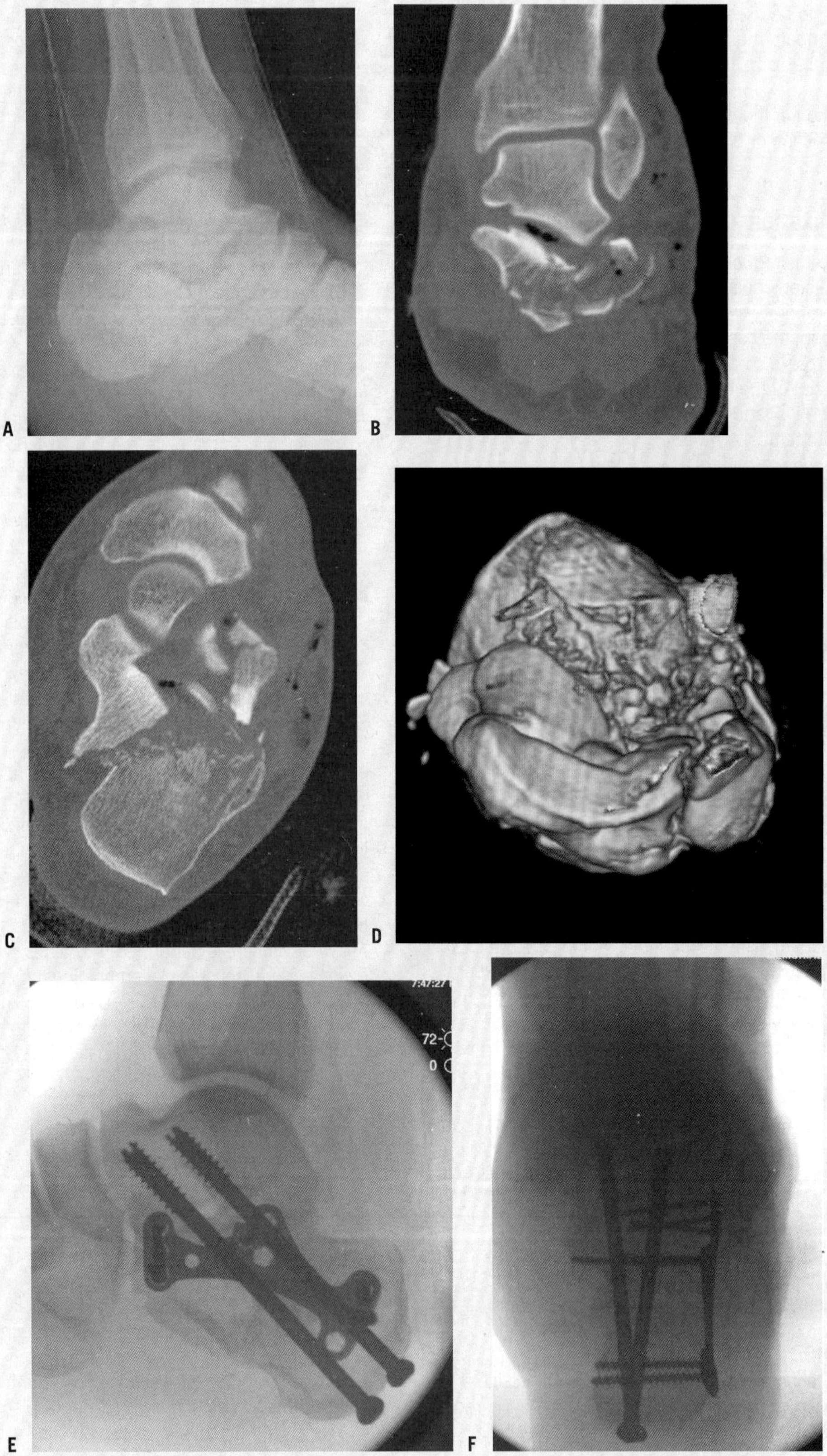

TECH FIG 10 A. X-ray showing a highly comminuted Sanders IV fracture. **B.** Coronal CT demonstrating Sanders IV fracture. **C.** Axial CT. **D.** Reconstructed CT showing severe destruction to posterior facet. **E.** Lateral fluoroscopy demonstrating open reduction and internal fixation and primary subtalar fusion. Partially threaded cannulated screws are used to compress the subtalar joint. A single locking screw in each of the three main portions of the calcaneus allows for compression without deforming the calcaneus. **F.** Axial fluoroscopy demonstrating adequate alignment.

Pearls and Pitfalls

Indications	• Less invasive approaches require an accurate definition of the pathoanatomy and then matching the pathoanatomy with an operative plan. Only surgeons with significant previous experience with the extensile lateral approach should attempt the sinus tarsi and other minimal-incision approaches for joint depression fractures. • Extensile approaches should be used cautiously with open fractures. • Temporary pin fixation may allow for improved soft tissue results for Sanders III/IV fracture patterns.
Fracture Reduction	• With open approaches, the order of reduction is the same: superomedial fragment to tuberosity, posterior facet to superomedial fragment, anterolateral fragment to posterior facet, lateral wall. • Exact posterior facet reduction is difficult to achieve but required to achieve excellent results. Adjuncts of fluoroscopy and arthroscopy help visualize the highly congruent subtalar joint. • In Sanders III fractures, the intermediate piece can be fixated to the superomedial fragment with small buried lag screws or absorbable pins, thus converting it to a Sanders II pattern.
Fracture Reduction	• Extra-long, minifragment screws are essential to allow matching of screw and fragment size, especially in the posterior facet. • The application of a straight plate to the lateral calcaneal surface will avoid varus of the heel, in combination with pin manipulation of the tuberosity out of varus. Simply pulling the tuberosity to the plate does not always correct the varus. • Indication-specific plates exist for the sinus tarsi approach and make reduction and stabilization more reproducible.
Complications	• Strict foot elevation and elimination of movement until adequate wound healing is recommended.
Postoperative Care	• Reliable patients without diabetes can safely perform touchdown range-of-motion exercises to assist in recovery of subtalar motion.

POSTOPERATIVE CARE

- A well-padded bivalved, short-leg cast or splint is applied.
- The patient is instructed to maintain strict elevation as much as possible until the sutures are removed.
- In reliable nondiabetic patients, the cast can be discontinued and range-of-motion exercises begun once the wound is ready.
  - With the sinus tarsi approach, motion can be started between 1 and 2 weeks if the wound is healing well.
- Touchdown weight bearing to promote ankle and subtalar motion can be started at the same time.
- Physical therapy is prescribed on an individualized basis.
- At 6 weeks, a radiograph is obtained and weight bearing progressed as pain allows. Full weight bearing is expected by 12 weeks postoperatively.

OUTCOMES

- Despite appropriate care, most patients with a calcaneal fracture will lose some degree of foot function and have permanent symptoms.
- Although nonoperative treatment yields the fewest iatrogenic complications, it accepts malunion in nearly 100% and a higher incidence of later subtalar fusion.
- Overall, minimal-incision techniques with a sinus tarsi approach have similar clinical and radiographic outcomes to open treatment and internal fixation with an extensile lateral approach. However, the minimal-incision techniques have a lower risk of wound healing problems and infections.
- Symptom improvement can take up to a year to plateau.
- In a recent randomized study, visual analog pain scores between nonoperative and operative groups were similar, but nonoperative treatment resulted in a 5.5 times greater incidence of late subtalar fusion.
  - In that same study, females, nonworkmen's compensation cases, and nonmanual laborers had improved results with operative treatment.
  - Better results were also seen with an anatomic reduction versus a nonanatomic one.
- Soft tissue complications frequently lead to a poor result.
- Although extremely rare, amputations have been reported with extensile lateral approaches.
- Open techniques should be used cautiously in diabetic patients, although injuries such as fracture-dislocation are best treated with operative reduction and fixation.
  - In high-risk patients, the minimal-incision techniques appear to have a lower risk of wound healing and infectious complications.

COMPLICATIONS

- Severe crush deformities affect not only the subtalar joint but the midfoot and ankle as well. They can be difficult to reconstruct, so initial management to avoid such a malunion is recommended.
- Smoking, diabetes, and open fracture are the most significant risk factors for soft tissue complications.
- Infection occurs in about 2% of fractures treated operatively.
- Deep infection is managed with débridement and intravenous antibiotics based on culture results.
  - Retention of hardware (if providing bone stability) until bone healing is optimal.
  - Removal of the hardware to eradicate the infection once the bone is healed is needed.
- Posterior tibial nerve injury can result from the fracture and commonly presents with severe pain nonresponsive to narcotics in the postinjury period.
  - Administration of medications aimed at neuropathic pain is recommended, and consultation with a pain specialist is considered.
- Cushioned shoe inserts are often comforting to individuals with postfracture plantar heel pain. A rocker-bottom shoe can also reduce discomfort.
  - Orthotics can be used in patients with symptomatic posttraumatic arthrosis.

- Late implant-related symptoms are rare with percutaneous or small-incision techniques. If necessary, symptoms often improve with implant removal. They are lessened by the use of low-profile perimeter plates with the extensile lateral approach.
- Painful, posttraumatic arthrosis is managed first with analgesics and orthotics. If conservative measures fail, a subtalar fusion can be performed.
- In cases involving injured workers, the vast majority, if not all workers, who have sustained an isolated, unilateral calcaneus fracture are capable of getting back to gainful employment. Certain restrictions such as ladder climbing and working at heights may be necessary.

SUGGESTED READINGS

Abidi N, Dhawan S, Gruen GS, et al. Wound-healing risk factors after open reduction and internal fixation of calcaneal fractures. Foot Ankle Int 1998;19:856–861.

Berberian W, Sood A, Karanfilian B, et al. Displacement of the sustentacular fragment in intra-articular calcaneal fractures. J Bone Joint Surg Am 2013;95:995–1000.

Buckley R, Tough S, McCormack R, et al. Operative compared with nonoperative treatment of displaced intra-articular calcaneal fractures: a prospective, randomized, controlled multicenter trial. J Bone Joint Surg Am 2002;84(10):1733–1744.

Burdeaux BD. Reduction of calcaneal fractures by the McReynolds medial approach technique and its experimental basis. Clin Orthop Relat Res 1983;(177):87–103.

Carr JB. Mechanism and pathoanatomy of the intraarticular calcaneal fracture. Clin Orthop Relat Res 1993;(290):36–40.

Ebraheim N, Elgafy H, Sabry F, et al. Sinus tarsi approach with transarticular fixation for displaced intra-articular fractures of the calcaneus. Foot Ankle Int 2000;21:105–113.

Femino JE, Vaseenon T, Levin DA, et al. Modification of the sinus tarsi approach for open reduction and plate fixation of intra-articular calcaneus fractures: the limits of proximal extension based upon the vascular anatomy of the lateral calcaneal artery. Iowa Orthop J 2010;30:161–167.

Fernandez D, Koella C. Combined percutaneous and "minimal" internal fixation for displaced articular fractures of the calcaneus. Clin Orthop Relat Res 1993;290:108–116.

Gupta A, Ghalambor N, Nihal A, et al. The modified Palmer lateral approach for calcaneal fractures: wound healing and postoperative computed tomographic evaluation of fracture reduction. Foot Ankle Int 2003;24:744–753.

Johnson EE, Gebhardt JS. Surgical management of calcaneal fractures using bilateral incisions and minimal internal fixation. Clin Orthop Relat Res 1993;(290):117–124.

Kline AJ, Anderson RB, Davis WH, et al. Minimally invasive technique versus an extensile lateral approach for intra-articular calcaneal fractures. Foot Ankle Int 2013;34:773–780.

Levine DS, Helfet DL. An introduction to the minimally invasive osteosynthesis of intra-articular calcaneal fractures. Injury 2001;(32 suppl 1): SA51–SA54.

McReynolds I. Trauma to the os calcis and heel cord. In: Jahss M, ed. Disorders of the Foot. Philadelphia: W.B. Saunders, 1982:1497–1542.

Phisitkul P, Sullivan JP, Goetz JE, et al. Maximizing safety in screw placement for posterior facet fixation in calcaneus fractures: a cadaveric radio-anatomical study. Foot Ankle Int 2013;34(9):1279–1285.

Radnay CS, Clare MP, Sanders RW. Subtalar fusion after displaced intra-articular calcaneal fractures: does initial operative treatment matter? Surgical technique. J Bone Joint Surg Am 2010;(92 suppl 1)(pt 1):32–43.

Rammelt S, Amlang M, Barthel S, et al. Minimally-invasive treatment of calcaneal fractures. Injury 2004;(35 suppl 2):SB55–SB63.

Rammelt S, Gavlik J, Barthel S, et al. The value of subtalar arthroscopy in the management of intra-articular calcaneus fractures. Foot Ankle Int 2002;23:906–916.

Sanders R, Fortin P, DiPasquale T, et al. Operative treatment in 120 displaced intraarticular calcaneal fractures. Results using a prognostic computed tomography scan classification. Clin Orthop Relat Res 1993;(290):87–95.

Schepers T. The sinus tarsi approach in displaced intra-articular calcaneal fractures: a systematic review. Int Orthop 2011;35(5):697–703.

Stephenson J. Surgical treatment of displaced intraarticular fractures of the calcaneus. A combined lateral and medial approach. Clin Orthop Relat Res 1993;(290):68–75.

Thordarson DB, Krieger LE. Operative vs. nonoperative treatment of intra-articular fractures of the calcaneus: a prospective randomized trial. Foot Ankle Int 1996;17:2–9.

Tornetta P III. Percutaneous treatment of calcaneal fractures. Clin Orthop Relat Res 2000;(375):91–96.

Tornetta P III. The Essex-Lopresti reduction for calcaneal fractures revisited. J Orthop Trauma 1998;12:469–473.

Zwipp H, Tscherne H, Therman H, et al. Osteosynthesis of displaced intraarticular fractures of the calcaneus. Results in 123 cases. Clin Orthop Relat Res 1993;(290):76–86.

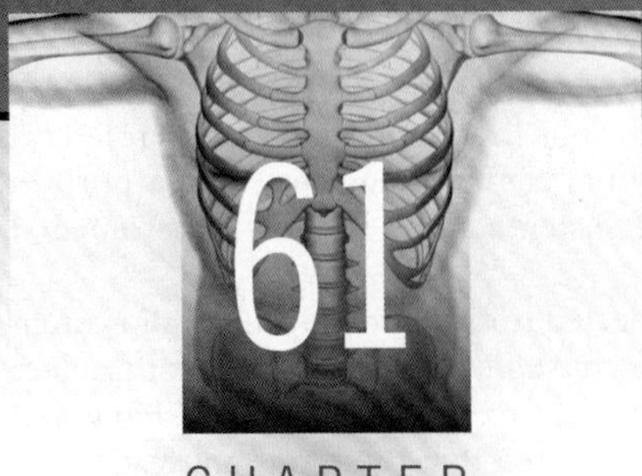

CHAPTER 61

Surgical Fixation of Calcaneal Fractures via the Sinus Tarsi Approach

Steven D. Steinlauf

DEFINITION

- An intra-articular calcaneus fracture is an injury that involves the joint surfaces of the calcaneus, usually with displacement.
- A fracture-dislocation of the calcaneus occurs when the superior lateral fragment of the posterior facet dislocates from beneath the talus to a position beneath the fibula or interposed between the fibula and the lateral talus. It carries a poor prognosis if treated nonoperatively. Therefore, all patients with this injury should be treated operatively, unless their medical condition precludes surgery.
- "Soft tissue" damage refers to the injury to the skin, adipose, tendinous, muscular, and nerve structures that surround the calcaneus and ranges from mild bruising to near-amputation in open fractures.
  - Fracture blisters and varying degrees of skin contusion occur most commonly.
  - "Wrinkle sign" refers to the skin wrinkles that appear when the injury swelling response is resolving.
- A primary fracture line is one that occurs early in the mechanism of the calcaneal fracture. There are two that occur, and, if their pathogenesis is understood, this can explain the majority of the pathology observed. This will be defined further in the Pathogenesis section.
  - Minimal-incision surgery refers to all surgical approaches other than the extensile lateral approach.
  - Anterior process fractures are injuries involving only the anterior portion of the calcaneus. When nondisplaced, they can be treated nonoperatively. Displaced fragments usually require surgery.
  - A fibular rim fracture represents an avulsion of the superior peroneal retinaculum and is indicative of peroneal tendon instability.

ANATOMY

- The calcaneus is the largest bone in the foot. It has a complex shape that makes exact surgical reconstruction difficult.
- The calcaneus functions to transmit weight-bearing forces of the leg into the foot.
- The articular facets of the calcaneus combined with the corresponding facets on the talus form the subtalar joint. This joint along with the calcaneocuboid joint has a shock absorber function, thus allowing the foot to accommodate to variations in terrain.
- The four articular facets of the calcaneus include posterior, anterior, middle, and cuboid. Exact articular alignment is required for full function of this four-joint complex.
- The internal structure of the calcaneus reflects its weight-bearing role.
  - There is particularly dense trabecular bone in the juxta-articular regions, especially below the posterior facet (the thalamic trabecular system).
  - The tendo Achilles insertion also has dense trabecular bone.
  - There exists a normal area of relatively little trabecular bone directly below the angle of Gissane called the *neutral triangle*. For this reason, filling this area with bone graft after fixation of a calcaneus fracture is rarely necessary.
- Cortical bone of 3 to 4 mm in thickness occurs in the superomedial region (sustentaculum area) and in the superolateral strut of bone that runs between the cuboid and posterior facets (anterolateral fragment). These regions of cortical bone will come into play when discussing the internal fixation of the calcaneus **(FIG 1)**.
- The soft tissues of the calcaneus are easily damaged by trauma. This is especially true in the case of displaced tongue and tuberosity fractures, which can lead to pressure necrosis of the posterior soft tissue. Management of this injury component is essential to avoid iatrogenic surgical complications. The peroneal tendons traverse the retrofibular groove and are located on the lateral aspect of the calcaneus.
- The sural nerve and its branches course along the lateral calcaneus and can be injured during any lateral exposure of the calcaneus. These branches include the lateral calcaneal nerves and a branch that connects the main sural nerve to

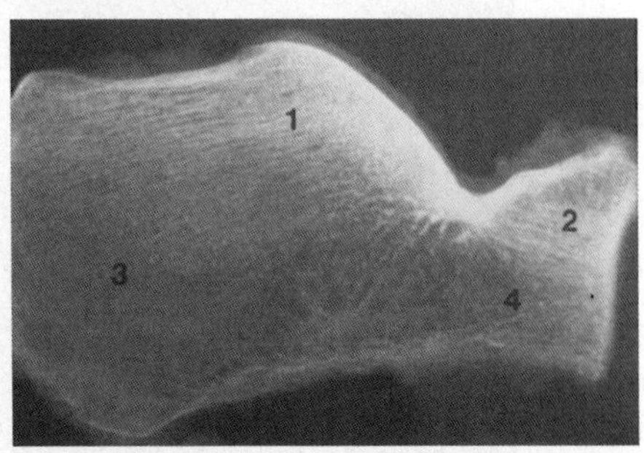

FIG 1 A lateral radiograph of a calcaneus specimen sectioned in the sagittal plane. The trabecular systems are visualized and numbered *1* to *4*. The densest bone is in the juxta-articular regions. Thick cortical bone also is present in the anterolateral fragment and medial wall in the sustentacular region. *1*, thalamic trabecular system; *2*, anterior apophyseal trabecular system; *3*, posterior plantar trabecular system; *4*, anterior plantar trabecular system. These regions provide optimal bone for internal fixation.

the superficial peroneal nerve at the level of the sinus tarsi. Thus, the smaller incisions used in the sinus tarsi approach must be performed with meticulous attention to detail.

- The blood supply to the lateral soft tissues of the calcaneus includes the lateral calcaneal artery, the lateral malleolar artery, and the lateral tarsal artery.
  - In both the extensile lateral exposure and the sinus tarsi approach, the lateral calcaneal artery is at risk for injury.

PATHOGENESIS

- Despite the seemingly infinite varieties of fractures that occur, stereotypic fracture lines, fragments, and displacements can be recognized.
- The calcaneus is fractured by a combination of shear and compression forces generated by the talus descending on the calcaneus.
- Two primary fracture lines occur.
  - The first occurs in the angle of Gissane and divides the calcaneus into anterior and posterior fragments. It can split either the middle or anterior facet, and the fracture continues on the lateral wall in an inverted Y shape **(FIG 2)**.
  - The second fracture divides the calcaneus into medial and lateral halves and shears the posterior facet into two or more fragments.
    - As the talus continues to compress the calcaneus, the lateral half of the posterior facet is impacted into the body of the calcaneus, with the recoil producing a step-off in the posterior facet.
    - This same fracture line commonly continues into the cuboid facet and, in combination with the first primary fracture line, produces the anterolateral and superomedial fragment.
    - In this way, these two fracture lines produce fracture components that include the superomedial fragment, anterolateral fragment, posterior facet, and tuberosity.
  - The posterior facet is fractured into a superolateral fragment, occasional central fragments, and a portion connected to the sustentaculum tali (the superomedial fragment).
  - The portion connected to the sustentaculum tali is often referred to as the *constant fragment* because of the fact that it is rarely displaced to a significant extent. However, a study has demonstrated that the "constant fragment" frequently has some displacement and fracture lines. This must be taken into consideration when planning fixation.
- Characteristic displacements of these components occur.
  - The tuberosity is driven up between the pieces of the posterior facet, can tilt into valgus or varus, and is usually translated laterally. The tuberosity acts as a wedge that prevents reduction of the posterior facet **(FIG 3A)**. (This wedge must be pulled distally to allow for accurate reduction of the posterior facet.)
  - The lateral posterior facet fragments are impacted and rotated plantarly into the body of the calcaneus **(FIG 3B)**.
  - The posterior facet breaks into one of three patterns, which form the basis of the Sanders classification:
    - Sanders type II: two main pieces **(FIG 3C)**
    - Sanders type III: three main pieces **(FIG 3D)**
    - Sanders type IV: multifragmentary
  - The superomedial fragment retains alignment to the talus by means of its ligamentous attachments but can be subtly displaced by overlap with the anterior portion of the calcaneus. This overlap occurs along the primary fracture line that occurs in the sinus tarsi.
  - The anterolateral fragment displaces superiorly a variable amount. It typically extends into the cuboid facet, with varying degrees of displacement **(FIG 3E)**.
- The lateral calcaneal wall is displaced outward in the area of the trochlear tubercle. This, in combination with tuberosity translation, accounts for the heel widening and peroneal impingement that occur.

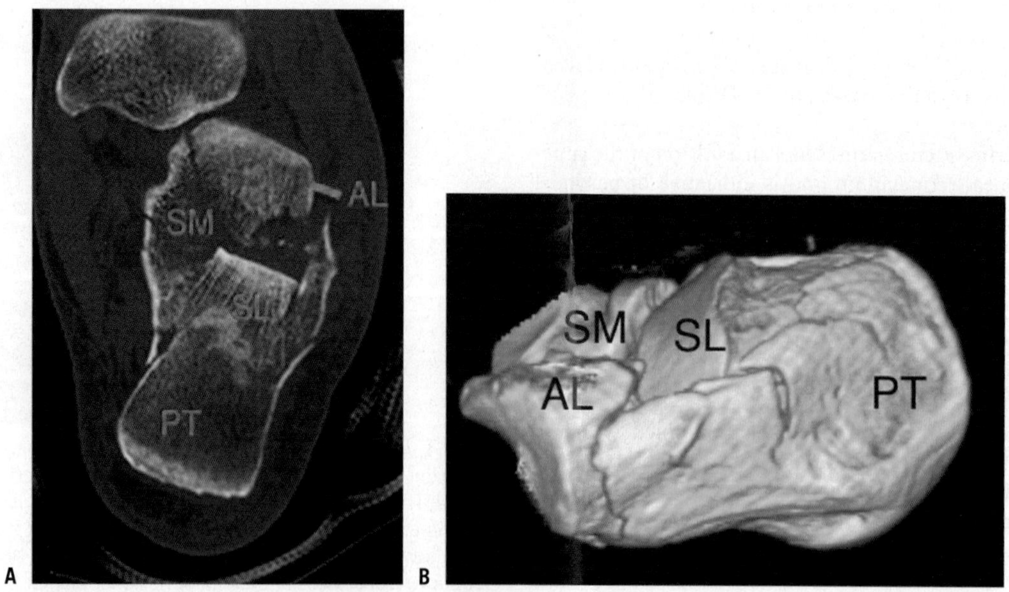

FIG 2 A,B. CT scans showing pattern of joint depression calcaneal fractures and main fragments. *SM*, superomedial fragment; *AL*, anterolateral fragment; *SL*, superolateral fragment; *PT*, posterior tuberosity.

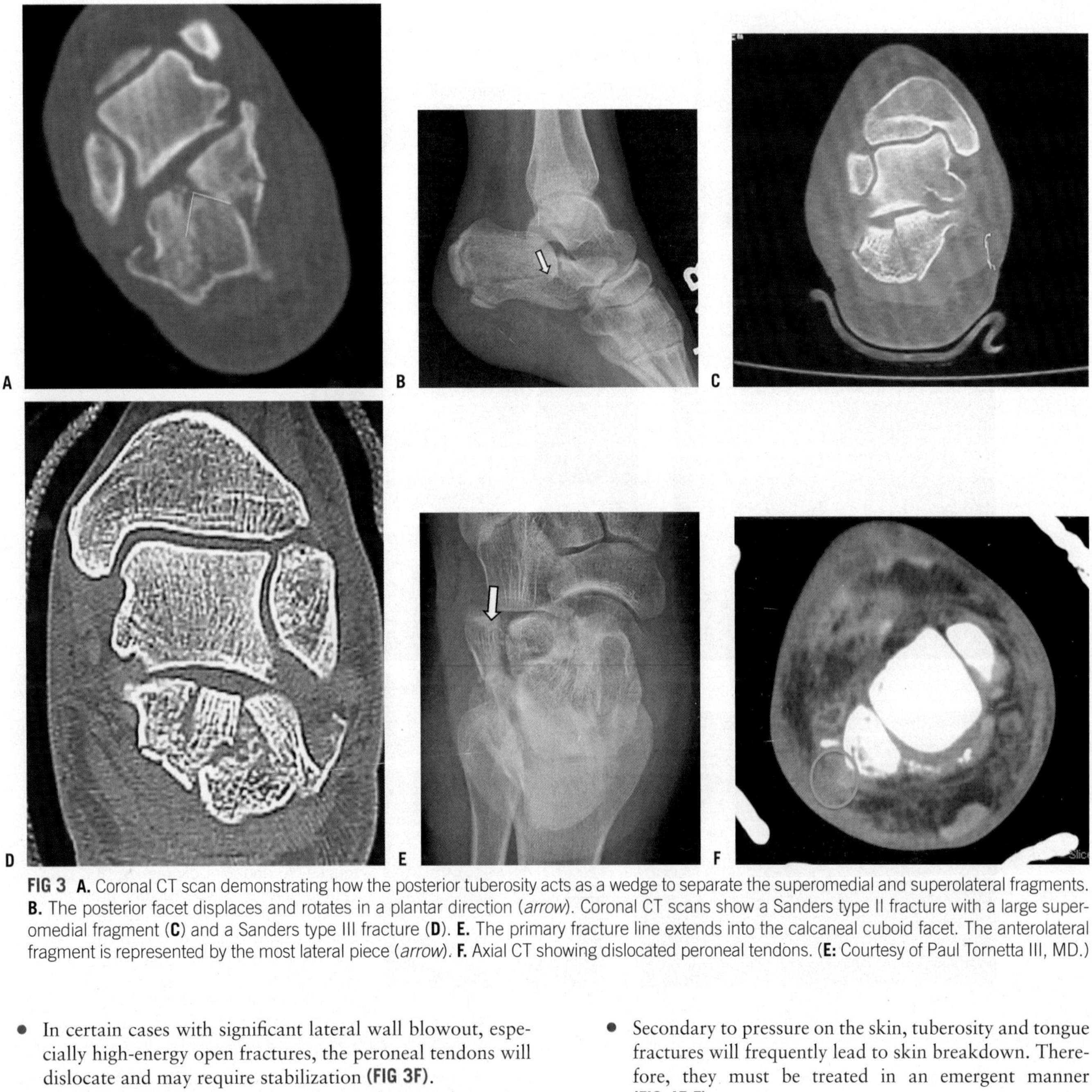

FIG 3 **A.** Coronal CT scan demonstrating how the posterior tuberosity acts as a wedge to separate the superomedial and superolateral fragments. **B.** The posterior facet displaces and rotates in a plantar direction (*arrow*). Coronal CT scans show a Sanders type II fracture with a large superomedial fragment (**C**) and a Sanders type III fracture (**D**). **E.** The primary fracture line extends into the calcaneal cuboid facet. The anterolateral fragment is represented by the most lateral piece (*arrow*). **F.** Axial CT showing dislocated peroneal tendons. (**E:** Courtesy of Paul Tornetta III, MD.)

- In certain cases with significant lateral wall blowout, especially high-energy open fractures, the peroneal tendons will dislocate and may require stabilization (**FIG 3F**).
- The first fracture types recognized were the joint depression and tongue-type patterns, which are readily identified on a lateral heel radiograph.
  - The tongue fracture maintains a connection between the tuberosity and the posterior facet, whereas the joint depression separates the fractured joint surface from the tuberosity (**FIG 4A,B**).
  - Because of this anatomy, certain tongue fractures have a large portion, or even the entire posterior facet, in continuity with the tuberosity (AO Orthopaedic Trauma Association 73 C1). Thus, reduction of the tuberosity will reduce indirectly the posterior facet and restore the angle of Böhler. This particular pattern is well suited for small incision or percutaneous techniques (**FIG 4C,D**).
  - Tuberosity fractures involve the insertion of the Achilles tendon. They do not involve the posterior facet.
- Secondary to pressure on the skin, tuberosity and tongue fractures will frequently lead to skin breakdown. Therefore, they must be treated in an emergent manner (**FIG 4E,F**).
- Reduction of a joint depression pattern is best performed with an open reduction.

NATURAL HISTORY

- An intra-articular fracture of the calcaneus is a serious injury that will diminish foot function.
- Nonoperative treatment is with early motion and delayed weight bearing 6 to 8 weeks after injury. This method has the least chance of iatrogenic injury.
- In a classic review by Lindsay and Dewar, only 17% of patients had no foot symptoms with long-term follow-up.
- The loss of ability to perform manual labor is common, with an average time off work of 4 to 6 months for laborers.

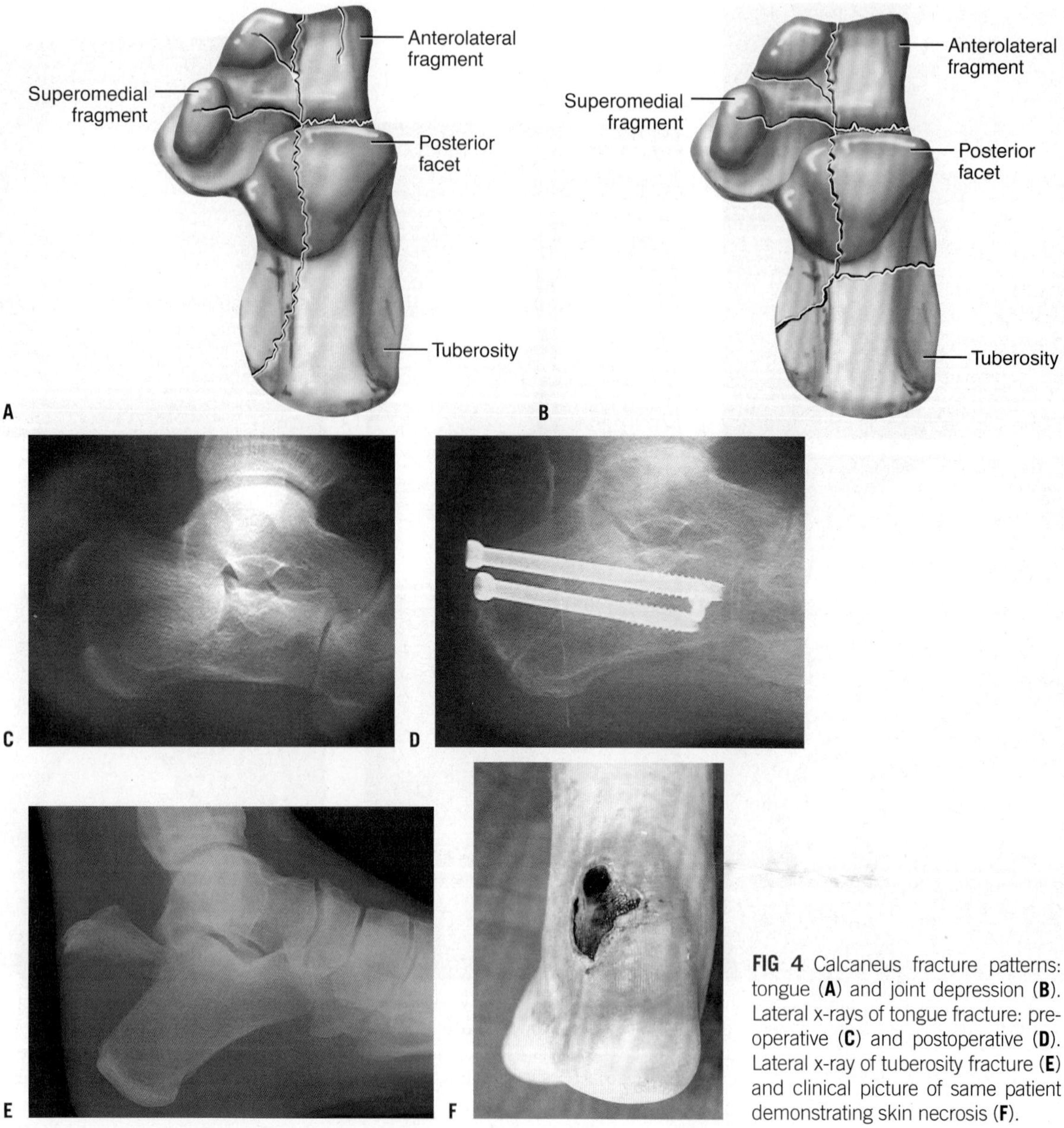

FIG 4 Calcaneus fracture patterns: tongue (**A**) and joint depression (**B**). Lateral x-rays of tongue fracture: preoperative (**C**) and postoperative (**D**). Lateral x-ray of tuberosity fracture (**E**) and clinical picture of same patient demonstrating skin necrosis (**F**).

- Loss of subtalar motion to varying extents will occur.
- Tibiotalar impingement and anterior ankle pain can be produced if the crush deformity is severe enough, leading to settling of the talus into the body of the calcaneus.
- It can take 18 to 24 months for the foot symptoms to maximally improve after this injury. Most improvement occurs in the first 12 months.
- The key concept here is that patients who continue to improve symptomatically can be observed until maximum improvement occurs.
- A randomized, prospective study found that the need for late subtalar arthrodesis is five to six times greater if nonoperative treatment is used on all injuries. The overall rate was approximately 17%.
  - If a subtalar fusion is used to treat posttraumatic arthrosis after a calcaneus fracture that was treated without surgery and allowed to go on to a malunion, the outcome is not as favorable as a subtalar fusion performed after a previous open treatment and internal fixation of the calcaneal fracture.

PATIENT HISTORY AND PHYSICAL FINDINGS

- The history is typically one of a fall or vehicle crash. However, calcaneal fractures can occur and are frequently misdiagnosed after minor trauma in older osteoporotic patients and in diabetics with neuropathy.
  - Important risk factors for operative treatment complications include smoking, diabetes, peripheral vascular disease, and steroid use.
  - The foot and ankle are visually inspected.
  - Swelling is graded as mild, moderate, or severe.
    - Operative treatment in the face of severe soft tissue swelling is prone to wound healing complications.

- Fracture blisters are graded as fluid-filled or blood-filled. If unhealed, fracture blisters are a source of skin bacterial colonization. Blood-filled blisters denote a deeper dermal injury.
- Skin contusion is noted.
- If present, the wrinkle sign is noted. It means the swelling is resolving and surgical incisions are less likely to experience complications.
- Open wounds are noted and, if present, represent a surgical emergency.

- The physician palpates the foot and ankle, looks for spine injuries or ipsilateral fractures, and performs a secondary survey for other injuries.
  - Spine injuries are said to accompany up to 10% of all calcaneal fractures.
- The physician assesses for compartment syndrome. Look for pain with passive flexion and extension of the toes, significant foot swelling, and elevated compartment pressure measurements (pressures within 30 mm Hg of diastolic pressure).
  - Compartment syndrome can occur in 5% to 10% of all calcaneal fractures.
- The physician performs a neurologic examination to check the sensory function of the foot and toes, including light touch and pinprick.
  - Calcaneal fractures, especially fractures with open wounds medially, can damage the posterior tibial nerve and vessels.
- Open fractures are assessed. These require irrigation and débridement. They will often require early plastic surgical intervention and may require free flap coverage. Early intervention may decrease the risk of infection.

IMAGING AND OTHER DIAGNOSTIC STUDIES

- Anteroposterior (AP) and lateral **(FIG 5A,B)** foot radiographs are the initial screening study.
  - The axial (Harris) view should also be obtained **(FIG 5C)**. This view will demonstrate the medial wall and show the relation of the superomedial fragment to the tuberosity.
  - Broden views are radiographs that focus on the subtalar joint. They are taken with the foot internally rotated and the x-ray beam angled to varying degrees cephalad **(FIG 5D,E)**. By using different degrees of cephalad angulation, different parts of the posterior facet may be

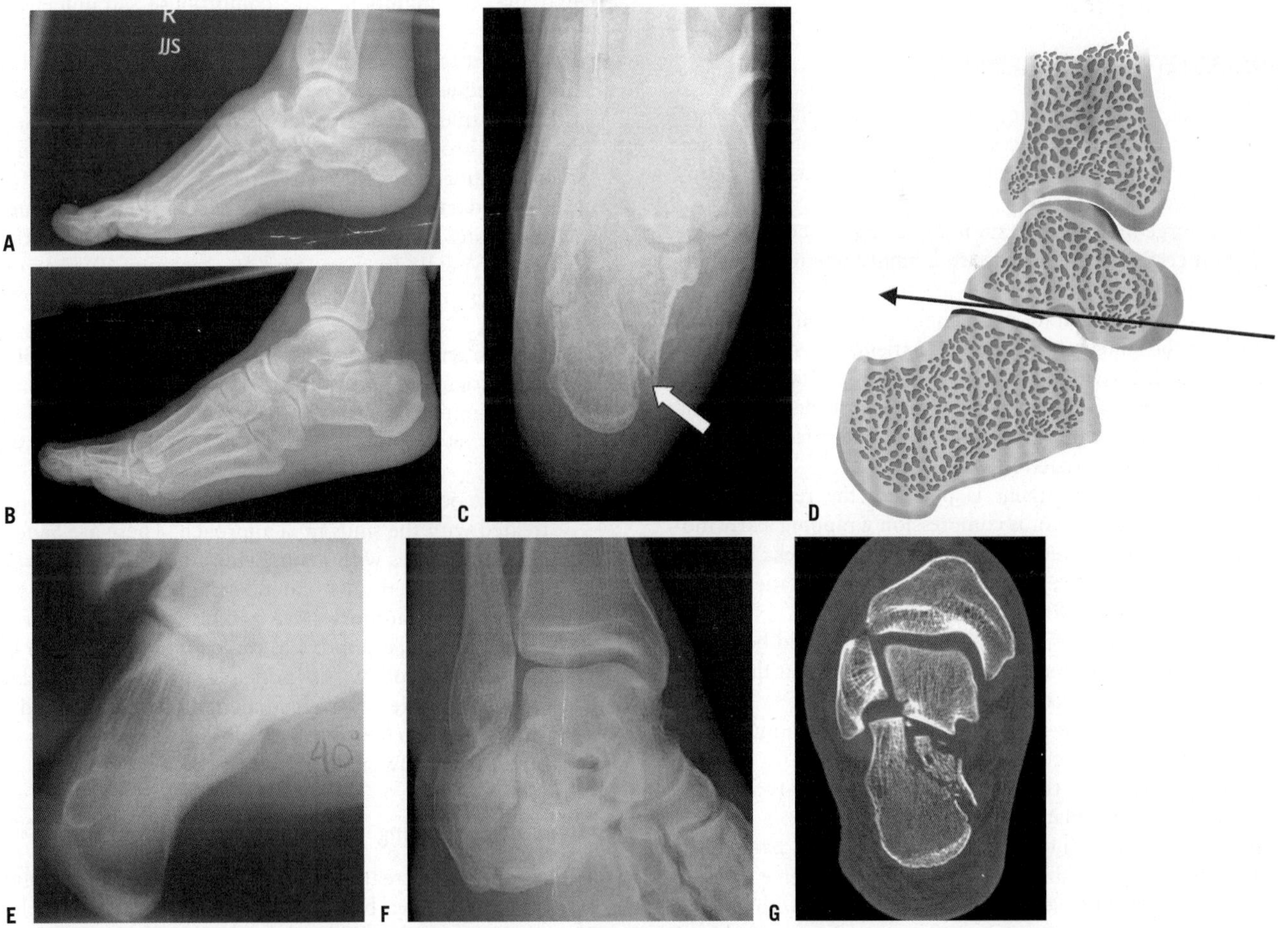

FIG 5 Lateral radiographs showing a severely displaced tongue-type Sanders type II fracture of the calcaneus with midfoot dislocation (**A**) and a Sanders type III fracture (**B**). **C.** The axial Harris view demonstrates displacement of the medial wall (*arrow*). Reduction of this pathoanatomy is the basis for the medial approach. **D.** Broden views are obtained by centering the x-ray beam on the posterior facet, internally rotating the foot, and directing the beam cephalad (*red arrow*). **E.** As the beam is aimed cephalad, more anterior portions of the posterior facet are visualized. Also, note the medial wall on profile. As the x-ray is tilted more, the view becomes a true Harris axial view (if the internal rotation is removed). **F.** Ankle mortise showing a fracture-dislocation. **G.** Coronal CT scan of the same patient with a fracture-dislocation.

imaged. They are best used intraoperatively to judge the reduction of the posterior facet and the medial wall of the calcaneus.
- Three views of the ankle are also helpful. The AP and mortise views can demonstrate fibular rim fractures (indicative of peroneal instability) and fracture-dislocations (superolateral fragment may be displaced into the lateral gutter) (**FIG 5F,G**).
- A computed tomography (CT) scan is ordered for all patients.
- If the fracture is displaced, a CT scan is needed to define the anatomy and plan surgery (see **FIG 3A,C,D,F**).
  - A CT scan with sagittal and coronal reconstructions is needed. This will best delineate the fragments and displacements.

DIFFERENTIAL DIAGNOSIS

- Lateral process of talus fracture
- Severe ankle sprain
  - In patients involved in low-energy trauma, calcaneal fractures can be missed by the emergency room physician. The treating doctor must look for a double-density sign (depressed superolateral fragment) (see **FIG 3B**) and flattening of Böhler angle.
- Subtalar dislocation

NONOPERATIVE MANAGEMENT

- The indications for nonoperative treatment include posterior facet displacement less than 2 mm and medical conditions such as severe peripheral vascular disease or poorly controlled diabetes.
- Some surgeons consider smoking a relative contraindication; it certainly predisposes to a higher wound complication rate.
- With the implementation of minimal-incision techniques, such as the sinus tarsi approach, patients considered to be at high risk for wound healing problems and infection can be offered surgery. Extensive literature exists demonstrating a lower risk of wound complications and infections when the sinus tarsi approach is used.
- If nonoperative treatment is pursued, the recommended nonoperative treatment is compression wrapping, early motion, and delayed weight bearing at 6 to 8 weeks after injury. This offers the least iatrogenic risk to the patient while optimizing chances for subtalar motion.
- During the first 2 to 3 weeks, the patient should be placed into a CAM boot or splint at all times to prevent the development of an equinus contracture.
- Once weight bearing is started, the patient continues with range-of-motion exercises.
  - Strengthening of the foot and ankle muscles is added as fracture consolidation progresses.
- A well-cushioned shoe usually offers the best pain relief. Two different shoe sizes may be needed in extreme cases.
  - A rocker bottom sole can be added to assist with the toe-off stance phase of gait.
- If posttraumatic arthrosis develops, various orthotics can be used in an attempt to relieve symptoms.
- Nonoperative treatment is not recommended for calcaneal fracture-dislocations, as a painful deformed foot is practically guaranteed if it is left unreduced.

SURGICAL MANAGEMENT

- The displaced intra-articular calcaneal fracture presents a difficult challenge.
- Foot pain and stiffness are common even with the best of treatment, and iatrogenic problems such as infection can result in loss of limb in extreme circumstances and, at the least, predispose to a poor result.
- Thus, a careful, individualized approach is recommended, with a priority on avoiding iatrogenic problems while attaining an anatomic alignment of the calcaneus.
- Indications include displacement of the posterior facet of more than 2 mm and calcaneus fracture-dislocation.
  - Research shows that certain patient groups, such as those receiving worker's compensation, are predisposed to a poor result with operative treatment but that does not obviate the benefits of obtaining anatomic foot alignment and lessening the chances of late subtalar fusion.
  - In addition, not all patients receiving worker's compensation do poorly, and some do return to gainful employment, although with restrictions in some settings.
- The choice of any surgical approach or technique should always have the goal of total anatomic restoration, although extreme comminution can compromise attainment of this goal.
- In an effort to decrease the risk of wound healing problems and subsequent infections, various surgeons have pursued open treatment and internal fixation of joint depression fractures through a minimal-incision technique using an incision centered over the sinus tarsi.
- This approach is ideally suited for Sanders type II fractures. With greater experience, surgeons can also treat certain Sanders type III fractures and Sanders type IV fractures undergoing fixation and primary subtalar fusion with this approach.
  - Open fractures are ideally treated with this more biologically friendly approach.
- Surgical timing is extremely important. Fractures should be treated prior to approximately 14 days, if the soft tissues will allow.
  - On rare occasions, a fracture as old as 3.5 weeks can be treated with the sinus tarsi approach. These are Sanders type II fractures with maintenance of height and a moderately displaced superolateral fragment.
- Although some authors have recently advocated for an extensile sinus tarsi approach, the chapter authors do not believe that this follows the principles of being biologically friendly. Therefore, it is recommended to use a standard sinus tarsi approach or the extensile lateral approach as discussed in the following text.

Preoperative Planning

- Once operative treatment has been elected, the surgical approach is chosen based on a number of factors, including the surgeon's training and experience and the pathoanatomy present.
- The timing of surgery differs between minimal-incision techniques and the extensile lateral approach. The timing is in general when the wrinkle sign develops and the soft tissue envelope is optimal.

- When using a sinus tarsi or similar minimal-incision approach, surgery should be performed in most cases before 2 weeks. If the soft tissue envelope is not ready in that time frame, then an extensile lateral approach should be used once the soft tissues are optimal.
- The extensile lateral approach can be performed up to 4 weeks after injury if necessary.
- The injury pathoanatomy is analyzed first by looking at the posterior facet pattern (Sanders type II, III, or IV), displacement, and location of the primary fracture line in the posterior facet.
  - Fractures that are more medial are more difficult to visualize, and more fragments involving the posterior facet are more difficult to fixate anatomically.
  - Fractures that separate the entire posterior facet and have a tongue pattern are amenable to percutaneous Essex-Lopresti techniques.
  - Conversely, joint depression fractures require open reduction of the posterior facet.
  - A highly comminuted Sanders type IV fracture should be treated with open reduction and primary fusion through a sinus tarsi or extensile lateral exposure.
- The other fracture components to be analyzed for displacement are the superomedial fragment, anterolateral fragment, and tuberosity. The surgical plan should address each of these pathologies for reduction strategy and fixation.
- When performing open reduction and internal fixation through a sinus tarsi approach, the posterior tuberosity must be distracted distally. During the preoperative planning, the method to achieve this must be determined so that appropriate equipment is available.
  - Distraction can be performed with a temporary external fixator placed medially or with various other distraction techniques involving a pin in the posterior tuberosity combined with a T-handle chuck or traction bow.
- In planning the sinus tarsi approach, it should be noted that there are multiple variations of this approach. General concepts need to be followed during the surgical approach:
  - Dissect carefully to avoid a communicating nerve branch between the sural and superficial peroneal nerves **(FIG 6)**
  - Carefully elevate the peroneal tendons laterally attempting to keep them in their sheath. This decreases scarring and pain.

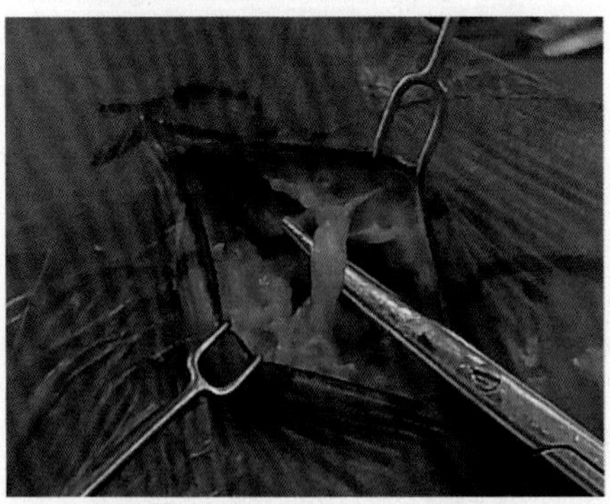

FIG 6 The connecting nerve branch between the sural nerve and the superficial peroneal nerve is commonly present in the region of the sinus tarsi incision, and efforts should be made to avoid damaging it.

- In planning the fixation technique and implants to be used, multiple factors contribute to the decision.
  - The size and integrity of the superomedial fragment is critical, as fixation techniques largely center on screw placement into its substance. A small or comminuted superomedial fragment makes rigid fixation harder to achieve and may call for alternative techniques.
  - A significantly displaced superomedial fragment may require a separate medial incision to assist with reduction and fixation.
  - Restoration of the superomedial fragment to the tuberosity will restore the calcaneal shape and make room for reduction of the displaced posterior facet fragments.
  - The superomedial fragment may be incarcerated in the sinus tarsi and subtly subluxated. This is recognized by the preoperative CT scan on the sagittal reconstructions and by the lack of congruence of the superomedial fragment with the undersurface of the talus.
    - Failure to correct this subluxation makes posterior facet reduction very difficult.
  - The anterolateral fragment should key into location just in front of the reduced posterior facet and restores lateral column length. This is assessed by assuring reconstruction of the hard cortical bone that represents the crucial angle of Gissane.
  - It can be fixed with either lag screws into the superomedial fragment or a plate.
  - Fractures splitting the posterior facet will require lag screws inserted from lateral to medial; they range in size from 2 to 4 mm, depending on the fractures present.
  - Sanders type III fractures are converted into two major pieces with the use of countersunk minifragment screws or bioabsorbable pins that fix the intermediate piece to the more medial or lateral piece.
  - The final internal fixation construct must secure the anterior calcaneus to the posterior facet/sustentacular portion and then to the posterior tuberosity.
  - This is accomplished with fracture-specific plates or multiple screws and minifragment plates.
- Plans must be made for imaging, most typically, fluoroscopy. This will allow control of the AP, lateral, axial, and Broden views intraoperatively.
  - Dry arthroscopy can also help visualize the posterior facet. It allows for more accurate reduction in fractures managed with either the extensile lateral or minimal-incision approaches.
    - Correlation between fluoroscopy and arthroscopy is critical to ensure accurate reduction.

Positioning

- The sinus tarsi approach can be performed supine with a bump under the ipsilateral hip or with the patient in the lateral decubitus position. The supine approach is easier **(FIG 7A)**. A thigh tourniquet is placed.
  - The injured leg is elevated on a stable base of sheets or foam. This allows for easier lateral imaging with fluoroscopy and easier medial external fixator placement, which may be used to assist with reduction. A radiolucent foot board is used.

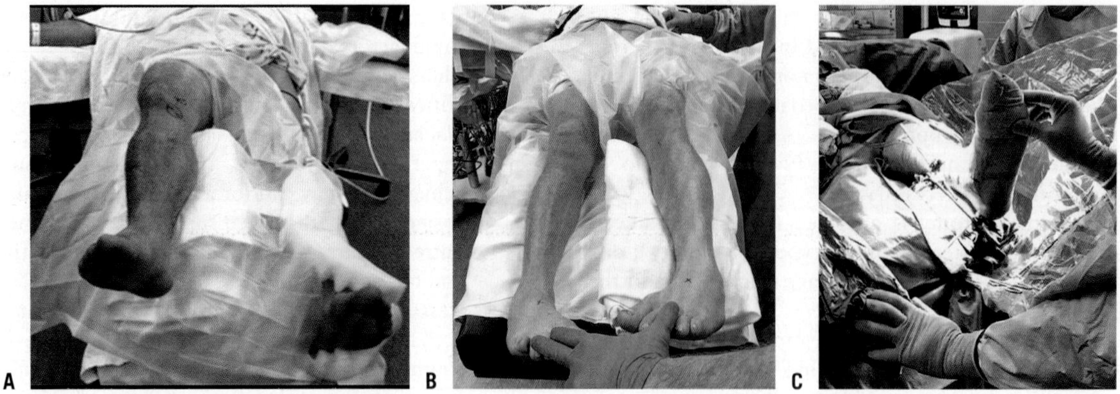

FIG 7 A. Supine position of patient for unilateral sinus tarsi approach. Leg is elevated on a blanket platform. **B.** For bilateral fractures, both legs are prepped at the same time with one slightly higher than the other. **C.** The slight offset allows for ease of external fixator placement and fluoroscopic imaging.

- For bilateral injuries treated with a sinus tarsi approach, the patient is placed supine **(FIG 7B,C)**.
- The fluoroscope is brought in from the side opposite the surgeon.
- The arthroscope is placed with the monitor on the same side as the C-arm toward the head of the bed.

Approach

- The sinus tarsi approach was developed as a logical evolution of previous minimally invasive techniques.
- Multiple minimal-incision techniques have been developed over the years in an effort to avoid the wound healing and infectious complications of the extensile lateral approach.
- A medial approach alone can be used. This approach does not allow for visualization of the posterior facet and is therefore suboptimal for joint depression fractures with displacement.
    - A medial approach can be combined with a sinus tarsi approach, but with newer techniques, the medial approach is not necessary, unless there is dislocation or significant displacement of a small sustentacular fragment.
- True minimal-incision fixation techniques without direct visualization of the posterior facet have also been described. These are best suited for fractures with minimal joint displacement that can be successfully reduced with fluoroscopic guidance alone. If the posterior facet cannot be adequately realigned closed, an open approach is necessary to reduce the risk of posttraumatic arthritis and to obtain an optimal functional result.
- Minimally invasive techniques for the management of tongue and tuberosity fractures exist but are beyond the scope of this chapter.
- The sinus tarsi approach will address most, but not all, calcaneal pathologies but requires a firm understanding of the fragments, displacements, and deforming forces present.
    - Sinus tarsi approaches allow adequate visualization of the posterior facet and can be used for all Sanders type II fractures **(FIG 8)**.
    - Sanders type III fractures that can be treated with this approach include those with central fragments that can be easily seen, manipulated, and fixed from the anterior exposure afforded by the sinus tarsi approach **(FIG 9)**.
    - Sanders type IV fractures undergoing open reduction internal fixation and primary fusion are ideally suited for the sinus tarsi approach.
    - Sanders type III fractures with posteriorly located central fragments should not be treated with a sinus tarsi approach **(FIG 10)**. These fractures are extremely difficult to reduce from the anterior approach, even with the assistance of an arthroscope and special instruments and implants.
        - In the end, a small incision with poor reduction does not lead to optimal results.
        - These fractures are better treated with an extensile lateral approach.
        - Sanders type III fractures should be treated only by surgeons with extensive knowledge of calcaneal fracture management.
- Sanders type II, III, and IV fractures with significant loss of height are nearly impossible to reduce after 2 weeks using anything other than an extensile lateral exposure (see **FIG 10**).

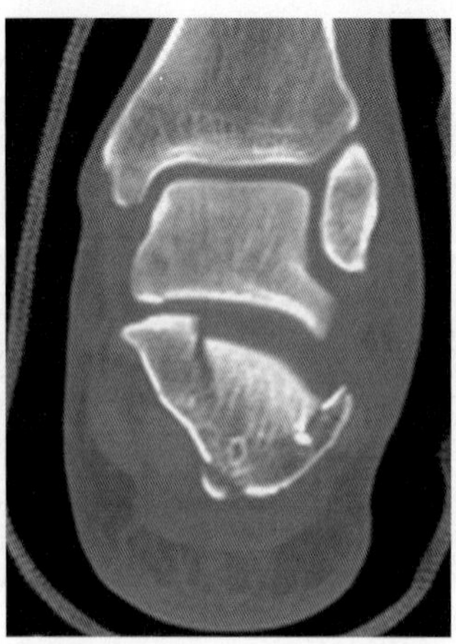

FIG 8 Sanders type II joint depression fracture.

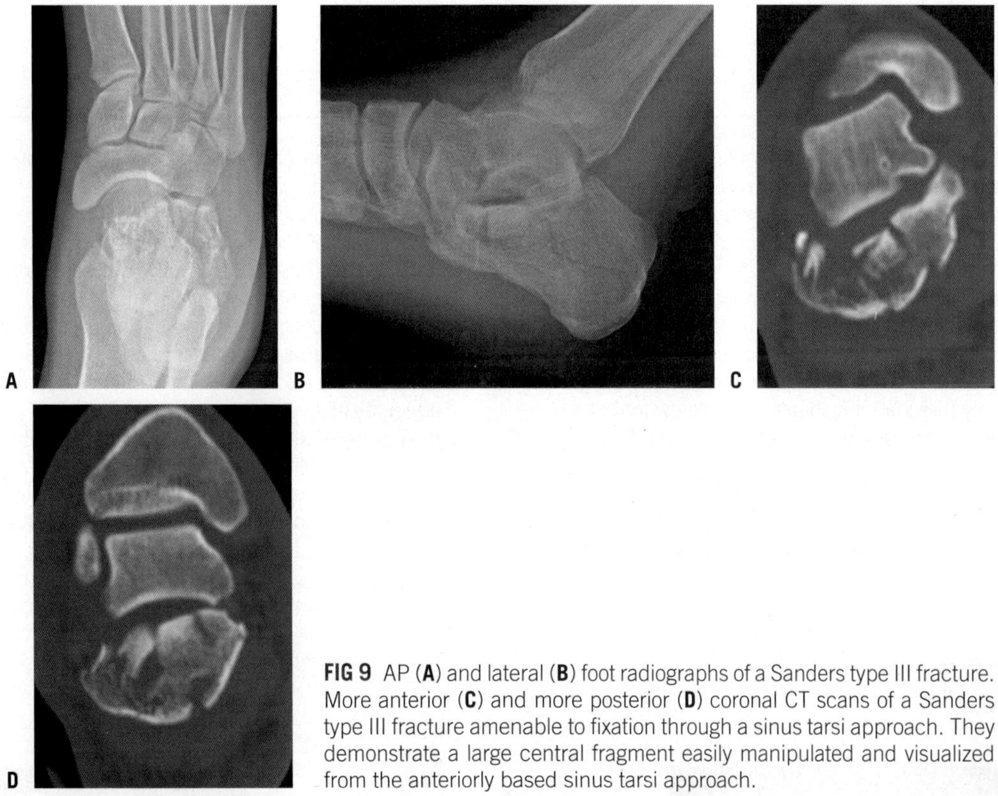

FIG 9 AP (**A**) and lateral (**B**) foot radiographs of a Sanders type III fracture. More anterior (**C**) and more posterior (**D**) coronal CT scans of a Sanders type III fracture amenable to fixation through a sinus tarsi approach. They demonstrate a large central fragment easily manipulated and visualized from the anteriorly based sinus tarsi approach.

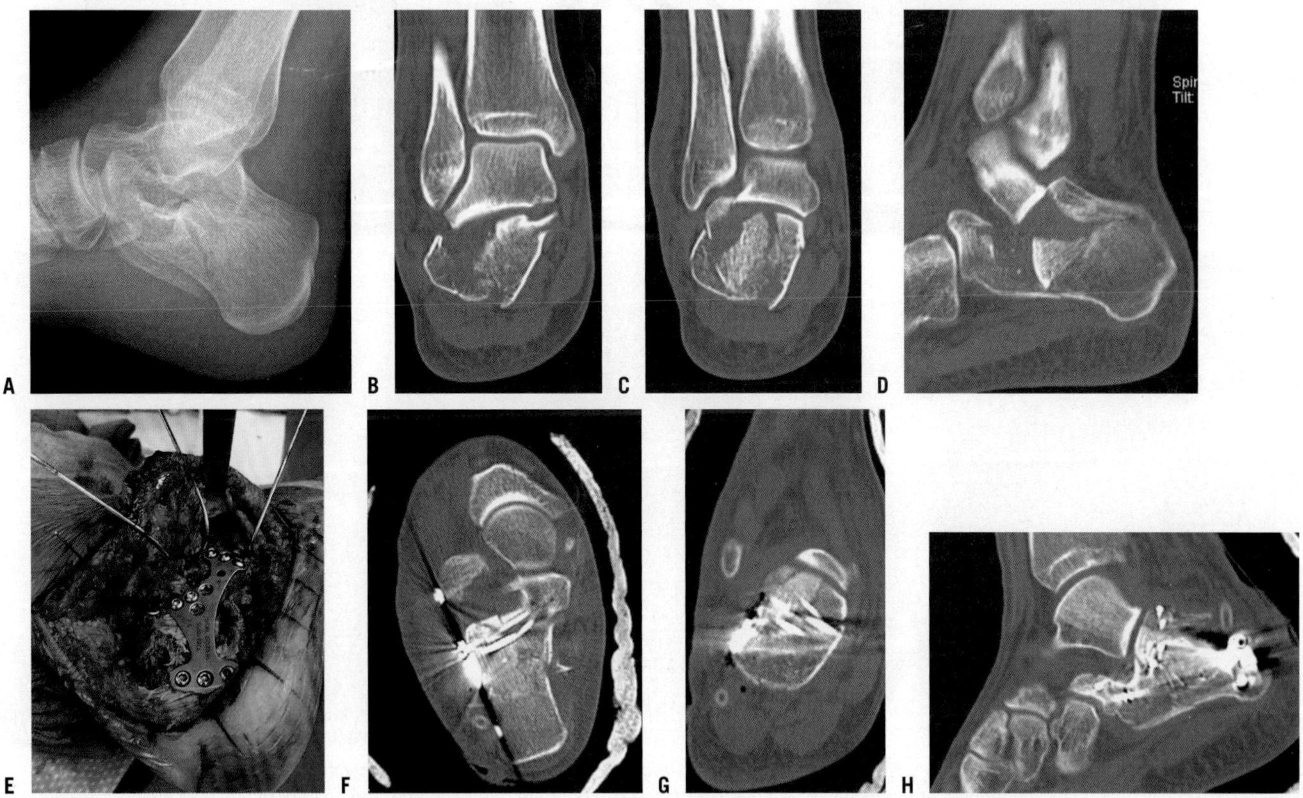

FIG 10 A. Lateral radiograph of 3-week-old Sanders type III fracture not suited for the sinus tarsi approach. **B–D.** CT scans demonstrating fracture with a superolateral fragment dislocated posterior lateral and a large central fragment significantly displaced. **E.** Intraoperative image of extensile lateral approach. **F–H.** Postoperative CT scans demonstrating adequate restoration of alignment.

PRELIMINARY REDUCTION

- In an effort to facilitate open treatment and internal fixation through a sinus tarsi approach, the posterior tuberosity must be reduced to the sustentacular fragment or at least pulled distally prior to attempting reduction of the posterior facet **(TECH FIG 1A–C)**.
  - If this is not performed, the posterior facet can be reduced but will be angled.
- Multiple techniques can be used. These include manual distraction, reduction, and then internal fixation with temporary wires or a fully threaded noncompression screw from the posterior tuberosity into the sustentacular fragment.
- The easiest and most reproducible maneuver to date has been application of a temporary, medially placed external fixator **(TECH FIG 1D–F)**.
- This is accomplished with a small pin to bar frame system and a universal clamp.
- A 4-mm half-pin is placed in the tibial metadiaphyseal region (bicortical), taking care not to injure the saphenous vein and nerve. The pin is placed from medial to lateral.
- A second 4-mm half-pin is placed from medial to lateral in the posterior tuberosity under fluoroscopic guidance.
  - The pin must be placed posterior to all fracture lines.
  - The pin should be placed posterior to where the plate will sit.
- Each pin is connected to a bar, and then the bars are connected with a universal clamp.
- A closed reduction is performed, bringing the posterior tuberosity out of varus or valgus and back to the appropriate height. Translation is also corrected. With fluoroscopic imaging, adequate alignment is achieved.
  - The external fixator may need adjustment throughout the case to facilitate reduction.
  - The fixator is usually disassembled after the anterior calcaneus and posterior facet have been reconstructed and just prior to fixation of the posterior tuberosity.
    - Height is usually maintained at this time.
    - Without the external fixator, the half-pin in the posterior tuberosity is then used to correct any varus or valgus prior to placing screws through the posterior plate.

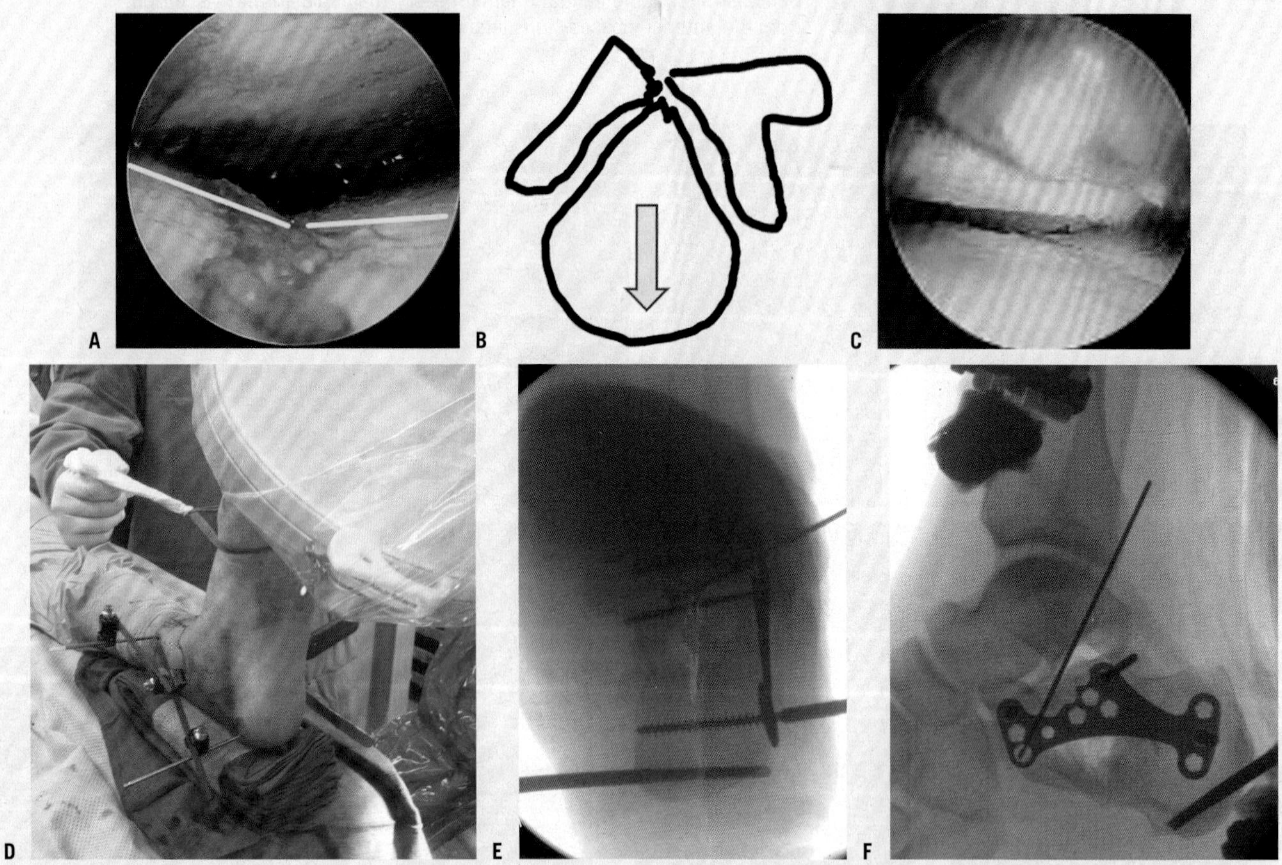

TECH FIG 1 **A.** Malreduced (angled) posterior facet secondary to wedging effect of the posterior tuberosity. **B.** Distraction of the posterior tuberosity is used to allow for adequate reduction of the posterior facet. **C.** Adequate reduction after the posterior facet was pulled distally. **D.** The medial external fixator is placed with fluoroscopic guidance to ensure that adequate axial alignment and height are achieved. **E.** The pin in the posterior tuberosity is placed perpendicular to the medial cortex. This allows for correction of alignment when the tuberosity is brought out to length. **F.** The pin in the tuberosity is placed posteriorly to where the plate will eventually sit and does not penetrate too far past the lateral cortex.

INCISION AND DISSECTION

- Different sinus tarsi incisions have been described in the literature. The lead author prefer a slightly longer, longitudinal incision. This allows for easier reduction and hardware placement with less tension on the skin. This ultimately leads to improved wound healing.
  - The incision starts 1 cm above the tip of the lateral malleolus and extends to 1 cm distal to the anterior process of the calcaneus. It is located just anterior to the peroneal tendon sheath **(TECH FIG 2A)**.
- After sharp dissection through the skin, bluntly dissect down, taking precautions not to injure any branches of the sural nerve. The extensor digitorum brevis is elevated anteriorly, and the joint capsule to the posterior facet is incised, exposing the displaced articular fragments and hematoma.
  - The lateral wall is exposed by elevating the peroneal tendons while attempting to keep them within their sheath **(TECH FIG 2B)**.
  - The calcaneofibular ligament is also elevated but left attached to the fibula.
- Multiple small fragments of the wall will need to be gently teased away from the overlying soft tissues and either placed into a sterile container with saline or simply impacted back into the body.
  - The entire lateral wall does not need to be removed as in the extensile lateral approach, secondary to adequate visualization of the displaced posterior facet from the sinus tarsi.
- If a plate is going to be used, which will fixate all portions of the calcaneus, then a path must be created along the lateral aspect of the posterior tuberosity. This is performed with a broad blunt elevator.
- The anterior portion of the calcaneus is similarly exposed with either sharp dissection or blunt elevator dissection below the peroneal tendons.
- The medial soft tissues can be freed up with a blunt, broad, curved elevator placed through the fracture from lateral.

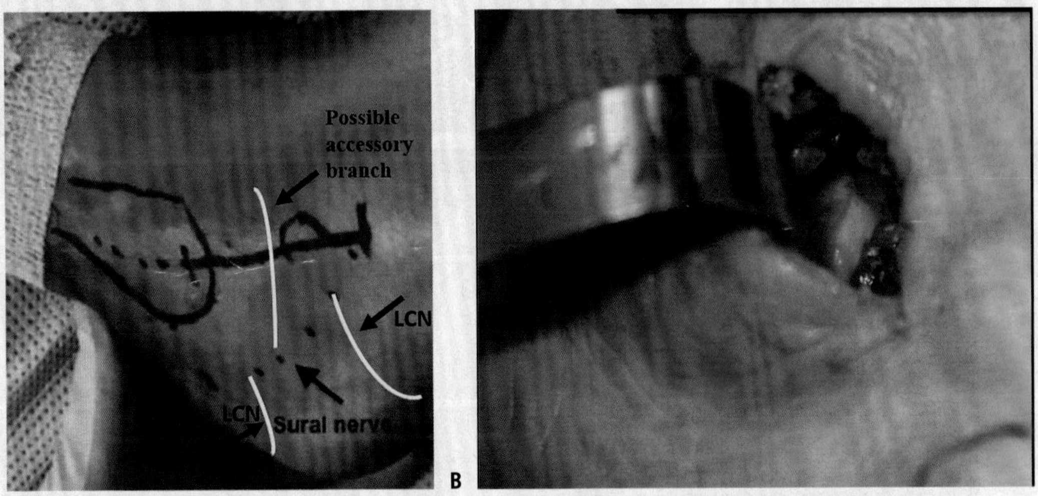

A B

TECH FIG 2 A. The sinus tarsi incision extends from 1 cm above the tip of the fibula to just beyond the anterior process *Dotted line* represents the sural nerve. *Yellow lines* represent branches of the sural nerve. **B.** Malleable retractors are used to protect the peroneal tendons. *LCN*, lateral calcaneal nerve.

REDUCTION AND FIXATION

Posterior Facet

Sanders Type II Fractures

- The posterior facet is reduced first. With the posterior tuberosity pulled distally by the external fixator, the posterior facet fragments are easily mobilized.
  - In Sanders type II part fractures, the superolateral fragment is elevated out of the body of the calcaneus with a broad elevator. Care is taken not to damage the cartilage. The fragment is then temporarily stabilized to the superomedial fragment with multiple wires.
- After reducing the superolateral fragment to the superomedial fragment, alignment is confirmed with both fluoroscopy with multiple Broden views and with dry arthroscopy. A 2.7-mm stubby 30-degree arthroscope is used **(TECH FIG 3A)**.
  - The fluoroscopy and arthroscopy images must correlate. If they do not, a translational or rotational malreduction exists **(TECH FIG 3B–L)**.
  - If reduction is anatomic or near anatomic, fixation is placed. If it is not, the reduction maneuvers are repeated until appropriate reduction is obtained. At that point, small lag screws are placed from the superolateral fragment into the superomedial fragment.
  - These vary from 2.0- to 3.0-mm cannulated or solid screws. An attempt is made to place them as parallel as possible to the posterior facet so that they engage good-quality bone

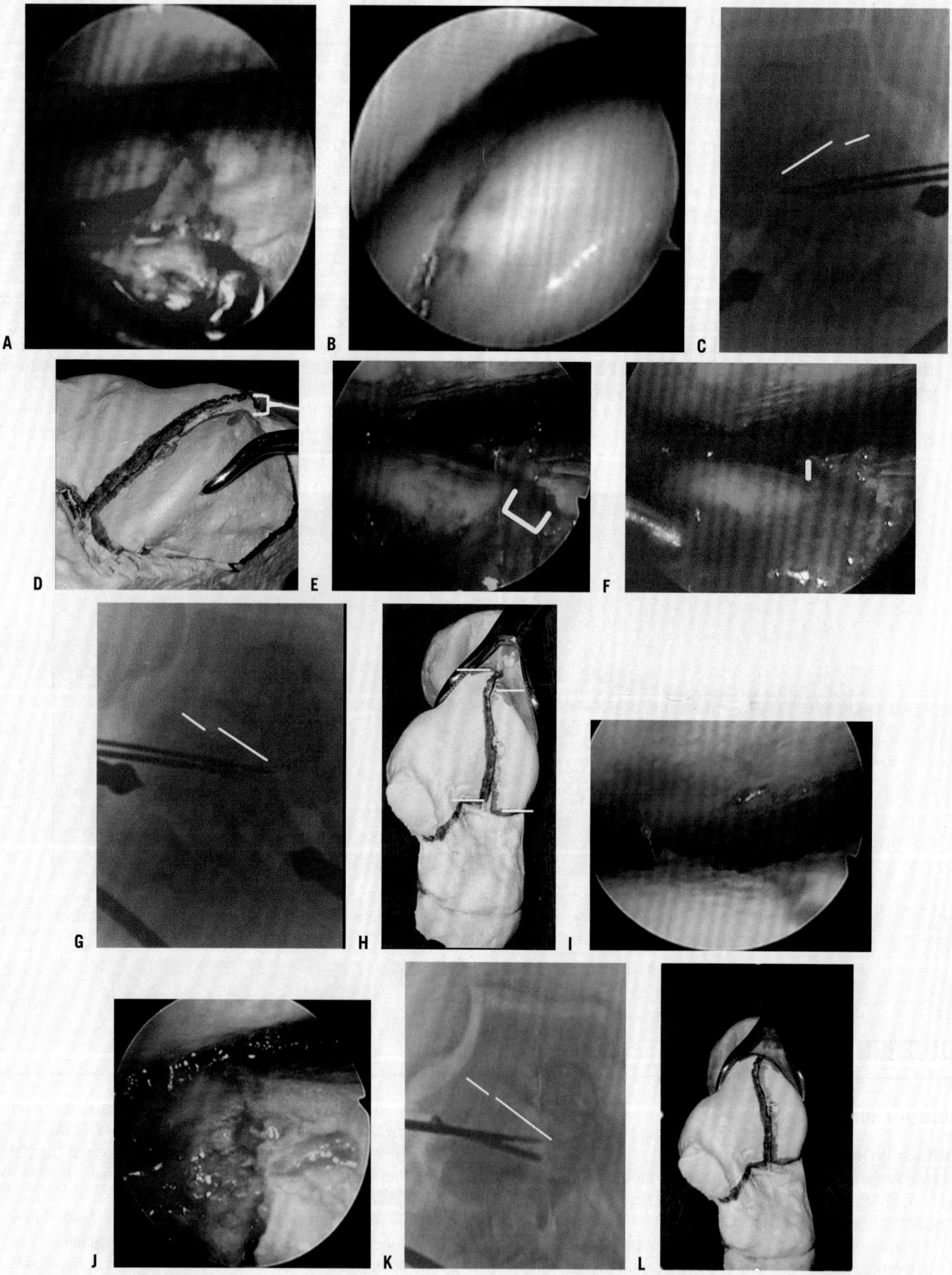

TECH FIG 3 **A.** Arthroscopic confirmation of adequate articular alignment. **B–K.** How to correlate dry arthroscopic data and fluoroscopic data. The two imaging modalities must both show adequate alignment to confirm truly anatomic alignment. **B.** Anterior view from arthroscope shows apparent anatomic alignment. **C.** Corresponding fluoroscopy showing a significant step-off. **D.** This results from a rotational deformity, as depicted on the sawbones model. **E,F.** These arthroscopic images show both a translational malalignment and a step-off. **G.** Corresponding fluoroscopic view. **H.** Sawbones model. Both deformities must be corrected. **I–K.** Revised arthroscopic reduction with corresponding fluoroscopy. **L.** Ideal reduction shown on a sawbones model. *Yellow lines* represent the articular surface in **C**, **G**, and **K**. *Brackets* and *lines* in **D**, **E**, **F**, and **H** highlight the joint displacement.

medially. This is performed by using a malleable retractor to retract the peroneal tenon sheath plantarly.
- Proper placement of these lag screws is crucial to avoid interference with the plate and screws that will be placed next.
- The goal is to place the screws into the good-quality bone of the sustentaculum. Be careful not to penetrate the medial articular surface.

Sanders Type III and IV Fractures

- In Sanders type III fractures **(TECH FIG 4A)**, a broad elevator is used to disimpact the displaced central and superolateral fragments out of the body, taking care not to damage the cartilage.
  - The central fragments are reduced to the sustentacular (superomedial) fragment and stabilized with temporary wires in most instances.
  - To facilitate this process, the superolateral fragment is displaced inferiorly and usually posteriorly **(TECH FIG 4B,C)**.
  - In other cases, the central fragment can be reduced to the superolateral fragment first and temporarily stabilized.
  - If reduction is adequate based on both fluoroscopy and dry arthroscopy, definitive fixation is performed.
  - Fixation can take the form of small absorbable pins, small Kirschner wires (K-wires) or countersunk small lag screws.
  - The fixation must be flush to the bony surface to allow for reduction of the reconstructed fragments with the third fragment.
  - After reducing and stabilizing the central fragment, the superolateral fragment is reduced to the reconstructed central and superomedial fragment and stabilized with small screws **(TECH FIG 4D–G)**.
- In Sanders type IV part fractures, the fragments are reduced and stabilized in a similar manner, but they do not have to be reduced anatomically if the subtalar joint is being primarily fused.

Fixation of the Reconstructed Posterior Facet to the Anterior Calcaneus and the Posterior Tuberosity

- Once the posterior facet is reconstructed, the anterior calcaneus must be reduced and fixated to the posterior facet reestablishing the crucial angle of Gissane. The reconstructed anterior portion and posterior facet are then reduced and fixated to the posterior tuberosity.
  - This can be accomplished with either multiple screws or a plate and screws. In simple terms, the three main portions of the calcaneus need to be brought together, and any manner of stable internal fixation is acceptable.
  - Most surgeons use a plate that connects all three segments. After determining plate size based on template placement under fluoroscopy, the final plate is placed through the incision while protecting and elevating the peroneal tendons. It is aligned into appropriate position, and the screws are placed **(TECH FIG 5A)**.

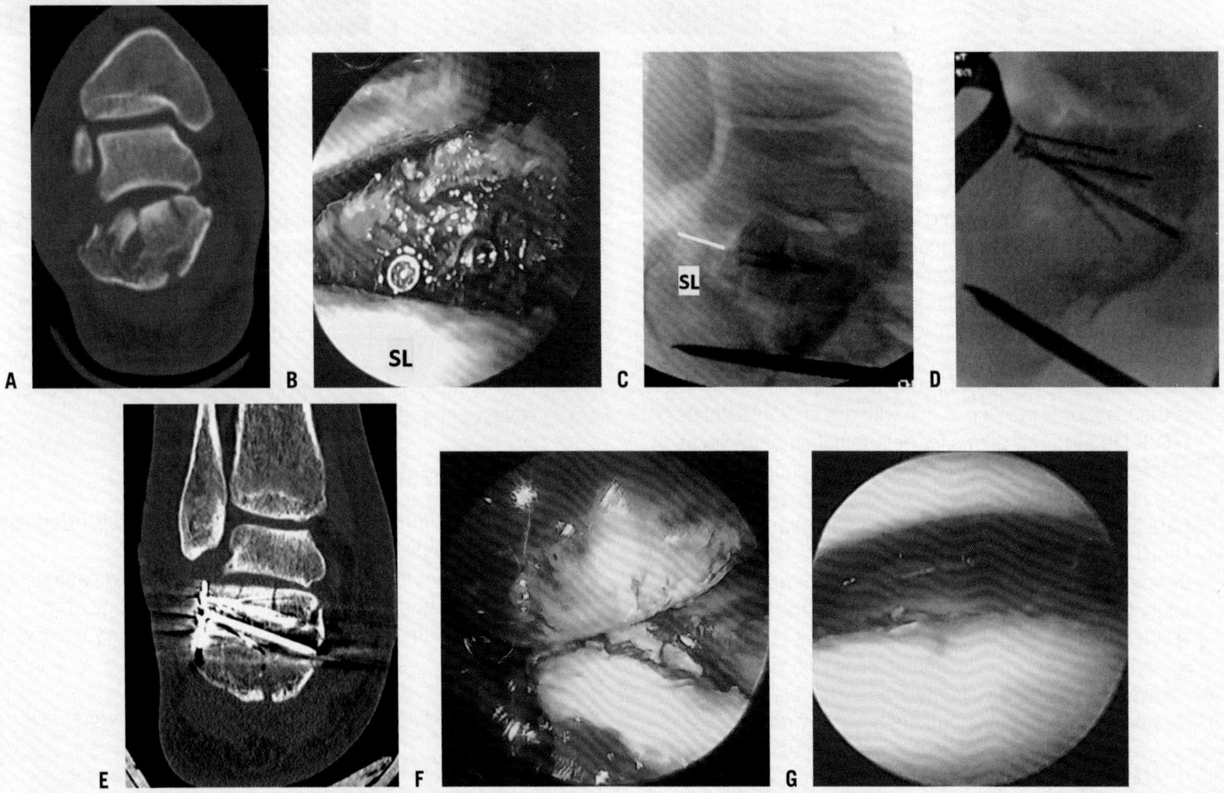

TECH FIG 4 **A.** Sanders type III fracture. **B.** The central fragment is reduced to the superomedial fragment by displacing the superolateral fragment inferiorly and posteriorly. It is stabilized with two small lag screws with the heads countersunk. **C.** The corresponding Broden view. *Yellow line*, displaced articular surface of the superolateral fragment. **D.** The superolateral fragment is then reduced to the reconstructed central and medial fragments. **E.** Postoperative CT demonstrates adequate alignment. **F,G.** Postfixation dry arthroscopy demonstrates adequate alignment at the joint level laterally and medially. *SL*, superolateral fragment.

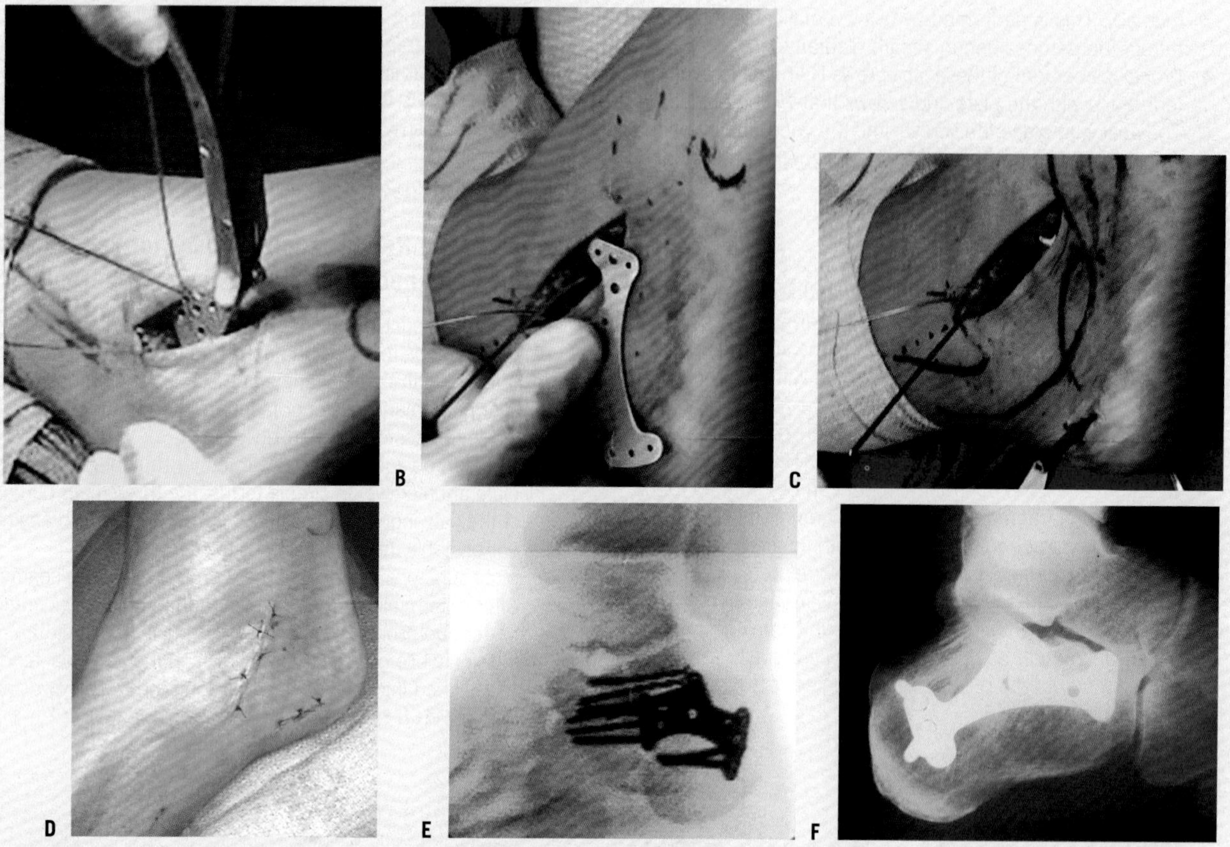

TECH FIG 5 **A.** Plate placement with specially designed holder. **B.** The template is placed in line with the indwelling plate to identify the location of the posterior screws. **C.** Posterior screw placement. **D.** Technique of making two or three small incisions for posterior screw placement. **E.** Final Broden view. **F.** Final lateral view.

- The first screw is placed into the anterior calcaneus just proximal to the calcaneocuboid joint. The anterior calcaneus is then reduced to the posterior facet, and screws are then placed to fixate the posterior facet. A second and, if necessary, third screw are then placed into the anterior portion of the calcaneal plate.
- The same sized template or a second plate of similar size is then laid over the skin in line with the implanted plate **(TECH FIG 5B)**. This allows for determination of the location of the holes in the plate overlying the posterior tuberosity.
- The posterior plate is accessed and screws are placed. Care is taken to protect the skin. Even though these holes should be posterior to the sural nerve, care is taken during dissection, drilling, and screw placement to avoid injury to the lateral calcaneal branches of the sural nerve **(TECH FIG 5C)**.
  - In the past, a single longitudinal incision was made over the posterior plate. Secondary to delayed wound healing, however, the authors have converted to using two or three small incisions over the posterior plate **(TECH FIG 5D)**. These heal better.
- A final axial fluoroscopic image is obtained prior to screw placement, and if adequate alignment is noted, two or three screws are placed through the plate. If adequate alignment is not noted, the original half-pin is used to manipulate the posterior tuberosity into appropriate position prior to screw placement. The varus–valgus alignment and the height must be correct.
- Nonlocking screws are usually sufficient, but in cases of comminution or poor bone quality, locking screws can be used.
- Final imaging is performed to confirm adequate hardware placement and reduction **(TECH FIG 5E,F)**.

Tendon Stabilization and Completion

- If the peroneal tendons are unstable, the incision is extended in line with the distal fibula.
- The tendons are then reduced and stabilized by repairing the superior peroneal retinaculum back to the fibular rim utilizing suture anchors. Groove deepening is rarely needed **(TECH FIG 6A)**.
- Bone grafting is usually not necessary.
- Vancomycin powder is placed on the hardware in high-risk patients.
- A layered closure is performed. A drain is not needed.
- A well-padded splint is placed holding the ankle in neutral.
- CT scan can be obtained postoperatively. This will help surgeons determine how well they executed their operative plan and help them fine-tune their skills **(TECH FIG 6B,C)**.

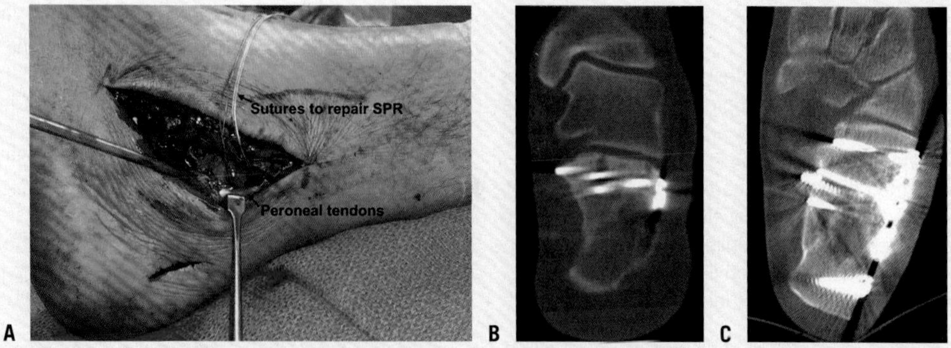

TECH FIG 6 A. Proximal extension of the sinus tarsi incision used to stabilize the peroneal tendons. The superior peroneal retinaculum is anchored back to the fibula with sutures. **B,C.** CT scan after surgery demonstrates maintenance of alignment at the articular surface and correction of varus. *SPR*, superior peroneal retinaculum.

HIGHLY COMMINUTED SANDERS TYPE IV FRACTURES

- Special consideration must be given to these high-energy fractures. Open reduction and internal fixation alone leads to very poor results in most cases. For this reason, open reduction and internal fixation is combined with primary subtalar fusion **(TECH FIG 7A–D)**.
- On rare occasions, in a young active patient with cartilage that has sustained minimal damage and in the extremely rare scenario in which anatomic alignment can be obtained, the authors have performed internal fixation without primary fusion. This has been possible in only a handful of cases, and future

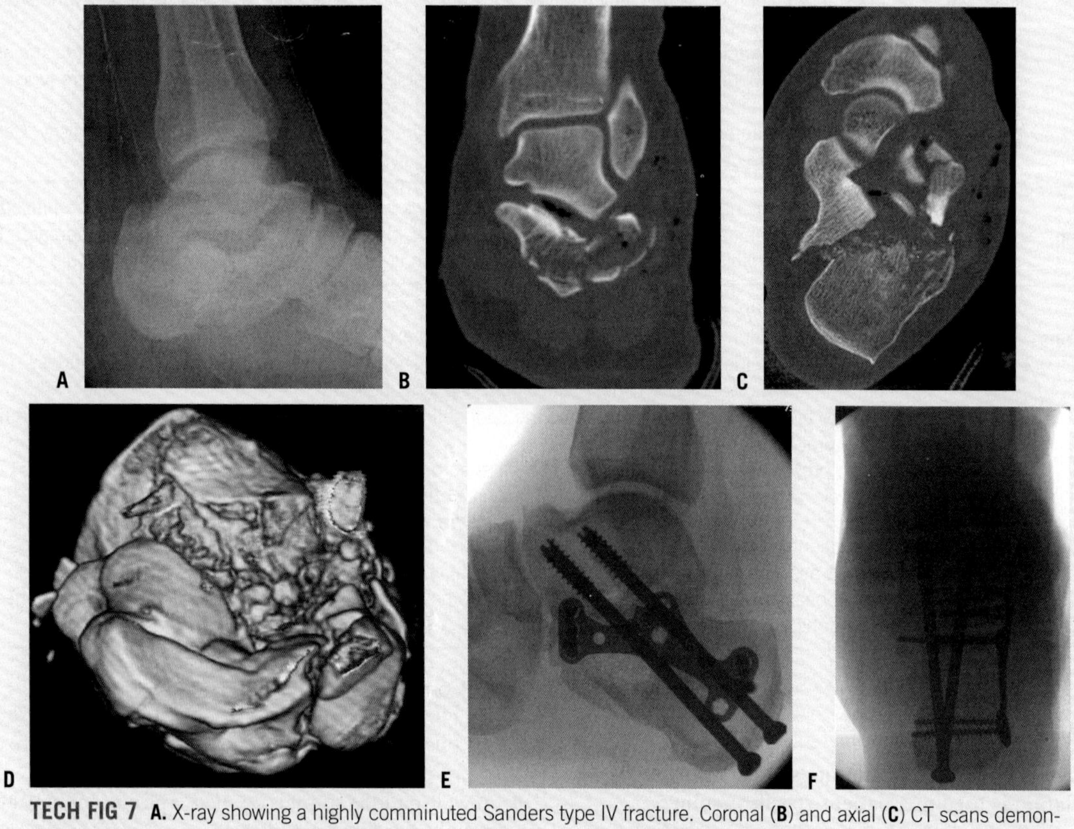

TECH FIG 7 A. X-ray showing a highly comminuted Sanders type IV fracture. Coronal (**B**) and axial (**C**) CT scans demonstrating Sanders type IV fracture. **D.** Reconstructed CT showing severe destruction to posterior facet. **E.** Lateral fluoroscopy demonstrating open reduction and internal fixation and primary subtalar fusion. Partially threaded cannulated screws are used to compress the subtalar joint. A single locking screw in each of the three main portions of the calcaneus allows for compression without deforming the calcaneus. **F.** Axial fluoroscopy demonstrating adequate alignment.

review of outcomes must be performed before this can be recommended to all surgeons.
- Whether the reduction and fixation are performed through a sinus tarsi approach or an extensile lateral approach, the technique is as noted earlier. The reduction of the body and the articular surfaces must be accomplished, as this is not an in situ fusion.
- The fusion is performed by removing cartilage from the opposing surfaces of the posterior and medial facets of the calcaneus and talus. The subchondral bone is then drilled, and cancellous bone graft is used to fill any voids. The fusion is then performed with two screws placed from the posterior tuberosity into the talus.
- The screws can be cannulated or solid, fully threaded or partially threaded, and are placed to miss the hardware already in position.
  - Advocates of fully threaded screws cite the benefit of avoiding compression and subsequent displacement.
  - Partially threaded screws can be used without the risk of leading to displacement by placing one locking screw in each of the three segments of the reconstructed calcaneus (anterior, posterior facet, and posterior tuberosity). This technique provides a stable calcaneus against which the talus can be compressed **(TECH FIG 7E,F)**.

Pearls and Pitfalls

Indications	• Less invasive approaches require an accurate definition of the pathoanatomy and then matching the pathoanatomy with an operative plan. Only surgeons with either significant previous experience with the extensile lateral approach or with extensive formal training in the sinus tarsi approach should attempt the sinus tarsi and other minimal-incision approaches for joint depression fractures. • The sinus tarsi approach is the preferred approach for patients with open fractures. • The sinus tarsi approach is the preferred approach for patients with risk factors for poor wound healing. This includes patients who smoke, diabetics, and patients with any other comorbidity that can affect wound healing and the risk of infection.
Fracture Reduction	• With the sinus tarsi approach, the first step is to place a temporary medial external fixator or to employ another method of distraction to pull the posterior tuberosity distally. • The posterior facet is then reconstructed. • Exact posterior facet reduction is difficult to achieve but required to achieve excellent results. Adjuncts of fluoroscopy and dry arthroscopy help visualize the highly congruent subtalar joint. • In Sanders type III fractures, the intermediate piece can be fixated to the superomedial fragment or the superolateral fragment with small buried lag screws, K-wires, or absorbable pins, thus converting it to a Sanders type II pattern. • The anterolateral fragment is then reduced to the posterior facet, lateral wall. • The reconstructed anterior calcaneus and posterior facet are then reduced to the posterior tuberosity. Care must be taken to ensure correct height and alignment prior to placing the screws through the posterior plate.
Fracture Stabilization	• Multiple fixation options are available. These include screws varying from 1.5 to 5.0 mm, K-wires of all sizes, absorbable pins, minifragment plates, and fracture-specific plates designed for the sinus tarsi approach. For fusion cases and cases in which only percutaneous screw fixation is used, large cannulated screws should be available.
Avoiding Complications	• Gentle handling of the soft tissues is essential. • The sinus tarsi incision must not be too small. This avoids excessive traction. • Extensile sinus tarsi incisions are not biologically friendly. There is no indication for these approaches. • Multiple small incisions posteriorly heal better than one long incision. • Take care to avoid injury to the sural nerve, the connecting nerve between the sural and superficial peroneal nerve, and the lateral calcaneal nerve branches. • Attempt to preserve the peroneal tendons in their sheath to avoid scarring and excessive stiffness. • Strict foot elevation and elimination of movement until adequate wound healing is recommended
Postoperative Care	• Reliable patients without neuropathy can safely perform touchdown weight bearing immediately. Range-of-motion exercises to assist in recovery of subtalar motion begin once the wound heals at approximately 2 weeks. • Full weight bearing begins at 6 weeks in patients who have stable plate fixation and adequate signs of healing on radiographs.

POSTOPERATIVE CARE

- Two doses of postoperative antibiotics are administered.
- Anticoagulation is used in a patient-specific manner.
  - Lower risk patients for venous thromboembolism are treated with 81-mg aspirin twice a day and, in some cases, sequential compression devices.
  - Higher risk patients are treated with more aggressive pharmacologic anticoagulation until they are adequately mobile.
- A well-padded splint is applied. The patient may be toe-touch weight bearing immediately.
- The patient is instructed to maintain strict elevation as much as possible until the sutures are removed.

- The splint can be discontinued, and range-of-motion exercises begun once the wound is ready. This usually is at 2 weeks but can take longer.
- The patient is converted from a splint to a tall CAM boot at 2 weeks. The patient sleeps in the CAM boot until 6 weeks to prevent equinus.
- Physical therapy is started once the wounds are healed to help regain motion.
- At 6 weeks, a radiograph is obtained and weight bearing progressed as pain and osseous healing allow. In patients with good-quality bone, stable fixation, and adequate healing, full weight bearing is allowed at 6 weeks. In all other patients, a graduated return to full weight bearing is pursued with full weight bearing being achieved at approximately 10 to 12 weeks.

OUTCOMES

- Despite appropriate care, most patients with a calcaneal fracture will lose some degree of foot function and have permanent symptoms.
- Although nonoperative treatment yields the fewest iatrogenic complications, it accepts malunion in nearly 100% and a higher incidence of later subtalar fusion.
- Overall, minimal-incision techniques with a sinus tarsi approach have similar clinical and radiographic outcomes to open treatment and internal fixation with an extensile lateral approach. However, the minimal-incision techniques have a lower risk of wound healing problems and infections.
- Symptom improvement can take up to a year to plateau.
- In a randomized study, visual analog pain scores between nonoperative and operative groups were similar, but nonoperative treatment resulted in a 5.5 times greater incidence of late subtalar fusion.
  - In that same study, females, nonworkmen's compensation cases, and nonmanual laborers had improved results with operative treatment.
  - Better results were also seen with an anatomic reduction versus a nonanatomic one.
- Soft tissue complications frequently lead to a poor result.
- In high-risk patients, the sinus tarsi approach has a lower risk of wound healing and infectious complications.

COMPLICATIONS

- The complications of nonoperative treatment include malunion, persistent foot pain, and a higher chance of later subtalar fusion.
- Severe crush deformities affect not only the subtalar joint but also the midfoot and ankle as well. They can be difficult to reconstruct, so initial management to avoid such a malunion is recommended.
- Smoking, diabetes, and open fracture are the most significant risk factors for soft tissue complications.
- Infection occurs in about 2% of fractures treated operatively.
- Deep infection is managed with débridement and intravenous antibiotics based on culture results.
  - Retention of hardware (if providing bone stability) until bone healing is optimal
  - Removal of the hardware to eradicate the infection once the bone is healed is needed.
- To decrease the risk of deep infection, open fractures are managed with irrigation and débridement, possible antibiotic spacers, and early plastic surgery intervention. The sinus tarsi approach is ideal in patients with a medial wound.
- Posterior tibial nerve injury can result from the fracture and commonly presents with severe pain nonresponsive to narcotics in the postinjury period.
  - Administration of medications aimed at neuropathic pain is recommended, and consultation with a pain specialist is considered.
- Cushioned shoe inserts are often comforting to individuals with postfracture plantar heel pain. A rocker bottom shoe can also reduce discomfort.
  - Orthotics can be used in patients with symptomatic posttraumatic arthrosis.
- Late implant-related symptoms can occur with the sinus tarsi approach. They present as pain over the peroneal tendons and lateral plate and screws. If necessary, symptoms often improve with implant removal and peroneal tenolysis.
  - Painful, posttraumatic arthrosis is managed first with analgesics and orthotics. If conservative measures fail, a subtalar fusion can be performed. After a sinus tarsi approach with anatomic reduction, this can possibly be performed arthroscopically.
- In cases involving injured workers, nearly all who have sustained an isolated, unilateral calcaneus fracture are capable of getting back to gainful employment. Certain restrictions, such as avoiding ladder and working at heights, may be necessary.

SUGGESTED READINGS

Basile A, Albo F, Via AG. Comparison between sinus tarsi approach and extensile lateral approach for treatment of closed displaced intra-articular calcaneal fractures: a multicenter prospective study. J Foot Ankle Surg 2016;55(3):513–521.

Berberian W, Sood A, Karanfilian B, et al. Displacement of the sustentacular fragment in intra-articular calcaneal fractures. J Bone Joint Surg Am 2013;95(11):995–1000.

Carr JB. Surgical treatment of intra-articular calcaneal fractures: a review of small incision approaches. J Orthop Trauma 2005;19(2):109–117.

Ebraheim N, Elgafy H, Sabry F, et al. Sinus tarsi approach with trans-articular fixation for displaced intra-articular fractures of the calcaneus. Foot Ankle Int 2000;21(2):105–113.

Femino JE, Vaseenon T, Levin DA, et al. Modification of the sinus tarsi approach for open reduction and plate fixation of intra-articular calcaneus fractures: the limits of proximal extension based upon the vascular anatomy of the lateral calcaneal artery. Iowa Orthop J 2010;30:161–167.

Kikuchi C, Charlton TP, Thordarson DB. Limited sinus tarsi approach for intra-articular calcaneus fractures. Foot Ankle Int 2013;34(12): 1689–1694.

Kline AJ, Anderson RB, Davis WH, et al. Minimally invasive technique versus an extensile lateral approach for intra-articular calcaneal fractures. Foot Ankle Int 2013;34(6):773–780.

Kwon JY, Guss D, Lin DE, et al. Effect of delay to definitive surgical fixation on wound complications in the treatment of closed, intra-articular calcaneus fractures. Foot Ankle Int 2015;36(5):508–517.

Levine DS, Helfet DL. An introduction of the minimally invasive osteosynthesis of intra-articular calcaneal fractures. Injury 2001;32(suppl 1):SA51–SA54.

Li S. Wound and sural nerve complications of the sinus tarsi approach for calcaneus fractures. Foot Ankle Int 2018;39(9):1106–1112.

Mehta CR, An VVG, Phan K, et al. Extensile lateral versus sinus tarsi approach for displaced, intra-articular calcaneal fractures: a meta-analysis. J Orthop Surg Res 2018;13(1):243.

Nosewicz T, Knupp M, Barg A, et al. Mini-open sinus tarsi approach with percutaneous screw fixation of displaced calcaneal fractures: a prospective computed tomography-based study. Foot Ankle Int 2012;33(11):925–933.

Park CH, Yoon DH. Role of subtalar arthroscopy in operative treatment of sanders type 2 calcaneal fractures using a sinus tarsi approach. Foot Ankle Int 2018;39(4):443–449.

Phisitkul P, Sullivan JP, Goetz JE, et al. Maximizing safety in screw placement for posterior facet fixation in calcaneus fractures: a cadaveric radio-anatomical study. Foot Ankle Int 2013;34(9):1279–1285.

Radnay CS, Clare MP, Sanders RW. Subtalar fusion after displaced intra-articular calcaneal fractures: does initial operative treatment matter? Surgical technique. J Bone Joint Surg Am 2010;92(suppl 1, pt 1): 32–43.

Rammelt S, Amlang M, Barthel S, et al. Minimally-invasive treatment of calcaneal fractures. Injury 2004;35(suppl 2):SB55–SB63.

Rammelt S, Amlang M, Barthel S, et al. Percutaneous treatment of less severe intraarticular calcaneal fractures. Clin Orthop Relat Res 2010;468(4):983–990.

Rammelt S, Gavlik JM, Barthel S, et al. The value of subtalar arthroscopy in the management of intra-articular calcaneus fractures. Foot Ankle Int 2002;23(10):906–916.

Sanders R. Displaced intra-articular fractures of the calcaneus. J Bone Joint Surg Am 2000;82(2):225–250.

Schepers T. The sinus tarsi approach in displaced intra-articular calcaneal fractures: a systematic review. Int Orthop 2011;35(5):697–703.

Schepers T, Backes M, Dingemans SA, et al. Similar anatomical reduction and lower complication rates with the sinus tarsi approach compared with the extended lateral approach in displaced intra-articular calcaneal fractures. J Orthop Trauma 2017;31(6):293–298.

Scott AT, Pacholke DA, Hamid KS. Radiographic and CT assessment of reduction of calcaneus fractures using a limited sinus tarsi incision. Foot Ankle Int 2016;37(9):950–957.

Smyth NA, Zachwieja EC, Buller LT, et al. Surgical approaches to the calcaneus and the sural nerve: there is no safe zone. Foot Ankle Surg 2018;24(6):517–520.

Thordarson DB, Latteier M. Open reduction and internal fixation of calcaneal fractures with a low profile titanium calcaneal perimeter plate. Foot Ankle Int 2003;24(3):217–221.

Tornetta P III. Percutaneous treatment of calcaneal fractures. Clin Orthop Relat Res 2000;(375):91–96.

Zeng Z, Yuan L, Zheng S, et al. Minimally invasive versus extensile lateral approach for Sanders type II and III calcaneal fractures: a meta-analysis of randomized controlled trials. Int J Surg 2018;50:146–153.

CHAPTER 62

Open Reduction and Internal Fixation of Lisfranc Injury

Michael P. Clare and Roy W. Sanders

DEFINITION

- A Lisfranc injury refers to bony or ligamentous compromise of the tarsometatarsal and intercuneiform joint complex and includes a spectrum of injuries ranging from a stable, partial sprain to a grossly displaced and unstable fracture or fracture-dislocation of the midfoot.

ANATOMY

- The bony elements of the medial three tarsometatarsal joints (medial, middle, and lateral cuneiforms and first, second, and third metatarsal bases) feature a unique trapezoidal shape in cross-section, creating a concave arrangement plantarly resembling a Roman arch **(FIG 1A)**.
- The second metatarsal is recessed between the medial and lateral cuneiforms in the axial plane and is positioned at the apex of the Roman arch in the coronal plane. It thus functions as the keystone of the entire midfoot complex **(FIG 1B)**.

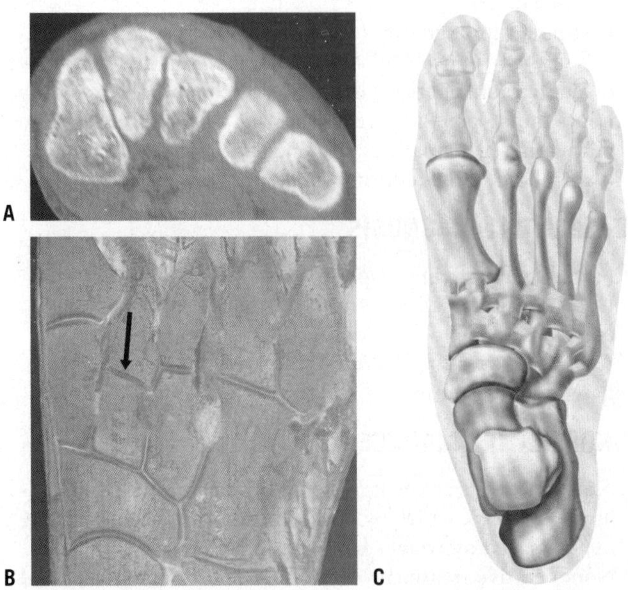

FIG 1 A. Axial CT image depicting the Roman arch configuration of the tarsometatarsal joints. **B.** Anatomic specimen demonstrating the keystone of the Roman arch: The second metatarsal base is recessed between the medial and lateral cuneiforms (*black arrow*). **C.** Dorsal and plantar tarsometatarsal, intermetatarsal, and intercuneiform ligaments stabilizing the articulations of the midfoot.

- The tarsometatarsal joints are stabilized by dorsal and plantar tarsometatarsal ligaments.
  - Dorsal and plantar intermetatarsal ligaments provide further stability between the second through fifth metatarsal bases.
  - There are no intermetatarsal ligaments between the first and second metatarsals, which may predispose the area to injury.
  - The Lisfranc ligament courses from the plantar portion of the medial cuneiform to the base of the second metatarsal **(FIG 1C)**.
- The unique bony arrangement of the medial midfoot imparts inherent bony stability to the medial and middle columns of the foot, which in combination with the stout plantar ligaments prevents plantar displacement of the metatarsal bases and facilitates the weight-bearing function of the first ray **(FIG 2)**.
- The medial three tarsometatarsal joints and the adjacent intercuneiform and naviculocuneiform articulations (medial and middle columns) have limited inherent motion, making these joints nonessential to normal foot function and therefore relatively expendable.
  - The medial column refers to the first tarsometatarsal and navicular–medial cuneiform articulations; the middle column includes the second and third tarsometatarsal joints and articulations between the navicular and middle and lateral cuneiforms, respectively.
- The fourth and fifth tarsometatarsal (lateral column) joints have distinctly more inherent motion and are critical in accommodation of the foot to uneven surfaces.
  - These joints are considered essential joints to normal foot function and therefore nonexpendable.

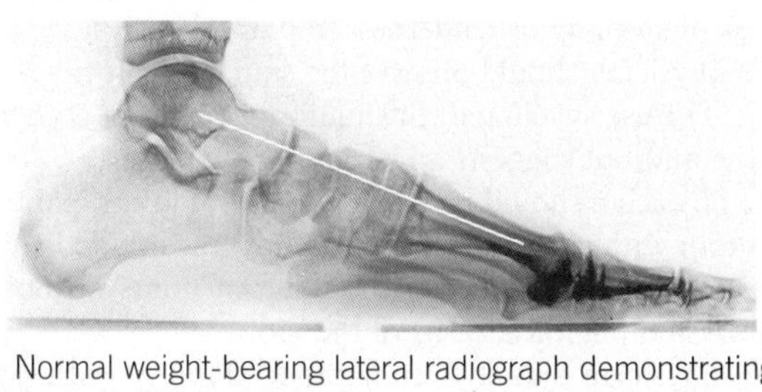

FIG 2 Normal weight-bearing lateral radiograph demonstrating normal alignment of the medial column and the weight-bearing first ray (*white line*).

PATHOGENESIS

- Lisfranc injuries are generally the result of a high-energy injury, such as a fall from a height or a high-speed motor vehicle accident, but depending on the position of the foot, they may also result from a lower energy injury, such as a slip and ground-level fall.
- These injuries result from a combination of axial load and dorsiflexion, plantarflexion, abduction, or adduction (or variable combinations thereof) of the midfoot.
- The pathoanatomy is individually specific and highly variable and may consist of a pure ligamentous injury, a pure bony injury (fracture), or a combination.
- Although the injury classically includes the first, second, and third tarsometatarsal joints, there may be involvement of all five tarsometatarsal articulations, extension into the intercuneiform joints, or even fracture lines into the navicular or cuboid proximally or metatarsal shafts or necks distally.
- In pure ligamentous patterns, the stability of the injury depends on the status of the plantar tarsometatarsal ligaments. Disruption of these stout structures makes the injury unstable.
- Partial injuries (sprains) occur as a result of lower energy and are more common with axial load and plantarflexion, such as in competitive sports.
  - In this instance, by definition, the plantar tarsometatarsal ligaments remain intact, making the injury stable.

NATURAL HISTORY

- Stable injuries (partial sprains, extra-articular fractures) often require prolonged recovery time. When accurately diagnosed, however, patients with these injuries can generally expect full recovery and return to activity with minimal long-term implications.[8]
- Unstable injuries that are misdiagnosed or inadequately treated generally go on to a poor result with persistent pain, activity limitations, and progressive posttraumatic arthritis in the involved joints,[3,4] necessitating arthrodesis as salvage.[5,11]
- A high index of suspicion must therefore be maintained; historically, up to 20% of unstable Lisfranc injuries are misdiagnosed on plain radiographs.[4]

PATIENT HISTORY AND PHYSICAL FINDINGS

- The physician should obtain a history of trauma and details of the exact injury mechanism (position of foot, direction of force, extent of energy involved).
- The physician should observe any initial swelling and inability to bear weight.
- A thorough examination of the involved foot and ankle also includes assessment of associated injuries and any other areas of swelling or tenderness to palpation.
- The physician should observe the skin and soft tissue envelope. Diffuse swelling of the midfoot or plantar ecchymosis at the midfoot suggests a Lisfranc injury.
- The physician should palpate the midfoot joints; pain at the midfoot with palpation suggests a Lisfranc injury. Palpation should be performed over the midfoot joints on both the dorsal and plantar aspects of the foot.
- The physician should test midfoot stability with passive flexion of the metatarsal heads and passive abduction and adduction through the forefoot. Pain at the tarsometatarsal joint region with passive forefoot range of motion suggests a Lisfranc injury.

IMAGING AND OTHER DIAGNOSTIC STUDIES

- Initial radiographic evaluation consists of non–weight-bearing anteroposterior (AP), oblique, and lateral views of the foot, which, depending on the extent of intra-articular displacement, may provide sufficient diagnostic information **(FIG 3A–C)**.
- Fluoroscopic stress views may be helpful in more subtle injuries; however, these studies are painful and generally require anesthesia.
- We therefore prefer weight-bearing radiographs of the foot for more subtle injuries **(FIG 3D–H)**; comparison weight-bearing radiographs of the contralateral foot may also be obtained where necessary.
  - The weight-bearing AP view of the foot will demonstrate intra-articular displacement through the first and second tarsometatarsal joints (so-called Lisfranc joint), intercuneiform joint, and naviculocuneiform joint; fractures through the first and second metatarsal bases, medial and middle cuneiforms, and proximal extension into the navicular; and the extent of columnar shortening or asymmetry.
    - The medial border of the second metatarsal should align with the medial border of the middle cuneiform (see **FIG 3D**).
  - The oblique view will reveal intra-articular displacement through the third, fourth, and fifth tarsometatarsal joints and fractures of the third, fourth, and fifth metatarsal bases, lateral cuneiform, and cuboid.
    - The medial borders of the third and fourth metatarsals should align with the medial borders of the lateral cuneiform and cuboid, respectively (see **FIG 3E**).
  - The lateral view may reveal dorsal–plantar displacement of fractures or dislocations as well as any flattening of the medial longitudinal arch, thereby reflecting the status of the weight-bearing medial column and first ray (see **FIG 3F**).
- Computed tomography (CT) scanning may also be beneficial in the instance of a subtle Lisfranc injury, particularly in a polytrauma patient or a patient with multiple extremity injuries that preclude weight-bearing radiographs, and in delineating proximal fracture line extension into the navicular, cuboid, or cuneiforms **(FIG 4)**.

DIFFERENTIAL DIAGNOSIS

- Partial Lisfranc injury (sprain)
- Isolated metatarsal fracture
- Navicular–cuneiform fracture
- Anterior process of calcaneus fracture
- Lateral ankle sprain

NONOPERATIVE MANAGEMENT

- Nonoperative treatment is indicated for partial Lisfranc injuries (sprains), which by definition are stable and therefore nondisplaced on weight-bearing radiographs.
- Nonoperative treatment is also indicated for nondisplaced or minimally displaced extra-articular metatarsal base fractures with no intra-articular involvement (displacement) on weight-bearing radiographs.
- Because of the often-subtle nature of Lisfranc injuries and the negative consequences of misdiagnosis, if the findings are inconclusive, weight-bearing radiographs may be repeated 2 to 3 weeks after the injury when the patient may be more able to perform the examination.

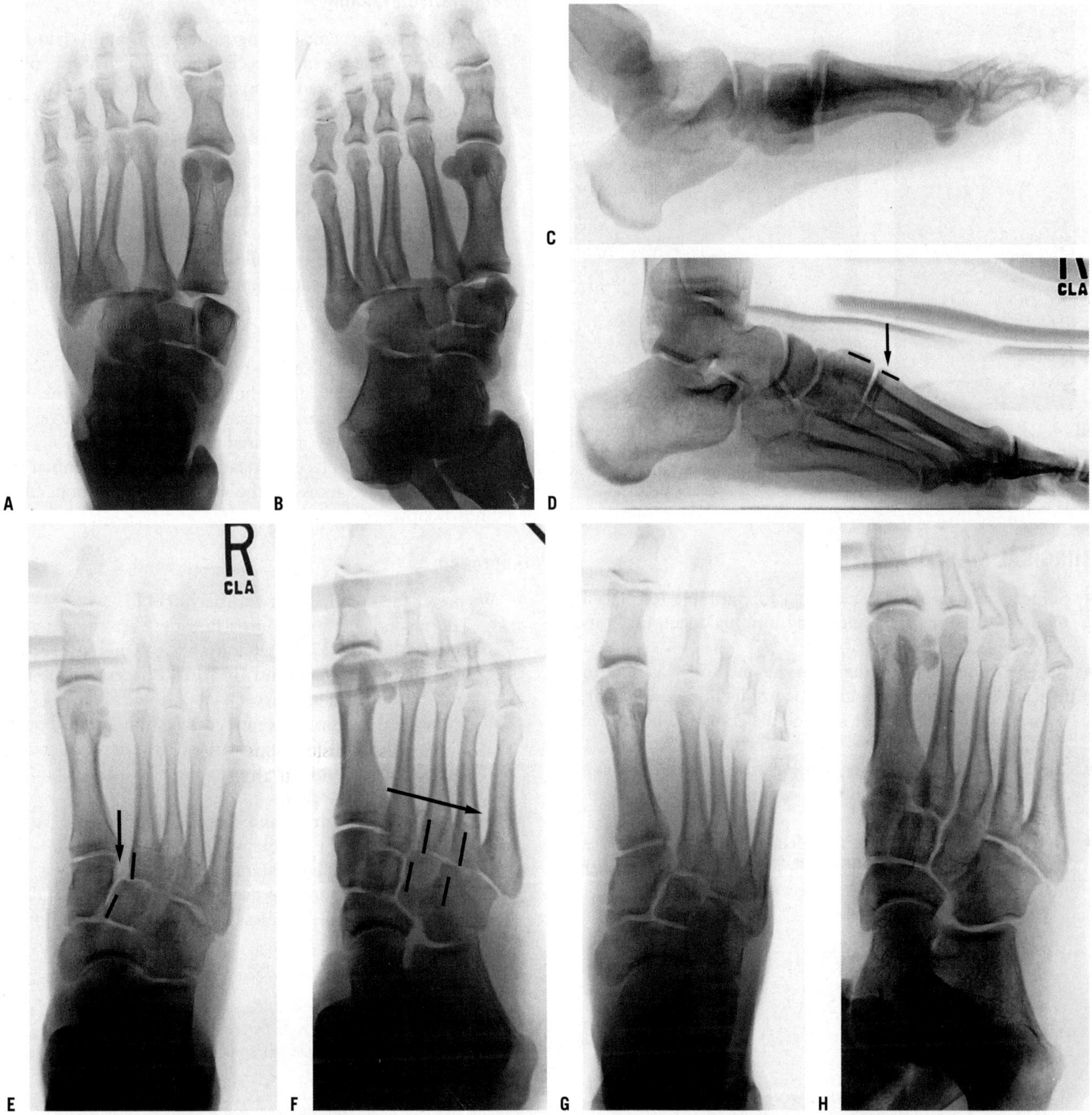

FIG 3 Non–weight-bearing AP (**A**), oblique (**B**), and lateral (**C**) radiographs of grossly unstable, purely ligamentous, Lisfranc dislocation involving all five tarsometatarsal articulations. Marked lateral subluxation through all five tarsometatarsal joints is evident on the AP and oblique views, and significant dorsal displacement is evident on the lateral view. Weight-bearing lateral (**D**), AP (**E**), and oblique (**F**) and non–weight-bearing (**G**) and oblique (**H**) radiographs of more subtle Lisfranc injury. Lateral and plantar subluxations (*black arrows*) are evident on the weight-bearing radiographs, and displacement of normal radiographic landmarks (*black lines*) confirms injury.

- Nonoperative management consists of immobilization in a venous compression stocking and prefabricated fracture boot.
  - The patient is allowed to bear weight to tolerance, and early progression to range of motion is encouraged.
  - The patient continues in the fracture boot for 5 to 6 weeks, at which point maintenance of alignment or radiographic union is confirmed on repeat weight-bearing radiographs.
  - The patient is then allowed to wear regular shoes, and activities are advanced as tolerated thereafter.
- Full recovery and return to sports or other rigorous activity may require up to 3 to 4 months.
- In patients with high risks of surgery, stress positive injuries that are aligned in a cast based on CT scans may be treated non–weight bearing for 10 to 12 weeks with deep vein thrombosis prophylaxis. Recovery is slow, but if the joints are all well aligned, the expected outcome is acceptable.

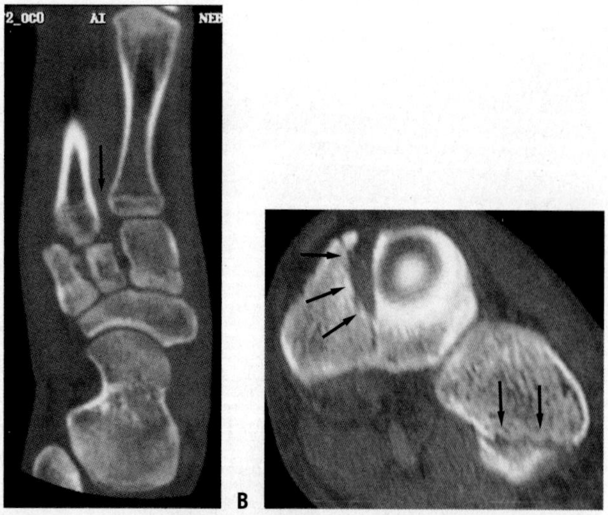

A B

FIG 4 CT scan showing displacement (*single black arrow*) through the second tarsometatarsal and intercuneiform articulations (**A**) and intra-articular fractures of navicular and cuboid (**B**, *black arrows*) in a different patient.

SURGICAL MANAGEMENT

- Surgical management is indicated for unstable (displaced) injuries of the midfoot, including pure ligamentous, bony, or variable combinations.
- Recent studies suggest that pure ligamentous Lisfranc injuries are best managed with open reduction and primary arthrodesis of the medial and middle columns, but others prefer firm fixation.[4,7,10,12]
- Any dislocation producing tension on the overlying skin and soft tissue envelope should be immediately reduced and immobilized **(FIG 5)**.
- Definitive surgery is generally delayed until adequate resolution of soft tissue swelling allows for safe surgery. This may take 7 to 14 days.

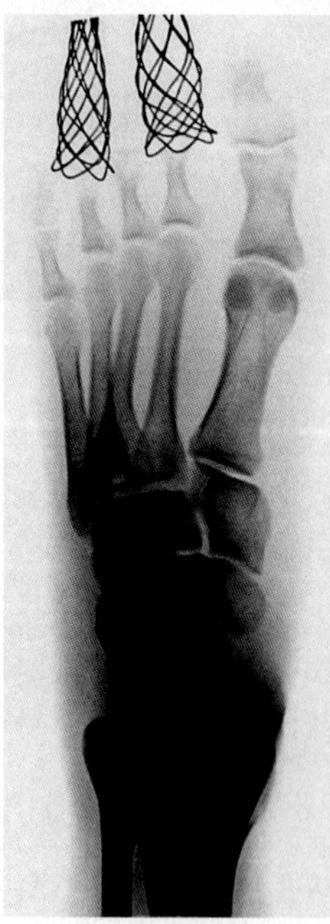

FIG 5 Closed reduction of Lisfranc dislocation; displaced fragments were tenting skin.

Preoperative Planning

- The injury and weight-bearing radiographs and CT images are reviewed and the injury is classified,[9] which allows planning for the anticipated pathoanatomy of the injury.
- It is critical to evaluate the intercuneiform region and the navicular–cuneiform joints as these are often injured. If they are unstable, fixation will begin proximally and proceed distally.
- Pure ligamentous injuries require rigid fixation with either screws or plates for the medial and middle column joints and Kirschner wire fixation for the lateral column joints; bony injury patterns, particularly those with more comminution, may require minifragment bridge plate fixation.[1,6]

Positioning

- The patient is placed supine with a bolster beneath the ipsilateral hip. Protective padding is placed around the contralateral limb, primarily to protect the peroneal nerve, and the contralateral limb is secured to the table.
- A sterile bolster is placed beneath the operative limb at the knee to facilitate access to the midfoot and intraoperative fluoroscopy.

Approach

- We prefer the dual-incision approach **(FIG 6)**.
  - The medial incision courses directly over the extensor hallucis longus (EHL) tendon and is centered over the first tarsometatarsal joint. It affords access to the first and second tarsometatarsal joints.
  - The lateral incision is centered over the lateral border of the third tarsometatarsal joint. If extended, it also provides exposure to the fourth and fifth tarsometatarsal joints where necessary.
- A third, more proximal and lateral, incision may be required to stabilize the cuboid where necessary.
- Because of the limited soft tissue envelope overlying the midfoot, the importance of meticulous soft tissue handling and maintaining full-thickness soft tissue flaps cannot be overemphasized.

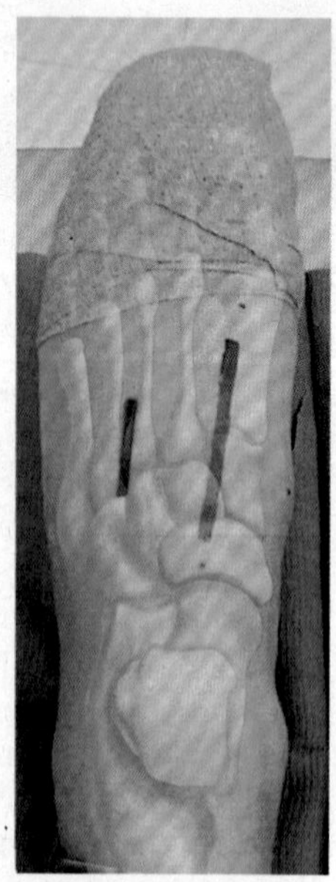

FIG 6 Planned incisions for dual-incision approach.

MEDIAL INCISION

- The medial incision is made directly over the EHL tendon and is centered over the first tarsometatarsal joint.
  - The tendon sheath is incised dorsally, and the EHL is retracted laterally **(TECH FIG 1A)**.
- The floor of the tendon sheath is then incised and subperiosteal dissection commences medially, extending to the medial margin of the first tarsometatarsal joint and producing a full-thickness flap.
- Subperiosteal dissection then extends laterally to the lateral margin of the second tarsometatarsal joint, again producing a full-thickness flap while preserving the adjacent neurovascular bundle within the soft tissue flap **(TECH FIG 1B)**.
- The status is noted of each of the tarsometatarsal and intercuneiform joint capsules dorsally and therefore the extent of instability of each joint **(TECH FIG 1C,D)**.
- We prefer using the medial (EHL) incision for access to the second tarsometatarsal and intercuneiform joints, even if the first tarsometatarsal joint is not involved because the neurovascular bundle remains protected within the full-thickness flap.

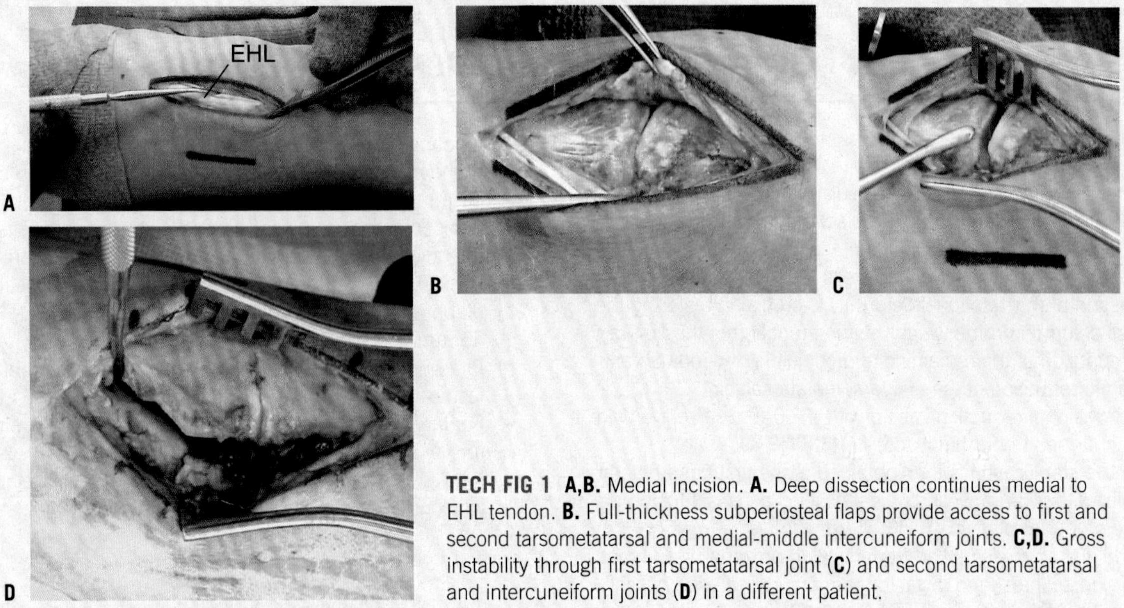

TECH FIG 1 A,B. Medial incision. **A.** Deep dissection continues medial to EHL tendon. **B.** Full-thickness subperiosteal flaps provide access to first and second tarsometatarsal and medial-middle intercuneiform joints. **C,D.** Gross instability through first tarsometatarsal joint (**C**) and second tarsometatarsal and intercuneiform joints (**D**) in a different patient.

LATERAL INCISION

- The lateral incision is made overlying the lateral border of the third tarsometatarsal joint. A Freer elevator can be inserted beneath the full-thickness flap of the medial incision to confirm proper location of the incision where necessary.
- Dissection extends through the overlying extensor retinaculum, exposing the extensor digitorum longus tendon and medial margin of the extensor digitorum brevis muscle, both of which are retracted laterally, thereby exposing the third tarsometatarsal joint **(TECH FIG 2)**.
- The extensor hallucis brevis muscle is identified and elevated medially, thereby exposing the second metatarsal shaft and lateral portion of the second tarsometatarsal joint, providing protection to the adjacent neurovascular bundle.
- The lateral incision may be extended proximally and distally to facilitate exposure of the fourth and fifth tarsometatarsal joints where necessary.
- Again, the status is noted of each of the tarsometatarsal and intercuneiform joint capsules dorsally and therefore the extent of instability of each joint.

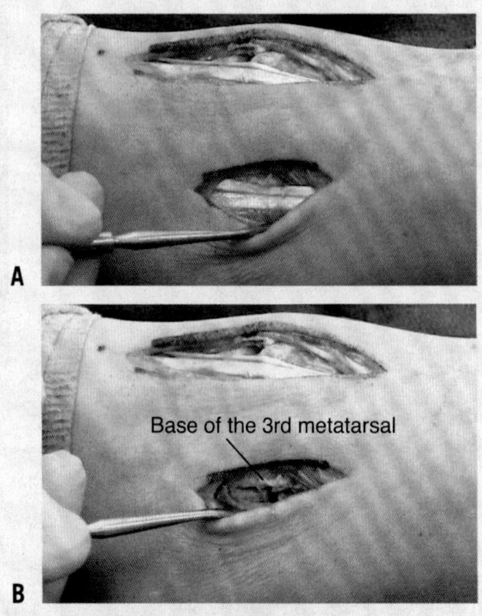

TECH FIG 2 Lateral incision. Deep dissection continues medial to extensor digitorum communis tendon and extensor digitorum brevis muscle (**A**) and exposes the third tarsometatarsal and the lateral portion of the second tarsometatarsal (not visualized here) joints (**B**).

ARTICULAR SURFACE ASSESSMENT AND DECISION MAKING

- The fracture lines and articular surface of the involved joints are then débrided of residual hematoma and assessed for chondral damage.
- If more than 50% of the articular surface of the medial and middle column joints is involved, primary arthrodesis should be considered, although this is controversial.
- Arthrodesis of the fourth and fifth tarsometatarsal joints should be avoided if possible.
- If primary arthrodesis is elected, the involved joints are meticulously débrided of residual articular cartilage, preserving the underlying subchondral plate.
  - The joints are irrigated and the subchondral plate is perforated with a 2.0-mm drill bit to stimulate vascular ingrowth.
  - Supplemental allograft or bone void filler may place within the involved joint spaces.

PROVISIONAL REDUCTION AND DEFINITIVE STABILIZATION

First Tarsometatarsal Joint

- The provisional reduction begins medially at the first tarsometatarsal joint if injured. Although the exact reduction maneuver may vary depending on the injury pattern, the first metatarsal is typically supinated (externally rotated) relative to the medial cuneiform.
- Correction of this rotational deformity is crucial in restoring the medial column and the weight-bearing function of the first ray. The reduction of the remaining midfoot joints depends on an anatomic reduction of the first tarsometatarsal joint.
- The provisional reduction is held with a 2.0-mm Kirschner wire and confirmed under fluoroscopy **(TECH FIG 3A)**.
- Definitive stabilization is then obtained at the first tarsometatarsal joint with 3.5-mm solid cortical position screws if fusion is not being performed **(TECH FIG 3B–D)**.
  - The first screw is placed from distal to proximal, starting at the dorsal crest and distal to the metaphyseal–diaphyseal junction, and is angled toward the plantar–proximal cortex of the medial cuneiform; this screw is generally 45 to 50 mm long.
  - A second screw is placed from proximal to distal starting at the edge of the naviculocuneiform joint and similarly angled to exit at the plantar cortex distal to the metaphyseal–diaphyseal junction. This screw typically measures 40 to 45 mm.
  - In a primary arthrodesis, these screws are placed in lag fashion.
  - For larger patients, 4.0-mm cortical screws may be used for further stability.
  - If a fusion is being performed, then lag screw or plate fixation is used.

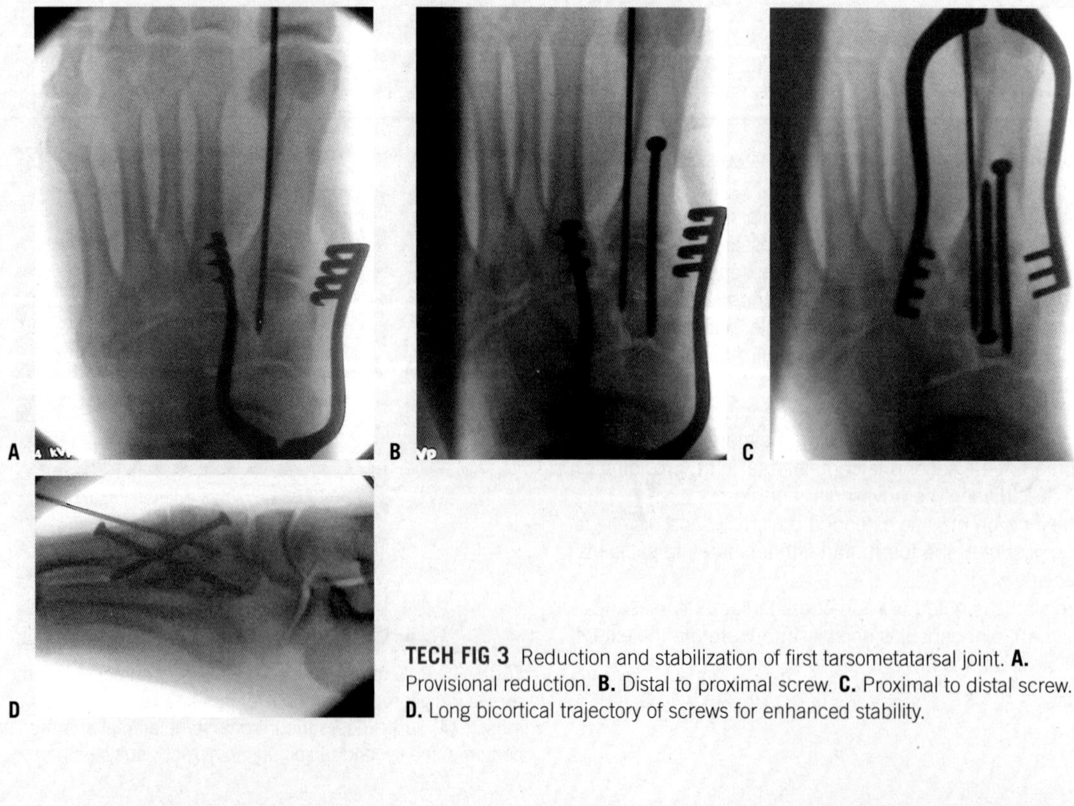

TECH FIG 3 Reduction and stabilization of first tarsometatarsal joint. **A.** Provisional reduction. **B.** Distal to proximal screw. **C.** Proximal to distal screw. **D.** Long bicortical trajectory of screws for enhanced stability.

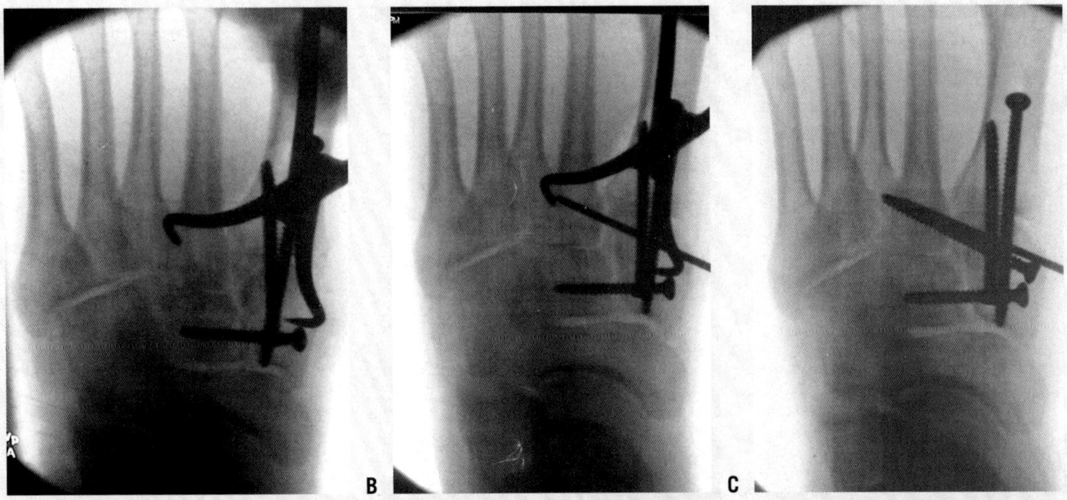

A B C

TECH FIG 4 Reduction and stabilization of Lisfranc joint. **A.** Pointed reduction forceps. **B.** Supplemental Kirschner wire. **C.** Screw fixation. Trajectory of screw mirrors the normal path of ligamentous structures. Intercuneiform joint was previously reduced and stabilized as initial step.

Lisfranc Joint

- A pointed reduction forceps is then placed from the medial cuneiform to the lateral border of the second metatarsal to anatomically reduce the so-called Lisfranc joint; care is taken to ensure accurate dorsal–plantar alignment of the second tarsometatarsal joint.
- The reduction is confirmed under fluoroscopy, and a 2.0-mm Kirschner wire that mirrors the intended path of the screw is placed to provide further rotational control **(TECH FIG 4A,B)**.
- There is typically a distinct cortical "shelf" on the medial cuneiform that provides an excellent buttress for screw purchase.
  - A 3.5-mm cortical screw is placed through a stab incision overlying this cortical shelf medially, angling toward the proximal metaphysis of the second metatarsal; for a primary arthrodesis, this screw is placed in lag fashion **(TECH FIG 4C)**.

Other Joints

- If the intercuneiform joint is involved, it is first reduced and stabilized before stabilizing the Lisfranc joint **(TECH FIG 5A)**. Alternatively, this joint may also be reduced and stabilized before stabilizing the first tarsometatarsal joint.
  - A 3.5-mm cortical screw is again used, coursing parallel to the plane of the naviculocuneiform joint. It is placed in lag fashion for a primary arthrodesis.
  - Care is taken not to violate the articulation between the middle and lateral cuneiform.
- The second tarsometatarsal joint is then provisionally reduced and provisionally stabilized with a 1.6-mm Kirschner wire.
  - Definitive fixation is obtained with a countersunk 2.7-mm cortical screw from distal to proximal; it is placed in lag fashion for a primary arthrodesis **(TECH FIG 5B)**.
  - For larger patients, 3.5-mm cortical screws may be used for further stability.

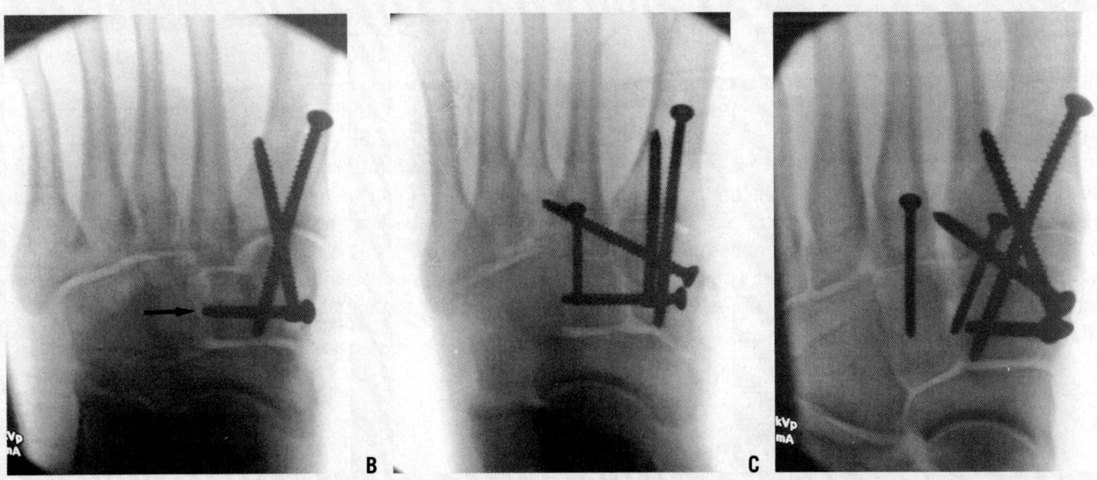

A B C

TECH FIG 5 **A.** Reduction and stabilization of intercuneiform joint (*single black arrow*). **B.** Reduction and stabilization of second tarsometatarsal joint. **C.** Reduction and stabilization of third tarsometatarsal joint. *(continued)*

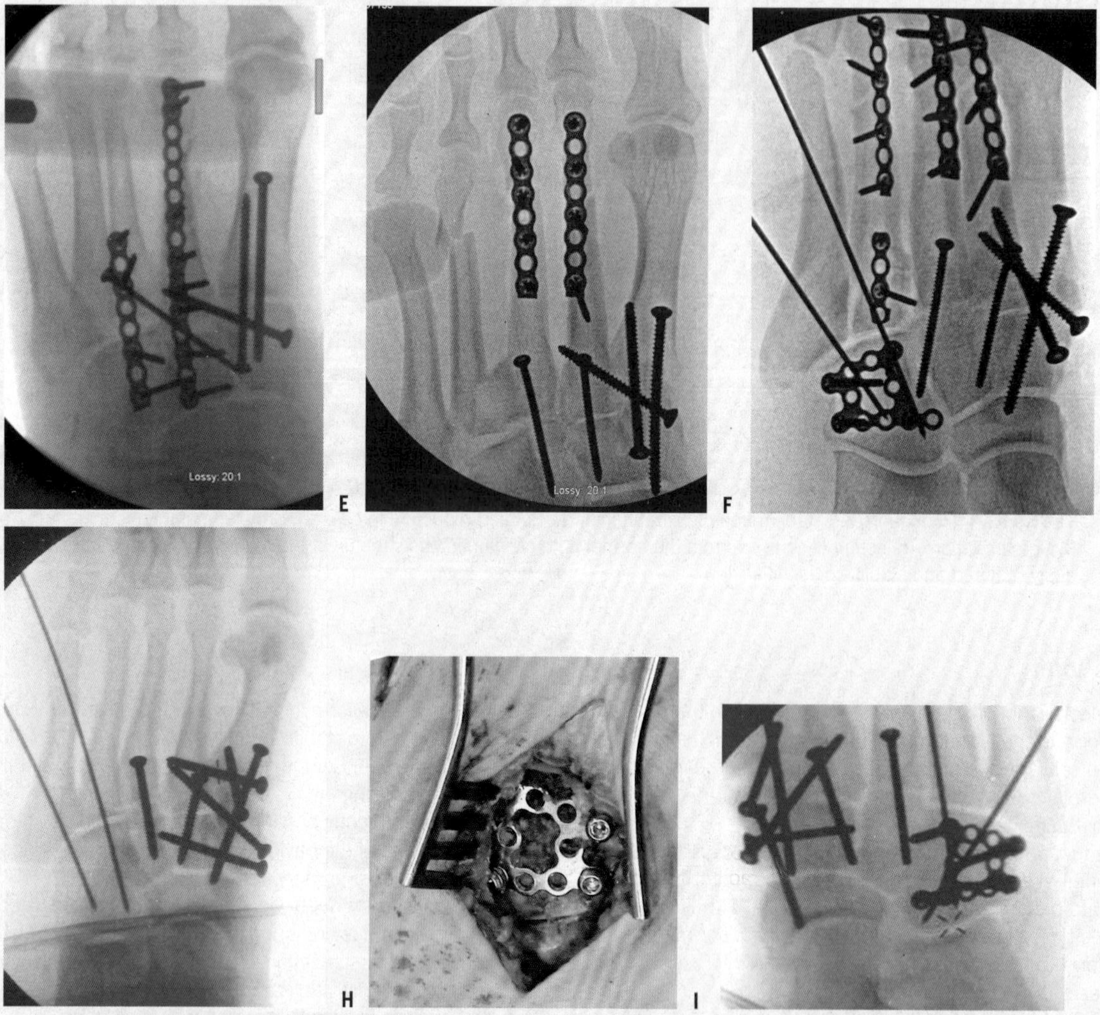

D E F G H I

TECH FIG 5 *(continued)* **D.** Comminuted second metatarsal and second and third tarsometatarsal joints. **E,F.** Second and third metatarsals and segmental fourth metatarsal in a different patient. **G.** Kirschner wire fixation of fourth and fifth tarsometatarsal joints. **H.** Reduction and stabilization of cuboid through separate proximal–lateral incision. **I.** Fluoroscopic image.

- The third tarsometatarsal joint is reduced and stabilized in identical fashion **(TECH FIG 5C)**.
- For a metatarsal base fracture or fracture-dislocation pattern precluding transarticular fixation, bridge plate fixation may be required.
  - We prefer a low-profile 2.4-mm plate and 2.4-mm cortical screws **(TECH FIG 5D–F)**. Multiple precontoured plates are also available for tarsometatarsal fixation.
- The fourth and fifth tarsometatarsal joints are then reduced and definitively stabilized with 1.6-mm Kirschner wires.
  - Because the intermetatarsal ligaments between the third, fourth, and fifth metatarsals are often preserved, these joints may anatomically reduce indirectly, thereby allowing percutaneous stabilization.
  - The Kirschner wires are contoured and buried beneath the skin layer through separate stab incisions, which facilitates removal at 6 weeks postoperatively, either in the office under local anesthesia or in the operating room under sedation **(TECH FIG 5G)**.
- For a cuboid fracture, the cuboid is reduced and definitively stabilized to ensure restoration of lateral column length before stabilizing the fourth and fifth tarsometatarsal joints; by definition, this is then an open reduction **(TECH FIG 5H)**.
- Final fluoroscopic images are obtained, confirming articular reduction and implant placement **(TECH FIG 5I)**.

CLOSURE

- The wounds are irrigated, and closure commences with the medial incision. The floor of the EHL tendon sheath (and subperiosteal flaps) is closed with 2-0 absorbable suture, thereby sealing the intra-articular surfaces of the first and second tarsometatarsal joints and intercuneiform joints.
- The EHL tendon sheath is closed in similar fashion, thereby sealing the tendon **(TECH FIG 6A)**.
- The remainder of the incision is closed in layered fashion with subcutaneous 2-0 absorbable suture and 3-0 monofilament suture for the skin layer using the modified Allgöwer-Donati technique **(TECH FIG 6B)**.
- The tourniquet is deflated, and sterile dressings are placed, followed by a bulky Jones dressing and Weber splint.

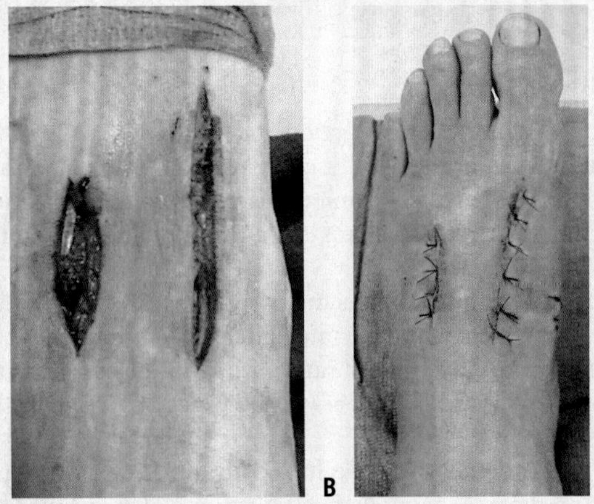

TECH FIG 6 Wound closure. **A.** Deep-layered closure sealing intra-articular contents and EHL tendon. **B.** Skin closure with modified Allgöwer-Donati technique.

TECHNIQUES

Pearls and Pitfalls

Misdiagnosis of Proximal Joint Injuries (Medial, Middle, or Lateral Cuneiform; Intercuneiform Joint; Cuboid Fracture)	• Because of the highly variable injury patterns, a high index of suspicion must be maintained. Injury radiographs must be closely scrutinized preoperatively for proximal joint involvement. If radiographs are inconclusive, CT evaluation is warranted. During surgery, the status is noted of each of the intercuneiform joint capsules dorsally and therefore the extent of instability of each joint.
Correcting Plantar Displacement or Malalignment of the First and Second Tarsometatarsal Joints	• Strict attention is paid to dorsal–plantar alignment of the first and second metatarsals and their respective cuneiforms because plantar displacement or malalignment greater than 2 mm may affect the weight-bearing metatarsal cascade, potentially resulting in a transfer (metatarsalgia) lesion.
Correcting Supination Malrotation of First Tarsometatarsal Joint	• There is typically a distinct dorsal crest on both the first metatarsal and medial cuneiform. They should be precisely aligned to ensure an accurate reduction.
Definitive Fixation of First Tarsometatarsal Joint	• Because of the hard cortical bone at the diaphysis of the first metatarsal, the screw head of the distal to proximal screw is specifically countersunk to avoid compromise of the dorsal cortex and loss of fixation.
Definitive Fixation of Lisfranc Joint	• With fixation of the Lisfranc joint, the screw must angle slightly dorsally (relative to the plantar foot) to accommodate the normal "Roman arch" configuration in the coronal plane.

POSTOPERATIVE CARE

- The patient is converted to a venous compression stocking and prefabricated fracture boot, and early progression to motion is initiated. The long extensor tendons (EHL and extensor digitorum) tend to become adhesed within their respective tendon sheaths with prolonged immobilization, such that particular attention is directed toward early passive motion of the toes to prevent tendon adhesions and secondary stiffness/contractures in the metatarsophalangeal joints.
  - The Kirschner wires traversing the lateral column joints are removed 6 weeks postoperatively.
- Weight bearing is not permitted until 8 to 10 weeks postoperatively, at which point weight-bearing radiographs are obtained to confirm maintenance of reduction.
  - The patient is gradually allowed to resume regular shoes, and activity is advanced as tolerated thereafter.

- The exact same postoperative protocol is followed for a primary arthrodesis.
- We do not routinely remove hardware unless symptomatic or specifically requested by the patient, in which case the implants may be removed at 1 year after surgery.

OUTCOMES

- Outcomes after open reduction and internal fixation of Lisfranc injuries are generally good overall, as patients have relatively few activity limitations. An accurate diagnosis and anatomic reduction are crucial to ensuring satisfactory results.[6]
- Outcomes for pure ligamentous patterns are less predictable after open reduction and internal fixation; these patients tend to have higher rates of posttraumatic arthritis.[6] Primary arthrodesis appears to be especially beneficial in this situation.[2,7,10,12]
- Late arthrodesis as salvage for posttraumatic arthritis provides predictable pain relief and functional improvement.[5,10]

COMPLICATIONS

- Delayed wound healing, wound dehiscence, deep infection
- Malunion or nonunion
- Late displacement (premature implant removal)
- Neurovascular compromise
- Chronic pain

REFERENCES

1. Arntz CT, Veith RG, Hansen ST. Fractures and fracture-dislocations of the tarsometatarsal joint. J Bone Joint Surg Am 1988;70A:154–162.
2. Clare MP. Lisfranc injuries. Curr Rev Musculoskelet Med 2017;10:81–85.
3. Curtis M, Myerson M, Szura B. Tarsometatarsal injuries in the athlete. Am J Sports Med 1994;21:497–502.
4. Goossens M, DeStoop N. Lisfranc's fracture-dislocations: etiology, radiology, and results of treatment. Clin Orthop Relat Res 1983;176:154–162.
5. Komenda GA, Myerson MS, Biddinger KR. Results of arthrodesis of the tarsometatarsal joints after traumatic injury. J Bone Joint Surg Am 1996;78A:1665–1676.
6. Kuo RS, Tejwani NC, DiGiovanni CW, et al. Outcome after open reduction and internal fixation of Lisfranc joint injuries. J Bone Joint Surg Am 2000;82:1609–1618.
7. Ly TV, Coetzee JC. Treatment of primarily ligamentous Lisfranc joint injuries: primary arthrodesis compared with open reduction and internal fixation: a prospective, randomized study. J Bone Joint Surg Am 2006;88A:514–520.
8. Meyer SA, Callaghan JJ, Albright JP, et al. Midfoot sprains in collegiate football players. Am J Sports Med 1994;22:392–401.
9. Myerson MS, Fisher TR, Burgess RA, et al. Fracture-dislocations of the tarsometatarsal joints: end results correlated with pathology and treatment. Foot Ankle 1986;6:225–242.
10. Reinhardt KR, Oh LS, Schottel P, et al. Treatment of Lisfranc fracture-dislocations with primary partial arthrodesis. Foot Ankle Int 2012;33:50–56.
11. Sangeorzan BJ, Veith RG, Hansen ST. Salvage of Lisfranc's tarsometatarsal joint by arthrodesis. Foot Ankle 1990;4:193–200.
12. Weatherford BM, Bohay DR, Anderson JG. Open reduction and internal fixation versus primary arthrodesis of Lisfranc injuries. Foot Ankle Clin 2017;22:1–14.

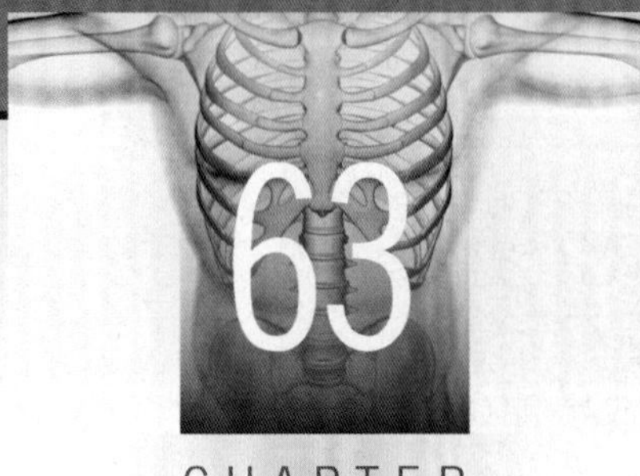

CHAPTER

Open Reduction and Internal Fixation of Jones Fractures

Max P. Michalski, John Y. Kwon, Elizabeth A. Martin, and Christopher Chiodo

DEFINITION

- Throughout the literature, the term *Jones fracture* has been used indiscriminately to describe fifth metatarsal base fractures that occur distal to the tuberosity of the bone. Various descriptions in the literature and continued use of the eponym have created historic confusion regarding definition of the Jones fracture.
- In 1984, Torg et al[42] reported a radiographic classification for these fractures without reference to the intermetatarsal articulation. They described a 1.5-cm segment of bone distal to the tuberosity in which there may be three types of fractures:
  - Type 1: acute fracture characterized by a fracture line with sharp margins and no intramedullary sclerosis
  - Type 2: delayed union with widening of the fracture line and evidence of intramedullary sclerosis
  - Type 3: nonunion with obliteration of the medullary canal by sclerotic bone
- In 1993, Lawrence and Botte[24] described three distinct fracture morphologies. This classification was popularized by Dameron[6] **(FIG 1A)**:
  - Tuberosity avulsion fractures (zone 1)
  - Metaphyseal–diaphyseal fractures (zone 2)
  - Diaphyseal stress fractures (zone 3)
- A Jones fracture is currently defined as an acute injury at the metaphyseal–diaphyseal junction of the fifth metatarsal without extension distal to the fourth–fifth intermetatarsal articulation **(FIG 2)**.

ANATOMY

- Stability of the proximal fifth metatarsal is provided by the dorsal and plantar tarsometatarsal ligaments, intermetatarsal ligaments, the lateral band of the plantar aponeurosis, and the peroneus brevis.[24]
- There are two major tendinous insertions onto the fifth metatarsal base:
  - The peroneus brevis inserts onto the dorsal aspect of the fifth metatarsal tubercle.
  - The peroneus tertius inserts onto the dorsal aspect of the metatarsal at the proximal metaphyseal–diaphyseal junction.
- The plantar fascia has a strong insertion along the plantar aspect of the fifth metatarsal tubercle.
- The proximal metaphyseal–diaphyseal junction represents a watershed area of hypovascular blood supply.
  - The diaphysis is supplied by a single-nutrient artery that enters from the medial cortex at the junction of the proximal and middle thirds of the diaphysis. The base and tuberosity are supplied by secondary epiphyseal and metaphyseal arteries **(FIG 1B)**.[38,39]
- The sural nerve is in close proximity and should be protected during the surgical procedure.
  - The sural nerve branches into the lateral dorsal cutaneous nerve and an anastomotic branch to the intermediate branch of the superficial peroneal nerve. The lateral dorsal cutaneous nerve further divides into terminal dorsolateral and dorsomedial branches, which have been shown to run inferior to the superior border of the peroneus brevis tendon.[11]
  - A cadaveric study simulating percutaneous intramedullary fixation of the fifth metatarsal reported that the dorsolateral branch of the sural nerve was within 3 mm of the screw head in 80% of specimens.[8]
- The fifth metatarsal has a distinct lateroplantar curvature. There is a proximal straight segment of the bone that has

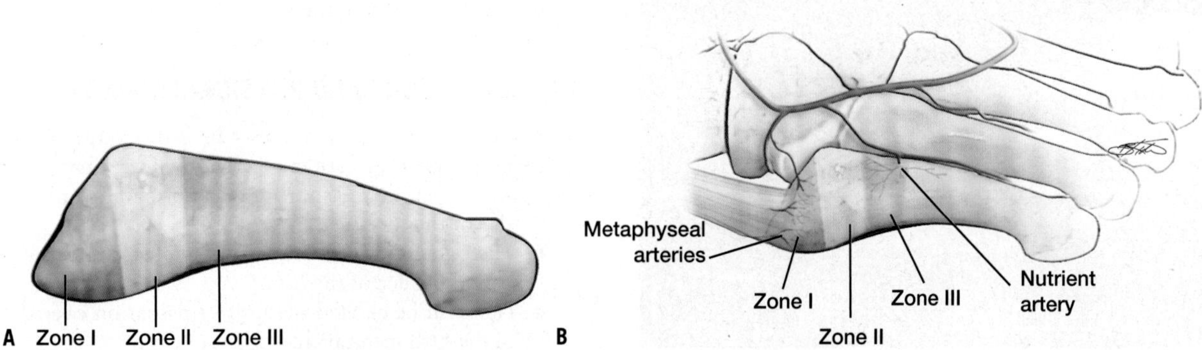

FIG 1 **A.** The three anatomic and clinical zones for fractures of the proximal fifth metatarsal. **B.** Vascular supply to the proximal fifth metatarsal with watershed supply to zone II.

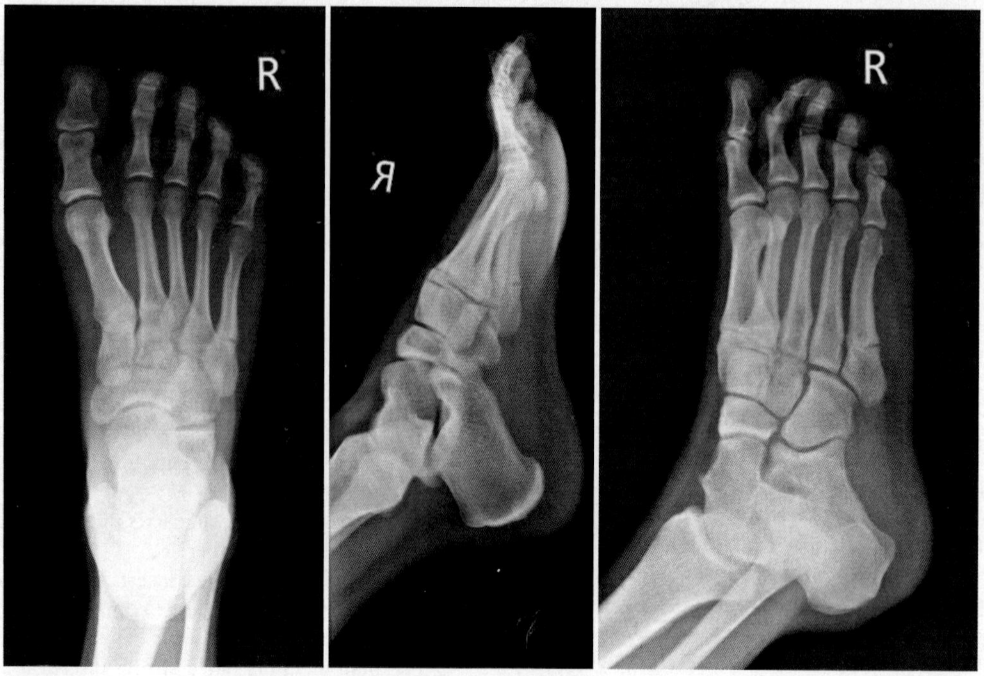

FIG 2 Acute Jones fracture. The fracture line is at the junction of zones 1 and 2; there is no cortical hypertrophy or periosteal reaction.

a mean length of 51.9 mm that can more readily accept an intramedullary screw (**FIG 3**).[31]

- The medullary canal is elliptical in cross-section, wider in the sagittal than the coronal plane.
- The average coronal and sagittal diameter of the medullary canal 40 mm distal to the tuberosity is 5.0 and 7.0 mm, respectively.
- Curvature and medullary canal diameter of the fifth metatarsal have implications when intramedullary fixation is used.

PATHOGENESIS

- In 1902, Sir Robert Jones[18] was the first to describe metatarsal fractures at the base of the fifth metatarsal as a result of "indirect violence."
  - Jones theorized, based on his own injury, that acute proximal fifth metatarsal fractures are the result of an abduction force on the forefoot while the ankle is plantarflexed.

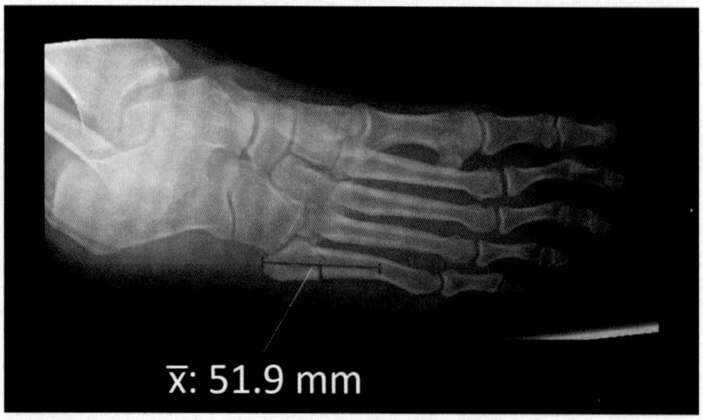

FIG 3 The average straight segment of the proximal metatarsal canal is 51.9 mm.

- Dameron[5] theorized that acute fractures are the result of tensile forces along the lateral border of the metatarsal with propagation medially between the peroneus brevis and peroneus tertius.

NATURAL HISTORY

- The natural history and outcomes of treatment are difficult to extrapolate from the current literature as many published reports included a mixture of acute metadiaphyseal and diaphyseal stress fractures.
- There is an increased risk of delayed or nonunion due to the watershed blood supply at the metaphyseal–diaphyseal junction.
- An early report by Clapper et al[4] found 100% healing of tuberosity fractures but only 72% healing in Jones fractures treated in a cast with 8 weeks of non–weight bearing. Torg et al[42] reported 93% healing with nonoperative management of Jones fractures.
- More recent studies have examined nonoperative versus operative treatment with some authors advocating surgical management even in the nonathlete given increased healing rates and faster recovery times.[29,33,35]

PATIENT HISTORY AND PHYSICAL FINDINGS

- Acutely, the patient may describe a traumatic incident or participation in an athletic activity where, after a particular maneuver, there is abrupt onset of pain over the lateral border of the foot.
  - The patient may have swelling and ecchymosis over the lateral border of the foot.
  - Pain will be elicited with direct palpation over the base of the fifth metatarsal.
- In the chronic setting, patients will frequently report a prodrome of symptoms before an acute worsening of symptoms.

- Patient-related factors may contribute to the risk of fracture, refracture, and nonunion. These may include cavovarus alignment, prominence of the fifth metatarsal head, increased body mass index, low vitamin D, and a history of narrow-width athletic shoes.[1]
- Physical examination should include the following:
  - Evaluation of hindfoot alignment. Many patients have varus alignment that predisposes to fifth metatarsal fracture.[34]
  - Palpation over the base of the fifth metatarsal. Pain in this region increases suspicion of injury.
  - Pain with palpation over the tarsometatarsal joint complex, passive dorsiflexion/plantarflexion, and attempted single-leg heel lift. Pain with of any of these findings indicates possible injury to the Lisfranc complex.
  - Examination of the lateral ankle ligamentous complex for instability

IMAGING AND OTHER DIAGNOSTIC STUDIES

- Radiographs of the affected foot, including anteroposterior (AP), lateral, and internal oblique views, are sufficient to diagnose an acute Jones fracture.
  - Location of fracture is used to distinguish between tuberosity avulsions and Jones fractures.
  - Sclerotic changes help delineate between acute versus chronic stress injury.
- Radiographic parameters:
  - AP radiograph: Elite athletes with Jones fractures have been found to have decreased talar-first, talar-second, and talar-fifth metatarsal angles.[2]
  - Oblique radiograph: A plantar gap greater than 1 mm has prognostic value with an increased likelihood of failing surgical intervention in patients with stress fractures.[25,26]
  - Lateral radiograph: Evaluate calcaneal pitch and Meary angle to evaluate cavovarus alignment.[34]
- Weight-bearing radiographs of the affected foot, if possible, are helpful to rule out an occult Lisfranc injury.
- Computed tomography and magnetic resonance imaging are typically unnecessary but sometimes used to evaluate for concomitant pathology or subsequent fracture healing.

DIFFERENTIAL DIAGNOSIS

- Tuberosity avulsion fracture
- Lisfranc sprain or subluxation
- Painful os peroneum syndrome[40]
- Cuboid fracture
- Lateral ankle ligamentous injury
- Peroneal tendon subluxation/rupture

NONOPERATIVE MANAGEMENT

- Recent literature has shown prolonged union rates and time to weight bearing with nonoperative treatment compared to surgical intervention.
  - The traditional nonoperative protocol involved non-weight bearing in a short-leg cast or CAM boot for 6 to 8 weeks followed by progressive weight bearing in a walker boot for an additional 4 to 6 weeks.[36]
    - More aggressive nonoperative protocols allow return to weight bearing as early as 2 weeks for acute zone II injuries.
- One pooled analysis of 26 studies (630 fractures) reported union rates with nonoperative treatment of 76% and 44% in acute and delayed presentations, respectively.[35]
- Low-pulsed ultrasound or pulsed electromagnetic stimulation may be considered as an adjunct to augment healing in operative and nonoperative protocols.[15,41]

SURGICAL MANAGEMENT

- The indications for surgical fixation of an acute Jones fracture continue to evolve.
  - Surgery has been advocated for elite athletes, fracture displacement greater than 2 to 3 mm, no progression of healing after 3 months of conservative treatment, sclerosis at the fracture site, and those not willing to accept nonoperative treatment.[3]
- High-performance athletes or individuals desiring a quicker return to activity may benefit from intramedullary screw fixation, as this provides a more predictable and shorter recovery period.
  - This treatment also eliminates possibility of two recovery periods if nonunion develops from nonoperative treatment.[36]
    - Hunt and Anderson[17] reported a series of nonunions and refractures in elite athletes. In this series, five elite athletes attempted nonoperative treatment for an average of 49.6 weeks before eventually undergoing operative fixation.
  - Prior reports show high union rates and low complication rates with acute fixation.[7,28,33]
- Multiple fixation techniques have been described including intramedullary screws, tension band wiring, lateral hook plating, plantar lateral plating, and inlay grafting without fixation.
- A brief summary of biomechanical and clinical data comparing fixation techniques and implants
  - No significant difference in load to failure when comparing 4.5- and 5.5-mm screws.[37]
  - Screws less than 4.5 mm have been associated with increased risk of delayed and nonunion.[12]
  - Conventional partially threaded screws improved fracture site compression and less angulation but offered no improvement in fracture site stiffness compared with tapered variable pitch screws.[32]
  - Plantar lateral plating has higher cycles to failure and less plantar gapping compared to 5.5 mm cannulated screws in vitro.[16]
  - Intramedullary screw fixation provides greater bending stiffness and resistance to early torsional loading compared to lateral hook plating.[9]
  - No difference found in union rates or clinical results between Jones fracture–specific screw and traditional screws.[27]

Goals of Treatment

- Reduction of fracture
- Minimize soft tissue trauma.
- Protect at-risk structures.
  - Sural nerve, peroneus brevis tendon, peroneus tertius tendon, lateral anchor of extensor retinaculum
- Reinforce postoperative weight-bearing precautions.

- Prevent iatrogenic complications.
  - Malreduction
  - Inadequate hardware length (failure to cross fracture site with intramedullary screw threads)
  - Failure to débride sclerotic bone in nonunion
  - Intraoperative fracture

Positioning

- The patient may be positioned lateral (described in this chapter) or supine on a radiolucent table.
  - Lateral position allows the surgeon to have his or her hands free with the foot stabilized.
- A C-arm image intensifier is used to assist in the operative procedure.
  - Mini C-arm can be inverted to be used as an operating surface.
  - Standard C-arm can be used and should be positioned contralateral to the surgeon **(FIG 4)**.
- A tourniquet is not required but may be used based on surgeon preference.

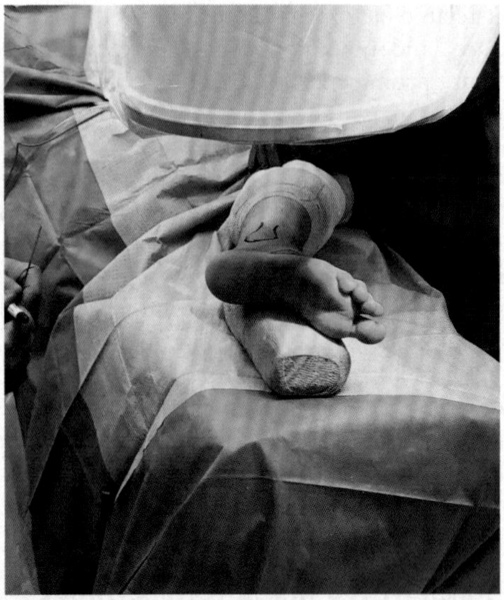

FIG 4 Lateral positioning with standard C-arm positioned on the contralateral side.

TECHNIQUES

PERCUTANEOUS INTRAMEDULLARY SCREW FIXATION

Incision and Dissection

- Use a guidewire and fluoroscopy to identify the projected screw trajectory **(TECH FIG 1A,B)**.
- The incision should begin approximately 2 cm proximal to the tip of the fifth metatarsal tuberosity, in line with the previously identified screw trajectory **(TECH FIG 1C)**.
- Blunt dissection is used to expose the tuberosity and protect the sural nerve **(TECH FIG 1D)**.
- The sural nerve and peroneus brevis tendons may be encountered in the wound and should be protected.

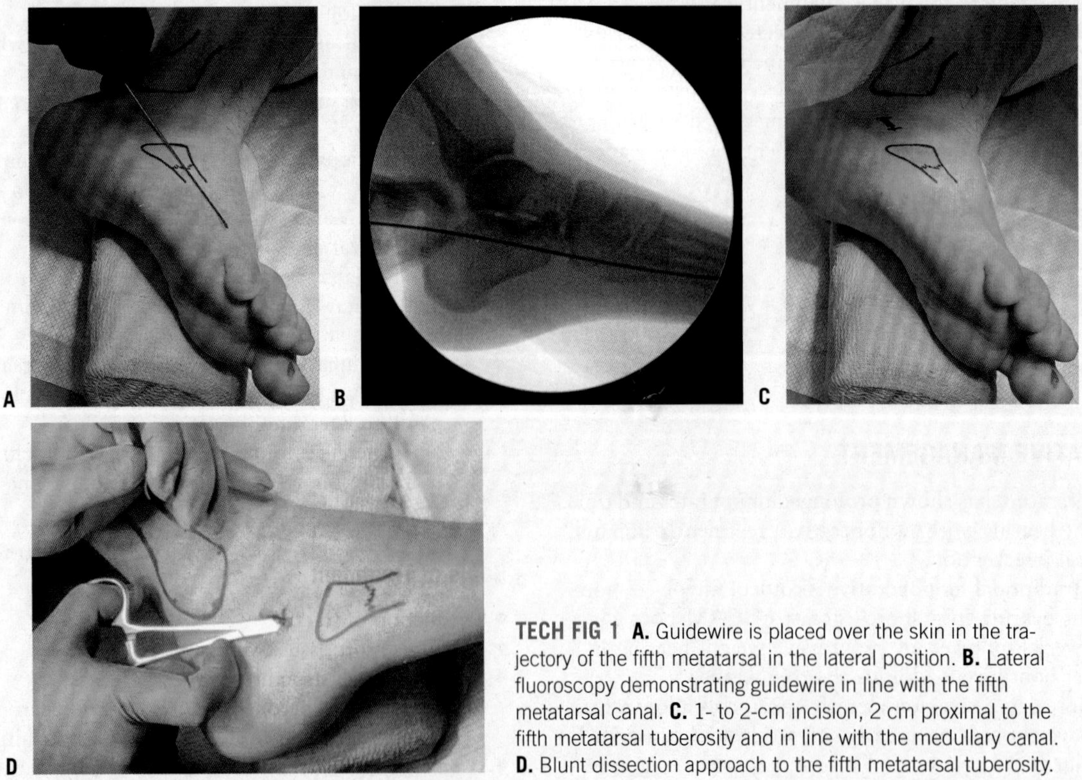

TECH FIG 1 A. Guidewire is placed over the skin in the trajectory of the fifth metatarsal in the lateral position. **B.** Lateral fluoroscopy demonstrating guidewire in line with the fifth metatarsal canal. **C.** 1- to 2-cm incision, 2 cm proximal to the fifth metatarsal tuberosity and in line with the medullary canal. **D.** Blunt dissection approach to the fifth metatarsal tuberosity.

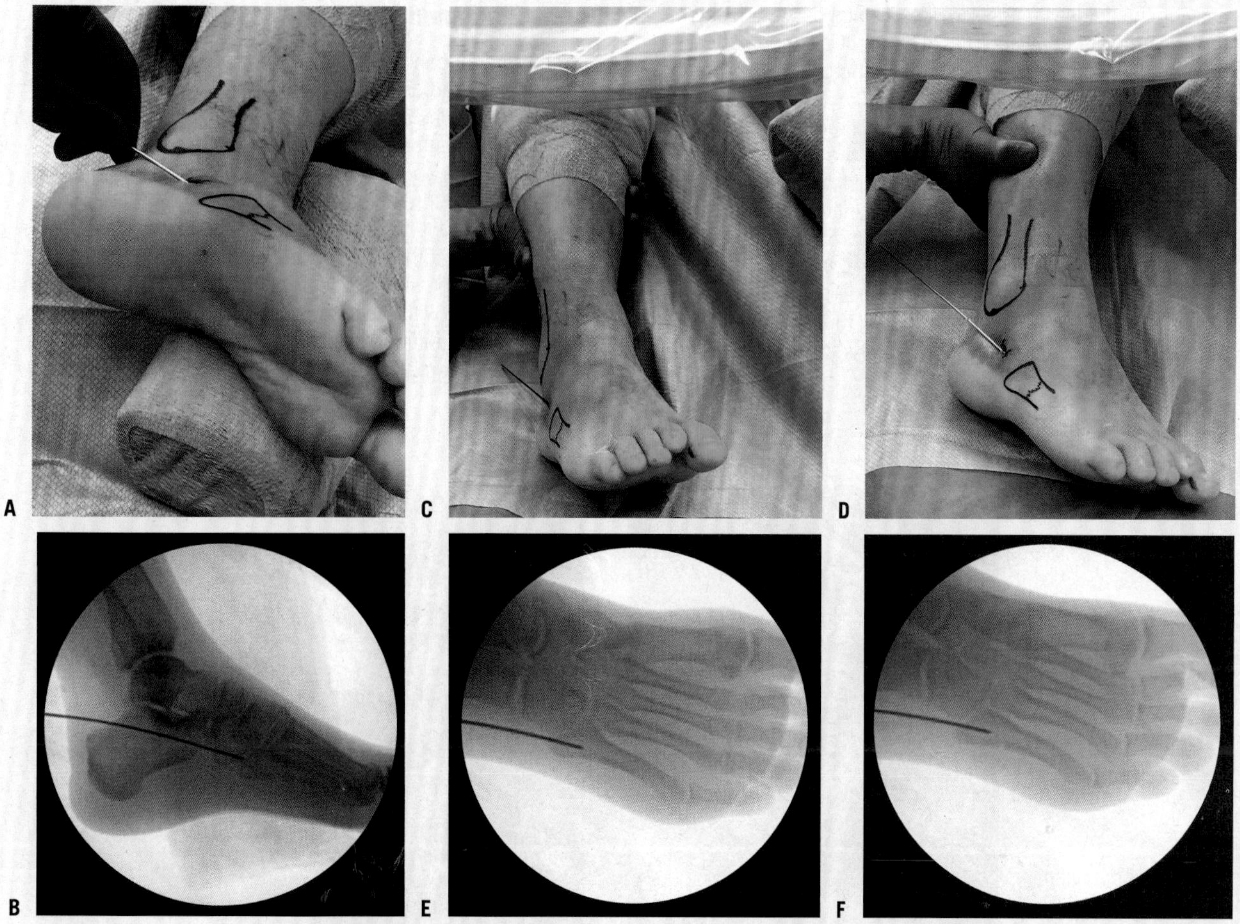

TECH FIG 2 A. Insertion of the guidewire. **B.** Lateral fluoroscopic image confirming appropriate start site. **C,D.** Positioning for AP and internal oblique fluoroscopy without movement of the C-arm. **E,F.** AP and internal oblique fluoroscopy of the guidewire entering at the "high and inside" start site.

Guidewire Placement, Cannulated Drilling, and Tap Insertion

- The correct entry site is in line with the medullary canal, just medial to the tip of the tuberosity.
- This is typically in the dorsomedial or "high and inside" aspect of the tuberosity.
- The correct starting position is confirmed with a guidewire using fluoroscopy **(TECH FIG 2A,B)**.
- Gently advance the guidewire with a mallet or oscillating wire driver to secure the insertion site and then obtain oblique and AP radiographs **(TECH FIG 2C–F)**.
- Advance the guidewire down the medullary canal. This should be performed under biplanar C-arm guidance to ensure proper positioning and length **(TECH FIG 3)**.
  - Technique tip: Gently advance the guidewire into the cortex without perforating, this will prevent the guidewire from backing out while drilling and tapping.

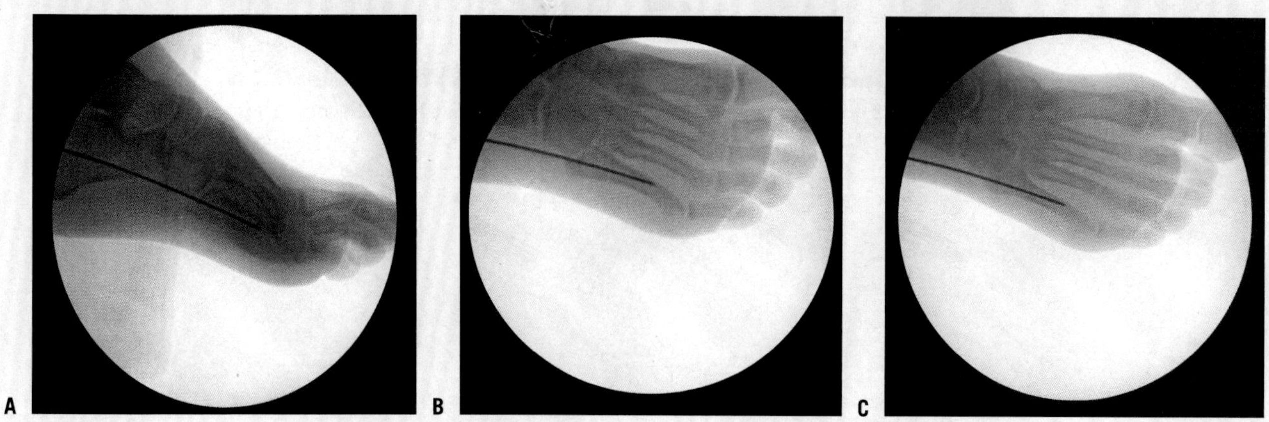

TECH FIG 3 A–C. Advancement of the guidewire utilizing lateral, internal oblique, and AP fluoroscopy.

- Leaving the guidewire in place, insert a soft tissue protector.
- Insert cannulated drill and drill to depth of planned screw using frequent fluoroscopic images to ensure no cortical perforation **(TECH FIG 4A,B)**.
  - Take a fluoroscopic image during drill removal to ensure the guidewire is not being retracted with the drill.
- Advance the cannulated tap over the guidewire, starting with a smaller size and increasing diameter until there is adequate distal bite. Often, this is characterized by rotation of the forefoot with advancement of the tap **(TECH FIG 4C,D)**.
  - Frequently assess the fracture reduction while tapping as significant gapping can occur during this step.[19]
  - Consider placement of a temporary Kirschner wire to prevent iatrogenic gapping.

Screw Placement

- Screw length can be easily approximated by overlying the screw on the skin and using fluoroscopy **(TECH FIG 5A,B)**.
  - This provides a more accurate length estimation and can be used to ensure all threads will cross the fracture site.
- The guidewire and soft tissue protector are removed, and a solid, partially threaded screw is inserted **(TECH FIG 5C–E)**.
  - Use frequent fluoroscopy to monitor fracture reduction and confirm that there is no cortical perforation.
    - Once the screw is seated, obtain AP, lateral, and oblique images with the screwdriver in the screw. If removed, it can be difficult to localize the screw head if advancement is required.

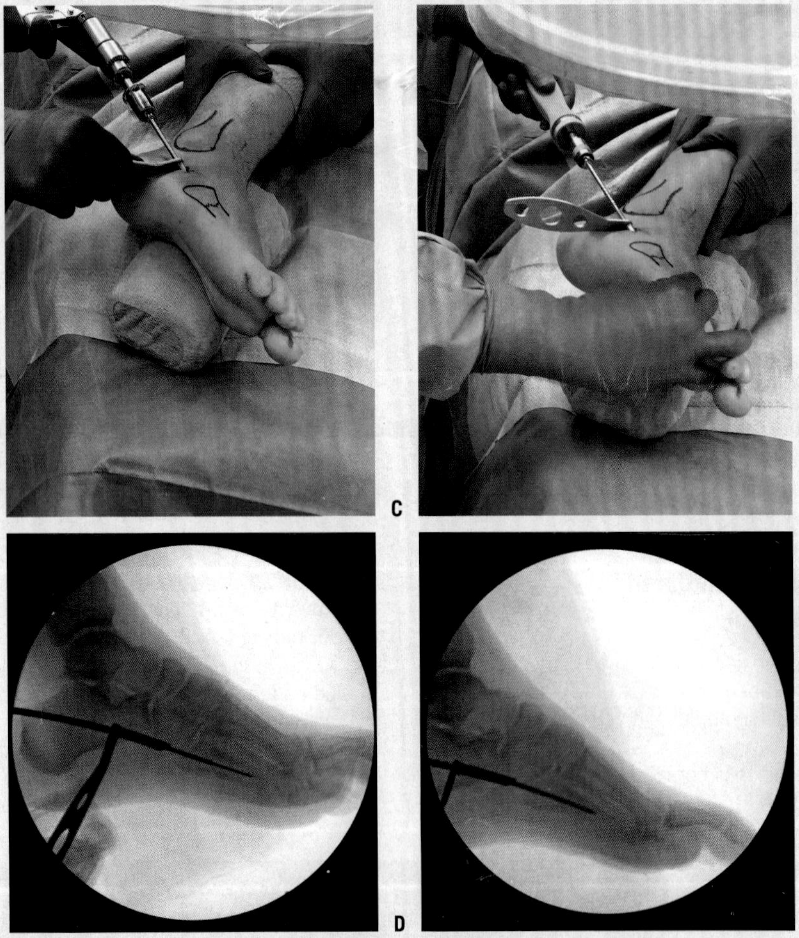

A B C D

TECH FIG 4 **A,B.** Insertion of the soft tissue protector and cannulated drill bit under fluoroscopy. **C,D.** Tapping the medullary canal under fluoroscopic guidance.

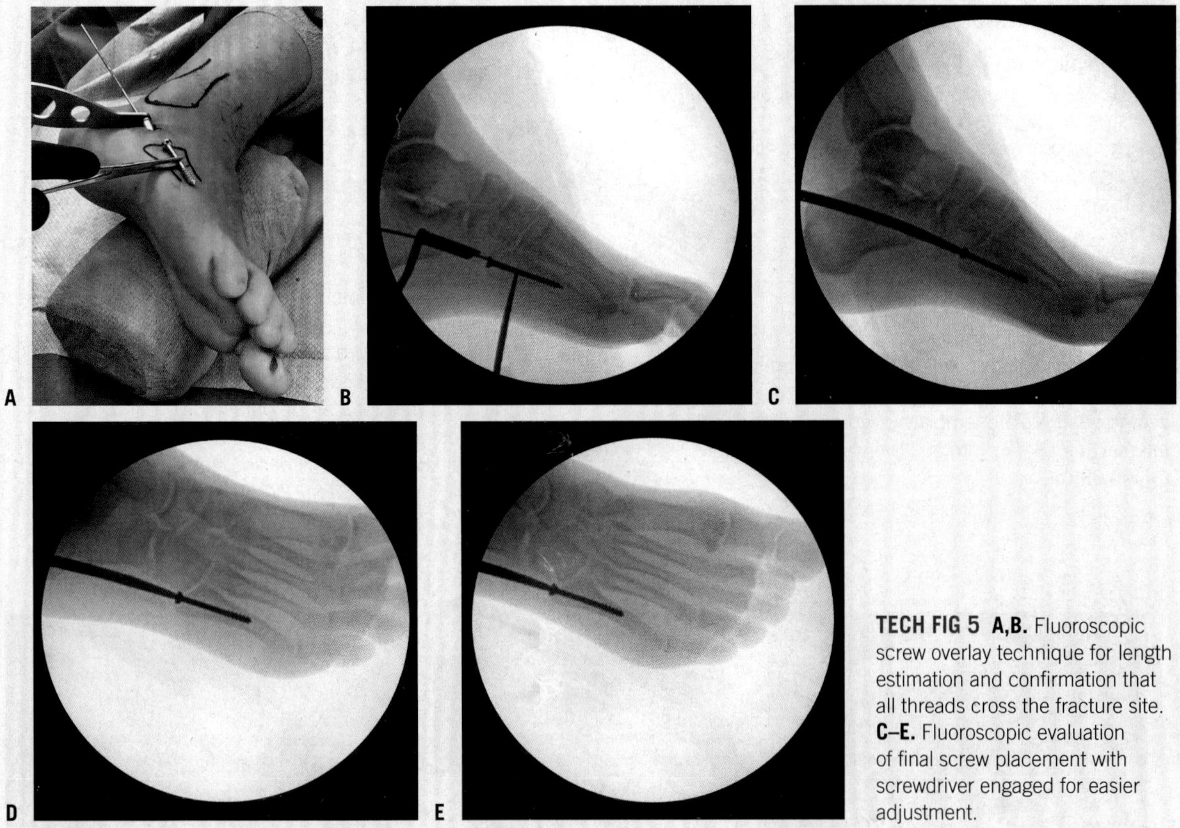

TECH FIG 5 A,B. Fluoroscopic screw overlay technique for length estimation and confirmation that all threads cross the fracture site. **C–E.** Fluoroscopic evaluation of final screw placement with screwdriver engaged for easier adjustment.

PERCUTANEOUS INTRAMEDULLARY SCREW FIXATION WITH LOCAL BONE GRAFT

- The procedure is performed as described for percutaneous intramedullary screw fixation.[23]
- Once the medullary canal has been overdrilled over the guidewire, the wire is removed.
- A slender curette is advanced to the depth of the fracture and manipulated to débride sclerotic bone and transfer local autograft to the fracture site.
- Care should be taken to limit procurement of bone to within 7 mm of the fracture site.
- Once the local bone grafting has been completed, the wire is reintroduced into the canal.
- The intramedullary screw is placed as described for percutaneous intramedullary screw fixation.
- Alternatively, another technique is to make a secondary incision directly over the nonunion site to directly débride the nonunion and bone graft the site, which is described in the following text.

OPEN REDUCTION INTERNAL PLATE FIXATION WITH PLATE FIXATION AND CALCANEAL BONE GRAFTING FOR NONUNION

Calcaneal Bone Graft

- A 1-cm incision along posterolateral heel
- Blunt dissection down to calcaneus to avoid iatrogenic injury to the sural nerve
- Bone graft harvester inserted or drilled into calcaneus to obtain cancellous autograft
  - If more graft is needed, reinsert graft harvester at a different trajectory to gather more cancellous bone.
- Alternatively, a 4.5-mm drill guide can be used to obtain cancellous cores for grafting.

Incision and Dissection

- Localize the nonunion with fluoroscopy.
- Make a 3- to 4-cm incision along lateral border of the fifth metatarsal overlying the nonunion site.
  - Take caution not to injure the sural nerve.
- Identify and débride nonunion site **(TECH FIG 6A)**.
  - A 1.5-mm drill bit may be used to drill through sclerotic bone.

Reduction and Plate Insertion

- Place graft into nonunion site.
- Obtain reduction with a pointed reduction clamp and verify on multiplanar fluoroscopy.
- Place and secure plate template or guide onto the fifth metatarsal and secure with an olive wire and guidewire **(TECH FIG 6B,C)**.
- In this illustrated case, a hook plate was used.
  - Intramedullary screw fixation is an acceptable alternative.
- With the hook plate guide secured, predrill the plate hooks with a drill pin.
- Remove the hook plate guide and distal olive wire, leaving the guidewire in place.
- Insert the hook plate using the guidewire for the proper trajectory.
  - Impact hooks into the tuberosity to generate compression of the fracture site.
- Place an olive wire into the distal plate and remove the hook plate inserter.
- Overdrill the guidewire with a cannulated drill and insert a cannulated partially threaded screw for further compression.
- Further compression can be obtained by removing the olive wire and using a dynamic compression hole.
- Insert additional screws as desired for stability and obtain final fluoroscopic images **(TECH FIG 6D–F)**.

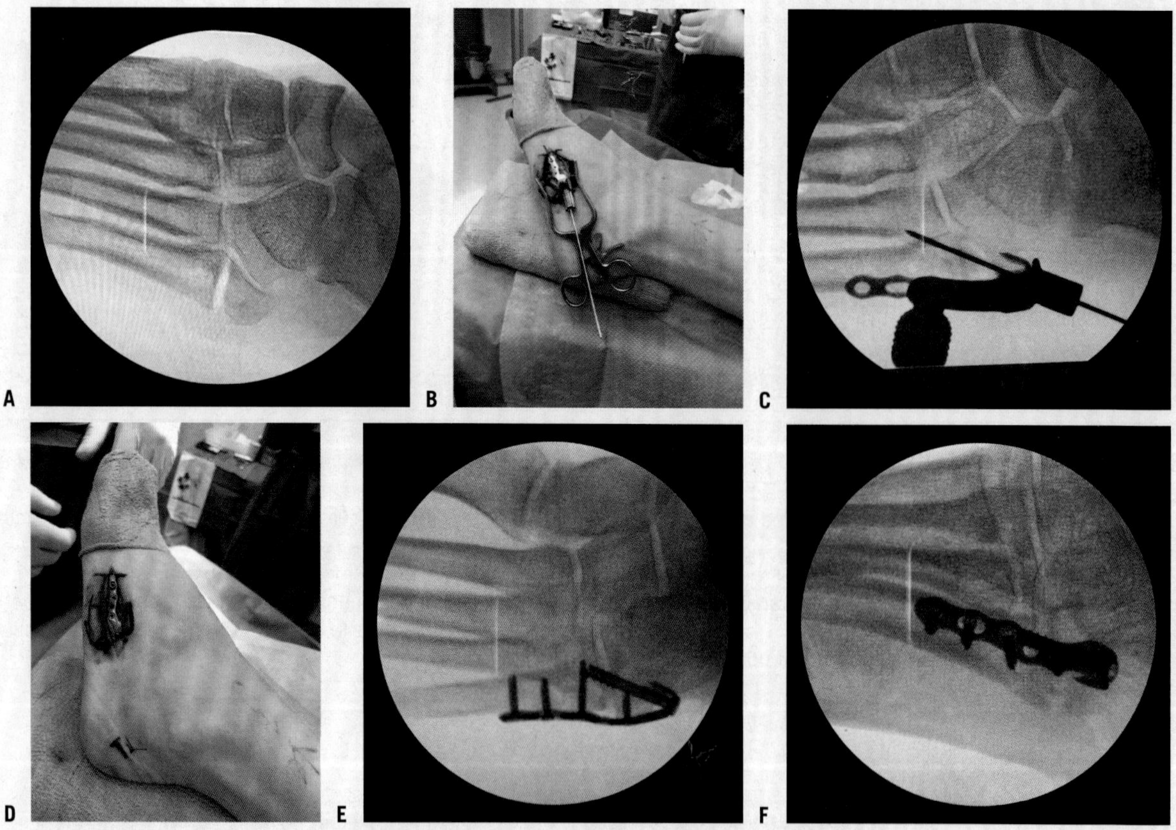

TECH FIG 6 **A.** Fluoroscopic view of nonunion site following débridement. **B,C.** Clinical and fluoroscopic view of guidewire insertion through plate template. **D–F.** Clinical and fluoroscopic images of final plate fixation.

Pearls and Pitfalls

Indications	• Current literature supports expanding surgical indications for fifth metatarsal fractures.
Deformity	• Concomitant surgical correction of hindfoot varus may be indicated if present.
Start Point	• A "high and inside" guide pin start point on the tuberosity is ideal.
Intramedullary Screws	• Use the largest diameter screw possible to fill cortex and obtain endosteal purchase without fracturing the cortex. • Screws should not extend past curve of metatarsal as this may cause fracture distraction and/or iatrogenic distal fracture. • Partially threaded screws should have all threads cross the fracture site.
Postoperative	• Refrain from return to athletics until fracture has healed symptomatically and radiographically.

POSTOPERATIVE CARE

- Traditional protocol
  - Immobilization in a walker boot and non–weight bearing for 6 weeks
    - Casting can be implemented if patient compliance is a concern.
  - During this period, range of motion and gentle strengthening may be allowed.
  - Progressive weight bearing and boot removal are allowed when radiographic evidence of healing is observed.
  - Return to full activity, especially competitive athletics, is allowed only when complete healing is observed on radiographs in AP, lateral, and oblique planes, and when symptoms allow.
- More aggressive protocols have been described with weight bearing as early as 2 weeks[20] to 4 weeks.[30]
  - Return to high-impact activities after clinical union but prior to radiographic union increases the risk for intramedullary screw failure.[22]
- Functional bracing or orthosis is recommended for individuals returning to athletic activities.[14]
  - Clinical hindfoot varus may be managed postoperatively with lateral hindfoot wedge orthotic inserts to correct the deformity and reduce the stress on the lateral aspect of the midfoot.[34]
- In athletes, consideration should be given to leaving screws in place until after the end of the athletic career to prevent refracture.[12]
- Pulsed electromagnetic fields for treatment of Jones fracture nonunions have been shown to decrease time to radiographic union from 14.7 to 8.9 weeks compared to placebo in addition to increased local growth factors.[41]

OUTCOMES

- Portland et al[33] treated 15 patients, including nonathletes, with acute Jones fractures and achieved 100% union at an average of 6.25 weeks.
- Union rates in a pooled analysis of 26 studies (22 level IV and 1 randomized controlled trial)[35]
  - Acute fractures: operative (96%), nonoperative (76%)
  - Delayed unions: operative (97%), nonoperative (44%)
  - Nonunions: operative (97%)
- Return to play in elite athletes
  - 25 National Football League players treated with intramedullary screw, demineralize bone matrix (DBM), bone marrow aspirate concentration (BMAC), and bone stimulator[21]
    - 100% return to play
    - In season, surgery had average return to play at 8.7 weeks.
  - 21 athletes with refractures treated with intramedullary screw, autograft, and augments[17]
    - 100% union
    - Return to previous level of competition at 12.3 weeks
  - 28 Union of European Football Associations soccer players treated with intramedullary screw[10]
    - 76% union, average return to play 80 days
    - 25% refracture rate

COMPLICATIONS

- Nonunion
  - Strict weight-bearing precautions in both operative and nonoperative treatment are important to prevent nonunion.
  - Use of a screw less than 4.5 mm has been associated with an increased risk of nonunion.[12]
  - Elite athletes returning to high impact prior to radiographic union has been associated with nonunion and refracture.
  - When treating nonunions, undersized inlay grafts and incomplete débridement of sclerotic bone is associated with failure.[43]
- Sural neurapraxia
  - Temporary neurapraxia has been reported but resolved in less than 6 weeks.[1,13]
- Deep infection
- Painful hardware

REFERENCES

1. Bernstein DT, Mitchell RJ, McCulloch PC, et al. Treatment of proximal fifth metatarsal fractures and refractures with plantar plating in elite athletes. Foot Ankle Int 2018;39:1410–1415. doi:10.1177/1071100718791835.
2. Carreira DS, Sandilands SM. Radiographic factors and effect of fifth metatarsal Jones and diaphyseal stress fractures on participation in the NFL. Foot Ankle Int 2013;34:518–522. doi:10.1177/1071100713477616.
3. Chuckpaiwong B, Queen RM, Easley ME, et al. Distinguishing Jones and proximal diaphyseal fractures of the fifth metatarsal. Clin Orthop Relat Res 2008;466:1966–1970. doi:10.1007/s11999-008-0222-7.

4. Clapper MF, O'Brien TJ, Lyons PM. Fractures of the fifth metatarsal. Analysis of a fracture registry. Clin Orthop Relat Res 1995;(315): 238–241.
5. Dameron TB Jr. Fractures and anatomical variations of the proximal portion of the fifth metatarsal. J Bone Joint Surg Am 1975;57: 788–792.
6. Dameron TB Jr. Fractures of the proximal fifth metatarsal: selecting the best treatment option. J Am Acad Orthop Surg 1995;3: 110–114.
7. DeLee JC, Evans JP, Julian J. Stress fracture of the fifth metatarsal. Am J Sports Med 1983;11:349–353. doi:10.1177/036354658301100513.
8. Donley BG, McCollum MJ, Murphy GA, et al. Risk of sural nerve injury with intramedullary screw fixation of fifth metatarsal fractures: a cadaver study. Foot Ankle Int 1999;20:182–184. doi:10.1177/107110079902000308.
9. Duplantier NL, Mitchell RJ, Zambrano S, et al. A biomechanical comparison of fifth metatarsal Jones fracture fixation methods. Am J Sports Med 2018;46:1220–1227. doi:10.1177/0363546517753376.
10. Ekstrand J, van Dijk CN. Fifth metatarsal fractures among male professional footballers: a potential career-ending disease. Br J Sports Med 2013;47:754–758. doi:10.1136/bjsports-2012-092096.
11. Fansa AM, Smyth NA, Murawski CD, et al. The lateral dorsal cutaneous branch of the sural nerve: clinical importance of the surgical approach to proximal fifth metatarsal fracture fixation. Am J Sports Med 2012;40:1895–1898. doi:10.1177/0363546512448320.
12. Glasgow MT, Naranja RJ Jr, Glasgow SG, et al. Analysis of failed surgical management of fractures of the base of the fifth metatarsal distal to the tuberosity: the Jones fracture. Foot Ankle Int 1996;17: 449–457. doi:10.1177/107110079601700803.
13. Habbu RA, Marsh RS, Anderson JG, et al. Closed intramedullary screw fixation for nonunion of fifth metatarsal Jones fracture. Foot Ankle Int 2011;32:603–608. doi:10.3113/FAI.2011.0603.
14. Hartog C, Centmaier-Molnar V, Patzwahl R, et al. Bizarre parosteal osteochondromatous proliferation of the metatarsal bone [in German]. Orthopade 2016;45:901–905. doi:10.1007/s00132-016-3317-y.
15. Holmes GB Jr. Treatment of delayed unions and nonunions of the proximal fifth metatarsal with pulsed electromagnetic fields. Foot Ankle Int 1994;15:552–556. doi:10.1177/107110079401501006.
16. Huh J, Glisson RR, Matsumoto T, et al. Biomechanical comparison of intramedullary screw versus low-profile plate fixation of a Jones fracture. Foot Ankle Int 2016;37:411–418. doi:10.1177 /1071100715619678.
17. Hunt KJ, Anderson RB. Treatment of Jones fracture nonunions and refractures in the elite athlete: outcomes of intramedullary screw fixation with bone grafting. Am J Sports Med 2011;39:1948–1954. doi:10.1177/0363546511408868.
18. Jones R. I. Fracture of the base of the fifth metatarsal bone by indirect violence. Ann Surg 1902;35:697–700.2.
19. Kaiser PB, Riedel MD, Qudsi RA, et al. Iatrogenic fracture gapping during fixation of Jones fractures: anatomic and mechanical considerations in a cadaveric model. Injury 2018;49:1485–1490. doi:10.1016/j.injury.2018.04.024.
20. Lareau CR, Anderson RB. Jones fractures: pathophysiology and treatment. JBJS Rev 2015;3:01874474-201503070-00004. doi:10.2106/ JBJS.RVW.N.00100.
21. Lareau CR, Hsu AR, Anderson RB. Return to play in National Football League players after operative jones fracture treatment. Foot Ankle Int 2016;37:8–16. doi:10.1177/1071100715603983.
22. Larson CM, Almekinders LC, Taft TN, et al. Intramedullary screw fixation of Jones fractures. Analysis of failure. Am J Sports Med 2002;30:55–60. doi:10.1177/03635465020300012301.
23. Lawrence SJ. Technique tip: local bone grafting technique for Jones fracture management with intramedullary screw fixation. Foot Ankle Int 2004;25:920–921. doi:10.1177/107110070402501213.
24. Lawrence SJ, Botte MJ. Jones' fractures and related fractures of the proximal fifth metatarsal. Foot Ankle 1993;14:358–365.
25. Lee KT, Park YU, Jegal H, et al. Prognostic classification of fifth metatarsal stress fracture using plantar gap. Foot Ankle Int 2013;34: 691–696. doi:10.1177/1071100713475349.
26. Lee KT, Park YU, Young KW, et al. The plantar gap: another prognostic factor for fifth metatarsal stress fracture. Am J Sports Med 2011;39:2206–2211. doi:10.1177/0363546511414856.
27. Metzl J, Olson K, Davis WH, et al. A clinical and radiographic comparison of two hardware systems used to treat jones fracture of the fifth metatarsal. Foot Ankle Int 2013;34:956–961. doi:10.1177/1071100713483100.
28. Mindrebo N, Shelbourne KD, Van Meter CD, et al. Outpatient percutaneous screw fixation of the acute Jones fracture. Am J Sports Med 1993;21:720–723. doi:10.1177/036354659302100514.
29. Mologne TS, Lundeen JM, Clapper MF, et al. Early screw fixation versus casting in the treatment of acute Jones fractures. Am J Sports Med 2005;33:970–975. doi:10.1177/0363546504272262.
30. Murawski CD, Kennedy JG. Percutaneous internal fixation of proximal fifth metatarsal jones fractures (zones II and III) with Charlotte Carolina screw and bone marrow aspirate concentrate: an outcome study in athletes. Am J Sports Med 2011;39:1295–1301. doi:10.1177/0363546510393306.
31. Ochenjele G, Ho B, Switaj PJ, et al. Radiographic study of the fifth metatarsal for optimal intramedullary screw fixation of Jones fracture. Foot Ankle Int 2015;36:293–301. doi:10.1177/1071100714553467.
32. Orr JD, Glisson RR, Nunley JA. Jones fracture fixation: a biomechanical comparison of partially threaded screws versus tapered variable pitch screws. Am J Sports Med 2012;40:691–698. doi:10.1177/0363546511428870.
33. Portland G, Kelikian A, Kodros S. Acute surgical management of Jones' fractures. Foot Ankle Int 2003;24:829–833. doi:10.1177/107110070302401104.
34. Raikin SM, Slenker N, Ratigan B. The association of a varus hindfoot and fracture of the fifth metatarsal metaphyseal-diaphyseal junction: the Jones fracture. Am J Sports Med 2008;36:1367–1372. doi:10.1177/0363546508314401.
35. Roche AJ, Calder JD. Treatment and return to sport following a Jones fracture of the fifth metatarsal: a systematic review. Knee Surg Sports Traumatol Arthrosc 2013;21:1307–1315. doi:10.1007/s00167-012-2138-8.
36. Rosenberg GA, Sferra JJ. Treatment strategies for acute fractures and nonunions of the proximal fifth metatarsal. J Am Acad Orthop Surg 2000;8:332–338.
37. Shah SN, Knoblich GO, Lindsey DP, et al. Intramedullary screw fixation of proximal fifth metatarsal fractures: a biomechanical study. Foot Ankle Int 2001;22:581–584. doi:10.1177/107110070102200709.
38. Shereff MJ, Yang QM, Kummer FJ, et al. Vascular anatomy of the fifth metatarsal. Foot Ankle 1991;11:350–353.
39. Smith JW, Arnoczky SP, Hersh A. The intraosseous blood supply of the fifth metatarsal: implications for proximal fracture healing. Foot Ankle 1992;13:143–152.
40. Sobel M, Pavlov H, Geppert MJ, et al. Painful os peroneum syndrome: a spectrum of conditions responsible for plantar lateral foot pain. Foot Ankle Int 1994;15:112–124. doi:10.1177/107110079401500306.
41. Streit A, Watson BC, Granata JD, et al. Effect on clinical outcome and growth factor synthesis with adjunctive use of pulsed electromagnetic fields for fifth metatarsal nonunion fracture: a double-blind randomized study. Foot Ankle Int 2016;37:919–923. doi:10.1177/1071100716652621.
42. Torg JS, Balduini FC, Zelko RR, et al. Fractures of the base of the fifth metatarsal distal to the tuberosity. Classification and guidelines for non-surgical and surgical management. J Bone Joint Surg Am 1984;66:209–214.
43. Wright RW, Fischer DA, Shively RA, et al. Refracture of proximal fifth metatarsal (Jones) fracture after intramedullary screw fixation in athletes. Am J Sports Med 2000;28:732–736. doi:10.1177/03635 465000280051901.

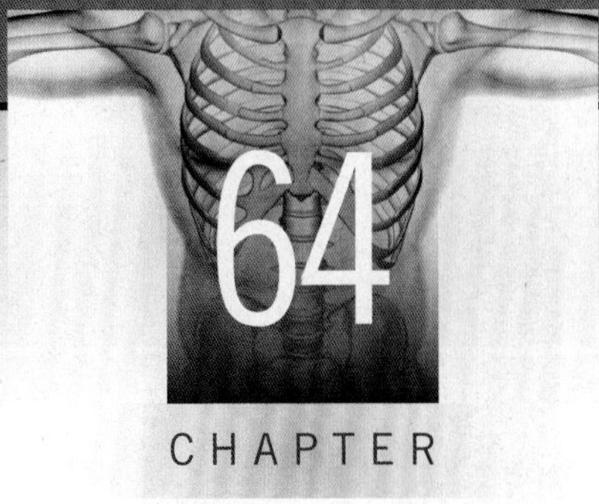

Foot Amputations

Israel Dudkiewicz, Martin M. Malawer, and Jacob Bickels

BACKGROUND

- Malignant tumors around the foot requiring amputation are rare and pose a considerable challenge because of the impact of surgical planning on functional outcomes in terms of weight bearing, stability, and gait.
- The functional anatomy of the foot is based on a complexed three-dimensional structure of multiple small bones with unique structure, ligaments, muscles, and neurovascular bundles, all of which are packed in a small volume. Therefore, even resection of a relatively small area may have a profound impact on function.
- The foot is composed of functional compartments that, unlike the thigh and leg, are not defined by thick fascial walls. Malignant tumors usually cross these compartments, and their wide resection may end in a devastating functional result.
- Level of amputation done for a high-grade sarcoma should carefully be planned to achieve wide margins of resection; marginal margins are unacceptable **(FIG 1)**. As a rule, distal amputations have a lesser impact on gait.
  - Special attention should be given to preserve the maximal possible length of the first ray, which bears approximately 50% of the weight with toe-off during each gait cycle.

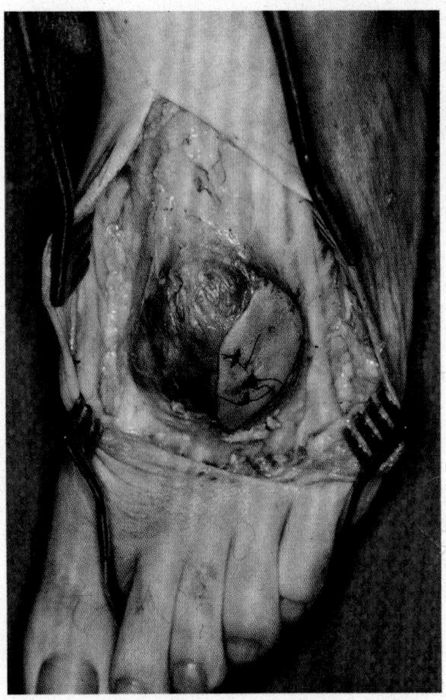

FIG 1 Soft tissue sarcoma of the foot. Wide margins of resection, 2 cm from the closest tumoral margin, can be achieved by Lisfranc or Chopart amputation.

ANATOMIC AND FUNCTIONAL CONSIDERATIONS

- The extent of a foot amputation that is done for oncologic reasons is first dictated by the anatomic boundaries of the tumor. However, familiarity with the unique biomechanical complexity of the foot may modify the line of resection and technique of reconstruction to minimize the impairment of normal gait **(FIG 2)**.
- The human foot is unique because its various bones and supporting ligamentous elements form stiff arches, longitudinal and transverse as well as having flexible components: The first ray provides the support required for the toe-off, whereas the integrity of the mobile fifth ray is essential for walking on an uneven ground.
  - Amputation of the metatarsal heads or any proximal component may result in altered weight bearing and loss of cosmesis, most of which can be managed by the use of modified shoes and orthoses.
- Resection of the middle rays results in insignificant loss of function and acceptable cosmesis **(FIG 3)**. The only net result is narrowing of the forefoot, which can be easily compensated for with shoe modifications.
- Transverse amputations done proximal to the insertion site of the tibialis anterior tendon may result in an unbalanced contracture of the Achilles tendon and equinus deformity of the foot.
  - An amputation at the Lisfranc joint will preserve the dorsiflexors and the plantar flexors.
  - These amputation levels usually allow reasonable functional but require shoe-wear modifications and forefoot fillers.
  - If the metatarsal bases can be preserved using a transmetatarsal amputation, the functional outcome is improved.
- The transverse tarsal joint (Chopart joint) includes the talonavicular and calcaneocuboid joints.
  - An amputation at this level preserves the plantar flexors but sacrifices the dorsiflexors, often resulting in an equinus contracture due to unopposed action of the Achilles tendon.
  - The advantage of a Chopart amputation over a Syme amputation is the maintenance of hindfoot height. This is an end-bearing residual limb, and the patient can negotiate short distances without modified shoe wear or prosthetic fitting. Syme amputation, on the other hand, necessitates the use of a prosthesis for weight bearing and ambulation. These patients, however, may benefit better reciprocal gait when compared to those who underwent Chopart amputation.

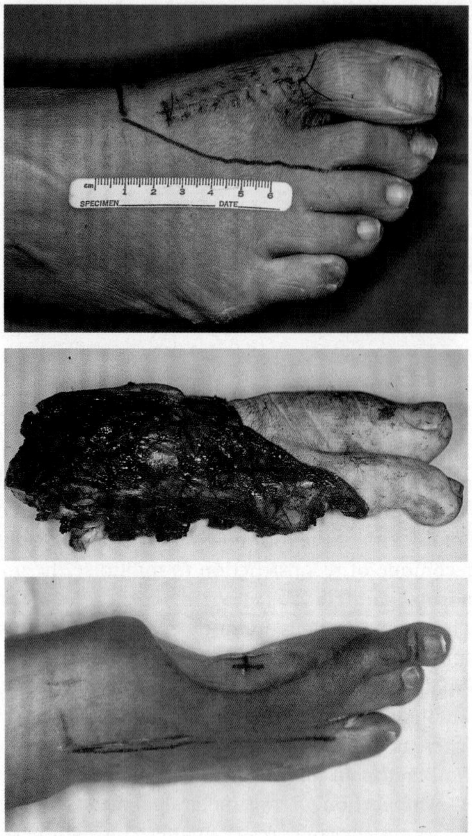

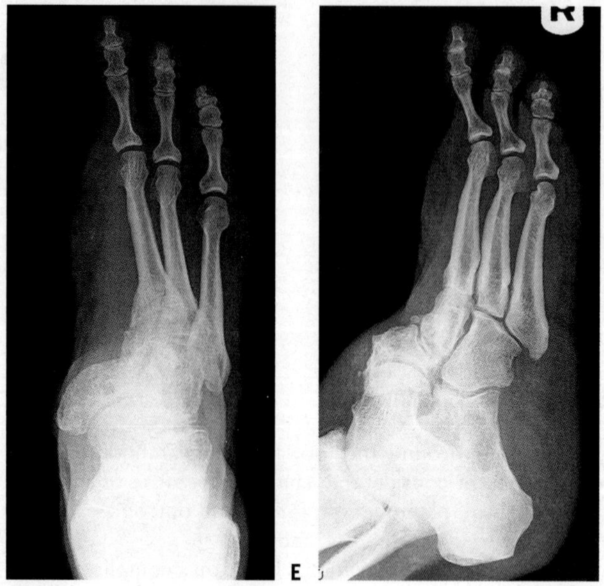

FIG 2 Anatomic location of tumors around the foot may dictate amputation type, different from the conventional transmetatarsal, Lisfranc, and Chopart amputations. **A.** Incision line planned for resection of a soft tissue sarcoma at the base of the first toe. **B.** Surgical specimen. **C.** Postoperative photograph showing the planned field of radiation. **D,E.** Postoperative plain radiographs. Modified shoes and orthoses are required for weight bearing and ambulation.

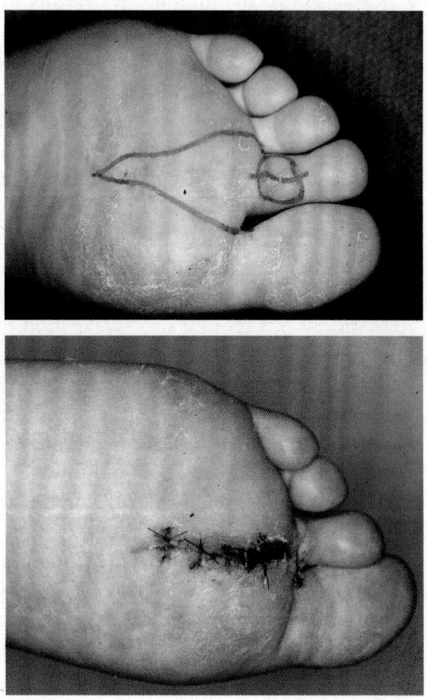

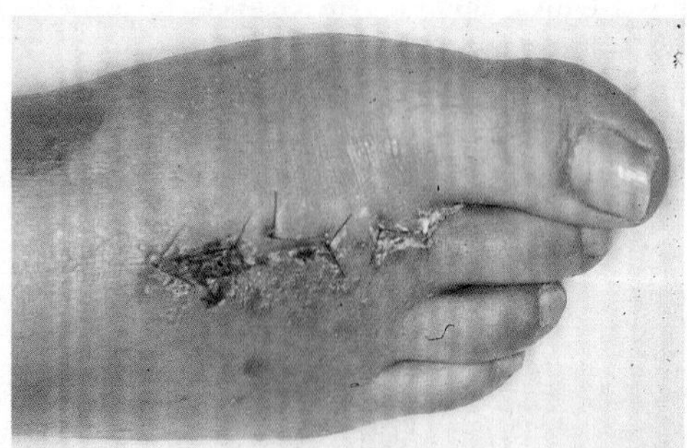

FIG 3 **A.** Planned line of incision for amputation of the second toe, done for a high-grade soft tissue sarcoma. **B,C.** Following amputation, loss of cosmesis, and impairment of function are minimal.

INDICATIONS

- The most common indications for foot amputations are soft tissue sarcomas and extensive tumors of skin.
- Primary and metastatic tumors requiring amputation at that site are rare.

IMAGING AND OTHER STAGING STUDIES

- Physical examination should include evaluation of vascularity and lymphadenopathy along the ipsilateral extremity and groin.
- Plain radiographs are required to evaluate the general foot morphology.
- Magnetic resonance imaging (MRI) is the modality of choice for evaluating the extent of bone destruction and soft tissue extension. It provides the data required for determination of the amputation type and its extent **(FIG 4)**.

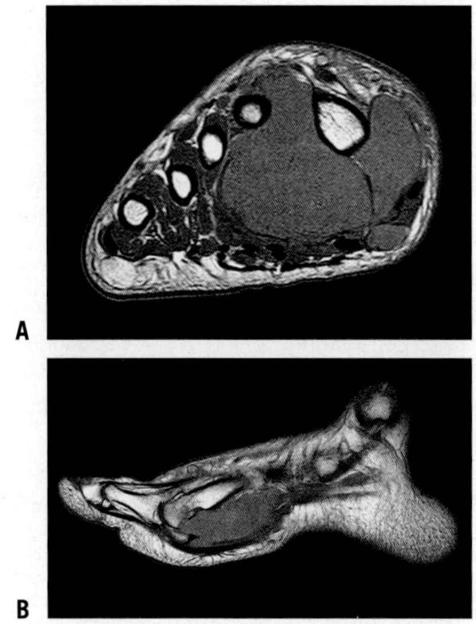

FIG 4 Axial (**A**) and sagittal (**B**) MRIs showing high-grade soft tissue sarcoma of occupying the first intermetatarsal space and extending to the midfoot. Chopart amputation was done to achieve wide margins of resection.

SURGICAL MANAGEMENT

Positioning

- The patient is placed supine on the operating table. A tourniquet is placed over adequate padding.

Approach

- Ray resections are performed through a longitudinal dorsal incision in line with the involved metatarsal. At the metatarsophalangeal joint, the incision is carried plantarly in a curvilinear fashion around the joint, this tissue is then used to reconstruct the resulting web space between the adjacent digits **(FIG 5A)**.
- Lisfranc, transmetatarsal, and Chopart amputations are performed through a midfoot incision, with a long plantar flap **(FIG 5B–D)**.
- It is important to maintain as much plantar skin as possible for the purpose of reconstruction because it is thick and has specialized columns of plantar fat to support and pad weight bearing.

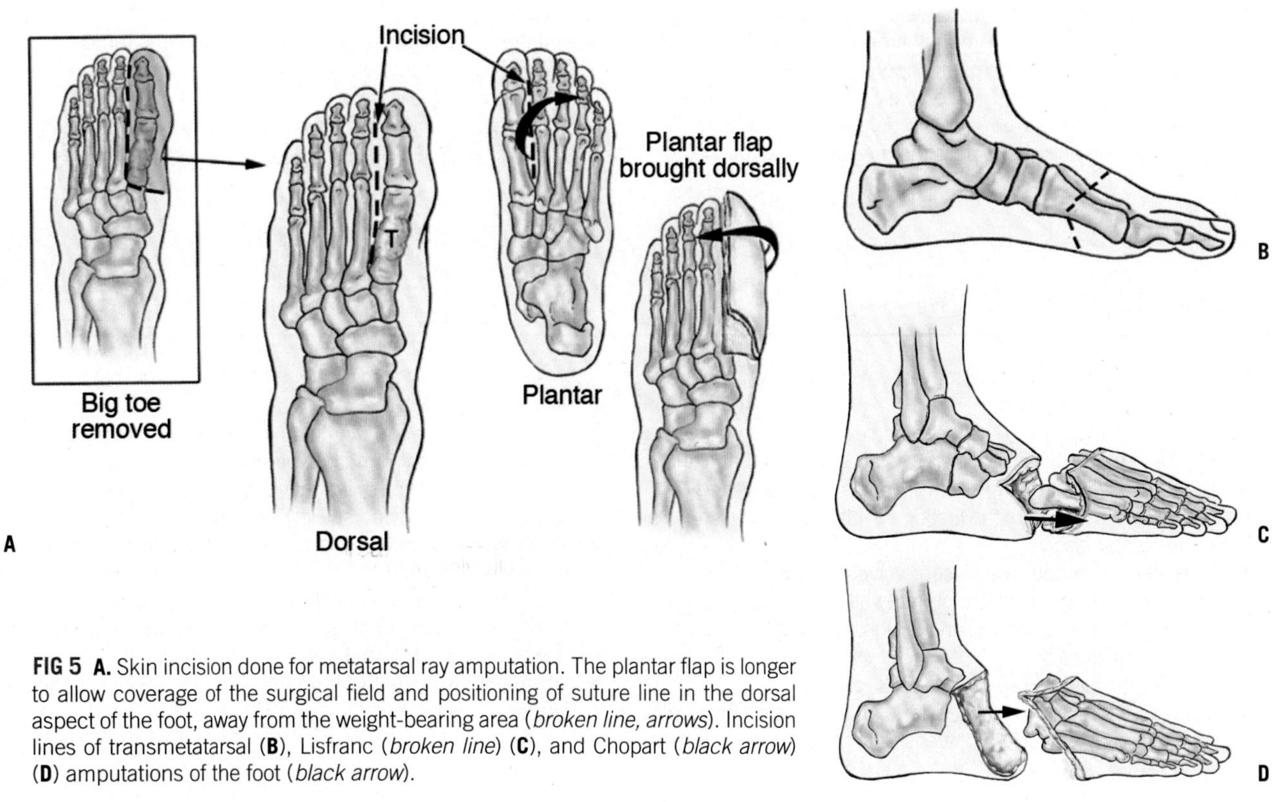

FIG 5 **A.** Skin incision done for metatarsal ray amputation. The plantar flap is longer to allow coverage of the surgical field and positioning of suture line in the dorsal aspect of the foot, away from the weight-bearing area (*broken line, arrows*). Incision lines of transmetatarsal (**B**), Lisfranc (*broken line*) (**C**), and Chopart (*black arrow*) (**D**) amputations of the foot (*black arrow*).

RAY AMPUTATION

- The sensory nerves are identified just beneath the skin and are pulled distally and transected sharply with a scalpel.
- The extensor tendon is also transected sharply near the tarsometatarsal joint.
- The digital nerves are identified along with the vascular bundle.
  - If involved or adherent to the tumor pseudocapsule, they are ligated proximally.
- The lumbrical and interosseous muscles are transected proximally, exposing the base of the metatarsal.
  - An oscillating saw is used to transect the metatarsal, or the metatarsal is disarticulated at the tarsometatarsal joint and elevated.
- The resection then is performed from proximal to distal.
- The flexor tendon is identified and transected.
- The entire metatarsal is then excised along with the adjacent soft tissue (lumbricals, intrinsics, and flexor extensor tendons).
- The dissection is then carried distally and plantarward.
- The capsular structures of the metatarsophalangeal joint are then separated from the underlying dermis, and the ray is removed.

TRANSMETATARSAL AMPUTATION

- The cutaneous branches of the terminal portions of the peroneal nerve are identified.
  - Traction is applied, pulling the nerve distally.
  - The nerve is transected sharply to allow it to retract proximally.
- The terminal branch of the dorsalis pedis is preserved, if possible, to maintain continuity of the anastomosis with the posterior tibial terminal arterial branch, thus maintaining the dorsalis pedis contribution of arterial flow through the arch.
- The extensor tendons are placed on a stretch, and this is best accomplished by flexing the forefoot and sharply dividing the tendons at the level of the skin incision, allowing the tendons to retract proximally.
- A beveled cut is made in the metatarsal heads by angling an oscillating saw 30 degrees from the perpendicular with the foot placed in neutral position on the operating table.
- A plantar flap is then fashioned by extending the incision through the skin approximately 45 degrees from the transverse dorsal incision obliquely across the medial and lateral foot to the level of approximately the metatarsal heads and then transversely across the skin just proximal to the metatarsal heads.
- The sensory nerve to the first ray is identified, traction is placed, and the nerve is transected sharply.
- The terminal branches in the medial plantar nerve are identified as well, placed on stretch, and sharply divided.
- The terminal branches of the medial plantar artery are identified, ligated, and divided. The superficial and deep flexor tendons are placed on stretch by dorsiflexing the forefoot through the metatarsal osteotomies and sharply dividing them, allowing them to retract proximally.
- No attempt is made to suture the extensor tendons to the flexor tendons.
- If there is a significant plantar extension of the tumor, a long plantar flap cannot be used. In this case, a fish-mouth configuration is preferable.
  - To achieve this, equal dorsal and plantar flaps are constructed, and the same operation is carried out as indicated earlier.

LISFRANC AMPUTATION

- The cutaneous branches of the terminal portions of the peroneal nerve are identified.
  - Traction is applied, pulling the nerve distally.
  - The nerve is transected sharply to allow it to retract proximally.
- The terminal branch of the dorsalis pedis artery is ligated and divided as it enters the first dorsal interspace and courses in the plantar fascia.
- The extensor tendons are placed on a stretch; this is best accomplished by flexing the forefoot and sharply dividing the tendons at the level of the skin incision, allowing the tendons to retract proximally.
- The Lisfranc joint is disarticulated sharply.
- A plantar flap is fashioned by extending the incision through the skin approximately 45 degrees from the transverse dorsal incision obliquely across the medial and lateral foot to the level of the distal.
- The sensory nerve to the first ray is identified, traction is placed, and the nerve is transected sharply.
- The terminal branches in the medial plantar nerve are identified, placed on stretch, and sharply divided.
- The terminal branches of the medial plantar artery are identified, ligated, and divided.
- The superficial and deep flexor tendons are placed on stretch by dorsiflexing the forefoot through the Lisfranc joint and sharply dividing them, allowing them to retract proximally.
- No attempt is made to suture the extensor tendons to the flexor tendons.

CHOPART AMPUTATION

- The dorsalis pedis artery and accompanying nerve are identified.
  - The dorsalis pedis artery is ligated and divided, and the sensory nerve is placed on stretch and transected sharply, allowing it to retract proximally.
- The capsule of the talonavicular joint is circumferentially divided, along with release of the posterior tibial tendon. This tendon is tagged for later use as it is brought through the interosseous membrane and reattached to the neck of the talus with suture anchors or through a hole drilled in the talus.
- The Achilles tendon is then suture-anchored to the neck of the talus and used to augment the tibialis anterior or posterior tibial tendon.
- A long plantar flap is preferred, but if the tumor invades the plantar flap, a fish-mouth incision is made with equal length dorsal and plantar flaps.
- To help prevent equinus contracture, the tibialis anterior is detached from the tarsal navicular with a cuff of soft tissue, preferably periosteum.
- A drill hole is made through the neck and head of the talus in an oblique fashion from dorsolateral to plantar medial.
- The tendon is then routed through this bone tunnel and sewn to itself or soft tissue as it exits through the tunnel **(TECH FIG 1)**.

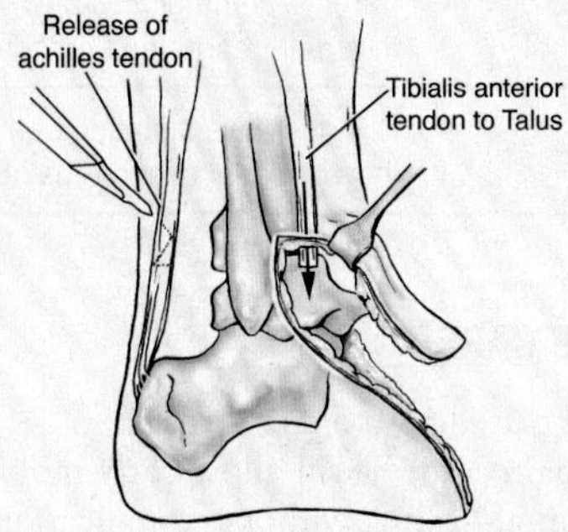

TECH FIG 1 Attachment of the tibialis anterior tendon (*black arrow*) into the neck of the talus through drill holes.

SYME AMPUTATION

- The incision extends from the anterior aspect of the lateral malleolus to the anterior aspect of the medial malleolus, continuing to the plantar skin. The incision at the plantar flap is made to the level of the calcaneocuboid joint.
- The soft tissues, including tendons, are incised and allowed to retract; the neurovascular bundle is identified and ligated.
- The talus and calcaneus are dissected sharply and removed. The skin around the Achilles tendon insertion site is thin, and dissection should be performed with caution.
- The flares of the malleoli are removed with an oscillating saw.
- The plantar fat pad is fixed to the end of the stump with nonabsorbable sutures into drill holes of the distal tibia and fibula.
- A drain is placed and the wound closed in layers; 3-0 nylon suture is used to repair the skin.
- A well-padded soft dressing is applied.

WOUND CLOSURE

- The tourniquet is deflated and meticulous hemostasis is obtained. Excessive use of cautery around the plantar flap is discouraged to minimize the damage to its vascularity.
- The end of the exposed bone should be contoured to leave smooth edges and prevent pressure on the overlying flaps.
- A small drain is positioned within the surgical field, and flaps are sutured meticulously **(TECH FIG 2)**.
- A bulky dressing is applied, maintaining even compression across the foot and stump.

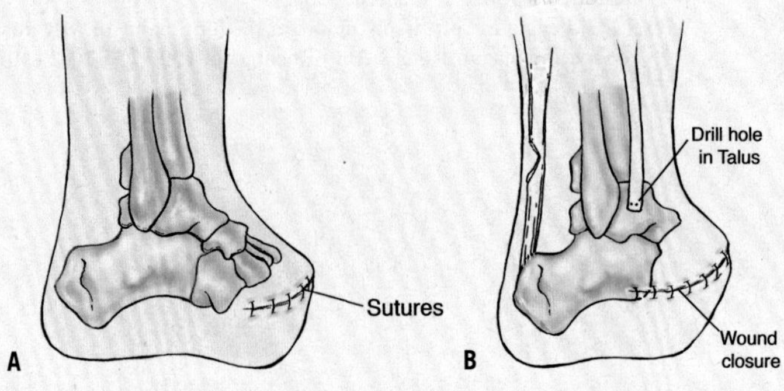

TECH FIG 2 A drain is positioned within the surgical field and flaps are meticulously sutured. Flap closure following Lisfranc amputation (**A**) and Chopart amputation (**B**).

Pearls and Pitfalls

Preoperative Evaluation	• Detailed imaging is mandatory to determine tumor extent and level of amputation.
Surgical Incision	• A long plantar flap results in a better end-bearing stump. The natural cascade of metatarsal lengths should be maintained.
Wound Healing Complications	• Meticulous flap closure, bulky and compressive wound dressing, and prevention of swelling around the stump are essential for wound healing.
Deep Infection	• Parenteral antibiotics and surgical débridement may be necessary to treat deep infections. Early diagnosis and treatment can affect outcome.
Contractures	• Postoperative splinting can help prevent contractures. Once a contracture occurs, it is treated with stretching if mild. Serial casting may be needed.

POSTOPERATIVE CARE

- Splinting may be used to avoid contractures.
- Postoperative pain control will allow early mobilization of the patient. Wound healing without complications and prevention of contractures, particularly equinus contractures, are vital.
  - Following ray resection, the patient is placed in a well-padded splint. Crutches are used until the sutures are removed. The patient may begin range-of-motion exercises and weight bearing as tolerated.
  - Toe amputation patients may ambulate in a postoperative shoe immediately.
  - The sutures are removed at 2 to 3 weeks. A wide comfort shoe is worn, and activities are progressed as tolerated.
- For the Lisfranc and transmetatarsal amputations, a rigid postoperative dressing is used. The wound is dressed with nonadherent dressing gauze.
- A gauze roll is used to bind the residual foot. Cotton padding is then placed in strips from the hindfoot to the forefoot from plantar to dorsal in an attempt to reduce the tension on the suture line.
  - The heel is well padded with cotton padding and then a plaster cast is applied. The cotton padding may have elastic in it for built-in stretch. The plaster is also applied from proximal and plantar to distal and dorsal to reduce the tension on the suture line. The plaster application should be firm but not tight. It should be placed in closed-toe fashion and should extend up to the proximal leg, maintaining the residual foot in the neutral position to a slightly dorsiflexed position.
  - This initial dressing is changed after 3 to 5 days. A similar plaster is applied for an additional 2 weeks. At the time of plaster removal, the sutures are removed.
  - The patient is given a prescription for a shoe filler. After 2.5 weeks, the patient's foot is placed in a buckle-wedge shoe for an additional 3 to 4 weeks. After that, shoe wear and progressive ambulation are encouraged.
- After a Chopart amputation, the cast is removed after 5 days, and the drain is removed. A second dressing and cast are applied for about 3 weeks. The second cast is removed, and the sutures are removed at the end of the 3 weeks. A third cast is applied and maintained for 6 to 8 weeks. After the final cast is removed, the patient begins physical therapy to begin range of motion, in particular dorsiflexion and plantarflexion excursion of the residual foot. A prosthetic measurement is taken.

COMPLICATIONS

- Wound infection
- Wound dehiscence
- Chronic pain syndrome
- Equinus contracture

SUGGESTED READINGS

Berenji M, Kwok-Oleksy C, Dang BN, et al. Chopart's amputation for resection of clear cell sarcoma of the foot: a case report and review of the literature. J Foot Ankle Surg 2009;48(6):677–683.

Chou LB, Malawer MM. Analysis of surgical treatment of 33 foot and ankle tumors. Foot Ankle Int 1994;15:175–181.

Furtado S, Grimer RJ, Cool P, et al. Physical functioning, pain and quality of life after amputation for musculoskeletal tumours: a national survey. Bone Joint J 2015;97-B(9):1284–1290.

Lin PP, Guzel VB, Pisters PW, et al. Surgical management of soft tissue sarcomas of the hand and foot. Cancer 2002;95(4):852–861.

Özger H, Alpan B, Aycan OE, et al. Management of primary malignant bone and soft tissue tumors of foot and ankle: is it worth salvaging? J Surg Oncol 2018;117(2):307–320.

Seale KS, Lange TA, Monson D, et al. Soft tissue tumors of the foot and ankle. Foot Ankle 1988;9:19–27.

Sundberg SB, Carlson WO, Johnson KA. Metastatic lesions of the foot and ankle. Foot Ankle 1982;3:167–169.

Wetzel LH, Levine E. Soft-tissue tumors of the foot: value of MR imaging for specific diagnosis. AJR Am J Roentgenol 1990;155:1025–1030.

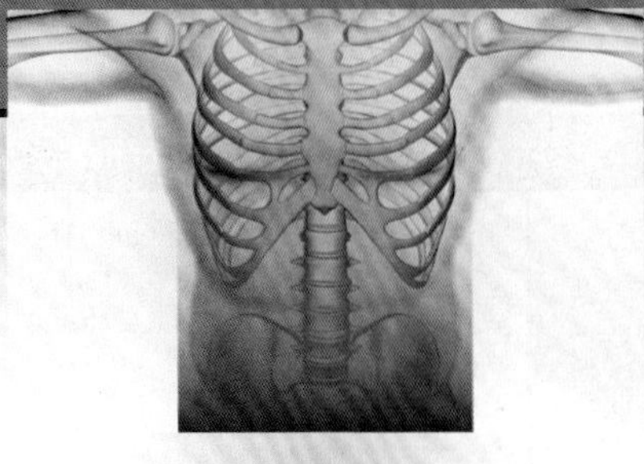

Exam Table for Pelvis and Lower Extremity Trauma

Examination	Technique	Illustration	Grading and Significance
Effusion	The examiner palpates and performs ballottement of the patella. Smaller effusions can be detected by compressing fluid from the suprapatellar pouch.	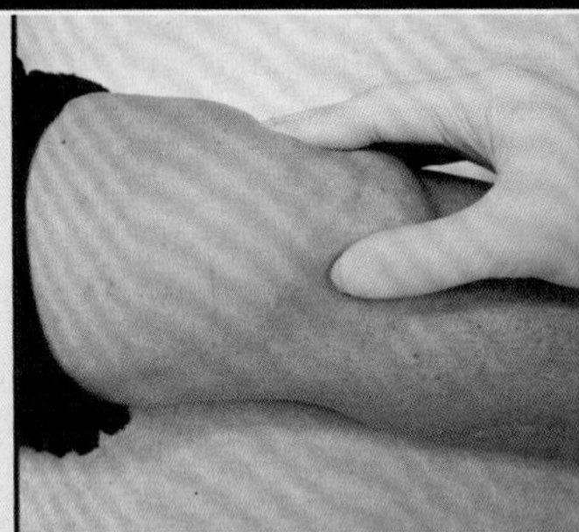	Trace, mild, moderate, or large. Presence of an effusion is indirect evidence of intra-articular injury. Most commonly graded subjectively as mild, moderate, or larger; new onset of effusion after injury localizes injury to within the capsule of the knee.
Heel strike	Light blows of the fist or heel of hand to the heel of the injured leg	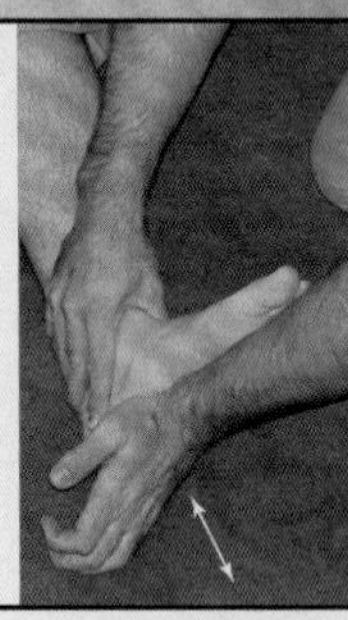	Groin pain that did not exist at rest implies hip fracture.
Iliac wing compression	The examiner can test for stability of the pelvic ring by placing the palms of the hands on the outside of the iliac wings and pushing the two wings together.	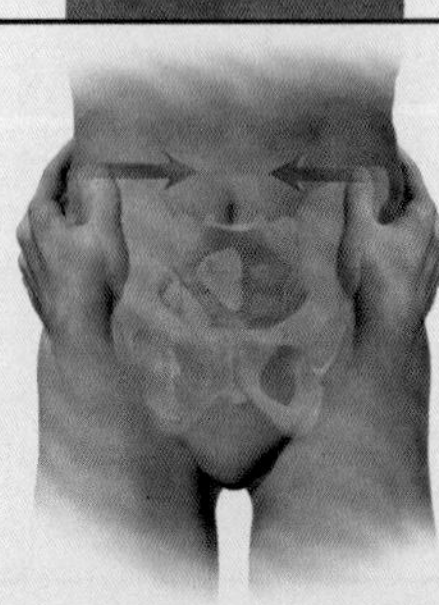	This should be avoided if radiology demonstrates displacement.
Lower extremity rotation	In a patient with a suspected femoral neck fracture, gentle internal and external rotation at the leg is all that is needed to elicit pain.	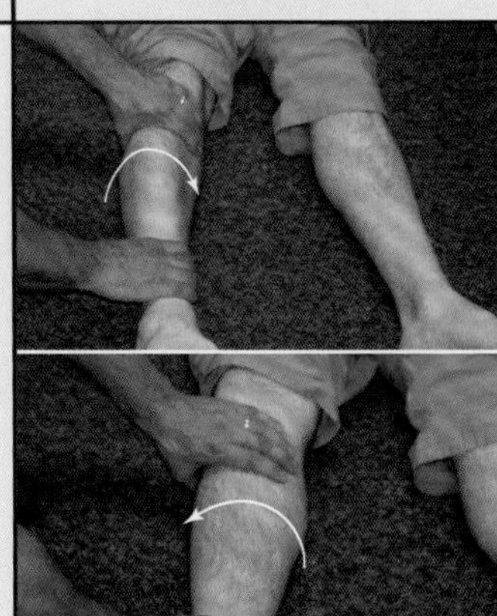	Pain in the groin is concerning for femoral neck fracture but may also be caused by fractures of the anterior pelvic ring.

(continued)

Examination	Technique	Illustration	Grading and Significance
Midfoot joint palpation	Direct palpation of each of the midfoot joints, particularly the medial column of the foot	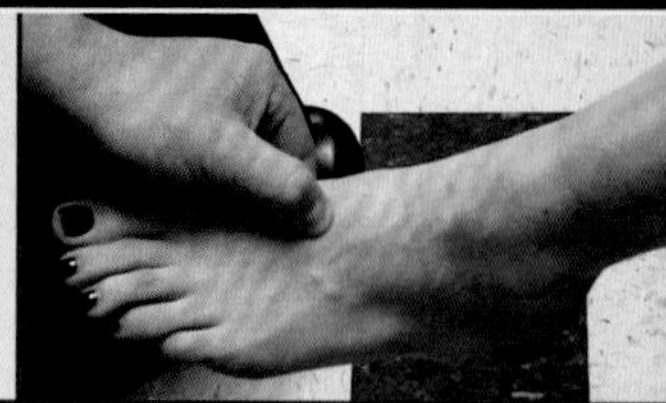	Presence or absence of pain. The presence of pain at the midfoot with palpation suggests a Lisfranc injury.
Midfoot stability	Gentle passive dorsiflexion and plantarflexion of each of the metatarsal heads; gentle passive abduction and adduction through the forefoot	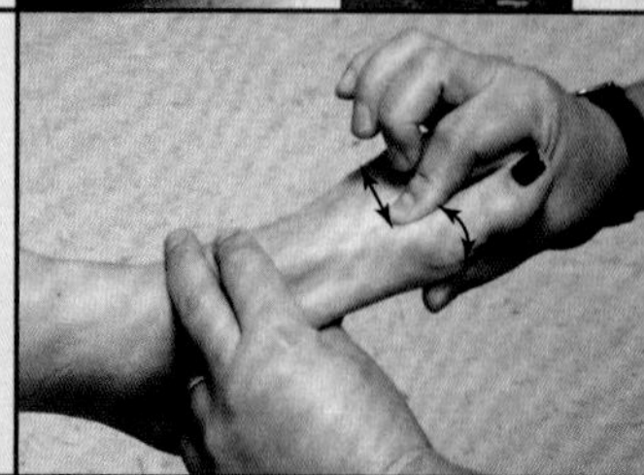	Presence or absence of pain. The presence of pain at the tarsometatarsal joint region with passive forefoot range of motion suggests a Lisfranc injury.
Patellar palpation	The patella, quadriceps tendon, and patellar tendon are palpated for defects. The examiner notes inferior or superior patellar displacement in comparison to the unaffected side.	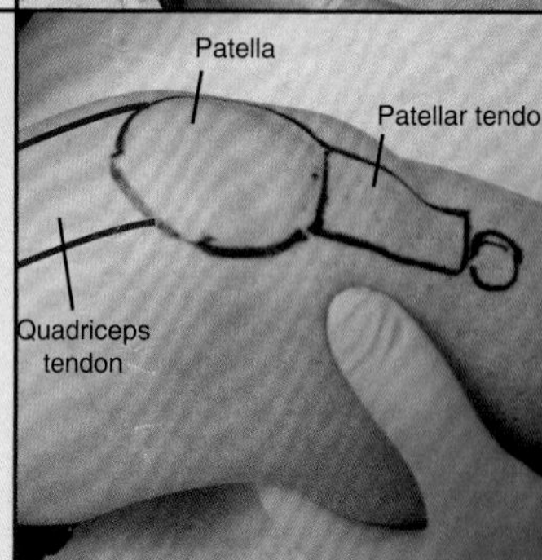	Patella baja is an inferiorly displaced patella seen with quadriceps tendon rupture; patella alta is a high-riding patella associated with patellar tendon rupture. The placement of the patella and palpation of defects with the patella, quadriceps tendon, or patellar tendon can help differentiate between patellar fracture and ligamentous extensor disruption.
Pelvic instability: external rotation	Legs are positioned flexed, abducted, and externally rotated. Hands are placed on the iliac crests, and an anteroposterior force is applied.	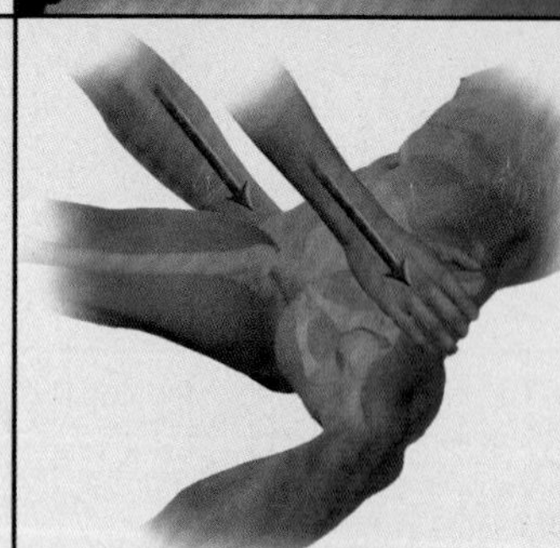	Palpable widening of the pelvis or increased sacroiliac joint space or symphyseal widening is seen on simultaneous fluoroscopic images with the C-arm.
Pelvic instability: internal rotation	Legs are positioned extended and internally rotated. Hands are positioned lateral to iliac crests, and a lateral-to-medial compressive force is applied.	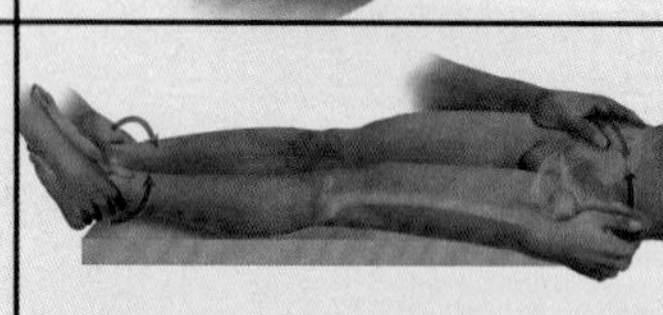	Palpable instability of the pelvis or a decrease in sacroiliac joint space or symphyseal diastasis is seen on simultaneous C-arm images.
Pelvic instability: vertical instability	Legs are positioned extended. While one extremity is supported at the heel, traction is applied to the other.	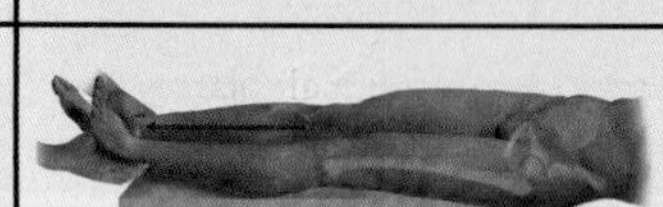	A visual change in leg-length discrepancy can be seen in some cases. Otherwise, simultaneous C-arm images may disclose one acetabulum or iliac crest at a different level than the other.

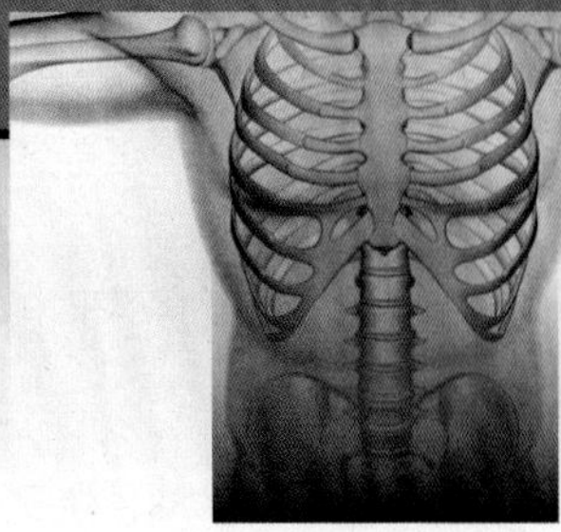

Index

Page numbers followed by *f* and *t* indicate figures and tables, respectively.

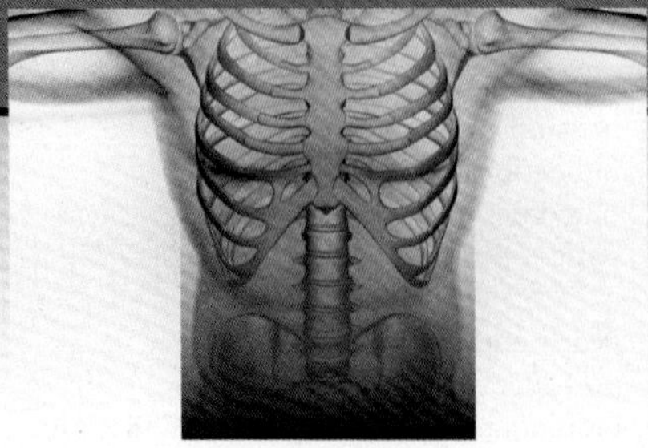

Index

Page numbers followed by *f* and *t* indicate figures and tables, respectively.

D

E

F

G

H

Q

R

S